QUICK LOOK DRUG BOOK

2008

Leonard L. Lance, RPh, BSPharm
Senior Editor
Pharmacist
Lexi-Comp, Inc.
Hudson, Ohio

Charles F. Lacy, MS, PharmD, FCSHP
Editor
Vice President for Executive Affairs
Professor, Pharmacy Practice
Professor, Business Leadership
University of Southern Nevada
Las Vegas, Nevada

Morton P. Goldman, PharmD, BCPS, FCCP
Associate Editor
Director of Pharmacotherapy Services
Department of Pharmacy
Cleveland Clinic Foundation
Cleveland, Ohio

Lora L. Armstrong, PharmD, BCPS
Associate Editor
Vice President, Clinical Affairs
Pharmacy & Therapeutics Formulary Process
Clinical Program Oversight
CaremarkRx
Northbrook, Illinois

Wolters Kluwer | Lippincott Williams & Wilkins
Health

Philadelphia • Baltimore • New York • London
Buenos Aires • Hong Kong • Sydney • Tokyo

QUICK LOOK DRUG BOOK

2008

Leonard L. Lance, RPh, BSPharm
Senior Editor
Pharmacist
Lexi-Comp, Inc.
Hudson, Ohio

Charles F. Lacy, MS, PharmD, FCSHP
Editor
Vice President for Executive Affairs
Professor, Pharmacy Practice
Professor, Business Leadership
University of Southern Nevada
Las Vegas, Nevada

Morton P. Goldman, PharmD, BCPS, FCCP
Associate Editor
Director of Pharmacotherapy Services
Department of Pharmacy
Cleveland Clinic Foundation
Cleveland, Ohio

Lora L. Armstrong, PharmD, BCPS
Associate Editor
Vice President, Clinical Affairs
Pharmacy & Therapeutics Formulary Process
Clinical Program Oversight
CaremarkRx
Northbrook, Illinois

NOTICE

LEXI-COMP
1100 Terex Road
Hudson, Ohio 44236
(330) 650-6506

TABLE OF CONTENTS

Visit the Point http://thepoint.lww.com/QL2008 for exclusive access to:

Apothecary/Metric Conversions

Pounds/Kilograms Conversion

Temperature Conversion

Pharmaceutical Manufacturers and Distributors

Vitamin Products

Refer to the inside front cover of this book for your online access code.

ABOUT THE AUTHORS

Leonard L. Lance, RPh, BSPharm

Leonard L. (Bud) Lance has been directly involved in the pharmaceutical industry since receiving his bachelor's degree in pharmacy from Ohio Northern University in 1970. Upon graduation from ONU, Mr Lance spent four years as a navy pharmacist in various military assignments and was instrumental in the development and operation of the first whole hospital I.V. admixture program in a military (Portsmouth Naval Hospital) facility. His last 15 months in the Navy were spent on the USS Independence CV-62.

After completing his military service, he entered the retail pharmacy field and has managed both an independent and a home I.V. franchise pharmacy operation. Since the late 1970s, Mr Lance has focused much of his interest on using computers to improve pharmacy service. The independent pharmacy he worked for was one of the first retail pharmacies in the State of Ohio to computerize (1977).

His love for computers and pharmacy led him to Lexi-Comp, Inc. in 1988. He was the first pharmacist at Lexi-Comp and helped develop Lexi-Comp's first drug database in 1989 and was involved in the editing and publishing of Lexi-Comp's first *Drug Information Handbook* in 1990.

As a result of his strong publishing interest, he presently serves in the capacity of pharmacy editor and technical advisor as well as pharmacy (information) database coordinator for Lexi-Comp. Along with the *Quick Look Drug Book*, he provides technical support to Lexi-Comp's *Drug Information Handbook for the Allied Health Professional* and Lexi-Comp's reference publications. Mr Lance also assists over 300 major hospitals in producing their own formulary (pharmacy) publications through Lexi-Comp's custom publishing service. Mr Lance is also Manager of the Dosage Forms database in the Medical Sciences Division at Lexi-Comp.

Mr Lance is past president (1984) of the Summit Pharmaceutical Association (SPA). He is also a member of the Ohio Pharmacists Association (OPA), the American Pharmaceutical Association (APhA), and the American Society of Health-System Pharmacists (ASHP).

Charles F. Lacy, PharmD, FCSHP

Dr Lacy is the Vice President for Information Technologies, Professor of Pharmacy Practice, and Professor of Business Leadership at the University of Southern Nevada. In his capacity at the university, Dr Lacy oversees the directors of the Library and Learning Resources Center and the University Information Systems. Additionally, Dr Lacy is a co-founder of the University. Currently, Dr Lacy is also the Director of International Programs for the university, which includes the College of Pharmacy, the College of Business Administration, and the College of Nursing. Previously, Dr Lacy was the Facilitative Officer for Clinical Programs for the College of Pharmacy where he managed the clinical curriculum, clinical faculty activities, student experiential programs, pharmacy residency programs, and the college's continuing education programs.

Prior to co-founding the Nevada College of Pharmacy, Dr Lacy was the Clinical Coordinator for the Department of Pharmacy at Cedars-Sinai Medical Center. With 20 years of clinical experience, he has developed a reputation as an acknowledged expert in drug information, pharmacy practice, and critical care drug therapy.

Dr Lacy received his doctorate from the University of Southern California School of Pharmacy. Presently, Dr Lacy holds teaching affiliations with the University of Southern Nevada, the University of Southern California, the University of the Pacific School of Pharmacy, Western University of Health Sciences School of Pharmacy, Hokkaido College of Pharmacy in Otaru, Japan, and the University of Alberta at Edmonton, School of Pharmacy and Health Sciences.

Dr Lacy is an active member of numerous professional associations including the American Society of Health-System Pharmacists (ASHP), the American College of Clinical Pharmacy (ACCP), the American Society of Consultant Pharmacists (ASCP), the American Association of Colleges of Pharmacy (AACP), American Pharmacists Association (APhA), and the California Society of Hospital Pharmacists (CSHP), through which he has chaired many committees and subcommittees.

Morton P. Goldman, PharmD, BCPS, FCCP

Dr Goldman received his bachelor's degree in pharmacy from the University of Pittsburgh, College of Pharmacy and his Doctor of Pharmacy degree from the University of Cincinnati, Division of Graduate Studies and Research. He completed his concurrent 2-year hospital pharmacy residency at the VA Medical Center in Cincinnati. Dr Goldman is presently the Director of Pharmacotherapy Services for the Department of Pharmacy at the Cleveland Clinic Foundation (CCF) after having spent over 4 years at CCF as an Infectious Disease pharmacist and 10 years as Clinical Manager/Assistant Director. He holds faculty appointments from The University of Toledo, College of Pharmacy and Case Western Reserve University, College of Medicine and is the Pharmacology Curriculum Director Coordinator for the new Cleveland Clinic Lerner College of Medicine. Dr Goldman is a Board-Certified Pharmacotherapy Specialist (BCPS) with added qualifications in infectious diseases.

In his capacity as Director of Pharmacotherapy Services at CCF, Dr Goldman remains actively involved in patient care and clinical research with the Department of Infectious Disease, as well as the continuing education of the medical and pharmacy staff. He is an editor of CCF's *Guidelines for Antibiotic Use* and participates in their annual Antimicrobial Review retreat. He is a member of the Pharmacy and Therapeutics Committee and many of its subcommittees. Dr Goldman has authored numerous journal articles and lectures locally and nationally on infectious diseases topics and current drug therapies. He is currently a reviewer for the *Clinical Infectious Diseases* and the *Journal of the American Medical Association*, an editorial board member of the *Journal of Infectious Disease Pharmacotherapy*, and coauthor of the *Infectious Diseases Handbook*, the *Drug Information Handbook*, and the *Drug Information Handbook for the Allied Health Professional* produced by Lexi-Comp, Inc. He also provides technical support to Lexi-Comp's Clinical Reference Library™ publications.

Dr Goldman is an active member of the Ohio College of Clinical Pharmacy, the Society of Infectious Disease Pharmacists, the American College of Clinical Pharmacy (and is a Fellow of the College), and the American Society of Health-Systems Pharmacists.

Lora Armstrong, PharmD, BCPS

Dr Armstrong received her bachelor's degree in pharmacy from Ferris State University and her Doctor of Pharmacy degree from Midwestern University. Dr Armstrong is a Board-Certified Pharmacotherapy Specialist (BCPS).

In her current position, Dr Armstrong serves as Vice President of Clinical Affairs with responsibility for the National Pharmacy & Therapeutics Committee process, Clinical Program Oversight process, and Pharmaceutical Pipeline Services at Caremark. Caremark is a prescription benefit management company (PBM). Dr Armstrong is also responsible for monitoring drug surveillance and communicating Pharmacy & Therapeutics Committee Formulary information to Caremark's internal and external customers.

Prior to joining Caremark, Inc, Dr Armstrong served as the Director of Drug Information Services at the University of Chicago Hospitals. She obtained 17 years of experience in a variety of clinical settings including critical care, hematology, oncology, infectious diseases, and clinical pharmacokinetics. Dr Armstrong played an active role in the education and training of medical, pharmacy, and nursing staff. She coordinated the Drug Information Center, the medical center's Adverse Drug Reaction Monitoring Program, and the continuing Education Program for pharmacists. She also maintained the hospital's strict formulary program and was the editor of the University of Chicago Hospitals' *Formulary of Accepted Drugs* and the drug information center's monthly newsletter *Topics in Drug Therapy*.

Dr Armstrong is an active member of the Academy of Managed Care Pharmacy (AMCP), the American Society of Health-Systems Pharmacists (ASHP), the American Pharmaceutical Association (APhA), the American College of Clinical Pharmacy (ACCP), and the Pharmacy & Therapeutics Society (P & T Society). Dr Armstrong wrote the chapter entitled "Drugs and Hormones Used in Endocrinology" in the 4th edition of the textbook *Endocrinology*. She is an Adjunct Clinical Instructor of Pharmacy Practice at Midwestern University. Dr Armstrong currently serves on the Drug Information Advisory Board for pharmacist.com and on the American Pharmaceutical Association Scientific Review Panel for Evaluations of Drug Interactions (EDI).

EDITORIAL ADVISORY PANEL

PREFACE

Working with clinical pharmacists, hospital pharmacy and therapeutics committees, and hospital drug information centers, the editors of this handbook have directly assisted in the development and production of hospital-specific formulary documentation for several hundred major medical institutions in the United States and Canada. The resultant documentation provides pertinent detail concerning use of medications within the hospital and other clinical settings. The most current information on medications has been extracted, reviewed, coalesced, and cross-referenced by the editors to create this *Quick Look Drug Book*.

Thus, this handbook gives the user quick access to data on over 1600 medications with cross-referencing to over 5700 U.S. and Canadian brand or trade names. Selection of the included medications was based on the analysis of those medications offered in a wide range of hospital formularies. The concise standardized format for data used in this handbook was developed to ensure a consistent presentation of information for all medications.

All generic drug names and synonyms appear in lower case, whereas brand or trade names appear in upper/lower case with the proper trademark information. These three items appear as individual entries in the alphabetical listing of drugs and, thus, there is no requirement for an alphabetical index of drugs.

The Indication/Therapeutic Category Index is an expedient mechanism for locating the medication of choice along with its classification. This index will help the user, with knowledge of the disease state, to identify medications which are most commonly used in treatment. All disease states are cross-referenced to a varying number of medications with the most frequently used medication(s) noted.

— L.L. Lance

ACKNOWLEDGMENTS

The *Quick Look Drug Book* exists in its present form as the result of the concerted efforts of the following individuals: Robert D. Kerscher, publisher and chief executive officer of Lexi-Comp, Inc; Steven Kerscher, president and chief operating officer; Mark F. Bonfiglio, BS, PharmD, RPh, chief content officer; Stacy S. Robinson, editorial manager; Cynthia Forney, drug identification database manager; Ginger S. Stein, project manager; David C. Marcus, chief information officer; Leslie Jo Hoppes, pharmacology database manager; and Alexandra Hart, composition specialist.

Special acknowledgment goes to all Lexi-Comp staff for their contributions to this handbook.

USE OF THE HANDBOOK

The *Quick Look Drug Book* is organized into a drug information section, an appendix, and an indication/therapeutic category index.

The drug information section of the handbook, wherein all drugs are listed alphabetically, details information pertinent to each drug. Extensive cross-referencing is provided by brand name and synonyms.

Drug information is presented in a consistent format and for quick reference will provide the following:

Generic Name	U.S. Adopted Name (USAN) or International Nonproprietary Name (INN)
	If a drug product is only available in Canada, a *(Canada only)* will be attached to that product and will appear with every occurrence of that drug throughout the book
Pronunciation Guide	Subjective aid for pronouncing drug names
Sound-Alike/Look-Alike Issues	Lists drugs with similar sounding names or names that look alike
Synonyms	Official names and some slang
Tall-Man	"Tall-Man" lettering revisions recommended by the FDA
U.S./Canadian Brand Names	Common trade names used in the United States and Canada
Therapeutic Category	Lexi-Comp's own system of logical medication classification
Controlled Substance	Drug Enforcement Agency (DEA) classification for federally scheduled controlled substances
Use	Information pertaining to appropriate use of the drug
Usual Dosage	The amount of the drug to be typically given or taken during therapy
Dosage Forms	Information with regard to form, strength and availability of the drug **Note:** Please consult individual product labeling for additional formulation information (eg, excipients, preservatives).

Appendix

The appendix offers a compilation of tables, guidelines, and conversion information that can often be helpful when considering patient care.

Indication/Therapeutic Category Index

This index provides a listing of accepted drugs for various disease states thus focusing attention on selection of medications most frequently prescribed in relation to a clinical diagnosis. Diseases may have other nonofficial drugs for their treatment and this indication/therapeutic category index should not be used by itself to determine the appropriateness of a particular therapy. The listed indications may encompass varying degrees of severity and, since certain medications may not be appropriate for a given degree of severity, it should not be assumed that the agents listed for specific indications are interchangeable. Also included as a valuable reference is each medication's therapeutic category.

TALL-MAN LETTERS

Confusion between similar drug names is an important cause of medication errors. For years, The Institute for Safe Medication Practices (ISMP), has urged generic manufacturers use a combination of large and small letters as well as bolding (ie, chlorpro**MAZINE** and chlorpro**PAMIDE**) to help distinguish drugs with look-alike names, especially when they share similar strengths. Recently the FDA's Division of Generic Drugs began to issue recommendation letters to manufacturers suggesting this novel way to label their products to help reduce this drug name confusion. Although this project has had marginal success, the method has successfully eliminated problems with products such as diphenhydr**AMINE** and dimenhy**DRINATE**. Hospitals should also follow suit by making similar changes in their own labels, preprinted order forms, computer screens and printouts, and drug storage location labels.

In order for all involved to become more familiar with the FDA's suggestion, in this edition of the *Quick Look Drug Book* the "Tall-Man" lettering revisions will be listed in a field called **Tall-Man**.

The following is a list of product names and recommended FDA revisions.

Drug Product	Recommended Revision
acetazolamide	aceta**ZOLAMIDE**
acetohexamide	aceto**HEXAMIDE**
bupropion	bu**PROP**ion
buspirone	bus**PIR**one
chlorpromazine	chlorpro**MAZINE**
chlorpropamide	chlorpro**PAMIDE**
clomiphene	clomi**PHENE**
clomipramine	clomi**PRAMINE**
cycloserine	cyclo**SERINE**
cyclosporine	cyclo**SPORINE**
daunorubicin	**DAUNO**rubicin
dimenhydrinate	dimenhy**DRINATE**
diphenhydramine	diphenhydr**AMINE**
dobutamine	**DOBUT**amine
dopamine	**DOP**amine
doxorubicin	**DOXO**rubicin
glipizide	glipi**ZIDE**
glyburide	gly**BURIDE**
hydralazine	hydr**ALAZINE**
hydroxyzine	hydr**OXY**zine
medroxyprogesterone	medroxy**PROGESTER**one
methylprednisolone	methyl**PREDNIS**olone
methyltestosterone	methyl**TESTOSTER**one
nicardipine	ni**CAR**dipine
nifedipine	**NIFE**dipine
prednisolone	predniso**LONE**
prednisone	predni**SONE**

sulfadiazine	sulfa**DIAZINE**
sulfisoxazole	sulfi**SOXAZOLE**
tolazamide	**TOLAZ**amide
tolbutamide	**TOLBUT**amide
vinblastine	vin**BLAS**tine
vincristine	vin**CRIS**tine

Institute for Safe Medication Practices. "New Tall-Man Lettering Will Reduce Mix-Ups Due to Generic Drug Name Confusion," *ISMP Medication Safety Alert*, September 19, 2001. Available at: http://www.ismp.org.

Institute for Safe Medication Practices. "Prescription Mapping, Can Improve Efficiency While Minimizing Errors With Look-Alike Products," *ISMP Medication Safety Alert*, October 6, 1999. Available at: http://www.ismp.org.

U.S. Pharmacopeia, "USP Quality Review: Use Caution-Avoid Confusion," March 2001, No. 76. Available at: http://www.usp.org.

SAFE WRITING

Health professionals and their support personnel frequently produce handwritten copies of information they see in print; therefore, such information is subjected to even greater possibilities for error or misinterpretation on the part of others. Thus, particular care must be given to how drug names and strengths are expressed when creating written health care documents.

The following are a few examples of safe writing rules suggested by the Institute for Safe Medication Practices, Inc.*

1. There should be a space between a number and its units as it is easier to read. There should be no periods after the abbreviations mg or mL.

Correct	Incorrect
10 mg	10mg
100 mg	100mg

2. Never place a decimal and a zero after a whole number (2 mg is correct and 2.0 mg is incorrect). If the decimal point is not seen because it falls on a line or because individuals are working from copies where the decimal point is not seen, this causes a tenfold overdose.

3. Just the opposite is true for numbers less than one. Always place a zero before a naked decimal (0.5 mL is correct, .5 mL is **in**correct).

4. Never abbreviate the word "unit." The handwritten U or u, looks like a 0 (zero), and may cause a tenfold overdose error to be made.

5. IU is not a safe abbreviation for international units. The handwritten IU looks like IV. Write out international units or use int. units.

6. Q.D. is not a safe abbreviation for once daily, as when the Q is followed by a sloppy dot, it looks like QID which means four times daily.

7. O.D. is not a safe abbreviation for once daily, as it is properly interpreted as meaning "right eye" and has caused liquid medications such as saturated solution of potassium iodide and Lugol's solution to be administered incorrectly. There is no safe abbreviation for once daily. It must be written out in full.

8. Do not use chemical names such as 6-mercaptopurine or 6-thioguanine, as 6-fold overdoses have been given when these were not recognized as chemical names. The proper names of these drugs are mercaptopurine or thioguanine.

9. Do not abbreviate drug names (5FC, 6MP, 5-ASA, MTX, HCTZ CPZ, PBZ, etc) as they are misinterpreted and cause error.

10. Do not use the apothecary system or symbols.

11. Do not abbreviate microgram as μg; instead use mcg as there is less likelihood of misinterpretation.

12. When writing an outpatient prescription, write a complete prescription. A complete prescription can prevent the prescriber, the pharmacist, and/or the patient from making a mistake and can eliminate the need for further clarification. The legible prescriptions should contain:

   a. patient's full name

   b. for pediatric or geriatric patients: their age (or weight where applicable)

---

*From "Safe Writing" by Davis NM, PharmD and Cohen MR, MS, Lecturers and Consultants for Safe Medication Practices, 1143 Wright Drive, Huntingdon Valley, PA 19006. Phone: (215) 947-7566.

c.   drug name, dosage form and strength; if a drug is new or rarely prescribed, print this information

d.   number or amount to be dispensed

e.   complete instructions for the patient, including the purpose of the medication

f.   when there are recognized contraindications for a prescribed drug, indicate to the pharmacist that you are aware of this fact (ie, when prescribing a potassium salt for a patient receiving an ACE inhibitor, write "K serum leveling being monitored")

ALPHABETICAL LISTING OF DRUGS

1370-999-397 *see* anagrelide *on page 55*

A₁-PI *see* alpha₁-proteinase inhibitor *on page 32*

A200® Lice [US-OTC] *see* permethrin *on page 670*

A-200® Lice Treatment Kit [US-OTC] *see* pyrethrins and piperonyl butoxide *on page 734*

A-200® Maximum Strength [US-OTC] *see* pyrethrins and piperonyl butoxide *on page 734*

A and D® Original [US-OTC] *see* vitamin A and vitamin D *on page 893*

abacavir (a BAK a veer)

Synonyms abacavir sulfate; ABC

U.S./Canadian Brand Names Ziagen® [US/Can]

Therapeutic Category Nucleoside Reverse Transcriptase Inhibitor (NRTI)

Use Treatment of HIV infections in combination with other antiretroviral agents

Usual Dosage Oral:

Children: 3 months to 16 years: 8 mg/kg body weight twice daily (maximum: 300 mg twice daily) in combination with other antiretroviral agents

Adults: 300 mg twice daily or 600 mg once daily in combination with other antiretroviral agents

Dosage Forms

Solution, oral:

Ziagen®: 20 mg/mL

Tablet:

Ziagen®: 300 mg

abacavir and lamivudine (a BAK a veer & la MI vyoo deen)

Synonyms abacavir sulfate and lamivudine; lamivudine and abacavir

U.S./Canadian Brand Names Epzicom™ [US]; Kivexa™ [Can]

Therapeutic Category Antiretroviral Agent, Reverse Transcriptase Inhibitor (Nucleoside)

Use Treatment of HIV infections in combination with other antiretroviral agents

Usual Dosage Oral: Adults: HIV: One tablet (abacavir 600 mg and lamivudine 300 mg) once daily

Dosage Forms

Tablet:

Epzicom™: Abacavir 600 mg and lamivudine 300 mg

abacavir, lamivudine, and zidovudine (a BAK a veer, la MI vyoo deen, & zye DOE vyoo deen)

Synonyms azidothymidine, abacavir, and lamivudine; AZT, abacavir, and lamivudine; compound S, abacavir, and lamivudine; lamivudine, abacavir, and zidovudine; 3TC, abacavir, and zidovudine; ZDV, abacavir, and lamivudine; zidovudine, abacavir, and lamivudine

U.S./Canadian Brand Names Trizivir® [US]

Therapeutic Category Antiretroviral Agent, Nucleoside Reverse Transcriptase Inhibitor (NRTI)

Use Treatment of HIV infection (either alone or in combination with other antiretroviral agents) in patients whose regimen would otherwise contain the components of Trizivir®

Usual Dosage Oral: Adolescents and Adults: 1 tablet twice daily; **Note:** Not recommended for patients <40 kg

Dosage Forms

Tablet:

Trizivir®: Abacavir 300 mg, lamivudine 150 mg, and zidovudine 300 mg

abacavir sulfate *see* abacavir *on this page*

abacavir sulfate and lamivudine *see* abacavir and lamivudine *on this page*

abarelix (a ba REL iks)

Synonyms PPI-149; R-3827

Therapeutic Category Gonadotropin Releasing Hormone Antagonist

Use Palliative treatment of advanced prostate cancer; treatment is limited to men who are not candidates for LHRH therapy, refuse surgical castration, and have one or more of the following complications due to metastases or local encroachment: 1) risk of neurological compromise, 2) ureteral or bladder outlet obstruction, or 3) severe bone pain (persisting despite narcotic analgesia)

Usual Dosage I.M.: Male prostate cancer: 100 mg administered on days 1, 15, 29 (week 4), then every 4 weeks

abatacept (ab a TA sept)
Synonyms CTLA-4Ig
U.S./Canadian Brand Names Orencia® [US]
Therapeutic Category Antirheumatic, Disease Modifying
Use Treatment of rheumatoid arthritis not responsive to other disease-modifying antirheumatic drugs (DMARD); may be used as monotherapy or in combination with other DMARDs (**not** in combination with anakinra or TNF-blocking agents)
Usual Dosage I.V.: Adults: Dosing is according to body weight: Repeat dose at 2 weeks and 4 weeks after initial dose, and every 4 weeks thereafter:
<60 kg: 500 mg
60-100 kg: 750 mg
>100 kg: 1000 mg
Dosage Forms
Injection, powder for reconstitution [preservative free]:
Orencia®: 250 mg

Abbokinase® [US] *see* urokinase *on page 879*

abbott-43818 *see* leuprolide *on page 497*

ABC *see* abacavir *on previous page*

ABCD *see* amphotericin B cholesteryl sulfate complex *on page 50*

abciximab (ab SIK si mab)
Synonyms C7E3; 7E3
U.S./Canadian Brand Names ReoPro® [US/Can]
Therapeutic Category Platelet Aggregation Inhibitor
Use Prevention of acute cardiac ischemic complications in patients at high risk for abrupt closure of the treated coronary vessel and patients at risk of restenosis; an adjunct with heparin to prevent cardiac ischemic complications in patients with unstable angina not responding to conventional therapy when a percutaneous coronary intervention (PCI) is scheduled within 24 hours
Usual Dosage
Acute coronary syndromes: PCI: I.V.: 0.25 mg/kg bolus administered 10-60 minutes before the start of intervention followed by an infusion of 0.125 mcg/kg/minute (to a maximum of 10 mcg/minute) for 12 hours
Patients with unstable angina not responding to conventional medical therapy and who are planning to undergo percutaneous coronary intervention within 24 hours may be treated with abciximab 0.25 mg/kg intravenous bolus followed by an 18- to 24-hour intravenous infusion of 10 mcg/minute, concluding 1 hour after the percutaneous coronary intervention.
Dosage Forms
Injection, solution:
ReoPro®: 2 mg/mL (5 mL)

Abelcet® [US/Can] *see* amphotericin B lipid complex *on page 52*

Abenol® [Can] *see* acetaminophen *on page 5*

ABI-007 *see* paclitaxel (protein bound) *on page 646*

Abilify® [US] *see* aripiprazole *on page 73*

Abilify® Discmelt™ [US] *see* aripiprazole *on page 73*

ABLC *see* amphotericin B lipid complex *on page 52*

A/B Otic [US] *see* antipyrine and benzocaine *on page 61*

Abraxane® [US] *see* paclitaxel (protein bound) *on page 646*

Abreva® [US-OTC] *see* docosanol *on page 273*

absorbable cotton *see* cellulose, oxidized regenerated *on page 167*

absorbable gelatin sponge *see* gelatin (absorbable) *on page 386*

Absorbine® Antifungal (Discontinued) *see* tolnaftate *on page 849*

Absorbine® Jock Itch (Discontinued) *see* tolnaftate *on page 849*

ABX-EGF *see* panitumumab *on page 650*

AC 2993 *see* exenatide *on page 338*

acamprosate (a kam PROE sate)
Synonyms acamprosate calcium; calcium acetylhomotaurinate
U.S./Canadian Brand Names Campral® [US/Can]
Therapeutic Category GABA Agonist/Glutamate Antagonist
Use Maintenance of alcohol abstinence
Usual Dosage Oral: Adults: Alcohol abstinence: 666 mg 3 times/day (a lower dose may be effective in some patients)
Dosage Forms
Tablet, enteric coated, delayed release:
Campral®: 333 mg

acamprosate calcium *see* acamprosate *on this page*

acarbose (AY car bose)
Sound-Alike/Look-Alike Issues
Precose® may be confused with PreCare®
U.S./Canadian Brand Names Prandase® [Can]; Precose® [US]
Therapeutic Category Antidiabetic Agent, Oral
Use
Monotherapy, as indicated as an adjunct to diet to lower blood glucose in patients with type 2 diabetes mellitus (noninsulin dependent, NIDDM) whose hyperglycemia cannot be managed on diet alone
Combination with a sulfonylurea, metformin, or insulin in patients with type 2 diabetes mellitus (noninsulin dependent, NIDDM) when diet plus acarbose do not result in adequate glycemic control. The effect of acarbose to enhance glycemic control is additive to that of other hypoglycemic agents when used in combination.
Usual Dosage Oral:
Adults: Dosage must be individualized on the basis of effectiveness and tolerance while not exceeding the maximum recommended dose
Initial dose: 25 mg 3 times/day with the first bite of each main meal
Maintenance dose: Should be adjusted at 4- to 8-week intervals based on 1-hour postprandial glucose levels and tolerance. Dosage may be increased from 25 mg 3 times/day to 50 mg 3 times/day. Some patients may benefit from increasing the dose to 100 mg 3 times/day.
Maintenance dose ranges: 50-100 mg 3 times/day.
Maximum dose:
≤60 kg: 50 mg 3 times/day
>60 kg: 100 mg 3 times/day
Patients receiving sulfonylureas: Acarbose given in combination with a sulfonylurea will cause a further lowering of blood glucose and may increase the hypoglycemic potential of the sulfonylurea. If hypoglycemia occurs, appropriate adjustments in the dosage of these agents should be made.
Dosage Forms
Tablet:
Precose®: 25 mg, 50 mg, 100 mg

A-Caro-25 [US] *see* beta-carotene *on page 107*

Accolate® [US/Can] *see* zafirlukast *on page 902*

AccuHist® [US] *see* brompheniramine and pseudoephedrine *on page 120*

AccuHist® PDX Drops [US] *see* brompheniramine, pseudoephedrine, and dextromethorphan *on page 122*

AccuHist® Pediatric (Discontinued) *see* brompheniramine and pseudoephedrine *on page 120*

AccuNeb® [US] *see* albuterol *on page 23*

Accupril® [US/Can] *see* quinapril *on page 739*

Accuretic® [US/Can] *see* quinapril and hydrochlorothiazide *on page 739*

Accutane® [US/Can] *see* isotretinoin *on page 477*

Accuzyme® [US] *see* papain and urea *on page 652*

ACE *see* captopril *on page 145*

acebutolol (a se BYOO toe lole)
Sound-Alike/Look-Alike Issues
Sectral® may be confused with Factrel®, Seconal®, Septra®

Synonyms acebutolol hydrochloride

U.S./Canadian Brand Names Apo-Acebutolol® [Can]; Gen-Acebutolol [Can]; Monitan® [Can]; Novo-Acebutolol [Can]; Nu-Acebutolol [Can]; Rhotral [Can]; Rhoxal-acebutolol [Can]; Sandoz-Acebutolol [Can]; Sectral® [US/Can]

Therapeutic Category Antiarrhythmic Agent, Class II; Beta-Adrenergic Blocker

Use Treatment of hypertension; management of ventricular arrhythmias

Usual Dosage Oral: Adults:
Hypertension: 400-800 mg/day (larger doses may be divided); maximum: 1200 mg/day; usual dose range (JNC 7): 200-800 mg/day in 2 divided doses
Ventricular arrhythmias: Initial: 400 mg/day in divided doses; maintenance: 600-1200 mg/day in divided doses

Dosage Forms
Capsule, as hydrochloride: 200 mg, 400 mg
Sectral®: 200 mg, 400 mg

acebutolol hydrochloride *see* acebutolol *on previous page*

Aceon® [US] *see* perindopril erbumine *on page 669*

Acephen™ [US-OTC] *see* acetaminophen *on this page*

Acerola [US-OTC] *see* ascorbic acid *on page 76*

Acetadote® [US] *see* acetylcysteine *on page 15*

Aceta-Gesic [US-OTC] *see* acetaminophen and phenyltoloxamine *on page 8*

acetaminophen (a seet a MIN oh fen)

Sound-Alike/Look-Alike Issues
Acephen™ may be confused with AcipHex®
FeverAll® may be confused with Fiberall®
Tylenol® may be confused with atenolol, timolol, Tuinal®, Tylox®

Synonyms APAP; n-acetyl-p-aminophenol; paracetamol

U.S./Canadian Brand Names Abenol® [Can]; Acephen™ [US-OTC]; Apo-Acetaminophen® [Can]; Apra Children's [US-OTC]; Aspirin Free Anacin® Maximum Strength [US-OTC]; Atasol® [Can]; Cetafen Extra® [US-OTC]; Cetafen® [US-OTC]; Comtrex® Sore Throat Maximum Strength [US-OTC]; FeverAll® [US-OTC]; Genapap™ Children [US-OTC]; Genapap™ Extra Strength [US-OTC]; Genapap™ Infant [US-OTC]; Genapap™ [US-OTC]; Genebs Extra Strength [US-OTC]; Genebs [US-OTC]; Infantaire [US-OTC]; Mapap Children's [US-OTC]; Mapap Extra Strength [US-OTC]; Mapap Infants [US-OTC]; Mapap [US-OTC]; Nortemp Children's [US-OTC]; Novo-Gesic [Can]; Pain Eze [US-OTC]; Pediatrix [Can]; Silapap® Children's [US-OTC]; Silapap® Infants [US-OTC]; Tempra® [Can]; Tycolene Maximum Strength [US-OTC]; Tycolene [US-OTC]; Tylenol® 8 Hour [US-OTC]; Tylenol® Arthritis Pain [US-OTC]; Tylenol® Children's with Flavor Creator [US-OTC]; Tylenol® Children's [US-OTC]; Tylenol® Extra Strength [US-OTC]; Tylenol® Infants [US-OTC]; Tylenol® Junior [US-OTC]; Tylenol® [US-OTC/Can]; Valorin Extra [US-OTC]; Valorin [US-OTC]

Therapeutic Category Analgesic, Nonnarcotic; Antipyretic

Use Treatment of mild-to-moderate pain and fever (antipyretic/analgesic); does not have antirheumatic or antiinflammatory effects

Usual Dosage Oral, rectal:
Children <12 years: 10-15 mg/kg/dose every 4-6 hours as needed; do **not** exceed 5 doses (2.6 g) in 24 hours; alternatively, the following age-based doses may be used:
0-3 months: 40 mg
4-11 months: 80 mg
1-2 years: 120 mg
2-3 years: 160 mg
4-5 years: 240 mg
6-8 years: 320 mg
9-10 years: 400 mg
11 years: 480 mg
Note: Higher rectal doses have been studied for use in preoperative pain control in children. However, specific guidelines are not available and dosing may be product dependent. The safety and efficacy of alternating acetaminophen and ibuprofen dosing has not been established.
Adults: 325-650 mg every 4-6 hours or 1000 mg 3-4 times/day; do **not** exceed 4 g/day

Dosage Forms
Caplet: 500 mg
Cetafen Extra® Strength [OTC], Genapap™ Extra Strength [OTC], Genebs Extra Strength [OTC], Mapap Extra Strength [OTC], Tycolene Maximum Strength [OTC], Tylenol® Extra Strength [OTC]: 500 mg
Caplet, extended release:
Tylenol® 8 Hour [OTC], Tylenol® Arthritis Pain [OTC]: 650 mg
Capsule: 500 mg
(Continued)

5

acetaminophen *(Continued)*

Elixir: 160 mg/5 mL
  Apra Children's [OTC]: 160 mg/5 mL
  Mapap Children's [OTC]: 160 mg/5 mL
Gelcap: 500 mg
  Mapap Extra Strength [OTC], Tylenol® Extra Strength [OTC]: 500 mg
Geltab: 500 mg
  Tylenol® Extra Strength [OTC]: 500 mg
Liquid, oral: 500 mg/15 mL
  Comtrex® Sore Throat Maximum Strength [OTC], Tylenol® Extra Strength [OTC]: 500 mg/15 mL
  Genapap™ Children [OTC], Silapap® [OTC]: 160 mg/5 mL
Solution, oral: 160 mg/5 mL
Solution, oral [drops]: 80 mg/0.8 mL
  Genapap™ Infant [OTC], Infantaire [OTC], Silapap® Infant's [OTC]: 80 mg/0.8 mL
  Little Fevers™ [OTC]: 80 mg/1 mL
Suppository, rectal: 120 mg, 325 mg, 650 mg
  Acephen® [OTC]: 120 mg, 325 mg, 650 mg
  FeverAll® [OTC]: 80 mg, 120 mg, 325 mg, 650 mg
  Mapap [OTC]: 125 mg, 650 mg
Suspension, oral: 160 mg/5 mL
  Mapap Children's [OTC], Nortemp Children's [OTC], Tylenol® Children's [OTC], Tylenol® Children's with Flavor Creator [OTC]: 160 mg/5 mL
Suspension, oral [drops]: 80 mg/0.8 mL
  Mapap Infants [OTC], Tylenol® Infants [OTC]: 80 mg/0.8 mL
Tablet: 325 mg, 500 mg
  Aspirin Free Anacin® Extra Strength [OTC], Genapap™ Extra Strength [OTC], Genebs Extra Strength [OTC], Mapap Extra Strength [OTC], Redutemp® [OTC], Tylenol® Extra Strength [OTC], Valorin Extra [OTC]: 500 mg
  Cetafen® [OTC], Genapap™ [OTC], Genebs [OTC], Mapap [OTC], Tylenol® [OTC], Valorin [OTC]: 325 mg
Tablet, chewable: 80 mg
  Genapap™ Children [OTC], Mapap Children's [OTC]: 80 mg
  Mapap Junior Strength [OTC]: 160 mg
Tablet, orally disintegrating: 80 mg, 160 mg
  Tylenol® Children's Meltaways [OTC]: 80 mg
  Tylenol® Junior Meltaways [OTC]: 160 mg

acetaminophen and butalbital *see* butalbital and acetaminophen *on page 131*

acetaminophen and chlorpheniramine *see* chlorpheniramine and acetaminophen *on page 177*

acetaminophen and codeine *(a seet a MIN oh fen & KOE deen)*

Sound-Alike/Look-Alike Issues
  Capital® may be confused with Capitrol®
  Tylenol® may be confused with atenolol, timolol, Tuinal®, Tylox®
Synonyms codeine and acetaminophen
U.S./Canadian Brand Names Capital® and Codeine [US]; ratio-Emtec [Can]; ratio-Lenoltec [Can]; Triatec-30 [Can]; Triatec-8 Strong [Can]; Triatec-8 [Can]; Tylenol® Elixir with Codeine [Can]; Tylenol® No. 1 Forte [Can]; Tylenol® No. 1 [Can]; Tylenol® No. 2 with Codeine [Can]; Tylenol® No. 3 with Codeine [Can]; Tylenol® No. 4 with Codeine [Can]; Tylenol® With Codeine [US]
Therapeutic Category Analgesic, Narcotic
Controlled Substance C-III; C-V
Use Relief of mild-to-moderate pain
Usual Dosage Doses should be adjusted according to severity of pain and response of the patient. Adult doses ≥60 mg codeine fail to give commensurate relief of pain but merely prolong analgesia and are associated with an appreciably increased incidence of side effects. Oral:
Children: Analgesic:
  Codeine: 0.5-1 mg codeine/kg/dose every 4-6 hours
  Acetaminophen: 10-15 mg/kg/dose every 4 hours up to a maximum of 2.6 g/24 hours for children <12 years;
  alternatively, the following can be used:
    3-6 years: 5 mL 3-4 times/day as needed of elixir
    7-12 years: 10 mL 3-4 times/day as needed of elixir
    >12 years: 15 mL every 4 hours as needed of elixir
Adults:
  Antitussive: Based on codeine (15-30 mg/dose) every 4-6 hours (maximum: 360 mg/24 hours based on codeine component)
  Analgesic: Based on codeine (30-60 mg/dose) every 4-6 hours (maximum: 4000 mg/24 hours based on acetaminophen component)

Dosage Forms [CAN] = Canadian brand name
Caplet:
ratio-Lenoltec No. 1 [CAN], Tylenol No. 1 [CAN]: Acetaminophen 300 mg, codeine 8 mg, and caffeine 15 mg [not available in the U.S.]
Tylenol No. 1 Forte [CAN]: Acetaminophen 500 mg, codeine 8 mg, and caffeine 15 mg [not available in the U.S.]
Elixir, oral [C-V]: Acetaminophen 120 mg and codeine 12 mg per 5 mL
Tylenol Elixir with Codeine [CAN]: Acetaminophen 160 mg and codeine 8 mg per 5 mL [not available in the U.S.]
Suspension, oral [C-V]: Acetaminophen 120 mg and codeine 12 mg per 5 mL
Capital® and Codeine [C-V]: Acetaminophen 120 mg and codeine 12 mg per 5 mL
Tablet [C-III]: Acetaminophen 300 mg and codeine 15 mg; acetaminophen 300 mg and codeine 30 mg; acetaminophen 300 mg and codeine 60 mg
ratio-Emtec [CAN], Triatec-30 [CAN]: Acetaminophen 300 mg and codeine 30 mg [not available in the U.S.]
ratio-Lenoltec No. 1 [CAN]: Acetaminophen 300 mg, codeine 8 mg, and caffeine 15 mg [not available in the U.S.]
ratio-Lenoltec No. 2 [CAN], Tylenol No. 2 with Codeine [CAN]: Acetaminophen 300 mg, codeine 15 mg, and caffeine 15 mg [not available in the U.S.]
ratio-Lenoltec No. 3 [CAN], Tylenol No. 3 with Codeine [CAN]: Acetaminophen 300 mg, codeine 30 mg, and caffeine 15 mg [not available in the U.S.]
ratio-Lenoltec No. 4 [CAN], Tylenol No. 4 with Codeine [CAN]: Acetaminophen 300 mg and codeine 60 mg [not available in the U.S.]
Triatec-8 [CAN]: Acetaminophen 325 mg, codeine 8 mg, and caffeine 30 mg [not available in the U.S.]
Triatec-8 Strong [CAN]: Acetaminophen 500 mg, codeine 8 mg, and caffeine 30 mg [not available in the U.S.]
Tylenol® with Codeine No. 3: Acetaminophen 300 mg and codeine 30 mg
Tylenol® with Codeine No. 4: Acetaminophen 300 mg and codeine 60 mg

acetaminophen and diphenhydramine (a seet a MIN oh fen & dye fen HYE dra meen)

Sound-Alike/Look-Alike Issues
Excedrin® may be confused with Dexatrim®, Dexedrine®
Percogesic® may be confused with paregoric, Percodan®
Tylenol® may be confused with atenolol, timolol, Tuinal®, Tylox®
Synonyms diphenhydramine and acetaminophen
U.S./Canadian Brand Names Excedrin® P.M. [US-OTC]; Goody's PM® [US-OTC]; Legatrin PM® [US-OTC]; Percogesic® Extra Strength [US-OTC]; Tylenol® PM [US-OTC]; Tylenol® Severe Allergy [US-OTC]
Therapeutic Category Analgesic, Nonnarcotic
Use Aid in the relief of insomnia accompanied by minor pain
Usual Dosage Oral: Adults: 50 mg of diphenhydramine HCl (76 mg diphenhydramine citrate) at bedtime or as directed by physician; do not exceed recommended dosage; not for use in children <12 years of age
Dosage Forms
Caplet: Acetaminophen 500 mg and diphenhydramine 25 mg
Excedrin® P.M. [OTC]: Acetaminophen 500 mg and diphenhydramine 38 mg
Legatrin PM® [OTC]: Acetaminophen 500 mg and diphenhydramine 50 mg
Percogesic® Extra Strength [OTC], Tylenol® PM [OTC]: Acetaminophen 500 mg and diphenhydramine 25 mg
Tylenol® Severe Allergy [OTC]: Acetaminophen 500 mg and diphenhydramine 12.5 mg
Gelcap:
Tylenol® PM [OTC]: Acetaminophen 500 mg and diphenhydramine 25 mg
Geltab: Acetaminophen 500 mg and diphenhydramine 25 mg
Excedrin® P.M. [OTC]: Acetaminophen 500 mg and diphenhydramine 38 mg
Tylenol® PM [OTC]: Acetaminophen 500 mg and diphenhydramine 25 mg
Liquid:
Tylenol® PM [OTC]: Acetaminophen 500 mg and diphenhydramine 25 mg per 15 mL
Powder for oral solution:
Goody's PM® [OTC]: Acetaminophen 500 mg and diphenhydramine 38 mg
Tablet: Acetaminophen 500 mg and diphenhydramine 25 mg
Excedrin® P.M. [OTC]: Acetaminophen 500 mg and diphenhydramine 38 mg

acetaminophen and hydrocodone see hydrocodone and acetaminophen on page 427

acetaminophen and oxycodone see oxycodone and acetaminophen on page 641

acetaminophen and pentazocine see pentazocine and acetaminophen on page 666

acetaminophen and phenyltoloxamine (a seet a MIN oh fen & fen il to LOKS a meen)
Sound-Alike/Look-Alike Issues
Percogesic® may be confused with paregoric, Percodan®
Synonyms phenyltoloxamine citrate and acetaminophen
U.S./Canadian Brand Names Aceta-Gesic [US-OTC]; Alpain [US]; Dologesic® [US]; Flextra 650 [US]; Flextra-DS [US]; Genesec™ [US-OTC]; Hyflex-DS® [US]; Lagesic™ [US]; Percogesic® [US-OTC]; Phenagesic [US-OTC]; Phenylgesic [US-OTC]; RhinoFlex 650 [US]; RhinoFlex™ [US]; Staflex [US]
Therapeutic Category Analgesic, Nonnarcotic
Use Relief of mild pain
Usual Dosage Oral:
Analgesic: Based on acetaminophen component:
Children: 10-15 mg/kg/dose every 4-6 hours as needed (maximum: 5 doses/24 hours)
Adults: 325-650 mg every 4-6 hours as needed (maximum: 4 g/day)
Product-specific labeling:
Flextra-650:
Children 6 to <12 years: 1/2 tablet every 6 hours (maximum: 2 tablets/day)
Children ≥12 years and Adults: 1/2-1 tablet every 6 hours (maximum: 4 tablets/day)
Flextra-DS, Hyflex-DS®, RhinoFlex™, RhinoFlex™-650:
Children 6 to <12 years: 1/2 tablet every 4 hours (maximum: 2.5 tablets/day)
Children ≥12 years and Adults: 1/2-1 tablet every 4 hours (maximum: 5 tablets/day)
Percogesic®:
Children 6-12 years: 1 tablet every 4 hours (maximum: 4 tablets/24 hours)
Adults: 1-2 tablets every 4 hours (maximum: 8 tablets/24 hours)
Dosage Forms
Caplet:
Alpain: Acetaminophen 500 mg and phenyltoloxamine citrate 60 mg
Dologesic®: Acetaminophen 500 mg and phenyltoloxamine citrate 30 mg
Staflex: Acetaminophen 500 mg and phenyltoloxamine citrate 55 mg
Caplet, extended release [scored]:
Lagesic™: Acetaminphen 600 mg and phenyltoloxamine citrate 66 mg
Capsule:
Dologesic®: Acetaminophen 500 mg and phenyltoloxamine citrate 30 mg
Liquid:
Dologesic®: Acetaminophen 500 mg and phenyltoloxamine citrate 30 mg per 15 mg
Tablet: Acetaminophen 325 mg and phenyltoloxamine citrate 30 mg
Aceta-Gesic [OTC], Genasec™ [OTC], Percogesic® [OTC], Phenagesic [OTC], Phenylgesic [OTC]: Acetaminophen 325 mg and phenyltoloxamine citrate 30 mg
Flextra-650: Acetaminophen 650 mg and phenyltoloxamine citrate 60 mg
Flextra-DS, Hyflex-DS®, RhinoFlex™: Acetaminophen 500 mg and phenyltoloxamine citrate 50 mg
RhinoFlex™-650: Acetaminophen 650 mg and phenyltoloxamine citrate 50 mg

acetaminophen and propoxyphene see propoxyphene and acetaminophen on page 723

acetaminophen and pseudoephedrine (a seet a MIN oh fen & soo doe e FED rin)
Sound-Alike/Look-Alike Issues
Ornex® may be confused with Orexin®, Orinase®
Sudafed® may be confused with Sufenta®
Tylenol® may be confused with atenolol, timolol, Tuinal®, Tylox®
Synonyms pseudoephedrine and acetaminophen
U.S./Canadian Brand Names Allerest® Allergy and Sinus Relief [US-OTC]; Contac® Cold and Sore Throat, Non Drowsy, Extra Strength [Can]; Dristan® N.D. [Can]; Dristan® N.D., Extra Strength [Can]; Genapap™ Sinus Maximum Strength [US-OTC]; Mapap Sinus Maximum Strength [US-OTC]; Medi-Synal [US-OTC]; Oranyl Plus [US-OTC]; Ornex® Maximum Strength [US-OTC]; Ornex® [US-OTC]; Sinutab® Non Drowsy [Can]; Sudafed® Head Cold and Sinus Extra Strength [Can]; Sudafed® Multi-Symptom Sinus and Cold [US-OTC]; Tylenol® Cold Daytime, Children's [US-OTC]; Tylenol® Cold, Infants [US-OTC]; Tylenol® Decongestant [Can]; Tylenol® Sinus Daytime [US-OTC]; Tylenol® Sinus [Can]
Therapeutic Category Decongestant/Analgesic
Use Relief of mild-to-moderate pain; relief of congestion
Usual Dosage Oral:
Analgesic: Based on acetaminophen component:
Children: 10-15 mg/kg/dose every 4-6 hours as needed; do **not** exceed 5 doses in 24 hours
Adults: 325-650 mg every 4-6 hours as needed; do **not** exceed 4 g/day
Decongestant: Based on pseudoephedrine component:
Children:
2-6 years: 15 mg every 4 hours; do **not** exceed 90 mg/day

6-12 years: 30 mg every 4 hours; do **not** exceed 180 mg/day
Children >12 years and Adults: 60 mg every 4 hours; do **not** exceed 360 mg/day

Product labeling:
Children's Tylenol® Cold Daytime: Children:
2-5 years (24-47 lb): 1 teaspoonful every 4-6 hours (maximum: 4 doses/24 hours)
6-11 years (48-95 lb): 2 teaspoonfuls every 4-6 hours (maximum: 4 doses/24 hours)
Infants' Tylenol® Cold: Children 2-3 years (24-35 lb): 1.6 mL every 4-6 hours (maximum: 4 doses/24 hours)
Sudafed® Multi-Symptom Sinus and Cold: Children ≥12 years and Adults: 2 capsules every 4-6 hours (maximum: 8 capsules/24 hours)
Tylenol® Sinus Daytime: Children ≥12 years and Adults: 2 caplets or gelcaps every 4-6 hours (maximum: 8 caplets or gelcaps/24 hours)

Dosage Forms
Caplet:
Allerest® Allergy and Sinus Relief, Ornex®: Acetaminophen 325 mg and pseudoephedrine hydrochloride 30 mg
Mapap Sinus Maximum Strength, Ornex® Maximum Strength, Tylenol® Sinus Daytime: Acetaminophen 500 mg and pseudoephedrine hydrochloride 30 mg
Capsule, liquid:
Sudafed® Multi-Symptom Sinus and Cold: Acetaminophen 325 mg and pseudoephedrine hydrochloride 30 mg
Gelcap:
Tylenol® Sinus Daytime: Acetaminophen 500 mg and pseudoephedrine hydrochloride 30 mg
Liquid:
Childrens Tylenol® Cold Daytime: Acetaminophen 160 mg and pseudoephedrine hydrochloride 15 mg per 5 mL
Tablet:
Medi-Synal: Acetaminophen 325 mg and pseudoephedrine hydrochloride 30 mg
Oranyl Plus: Acetaminophen 500 mg and pseudoephedrine hydrochloride 30 mg

acetaminophen and tramadol (a seet a MIN oh fen & TRA ma dole)
Synonyms APAP and tramadol; tramadol hydrochloride and acetaminophen
U.S./Canadian Brand Names Tramacet [Can]; Ultracet™ [US]
Therapeutic Category Analgesic, Miscellaneous; Analgesic, Nonnarcotic
Use Short-term (≤5 days) management of acute pain
Usual Dosage Oral: Adults: Acute pain: Two tablets every 4-6 hours as needed for pain relief (maximum: 8 tablets/day); treatment should not exceed 5 days
Dosage Forms
Tablet: Acetaminophen 325 mg and tramadol 37.5 mg
Ultracet™: Acetaminophen 325 mg and tramadol 37.5 mg

acetaminophen, aspirin, and caffeine (a seet a MIN oh fen, AS pir in, & KAF een)
Sound-Alike/Look-Alike Issues
Excedrin® may be confused with Dexatrim®, Dexedrine®
Synonyms aspirin, acetaminophen, and caffeine; aspirin, caffeine, and acetaminophen; caffeine, acetaminophen, and aspirin; caffeine, aspirin, and acetaminophen
U.S./Canadian Brand Names Excedrin® Extra Strength [US-OTC]; Excedrin® Migraine [US-OTC]; Fem-Prin® [US-OTC]; Genaced™ [US-OTC]; Goody's® Extra Strength Headache Powder [US-OTC]; Goody's® Extra Strength Pain Relief [US-OTC]; Pain-Off [US-OTC]; Vanquish® Extra Strength Pain Reliever [US-OTC]
Therapeutic Category Analgesic, Nonnarcotic
Use Relief of mild-to-moderate pain; mild-to-moderate pain associated with migraine headache
Usual Dosage Oral: Adults:
Analgesic:
Based on **acetaminophen** component:
Mild-to-moderate pain: 325-650 mg every 4-6 hours as needed; do **not** exceed 4 g/day
Mild-to-moderate pain associated with migraine headache: 500 mg/dose (in combination with 500 mg aspirin and 130 mg caffeine) every 6 hours while symptoms persist; do not use for longer than 48 hours
Based on **aspirin** component:
Mild-to-moderate pain: 325-650 mg every 4-6 hours as needed; do **not** exceed 4 g/day
Mild-to-moderate pain associated with migraine headache: 500 mg/dose (in combination with 500 mg acetaminophen and 130 mg caffeine) every 6 hours; do not use for longer than 48 hours

Product labeling:
Excedrin® Extra Strength, Excedrin® Migraine: Children >12 years and Adults: 2 doses every 6 hours (maximum: 8 doses/24 hours)
Note: When used for migraine, do not use for longer than 48 hours
(Continued)

acetaminophen, aspirin, and caffeine *(Continued)*

Goody's® Extra Strength Headache Powder: Children >12 years and Adults: 1 powder, placed on tongue or dissolved in water, every 4-6 hours (maximum: 4 powders/24 hours)

Goody's® Extra Strength Pain Relief Tablets: Children >12 years and Adults: 2 tablets every 4-6 hours (maximum: 8 tablets/24 hours)

Vanquish® Extra Strength Pain Reliever: Children >12 years and Adults: 2 tablets every 4 hours (maximum: 12 tablets/24 hours)

Dosage Forms

Caplet: Acetaminophen 250 mg, aspirin 250 mg, and caffeine 65 mg; acetaminophen 194 mg, aspirin 227 mg, and caffeine 33 mg

Excedrin® Extra Strength [OTC], Excedrin® Migraine [OTC]: Acetaminophen 250 mg, aspirin 250 mg, and caffeine 65 mg

Vanquish® Extra Strength Pain Reliever [OTC]: Acetaminophen 194 mg, aspirin 227 mg, and caffeine 33 mg

Geltab: Acetaminophen 250 mg, aspirin 250 mg, and caffeine 65 mg

Excedrin® Extra Strength [OTC], Excedrin® Migraine [OTC]: Acetaminophen 250 mg, aspirin 250 mg, and caffeine 65 mg

Powder: Acetaminophen 260 mg, aspirin 520 mg, and caffeine 32.5 mg

Goody's® Extra Strength Headache Powder [OTC]: Acetaminophen 260 mg, aspirin 520 mg, and caffeine 32.5 mg

Tablet:

Excedrin® Extra Strength [OTC], Excedrin® Migraine [OTC], Genaced™ [OTC], Pain-Off [OTC]: Acetaminophen 250 mg, aspirin 250 mg, and caffeine 65 mg

Fem-Prin® [OTC]: Acetaminophen 194.4 mg, aspirin 226.8 mg, and caffeine 32.4 mg

Goody's® Extra Strength Pain Relief [OTC]: Acetaminophen 130 mg, aspirin 260 mg, and caffeine 16.25 mg

acetaminophen, butalbital, and caffeine *see* butalbital, acetaminophen, and caffeine *on page 130*

acetaminophen, caffeine, and dihydrocodeine

(a seet a MIN oh fen, KAF een, & dye hye droe KOE deen)

Synonyms caffeine, dihydrocodeine, and acetaminophen; dihydrocodeine bitartrate, acetaminophen, and caffeine

U.S./Canadian Brand Names Panlor® DC [US]; Panlor® SS [US]; ZerLor™ [US]

Therapeutic Category Analgesic Combination (Opioid)

Controlled Substance C-III

Use Relief of moderate to moderately-severe pain

Usual Dosage Oral: Adults: Relief of pain:

Panlor® DC: 2 capsules every 4 hours as needed; adjust dose based on severity of pain (maximum dose: 10 capsules/24 hours)

Panlor® SS, ZerLor™: 1 tablet every 4 hours as needed; adjust dose based on severity of pain (maximum dose: 5 tablets/24 hours)

Dosage Forms

Capsule:

Panlor® DC: Acetaminophen 356.4 mg, caffeine 30 mg, and dihydrocodeine 16 mg

Tablet:

Panlor® SS, ZerLor™: Acetaminophen 712.8 mg, caffeine 60 mg, and dihydrocodeine 32 mg

acetaminophen, caffeine, codeine, and butalbital *see* butalbital, acetaminophen, caffeine, and codeine *on page 130*

acetaminophen, caffeine, hydrocodone, chlorpheniramine, and phenylephrine *see* hydrocodone, chlorpheniramine, phenylephrine, acetaminophen, and caffeine *on page 431*

acetaminophen, chlorpheniramine, and pseudoephedrine

(a seet a MIN oh fen, klor fen IR a meen, & soo doe e FED rin)

Sound-Alike/Look-Alike Issues

Thera-Flu® may be confused with Tamiflu®, Thera-Flur-N®

Tylenol® may be confused with atenolol, timolol, Tuinal®, Tylox®

Synonyms acetaminophen, pseudoephedrine, and chlorpheniramine; chlorpheniramine, acetaminophen, and pseudoephedrine; chlorpheniramine, pseudoephedrine, and acetaminophen; pseudoephedrine, acetaminophen, and chlorpheniramine; pseudoephedrine, chlorpheniramine, and acetaminophen

U.S./Canadian Brand Names Actifed® Cold and Sinus [US-OTC]; Comtrex® Flu Therapy Nighttime [US-OTC]; Drinex [US-OTC]; Kolephrin® [US-OTC]; Sinutab® Sinus & Allergy [Can]; Sinutab® Sinus Allergy Maximum Strength [US-OTC]; Tylenol® Allergy Sinus [Can]

Therapeutic Category Antihistamine/Decongestant/Analgesic

Use Temporary relief of sinus symptoms

Usual Dosage Oral:
Analgesic: Based on **acetaminophen** component:
Children: 10-15 mg/kg/dose every 4-6 hours as needed; do **not** exceed 5 doses in 24 hours
Adults: 325-650 mg every 4-6 hours as needed; do **not** exceed 4 g/day
Antihistamine: Based on **chlorpheniramine maleate** component:
Children:
2-6 years: 1 mg every 4-6 hours (maximum: 6 mg/24 hours)
6-12 years: 2 mg every 4-6 hours (maximum: 12 mg/24 hours)
Children >12 years and Adults: 4 mg every 4-6 hours (maximum: 24 mg/24 hours)
Decongestant: Based on **pseudoephedrine** component:
Children:
2-6 years: 15 mg every 4 hours (maximum: 90 mg/24 hours)
6-12 years: 30 mg every 4 hours (maximum: 180 mg/24 hours)
Children >12 years and Adults: 60 mg every 4 hours (maximum: 360 mg/24 hours)

Product labeling:
Sinutab® Sinus Allergy Maximum Strength: Children >12 years and Adults: 2 tablets/caplets every 6 hours (maximum: 8 doses/24 hours)

Dosage Forms
Caplet: Acetaminophen 325 mg, chlorpheniramine 2 mg, and pseudoephedrine 30 mg
Actifed® Cold and Sinus [OTC], Sinutab® Sinus Allergy Maximum Strength [OTC]: Acetaminophen 500 mg, chlorpheniramine 2 mg, and pseudoephedrine 30 mg
Kolephrin® [OTC]: Acetaminophen 325 mg, chlorpheniramine 2 mg, and pseudoephedrine 30 mg
Liquid:
Comtrex® Flu Therapy Nighttime [OTC]: Acetaminophen 100 mg, chlorpheniramine 4 mg, and pseudoephedrine 60 mg per 30 mL
Tablet:
Drinex: Acetaminophen 650 mg, chlorpheniramine maleate 4 mg, and pseudoephedrine hydrochloride 60 mg

acetaminophen, codeine, and doxylamine *(Canada only)*
(a seet a MIN oh fen, KOE deen, & dox IL a meen)
Synonyms codeine, doxylamine, and acetaminophen; doxylamine succinate, codeine phosphate, and acetaminophen
U.S./Canadian Brand Names Mersyndol® With Codeine [Can]
Therapeutic Category Analgesic, Opioid; Antihistamine
Controlled Substance CDSA-1
Use Relief of headache, cold symptoms, neuralgia, and muscular aches/pain
Usual Dosage Oral: Children >12 years and Adults: 1-2 tablets every 4 hours as needed; total dose should not exceed 12 tablets in a 24-hour period
Dosage Forms [CAN] = Canadian brand name
Tablet:
Mersyndol® With Codeine [CAN]: Acetaminophen 325 mg, codeine 8 mg, and doxylamine 5 mg [not available in the U.S.]

acetaminophen, dextromethorphan, and phenylephrine
(a seet a MIN oh fen, deks troe meth OR fan, & fen il EF rin)
Synonyms dextromethorphan hydrobromide, acetaminophen, and phenylephrine hydrochloride; phenylephrine, acetaminophen, and dextromethorphan; phenylephrine, dextromethorphan, and acetaminophen
U.S./Canadian Brand Names Alka-Seltzer Plus® Day Cold [US-OTC]; Tylenol® Cold Head Congestion Daytime [US-OTC]; Tylenol® Cold Multi-Symptom Daytime [US-OTC]; Vicks® DayQuil® Cold/Flu Multi-Symptom Relief [US-OTC]
Therapeutic Category Analgesic, Miscellaneous; Antitussive; Decongestant
Use Temporary relief of common cold and flu symptoms (eg, pain, fever, cough, congestion)
Usual Dosage Product labeling: Oral:
Alka-Seltzer Plus® Day Cold: Children ≥12 years and Adults: 2 capsules or 20 mL every 4 hours (maximum: 6 doses/24 hours)
Tylenol® Cold Head Congestion Daytime: Children ≥12 years and Adults: 2 caplets every 4 hours (maximum: 6 doses/24 hours)
Tylenol® Cold Multi-Symptom Daytime: Children ≥12 years and Adults: 2 caplets/gelcaps or 30 mL every 4 hours (maximum: 6 doses/24 hours)
Tylenol® Plus Infants Cold & Cough: Children 2-3 years (≥24 lbs): 1.6 mL every 4 hours as needed (maximum: 5 doses/24 hours)
Vicks® DayQuil® Cold/Flu Multi-Symptom Relief LiquiCaps: Children ≥12 years and Adults: 2 capsules every 4 hours (maximum: 6 doses/24 hours)
(Continued)

acetaminophen, dextromethorphan, and phenylephrine *(Continued)*

Vicks® DayQuil® Cold/Flu Multi-Symptom Relief Liquid:
Children 6-11 years: 15 mL every 4 hours, up to 5 doses/day (maximum: 75 mL/24 hours)
Children ≥12 years and Adults: 30 mL every 4 hours (maximum: 6 doses/24 hours)

Dosage Forms
  Caplet:
    Mapap® Multi-Symptom Cold [OTC], Tylenol® Cold Head Congestion Daytime [OTC], Tylenol® Cold Multi-Symptom Daytime [OTC]: Acetaminophen 325 mg, dextromethorphan 10 mg, and phenylephrine 5 mg
  Capsule, liquid gel:
    Alka-Seltzer Plus® Day Cold [OTC]: Acetaminophen 325 mg, dextromethorphan 10 mg, and phenylephrine 5 mg
  Capsule, liquicap:
    Vicks® DayQuil® Cold/Flu Multi-Symptom Relief [OTC]: Acetaminophen 325 mg, dextromethorphan 10 mg, and phenylephrine 5 mg
  Gelcap:
    Tylenol® Cold Multi-Symptom Daytime [OTC]: Acetaminophen 325 mg, dextromethorphan 10 mg, and phenylephrine 5 mg
  Liquid:
    Alka-Seltzer Plus® Day Cold [OTC]: Acetaminophen 162.5 mg, dextromethorphan 5 mg, and phenylephrine 2.5 mg per 5 mL
    Tylenol® Cold Multi-Symptom Daytime [OTC], Vicks® DayQuil® Cold/Flu Multi-Symptom Relief [OTC]: Acetaminophen 325 mg, dextromethorphan 10 mg, and phenylephrine 5 mg per 15 mL

acetaminophen, dextromethorphan, and pseudoephedrine

(a seet a MIN oh fen, deks troe meth OR fan, & soo doe e FED rin)

Sound-Alike/Look-Alike Issues
  Sudafed® may be confused with Sufenta®
  Thera-Flu® may be confused with Tamiflu®, Thera-Flur-N®
  Tylenol® may be confused with atenolol, timolol, Tuinal®, Tylox®

Synonyms dextromethorphan, acetaminophen, and pseudoephedrine; pseudoephedrine, acetaminophen, and dextromethorphan; pseudoephedrine, dextromethorphan, and acetaminophen

U.S./Canadian Brand Names Contac® Complete [Can]; Contac® Cough, Cold and Flu Day & Night™ [Can]; Sudafed® Cold & Cough Extra Strength [Can]; Sudafed® Severe Cold [US-OTC]; Tylenol® Cold Day Non-Drowsy [US-OTC]; Tylenol® Cold Daytime [Can]; Tylenol® Flu Non-Drowsy Maximum Strength [US-OTC]

Therapeutic Category Cold Preparation

Use Treatment of mild-to-moderate pain and fever; symptomatic relief of cough and congestion

Usual Dosage Oral:
  Analgesic: Based on acetaminophen component:
    Children: 10-15 mg/kg/dose every 4-6 hours as needed; do **not** exceed 5 doses/24 hours
    Adults: 325-650 mg every 4-6 hours as needed; do **not** exceed 4 g/day
  Cough suppressant: Based on dextromethorphan component:
    Children 6-12 years: 15 mg every 6-8 hours; do **not** exceed 60 mg/24 hours
    Children >12 years and Adults: 10-20 mg every 4-8 hours **or** 30 mg every 8 hours; do **not** exceed 120 mg/24 hours
  Decongestant: Based on pseudoephedrine component:
    Children:
      2-6 years: 15 mg every 4 hours (maximum: 90 mg/24 hours)
      6-12 years: 30 mg every 4 hours (maximum: 180 mg/24 hours)
      Children >12 years and Adults: 60 mg every 4 hours (maximum: 360 mg/24 hours)

  Product labeling:
    Infants' Tylenol® Cold Plus Cough Concentrated Drops: Children 2-3 years (24-55 lb): 2 dropperfuls every 4-6 hours (maximum: 4 doses/24 hours)
    Sudafed® Severe Cold, Tylenol® Flu Non-Drowsy Maximum Strength: Children >12 years and Adults: 2 doses every 6 hours (maximum: 8 doses/24 hours)
    Tylenol® Cold Non-Drowsy:
      Children 6-11 years: 1 dose every 6 hours (maximum: 4 doses/24 hours)
      Children ≥12 years and Adults: 2 doses every 6 hours (maximum: 8 doses/24 hours)

Dosage Forms
  Caplet:
    Sudafed® Severe Cold [OTC], Tylenol® Cold Day Non-Drowsy [OTC]: Acetaminophen 325 mg, dextromethorphan 15 mg, and pseudoephedrine 30 mg
  Gelcap:
    Tylenol® Flu Non-Drowsy Maximum Strength [OTC]: Acetaminophen 500 mg, dextromethorphan 15 mg, and pseudoephedrine 30 mg

acetaminophen, dichloralphenazone, and isometheptene *see* acetaminophen, isometheptene, and dichloralphenazone *on this page*

acetaminophen, isometheptene, and dichloralphenazone
(a seet a MIN oh fen, eye soe me THEP teen, & dye KLOR al FEN a zone)
Sound-Alike/Look-Alike Issues
Midrin® may be confused with Mydfrin®
Synonyms acetaminophen, dichloralphenazone, and isometheptene; dichloralphenazone, acetaminophen, and isometheptene; dichloralphenazone, isometheptene, and acetaminophen; isometheptene, acetaminophen, and dichloralphenazone; isometheptene, dichloralphenazone, and acetaminophen
U.S./Canadian Brand Names Midrin® [US]; Migratine [US]
Therapeutic Category Analgesic, Nonnarcotic
Controlled Substance C-IV
Use Relief of migraine and tension headache
Usual Dosage Oral: Adults:
Migraine headache: 2 capsules to start, followed by 1 capsule every hour until relief is obtained (maximum: 5 capsules/12 hours)
Tension headache: 1-2 capsules every 4 hours (maximum: 8 capsules/24 hours)
Dosage Forms
Capsule: Acetaminophen 325 mg, isometheptene 65 mg
Midrin®, Migratine: Acetaminophen 325 mg, isometheptene 65 mg, and dichloralphenazone 100 mg

acetaminophen, pseudoephedrine, and chlorpheniramine *see* acetaminophen, chlorpheniramine, and pseudoephedrine *on page 10*

Acetasol® HC [US] *see* acetic acid, propylene glycol diacetate, and hydrocortisone *on next page*

acetazolamide (a set a ZOLE a mide)
Sound-Alike/Look-Alike Issues
acetaZOLAMIDE may be confused with acetoHEXAMIDE
Diamox® Sequels® may be confused with Diabinese®, Dobutrex®, Trimox®
Tall-Man acetaZOLAMIDE
U.S./Canadian Brand Names Apo-Acetazolamide® [Can]; Diamox® Sequels® [US]; Diamox® [Can]
Therapeutic Category Anticonvulsant; Carbonic Anhydrase Inhibitor
Use Treatment of glaucoma (chronic simple open-angle, secondary glaucoma, preoperatively in acute angle-closure); drug-induced edema or edema due to congestive heart failure (adjunctive therapy); centrencephalic epilepsies (immediate release dosage form); prevention or amelioration of symptoms associated with acute mountain sickness
Usual Dosage Note: I.M. administration is not recommended because of pain secondary to the alkaline pH
Children:
Glaucoma:
Oral: 8-30 mg/kg/day or 300-900 mg/m^2/day divided every 8 hours
I.V.: 20-40 mg/kg/24 hours divided every 6 hours, not to exceed 1 g/day
Edema: Oral, I.V.: 5 mg/kg or 150 mg/m^2 once every day
Epilepsy: Oral: 8-30 mg/kg/day in 1-4 divided doses, not to exceed 1 g/day; extended release capsule is not recommended for treatment of epilepsy
Adults:
Glaucoma:
Chronic simple (open-angle): Oral: 250 mg 1-4 times/day or 500 mg extended release capsule twice daily
Secondary, acute (closed-angle): I.V.: 250-500 mg, may repeat in 2-4 hours to a maximum of 1 g/day
Edema: Oral, I.V.: 250-375 mg once daily
Epilepsy: Oral: 8-30 mg/kg/day in 1-4 divided doses; **extended release capsule is not recommended for treatment of epilepsy**
Mountain sickness: Oral: 250 mg every 8-12 hours (or 500 mg extended release capsules every 12-24 hours)
Therapy should begin 24-48 hours before and continue during ascent and for at least 48 hours after arrival at the high altitude
Note: In situations of rapid ascent (such as rescue or military operations), 1000 mg/day is recommended.
Dosage Forms
Capsule, extended release:
Diamox® Sequels®: 500 mg
Injection, powder for reconstitution: 500 mg
Tablet: 125 mg, 250 mg

acetic acid (a SEE tik AS id)
Sound-Alike/Look-Alike Issues
VoSol® may be confused with Vexol®
Synonyms ethanoic acid
Therapeutic Category Antibacterial, Otic; Antibacterial, Topical
Use Irrigation of the bladder; treatment of superficial bacterial infections of the external auditory canal
Usual Dosage
Irrigation (**Note:** Dosage of an irrigating solution depends on the capacity or surface area of the structure being irrigated):
For continuous irrigation of the urinary bladder with 0.25% acetic acid irrigation, the rate of administration will approximate the rate of urine flow; usually 500-1500 mL/24 hours
For periodic irrigation of an indwelling urinary catheter to maintain patency, about 50 mL of 0.25% acetic acid irrigation is required
Otic: Insert saturated wick; keep moist 24 hours; remove wick and instill 5 drops 3-4 times/day
Dosage Forms
Solution for irrigation: 0.25% (250 mL, 500 mL, 1000 mL)
Solution, otic: 2% (15 mL)

acetic acid, hydrocortisone, and propylene glycol diacetate *see* acetic acid, propylene glycol diacetate, and hydrocortisone *on this page*

acetic acid, propylene glycol diacetate, and hydrocortisone
(a SEE tik AS id, PRO pa leen GLY kole dye AS e tate, & hye droe KOR ti sone)
Synonyms acetic acid, hydrocortisone, and propylene glycol diacetate; hydrocortisone, acetic acid, and propylene glycol diacetate; propylene glycol diacetate, acetic acid, and hydrocortisone
U.S./Canadian Brand Names Acetasol® HC [US]; VoSol® HC [US]
Therapeutic Category Antibiotic/Corticosteroid, Otic
Use Treatment of superficial infections of the external auditory canal caused by organisms susceptible to the action of the antimicrobial, complicated by swelling
Usual Dosage Otic: Children ≥3 years and Adults: Instill 3-5 drops in ear(s) every 4-6 hours
Dosage Forms
Solution, otic drops: Acetic acid 2%, propylene glycol diacetate 3%, and hydrocortisone 1% (10 mL)
Acetasol® HC, VoSol® HC: Acetic acid 2%, propylene glycol diacetate 3%, and hydrocortisone 1% (10 mL)

acetohydroxamic acid (a SEE toe hye droks am ik AS id)
Sound-Alike/Look-Alike Issues
Lithostat® may be confused with Lithobid®
Synonyms AHA
U.S./Canadian Brand Names Lithostat® [US/Can]
Therapeutic Category Urinary Tract Product
Use Adjunctive therapy in chronic urea-splitting urinary infection
Usual Dosage Oral:
Children: Initial: 10 mg/kg/day
Adults: 250 mg 3-4 times/day for a total daily dose of 10-15 mg/kg/day
Dosage Forms
Tablet:
Lithostat®: 250 mg

Acetoxyl® [Can] *see* benzoyl peroxide *on page 103*
acetoxymethylprogesterone *see* medroxyprogesterone *on page 537*

acetylcholine (a se teel KOE leen)
Sound-Alike/Look-Alike Issues
acetylcholine may be confused with acetylcysteine
Synonyms acetylcholine chloride
U.S./Canadian Brand Names Miochol-E® [US/Can]
Therapeutic Category Cholinergic Agent
Use Produces complete miosis in cataract surgery, keratoplasty, iridectomy, and other anterior segment surgery where rapid miosis is required
Usual Dosage Intraocular: Adults: 0.5-2 mL of 1% injection (5-20 mg) instilled into anterior chamber before or after securing one or more sutures
Dosage Forms
Powder for intraocular solution:
Miochol®-E: 1:100 [20 mg; packaged with diluent (2 mL)]

acetylcholine chloride *see acetylcholine on previous page*

acetylcysteine (a se teel SIS teen)
Sound-Alike/Look-Alike Issues
acetylcysteine may be confused with acetylcholine
Mucomyst® may be confused with Mucinex®
Synonyms acetylcysteine sodium; mercapturic acid; NAC; *n*-acetylcysteine; *n*-acetyl-L-cysteine
U.S./Canadian Brand Names Acetadote® [US]; Acetylcysteine Solution [Can]; Mucomyst® [Can]; Parvolex® [Can]
Therapeutic Category Mucolytic Agent
Use Adjunctive mucolytic therapy in patients with abnormal or viscid mucous secretions in acute and chronic bronchopulmonary diseases; pulmonary complications of surgery and cystic fibrosis; diagnostic bronchial studies; antidote for acute acetaminophen toxicity
Usual Dosage
Acetaminophen poisoning: Children and Adults:
Oral: 140 mg/kg; followed by 17 doses of 70 mg/kg every 4 hours; repeat dose if emesis occurs within 1 hour of administration; therapy should continue until acetaminophen levels are undetectable and there is no evidence of hepatotoxicity.
I.V. (Acetadote®): Loading dose: 150 mg/kg over 60 minutes. Loading dose is followed by 2 additional infusions: Initial maintenance dose of 50 mg/kg infused over 4 hours, followed by a second maintenance dose of 100 mg/kg infused over 16 hours. To avoid fluid overload in patients <40 kg and those requiring fluid restriction, decrease volume of D_5W proportionally. Total dosage: 300 mg/kg administered over 21 hours.
Experts suggest that the duration of acetylcysteine administration may vary depending upon serial acetaminophen levels and liver function tests obtained during treatment. In general, patients without measurable acetaminophen levels and without significant LFT elevations (>3 times the ULN) can safely stop acetylcysteine after ≤24 hours of treatment. The patients who still have detectable levels of acetaminophen, and/or LFT elevations (>1000 units/L) continue to benefit from addition acetylcysteine administration

Adjuvant therapy in respiratory conditions: **Note:** Patients should receive an aerosolized bronchodilator 10-15 minutes prior to acetylcysteine.
Inhalation, nebulization (face mask, mouth piece, tracheostomy): Acetylcysteine 10% and 20% solution (dilute 20% solution with sodium chloride or sterile water for inhalation); 10% solution may be used undiluted
Infants: 1-2 mL of 20% solution or 2-4 mL of 10% solution until nebulized given 3-4 times/day
Children and Adults: 3-5 mL of 20% solution or 6-10 mL of 10% solution until nebulized given 3-4 times/day; dosing range: 1-10 mL of 20% solution or 2-20 mL of 10% solution every 2-6 hours
Inhalation, nebulization (tent, croupette): Children and Adults: Dose must be individualized; may require up to 300 mL solution/treatment
Direct instillation: Adults:
Into tracheostomy: 1-2 mL of 10% to 20% solution every 1-4 hours
Through percutaneous intratracheal catheter: 1-2 mL of 20% or 2-4 mL of 10% solution every 1-4 hours via syringe attached to catheter
Diagnostic bronchogram: Nebulization or intratracheal: Adults: 1-2 mL of 20% solution or 2-4 mL of 10% solution administered 2-3 times prior to procedure
Dosage Forms
Injection, solution:
Acetadote®: 20% [200 mg/mL] (30 mL)
Solution, inhalation/oral: 10% [100 mg/mL]; 20% [200 mg/mL]

acetylcysteine sodium *see acetylcysteine on this page*

Acetylcysteine Solution [Can] *see acetylcysteine on this page*

acetylsalicylic acid *see aspirin on page 78*

Aches-N-Pain® *(Discontinued) see ibuprofen on page 444*

achromycin *see tetracycline on page 831*

aciclovir *see acyclovir on page 17*

Acid Gone [US-OTC] *see aluminum hydroxide and magnesium carbonate on page 36*

Acid Gone Extra Strength [US-OTC] *see aluminum hydroxide and magnesium carbonate on page 36*

acidulated phosphate fluoride *see fluoride on page 361*

Aci-jel® *(Discontinued) see acetic acid on previous page*

Acilac [Can] *see lactulose on page 489*

AcipHex® [US/Can] *see rabeprazole on page 741*

acitretin (a si TRE tin)

Sound-Alike/Look-Alike Issues
Soriatane® may be confused with Loxitane®
U.S./Canadian Brand Names Soriatane® [US/Can]
Therapeutic Category Retinoid-like Compound
Use Treatment of severe psoriasis
Usual Dosage Oral: Adults: Individualization of dosage is required to achieve maximum therapeutic response while minimizing side effects
Initial therapy: Therapy should be initiated at 25-50 mg/day, given as a single dose with the main meal
Maintenance doses of 25-50 mg/day may be given after initial response to treatment; the maintenance dose should be based on clinical efficacy and tolerability
Dosage Forms
  Capsule:
    Soriatane®: 10 mg, 25 mg

Aclasta® [Can] *see* zoledronic acid *on page 907*

Aclovate® [US] *see* alclometasone *on page 24*

acrivastine and pseudoephedrine (AK ri vas teen & soo doe e FED rin)

Synonyms pseudoephedrine hydrochloride and acrivastine
U.S./Canadian Brand Names Semprex®-D [US]
Therapeutic Category Antihistamine/Decongestant Combination
Use Temporary relief of nasal congestion, decongest sinus openings, running nose, itching of nose or throat, and itchy, watery eyes due to hay fever or other upper respiratory allergies
Usual Dosage Oral: Adults: 1 capsule 3-4 times/day
Dosage Forms
  Capsule:
    Semprex®-D: Acrivastine 8 mg and pseudoephedrine 60 mg

ACT *see* dactinomycin *on page 228*

ACT® [US-OTC] *see* fluoride *on page 361*

Act-D *see* dactinomycin *on page 228*

Actagen® Syrup (Discontinued) *see* triprolidine and pseudoephedrine *on page 869*

Actagen® Tablet (Discontinued) *see* triprolidine and pseudoephedrine *on page 869*

Act-A-Med® (Discontinued) *see* triprolidine and pseudoephedrine *on page 869*

ACTH *see* corticotropin *on page 216*

ActHIB® [US/Can] *see Haemophilus* B conjugate vaccine *on page 411*

Acthrel® [US] *see* corticorelin *on page 216*

Acticin® [US] *see* permethrin *on page 670*

Actidose-Aqua® [US-OTC] *see* charcoal *on page 171*

Actidose® with Sorbitol [US-OTC] *see* charcoal *on page 171*

Actifed® [Can] *see* triprolidine and pseudoephedrine *on page 869*

Actifed® Allergy Tablet (Night) (Discontinued) *see* diphenhydramine and pseudoephedrine *on page 266*

Actifed® Cold and Allergy [US-OTC] [reformulation] *see* chlorpheniramine and phenylephrine *on page 177*

Actifed® Cold and Allergy (Discontinued) *see* triprolidine and pseudoephedrine *on page 869*

Actifed® Cold and Sinus [US-OTC] *see* acetaminophen, chlorpheniramine, and pseudoephedrine *on page 10*

Actigall® [US] *see* ursodiol *on page 879*

Actimmune® [US/Can] *see* interferon gamma-1b *on page 465*

actinomycin *see* dactinomycin *on page 228*

actinomycin D *see* dactinomycin *on page 228*

actinomycin Cl *see* dactinomycin *on page 228*

Actiq® [US/Can] *see* fentanyl *on page 346*

Activase® [US] *see* alteplase *on page 34*

Activase® rt-PA [Can] *see* alteplase *on page 34*

activated carbon *see* charcoal *on page 171*

activated charcoal *see* charcoal *on page 171*

activated dimethicone *see* simethicone *on page 786*

activated ergosterol *see* ergocalciferol *on page 305*

activated methylpolysiloxane *see* simethicone *on page 786*

activated protein C, human, recombinant *see* drotrecogin alfa *on page 285*

Activella® [US] *see* estradiol and norethindrone *on page 316*

Actonel® [US/Can] *see* risedronate *on page 760*

Actonel® and Calcium [US] *see* risedronate and calcium *on page 760*

Actoplus Met™ [US] *see* pioglitazone and metformin *on page 685*

Actos® [US/Can] *see* pioglitazone *on page 684*

ACT® Plus [US-OTC] *see* fluoride *on page 361*

ACT® x2™ [US-OTC] *see* fluoride *on page 361*

Acular® [US/Can] *see* ketorolac *on page 483*

Acular LS™ [US/Can] *see* ketorolac *on page 483*

Acular® PF [US] *see* ketorolac *on page 483*

ACV *see* acyclovir *on this page*

acycloguanosine *see* acyclovir *on this page*

acyclovir (ay SYE kloe veer)

Sound-Alike/Look-Alike Issues
Zovirax® may be confused with Zostrix®, Zyvox™

Synonyms aciclovir; ACV; acycloguanosine

U.S./Canadian Brand Names Apo-Acyclovir® [Can]; Gen-Acyclovir [Can]; Nu-Acyclovir [Can]; ratio-Acyclovir [Can]; Zovirax® [US/Can]

Therapeutic Category Antiviral Agent

Use Treatment of genital herpes simplex virus (HSV), herpes labialis (cold sores), herpes zoster (shingles), HSV encephalitis, neonatal HSV, mucocutaneous HSV in immunocompromised patients, varicella-zoster (chickenpox)

Usual Dosage Note: Obese patients should be dosed using ideal body weight

Genital HSV:
I.V.: Children ≥12 years and Adults (immunocompetent): Initial episode, severe: 5 mg/kg every 8 hours for 5-7 days
Oral: Adults:
Initial episode: 200 mg every 4 hours while awake (5 times/day) for 10 days (per manufacturer's labeling); 400 mg 3 times/day for 5-10 days has also been reported
Recurrence: 200 mg every 4 hours while awake (5 times/day) for 5 days (per manufacturer's labeling; begin at earliest signs of disease); 400 mg 3 times/day for 5 days has also been reported
Chronic suppression: 400 mg twice daily or 200 mg 3-5 times/day, for up to 12 months followed by re-evaluation (per manufacturer's labeling); 400-1200 mg/day in 2-3 divided doses has also been reported
Topical: Adults (immunocompromised): Ointment: Initial episode: ¹/₂" ribbon of ointment for a 4" square surface area every 3 hours (6 times/day) for 7 days

Herpes labialis (cold sores): Topical: Children ≥12 years and Adults: Cream: Apply 5 times/day for 4 days

Herpes zoster (shingles):
Oral: Adults (immunocompetent): 800 mg every 4 hours (5 times/day) for 7-10 days
I.V.:
Children <12 years (immunocompromised): 20 mg/kg/dose every 8 hours for 7 days
Children ≥12 years and Adults (immunocompromised): 10 mg/kg/dose or 500 mg/m²/dose every 8 hours for 7 days

HSV encephalitis: I.V.:
Children 3 months to 12 years: 20 mg/kg/dose every 8 hours for 10 days (per manufacturer's labeling); dosing for 14-21 days also reported
Children ≥12 years and Adults: 10 mg/kg/dose every 8 hours for 10 days (per manufacturer's labeling); 10-15 mg/kg/dose every 8 hours for 14-21 days also reported

Mucocutaneous HSV:
I.V.:
Children <12 years (immunocompromised): 10 mg/kg/dose every 8 hours for 7 days
(Continued)

acyclovir *(Continued)*

Children ≥12 years and Adults (immunocompromised): 5 mg/kg/dose every 8 hours for 7 days (per manufacturer's labeling); dosing for up to 14 days also reported

Topical: Ointment: Adults (nonlife-threatening, immunocompromised): ½" ribbon of ointment for a 4" square surface area every 3 hours (6 times/day) for 7 days

Neonatal HSV: I.V.: Neonate: Birth to 3 months: 10 mg/kg/dose every 8 hours for 10 days (manufacturer's labeling); 15 mg/kg/dose or 20 mg/kg/dose every 8 hours for 14-21 days has also been reported

Varicella-zoster (chickenpox): Begin treatment within the first 24 hours of rash onset:
Oral:
Children ≥2 years and ≤40 kg (immunocompetent): 20 mg/kg/dose (up to 800 mg/dose) 4 times/day for 5 days
Children >40 kg and Adults (immunocompetent): 800 mg/dose 4 times a day for 5 days

Dosage Forms
Capsule: 200 mg
Zovirax®: 200 mg
Cream, topical:
Zovirax®: 5% (2 g, 5 g)
Injection, powder for reconstitution: 500 mg, 1000 mg
Injection, solution [preservative free]: 25 mg/mL (20 mL, 40 mL); 50 mg/mL (10 mL, 20 mL)
Ointment, topical:
Zovirax®: 5% (15 g)
Suspension, oral: 200 mg/5 mL
Zovirax®: 200 mg/5 mL
Tablet: 400 mg, 800 mg
Zovirax®: 400 mg, 800 mg

Aczone™ **[US]** *see* dapsone *on page 231*

Adacel™ **[US/Can]** *see* diphtheria, tetanus toxoids, and acellular pertussis vaccine *on page 269*

Adagen® **[US/Can]** *see* pegademase (bovine) *on page 657*

Adalat® **XL**® **[Can]** *see* nifedipine *on page 605*

Adalat® **CC [US]** *see* nifedipine *on page 605*

Adalat® *(Discontinued) see* nifedipine *on page 605*

adalimumab *(a da LIM yoo mab)*
Sound-Alike/Look-Alike Issues
Humira® may be confused with Humulin®
Synonyms antitumor necrosis factor apha (human); D2E7; human antitumor necrosis factor alpha
U.S./Canadian Brand Names Humira® [US/Can]
Therapeutic Category Antirheumatic, Disease Modifying; Monoclonal Antibody
Use
Treatment of active rheumatoid arthritis, active psoriatic arthritis (moderate-to-severe), or ankylosing spondylitis; may be used alone or in combination with disease-modifying antirheumatic drugs (DMARDs).
Treatment of moderate-to-severe active Crohn disease which has inadequate response to conventional treatment, or which has lost response to or is intolerant of infliximab
Usual Dosage SubQ: Adults:
Rheumatoid arthritis: 40 mg every other week; may be administered with other DMARDs; patients not taking methotrexate may increase dose to 40 mg/week
Ankylosing spondylitis, psoriatic arthritis: 40 mg every other week
Dosage Forms
Injection, solution [preservative free]:
Humira®: 40 mg/0.8 mL (1 mL)

adamantanamine hydrochloride *see* amantadine *on page 38*

adapalene *(a DAP a leen)*
U.S./Canadian Brand Names Differin® XP [Can]; Differin® [US/Can]
Therapeutic Category Acne Products
Use Treatment of acne vulgaris
Usual Dosage Topical: Children >12 years and Adults: Apply once daily at bedtime; therapeutic results should be noticed after 8-12 weeks of treatment

Dosage Forms
 Cream, topical:
  Differin®: 0.1% (15 g, 45 g)
 Gel, topical:
  Differin®: 0.1% (15 g, 45 g); 0.3% (45 g)

Adderall® [US] *see* dextroamphetamine and amphetamine *on page 246*

Adderall XR® [US/Can] *see* dextroamphetamine and amphetamine *on page 246*

adefovir (a DEF o veer)
 Synonyms adefovir dipivoxil
 U.S./Canadian Brand Names Hepsera™ [US/Can]
 Therapeutic Category Antiretroviral Agent, Nonnucleoside Reverse Transcriptase Inhibitor (NNRTI)
 Use Treatment of chronic hepatitis B with evidence of active viral replication (based on persistent elevation of ALT/AST or histologic evidence), including patients with lamivudine-resistant hepatitis B
 Usual Dosage Oral: Adults: 10 mg once daily
 Dosage Forms
  Tablet:
   Hepsera®: 10 mg

adefovir dipivoxil *see* adefovir *on this page*

ADEKs [US-OTC] *see* vitamins (multiple/pediatric) *on page 896*

Adenocard® [US/Can] *see* adenosine *on this page*

Adenoscan® [US/Can] *see* adenosine *on this page*

adenosine (a DEN oh seen)
 Synonyms 9-beta-d-ribofuranosyladenine
 U.S./Canadian Brand Names Adenocard® [US/Can]; Adenoscan® [US/Can]; Adenosine Injection, USP [Can]
 Therapeutic Category Antiarrhythmic Agent, Class IV; Diagnostic Agent
 Use
  Adenocard®: Treatment of paroxysmal supraventricular tachycardia (PSVT) including that associated with accessory bypass tracts (Wolff-Parkinson-White syndrome); when clinically advisable, appropriate vagal maneuvers should be attempted prior to adenosine administration; **not effective in atrial flutter, atrial fibrillation, or ventricular tachycardia**
  Adenoscan®: Pharmacologic stress agent used in myocardial perfusion thallium-201 scintigraphy
 Usual Dosage
  Adenocard®: **Rapid I.V. push (over 1-2 seconds) via peripheral line:**
  Infants and Children:
   Manufacturer's recommendation:
    <50 kg: 0.05-0.1 mg/kg. If conversion of PSVT does not occur within 1-2 minutes, may increase dose by 0.05-0.1 mg/kg. May repeat until sinus rhythm is established or to a maximum single dose of 0.3 mg/kg or 12 mg. Follow each dose with normal saline flush.
    ≥50 kg: Refer to Adult dosing
   Pediatric advanced life support (PALS): Treatment of SVT: I.V., I.O.: 0.1 mg/kg; if not effective, administer 0.2 mg/kg of PSVT; medium dose required: 0.15 mg/kg; maximum single dose: 12 mg. Follow each dose with normal saline flush.
  Adults: 6 mg; if not effective within 1-2 minutes, 12 mg may be given; may repeat 12 mg bolus if needed
  Maximum single dose: 12 mg
  Follow each I.V. bolus of adenosine with normal saline flush
  Note: Preliminary results in adults suggest adenosine may be administered via a central line at lower doses (ie, initial adult dose: 3 mg).

  Adenoscan®: Stress testing: Continuous I.V. infusion via peripheral line: 140 mcg/kg/minute for 6 minutes using syringe or columetric infusion pump; total dose: 0.84 mg/kg. Thallium-201 is injected at midpoint (3 minutes) of infusion.
 Dosage Forms
  Injection, solution [preservative free]: 3 mg/mL (2 mL, 4 mL)
   Adenocard®: 3 mg/mL (2 mL, 4 mL)
   Adenoscan®: 3 mg/mL (20 mL, 30 mL)

Adenosine Injection, USP [Can] *see* adenosine *on this page*

Adept® [US] *see* icodextrin *on page 446*

ADH *see* vasopressin *on page 886*

Adipex-P® [US] *see* phentermine *on page 674*

Adlone® **Injection** *(Discontinued)* *see* methylprednisolone *on page 559*

Adoxa® **[US]** *see* doxycycline *on page 281*

Adrenalin® **[US/Can]** *see* epinephrine *on page 300*

adrenaline *see* epinephrine *on page 300*

adrenocorticotropic hormone *see* corticotropin *on page 216*

adria *see* doxorubicin *on page 280*

Adriamycin® **[US/Can]** *see* doxorubicin *on page 280*

Adrucil® **[US]** *see* fluorouracil *on page 363*

adsorbent charcoal *see* charcoal *on page 171*

Adsorbocarpine® **Ophthalmic** *(Discontinued)* *see* pilocarpine *on page 682*

Adsorbonac® *(Discontinued)* *see* sodium chloride *on page 792*

Adsorbotear® **Ophthalmic Solution** *(Discontinued)* *see* artificial tears *on page 75*

Advair Diskus® **[US/Can]** *see* fluticasone and salmeterol *on page 367*

Advair® **HFA [US]** *see* fluticasone and salmeterol *on page 367*

Advanced Formula Oxy® **Sensitive Gel** *(Discontinued)* *see* benzoyl peroxide *on page 103*

Advanced NatalCare® **[US]** *see* vitamins (multiple/prenatal) *on page 896*

Advanced-RF NatalCare® **[US]** *see* vitamins (multiple/prenatal) *on page 896*

Advantage-S™ **[US-OTC]** *see* nonoxynol 9 *on page 610*

Advate [US] *see* antihemophilic factor (recombinant) *on page 59*

Advicor® **[US/Can]** *see* niacin and lovastatin *on page 603*

Advil® **[US-OTC/Can]** *see* ibuprofen *on page 444*

Advil® **Allergy Sinus [US]** *see* ibuprofen, pseudoephedrine, and chlorpheniramine *on page 445*

Advil® **Children's [US-OTC]** *see* ibuprofen *on page 444*

Advil® **Cold and Sinus Plus [Can]** *see* ibuprofen, pseudoephedrine, and chlorpheniramine *on page 445*

Advil® **Cold, Children's [US-OTC]** *see* pseudoephedrine and ibuprofen *on page 729*

Advil® **Cold & Sinus [US-OTC/Can]** *see* pseudoephedrine and ibuprofen *on page 729*

Advil® **Infants' [US-OTC]** *see* ibuprofen *on page 444*

Advil® **Junior [US-OTC]** *see* ibuprofen *on page 444*

Advil® **Migraine [US-OTC]** *see* ibuprofen *on page 444*

Advil® **Multi-Symptom Cold [US]** *see* ibuprofen, pseudoephedrine, and chlorpheniramine *on page 445*

Aerius® **[Can]** *see* desloratadine *on page 238*

Aeroaid® *(Discontinued)*

AeroBid® **[US]** *see* flunisolide *on page 359*

AeroBid®**-M [US]** *see* flunisolide *on page 359*

Aerodine® *(Discontinued)* *see* povidone-iodine *on page 704*

aerohist plus™ **[US]** *see* chlorpheniramine, phenylephrine, and methscopolamine *on page 181*

aeroKid™ **[US]** *see* chlorpheniramine, phenylephrine, and methscopolamine *on page 181*

Aerospan™ **[US]** *see* flunisolide *on page 359*

Afeditab™ **CR [US]** *see* nifedipine *on page 605*

A-Free Prenatal [US] *see* vitamins (multiple/prenatal) *on page 896*

Afrin® **Children's Nose Drops** *(Discontinued)* *see* oxymetazoline *on page 643*

Afrin® **Extra Moisturizing [US-OTC]** *see* oxymetazoline *on page 643*

Afrinol® *(Discontinued)* *see* pseudoephedrine *on page 727*

Afrin® **Original [US-OTC]** *see* oxymetazoline *on page 643*

Afrin® **Saline Mist** *(Discontinued)* *see* sodium chloride *on page 792*

Afrin® **Severe Congestion [US-OTC]** *see* oxymetazoline *on page 643*

Afrin® **Sinus [US-OTC]** *see* oxymetazoline *on page 643*

Aftate® **Antifungal** *(Discontinued)* *see* tolnaftate *on page 849*

AG *see* aminoglutethimide *on page 42*

agalsidase alfa *(Canada only)* (aye GAL si days AL fa)
Sound-Alike/Look-Alike Issues
  agalsidase alfa may be confused with agalsidase beta, alglucerase, alglucosidase alfa
Synonyms agalsidase alpha; alpha-galactosidase-A (gene-activated)
U.S./Canadian Brand Names Replagal™ [Can]
Therapeutic Category Enzyme
Use Replacement therapy for Fabry disease
Usual Dosage Note: Premedication with oral antihistamines and corticosteroids may alleviate infusion-related reactions associated with agalsidase alfa.
  I.V.: Children and Adults: Fabry disease: 0.2 mg/kg every 2 weeks
Dosage Forms [CAN] = Canadian brand name
  Injection, solution [preservative free]:
  Replagal™ [CAN]: 1 mg/1mL (3.5 mL) [not available in the U.S.]

agalsidase alpha *see* agalsidase alfa *(Canada only) on this page*

agalsidase beta (aye GAL si days BAY ta)
Sound-Alike/Look-Alike Issues
  agalsidase beta may be confused with agalsidase alfa, alglucerase, alglucosidase alfa
Synonyms alpha-galactosidase-A (human, recombinant); r-h α-GAL
U.S./Canadian Brand Names Fabrazyme® [US/Can]
Therapeutic Category Enzyme
Use Replacement therapy for Fabry disease
Usual Dosage I.V.: Children ≥8 years and Adults: 1 mg/kg every 2 weeks
Dosage Forms
  Injection, powder for reconstitution:
  Fabrazyme®: 5 mg, 35 mg

Agenerase® **[US/Can]** *see* amprenavir *on page 54*

Aggrastat® **[US/Can]** *see* tirofiban *on page 846*

Aggrenox® **[US/Can]** *see* aspirin and dipyridamole *on page 79*

AGN 1135 *see* rasagiline *on page 745*

AgNO₃ *see* silver nitrate *on page 785*

Agrylin® **[US/Can]** *see* anagrelide *on page 55*

AGT *see* aminoglutethimide *on page 42*

AHA *see* acetohydroxamic acid *on page 14*

AH-Chew® **[US]** *see* chlorpheniramine, phenylephrine, and methscopolamine *on page 181*

AH-Chew® **II [US]** *see* chlorpheniramine, phenylephrine, and methscopolamine *on page 181*

Ah-Chew D® **[US]** *see* phenylephrine *on page 675*

AHF (human) *see* antihemophilic factor (human) *on page 58*

AHF (human) *see* antihemophilic factor/von Willebrand factor complex (human) *on page 60*

AHF (recombinant) *see* antihemophilic factor (recombinant) *on page 59*

Ahist™ **[US]** *see* chlorpheniramine *on page 177*

AICC *see* antiinhibitor coagulant complex *on page 61*

Airet® *(Discontinued)* *see* albuterol *on page 23*

Airomir [Can] *see* albuterol *on page 23*

AKBeta® *(Discontinued)* *see* levobunolol *on page 499*

Ak-Chlor® **Ophthalmic** *(Discontinued)* *see* chloramphenicol *on page 173*

AK-Con™ **[US]** *see* naphazoline *on page 590*

AK-Dilate® **[US]** *see* phenylephrine *on page 675*

AK-Fluor® **[US]** *see* fluorescein *on page 361*

Ak-Homatropine® **Ophthalmic** *(Discontinued)* *see* homatropine *on page 421*

Akineton® **[US/Can]** *see* biperiden *on page 112*

AK-Nefrin *(Discontinued)* *see* phenylephrine *on page 675*

Akne-Mycin® **[US]** *see* erythromycin *on page 309*

AK-Pentolate® *(Discontinued) see* cyclopentolate *on page 221*

AK-Poly-Bac™ **[US]** *see* bacitracin and polymyxin B *on page 91*

AK-Pred® **[US]** *see* prednisolone (ophthalmic) *on page 709*

AK-Spore® **H.C. Ophthalmic** *(Discontinued) see* bacitracin, neomycin, polymyxin B, and hydrocortisone *on page 92*

AK-Spore® **H.C. Otic** *(Discontinued) see* neomycin, polymyxin B, and hydrocortisone *on page 597*

AK-Spore® **Ophthalmic Ointment** *(Discontinued) see* bacitracin, neomycin, and polymyxin B *on page 91*

AK-Taine® *(Discontinued) see* proparacaine *on page 721*

AKTob® **[US]** *see* tobramycin *on page 846*

AK-Tracin® *(Discontinued) see* bacitracin *on page 91*

AK-Trol® **Ophthalmic Ointment** *(Discontinued) see* neomycin, polymyxin B, and dexamethasone *on page 597*

AK-Trol® **Ophthalmic Suspension** *(Discontinued) see* neomycin, polymyxin B, and dexamethasone *on page 597*

Akwa Tears® **[US-OTC]** *see* artificial tears *on page 75*

Alamag [US-OTC] *see* aluminum hydroxide and magnesium hydroxide *on page 37*

Alamag Plus [US-OTC] *see* aluminum hydroxide, magnesium hydroxide, and simethicone *on page 37*

Alamast® **[US/Can]** *see* pemirolast *on page 660*

Alavert® **[US-OTC]** *see* loratadine *on page 517*

Alavert™ **Allergy and Sinus [US-OTC]** *see* loratadine and pseudoephedrine *on page 518*

Alaway™ **[US-OTC]** *see* ketotifen *on page 484*

Alazide® *(Discontinued) see* hydrochlorothiazide and spironolactone *on page 426*

Albalon® **[US]** *see* naphazoline *on page 590*

Albalon-A® **Ophthalmic** *(Discontinued)*

albendazole (al BEN da zole)

U.S./Canadian Brand Names Albenza® [US]
Therapeutic Category Anthelmintic
Use Treatment of parenchymal neurocysticercosis caused by *Taenia solium* and cystic hydatid disease of the liver, lung, and peritoneum caused by *Echinococcus granulosus*
Usual Dosage Oral: Children and Adults:
Neurocysticercosis:
<60 kg: 15 mg/kg/day in 2 divided doses (maximum: 800 mg/day) for 8-30 days
≥60 kg: 400 mg twice daily for 8-30 days
Note: Give concurrent anticonvulsant and steroid therapy during first week.
Hydatid:
<60 kg: 15 mg/kg/day in 2 divided doses (maximum: 800 mg/day)
≥60 kg: 400 mg twice daily
Note: Administer dose for three 28-day cycles with a 14-day drug-free interval in between.
Dosage Forms
Tablet:
Albenza®: 200 mg

Albenza® **[US]** *see* albendazole *on this page*

Albert® **Glyburide [Can]** *see* glyburide *on page 396*

Albert® **Pentoxifylline [Can]** *see* pentoxifylline *on page 667*

Albert® **Tiafen [Can]** *see* tiaprofenic acid *(Canada only) on page 840*

Albumarc® **[US]** *see* albumin *on this page*

albumin (al BYOO min)

Sound-Alike/Look-Alike Issues
Albutein® may be confused with albuterol
Buminate® may be confused with bumetanide

Synonyms albumin (human); normal human serum albumin; normal serum albumin (human); salt-poor albumin; SPA

U.S./Canadian Brand Names Albumarc® [US]; Albuminar® [US]; AlbuRx™ [US]; Albutein® [US]; Buminate® [US]; Flexbumin [US]; Plasbumin® [US]; Plasbumin®-25 [Can]; Plasbumin®-5 [Can]

Therapeutic Category Blood Product Derivative

Use Plasma volume expansion and maintenance of cardiac output in the treatment of certain types of shock or impending shock; may be useful for burn patients, ARDS, and cardiopulmonary bypass; other uses considered by some investigators (but not proven) are retroperitoneal surgery, peritonitis, and ascites; unless the condition responsible for hypoproteinemia can be corrected, albumin can provide only symptomatic relief or supportive treatment

Usual Dosage I.V.:

5% should be used in hypovolemic patients or intravascularly-depleted patients

25% should be used in patients in whom fluid and sodium intake must be minimized

Dose depends on condition of patient:

Children: Hypovolemia: 0.5-1 g/kg/dose (10-20 mL/kg/dose of albumin 5%); maximum dose: 6 g/kg/day

Adults: Usual dose: 25 g; initial dose may be repeated in 15-30 minutes if response is inadequate; no more than 250 g should be administered within 48 hours

Hypoproteinemia: 0.5-1 g/kg/dose; repeat every 1-2 days as calculated to replace ongoing losses

Hypovolemia: 5% albumin: 0.5-1 g/kg/dose; repeat as needed. **Note:** May be considered after inadequate response to crystalloid therapy and when nonprotein colloids are contraindicated. The volume administered and the speed of infusion should be adapted to individual response.

Dosage Forms

Injection, solution [preservative free; human]:

Albuminar®: 5% [50 mg/mL] (50 mL, 250 mL, 500 mL); 25% [250 mg/mL] (20 mL, 50 mL, 100 mL)

AlbuRx™: 5% [50 mg/mL] (250 mL, 500 mL); 25% [250 mg/mL] (50 mL, 100 mL)

Albutein®: 5% [50 mg/mL] (250 mL, 500 mL); 25% [250 mg/mL] (50 mL, 100 mL)

Buminate®: 5% [50 mg/mL] (250 mL, 500 mL); 25% [250 mg/mL] (20 mL, 50 mL, 100 mL)

Flexbumin: 25% [250 mg/mL] (50 mL, 100 mL)

Human Albumin Grifols®: 25% [250 mg/mL] (50 mL, 100 mL)

Plasbumin®: 5% [50 mg/mL] (50 mL, 250 mL); 25% [250 mg/mL] (20 mL, 50 mL, 100 mL)

Albuminar® [US] *see albumin* *on previous page*

albumin-bound paclitaxel *see paclitaxel (protein bound)* *on page 646*

albumin (human) *see albumin* *on previous page*

Albumisol® (Discontinued) *see albumin* *on previous page*

Albunex® (Discontinued) *see albumin* *on previous page*

AlbuRx™ [US] *see albumin* *on previous page*

Albutein® [US] *see albumin* *on previous page*

albuterol (al BYOO ter ole)

Sound-Alike/Look-Alike Issues

albuterol may be confused with Albutein®, atenolol

Proventil® may be confused with Bentyl®, Prilosec® Prinivil®

salbutamol may be confused with salmeterol

Ventolin® may be confused with phentolamine, Benylin®, Vantin®

Volmax® may be confused with Flomax®

Synonyms albuterol sulfate; salbutamol; salbutamol sulphate

U.S./Canadian Brand Names AccuNeb® [US]; Airomir [Can]; Alti-Salbutamol [Can]; Apo-Salvent® CFC Free [Can]; Apo-Salvent® Respirator Solution [Can]; Apo-Salvent® Sterules [Can]; Apo-Salvent® [Can]; Gen-Salbutamol [Can]; PMS-Salbutamol [Can]; ProAir™ HFA [US]; Proventil® HFA [US]; Proventil® [US]; ratio-Inspra-Sal [Can]; ratio-Salbutamol [Can]; Rhoxal-salbutamol [Can]; Salbu-2 [Can]; Salbu-4 [Can]; Ventolin® Diskus [Can]; Ventolin® HFA [US/Can]; Ventolin® [Can]; Ventrodisk [Can]; VoSpire ER® [US]

Therapeutic Category Adrenergic Agonist Agent

Use Bronchodilator in reversible airway obstruction due to asthma or COPD; prevention of exercise-induced bronchospasm

Usual Dosage

Oral:

Children: Bronchospasm (treatment):

2-6 years: 0.1-0.2 mg/kg/dose 3 times/day; maximum dose not to exceed 12 mg/day (divided doses)

6-12 years: 2 mg/dose 3-4 times/day; maximum dose not to exceed 24 mg/day (divided doses)

Extended release: 4 mg every 12 hours; maximum dose not to exceed 24 mg/day (divided doses)

Children >12 years and Adults: Bronchospasm (treatment): 2-4 mg/dose 3-4 times/day; maximum dose not to exceed 32 mg/day (divided doses)

(Continued)

albuterol (Continued)

Extended release: 8 mg every 12 hours; maximum dose not to exceed 32 mg/day (divided doses). A 4 mg dose every 12 hours may be sufficient in some patients, such as adults of low body weight.

Inhalation: MDI 90 mcg/puff:

Children ≤12 years:

Bronchospasm (acute): 4-8 puffs every 20 minutes for 3 doses, then every 1-4 hours; spacer/holding-chamber device should be used

Exercise-induced bronchospasm (prophylaxis): 1-2 puffs 5 minutes prior to exercise

Children >12 years and Adults:

Bronchospasm (acute): 4-8 puffs every 20 minutes for up to 4 hours, then every 1-4 hours as needed

Exercise-induced bronchospasm (prophylaxis): 2 puffs 5-30 minutes prior to exercise

Children ≥4 years and Adults: Bronchospasm (chronic treatment): 1-2 inhalations every 4-6 hours; maximum: 12 inhalations/day

NIH guidelines: 2 puffs 3-4 times a day as needed; may double dose for mild exacerbations

Nebulization:

Children ≤12 years:

Bronchospasm (treatment): 0.05 mg/kg every 4-6 hours; minimum dose: 1.25 mg, maximum dose: 2.5 mg

2-12 years: AccuNeb®: 0.63 mg or 1.25 mg 3-4 times/day, as needed, delivered over 5-15 minutes

Children >40 kg, patients with more severe asthma, or children 11-12 years: May respond better with a 1.25 mg dose

Bronchospasm (acute): Solution 0.5%: 0.15 mg/kg (minimum dose: 2.5 mg) every 20 minutes for 3 doses, then 0.15-0.3 mg/kg (up to 10 mg) every 1-4 hours as needed; may also use 0.5 mg/kg/hour by continuous infusion. Continuous nebulized albuterol at 0.3 mg/kg/hour has been used safely in the treatment of severe status asthmaticus in children; continuous nebulized doses of 3 mg/kg/hour ± 2.2 mg/kg/hour in children whose mean age was 20.7 months resulted in no cardiac toxicity; the optimal dosage for continuous nebulization remains to be determined.

Note: Use of the 0.5% solution should be used for bronchospasm (acute or treatment) in children <15 kg. AccuNeb® has not been studied for the treatment of acute bronchospasm; use of the 0.5% concentrated solution may be more appropriate.

Children >12 years and Adults:

Bronchospasm (treatment): 2.5 mg, diluted to a total of 3 mL, 3-4 times/day over 5-15 minutes

NIH guidelines: 1.25-5 mg every 4-8 hours

Bronchospasm (acute) in intensive care patients: 2.5-5 mg every 20 minutes for 3 doses, then 2.5-10 mg every 1-4 hours as needed, **or** 10-15 mg/hour continuously

Dosage Forms [CAN] = Canadian brand name

Aerosol, for oral inhalation [contains chlorofluorocarbon]: 90 mcg/metered inhalation (17 g)

Proventil®: 90 mcg/metered inhalation (17 g)

Aerosol, for oral inhalation [chlorofluorocarbon free]: 90 mcg/metered inhalation (8.5 g)

ProAir™ HFA: 90 mcg/metered inhalation (8.5 g)

Proventil® HFA: 90 mcg/metered inhalation (6.7 g)

Ventolin® HFA: 90 mcg/metered inhalation (18 g)

Injection, solution, as sulphate:

Ventolin® I.V. [CAN]: 1 mg/1mL (5 mL) [not available in U.S.]

Solution for nebulization: 0.042% (3 mL); 0.083% (3 mL); 0.5% (0.5 mL, 20 mL)

AccuNeb® [preservative free]: 0.63 mg/3 mL (3 mL) [0.021%]; 1.25 mg/3 mL (3 mL) [0.042%]

Proventil®: 0.083% (3 mL) [preservative free]; 0.5% (20 mL) [contains benzalkonium chloride]

Syrup: 2 mg/5 mL

Tablet: 2 mg, 4 mg

Tablet, extended release: 4 mg, 8 mg

VoSpire ER™: 4 mg, 8 mg

albuterol and ipratropium see ipratropium and albuterol on page 471

albuterol sulfate see albuterol on previous page

Alcaine® [US/Can] see proparacaine on page 721

Alcalak [US-OTC] see calcium carbonate on page 138

alclometasone (al kloe MET a sone)

Sound-Alike/Look-Alike Issues

Aclovate® may be confused with Accolate®

Synonyms alclometasone dipropionate

U.S./Canadian Brand Names Aclovate® [US]

Therapeutic Category Corticosteroid, Topical

Use Treatment of inflammation of corticosteroid-responsive dermatosis (low to medium potency topical corticosteroid)

Usual Dosage Topical: Apply a thin film to the affected area 2-3 times/day. Therapy should be discontinued when control is achieved; if no improvement is seen, reassessment of diagnosis may be necessary.

Dosage Forms
Cream: 0.05% (15 g, 45 g, 60 g)
Aclovate®: 0.05% (15 g, 45 g, 60 g)
Ointment: 0.05% (15 g, 45 g, 60 g)
Aclovate®: 0.05% (15 g, 45 g, 60 g)

alclometasone dipropionate *see* alclometasone *on previous page*

alcohol, absolute *see* alcohol (ethyl) *on this page*

alcohol, dehydrated *see* alcohol (ethyl) *on this page*

alcohol (ethyl) (AL koe hol, ETH il)
Sound-Alike/Look-Alike Issues
ethanol may be confused with Ethyol®, Ethamolin®
Synonyms alcohol, absolute; alcohol, dehydrated; ethanol; ethyl alcohol; EtOH
U.S./Canadian Brand Names Biobase-G™ [Can]; Biobase™ [Can]; EpiClenz™ [US-OTC]; Gel-Stat™ [US-OTC]; GelRite [US-OTC]; Isagel® [US-OTC]; Lavacol® [US-OTC]; Prevacare® [US-OTC]; Protection Plus® [US-OTC]; Purell® 2 in 1 [US-OTC]; Purell® with Aloe [US-OTC]; Purell® [US-OTC]
Therapeutic Category Intravenous Nutritional Therapy; Pharmaceutical Aid
Use Topical anti-infective; pharmaceutical aid; therapeutic neurolysis (nerve or ganglion block); replenishment of fluid and carbohydrate calories
Usual Dosage
Oral: **Note:** Oral dosing is not recommended outside of a hospital setting: Initial dose: 600 mg/kg [equivalent to 1.8 mL/kg using a 43% solution]
Maintenance dose:
Nondrinker: 66 mg/kg/hour [equivalent to 0.2 mL/kg/hour using a 43% solution]
Chronic drinker: 154 mg/kg/hour [equivalent to 0.46 mL/kg/hour using a 43% solution]
I.V.: Initial: 600 mg/kg [equivalent to 7.6 mL/kg using a 10% solution]
Maintenance dose:
Nondrinker: 66 mg/kg/hour [equivalent to 0.83 mL/kg/hour using a 10% solution]
Chronic drinker: 154 mg/kg/hour [equivalent to 1.96 mL/kg/hour using a 10% solution]
Antiseptic: Children and Adults: Liquid denatured alcohol: Topical: Apply 1-3 times/day as needed
Therapeutic neurolysis (nerve or ganglion block): Adults: Dehydrated alcohol injection: Intraneural: Dosage variable depending upon the site of injection (eg, trigeminal neuralgia: 0.05-0.5 mL as a single injection per interspace vs subarachnoid injection: 0.5-1 mL as a single injection per interspace); single doses >1.5 mL are seldom required
Replenishment of fluid and carbohydrate calories: Adults: Dehydrated alcohol infusion: Alcohol 5% and dextrose 5%: 1-2 L/day by slow infusion
Dosage Forms
Foam, topical:
Epi-Clenz™: 62% (240 mL, 480 mL)
Gel, topical:
Epi-Clenz™: 70% (45 mL, 120 mL, 480 mL)
GelRite: 67% (120 mL, 480 mL, 800 mL)
Gel-Stat™: 62% (120 mL, 480 mL)
Isagel®: 60% (59 mL, 118 mL, 621 mL, 800 mL)
Prevacare®: 60% (120 mL, 240 mL, 960 mL, 1200 mL, 1500 mL)
Protection Plus®: 62% (800 mL)
Purell®: 62% (15 mL, 30 mL, 59 mL, 120 mL, 236 mL, 250 mL, 360 mL, 500 mL, 800 mL, 1000 mL, 2000 mL)
Purell® Moisture Therapy: 62% (75 mL)
Purell® with Aloe: 62% (15 mL, 59 mL, 236 mL, 360 mL, 800 mL, 1000 mL, 2000 mL)
Infusion [in D_5W, dehydrated]: Alcohol 5% (1000 mL); alcohol 10% (1000 mL)
Injection, solution [dehydrated]: 98% (1 mL, 5 mL)
Liquid, topical [denatured]: 70% (3840 mL)
Lavacol® [OTC]: 70% (473 mL)
Lotion, topical:
Purell® 2 in 1: 62% (60 mL, 360 mL, 1000 mL)
Towlettes, topical:
Isagel®: 60% (50s, 300s)
Purell®: 62% (35s, 175s)

Alcomicin® [Can] *see* gentamicin *on page 390*

Alconefrin® Nasal Solution (Discontinued) *see* phenylephrine *on page 675*

Aldactazide® **[US]** *see* hydrochlorothiazide and spironolactone *on page 426*

Aldactazide 25® **[Can]** *see* hydrochlorothiazide and spironolactone *on page 426*

Aldactazide 50® **[Can]** *see* hydrochlorothiazide and spironolactone *on page 426*

Aldactone® **[US/Can]** *see* spironolactone *on page 804*

Aldara™ **[US/Can]** *see* imiquimod *on page 450*

aldesleukin (al des LOO kin)

Sound-Alike/Look-Alike Issues
aldesleukin may be confused with oprelvekin
Proleukin® may be confused with oprelvekin

Synonyms epidermal thymocyte activating factor; ETAF; IL-2; interleukin-2; lymphocyte mitogenic factor; NSC-373364; T-cell growth factor; TCGF; thymocyte stimulating factor

U.S./Canadian Brand Names Proleukin® [US/Can]

Therapeutic Category Biological Response Modulator

Use Treatment of metastatic renal cell cancer, melanoma

Usual Dosage Refer to individual protocols.
I.V.:
Renal cell carcinoma: 600,000 int. units/kg every 8 hours for a maximum of 14 doses; repeat after 9 days for a total of 28 doses per course. Retreat if needed 7 weeks after previous course.
Melanoma:
Single-agent use: 600,000 int. units/kg every 8 hours for a maximum of 14 doses; repeat after 9 days for a total of 28 doses per course. Retreat if needed 7 weeks after previous course.
In combination with cytotoxic agents: 24 million int. units/m^2 days 12-16 and 19-23
SubQ:
Single-agent doses: 3-18 million int. units/day for 5 days each week, up to 6 weeks
In combination with interferon:
5 million int. units/m^2 3 times/week
1.8 million int. units/m^2 twice daily 5 days/week for 6 weeks

Dosage Forms
Injection, powder for reconstitution:
Proleukin®: 22 x 10^6 int. units

Aldex™ **[US]** *see* guaifenesin and phenylephrine *on page 404*

Aldex® D [US] *see* phenylephrine and pyrilamine *on page 677*

Aldex® DM [US] *see* phenylephrine, pyrilamine, and dextromethorphan *on page 679*

Aldomet® *(Discontinued)* *see* methyldopa *on page 557*

Aldoril® **[US]** *see* methyldopa and hydrochlorothiazide *on page 557*

Aldoril® D50 *(Discontinued)* *see* methyldopa and hydrochlorothiazide *on page 557*

Aldroxicon I [US-OTC] *see* aluminum hydroxide, magnesium hydroxide, and simethicone *on page 37*

Aldroxicon II [US-OTC] *see* aluminum hydroxide, magnesium hydroxide, and simethicone *on page 37*

Aldurazyme® **[US/Can]** *see* laronidase *on page 494*

alefacept (a LE fa sept)

Synonyms B 9273; BG 9273; human LFA-3/IgG(1) fusion protein; LFA-3/IgG(1) fusion protein, human

U.S./Canadian Brand Names Amevive® [US/Can]

Therapeutic Category Monoclonal Antibody

Use Treatment of moderate to severe chronic plaque psoriasis in adults who are candidates for systemic therapy or phototherapy

Usual Dosage Adults:
I.M.: 15 mg once weekly; usual duration of treatment: 12 weeks
A second course of treatment may be initiated at least 12 weeks after completion of the initial course of treatment, provided CD4+ T-lymphocyte counts are within the normal range.
Note: CD4+ T-lymphocyte counts should be monitored before initiation of treatment and every 2 weeks during therapy. Dosing should be withheld if CD4+ counts are <250 cells/μL, and dosing should be permanently discontinued if CD4+ lymphocyte counts remain at <250 cell/μL for longer than 1 month.

Dosage Forms
Injection, powder for reconstitution [I.M. administration]:
Amevive®: 15 mg

alemtuzumab (ay lem TU zoo mab)

Synonyms C1H; campath-1H; DNA-derived humanized monoclonal antibody; humanized IgG1 anti-CD52 monoclonal antibody; NSC-715969

U.S./Canadian Brand Names Campath® [US]; MabCampath® [Can]

Therapeutic Category Antineoplastic Agent, Monoclonal Antibody

Use Treatment of B-cell chronic lymphocytic leukemia (B-CLL)

Usual Dosage Note: Dose escalation is required; usually accomplished in 3-7 days. Do not exceed single doses >30 mg or cumulative doses >90 mg/week. Pretreatment (with acetaminophen and an oral antihistamine) is recommended prior to the first dose, with dose escalations, and as clinically indicated; I.V. hydrocortisone may be used for severe infusion-related reactions.

I.V. infusion, SubQ (unlabeled route): Adults: B-CLL:
  Initial: 3 mg/day beginning on day 1; when tolerated, increase to 10 mg/day; when tolerated, increase to maintenance dose of 30 mg/day 3 times/week on alternate days for up to 12 weeks
  Maximum dose/day: 30 mg; maximum cumulative dose/week: 90 mg

Dosage Forms
  Injection, solution [vial; preservative free]:
  Campath®: 30 mg/mL (1 mL)

alendronate (a LEN droe nate)

Sound-Alike/Look-Alike Issues
  Fosamax® may be confused with Flomax®

Synonyms alendronate sodium

U.S./Canadian Brand Names Apo-Alendronate® [Can]; CO Alendronate [Can]; Fosamax® [US/Can]; Gen-Alendronate [Can]; Novo-Alendronate [Can]; PMS-Alendronate [Can]; ratio-Alendronate [Can]; Riva-Alendronate [Can]; Sandoz Alendronate [Can]

Therapeutic Category Bisphosphonate Derivative

Use Treatment and prevention of osteoporosis in postmenopausal females; treatment of osteoporosis in males; Paget disease of the bone in patients who are symptomatic, at risk for future complications, or with alkaline phosphatase ≥2 times the upper limit of normal; treatment of glucocorticoid-induced osteoporosis in males and females with low bone mineral density who are receiving a daily dosage ≥7.5 mg of prednisone (or equivalent)

Usual Dosage Oral: Adults: **Note:** Patients treated with glucocorticoids and those with Paget disease should receive adequate amounts of calcium and vitamin D.
  Osteoporosis in postmenopausal females:
  Prophylaxis: 5 mg once daily **or** 35 mg once weekly
  Treatment: 10 mg once daily **or** 70 mg once weekly
  Osteoporosis in males: 10 mg once daily **or** 70 mg once weekly
  Osteoporosis secondary to glucocorticoids in males and females: Treatment: 5 mg once daily; a dose of 10 mg once daily should be used in postmenopausal females who are not receiving estrogen.
  Paget disease of bone in males and females: 40 mg once daily for 6 months
  Retreatment: Relapses during the 12 months following therapy occurred in 9% of patients who responded to treatment. Specific retreatment data are not available. Following a 6-month post-treatment evaluation period, retreatment with alendronate may be considered in patients who have relapsed based on increases in serum alkaline phosphatase, which should be measured periodically. Retreatment may also be considered in those who failed to normalize their serum alkaline phosphatase.

Dosage Forms Note: Strength expressed as free acid
  Solution, oral:
  Fosamax®: 70 mg/75 mL
  Tablet:
  Fosamax®: 5 mg, 10 mg, 35 mg, 40 mg, 70 mg

alendronate and cholecalciferol (a LEN droe nate & kole e kal SI fer ole)

Synonyms alendronate sodium and cholecalciferol; cholecalciferol and alendronate; vitamin D_3 and alendronate

U.S./Canadian Brand Names Fosamax Plus D™ [US]; Fosavance [Can]

Therapeutic Category Bisphosphonate Derivative; Vitamin D Analog

Use Treatment of osteoporosis in postmenopausal females; increase bone mass in males with osteoporosis

Usual Dosage Oral: Adults: One tablet (alendronate 70 mg/cholecalciferol 2800 int. units **or** alendronate 70 mg/cholecalciferol 5600 int. units) once weekly. Appropriate dose in most osteoporotic women or men: Alendronate 70 mg/cholecalciferol 5600 int. units once weekly.

Dosage Forms
  Tablet:
  Fosamax Plus D™ 70/2800: Alendronate 70 mg and cholecalciferol 2800 int. units
  Fosamax Plus D™ 70/5600: Alendronate 70 mg and cholecalciferol 5600 int. units

alendronate sodium *see* alendronate *on previous page*

alendronate sodium and cholecalciferol *see* alendronate and cholecalciferol *on previous page*

Alenic Alka [US-OTC] *see* aluminum hydroxide and magnesium carbonate *on page 36*

Alenic Alka Tablet [US-OTC] *see* aluminum hydroxide and magnesium trisilicate *on page 37*

Aler-Cap [US-OTC] *see* diphenhydramine *on page 265*

Aler-Dryl [US-OTC] *see* diphenhydramine *on page 265*

Aler-Tab [US-OTC] *see* diphenhydramine *on page 265*

Alertec® [Can] *see* modafinil *on page 575*

Alesse® [US/Can] *see* ethinyl estradiol and levonorgestrel *on page 325*

Aleve® [US-OTC] *see* naproxen *on page 591*

Aleve® Cold & Sinus [US-OTC] *see* naproxen and pseudoephedrine *on page 592*

Aleve® Sinus & Headache [US-OTC] *see* naproxen and pseudoephedrine *on page 592*

Alfenta® [US/Can] *see* alfentanil *on this page*

alfentanil (al FEN ta nil)

Sound-Alike/Look-Alike Issues
alfentanil may be confused with Anafranil®, fentanyl, remifentanil, sufentanil
Alfenta® may be confused with Sufenta®
Synonyms alfentanil hydrochloride
U.S./Canadian Brand Names Alfentanil Injection, USP [Can]; Alfenta® [US/Can]
Therapeutic Category Analgesic, Narcotic; General Anesthetic
Controlled Substance C-II
Use Analgesic adjunct given by continuous infusion or in incremental doses in maintenance of anesthesia with barbiturate or N_2O or a primary anesthetic agent for the induction of anesthesia in patients undergoing general surgery in which endotracheal intubation and mechanical ventilation are required
Usual Dosage Doses should be titrated to appropriate effects; wide range of doses is dependent upon desired degree of analgesia/anesthesia
Adults: Dose should be based on ideal body weight.
Dosage Forms
Injection, solution [preservative free]: 500 mcg/mL (2 mL, 5 mL, 10 mL)
Alfenta®: 500 mcg/mL (2 mL, 5 mL, 10 mL, 20 mL)

alfentanil hydrochloride *see* alfentanil *on this page*

Alfentanil Injection, USP [Can] *see* alfentanil *on this page*

Alferon® N [US/Can] *see* interferon alfa-n3 *on page 464*

alfuzosin (al FYOO zoe sin)

Synonyms alfuzosin hydrochloride
U.S./Canadian Brand Names Uroxatral® [US]; Xatral [Can]
Therapeutic Category Alpha-Adrenergic Blocking Agent
Use Treatment of the functional symptoms of benign prostatic hyperplasia (BPH)
Usual Dosage Oral: Adults: 10 mg once daily
Dosage Forms
Tablet, extended release:
Uroxatral™: 10 mg

alfuzosin hydrochloride *see* alfuzosin *on this page*

alglucerase (al GLOO ser ase)

Sound-Alike/Look-Alike Issues
alglucerase may be confused with agalsidase alfa, agalsidase beta, alglucosidase alfa
Ceredase® may be confused with Cerezyme®
Synonyms glucocerebrosidase
U.S./Canadian Brand Names Ceredase® [US]
Therapeutic Category Enzyme
Use Replacement therapy for Gaucher disease (type 1)
Usual Dosage I.V.: Children and Adults: Initial: 30-60 units/kg every 2 weeks; dosing is individualized based on disease severity; average dose: 60 units/kg every 2 weeks. Range: 2.5 units/kg 3 times/week to 60 units/kg once weekly to every 4 weeks. Once patient response is well established, dose may be reduced every 3-6 months to determine maintenance therapy.

Dosage Forms
Injection, solution [preservative free]:
Ceredase®: 80 units/mL (5 mL)

alglucosidase *see* alglucosidase alfa *on this page*

alglucosidase alfa (al gloo KOSE i dase AL fa)

Sound-Alike/Look-Alike Issues
alglucosidase alfa may be confused with agalsidase alfa, agalsidase beta, alglucerase
Synonyms alglucosidase; GAA; rhGAA
U.S./Canadian Brand Names Myozyme® [US]
Therapeutic Category Enzyme
Use Replacement therapy for Pompe disease (infantile onset)
Usual Dosage I.V.: Children 1 month to 3.5 years (at first infusion): 20 mg/kg over ~4 hours every 2 weeks
Dosage Forms
Injection, powder for reconstitution [preservative free]:
Myozyme®: 50 mg

Alimta® [US/Can] *see* pemetrexed *on page 660*

Alinia® [US] *see* nitazoxanide *on page 606*

aliskiren (a lis KYE ren)

Synonyms aliskiren hemifumarate; SPP100
U.S./Canadian Brand Names Tekturna® [US]
Therapeutic Category Renin Inhibitor
Use Treatment of hypertension, alone or in combination with other antihypertensive agents
Usual Dosage Oral: Adults: Initial: 150 mg once daily; may increase to 300 mg once daily (maximum: 300 mg/day). **Note:** Prior to initiation, correct hypovolemia and/or closely monitor volume status in patients on concurrent diuretics during treatment initiation.
Dosage Forms
Tablet:
Tekturna®: 150 mg, 300 mg

aliskiren hemifumarate *see* aliskiren *on this page*

alitretinoin (a li TRET i noyn)

Sound-Alike/Look-Alike Issues
Panretin® may be confused with pancreatin
U.S./Canadian Brand Names Panretin® [US/Can]
Therapeutic Category Antineoplastic Agent, Miscellaneous; Retinoic Acid Derivative
Use Orphan drug: Topical treatment of cutaneous lesions in AIDS-related Kaposi sarcoma
Usual Dosage Topical: Apply gel twice daily to cutaneous lesions
Dosage Forms
Gel:
Panretin®: 0.1% (60 g tube)

Alka-Mints® [US-OTC] *see* calcium carbonate *on page 138*

Alka-Seltzer Plus® Day Cold [US-OTC] *see* acetaminophen, dextromethorphan, and phenylephrine *on page 11*

Alkeran® [US/Can] *see* melphalan *on page 539*

Allanfil 405 [US] *see* chlorophyllin, papain, and urea *on page 175*

Allanfil Spray [US] *see* chlorophyllin, papain, and urea *on page 175*

AllanFol RX [US] *see* folic acid, cyanocobalamin, and pyridoxine *on page 371*

AllanHist PDX [US] *see* brompheniramine, pseudoephedrine, and dextromethorphan *on page 122*

AllanTan Pediatric [US] *see* chlorpheniramine and phenylephrine *on page 177*

AllanVan-DM [US] *see* phenylephrine, pyrilamine, and dextromethorphan *on page 679*

AllanVan-S [US] *see* phenylephrine and pyrilamine *on page 677*

Allanzyme [US] *see* papain and urea *on page 652*

Allanzyme 650 [US] *see* papain and urea *on page 652*

Allbee® C-800 [US-OTC] *see* vitamin B complex combinations *on page 894*

Allbee® C-800 + Iron [US-OTC] *see* vitamin B complex combinations *on page 894*

Allbee® with C [US-OTC] *see* vitamin B complex combinations *on page 894*

Allegra® [US/Can] *see* fexofenadine *on page 351*

Allegra® 60 mg Capsule (Discontinued) *see* fexofenadine *on page 351*

Allegra-D® [Can] *see* fexofenadine and pseudoephedrine *on page 351*

Allegra-D® 12 Hour [US] *see* fexofenadine and pseudoephedrine *on page 351*

Allegra-D® 24 Hour [US] *see* fexofenadine and pseudoephedrine *on page 351*

Aller-Chlor® [US-OTC] *see* chlorpheniramine *on page 177*

Allercon® Tablet (Discontinued) *see* triprolidine and pseudoephedrine *on page 869*

Allerdryl® [Can] *see* diphenhydramine *on page 265*

Allerest® 12 Hour Nasal Solution (Discontinued) *see* oxymetazoline *on page 643*

Allerest® Allergy and Sinus Relief [US-OTC] *see* acetaminophen and pseudoephedrine *on page 8*

Allerest® Eye Drops (Discontinued) *see* naphazoline *on page 590*

Allerest® Maximum Strength Allergy and Hay Fever [US-OTC] *see* chlorpheniramine and pseudoephedrine *on page 178*

Allerfrim® [US-OTC] *see* triprolidine and pseudoephedrine *on page 869*

Allerfrin® Syrup (Discontinued) *see* triprolidine and pseudoephedrine *on page 869*

Allerfrin® Tablet (Discontinued) *see* triprolidine and pseudoephedrine *on page 869*

Allerfrin® with Codeine (Discontinued) *see* triprolidine, pseudoephedrine, and codeine *(Canada only) on page 869*

Allergen® [US] *see* antipyrine and benzocaine *on page 61*

AllerMax® [US-OTC] *see* diphenhydramine *on page 265*

Allernix [Can] *see* diphenhydramine *on page 265*

AlleRx™-D [US] *see* pseudoephedrine and methscopolamine *on page 730*

AlleRx™ Dose Pack [US] *see* chlorpheniramine, pseudoephedrine, and methscopolamine *on page 184*

Allerx™ Suspension [US] *see* chlorpheniramine and phenylephrine *on page 177*

Allfen-DM [US] *see* guaifenesin and dextromethorphan *on page 402*

Allfen Jr [US] *see* guaifenesin *on page 401*

Allfen (reformulation) [US] *see* guaifenesin and potassium guaiacolsulfonate *on page 405*

Alli™ [US-OTC] *see* orlistat *on page 633*

Alloprin® [Can] *see* allopurinol *on this page*

allopurinol (al oh PURE i nole)

Sound-Alike/Look-Alike Issues
allopurinol may be confused with Apresoline
Zyloprim® may be confused with Xylo-Pfan®, ZORprin®

Synonyms allopurinol sodium

U.S./Canadian Brand Names Alloprin® [Can]; Aloprim™ [US]; Apo-Allopurinol® [Can]; Novo-Purol [Can]; Zyloprim® [US/Can]

Therapeutic Category Xanthine Oxidase Inhibitor

Use
Oral: Prevention of attack of gouty arthritis and nephropathy; treatment of secondary hyperuricemia which may occur during treatment of tumors or leukemia; prevention of recurrent calcium oxalate calculi

I.V.: Treatment of elevated serum and urinary uric acid levels when oral therapy is not tolerated in patients with leukemia, lymphoma, and solid tumor malignancies who are receiving cancer chemotherapy

Usual Dosage
Oral: Doses >300 mg should be given in divided doses.
  Children ≤10 years: Secondary hyperuricemia associated with chemotherapy: 10 mg/kg/day in 2-3 divided doses **or** 200-300 mg/m^2/day in 2-4 divided doses, maximum: 800 mg/24 hours
    Alternative (manufacturer labeling): <6 years: 150 mg/day in 3 divided doses; 6-10 years: 300 mg/day in 2-3 divided doses
  Children >10 years and Adults:
    Secondary hyperuricemia associated with chemotherapy: 600-800 mg/day in 2-3 divided doses for prevention of acute uric acid nephropathy for 2-3 days starting 1-2 days before chemotherapy

Gout: Mild: 200-300 mg/day; Severe: 400-600 mg/day; to reduce the possibility of acute gouty attacks, initiate dose at 100 mg/day and increase weekly to recommended dosage.

Recurrent calcium oxalate stones: 200-300 mg/day in single or divided doses

I.V.: Hyperuricemia secondary to chemotherapy: Intravenous daily dose can be given as a single infusion or in equally divided doses at 6-, 8-, or 12-hour intervals. A fluid intake sufficient to yield a daily urinary output of at least 2 L in adults and the maintenance of a neutral or, preferably, slightly alkaline urine are desirable.

Children ≤10 years: Starting dose: 200 mg/m^2/day

Children >10 years and Adults: 200-400 mg/m^2/day (maximum: 600 mg/day)

Dosage Forms
Injection, powder for reconstitution: 500 mg
Aloprim™: 500 mg
Tablet: 100 mg, 300 mg
Zyloprim®: 100 mg, 300 mg

allopurinol sodium see allopurinol on previous page

all-*trans*-retinoic acid see tretinoin (oral) on page 860

Almacone® [US-OTC] see aluminum hydroxide, magnesium hydroxide, and simethicone on page 37

Almacone Double Strength® [US-OTC] see aluminum hydroxide, magnesium hydroxide, and simethicone on page 37

Almora® [US-OTC] see magnesium gluconate on page 526

almotriptan (al moh TRIP tan)

Sound-Alike/Look-Alike Issues
Axert™ may be confused with Antivert®
Synonyms almotriptan malate
U.S./Canadian Brand Names Axert™ [US/Can]
Therapeutic Category Serotonin 5-HT$_{1D}$ Receptor Agonist
Use Acute treatment of migraine with or without aura
Usual Dosage Oral: Adults: Migraine: Initial: 6.25-12.5 mg in a single dose; if the headache returns, repeat the dose after 2 hours; no more than 2 doses in 24-hour period
Note: If the first dose is ineffective, diagnosis needs to be reevaluated. Safety of treating more than 4 migraines/month has not been established.
Dosage Forms
Tablet:
Axert™: 6.25 mg, 12.5 mg

almotriptan malate see almotriptan on this page

Alocril® [US/Can] see nedocromil (ophthalmic) on page 595

Aloe Vesta® 2-n-1 Antifungal [US-OTC] see miconazole on page 566

Alomide® [US/Can] see lodoxamide on page 514

Alophen® [US-OTC] see bisacodyl on page 112

Aloprim™ [US] see allopurinol on previous page

Alor® 5/500 *(Discontinued)* see hydrocodone and aspirin on page 428

Alora® [US] see estradiol on page 313

alosetron (a LOE se tron)

Sound-Alike/Look-Alike Issues
Lotronex® may be confused with Lovenox®, Protonix®
U.S./Canadian Brand Names Lotronex® [US]
Therapeutic Category 5-HT$_3$ Receptor Antagonist
Use Treatment of women with severe diarrhea-predominant irritable bowel syndrome (IBS) who have failed to respond to conventional therapy
Usual Dosage Oral: Adults: Female: Initial: 0.5 mg twice daily for 4 weeks, with or without food; if tolerated, but response is inadequate, may be increased after 4 weeks to 1 mg twice daily. If response is inadequate after 4 weeks of 1 mg twice-daily dosing, discontinue treatment.
Note: Discontinue immediately if constipation or signs/symptoms of ischemic colitis occur. Do not reinitiate in patients who develop ischemic colitis.
Dosage Forms
Tablet:
Lotronex®: 0.5 mg, 1 mg

Aloxi® **[US]** *see* palonosetron *on page 647*

Alpain [US] *see* acetaminophen and phenyltoloxamine *on page 8*

alpha₁-antitrypsin *see* alpha₁-proteinase inhibitor *on this page*

alpha₁-PI *see* alpha₁-proteinase inhibitor *on this page*

alpha₁-proteinase inhibitor, human *see* alpha₁-proteinase inhibitor *on this page*

alpha₁-proteinase inhibitor (al fa won PRO tee in ase in HI bi tor)

Synonyms alpha₁-antitrypsin; α₁-PI; alpha₁-proteinase inhibitor, human; A₁-PI

U.S./Canadian Brand Names Aralast [US]; Prolastin® [US/Can]; Zemaira® [US]

Therapeutic Category Antitrypsin Deficiency Agent

Use Replacement therapy in congenital alpha₁-antitrypsin deficiency with clinical emphysema

Usual Dosage I.V.: Adults: 60 mg/kg once weekly

Dosage Forms

Injection, powder for reconstitution [preservative free]:

Aralast, Aralast NP, Prolastin®: 500 mg, 1000 mg

Zemaira®: 1000 mg

alpha-galactosidase (AL fa ga lak TOE si days)

Synonyms *Aspergillus niger*

U.S./Canadian Brand Names beano® [US-OTC]

Therapeutic Category Enzyme

Use Prevention of flatulence and bloating attributed to a variety of grains, cereals, nuts, and vegetables containing the sugars raffinose, stachyose, and/or verbascose

Usual Dosage Oral: Children ≥12 years and Adults:

Drops: Take 5 drops per serving of problem food; adjust according to number of problem foods per meal; usual dose/meal: 10-15 drops

Tablet: One tablet per serving of problem food; adjust according to number of problem foods per meal; usual dose/meal: 2-3 tablets

Dosage Forms

Drops:

beano® Drops: 150 galactosidase units/5 drops

Tablet:

beano®: 150 galactosidase units/5 tablets

alpha-galactosidase-A (gene-activated) *see* agalsidase alfa *(Canada only) on page 21*

alpha-galactosidase-A (human, recombinant) *see* agalsidase beta *on page 21*

Alphagan® **[Can]** *see* brimonidine *on page 118*

Alphagan® **(Discontinued)** *see* brimonidine *on page 118*

Alphagan® **P [US]** *see* brimonidine *on page 118*

Alphamul® **(Discontinued)** *see* castor oil *on page 157*

Alphanate® **[US]** *see* antihemophilic factor/von Willebrand factor complex (human) *on page 60*

AlphaNine® **SD [US]** *see* factor IX *on page 340*

Alphaquin HP® **[US]** *see* hydroquinone *on page 437*

Alph-E [US-OTC] *see* vitamin E *on page 894*

Alph-E-Mixed [US-OTC] *see* vitamin E *on page 894*

alprazolam (al PRAY zoe lam)

Sound-Alike/Look-Alike Issues

alprazolam may be confused with alprostadil, lorazepam, triazolam

Xanax® may be confused with Lanoxin®, Tenex®, Tylox®, Xopenex®, Zantac®, Zyrtec®

U.S./Canadian Brand Names Alprazolam Intensol® [US]; Alti-Alprazolam [Can]; Apo-Alpraz® TS [Can]; Apo-Alpraz® [Can]; Gen-Alprazolam [Can]; Niravam™ [US]; Novo-Alprazol [Can]; Nu-Alprax [Can]; Xanax TS™ [Can]; Xanax XR® [US]; Xanax® [US/Can]

Therapeutic Category Benzodiazepine

Controlled Substance C-IV

Use Treatment of generalized anxiety disorder (GAD); panic disorder, with or without agoraphobia; anxiety associated with depression

Usual Dosage Oral: **Note:** Treatment >4 months should be reevaluated to determine the patient's continued need for the drug

Adults:

Anxiety: Immediate release: Effective doses are 0.5-4 mg/day in divided doses; the manufacturer recommends starting at 0.25-0.5 mg 3 times/day; titrate dose upward; maximum: 4 mg/day. Patients requiring doses >4 mg/day should be increased cautiously. Periodic reassessment and consideration of dosage reduction is recommended.

Anxiety associated with depression: Immediate release: Average dose required: 2.5-3 mg/day in divided doses

Panic disorder:

Immediate release: Initial: 0.5 mg 3 times/day; dose may be increased every 3-4 days in increments ≤1 mg/day. Mean effective dosage: 5-6 mg/day; many patients obtain relief at 2 mg/day, as much as 10 mg/day may be required

Extended release: 0.5-1 mg once daily; may increase dose every 3-4 days in increments ≤1 mg/day (range: 3-6 mg/day)

Switching from immediate release to extended release: Patients may be switched to extended release tablets by taking the total daily dose of the immediate release tablets and giving it once daily using the extended release preparation.

Preoperative sedation: 0.5 mg in evening at bedtime and 0.5 mg 1 hour before procedure

Dose reduction: Abrupt discontinuation should be avoided. Daily dose may be decreased by 0.5 mg every 3 days, however, some patients may require a slower reduction. If withdrawal symptoms occur, resume previous dose and discontinue on a less rapid schedule.

Dosage Forms

Solution, oral [concentrate]:

Alprazolam Intensol®: 1 mg/mL

Tablet: 0.25 mg, 0.5 mg, 1 mg, 2 mg

Xanax®: 0.25 mg, 0.5 mg, 1 mg, 2 mg

Tablet, extended release: 0.5 mg, 1 mg, 2 mg, 3 mg

Xanax XR®: 0.5 mg, 1 mg, 2 mg, 3 mg

Tablet, orally disintegrating [scored]:

Niravam™: 0.25 mg, 0.5 mg, 1 mg, 2 mg

Alprazolam Intensol® [US] *see alprazolam on previous page*

alprostadil (al PROS ta dill)

Sound-Alike/Look-Alike Issues

alprostadil may be confused with alprazolam

Synonyms PGE_1; prostaglandin E_1

U.S./Canadian Brand Names Caverject Impulse® [US]; Caverject® [US/Can]; Edex® [US]; Muse® Pellet [Can]; Muse® [US]; Prostin VR Pediatric® [US]; Prostin® VR [Can]

Therapeutic Category Prostaglandin

Use

Prostin VR Pediatric®: Temporary maintenance of patency of ductus arteriosus in neonates with ductal-dependent congenital heart disease until surgery can be performed. These defects include cyanotic (eg, pulmonary atresia, pulmonary stenosis, tricuspid atresia, Fallot tetralogy, transposition of the great vessels) and acyanotic (eg, interruption of aortic arch, coarctation of aorta, hypoplastic left ventricle) heart disease.

Caverject®: Treatment of erectile dysfunction of vasculogenic, psychogenic, or neurogenic etiology; adjunct in the diagnosis of erectile dysfunction

Edex®, Muse®: Treatment of erectile dysfunction of vasculogenic, psychogenic, or neurogenic etiology

Usual Dosage

Patent ductus arteriosus (Prostin VR Pediatric®):

I.V. continuous infusion into a large vein, or alternatively through an umbilical artery catheter placed at the ductal opening: 0.05-0.1 mcg/kg/minute with therapeutic response, rate is reduced to lowest effective dosage; with unsatisfactory response, rate is increased gradually; maintenance: 0.01-0.4 mcg/kg/minute

PGE_1 is usually given at an infusion rate of 0.1 mcg/kg/minute, but it is often possible to reduce the dosage to $1/2$ or even $1/10$ without losing the therapeutic effect. The mixing schedule is as follows. Infusion rates deliver 0.1 mcg/kg/minute. **Note:** 500 mcg equals 1 ampul.

For a concentration of 2 mcg/mL, add 500 mcg to 250 mL; infuse at 0.05 mL/kg/minute (72 mL/kg/24 hours)

For a concentration of 5 mcg/mL, add 500 mcg to 100 mL; infuse at 0.02 mL/kg/minute (28.8 mL/kg/24 hours)

For a concentration of 10 mcg/mL, add 500 mcg to 50 mL; infuse at 0.01 mL/kg/minute (14.4 mL/kg/24 hours)

For a concentration of 20 mcg/mL, add 500 mcg to 25 mL; infuse at 0.005 mL/kg/minute (7.2 mL/kg/24 hours)

Therapeutic response is indicated by increased pH in those with acidosis or by an increase in oxygenation (PO_2) usually evident within 30 minutes

(Continued)

alprostadil *(Continued)*

Erectile dysfunction:
Caverject®, Edex®: Intracavernous: Individualize dose by careful titration; doses >40 mcg (Edex®) or >60 mcg (Caverject®) are not recommended: Initial dose must be titrated in physicians office. Patient must stay in the physician's office until complete detumescence occurs; if there is no response, then the next higher dose may be given within 1 hour; if there is still no response, a 1-day interval before giving the next dose is recommended; increasing the dose or concentration in the treatment of impotence results in increasing pain and discomfort

Vasculogenic, psychogenic, or mixed etiology: Initiate dosage titration at 2.5 mcg, increasing by 2.5 mcg to a dose of 5 mcg and then in increments of 5-10 mcg depending on the erectile response until the dose produces an erection suitable for intercourse, not lasting >1 hour; if there is absolutely no response to initial 2.5 mcg dose, the second dose may be increased to 7.5 mcg, followed by increments of 5-10 mcg

Neurogenic etiology (eg, spinal cord injury): Initiate dosage titration at 1.25 mcg, increasing to a dose of 2.5 mcg and then 5 mcg; increase further in increments 5 mcg until the dose is reached that produces an erection suitable for intercourse, not lasting >1 hour

Maintenance: Once appropriate dose has been determined, patient may self-administer injections at a frequency of no more than 3 times/week with at least 24 hours between doses

Muse® Pellet: Intraurethral:

Initial: 125-250 mcg

Maintenance: Administer as needed to achieve an erection; duration of action is about 30-60 minutes; use only two systems per 24-hour period

Dosage Forms
Injection, powder for reconstitution: 10 mcg, 20 mcg, 40 mcg

Caverject®: 20 mcg, 40 mcg

Caverject Impulse®: 10 mcg, 20 mcg

Edex®: 10 mcg, 20 mcg, 40 mcg

Injection, solution: 500 mcg/mL (1 mL)

Prostin VR Pediatric®: 500 mcg/mL (1 mL)

Pellet, urethral: 125 mcg, 250 mcg, 500 mcg, 1000 mcg

Muse®: 125 mcg (6s), 250 mcg (6s), 500 mcg (6s), 1000 mcg (6s)

Alrex® [US/Can] *see* loteprednol *on page 519*

AL-Rr® Oral (Discontinued) *see* chlorpheniramine *on page 177*

Altabax™ [US] *see* retapamulin *on page 751*

Altace® [US/Can] *see* ramipril *on page 743*

Altace® HCT [Can] *see* ramipril and hydrochlorothiazide *(Canada only) on page 743*

Altachlore [US-OTC] *see* sodium chloride *on page 792*

Altafrin [US] *see* phenylephrine *on page 675*

Altamist [US-OTC] *see* sodium chloride *on page 792*

Altarussin DM [US-OTC] *see* guaifenesin and dextromethorphan *on page 402*

Altaryl [US-OTC] *see* diphenhydramine *on page 265*

alteplase *(AL te plase)*

Sound-Alike/Look-Alike Issues
alteplase may be confused with Altace®

"tPA" abbreviation should not be used when writing orders for this medication; has been misread as TNKase (tenecteplase)

Synonyms alteplase, recombinant; alteplase, tissue plasminogen activator, recombinant; tPA

U.S./Canadian Brand Names Activase® rt-PA [Can]; Activase® [US]; Cathflo® Activase® [US/Can]

Therapeutic Category Fibrinolytic Agent

Use Management of acute myocardial infarction for the lysis of thrombi in coronary arteries; management of acute ischemic stroke

Acute myocardial infarction (AMI): Chest pain ≥20 minutes, ≤12-24 hours; S-T elevation ≥0.1 mV in at least two ECG leads

Acute pulmonary embolism (APE): Age ≤75 years: Documented massive pulmonary embolism by pulmonary angiography or echocardiography or high probability lung scan with clinical shock

Cathflo® Activase®: Restoration of central venous catheter function

Usual Dosage
I.V.:

Coronary artery thrombi: Front loading dose (weight-based):

Patients >67 kg: Total dose: 100 mg over 1.5 hours; infuse 15 mg over 1-2 minutes. Infuse 50 mg over 30 minutes. Infuse remaining 35 mg of alteplase over the next hour. See "Note."

Patients ≤67 kg: Infuse 15 mg I.V. bolus over 1-2 minutes, then infuse 0.75 mg/kg (not to exceed 50 mg) over next 30 minutes, followed by 0.5 mg/kg over next 60 minutes (not to exceed 35 mg). See "Note."

Note: Concurrently, begin heparin 60 units/kg bolus (maximum: 4000 units) followed by continuous infusion of 12 units/kg/hour (maximum: 1000 units/hour) and adjust to aPTT target of 1.5-2 times the upper limit of control.

Acute pulmonary embolism: 100 mg over 2 hours.

Acute ischemic stroke: Doses should be given within the first 3 hours of the onset of symptoms; recommended total dose: 0.9 mg/kg (maximum dose should not exceed 90 mg) infused over 60 minutes.

Load with 0.09 mg/kg (10% of the 0.9 mg/kg dose) as an I.V. bolus over 1 minute, followed by 0.81 mg/kg (90% of the 0.9 mg/kg dose) as a continuous infusion over 60 minutes. Heparin should not be started for 24 hours or more after starting alteplase for stroke.

Intracatheter: Central venous catheter clearance: Cathflo® Activase® 1 mg/mL:

Patients <30 kg: 110% of the internal lumen volume of the catheter, not to exceed 2 mg/2 mL; retain in catheter for 0.5-2 hours; may instill a second dose if catheter remains occluded

Patients ≥30 kg: 2 mg (2 mL); retain in catheter for 0.5-2 hours; may instill a second dose if catheter remains occluded

Advisory Panel to the Society for Cardiovascular and Interventional Radiology on Thrombolytic Therapy recommendation: ≤2 mg/hour and subtherapeutic heparin (aPTT <1.5 times baseline)

Dosage Forms

Injection, powder for reconstitution, recombinant:

Activase®: 50 mg [29 million int. units]; 100 mg [58 million int. units]

Cathflo® Activase®: 2 mg

alteplase, recombinant *see* alteplase *on previous page*

alteplase, tissue plasminogen activator, recombinant *see* alteplase *on previous page*

ALternaGel® [US-OTC] *see* aluminum hydroxide *on next page*

Alti-Alprazolam [Can] *see* alprazolam *on page 32*

Alti-Amiodarone [Can] *see* amiodarone *on page 43*

Alti-Amoxi-Clav [Can] *see* amoxicillin and clavulanate potassium *on page 49*

Alti-Azathioprine [Can] *see* azathioprine *on page 87*

Alti-Captopril [Can] *see* captopril *on page 145*

Alti-Clindamycin [Can] *see* clindamycin *on page 198*

Alti-Clobazam [Can] *see* clobazam *(Canada only) on page 201*

Alti-Clonazepam [Can] *see* clonazepam *on page 204*

Alti-Desipramine [Can] *see* desipramine *on page 238*

Alti-Diltiazem CD [Can] *see* diltiazem *on page 261*

Alti-Divalproex [Can] *see* valproic acid and derivatives *on page 881*

Alti-Domperidone [Can] *see* domperidone *(Canada only) on page 276*

Alti-Doxazosin [Can] *see* doxazosin *on page 278*

Alti-Flunisolide [Can] *see* flunisolide *on page 359*

Alti-Fluoxetine [Can] *see* fluoxetine *on page 364*

Alti-Flurbiprofen [Can] *see* flurbiprofen *on page 366*

Alti-Fluvoxamine [Can] *see* fluvoxamine *on page 370*

Alti-Ipratropium [Can] *see* ipratropium *on page 470*

Alti-Metformin [Can] *see* metformin *on page 548*

Alti-Minocycline [Can] *see* minocycline *on page 571*

Alti-Moclobemide [Can] *see* moclobemide *(Canada only) on page 575*

Alti-MPA [Can] *see* medroxyprogesterone *on page 537*

Alti-Nadolol [Can] *see* nadolol *on page 586*

Alti-Nortriptyline [Can] *see* nortriptyline *on page 613*

Alti-Ranitidine [Can] *see* ranitidine *on page 744*

Alti-Salbutamol [Can] *see* albuterol *on page 23*

Alti-Sotalol [Can] *see* sotalol *on page 802*

Alti-Sulfasalazine [Can] *see* sulfasalazine *on page 814*

Alti-Terazosin [Can] *see* terazosin *on page 826*

Alti-Ticlopidine [Can] *see* ticlopidine *on page 842*

Alti-Timolol [Can] *see* timolol *on page 843*

Alti-Trazodone [Can] *see* trazodone *on page 859*

Alti-Verapamil [Can] *see* verapamil *on page 887*

Alti-Zopiclone [Can] *see* zopiclone *(Canada only) on page 909*

Altocor™ *(Discontinued)* *see* lovastatin *on page 520*

Altoprev® [US] *see* lovastatin *on page 520*

altretamine (al TRET a meen)
 Synonyms hexamethylmelamine; HEXM; HMM; HXM; NSC-13875
 U.S./Canadian Brand Names Hexalen® [US/Can]
 Therapeutic Category Antineoplastic Agent
 Use Palliative treatment of persistent or recurrent ovarian cancer
 Usual Dosage Refer to individual protocols. Oral: Adults: Ovarian cancer: 260 mg/m^2/day in 4 divided doses
  for 14 or 21 days of a 28-day cycle
 Dosage Forms
  Gelcap:
   Hexalen®: 50 mg

Alu-Cap® *(Discontinued)* *see* aluminum hydroxide *on this page*

Aludrox® *(Discontinued)* *see* aluminum hydroxide and magnesium hydroxide *on next page*

aluminum chloride hexahydrate (a LOO mi num KLOR ide heks a HYE drate)
 Sound-Alike/Look-Alike Issues
  Drysol™ may be confused with Drisdol®
 U.S./Canadian Brand Names Certain Dri® [US-OTC]; Drysol™ [US]; Xerac AC™ [US]
 Therapeutic Category Topical Skin Product
 Use Astringent in the management of hyperhidrosis
 Usual Dosage Topical: Adults: Apply once daily at bedtime; once excessive sweating has stopped, may
  decrease to once or twice weekly, or as needed. Wash treated area in the morning.
 Dosage Forms
  Solution, topical:
   Certain Dri® [OTC]: 12% (36 mL)
   Drysol™: 20% (35 mL, 37.5 mL, 60 mL)
   Xerac AC™: 6.25% (35 mL, 60 mL)

aluminum hydroxide (a LOO mi num hye DROKS ide)
 U.S./Canadian Brand Names ALternaGel® [US-OTC]; Amphojel® [Can]; Basaljel® [Can]; Dermagran® [US-
  OTC]
 Therapeutic Category Antacid
 Use Treatment of hyperacidity; hyperphosphatemia; temporary protection of minor cuts, scrapes, and burns
 Usual Dosage
  Oral:
   Hyperphosphatemia:
    Children: 50-150 mg/kg/24 hours in divided doses every 4-6 hours, titrate dosage to maintain serum
     phosphorus within normal range
    Adults: Initial: 300-600 mg 3 times/day with meals
   Antacid: Adults: 600-1200 mg between meals and at bedtime
   Topical: Apply to affected area as needed; reapply at least every 12 hours
 Dosage Forms
  Ointment:
   Dermagran® [OTC]: 0.275% (120 g)
  Suspension, oral: 320 mg/5 mL
   ALternaGel® [OTC]: 600 mg/5 mL

aluminum hydroxide and magnesium carbonate
 (a LOO mi num hye DROKS ide & mag NEE zhum KAR bun nate)
 Synonyms magnesium carbonate and aluminum hydroxide
 U.S./Canadian Brand Names Acid Gone Extra Strength [US-OTC]; Acid Gone [US-OTC]; Alenic Alka [US-
  OTC]; Gaviscon® Extra Strength [US-OTC]; Gaviscon® Liquid [US-OTC]; Genaton™ [US-OTC]
 Therapeutic Category Antacid
 Use Temporary relief of symptoms associated with gastric acidity

Usual Dosage Oral: Adults:
Liquid:
Gaviscon® Regular Strength: 15-30 mL 4 times/day after meals and at bedtime
Gaviscon® Extra Strength Relief: 15-30 mL 4 times/day after meals
Tablet (Gaviscon® Extra Strength Relief): Chew 2-4 tablets 4 times/day
Dosage Forms
Liquid: Aluminum hydroxide 31.7 mg and magnesium carbonate 119.3 mg per 5 mL; aluminum hydroxide 84.6 mg and magnesium carbonate 79.1 mg per 5 mL
Acid Gone [OTC], Alenic Alka [OTC], Gaviscon® [OTC], Genaton™ [OTC]: Aluminum hydroxide 31.7 mg and magnesium carbonate 119.3 mg per 5 mL
Gaviscon® Extra Strength [OTC]: Aluminum hydroxide 84.6 mg and magnesium carbonate 79.1 mg per 5 mL
Tablet, chewable: Aluminum hydroxide 160 mg and magnesium carbonate 105 mg
Acid Gone Extra Strength [OTC], Gaviscon® Extra Strength [OTC]: Aluminum hydroxide 160 mg and magnesium carbonate 105 mg

aluminum hydroxide and magnesium hydroxide
(a LOO mi num hye DROKS ide & mag NEE zhum hye DROK side)
Sound-Alike/Look-Alike Issues
Maalox® may be confused with Maox®, Monodox®
Synonyms magnesium hydroxide and aluminum hydroxide
U.S./Canadian Brand Names Alamag [US-OTC]; Diovol® Ex [Can]; Diovol® [Can]; Gelusil® Extra Strength [Can]; Mylanta™ [Can]; Rulox [US-OTC]
Therapeutic Category Antacid
Use Antacid, hyperphosphatemia in renal failure
Usual Dosage Oral: 5-10 mL 4-6 times/day, between meals and at bedtime; may be used every hour for severe symptoms
Dosage Forms
Suspension: Aluminum hydroxide 225 mg and magnesium hydroxide 200 mg per 5 mL
Alamag [OTC], Rulox [OTC]: Aluminum hydroxide 225 mg and magnesium hydroxide 200 mg per 5 mL
Tablet, chewable:
Alamag [OTC]: Aluminum hydroxide 300 mg and magnesium hydroxide 150 mg

aluminum hydroxide and magnesium trisilicate
(a LOO mi num hye DROKS ide & mag NEE zhum trye SIL i kate)
Synonyms magnesium trisilicate and aluminum hydroxide
U.S./Canadian Brand Names Alenic Alka Tablet [US-OTC]; Gaviscon® Tablet [US-OTC]; Genaton Tablet [US-OTC]
Therapeutic Category Antacid
Use Temporary relief of hyperacidity
Usual Dosage Oral: Adults: Chew 2-4 tablets 4 times/day or as directed by healthcare provider
Dosage Forms
Tablet, chewable: Aluminum hydroxide 80 mg and magnesium trisilicate 20 mg
Alenic Alka [OTC], Gaviscon® [OTC], Genaton [OTC]: Aluminum hydroxide 80 mg and magnesium trisilicate 20 mg

aluminum hydroxide, magnesium hydroxide, and simethicone
(a LOO mi num hye DROKS ide, mag NEE zhum hye DROKS ide, & sye METH i kone)
Sound-Alike/Look-Alike Issues
Maalox® may be confused with Maox®, Monodox®
Mylanta® may be confused with Mynatal®
Synonyms magnesium hydroxide, aluminum hydroxide, and simethicone; simethicone, aluminum hydroxide, and magnesium hydroxide
U.S./Canadian Brand Names Alamag Plus [US-OTC]; Aldroxicon I [US-OTC]; Aldroxicon II [US-OTC]; Almacone Double Strength® [US-OTC]; Almacone® [US-OTC]; Diovol Plus® [Can]; Gelusil® [US-OTC/Can]; Maalox® Max [US-OTC]; Maalox® [US-OTC]; Mi-Acid Maximum Strength [US-OTC]; Mi-Acid [US-OTC]; Mintox Extra Strength [US-OTC]; Mintox Plus [US-OTC]; Mylanta® Double Strength [Can]; Mylanta® Extra Strength [Can]; Mylanta® Liquid [US-OTC]; Mylanta® Maximum Strength Liquid [US-OTC]; Mylanta® Regular Strength [Can]
Therapeutic Category Antacid; Antiflatulent
Use Temporary relief of hyperacidity associated with gas; may also be used for indications associated with other antacids
Usual Dosage Oral: Adults: 10-20 mL or 2-4 tablets 4-6 times/day between meals and at bedtime; may be used every hour for severe symptoms
(Continued)

aluminum hydroxide, magnesium hydroxide, and simethicone (Continued)

Dosage Forms

Liquid: Aluminum hydroxide 200 mg, magnesium hydroxide 200 mg, and simethicone 20 mg per 5 mL; aluminum hydroxide 400 mg, magnesium hydroxide 400 mg, and simethicone 40 mg per 5 mL

Aldroxicon I [OTC], Almacone® [OTC], Maalox® [OTC], Mi-Acid [OTC], Mylanta® [OTC]: Aluminum hydroxide 200 mg, magnesium hydroxide 200 mg, and simethicone 20 mg per 5 mL

Aldroxicon II [OTC], Almacone Double Strength [OTC], Maalox® Max® [OTC], Mi-Acid Maximum Strength [OTC], Mylanta® Maximum Strength [OTC]: Aluminum hydroxide 400 mg, magnesium hydroxide 400 mg, and simethicone 40 mg per 5 mL

Mintox Extra Strength [OTC]: Aluminum hydroxide 500 mg, magnesium hydroxide 450 mg, and simethicone 40 mg per 5 mL

Suspension:

Alamag Plus [OTC]: Aluminum hydroxide 225 mg, magnesium hydroxide 200 mg, and simethicone 25 mg per 5 mL

Tablet, chewable: Aluminum hydroxide 200 mg, magnesium hydroxide 200 mg, and simethicone 25 mg

Alamag Plus [OTC], Gelusil® [OTC], Mintox Plus [OTC]: Aluminum hydroxide 200 mg, magnesium hydroxide 200 mg, and simethicone 25 mg

Almacone® [OTC]: Aluminum hydroxide 200 mg, magnesium hydroxide 200 mg, and simethicone 20 mg

aluminum sucrose sulfate, basic see sucralfate on page 808

aluminum sulfate and calcium acetate (a LOO mi num SUL fate & KAL see um AS e tate)

Synonyms calcium acetate and aluminum sulfate

U.S./Canadian Brand Names Domeboro® [US-OTC]; Gordon Boro-Packs [US-OTC]; Pedi-Boro® [US-OTC]

Therapeutic Category Topical Skin Product

Use Astringent wet dressing for relief of inflammatory conditions of the skin; reduce weeping that may occur in dermatitis

Usual Dosage Topical: Soak affected area in the solution 2-4 times/day for 15-30 minutes or apply wet dressing soaked in the solution for more extended periods; rewet dressing with solution 2-4 times/day every 15-30 minutes

Dosage Forms

Powder, for topical solution:

Domeboro® [OTC]: Aluminum sulfate 1191 mg and calcium acetate 938 mg per packet (12s, 100s)

Gordon Boro-Packs: Aluminum sulfate 49% and calcium acetate 51% per packet (100s)

Pedi-Boro® [OTC]: Aluminum sulfate 49% and calcium acetate 51% per packet (12s, 100s)

Alupent® [US] see metaproterenol on page 548

Alupent® Inhalation Solution (Discontinued) see metaproterenol on page 548

Alu-Tab® (Discontinued) see aluminum hydroxide on page 36

Alvesco® [Can] see ciclesonide on page 188

amantadine (a MAN ta deen)

Sound-Alike/Look-Alike Issues

amantadine may be confused with ranitidine, rimantadine

Symmetrel® may be confused with Synthroid®

Synonyms adamantanamine hydrochloride; amantadine hydrochloride

U.S./Canadian Brand Names Endantadine® [Can]; PMS-Amantadine [Can]; Symmetrel® [US/Can]

Therapeutic Category Anti-Parkinson Agent (Dopamine Agonist); Antiviral Agent

Use Prophylaxis and treatment of influenza A viral infection (per manufacturer labeling; also refer to current CDC guidelines for recommendations during current flu season); treatment of parkinsonism; treatment of drug-induced extrapyramidal symptoms

Usual Dosage Oral:

Children:

Influenza A treatment:

1-9 years: 5 mg/kg/day in 2 divided doses (manufacturers range: 4.4-8.8 mg/kg/day); maximum dose: 150 mg/day

≥10 years and <40 kg: 5 mg/kg/day; maximum dose: 150 mg/day

≥10 years and ≥40 kg: 100 mg twice daily

Note: Initiate within 24-48 hours after onset of symptoms; discontinue as soon as possible based on clinical response (generally within 3-5 days or within 24-48 hours after symptoms disappear)

Influenza A prophylaxis: Refer to "Influenza A treatment" dosing

Note: Continue treatment throughout the peak influenza activity in the community or throughout the entire influenza season in patients who cannot be vaccinated. Development of immunity following vaccination takes ~2 weeks; amantadine therapy should be considered for high-risk patients from the time of vaccination until immunity has developed. For children <9 years receiving influenza vaccine for the first time, amantadine prophylaxis should continue for 6 weeks (4 weeks after the first dose and 2 weeks after the second dose)

Adults:

Drug-induced extrapyramidal symptoms: 100 mg twice daily; may increase to 300-400 mg/day, if needed

Influenza A viral infection: 100 mg twice daily; initiate within 24-48 hours after onset of symptoms; discontinue as soon as possible based on clinical response (generally within 3-5 days or within 24-48 hours after symptoms disappear)

Influenza A prophylaxis: 100 mg twice daily

Note: Continue treatment throughout the peak influenza activity in the community or throughout the entire influenza season in patients who cannot be vaccinated. Development of immunity following vaccination takes ~2 weeks; amantadine therapy should be considered for high-risk patients from the time of vaccination until immunity has developed

Dosage Forms
Capsule: 100 mg
Syrup: 50 mg/5 mL
Tablet: 100 mg
Symmetrel®: 100 mg

amantadine hydrochloride *see* amantadine *on previous page*

Amaphen® *(Discontinued)*

Amaryl® [US/Can] *see* glimepiride *on page 393*

Amatine® [Can] *see* midodrine *on page 569*

ambenonium (am be NOE nee um)
Synonyms ambenonium chloride
U.S./Canadian Brand Names Mytelase® [US/Can]
Therapeutic Category Cholinergic Agent
Use Treatment of myasthenia gravis
Usual Dosage Oral: Adults: 5-25 mg 3-4 times/day
Dosage Forms
Caplet [scored]:
Mytelase®: 10 mg

ambenonium chloride *see* ambenonium *on this page*

Ambi 10® *(Discontinued)* *see* benzoyl peroxide *on page 103*

Ambien® [US] *see* zolpidem *on page 908*

Ambien CR™ [US] *see* zolpidem *on page 908*

Ambifed-G [US] *see* guaifenesin and pseudoephedrine *on page 406*

Ambifed-G DM [US] *see* guaifenesin, pseudoephedrine, and dextromethorphan *on page 408*

Ambi® Skin Tone *(Discontinued)* *see* hydroquinone *on page 437*

AmBisome® [US/Can] *see* amphotericin B liposomal *on page 52*

ambrisentan (am bri SEN tan)
Synonyms BSF208075
U.S./Canadian Brand Names Letairis™ [US]
Therapeutic Category Endothelin Antagonist
Use Treatment of pulmonary artery hypertension (PAH) World Health Organization (WHO) Group I in patients with WHO Class II or III symptoms to improve exercise capacity and decrease the rate of clinical deterioration
Usual Dosage Oral: Adults: Initial: 5 mg once daily; as tolerated, increase to maximum 10 mg once daily
Dosage Forms
Tablet:
Letairis™: 5 mg, 10 mg

amcinonide (am SIN oh nide)
U.S./Canadian Brand Names Amcort® [Can]; Cyclocort® [Can]; ratio-Amcinonide [Can]; Taro-Amcinonide [Can]
Therapeutic Category Corticosteroid, Topical
Use Relief of the inflammatory and pruritic manifestations of corticosteroid-responsive dermatoses (high potency corticosteroid)
(Continued)

º **amcinonide** *(Continued)*

Usual Dosage Topical: Adults: Apply in a thin film 2-3 times/day. Therapy should be discontinued when control is achieved; if no improvement is seen, reassessment of diagnosis may be necessary.

Dosage Forms
Cream: 0.1% (15 g, 30 g, 60 g)
Lotion: 0.1% (60 mL)
Ointment: 0.1% (30 g, 60 g)

Amcort® **[Can]** *see* amcinonide *on previous page*

Amcort® **Injection** *(Discontinued)*

Amdry-D [US] *see* pseudoephedrine and methscopolamine *on page 730*

Amerge® **[US/Can]** *see* naratriptan *on page 592*

Americaine® **[US-OTC]** *see* benzocaine *on page 101*

Americaine® **Anesthetic Lubricant** *(Discontinued) see* benzocaine *on page 101*

Americaine® **Hemorrhoidal [US-OTC]** *see* benzocaine *on page 101*

A-methapred *see* methylprednisolone *on page 559*

amethocaine hydrochloride *see* tetracaine *on page 831*

amethopterin *see* methotrexate *on page 553*

Ametop™ **[Can]** *see* tetracaine *on page 831*

Amevive® **[US/Can]** *see* alefacept *on page 26*

amfepramone *see* diethylpropion *on page 256*

AMG 073 *see* cinacalcet *on page 190*

Amibid DM *(Discontinued) see* guaifenesin and dextromethorphan *on page 402*

Amibid LA *(Discontinued) see* guaifenesin *on page 401*

Amicar® **[US]** *see* aminocaproic acid *on page 42*

Amidal *(Discontinued) see* guaifenesin and phenylephrine *on page 404*

Amidate® **[US/Can]** *see* etomidate *on page 335*

Amidrine *(Discontinued) see* acetaminophen, isometheptene, and dichloralphenazone *on page 13*

amifostine (am i FOS teen)
Sound-Alike/Look-Alike Issues
Ethyol® may be confused with ethanol
Synonyms ethiofos; gammaphos; WR-2721; YM-08310
U.S./Canadian Brand Names Ethyol® [US/Can]
Therapeutic Category Antidote
Use Reduce the incidence of moderate to severe xerostomia in patients undergoing postoperative radiation treatment for head and neck cancer, where the radiation port includes a substantial portion of the parotid glands; reduce the cumulative renal toxicity associated with repeated administration of cisplatin
Usual Dosage Note: Antiemetic medication, including dexamethasone 20 mg I.V. and a serotonin 5-HT$_3$ receptor antagonist, is recommended prior to and in conjunction with amifostine.
Adults:
Cisplatin-induced renal toxicity, reduction: I.V.: 740-910 mg/m^2 once daily 30 minutes prior to cytotoxic therapy
Note: Doses >740 mg/m^2 are associated with a higher incidence of hypotension and may require interruption of therapy or dose modification for subsequent cycles. For 910 mg/m^2 doses, the manufacturer suggests the following blood pressure-based adjustment schedule:
The infusion of amifostine should be interrupted if the systolic blood pressure decreases significantly from baseline, as defined below:
Decrease of 20 mm Hg if baseline systolic blood pressure <100
Decrease of 25 mm Hg if baseline systolic blood pressure 100-119
Decrease of 30 mm Hg if baseline systolic blood pressure 120-139
Decrease of 40 mm Hg if baseline systolic blood pressure 140-179
Decrease of 50 mm Hg if baseline systolic blood pressure ≥180
If the blood pressure returns to normal within 5 minutes (assisted by fluid administration and postural management) and the patient is asymptomatic, the infusion may be restarted so that the full dose of amifostine may be administered. If the full dose of amifostine cannot be administered, the dose of amifostine for subsequent cycles should be 740 mg/m^2.
Xerostomia from head and neck cancer, reduction: I.V.: 200 mg/m^2/day during radiation therapy

Dosage Forms
  Injection, powder for reconstitution:
   Ethyol®: 500 mg

Amigesic® [US/Can] *see* salsalate *on page 775*

amikacin (am i KAY sin)
Sound-Alike/Look-Alike Issues
   amikacin may be confused with Amicar®, anakinra
   Amikin® may be confused with Amicar®
Synonyms amikacin sulfate
U.S./Canadian Brand Names Amikacin Sulfate Injection, USP [Can]; Amikin® [US/Can]
Therapeutic Category Aminoglycoside (Antibiotic)
Use Treatment of serious infections (bone infections, respiratory tract infections, endocarditis, and septicemia) due to organisms resistant to gentamicin and tobramycin, including *Pseudomonas*, *Proteus*, *Serratia*, and other gram-negative bacilli; documented infection of mycobacterial organisms susceptible to amikacin
Usual Dosage Note: Individualization is critical because of the low therapeutic index
  Use of ideal body weight (IBW) for determining the mg/kg/dose appears to be more accurate than dosing on the basis of total body weight (TBW)
   In morbid obesity, dosage requirement may best be estimated using a dosing weight of IBW + 0.4 (TBW - IBW)
   Initial and periodic peak and trough plasma drug levels should be determined, particularly in critically-ill patients with serious infections or in disease states known to significantly alter aminoglycoside pharmacokinetics (eg, cystic fibrosis, burns, or major surgery)
  Usual dosage range:
   Infants and Children: I.M., I.V.: 5-7.5 mg/kg/dose every 8 hours
   Adults: I.M., I.V.: 5-7.5 mg/kg/dose every 8 hours
   Note: Some clinicians suggest a daily dose of 15-20 mg/kg for all patients with normal renal function. This dose is at least as efficacious with similar, if not less, toxicity than conventional dosing.
  Indication-specific dosing:
   Adults: I.V.:
    Hospital-acquired pneumonia (HAP): 20 mg/kg/day with antipseudomonal beta-lactam or carbapenem (American Thoracic Society/ATS guidelines)
    Meningitis *(Pseudomonas aeruginosa):* 5 mg/kg every 8 hours (administered with another bacteriocidal drug)
    Mycobacterium fortuitum, M. chelonae, or M. abscessus: 10-15 mg/kg twice daily for at least 2 weeks with high dose cefoxitin
Dosage Forms
  Injection, solution: 50 mg/mL (2 mL, 4 mL); 250 mg/mL (2 mL, 4 mL)
   Amikin®: 50 mg/mL (2 mL); 250 mg/mL (2 mL, 4 mL)

amikacin sulfate *see* amikacin *on this page*

Amikacin Sulfate Injection, USP [Can] *see* amikacin *on this page*

Amikin® [US/Can] *see* amikacin *on this page*

amiloride (a MIL oh ride)
Sound-Alike/Look-Alike Issues
   amiloride may be confused with amiodarone, amlodipine, amrinone
Synonyms amiloride hydrochloride
U.S./Canadian Brand Names Apo-Amiloride® [Can]
Therapeutic Category Diuretic, Potassium Sparing
Use Counteracts potassium loss induced by other diuretics in the treatment of hypertension or edematous conditions including CHF, hepatic cirrhosis, and hypoaldosteronism; usually used in conjunction with more potent diuretics such as thiazides or loop diuretics
Usual Dosage Oral:
   Children: Although safety and efficacy in children have not been established by the FDA, a dosage of 0.625 mg/kg/day has been used in children weighing 6-20 kg.
   Adults: 5-10 mg/day (up to 20 mg)
   Hypertension (JNC 7): 5-10 mg/day in 1-2 divided doses
Dosage Forms
  Tablet: 5 mg

amiloride and hydrochlorothiazide (a MIL oh ride & hye droe klor oh THYE a zide)

Synonyms hydrochlorothiazide and amiloride

U.S./Canadian Brand Names Apo-Amilzide® [Can]; Gen-Amilazide [Can]; Moduret [Can]; Novamilor [Can]; Nu-Amilzide [Can]

Therapeutic Category Diuretic, Combination

Use Potassium-sparing diuretic; antihypertensive

Usual Dosage Oral: Adults: Start with 1 tablet/day, then may be increased to 2 tablets/day if needed; usually given in a single dose

Dosage Forms
Tablet: 5/50: Amiloride 5 mg and hydrochlorothiazide 50 mg

amiloride hydrochloride *see* amiloride *on previous page*

Aminate Fe-90 [US] *see* vitamins (multiple/prenatal) *on page 896*

2-amino-6-mercaptopurine *see* thioguanine *on page 837*

2-amino-6-methoxypurine arabinoside *see* nelarabine *on page 595*

2-amino-6-trifluoromethoxy-benzothiazole *see* riluzole *on page 759*

aminobenzylpenicillin *see* ampicillin *on page 53*

aminocaproic acid (a mee noe ka PROE ik AS id)

Sound-Alike/Look-Alike Issues
Amicar® may be confused with amikacin, Amikin®, Omacor®

Synonyms epsilon aminocaproic acid

U.S./Canadian Brand Names Amicar® [US]

Therapeutic Category Hemostatic Agent

Use Treatment of excessive bleeding from fibrinolysis

Usual Dosage Oral, I.V.: Adults: Acute bleeding syndrome: 4-5 g during the first hour, followed by 1 g/hour for 8 hours or until bleeding controlled (maximum daily dose: 30 g)

Dosage Forms
Injection, solution: 250 mg/mL (20 mL)
Amicar®: 250 mg/mL (20 mL)
Solution, oral: 1.25 g/5 mL (480 mL)
Syrup:
Amicar®: 1.25 g/5 mL
Tablet [scored]: 500 mg, 1000 mg
Amicar®: 500 mg, 1000 mg

Amino-Cerv™ [US] *see* urea *on page 877*

aminoglutethimide (a mee noe gloo TETH i mide)

Sound-Alike/Look-Alike Issues
Cytadren® may be confused with cytarabine

Synonyms AG; AGT; BA-16038; eliptin

U.S./Canadian Brand Names Cytadren® [US]

Therapeutic Category Antineoplastic Agent

Use Suppression of adrenal function in selected patients with Cushing syndrome

Usual Dosage Oral: Adults: Adrenal suppression: 250 mg every 6 hours may be increased at 1- to 2-week intervals to a total of 2 g/day

Dosage Forms
Tablet [scored]:
Cytadren®: 250 mg

aminolevulinic acid (a MEE noh lev yoo lin ik AS id)

Synonyms aminolevulinic acid hydrochloride

U.S./Canadian Brand Names Levulan® Kerastick® [US]; Levulan® [Can]

Therapeutic Category Photosensitizing Agent, Topical; Porphyrin Agent, Topical

Use Treatment of minimally to moderately thick actinic keratoses (grade 1 or 2) of the face or scalp; to be used in conjunction with blue light illumination

Usual Dosage Topical: Adults: Apply to actinic keratoses (**not** perilesional skin) followed 14-18 hours later by blue light illumination. Application/treatment may be repeated at a treatment site after 8 weeks.

Dosage Forms
Powder for topical solution:
Levulan® Kerastick®: 20% (6s)

aminolevulinic acid hydrochloride *see* aminolevulinic acid *on previous page*

aminophylline (am in OFF i lin)
Sound-Alike/Look-Alike Issues
aminophylline may be confused with amitriptyline, ampicillin
Synonyms theophylline ethylenediamine
U.S./Canadian Brand Names Phyllocontin® [Can]; Phyllocontin®-350 [Can]
Therapeutic Category Theophylline Derivative
Use Bronchodilator in reversible airway obstruction due to asthma or COPD; increase diaphragmatic contractility
Usual Dosage
Treatment of acute bronchospasm: I.V.:
Loading dose (in patients not currently receiving aminophylline or theophylline): 6 mg/kg (based on aminophylline) administered I.V. over 20-30 minutes; administration rate should not exceed 25 mg/minute (aminophylline)
Approximate I.V. maintenance dosages are based upon **continuous infusions**; bolus dosing (often used in children <6 months of age) may be determined by multiplying the hourly infusion rate by 24 hours and dividing by the desired number of doses/day
6 weeks to 6 months: 0.5 mg/kg/hour
6 months to 1 year: 0.6-0.7 mg/kg/hour
1-9 years: 1 mg/kg/hour
9-16 years and smokers: 0.8 mg/kg/hour
Adults, nonsmoking: 0.5 mg/kg/hour
Older patients and patients with cor pulmonale: 0.3 mg/kg/hour
Patients with congestive heart failure: 0.1-0.2 mg/kg/hour
Dosage should be adjusted according to serum level measurements during the first 12- to 24-hour period.
Bronchodilator: Oral: Children ≥45 kg and Adults: Initial: 380 mg/day (equivalent to theophylline 300 mg/day) in divided doses every 6-8 hours; may increase dose after 3 days; maximum dose: 928 mg/day (equivalent to theophylline 800 mg/day)
Dosage Forms
Injection, solution: 25 mg/mL (10 mL, 20 mL)
Tablet: 100 mg, 200 mg

aminosalicylate sodium *see* aminosalicylic acid *on this page*

aminosalicylic acid (a mee noe sal i SIL ik AS id)
Synonyms aminosalicylate sodium; 4-aminosalicylic acid; para-aminosalicylate sodium; PAS; sodium PAS
U.S./Canadian Brand Names Paser® [US]
Therapeutic Category Nonsteroidal Antiinflammatory Drug (NSAID)
Use Adjunctive treatment of tuberculosis used in combination with other antitubercular agents
Usual Dosage Oral: Tuberculosis:
Children: 200-300 mg/kg/day in 3-4 equally divided doses
Adults: 150 mg/kg/day in 2-3 equally divided doses
Dosage Forms
Granules, delayed release:
Paser®: 4 g/packet

4-aminosalicylic acid *see* aminosalicylic acid *on this page*
5-aminosalicylic acid *see* mesalamine *on page 546*
Aminoxin [US-OTC] *see* pyridoxine *on page 735*

amiodarone (a MEE oh da rone)
Sound-Alike/Look-Alike Issues
amiodarone may be confused with amiloride, amrinone
Cordarone® may be confused with Cardura®, Cordran®
Synonyms amiodarone hydrochloride
U.S./Canadian Brand Names Alti-Amiodarone [Can]; Amiodarone Hydrochloride for Injection® [Can]; Apo-Amiodarone® [Can]; Cordarone® [US/Can]; Gen-Amiodarone [Can]; Novo-Amiodarone [Can]; Pacerone® [US]; PMS-Amiodarone [Can]; Rhoxal-amiodarone [Can]; Sandoz-Amiodarone [Can]
Therapeutic Category Antiarrhythmic Agent, Class III
Use Management of life-threatening recurrent ventricular fibrillation (VF) or hemodynamically-unstable ventricular tachycardia (VT) refractory to other antiarrhythmic agents or in patients intolerant of other agents used for these conditions
(Continued)

amiodarone *(Continued)*

Usual Dosage Note: Lower loading and maintenance doses are preferable in women and all patients with low body weight.

Oral: Adults: Ventricular arrhythmias: 800-1600 mg/day in 1-2 doses for 1-3 weeks, then when adequate arrhythmia control is achieved, decrease to 600-800 mg/day in 1-2 doses for 1 month; maintenance: 400 mg/day. Lower doses are recommended for supraventricular arrhythmias.

I.V.:

Children:

Pulseless VF or VT (PALS dosing): 5 mg/kg rapid I.V. bolus or I.O.; repeat up to a maximum dose of 15 mg/kg (300 mg)

Perfusing tachycardias (PALS dosing): Loading dose: 5 mg/kg I.V. over 20-60 minutes or I.O.; may repeat up to maximum dose of 15 mg/kg/day

Adults:

Breakthrough VF or VT: 150 mg supplemental doses in 100 mL D_5W over 10 minutes

Pulseless VF or VT: I.V. push: Initial: 300 mg in 20-30 mL NS or D_5W; if VF or VT recurs, supplemental dose of 150 mg followed by infusion of 1 mg/minute for 6 hours, then 0.5 mg/minute (maximum daily dose: 2.1 g)

Note: When switching from I.V. to oral therapy, use the following as a guide:

<1-week I.V. infusion: 800-1600 mg/day

1- to 3-week I.V. infusion: 600-800 mg/day

>3-week I.V. infusion: 400 mg/day

Recommendations for conversion to intravenous amiodarone after oral administration: During long-term amiodarone therapy (ie, ≥4 months), the mean plasma-elimination half-life of the active metabolite of amiodarone is 61 days. Replacement therapy may not be necessary in such patients if oral therapy is discontinued for a period <2 weeks, since any changes in serum amiodarone concentrations during this period may **not** be clinically significant.

Dosage Forms

Injection, solution: 50 mg/mL (3 mL, 9 mL, 18 mL)

Tablet [scored]: 200 mg, 400 mg

Cordarone®: 200 mg

Pacerone®: 100 mg [not scored], 200 mg, 400 mg

amiodarone hydrochloride *see* amiodarone *on previous page*

Amiodarone Hydrochloride for Injection® [Can] *see* amiodarone *on previous page*

Ami-Tex LA *(Discontinued)* *see* guaifenesin and phenylephrine *on page 404*

Amitiza™ [US] *see* lubiprostone *on page 522*

Amitone® *(Discontinued)* *see* calcium carbonate *on page 138*

amitriptyline *(a mee TRIP ti leen)*

Sound-Alike/Look-Alike Issues

amitriptyline may be confused with aminophylline, imipramine, nortriptyline

Elavil® may be confused with Aldoril®, Eldepryl®, enalapril, Equanil®, Mellaril®, Oruvail®, Plavix®

Synonyms amitriptyline hydrochloride

U.S./Canadian Brand Names Apo-Amitriptyline® [Can]; Levate® [Can]; Novo-Triptyn [Can]; PMS-Amitriptyline [Can]

Therapeutic Category Antidepressant, Tricyclic (Tertiary Amine)

Use Relief of symptoms of depression

Usual Dosage Oral:

Adolescents: Depressive disorders: Initial: 25-50 mg/day; may administer in divided doses; increase gradually to 100 mg/day in divided doses

Adults: Depression: 50-150 mg/day single dose at bedtime or in divided doses; dose may be gradually increased up to 300 mg/day

Dosage Forms

Tablet: 10 mg, 25 mg, 50 mg, 75 mg, 100 mg, 150 mg

amitriptyline and chlordiazepoxide *(a mee TRIP ti leen & klor dye az e POKS ide)*

Synonyms chlordiazepoxide and amitriptyline hydrochloride

U.S./Canadian Brand Names Limbitrol® DS [US]; Limbitrol® [US/Can]

Therapeutic Category Antidepressant, Tricyclic (Tertiary Amine)

Controlled Substance C-IV

Use Treatment of moderate to severe anxiety and/or agitation and depression

Usual Dosage Initial: 3-4 tablets in divided doses; this may be increased to 6 tablets/day as required; some patients respond to smaller doses and can be maintained on 2 tablets

Dosage Forms
Tablet: 12.5/5: Amitriptyline 12.5 mg and chlordiazepoxide 5 mg; 25/10: Amitriptyline 25 mg and chlordiaze-poxide 10 mg
Limbitrol®: 12.5/5: Amitriptyline 12.5 mg and chlordiazepoxide 5 mg
Limbitrol® DS: 25/10: Amitriptyline 25 mg and chlordiazepoxide 10 mg

amitriptyline and perphenazine (a mee TRIP ti leen & per FEN a zeen)
Synonyms perphenazine and amitriptyline hydrochloride
U.S./Canadian Brand Names Etrafon® [Can]
Therapeutic Category Antidepressant/Phenothiazine
Use Treatment of patients with moderate to severe anxiety and depression
Usual Dosage Oral: 1 tablet 2-4 times/day
Dosage Forms
Tablet:
Generics:
2-10: Amitriptyline 10 mg and perphenazine 2 mg
2-25: Amitriptyline 25 mg and perphenazine 2 mg
4-10: Amitriptyline 10 mg and perphenazine 4 mg
4-25: Amitriptyline 25 mg and perphenazine 4 mg
4-50: Amitriptyline 50 mg and perphenazine 4 mg

amitriptyline hydrochloride *see* amitriptyline *on previous page*

AMJ 9701 *see* palifermin *on page 646*

AmLactin® [US-OTC] *see* lactic acid and ammonium hydroxide *on page 487*

amlexanox (am LEKS an oks)
U.S./Canadian Brand Names Aphthasol® [US]
Therapeutic Category Antiinflammatory Agent, Locally Applied
Use Treatment of aphthous ulcers (ie, canker sores)
Usual Dosage Topical: Administer (0.5 cm - ¼") directly on ulcers 4 times/day following oral hygiene, after meals, and at bedtime
Dosage Forms
Paste:
Aphthasol®: 5% (5 g)

amlodipine (am LOE di peen)
Sound-Alike/Look-Alike Issues
amlodipine may be confused with amiloride
Norvasc® may be confused with Navane®, Norvir®, Vascor®
Synonyms amlodipine besylate
U.S./Canadian Brand Names Norvasc® [US/Can]
Therapeutic Category Calcium Channel Blocker
Use Treatment of hypertension; treatment of symptomatic chronic stable angina, vasospastic (Prinzmetal) angina (confirmed or suspected); prevention of hospitalization due to angina with documented CAD (limited to patients without heart failure or ejection fraction <40%)
Usual Dosage Oral:
Children 6-17 years: Hypertension: 2.5-5 mg once daily
Adults:
Hypertension: Initial dose: 5 mg once daily; maximum dose: 10 mg once daily. In general, titrate in 2.5 mg increments over 7-14 days. Usual dosage range (JNC 7): 2.5-10 mg once daily.
Angina: Usual dose: 5-10 mg
Dosage Forms
Tablet: 2.5 mg, 5 mg, 10 mg
Norvasc®: 2.5 mg, 5 mg, 10 mg

amlodipine and atorvastatin (am LOW di peen & a TORE va sta tin)
Synonyms atorvastatin calcium and amlodipine besylate
U.S./Canadian Brand Names Caduet® [US/Can]
Therapeutic Category Antilipemic Agent, HMG-CoA Reductase Inhibitor; Calcium Channel Blocker
Use For use when treatment with both amlodipine and atorvastatin is appropriate:
Amlodipine: Treatment of hypertension; treatment of symptomatic chronic stable angina, vasospastic (Prinzmetal) angina (confirmed or suspected); prevention of hospitalization due to angina with documented CAD (limited to patients without heart failure or ejection fraction <40%)
(Continued)

45

amlodipine and atorvastatin *(Continued)*

Atorvastatin: Treatment of dyslipidemias or primary prevention of cardiovascular disease (atherosclerotic) as detailed here:

Primary prevention of cardiovascular disease (high-risk for CVD): To reduce the risk of MI or stroke in patients without evidence of heart disease who have multiple CVD risk factors or type 2 diabetes. Treatment reduces the risk for angina or revascularization procedures in patients with multiple risk factors.

Treatment of dyslipidemias: To reduce elevations in total cholesterol, LDL-C, apolipoprotein B, and triglycerides in patients with elevations of one or more components, and/or to increase HDL-C as present in heterozygous hypercholesterolemia (Fredrickson type IIa hyperlipidemias); treatment of primary dysbetalipoproteinemia (Fredrickson type III), elevated serum TG levels (Fredrickson type IV), and homozygous familial hypercholesterolemia

Treatment of heterozygous familial hypercholesterolemia (HeFH) in adolescent patients (10-17 years of age, females >1 year postmenarche) having LDL-C ≥190 mg/dL or LDL-C ≥160 mg/dL with positive family history of premature cardiovascular disease (CVD) or with two or more CVD risk factors.

Usual Dosage Oral:

Amlodipine:

Children >10 years: Hypertension: 2.5-5 mg once daily. **Note:** Use in ages >10 years because of atorvastatin content.

Adults:

Hypertension: Initial dose: 5 mg once daily; maximum dose: 10 mg once daily; in general, titrate in 2.5 mg increments over 7-14 days. Usual dosage range (JNC 7): 2.5-10 mg once daily

Angina: Usual dose: 5-10 mg; most patients require 10 mg for adequate effect

Atorvastatin:

Children 10-17 years (females >1 year postmenarche): HeFH: 10 mg once daily (maximum: 20 mg/day)

Adults:

Hyperlipidemias: Initial: 10-20 mg once daily; patients requiring >45% reduction in LDL-C may be started at 40 mg once daily; range: 10-80 mg once daily

Primary prevention of CVD: 10 mg once daily

Dosage Forms

Tablet:

Caduet®:

2.5/10: Amlodipine 2.5 mg and atorvastatin 10 mg

2.5/20: Amlodipine 2.5 mg and atorvastatin 20 mg

2.5/40: Amlodipine 2.5 mg and atorvastatin 40 mg

5/10: Amlodipine 5 mg and atorvastatin 10 mg

5/20: Amlodipine 5 mg and atorvastatin 20 mg

5/40: Amlodipine 5 mg and atorvastatin 40 mg

5/80: Amlodipine 5 mg and atorvastatin 80 mg

10/10: Amlodipine 10 mg and atorvastatin 10 mg

10/20: Amlodipine 10 mg and atorvastatin 20 mg

10/40: Amlodipine 10 mg and atorvastatin 40 mg

10/80: Amlodipine 10 mg and atorvastatin 80 mg

amlodipine and benazepril (am LOE di peen & ben AY ze pril)

Synonyms benazepril hydrochloride and amlodipine besylate

U.S./Canadian Brand Names Lotrel® [US]

Therapeutic Category Antihypertensive Agent, Combination

Use Treatment of hypertension

Usual Dosage Oral: Adults: 2.5-10 mg (amlodipine) and 10-40 mg (benazepril) once daily; maximum: Amlodipine: 10 mg/day; benazepril: 40 mg/day

Dosage Forms

Capsule:

2.5/10: Amlodipine 2.5 mg and benazepril 10 mg

5/10: Amlodipine 5 mg and benazepril 10 mg

5/20: Amlodipine 5 mg and benazepril 20 mg

10/20: Amlodipine 10 mg and benazepril 20 mg

Lotrel®:

2.5/10: Amlodipine 2.5 and benazepril 10 mg

5/10: Amlodipine 5 mg and benazepril 10 mg

5/20: Amlodipine 5 mg and benazepril 20 mg

5/40: Amlodipine 5 mg and benazepril 40 mg

10/20: Amlodipine 10 mg and benazepril 20 mg

10/40: Amlodipine 10 mg and benazepril 40 mg

amlodipine and valsartan (am LOE di peen & val SAR tan)
Synonyms amlodipine besylate and valsartan; valsartan and amlodipine
U.S./Canadian Brand Names Exforge® [US]
Therapeutic Category Angiotensin II Receptor Blocker Combination; Antihypertensive Agent, Combination; Calcium Channel Blocker
Use Treatment of hypertension
Usual Dosage Oral: Dose is individualized; combination product may be substituted for individual components in patients currently maintained on both agents separately or in patients not adequately controlled with monotherapy (using one of the agents or an agent within same antihypertensive class).
Adults: Hypertension: Amlodipine 5-10 mg and valsartan 160-320 mg once daily; dose may be titrated after 3-4 weeks of therapy. Maximum recommended doses: Amlodipine 10 mg/day; valsartan 320 mg/day.
Dosage Forms
Tablet:
Exforge®:
5/160: Amlodipine 5 mg and valsartan 160 mg
5/320 mg: Amlodipine 5 mg and valsartan 320 mg
10/160: Amlodipine 10 mg and valsartan 160 mg
10/320: Amlodipine 10 mg and valsartan 320 mg

amlodipine besylate see amlodipine on page 45

amlodipine besylate and valsartan see amlodipine and valsartan on this page

Ammens® Medicated Deodorant [US-OTC] see zinc oxide on page 906

ammonapse see sodium phenylbutyrate on page 796

ammonia spirit (aromatic) (a MOE nee ah SPEAR it, air oh MAT ik)
Synonyms smelling salts
Therapeutic Category Respiratory Stimulant
Use Respiratory and circulatory stimulant; treatment of fainting
Usual Dosage Used as "smelling salts" to treat or prevent fainting
Dosage Forms
Solution for inhalation [ampul]: 1.7% to 2.1% (0.33 mL)

ammonium chloride (a MOE nee um KLOR ide)
Therapeutic Category Electrolyte Supplement, Oral
Use Treatment of hypochloremic states or metabolic alkalosis
Usual Dosage Metabolic alkalosis: The following equations represent different methods of correction utilizing either the serum HCO_3^-, the serum chloride, or the base excess
Dosing of mEq NH_4Cl via the chloride-deficit method (hypochloremia):
Dose of mEq NH_4Cl = [0.2 L/kg x body weight (kg)] x [103 - observed serum chloride]; administer 50% of dose over 12 hours, then reevaluate
Note: 0.2 L/kg is the estimated chloride volume of distribution and 103 is the average normal serum chloride concentration (mEq/L)
Dosing of mEq NH_4Cl via the bicarbonate-excess method (refractory hypochloremic metabolic alkalosis):
Dose of NH_4Cl = [0.5 L/kg x body weight (kg)] x (observed serum HCO_3^- - 24); administer 50% of dose over 12 hours, then reevaluate
Note: 0.5 L/kg is the estimated bicarbonate volume of distribution and 24 is the average normal serum bicarbonate concentration (mEq/L)
These equations will yield different requirements of ammonium chloride
Dosage Forms
Injection, solution: Ammonium 5 mEq/mL and chloride 5 mEq/mL (20 mL)

ammonium lactate see lactic acid and ammonium hydroxide on page 487

Ammonul® [US] see sodium phenylacetate and sodium benzoate on page 795

Amnesteem™ [US] see isotretinoin on page 477

amobarbital (am oh BAR bi tal)
Synonyms amobarbital sodium; amylobarbitone
U.S./Canadian Brand Names Amytal® [US]
Therapeutic Category Barbiturate
Controlled Substance C-II
Use Hypnotic in short-term treatment of insomnia; reduce anxiety and provide sedation preoperatively
(Continued)

amobarbital *(Continued)*

Usual Dosage
Children:
Sedative: I.M., I.V.: 6-12 years: Manufacturer's dosing range: 65-500 mg
Hypnotic: I.M.: 2-3 mg/kg (maximum: 500 mg)
Adults:
Hypnotic: I.M., I.V.: 65-200 mg at bedtime (maximum I.M. dose: 500 mg)
Sedative: I.M., I.V.: 30-50 mg 2-3 times/day
Dosage Forms
Injection, powder for reconstitution:
Amytal®: 500 mg

amobarbital sodium *see* amobarbital *on previous page*

Amoclan [US] *see* amoxicillin and clavulanate potassium *on next page*

AMO Vitrax® *(Discontinued)* *see* hyaluronate and derivatives *on page 423*

amoxapine (a MOKS a peen)

Sound-Alike/Look-Alike Issues
amoxapine may be confused with amoxicillin, Amoxil®
Asendin may be confused with aspirin
Therapeutic Category Antidepressant, Tricyclic (Secondary Amine)
Use Treatment of depression, psychotic depression, depression accompanied by anxiety or agitation
Usual Dosage Oral:
Adolescents: Initial: 25-50 mg/day; increase gradually to 100 mg/day; may administer as divided doses or as a single dose at bedtime
Adults: Initial: 25 mg 2-3 times/day, if tolerated, dosage may be increased to 100 mg 2-3 times/day; may be given in a single bedtime dose when dosage <300 mg/day
Maximum daily dose:
Inpatient: 600 mg
Outpatient: 400 mg
Dosage Forms
Tablet: 25 mg, 50 mg, 100 mg, 150 mg

amoxicillin (a moks i SIL in)

Sound-Alike/Look-Alike Issues
amoxicillin may be confused with amoxapine, Amoxil®, Atarax®
Amoxil® may be confused with amoxapine, amoxicillin
Synonyms amoxicillin trihydrate; amoxycillin; *p*-hydroxyampicillin
U.S./Canadian Brand Names Amoxil® [US]; Apo-Amoxi® [Can]; Gen-Amoxicillin [Can]; Lin-Amox [Can]; Novamoxin® [Can]; Nu-Amoxi [Can]; PHL-Amoxicillin [Can]; PMS-Amoxicillin [Can]
Therapeutic Category Penicillin
Use Treatment of otitis media, sinusitis, and infections caused by susceptible organisms involving the respiratory tract, skin, and urinary tract; prophylaxis of infective endocarditis in patients undergoing surgical or dental procedures; as part of a multidrug regimen for *H. pylori* eradication
Usual Dosage
Usual dosage range:
Children ≤3 months: Oral: 20-30 mg/kg/day divided every 12 hours
Children >3 months and <40 kg: Oral: 20-50 mg/kg/day in divided doses every 8-12 hours
Adults: Oral: 250-500 mg every 8 hours or 500-875 mg twice daily
Indication-specific dosing:
Children >3 months and <40 kg: Oral:
Acute otitis media: 80-90 mg/kg/day divided every 12 hours
Anthrax exposure (CDC guidelines): Note: Postexposure prophylaxis only with documented susceptible organisms: 80 mg/kg/day in divided doses every 8 hours (maximum: 500 mg/dose)
Community-acquired pneumonia:
4 months to <5 years: 80-100 mg/kg/day divided every 8 hours
5-15 years: 100 mg/kg/day divided every 8 hours; **Note:** Treatment with a macrolide or doxycycline (if age >8 years) is preferred due to higher prevalence of atypical pathogens in this age group
Ear, nose, throat, genitourinary tract, or skin/skin structure infections:
Mild to moderate: 25 mg/kg/day in divided doses every 12 hours **or** 20 mg/kg/day in divided doses every 8 hours
Severe: 45 mg/kg/day in divided doses every 12 hours **or** 40 mg/kg/day in divided doses every 8 hours
Endocarditis (subacute bacterial) prophylaxis: 50 mg/kg 1 hour before procedure

Lower respiratory tract infections: 45 mg/kg/day in divided doses every 12 hours **or** 40 mg/kg/day in divided doses every 8 hours

Lyme disease: 25-50 mg/kg/day divided every 8 hours (maximum: 500 mg)

Adults: Oral:

Anthrax exposure (CDC guidelines): Note: Postexposure prophylaxis in pregnant or nursing women only with documented susceptible organisms: 500 mg every 8 hours

Ear, nose, throat, genitourinary tract, or skin/skin structure infections:

Mild to moderate: 500 mg every 12 hours **or** 250 mg every 8 hours

Severe: 875 mg every 12 hours **or** 500 mg every 8 hours

***Helicobacter pylori* eradication:** 1000 mg twice daily; requires combination therapy with at least one other antibiotic and an acid-suppressing agent (proton pump inhibitor or H_2 blocker)

Infective endocarditis prophylaxis: 2 g 30-60 minutes before procedure

Lower respiratory tract infections: 875 mg every 12 hours **or** 500 mg every 8 hours

Lyme disease: 500 mg every 6-8 hours (depending on size of patient) for 21-30 days

Dosage Forms

Capsule: 250 mg, 500 mg

Amoxil®: 500 mg

Powder for oral suspension: 125 mg/5 mL, 200 mg/5 mL, 250 mg/5 mL, 400 mg/5 mL

Amoxil®: 250 mg/5 mL, 400 mg/5 mL

Powder for oral suspension [drops]: 50 mg/mL

Amoxil®: 50 mg/mL

Tablet: 500 mg, 875 mg

Amoxil®: 500 mg, 875 mg

Tablet, chewable: 125 mg, 200 mg, 250 mg, 400 mg

Amoxil®: 200 mg, 400 mg

amoxicillin and clavulanate potassium (a moks i SIL in & klav yoo LAN ate poe TASS ee um)

Sound-Alike/Look-Alike Issues

Augmentin® may be confused with Azulfidine®

Synonyms amoxicillin and clavulanic acid; clavulanic acid and amoxicillin

U.S./Canadian Brand Names Alti-Amoxi-Clav [Can]; Amoclan [US]; Apo-Amoxi-Clav® [Can]; Augmentin ES-600® [US]; Augmentin XR® [US]; Augmentin® [US/Can]; Clavulin® [Can]; Novo-Clavamoxin [Can]; ratio-Aclavulanate [Can]

Therapeutic Category Penicillin

Use Treatment of otitis media, sinusitis, and infections caused by susceptible organisms involving the lower respiratory tract, skin and skin structure, and urinary tract; spectrum same as amoxicillin with additional coverage of beta-lactamase producing *B. catarrhalis*, *H. influenzae*, *N. gonorrhoeae*, and *S. aureus* (not MRSA). The expanded coverage of this combination makes it a useful alternative when amoxicillin resistance is present and patients cannot tolerate alternative treatments.

Usual Dosage Note: Dose is based on the amoxicillin component

Usual dosage range:

Infants <3 months: Oral: 30 mg/kg/day divided every 12 hours using the 125 mg/5 mL suspension

Children ≥3 months and <40 kg: Oral: 20-90 mg/kg/day divided every 8-12 hours

Children >40 kg and Adults: Oral: 250-500 mg every 8 hours or 875 mg every 12 hours

Indication-specific dosing:

Children ≥3 months and <40 kg: Oral:

Lower respiratory tract infections, severe infections, sinusitis: 45 mg/kg/day divided every 12 hours **or** 40 mg/kg/day divided every 8 hours

Mild-to-moderate infections: 25 mg/kg/day divided every 12 hours or 20 mg/kg/day divided every 8 hours

Otitis media (Augmentin® ES-600): 90 mg/kg/day divided every 12 hours for 10 days in children with severe illness and when coverage for β-lactamase-positive *H. influenzae* and *M. catarrhalis* is needed.

Children ≥16 years and Adults: Oral:

Acute bacterial sinusitis: Extended release tablet: Two 1000 mg tablets every 12 hours for 10 days

Bite wounds (animal/human): 875 mg every 12 hours **or** 500 mg every 8 hours

Chronic obstructive pulmonary disease: 875 mg every 12 hours **or** 500 mg every 8 hours

Diabetic foot: Extended release tablet: Two 1000 mg tablets every 12 hours for 7-14 days

Diverticulitis, perirectal abscess: Extended release tablet: Two 1000 mg tablets every 12 hours for 7-10 days

Erysipelas: 875 mg every 12 hours **or** 500 mg every 8 hours

Febrile neutropenia: 875 mg every 12 hours

Pneumonia:

Aspiration: 875 mg every 12 hours

Community-acquired: Extended release tablet: Two 1000 mg tablets every 12 hours for 7-10 days

Pyelonephritis (acute, uncomplicated): 875 mg every 12 hours **or** 500 mg every 8 hours

Skin abscess: 875 mg every 12 hours

(Continued)

amoxicillin and clavulanate potassium *(Continued)*

Dosage Forms

Powder for oral suspension: 200: Amoxicillin 200 mg and clavulanate potassium 28.5 mg per 5 mL; 400: Amoxicillin 400 mg and clavulanate potassium 57 mg per 5 mL; 600: Amoxicillin 600 mg and clavulanate potassium 42.9 mg per 5 mL

Amoclan:

200: Amoxicillin 200 mg and clavulanate potassium 28.5 mg per 5 mL

400: Amoxicillin 400 mg and clavulanate potassium 57 mg per 5 mL

Augmentin®:

125: Amoxicillin 125 mg and clavulanate potassium 31.25 mg per 5 mL

200: Amoxicillin 200 mg and clavulanate potassium 28.5 mg per 5 mL

250: Amoxicillin 250 mg and clavulanate potassium 62.5 mg per 5 mL

400: Amoxicillin 400 mg and clavulanate potassium 57 mg per 5 mL

Augmentin ES-600®: Amoxicillin 600 mg and clavulanate potassium 42.9 mg per 5 mL

Tablet: 500: Amoxicillin 500 mg and clavulanate potassium 125 mg; 875: Amoxicillin 875 mg and clavulanate potassium 125 mg

Augmentin®:

250: Amoxicillin 250 mg and clavulanate potassium 125 mg

500: Amoxicillin 500 mg and clavulanate potassium 125 mg

875: Amoxicillin 875 mg and clavulanate potassium 125 mg

Tablet, chewable: 200: Amoxicillin 200 mg and clavulanate potassium 28.5 mg; 400: Amoxicillin 400 mg and clavulanate potassium 57 mg

Augmentin®:

250: Amoxicillin 250 mg and clavulanate potassium 62.5 mg

Tablet, extended release:

Augmentin XR®: Amoxicillin 1000 mg and clavulanate acid 62.5 mg

amoxicillin and clavulanic acid *see* amoxicillin and clavulanate potassium *on previous page*

amoxicillin, lansoprazole, and clarithromycin *see* lansoprazole, amoxicillin, and clarithromycin *on page 493*

amoxicillin trihydrate *see* amoxicillin *on page 48*

Amoxil® [US] *see* amoxicillin *on page 48*

amoxycillin *see* amoxicillin *on page 48*

Amphadase™ [US] *see* hyaluronidase *on page 424*

amphetamine and dextroamphetamine *see* dextroamphetamine and amphetamine *on page 246*

Amphocin® *(Discontinued)* *see* amphotericin B (conventional) *on next page*

Amphojel® [Can] *see* aluminum hydroxide *on page 36*

Amphojel® *(Discontinued)* *see* aluminum hydroxide *on page 36*

Amphotec® [US/Can] *see* amphotericin B cholesteryl sulfate complex *on this page*

amphotericin B cholesteryl sulfate complex

(am foe TER i sin bee kole LES te ril SUL fate KOM plecks)

Synonyms ABCD; amphotericin B colloidal dispersion

U.S./Canadian Brand Names Amphotec® [US/Can]

Therapeutic Category Antifungal Agent

Use Treatment of invasive aspergillosis in patients who have failed amphotericin B deoxycholate treatment, or who have renal impairment or experience unacceptable toxicity which precludes treatment with amphotericin B deoxycholate in effective doses.

Usual Dosage I.V.: Children and Adults:

Premedication: For patients who experience chills, fever, hypotension, nausea, or other nonanaphylactic infusion-related immediate reactions, premedicate with the following drugs, 30-60 minutes prior to drug administration: a nonsteroidal (eg, ibuprofen, choline magnesium trisalicylate) with or without diphenhydramine; **or** acetaminophen with diphenhydramine; **or** hydrocortisone 50-100 mg. If the patient experiences rigors during the infusion, meperidine may be administered.

Range: 3-4 mg/kg/day (infusion of 1 mg/kg/hour); maximum: 7.5 mg/kg/day

Dosage Forms

Injection, powder for reconstitution:

Amphotec®: 50 mg, 100 mg

amphotericin B colloidal dispersion *see* amphotericin B cholesteryl sulfate complex *on this page*

amphotericin B (conventional) (am foe TER i sin bee con VEN sha nal)
Synonyms amphotericin B desoxycholate
U.S./Canadian Brand Names Fungizone® [Can]
Therapeutic Category Antifungal Agent
Use Treatment of severe systemic and central nervous system infections caused by susceptible fungi such as *Candida* species, *Histoplasma capsulatum*, *Cryptococcus neoformans*, *Aspergillus* species, *Blastomyces dermatitidis*, *Torulopsis glabrata*, and *Coccidioides immitis*; fungal peritonitis; irrigant for bladder fungal infections; used in fungal infection in patients with bone marrow transplantation, amebic meningoencephalitis, ocular aspergillosis (intraocular injection), candidal cystitis (bladder irrigation), chemoprophylaxis (low-dose I.V.), immunocompromised patients at risk of aspergillosis (intranasal/nebulized), refractory meningitis (intrathecal), coccidioidal arthritis (intra-articular/I.M.).

Low-dose amphotericin B has been administered after bone marrow transplantation to reduce the risk of invasive fungal disease.

Usual Dosage
Premedication: For patients who experience infusion-related immediate reactions, premedicate with the following drugs 30-60 minutes prior to drug administration: NSAID (with or without diphenhydramine) **or** acetaminophen with diphenhydramine **or** hydrocortisone 50-100 mg. If the patient experiences rigors during the infusion, meperidine may be administered.

Usual dosage ranges:
Infants and Children:
Test dose: I.V.: 0.1 mg/kg/dose to a maximum of 1 mg; infuse over 30-60 minutes. Many clinicians believe a test dose is unnecessary.
Maintenance dose: 0.25-1 mg/kg/day given once daily; infuse over 2-6 hours. Once therapy has been established, amphotericin B can be administered on an every-other-day basis at 1-1.5 mg/kg/dose; cumulative dose: 1.5-2 g over 6-10 weeks.
Duration of therapy: Varies with nature of infection, usual duration is 4-12 weeks or cumulative dose of 1-4 g
Adults:
Test dose: 1 mg infused over 20-30 minutes. Many clinicians believe a test dose is unnecessary.
Maintenance dose: Usual: 0.05-1.5 mg/kg/day; 1-1.5 mg/kg over 4-6 hours every other day may be given once therapy is established; aspergillosis, rhinocerebral mucormycosis, often require 1-1.5 mg/kg/day; do not exceed 1.5 mg/kg/day

Indication-specific dosing:
Children: **Meningitis, coccidioidal or cryptococcal:** I.T.: 25-100 mcg every 48-72 hours; increase to 500 mcg as tolerated
Adults:
Aspergillosis, disseminated: I.V.: 0.6-0.7 mg/kg/day for 3-6 months
Bone marrow transplantation (prophylaxis): I.V.: Low-dose amphotericin B 0.1-0.25 mg/kg/day has been administered after bone marrow transplantation to reduce the risk of invasive fungal disease.
Candidemia (neutropenic or nonneutropenic): I.V.: 0.6-1 mg/kg/day until 14 days after last positive blood culture and resolution of signs and symptoms
Candidiasis, chronic, disseminated: I.V.: 0.6-0.7 mg/kg/day for 3-6 months and resolution of radiologic lesions
Cystitis: Candidal: Bladder irrigation: Irrigate with 50 mcg/mL solution instilled periodically or continuously for 5-10 days or until cultures are clear
Dematiaceous fungi: I.V.: 0.7 mg/kg/day in combination with an azole
Endocarditis: I.V.: 0.6-1 mg/kg/day (with or without flucytosine) for 1 week, then 0.8 mg/kg/day every other day for 6-8 weeks postoperatively
Endophthalmitis, fungal: I.V.: 0.7-1 mg/kg/day (with or without flucytosine) for at least 4 weeks
Esophagitis: I.V.: 0.3-0.7 mg/kg/day for 14-21 after clinical improvement
Histoplasmosis: Chronic, severe pulmonary or disseminated: I.V.: 0.5-1 mg/kg/day for 7 days, then 0.8 mg/kg every other day (or 3 times/week) until total dose of 10-15 mg/kg; may continue itraconazole as suppressive therapy (lifelong for immunocompromised patients)
Meningitis:
Candidal: I.V.: 0.7-1 mg/kg/day (with or without flucytosine) for at least 4 weeks
Cryptococcal or Coccidioides: I.T.: Initial: 25-300 mcg every 48-72 hours; increase to 500 mcg to 1 mg as tolerated; maximum total dose: 15 mg has been suggested
Histoplasma: I.V.: 0.5-1 mg/kg/day for 7 days, then 0.8 mg/kg every other day (or 3 times/week) for 3 months total duration; follow with fluconazole suppressive therapy for up to 12 months
Meningoencephalitis, cryptococcal: I.V.:
HIV positive: 0.7-1 mg/kg/day (plus flucytosine 100 mg/kg/day) for 2 weeks, then change to oral fluconazole for at least 10 weeks; alternatively, amphotericin and flucytosine may be continued uninterrupted for 6-10 weeks
HIV negative: 0.5-0.7 mg/kg/day (plus flucytosine) for 2 weeks
Osteomyelitis: Candidal: I.V.: 0.5-1 mg/kg/day for 6-10 weeks
Penicillium marneffei: I.V.: 0.6 mg/kg/day for 2 weeks
(Continued)

amphotericin B (conventional) *(Continued)*

Pneumonia: Cryptococcal (mild to moderate): I.V.:
HIV positive: 0.5-1 mg/kg/day
HIV negative: 0.5-0.7 mg/kg/day (plus flucytosine) for 2 weeks
Sporotrichosis: Pulmonary, meningeal, osteoarticular, or disseminated: I.V.: Total dose of 1-2 g, then change to oral itraconazole or fluconazole for suppressive therapy
Dosage Forms
Injection, powder for reconstitution: 50 mg

amphotericin B desoxycholate *see* amphotericin B (conventional) *on previous page*

amphotericin B lipid complex (am foe TER i sin bee LIP id KOM pleks)

Synonyms ABLC
U.S./Canadian Brand Names Abelcet® [US/Can]
Therapeutic Category Antifungal Agent
Use Treatment of aspergillosis or any type of progressive fungal infection in patients who are refractory to or intolerant of conventional amphotericin B therapy
Usual Dosage I.V.: Children and Adults:
Premedication: For patients who experience infusion-related immediate reactions, premedicate with the following drugs, 30-60 minutes prior to drug administration: a nonsteroidal antiinflammatory agent ± diphenhydramine; **or** acetaminophen with diphenhydramine; **or** hydrocortisone 50-100 mg. If the patient experiences rigors during the infusion, meperidine may be administered.
Range: 2.5-5 mg/kg/day as a single infusion
Dosage Forms
Injection, suspension [preservative free]:
Abelcet®: 5 mg/mL (20 mL)

amphotericin B liposomal (am foe TER i sin bee lye po SO mal)

Synonyms L-AmB
U.S./Canadian Brand Names AmBisome® [US/Can]
Therapeutic Category Antifungal Agent, Systemic
Use Empirical therapy for presumed fungal infection in febrile, neutropenic patients; treatment of patients with *Aspergillus* species, *Candida* species, and/or *Cryptococcus* species infections refractory to amphotericin B desoxycholate, or in patients where renal impairment or unacceptable toxicity precludes the use of amphotericin B desoxycholate; treatment of cryptococcal meningitis in HIV-infected patients; treatment of visceral leishmaniasis
Usual Dosage
Usual dosage range:
Children: I.V.: 3-5 mg/kg/day
Adults: I.V.: 2-6 mg/kg/day; **Note:** Higher doses (15 mg/kg/day) have been used clinically.
Note: Premedication: For patients who experience nonanaphylactic infusion-related immediate reactions, premedicate with the following drugs 30-60 minutes prior to drug administration: A nonsteroidal antiinflammatory agent ± diphenhydramine; **or** acetaminophen with diphenhydramine; **or** hydrocortisone 50-100 mg. If the patient experiences rigors during the infusion, meperidine may be administered.

Indication-specific dosing:
Children: I.V.:
Candidal infection:
Endocarditis: 3-6 mg/kg/day with flucytosine 25-37.5 mg/kg 4 times daily
Meningitis: 5 mg/kg/day with flucytosine 100 mg/kg/day
Cryptococcal meningitis (HIV-positive): 6 mg/kg/day
Note: IDSA guidelines (April, 2000) report doses of 3-6 mg/kg/day, noting that 4 mg/kg/day was effective in a small, open-label trial. The manufacturer's labeled dose of 6 mg/kg/day was approved in June, 2000.
Empiric therapy: 3 mg/kg/day
Systemic fungal infections *(Aspergillus, Candida, Cryptococcus)*: 3-5 mg/kg/day
Visceral leishmaniasis:
Immunocompetent: 3 mg/kg/day on days 1-5, and 3 mg/kg/day on days 14 and 21; a repeat course may be given in patients who do not achieve parasitic clearance
Note: Alternate regimen of 10 mg/kg/day for 2 days has been reportedly effective.
Immunocompromised: 4 mg/kg/day on days 1-5, and 4 mg/kg/day on days 10, 17, 24, 31, and 38
Adults: I.V.:
Candidal infection:
Endocarditis: 3-6 mg/kg/day with flucytosine 25-37.5 mg/kg 4 times daily
Meningitis: 5 mg/kg/day with flucytosine 100 mg/kg/day

Cryptococcal meningitis (HIV-positive): 6 mg/kg/day
  Note: IDSA guidelines (April, 2000) report doses of 3-6 mg/kg/day, noting that 4 mg/kg/day was effective in a small, open-label trial. The manufacturer's labeled dose of 6 mg/kg/day was approved in June, 2000.
Empiric therapy: 3 mg/kg/day
Fungal sinusitis: 5-7.5 mg/kg/day
  Note: Use azole antifungal if causative organism is *Pseudallescheria boydii* (*Scedosporium* sp).
Systemic fungal infections *(Aspergillus, Candida, Cryptococcus)*: 3-5 mg/kg/day
Visceral leishmaniasis:
  Immunocompetent: 3 mg/kg/day on days 1-5, and 3 mg/kg/day on days 14 and 21; a repeat course may be given in patients who do not achieve parasitic clearance
  Note: Alternate regimen of 2 mg/kg/day for 5 days has been reportedly effective.
  Immunocompromised: 4 mg/kg/day on days 1-5, and 4 mg/kg/day on days 10, 17, 24, 31, and 38
Dosage Forms
  Injection, powder for reconstitution:
  AmBisome®: 50 mg

ampicillin (am pi SIL in)
Sound-Alike/Look-Alike Issues
  ampicillin may be confused with aminophylline
Synonyms aminobenzylpenicillin; ampicillin sodium; ampicillin trihydrate
U.S./Canadian Brand Names Apo-Ampi® [Can]; Novo-Ampicillin [Can]; Nu-Ampi [Can]
Therapeutic Category Penicillin
Use Treatment of susceptible bacterial infections (nonbeta-lactamase-producing organisms); treatment or prophylaxis of infective endocarditis; susceptible bacterial infections caused by streptococci, pneumococci, nonpenicillinase-producing staphylococci, *Listeria*, meningococci; some strains of *H. influenzae*, *Salmonella*, *Shigella*, *E. coli*, *Enterobacter*, and *Klebsiella*
Usual Dosage
  Usual dosage range:
    Infants and Children:
      Oral: 50-100 mg/kg/day in doses divided every 6 hours (maximum: 2-4 g/day)
      I.M., I.V.: 100-400 mg/kg/day in divided doses every 6 hours (maximum: 12 g/day)
    Adults: Oral, I.M., I.V.: 250-500 mg every 6 hours
  Indication-specific dosing:
    Infants and Children:
      Endocarditis prophylaxis:
        Dental, oral, respiratory tract, or esophageal procedures: I.M., I.V.: 50 mg/kg within 30 minutes prior to procedure in patients unable to take oral amoxicillin
        Genitourinary and gastrointestinal tract (except esophageal) procedures: I.M., I.V.:
          High-risk patients: 50 mg/kg (maximum: 2 g) within 30 minutes prior to procedure, followed by ampicillin 25 mg/kg (or amoxicillin 25 mg/kg orally) 6 hours later; must be used in combination with gentamicin.
          Moderate-risk patients: 50 mg/kg within 30 minutes prior to procedure
      Mild-to-moderate infections:
        Oral: 50-100 mg/kg/day in doses divided every 6 hours (maximum: 2-4 g/day)
        I.M., I.V.: 100-150 mg/kg/day in divided doses every 6 hours (maximum: 2-4 g/day)
      Severe infections, meningitis: I.M., I.V.: 200-400 mg/kg/day in divided doses every 6 hours (maximum: 6-12 g/day)
    Adults:
      Actinomycosis: I.V.: 50 mg/kg/day for 4-6 weeks then oral amoxicillin
      Cholangitis (acute): I.V.: 2 g every 4 hours with gentamicin
      Diverticulitis: I.M., I.V.: 2 g every 6 hours with metronidazole
      Endocarditis:
        Infective: I.V.: 12 g/day via continuous infusion or divided every 4 hours
        Prophylaxis: Dental, oral, respiratory tract, or esophageal procedures: I.M., I.V.: 2 g within 30 minutes prior to procedure in patients unable to take oral amoxicillin
        Genitourinary and gastrointestinal tract (except esophageal) procedures:
          High-risk patients: I.M., I.V.: 2 g within 30 minutes prior to procedure, followed by ampicillin 1 g (or amoxicillin 1g orally) 6 hours later; must be used in combination with gentamicin.
          Moderate-risk patients: I.M., I.V.: 2 g within 30 minutes prior to procedure
      Group B strep prophylaxis (intrapartum): I.V.: 2 g initial dose, then 1 g every 4 hours until delivery
      Listeria **infections:** I.V.: 200 mg/kg/day divided every 6 hours
      Sepsis/meningitis: I.M., I.V.: 150-250 mg/kg/day divided every 3-4 hours (range: 6-12 g/day)
      Urinary tract infections (enterococcus suspected): I.V.: 1-2 g every 6 hours with gentamicin
Dosage Forms
  Capsule: 250 mg, 500 mg
  Injection, powder for reconstitution: 125 mg, 250 mg, 500 mg, 1 g, 2 g, 10 g
  Powder for oral suspension: 125 mg/5 mL, 250 mg/5 mL

ampicillin and sulbactam (am pi SIL in & SUL bak tam)

Synonyms sulbactam and ampicillin

U.S./Canadian Brand Names Unasyn® [US/Can]

Therapeutic Category Penicillin

Use Treatment of susceptible bacterial infections involved with skin and skin structure, intraabdominal infections, gynecological infections; spectrum is that of ampicillin plus organisms producing beta-lactamases such as *S. aureus*, *H. influenzae*, *E. coli*, *Klebsiella*, *Acinetobacter*, *Enterobacter*, and anaerobes

Usual Dosage Note: Unasyn® (ampicillin/sulbactam) is a combination product. Dosage recommendations for Unasyn® are based on the ampicillin component.

Usual dosage range:

Children ≥1 year: I.V.: 100-400 mg ampicillin/kg/day divided every 6 hours (maximum: 8 g ampicillin/day, 12 g Unasyn®). **Note:** The American Academy of Pediatrics recommends a dose of up to 300 mg/kg/day for severe infection in infants >1 month of age.

Adults: I.M., I.V.: 1-2 g ampicillin (1.5-3 g Unasyn®) every 6 hours (maximum: 8 g ampicillin/day, 12 g Unasyn®)

Indication-specific dosing:

Children:

Epiglottitis: I.V.: 100-200 mg ampicillin/kg/day divided in 4 doses

Mild-to-moderate infections: I.M., I.V.: 100-200 mg ampicillin/kg/day (150-300 mg Unasyn®) divided every 6 hours (maximum: 8 g ampicillin/day, 12 g Unasyn®)

Peritonsillar and retropharyngeal abscess: I.V.: 50 mg ampicillin/kg/dose every 6 hours

Severe infections: I.M., I.V.: 200-400 mg ampicillin/kg/day divided every 6 hours (maximum: 8 g ampicillin/day, 12 g Unasyn®)

Adults: Doses expressed as ampicillin/sulbactam combination:

Amnionitis, cholangitis, diverticulitis, endometritis, endophthalmitis, epididymitis/orchitis, liver abscess, osteomyelitis (diabetic foot), peritonitis: I.V.: 3 g every 6 hours

Endocarditis: I.V.: 3 g every 6 hours with gentamicin or vancomycin for 4-6 weeks

Orbital cellulitis: I.V.: 1.5 g every 6 hours

Parapharyngeal space infections: I.V.: 3 g every 6 hours

Pasteurella multocida **(human, canine/feline bites):** I.V.: 1.5-3 g every 6 hours

Pelvic inflammatory disease: I.V.: 3 g every 6 hours with doxycycline

Peritonitis (CAPD): Intraperitoneal:

Anuric, intermittent: 3 g every 12 hours

Anuric, continuous: Loading dose: 1.5 g; maintenance dose: 150 mg

Pneumonia:

Aspiration, community-acquired: I.V.: 1.5-3 g every 6 hours

Hospital-acquired: I.V.: 3 g every 6 hours

Urinary tract infections, pyelonephritis: I.V.: 3 g every 6 hours for 14 days

Dosage Forms

Injection, powder for reconstitution: 1.5 g [ampicillin 1 g and sulbactam 0.5 g]; 3 g [ampicillin 2 g and sulbactam 1 g]; 15 g [ampicillin 10 g and sulbactam 5 g]

Unasyn®: 1.5 g [ampicillin 1 g and sulbactam 0.5 g]; 3 g [ampicillin 2 g and sulbactam 1 g]; 15 g [ampicillin 10 g and sulbactam 5 g]; 15 g [ampicillin 10 g and sulbactam 5 g

ampicillin sodium *see* ampicillin *on previous page*

ampicillin trihydrate *see* ampicillin *on previous page*

amprenavir (am PREN a veer)

U.S./Canadian Brand Names Agenerase® [US/Can]

Therapeutic Category Protease Inhibitor

Use Treatment of HIV infections in combination with at least two other antiretroviral agents; oral solution should only be used when capsules or other protease inhibitors are not therapeutic options

Usual Dosage Oral: **Note:** Capsule and oral solution are **not** interchangeable on a mg-per-mg basis.

Capsule:

Children 4-12 years **or** 13-16 years (<50 kg): 20 mg/kg twice daily or 15 mg/kg 3 times daily; maximum: 2400 mg/day

Children >13 years (≥50 kg) and Adults: 1200 mg twice daily

Note: Dosage adjustments for amprenavir when administered in combination therapy:

Efavirenz: Adjustments necessary for both agents:

Amprenavir 1200 mg 3 times/day (single protease inhibitor) **or**

Amprenavir 1200 mg twice daily plus ritonavir 200 mg twice daily

Ritonavir: Adjustments necessary for both agents:

Amprenavir 1200 mg plus ritonavir 200 mg once daily **or**

Amprenavir 600 mg plus ritonavir 100 mg twice daily

Note: Oral solution of ritonavir and amprenavir should not be coadministered.

Solution:
Children 4-12 years **or** 13-16 years (<50 kg): 22.5 mg/kg twice daily or 17 mg/kg 3 times daily; maximum: 2800 mg/day
Children >13 years (≥50 kg) and Adults: 1400 mg twice daily
Dosage Forms
Capsule:
Agenerase®: 50 mg
Solution, oral:
Agenerase®: 15 mg/mL

AMPT *see* metyrosine *on page 565*

amrinone lactate *see* inamrinone *on page 452*

Amvisc® *(Discontinued)* *see* hyaluronate and derivatives *on page 423*

Amvisc® Plus *(Discontinued)* *see* hyaluronate and derivatives *on page 423*

amyl nitrite (AM il NYE trite)
Synonyms isoamyl nitrite
Therapeutic Category Vasodilator
Use Coronary vasodilator in angina pectoris; adjunct in treatment of cyanide poisoning; produce changes in the intensity of heart murmurs
Usual Dosage Nasal inhalation:
Cyanide poisoning: Children and Adults: Inhale the vapor from a 0.3 mL crushed ampul every minute for 15-30 seconds until I.V. sodium nitrite infusion is available
Angina: Adults: 1-6 inhalations from 1 crushed ampul; may repeat in 3-5 minutes
Dosage Forms
Vapor for inhalation [crushable covered glass capsules]: Amyl nitrite USP (0.3 mL)

amyl nitrite, sodium thiosulfate, and sodium nitrite *see* sodium nitrite, sodium thiosulfate, and amyl nitrite *on page 794*

amylobarbitone *see* amobarbital *on page 47*

Amytal® [US] *see* amobarbital *on page 47*

AN100226 *see* natalizumab *on page 593*

Anabolin® *(Discontinued)* *see* nandrolone *on page 590*

Anacin® PM Aspirin Free *(Discontinued)* *see* acetaminophen and diphenhydramine *on page 7*

Anadrol® [US] *see* oxymetholone *on page 643*

Anafranil® [US/Can] *see* clomipramine *on page 203*

anagrelide (an AG gre lide)
Synonyms 1370-999-397; anagrelide hydrochloride; BL4162A; 6,7-dichloro-1,5-dihydroimidazo [2,1b] quinazolin-2(3H)-one monohydrochloride
U.S./Canadian Brand Names Agrylin® [US/Can]; Gen-Anagrelide [Can]; PMS-Anagrelide [Can]; Rhoxal-anagrelide [Can]; Sandoz-Anagrelide [Can]
Therapeutic Category Platelet Reducing Agent
Use Treatment of essential thrombocythemia (ET) and thrombocythemia associated with myeloproliferative disorders
Usual Dosage Note: Maintain for ≥1 week, then adjust to the lowest effective dose to reduce and maintain platelet count <600,000/μL ideally to the normal range; the dose must not be increased by >0.5 mg/day in any 1 week; maximum dose: 10 mg/day or 2.5 mg/dose
Oral:
Children: Initial: 0.5 mg/day (range: 0.5 mg 1-4 times/day)
Adults: 0.5 mg 4 times/day or 1 mg twice daily
Dosage Forms
Capsule: 0.5 mg, 1 mg
Agrylin®: 0.5 mg, 1 mg

anagrelide hydrochloride *see* anagrelide *on this page*

anakinra (an a KIN ra)
Sound-Alike/Look-Alike Issues
anakinra may be confused with amikacin
(Continued)

anakinra *(Continued)*

Synonyms IL-1Ra; interleukin-1 receptor antagonist
U.S./Canadian Brand Names Kineret® [US/Can]
Therapeutic Category Antirheumatic, Disease Modifying
Use Treatment of moderately- to severely-active rheumatoid arthritis in adult patients who have failed one or more disease-modifying antirheumatic drugs (DMARDs); may be used alone or in combination with DMARDs (other than tumor necrosis factor-blocking agents)
Usual Dosage SubQ: Adults: Rheumatoid arthritis: 100 mg once daily (administer at approximately the same time each day)
Dosage Forms
  Injection, solution [preservative free]:
  Kineret®: 100 mg/0.67 mL (1 mL)

Ana-Kit® [US] *see* epinephrine and chlorpheniramine *on page 302*

Analpram-HC® [US] *see* pramoxine and hydrocortisone *on page 707*

AnaMantle® HC [US] *see* lidocaine and hydrocortisone *on page 507*

Anamine® Syrup *(Discontinued)* *see* chlorpheniramine and pseudoephedrine *on page 178*

Anandron® [Can] *see* nilutamide *on page 606*

Anaplex® DM [US] *see* brompheniramine, pseudoephedrine, and dextromethorphan *on page 122*

Anaplex® DMX [US] *see* brompheniramine, pseudoephedrine, and dextromethorphan *on page 122*

Anaplex® Liquid *(Discontinued)* *see* chlorpheniramine and pseudoephedrine *on page 178*

Anaprox® [US/Can] *see* naproxen *on page 591*

Anaprox® DS [US/Can] *see* naproxen *on page 591*

Anaspaz® [US] *see* hyoscyamine *on page 441*

anastrozole *(an AS troe zole)*

Synonyms ICI-D1033; NSC-719344; ZD1033
U.S./Canadian Brand Names Arimidex® [US/Can]
Therapeutic Category Antineoplastic Agent
Use Treatment of locally-advanced or metastatic breast cancer (ER-positive or hormone receptor unknown) in postmenopausal women; treatment of advanced breast cancer in postmenopausal women with disease progression following tamoxifen therapy; adjuvant treatment of early ER-positive breast cancer in postmenopausal women
Usual Dosage Oral (refer to individual protocols): Adults: Breast cancer: 1 mg once daily
Dosage Forms
  Tablet:
  Arimidex®: 1 mg

Anatrast [US] *see* barium *on page 94*

Anbesol® [US-OTC] *see* benzocaine *on page 101*

Anbesol® Baby [US-OTC/Can] *see* benzocaine *on page 101*

Anbesol® Cold Sore Therapy [US-OTC] *see* benzocaine *on page 101*

Anbesol® Jr. [US-OTC] *see* benzocaine *on page 101*

Anbesol® Maximum Strength [US-OTC] *see* benzocaine *on page 101*

Ancobon® [US/Can] *see* flucytosine *on page 357*

Andehist DM NR [US] *see* brompheniramine, pseudoephedrine, and dextromethorphan *on page 122*

Andehist DM NR Drops *(Discontinued)* *see* carbinoxamine, pseudoephedrine, and dextromethorphan *on page 152*

Andehist NR Drops *(Discontinued)* *see* carbinoxamine and pseudoephedrine *on page 151*

Andehist NR Syrup [US] *see* brompheniramine and pseudoephedrine *on page 120*

Andriol® [Can] *see* testosterone *on page 828*

Androcur® [Can] *see* cyproterone *(Canada only) on page 225*

Androcur® Depot [Can] *see* cyproterone *(Canada only) on page 225*

Androderm® [US/Can] *see* testosterone *on page 828*

AndroGel® [US/Can] *see* testosterone *on page 828*

Android® [US] *see* methyltestosterone *on page 560*

Andro-L.A.® Injection *(Discontinued)* *see* testosterone *on page 828*

Androlone®-D *(Discontinued)* *see* nandrolone *on page 590*

Androlone® *(Discontinued)* *see* nandrolone *on page 590*

Andropository [Can] *see* testosterone *on page 828*

Andropository® Injection *(Discontinued)* *see* testosterone *on page 828*

Androvite® [US-OTC] *see* vitamins (multiple/oral) *on page 895*

Anectine® [US] *see* succinylcholine *on page 808*

Anestacon® [US] *see* lidocaine *on page 504*

aneurine hydrochloride *see* thiamine *on page 836*

Anexate® [Can] *see* flumazenil *on page 358*

Anexsia® [US] *see* hydrocodone and acetaminophen *on page 427*

Anextuss [US] *see* guaifenesin, dextromethorphan, and phenylephrine *on page 407*

Angeliq® [US/Can] *see* drospirenone and estradiol *on page 285*

Angiofluor™ **Lite [US]** *see* fluorescein *on page 361*

Angiomax® [US/Can] *see* bivalirudin *on page 115*

anidulafungin (ay nid yoo la FUN jin)
Synonyms LY303366
U.S./Canadian Brand Names Eraxis™ [US]
Therapeutic Category Antifungal Agent, Parenteral; Echinocandin
Use Treatment of candidemia and other forms of *Candida* infections (including those of intraabdominal, peritoneal, and esophageal locus)
Usual Dosage I.V.: Adults:
Candidemia, intraabdominal or peritoneal candidiasis: 200 mg loading dose on day 1, followed by 100 mg daily for at least 14 days after last positive culture
Esophageal candidiasis: 100 mg loading dose on day 1, followed by 50 mg daily for at least 14 days and for at least 7 days after symptom resolution
Dosage Forms
Injection, powder for reconstitution [preservative-free]:
Eraxis™: 50 mg

Anodynos-DHC® *(Discontinued)* *see* hydrocodone and acetaminophen *on page 427*

Anolor 300 [US] *see* butalbital, acetaminophen, and caffeine *on page 130*

Anoquan® *(Discontinued)*

Ansaid® [Can] *see* flurbiprofen *on page 366*

Ansaid® *(Discontinued)* *see* flurbiprofen *on page 366*

ansamycin *see* rifabutin *on page 757*

Antabuse® [US] *see* disulfiram *on page 271*

Antara™ **[US]** *see* fenofibrate *on page 345*

Antazoline-V® Ophthalmic *(Discontinued)*

Anthra-Derm® *(Discontinued)* *see* anthralin *on this page*

Anthraforte® [Can] *see* anthralin *on this page*

anthralin (AN thra lin)
Synonyms dithranol
U.S./Canadian Brand Names Anthraforte® [Can]; Anthranol® [Can]; Anthrascalp® [Can]; Dritho-Scalp® [US]; Micanol® [Can]; Psoriatec™ [US]
Therapeutic Category Keratolytic Agent
Use Treatment of psoriasis (quiescent or chronic psoriasis)
Usual Dosage Topical: Adults: Generally, apply once a day or as directed. The irritant potential of anthralin is directly related to the strength being used and each patient's individual tolerance. Always commence treatment using a short, daily contact time (5-10 minutes) for at least 1 week using the lowest strength possible. Contact time may be gradually increased (to 20-30 minutes) as tolerated.
Skin application: Apply sparingly only to psoriatic lesions and rub gently and carefully into the skin until absorbed. Avoid applying an excessive quantity which may cause unnecessary soiling and staining of the clothing or bed linen.
(Continued)

anthralin *(Continued)*

Scalp application: Comb hair to remove scalar debris, wet hair and, after suitably parting, rub cream well into the lesions, taking care to prevent the cream from spreading onto the forehead,

Remove by washing or showering; optimal period of contact will vary according to the strength used and the patient's response to treatment. Continue treatment until the skin is entirely clear (ie, when there is nothing to feel with the fingers and the texture is normal).

Dosage Forms
Cream:
Dritho-Scalp®: 0.5% (50 g)
Psoriatec™: 1% (50 g)

Anthranol® [Can] *see* anthralin *on previous page*

Anthrascalp® [Can] *see* anthralin *on previous page*

anthrax vaccine, adsorbed (AN thraks vak SEEN ad SORBED)

Synonyms AVA
U.S./Canadian Brand Names BioThrax™ [US]
Therapeutic Category Vaccine
Use Immunization against *Bacillus anthracis*. Recommended for individuals who may come in contact with animal products which come from anthrax endemic areas and may be contaminated with *Bacillus anthracis* spores; recommended for high-risk persons such as veterinarians and other handling potentially infected animals. Routine immunization for the general population is not recommended.

The Department of Defense is implementing an anthrax vaccination program against the biological warfare agent anthrax, which will be administered to all active duty and reserve personnel.
Usual Dosage SubQ: Children ≥18 years and Adults:
Primary immunization: Three injections of 0.5 mL each given 2 weeks apart, followed by three additional injections given at 6, 12, and 18 months; it is not necessary to restart the series if a dose is not given on time; resume as soon as practical
Subsequent booster injections: 0.5 mL at 1-year intervals are recommended for immunity to be maintained
Dosage Forms
Injection, suspension:
BioThrax™: 5 mL

anti-4 alpha integrin *see* natalizumab *on page 593*

131 I anti-B1 antibody *see* tositumomab and iodine I 131 tositumomab *on page 852*

131 I-anti-B1 monoclonal antibody *see* tositumomab and iodine I 131 tositumomab *on page 852*

Antiben® *(Discontinued)* *see* antipyrine and benzocaine *on page 61*

anti-CD11a *see* efalizumab *on page 292*

anti-CD20 monoclonal antibody *see* rituximab *on page 762*

anti-CD20-murine monoclonal antibody I-131 *see* tositumomab and iodine I 131 tositumomab *on page 852*

antidigoxin fab fragments, ovine *see* digoxin immune Fab *on page 258*

antidiuretic hormone *see* vasopressin *on page 886*

antihemophilic factor (human) (an tee hee moe FIL ik FAK tor HYU man)

Synonyms AHF (human); factor VIII (human)
U.S./Canadian Brand Names Hemofil M [US/Can]; Koāte®-DVI [US]; Monarc-M™ [US]; Monoclate-P® [US]
Therapeutic Category Blood Product Derivative
Use Prevention and treatment of hemorrhagic episodes in patients with hemophilia A (classic hemophilia); perioperative management of hemophilia A; can be of significant therapeutic value in patients with acquired factor VIII inhibitors not exceeding 10 Bethesda units/mL
Usual Dosage I.V.: Children and Adults: Individualize dosage based on coagulation studies performed prior to treatment and at regular intervals during treatment. In general, administration of factor VIII 1 int. unit/kg will increase circulating factor VIII levels by ~2 int. units/dL. (General guidelines presented; consult individual product labeling for specific dosing recommendations.)

Dosage based on desired factor VIII increase (%):
To calculate dosage needed based on desired factor VIII increase (%):
Body weight (kg) x 0.5 int. units/kg x desired factor VIII increase (%) = int. units factor VIII required
For example:
50 kg x 0.5 int. units/kg x 30 (% increase) = 750 int. units factor VIII

Dosage based on expected factor VIII increase (%):
It is also possible to calculate the **expected** % factor VIII increase:
(# int. units administered x 2%/int. units/kg) divided by body weight (kg) = expected % factor VIII increase
For example:
(1400 int. units x 2%/int. units/kg) divided by 70 kg = 40%

General guidelines:
Minor hemorrhage: 10-20 int. units/kg as a single dose to achieve FVIII plasma level ~20% to 40% of normal. Mild superficial or early hemorrhages may respond to a single dose; may repeat dose every 12-24 hours for 1-3 days until bleeding is resolved or healing achieved.

Moderate hemorrhage/minor surgery: 15-25 int. units/kg to achieve FVIII plasma level 30% to 50% of normal. If needed, may continue with a maintenance dose of 10-15 int. units/kg every 8-12 hours.

Major to life-threatening hemorrhage: Initial dose 40-50 int. units/kg, followed by a maintenance dose of 20-25 int. units/kg every 8-12 hours until threat is resolved, to achieve FVIII plasma level 80% to 100% of normal.

Major surgery: 50 int. units/kg given preoperatively to raise factor VIII level to 100% before surgery begins. May repeat as necessary after 6-12 hours initially and for a total of 10-14 days until healing is complete. Intensity of therapy may depend on type of surgery and postoperative regimen.

Bleeding prophylaxis: May be administered on a regular basis for bleeding prophylaxis. Doses of 24-40 int. units/kg 3 times/week have been reported in patients with severe hemophilia to prevent joint bleeding.

If bleeding is not controlled with adequate dose, test for presence of inhibitor. It may not be possible or practical to control bleeding if inhibitor titers are >10 Bethesda units/mL.

Dosage Forms
Injection, powder for reconstitution:
Hemofil M: Vial labeled with international units
Koate®-DVI: ~250 int. units, ~500 int. units, ~1000 int. units
Monarc-M™: Vial labeled with international units
Monoclate-P®: ~250 int. units, ~500 int. units, ~1000 int. units, ~1500 int. units

antihemophilic factor (recombinant) (an tee hee moe FIL ik FAK tor ree KOM be nant)
Synonyms AHF (recombinant); factor VIII (recombinant); rAHF

U.S./Canadian Brand Names Advate [US]; Helixate® FS [US/Can]; Kogenate® FS [US/Can]; Kogenate® [Can]; Recombinate [US/Can]; ReFacto® [US/Can]

Therapeutic Category Blood Product Derivative

Use Prevention and treatment of hemorrhagic episodes in patients with hemophilia A (classic hemophilia); perioperative management of hemophilia A; can be of significant therapeutic value in patients with acquired factor VIII inhibitors ≤10 Bethesda units/mL

Usual Dosage I.V.: Children and Adults: Individualize dosage based on coagulation studies performed prior to treatment and at regular intervals during treatment. In general, administration of factor VIII 1 int. unit/kg will increase circulating factor VIII levels by ~2 int. units/dL. (General guidelines presented; consult individual product labeling for specific dosing recommendations.)

Dosage based on desired factor VIII increase (%):
To calculate dosage needed based on desired factor VIII increase (%):
[Body weight (kg) x desired factor VIII increase (%)] divided by 2%/int. units/kg = int. units factor VIII required
For example:
50 kg x 30 (% increase) divided by 2%/int. units/kg = 750 int. units factor VIII

Dosage based on expected factor VIII increase (%):
It is also possible to calculate the **expected** % factor VIII increase:
(# int. units administered x 2%/int. units/kg) divided by body weight (kg) = expected % factor VIII increase
For example:
(1400 int. units x 2%/int. units/kg) divided by 70 kg = 40%

General guidelines:
Minor hemorrhage: 10-20 int. units/kg as a single dose to achieve FVIII plasma level ~20% to 40% of normal. Mild superficial or early hemorrhages may respond to a single dose; may repeat dose every 12-24 hours for 1-3 days until bleeding is resolved or healing achieved.

Moderate hemorrhage/minor surgery: 15-30 int. units/kg to achieve FVIII plasma level 30% to 60% of normal. May repeat 1 dose at 12-24 hours if needed. Some products suggest continuing for ≥3 days until pain and disability are resolved

Major to life-threatening hemorrhage: Initial dose 40-50 int. units/kg followed by a maintenance dose of 20-25 int. units/kg every 8-12 hours until threat is resolved, to achieve FVIII plasma level 80% to 100% of normal.

Major surgery: 50 int. units/kg given preoperatively to raise factor VIII level to 100% before surgery begins. May repeat as necessary after 6-12 hours initially and for a total of 10-14 days until healing is complete. Intensity of therapy may depend on type of surgery and postoperative regimen.

(Continued)

antihemophilic factor (recombinant) *(Continued)*

Bleeding prophylaxis: May be administered on a regular basis for bleeding prophylaxis. Doses of 24-40 int. units/kg 3 times/week have been reported in patients with severe hemophilia to prevent joint bleeding.

If bleeding is not controlled with adequate dose, test for presence of inhibitor. It may not be possible or practical to control bleeding if inhibitor titers >10 Bethesda units/mL.

Dosage Forms

Injection, powder for reconstitution, recombinant [preservative free]:

Advate: 250 int. units, 500 int. units, 1000 int. units, 1500 int. units, 3000 int. units

Helixate® FS, Kogenate® FS, Recombinate: 250 int. units, 500 int. units, 1000 int. units

ReFacto®: 250 int. units, 500 units, 1000 int. units, 2000 int. units

antihemophilic factor/von Willebrand factor complex (human)

(an tee hee moe FIL ik FAK tor von WILL le brand FAK tor KOM plex HYU man)

Synonyms AHF (human); factor VIII (human); FVIII/vWF; vWF:RCof

U.S./Canadian Brand Names Alphanate® [US]; Humate-P® [US/Can]

Therapeutic Category Antihemophilic Agent; Blood Product Derivative

Use

Prevention and treatment of hemorrhagic episodes in patients with hemophilia A (classical hemophilia) (Alphanate®, Humate-P®) or acquired factor VIII deficiency (Alphanate®)

Prophylaxis with surgical and/or invasive procedures in patients with vWD when desmopressin is either ineffective or contraindicated (Alphanate®, Humate-P®)

Treatment of spontaneous or trauma-induced bleeding, as well as prevention of excessive bleeding during and after surgery, in patients with von Willebrand disease (vWD) (mild, moderate, or severe) where use of desmopressin is known or suspected to be inadequate (Humate-P®)

Usual Dosage

Hemophilia A: General guidelines (consult specific product labeling): Children and Adults: I.V.:

Individualize dosage based on coagulation studies performed prior to treatment and at regular intervals during treatment; in general, administration of factor VIII 1 int. unit/kg will increase circulating factor VIII levels by ~2 int. units/dL.

Minor hemorrhage: Loading dose: FVIII:C 15 int. units/kg to achieve FVIII:C plasma level ~30% of normal. If second infusion is needed, half the loading dose may be given once or twice daily for 1-2 days.

Moderate hemorrhage: Loading dose: FVIII:C 25 int. units/kg to achieve FVIII:C plasma level ~50% of normal; Maintenance: FVIII:C 15 int. units/kg every 8-12 hours for 1-2 days in order to maintain FVIII:C plasma levels at 30% of normal. Repeat the same dose once or twice daily for up to 7 days or until adequate wound healing.

Life-threatening hemorrhage/major surgery: Loading dose: FVIII:C 40-50 int. units/kg; Maintenance: FVIII:C 20-25 int. units/kg every 8 hours to maintain FVIII:C plasma levels at 80% to 100% of normal for 7 days. Continue same dose once or twice daily for another 7 days in order to maintain FVIII:C levels at 30% to 50% of normal.

von Willebrand disease (vWD): Treatment (Humate-P®): Children and Adults: I.V.: Individualize dosage based on coagulation studies performed prior to treatment and at regular intervals during treatment; in general, administration of factor VIII 1 int. unit/kg would be expected to raise circulating vWF:RCof ~5 int. units/dL

Type 1, mild (if desmopressin is not appropriate): Major hemorrhage:

Loading dose: vWF:RCof 40-60 int. units/kg

Maintenance dose: vWF:RCof 40-50 int. units/kg every 8-12 hours for 3 days, keeping vWF:RCof nadir >50%; follow with 40-50 int. units/kg daily for up to 7 days

Type 1, moderate or severe:

Minor hemorrhage: vWF:RCof 40-50 int. units/kg for 1-2 doses

Major hemorrhage:

Loading dose: vWF:RCof 50-75 int. units/kg

Maintenance dose: vWF:RCof 40-60 int. units/kg every 8-12 hours for 3 days to keep the vWF:RCof nadir >50%, then 40-60 int. units/kg daily for a total of up to 7 days

Types 2 and 3:

Minor hemorrhage: vWF:RCof 40-50 int. units/kg for 1-2 doses

Major hemorrhage:

Loading dose: vWF:RCof 60-80 int. units/kg

Maintenance dose: vWF:RCof 40-60 int. units/kg every 8-12 hours for 3 days, keeping the vWF:RCof nadir >50%; follow with 40-60 int. units/kg daily for a total of up to 7 days

von Willebrand disease (vWD): Surgery/procedure prophylaxis (except patients with type 3 undergoing major surgery) (Alphanate®):

Children: I.V.:

Preoperative dose: vWF:RCoF 75 int. units /kg 1 hour prior to surgery

Maintenance dose: vWF:RCoF 50-75 int. units/kg every 8-12 hours as clinically needed. May reduce dose after third postoperative day; continue treatment until healing is complete.

Adults: I.V.:
Preoperative dose: vWF:RCoF 60 int. units /kg 1 hour prior to surgery
Maintenance dose: vWF:RCoF 40-60 int. units/kg every 8-12 hours as clinically needed. May reduce dose after third postoperative day; continue treatment until healing is complete. For minor procedures, maintain vWF of 40% to 50% during postoperative days 1-3; for major procedures maintain vWF of 40% to 50% for ≥3-7 days.

von Willebrand disease (vWD): Surgery/procedure prevention of bleeding (Humate-P®): Children and Adults: I.V.:

Emergency surgery: Administer 50-60 int units/kg; monitor trough coagulation factor levels for subsequent doses

Surgical management (nonemergency):
Loading dose calculation based on baseline target vWF:RCo: (Target peak vWF:RCo - Baseline vWF:RCo) x weight (in kg) / IVR = int. units vWF:RCo required. Administer loading dose 1-2 hours prior to surgery. **Note:** If IVR not available, assume 2 int. units/kg.
Target concentrations for vWF:RCo following loading dose:
Major surgery: 100 int. units/dL
Minor surgery: 50-60 int. units/dL
Maintenance dose: Initial: 1/2 loading dose followed by dosing determined by target tough concentrations, generally every 8-12 hours.
Target maintenance trough vWF:RCo concentrations:
Major surgery: >50 int. units/dL for up to 3 days,followed by >30 int. units/dL for a minimum total treatment of 72 hours
Minor surgery: ≥30 int. units/dL for a minimum duration of 48 hours
Oral surgery: ≥30 int. units/dL for a minimum duration of 8-12 hours

Dosage Forms
Injection, powder for reconstitution:
Alphanate®: Vial labeled with international units [human derived]
Humate-P®: FVIII 250 int. units and vWF:RCof 600 int. units [human derived]; FVIII 500 int. units and vWF:RCof 1200 int. units [human derived]; FVIII 1000 int. units and vWF:RCof 2400 int. units [human derived]

Antihist-1® *(Discontinued)* see clemastine on page 198

antiinhibitor coagulant complex (an tee in HI bi tor coe AG yoo lant KOM pleks)
Synonyms AICC; coagulant complex inhibitor
U.S./Canadian Brand Names Feiba VH Immuno [Can]; Feiba VH [US]
Therapeutic Category Hemophilic Agent
Use Hemophilia A & B patients with factor VIII inhibitors who are to undergo surgery or those who are bleeding
Usual Dosage I.V.: Children and Adults:
Autoplex® T: Dosage range: 25-100 factor VIII correctional units per kg depending on the severity of hemorrhage; may repeat in ~6 hours if needed. Adjust dose based on patient response.
Feiba VH: General dosing guidelines: 50-100 units/kg (maximum 200 units/kg)
Joint hemorrhage: 50 units/kg every 12 hours; may increase to 100 units/kg; continue until signs of clinical improvement occur
Mucous membrane bleeding: 50 units/kg every 6 hours; may increase to 100 units/kg (maximum: 2 administrations/day or 200 units/kg/day
Soft tissue hemorrhage: 100 units/kg every 12 hours (maximum: 200 units/kg/day)
Other severe hemorrhage: 100 units/kg every 12 hours; may be used every 6 hours if needed; continue until clinical improvement

Dosage Forms
Injection, powder for reconstitution:
Feiba VH: Each bottle is labeled with Immuno units of factor VIII [heparin free; contains sodium 8 mg/mL]

Antilirium® *(Discontinued)* see physostigmine on page 681
Antiminth® *(Discontinued)* see pyrantel pamoate on page 733
Antiphlogistine Rub A-535 No Odour [Can] see trolamine on page 870

antipyrine and benzocaine (an tee PYE reen & BEN zoe kane)
Synonyms benzocaine and antipyrine
U.S./Canadian Brand Names A/B Otic [US]; Allergen® [US]; Auralgan® [Can]; Aurodex [US]
Therapeutic Category Otic Agent, Analgesic; Otic Agent, Ceruminolytic
Use Temporary relief of pain and reduction of swelling associated with acute congestive and serous otitis media, swimmer's ear, otitis externa; facilitates ear wax removal
(Continued)

antipyrine and benzocaine *(Continued)*

Usual Dosage Otic: Children and Adults: Fill ear canal; moisten cotton pledget, place in external ear, repeat every 1-2 hours until pain and congestion are relieved; for ear wax removal instill drops 3-4 times/day for 2-3 days

Dosage Forms
Solution, otic [drops]: Antipyrine 5.4% and benzocaine 1.4% (10 mL)
A/B Otic, Allergen®, Aurodex, Auroto: Antipyrine 5.4% and benzocaine 1.4% (15 mL)

Antispas® Injection *(Discontinued)* see dicyclomine *on page 255*

antithrombin III (an tee THROM bin three)

Synonyms AT-III; heparin cofactor I
U.S./Canadian Brand Names Thrombate III® [US/Can]
Therapeutic Category Blood Product Derivative
Use Treatment of hereditary antithrombin III deficiency in connection with surgical procedures, obstetrical procedures, or thromboembolism
Usual Dosage Adults:
Initial dose: Dosing is individualized based on pretherapy AT-III levels. The initial dose should raise antithrombin III levels (AT-III) to 120% and may be calculated based on the following formula:

[desired AT-III level % - baseline AT-III level %] x body weight (kg)
divided by 1.4%/int. units/kg

For example, if a 70 kg adult patient had a baseline AT-III level of 57%, the initial dose would be [(120% - 57%) x 70] divided by 1.4 = 3150 int. units

Maintenance dose: Subsequent dosing should be targeted to keep levels between 80% to 120% which may be achieved by administering 60% of the initial dose every 24 hours. Adjustments may be made by adjusting dose or interval. Maintain level within normal range for 2-8 days depending on type of procedure.

Dosage Forms
Injection, powder for reconstitution [preservative free]:
Thrombate III®: 500 int. units, 1000 int. units

antithymocyte globulin (equine) (an te THY moe site GLOB yu lin, E kwine)

Sound-Alike/Look-Alike Issues
Atgam® may be confused with Ativan®
Synonyms antithymocyte immunoglobulin; ATG; horse antihuman thymocyte gamma globulin; lymphocyte immune globulin
U.S./Canadian Brand Names Atgam® [US/Can]
Therapeutic Category Immunosuppressant Agent
Use Prevention and treatment of acute renal allograft rejection; treatment of moderate to severe aplastic anemia in patients not considered suitable candidates for bone marrow transplantation
Usual Dosage An intradermal skin test is recommended prior to administration of the initial dose of ATG; use 0.1 mL of a 1:1000 dilution of ATG in normal saline. A positive skin reaction consists of a wheal ≥10 mm in diameter. If a positive skin test occurs, the first infusion should be administered in a controlled environment with intensive life support immediately available. A systemic reaction precludes further administration of the drug. The absence of a reaction does **not** preclude the possibility of an immediate sensitivity reaction.

Premedication with diphenhydramine, hydrocortisone, and acetaminophen is recommended prior to first dose.
Children: I.V.:
Aplastic anemia protocol: 10-20 mg/kg/day for 8-14 days; then administer every other day for 7 more doses; addition doses may be given every other day for 21 total doses in 28 days
Renal allograft: 5-25 mg/kg/day
Adults: I.V.:
Aplastic anemia protocol: 10-20 mg/kg/day for 8-14 days, then administer every other day for 7 more doses, for a total of 21 doses in 28 days
Renal allograft:
Rejection prophylaxis: 15 mg/kg/day for 14 days followed by 14 days of alternative day therapy at the same dose; the first dose should be administered within 24 hours before or after transplantation
Rejection treatment: 10-15 mg/kg/day for 14 days, then administer every other day for 10-14 days up to 21 doses in 28 days
Dosage Forms
Injection, solution:
Atgam®: 50 mg/mL (5 mL)

antithymocyte globulin (rabbit) <small>(an te THY moe site GLOB yu lin RAB bit)</small>
U.S./Canadian Brand Names Thymoglobulin® [US]
Therapeutic Category Immunosuppressant Agent
Use Treatment of acute rejection of renal transplant; used in conjunction with concomitant immunosuppression
Usual Dosage I.V.: 1.5 mg/kg/day for 7-14 days
Dosage Forms
Injection, powder for reconstitution:
Thymoglobulin®: 25 mg

antithymocyte immunoglobulin *see* antithymocyte globulin (equine) *on previous page*

antitumor necrosis factor apha (human) *see* adalimumab *on page 18*

Anti-Tuss® Expectorant *(Discontinued)* *see* guaifenesin *on page 401*

anti-VEGF monoclonal antibody *see* bevacizumab *on page 110*

antivenin *(Crotalidae)* polyvalent <small>(an tee VEN in (kroe TAL ih die) pol i VAY lent)</small>
Synonyms crotalidae antivenin; crotaline antivenin, polyvalent; North and South American antisnake-bite serum; pit viper antivenin; snake (pit vipers) antivenin
U.S./Canadian Brand Names CroFab™ [Ovine] [US]
Therapeutic Category Antivenin
Use Neutralization of venoms of North and South American crotalids: Rattlesnake, copperhead, cottonmouth, tropical moccasins, fer-de-lance, bushmaster
Usual Dosage Children and Adults: Crotalid envenomation:
Antivenin polyvalent (equine): I.M., I.V.: Initial sensitivity test: 0.02-0.03 mL of a 1:10 dilution of normal horse serum or antivenin given intracutaneously; also give a control test using normal saline in the opposite extremity. A positive reaction occurs within 5-30 minutes. A negative reaction does not rule out the possibility of an immediate or delayed reaction with treatment.
Minimal envenomation: 20-40 mL (2-4 vials)
Moderate envenomation: 50-90 mL (5-9 vials)
Severe envenomation: 100-150 mL (10-15 vials) or more
Note: The entire initial dose of antivenin should be administered as soon as possible to be most effective (within 4 hours after the bite). I.V. is the preferred route of administration. When administered I.V., infuse the initial 5-10 mL dilution over 3-5 minutes while carefully observing the patient for signs and symptoms of sensitivity reactions. If no reaction occurs, continue infusion at a safe I.V. fluid delivery rate. Additional doses of antivenin are based on clinical response to the initial dose. If swelling continues to progress, symptoms increase in severity, hypotension occurs, or decrease in hematocrit appears, an additional 10-50 mL (1-5 vials) should be administered.
Antivenin polyvalent (ovine): I.V.: Minimal or moderate envenomation:
Initial dose: 4-6 vials, dependent upon patient response. Treatment should begin within 6 hours of snakebite; monitor for 1 hour following infusion. Repeat with an additional 4-6 vials if control is not achieved with initial dose. Continue to treat with 4- to 6-vial doses until complete arrest of local manifestations, coagulation tests, and systemic signs are normal. Administer I.V. over 60 minutes at a rate of 25-50 mL/hour for the first 10 minutes. If no allergic reaction is observed, increase rate to 250 mL/hour. Monitor closely
Maintenance dose: Once control is achieved, administer 2 vials every 6 hours for up to 18 hours; optimal dosing past 18 hours has not been established; however, treatment may be continued if deemed necessary based on the patient's condition
Dosage Forms
Injection, powder for reconstitution:
CroFab™: Derived from *Crotalus adamanteus, C. atrox, C. scutulatus,* and *Agkistrodon piscivorus* snake venoms

antivenin *(Latrodectus mactans)* <small>(an tee VEN in lak tro DUK tus MAK tans)</small>
Synonyms black widow spider species antivenin (*Latrodectus mactans*)
Therapeutic Category Antivenin
Use Treatment of patients with symptoms of black widow spider bites
Usual Dosage
Skin test: Intradermal: Children and Adults: 0.02 mL of a 1:10 dilution in NS (also use a control solution of NS); evaluate in 10 minutes. Positive reaction is urticarial wheal surrounded by zone of erythema
Conjunctival test: Ophthalmic:
Children: Instill 1 drop of a 1:100 dilution into the conjunctival sac
Adults: Instill 1 drop of a 1:10 dilution into the conjunctival sac
Note: Itching of the eye and/or reddening of conjunctiva indicates a positive reaction, usually occurring within 10 minutes.
Desensitization: Children and Adults: **Note:** In separate vials or syringes, prepare 1:10 and 1:100 dilutions of antivenin in NS.
(Continued)

antivenin *(Latrodectus mactans)* *(Continued)*

SubQ: Inject 0.1, 0.2, and 0.5 mL of the 1:100 dilution at 15- to 30- minute intervals. Proceed with the next dose only if no reaction has occurred following the previous. Repeat procedure using the 1:10 dilution and then undiluted antivenin.

If a reaction occurs, apply tourniquet proximal to the injection site and administer epinephrine 1:1000. Wait at least 30 minutes, then administer another antivenin injection at the last dose which did not evoke a reaction.

If no reaction has occurred following 0.5 mL of undiluted antivenin, continue the dose at 15 minute intervals until entire dose has been administered.

Treatment of symptoms due to black widow spider bite: Administer only following the skin test or conjunctival test:

Children <12 years: I.V.: 2.5 mL

Children >12 years and Adults: I.M., I.V.: 2.5 mL

Dosage Forms

Injection, powder for reconstitution:

6000 antivenin units

antivenin *(Micrurus fulvius)* (an tee VEN in mye KRU rus FUL vee us)

Synonyms North American coral snake antivenin

Therapeutic Category Antivenin

Use Neutralization of venoms of Eastern coral snake and Texas coral snake

Usual Dosage I.V.: Children and Adults: 3-5 vials by slow injection (dependent on severity of signs/symptoms; some patients may need more than 10 vials)

Antivenin Polyvalent [Equine] *(Discontinued)* see antivenin *(Crotalidae)* polyvalent *on previous page*

Antivert® **[US]** *see* meclizine *on page 535*

Antizol® **[US]** *see* fomepizole *on page 373*

Antrizine® *(Discontinued)* see meclizine *on page 535*

Anturane® *(Discontinued)* see sulfinpyrazone *on page 814*

Anucort-HC® **[US]** *see* hydrocortisone (rectal) *on page 433*

Anu-Med [US-OTC] *see* phenylephrine *on page 675*

Anusol-HC® **[US]** *see* hydrocortisone (rectal) *on page 433*

Anusol® **HC-1 [US-OTC]** *see* hydrocortisone (rectal) *on page 433*

Anusol® **Ointment [US-OTC]** *see* pramoxine *on page 706*

Anuzinc [Can] *see* zinc sulfate *on page 906*

Anxanil® **Oral** *(Discontinued)* see hydroxyzine *on page 440*

Anzemet® **[US/Can]** *see* dolasetron *on page 274*

Apacet® *(Discontinued)* see acetaminophen *on page 5*

APAP *see* acetaminophen *on page 5*

APAP and tramadol *see* acetaminophen and tramadol *on page 9*

Apaphen® *(Discontinued)* see acetaminophen and phenyltoloxamine *on page 8*

Apatate® **[US-OTC]** *see* vitamin B complex combinations *on page 894*

ApexiCon™ **[US]** *see* diflorasone *on page 257*

ApexiCon™ **E [US]** *see* diflorasone *on page 257*

Aphrodyne® **[US]** *see* yohimbine *on page 901*

Aphthasol® **[US]** *see* amlexanox *on page 45*

Apidra® **[US/Can]** *see* insulin glulisine *on page 458*

A.P.L.® *(Discontinued)* see chorionic gonadotropin (human) *on page 187*

Aplisol® **[US]** *see* tuberculin tests *on page 872*

Aplitest® *(Discontinued)* see tuberculin tests *on page 872*

aplonidine *see* apraclonidine *on page 70*

Apo-Acebutolol® **[Can]** *see* acebutolol *on page 4*

Apo-Acetaminophen® **[Can]** *see* acetaminophen *on page 5*

Apo-Acetazolamide® **[Can]** *see* acetazolamide *on page 13*

Apo-Acyclovir® **[Can]** *see* acyclovir *on page 17*

Apo-Alendronate® [Can] *see* alendronate *on page 27*

Apo-Allopurinol® [Can] *see* allopurinol *on page 30*

Apo-Alpraz® [Can] *see* alprazolam *on page 32*

Apo-Alpraz® TS [Can] *see* alprazolam *on page 32*

Apo-Amiloride® [Can] *see* amiloride *on page 41*

Apo-Amilzide® [Can] *see* amiloride and hydrochlorothiazide *on page 42*

Apo-Amiodarone® [Can] *see* amiodarone *on page 43*

Apo-Amitriptyline® [Can] *see* amitriptyline *on page 44*

Apo-Amoxi® [Can] *see* amoxicillin *on page 48*

Apo-Amoxi-Clav® [Can] *see* amoxicillin and clavulanate potassium *on page 49*

Apo-Ampi® [Can] *see* ampicillin *on page 53*

Apo-Atenidone® [Can] *see* atenolol and chlorthalidone *on page 81*

Apo-Atenol® [Can] *see* atenolol *on page 80*

Apo-Azathioprine® [Can] *see* azathioprine *on page 87*

Apo-Azithromycin® [Can] *see* azithromycin *on page 88*

Apo-Baclofen® [Can] *see* baclofen *on page 92*

Apo-Beclomethasone® [Can] *see* beclomethasone *on page 97*

Apo-Benazepril® [Can] *see* benazepril *on page 98*

Apo-Benztropine® [Can] *see* benztropine *on page 105*

Apo-Benzydamine® [Can] *see* benzydamine *(Canada only)* *on page 105*

Apo-Bisacodyl® [Can] *see* bisacodyl *on page 112*

Apo-Bisoprolol® [Can] *see* bisoprolol *on page 114*

Apo-Brimonidine® [Can] *see* brimonidine *on page 118*

Apo-Bromazepam® [Can] *see* bromazepam *(Canada only)* *on page 119*

Apo-Bromocriptine® [Can] *see* bromocriptine *on page 119*

Apo-Buspirone® [Can] *see* buspirone *on page 129*

Apo-Butorphanol® [Can] *see* butorphanol *on page 132*

Apo-Cal® [Can] *see* calcium carbonate *on page 138*

Apo-Calcitonin® [Can] *see* calcitonin *on page 135*

Apo-Capto® [Can] *see* captopril *on page 145*

Apo-Carbamazepine® [Can] *see* carbamazepine *on page 147*

Apo-Carvedilol® [Can] *see* carvedilol *on page 155*

Apo-Cefaclor® [Can] *see* cefaclor *on page 157*

Apo-Cefadroxil® [Can] *see* cefadroxil *on page 158*

Apo-Cefoxitin® [Can] *see* cefoxitin *on page 161*

Apo-Cefprozil® [Can] *see* cefprozil *on page 162*

Apo-Cefuroxime® [Can] *see* cefuroxime *on page 165*

Apo-Cephalex® [Can] *see* cephalexin *on page 167*

Apo-Cetirizine® [Can] *see* cetirizine *on page 169*

Apo-Chlorax® [Can] *see* clidinium and chlordiazepoxide *on page 198*

Apo-Chlordiazepoxide® [Can] *see* chlordiazepoxide *on page 173*

Apo-Chlorpropamide® [Can] *see* chlorpropamide *on page 185*

Apo-Chlorthalidone® [Can] *see* chlorthalidone *on page 185*

Apo-Cilazapril® [Can] *see* cilazapril *(Canada only)* *on page 189*

Apo-Cimetidine® [Can] *see* cimetidine *on page 189*

Apo-Ciproflox® [Can] *see* ciprofloxacin *on page 190*

Apo-Citalopram® [Can] *see* citalopram *on page 194*

Apo-Clindamycin® [Can] *see* clindamycin *on page 198*

Apo-Clobazam® [Can] *see* clobazam *(Canada only)* *on page 201*

Apo-Clomipramine® **[Can]** *see* clomipramine *on page 203*

Apo-Clonazepam® **[Can]** *see* clonazepam *on page 204*

Apo-Clonidine® **[Can]** *see* clonidine *on page 204*

Apo-Clorazepate® **[Can]** *see* clorazepate *on page 206*

Apo-Cloxi® **[Can]** *see* cloxacillin *on page 207*

Apo-Clozapine® **[Can]** *see* clozapine *on page 207*

Apo-Cromolyn® **[Can]** *see* cromolyn sodium *on page 218*

Apo-Cyclobenzaprine® **[Can]** *see* cyclobenzaprine *on page 221*

Apo-Cyproterone® **[Can]** *see* cyproterone *(Canada only) on page 225*

Apo-Desipramine® **[Can]** *see* desipramine *on page 238*

Apo-Desmopressin® **[Can]** *see* desmopressin acetate *on page 239*

Apo-Dexamethasone® **[Can]** *see* dexamethasone (systemic) *on page 241*

Apo-Diazepam® **[Can]** *see* diazepam *on page 251*

Apo-Diclo® **[Can]** *see* diclofenac *on page 253*

Apo-Diclo Rapide® **[Can]** *see* diclofenac *on page 253*

Apo-Diclo SR® **[Can]** *see* diclofenac *on page 253*

Apo-Diflunisal® **[Can]** *see* diflunisal *on page 257*

Apo-Digoxin® **[Can]** *see* digoxin *on page 257*

Apo-Diltiaz® **[Can]** *see* diltiazem *on page 261*

Apo-Diltiaz CD® **[Can]** *see* diltiazem *on page 261*

Apo-Diltiaz® **Injectable [Can]** *see* diltiazem *on page 261*

Apo-Diltiaz SR® **[Can]** *see* diltiazem *on page 261*

Apo-Diltiaz TZ® **[Can]** *see* diltiazem *on page 261*

Apo-Dimenhydrinate® **[Can]** *see* dimenhydrinate *on page 262*

Apo-Dipyridamole FC® **[Can]** *see* dipyridamole *on page 270*

Apo-Divalproex® **[Can]** *see* valproic acid and derivatives *on page 881*

Apo-Docusate-Sodium® **[Can]** *see* docusate *on page 273*

Apo-Domperidone® **[Can]** *see* domperidone *(Canada only) on page 276*

Apo-Doxazosin® **[Can]** *see* doxazosin *on page 278*

Apo-Doxepin® **[Can]** *see* doxepin *on page 279*

Apo-Doxy® **[Can]** *see* doxycycline *on page 281*

Apo-Doxy Tabs® **[Can]** *see* doxycycline *on page 281*

Apo-Erythro Base® **[Can]** *see* erythromycin *on page 309*

Apo-Erythro E-C® **[Can]** *see* erythromycin *on page 309*

Apo-Erythro-ES® **[Can]** *see* erythromycin *on page 309*

Apo-Erythro-S® **[Can]** *see* erythromycin *on page 309*

Apo-Etodolac® **[Can]** *see* etodolac *on page 335*

Apo-Famciclovir [Can] *see* famciclovir *on page 341*

Apo-Famotidine® **[Can]** *see* famotidine *on page 341*

Apo-Famotidine® **Injectable [Can]** *see* famotidine *on page 341*

Apo-Fenofibrate® **[Can]** *see* fenofibrate *on page 345*

Apo-Feno-Micro® **[Can]** *see* fenofibrate *on page 345*

Apo-Ferrous Gluconate® **[Can]** *see* ferrous gluconate *on page 349*

Apo-Ferrous Sulfate® **[Can]** *see* ferrous sulfate *on page 350*

Apo-Flavoxate® **[Can]** *see* flavoxate *on page 354*

Apo-Flecainide® **[Can]** *see* flecainide *on page 354*

Apo-Floctafenine® **[Can]** *see* floctafenine *(Canada only) on page 355*

Apo-Fluconazole® **[Can]** *see* fluconazole *on page 356*

Apo-Flunarizine® **[Can]** *see* flunarizine *(Canada only) on page 359*

Apo-Flunisolide® [Can] *see* flunisolide *on page 359*
Apo-Fluoxetine® [Can] *see* fluoxetine *on page 364*
Apo-Fluphenazine® [Can] *see* fluphenazine *on page 365*
Apo-Fluphenazine Decanoate® [Can] *see* fluphenazine *on page 365*
Apo-Flurazepam® [Can] *see* flurazepam *on page 366*
Apo-Flurbiprofen® [Can] *see* flurbiprofen *on page 366*
Apo-Flutamide® [Can] *see* flutamide *on page 367*
Apo-Fluvoxamine® [Can] *see* fluvoxamine *on page 370*
Apo-Folic® [Can] *see* folic acid *on page 371*
Apo-Fosinopril® [Can] *see* fosinopril *on page 376*
Apo-Furosemide® [Can] *see* furosemide *on page 379*
Apo-Gabapentin® [Can] *see* gabapentin *on page 380*
Apo-Gain® [Can] *see* minoxidil *on page 572*
Apo-Gemfibrozil® [Can] *see* gemfibrozil *on page 387*
Apo-Gliclazide® [Can] *see* gliclazide *(Canada only) on page 393*
Apo-Glyburide® [Can] *see* glyburide *on page 396*
Apo-Haloperidol® [Can] *see* haloperidol *on page 413*
Apo-Haloperidol LA® [Can] *see* haloperidol *on page 413*
Apo-Hydralazine® [Can] *see* hydralazine *on page 425*
Apo-Hydro® [Can] *see* hydrochlorothiazide *on page 426*
Apo-Hydroxyquine® [Can] *see* hydroxychloroquine *on page 438*
Apo-Hydroxyurea® [Can] *see* hydroxyurea *on page 439*
Apo-Hydroxyzine® [Can] *see* hydroxyzine *on page 440*
Apo-Ibuprofen® [Can] *see* ibuprofen *on page 444*
Apo-Imipramine® [Can] *see* imipramine *on page 449*
Apo-Indapamide® [Can] *see* indapamide *on page 452*
Apo-Indomethacin® [Can] *see* indomethacin *on page 454*
Apo-Ipravent® [Can] *see* ipratropium *on page 470*
Apo-ISDN® [Can] *see* isosorbide dinitrate *on page 476*
Apo-ISMN [Can] *see* isosorbide mononitrate *on page 476*
Apo-K® [Can] *see* potassium chloride *on page 700*
Apo-Keto® [Can] *see* ketoprofen *on page 482*
Apo-Ketoconazole® [Can] *see* ketoconazole *on page 482*
Apo-Keto-E® [Can] *see* ketoprofen *on page 482*
Apo-Ketorolac® [Can] *see* ketorolac *on page 483*
Apo-Ketorolac Injectable® [Can] *see* ketorolac *on page 483*
Apo-Keto SR® [Can] *see* ketoprofen *on page 482*
Apo-Ketotifen® [Can] *see* ketotifen *on page 484*
Apokyn® [US] *see* apomorphine *on next page*
Apo-Labetalol® [Can] *see* labetalol *on page 486*
Apo-Lactulose® [Can] *see* lactulose *on page 489*
Apo-Lamotrigine® [Can] *see* lamotrigine *on page 490*
Apo-Leflunomide® [Can] *see* leflunomide *on page 495*
Apo-Levobunolol® [Can] *see* levobunolol *on page 499*
Apo-Levocarb® [Can] *see* levodopa and carbidopa *on page 500*
Apo-Levocarb® CR [Can] *see* levodopa and carbidopa *on page 500*
Apo-Lisinopril® [Can] *see* lisinopril *on page 512*
Apo-Lithium® Carbonate [Can] *see* lithium *on page 513*
Apo-Lithium® Carbonate SR [Can] *see* lithium *on page 513*

Apo-Loperamide® **[Can]** *see* loperamide *on page 515*

Apo-Loratadine® **[Can]** *see* loratadine *on page 517*

Apo-Lorazepam® **[Can]** *see* lorazepam *on page 518*

Apo-Lovastatin® **[Can]** *see* lovastatin *on page 520*

Apo-Loxapine® **[Can]** *see* loxapine *on page 521*

Apo-Medroxy® **[Can]** *see* medroxyprogesterone *on page 537*

Apo-Mefenamic® **[Can]** *see* mefenamic acid *on page 537*

Apo-Mefloquine® **[Can]** *see* mefloquine *on page 538*

Apo-Megestrol® **[Can]** *see* megestrol *on page 538*

Apo-Meloxicam® **[Can]** *see* meloxicam *on page 539*

Apo-Metformin® **[Can]** *see* metformin *on page 548*

Apo-Methazide® **[Can]** *see* methyldopa and hydrochlorothiazide *on page 557*

Apo-Methazolamide® **[Can]** *see* methazolamide *on page 551*

Apo-Methoprazine® **[Can]** *see* methotrimeprazine *(Canada only) on page 554*

Apo-Methotrexate® **[Can]** *see* methotrexate *on page 553*

Apo-Methyldopa® **[Can]** *see* methyldopa *on page 557*

Apo-Methylphenidate® **[Can]** *see* methylphenidate *on page 558*

Apo-Methylphenidate® **SR [Can]** *see* methylphenidate *on page 558*

Apo-Metoclop® **[Can]** *see* metoclopramide *on page 561*

Apo-Metoprolol® **[Can]** *see* metoprolol *on page 562*

Apo-Metronidazole® **[Can]** *see* metronidazole *on page 563*

Apo-Midazolam® **[Can]** *see* midazolam *on page 568*

Apo-Midodrine® **[Can]** *see* midodrine *on page 569*

Apo-Minocycline® **[Can]** *see* minocycline *on page 571*

Apo-Misoprostol® **[Can]** *see* misoprostol *on page 573*

Apo-Moclobemide® **[Can]** *see* moclobemide *(Canada only) on page 575*

apomorphine (a poe MOR feen)

Synonyms apomorphine hydrochloride; apomorphine hydrochloride hemihydrate

U.S./Canadian Brand Names Apokyn® [US]

Therapeutic Category Anti-Parkinson Agent (Dopamine Agonist)

Use Treatment of hypomobility, "off" episodes with Parkinson disease

Usual Dosage SubQ: Adults: Begin antiemetic therapy 3 days prior to initiation and continue for 2 months before reassessing need.

Parkinson disease, "off" episode: Initial test dose 2 mg, **medical supervision required; see "Note".** Subsequent dosing is based on both tolerance and response to initial test dose.

If patient tolerates test dose and responds: Starting dose: 2 mg as needed; may increase dose in 1 mg increments every few days; maximum dose: 6 mg

If patient tolerates but does not respond to 2 mg test dose: Second test dose: 4 mg

If patient tolerates and responds to 4 mg test dose: Starting dose: 3 mg, as needed for "off" episodes; may increase dose in 1 mg increments every few days; maximum dose 6 mg

If patient does not tolerate 4 mg test dose: Third test dose: 3 mg

If patient tolerates 3 mg test dose: Starting dose: 2 mg as needed for "off" episodes; may increase dose in 1 mg increments to a maximum of 3 mg

If therapy is interrupted for >1 week, restart at 2 mg and gradually titrate dose.

Note: Medical supervision is required for all test doses with standing and supine blood pressure monitoring predose and 20-, 40-, and 60 minutes postdose. If subsequent test doses are required, wait >2 hours before another test dose is given; next test dose should be timed with another "off" episode. If a single dose is ineffective for a particular "off" episode, then a second dose should not be given. The average dosing frequency was 3 times/day in the development program with limited experience in dosing >5 times/day and with total daily doses >20 mg. Apomorphine is intended to treat the "off" episodes associated with levodopa therapy of Parkinson disease and has not been studied in levodopa-naive Parkinson patients.

Dosage Forms

Injection, solution:

Apokyn®: 10 mg/mL (2 mL, 3 mL)

apomorphine hydrochloride *see* apomorphine *on previous page*

apomorphine hydrochloride hemihydrate *see* apomorphine *on previous page*

Apo-Nabumetone® **[Can]** *see* nabumetone *on page 585*

Apo-Nadol® **[Can]** *see* nadolol *on page 586*

Apo-Napro-Na® **[Can]** *see* naproxen *on page 591*

Apo-Napro-Na DS® **[Can]** *see* naproxen *on page 591*

Apo-Naproxen® **[Can]** *see* naproxen *on page 591*

Apo-Naproxen EC® **[Can]** *see* naproxen *on page 591*

Apo-Naproxen SR® **[Can]** *see* naproxen *on page 591*

Apo-Nifed® **[Can]** *see* nifedipine *on page 605*

Apo-Nifed PA® **[Can]** *see* nifedipine *on page 605*

Apo-Nitrazepam® **[Can]** *see* nitrazepam *(Canada only) on page 607*

Apo-Nitrofurantoin® **[Can]** *see* nitrofurantoin *on page 607*

Apo-Nizatidine® **[Can]** *see* nizatidine *on page 610*

Apo-Norflox® **[Can]** *see* norfloxacin *on page 612*

Apo-Nortriptyline® **[Can]** *see* nortriptyline *on page 613*

Apo-Oflox® **[Can]** *see* ofloxacin *on page 625*

Apo-Ofloxacin® **[Can]** *see* ofloxacin *on page 625*

Apo-Omeprazole® **[Can]** *see* omeprazole *on page 629*

Apo-Ondansetron® **[Can]** *see* ondansetron *on page 630*

Apo-Orciprenaline® **[Can]** *see* metaproterenol *on page 548*

Apo-Oxaprozin® **[Can]** *see* oxaprozin *on page 637*

Apo-Oxazepam® **[Can]** *see* oxazepam *on page 637*

Apo-Oxybutynin® **[Can]** *see* oxybutynin *on page 639*

Apo-Paclitaxel® **[Can]** *see* paclitaxel *on page 645*

Apo-Paroxetine® **[Can]** *see* paroxetine *on page 654*

Apo-Pentoxifylline SR® **[Can]** *see* pentoxifylline *on page 667*

Apo-Pen VK® **[Can]** *see* penicillin V potassium *on page 664*

Apo-Perindopril® **[Can]** *see* perindopril erbumine *on page 669*

Apo-Perphenazine® **[Can]** *see* perphenazine *on page 670*

Apo-Pimozide® **[Can]** *see* pimozide *on page 683*

Apo-Pindol® **[Can]** *see* pindolol *on page 683*

Apo-Piroxicam® **[Can]** *see* piroxicam *on page 687*

Apo-Pramipexole [Can] *see* pramipexole *on page 706*

Apo-Pravastatin® **[Can]** *see* pravastatin *on page 707*

Apo-Prazo® **[Can]** *see* prazosin *on page 708*

Apo-Prednisone® **[Can]** *see* prednisone *on page 710*

Apo-Primidone® **[Can]** *see* primidone *on page 714*

Apo-Procainamide® **[Can]** *see* procainamide *on page 715*

Apo-Prochlorperazine® **[Can]** *see* prochlorperazine *on page 716*

Apo-Propafenone® **[Can]** *see* propafenone *on page 721*

Apo-Propranolol® **[Can]** *see* propranolol *on page 724*

Apo-Quinidine® **[Can]** *see* quinidine *on page 740*

Apo-Quinine® **[Can]** *see* quinine *on page 740*

Apo-Ramipril® **[Can]** *see* ramipril *on page 743*

Apo-Ranitidine® **[Can]** *see* ranitidine *on page 744*

Apo-Risperidone® **[Can]** *see* risperidone *on page 760*

Apo-Salvent® **[Can]** *see* albuterol *on page 23*

Apo-Salvent® **CFC Free [Can]** *see* albuterol *on page 23*

Apo-Salvent® **Respirator Solution [Can]** *see* albuterol *on page 23*

Apo-Salvent® **Sterules [Can]** *see* albuterol *on page 23*

Apo-Selegiline® **[Can]** *see* selegiline *on page 780*

Apo-Sertraline® **[Can]** *see* sertraline *on page 783*

Apo-Simvastatin® **[Can]** *see* simvastatin *on page 787*

Apo-Sotalol® **[Can]** *see* sotalol *on page 802*

Apo-Sulfatrim® **[Can]** *see* sulfamethoxazole and trimethoprim *on page 813*

Apo-Sulfatrim® **DS [Can]** *see* sulfamethoxazole and trimethoprim *on page 813*

Apo-Sulfatrim® **Pediatric [Can]** *see* sulfamethoxazole and trimethoprim *on page 813*

Apo-Sulfinpyrazone® **[Can]** *see* sulfinpyrazone *on page 814*

Apo-Sulin® **[Can]** *see* sulindac *on page 815*

Apo-Sumatriptan® **[Can]** *see* sumatriptan *on page 815*

Apo-Tamox® **[Can]** *see* tamoxifen *on page 819*

Apo-Temazepam® **[Can]** *see* temazepam *on page 823*

Apo-Terazosin® **[Can]** *see* terazosin *on page 826*

Apo-Tetra® **[Can]** *see* tetracycline *on page 831*

Apo-Theo LA® **[Can]** *see* theophylline *on page 834*

Apo-Tiaprofenic® **[Can]** *see* tiaprofenic acid *(Canada only) on page 840*

Apo-Ticlopidine® **[Can]** *see* ticlopidine *on page 842*

Apo-Timol® **[Can]** *see* timolol *on page 843*

Apo-Timop® **[Can]** *see* timolol *on page 843*

Apo-Tizanidine® **[Can]** *see* tizanidine *on page 846*

Apo-Tolbutamide® **[Can]** *see* tolbutamide *on page 849*

Apo-Trazodone® **[Can]** *see* trazodone *on page 859*

Apo-Trazodone D® **[Can]** *see* trazodone *on page 859*

Apo-Triazide® **[Can]** *see* hydrochlorothiazide and triamterene *on page 427*

Apo-Triazo® **[Can]** *see* triazolam *on page 864*

Apo-Trifluoperazine® **[Can]** *see* trifluoperazine *on page 865*

Apo-Trihex® **[Can]** *see* trihexyphenidyl *on page 866*

Apo-Trimebutine® **[Can]** *see* trimebutine *(Canada only) on page 866*

Apo-Trimethoprim® **[Can]** *see* trimethoprim *on page 867*

Apo-Trimip® **[Can]** *see* trimipramine *on page 868*

Apo-Valproic® **[Can]** *see* valproic acid and derivatives *on page 881*

Apo-Verap® **[Can]** *see* verapamil *on page 887*

Apo-Verap® **SR [Can]** *see* verapamil *on page 887*

Apo-Warfarin® **[Can]** *see* warfarin *on page 899*

Apo-Zidovudine® **[Can]** *see* zidovudine *on page 904*

Apo-Zopiclone® **[Can]** *see* zopiclone *(Canada only) on page 909*

APPG *see* penicillin G procaine *on page 663*

Apra Children's [US-OTC] *see* acetaminophen *on page 5*

apraclonidine (a pra KLOE ni deen)

Sound-Alike/Look-Alike Issues
Iopidine® may be confused with indapamide, iodine, Lodine®
Synonyms aplonidine; apraclonidine hydrochloride; p-aminoclonidine
U.S./Canadian Brand Names Iopidine® [US/Can]
Therapeutic Category Alpha$_2$-Adrenergic Agonist Agent, Ophthalmic
Use Prevention and treatment of postsurgical intraocular pressure (IOP) elevation; short-term, adjunctive therapy in patients who require additional reduction of IOP
Usual Dosage Ophthalmic: Adults:
0.5%: Instill 1-2 drops in the affected eye(s) 3 times/day

1%: Instill 1 drop in operative eye 1 hour prior to anterior segment laser surgery, second drop in eye immediately upon completion of procedure

Dosage Forms
Solution, ophthalmic:
Iopidine®: 0.5% (5 mL, 10 mL); 1% (0.1 mL)

apraclonidine hydrochloride *see* apraclonidine *on previous page*

aprepitant (ap RE pi tant)
Synonyms L 754030; MK 869
U.S./Canadian Brand Names Emend® [US]
Therapeutic Category Antiemetic
Use Prevention of acute and delayed nausea and vomiting associated with moderately- and highly-emetogenic chemotherapy in combination with a corticosteroid and 5-HT₃ receptor antagonist; prevention of postoperative nausea and vomiting (PONV)
Usual Dosage Oral: Adults:
Prevention of chemotherapy induced nausea/vomiting: 125 mg on day 1, followed by 80 mg on days 2 and 3 in combination with a corticosteroid and 5-HT₃ receptor antagonist
In clinical trials, the following regimens were used:
For highly-emetogenic chemotherapy:
Aprepitant: Oral: 125 mg on day 1, followed by 80 mg on days 2 and 3
Dexamethasone: Oral: 12 mg on day 1, followed 8 mg on days 2, 3, and 4
Ondansetron: I.V.: 32 mg on day 1
For moderately-emetogenic chemotherapy:
Aprepitant: Oral: 125 mg on day 1, followed by 80 mg on days 2 and 3
Dexamethasone: Oral: 12 mg on day 1 only
Ondansetron: Oral: Two 8 mg doses on day 1 only
Prevention of PONV: 40 mg within 3 hours prior to induction
Dosage Forms
Capsule:
Emend®: 40 mg, 80 mg, 125 mg
Combination package: Capsule 80 mg (2s), capsule 125 mg (1s)

Apresoline® [Can] *see* hydralazine *on page 425*
Apresoline® (Discontinued) *see* hydralazine *on page 425*
Apri® [US] *see* ethinyl estradiol and desogestrel *on page 322*
Aprodine® [US-OTC] *see* triprolidine and pseudoephedrine *on page 869*

aprotinin (a proe TYE nin)
U.S./Canadian Brand Names Trasylol® [US/Can]
Therapeutic Category Hemostatic Agent
Use Prevention of perioperative blood loss in patients who are at increased risk for blood loss and blood transfusions in association with cardiopulmonary bypass in coronary artery bypass graft surgery
Usual Dosage Adults:
Test dose: **All** patients should receive a 1 mL (1.4 mg) I.V. test dose at least 10 minutes prior to the loading dose to assess the potential for allergic reactions. **Note:** To avoid physical incompatibility with heparin when adding to pump-prime solution, each agent should be added during recirculation to assure adequate dilution.
Regimen A (standard dose):
2 million KIU (280 mg; 200 mL) loading dose I.V. over 20-30 minutes
2 million KIU (280 mg; 200 mL) into pump prime volume
500,000 KIU/hour (70 mg/hour; 50 mL/hour) I.V. during operation
Regimen B (low dose):
1 million KIU (140 mg; 100 mL) loading dose I.V. over 20-30 minutes
1 million KIU (140 mg; 100 mL) into pump prime volume
250,000 KIU/hour (35 mg/hour; 25 mL/hour) I.V. during operation
Dosage Forms
Injection, solution:
Trasylol®: 1.4 mg/mL [10,000 KIU/mL] (100 mL, 200 mL)

Aptivus® [US/Can] *see* tipranavir *on page 845*
Aquacare® [US-OTC] *see* urea *on page 877*
Aquachloral® Supprettes® [US] *see* chloral hydrate *on page 172*
Aquacort® [Can] *see* hydrocortisone (topical) *on page 434*

AquADEKs™ **[US-OTC]** *see* vitamins (multiple/pediatric) *on page 896*

AquaLase™ **[US]** *see* balanced salt solution *on page 93*

AquaMEPHYTON® **[Can]** *see* phytonadione *on page 681*

AquaMEPHYTON® *(Discontinued)* *see* phytonadione *on page 681*

Aquanil™ **HC [US-OTC]** *see* hydrocortisone (topical) *on page 434*

Aquaphilic® **With Carbamide [US-OTC]** *see* urea *on page 877*

Aquaphyllin® *(Discontinued)* *see* theophylline *on page 834*

AquaSite® **[US-OTC]** *see* artificial tears *on page 75*

Aquasol A® **[US]** *see* vitamin A *on page 892*

Aquasol E® **[US-OTC]** *see* vitamin E *on page 894*

Aquatab® **C** *(Discontinued)* *see* guaifenesin, pseudoephedrine, and dextromethorphan *on page 408*

Aquatab® **D** *(Discontinued)* *see* guaifenesin and pseudoephedrine *on page 406*

Aquatab® **DM** *(Discontinued)* *see* guaifenesin and dextromethorphan *on page 402*

AquaTar® *(Discontinued)* *see* coal tar *on page 208*

Aquatensen® **[Can]** *see* methyclothiazide *on page 556*

Aquavit-E® **[US-OTC]** *see* vitamin E *on page 894*

aqueous procaine penicillin G *see* penicillin G procaine *on page 663*

Aquoral™ **[US]** *see* saliva substitute *on page 774*

ara-C *see* cytarabine *on page 226*

arabinosylcytosine *see* cytarabine *on page 226*

Aralast [US] *see* alpha$_1$-proteinase inhibitor *on page 32*

Aralen® **[US/Can]** *see* chloroquine *on page 176*

Aranelle™ **[US]** *see* ethinyl estradiol and norethindrone *on page 328*

Aranesp® **[US/Can]** *see* darbepoetin alfa *on page 232*

Arava® **[US/Can]** *see* leflunomide *on page 495*

Arduan® *(Discontinued)*

Aredia® **[US/Can]** *see* pamidronate *on page 647*

arformoterol (ar for MOE ter ol)

Synonyms arformoterol tartrate; (R,R)-formoterol L-tartrate
U.S./Canadian Brand Names Brovana™ [US]
Therapeutic Category Beta$_2$-Adrenergic Agonist
Use Long-term maintenance treatment of bronchoconstriction in chronic obstructive pulmonary disease (COPD), including chronic bronchitis and emphysema
Usual Dosage Nebulization: Adults: COPD: 15 mcg twice daily; maximum: 30 mcg/day
Dosage Forms
  Solution for nebulization:
    Brovana™: 15 mcg/2 mL (30s)

arformoterol tartrate *see* arformoterol *on this page*

argatroban (ar GA troh ban)

Sound-Alike/Look-Alike Issues
  argatroban may be confused with Aggrastat®
Therapeutic Category Anticoagulant, Thrombin Inhibitor
Use Prophylaxis or treatment of thrombosis in adults with heparin-induced thrombocytopenia; adjunct to percutaneous coronary intervention (PCI) in patients who have or are at risk of thrombosis associated with heparin-induced thrombocytopenia
Usual Dosage I.V.: Adults:
  Heparin-induced thrombocytopenia:
    Initial dose: 2 mcg/kg/minute
    Maintenance dose: Measure aPTT after 2 hours, adjust dose until the steady-state aPTT is 1.5-3.0 times the initial baseline value, not exceeding 100 seconds; dosage should not exceed 10 mcg/kg/minute
    Conversion to oral anticoagulant: Because there may be a combined effect on the INR when argatroban is combined with warfarin, loading doses of warfarin should not be used. Warfarin therapy should be started at the expected daily dose.

Patients receiving ≤2 mcg/kg/minute of argatroban: Argatroban therapy can be stopped when the combined INR on warfarin and argatroban is >4; repeat INR measurement in 4-6 hours; if INR is below therapeutic level, argatroban therapy may be restarted. Repeat procedure daily until desired INR on warfarin alone is obtained.

Patients receiving >2 mcg/kg/minute of argatroban: Reduce dose of argatroban to 2 mcg/kg/minute; measure INR for argatroban and warfarin 4-6 hours after dose reduction; argatroban therapy can be stopped when the combined INR on warfarin and argatroban is >4. Repeat INR measurement in 4-6 hours; if INR is below therapeutic level, argatroban therapy may be restarted. Repeat procedure daily until desired INR on warfarin alone is obtained.

Note: Critically-ill patients with normal hepatic function became excessively anticoagulated with FDA-approved or lower starting doses of argatroban. Doses between 0.15-1.3 mcg/kg/minute were required to maintain aPTTs in the target range. Another report of a cardiac patient with anasarca secondary to acute renal failure had a reduction in argatroban clearance similar to patients with hepatic dysfunction. Reduced clearance may have been attributed to reduced perfusion to the liver. Consider reducing starting dose to 0.5-1 mcg/kg/minute in critically-ill patients who may have impaired hepatic perfusion (eg, patients requiring vasopressors, having decreased cardiac output, having fluid overload). In a retrospective review of critical care patients, patients with three organ system failure required 0.5 mcg/kg/minute. The mean argatroban dose of ICU patients was 0.9 mcg/kg/minute.

Percutaneous coronary intervention (PCI):
Initial: Begin infusion of 25 mcg/kg/minute and administer bolus dose of 350 mcg/kg (over 3-5 minutes). ACT should be checked 5-10 minutes after bolus infusion; proceed with procedure if ACT >300 seconds. Following initial bolus:
ACT <300 seconds: Give an additional 150 mcg/kg bolus, and increase infusion rate to 30 mcg/kg/minute (recheck ACT in 5-10 minutes)
ACT >450 seconds: Decrease infusion rate to 15 mcg/kg/minute (recheck ACT in 5-10 minutes)
Once a therapeutic ACT (300-450 seconds) is achieved, infusion should be continued at this dose for the duration of the procedure.
If dissection, impending abrupt closure, thrombus formation during PCI, or inability to achieve ACT >300 sec: An additional bolus of 150 mcg/kg, followed by an increase in infusion rate to 40 mcg/kg/minute may be administered.

Note: Post-PCI anticoagulation, if required, may be achieved by continuing infusion at a reduced dose of 2-10 mcg/kg/minute, with close monitoring of aPTT.

Dosage Forms
Injection, solution:
100 mg/mL (2.5 mL)

arginine (AR ji neen)
Synonyms arginine hydrochloride
U.S./Canadian Brand Names R-Gene® [US]
Therapeutic Category Diagnostic Agent
Use Pituitary function test (growth hormone)
Usual Dosage I.V.: Pituitary function test:
Children: 500 mg/kg/dose administered over 30 minutes
Adults: 30 g (300 mL) administered over 30 minutes
Dosage Forms
Injection, solution:
R-Gene®: 10% [100 mg/mL = 950 mOsm/L] (300 mL)

arginine hydrochloride *see* arginine *on this page*

8-arginine vasopressin *see* vasopressin *on page 886*

Aricept® [US/Can] *see* donepezil *on page 276*

Aricept® ODT [US] *see* donepezil *on page 276*

Aricept® RDT [Can] *see* donepezil *on page 276*

Arimidex® [US/Can] *see* anastrozole *on page 56*

aripiprazole (ay ri PIP ray zole)
Sound-Alike/Look-Alike Issues
aripiprazole may be confused with rabeprazole
Synonyms BMS 337039; OPC-14597
U.S./Canadian Brand Names Abilify® Discmelt™ [US]; Abilify® [US]
Therapeutic Category Antipsychotic Agent, Quinolone
Use Treatment of schizophrenia; stabilization and maintenance therapy of bipolar disorder (with acute manic or mixed episodes); agitation associated with schizophrenia or bipolar mania
(Continued)

aripiprazole *(Continued)*

Usual Dosage Note: Oral solution may be substituted for the oral tablet on a mg-per-mg basis, up to 25 mg. Patients receiving 30 mg tablets should be given 25 mg oral solution. Orally disintegrating tablets (Abilify® Discmelt™) are bioequivalent to the immediate release tablets (Abilify®).

Adults:

Acute agitation (schizophrenia/bipolar mania): I.M.: 9.75 mg as a single dose (range: 5.25-15 mg); repeated doses may be given at ≥2-hour intervals to a maximum of 30 mg/day. **Note:** If ongoing therapy with aripiprazole is necessary, transition to oral therapy as soon as possible.

Schizophrenia: Oral: 10-15 mg once daily; may be increased to a maximum of 30 mg once daily (efficacy at dosages above 10-15 mg has not been shown to be increased). Dosage titration should not be more frequent than every 2 weeks.

Bipolar disorder (acute manic or mixed episodes): Oral:

Stabilization: 30 mg once daily; may require a decrease to 15 mg based on tolerability (15% of patients had dose decreased); safety of doses >30 mg/day has not been evaluated

Maintenance: Continue stabilization dose for up to 6 weeks; efficacy of continued treatment >6 weeks has not been established

Dosage Forms

Injection, solution:

Abilify®: 7.5 mg/mL (1.3 mL)

Solution, oral:

Abilify®: 1 mg/mL

Tablet:

Abilify®: 2 mg, 5 mg, 10 mg, 15 mg, 20 mg, 30 mg

Tablet, orally disintegrating:

Abilify® Discmelt™: 10 mg, 15 mg

Aristocort® A [US] *see* triamcinolone (topical) *on page 863*

Aristospan® [US/Can] *see* triamcinolone (systemic) *on page 862*

Arixtra® [US/Can] *see* fondaparinux *on page 373*

A.R.M® [US-OTC] *see* chlorpheniramine and pseudoephedrine *on page 178*

Arm-a-Med® Isoproterenol *(Discontinued)* *see* isoproterenol *on page 475*

Arm-a-Med® Metaproterenol *(Discontinued)*

Armour® Thyroid [US] *see* thyroid *on page 839*

Aromasin® [US/Can] *see* exemestane *on page 337*

Arranon® [US] *see* nelarabine *on page 595*

Arrestin® *(Discontinued)* *see* trimethobenzamide *on page 867*

arsenic trioxide *(AR se nik tri OKS id)*

Synonyms As_2O_3; NSC-706363

U.S./Canadian Brand Names Trisenox® [US]

Therapeutic Category Antineoplastic Agent, Miscellaneous

Use Induction of remission and consolidation in patients with relapsed or refractory acute promyelocytic leukemia (APL) which is specifically characterized by t(15;17) translocation or PML/RAR-alpha gene expression

Usual Dosage I.V.: Children >5 years and Adults:

Induction: 0.15 mg/kg/day; administer daily until bone marrow remission; maximum induction: 60 doses

Consolidation: 0.15 mg/kg/day starting 3-6 weeks after completion of induction therapy; maximum consolidation: 25 doses over 5 weeks

Dosage Forms

Injection, solution [preservative free]:

Trisenox®: 1 mg/mL (10 mL)

Artane® *(Discontinued)* *see* trihexyphenidyl *on page 866*

Artha-G® *(Discontinued)* *see* salsalate *on page 775*

ArthriCare® for Women Extra Moisturizing *(Discontinued)* *see* capsaicin *on page 145*

ArthriCare® for Women Multi-Action *(Discontinued)* *see* capsaicin *on page 145*

ArthriCare® for Women Silky Dry *(Discontinued)* *see* capsaicin *on page 145*

ArthriCare® for Women Ultra Strength *(Discontinued)* *see* capsaicin *on page 145*

Arthropan® *(Discontinued)*

Arthrotec® [US/Can] *see* diclofenac and misoprostol *on page 254*

articaine and epinephrine (AR ti kane & ep i NEF rin)

Synonyms epinephrine and articaine hydrochloride

U.S./Canadian Brand Names Astracaine® with epinephrine 1:200,000 [Can]; Astracaine® with epinephrine forte 1:100,000 [Can]; Septanest® N [Can]; Septanest® SP [Can]; Septocaine® with epinephrine 1:100,000 [US]; Septocaine® with epinephrine 1:200,000 [US]; Ultracaine® D-S Forte [Can]; Ultracaine® D-S [Can]; Zorcaine™ [US/Can]

Therapeutic Category Local Anesthetic

Use Local, infiltrative, or conductive anesthesia in both simple and complex dental and periodontal procedures

Usual Dosage Summary of recommended volumes and concentrations for various types of anesthetic procedures; dosages (administered by submucosal injection and/or nerve block) apply to normal healthy adults:

Infiltration: Injection volume of 4% solution: 0.5-2.5 mL; total dose: 20-100 mg
Nerve block: Injection volume of 4% solution: 0.5-3.4 mL; total dose: 20-136 mg
Oral surgery: Injection volume of 4% solution: 1-5.1 mL; total dose: 40-204 mg
Note: These dosages are guides only; other dosages may be used; however, do not exceed maximum recommended dose

Dosage Forms [CAN] = Canadian brand name

Injection, solution:
Septocaine® with epinephrine 1:100,000: Articaine 4% and epinephrine 1:100,000 (1.7 mL)
Septocaine® with epinephrine 1:200,000: Articaine 4% and epinephrine 1:200,000 (1.7 mL)
Ultracaine DS® [CAN]: Articaine 4% and epinephrine 1:200,000 (1.7 mL) [not available in the U.S.]
Ultracaine DS Forte® [CAN]: Articaine 4% and epinephrine 1:100,000 (1.7 mL) [not available in the U.S.]
Zorcaine™: Articaine 4% and epinephrine 1:100,000 (1.7 mL)

artificial tears (ar ti FISH il tears)

Sound-Alike/Look-Alike Issues
Isopto® Tears may be confused with Isoptin®
Murocel® may be confused with Murocoll-2®

Synonyms hydroxyethylcellulose; polyvinyl alcohol

U.S./Canadian Brand Names Akwa Tears® [US-OTC]; AquaSite® [US-OTC]; Bion® Tears [US-OTC]; HypoTears PF [US-OTC]; HypoTears [US-OTC]; Liquifilm® Tears [US-OTC]; Moisture® Eyes PM [US-OTC]; Moisture® Eyes [US-OTC]; Murine® Tears [US-OTC]; Murocel® [US-OTC]; Nature's Tears® [US-OTC]; Nu-Tears® II [US-OTC]; Nu-Tears® [US-OTC]; OcuCoat® PF [US-OTC]; OcuCoat® [US-OTC]; Puralube® Tears [US-OTC]; Refresh Plus® [US-OTC]; Refresh Tears® [US-OTC]; Refresh® [US-OTC]; Soothe® [US-OTC]; Systane® Free [US-OTC]; Systane® [US-OTC]; Teardrops® [Can]; Teargen® II [US-OTC]; Teargen® [US-OTC]; Tearisol® [US-OTC]; Tears Again® [US-OTC]; Tears Naturale® Free [US-OTC]; Tears Naturale® II [US-OTC]; Tears Naturale® [US-OTC]; Tears Plus® [US-OTC]; Tears Renewed® [US-OTC]; Ultra Tears® [US-OTC]; Viva-Drops® [US-OTC]

Therapeutic Category Ophthalmic Agent, Miscellaneous

Use Ophthalmic lubricant; for relief of dry eyes and eye irritation

Usual Dosage Ophthalmic: Children and Adults: Use as needed to relieve symptoms, 1-2 drops into eye(s) 3-4 times/day

Dosage Forms
Solution, ophthalmic: 15 mL and 30 mL dropper bottles
Akwa Tears® [OTC], AquaSite® [OTC], Bion® Tears [OTC], HypoTears PF [OTC], HypoTears [OTC], Isopto® Tears [OTC], Liquifilm® Tears [OTC], Moisture® Eyes PM [OTC], Moisture® Eyes [OTC], Murine® Tears [OTC], Murocel® [OTC], Nature's Tears® [OTC], Nu-Tears® II [OTC], Nu-Tears® [OTC], OcuCoat® PF [OTC], OcuCoat® [OTC], Puralube® Tears [OTC], Refresh® [OTC], Refresh Plus [OTC], Refresh Tears® [OTC], Teargen® [OTC], Teargen® II [OTC], Tearisol® [OTC], Tears Again® [OTC], Tears Naturale® Free [OTC], Tears Naturale® II [OTC], Tears Naturale® [OTC], Tears Plus® [OTC], Tears Renewed® [OTC], Ultra Tears® [OTC], Viva-Drops® [OTC]: 15 mL and 30 mL dropper bottles

As$_2$O$_3$ see arsenic trioxide *on previous page*

ASA see aspirin *on page 78*

5-ASA see mesalamine *on page 546*

Asacol® [US/Can] see mesalamine *on page 546*

Asacol® 800 [Can] see mesalamine *on page 546*

A.S.A.® (Discontinued) see aspirin *on page 78*

Asaphen [Can] see aspirin *on page 78*

Asaphen E.C. [Can] see aspirin *on page 78*

Asco-Caps [US-OTC] see ascorbic acid *on next page*

Ascocid® [US-OTC] see ascorbic acid *on next page*

Ascomp® with Codeine [US] *see* butalbital, aspirin, caffeine, and codeine *on page 131*

ascorbic acid (a SKOR bik AS id)

Synonyms vitamin C

U.S./Canadian Brand Names Acerola [US-OTC]; Asco-Caps [US-OTC]; Asco-Tabs [US-OTC]; Ascocid® [US-OTC]; C-Gel [US-OTC]; C-Gram [US-OTC]; C-Time [US-OTC]; Cecon® [US-OTC]; Cemill [US-OTC]; Cenolate® [US]; Chew-C [US-OTC]; Dull-C® [US-OTC]; Mild-C® [US-OTC]; One Gram C [US-OTC]; Proflavanol C™ [Can]; Revitalose C-1000® [Can]; Time-C [US-OTC]; Time-C-Bio [US-OTC]; Vicks® Vitamin C [US-OTC]; Vita-C® [US-OTC]

Therapeutic Category Vitamin, Water Soluble

Use Prevention and treatment of scurvy; acidify the urine

Usual Dosage Oral, I.M., I.V., SubQ:

Recommended daily allowance (RDA):
  <6 months: 30 mg
  6 months to 1 year: 35 mg
  1-3 years: 15 mg; upper limit of intake should not exceed 400 mg/day
  4-8 years: 25 mg; upper limit of intake should not exceed 650 mg/day
  9-13 years: 45 mg; upper limit of intake should not exceed 1200 mg/day
  14-18 years: Upper limit of intake should not exceed 1800 mg/day
   Male: 75 mg
   Female: 65 mg
  Adults: Upper limit of intake should not exceed 2000 mg/day
   Male: 90 mg
   Female: 75 mg
  Pregnant female:
   ≤18 years: 80 mg; upper limit of intake should not exceed 1800 mg/day
   19-50 years: 85 mg; upper limit of intake should not exceed 2000 mg/day
  Lactating female:
   ≤18 years: 15 mg; upper limit of intake should not exceed 1800 mg/day
   19-50 years: 20 mg; upper limit of intake should not exceed 2000 mg/day
  Adult smoker: Add an additional 35 mg/day

Children:
  Scurvy: 100-300 mg/day in divided doses for at least 2 weeks
  Urinary acidification: 500 mg every 6-8 hours
  Dietary supplement: 35-100 mg/day

Adults:
  Scurvy: 100-250 mg 1-2 times/day for at least 2 weeks
  Urinary acidification: 4-12 g/day in 3-4 divided doses
  Prevention and treatment of colds: 1-3 g/day
  Dietary supplement: 50-200 mg/day

Dosage Forms

Caplet: 1000 mg

Caplet, timed release: 500 mg, 1000 mg

Capsule:
  Mild-C® [OTC]: 500 mg

Capsule, softgel:
  C-Gel [OTC]: 1000 mg

Capsule, sustained release:
  C-Time [OTC]: 500 mg

Capsule, timed release: 500 mg
  Asco-Caps [OTC]: 500 mg, 1000 mg
  Time-C® [OTC]: 500 mg

Crystals for solution, oral: 4 g/teaspoonful
  Mild-C® [OTC]: 3600 mg/teaspoonful
  Vita-C® [OTC]: 4 g/teaspoonful

Injection, solution: 500 mg/mL (50 mL)
  Cenolate® [OTC]: 500 mg/mL (1 mL, 2 mL)

Liquid, oral: 500 mg/5 mL

Lozenge:
  Vicks® Vitamin C [OTC]: 25 mg

Powder, for solution, oral:
  Ascocid® [OTC]: 4000 mg/5 mL; 4300 mg/5 mL; 5000 mg/5 mL
  Dull-C® [OTC]: 4 g/teaspoonful

Solution, oral:
  Cecon® [OTC]: 90 mg/mL

Tablet: 100 mg, 250 mg, 500 mg, 1000 mg
  Asco-Tabs [OTC]: 1000 mg
  Ascocid® [OTC]: 500 mg
  C-Gram [OTC]: 1000 mg
  One Gram C [OTC]: 1000 mg
Tablet, chewable: 250 mg, 500 mg
  Acerola [OTC]: 500 mg
  Chew-C [OTC]: 500 mg
  Mild-C® [OCT]: 250 mg
Tablet, timed release: 500 mg, 1000 mg
  Cemill [OTC]: 500 mg, 1000 mg
  Mild-C® [OTC]: 1000 mg
  Time-C-Bio [OTC]: 500 mg

ascorbic acid and ferrous sulfate *see* ferrous sulfate and ascorbic acid *on page 350*

Ascorbicap® *(Discontinued)* *see* ascorbic acid *on previous page*

Asco-Tabs [US-OTC] *see* ascorbic acid *on previous page*

Ascriptin® [US-OTC] *see* aspirin *on next page*

Ascriptin® Maximum Strength [US-OTC] *see* aspirin *on next page*

Asendin® *(Discontinued)* *see* amoxapine *on page 48*

Asmalix® *(Discontinued)* *see* theophylline *on page 834*

Asmanex® Twisthaler® [US] *see* mometasone *on page 576*

asparaginase (a SPEAR a ji nase)
Sound-Alike/Look-Alike Issues
  asparaginase may be confused with pegaspargase
  Elspar® may be confused with Elaprase™
Synonyms *E. coli* asparaginase; *Erwinia* asparaginase; L-asparaginase; NSC-106977 (*Erwinia*); NSC-109229 (*E. coli*)
U.S./Canadian Brand Names Elspar® [US/Can]; Kidrolase® [Can]
Therapeutic Category Antineoplastic Agent
Use Treatment of acute lymphocytic leukemia
Usual Dosage Refer to individual protocols.
  Children:
  I.V.:
    Infusion for induction: 1000 units/kg/day for 10 days
    Consolidation: 6000-10,000 units/m^2/day for 14 days
    I.M.: 6000 units/m^2 on days 4, 7, 10, 13, 16, 19, 22, 25, 28
  Adults:
    I.V. infusion single agent for induction:
    200 units/kg/day for 28 days **or**
    5000-10,000 units/m^2/day for 7 days every 3 weeks **or**
    10,000-40,000 units every 2-3 weeks
    I.M. as single agent: 6000-12,000 units/m^2; reconstitution to 10,000 units/mL may be necessary

Test dose: A test dose is often recommended prior to the first dose of asparaginase, or prior to restarting therapy after a hiatus of several days. Most commonly, 0.1 mL of a 20 units/mL (2 units) asparaginase dilution is injected intradermally, and the patient observed for at least 1 hour. False-negative rates of up to 80% to test doses of 2-50 units are reported.

Some practitioners recommend an asparaginase desensitization regimen for patients who react to a test dose, or are being retreated following a break in therapy. Doses are doubled and given every 10 minutes until the total daily dose for that day has been administered. One schedule begins with a total of 1 unit given I.V. and doubles the dose every 10 minutes until the total amount given is the planned dose for that day. For example, if a patient was to receive a total dose of 4000 units, he/she would receive injections 1 through 12 during the desensitization.

Dosage Forms
Injection, powder for reconstitution:
  Elspar®: 10,000 units

aspart insulin *see* insulin aspart *on page 457*

A-Spas® *(Discontinued)* *see* hyoscyamine *on page 441*

Aspercin [US-OTC] *see* aspirin *on next page*

Aspercreme® [US-OTC] *see* trolamine *on page 870*

Aspergillus niger see alpha-galactosidase *on page 32*

Aspergum® [US-OTC] *see* aspirin *on this page*

aspirin (AS pir in)
Sound-Alike/Look-Alike Issues
aspirin may be confused with Afrin®, Asendin®
Ascriptin® may be confused with Aricept®
Ecotrin® may be confused with Akineton®, Edecrin®, Epogen®
Halfprin® may be confused with Halfan®, Haltran®
ZORprin® may be confused with Zyloprim®

Synonyms acetylsalicylic acid; ASA

U.S./Canadian Brand Names Asaphen E.C. [Can]; Asaphen [Can]; Ascriptin® Maximum Strength [US-OTC]; Ascriptin® [US-OTC]; Aspercin [US-OTC]; Aspergum® [US-OTC]; Aspirtab [US-OTC]; Bayer® Aspirin Extra Strength [US-OTC]; Bayer® Aspirin Regimen Adult Low Dose [US-OTC]; Bayer® Aspirin Regimen Children's [US-OTC]; Bayer® Aspirin Regimen Regular Strength [US-OTC]; Bayer® Genuine Aspirin [US-OTC]; Bayer® Plus Extra Strength [US-OTC]; Bayer® Women's Aspirin Plus Calcium [US-OTC]; Buffasal [US-OTC]; Bufferin® Extra Strength [US-OTC]; Bufferin® [US-OTC]; Buffinol [US-OTC]; Easprin® [US]; Ecotrin® Low Strength [US-OTC]; Ecotrin® Maximum Strength [US-OTC]; Ecotrin® [US-OTC]; Entrophen® [Can]; Genacote™ [US-OTC]; Halfprin® [US-OTC]; Novasen [Can]; St. Joseph® Adult Aspirin [US-OTC]; ZORprin® [US]

Therapeutic Category Analgesic, Nonnarcotic; Antiplatelet Agent; Antipyretic; Nonsteroidal Antiinflammatory Drug (NSAID)

Use Treatment of mild-to-moderate pain, inflammation, and fever; may be used as prophylaxis of myocardial infarction; prophylaxis of stroke and/or transient ischemic episodes; management of rheumatoid arthritis, rheumatic fever, osteoarthritis, and gout (high dose); adjunctive therapy in revascularization procedures (coronary artery bypass graft [CABG], percutaneous transluminal coronary angioplasty [PTCA], carotid endarterectomy), stent implantation

Usual Dosage
Children:
Analgesic and antipyretic: Oral, rectal: 10-15 mg/kg/dose every 4-6 hours, up to a total of 4 g/day
Antiinflammatory: Oral: Initial: 60-90 mg/kg/day in divided doses; usual maintenance: 80-100 mg/kg/day divided every 6-8 hours; monitor serum concentrations
Antiplatelet effects: Adequate pediatric studies have not been performed; pediatric dosage is derived from adult studies and clinical experience and is not well established; suggested doses have ranged from 3-5 mg/kg/day to 5-10 mg/kg/day given as a single daily dose. Doses are rounded to a convenient amount (eg, $\frac{1}{2}$ of 80 mg tablet).
Mechanical prosthetic heart valves: 6-20 mg/kg/day given as a single daily dose (used in combination with an oral anticoagulant in children who have systemic embolism despite adequate oral anticoagulation therapy (INR 2.5-3.5) and used in combination with low-dose anticoagulation (INR 2-3) and dipyridamole when full-dose oral anticoagulation is contraindicated)
Blalock-Taussig shunts: 3-5 mg/kg/day given as a single daily dose
Kawasaki disease: Oral: 80-100 mg/kg/day divided every 6 hours; monitor serum concentrations; after fever resolves: 3-5 mg/kg/day once daily; in patients without coronary artery abnormalities, give lower dose for at least 6-8 weeks or until ESR and platelet count are normal; in patients with coronary artery abnormalities, low-dose aspirin should be continued indefinitely
Antirheumatic: Oral: 60-100 mg/kg/day in divided doses every 4 hours
Adults:
Analgesic and antipyretic: Oral, rectal: 325-650 mg every 4-6 hours up to 4 g/day
Antiinflammatory: Oral: Initial: 2.4-3.6 g/day in divided doses; usual maintenance: 3.6-5.4 g/day; monitor serum concentrations
Myocardial infarction prophylaxis: 75-325 mg/day; use of a lower aspirin dosage has been recommended in patients receiving ACE inhibitors
Acute myocardial infarction: 160-325 mg/day (have patient chew tablet if not taking aspirin before presentation)
CABG: 75-325 mg/day starting 6 hours following procedure; if bleeding prevents administration at 6 hours after CABG, initiate as soon as possible
PTCA: Initial: 80-325 mg/day starting 2 hours before procedure; longer pretreatment durations (up to 24 hours) should be considered if lower dosages (80-100 mg) are used
Stent implantation: Oral: 325 mg 2 hours prior to implantation and 160-325 mg daily thereafter
Carotid endarterectomy: 81-325 mg/day preoperatively and daily thereafter
Acute stroke: 160-325 mg/day, initiated within 48 hours (in patients who are not candidates for thrombolytics and are not receiving systemic anticoagulation)
Stroke prevention/TIA: 30-325 mg/day (dosages up to 1300 mg/day in 2-4 divided doses have been used in clinical trials)

Dosage Forms
Caplet: 81 mg, 325 mg, 500 mg
Bayer® Aspirin Regimen Regular Strength [OTC], Bayer® Genuine Aspirin [OTC]: 325 mg
Bayer® Aspirin Extra Strength [OTC], Bayer® Plus Extra Strength [OTC]: 500 mg
Bayer® Women's Aspirin Plus Calcium [OTC]: 81 mg
Caplet, buffered: 500 mg
Ascriptin® Maximum Strength [OTC]: 500 mg
Gum:
Aspergum® [OTC]: 227 mg
Suppository, rectal: 300 mg, 600 mg
Tablet: 325 mg
Aspercin [OTC], Aspirtab [OTC], Bayer® Genuine Aspirin [OTC]: 325 mg
Tablet, buffered: 325 mg
Ascriptin® [OTC], Bufferin® [OTC], Buffasal [OTC], Buffinol [OTC]: 325 mg
Bufferin® Extra Strength [OTC]: 500 mg
Tablet, chewable: 81 mg
Bayer® Aspirin Regimen Children's [OTC], St. Joseph® Adult Aspirin [OTC]: 81 mg
Tablet, controlled release: 800 mg
ZORprin®: 800 mg
Tablet, delayed release, enteric coated:
Easprin®: 975 mg
Tablet, enteric coated: 81 mg, 325 mg, 500 mg, 650 mg, 975 mg
Bayer® Aspirin Regimen Adult Low Dose [OTC], Ecotrin® Low Strength [OTC], St. Joseph Adult Aspirin [OTC], Sureprin 81™ [OTC]: 81 mg
Ecotrin® [OTC], Genacote™ [OTC]: 325 mg
Ecotrin® Maximum Strength [OTC]: 500 mg
Halfprin® [OTC]: 81 mg, 162 mg

aspirin, acetaminophen, and caffeine *see* acetaminophen, aspirin, and caffeine *on page 9*

aspirin and carisoprodol *see* carisoprodol and aspirin *on page 154*

aspirin and dipyridamole (AS pir in & dye peer ID a mole)
Sound-Alike/Look-Alike Issues
Aggrenox® may be confused with Aggrastat®
Synonyms aspirin and extended-release dipyridamole; dipyridamole and aspirin
U.S./Canadian Brand Names Aggrenox® [US/Can]
Therapeutic Category Antiplatelet Agent
Use Reduction in the risk of stroke in patients who have had transient ischemia of the brain or completed ischemic stroke due to thrombosis
Usual Dosage Oral: Adults: 1 capsule (dipyridamole 200 mg, aspirin 25 mg) twice daily.
Dosage Forms
Capsule:
Aggrenox®: Aspirin 25 mg (immediate release) and dipyridamole 200 mg (extended release)

aspirin and extended-release dipyridamole *see* aspirin and dipyridamole *on this page*

aspirin and hydrocodone *see* hydrocodone and aspirin *on page 428*

aspirin and meprobamate *see* meprobamate and aspirin *on page 544*

aspirin and oxycodone *see* oxycodone and aspirin *on page 642*

aspirin, caffeine, and acetaminophen *see* acetaminophen, aspirin, and caffeine *on page 9*

aspirin, caffeine, and butalbital *see* butalbital, aspirin, and caffeine *on page 131*

aspirin, caffeine, and propoxyphene *see* propoxyphene, aspirin, and caffeine *on page 723*

aspirin, caffeine, codeine, and butalbital *see* butalbital, aspirin, caffeine, and codeine *on page 131*

aspirin, carisoprodol, and codeine *see* carisoprodol, aspirin, and codeine *on page 154*

Aspirin Free Anacin® *(Discontinued)* *see* acetaminophen *on page 5*

Aspirin Free Anacin® Maximum Strength [US-OTC] *see* acetaminophen *on page 5*

aspirin, orphenadrine, and caffeine *see* orphenadrine, aspirin, and caffeine *on page 634*

Aspirtab [US-OTC] *see* aspirin *on previous page*

Astelin® [US/Can] *see* azelastine *on page 88*

AsthmaHaler® Mist *(Discontinued)* *see* epinephrine *on page 300*

AsthmaNefrin® *(Discontinued)* *see* epinephrine *on page 300*

Astracaine® **with epinephrine 1:200,000 [Can]** *see* articaine and epinephrine *on page 75*

Astracaine® **with epinephrine forte 1:100,000 [Can]** *see* articaine and epinephrine *on page 75*

Astramorph/PF™ **[US]** *see* morphine sulfate *on page 578*

AT-III *see* antithrombin III *on page 62*

Atacand® **[US/Can]** *see* candesartan *on page 143*

Atacand HCT™ **[US]** *see* candesartan and hydrochlorothiazide *on page 144*

Atacand® **Plus [Can]** *see* candesartan and hydrochlorothiazide *on page 144*

Atapryl® *(Discontinued)*

Atarax® **[Can]** *see* hydroxyzine *on page 440*

Atarax® *(Discontinued)* *see* hydroxyzine *on page 440*

Atasol® **[Can]** *see* acetaminophen *on page 5*

atazanavir (at a za NA veer)

Synonyms atazanavir sulfate; BMS-232632

U.S./Canadian Brand Names Reyataz® [US/Can]

Therapeutic Category Antiretroviral Agent, Protease Inhibitor

Use Treatment of HIV-1 infections in combination with at least two other antiretroviral agents

Note: In patients with prior virologic failure, coadministration with ritonavir is recommended.

Usual Dosage Oral: Adolescents ≥16 years and Adults:

Antiretroviral-naive patients: 400 mg once daily; administer with food

Antiretroviral-experienced patients: 300 mg once daily **plus** ritonavir 100 mg once daily; administer with food

Coadministration with efavirenz:

Antiretroviral-naive patients: It is recommended that atazanavir 300 mg plus ritonavir 100 mg be given with efavirenz 600 mg (all as a single daily dose); administer with food

Antiretroviral-experienced patients: Recommendations have not been established.

Coadministration with didanosine buffered formulations: Administer atazanavir 2 hours before or 1 hour after didanosine buffered formulations

Coadministration with tenofovir: The manufacturer recommends that atazanavir 300 mg plus ritonavir 100 mg be given with tenofovir 300 mg (all as a single daily dose); administer with food

Dosage Forms

Capsule:

Reyataz®: 100 mg, 150 mg, 200 mg, 300 mg

atazanavir sulfate *see* atazanavir *on this page*

atenolol (a TEN oh lole)

Sound-Alike/Look-Alike Issues

atenolol may be confused with albuterol, Altenol®, timolol, Tylenol®

Tenormin® may be confused with Imuran®, Norpramin®, thiamine, Trovan®

U.S./Canadian Brand Names Apo-Atenol® [Can]; Gen-Atenolol [Can]; Novo-Atenol [Can]; Nu-Atenol [Can]; PMS-Atenolol [Can]; RAN™-Atenolol [Can]; Rhoxal-atenolol [Can]; Riva-Atenolol [Can]; Sandoz-Atenolol [Can]; Tenolin [Can]; Tenormin® [US/Can]

Therapeutic Category Beta-Adrenergic Blocker

Use Treatment of hypertension, alone or in combination with other agents; management of angina pectoris, postmyocardial infarction patients

Usual Dosage

Oral:

Children: Hypertension: 0.5-1 mg/kg/dose given daily; range of 0.5-1.5 mg/kg/day; maximum dose: 2 mg/kg/day up to 100 mg/day

Adults:

Hypertension: 25-50 mg once daily, may increase to 100 mg/day. Doses >100 mg are unlikely to produce any further benefit.

Angina pectoris: 50 mg once daily, may increase to 100 mg/day. Some patients may require 200 mg/day.

Postmyocardial infarction: Follow I.V. dose with 100 mg/day or 50 mg twice daily for 6-9 days postmyocardial infarction.

I.V.:

Hypertension: Dosages of 1.25-5 mg every 6-12 hours have been used in short-term management of patients unable to take oral enteral beta-blockers

Postmyocardial infarction: Early treatment: 5 mg slow I.V. over 5 minutes; may repeat in 10 minutes. If both doses are tolerated, may start oral atenolol 50 mg every 12 hours or 100 mg/day for 6-9 days postmyocardial infarction.

Dosage Forms
Injection, solution:
Tenormin®: 0.5 mg/mL (10 mL)
Tablet: 25 mg, 50 mg, 100 mg
Tenormin®: 25 mg, 50 mg, 100 mg

atenolol and chlorthalidone (a TEN oh lole & klor THAL i done)

Synonyms chlorthalidone and atenolol
U.S./Canadian Brand Names Apo-Atenidone® [Can]; Tenoretic® [US/Can]
Therapeutic Category Antihypertensive Agent, Combination
Use Treatment of hypertension with a cardioselective beta-blocker and a diuretic
Usual Dosage Oral: Adults: Initial (based on atenolol component): 50 mg once daily, then individualize dose until optimal dose is achieved
Dosage Forms
Tablet: 50: Atenolol 50 mg and chlorthalidone 25 mg; 100: Atenolol 100 mg and chlorthalidone 25 mg
Tenoretic®: 50: Atenolol 50 mg and chlorthalidone 25 mg; 100: Atenolol 100 mg and chlorthalidone 25 mg

ATG see antithymocyte globulin (equine) on page 62

Atgam® [US/Can] see antithymocyte globulin (equine) on page 62

Ativan® [US/Can] see lorazepam on page 518

ATNAA [US] see atropine and pralidoxime on page 84

Atolone® Oral (Discontinued)

atomoxetine (AT oh mox e teen)

Synonyms atomoxetine hydrochloride; LY139603; methylphenoxy-benzene propanamine; tomoxetine
U.S./Canadian Brand Names Strattera® [US/Can]
Therapeutic Category Norepinephrine Reuptake Inhibitor, Selective
Use Treatment of attention deficit/hyperactivity disorder (ADHD)
Usual Dosage Oral: **Note:** Atomoxetine may be discontinued without the need for tapering dose.
Children and Adolescents ≤70 kg: ADHD: Initial: 0.5 mg/kg/day, increase after minimum of 3 days to ~1.2 mg/kg/day; may administer as either a single daily dose or 2 evenly divided doses in morning and late afternoon/early evening. Maximum daily dose: 1.4 mg/kg or 100 mg, whichever is less.
Dosage adjustment in patients receiving strong CYP2D6 inhibitors (eg, paroxetine, fluoxetine, quinidine), do not exceed 1.2 mg/kg/day; dose adjustments should occur only after 4 weeks.
Children and Adolescents >70 kg and Adults: ADHD: Initial: 40 mg/day, increased after minimum of 3 days to ~80 mg/day; may administer as either a single daily dose or two evenly divided doses in morning and late afternoon/early evening. May increase to 100 mg in 2-4 additional weeks to achieve optimal response.
Dosage adjustment in patients receiving strong CYP2D6 inhibitors (eg, paroxetine, fluoxetine, quinidine), do not exceed 80 mg/day; dose adjustments should occur only after 4 weeks.
Dosage Forms
Capsule:
Strattera®: 10 mg, 18 mg, 25 mg, 40 mg, 60 mg, 80 mg, 100 mg

atomoxetine hydrochloride see atomoxetine on this page

atorvastatin (a TORE va sta tin)

Sound-Alike/Look-Alike Issues
Lipitor® may be confused with Levatol®
U.S./Canadian Brand Names Lipitor® [US/Can]
Therapeutic Category HMG-CoA Reductase Inhibitor
Use Treatment of dyslipidemias or primary prevention of cardiovascular disease (atherosclerotic) as detailed below:

Primary prevention of cardiovascular disease (high-risk for CVD): To reduce the risk of MI or stroke in patients without evidence of heart disease who have multiple CVD risk factors or type 2 diabetes. Treatment reduces the risk for angina or revascularization procedures in patients with multiple risk factors.
Secondary prevention of cardiovascular disease: To reduce the risk of MI, stroke, revascularization procedures, and angina in patients with evidence of heart disease. To reduce the risk of hospitalization for heart failure.
Treatment of dyslipidemias: To reduce elevations in total cholesterol, LDL-C, apolipoprotein B, and triglycerides in patients with elevations of one or more components, and/or to increase HDL-C as present in
(Continued)

atorvastatin *(Continued)*

Fredrickson type IIa, IIb, III, and IV hyperlipidemias; treatment of primary dysbetalipoproteinemia, homozygous familial hypercholesterolemia

Treatment of heterozygous familial hypercholesterolemia (HeFH) in adolescent patients (10-17 years of age, females >1 year postmenarche) having LDL-C ≥190 mg/dL or LDL-C ≥160 mg/dL with positive family history of premature cardiovascular disease (CVD) or with two or more CVD risk factors.

Usual Dosage Oral: **Note:** Doses should be individualized according to the baseline LDL-cholesterol levels, the recommended goal of therapy, and patient response; adjustments should be made at intervals of 2-4 weeks

Children 10-17 years (females >1 year postmenarche): HeFH: 10 mg once daily (maximum: 20 mg/day)

Adults:

Hyperlipidemias: Initial: 10-20 mg once daily; patients requiring >45% reduction in LDL-C may be started at 40 mg once daily; range: 10-80 mg once daily

Primary prevention of CVD: 10 mg once daily

Dosage Forms

Tablet:

Lipitor®: 10 mg, 20 mg, 40 mg, 80 mg

atorvastatin calcium and amlodipine besylate *see* amlodipine and atorvastatin *on page 45*

atovaquone (a TOE va kwone)

U.S./Canadian Brand Names Mepron® [US/Can]

Therapeutic Category Antiprotozoal

Use Acute oral treatment of mild-to-moderate *Pneumocystis carinii* pneumonia (PCP) in patients who are intolerant to co-trimoxazole; prophylaxis of PCP in patients intolerant to co-trimoxazole; treatment/suppression of *Toxoplasma gondii* encephalitis; primary prophylaxis of HIV-infected persons at high risk for developing *Toxoplasma gondii* encephalitis

Usual Dosage Oral: Adolescents 13-16 years and Adults:

Prevention of PCP: 1500 mg once daily with food

Treatment of mild-to-moderate PCP: 750 mg twice daily with food for 21 days

Dosage Forms

Suspension, oral:

Mepron®: 750 mg/5 mL

atovaquone and proguanil (a TOE va kwone & pro GWA nil)

Synonyms proguanil and atovaquone

U.S./Canadian Brand Names Malarone® Pediatric [Can]; Malarone® [US/Can]

Therapeutic Category Antimalarial Agent

Use Prevention or treatment of acute, uncomplicated *P. falciparum* malaria

Usual Dosage Oral:

Children (dosage based on body weight):

Prevention of malaria: Start 1-2 days prior to entering a malaria-endemic area, continue throughout the stay and for 7 days after returning. Take as a single dose, once daily.

11-20 kg: Atovaquone/proguanil 62.5 mg/25 mg

21-30 kg: Atovaquone/proguanil 125 mg/50 mg

31-40 kg: Atovaquone/proguanil 187.5 mg/75 mg

>40 kg: Atovaquone/proguanil 250 mg/100 mg

Treatment of acute malaria: Take as a single dose, once daily for 3 consecutive days.

5-8 kg: Atovaquone/proguanil 125 mg/50 mg

9-10 kg: Atovaquone/proguanil 187.5 mg/75 mg

11-20 kg: Atovaquone/proguanil 250 mg/100 mg

21-30 kg: Atovaquone/proguanil 500 mg/200 mg

31-40 kg: Atovaquone/proguanil 750 mg/300 mg

>40 kg: Atovaquone/proguanil 1 g/400 mg

Adults:

Prevention of malaria: Atovaquone/proguanil 250 mg/100 mg once daily; start 1-2 days prior to entering a malaria-endemic area, continue throughout the stay and for 7 days after returning

Treatment of acute malaria: Atovaquone/proguanil 1 g/400 mg as a single dose, once daily for 3 consecutive days

Dosage Forms

Tablet:

Malarone®: Atovaquone 250 mg and proguanil 100 mg

Tablet, pediatric:

Malarone®: Atovaquone 62.5 mg and proguanil 25 mg

Atozine® Oral **(Discontinued)** *see* hydroxyzine *on page 440*

ATRA *see* tretinoin (oral) *on page 860*

atracurium (a tra KYOO ree um)
Synonyms atracurium besylate
U.S./Canadian Brand Names Atracurium Besylate Injection [Can]
Therapeutic Category Skeletal Muscle Relaxant
Use Adjunct to general anesthesia to facilitate endotracheal intubation and to relax skeletal muscles during surgery; to facilitate mechanical ventilation in ICU patients; does not relieve pain or produce sedation
Usual Dosage I.V. (not to be used I.M.): Dose to effect; doses must be individualized due to interpatient variability; use ideal body weight for obese patients
Children 1 month to 2 years: Initial: 0.3-0.4 mg/kg followed by maintenance doses as needed to maintain neuromuscular blockade
Children >2 years to Adults: 0.4-0.5 mg/kg, then 0.08-0.1 mg/kg 20-45 minutes after initial dose to maintain neuromuscular block, followed by repeat doses of 0.08-0.1 mg/kg at 15- to 25-minute intervals
Initial dose after succinylcholine for intubation (balanced anesthesia): Adults: 0.2-0.4 mg/kg
Pretreatment/priming: 10% of intubating dose given 3-5 minutes before initial dose

Continuous infusion:
Surgery: Initial: 9-10 mcg/kg/minute at initial signs of recovery from bolus dose; block usually maintained by a rate of 5-9 mcg/kg/minute under balanced anesthesia
ICU: Block usually maintained by rate of 11-13 mcg/kg/minute (rates for pediatric patients may be higher)
Dosage Forms
Injection: 10 mg/mL (10 mL)
Injection [preservative free]: 10 mg/mL (5 mL)

atracurium besylate *see* atracurium *on this page*

Atracurium Besylate Injection [Can] *see* atracurium *on this page*

Atripla™ [US] *see* efavirenz, emtricitabine, and tenofovir *on page 293*

Atropair® (Discontinued) *see* atropine *on this page*

AtroPen® [US] *see* atropine *on this page*

atropine (A troe peen)
Synonyms atropine sulfate
U.S./Canadian Brand Names AtroPen® [US]; Atropine-Care® [US]; Dioptic's Atropine Solution [Can]; Isopto® Atropine [US/Can]; Sal-Tropine™ [US]
Therapeutic Category Anticholinergic Agent
Use
Injection: Preoperative medication to inhibit salivation and secretions; treatment of symptomatic sinus bradycardia; AV block (nodal level); ventricular asystole; antidote for anticholinesterase inhibitor poisoning (carbamate insecticides, nerve agents, organophosphate insecticides)
Ophthalmic: Produce mydriasis and cycloplegia for examination of the retina and optic disc and accurate measurement of refractive errors; uveitis
Oral: Inhibit salivation and secretions
Usual Dosage
Neonates, Infants, and Children: Doses <0.1 mg have been associated with paradoxical bradycardia.
Inhibit salivation and secretions (preanesthesia): Oral, I.M., I.V., SubQ:
<5 kg: 0.02 mg/kg/dose 30-60 minutes preop then every 4-6 hours as needed. Use of a minimum dosage of 0.1 mg in neonates <5 kg will result in dosages >0.02 mg/kg. There is no documented minimum dosage in this age group.
>5 kg: 0.01-0.02 mg/kg/dose to a maximum 0.4 mg/dose 30-60 minutes preop; minimum dose: 0.1 mg
Alternate dosing:
3-7 kg (7-16 lb): 0.1 mg
8-11 kg (17-24 lb): 0.15 mg
11-18 kg (24-40 lb): 0.2 mg
18-29 kg (40-65 lb): 0.3 mg
>30 kg (>65 lb): 0.4 mg
Bradycardia: I.V., intratracheal: 0.02 mg/kg, minimum dose 0.1 mg, maximum single dose: 0.5 mg in children and 1 mg in adolescents; may repeat in 5-minute intervals to a maximum total dose of 1 mg in children or 2 mg in adolescents. (**Note:** For intratracheal administration, the dosage must be diluted with normal saline to a total volume of 1-5 mL). When treating bradycardia in neonates, reserve use for those patients unresponsive to improved oxygenation and epinephrine.
Children: Organophosphate or carbamate poisoning:
I.V.: 0.03-0.05 mg/kg every 10-20 minutes until atropine effect, then every 1-4 hours for at least 24 hours
(Continued)

atropine *(Continued)*

I.M. (AtroPen®): Mild symptoms: Administer dose listed below as soon as exposure is known or suspected. If severe symptoms develop after first dose, 2 additional doses should be repeated in 10 minutes; do not administer more than 3 doses. Severe symptoms: Immediately administer 3 doses as follows:

<6.8 kg (15 lb): Use of **AtroPen® formulation not recommended;** administer atropine 0.05 mg/kg

6.8-18 kg (15-40 lb): 0.5 mg/dose

18-41 kg (40-90 lb): 1 mg/dose

>41 kg (>90 lb): 2 mg/dose

Adults (doses <0.5 mg have been associated with paradoxical bradycardia):

Asystole or pulseless electrical activity:

I.V.: 1 mg; repeat in 3-5 minutes if asystole persists; total dose of 0.04 mg/kg.

Intratracheal: Administer 2-2.5 times the recommended I.V. dose; dilute in 10 mL NS or distilled water. **Note:** Absorption is greater with distilled water, but causes more adverse effects on PaO_2.

Inhibit salivation and secretions (preanesthesia):

I.M., I.V., SubQ: 0.4-0.6 mg 30-60 minutes preop and repeat every 4-6 hours as needed

Oral: 0.4 mg; may repeat in 4 hours if necessary; 0.4 mg initial dose may be exceeded in certain cases and may repeat in 4 hours if necessary

Bradycardia: I.V.: 0.5-1 mg every 5 minutes, not to exceed a total of 3 mg or 0.04 mg/kg; may give intratracheally in 10 mL NS (intratracheal dose should be 2-2.5 times the I.V. dose)

Neuromuscular blockade reversal: I.V.: 25-30 mcg/kg 30-60 seconds before neostigmine or 7-10 mcg/kg 30-60 seconds before edrophonium

Organophosphate or carbamate poisoning:

I.V.: 2 mg, followed by 2 mg every 5-60 minutes until adequate atropinization has occurred; initial doses of up to 6 mg may be used in life-threatening cases

I.M. (AtroPen®): Mild symptoms: Administer 2 mg as soon as exposure is known or suspected. If severe symptoms develop after first dose, 2 additional doses should be repeated in 10 minutes; do not administer more than 3 doses. Severe symptoms: Immediately administer three 2 mg doses.

Mydriasis, cycloplegia (preprocedure): Ophthalmic (1% solution): Instill 1-2 drops 1 hour before procedure.

Uveitis: Ophthalmic:

1% solution: Instill 1-2 drops 4 times/day

Ointment: Apply a small amount in the conjunctival sac up to 3 times/day; compress the lacrimal sac by digital pressure for 1-3 minutes after instillation

Dosage Forms

Injection, solution: 0.05 mg/mL (5 mL); 0.1 mg/mL (5 mL, 10 mL); 0.4 mg/0.5 mL (0.5 mL); 0.4 mg/mL (0.5 mL, 1 mL, 20 mL); 1 mg/mL (1 mL)

AtroPen®: 0.25 mg/0.3 mL (0.3 mL); 0.5 mg/0.7 mL (0.7 mL); 1 mg/0.7 mL (0.7 mL); 2 mg/0.7 mL (0.7 mL) [prefilled autoinjector]

Ointment, ophthalmic: 1% (3.5 g)

Solution, ophthalmic: 1% (2 mL, 5 mL, 15 mL)

Atropine-Care®: 1% (2 mL) [contains benzalkonium chloride]

Isopto® Atropine: 1% (5 mL, 15 mL) [contains benzalkonium chloride]

Tablet:

Sal-Tropine™: 0.4 mg

atropine and difenoxin *see* difenoxin and atropine *on page 256*

atropine and diphenoxylate *see* diphenoxylate and atropine *on page 267*

atropine and pralidoxime (A troe peen & pra li DOKS eem)

Synonyms atropine and pralidoxime chloride; pralidoxime and atropine

U.S./Canadian Brand Names ATNAA [US]; Duodote™ [US]

Therapeutic Category Anticholinergic Agent; Antidote

Use

ATNAA: Treatment of poisoning by susceptible organophosphorous nerve agents having anticholinesterase activity for self or buddy-administration by military personnel

Duodote™: Treatment of poisoning by organophosphorous nerve agents (eg, tabun, sarin, soman) or organophosphorous insecticide for use by trained emergency medical services personnel

Usual Dosage I.M.: Adults: Organophosphorous poisoning: **Note:** If suspected, antidotal therapy should be given immediately as soon as symptoms appear (critical to administer immediately in case of soman exposure). Definitive medical care should be sought after any injection given. One injection only may be given as self-aid. If repeat injections needed, administration must be done by another trained individual. Emergency medical personnel who have self-administered a dose must determine capacity to continue to provide care.

ATNAA:
Mild symptoms (some or all mild symptoms): Self-Aid or Buddy-Aid: 1 injection (wait 10-15 minutes for effect); if patient is able to ambulate, and knows who and where they are, then no more injections are needed. If symptoms still present: Buddy-Aid: May repeat 1-2 more injections

Severe symptoms (if most or all): Buddy-Aid: If no self-aid given, 3 injections in rapid succession; if 1 self-aid injection given, 2 injections in rapid succession

Maximum cumulative dose: 3 injections

Symptoms provided by manufacturer in ATNAA product labeling to guide therapy:

Mild symptoms: Breathing difficulties, chest tightness, coughing, difficulty in seeing, drooling, headache, localized sweating and muscular twitching, miosis, nausea (with or without vomiting), runny nose, stomach cramps, tachycardia (followed by bradycardia), wheezing

Severe symptoms: Bradycardia, confused/strange behavior, convulsions, increased wheezing and breathing difficulties, involuntary urination/defecation, miosis (severe), muscular twitching/generalized weakness (severe), red/teary eyes, respiratory failure, unconsciousness, vomiting

Duodote™:
Mild symptoms (≥2 mild symptoms): 1 injection (wait 10-15 minutes for effect); if after 10-15 minutes no severe symptoms emerge, no further injections are indicated; if any severe symptoms emerge at any point following initial injection, repeat dose by giving 2 additional injections in rapid succession. Transport to medical care facility.

Severe symptoms (≥1 severe symptom): 3 injections in rapid succession. Transport to medical care facility.

Maximum cumulative dose: 3 injections unless medical care support (eg, hospital, respiratory support) is available

Symptoms provided by manufacturer in Duodote™ product labeling to guide therapy:

Mild symptoms: Airway secretions increased, blurred vision, bradycardia, breathing difficulties, chest tightness, drooling miosis, nausea, vomiting, runny nose, salivation, stomach cramps (acute onset), tachycardia, teary eyes, tremors/muscular twitching, wheezing/coughing

Severe symptoms: Breathing difficulties (severe), confused/strange behavior, convulsions, copious secretions from lung or airway, involuntary urination/defecation, muscular twitching/generalized weakness (severe)

Dosage Forms
Injection, solution:
ATNAA, Duodote™: Atropine 2.1 mg/0.7 mL and pralidoxime chloride 600 mg/2 mL [contains benzyl alcohol; prefilled auto-injector]

atropine and pralidoxime chloride *see* atropine and pralidoxime *on previous page*

Atropine-Care® [US] *see* atropine *on page 83*

atropine, hyoscyamine, scopolamine, and phenobarbital *see* hyoscyamine, atropine, scopolamine, and phenobarbital *on page 442*

atropine soluble tablet *(Discontinued)*

atropine sulfate *see* atropine *on page 83*

atropine sulfate and edrophonium chloride *see* edrophonium and atropine *on page 292*

Atropisol® *(Discontinued)* *see* atropine *on page 83*

Atrovent® [US/Can] *see* ipratropium *on page 470*

Atrovent® HFA [US/Can] *see* ipratropium *on page 470*

Attenuvax® [US] *see* measles virus vaccine (live) *on page 534*

Atuss® HD [US] *see* pseudoephedrine, hydrocodone, and chlorpheniramine *on page 731*

Atuss® HX [US] *see* hydrocodone and guaifenesin *on page 429*

Augmentin® [US/Can] *see* amoxicillin and clavulanate potassium *on page 49*

Augmentin ES-600® [US] *see* amoxicillin and clavulanate potassium *on page 49*

Augmentin XR® [US] *see* amoxicillin and clavulanate potassium *on page 49*

Auralgan® [Can] *see* antipyrine and benzocaine *on page 61*

auranofin (au RANE oh fin)
Sound-Alike/Look-Alike Issues
Ridaura® may be confused with Cardura®
U.S./Canadian Brand Names Ridaura® [US/Can]
Therapeutic Category Gold Compound
Use Management of active stage of classic or definite rheumatoid arthritis in patients who do not respond to or tolerate other agents; psoriatic arthritis; adjunctive or alternative therapy for pemphigus
(Continued)

auranofin *(Continued)*

Usual Dosage Oral:

Children: Initial: 0.1 mg/kg/day divided daily; usual maintenance: 0.15 mg/kg/day in 1-2 divided doses; maximum: 0.2 mg/kg/day in 1-2 divided doses

Adults: 6 mg/day in 1-2 divided doses; after 3 months may be increased to 9 mg/day in 3 divided doses; if still no response after 3 months at 9 mg/day, discontinue drug

Dosage Forms

Capsule:

Ridaura®: 3 mg

Aurodex [US] *see* antipyrine and benzocaine *on page 61*

Autoplex® T *(Discontinued)* *see* antiinhibitor coagulant complex *on page 61*

AVA *see* anthrax vaccine, adsorbed *on page 58*

Avagard™ [US-OTC] *see* chlorhexidine gluconate *on page 174*

Avage™ [US] *see* tazarotene *on page 821*

Avalide® [US/Can] *see* irbesartan and hydrochlorothiazide *on page 472*

Avandamet® [US/Can] *see* rosiglitazone and metformin *on page 767*

Avandaryl™ [US] *see* rosiglitazone and glimepiride *on page 767*

Avandia® [US/Can] *see* rosiglitazone *on page 767*

Avapro® [US/Can] *see* irbesartan *on page 471*

Avapro® HCT *see* irbesartan and hydrochlorothiazide *on page 472*

AVAR™ [US] *see* sulfur and sulfacetamide *on page 815*

AVAR™-e [US] *see* sulfur and sulfacetamide *on page 815*

AVAR™-e Green [US] *see* sulfur and sulfacetamide *on page 815*

AVAR™ Green [US] *see* sulfur and sulfacetamide *on page 815*

Avastin® [US/Can] *see* bevacizumab *on page 110*

Avaxim® [Can] *see* hepatitis A vaccine *on page 417*

Avaxim®-Pediatric [Can] *see* hepatitis A vaccine *on page 417*

Avelox® [US/Can] *see* moxifloxacin *on page 581*

Avelox® I.V. [US/Can] *see* moxifloxacin *on page 581*

Aventyl® [Can] *see* nortriptyline *on page 613*

Aventyl® HCl *(Discontinued)* *see* nortriptyline *on page 613*

Aviane™ [US] *see* ethinyl estradiol and levonorgestrel *on page 325*

avian influenza virus vaccine *see* influenza virus vaccine (H5N1) *on page 456*

Avinza® [US] *see* morphine sulfate *on page 578*

Avita® [US] *see* tretinoin (topical) *on page 861*

Avitene® [US] *see* collagen hemostat *on page 213*

Avitene® Flour [US] *see* collagen hemostat *on page 213*

Avitene® Ultrafoam [US] *see* collagen hemostat *on page 213*

Avitene® UltraWrap™ [US] *see* collagen hemostat *on page 213*

Avlosulfon® *(Discontinued)* *see* dapsone *on page 231*

Avodart™ [US/Can] *see* dutasteride *on page 287*

Avonex® [US/Can] *see* interferon beta-1a *on page 464*

Axert™ [US/Can] *see* almotriptan *on page 31*

Axid® [US/Can] *see* nizatidine *on page 610*

Axid® AR [US-OTC] *see* nizatidine *on page 610*

AY-25650 *see* triptorelin *on page 870*

Aygestin® [US] *see* norethindrone *on page 611*

Ayr® Baby Saline [US-OTC] *see* sodium chloride *on page 792*

Ayr® Saline [US-OTC] *see* sodium chloride *on page 792*

Ayr® Saline No-Drip [US-OTC] *see* sodium chloride *on page 792*

5-aza-2'-deoxycytidine *see* decitabine *on page 234*

5-azaC *see* decitabine *on page 234*

azacitidine (ay za SYE ti deen)
Synonyms AZA-CR; azacytidine; 5-azacytidine; 5-AZC; ladakamycin; NSC-102816
U.S./Canadian Brand Names Vidaza® [US]
Therapeutic Category Antineoplastic Agent, Antimetabolite (Pyrimidine)
Use Treatment of myelodysplastic syndrome (MDS)
Usual Dosage I.V., SubQ: Adults: MDS: 75 mg/m^2/day for 7 days repeated every 4 weeks. Dose may be increased to 100 mg/m^2/day if no benefit is observed after 2 cycles and no toxicity other than nausea and vomiting have occurred. Treatment is recommended for at least 4 cycles; treatment may be continued as long as patient continues to benefit.
Dosage Forms
Injection, powder for suspension:
Vidaza®: 100 mg

AZA-CR *see* azacitidine *on this page*

Azactam® [US/Can] *see* aztreonam *on page 90*

azacytidine *see* azacitidine *on this page*

5-azacytidine *see* azacitidine *on this page*

Azasan® [US] *see* azathioprine *on this page*

Azasite™ [US] *see* azithromycin *on next page*

azatadine *(Canada only)* (a ZA ta deen)
Synonyms azatadine maleate
U.S./Canadian Brand Names Optimine® [Can]
Therapeutic Category Antihistamine
Use Treatment of perennial and seasonal allergic rhinitis and chronic urticaria
Usual Dosage Oral: Children >12 years and Adults: 1-2 mg twice daily
Dosage Forms Tablet, as maleate: 1 mg

azatadine maleate *see* azatadine *(Canada only)* *on this page*

azathioprine (ay za THYE oh preen)
Sound-Alike/Look-Alike Issues
azathioprine may be confused with azatadine, azidothymidine, Azulfidine®
Imuran® may be confused with Elmiron®, Enduron®, Imdur®, Inderal®, Tenormin®
Synonyms azathioprine sodium
U.S./Canadian Brand Names Alti-Azathioprine [Can]; Apo-Azathioprine® [Can]; Azasan® [US]; Gen-Azathioprine [Can]; Imuran® [US/Can]; Novo-Azathioprine [Can]
Therapeutic Category Immunosuppressant Agent
Use Adjunctive therapy in prevention of rejection of kidney transplants; active rheumatoid arthritis
Usual Dosage I.V. dose is equivalent to oral dose (dosing should be based on ideal body weight):
Adults:
Renal transplantation: Oral, I.V.: Initial: 3-5 mg/kg/day usually given as a single daily dose, then 1-3 mg/kg/day maintenance
Rheumatoid arthritis: Oral:
Initial: 1 mg/kg/day given once daily or divided twice daily for 6-8 weeks; increase by 0.5 mg/kg every 4 weeks until response or up to 2.5 mg/kg/day; an adequate trial should be a minimum of 12 weeks
Maintenance dose: Reduce dose by 0.5 mg/kg every 4 weeks until lowest effective dose is reached; optimum duration of therapy not specified; may be discontinued abruptly
Dosage Forms
Injection, powder for reconstitution: 100 mg
Tablet [scored]: 50 mg
Azasan®: 75 mg, 100 mg
Imuran®: 50 mg

azathioprine sodium *see* azathioprine *on this page*

5-AZC *see* azacitidine *on this page*

Azdone® *(Discontinued)* *see* hydrocodone and aspirin *on page 428*

azelaic acid (a zeh LAY ik AS id)

U.S./Canadian Brand Names Azelex® [US]; Finacea® [US/Can]

Therapeutic Category Topical Skin Product

Use Topical treatment of inflammatory papules and pustules of mild-to-moderate rosacea; mild-to-moderate intlammatory acne vulgaris

Finacea®: Not FDA-approved for the treatment of acne

Usual Dosage Topical:

Adolescents ≥12 years and Adults: Acne vulgaris: Cream 20%: After skin is thoroughly washed and patted dry, gently but thoroughly massage a thin film of azelaic acid cream into the affected areas twice daily, in the morning and evening. The duration of use can vary and depends on the severity of the acne. In the majority of patients with inflammatory lesions, improvement of the condition occurs within 4 weeks.

Adults: Rosacea: Gel 15%: Massage gently into affected areas of the face twice daily; use beyond 12 weeks has not been studied

Dosage Forms

Cream:

Azelex®: 20% (30 g, 50 g)

Gel:

Finacea®: 15% (30 g)

azelastine (a ZEL as teen)

Sound-Alike/Look-Alike Issues

Optivar® may be confused with Optiray®

Synonyms azelastine hydrochloride

U.S./Canadian Brand Names Astelin® [US/Can]; Optivar® [US]

Therapeutic Category Antihistamine; Antihistamine, Ophthalmic

Use

Nasal spray: Treatment of the symptoms of seasonal allergic rhinitis such as rhinorrhea, sneezing, and nasal pruritus in children ≥5 years of age and adults; treatment of the symptoms of vasomotor rhinitis in children ≥12 years of age and adults

Ophthalmic: Treatment of itching of the eye associated with seasonal allergic conjunctivitis in children ≥3 years of age and adults

Usual Dosage

Children 5-11 years: Seasonal allergic rhinitis: Intranasal: 1 spray each nostril twice daily

Children ≥3 years and Adults: Itching eyes due to seasonal allergic conjunctivitis: Ophthalmic: Instill 1 drop into affected eye(s) twice daily

Children ≥12 years and Adults:

Seasonal allergic rhinitis: Intranasal: 1-2 sprays (137 mcg/spray) each nostril twice daily

Vasomotor rhinitis: Intranasal: 2 sprays each nostril twice daily.

Dosage Forms

Solution, intranasal [spray]:

Astelin®: 1 mg/mL [137 mcg/spray] (30 mL)

Solution, ophthalmic:

Optivar®: 0.05% (6 mL)

azelastine hydrochloride *see* azelastine *on this page*

Azelex® [US] *see* azelaic acid *on this page*

azidothymidine *see* zidovudine *on page 904*

azidothymidine, abacavir, and lamivudine *see* abacavir, lamivudine, and zidovudine *on page 2*

Azilect® [US] *see* rasagiline *on page 745*

azithromycin (az ith roe MYE sin)

Sound-Alike/Look-Alike Issues

azithromycin may be confused with erythromycin

Zithromax® may be confused with Zinacef®

Synonyms azithromycin dihydrate; azithromycin hydrogen citrate; azithromycin monohydrate; Zithromax® TRI-PAK™; Zithromax® Z-PAK®

U.S./Canadian Brand Names Apo-Azithromycin® [Can]; Azasite™ [US]; CO Azithromycin [Can]; Dom-Azithromycin [Can]; GMD-Azithromycin [Can]; Novo-Azithromycin [Can]; PHL-Azithromycin [Can]; PMS-Azithromycin [Can]; ratio-Azithromycin [Can]; Sandoz-Azithromycin [Can]; Zithromax® [US/Can]; Zmax™ [US]

Therapeutic Category Macrolide (Antibiotic)

Use

Oral, I.V.: Treatment of acute otitis media due to *H. influenzae*, *M. catarrhalis*, or *S. pneumoniae*; pharyngitis/tonsillitis due to *S. pyogenes*; treatment of mild-to-moderate upper and lower respiratory tract infections,

infections of the skin and skin structure, community-acquired pneumonia, pelvic inflammatory disease (PID), sexually-transmitted diseases (urethritis/cervicitis), pharyngitis/tonsillitis (alternative to first-line therapy), and genital ulcer disease (chancroid) due to susceptible strains of *C. trachomatis*, *M. catarrhalis*, *H. influenzae*, *S. aureus*, *S. pneumoniae*, *Mycoplasma pneumoniae*, and *C. psittaci*; acute bacterial exacerbations of chronic obstructive pulmonary disease (COPD) due to *H. influenzae*, *M. catarrhalis*, or *S. pneumoniae*; acute bacterial sinusitis

Ophthalmic: Bacterial conjunctivitis

Usual Dosage Note: Extended release suspension (Zmax™) is not interchangeable with immediate release formulations. Use should be limited to approved indications. All doses are expressed as immediate release azithromycin unless otherwise specified.

Usual dosage range:
Children ≥6 months: Oral: 5-12 mg/kg given once daily (maximum: 500 mg/day) **or** 30 mg/kg as a single dose (maximum: 1500 mg)
Children ≥1 year and Adults: Ophthalmic: Instill 1 drop into affected eye(s) twice daily (8-12 hours apart) for 2 days, then 1 drop once daily for 5 days
Adolescents ≥16 years and Adults:
Oral: 250-600 mg once daily **or** 1-2 g as a single dose
I.V.: 250-500 mg once daily

Indication-specific dosing:
Children: Oral:
Bacterial sinusitis: 10 mg/kg once daily for 3 days (maximum: 500 mg/day)
Community-acquired pneumonia: 10 mg/kg on day 1 (maximum: 500 mg/day) followed by 5 mg/kg/day once daily on days 2-5 (maximum: 250 mg/day)
Otitis media:
1-day regimen: 30 mg/kg as a single dose (maximum: 1500 mg)
3-day regimen: 10 mg/kg once daily for 3 days (maximum: 500 mg/day)
5-day regimen: 10 mg/kg on day 1 (maximum: 500 mg/day) followed by 5 mg/kg/day once daily on days 2-5 (maximum: 250 mg/day)
Pharyngitis, tonsillitis: Children ≥2 years: 12 mg/kg/day once daily for 5 days (maximum: 500 mg/day)
Pertussis (CDC guidelines):
Children <6 months: 10 mg/kg/day for 5 days
Children ≥6 months: 10 mg/kg on day 1 (maximum: 500 mg/day) followed by 5 mg/kg/day once daily on days 2-5 (maximum: 250 mg/day)
Children ≥1 year and Adults: Ophthalmic:
Bacterial conjunctivitis: Instill 1 drop into affected eye(s) twice daily (8-12 hours apart) for 2 days, then 1 drop once daily for 5 days
Adolescents ≥16 years and Adults:
Bacterial sinusitis: Oral: 500 mg/day for a total of 3 days
Extended release suspension (Zmax™): 2 g as a single dose
Chancroid due to *H. ducreyi*: Oral: 1 g as a single dose
Community-acquired pneumonia:
Oral (Zmax™): 2 g as a single dose
I.V.: 500 mg as a single dose for at least 2 days, follow I.V. therapy by the oral route with a single daily dose of 500 mg to complete a 7- to 10-day course of therapy.
Mild-to-moderate respiratory tract, skin, and soft tissue infections: Oral: 500 mg in a single loading dose on day 1 followed by 250 mg/day as a single dose on days 2-5
Alternative regimen: Bacterial exacerbation of COPD: 500 mg/day for a total of 3 days
Pelvic inflammatory disease (PID): I.V.: 500 mg as a single dose for 1-2 days, follow I.V. therapy by the oral route with a single daily dose of 250 mg to complete a 7-day course of therapy
Pertussis (CDC guidelines): Oral: 500 mg on day 1 followed by 250 mg/day on days 2-5 (maximum: 500 mg/day)
Urethritis/cervicitis: Oral:
Due to C. trachomatis: 1 g as a single dose
Due to N. gonorrhoeae: 2 g as a single dose

Dosage Forms
Injection, powder for reconstitution: 500 mg
Zithromax®: 500 mg
Injection, powder for reconstitution, as hydrogencitrate: 500 mg
Injection, powder for reconstitution, as monohydrate: 500 mg
Microspheres for oral suspension, extended release:
Zmax™: 2 g
Powder for oral suspension, as monohydrate: 100 mg/5 mL (15 mL); 200 mg/5 mL (15 mL, 22.5 mL, 30 mL)
Powder for oral suspension, immediate release:
Zithromax®: 100 mg/5 mL, 200 mg/5 mL, 1 g
(Continued)

azithromycin *(Continued)*

Solution, ophthalmic:
Azasite™: 1% (2.5 mL)
Tablet: 250 mg, 500 mg, 600 mg
Zithromax®: 250 mg, 500 mg, 600 mg
Zithromax® TRI-PAK™ [unit-dose pack]: 500 mg (3s)
Zithromax® Z-PAK® [unit-dose pack]: 250 mg (6s)

azithromycin dihydrate *see* azithromycin *on page 88*

azithromycin hydrogen citrate *see* azithromycin *on page 88*

azithromycin monohydrate *see* azithromycin *on page 88*

Azmacort® [US] *see* triamcinolone (inhalation, oral) *on page 862*

AZO-Gesic® [US-OTC] *see* phenazopyridine *on page 671*

Azopt® [US/Can] *see* brinzolamide *on page 118*

AZO-Standard® [US-OTC] *see* phenazopyridine *on page 671*

AZO-Standard® Maximum Strength [US-OTC] *see* phenazopyridine *on page 671*

AZT™ [Can] *see* zidovudine *on page 904*

AZT, abacavir, and lamivudine *see* abacavir, lamivudine, and zidovudine *on page 2*

azthreonam *see* aztreonam *on this page*

aztreonam *(AZ tree oh nam)*

Sound-Alike/Look-Alike Issues
aztreonam may be confused with azidothymidine
Synonyms azthreonam
U.S./Canadian Brand Names Azactam® [US/Can]
Therapeutic Category Antibiotic, Miscellaneous
Use Treatment of patients with urinary tract infections, lower respiratory tract infections, septicemia, skin/skin structure infections, intra-abdominal infections, and gynecological infections caused by susceptible gram-negative bacilli
Usual Dosage
Children >1 month: I.M., I.V.:
Mild-to-moderate infections: I.M., I.V.: 30 mg/kg every 8 hours
Moderate-to-severe infections: I.M., I.V.: 30 mg/kg every 6-8 hours; maximum: 120 mg/kg/day (8 g/day)
Cystic fibrosis: I.V.: 50 mg/kg/dose every 6-8 hours (ie, up to 200 mg/kg/day); maximum: 8 g/day
Adults:
Urinary tract infection: I.M., I.V.: 500 mg to 1 g every 8-12 hours
Moderately-severe systemic infections: 1 g I.V. or I.M. or 2 g I.V. every 8-12 hours
Severe systemic or life-threatening infections (especially caused by *Pseudomonas aeruginosa*): I.V.: 2 g every 6-8 hours; maximum: 8 g/day
Meningitis (gram-negative): I.V.: 2 g every 6-8 hours
Dosage Forms
Infusion [premixed]:
Azactam®: 1 g (50 mL); 2 g (50 mL)
Injection, powder for reconstitution:
Azactam®: 500 mg, 1 g, 2 g

Azulfidine® [US] *see* sulfasalazine *on page 814*

Azulfidine® EN-tabs® [US] *see* sulfasalazine *on page 814*

B1 *see* tositumomab and iodine I 131 tositumomab *on page 852*

B1 antibody *see* tositumomab and iodine I 131 tositumomab *on page 852*

B-D™ Glucose [US-OTC] *see* glucose (instant) *on page 395*

B2036-PEG *see* pegvisomant *on page 659*

B 9273 *see* alefacept *on page 26*

BA-16038 *see* aminoglutethimide *on page 42*

Babee® Cof Syrup [US-OTC] *see* dextromethorphan *on page 247*

BabyBIG® [US] *see* botulism immune globulin (intravenous-human) *on page 117*

BAC *see* benzalkonium chloride *on page 100*

Bacid® [US-OTC/Can] *see* Lactobacillus *on page 488*

Baciguent® [US-OTC/Can] *see* bacitracin *on this page*

BaciiM® [US] *see* bacitracin *on this page*

Baciject® [Can] *see* bacitracin *on this page*

bacillus calmette-Guérin (BCG) live *see* BCG vaccine *on page 96*

bacitracin (bas i TRAY sin)

Sound-Alike/Look-Alike Issues
bacitracin may be confused with Bactrim®, Bactroban®

U.S./Canadian Brand Names Baciguent® [US-OTC/Can]; BaciiM® [US]; Baciject® [Can]

Therapeutic Category Antibiotic, Miscellaneous; Antibiotic, Ophthalmic; Antibiotic, Topical

Use Treatment of susceptible bacterial infections mainly; has activity against gram-positive bacilli; due to toxicity risks, systemic and irrigant uses of bacitracin should be limited to situations where less toxic alternatives would not be effective

Usual Dosage Do not administer I.V.:
Infants: I.M.:
≤2.5 kg: 900 units/kg/day in 2-3 divided doses
>2.5 kg: 1000 units/kg/day in 2-3 divided doses
Children: I.M.: 800-1200 units/kg/day divided every 8 hours
Adults: Oral: Antibiotic-associated colitis: 25,000 units 4 times/day for 7-10 days
Children and Adults:
Topical: Apply 1-5 times/day
Ophthalmic, ointment: Instill $1/4$" to $1/2$" ribbon every 3-4 hours into conjunctival sac for acute infections, or 2-3 times/day for mild-to-moderate infections for 7-10 days
Irrigation, solution: 50-100 units/mL in normal saline, lactated Ringer's, or sterile water for irrigation; soak sponges in solution for topical compresses 1-5 times/day or as needed during surgical procedures

Dosage Forms
Injection, powder for reconstitution: 50,000 units
BaciiM®: 50,000 units
Ointment, ophthalmic: 500 units/g (3.5 g)
Ointment, topical: 500 units/g (0.9 g, 15 g, 30 g, 120 g, 454 g)
Baciguent® [OTC]: 500 units/g (15 g, 30 g)

bacitracin and polymyxin B (bas i TRAY sin & pol i MIKS in bee)

Sound-Alike/Look-Alike Issues
Betadine® may be confused with Betagan®, betaine

Synonyms polymyxin B and bacitracin

U.S./Canadian Brand Names AK-Poly-Bac™ [US]; LID-Pack® [Can]; Optimyxin® [Can]; Polysporin® [US-OTC]

Therapeutic Category Antibiotic, Ophthalmic; Antibiotic, Topical

Use Treatment of superficial infections caused by susceptible organisms

Usual Dosage Children and Adults:
Ophthalmic ointment: Instill $1/2$" ribbon in the affected eye(s) every 3-4 hours for acute infections or 2-3 times/day for mild-to-moderate infections for 7-10 days
Topical ointment/powder: Apply to affected area 1-4 times/day; may cover with sterile bandage if needed

Dosage Forms
Ointment, ophthalmic: Bacitracin 500 units and polymyxin B 10,000 units per g (3.5 g)
AK-Poly-Bac™: Bacitracin 500 units and polymyxin 10,000 units per g (3.5 g)
Ointment, topical: Bacitracin 500 units and polymyxin B 10,000 units per g in white petrolatum (15 g, 30 g)
Polysporin®: Bacitracin 500 units and polymyxin B 10,000 units per g (0.9 g, 15 g, 30 g)
Powder, topical:
Polysporin®: Bacitracin 500 units and polymyxin B 10,000 units per g (10 g)

bacitracin, neomycin, and polymyxin B

(bas i TRAY sin, nee oh MYE sin, & pol i MIKS in bee)

Synonyms neomycin, bacitracin, and polymyxin B; polymyxin B, bacitracin, and neomycin; triple antibiotic

U.S./Canadian Brand Names Neosporin® Neo To Go® [US-OTC]; Neosporin® Ophthalmic Ointment [Can]; Neosporin® Topical [US-OTC]

Therapeutic Category Antibiotic, Ophthalmic; Antibiotic, Topical

Use Helps prevent infection in minor cuts, scrapes, and burns; short-term treatment of superficial external ocular infections caused by susceptible organisms

Usual Dosage Children and Adults:
Ophthalmic: Ointment: Instill $1/2$" into the conjunctival sac every 3-4 hours for 7-10 days for acute infections
Topical: Apply 1-3 times/day to infected area; may cover with sterile bandage as needed

(Continued)

91

bacitracin, neomycin, and polymyxin B *(Continued)*

Dosage Forms
Ointment, ophthalmic: Bacitracin 400 units, neomycin 3.5 mg, and polymyxin B 10,000 units per g (3.5 g)
Ointment, topical: Bacitracin 400 units, neomycin 3.5 mg, and polymyxin B 5000 units per g (0.9 g, 15 g, 30 g, 454 g)
Neosporin® [OTC]: Bacitracin 400 units, neomycin 3.5 mg, and polymyxin B 5000 units per g (15 g, 30 g)
Neosporin® Neo To Go® [OTC]: Bacitracin 400 units, neomycin 3.5 mg, and polymyxin B 5000 units per g (0.9 g)

bacitracin, neomycin, polymyxin B, and hydrocortisone

(bas i TRAY sin, nee oh MYE sin, pol i MIKS in bee, & hye droe KOR ti sone)
Synonyms hydrocortisone, bacitracin, neomycin, and polymyxin B; neomycin, bacitracin, polymyxin B, and hydrocortisone; polymyxin B, bacitracin, neomycin, and hydrocortisone
U.S./Canadian Brand Names Cortisporin® Ointment [US]; Cortisporin® Topical Ointment [Can]
Therapeutic Category Antibiotic/Corticosteroid, Ophthalmic; Antibiotic/Corticosteroid, Topical
Use Prevention and treatment of susceptible inflammatory conditions where bacterial infection (or risk of infection) is present
Usual Dosage Children and Adults:
Ophthalmic: Ointment: Instill ½" ribbon to inside of lower lid every 3-4 hours until improvement occurs
Topical: Apply sparingly 2-4 times/day. Therapy should be discontinued when control is achieved; if no improvement is seen, reassessment of diagnosis may be necessary.
Dosage Forms
Ointment, ophthalmic: Bacitracin 400 units, neomycin sulfate 3.5 mg, polymyxin B 10,000 units, and hydrocortisone 10 mg per g (3.5 g)
Ointment, topical:
Cortisporin®: Bacitracin 400 units, neomycin 3.5 mg, polymyxin B 5000 units, and hydrocortisone 10 mg per g (15 g)

bacitracin, neomycin, polymyxin B, and pramoxine

(bas i TRAY sin, nee oh MYE sin, pol i MIKS in bee, & pra MOKS een)
Synonyms neomycin, bacitracin, polymyxin B, and pramoxine; polymyxin B, neomycin, bacitracin, and pramoxine; pramoxine, neomycin, bacitracin, and polymyxin B
U.S./Canadian Brand Names Neosporin® + Pain Relief Ointment [US-OTC]; Tri Biozene [US-OTC]
Therapeutic Category Antibiotic, Topical
Use Prevention and treatment of susceptible superficial topical infections and provide temporary relief of pain or discomfort
Usual Dosage Children ≥2 years and Adults: Apply 1-3 times/day to infected areas; cover with sterile bandage if needed
Dosage Forms
Ointment, topical: Bacitracin 500 units, neomycin 3.5 mg, polymyxin B 10,000 units, and pramoxine 10 mg (15 g, 30 g)
Neosporin® + Pain Relief Ointment [OTC]: Bacitracin 500 units, neomycin 3.5 mg, polymyxin B 10,000 units, and pramoxine 10 mg (15 g, 30 g)
Tri Biozene: Bacitracin 500 units, neomycin 3.5 mg, polymyxin B 10,000 units, and pramoxine 10 mg (15 g)

baclofen (BAK loe fen)

Sound-Alike/Look-Alike Issues
baclofen may be confused with Bactroban®
Lioresal® may be confused with lisinopril, Lotensin®
U.S./Canadian Brand Names Apo-Baclofen® [Can]; Gen-Baclofen [Can]; Lioresal® [US/Can]; Liotec [Can]; Nu-Baclo [Can]; PMS-Baclofen [Can]
Therapeutic Category Skeletal Muscle Relaxant
Use Treatment of reversible spasticity associated with multiple sclerosis or spinal cord lesions
Orphan drug: Intrathecal: Treatment of intractable spasticity caused by spinal cord injury, multiple sclerosis, and other spinal disease (spinal ischemia or tumor, transverse myelitis, cervical spondylosis, degenerative myelopathy)
Usual Dosage
Oral (avoid abrupt withdrawal of drug):
Children:
2-7 years: Initial: 10-15 mg/24 hours divided every 8 hours; titrate dose every 3 days in increments of 5-15 mg/day to a maximum of 40 mg/day
≥8 years: Maximum: 60 mg/day in 3 divided doses
Adults: 5 mg 3 times/day, may increase 5 mg/dose every 3 days to a maximum of 80 mg/day
Hiccups: Adults: Usual effective dose: 10-20 mg 2-3 times/day

Intrathecal: Children and Adults:
Test dose: 50-100 mcg, doses >50 mcg should be given in 25 mcg increments, separated by 24 hours. A screening dose of 25 mcg may be considered in very small patients. Patients not responding to screening dose of 100 mcg should not be considered for chronic infusion/implanted pump.
Maintenance: After positive response to test dose, a maintenance intrathecal infusion can be administered via an implanted intrathecal pump. Initial dose via pump: Infusion at a 24-hour rate dosed at twice the test dose. Avoid abrupt discontinuation.

Dosage Forms
Injection, solution, intrathecal [preservative free]:
Lioresal®: 50 mcg/mL (1 mL); 500 mcg/mL (20 mL); 2000 mcg/mL (5 mL, 20 mL)
Tablet: 10 mg, 20 mg

BactoShield® **CHG [US-OTC]** *see* chlorhexidine gluconate *on page 174*

BactoShield® *(Discontinued)* *see* chlorhexidine gluconate *on page 174*

Bactrim™ **[US]** *see* sulfamethoxazole and trimethoprim *on page 813*

Bactrim™ **DS [US]** *see* sulfamethoxazole and trimethoprim *on page 813*

Bactrim™ **I.V. Infusion** *(Discontinued)* *see* sulfamethoxazole and trimethoprim *on page 813*

Bactroban® **[US/Can]** *see* mupirocin *on page 582*

Bactroban® **Nasal [US]** *see* mupirocin *on page 582*

baking soda *see* sodium bicarbonate *on page 791*

BAL *see* dimercaprol *on page 263*

Balacet 325™ **[US]** *see* propoxyphene and acetaminophen *on page 723*

balanced salt solution (BAL anced salt soe LOO shun)

U.S./Canadian Brand Names AquaLase™ [US]; BSS Plus® [US/Can]; BSS® [US/Can]; Eye-Stream® [Can]
Therapeutic Category Ophthalmic Agent, Miscellaneous
Use
Irrigation solution for ophthalmic surgery:
AquaLase™, BSS®: Intraocular or extraocular irrigating solution
BSS® Plus: Intraocular irrigating solution
Irrigation solution for eyes, ears, nose, or throat
Usual Dosage Adults: Ophthalmic irrigation: Based on standard for each surgical procedure
Dosage Forms
Solution, irrigation [preservative free]: Sodium chloride 0.64%, potassium chloride 0.075%, calcium chloride 0.048%, magnesium chloride 0.03%, sodium acetate 0.39%, sodium citrate 0.17% (500 mL)
Solution, ophthalmic [irrigation; preservative free]: Sodium chloride 0.64%, potassium chloride 0.075%, calcium chloride 0.048%, magnesium chloride 0.03%, sodium acetate 0.39%, sodium citrate 0.17% (18 mL, 500 mL)
AquaLase™: Sodium chloride 0.64%, potassium chloride 0.075%, calcium chloride 0.048%, magnesium chloride 0.03%, sodium acetate 0.39%, sodium citrate 0.17% (90 mL)
BSS®: Sodium chloride 0.64%, potassium chloride 0.075%, calcium chloride 0.048%, magnesium chloride 0.03%, sodium acetate 0.39%, sodium citrate 0.17% (15 mL, 30 mL, 250 mL, 500 mL)
BSS Plus®: Sodium chloride 0.71%, potassium chloride 0.038%, calcium chloride 0.015%, magnesium chloride 0.02%, sodium phosphate 0.042%, sodium bicarbonate 0.21%, dextrose 0.092%, glutathione 0.018% (250 mL, 500 mL)

Baldex® *(Discontinued)*

BAL in Oil® **[US]** *see* dimercaprol *on page 263*

Balmex® **[US-OTC]** *see* zinc oxide *on page 906*

Balminil Decongestant [Can] *see* pseudoephedrine *on page 727*

Balminil DM D [Can] *see* pseudoephedrine and dextromethorphan *on page 728*

Balminil DM + Decongestant + Expectorant [Can] *see* guaifenesin, pseudoephedrine, and dextromethorphan *on page 408*

Balminil DM E [Can] *see* guaifenesin and dextromethorphan *on page 402*

Balminil Expectorant [Can] *see* guaifenesin *on page 401*

Balnetar® **[US-OTC/Can]** *see* coal tar *on page 208*

balsalazide (bal SAL a zide)

Sound-Alike/Look-Alike Issues
Colazal® may be confused with Clozaril®
(Continued)

balsalazide *(Continued)*

Synonyms balsalazide disodium
U.S./Canadian Brand Names Colazal® [US]
Therapeutic Category 5-Aminosalicylic Acid Derivative; Antiinflammatory Agent
Use Treatment of mild-to-moderate active ulcerative colitis
Usual Dosage Oral: Adults: 2.25 g (three 750 mg capsules) 3 times/day for 8-12 weeks
Dosage Forms
  Capsule:
    Colazal®: 750 mg

balsalazide disodium *see* balsalazide *on previous page*

balsam peru, trypsin, and castor oil *see* trypsin, balsam peru, and castor oil *on page 872*

Baltussin [US] *see* dihydrocodeine, chlorpheniramine, and phenylephrine *on page 259*

Balziva™ [US] *see* ethinyl estradiol and norethindrone *on page 328*

Band-Aid® Hurt-Free™ Antiseptic Wash [US-OTC] *see* lidocaine *on page 504*

Banophen® [US-OTC] *see* diphenhydramine *on page 265*

Banophen® Anti-Itch [US-OTC] *see* diphenhydramine *on page 265*

Banophen® Decongestant Capsule *(Discontinued)* *see* diphenhydramine and pseudoephedrine *on page 266*

Baraclude® [US/Can] *see* entecavir *on page 299*

Barbidonna® *(Discontinued)* *see* hyoscyamine, atropine, scopolamine, and phenobarbital *on page 442*

Barbita® *(Discontinued)* *see* phenobarbital *on page 672*

Barc™ Liquid *(Discontinued)*

Baricon™ [US] *see* barium *on this page*

Baridium® [US-OTC] *see* phenazopyridine *on page 671*

barium *(BA ree um)*

Synonyms barium sulfate
U.S./Canadian Brand Names Anatrast [US]; Bar-Test [US]; Baricon™ [US]; Baro-Cat® [US]; Barobag® [US]; Barosperse® [US]; CheeTah® [US]; E-Z-Cat® Dry [US]; E-Z-Cat® [US]; E-Z-Disk™ [US]; Enhancer [US]; Entero Vu™ [US]; Entrobar® [US]; EntroEase® [US]; Esopho-Cat® [US]; HD 200® Plus [US]; Intropaste [US]; Liqui-Coat HD® [US]; Liquid Barosperse® [US]; Medebar® Plus [US]; Prepcat [US]; Readi-Cat® 2 [US]; Readi-Cat® [US]; Tomocat® 1000 [US]; Tomocat® [US]; Tonojug [US]; Tonopaque [US]; Varibar® Honey [US]; Varibar® Nectar [US]; Varibar® Pudding [US]; Varibar® Thin Honey [US]; Varibar® Thin Liquid [US]; VoLumen™ [US]
Therapeutic Category Radiopaque Agents
Use Diagnostic aid for computed tomography or x-ray examinations of the GI tract
Dosage Forms
  Cream, oral:
    Esopho-Cat®: 3% w/w
  Paste, oral:
    Varibar® Pudding: 40% w/v
  Powder for suspension, oral:
    Baricon™, Enhancer, HD 200® Plus: 98% w/w
    E-Z-Cat® Dry: 2% w/w
    Tonopaque: 95% w/w
    Varibar® Thin Liquid: 40% w/w
  Powder for suspension, oral/rectal:
    Barosperse®, Tonojug: 95% w/w
  Powder for suspension, rectal:
    Barobag®: 97% w/w
  Suspension, oral:
    Entero Vu™: 24% w/v
    EntroEase®: 13% w/v
    E-Z-Cat®: 4.9% w/v
    Liqui-Coat HD®: 210% w/v
    Readi-Cat® 2: 2.1% w/v
    Varibar® Honey, Varibar® Nectar, Varibar® Thin Honey: 40% w/v
    VoLumen™: 0.1% w/v

Suspension, oral/rectal:
Baro-Cat®, Prepcat: 1.5% w/v
CheeTah®: 2.2% w/w
Liquid Barosperse®: 60% w/v
Readi-Cat®: 1.3% w/v
Readi-Cat® 2: 2.1% w/v
Tomocat®, Tomocat® 1000: 5% w/v
Suspension, paste:
Anatrast: 100% w/v
Intropaste: 70% w/v
Suspension, rectal:
Entrobar®: 50% w/v
Medebar® Plus: 100% w/v
Tablet, oral, as sulfate:
Bar-Test, E-Z-Disk™: 648 mg

barium sulfate *see* barium *on previous page*

Barobag® [US] *see* barium *on previous page*

Baro-Cat® [US] *see* barium *on previous page*

Barosperse® [US] *see* barium *on previous page*

Bar-Test [US] *see* barium *on previous page*

Basaljel® [Can] *see* aluminum hydroxide *on page 36*

base ointment *see* zinc oxide *on page 906*

basiliximab (ba si LIK si mab)
U.S./Canadian Brand Names Simulect® [US/Can]
Therapeutic Category Immunosuppressant Agent
Use Prophylaxis of acute organ rejection in renal transplantation
Usual Dosage Note: Patients previously administered basiliximab should only be reexposed to a subsequent course of therapy with extreme caution.
I.V.:
Children <35 kg: Renal transplantation: 10 mg within 2 hours prior to transplant surgery, followed by a second 10 mg dose 4 days after transplantation; the second dose should be withheld if complications occur (including severe hypersensitivity reactions or graft loss)
Children ≥35 kg and Adults: Renal transplantation: 20 mg within 2 hours prior to transplant surgery, followed by a second 20 mg dose 4 days after transplantation; the second dose should be withheld if complications occur (including severe hypersensitivity reactions or graft loss)
Dosage Forms
Injection, powder for reconstitution [preservative free]:
Simulect®: 10 mg, 20 mg

Bausch & Lomb® Computer Eye Drops [US-OTC] *see* glycerin *on page 397*

BAY 43-9006 *see* sorafenib *on page 802*

Bayer® Aspirin Extra Strength [US-OTC] *see* aspirin *on page 78*

Bayer® Aspirin Regimen Adult Low Dose [US-OTC] *see* aspirin *on page 78*

Bayer® Aspirin Regimen Children's [US-OTC] *see* aspirin *on page 78*

Bayer® Aspirin Regimen Regular Strength [US-OTC] *see* aspirin *on page 78*

Bayer® Genuine Aspirin [US-OTC] *see* aspirin *on page 78*

Bayer® Plus Extra Strength [US-OTC] *see* aspirin *on page 78*

Bayer® Women's Aspirin Plus Calcium [US-OTC] *see* aspirin *on page 78*

BayGam® [Can] *see* immune globulin (intramuscular) *on page 450*

BayGam® (Discontinued) *see* immune globulin (intramuscular) *on page 450*

BayHepB® (Discontinued) *see* hepatitis B immune globulin *on page 417*

BayRab® (Discontinued) *see* rabies immune globulin (human) *on page 741*

BayRho-D® Full Dose (Discontinued) *see* Rh₀(D) immune globulin *on page 753*

BayRho-D® Mini Dose (Discontinued) *see* Rh₀(D) immune globulin *on page 753*

BayTet™ (Discontinued) *see* tetanus immune globulin (human) *on page 829*

Baza® Antifungal [US-OTC] *see* miconazole *on page 566*

Baza® Clear [US-OTC] *see* vitamin A and vitamin D *on page 893*

β,β-dimethylcysteine *see* penicillamine *on page 661*

B-Caro-T™ [US] *see* beta-carotene *on page 107*

BCG, live *see* BCG vaccine *on this page*

BCG vaccine (bee see jee vak SEEN)

Synonyms bacillus calmette-Guérin (BCG) live; BCG, live; BCG vaccine U.S.P. *(percutaneous use product)*

U.S./Canadian Brand Names ImmuCyst® [Can]; Oncotice™ [Can]; Pacis™ [Can]; TheraCys® [US]; TICE® BCG [US]

Therapeutic Category Biological Response Modulator

Use Immunization against tuberculosis and immunotherapy for cancer; treatment and prophylaxis of carcinoma *in situ* of the bladder; prophylaxis of primary or recurrent superficial papillary tumors following transurethral resection

Usual Dosage

Immunization against tuberculosis: Percutaneous: **Note:** Initial lesion usually appears after 10-14 days consisting of small, red papule at injection site and reaches maximum diameter of 3 mm in 4-6 weeks.

Children <1 month: 0.2-0.3 mL (half-strength dilution). Administer tuberculin test (5 TU) after 2-3 months; repeat vaccination after 1 year of age for negative tuberculin test if indications persist.

Children >1 month and Adults: 0.2-0.3 mL (full strength dilution); conduct postvaccinal tuberculin test (5 TU of PPD) in 2-3 months; if test is negative, repeat vaccination.

Immunotherapy for bladder cancer: Intravesicular Adults:

TheraCys®: One dose instilled into bladder (for 2 hours) once weekly for 6 weeks followed by one treatment at 3, 6, 12, 18, and 24 months after initial treatment

TICE® BCG: One dose instilled into the bladder (for 2 hours) once weekly for 6 weeks followed by once monthly for 6-12 months

Dosage Forms

Injection, powder for reconstitution, intravesical [preservative free]:

TheraCys®: 81 mg

TICE® BCG: 50 mg

Injection, powder for reconstitution, percutaneous [preservative free]:

BCG Vaccine U.S.P.: 50 mg

BCG vaccine U.S.P. *(percutaneous use product)* *see* BCG vaccine *on this page*

BCI-Fluoxetine [Can] *see* fluoxetine *on page 364*

BCI-Gabapentin [Can] *see* gabapentin *on page 380*

BCI-Metformin [Can] *see* metformin *on page 548*

BCI-Ranitidine [Can] *see* ranitidine *on page 744*

BCI-Simvastatin [Can] *see* simvastatin *on page 787*

BCNU *see* carmustine *on page 155*

B complex combinations *see* vitamin B complex combinations *on page 894*

beano® [US-OTC] *see* alpha-galactosidase *on page 32*

Bebulin® VH [US] *see* factor IX complex (human) *on page 341*

becaplermin (be KAP ler min)

Sound-Alike/Look-Alike Issues

Regranex® may be confused with Granulex®, Repronex®

Synonyms recombinant human platelet-derived growth factor B; rPDGF-BB

U.S./Canadian Brand Names Regranex® [US/Can]

Therapeutic Category Topical Skin Product

Use Debridement adjunct for the treatment of diabetic ulcers that occur on the lower limbs and feet

Usual Dosage Topical: Adults:

Diabetic ulcers: Apply appropriate amount of gel once daily with a cotton swab or similar tool, as a coating over the ulcer

The amount of becaplermin to be applied will vary depending on the size of the ulcer area. To calculate the length of gel applied to the ulcer, measure the greatest length of the ulcer by the greatest width of the ulcer in inches. Tube size will determine the formula used in the calculation. For a 15 or 7.5 g tube, multiply length x width x 0.6. For a 2 g tube, multiply length x width x 1.3.

Note: If the ulcer does not decrease in size by ~30% after 10 weeks of treatment or complete healing has not occurred in 20 weeks, continued treatment with becaplermin gel should be reassessed.

Dosage Forms

Gel, topical:

Regranex®: 0.01% (2 g, 15 g)

beclomethasone (be kloe METH a sone)

Sound-Alike/Look-Alike Issues
Vanceril® may be confused with Vancenase®
Synonyms beclomethasone dipropionate
U.S./Canadian Brand Names Apo-Beclomethasone® [Can]; Beconase® AQ [US]; Gen-Beclo [Can]; Nu-Beclomethasone [Can]; Propaderm® [Can]; QVAR® [US/Can]; Rivanase AQ [Can]; Vanceril® AEM [Can]
Therapeutic Category Adrenal Corticosteroid
Use
Oral inhalation: Maintenance and prophylactic treatment of asthma; includes those who require corticosteroids and those who may benefit from a dose reduction/elimination of systemically-administered corticosteroids. Not for relief of acute bronchospasm.
Nasal aerosol: Symptomatic treatment of seasonal or perennial rhinitis; prevent recurrence of nasal polyps following surgery.
Usual Dosage Nasal inhalation and oral inhalation dosage forms are not to be used interchangeably
Inhalation, nasal: Rhinitis, nasal polyps (Beconase® AQ): Children ≥6 years and Adults: 1-2 inhalations each nostril twice daily; total dose 168-336 mcg/day
Inhalation, oral: Asthma (doses should be titrated to the lowest effective dose once asthma is controlled) (QVAR®):
Children 5-11 years: Initial: 40 mcg twice daily; maximum dose: 80 mcg twice daily
Children ≥12 years and Adults:
Patients previously on bronchodilators only: Initial dose 40-80 mcg twice daily; maximum dose: 320 mcg twice day
Patients previously on inhaled corticosteroids: Initial dose 40-160 mcg twice daily; maximum dose: 320 mcg twice daily
NIH Asthma Guidelines (NAEPP, 2002; NIH, 1997): HFA formulation (eg, QVAR®): Administer in divided doses:
Children ≤12 years:
"Low" dose: 80-160 mcg/day
"Medium" dose: 160-320 mcg/day
"High" dose: >320 mcg/day
Children >12 years and Adults:
"Low" dose: 80-240 mcg/day
"Medium" dose: 240-480 mcg/day
"High" dose: >480 mcg/day
Dosage Forms
Aerosol for oral inhalation:
QVAR®: 40 mcg/inhalation (7.3 g); 80 mcg/inhalation (7.3 g)
Suspension, intranasal, aqueous [spray]:
Beconase® AQ: 42 mcg/inhalation (25 g)

beclomethasone dipropionate *see beclomethasone on this page*

Beclovent® *(Discontinued) see beclomethasone on this page*

Beconase® AQ [US] *see beclomethasone on this page*

Beconase® *(Discontinued) see beclomethasone on this page*

Becotin® Pulvules® *(Discontinued)*

Beepen-VK® *(Discontinued) see penicillin V potassium on page 664*

behenyl alcohol *see docosanol on page 273*

Belix® Oral *(Discontinued) see diphenhydramine on page 265*

belladonna alkaloids with phenobarbital *see hyoscyamine, atropine, scopolamine, and phenobarbital on page 442*

belladonna and opium (bel a DON a & OH pee um)

Synonyms opium and belladonna
U.S./Canadian Brand Names B&O Supprettes® [US]
Therapeutic Category Analgesic, Narcotic
Controlled Substance C-II
Use Relief of moderate-to-severe pain associated with ureteral spasms not responsive to nonopioid analgesics and to space intervals between injections of opiates
Usual Dosage Rectal: Children >12 years and Adults: 1 suppository 1-2 times/day, up to 4 doses/day
Dosage Forms
Suppository: #15 A: Belladonna extract 16.2 mg and opium 30 mg; #16 A: Belladonna extract 16.2 mg and opium 60 mg
(Continued)

belladonna and opium *(Continued)*

B&O Supprettes®: #15 A: Belladonna extract 16.2 mg and opium 30 mg; #16 A: Belladonna extract 16.2 mg and opium 60 mg

belladonna, phenobarbital, and ergotamine

(bel a DON a, fee noe BAR bi tal, & er GOT a meen)

Synonyms ergotamine tartrate, belladonna, and phenobarbital; phenobarbital, belladonna, and ergotamine tartrate

U.S./Canadian Brand Names Bellamine S [US]; Bellergal® Spacetabs® [Can]; Eperbel-S [US]; Spastrin® [US]

Therapeutic Category Ergot Derivative

Use Management and treatment of menopausal disorders, GI disorders, and recurrent throbbing headache

Usual Dosage Oral: Adults: 1 tablet each morning and evening

Bellamine S [US] *see* belladonna, phenobarbital, and ergotamine *on this page*

Bellatal® *(Discontinued)* *see* hyoscyamine, atropine, scopolamine, and phenobarbital *on page 442*

Bellergal-S® *(Discontinued)*

Bellergal® Spacetabs® [Can] *see* belladonna, phenobarbital, and ergotamine *on this page*

Bel-Tabs *(Discontinued)* *see* belladonna, phenobarbital, and ergotamine *on this page*

Benadryl® [Can] *see* diphenhydramine *on page 265*

Benadryl-D™ Allergy and Sinus Fastmelt™ [US-OTC] *see* diphenhydramine and pseudoephedrine *on page 266*

Benadryl-D™ Children's Allergy and Sinus [US-OTC] *see* diphenhydramine and pseudoephedrine *on page 266*

Benadryl® Allergy [US-OTC] *see* diphenhydramine *on page 265*

Benadryl® Children's Allergy [US-OTC] *see* diphenhydramine *on page 265*

Benadryl® Children's Allergy and Cold Fastmelt™ [US-OTC] *see* diphenhydramine and pseudoephedrine *on page 266*

Benadryl® Children's Allergy Fastmelt® [US-OTC] *see* diphenhydramine *on page 265*

Benadryl® Children's Dye-Free Allergy [US-OTC] *see* diphenhydramine *on page 265*

Benadryl® Injection [US] *see* diphenhydramine *on page 265*

Benadryl® Itch Stopping [US-OTC] *see* diphenhydramine *on page 265*

Benadryl® Itch Stopping Extra Strength [US-OTC] *see* diphenhydramine *on page 265*

Ben-Allergin-50® Injection *(Discontinued)* *see* diphenhydramine *on page 265*

Ben-Aqua® *(Discontinued)* *see* benzoyl peroxide *on page 103*

benazepril (ben AY ze pril)

Sound-Alike/Look-Alike Issues

benazepril may be confused with Benadryl®

Lotensin® may be confused with Lioresal®, lovastatin

Synonyms benazepril hydrochloride

U.S./Canadian Brand Names Apo-Benazepril® [Can]; Lotensin® [US/Can]

Therapeutic Category Angiotensin-Converting Enzyme (ACE) Inhibitor

Use Treatment of hypertension, either alone or in combination with other antihypertensive agents

Usual Dosage Oral: Hypertension:

Children ≥6 years: Initial: 0.2 mg/kg/day (up to 10 mg/day) as monotherapy; dosing range: 0.1-0.6 mg/kg/day (maximum dose: 40 mg/day)

Adults: Initial: 10 mg/day in patients not receiving a diuretic; 20-40 mg/day as a single dose or 2 divided doses; the need for twice-daily dosing should be assessed by monitoring peak (2-6 hours after dosing) and trough responses.

Note: Patients taking diuretics should have them discontinued 2-3 days prior to starting benazepril. If they cannot be discontinued, then initial dose should be 5 mg; restart after blood pressure is stabilized if needed.

Dosage Forms

Tablet: 5 mg, 10 mg, 20 mg, 40 mg

Lotensin®: 5 mg, 10 mg, 20 mg, 40 mg

benazepril and hydrochlorothiazide (ben AY ze pril & hye droe klor oh THYE a zide)
Synonyms hydrochlorothiazide and benazepril
U.S./Canadian Brand Names Lotensin® HCT [US]
Therapeutic Category Antihypertensive Agent, Combination
Use Treatment of hypertension
Usual Dosage Oral: Dose is individualized (range: benazepril: 5-20 mg; hydrochlorothiazide: 6.25-25 mg/day)
Dosage Forms
  Tablet:
  Generics:
  5/6.25: Benazepril 5 mg and hydrochlorothiazide 6.25 mg
  10/12.5: Benazepril 10 mg and hydrochlorothiazide 12.5 mg
  20/12.5: Benazepril 20 mg and hydrochlorothiazide 12.5 mg
  20/25: Benazepril 20 mg and hydrochlorothiazide 25 mg
  Brands:
  Lotensin® HCT 5/6.25: Benazepril 5 mg and hydrochlorothiazide 6.25 mg
  Lotensin® HCT 10/12.5: Benazepril 10 mg and hydrochlorothiazide 12.5 mg
  Lotensin® HCT 20/12.5: Benazepril 20 mg and hydrochlorothiazide 12.5 mg
  Lotensin® HCT 20/25: Benazepril 20 mg and hydrochlorothiazide 25 mg

benazepril hydrochloride *see* benazepril *on previous page*

benazepril hydrochloride and amlodipine besylate *see* amlodipine and benazepril *on page 46*

bendroflumethiazide and nadolol *see* nadolol and bendroflumethiazide *on page 586*

BeneFix® [US/Can] *see* factor IX *on page 340*

Beneflur® [Can] *see* fludarabine *on page 357*

Benemid® *(Discontinued)* *see* probenecid *on page 714*

Benicar® [US] *see* olmesartan *on page 627*

Benicar HCT® [US] *see* olmesartan and hydrochlorothiazide *on page 627*

Benoquin® [US] *see* monobenzone *on page 577*

Benoxyl® [Can] *see* benzoyl peroxide *on page 103*

benserazide and levodopa *(Canada only)* (ben SER a zide & lee voe DOE pa)
Synonyms levodopa and benserazide
U.S./Canadian Brand Names Prolopa® [Can]
Therapeutic Category Anti-Parkinson Agent (Dopamine Agonist)
Use Treatment of Parkinson disease (except drug-induced parkinsonism)
Usual Dosage Oral: Adults: **Note:** Dosage expressed as levodopa/benserazide:
  Initial: 100/25 mg 1-2 times/day, increase every 3-4 days until therapeutic effect; optimal dosage: 400/100 mg to 800/200 mg/day divided into 4-6 doses
  Note: 200/50 mg used only when maintenance therapy is reached and not to exceed levodopa 1000-1200 mg/benserazide 250-300 mg per day
  Patients previously on levodopa: Allow 12 hours or more to lapse between last dose of levodopa; start at 15% of previous levodopa dosage
  Note: Dosages should be introduced gradually, individualized, and continued for 3-6 weeks before assessing benefit. Decrease dosage in patients with dystonia.
Dosage Forms [CAN] = Canadian brand name
  Capsule:
  Prolopa® [CAN]:
  50-12.5: Levodopa 50 mg and benserazide 12.5 mg [not available in the U.S.]
  100-25: Levodopa 100 mg and benserazide 25 mg [not available in the U.S.]
  200-50: Levodopa 200 mg and benserazide 50 mg [not available in the U.S.]

Ben-Tann [US] *see* diphenhydramine *on page 265*

bentoquatam (BEN toe kwa tam)
Synonyms quaternium-18 bentonite
U.S./Canadian Brand Names IvyBlock® [US-OTC]
Therapeutic Category Protectant, Topical
Use Skin protectant for the prevention of allergic contact dermatitis to poison oak, ivy, and sumac
Usual Dosage Topical: Children >6 years and Adults: Apply to skin 15 minutes prior to potential exposure to poison ivy, poison oak, or poison sumac, and reapply every 4 hours
(Continued)

bentoquatam *(Continued)*
Dosage Forms
Lotion:
IvyBlock® [OTC]: 5% (120 mL)

Bentyl® [US] *see* dicyclomine *on page 255*

Bentyl® Injection *(Discontinued)* *see* dicyclomine *on page 255*

Bentylol® [Can] *see* dicyclomine *on page 255*

Benuryl™ [Can] *see* probenecid *on page 714*

Benylin® 3.3 mg-D-E [Can] *see* guaifenesin, pseudoephedrine, and codeine *on page 408*

Benylin® D for Infants [Can] *see* pseudoephedrine *on page 727*

Benylin® Adult *(Discontinued)* *see* dextromethorphan *on page 247*

Benylin® Cough Syrup *(Discontinued)* *see* diphenhydramine *on page 265*

Benylin® DM-D [Can] *see* pseudoephedrine and dextromethorphan *on page 728*

Benylin® DM-D-E [Can] *see* guaifenesin, pseudoephedrine, and dextromethorphan *on page 408*

Benylin® DM *(Discontinued)* *see* dextromethorphan *on page 247*

Benylin® DM-E [Can] *see* guaifenesin and dextromethorphan *on page 402*

Benylin® E Extra Strength [Can] *see* guaifenesin *on page 401*

Benylin® Expectorant *(Discontinued)* *see* guaifenesin and dextromethorphan *on page 402*

Benylin® Pediatric *(Discontinued)* *see* dextromethorphan *on page 247*

Benzac® AC [US/Can] *see* benzoyl peroxide *on page 103*

Benzac® AC Gel *(Discontinued)* *see* benzoyl peroxide *on page 103*

Benzac® AC Wash [US] *see* benzoyl peroxide *on page 103*

BenzaClin® [US/Can] *see* clindamycin and benzoyl peroxide *on page 200*

Benzac® W *(Discontinued)* *see* benzoyl peroxide *on page 103*

Benzac® W Gel [Can] *see* benzoyl peroxide *on page 103*

Benzac® W Wash [US/Can] *see* benzoyl peroxide *on page 103*

Benzagel® [US] *see* benzoyl peroxide *on page 103*

Benzagel® Wash *(Discontinued)* *see* benzoyl peroxide *on page 103*

benzalkonium chloride (benz al KOE nee um KLOR ide)
Sound-Alike/Look-Alike Issues
Benza® may be confused with Benzac®
Synonyms BAC
U.S./Canadian Brand Names HandClens® [US-OTC]; Pedi-Pro® [US]; Pronto® Plus Lice Egg Remover Kit [US-OTC]; Zephiran® [US-OTC]
Therapeutic Category Antibacterial, Topical
Use Surface antiseptic and germicidal preservative
Usual Dosage Thoroughly rinse anionic detergents and soaps from the skin or other areas prior to use of solutions because they reduce the antibacterial activity of BAC. To protect metal instruments stored in BAC solution, add crushed Anti-Rust Tablets, 4 tablets/quart, to antiseptic solution, change solution at least once weekly. Not to be used for storage of aluminum or zinc instruments, instruments with lenses fastened by cement, lacquered catheters, or some synthetic rubber goods.
Dosage Forms
Lotion, topical [foam]:
HandClens®: 0.13% (50 mL, 240 mL, 1800 mL)
Lotion, topical [spray]:
HandClens®: 0.13% (15 mL)
Powder, topical:
Pedi-Pro®: 1% (60 g)
Solution, topical:
Pronto® Plus Lice Egg Remover Kit: 0.1% (60 mL)
Zephiran® [OTC]: 1:750 (240 mL, 3840 mL)

Benzamycin® [US] *see* erythromycin and benzoyl peroxide *on page 310*

Benzamycin® Pak [US] *see* erythromycin and benzoyl peroxide *on page 310*

Benzashave® **[US]** *see* benzoyl peroxide *on page 103*

benzathine benzylpenicillin *see* penicillin G benzathine *on page 661*

benzathine penicillin G *see* penicillin G benzathine *on page 661*

Benzedrex® **[US-OTC]** *see* propylhexedrine *on page 725*

benzene hexachloride *see* lindane *on page 509*

benzhexol hydrochloride *see* trihexyphenidyl *on page 866*

Benziq™ **[US]** *see* benzoyl peroxide *on page 103*

Benziq™ **LS [US]** *see* benzoyl peroxide *on page 103*

benzmethyzin *see* procarbazine *on page 716*

benzocaine (BEN zoe kane)

Sound-Alike/Look-Alike Issues
Orabase®-B may be confused with Orinase®

Synonyms ethyl aminobenzoate

U.S./Canadian Brand Names Americaine® Hemorrhoidal [US-OTC]; Americaine® [US-OTC]; Anbesol® Baby [US-OTC/Can]; Anbesol® Cold Sore Therapy [US-OTC]; Anbesol® Jr. [US-OTC]; Anbesol® Maximum Strength [US-OTC]; Anbesol® [US-OTC]; Benzodent® [US-OTC]; Cepacol® Sore Throat [US-OTC]; Chiggerex® [US-OTC]; Chiggertox® [US-OTC]; Cylex® [US-OTC]; Dent's Extra Strength Toothache [US-OTC]; Dent's Maxi-Strength Toothache [US-OTC]; Dentapaine [US-OTC]; Dermoplast® Antibacterial [US-OTC]; Dermoplast® Pain Relieving [US-OTC]; Detane® [US-OTC]; Foille® [US-OTC]; HDA® Toothache [US-OTC]; Hurricaine® [US-OTC]; Ivy-Rid® [US-OTC]; Kanka® Soft Brush™ [US-OTC]; Lanacane® Maximum Strength [US-OTC]; Lanacane® [US-OTC]; Mycinettes® [US-OTC]; Orabase® with Benzocaine [US-OTC]; Orajel PM® [US-OTC]; Orajel® Baby Teething Daytime and Nighttime [US-OTC]; Orajel® Baby Teething Nighttime [US-OTC]; Orajel® Baby Teething [US-OTC]; Orajel® Denture Plus [US-OTC]; Orajel® Maximum Strength [US-OTC]; Orajel® Medicated Toothache [US-OTC]; Orajel® Mouth Sore [US-OTC]; Orajel® Multi-Action Cold Sore [US-OTC]; Orajel® Ultra Mouth Sore [US-OTC]; Oticaine [US]; Otocaine™ [US]; Outgro® [US-OTC]; Red Cross™ Canker Sore [US-OTC]; Rid-A-Pain Dental Drops [US-OTC]; Skeeter Stik [US-OTC]; Sting-Kill [US-OTC]; Tanac® [US-OTC]; Thorets [US-OTC]; Trocaine® [US-OTC]; Zilactin Baby® [Can]; Zilactin Toothache and Gum Pain® [US-OTC]; Zilactin®-B [US-OTC/Can]

Therapeutic Category Local Anesthetic

Use Temporary relief of pain associated with pruritic dermatosis, pruritus, minor burns, acute congestive and serous otitis media, swimmer's ear, otitis externa, bee stings, insect bites; mouth and gum irritations (toothache, minor sore throat pain, canker sores, dentures, orthodontia, teething, mucositis, stomatitis); sunburn; hemorrhoids; anesthetic lubricant for passage of catheters and endoscopic tubes

Usual Dosage Note: These are general dosing guidelines; Refer to specific product labeling for dosing instructions.

Children ≥4 months: Topical (oral): Teething pain: 7.5% to 10%: Apply to affected gum area up to 4 times daily

Children ≥2 years and Adults:
Topical:
Bee stings, insect bites, minor burns, sunburn: 5% to 20%: Apply to affected area 3-4 times a day as needed. In cases of bee stings, remove stinger before treatment.
Lubricant for passage of catheters and instruments: 20%: Apply evenly to exterior of instrument prior to use.
Topical (oral): Mouth and gum irritation: 10% to 20%: Apply thin layer to affected area up to 4 times daily
Children ≥5 years and Adults: Oral: Sore throat: Allow one lozenge (10-15 mg) to dissolve slowly in mouth; may repeat every 2 hours as needed
Children ≥12 years and Adults: Rectal: Hemorrhoids: 5% to 20%: Apply externally to affected area up to 6 times daily
Adults: Otic: 20%: Instill 4-5 drops into external auditory canal; may repeat in 1-2 hours if needed

Dosage Forms
Aerosol, oral spray:
Hurricaine® [OTC]: 20% (60 mL)
Aerosol, topical spray:
Americaine® [OTC]: 20% (60 mL)
Dermoplast® Antibacterial [OTC]: 20% (83 mL)
Dermoplast® Pain Relieving [OTC]: 20% (60 mL, 83 mL)
Foille® [OTC]: 5% (92 g)
Ivy-Rid® [OTC]: 2% (83 mL)
Lanacane® Maximum Strength [OTC], Solarcaine® [OTC]: 20% (120 mL)
Combination package:
Orajel® Baby Daytime and Nighttime [OTC]:
Gel, oral [Daytime Regular Formula]: 7.5% (5.3 g)
Gel, oral [Nighttime Formula]: 10% (5.3 g)
(Continued)

benzocaine *(Continued)*

Cream, oral:
Benzodent® [OTC]: 20% (7.5 g, 30 g)
Orajel PM® [OTC]: 20% (5.3 g, 7 g)
Cream, topical:
Lanacane® [OTC]: 6% (30 g, 60 g)
Lanacane® Maximum Strength [OTC]: 20% (30 g)
Gel, oral:
Anbesol® [OTC], Zilactin®-B [OTC]: 10% (7.5 g)
Anbesol® Baby [OTC]: 7.5% (7.5 g)
Anbesol® Jr. [OTC]: 10% (7 g)
Anbesol® Maximum Strength [OTC]: 20% (7.5 g, 10 g)
Dentapaine [OTC]: 20% (11 g)
HDA® Toothache [OTC]: 6.5% (15 mL)
Hurricaine® [OTC]: 20% (5 g, 30 g)
Kanka® Soft Brush™ [OTC]: 20% (2 mL)
Little Teethers® [OTC]: 7.5% (9.4 g)
Orabase® with Benzocaine® [OTC]: 20% (7 g)
Orajel® [OTC]: 10% (5.3 g, 7 g, 9.4 g)
Orajel® Baby Teething [OTC]: 7.5% (9.4 g, 11.9 g)
Orajel® Baby Teething Nighttime [OTC]: 10% (5.3 g)
Orajel® Denture Plus [OTC]: 15% (9 g)
Orajel® Maximum Strength [OTC]: 20% (5.3 g, 7 g, 9.4 g, 11.9 g)
Orajel® Mouth Sore [OTC]: 20% (5.3 g, 9.4 g, 11.9 g)
Orajel® Multi-Action Cold Sore [OTC]: 20% (9.4 g)
Orajel® Ultra Mouth Sore [OTC]: 15% (9.4 g)
Gel, topical:
Detane® [OTC]: 7.5% (15 g)
Liquid, oral:
Anbesol® [OTC]: 10%
Anbesol® Maximum Strength [OTC], Hurricaine® [OTC], Orajel® Maximum Strength [OTC]: 20%
Orajel® Baby Teething [OTC]: 7.5%
Liquid, oral drop:
Dent's Maxi-Strength Toothache [OTC]: 20%
Rid-A-Pain Dental Drops [OTC]: 6.3%
Liquid, topical:
Chiggertox® [OTC]: 2% (30 mL)
Outgro® [OTC]: 20% (9 mL)
Skeeter Stik [OTC]: 5% (14 mL)
Tanac® [OTC]: 10% (13 mL)
Lozenge: 6 mg (18s), 15 mg (10s)
Cepacol® Sore Throat [OTC]: 10 mg (16s, 18s)
Cylex® [OTC]: 15 mg
Mycinettes® [OTC]: 15 mg (12s)
Thorets [OTC]: 18 mg (500s)
Trocaine® [OTC]: 10 mg (40s, 400s)
Ointment, oral:
Anbesol® Cold Sore Therapy [OTC]: 20% (7.1 g)
Red Cross™ Canker Sore [OTC]: 20% (7.5 g)
Ointment, rectal:
Americaine® Hemorrhoidal [OTC]: 20% (30 g)
Ointment, topical:
Chiggerex® [OTC]: 2% (50 g)
Foille® [OTC]: 5% (3.5 g, 14 g, 28 g)
Pads, topical:
Sting-Kill [OTC]: 20% (8s)
Paste, oral:
Orabase® with Benzocaine [OTC]: 20% (6 g)
Solution, otic drops: 20% (15 mL)
Oticaine, Otocaine™: 20% (15 mL)
Swabs, oral:
Hurricaine® [OTC]: 20% (6s, 100s)
Orajel® Baby Teething [OTC]: 7.5% (12s)
Orajel® Medicated Mouth Sore [OTC], Orajel® Medicated Toothache [OTC]: 20% (8s, 12s)
Zilactin® Toothache and Gum Pain [OTC]: 20% (8s)

Swabs, topical:
Sting-Kill [OTC]: 20% (5s)
Wax, oral:
Dent's Extra Strength Toothache Gum [OTC]: 20% (1 g)

benzocaine and antipyrine *see* antipyrine and benzocaine *on page 61*

benzocaine, butamben, and tetracaine (BEN zoe kane, byoo TAM ben, & TET ra kane)
Synonyms benzocaine, butamben, and tetracaine hydrochloride; benzocaine, butyl aminobenzoate, and tetracaine; butamben, tetracaine, and benzocaine; tetracaine, benzocaine, and butamben
U.S./Canadian Brand Names Cetacaine® [US]; Exactacain™ [US]
Therapeutic Category Local Anesthetic
Use Topical anesthetic to control pain in surgical or endoscopic procedures; anesthetic for accessible mucous membranes except for the eyes
Usual Dosage Topical anesthetic: **Note:** Decrease dose in the acutely-ill patient:
Adults:
Cetacaine®:
Aerosol: Apply for ≤1 second; use of sprays >2 seconds is contraindicated
Gel: Apply ~0.5 inch (13 mm) x 3/16 inch (5 mm); application of >1 inch (26 cm) x 3/16 inch (5 mm) is contraindicated
Liquid: Apply 6-7 drops (0.2 mL); application of >12-14 drops (0.4 mL) is contraindicated
Exactacain™: 3 metered sprays (use of >6 metered sprays is contraindicated)
Dosage Forms
Aerosol, topical [spray]:
Cetacaine®: Benzocaine 14%, butamben 2%, and tetracaine 2% (56 g)
Exactacain™: Benzocaine 14%, butamben 2%, and tetracaine 2% (60 g)
Gel, topical:
Cetacaine®: Benzocaine 14%, butamben 2%, and tetracaine 2% (29 g)
Liquid, topical:
Cetacaine®: Benzocaine 14%, butamben 2%, and tetracaine 2% (56 g)

benzocaine, butamben, and tetracaine hydrochloride *see* benzocaine, butamben, and tetracaine *on this page*

benzocaine, butyl aminobenzoate, and tetracaine *see* benzocaine, butamben, and tetracaine *on this page*

Benzocol® *(Discontinued)* *see* benzocaine *on page 101*

Benzodent® [US-OTC] *see* benzocaine *on page 101*

benzoin (BEN zoin)
Synonyms gum benjamin
U.S./Canadian Brand Names Benz-Protect Swabs™ [US-OTC]; Sprayzoin™ [US-OTC]
Therapeutic Category Pharmaceutical Aid; Protectant, Topical
Use Protective application for irritations of the skin; sometimes used in boiling water as steam inhalants for its expectorant and soothing action
Usual Dosage Apply 1-2 times/day
Dosage Forms
Tincture: Benzoin USP [OTC] (60 mL); Benzoin Compound USP [OTC] (30 mL, 60 mL, 120 mL, 480 mL)
Tincture [swab]:
Benz-Protect Swabs™ [OTC]: Benzoin Compound USP (50s)
Tincture [spray]: Benzoin USP [OTC] (120 mL)
Sprayzoin™ [OTC]: Benzoin Compound USP (120 mL)

benzonatate (ben ZOE na tate)
U.S./Canadian Brand Names Tessalon® [US/Can]
Therapeutic Category Antitussive
Use Symptomatic relief of nonproductive cough
Usual Dosage Oral: Children >10 years and Adults: 100 mg 3 times/day or every 4 hours up to 600 mg/day
Dosage Forms
Capsule, softgel: 100 mg, 200 mg
Tessalon®: 100 mg, 200 mg

benzoyl peroxide (BEN zoe il peer OKS ide)
Sound-Alike/Look-Alike Issues
Benoxyl® may be confused with Brevoxyl®, Peroxyl®
(Continued)

benzoyl peroxide *(Continued)*

Benzac® may be confused with Benza®
Brevoxyl® may be confused with Benoxyl®
Fostex® may be confused with pHisoHex®

U.S./Canadian Brand Names Acetoxyl® [Can]; Benoxyl® [Can]; Benzac® AC Wash [US]; Benzac® AC [US/Can]; Benzac® W Gel [Can]; Benzac® W Wash [US/Can]; Benzagel® [US]; Benzashave® [US]; Benziq™ LS [US]; Benziq™ [US]; Brevoxyl® Cleansing [US]; Brevoxyl® Wash [US]; Brevoxyl® [US]; Clearplex [US-OTC]; Clinac™ BPO [US]; Del Aqua® [US]; Desquam-E™ [US]; Desquam-X® [US/Can]; Exact® Acne Medication [US-OTC]; Fostex® 10% BPO [US-OTC]; Loroxide® [US-OTC]; Neutrogena® Acne Mask [US-OTC]; Neutrogena® On The Spot® Acne Treatment [US-OTC]; Oxy 10® Balance Spot Treatment [US-OTC]; Oxy 10® Balanced Medicated Face Wash [US-OTC]; Oxyderm™ [Can]; Palmer's® Skin Success Acne [US-OTC]; PanOxyl® Aqua Gel [US]; PanOxyl® Bar [US-OTC]; PanOxyl® [US/Can]; PanOxyl®-AQ [US]; Seba-Gel™ [US]; Solugel® [Can]; Triaz® Cleanser [US]; Triaz® [US]; Zapzyt® [US-OTC]; Zoderm® [US]

Therapeutic Category Acne Products

Use Adjunctive treatment of mild-to-moderate acne vulgaris and acne rosacea

Usual Dosage Children and Adults:

Cleansers: Wash once or twice daily; control amount of drying or peeling by modifying dose frequency or concentration

Topical: Apply sparingly once daily; gradually increase to 2-3 times/day if needed. If excessive dryness or peeling occurs, reduce dose frequency or concentration; if excessive stinging or burning occurs, remove with mild soap and water; resume use the next day.

Dosage Forms

Cream, topical:
BenzaShave®: 5% (120 g); 10% (120 g)
Exact® Acne Medication [OTC]: 5% (18 g)
Neutrogena® Acne Mask [OTC]: 5% (60 g)
Neutrogena® On The Spot® Acne Treatment [OTC]: 2.5% (22.5 g)
Zoderm®: 4.5% (125 mL); 6.5% (125 mL); 8.5% (125 mL)

Emulsion, topical [cleanser]:
Zoderm®: 4.5% (400 mL); 6.5% (400 mL); 8.5% (400 mL)

Gel, topical: 2.5% (60 g); 5% (45 g, 60 g, 90 g); 10% (45 g, 60 g, 90 g)
Benzac® AC [water based]: 5% (60 g); 10% (60 g)
Benzagel®: 5% (45 g); 10% (45 g)
Benziq™: 5.25% (50 g)
Benziq™ LS: 2.75% (50 g)
Brevoxyl®: 4% (43 g, 90 g); 8% (43 g, 90 g)
Clearplex [OTC]: 5% (45 g); 10% (45 g)
Clinac™ BPO: 7% (45 g)
Desquam-E™ [water based]: 2.5% (42.5 g); 5% (42.5 g) [emollient gel]
Desquam-X®: 5% (42.5 g, 90 g); 10% (42.5 g, 90 g)
Fostex® 10% BPO [OTC]: 10% (45 g)
Oxy 10® Balance Spot Treatment [OTC]: 5% (30 g); 10% (30 g)
PanOxyl® [alcohol based]: 5% (57 g, 113 g); 10% (57 g, 113 g)
PanOxyl® AQ [water based]: 2.5% (57 g, 113 g); 5% (57 g, 113 g); 10% (57 g, 113 g)
PanOxyl® Aqua Gel [water based]: 10% (42.5 g)
Seba-Gel™: 5% (90 g); 10% (90 g)
Triaz® Cleanser: 3% (170 g, 340 g); 6% (170 g, 340 g); 10% (170 g, 340 g)
Zapzyt® [OTC]: 10% (30 g)
Zoderm®: 4.5% (125 mL); 6.5% (125 mL); 8.5% (125 mL)

Liquid, topical: 2.5% (240 mL); 5% (120 mL, 150 mL, 240 mL); 10% (150 mL, 240 mL)
Benzac® AC Wash [water based]: 5% (240 mL); 10% (240 mL)
Benzac® W Wash [water based]: 5% (240 mL)
Benziq™ [wash]: 5.25% (175 g)
Del-Aqua®: 5% (45 mL); 10% (45 mL)
Desquam-X®: 5% (150 mL)
Oxy-10® Balance Medicated Face Wash [OTC]: 10% (240 mL)

Lotion, topical: 5% (30 mL); 10% (30 mL)
Brevoxyl® Cleansing: 4% (297 g); 8% (297 g)
Brevoxyl® Wash: 4% (170 g); 8% (170 g)
Fostex® 10% BPO [OTC]: 10% (150 mL)
Palmer's® Skin Success Acne [OTC]: 10% (30 mL)

Pad, topical:
Triaz®: 3% (30s, 60s); 6% (30s, 60s); 9% (30s)
Zoderm®: 4.5% (30s); 6.5% (30s); 8.5% (30s)

Soap, topical [bar]:
Fostex® 10% BPO [OTC]: 10% (113 g)
PanOxyl® Bar [OTC]: 5% (113 g); 10% (113 g)

benzoyl peroxide and clindamycin *see* clindamycin and benzoyl peroxide *on page 200*

benzoyl peroxide and erythromycin *see* erythromycin and benzoyl peroxide *on page 310*

benzoyl peroxide and hydrocortisone (BEN zoe il peer OKS ide & hye droe KOR ti sone)
Synonyms hydrocortisone and benzoyl peroxide
U.S./Canadian Brand Names Vanoxide-HC® [US/Can]
Therapeutic Category Acne Products
Use Treatment of acne vulgaris and oily skin
Usual Dosage Topical: Adolescents and Adults: Shake well; apply thin film 1-3 times/day, gently massage into skin
Dosage Forms
  Lotion:
  Vanoxide-HC®: Benzoyl peroxide 5% and hydrocortisone 0.5% (25 mL)

benzphetamine (benz FET a meen)
Synonyms benzphetamine hydrochloride
U.S./Canadian Brand Names Didrex® [US/Can]
Therapeutic Category Anorexiant
Controlled Substance C-III
Use Short-term (few weeks) adjunct in exogenous obesity
Usual Dosage Oral: Children ≥12 years and Adults: Dose should be individualized based on patient response: Initial: 25-50 mg once daily; titrate to 25-50 mg 1-3 times/day; once-daily dosing should be administered midmorning or midafternoon; maximum dose: 50 mg 3 times/day
Dosage Forms
  Tablet: 50 mg
  Didrex®: 50 mg

benzphetamine hydrochloride *see* benzphetamine *on this page*

Benz-Protect Swabs™ [US-OTC] *see* benzoin *on page 103*

benztropine (BENZ troe peen)
Sound-Alike/Look-Alike Issues
  benztropine may be confused with bromocriptine
Synonyms benztropine mesylate
U.S./Canadian Brand Names Apo-Benztropine® [Can]; Cogentin® [US]
Therapeutic Category Anti-Parkinson Agent; Anticholinergic Agent
Use Adjunctive treatment of Parkinson disease; treatment of drug-induced extrapyramidal symptoms (except tardive dyskinesia)
Usual Dosage Use in children ≤3 years of age should be reserved for life-threatening emergencies
  Drug-induced extrapyramidal symptom: Oral, I.M., I.V.:
  Children >3 years: 0.02-0.05 mg/kg/dose 1-2 times/day
  Adults: 1-4 mg/dose 1-2 times/day
  Acute dystonia: Adults: I.M., I.V.: 1-2 mg
  Parkinsonism: Adults: Oral: 0.5-6 mg/day in 1-2 divided doses; if one dose is greater, administer at bedtime; titrate dose in 0.5 mg increments at 5- to 6-day intervals
Dosage Forms
  Injection, solution:
  Cogentin®: 1 mg/mL (2 mL)
  Tablet: 0.5 mg, 1 mg, 2 mg

benztropine mesylate *see* benztropine *on this page*

benzydamine *(Canada only)* (ben ZID a meen)
Synonyms benzydamine hydrochloride
U.S./Canadian Brand Names Apo-Benzydamine® [Can]; Dom-Benzydamine [Can]; Novo-Benzydamine [Can]; PMS-Benzydamine [Can]; ratio-Benzydamine [Can]; Sun-Benz® [Can]; Tantum® [Can]
Therapeutic Category Analgesic, Topical
Use Symptomatic treatment of pain associated with acute pharyngitis; treatment of pain associated with radiation-induced oropharyngeal mucositis
(Continued)

105

benzydamine *(Canada only)* *(Continued)*

Usual Dosage Oral rinse: Adults:

Acute pharyngitis: Gargle with 15 mL of undiluted solution every $1^1/_2$-3 hours until symptoms resolve. Patient should expel solution from mouth following use; solution should not be swallowed.

Mucositis: 15 mL of undiluted solution as a gargle or rinse 3-4 times/day; contact should be maintained for at least 30 seconds, followed by expulsion from the mouth. Clinical studies maintained contact for ~2 minutes, up to 8 times/day. Patient should not swallow the liquid. Begin treatment 1day prior to initiation of radiation therapy and continue daily during treatment. Continue oral rinse treatments after the completion of radiation therapy until desired result/healing is achieved.

Dosage Forms [CAN] = Canadian brand name

Oral rinse: 0.15% (100 mL, 250 mL) [not available in the U.S.]

Apo-Benzydamine® [CAN], Dom-Benzydamine [CAN], Novo-Benzydamine [CAN], PMS-Benzydamine [CAN], ratio-Benzydamine [CAN], Sun-Benz® [CAN], Tantum® [CAN]: 0.15% (100 mL, 250 mL) [not available in the U.S.]

benzydamine hydrochloride *see* benzydamine *(Canada only) on previous page*

benzylpenicillin benzathine *see* penicillin G benzathine *on page 661*

benzylpenicillin potassium *see* penicillin G (parenteral/aqueous) *on page 662*

benzylpenicillin sodium *see* penicillin G (parenteral/aqueous) *on page 662*

benzylpenicilloyl-polylysine (BEN zil pen i SIL oyl pol i LIE seen)

Synonyms penicilloyl-polylysine; PPL

Therapeutic Category Diagnostic Agent

Use Adjunct in assessing the risk of administering penicillin (penicillin or benzylpenicillin) in adults with a history of clinical penicillin hypersensitivity

Usual Dosage PPL is administered by a scratch technique or by intradermal injection. For initial testing, PPL should always be applied via the scratch technique. **Do not administer intradermally to patients who have positive reactions to a scratch test.** PPL test alone does not identify those patients who react to a minor antigenic determinant and does not appear to predict reliably the occurrence of late reactions.

Scratch test: Use scratch technique with a 20-gauge needle to make 3-5 mm nonbleeding scratch on epidermis, apply a small drop of solution to scratch, rub in gently with applicator or toothpick. A positive reaction consists of a pale wheal surrounding the scratch site which develops within 10 minutes and ranges from 5-15 mm or more in diameter.

Intradermal test: Use intradermal test with a tuberculin syringe with a 26- to 30-gauge short bevel needle; a dose of 0.01-0.02 mL is injected intradermally. A control of 0.9% sodium chloride should be injected at least 1.5" from the PPL test site. Most skin responses to the intradermal test will develop within 5-15 minutes.

Interpretation:

(-) Negative: No reaction

(±) Ambiguous: Wheal only slightly larger than original bleb with or without erythematous flare and larger than control site

(+) Positive: Itching and marked increase in size of original bleb

Control site should be reactionless

beractant (ber AKT ant)

Sound-Alike/Look-Alike Issues

Survanta® may be confused with Sufenta®

Synonyms bovine lung surfactant; natural lung surfactant

U.S./Canadian Brand Names Survanta® [US/Can]

Therapeutic Category Lung Surfactant

Use Prevention and treatment of respiratory distress syndrome (RDS) in premature infants

Prophylactic therapy: Body weight <1250 g in infants at risk for developing, or with evidence of, surfactant deficiency (administer within 15 minutes of birth)

Rescue therapy: Treatment of infants with RDS confirmed by x-ray and requiring mechanical ventilation (administer as soon as possible - within 8 hours of age)

Usual Dosage

Prophylactic treatment: Administer 100 mg phospholipids (4 mL/kg) intratracheal as soon as possible; as many as 4 doses may be administered during the first 48 hours of life, no more frequently than 6 hours apart. The need for additional doses is determined by evidence of continuing respiratory distress; if the infant is still intubated and requiring at least 30% inspired oxygen to maintain a PaO_2 ≤80 torr.

Rescue treatment: Administer 100 mg phospholipids (4 mL/kg) as soon as the diagnosis of RDS is made; may repeat if needed, no more frequently than every 6 hours to a maximum of 4 doses

Dosage Forms

Suspension, intratracheal [preservative free; bovine derived]:

Survanta®: 25 mg/mL

Berocca® *(Discontinued)*

Berocca® Plus *(Discontinued)*

Berotec® [Can] *see* fenoterol *(Canada only)* on page 346

Berubigen® *(Discontinued)* *see* cyanocobalamin on page 220

Betacaine® [Can] *see* lidocaine on page 504

beta-carotene (BAY ta KARE oh teen)
  U.S./Canadian Brand Names A-Caro-25 [US]; B-Caro-T™ [US]; Lumitene™ [US]
  Therapeutic Category Vitamin, Fat Soluble
  Usual Dosage Oral:
    Children <14 years: 30-150 mg/day
    Adults: 30-300 mg/day
  Dosage Forms
    Capsule, softgel: 10,000 int. units (6 mg); 25,000 int. units (15 mg)
     A-Caro-25: 25,000 int. units (15 mg)
     B-Caro-T™: 25,000 int. units (15 mg)
    Capsule:
     Lumitene™: 50,000 int. units (30 mg)
    Tablet: 10,000 int. units

Betachron® *(Discontinued)* *see* propranolol on page 724

Betaderm [Can] *see* betamethasone (topical) on page 109

Betadine® [US-OTC/Can] *see* povidone-iodine on page 704

Betadine® First Aid Antibiotics + Moisturizer *(Discontinued)* *see* bacitracin and polymyxin B on page 91

Betadine® Ophthalmic [US] *see* povidone-iodine on page 704

9-beta-d-ribofuranosyladenine *see* adenosine on page 19

Betagan® [US/Can] *see* levobunolol on page 499

Beta-HC® [US] *see* hydrocortisone (topical) on page 434

betahistine *(Canada only)* (bay ta HISS teen)
  Synonyms betahistine dihydrochloride
  U.S./Canadian Brand Names Serc® [Can]
  Therapeutic Category Antihistamine
  Use Treatment of Ménière disease (to decrease episodes of vertigo)
  Usual Dosage Oral: Adults: 8-16 mg 3 times/day; administration with meals is recommended
  Dosage Forms [CAN] = Canadian brand name
    Tablet:
     Serc® [CAN]: 16 mg, 24 mg [not available in the U.S.]

betahistine dihydrochloride *see* betahistine *(Canada only)* on this page

betaine (BAY ta een)
  Sound-Alike/Look-Alike Issues
    betaine may be confused with Betadine®
    Cystadane® may be confused with cysteamine, cysteine
  Synonyms betaine anhydrous
  U.S./Canadian Brand Names Cystadane® [US/Can]
  Therapeutic Category Homocystinuria Agent
  Use Treatment of homocystinuria (eg, deficiencies or defects in cystathionine beta-synthase [CBS], 5,10-methylene tetrahydrofolate reductase [MTHFR], and cobalamin cofactor metabolism [CBL])
  Usual Dosage Oral:
    Children <3 years: Initial dose: 100 mg/kg/day given once daily or in 2 divided doses; increase weekly by 50 mg/kg increments, as needed
    Children ≥3 years and Adults: Usual dose: 6 g/day administered in divided doses of 3 g twice daily; dosages of up to 20 g/day have been necessary to control homocysteine levels in some patients
    Note: Dosage in all patients can be gradually increased until plasma total homocysteine is undetectable or present only in small amounts. One study in six patients with CBS deficiency, ranging from 6-17 years of age, showed minimal benefit from exceeding a twice daily dosing schedule and a 150 mg/kg/day dosage.
  (Continued)

betaine *(Continued)*

Dosage Forms
Powder for oral solution, anhydrous:
Cystadane®: 1 g/scoop

betaine anhydrous *see* betaine *on previous page*

Betaject™ [Can] *see* betamethasone (systemic) *on this page*

Betalin® S *(Discontinued)* *see* thiamine *on page 836*

Betaloc® [Can] *see* metoprolol *on page 562*

Betaloc® Durules® [Can] *see* metoprolol *on page 562*

BetaMed [US-OTC] *see* pyrithione zinc *on page 737*

betamethasone and clotrimazole (bay ta METH a sone & kloe TRIM a zole)

Sound-Alike/Look-Alike Issues
Lotrisone® may be confused with Lotrimin®
Synonyms clotrimazole and betamethasone
U.S./Canadian Brand Names Lotriderm® [Can]; Lotrisone® [US]
Therapeutic Category Antifungal/Corticosteroid
Use Topical treatment of various dermal fungal infections (including tinea pedis, cruris, and corpora in patients ≥17 years of age)
Usual Dosage Topical: Children ≥17 years and Adults:
Allergic or inflammatory diseases: Apply to affected area twice daily, morning and evening
Tinea corporis, tinea cruris: Massage into affected area twice daily, morning and evening; do not use for longer than 2 weeks; re-evaluate after 1 week if no clinical improvement; do not exceed 45 g cream/week or 45 mL lotion/week
Tinea pedis: Massage into affected area twice daily, morning and evening; do not use for longer than 4 weeks; reevaluate after 2 weeks if no clinical improvement; do not exceed 45 g cream/week or 45 mL lotion/week
Dosage Forms
Cream: Betamethasone 0.05% and clotrimazole 1% (15 g, 45 g)
Lotrisone®: Betamethasone 0.05% and clotrimazole 1% (15 g, 45 g)
Lotion: Betamethasone 0.05% and clotrimazole 1% (30 mL)
Lotrisone®: Betamethasone 0.05% and clotrimazole 1% (30 mL)

betamethasone dipropionate *see* betamethasone (topical) *on next page*

betamethasone dipropionate and calcipotriene hydrate *see* calcipotriene and betamethasone *on page 135*

betamethasone dipropionate, augmented *see* betamethasone (topical) *on next page*

betamethasone sodium phosphate *see* betamethasone (systemic) *on this page*

betamethasone (systemic) (bay ta METH a sone sis TEM ik)

Synonyms betamethasone sodium phosphate
U.S./Canadian Brand Names Betaject™ [Can]; Celestone® Soluspan® [US/Can]; Celestone® [US]
Therapeutic Category Adrenal Corticosteroid
Use Antiinflammatory; immunosuppressant agent; corticosteroid replacement
Usual Dosage Base dosage on severity of disease and patient response
Children: Use lowest dose listed as initial dose for adrenocortical insufficiency (physiologic replacement)
I.M.: 0.0175-0.125 mg base/kg/day divided every 6-12 hours **or** 0.5-7.5 mg base/m^2/day divided every 6-12 hours
Oral: 0.0175-0.25 mg/kg/day divided every 6-8 hours **or** 0.5-7.5 mg/m^2/day divided every 6-8 hours
Adolescents and Adults:
Oral: 2.4-4.8 mg/day in 2-4 doses; range: 0.6-7.2 mg/day
I.M.: Betamethasone sodium phosphate and betamethasone acetate: 0.6-9 mg/day (generally, $^1/_3$ to $^1/_2$ of oral dose) divided every 12-24 hours
Adults:
Intrabursal, intra-articular, intradermal: 0.25-2 mL
Intralesional: Rheumatoid arthritis/osteoarthritis:
Very large joints: 1-2 mL
Large joints: 1 mL
Medium joints: 0.5-1 mL
Small joints: 0.25-0.5 mL

Dosage Forms
Injection, suspension:
Celestone® Soluspan®: Betamethasone sodium phosphate 3 mg and betamethasone acetate 3 mg per 1 mL (5 mL) [6 mg/mL]
Solution:
Celestone®: 0.6 mg/5 mL

betamethasone (topical) (bay ta METH a sone TOP i kal)

Sound-Alike/Look-Alike Issues
Luxiq® may be confused with Lasix®

Synonyms betamethasone dipropionate; betamethasone dipropionate, augmented; betamethasone valerate; flubenisolone

U.S./Canadian Brand Names Beta-Val® [US]; Betaderm [Can]; Betnesol® [Can]; Betnovate® [Can]; Diprolene® AF [US]; Diprolene® Glycol [Can]; Diprolene® [US]; Diprosone® [Can]; Ectosone [Can]; Luxiq® [US]; Maxivate® [US]; Prevex® B [Can]; Taro-Sone® [Can]; Topilene® [Can]; Topisone® [Can]; Valisone® Scalp Lotion [Can]

Therapeutic Category Corticosteroid, Topical

Use Inflammatory dermatoses such as seborrheic or atopic dermatitis, neurodermatitis, anogenital pruritus, psoriasis, inflammatory phase of xerosis

Usual Dosage Topical:
≥13 years: Use minimal amount for shortest period of time to avoid HPA axis suppression
Gel, augmented formulation: Apply once or twice daily; rub in gently. **Note:** Do not exceed 2 weeks of treatment or 50 g/week.
Lotion: Apply a few drops twice daily
Augmented formulation: Apply a few drops once or twice daily; rub in gently. **Note:** Do not exceed 2 weeks of treatment or 50 mL/week.
Cream/ointment: Apply one or twice daily.
Augmented formulation: Apply once or twice daily. **Note:** Do not exceed 2 weeks of treatment or 45 g/week.
Adults:
Foam: Apply to the scalp twice daily, once in the morning and once at night
Gel, augmented formulation: Apply once or twice daily; rub in gently. **Note:** Do not exceed 2 weeks of treatment or 50 g/week.
Lotion: Apply a few drops twice daily
Augmented formulation: Apply a few drops once or twice daily; runb in gently. **Note:** Do not exceed 2 weeks of treatment or 50 mL/week.
Cream/ointment: Apply once or twice daily
Augmented formulation: Apply once or twice daily. **Note:** Do not exceed 2 weeks of treatment or 45 g/week.

Dosage Forms
Aerosol, topical [foam]:
Luxiq®: 0.12% (50 g, 100 g, 150 g)
Cream, topical: 0.05% (15 g, 45 g; 50 g [augmented])
Beta-Val®: 0.1% (15 g, 45 g)
Diprolene® AF: 0.05% (15 g, 50 g)
Gel, topical: 0.05% (15 g, 50 g)
Lotion, topical: 0.05% (30 mL, 60 mL); 0.1% (60 mL)
Beta-Val®: 0.1% (60 mL)
Diprolene®: 0.05% (30 mL, 60 mL)
Ointment, topical: 0.05% (15 g, 45 g), 0.1% (15 g, 45 g)
Diprolene®: 0.05% (15 g, 50 g)

betamethasone valerate *see* betamethasone (topical) *on this page*

Betapace® [US] *see* sotalol *on page 802*

Betapace AF® [US/Can] *see* sotalol *on page 802*

Betasept® [US-OTC] *see* chlorhexidine gluconate *on page 174*

Betaseron® [US/Can] *see* interferon beta-1b *on page 465*

Betatar® Gel [US-OTC] *see* coal tar *on page 208*

Beta-Val® [US] *see* betamethasone (topical) *on this page*

Betaxin® [Can] *see* thiamine *on page 836*

betaxolol (be TAKS oh lol)

Sound-Alike/Look-Alike Issues
betaxolol may be confused with bethanechol, labetalol
Betoptic® S may be confused with Betagan®
(Continued)

betaxolol *(Continued)*

Synonyms betaxolol hydrochloride

U.S./Canadian Brand Names Betoptic® S [US/Can]; Kerlone® [US]; Sandoz-Betaxolol [Can]

Therapeutic Category Beta-Adrenergic Blocker

Use Treatment of chronic open-angle glaucoma and ocular hypertension; management of hypertension

Usual Dosage

Children and Adults: Ophthalmic suspension (Betoptic®): Instill 1 drop into affected eye(s) twice daily.

Adults:

Ophthalmic solution: Instill 1-2 drops into affected eye(s) twice daily.

Oral: 5-10 mg/day; may increase dose to 20 mg/day after 7-14 days if desired response is not achieved.

Dosage Forms

Solution, ophthalmic: 0.5% (5 mL, 10 mL, 15 mL)

Suspension, ophthalmic:

Betoptic® S: 0.25% (5 mL, 10 mL, 15 mL)

Tablet: 10 mg, 20 mg

Kerlone®: 10 mg, 20 mg

betaxolol hydrochloride *see* betaxolol *on previous page*

bethanechol *(be THAN e kole)*

Sound-Alike/Look-Alike Issues

bethanechol may be confused with betaxolol

Synonyms bethanechol chloride

U.S./Canadian Brand Names Duvoid® [Can]; Myotonachol® [Can]; PMS-Bethanechol [Can]; Urecholine® [US]

Therapeutic Category Cholinergic Agent

Use Treatment of acute postoperative and postpartum nonobstructive (functional) urinary retention; treatment of neurogenic atony of the urinary bladder with retention

Usual Dosage Adults: Urinary retention, neurogenic bladder, and/or bladder atony:

Oral: Initial: 10-50 mg 2-4 times/day (some patients may require dosages of 50-100 mg 4 times/day). To determine effective dose, may initiate at a dose of 5-10 mg, with additional doses of 5-10 mg hourly until an effective cumulative dose is reached. Cholinergic effects at higher oral dosages may be cumulative.

SubQ: Initial: 2.575 mg, may repeat in 15-30 minutes (maximum cumulative initial dose: 10.3 mg); subsequent doses may be given 3-4 times daily as needed (some patients may require more frequent dosing at 2.5- to 3-hour intervals). Chronic neurogenic atony may require doses of 7.5-10 every 4 hours.

Dosage Forms [CAN] = Canadian brand name

Tablet: 5 mg, 10 mg, 25 mg, 50 mg

Duvoid® [CAN]: 10 mg, 25 mg, 50 mg [not available in U.S.]

Urecholine®: 5 mg, 10 mg, 25 mg, 50 mg

bethanechol chloride *see* bethanechol *on this page*

Betimol® [US] *see* timolol *on page 843*

Betnesol® [Can] *see* betamethasone (topical) *on previous page*

Betnovate® [Can] *see* betamethasone (topical) *on previous page*

Betoptic® S [US/Can] *see* betaxolol *on previous page*

bevacizumab *(be vuh SIZ uh mab)*

Sound-Alike/Look-Alike Issues

bevacizumab may be confused with cetuximab

Synonyms anti-VEGF monoclonal antibody; NSC-704865; rhuMAb-VEGF

U.S./Canadian Brand Names Avastin® [US/Can]

Therapeutic Category Antineoplastic Agent, Monoclonal Antibody; Vaccine, Recombinant

Use Treatment of metastatic colorectal cancer; treatment of nonsquamous, nonsmall cell lung cancer

Usual Dosage I.V.: Adults:

Colorectal cancer: 5 or 10 mg/kg every 2 weeks (5 mg/kg in combination with fluorouracil based or irinotecan/fluorouracil/leucovorin treatment; 10 mg/kg when given in combination with FOLFOX4 regimen)

Lung cancer, nonsquamous cell nonsmall cell: 15 mg/kg every 3 weeks

Dosage Forms

Injection, solution [preservative free]:

Avastin®: 25 mg/mL (4 mL, 16 mL)

bexarotene (beks AIR oh teen)
  U.S./Canadian Brand Names Targretin® [US/Can]
  Therapeutic Category Retinoic Acid Derivative; Vitamin A Derivative; Vitamin, Fat Soluble
  Use
    Oral: Treatment of cutaneous manifestations of cutaneous T-cell lymphoma in patients who are refractory to
      at least one prior systemic therapy
    Topical: Treatment of cutaneous lesions in patients with refractory cutaneous T-cell lymphoma (stage 1A and
      1B) or who have not tolerated other therapies
  Usual Dosage Adults:
    Oral: 300-400 mg/m^2/day taken as a single daily dose.
    Topical: Apply once every other day for first week, then increase on a weekly basis to once daily, 2 times/day,
      3 times/day, and finally 4 times/day, according to tolerance
  Dosage Forms
    Capsule:
      Targretin®: 75 mg
    Gel:
      Targretin®: 1% (60 g)

Bextra® **(Discontinued)**

Bexxar® **[US]** see tositumomab and iodine I 131 tositumomab on page 852

bezafibrate (Canada only) (be za FYE brate)
  U.S./Canadian Brand Names Bezalip® [Can]; PMS-Bezafibrate [Can]
  Therapeutic Category Antihyperlipidemic Agent, Miscellaneous
  Use Adjunct to diet and other therapeutic measures for treatment of type IIa and IIb mixed hyperlipidemia, to
    regulate lipid and apoprotein levels (reduce serum TG, LDL-cholesterol, and apolipoprotein B, increase HDL-
    cholesterol and apolipoprotein A); treatment of adult patients with high to very high triglyceride levels
    (Fredrickson classification type IV and V hyperlipidemias) who are at high risk of sequelae and complications
    from their dyslipidemia
  Usual Dosage Oral: Adults:
    Immediate release: 200 mg 2-3 times/day; may reduce to 200 mg twice daily in patients with good response
    Sustained release: 400 mg once daily
  Dosage Forms [CAN] = Canadian brand name
    Tablet, immediate release: 200 mg [not available in the U.S.]
      PMA-Bezafibrate [CAN]: 200 mg [not available in the U.S.]
    Tablet, sustained release:
      Bezalip® [CAN]: 400 mg [not available in the U.S.]

Bezalip® **[Can]** see bezafibrate (Canada only) on this page

BG 9273 see alefacept on page 26

Biavax® **II** **(Discontinued)**

Biaxin® **[US/Can]** see clarithromycin on page 196

Biaxin® **XL [US/Can]** see clarithromycin on page 196

bicalutamide (bye ka LOO ta mide)
  Synonyms CDX; ICI-176334; NC-722665
  U.S./Canadian Brand Names Casodex® [US/Can]; CO Bicalutamide [Can]; Novo-Bicalutamide [Can]; PMS-
    Bicalutamide [Can]; ratio-Bicalutamide [Can]; Sandoz-Bicalutamide [Can]
  Therapeutic Category Androgen
  Use In combination therapy with LHRH agonist analogues in treatment of metastatic prostate cancer
  Usual Dosage Oral: Adults: Metastatic prostate cancer: 50 mg once daily (in combination with an LHRH
    analogue)
  Dosage Forms
    Tablet:
      Casodex®: 50 mg

Bicillin® **L-A [US/Can]** see penicillin G benzathine on page 661

Bicillin® **C-R [US]** see penicillin G benzathine and penicillin G procaine on page 662

Bicillin® **C-R 900/300 [US]** see penicillin G benzathine and penicillin G procaine on page 662

BiCNU® **[US/Can]** see carmustine on page 155

Bidhist [US] see brompheniramine on page 120

BiDil® **[US]** *see* isosorbide dinitrate and hydralazine *on page 476*

BIG-IV *see* botulism immune globulin (intravenous-human) *on page 117*

Biltricide® **[US/Can]** *see* praziquantel *on page 708*

bimatoprost (bi MAT oh prost)
U.S./Canadian Brand Names Lumigan® [US/Can]
Therapeutic Category Ophthalmic Agent, Miscellaneous
Use Reduction of intraocular pressure (IOP) in patients with open-angle glaucoma or ocular hypertension
Usual Dosage Ophthalmic: Adults: Open-angle glaucoma or ocular hypertension: Instill 1 drop into affected eye(s) once daily in the evening; do not exceed once-daily dosing (may decrease IOP-lowering effect). If used with other topical ophthalmic agents, separate administration by at least 5 minutes.
Dosage Forms
  Solution, ophthalmic:
    Lumigan®: 0.03% (2.5 mL, 5 mL, 7.5 mL)

Biobase™ **[Can]** *see* alcohol (ethyl) *on page 25*

Biobase-G™ **[Can]** *see* alcohol (ethyl) *on page 25*

Bioclate® *(Discontinued)* *see* antihemophilic factor (recombinant) *on page 59*

Biodine® *(Discontinued)* *see* povidone-iodine *on page 704*

Biolon™ *(Discontinued)* *see* hyaluronate and derivatives *on page 423*

Bion® Tears **[US-OTC]** *see* artificial tears *on page 75*

Biopatch® *(Discontinued)* *see* chlorhexidine gluconate *on page 174*

BioQuin® Durules™ **[Can]** *see* quinidine *on page 740*

Bio-Statin® **[US]** *see* nystatin *on page 623*

BioThrax™ **[US]** *see* anthrax vaccine, adsorbed *on page 58*

Biozyme-C® *(Discontinued)* *see* collagenase *on page 213*

biperiden (bye PER i den)
Synonyms biperiden hydrochloride; biperiden lactate
U.S./Canadian Brand Names Akineton® [US/Can]
Therapeutic Category Anti-Parkinson Agent; Anticholinergic Agent
Use Adjunct in the therapy of all forms of parkinsonism; control of extrapyramidal symptoms secondary to antipsychotics
Usual Dosage Oral: Adults:
  Parkinsonism: 2 mg 3-4 times/day
  Extrapyramidal: 2 mg 1-3 times/day
Dosage Forms
  Tablet:
    Akineton®: 2 mg

biperiden hydrochloride *see* biperiden *on this page*

biperiden lactate *see* biperiden *on this page*

Biphentin® **[Can]** *see* methylphenidate *on page 558*

bird flu vaccine *see* influenza virus vaccine (H5N1) *on page 456*

Bisac-Evac™ **[US-OTC]** *see* bisacodyl *on this page*

bisacodyl (bis a KOE dil)
Sound-Alike/Look-Alike Issues
  Doxidan® may be confused with doxepin
  Modane® may be confused with Matulane®, Moban®
U.S./Canadian Brand Names Alophen® [US-OTC]; Apo-Bisacodyl® [Can]; Bisac-Evac™ [US-OTC]; Bisolax™ [US-OTC]; Carter's Little Pills® [Can]; Correctol® Tablets [US-OTC]; Dacodyl™ [US-OTC]; Doxidan® [US-OTC]; Dulcolax® [US-OTC/Can]; ex-lax® Ultra [US-OTC]; Fematrol [US-OTC]; Femilax™ [US-OTC]; Fleet® Bisacodyl [US-OTC]; Fleet® Stimulant Laxative [US-OTC]; Gentlax® [Can]; Veracolate [US-OTC]
Therapeutic Category Laxative
Use Treatment of constipation; colonic evacuation prior to procedures or examination
Usual Dosage
  Children:
    Oral: >6 years: 5-10 mg (0.3 mg/kg) at bedtime or before breakfast

Rectal suppository:
    <2 years: 5 mg as a single dose
    >2 years: 10 mg
  Adults:
    Oral: 5-15 mg as single dose (up to 30 mg when complete evacuation of bowel is required)
    Rectal suppository: 10 mg as single dose

Dosage Forms
  Solution, rectal [enema]:
    Fleet® Bisacodyl [OTC]: 10 mg/30 mL (37 mL)
  Suppository, rectal: 10 mg
    Bisac-Evac™ [OTC], Bisolax™ [OTC], Dulcolax® [OTC]: 10 mg
  Tablet [enteric coated]: 5 mg
    Alophen® [OTC], Bisac-Evac™ [OTC], Correctol® [OTC], Dacodyl™ [OTC], Dulcolax® [OTC], ex-lax® Ultra [OTC], Fematrol [OTC], Femilax™ [OTC], Veracolate [OTC]: 5 mg
  Tablet, delayed release: 5 mg
    Doxidan® [OTC], Fleet® Stimulant Laxative [OTC]: 5 mg

Bisacodyl Uniserts® *(Discontinued)* see bisacodyl *on previous page*

bis-chloronitrosourea *see carmustine on page 155*

Bismatrol [US-OTC] *see bismuth on this page*

Bismatrol Maximum Strength [US-OTC] *see bismuth on this page*

bismuth (BIZ muth)

Sound-Alike/Look-Alike Issues
    Kaopectate® may be confused with Kayexalate®

Synonyms bismuth subsalicylate; pink bismuth

U.S./Canadian Brand Names Bismatrol Maximum Strength [US-OTC]; Bismatrol [US-OTC]; Diotame® [US-OTC]; Kao-Tin [US-OTC]; Kaopectate® Extra Strength [US-OTC]; Kaopectate® [US-OTC]; Kapectolin [US-OTC]; Maalox® Total Stomach Relief® [US-OTC]; Peptic Relief [US-OTC]; Pepto Relief [US-OTC]; Pepto-Bismol® Maximum Strength [US-OTC]; Pepto-Bismol® [US-OTC]

Therapeutic Category Antidiarrheal

Use Subsalicylate formulation: Symptomatic treatment of mild, nonspecific diarrhea; control of traveler's diarrhea (enterotoxigenic *Escherichia coli*); as part of a multidrug regimen for *H. pylori* eradication to reduce the risk of duodenal ulcer recurrence

Usual Dosage Oral:
    Treatment of nonspecific diarrhea, control/relieve traveler's diarrhea: Subsalicylate (doses based on 262 mg/15 mL liquid or 262 mg tablets):
    Children: Up to 8 doses/24 hours:
      3-6 years: $^1/_3$ tablet or 5 mL every 30 minutes to 1 hour as needed
      6-9 years: $^2/_3$ tablet or 10 mL every 30 minutes to 1 hour as needed
      9-12 years: 1 tablet or 15 mL every 30 minutes to 1 hour as needed
    Children >12 years and Adults: 2 tablets or 30 mL every 30 minutes to 1 hour as needed up to 8 doses/24 hours
    Helicobacter pylori eradication: Subsalicylate: Adults: 524 mg 4 times/day with meals and at bedtime; requires combination therapy

Dosage Forms
  Caplet:
    Kaopectate® [OTC]: 262 mg
    Pepto-Bismol® [OTC]: 262 mg
  Liquid: 262 mg/15 mL
    Bismatrol [OTC], Diotame® [OTC], Kaopectate® [OTC], Kao-Tin [OTC], Peptic Relief [OTC], Pepto-Bismol® [OTC]: 262 mg/15 mL
    Bismatrol Maximum Strength [OTC], Kaopectate® Extra Strength [OTC], Maalox® Total Stomach Relief® [OTC], Pepto-Bismol® Maximum Strength [OTC]: 525 mg/15 mL
  Suspension: 262 mg/15 mL
    Kapectolin [OTC]: 262 mg/15 mL
  Tablet, chewable: 262 mg
    Bismatrol [OTC], Diotame® [OTC], Peptic Relief [OTC], Pepto Relief [OTC], Pepto-Bismol® [OTC]: 262 mg

bismuth, metronidazole, and tetracycline (BIZ muth, me troe NI da zole, & tet ra SYE kleen)

Synonyms bismuth subcitrate potassium, tetracycline, and metronidazole; bismuth subsalicylate, tetracycline, and metronidazole; metronidazole, bismuth subcitrate potassium, and tetracycline; metronidazole, bismuth subsalicylate, and tetracycline; tetracycline, metronidazole, and bismuth subcitrate potassium; tetracycline, metronidazole, and bismuth subsalicylate
(Continued)

bismuth, metronidazole, and tetracycline *(Continued)*

U.S./Canadian Brand Names Helidac® [US]; Pylera™ [US]

Therapeutic Category Antidiarrheal

Use As part of a multidrug regimen for *H. pylori* eradication to reduce the risk of duodenal ulcer recurrence in combination with an H_2 agonist (Helidac®) or omeprazole (Pylera™)

Usual Dosage Oral: Adults:

Helidac®: Two bismuth subsalicylate 262.4 mg tablets, 1 metronidazole 250 mg tablet, and 1 tetracycline 500 mg capsule 4 times/day at meals and bedtime, plus an H_2 antagonist (at the appropriate dose) for 14 days; follow with 8 oz of water; the H_2 antagonist should be continued for a total of 28 days

Pylera™: Three capsules 4 times/day after meals and at bedtime, plus omeprazole 20 mg twice daily for 10 days; follow each dose with 8 oz of water (each capsule contains bismuth subcitrate potassium 140 mg, metronidazole 125 mg, and tetracycline 125 mg)

Dosage Forms

Capsule:

Pylera™: Bismuth subcitrate potassium 140 mg, metronidazole 125 mg, and tetracycline hydrochloride 125 mg

Combination package:

Helidac® [each package contains 14 blister cards (2-week supply); each card contains the following]:

Capsule: Tetracycline: 500 mg (4)

Tablet, chewable: Bismuth subsalicylate]: 262.4 mg (8)

Tablet: Metronidazole: 250 mg (4)

bismuth subcitrate potassium, tetracycline, and metronidazole *See* bismuth, metronidazole, and tetracycline *on previous page*

bismuth subsalicylate *see* bismuth *on previous page*

bismuth subsalicylate, tetracycline, and metronidazole *See* bismuth, metronidazole, and tetracycline *on previous page*

Bisolax™ [US-OTC] *see* bisacodyl *on page 112*

bisoprolol *(bis OH proe lol)*

Sound-Alike/Look-Alike Issues

Zebeta® may be confused with DiaBeta®

Synonyms bisoprolol fumarate

U.S./Canadian Brand Names Apo-Bisoprolol® [Can]; Monocor® [Can]; Novo-Bisoprolol [Can]; Sandoz-Bisoprolol [Can]; Zebeta® [US/Can]

Therapeutic Category Beta-Adrenergic Blocker

Use Treatment of hypertension, alone or in combination with other agents

Usual Dosage Oral: Adults: 2.5-5 mg once daily, may be increased to 10 mg, and then up to 20 mg once daily, if necessary

Hypertension (JNC 7): 2.5-10 mg once daily

Dosage Forms

Tablet: 5 mg, 10 mg

Zebeta®: 5 mg, 10 mg

bisoprolol and hydrochlorothiazide *(bis OH proe lol & hye droe klor oh THYE a zide)*

Sound-Alike/Look-Alike Issues

Ziac® may be confused with Tiazac®, Zerit®

Synonyms hydrochlorothiazide and bisoprolol

U.S./Canadian Brand Names Ziac® [US/Can]

Therapeutic Category Antihypertensive Agent, Combination

Use Treatment of hypertension

Usual Dosage Oral: Adults: Dose is individualized, given once daily

Dosage Forms

Tablet: 2.5/6.25: Bisoprolol 2.5 mg and hydrochlorothiazide 6.25 mg; 5/6.25: Bisoprolol 5 mg and hydrochlorothiazide 6.25 mg; 10/6.25: Bisoprolol 10 mg and hydrochlorothiazide 6.25 mg

Ziac®: 2.5/6.25: Bisoprolol 2.5 mg and hydrochlorothiazide 6.25 mg; 5/6.25: Bisoprolol 5 mg and hydrochlorothiazide 6.25 mg; 10/6.25: Bisoprolol 10 mg and hydrochlorothiazide 6.25 mg

bisoprolol fumarate *see* bisoprolol *on this page*

bistropamide *see* tropicamide *on page 871*

bivalirudin (bye VAL i roo din)

Synonyms hirulog

U.S./Canadian Brand Names Angiomax® [US/Can]

Therapeutic Category Anticoagulant (Other)

Use Anticoagulant used in conjunction with aspirin for patients with unstable angina undergoing percutaneous transluminal coronary angioplasty (PTCA) or percutaneous coronary intervention (PCI) with provisional glycoprotein IIb/IIIa inhibitor; anticoagulant used in patients undergoing PCI with (or at risk of) heparin-induced thrombocytopenia (HIT) / thrombosis syndrome (HITTS)

Usual Dosage I.V.: Adults: Anticoagulant in patients undergoing PTCA/PCI or PCI with HITS/HITTS (treatment should be started just prior to procedure): Initial: Bolus: 0.75 mg/kg, followed by continuous infusion: 1.75 mg/kg/hour for the duration of procedure and up to 4 hours post-procedure if needed; determine ACT 5 minutes after bolus dose; may administer additional bolus of 0.3 mg/kg if necessary.

A glycoprotein IIb/IIIa inhibitor may be administered concomitantly during the procedure.

If needed, infusion may be continued beyond initial 4 hours at 0.2 mg/kg/hour for up to 20 hours.

Dosage Forms

Injection, powder for reconstitution:

Angiomax®: 250 mg

BL4162A *see* anagrelide *on page 55*

Black-Draught Tablets [US-OTC] *see* senna *on page 781*

black widow spider species antivenin (*Latrodectus mactans*) *see* antivenin *(Latrodectus mactans) on page 63*

BlemErase® Lotion *(Discontinued)* *see* benzoyl peroxide *on page 103*

Blenoxane® [US/Can] *see* bleomycin *on this page*

bleo *see* bleomycin *on this page*

bleomycin (blee oh MYE sin)

Sound-Alike/Look-Alike Issues

bleomycin may be confused with Cleocin®

Synonyms bleo; bleomycin sulfate; BLM; NSC-125066

U.S./Canadian Brand Names Blenoxane® [US/Can]; Bleomycin Injection, USP [Can]

Therapeutic Category Antineoplastic Agent

Use Treatment of squamous cell carcinomas, melanomas, sarcomas, testicular carcinoma, Hodgkin lymphoma, and non-Hodgkin lymphoma

Orphan drug: Sclerosing agent for malignant pleural effusion

Usual Dosage Maximum cumulative lifetime dose: 400 units; refer to individual protocols; 1 unit = 1 mg

May be administered I.M., I.V., SubQ, or intracavitary

Children and Adults:

Test dose for lymphoma patients: I.M., I.V., SubQ: Because of the possibility of an anaphylactoid reaction, ≤2 units of bleomycin for the first 2 doses; monitor vital signs every 15 minutes; wait a minimum of 1 hour before administering remainder of dose; if no acute reaction occurs, then the regular dosage schedule may be followed. **Note:** Test doses may produce false-negative results.

Single-agent therapy:

I.M./I.V./SubQ: Squamous cell carcinoma, lymphoma, testicular carcinoma: 0.25-0.5 units/kg (10-20 units/m^2) 1-2 times/week

CIV: 15 units/m^2 over 24 hours daily for 4 days

Pleural sclerosing: Intrapleural: 60 units as a single instillation (some recommend limiting the dose in the elderly to 40 units/m^2; usual maximum: 60 units). Dose may be repeated at intervals of several days if fluid continues to accumulate (mix in 50-100 mL of NS); may add lidocaine 100-200 mg to reduce local discomfort.

Dosage Forms

Injection, powder for reconstitution: 15 units, 30 units

Blenoxane®: 15 units, 30 units

Bleomycin Injection, USP [Can] *see* bleomycin *on this page*

bleomycin sulfate *see* bleomycin *on this page*

Bleph®-10 [US] *see* sulfacetamide *on page 810*

Blephamide® [US/Can] *see* sulfacetamide and prednisolone *on page 811*

Blis-To-Sol® [US-OTC] *see* tolnaftate *on page 849*

BLM *see* bleomycin *on this page*

Blocadren® [US] *see* timolol *on page 843*

BMS-232632 *see* atazanavir *on page 80*

BMS 337039 *see* aripiprazole *on page 73*

BMS-354825 *see* dasatinib *on page 233*

Bonamine™ [Can] *see* meclizine *on page 535*

Bondronat® [Can] *see* ibandronate *on page 443*

Bonefos® [Can] *see* clodronate *(Canada only) on page 202*

Bonine® [US-OTC/Can] *see* meclizine *on page 535*

Boniva® [US] *see* ibandronate *on page 443*

Bontril® [Can] *see* phendimetrazine *on page 671*

Bontril PDM® [US] *see* phendimetrazine *on page 671*

Bontril® Slow-Release [US] *see* phendimetrazine *on page 671*

Boostrix® [US] *see* diphtheria, tetanus toxoids, and acellular pertussis vaccine *on page 269*

bortezomib (bore TEZ oh mib)
Synonyms LDP-341; MLN341; NSC-681239; PS-341
U.S./Canadian Brand Names Velcade® [US/Can]
Therapeutic Category Proteasome Inhibitor
Use Treatment of relapsed or refractory multiple myeloma; relapsed or refractory mantle cell lymphoma
Usual Dosage I.V.: Adults: Multiple myeloma: 1.3 mg/m² twice weekly for 2 weeks on days 1, 4, 8, 11 of a 21-day treatment regimen. Consecutive doses should be separated by at least 72 hours. Therapy extending beyond 8 cycles may be given once weekly for 4 weeks (days 1, 8, 15, and 22), followed by a 13-day rest (days 22 through 35).
Dosage Forms
Injection, powder for reconstitution [preservative free]:
Velcade®: 3.5 mg

bosentan (boe SEN tan)
U.S./Canadian Brand Names Tracleer® [US/Can]
Therapeutic Category Endothelin Antagonist
Use Treatment of pulmonary artery hypertension (PAH) (WHO Group I) in patients with World Health Organization (WHO) Class III or IV symptoms to improve exercise capacity and decrease the rate of clinical deterioration
Usual Dosage Oral: Adolescents >12 years and ≥40 kg and Adults: Initial: 62.5 mg twice daily for 4 weeks; increase to maintenance dose of 125 mg twice daily; adults <40 kg should be maintained at 62.5 mg twice daily. Doses >125 mg twice daily do not appear to confer additional clinical benefit but may increase risk of liver toxicity.
Note: When discontinuing treatment, consider a reduction in dosage to 62.5 mg twice daily for 3-7 days (to avoid clinical deterioration).
Dosage Forms
Tablet:
Tracleer®: 62.5 mg, 125 mg

B&O Supprettes® [US] *see* belladonna and opium *on page 97*

Botox® [US/Can] *see* botulinum toxin type A *on this page*

Botox® Cosmetic [US/Can] *see* botulinum toxin type A *on this page*

botulinum toxin type A (BOT yoo lin num TOKS in type aye)
Synonyms BTX-A
U.S./Canadian Brand Names Botox® Cosmetic [US/Can]; Botox® [US/Can]
Therapeutic Category Ophthalmic Agent, Toxin
Use Treatment of strabismus and blepharospasm associated with dystonia (including benign essential blepharospasm or VII nerve disorders in patients ≥12 years of age); cervical dystonia (spasmodic torticollis) in patients ≥16 years of age; temporary improvement in the appearance of lines/wrinkles of the face (moderate to severe glabellar lines associated with corrugator and/or procerus muscle activity) in adult patients ≤65 years of age; treatment of severe primary axillary hyperhidrosis in adults not adequately controlled with topical treatments
Orphan drug: Treatment of dynamic muscle contracture in pediatric cerebral palsy patients
Usual Dosage
Cervical dystonia: Children ≥16 years and Adults: I.M.: For dosing guidance, the mean dose is 236 units (25th to 75th percentile range 198-300 units) divided among the affected muscles in patients previously treated

with botulinum toxin. Initial dose in previously untreated patients should be lower. Sequential dosing should be based on the patient's head and neck position, localization of pain, muscle hypertrophy, patient response, and previous adverse reactions. The total dose injected into the sternocleidomastoid muscles should be ≤100 units to decrease the occurrence of dysphagia.

Blepharospasm: Children ≥12 years and Adults: I.M.: Initial dose: 1.25-2.5 units injected into the medial and lateral pretarsal orbicularis oculi of the upper and lower lid; dose may be increased up to twice the previous dose if the response from the initial dose lasted ≤2 months; maximum dose per site: 5 units; cumulative dose in a 30-day period: ≤200 units. Tolerance may occur if treatments are given more often than every 3 months, but the effect is not usually permanent.

Strabismus: Children ≥12 years and Adults: I.M.:
Initial dose:
Vertical muscles and for horizontal strabismus <20 prism diopters: 1.25-2.5 units in any one muscle
Horizontal strabismus of 20-50 prism diopters: 2.5-5 units in any one muscle
Persistent VI nerve palsy >1 month: 1.5-2.5 units in the medial rectus muscle
Reexamine patients 7-14 days after each injection to assess the effect of that dose. Subsequent doses for patients experiencing incomplete paralysis of the target may be increased up to twice the previous administered dose. The maximum recommended dose as a single injection for any one muscle is 25 units. Do not administer subsequent injections until the effects of the previous dose are gone.

Primary axillary hyperhidrosis: Adults ≥18 years: Intradermal: 50 units/axilla. Injection area should be defined by standard staining techniques. Injections should be evenly distributed into multiple sites (10-15), administered in 0.1-0.2 mL aliquots, ~1-2 cm apart.

Reduction of glabellar lines: Adults ≤65 years: I.M.: An effective dose is determined by gross observation of the patient's ability to activate the superficial muscles injected. The location, size and use of muscles may vary markedly among individuals. Inject 0.1 mL dose into each of five sites, two in each corrugator muscle and one in the procerus muscle (total dose 0.5 mL).

Dosage Forms
Injection, powder for reconstitution [preservative free]:
Botox®, Botox® Cosmetic: *Clostridium botulinum* toxin type A 100 units

botulinum toxin type B (BOT yoo lin num TOKS in type bee)

U.S./Canadian Brand Names Myobloc® [US]
Therapeutic Category Neuromuscular Blocker Agent, Toxin
Use Treatment of cervical dystonia (spasmodic torticollis)
Usual Dosage I.M.: Adults: Cervical dystonia: Initial: 2500-5000 units divided among the affected muscles in patients **previously treated** with botulinum toxin; initial dose in **previously untreated** patients should be lower. Subsequent dosing should be optimized according to patient's response.

Dosage Forms
Injection, solution [preservative free]:
Myobloc®: 5000 units/mL (0.5 mL, 1 mL, 2 mL)

botulism immune globulin (intravenous-human)

(BOT yoo lism i MYUN GLOB you lin, in tra VEE nus, YU man)
Synonyms BIG-IV
U.S./Canadian Brand Names BabyBIG® [US]
Therapeutic Category Immune Globulin
Use Treatment of infant botulism caused by toxin type A or B
Usual Dosage I.V.: Children <1 year: Infant botulism: 1 mL/kg (50 mg/kg) as a single dose; infuse at 0.5 mL/kg/hour (25 mg/kg/hour) for the first 15 minutes; if well tolerated, may increase to 1 mL/kg/hour (50 mg/kg/hour)

Dosage Forms
Injection, powder for reconstitution [preservative free]:
BabyBIG® [OTC]: ~100 mg

Boudreaux's® Butt Paste [US-OTC] *see* zinc oxide *on page 906*

bovine lung surfactant *see* beractant *on page 106*

Bravelle® [US/Can] *see* urofollitropin *on page 878*

Breathe Right® Saline [US-OTC] *see* sodium chloride *on page 792*

Breezee® Mist Antifungal *(Discontinued)* *see* miconazole *on page 566*

Breonesin® *(Discontinued)* *see* guaifenesin *on page 401*

Brethaire® *(Discontinued)* *see* terbutaline *on page 827*

Brevibloc® [US/Can] *see* esmolol *on page 311*

Brevicon® [US] *see* ethinyl estradiol and norethindrone *on page 328*

Brevicon® **0.5/35 [Can]** *see* ethinyl estradiol and norethindrone *on page 328*

Brevicon® **1/35 [Can]** *see* ethinyl estradiol and norethindrone *on page 328*

Brevital® **[Can]** *see* methohexital *on page 553*

Brevital® **Sodium [US]** *see* methohexital *on page 553*

Brevoxyl® **[US]** *see* benzoyl peroxide *on page 103*

Brevoxyl® **Cleansing [US]** *see* benzoyl peroxide *on page 103*

Brevoxyl® **Wash [US]** *see* benzoyl peroxide *on page 103*

Bricanyl® **[Can]** *see* terbutaline *on page 827*

Bricanyl® *(Discontinued) see* terbutaline *on page 827*

brimonidine (bri MOE ni deen)
Sound-Alike/Look-Alike Issues
brimonidine may be confused with bromocriptine
Synonyms brimonidine tartrate
U.S./Canadian Brand Names Alphagan® P [US]; Alphagan® [Can]; Apo-Brimonidine® [Can]; PMS-Brimonidine Tartrate [Can]; ratio-Brimonidine [Can]
Therapeutic Category Alpha₂-Adrenergic Agonist Agent, Ophthalmic
Use Lowering of intraocular pressure (IOP) in patients with open-angle glaucoma or ocular hypertension
Usual Dosage Ophthalmic: Children ≥2 years of age and Adults: Glaucoma: Instill 1 drop in affected eye(s) 3 times/day (approximately every 8 hours)
Dosage Forms
Solution, ophthalmic: 0.2% (5 mL, 10 mL, 15 mL)
Alphagan® P: 0.1% (5 mL, 10 mL, 15 mL); 0.15% (5 mL, 10 mL, 15 mL)

brimonidine and timolol (Canada only) (bri MOE ni deen & TIM oh lol)
Synonyms brimonidine tartrate and timolol maleate; timolol and brimonidine
U.S./Canadian Brand Names Combigan® [Can]
Therapeutic Category Alpha₂ Agonist, Ophthalmic; Beta Blocker, Nonselective; Ophthalmic Agent, Antiglaucoma
Use Control of intraocular pressure (IOP) in patients with chronic open-angle glaucoma or ocular hypertension, who have inadequately responded to monotherapy and in whom combination therapy is warranted
Usual Dosage Ophthalmic: Adults: Instill 1 drop into affected eye(s) every 12 hours
Dosage Forms [CAN] = Canadian brand name
Solution, ophthalmic:
Combigan® [CAN]: Brimonidine 0.2% and timolol 0.5%: (2.5 mL, 5 mL,10 mL) [contains benzalkonium chloride] [not available in the U.S.]

brimonidine tartrate *see* brimonidine *on this page*

brimonidine tartrate and timolol maleate *see* brimonidine and timolol *(Canada only) on this page*

brinzolamide (brin ZOH la mide)
U.S./Canadian Brand Names Azopt® [US/Can]
Therapeutic Category Carbonic Anhydrase Inhibitor
Use Lowers intraocular pressure in patients with ocular hypertension or open-angle glaucoma
Usual Dosage Ophthalmic: Adults: Instill 1 drop in affected eye(s) 3 times/day
Dosage Forms
Suspension, ophthalmic:
Azopt®: 1% (5 mL, 10 mL, 15 mL)

Brioschi® **[US-OTC]** *see* sodium bicarbonate *on page 791*

British anti-lewisite *see* dimercaprol *on page 263*

BRL 43694 *see* granisetron *on page 400*

Bromaline® **[US-OTC]** *see* brompheniramine and pseudoephedrine *on page 120*

Bromaline® **DM [US-OTC]** *see* brompheniramine, pseudoephedrine, and dextromethorphan *on page 122*

Bromarest® *(Discontinued) see* brompheniramine *on page 120*

Bromatane DX [US] *see* brompheniramine, pseudoephedrine, and dextromethorphan *on page 122*

Bromaxefed RF *(Discontinued) see* brompheniramine and pseudoephedrine *on page 120*

bromazepam *(Canada only)* (broe MA ze pam)
U.S./Canadian Brand Names Apo-Bromazepam® [Can]; Gen-Bromazepam [Can]; Lectopam® [Can]; Novo-Bromazepam [Can]; Nu-Bromazepam [Can]; Pro Doc Limitee [Can]
Therapeutic Category Benzodiazepine; Sedative
Use Short-term, symptomatic treatment of anxiety
Usual Dosage Oral: Adults: Initial: 6-18 mg/day in equally divided doses; initial course of treatment should not last longer than 1 week; optimal dosage range: 6-30 mg/day
Dosage Forms [CAN] = Canadian brand name
  Tablet: 1.5 mg, 3 mg, 6 mg [not available in the U.S.]
  Apo-Bromazepam® [CAN], Gen-Bromazepam [CAN], Lectopam® [CAN], Novo-Bromazepam [CAN], Nu-Bromazepam [CAN]: 1.5 mg, 3 mg, 6 mg [not available in the U.S.]

Brombay® *(Discontinued)* see brompheniramine *on next page*

Brometane DX [US] see brompheniramine, pseudoephedrine, and dextromethorphan *on page 122*

Bromfed® *(Discontinued)* see brompheniramine and pseudoephedrine *on next page*

Bromfed-PD® *(Discontinued)* see brompheniramine and pseudoephedrine *on next page*

bromfenac (BROME fen ak)
Synonyms bromfenac sodium
U.S./Canadian Brand Names Xibrom™ [US]
Therapeutic Category Analgesic, Nonnarcotic; Nonsteroidal Antiinflammatory Drug (NSAID), Oral
Use Treatment of postoperative inflammation and reduction in ocular pain following cataract removal
Usual Dosage Ophthalmic: Adults: Instill 1 drop into affected eye(s) twice daily beginning 24 hours after surgery and continuing for 2 weeks postoperatively
Dosage Forms
  Solution, ophthalmic:
  Xibrom™: 0.09% (5 mL)

bromfenac sodium see bromfenac *on this page*

Bromfenex® [US] see brompheniramine and pseudoephedrine *on next page*

Bromfenex® PD [US] see brompheniramine and pseudoephedrine *on next page*

Bromhist DM [US] see brompheniramine, pseudoephedrine, and dextromethorphan *on page 122*

Bromhist-NR [US] see brompheniramine and pseudoephedrine *on next page*

Bromhist PDX [US] see brompheniramine, pseudoephedrine, and dextromethorphan *on page 122*

Bromhist Pediatric [US] see brompheniramine and pseudoephedrine *on next page*

bromocriptine (broe moe KRIP teen)
Sound-Alike/Look-Alike Issues
  bromocriptine may be confused with benztropine, brimonidine
  Parlodel® may be confused with pindolol, Provera®
Synonyms bromocriptine mesylate
U.S./Canadian Brand Names Apo-Bromocriptine® [Can]; Parlodel® [US/Can]; PMS-Bromocriptine [Can]
Therapeutic Category Anti-Parkinson Agent (Dopamine Agonist); Ergot Alkaloid and Derivative
Use Treatment of hyperprolactinemia associated with amenorrhea with or without galactorrhea, infertility, or hypogonadism; treatment of prolactin-secreting adenomas; treatment of acromegaly; treatment of Parkinson disease
Usual Dosage Oral:
Children: Hyperprolactinemia:
  11-15 years (based on limited information): Initial: 1.25-2.5 mg daily; dosage may be increased as tolerated to achieve a therapeutic response (range: 2.5-10 mg daily).
  ≥16 years: Refer to adult dosing
Adults:
  Parkinsonism: 1.25 mg twice daily, increased by 2.5 mg/day in 2- to 4-week intervals (usual dose range is 30-90 mg/day in 3 divided doses), though elderly patients can usually be managed on lower doses
  Acromegaly: Initial: 1.25-2.5 mg daily increasing by 1.25-2.5 mg daily as necessary every 3-7 days; usual dose: 20-30 mg/day (maximum: 100 mg/day)
  Hyperprolactinemia: Initial: 1.25-2.5 mg/day; may be increased by 2.5 mg/day as tolerated every 2-7 days until optimal response (range: 2.5-15 mg/day)
Dosage Forms
  Capsule: 5 mg
  Parlodel®: 5 mg
  Tablet: 2.5 mg
  Parlodel® SnapTabs®: 2.5 mg

bromocriptine mesylate *see* bromocriptine *on previous page*

Bromphen® *(Discontinued)* *see* brompheniramine *on this page*

Bromphenex DM [US] *see* brompheniramine, pseudoephedrine, and dextromethorphan *on page 122*

brompheniramine (brome fen IR a meen)

Synonyms brompheniramine maleate; brompheniramine tannate

U.S./Canadian Brand Names B-Vex [US]; Bidhist [US]; BroveX™ CT [US]; BroveX™ [US]; Lodrane® 12 Hour [US]; Lodrane® 24 [US]; Lodrane® XR [US]; LoHist-12 [US]; TanaCof-XR [US]

Therapeutic Category Antihistamine

Use Perennial and seasonal allergic rhinitis and other allergic symptoms including urticaria

Usual Dosage Allergic rhinitis, allergic symptoms, vasomotor rhinitis: Oral:

Children:

1-2 years (B-Vex, BroveX™): 1.25 mL every 12 hours (maximum: 2.5 mL/day)

2-6 years:

B-Vex, BroveX™: 2.5 mL every 12 hours (maximum: 5 mL/day)

BroveX™ CT: ½ tablet every 12 hours (maximum: 1 tablet/day)

Lodrane® XR, TanaCof-XR: 1.25 mL every 12 hours (maximum: 2.5 mL/day)

6-12 years:

B-Vex, BroveX™: 5 mL every 12 hours (maximum: 10 mL/day)

BroveX™ CT: ½ to 1 tablet every 12 hours (maximum: 2 tablets/day)

Lodrane® 12 Hour, LoHist-12: One tablet every 12 hours (maximum: 2 tablets/day)

Lodrane® 24: One capsule once daily

Lodrane® XR, TanaCof-XR: 2.5 mL every 12 hours (maximum: 5 mL/day)

>12 years (B-Vex, BroveX™, BroveX™ CT, Lodrane® 12 Hour, Lodrane® 24, Lodrane® XR, LoHist-12, TanaCof-XR): Refer to adult dosing

Adults:

B-Vex, BroveX™: 5-10 mL every 12 hours (maximum: 20 mL/day)

BroveX™ CT: 1-2 tablets every 12 hours (maximum: 4 tablets/day)

Lodrane® 12 Hour, LoHist: 1-2 tablets every 12 hours (maximum: 4 tablets/day)

Lodrane® 24: 1-2 capsules once daily

Lodrane® XR, TanaCof-XR: 5 mL every 12 hours (maximum: 10 mL/day)

Dosage Forms

Capsule, extended release:

Lodrane® 24: 12 mg [dye free]

Suspension, as tannate:

B-Vex, BroveX™: 12 mg/5 mL

Lodrane® XR: 8 mg/5 mL

TanaCof-XR: 8 mg/5 mL

Tablet, chewable:

BroveX™ CT: 12 mg [banana flavor]

Tablet, extended release:

Bidhist: 6 mg

Tablet, extended release [scored]:

Lodrane® 12 Hour, LoHist-12: 6 mg [dye free]

Tablet, timed release: 6 mg

brompheniramine and pseudoephedrine (brome fen IR a meen & soo doe e FED rin)

Sound-Alike/Look-Alike Issues

Bromfed® may be confused with Bromphen®

Synonyms brompheniramine maleate and pseudoephedrine hydrochloride; brompheniramine maleate and pseudoephedrine sulfate; pseudoephedrine and brompheniramine

U.S./Canadian Brand Names AccuHist® [US]; Andehist NR Syrup [US]; Bromaline® [US-OTC]; Bromfenex® PD [US]; Bromfenex® [US]; Bromhist Pediatric [US]; Bromhist-NR [US]; Brotapp [US]; Brovex SR [US]; Dimaphen [US-OTC]; Lodrane® 12D [US]; Lodrane® 24D [US]; Lodrane® D [US]; Lodrane® [US]; LoHist 12D [US]; LoHist LQ [US]; LoHist PD [US]; Respahist® [US]; Sildec Syrup [US]; Touro® Allergy [US]

Therapeutic Category Antihistamine/Decongestant Combination

Use Temporary relief of symptoms of seasonal and perennial allergic rhinitis, and vasomotor rhinitis, including nasal obstruction

Usual Dosage Oral:

Capsule, long acting:

Based on 60 mg pseudoephedrine:

Children 6-12 years: 1 capsule every 12 hours

Children ≥12 years and Adults: 1-2 capsules every 12 hours

Based on 120 mg pseudoephedrine: Children ≥12 years and Adults: 1 capsule every 12 hours

Liquid:

Based on brompheniramine 1 mg/pseudoephedrine 15 mg per 1 mL: Children:

1-3 months: 0.25 mL 4 times/day

3-6 months: 0.5 mL 4 times/day

6-12 months: 0.75 mL 4 times/day

12-24 months: 1 mL 4 times/day

Based on brompheniramine 1 mg/pseudoephedrine 15 mg per 5 mL: Children:

6-11 months (6-8 kg): 2.5 mL every 6-8 hours (maximum: 4 doses/24 hours)

12-23 months (8-10 kg): 3.75 mL every 6-8 hours (maximum: 4 doses/24 hours)

2-6 years: 5 mL every 6-8 hours (maximum: 4 doses/24 hours)

6-12 years: 10 mL every 6-8 hours (maximum: 4 doses/24 hours)

>12 years and Adults: 20 mg every 4 hours (maximum: 4 doses/24 hours)

Based on brompheniramine 4 mg/pseudoephedrine 30 mg:

Children 2-6 years: 2.5 mL 3 times/day

Children >6 years and Adults: 5 mL 3 times/day

Brompheniramine 4 mg/pseudoephedrine 45 mg per 5 mL:

Children 2-6 years: 2.5 mL 4 times/day

Children >6 years and Adults: 5 mL 4 times/day

Tablet, extended release: Based on pseudoephedrine 45 mg:

Children 6-12 years: 1 tablet every 12 hours

Children ≥12 years and Adults: 1-2 tablets every 12 hours

Dosage Forms

Caplet, extended release:

Histex® SR: Brompheniramine 10 mg and pseudoephedrine 120 mg

Capsule, extended release:

Bromfenex®: Brompheniramine 12 mg and pseudoephedrine 120 mg

Bromfenex® PD: Brompheniramine 6 mg and pseudoephedrine 60 mg

Lodrane® 24D: Brompheniramine 12 mg and pseudoephedrine 90 mg

Capsule, sustained release:

Brovex SR: Brompheniramine 9 mg and pseudoephedrine 90 mg

Respahist®: Brompheniramine 6 mg and pseudoephedrine 60 mg

Elixir:

Dimaphen: Brompheniramine 1 mg and pseudoephedrine 15 mg per 5 mL

Liquid: Brompheniramine 4 mg and pseudoephedrine 60 mg per 5 mL (480 mL)

Brotapp: Brompheniramine 1 mg and pseudoephedrine 15 mg per 5 mL

Lodrane®, LoHist LQ: Brompheniramine 4 mg and pseudoephedrine 60 mg per 5 mL

Liquid, oral [drops]:

AccuHist®, Bromhist NR, LoHist LQ: Brompheniramine 1 mg and pseudoephedrine 12.5 mg per 1 mL

Bromhist Pediatric: Brompheniramine 1 mg and pseudoephedrine 15 mg per 1 mL

Solution:

Bromaline® [OTC]: Brompheniramine 1 mg and pseudoephedrine 15 mg per 5 mL

Suspension:

Lodrane® D: Brompheniramine 8 mg and pseudoephedrine 90 mg per 5 mL

Syrup:

Andehist NR, Sildec: Brompheniramine 4 mg and pseudoephedrine 45 mg per 5 mL

Tablet, extended release:

Lodrane® 12D, LoHist 12D: Brompheniramine 6 mg and pseudoephedrine 45 mg

Tablet, prolonged release:

Touro® Allergy: Brompheniramine 6 mg and pseudoephedrine 45 mg

Tablet, sustained release: Brompheniramine 6 mg and pseudoephedrine 45 mg

brompheniramine maleate *see* brompheniramine *on previous page*

brompheniramine maleate and pseudoephedrine hydrochloride *see* brompheniramine and pseudoephedrine *on previous page*

brompheniramine maleate and pseudoephedrine sulfate *see* brompheniramine and pseudoephedrine *on previous page*

brompheniramine, pseudoephedrine, and dextromethorphan
(brome fen IR a meen, soo doe e FED rin, & deks troe meth OR fan)

Synonyms dextromethorphan hydrobromide, brompheniramine maleate, and pseudoephedrine hydrochloride; pseudoephedrine tannate, dextromethorphan tannate, and brompheniramine tannate

U.S./Canadian Brand Names AccuHist® PDX Drops [US]; AllanHist PDX [US]; Anaplex® DM [US]; Anaplex® DMX [US]; Andehist DM NR [US]; Bromaline® DM [US-OTC]; Bromatane DX [US]; Brometane DX [US]; Bromhist DM [US]; Bromhist PDX [US]; Bromphenex DM [US]; Bromplex DX [US]; Brotapp-DM [US]; Carbofed DM [US]; EndaCof-DM [US]; EndaCof-PD [US]; Histacol™ BD [US]; Myphetane DX [US]; PediaHist DM [US]

Therapeutic Category Antihistamine; Cough Preparation; Decongestant

Use Relief of cough and upper respiratory symptoms (including nasal congestion) associated with allergy or the common cold

Usual Dosage
Children:
1-3 months (AccuHist® PDX, EndaCof-PD): 0.25 mL 4 times/day
3-6 months (AccuHist® PDX, EndaCof-PD): 0.5 mL 4 times/day
6-12 months (AccuHist® PDX, EndaCof-PD): 0.75 mL 4 times/day
12-24 months (AccuHist® PDX, EndaCof-PD): 1 mL 4 times/day
2-6 years:
Anaplex® DM, EndaCof-DM: 1.25 mL every 4-6 hours (maximum: 4 doses/24 hours)
Anaplex® DMX: 1.25 mL every 12 hours (maximum: 2.5 mL/24 hours)
6-12 years:
Anaplex® DM, EndaCof-DM: 2.5 mL every 4-6 hours (maximum: 4 doses/24 hours)
Anaplex® DMX: 2.5 mL every 12 hours (maximum: 5 mL/24 hours)
Bromaline® DM, Dimaphen DM, Dimetapp® DM Children's Cough and Cold: 10 mL every 4-6 hours (maximum: 4 doses/24 hours)
Children ≥12 years and Adults:
Anaplex® DM: 5 mL every 4-6 hours (maximum: 4 doses/24 hours)
Anaplex® DMX: 5 mL every 12 hours (maximum: 10 mL/24 hours)
Bromaline® DM, Dimaphen DM, Dimetapp® DM Children's Cough and Cold: 20 mL every 4-6 hours (maximum: 4 doses/24 hours)

Dosage Forms
Elixir:
Bromaline® DM [OTC]: Brompheniramine 1 mg, pseudoephedrine 15 mg, and dextromethorphan 5 mg per 5 mL
Liquid:
Bromplex DM: Brompheniramine 4 mg, pseudoephedrine 60 mg, and dextromethorphan 30 mg per 5 mL
Brotapp-DM: Brompheniramine 1 mg, pseudoephedrine 15 mg, and dextromethorphan 5 mg per 5 mL
Solution, oral [drops]:
AccuHist® PDX, AllanHist PDX, Bromhist PDX, EndaCof-PD, Histacol™ BD: Brompheniramine 1 mg, pseudoephedrine 12.5 mg, and dextromethorphan 3 mg per 1 mL
Bromhist DM, PediaHist DM: Brompheniramine 1 mg, pseudoephedrine 15 mg, and dextromethorphan 4 mg per 1 mL
Suspension:
Anaplex® DMX: Brompheniramine 8 mg, pseudoephedrine 90 mg, and dextromethorphan 60 mg per 5 mL
Syrup:
Anaplex® DM, Bromphenex DM, EndaCof-DM: Brompheniramine 4 mg, pseudoephedrine 60 mg, and dextromethorphan 30 mg per 5 mL
Andehist DM NR, Carbofed DM, Sildec-DM: Brompheniramine 4 mg, pseudoephedrine 45 mg, and dextromethorphan 15 mg per 5 mL
Bromatane DX, Brometane DX, Myphetane DX: Brompheniramine 2 mg, pseudoephedrine 30 mg, and dextromethorphan 10 mg per 5 mL

brompheniramine tannate *see* brompheniramine *on page 120*

Brompheril® *(Discontinued) see* dexbrompheniramine and pseudoephedrine *on page 243*

Bromplex DX [US] *see* brompheniramine, pseudoephedrine, and dextromethorphan *on this page*

Bronchial® *(Discontinued) see* theophylline and guaifenesin *on page 835*

Bronchial Mist® *(Discontinued) see* epinephrine *on page 300*

Broncho Saline® *(Discontinued) see* sodium chloride *on page 792*

Bronitin® Mist *(Discontinued) see* epinephrine *on page 300*

Brontex® [US] *see* guaifenesin and codeine *on page 402*

Brotane® *(Discontinued) see* brompheniramine *on page 120*

Brotapp [US] *see* brompheniramine and pseudoephedrine *on page 120*

Brotapp-DM [US] *see* brompheniramine, pseudoephedrine, and dextromethorphan *on previous page*

Brovana™ [US] *see* arformoterol *on page 72*

BroveX™ [US] *see* brompheniramine *on page 120*

BroveX™ CT [US] *see* brompheniramine *on page 120*

Brovex SR [US] *see* brompheniramine and pseudoephedrine *on page 120*

BSF208075 *see* ambrisentan *on page 39*

BSS® [US/Can] *see* balanced salt solution *on page 93*

BSS Plus® [US/Can] *see* balanced salt solution *on page 93*

B-Tuss™ [US] *see* phenylephrine, hydrocodone, and chlorpheniramine *on page 678*

BTX-A *see* botulinum toxin type A *on page 116*

B-type natriuretic peptide (human) *see* nesiritide *on page 600*

Bubbli-Pred™ [US] *see* prednisolone (systemic) *on page 710*

Budeprion™ SR [US] *see* bupropion *on page 127*

budesonide (byoo DES oh nide)

U.S./Canadian Brand Names Entocort® EC [US]; Entocort® [Can]; Gen-Budesonide AQ [Can]; Pulmicort Flexhaler® [US]; Pulmicort Respules® [US]; Pulmicort Turbuhaler® [US]; Pulmicort® [Can]; Rhinocort® Aqua® [US]; Rhinocort® Turbuhaler® [Can]

Therapeutic Category Adrenal Corticosteroid

Use

Intranasal: Management of symptoms of seasonal or perennial rhinitis

Nebulization: Maintenance and prophylactic treatment of asthma

Oral capsule: Treatment of active Crohn disease (mild-to-moderate) involving the ileum and/or ascending colon; maintenance of remission (for up to 3 months) of Crohn disease (mild-to-moderate) involving the ileum and/or ascending colon

Oral inhalation: Maintenance and prophylactic treatment of asthma; includes patients who require corticosteroids and those who may benefit from systemic dose reduction/elimination

Usual Dosage

Nasal inhalation: (Rhinocort® Aqua®): Children ≥6 years and Adults: 64 mcg/day as a single 32 mcg spray in each nostril. Some patients who do not achieve adequate control may benefit from increased dosage. A reduced dosage may be effective after initial control is achieved.

Maximum dose: Children <12 years: 128 mcg/day; Adults: 256 mcg/day

Nebulization: Children 12 months to 8 years: Pulmicort Respules®: Titrate to lowest effective dose once patient is stable; start at 0.25 mg/day or use as follows:

Previous therapy of bronchodilators alone: 0.5 mg/day administered as a single dose or divided twice daily (maximum daily dose: 0.5 mg)

Previous therapy of inhaled corticosteroids: 0.5 mg/day administered as a single dose or divided twice daily (maximum daily dose: 1 mg)

Previous therapy of oral corticosteroids: 1 mg/day administered as a single dose or divided twice daily (maximum daily dose: 1 mg)

Oral inhalation:

Children ≥6 years:

Pulmicort® Turbuhaler®:

Previous therapy of bronchodilators alone: 200 mcg twice initially which may be increased up to 400 mcg twice daily

Previous therapy of inhaled corticosteroids: 200 mcg twice initially which may be increased up to 400 mcg twice daily

Previous therapy of oral corticosteroids: The highest recommended dose in children is 400 mcg twice daily

Pulmicort® Flexhaler®: Initial: 180 mcg twice daily (some patients may be initiated at 360 mcg twice daily); maximum 360 mcg twice daily

Adults:

Pulmicort® Turbuhaler®:

Previous therapy of bronchodilators alone: 200-400 mcg twice initially which may be increased up to 400 mcg twice daily

Previous therapy of inhaled corticosteroids: 200-400 mcg twice initially which may be increased up to 800 mcg twice daily

Previous therapy of oral corticosteroids: 400-800 mcg twice daily which may be increased up to 800 mcg twice daily

(Continued)

budesonide *(Continued)*

Pulmicort® Flexhaler®: Initial: 360 mcg twice daily (selected patients may be initiated at 180 mcg twice daily); maximum 720 mcg twice daily

NIH Guidelines (NIH, 1997) (give in divided doses twice daily):
Children:
"Low" dose: 100-200 mcg/day
"Medium" dose: 200-400 mcg/day (1-2 inhalations/day)
"High" dose: >400 mcg/day (>2 inhalation/day)
Adults:
"Low" dose: 200-400 mcg/day (1-2 inhalations/day)
"Medium" dose: 400-600 mcg/day (2-3 inhalations/day)
"High" dose: >600 mcg/day (>3 inhalation/day)

Oral: Adults: Crohn disease (active): 9 mg once daily in the morning for up to 8 weeks; recurring episodes may be treated with a repeat 8-week course of treatment
Note: Patients receiving CYP3A4 inhibitors should be monitored closely for signs and symptoms of hypercorticism; dosage reduction may be required. If switching from oral prednisolone, prednisolone dosage should be tapered while budesonide (Entocort™ EC) treatment is initiated.
Maintenance of remission: Following treatment of active disease (control of symptoms with CDAI <150), treatment may be continued at a dosage of 6 mg once daily for up to 3 months. If symptom control is maintained for 3 months, tapering of the dosage to complete cessation is recommended. Continued dosing beyond 3 months has not been demonstrated to result in substantial benefit.

Dosage Forms [CAN] = Canadian brand name
Capsule, enteric coated:
Entocort® EC: 3 mg
Powder for oral inhalation:
Pulmicort Flexhaler®: 90 mcg/inhalation (165 mg)
Pulmicort Flexhaler®: 180 mcg/inhalation (225 mg)
Pulmicort Turbuhaler®: 200 mcg/inhalation (104 g)
Pulmicort Turbuhaler® [CAN]: 100 mcg/inhalation, 200 mcg/inhalation, 400 mcg/inhalation [not available in the U.S.]
Suspension, intranasal [spray]:
Rhinocort® Aqua®: 32 mcg/inhalation (8.6 g)
Suspension for nebulization:
Pulmicort Respules®: 0.25 mg/2 mL, 0.5 mg/2 mL

budesonide and eformoterol *see* budesonide and formoterol *on this page*

budesonide and formoterol (byoo DES oh nide & for MOH te rol)

Synonyms budesonide and eformoterol; eformoterol and budesonide; formoterol fumarate dehydrate and budesonide
U.S./Canadian Brand Names Symbicort® [US/Can]
Therapeutic Category Beta$_2$-Adrenergic Agonist Agent; Corticosteroid, Inhalant (Oral)
Use Treatment of asthma in patients ≥12 years of age where combination therapy is indicated
Usual Dosage Oral inhalation: Children ≥12 years and Adults:
Symbicort® 80/4.5, Symbicort® 160/4.5: 2 inhalations twice daily. Patients currently receiving a low-to-medium dose inhaled corticosteroid may be started on the lower strength combination; those receiving a medium-to-high dose inhaled corticosteroid may be started on the higher strength combination. Consider the higher dose combination for patients not adequately controlled on the lower combination following 1-2 weeks of therapy. Do not use more than 2 inhalations twice daily of either strength.
Symbicort® Turbuhaler®: 1-2 inhalations once or twice daily
Maximum long-term maintenance dose: 4 inhalations/day; in periods of worsening asthma, this may be temporarily increased to 4 inhalations twice daily
Manufacturer's recommendation: Initial: Symbicort® 200 once or twice daily to establish symptom control. Following the establishment of response/symptom control: Titrate to the lowest dosage possible to maintain control (may substitute Symbicort® 100).
Dosage Forms [CAN] = Canadian brand name
Powder for oral inhalation:
Powder for oral inhalation:
Symbicort® 80/4.5: Budesonide 80 mcg and formoterol fumarate dehydrate 4.5 mcg per actuation (10.2 g) [120 metered inhalations]
Symbicort® 160/4.5: Budesonide 160 mcg and formoterol fumarate dehydrate 4.5 mcg per actuation (10.2 g) [120 metered inhalations]

Symbicort® 100 Turbuhaler® [CAN]: Budesonide 100 mcg and formoterol dehydrate 6 mcg per inhalation (available in 60 or 120 metered doses) [delivers ~80 mcg budesonide and 4.5 mcg formoterol per inhalation; contains lactose] [not available in the U.S]
Symbicort® 200 Turbuhaler® [CAN]: Budesonide 200 mcg and formoterol dehydrate 6 mcg per inhalation (available in 60 or 120 metered doses) [delivers ~160 mcg budesonide and 4.5 mcg formoterol per inhalation; contains lactose] [not available in the U.S]

Buffasal [US-OTC] *see* aspirin *on page 78*

Bufferin® [US-OTC] *see* aspirin *on page 78*

Bufferin® Extra Strength [US-OTC] *see* aspirin *on page 78*

Buffinol [US-OTC] *see* aspirin *on page 78*

bumetanide (byoo MET a nide)

Sound-Alike/Look-Alike Issues
bumetanide may be confused with Buminate®
Bumex® may be confused with Brevibloc®, Buprenex®, Permax®
U.S./Canadian Brand Names Bumex® [US/Can]; Burinex® [Can]
Therapeutic Category Diuretic, Loop
Use Management of edema secondary to congestive heart failure or hepatic or renal disease including nephrotic syndrome; may be used alone or in combination with antihypertensives in the treatment of hypertension; can be used in furosemide-allergic patients
Usual Dosage
Oral, I.M., I.V.:
Neonates: 0.01-0.05 mg/kg/dose every 24-48 hours
Infants and Children: 0.015-0.1 mg/kg/dose every 6-24 hours (maximum dose: 10 mg/day)
Adults:
Edema:
Oral: 0.5-2 mg/dose (maximum dose: 10 mg/day) 1-2 times/day
I.M., I.V.: 0.5-1 mg/dose; may repeat in 2-3 hours for up to 2 doses if needed (maximum dose: 10 mg/day)
Continuous I.V. infusion: Initial: 1 mg I.V. load then 0.5-2 mg/hour (ACC/AHA 2005 practice guidelines for chronic heart failure)
Hypertension: Oral: 0.5 mg daily (maximum dose: 5 mg/day); usual dosage range (JNC 7): 0.5-2 mg/day in 2 divided doses
Dosage Forms
Injection, solution: 0.25 mg/mL (2 mL, 4 mL, 10 mL)
Tablet: 0.5 mg, 1 mg, 2 mg
Bumex®: 0.5 mg, 1 mg, 2 mg

Bumex® [US/Can] *see* bumetanide *on this page*

Bumex® Injection *(Discontinued)* *see* bumetanide *on this page*

Buminate® [US] *see* albumin *on page 22*

Bupap [US] *see* butalbital and acetaminophen *on page 131*

Buphenyl® [US] *see* sodium phenylbutyrate *on page 796*

bupivacaine (byoo PIV a kane)

Sound-Alike/Look-Alike Issues
bupivacaine may be confused with mepivacaine, ropivacaine
Marcaine® may be confused with Narcan®
Synonyms bupivacaine hydrochloride
U.S./Canadian Brand Names Marcaine® Spinal [US]; Marcaine® [US/Can]; Sensorcaine® [US/Can]; Sensorcaine®-MPF Spinal [US]; Sensorcaine®-MPF [US]
Therapeutic Category Local Anesthetic
Use Local anesthetic (injectable) for peripheral nerve block, infiltration, sympathetic block, caudal or epidural block, retrobulbar block
Usual Dosage Dose varies with procedure, depth of anesthesia, vascularity of tissues, duration of anesthesia, and condition of patient. Do not use solutions containing preservatives for caudal or epidural block.
Children >12 years and Adults:
Local anesthesia: Infiltration: 0.25% infiltrated locally; maximum: 175 mg
Caudal block (preservative free): 15-30 mL of 0.25% or 0.5%
Epidural block (other than caudal block; preservative free): Administer in 3-5 mL increments, allowing sufficient time to detect toxic manifestations of inadvertent I.V. or I.T. administration: 10-20 mL of 0.25% or 0.5%
(Continued)

bupivacaine *(Continued)*

Surgical procedures requiring a high degree of muscle relaxation and prolonged effects **only**: 10-20 mL of 0.75% (**Note:** Not to be used in obstetrical cases)
Peripheral nerve block: 5 mL of 0.25 or 0.5%.; maximum: 400 mg/day
Sympathetic nerve block: 20-50 mL of 0.25%
Retrobulbar anesthesia: 2-4 mL of 0.75%
Adults: Spinal anesthesia: Preservative free solution of 0.75% bupivacaine in 8.25% dextrose:
Lower extremity and perineal procedures: 1 mL
Lower abdominal procedures: 1.6 mL
Normal vaginal delivery: 0.8 mL (higher doses may be required in some patients)
Cesarean section: 1-1.4 mL

Dosage Forms

Injection, solution [preservative free]: 0.25% (10 mL, 20 mL, 30 mL, 50 mL); 0.5% (10 mL, 20 mL, 30 mL); 0.75% (10 mL, 20 mL, 30 mL)
Marcaine® [OTC]: 0.25% (10 mL, 30 mL); 0.5% (10 mL, 30 mL); 0.75% (10 mL, 30 mL)
Sensorcaine®-MPF [OTC]: 0.25% (10 mL, 30 mL); 0.5% (10 mL, 30 mL); 0.75% (10 mL, 30 mL)
Injection, solution [preservative free]: 0.75% (2 mL)
Marcaine® Spinal [OTC]: 0.75% (2 mL)
Sensorcaine®-MPF Spinal [OTC]: 0.75% (2 mL)
Injection, solution:
Marcaine® [OTC], Sensorcaine® [OTC]: 0.25% (50 mL); 0.5% (50 mL)

bupivacaine and epinephrine (byoo PIV a kane & ep i NEF rin)

Synonyms epinephrine bitartrate and bupivacaine hydrochloride
U.S./Canadian Brand Names Marcaine® with Epinephrine [US]; Sensorcaine® with Epinephrine [US/Can]; Sensorcaine®-MPF with Epinephrine [US]
Therapeutic Category Local Anesthetic
Use Local anesthetic (injectable) for peripheral nerve block, infiltration, sympathetic block, caudal or epidural block, retrobulbar block
Usual Dosage Dose varies with procedure, depth of anesthesia, vascularity of tissues, duration of anesthesia, and condition of patient. Do not use solutions containing preservatives for caudal or epidural block.
Children >12 years and Adults:
Caudal block (preservative free): 15-30 mL of 0.25% or 0.5%
Epidural block (other than caudal block, preservative free): 10-20 mL of 0.25% or 0.5%. Administer in 3-5 mL increments, allowing sufficient time to detect toxic manifestations of inadvertent I.V. or I.T. administration. Surgical procedures requiring a high degree of muscle relaxation and prolonged effects only: 10-20 mL of 0.75% (**Note:** Not to be used in obstetrical cases)
Local anesthesia: Infiltration: 0.25% infiltrated locally (maximum: 175 mg of bupivacaine)
Peripheral nerve block: 5 mL of 0.25 or 0.5% (maximum: 400 mg/day of bupivacaine)
Retrobulbar anesthesia: 2-4 mL of 0.75%
Sympathetic nerve block: 20-50 mL of 0.25%
Infiltration and nerve block in maxillary and mandibular area: 9 mg (1.8 mL) of bupivacaine as a 0.5% solution with epinephrine 1:200,000 per injection site. A second dose may be administered if necessary to produce adequate anesthesia after allowing up to 10 minutes for onset. Up to a maximum of 90 mg of bupivacaine hydrochloride per dental appointment. The effective anesthetic dose varies with procedure, intensity of anesthesia needed, duration of anesthesia required, and physical condition of the patient; always use the lowest effective dose along with careful aspiration.

Dosage Forms

Injection, solution [preservative free]: Bupivacaine 0.25% and epinephrine 1:200,000 (10 mL, 30 mL); bupivacaine 0.5% and epinephrine 1:200,000 (1.8 mL, 10 mL, 30 mL)
Marcaine® with Epinephrine: Bupivacaine 0.25% and epinephrine 1:200,000 (10 mL, 30 mL); bupivacaine 0.5% and epinephrine 1:200,000 (1.8 mL, 3 mL, 10 mL, 30 mL); bupivacaine 0.75% and epinephrine 1:200,000 (30 mL)
Sensorcaine® MPF with Epinephrine: Bupivacaine 0.25% and epinephrine 1:200,000 (10 mL, 30 mL); bupivacaine 0.5% and epinephrine 1:200,000 (10 mL, 30 mL)
Injection, solution: Bupivacaine 0.25% and epinephrine 1:200,000 (50 mL); bupivacaine 0.5% and epinephrine 1:200,000 (50 mL)
Marcaine® with Epinephrine: Bupivacaine 0.25% and epinephrine 1:200,000 (50 mL); bupivacaine 0.5% and epinephrine 1:200,000 (50 mL)
Sensorcaine® with Epinephrine: Bupivacaine 0.25% and epinephrine 1:200,000 (50 mL); bupivacaine 0.5% and epinephrine 1:200,000 (50 mL)

bupivacaine and lidocaine *see* lidocaine and bupivacaine *on page 506*
bupivacaine hydrochloride *see* bupivacaine *on previous page*

Buprenex® **[US/Can]** *see* buprenorphine *on this page*

buprenorphine (byoo pre NOR feen)

Sound-Alike/Look-Alike Issues
Buprenex® may be confused with Brevibloc®, Bumex®
Synonyms buprenorphine hydrochloride
U.S./Canadian Brand Names Buprenex® [US/Can]; Subutex® [US/Can]
Therapeutic Category Analgesic, Narcotic
Controlled Substance Injection: C-V/C-III; Tablet: C-III
Use
Injection: Management of moderate to severe pain
Tablet: Treatment of opioid dependence
Usual Dosage Long-term use is not recommended
Note: These are guidelines and do not represent the maximum doses that may be required in all patients.
Doses should be titrated to pain relief/prevention. In high-risk patients (eg, elderly, debilitated, presence of
respiratory disease) and/or concurrent CNS depressant use, reduce dose by one-half. Buprenorphine has an
analgesic ceiling.
Acute pain (moderate to severe):
Children 2-12 years: I.M., slow I.V.: 2-6 mcg/kg every 4-6 hours
Children ≥13 years and Adults:
I.M.: Initial: Opiate-naive: 0.3 mg every 6-8 hours as needed; initial dose (up to 0.3 mg) may be repeated
once in 30-60 minutes after the initial dose if needed; usual dosage range: 0.15-0.6 mg every 4-8 hours as
needed
Slow I.V.: Initial: Opiate-naive: 0.3 mg every 6-8 hours as needed; initial dose (up to 0.3 mg) may be
repeated once in 30-60 minutes after the initial dose if needed
Sublingual: Children ≥16 years and Adults: Opioid dependence:
Induction: Range: 12-16 mg/day (doses during an induction study used 8 mg on day 1, followed by 16 mg on
day 2; induction continued over 3-4 days). Treatment should begin at least 4 hours after last use of heroin or
short-acting opioid, preferably when first signs of withdrawal appear. Titrating dose to clinical effectiveness
should be done as rapidly as possible to prevent undue withdrawal symptoms and patient drop-out during
the induction period.
Maintenance: Target dose: 16 mg/day; range: 4-24 mg/day; patients should be switched to the buprenor-
phine/naloxone combination product for maintenance and unsupervised therapy
Dosage Forms
Injection, solution: 0.3 mg/mL (1 mL)
Buprenex®: 0.3 mg/mL (1 mL)
Tablet, sublingual:
Subutex®: 2 mg, 8 mg

buprenorphine and naloxone (byoo pre NOR feen & nal OKS one)

Synonyms buprenorphine hydrochloride and naloxone hydrochloride dihydrate; naloxone and buprenorphine;
naloxone hydrochloride dihydrate and buprenorphine hydrochloride
U.S./Canadian Brand Names Suboxone® [US]
Therapeutic Category Analgesic, Narcotic
Controlled Substance C-III
Use Treatment of opioid dependence
Usual Dosage Sublingual: Children ≥16 years and Adults: Opioid dependence: **Note:** This combination
product is not recommended for use during the induction period; initial treatment should begin using bupre-
norphine oral tablets. Patients should be switched to the combination product for maintenance and unsuper-
vised therapy.
Maintenance: Target dose (based on buprenorphine content): 16 mg/day; range: 4-24 mg/day
Dosage Forms
Tablet, sublingual:
Suboxone®: Buprenorphine 2 mg and naloxone 0.5 mg; buprenorphine 8 mg and naloxone 2 mg

buprenorphine hydrochloride *see* buprenorphine *on this page*

buprenorphine hydrochloride and naloxone hydrochloride dihydrate *see* buprenorphine and
naloxone *on this page*

Buproban™ **[US]** *see* bupropion *on this page*

bupropion (byoo PROE pee on)

Sound-Alike/Look-Alike Issues
buPROPion may be confused with busPIRone
Wellbutrin SR® may be confused with Wellbutrin XL™
(Continued)

bupropion *(Continued)*

Wellbutrin XL™ may be confused with Wellbutrin SR®

Zyban® may be confused with Zagam®, Diovan®

Tall-Man buPROPion

U.S./Canadian Brand Names Budeprion™ SR [US]; Buproban™ [US]; Novo-Bupropion SR [Can]; Wellbutrin SR® [US]; Wellbutrin XL™ [US/Can]; Wellbutrin® [US/Can]; Zyban® [US/Can]

Therapeutic Category Antidepressant, Aminoketone

Use Treatment of major depressive disorder, including seasonal affective disorder (SAD); adjunct in smoking cessation

Usual Dosage Oral: Adults:

Depression:

Immediate release: 100 mg 3 times/day; begin at 100 mg twice daily; may increase to a maximum dose of 450 mg/day

Sustained release: Initial: 150 mg/day in the morning; may increase to 150 mg twice daily by day 4 if tolerated; target dose: 300 mg/day given as 150 mg twice daily; maximum dose: 400 mg/day given as 200 mg twice daily

Extended release: Initial: 150 mg/day in the morning; may increase as early as day 4 of dosing to 300 mg/day; maximum dose: 450 mg/day

SAD (Wellbutrin XL™): Initial: 150 mg/day in the morning; if tolerated, may increase after 1 week to 300 mg/day

Note: Prophylactic treatment should be reserved for those patients with frequent depressive episodes and/or significant impairment. Initiate treatment in the Autumn prior to symptom onset, and discontinue in early Spring with dose tapering to 150 mg/day for 2 weeks

Smoking cessation (Zyban®): Initiate with 150 mg once daily for 3 days; increase to 150 mg twice daily; treatment should continue for 7-12 weeks

Dosage Forms

Tablet: 75 mg [generic for Wellbutrin®], 100 mg [generic for Wellbutrin®]

Wellbutrin®: 75 mg, 100 mg

Tablet, extended release: 100 mg [generic for Wellbutrin® SR], 150 mg [generic for Wellbutrin® SR], 150 mg [generic for Zyban®], 200 mg [generic for Wellbutrin® SR], 300 mg [generic for Wellbutrin XL™]

Budeprion™ SR: 100 mg [generic for Wellbutrin® SR], 150 mg [generic for Wellbutrin® SR]

Budeprion XL®: 300 mg [generic for Wellbutrin® XL]

Buproban™: 150 mg [generic for Zyban®]

Wellbutrin XL™: 150 mg, 300 mg

Tablet, sustained release: 100 mg [generic for Wellbutrin® SR], 150 mg [generic for Wellbutrin® SR], 150 mg [generic for Zyban®], 200 mg [generic for Wellbutrin® SR]

Wellbutrin® SR: 100 mg, 150 mg, 200 mg

Zyban®: 150 mg

Burinex® [Can] *see* bumetanide *on page 125*

Burnamycin [US-OTC] *see* lidocaine *on page 504*

Burn Jel [US-OTC] *see* lidocaine *on page 504*

Burn-O-Jel [US-OTC] *see* lidocaine *on page 504*

Buscopan® [Can] *see* scopolamine derivatives *on page 778*

buserelin acetate *see* buserelin acetate *(Canada only) on this page*

buserelin acetate *(Canada only)* (BYOO se rel in AS e tate)

Sound-Alike/Look-Alike Issues

Suprefact® may be confused with Suprane®

Synonyms buserelin acetate

U.S./Canadian Brand Names Suprefact® Depot [Can]; Suprefact® [Can]

Therapeutic Category Luteinizing Hormone-Releasing Hormone Analog

Use Palliative treatment in patients with hormone-dependent advanced prostate cancer (stage D); treatment of endometriosis in women who do not require surgical intervention as first-line therapy (length of therapy is usually 6 months, but no longer than 9 months)

Usual Dosage Adults:

Prostate cancer: **Note:** Administration of an antiandrogen agent beginning 7 days prior to initiation of buserelin therapy and continuing for ~5 weeks with buserelin therapy is recommended in patients with prostate cancer.

SubQ:

Suprefact®: Initial: 500 mcg every 8 hours for 7 days. Maintenance: 200 mcg once daily

Suprefact Depot®

2-month: 6.3 mg implant injected into lateral abdominal wall every 8 weeks

3-month: 9.45 mg injected into lateral abdominal wall every 12 weeks
Intranasal (Suprefact®): Maintenance: 400 mcg (200 mcg into each nostril) 3 times/day
Endometriosis: Intranasal (Suprefact®): 400 mcg (200 mcg into each nostril) 3 times/day for 6-9 months
Dosage Forms [CAN] = Canadian brand name
Injection, solution:
Suprefact® [CAN]: 1 mg/mL (5.5 mL, 10 mL) [not available in U.S.]
Solution, intranasal:
Suprefact® [CAN]: 1mg/1mL (10 mL) [not available in U.S.]
Implant, subcutaneous:
Suprefact® [CAN] Depot: 6.3 mg, 9.45 mg [not available in U.S.]

BuSpar® [US/Can] *see* buspirone *on this page*

Buspirex [Can] *see* buspirone *on this page*

buspirone (byoo SPYE rone)
Sound-Alike/Look-Alike Issues
busPIRone may be confused with buPROPion
Synonyms buspirone hydrochloride
Tall-Man busPIRone
U.S./Canadian Brand Names Apo-Buspirone® [Can]; BuSpar® [US/Can]; Buspirex [Can]; Bustab® [Can]; Gen-Buspirone [Can]; Lin-Buspirone [Can]; Novo-Buspirone [Can]; Nu-Buspirone [Can]; PMS-Buspirone [Can]
Therapeutic Category Antianxiety Agent
Use Management of generalized anxiety disorder (GAD)
Usual Dosage Oral: Generalized anxiety disorder:
Children and Adolescents: Initial: 5 mg daily; increase in increments of 5 mg/day at weekly intervals as needed, to a maximum dose of 60 mg/day divided into 2-3 doses
Adults: 15 mg/day (7.5 mg twice daily); may increase in increments of 5 mg/day every 2-4 days to a maximum of 60 mg/day; target dose for most people is 30 mg/day (15 mg twice daily)
Dosage Forms
Tablet: 5 mg, 7.5 mg, 10 mg, 15 mg, 30 mg
BuSpar®: 5 mg, 10 mg, 15 mg, 30 mg

buspirone hydrochloride *see* buspirone *on this page*

Bustab® [Can] *see* buspirone *on this page*

busulfan (byoo SUL fan)
Sound-Alike/Look-Alike Issues
busulfan may be confused with Butalan®
Myleran® may be confused with Leukeran®, melphalan, Mylicon®
Synonyms NSC-750
U.S./Canadian Brand Names Busulfex® [US/Can]; Myleran® [US/Can]
Therapeutic Category Antineoplastic Agent
Use
Oral: Chronic myelogenous leukemia (CML); conditioning regimens for bone marrow transplantation
I.V.: Combination therapy with cyclophosphamide as a conditioning regimen prior to allogeneic hematopoietic progenitor cell transplantation for chronic myelogenous leukemia
Usual Dosage
Children:
For remission induction of CML: Oral: 0.06-0.12 mg/kg/day **or** 1.8-4.6 mg/m^2/day; titrate dosage to maintain leukocyte count above 40,000/mm^3; reduce dosage by 50% if the leukocyte count reaches 30,000-40,000/mm^3; discontinue drug if counts fall to ≤20,000/mm^3
BMT marrow-ablative conditioning regimen:
Oral: 1 mg/kg/dose (ideal body weight) every 6 hours for 16 doses
I.V.:
≤12 kg: 1.1 mg/kg/dose (ideal body weight) every 6 hours for 16 doses
>12 kg: 0.8 mg/kg/dose (ideal body weight) every 6 hours for 16 doses
Adjust dose to desired AUC [1125 μmol(min)] using the following formula:
Adjusted dose (mg) = Actual dose (mg) x [target AUC μmol(min) / actual AUC μmol(min)]
Adults:
For remission induction of CML: Oral: 4-8 mg/day (may be as high as 12 mg/day); Maintenance doses: 1-4 mg/day to 2 mg/week to maintain WBC 10,000-20,000 cells/mm^3
BMT marrow-ablative conditioning regimen:
Oral: 1 mg/kg/dose (ideal body weight) every 6 hours for 16 doses
(Continued)

busulfan (Continued)

I.V.: 0.8 mg/kg (ideal body weight or actual body weight, whichever is lower) every 6 hours for 4 days (a total of 16 doses)

Dosage Forms
Injection, solution:
Busulfex®: 6 mg/mL (10 mL)
Tablet:
Myleran®: 2 mg

Busulfex® [US/Can] *see* busulfan *on previous page*

butabarbital (byoo ta BAR bi tal)

Sound-Alike/Look-Alike Issues
butabarbital may be confused with butalbital
U.S./Canadian Brand Names Butisol Sodium® [US]
Therapeutic Category Barbiturate
Controlled Substance C-III
Use Sedative; hypnotic
Usual Dosage Oral:
Children: Preoperative sedation: 2-6 mg/kg/dose (maximum: 100 mg)
Adults:
Sedative: 15-30 mg 3-4 times/day
Hypnotic: 50-100 mg
Preop: 50-100 mg 1-1¹/₂ hours before surgery
Dosage Forms
Elixir:
Butisol Sodium®: 30 mg/5 mL
Tablet:
Butisol Sodium®: 30 mg, 50 mg

Butalan® (Discontinued)

butalbital, acetaminophen, and caffeine (byoo TAL bi tal, a seet a MIN oh fen, & KAF een)

Sound-Alike/Look-Alike Issues
Fioricet® may be confused with Fiorinal®, Lorcet®
Repan® may be confused with Riopan®
Synonyms acetaminophen, butalbital, and caffeine
U.S./Canadian Brand Names Anolor 300 [US]; Dolgic® LQ [US]; Dolgic® Plus [US]; Esgic-Plus™ [US]; Esgic® [US]; Fioricet® [US]; Medigesic® [US]; Repan® [US]; Zebutal™ [US]
Therapeutic Category Barbiturate/Analgesic
Use Relief of the symptomatic complex of tension or muscle contraction headache
Usual Dosage Oral: Adults: 1-2 tablets or capsules (or 15-30 mL elixir) every 4 hours; not to exceed 6 tablets or capsules (or 180 mL elixir) daily
Dosage Forms
Capsule:
Anolor 300, Esgic®, Medigesic®: Butalbital 50 mg, acetaminophen 325 mg, and caffeine 40 mg
Dolgic® Plus: Butalbital 50 mg, acetaminophen 750 mg, and caffeine 40 mg
Esgic-Plus™, Zebutal™: Butalbital 50 mg, acetaminophen 500 mg, and caffeine 40 mg
Solution:
Dolgic® LQ: Butalbital 50 mg, acetaminophen 325 mg, and caffeine 40 mg per 15 mL
Tablet: Butalbital 50 mg, acetaminophen 325 mg, and caffeine 40 mg; butalbital 50 mg, acetaminophen 500 mg, and caffeine 40 mg
Esgic®, Fioricet®, Repan®: Butalbital 50 mg, acetaminophen 325 mg, and caffeine 40 mg
Esgic-Plus™: Butalbital 50 mg, acetaminophen 500 mg, and caffeine 40 mg

butalbital, acetaminophen, caffeine, and codeine

(byoo TAL bi tal, a seet a MIN oh fen, KAF een, & KOE deen)
Sound-Alike/Look-Alike Issues
Fioricet® may be confused with Fiorinal®, Lorcet®
Synonyms acetaminophen, caffeine, codeine, and butalbital; caffeine, acetaminophen, butalbital, and codeine; codeine, acetaminophen, butalbital, and caffeine
U.S./Canadian Brand Names Fioricet® with Codeine [US]; Phrenilin® with Caffeine and Codeine [US]
Therapeutic Category Analgesic Combination (Opioid); Barbiturate
Controlled Substance C-III

Use Relief of symptoms of complex tension (muscle contraction) headache
Usual Dosage Oral: Adults: 1-2 capsules every 4 hours. Total daily dosage should not exceed 6 capsules.
Dosage Forms
Capsule: Butalbital 50 mg, acetaminophen 325 mg, caffeine 40 mg, and codeine 30 mg
Fioricet® with Codeine: Butalbital 50 mg, acetaminophen 325 mg, caffeine 40 mg, and codeine 30 mg
Phrenilin® with Caffeine and Codeine: Butalbital 50 mg, acetaminophen 325 mg, caffeine 40 mg, and codeine 30 mg

butalbital and acetaminophen (byoo TAL bi tal & a seet a MIN oh fen)
Synonyms acetaminophen and butalbital
U.S./Canadian Brand Names Bupap [US]; Cephadyn [US]; Phrenilin® Forte [US]; Phrenilin® [US]; Promacet [US]; Sedapap® [US]
Therapeutic Category Analgesic, Miscellaneous; Barbiturate
Use Relief of the symptomatic complex of tension or muscle contraction headache
Usual Dosage Oral: Adults: One tablet/capsule every 4 hours as needed (maximum dose: 6 tablets/day)
Phrenilin®: 1-2 tablets every 4 hours as needed (maximum 6 tablets in 24 hours)
Dosage Forms
Capsule:
Phrenilin® Forte: Butalbital 50 mg and acetaminophen 650 mg
Tablet:
Phrenilin®: Butalbital 50 mg and acetaminophen 325 mg
Bupap, Cephadyn, Promacet, Sedapap®: Butalbital 50 mg and acetaminophen 650 mg

butalbital, aspirin, and caffeine (byoo TAL bi tal, AS pir in, & KAF een)
Sound-Alike/Look-Alike Issues
Fiorinal® may be confused with Fioricet®, Florical®, Florinef®
Synonyms aspirin, caffeine, and butalbital; butalbital compound
U.S./Canadian Brand Names Fiorinal® [US/Can]
Therapeutic Category Barbiturate/Analgesic
Controlled Substance C-III
Use Relief of the symptomatic complex of tension or muscle contraction headache
Usual Dosage Oral: Adults: 1-2 tablets or capsules every 4 hours; not to exceed 6/day
Dosage Forms
Capsule: Butalbital 50 mg, aspirin 325 mg, and caffeine 40 mg
Fiorinal®: Butalbital 50 mg, aspirin 325 mg, and caffeine 40 mg
Tablet: Butalbital 50 mg, aspirin 325 mg, and caffeine 40 mg

butalbital, aspirin, caffeine, and codeine (byoo TAL bi tal, AS pir in, KAF een, & KOE deen)
Sound-Alike/Look-Alike Issues
Fiorinal® may be confused with Fioricet®, Florical®, Florinef®
Phrenilin® may be confused with Phenergan®, Trinalin®
Synonyms aspirin, caffeine, codeine, and butalbital; butalbital compound and codeine; codeine and butalbital compound; codeine, butalbital, aspirin, and caffeine
U.S./Canadian Brand Names Ascomp® with Codeine [US]; Fiorinal® With Codeine [US]; Fiorinal®-C 1/2 [Can]; Fiorinal®-C 1/4 [Can]; Tecnal C 1/2 [Can]; Tecnal C 1/4 [Can]
Therapeutic Category Analgesic, Narcotic; Barbiturate
Controlled Substance C-III
Use Mild-to-moderate pain when sedation is needed
Usual Dosage Oral: Adults: 1-2 capsules every 4 hours as needed for pain; up to 6/day
Dosage Forms
Capsule: Butalbital 50 mg, aspirin 325 mg, caffeine 40 mg, and codeine 30 mg
Ascomp® with Codeine, Fiorinal® with Codeine: Butalbital 50 mg, aspirin 325 mg, caffeine 40 mg, and codeine 30 mg

butalbital compound see butalbital, aspirin, and caffeine on this page

butalbital compound and codeine see butalbital, aspirin, caffeine, and codeine on this page

butamben, tetracaine, and benzocaine see benzocaine, butamben, and tetracaine on page 103

butenafine (byoo TEN a feen)
Sound-Alike/Look-Alike Issues
Lotrimin® may be confused with Lotrisone®, Otrivin®
(Continued)

butenafine *(Continued)*

Synonyms butenafine hydrochloride

U.S./Canadian Brand Names Lotrimin® Ultra™ [US-OTC]; Mentax® [US]

Therapeutic Category Antifungal Agent

Use Topical treatment of tinea pedis (athlete's foot), tinea cruris (jock itch), tinea corporis (ringworm), and tinea versicolor

Usual Dosage Topical: Children >12 years and Adults:

Tinea corporis, tinea cruris, or tinea versicolor: Apply once daily for 2 weeks to affected area and surrounding skin

Tinea pedis: Apply once daily for 4 weeks or twice daily for 7 days to affected area and surrounding skin (7-day regimen may have lower efficacy)

Dosage Forms

Cream:

Lotrimin® Ultra™ [OTC]: 1% (12 g, 24 g)

Mentax®: 1% (15 g, 30 g)

butenafine hydrochloride *see* butenafine *on previous page*

Buticaps® *(Discontinued)*

Butisol Sodium® [US] *see* butabarbital *on page 130*

butoconazole *(byoo toe KOE na zole)*

Synonyms butoconazole nitrate

U.S./Canadian Brand Names Femstat® One [Can]; Gynazole-1® [US/Can]

Therapeutic Category Antifungal Agent

Use Local treatment of vulvovaginal candidiasis

Usual Dosage Adults: Female: Gynazole-1®: Insert 1 applicatorful (~5 g) intravaginally as a single dose; treatment may need to be extended for up to 6 days in pregnant women (use in pregnancy during 2nd or 3rd trimester only)

Dosage Forms

Cream, vaginal:

Gynazole-1®: 2% (5 g)

butoconazole nitrate *see* butoconazole *on this page*

butorphanol *(byoo TOR fa nole)*

Sound-Alike/Look-Alike Issues

Stadol® may be confused with Haldol®, sotalol

Synonyms butorphanol tartrate

U.S./Canadian Brand Names Apo-Butorphanol® [Can]; PMS-Butorphanol [Can]; Stadol® [US]

Therapeutic Category Analgesic, Narcotic

Controlled Substance C-IV

Use

Parenteral: Management of moderate-to-severe pain; preoperative medication; supplement to balanced anesthesia; management of pain during labor

Nasal spray: Management of moderate-to-severe pain, including migraine headache pain

Usual Dosage Note: These are guidelines and do not represent the maximum doses that may be required in all patients. Doses should be titrated to pain relief/prevention. Butorphanol has an analgesic ceiling. Adults:

Parenteral:

Acute pain (moderate to severe):

I.M.: Initial: 2 mg, may repeat every 3-4 hours as needed; usual range: 1-4 mg every 3-4 hours as needed

I.V.: Initial: 1 mg, may repeat every 3-4 hours as needed; usual range: 0.5-2 mg every 3-4 hours as needed

Preoperative medication: I.M.: 2 mg 60-90 minutes before surgery

Supplement to balanced anesthesia: I.V.: 2 mg shortly before induction and/or an incremental dose of 0.5-1 mg (up to 0.06 mg/kg), depending on previously administered sedative, analgesic, and hypnotic medications

Pain during labor (fetus >37 weeks gestation and no signs of fetal distress):

I.M., I.V.: 1-2 mg; may repeat in 4 hours

Note: Alternative analgesia should be used for pain associated with delivery or if delivery is anticipated within 4 hours

Nasal spray:

Moderate to severe pain (including migraine headache pain): Initial: 1 spray (~1 mg per spray) in 1 nostril; if adequate pain relief is not achieved within 60-90 minutes, an additional 1 spray in 1 nostril may be given; may repeat initial dose sequence in 3-4 hours after the last dose as needed

Alternatively, an initial dose of 2 mg (1 spray in each nostril) may be used in patients who will be able to remain recumbent (in the event drowsiness or dizziness occurs); additional 2 mg doses should not be given for 3-4 hours

Note: In some clinical trials, an initial dose of 2 mg (as 2 doses 1 hour apart or 2 mg initially - 1 spray in each nostril) has been used, followed by 1 mg in 1 hour; side effects were greater at these dosages

Dosage Forms
Injection, solution [preservative free]: 1 mg/mL (1 mL); 2 mg/mL (1 mL, 2 mL)
Stadol®: 1 mg/mL (1 mL); 2 mg/mL (1 mL, 2 mL)
Injection, solution [with preservative]: 2 mg/mL (10 mL)
Stadol®: 2 mg/mL (10 mL)
Solution, intranasal [spray]: 10 mg/mL (2.5 mL)

butorphanol tartrate *see* butorphanol *on previous page*

B-Vex [US] *see* brompheniramine *on page 120*

B vitamin combinations *see* vitamin B complex combinations *on page 894*

BW-430C *see* lamotrigine *on page 490*

BW524W91 *see* emtricitabine *on page 295*

Byclomine® Injection *(Discontinued)* *see* dicyclomine *on page 255*

Bydramine® Cough Syrup *(Discontinued)* *see* diphenhydramine *on page 265*

Byetta™ [US] *see* exenatide *on page 338*

C1H *see* alemtuzumab *on page 27*

C2B8 *see* rituximab *on page 762*

C2B8 monoclonal antibody *see* rituximab *on page 762*

C7E3 *see* abciximab *on page 3*

C8-CCK *see* sincalide *on page 787*

311C90 *see* zolmitriptan *on page 908*

C225 *see* cetuximab *on page 170*

cabergoline (ca BER goe leen)
U.S./Canadian Brand Names Dostinex® [US/Can]
Therapeutic Category Ergot-like Derivative
Use Treatment of hyperprolactinemic disorders, either idiopathic or due to pituitary adenomas
Usual Dosage Oral: Initial dose: 0.25 mg twice weekly; the dose may be increased by 0.25 mg twice weekly up to a maximum of 1 mg twice weekly according to the patient's serum prolactin level. Dosage increases should not occur more rapidly than every 4 weeks. Once a normal serum prolactin level is maintained for 6 months, the dose may be discontinued and prolactin levels monitored to determine if cabergoline is still required. The durability of efficacy beyond 24 months of therapy has not been established.
Dosage Forms
Tablet: 0.5 mg
Dostinex®: 0.5 mg

Ca-DTPA *see* diethylene triamine penta-acetic acid *on page 256*

Caduet® [US/Can] *see* amlodipine and atorvastatin *on page 45*

CaEDTA *see* edetate calcium disodium *on page 290*

Caelyx® [Can] *see* doxorubicin (liposomal) *on page 281*

Cafatine-PB® *(Discontinued)* *see* ergotamine *on page 307*

Cafcit® [US] *see* caffeine *on this page*

Cafergor® [Can] *see* ergotamine and caffeine *on page 307*

Cafergot® [US] *see* ergotamine and caffeine *on page 307*

Cafetrate® *(Discontinued)* *see* ergotamine *on page 307*

caffeine (KAF een)
Synonyms caffeine and sodium benzoate; caffeine citrate; sodium benzoate and caffeine
U.S./Canadian Brand Names Cafcit® [US]; Enerjets [US-OTC]; No Doz® Maximum Strength [US-OTC]; Vivarin® [US-OTC]
Therapeutic Category Stimulant
Use
Caffeine citrate: Treatment of idiopathic apnea of prematurity
(Continued)

caffeine *(Continued)*

Caffeine and sodium benzoate: Treatment of acute respiratory depression (not a preferred agent)

Caffeine [OTC labeling]: Restore mental alertness or wakefulness when experiencing fatigue

Usual Dosage

Note: Caffeine citrate should not be interchanged with the caffeine sodium benzoate formulation.

Caffeine citrate: Neonates: Apnea of prematurity: Oral, I.V.:

Loading dose: 10-20 mg/kg as caffeine citrate (5-10 mg/kg as caffeine base). If theophylline has been administered to the patient within the previous 3 days, a full or modified loading dose (50% to 75% of a loading dose) may be given.

Maintenance dose: 5 mg/kg/day as caffeine citrate (2.5 mg/kg/day as caffeine base) once daily starting 24 hours after the loading dose. Maintenance dose is adjusted based on patient's response and serum caffeine concentrations.

Caffeine and sodium benzoate:

Children: Stimulant: I.M., I.V., SubQ: 8 mg/kg every 4 hours as needed

Children ≥12 years and Adults: OTC labeling (stimulant): Oral: 100-200 mg every 3-4 hours as needed

Adults: Respiratory depression: I.M., I.V.: 250 mg as a single dose; may repeat as needed. Maximum single dose should be limited to 500 mg; maximum amount in any 24-hour period should generally be limited to 2500 mg.

Dosage Forms

Caplet:

NoDoz® Maximum Strength [OTC], Vivarin® [OTC]: 200 mg

Injection, solution [preservative free]:

Cafcit®: 20 mg/mL (3 mL)

Injection, solution [with sodium benzoate]: Caffeine 125 mg/mL and sodium benzoate 125 mg/mL (2 mL); caffeine 121 mg/mL and sodium benzoate 129 mg/mL (2 mL)

Lozenge:

Enerjets® [OTC]: 75 mg

Solution, oral [preservative free]:

Cafcit®: 20 mg/mL

Tablet: 200 mg

Vivarin® [OTC]: 200 mg

caffeine, acetaminophen, and aspirin *see* acetaminophen, aspirin, and caffeine *on page 9*

caffeine, acetaminophen, butalbital, and codeine *see* butalbital, acetaminophen, caffeine, and codeine *on page 130*

caffeine and ergotamine *see* ergotamine and caffeine *on page 307*

caffeine and sodium benzoate *see* caffeine *on previous page*

caffeine, aspirin, and acetaminophen *see* acetaminophen, aspirin, and caffeine *on page 9*

caffeine citrate *see* caffeine *on previous page*

caffeine, dihydrocodeine, and acetaminophen *see* acetaminophen, caffeine, and dihydrocodeine *on page 10*

caffeine, hydrocodone, chlorpheniramine, phenylephrine, and acetaminophen *see* hydrocodone, chlorpheniramine, phenylephrine, acetaminophen, and caffeine *on page 431*

caffeine, orphenadrine, and aspirin *see* orphenadrine, aspirin, and caffeine *on page 634*

caffeine, propoxyphene, and aspirin *see* propoxyphene, aspirin, and caffeine *on page 723*

Caladryl® Clear [US-OTC] *see* pramoxine *on page 706*

CalaMycin® Cool and Clear [US-OTC] *see* pramoxine *on page 706*

Calan® [US/Can] *see* verapamil *on page 887*

Calan® SR [US] *see* verapamil *on page 887*

Calcarb 600 [US-OTC] *see* calcium carbonate *on page 138*

Calci-Chew® [US-OTC] *see* calcium carbonate *on page 138*

Calciday-667® *(Discontinued)* *see* calcium carbonate *on page 138*

Calciferol™ [US] *see* ergocalciferol *on page 305*

Calciferol™ Injection *(Discontinued)* *see* ergocalciferol *on page 305*

Calcijex® [US/Can] *see* calcitriol *on next page*

Calcimar® [Can] *see* calcitonin *on next page*

Calcimar® *(Discontinued)* *see* calcitonin *on next page*

Calci-Mix® [US-OTC] *see* calcium carbonate *on page 138*

Calcionate [US-OTC] *see calcium glubionate on page 140*

calcipotriene (kal si POE try een)
U.S./Canadian Brand Names Dovonex® [US]
Therapeutic Category Antipsoriatic Agent
Use Treatment of plaque psoriasis
Usual Dosage Topical: Adults: Apply in a thin film to the affected skin twice daily and rub in gently and completely
Dosage Forms
Cream:
Dovonex® [OTC]: 0.005% (60 g, 120 g)
Solution, topical:
Dovonex® [OTC]: 0.005% (60 mL)

calcipotriene and betamethasone (kal si POE try een & bay ta METH a sone)
Synonyms betamethasone dipropionate and calcipotriene hydrate; calcipotriol and betamethasone dipropionate
U.S./Canadian Brand Names Dovobet® [Can]; Taclonex® [US]
Therapeutic Category Corticosteroid, Topical; Vitamin D Analog
Use Treatment of psoriasis vulgaris
Usual Dosage Topical: Adults: Psoriasis vulgaris: Apply to affected area once daily for up to 4 weeks (maximum recommended dose: 100 g/week). Application to >30% of body surface area is not recommended.
Dosage Forms [CAN] = Canadian brand name
Cream, topical:
Dovobet® [CAN]: Calcipotriol 50 mcg and betamethasone 0.5 mg per gram (3 g, 30 g, 60 g, 100 g, 120 g) [not available in the U.S.]
Ointment, topical:
Taclonex®: Calcipotriene 0.005% and betamethasone 0.064% (60 g, 100 g)

calcipotriol and betamethasone dipropionate *see calcipotriene and betamethasone on this page*

Calcite-500 [Can] *see calcium carbonate on page 138*

calcitonin (kal si TOE nin)
Sound-Alike/Look-Alike Issues
calcitonin may be confused with calcitriol
Miacalcin® may be confused with Micatin®
Synonyms calcitonin (salmon)
U.S./Canadian Brand Names Apo-Calcitonin® [Can]; Calcimar® [Can]; Caltine® [Can]; Fortical® [US]; Miacalcin® NS [Can]; Miacalcin® [US]
Therapeutic Category Polypeptide Hormone
Use Calcitonin (salmon): Treatment of Paget disease of bone (osteitis deformans); adjunctive therapy for hypercalcemia; treatment of osteoporosis in women >5 years postmenopause
Usual Dosage Adults:
Paget disease (Miacalcin®): Initial: I.M., SubQ: 100 units/day; maintenance: 50 units/day or 50-100 units every 1-3 days
Hypercalcemia (Miacalcin®): Initial: I.M., SubQ: 4 units/kg every 12 hours; may increase up to 8 units/kg every 12 hours to a maximum of every 6 hours
Postmenopausal osteoporosis:
I.M., SubQ: Miacalcin®: 100 units/every other day
Intranasal: Fortical®, Miacalcin®: 200 units (1 spray) in one nostril daily
Dosage Forms
Injection, solution [calcitonin-salmon]:
Miacalcin®: 200 int. units/mL (2 mL)
Solution, intranasal [spray, calcitonin-salmon]:
Fortical®: 200 int. units/0.09 mL (3.7 mL)
Miacalcin®: 200 int. units/0.09 mL (3.7 mL)

calcitonin (salmon) *see calcitonin on this page*

Cal-Citrate® 250 [US-OTC] *see calcium citrate on page 140*

calcitriol (kal si TRYE ole)
Sound-Alike/Look-Alike Issues
calcitriol may be confused with calcifediol, Calciferol®, calcitonin
(Continued)

calcitriol *(Continued)*

Synonyms 1,25 dihydroxycholecalciferol

U.S./Canadian Brand Names Calcijex® [US/Can]; Rocaltrol® [US/Can]

Therapeutic Category Vitamin D Analog

Use Management of hypocalcemia in patients on chronic renal dialysis; management of secondary hyperparathyroidism in patients with chronic kidney disease (CKD); management of hypocalcemia in hypoparathyroidism and pseudohypoparathyroidism

Usual Dosage

Hypocalcemia in patients on chronic renal dialysis (manufacturer labeling): *Adults:*

Oral: 0.25 mcg/day or every other day (may require 0.5-1 mcg/day); increases should be made at 4- to 8-week intervals

I.V.: Initial: 1-2 mcg 3 times/week (0.02 mcg/kg) approximately every other day. Adjust dose at 2-4 week intervals; dosing range: 0.5-4 mcg 3 times/week

Hypocalcemia in hypoparathyroidism/pseudohypoparathyroidism (manufacturers labeling): Oral (evaluate dosage at 2- to 4-week intervals):

Children 1-5 years: 0.25-0.75 mcg once daily

Children ≥6 years and Adults: Initial: 0.25 mcg/day, range: 0.5-2 mcg once daily

Secondary hyperparathyroidism associated with moderate-to-severe CKD in patients not on dialysis (manufacturer labeling): Oral:

Children <3 years: Initial dose: 0.01-0.015 mcg/kg/day

Children ≥3 years and Adults: 0.25 mcg/day; may increase to 0.5 mcg/day

K/DOQI guidelines for vitamin D therapy in CKD:

Children:

CKD stage 2, 3: Oral:

<10 kg: 0.05 mcg every other day

10-20 kg: 0.1-0.15 mcg/day

>20 kg: 0.25 mcg/day

Note: Treatment should only be started with serum 25(OH) D >30 ng/mL, serum iPTH >70 pg/mL, serum calcium <10 mg/dL and serum phosphorus less than or equal to the age appropriate level.

CKD stage 4: Oral:

<10 kg: 0.05 mcg every other day

10-20 kg: 0.1-0.15 mcg/day

>20 kg: 0.25 mcg/day

Note: Treatment should only be started with serum 25(OH) D >30 ng/mL, serum iPTH >110 pg/mL, serum calcium <10 mg/dL and serum phosphorus less than or equal to the age appropriate level.

CKD stage 5: Oral, I.V.: **Note:** The following initial doses are based on plasma PTH and serum calcium levels for patients with serum phosphorus <5.5 mg/dL in adolescents or <6.5 in infants and children, and Ca-P product <55 in adolescents or <65 in infants and children <12 years. Adjust dose based on serum phosphate, calcium and PTH levels. Administer dose with each dialysis session (3 times/week). Intermittent I.V./oral administration is more effective than daily oral dosing.

Plasma PTH 300-500 pg/mL and serum Ca <10 mg/dL: 0.0075 mcg/kg (maximum: 0.25 mcg/day)

Plasma PTH >500-1000 pg/mL and serum Ca <10 mg/dL: 0.015 mcg/kg (maximum: 0.5 mcg/day)

Plasma PTH >1000 pg/mL and serum Ca <10.5 mg/dL: 0.025 mcg/kg (maximum: 1 mcg/day)

Adults:

CKD stage 3: Oral: 0.25 mcg/day. Treatment should only be started with serum 25(OH) D >30 ng/mL, serum iPTH >70 pg/mL, serum calcium <9.5 mg/dL and serum phosphorus <4.6 mg/dL

CKD stage 4: Oral: 0.25 mcg/day. Treatment should only be started with serum 25(OH) D >30 ng/mL, serum iPTH >110 pg/mL, serum calcium <9.5 mg/dL and serum phosphorus <4.6 mg/dL

CKD stage 5:

Peritoneal dialysis: Oral: Initial: 0.5-1 mcg 2-3 times/week or 0.25 mcg/day

Hemodialysis: **Note:** The following initial doses are based on plasma PTH and serum calcium levels for patients with serum phosphorus <5.5 mg/dL and Ca-P product <55. Adjust dose based on serum phosphate, calcium, and PTH levels. Intermittent I.V. administration may be more effective than daily oral dosing.

Plasma PTH 300-600 pg/mL and serum Ca <9.5 mg/dL: Oral, I.V.: 0.5-1.5 mcg

Plasma PTH 600-1000 pg/mL and serum Ca <9.5 mg/dL:

Oral: 1-4 mcg

I.V.: 1-3 mcg

Plasma PTH >1000 pg/mL and serum Ca <10 mg/dL:

Oral: 3-7 mcg

I.V.: 3-5 mcg

Dosage Forms

Capsule: 0.25 mcg, 0.5 mcg

Rocaltrol®: 0.25 mcg, 0.5 mcg

Injection, solution: 1 mcg/mL (1 mL)
Calcijex®: 1 mcg/mL (1 mL)
Solution, oral: 1 mcg/mL
Rocaltrol®: 1 mcg/mL

calcium acetate (KAL see um AS e tate)

Sound-Alike/Look-Alike Issues
PhosLo® may be confused with Phos-Flur®, ProSom™
U.S./Canadian Brand Names PhosLo® [US]
Therapeutic Category Electrolyte Supplement, Oral
Use
Oral: Control of hyperphosphatemia in end-stage renal failure; does not promote aluminum absorption
I.V.: Calcium supplementation in parenteral nutrition therapy
Usual Dosage
Dietary Reference Intake:
0-6 months: 210 mg/day
7-12 months: 270 mg/day
1-3 years: 500 mg/day
4-8 years: 800 mg/day
Adults, Male/Female:
9-18 years: 1300 mg/day
19-50 years: 1000 mg/day
≥51 years: 1200 mg/day
Female: Pregnancy/Lactating: Same as for Adults, Male/Female

Oral: Adults, on dialysis: Initial: 1334 mg with each meal, can be increased gradually to bring the serum phosphate value <6 mg/dL as long as hypercalcemia does not develop (usual dose: 2001-2868 mg calcium acetate with each meal); do not give additional calcium supplements
I.V.: Dose is dependent on the requirements of the individual patient; in central venous total parental nutrition (TPN), calcium is administered at a concentration of 5 mEq (10 mL)/L of TPN solution; the additive maintenance dose in neonatal TPN is 0.5 mEq calcium/kg/day (1 mL/kg/day)
Neonates: 70-200 mg/kg/day
Infants and Children: 70-150 mg/kg/day
Adolescents: 18-35 mg/kg/day
Dosage Forms
Gelcap:
PhosLo®: 667 mg [169 mg]

calcium acetate and aluminum sulfate see aluminum sulfate and calcium acetate on page 38

calcium acetylhomotaurinate see acamprosate on page 4

calcium and risedronate see risedronate and calcium on page 760

calcium and vitamin D (KAL see um & VYE ta min dee)

Synonyms vitamin D and calcium carbonate
U.S./Canadian Brand Names Cal-CYUM [US-OTC]; Caltrate® 600+ Soy™ [US-OTC]; Caltrate® 600+D [US-OTC]; Caltrate® ColonHealth™ [US-OTC]; Chew-Cal [US-OTC]; Liqua-Cal [US-OTC]; Os-Cal® 500+D [US-OTC]; Oysco 500+D [US-OTC]; Oysco D [US-OTC]; Oyst-Cal-D 500 [US-OTC]; Oyst-Cal-D [US-OTC]
Therapeutic Category Calcium Salt; Electrolyte Supplement, Oral; Vitamin, Fat Soluble
Use Dietary supplement, antacid
Usual Dosage Oral: Adults: Refer to individual monographs for dietary reference intake.
Dosage Forms
Capsule, softgel: Calcium 500 mg and vitamin D 500 int. units; calcium 600 mg and vitamin D 100 int. units; calcium 600 mg and vitamin D 200 int. units
Liqua-Cal: Calcium 600 mg and vitamin D 200 int. units
Tablet: Calcium 250 mg and vitamin D 125 int. units; calcium 500 mg and vitamin D 125 int. units; calcium 500 mg and vitamin D 200 int. units; calcium 600 mg and vitamin D 125 int. units; calcium 600 mg and vitamin D 200 int. units
Caltrate® 600+D: Calcium 600 mg and vitamin D 200 int. units
Caltrate® 600+ Soy™: Calcium 600 mg and vitamin D 200 int. units
Caltrate® ColonHealth™: Calcium 600 mg and vitamin D 200 int. units
Oysco D: Calcium 250 mg and vitamin D 125 int. units
Oysco 500+D: Calcium 500 mg and vitamin D 200 int. units
Oyst-Cal-D: Calcium 250 mg and vitamin D 125 int. units
Oyst-Cal-D 500: Calcium 500 mg and vitamin D 200 int. units
Tablet, chewable: Calcium 500 mg and vitamin D 100 int. units; calcium 600 mg and vitamin D 400 int. units
Os-Cal® 500+D: Calcium 500 mg and vitamin D 400 int. units
(Continued)

calcium and vitamin D *(Continued)*
Wafer, chewable:
Cal-CYUM: Calcium 519 mg and vitamin D 150 int. units (50s)
Chew-Cal: Calcium 333 mg and vitamin D 40 int. units (100s, 250s)

calcium carbonate (KAL see um KAR bun ate)
Sound-Alike/Look-Alike Issues
Florical® may be confused with Fiorinal®
Mylanta® may be confused with Mynatal®
Nephro-Calci® may be confused with Nephrocaps®
Os-Cal® may be confused with Asacol®
U.S./Canadian Brand Names Alcalak [US-OTC]; Alka-Mints® [US-OTC]; Apo-Cal® [Can]; Cal-Gest [US-OTC]; Cal-Mint [US-OTC]; Calcarb 600 [US-OTC]; Calci-Chew® [US-OTC]; Calci-Mix® [US-OTC]; Calcite-500 [Can]; Caltrate® 600 [US-OTC]; Caltrate® Select [Can]; Caltrate® [Can]; Children's Pepto [US-OTC]; Chooz® [US-OTC]; Florical® [US-OTC]; Maalox® Regular Chewable [US-OTC]; Mylanta® Children's [US-OTC]; Nephro-Calci® [US-OTC]; Nutralox® [US-OTC]; Os-Cal® [Can]; Oysco 500 [US-OTC]; Oyst-Cal 500 [US-OTC]; Rolaids® Softchews [US-OTC]; Titralac™ [US-OTC]; Tums® E-X [US-OTC]; Tums® Extra Strength Sugar Free [US-OTC]; Tums® Smoothies™ [US-OTC]; Tums® Ultra [US-OTC]; Tums® [US-OTC]
Therapeutic Category Antacid; Electrolyte Supplement, Oral
Use As an antacid; treatment and prevention of calcium deficiency or hyperphosphatemia (eg, osteoporosis, osteomalacia, mild/moderate renal insufficiency, hypoparathyroidism, postmenopausal osteoporosis, rickets); has been used to bind phosphate
Usual Dosage Oral (dosage is in terms of elemental calcium):
Dietary Reference Intake:
0-6 months: 210 mg/day
7-12 months: 270 mg/day
1-3 years: 500 mg/day
4-8 years: 800 mg/day
Adults, Male/Female:
9-18 years: 1300 mg/day
19-50 years: 1000 mg/day
≥51 years: 1200 mg/day
Female: Pregnancy/Lactating: Same as for Adults, Male/Female
Hypocalcemia (dose depends on clinical condition and serum calcium level): Dose expressed in mg of **elemental calcium**
Neonates: 50-150 mg/kg/day in 4-6 divided doses; not to exceed 1 g/day
Children: 45-65 mg/kg/day in 4 divided doses
Adults: 1-2 g or more/day in 3-4 divided doses
Antacid:
Children 2-5 years (24-47 lb): Elemental calcium 161 mg as needed; maximum 483 mg per 24 hours
Children 6-11 years (48-95 lb): Elemental calcium 322 mg as needed; maximum: 966 mg per 24 hours
Adults: Dosage based on acid-neutralizing capacity of specific product; generally, 1-2 tablets or 5-10 mL every 2 hours; maximum: 7000 mg calcium carbonate per 24 hours; specific product labeling should be consulted
Dietary supplementation: Adults: 500 mg to 2 g divided 2-4 times/day
Osteoporosis: Adults >51 years: 1200 mg/day
Dosage Forms
Capsule: 364 mg, 1250 mg
Calci-Mix® [OTC]: 1250 mg
Florical® [OTC]: 364 mg
Gum, chewing: 250 mg (30s)
Chooz® [OTC]: 500 mg
Powder: 4000 mg/teaspoonful
Suspension, oral: 1250 mg/5 mL
Tablet: 1250 mg, 1500 mg
Calcarb 600 [OTC], Caltrate® 600 [OTC], Nephro-Calci® [OTC]: 1500 mg
Florical® [OTC]: 364 mg
Oysco 500 [OTC], Oyst-Cal 500 [OTC]: 1250 mg
Tablet, chewable: 500 mg, 650 mg, 750 mg
Alcalak [OTC], Nutralox® [OTC], Titralac™ [OTC]: 420 mg
Alka-Mints® [OTC]: 850 mg
Cal-Gest [OTC], Tums® [OTC]: 500 mg
Calci-Chew® [OTC]: 1250 mg
Cal-Mint [OTC]: 650 mg
Children's Pepto [OTC], Mylanta® Children's [OTC]: 400 mg

Maalox® Regular [OTC]: 600 mg
Tums® E-X [OTC], Tums® Extra Strength Sugar Free [OTC], Tums® Smoothies™ [OTC]: 750 mg
Tums® Ultra® [OTC]: 1000 mg
Tablet, softchew: 1177 mg
Rolaids® [OTC]: 1177 mg

calcium carbonate and etidronate disodium see etidronate and calcium on page 334

calcium carbonate and magnesium hydroxide
(KAL see um KAR bun ate & mag NEE zhum hye DROKS ide)
Sound-Alike/Look-Alike Issues
Mylanta® may be confused with Mynatal®
Synonyms magnesium hydroxide and calcium carbonate
U.S./Canadian Brand Names Mi-Acid™ Double Strength [US-OTC]; Mylanta® Gelcaps® [US-OTC]; Mylanta® Supreme [US-OTC]; Mylanta® Ultra [US-OTC]; Rolaids® Extra Strength [US-OTC]; Rolaids® [US-OTC]
Therapeutic Category Antacid
Use Hyperacidity
Usual Dosage Oral: Adults: 2-4 tablets between meals, at bedtime, or as directed by healthcare provider
Dosage Forms
Gelcap:
Mylanta® Gelcaps® [OTC]: Calcium carbonate 550 mg and magnesium hydroxide 125 mg
Liquid:
Mylanta® Supreme [OTC]: Calcium carbonate 400 mg and magnesium hydroxide 135 mg per 5 mL
Tablet, chewable: Calcium carbonate 550 mg and magnesium hydroxide 110 mg; calcium carbonate 675 mg and magnesium hydroxide 135 mg; calcium carbonate 700 mg and magnesium hydroxide 300 mg
Mi-Acid™ Double Strength [OTC], Mylanta® Ultra [OTC]: Calcium carbonate 700 mg and magnesium hydroxide 300 mg
Rolaids® [OTC]: Calcium carbonate 550 mg and magnesium hydroxide 110 mg
Rolaids® Extra Strength [OTC]: Calcium carbonate 675 mg and magnesium hydroxide 135 mg

calcium carbonate and simethicone (KAL see um KAR bun ate & sye METH i kone)
Synonyms simethicone and calcium carbonate
U.S./Canadian Brand Names Gas Ban™ [US-OTC]; Titralac® Plus [US-OTC]
Therapeutic Category Antacid; Antiflatulent
Use Relief of acid indigestion, heartburn
Usual Dosage Oral (OTC labeling): Adults: Two tablets every 2-3 hours as needed (maximum: 19 tablets/24 hours)
Dosage Forms
Tablet, chewable:
Gas Ban™ [OTC]: Calcium carbonate 300 mg and simethicone 40 mg
Titralac® Plus [OTC]: Calcium carbonate 420 mg and simethicone 21 mg

calcium carbonate, magnesium hydroxide, and famotidine see famotidine, calcium carbonate, and magnesium hydroxide on page 342

calcium chloride (KAL see um KLOR ide)
Sound-Alike/Look-Alike Issues
Dosing issues:
Calcium chloride may be confused with calcium gluconate
Confusion with the different intravenous salt forms of calcium has occurred. There is a threefold difference in the primary cation concentration between calcium chloride (in which 1g = 13.6 mEq [270 mg] of elemental Ca++) and calcium gluconate (in which 1g = 4.65 mEq [90 mg] of elemental Ca++).
Prescribers should specify which salt form is desired. Dosages should be expressed either as mEq, mg, or grams of the salt form.
Therapeutic Category Electrolyte Supplement, Oral
Use Treatment of acute symptomatic hypocalcemia; cardiac disturbances of hyperkalemia or hypocalcemia; emergent treatment of hypocalcemic tetany; treatment of severe hypermagnesemia
Usual Dosage Note: Calcium chloride has 3 times more elemental calcium than calcium gluconate. Calcium chloride is 27% elemental calcium; calcium gluconate is 9% elemental calcium. One gram of calcium chloride is equal to 270 mg of elemental calcium; one gram of calcium gluconate is equal to 90 mg of elemental calcium. Dosages are expressed in terms of the calcium chloride salt based on a solution concentration of 100 mg/mL (10%) containing 1.4 mEq (27.3 mg)/mL elemental calcium.

Cardiac arrest in the presence of hyperkalemia or hypocalcemia, magnesium toxicity: I.V.:
Infants and Children: 20 mg/kg; may repeat in 10 minutes if necessary
(Continued)

calcium chloride (Continued)

Adolescents and Adults: 2-4 mg/kg, repeated every 10 minutes if necessary

Hypocalcemia: I.V.:

Children (manufacturer's recommendation): 2.7-5 mg/kg/dose every 4-6 hours

Alternative pediatric dosing: Infants and Children: 10-20 mg/kg/dose, repeat every 4-6 hours if needed

Adults: 500 mg to 1 g/dose repeated every 4-6 hours if needed

Hypocalcemic tetany: I.V.:

Neonates: Divided doses totaling approximately 170 mg/kg/24 hours

Infants and Children: 10 mg/kg over 5-10 minutes; may repeat after 6-8 hours or follow with an infusion with a maximum dose of 200 mg/kg/day; alternatively, higher doses of 35-50 mg/kg/dose repeated every 6-8 hours have been used

Adults: 1 g over 10-30 minutes; may repeat after 6 hours

Hypocalcemia secondary to citrated blood transfusion: I.V.: **Note:** Routine administration of calcium, in the absence of signs/symptoms of hypocalcemia, is generally not recommended. A number of recommendations have been published seeking to address potential hypocalcemia during massive transfusion of citrated blood; however, many practitioners recommend replacement only as guided by clinical evidence of hypocalcemia and/or serial monitoring of ionized calcium.

Neonates, Infants, and Children: Give 32 mg (0.45 mEq elemental calcium) for each 100 mL citrated blood infused

Adults: 200-500 mg per 500 mL of citrated blood (infused into another vein)

Dosage Forms

Injection, solution [preservative free]: 10% (10 mL)

Injection, solution [with preservative]: 10% (10 mL)

calcium citrate (KAL see um SIT rate)

Sound-Alike/Look-Alike Issues

Citracal® may be confused with Citrucel®

U.S./Canadian Brand Names Cal-Citrate® 250 [US-OTC]; Citracal® [US-OTC]; Osteocit® [Can]

Therapeutic Category Electrolyte Supplement, Oral

Use Antacid; treatment and prevention of calcium deficiency or hyperphosphatemia (eg, osteoporosis, osteomalacia, mild/moderate renal insufficiency, hypoparathyroidism, postmenopausal osteoporosis, rickets)

Usual Dosage Oral: Dosage is in terms of elemental calcium

Dietary Reference Intake:

0-6 months: 210 mg/day

7-12 months: 270 mg/day

1-3 years: 500 mg/day

4-8 years: 800 mg/day

Adults, Male/Female:

9-18 years: 1300 mg/day

19-50 years: 1000 mg/day

≥51 years: 1200 mg/day

Female: Pregnancy/Lactating: Same as for Adults, Male/Female

Dietary supplement: Usual dose: 500 mg to 2 g 2-4 times/day

Dosage Forms

Granules: 760 mg/teaspoonful

Tablet: Elemental calcium 200 mg, 250 mg

Cal-Citrate® [OTC]: Elemental calcium 250 mg

Citracal® [OTC]: 950 mg

calcium disodium edetate *see* edetate calcium disodium *on page 290*

Calcium Disodium Versenate® [US] *see* edetate calcium disodium *on page 290*

calcium EDTA *see* edetate calcium disodium *on page 290*

calcium glubionate (KAL see um gloo BYE oh nate)

Sound-Alike/Look-Alike Issues

calcium glubionate may be confused with calcium gluconate

U.S./Canadian Brand Names Calcionate [US-OTC]

Therapeutic Category Electrolyte Supplement, Oral

Use Dietary supplement

Usual Dosage Dosage is in terms of **elemental** calcium

Dietary Reference Intake:

0-6 months: 210 mg/day

7-12 months: 270 mg/day

1-3 years: 500 mg/day

4-8 years: 800 mg/day
Adults, Male/Female:
  9-18 years: 1300 mg/day
  19-50 years: 1000 mg/day
  ≥51 years: 1200 mg/day
Female: Pregnancy/Lactating: Same as for Adults, Male/Female
Dietary supplement: Oral:
  Infants <12 months: 1 teaspoonful 5 times a day; may mix with juice or formula
  Children <4 years: 2 teaspoonsful 3 times a day
  Children ≥4 years and Adults: 1 tablespoonful 3 times a day
  Pregnant or lactating women: 1 tablespoonful 4 times a day
Dosage Forms
Syrup:
Calcionate: 1.8 g/5 mL

calcium gluconate (KAL see um GLOO koe nate)
Sound-Alike/Look-Alike Issues
calcium gluconate may be confused with calcium glubionate
Therapeutic Category Electrolyte Supplement, Oral
Use Treatment and prevention of hypocalcemia; treatment of tetany, cardiac disturbances of hyperkalemia, cardiac resuscitation when epinephrine fails to improve myocardial contractions, hypocalcemia; calcium supplementation; hydrofluoric acid (HF) burns
Usual Dosage
Adequate Intake (as elemental calcium):
  0-6 months: 210 mg/day
  7-12 months: 270 mg/day
  1-3 years: 500 mg/day
  4-8 years: 800 mg/day
  9-18 years: 1300 mg/day
  Adults, Male/Female:
   19-50 years: 1000 mg/day
   ≥51 years: 1200 mg/day
  Female: Pregnancy/Lactating: Same as for Adults, Male/Female
Dosage note: Calcium chloride has 3 times more elemental calcium than calcium gluconate. Calcium chloride is 27% elemental calcium; calcium gluconate is 9% elemental calcium. One gram of calcium chloride is equal to 270 mg of elemental calcium; 1 gram of calcium gluconate is equal to 90 mg of elemental calcium. The following dosages are expressed in terms of the calcium gluconate salt based on a solution concentration of 100 mg/mL (10%) containing 0.465 mEq (9.3 mg)/mL elemental calcium:
Hypocalcemia: I.V.:
  Neonates: 200-800 mg/kg/day as a continuous infusion or in 4 divided doses (maximum: 1 g/dose)
  Infants and Children: 200-500 mg/kg/day as a continuous infusion or in 4 divided doses (maximum: 2-3 g/dose)
  Adults: 2-15 g/24 hours as a continuous infusion or in divided doses
Hypocalcemia: Oral:
  Children: 200-500 mg/kg/day divided every 6 hours
  Adults: 500 mg to 2 g 2-4 times/day
Hypocalcemia secondary to citrated blood infusion: I.V.: **Note:** Routine administration of calcium, in the absence of signs/symptoms of hypocalcemia, is generally not recommended. A number of recommendations have been published seeking to address potential hypocalcemia during massive transfusion of citrated blood; however, many practitioners recommend replacement only as guided by clinical evidence of hypocalcemia and/or serial monitoring of ionized calcium.
  Neonates, Infants, and Children: Give 98 mg (0.45 mEq **elemental** calcium) for each 100 mL citrated blood infused
  Adults: 500 mg to 1 g per 500 mL of citrated blood (infused into another vein). Single doses up to 2 g have also been recommended.
Hypocalcemic tetany: I.V.:
  Neonates, Infants, and Children: 100-200 mg/kg/dose over 5-10 minutes; may repeat every 6-8 hours **or** follow with an infusion of 500 mg/kg/day
  Adults: 1-3 g may be administered until therapeutic response occurs
Magnesium intoxication, cardiac arrest in the presence of hyperkalemia or hypocalcemia: I.V.:
  Infants and Children: 60-100 mg/kg/dose (maximum: 3 g/dose)
  Adults: 500-800 mg/dose (maximum: 3 g/dose)
Maintenance electrolyte requirements for total parenteral nutrition: I.V.: Daily requirements: Adults: 1.7-3.4 g/1000 kcal/24 hours
Dosage Forms
Injection, solution [preservative free]: 10% [100 mg/mL] (10 mL, 50 mL, 100 mL, 200 mL)
(Continued)

calcium gluconate (Continued)

Powder: 347 mg/tablespoonful
Tablet: 500 mg, 650 mg, 975 mg

calcium lactate (KAL see um LAK tate)

Therapeutic Category Electrolyte Supplement, Oral
Use Adjunct in prevention of postmenopausal osteoporosis; treatment and prevention of calcium depletion
Usual Dosage Oral (in terms of calcium lactate):
  Dietary Reference Intake (in terms of elemental calcium):
  0-6 months: 210 mg/day
  7-12 months: 270 mg/day
  1-3 years: 500 mg/day
  4-8 years: 800 mg/day
  9-18 years: 1300 mg/day
  Adults, Male/Female:
   19-50 years: 1000 mg/day
   ≥51 years: 1200 mg/day
  Female: Pregnancy/Lactating: Same as Adults, Male/Female
Dosage Forms
  Tablet: 650 mg

calcium leucovorin see leucovorin on page 496

calcium pantothenate see pantothenic acid on page 651

calcium phosphate (tribasic) (KAL see um FOS fate tri BAY sik)

Synonyms tricalcium phosphate
U.S./Canadian Brand Names Posture® [US-OTC]
Therapeutic Category Electrolyte Supplement, Oral
Use Dietary supplement
Usual Dosage Oral:
  Adequate Intake (as elemental calcium):
  0-6 months: 210 mg/day
  7-12 months: 270 mg/day
  1-3 years: 500 mg/day
  4-8 years: 800 mg/day
  9-18 years: 1300 mg/day
  Adults, Male/Female:
   19-50 years: 1000 mg/day
   ≥51 years: 1200 mg/day
  Female: Pregnancy/Lactating: Same as for Adults, Male/Female
  Dietary supplement: Adults: 2 tablets daily
Dosage Forms
  Caplet:
   Posture® [OTC]: Calcium 600 mg and phosphorus 280 mg

Cal-CYUM [US-OTC] see calcium and vitamin D on page 137

Caldecort® [US-OTC] see hydrocortisone (topical) on page 434

calfactant (kaf AKT ant)

U.S./Canadian Brand Names Infasurf® [US]
Therapeutic Category Lung Surfactant
Use Prevention of respiratory distress syndrome (RDS) in premature infants at high risk for RDS and for the treatment ("rescue") of premature infants who develop RDS

Prophylaxis: Therapy at birth with calfactant is indicated for premature infants <29 weeks of gestational age at significant risk for RDS. Should be administered as soon as possible, preferably within 30 minutes after birth.
Treatment: For infants ≤72 hours of age with RDS (confirmed by clinical and radiologic findings) and requiring endotracheal intubation.
Usual Dosage Intratracheal administration **only**: Each dose is 3 mL/kg body weight at birth; should be administered every 12 hours for a total of up to 3 doses
Dosage Forms
  Suspension, intratracheal [preservative free]:
   Infasurf®: 35 mg/mL

Cal-Gest [US-OTC] see calcium carbonate on page 138

Callergy Clear [US-OTC] *see* pramoxine *on page 706*

Calm-X® **Oral** *(Discontinued)* *see* dimenhydrinate *on page 262*

Cal-Mint [US-OTC] *see* calcium carbonate *on page 138*

Calmylin with Codeine [Can] *see* guaifenesin, pseudoephedrine, and codeine *on page 408*

Cal-Nate™ **[US]** *see* vitamins (multiple/prenatal) *on page 896*

Calphron® *(Discontinued)* *see* calcium acetate *on page 137*

Cal-Plus® *(Discontinued)* *see* calcium carbonate *on page 138*

Caltine® **[Can]** *see* calcitonin *on page 135*

Caltrate® **[Can]** *see* calcium carbonate *on page 138*

Caltrate® **600 [US-OTC]** *see* calcium carbonate *on page 138*

Caltrate® **600+D [US-OTC]** *see* calcium and vitamin D *on page 137*

Caltrate® **600+ Soy**™ **[US-OTC]** *see* calcium and vitamin D *on page 137*

Caltrate® **ColonHealth**™ **[US-OTC]** *see* calcium and vitamin D *on page 137*

Caltrate® **Jr.** *(Discontinued)* *see* calcium carbonate *on page 138*

Caltrate® **Select [Can]** *see* calcium carbonate *on page 138*

Camila™ **[US]** *see* norethindrone *on page 611*

Campath® **[US]** *see* alemtuzumab *on page 27*

campath-1H *see* alemtuzumab *on page 27*

Campho-Phenique® **[US-OTC]** *see* camphor and phenol *on this page*

camphor and phenol (KAM for & FEE nole)
Synonyms phenol and camphor
U.S./Canadian Brand Names Campho-Phenique® [US-OTC]
Therapeutic Category Topical Skin Product
Use Relief of pain and itching associated with minor burns, sunburn, minor cuts, insect bites, minor skin irritation; temporary relief of pain from cold sores
Usual Dosage Topical: Adults: Relief of pain/itching: Apply 1-3 times/day
Dosage Forms
Gel, topical:
Campho-Phenique® [OTC]: Camphor 10.8% and phenol 4.7% (7 g, 14 g)
Liquid, topical: Camphor 10.8% and phenol 4.7% (45 mL)
Campho-Phenique® [OTC]: Camphor 10.8% and phenol 4.7% (22.5 mL, 45 mL)

Campral® **[US/Can]** *see* acamprosate *on page 4*

Camptosar® **[US/Can]** *see* irinotecan *on page 472*

camptothecin-11 *see* irinotecan *on page 472*

Canasa™ **[US]** *see* mesalamine *on page 546*

Cancidas® **[US/Can]** *see* caspofungin *on page 156*

candesartan (kan de SAR tan)
Synonyms candesartan cilexetil
U.S./Canadian Brand Names Atacand® [US/Can]
Therapeutic Category Angiotensin II Receptor Antagonist
Use Alone or in combination with other antihypertensive agents in treating essential hypertension; treatment of heart failure (NYHA class II-IV)
Usual Dosage Oral: Adults:
Hypertension: Usual dose is 4-32 mg once daily; dosage must be individualized. Blood pressure response is dose-related over the range of 2-32 mg. The usual recommended starting dose of 16 mg once daily when it is used as monotherapy in patients who are not volume depleted. It can be administered once or twice daily with total daily doses ranging from 8-32 mg. Larger doses do not appear to have a greater effect and there is relatively little experience with such doses.
Congestive heart failure: Initial: 4 mg once daily; double the dose at 2-week intervals, as tolerated; target dose: 32 mg
Note: In selected cases, concurrent therapy with an ACE inhibitor may provide additional benefit.
Dosage Forms
Tablet:
Atacand®: 4 mg, 8 mg, 16 mg, 32 mg

candesartan and hydrochlorothiazide (kan de SAR tan & hye droe klor oh THYE a zide)

Synonyms candesartan cilexetil and hydrochlorothiazide
U.S./Canadian Brand Names Atacand HCT™ [US]; Atacand® Plus [Can]
Therapeutic Category Antihypertensive Agent, Combination
Use Treatment of hypertension; combination product should not be used for initial therapy
Usual Dosage Oral: Adults: Replacement therapy: Combination product can be substituted for individual agents; maximum therapeutic effect would be expected within 4 weeks

Usual dosage range:
Candesartan: 16-32 mg/day, given once daily or twice daily in divided doses
Hydrochlorothiazide: 12.5-25 mg once daily
Dosage Forms
Tablet:
Atacand HCT™: 16-12.5: Candesartan 16 mg and hydrochlorothiazide 12.5 mg; 32-12.5: Candesartan 32 mg and hydrochlorothiazide 12.5 mg

candesartan cilexetil *see* candesartan *on previous page*

candesartan cilexetil and hydrochlorothiazide *see* candesartan and hydrochlorothiazide *on this page*

Candida albicans (Monilia) (KAN dee da AL bi kans mo NIL ya)

Synonyms *Monilia* skin test
U.S./Canadian Brand Names Candin® [US]
Therapeutic Category Diagnostic Agent
Use Screen for detection of nonresponsiveness to antigens in immunocompromised individuals
Usual Dosage Intradermal: 0.1 mL, examine reaction site in 24-48 hours; induration of ≥5 mm in diameter is a positive reaction
Dosage Forms
Injection, solution:
Candin®: 0.1 mL/dose (1 mL)

Candin® [US] *see Candida albicans (Monilia) on this page*

Candistatin® [Can] *see* nystatin *on page 623*

Canesten® Topical [Can] *see* clotrimazole *on page 206*

Canesten® Vaginal [Can] *see* clotrimazole *on page 206*

Cankaid® [US-OTC] *see* carbamide peroxide *on page 148*

cannabidiol and tetrahydrocannabinol *see* tetrahydrocannabinol and cannabidiol *(Canada only) on page 832*

Canthacur® [Can] *see* cantharidin *(Canada only) on this page*

cantharidin *(Canada only)* (kan THAR e din)

U.S./Canadian Brand Names Canthacur® [Can]; Cantharone® [Can]
Therapeutic Category Keratolytic Agent
Use Removal of ordinary and periungual warts
Usual Dosage Apply directly to lesion, cover with nonporous tape, remove tape in 24 hours, reapply if necessary

Cantharone® [Can] *see* cantharidin *(Canada only) on this page*

Cantil® [Can] *see* mepenzolate *on page 542*

Cantil® *(Discontinued)* *see* mepenzolate *on page 542*

Capastat® Sulfate [US] *see* capreomycin *on next page*

capecitabine (ka pe SITE a been)

Sound-Alike/Look-Alike Issues
Xeloda® may be confused with Xenical®
Synonyms NSC-712807
U.S./Canadian Brand Names Xeloda® [US/Can]
Therapeutic Category Antineoplastic Agent, Antimetabolite
Use Treatment of metastatic colorectal cancer; adjuvant therapy of Dukes C colon cancer; treatment of metastatic breast cancer
Usual Dosage Oral: Adults: 1250 mg/m^2 twice daily (morning and evening) for 2 weeks, every 21-28 days

Adjuvant therapy of Dukes C colon cancer: Recommended for a total of 24 weeks (8 cycles of 2 weeks of drug administration and 1 week rest period.

Dosage Forms
Tablet:
Xeloda®: 150 mg, 500 mg

Capex™ **[US/Can]** *see* fluocinolone *on page 359*

Caphasol [US] *see* saliva substitute *on page 774*

Capital® **and Codeine [US]** *see* acetaminophen and codeine *on page 6*

Capitrol® *(Discontinued)*

Capoten® **[US/Can]** *see* captopril *on this page*

Capozide® **[US/Can]** *see* captopril and hydrochlorothiazide *on next page*

capreomycin (kap ree oh MYE sin)
Sound-Alike/Look-Alike Issues
Capastat® may be confused with Cepastat®
Synonyms capreomycin sulfate
U.S./Canadian Brand Names Capastat® Sulfate [US]
Therapeutic Category Antibiotic, Miscellaneous
Use Treatment of tuberculosis in conjunction with at least one other antituberculosis agent
Usual Dosage I.M., I.V.:
Infants and Children: 15-30 mg/kg/day, up to 1 g/day maximum
Adults: 1 g/day (not to exceed 20 mg/kg/day) for 60-120 days, followed by 1 g 2-3 times/week
Dosage Forms
Injection, powder for reconstitution:
Capastat® Sulfate: 1 g

capreomycin sulfate *see* capreomycin *on this page*

Capsagel® **[US-OTC]** *see* capsaicin *on this page*

capsaicin (kap SAY sin)
Sound-Alike/Look-Alike Issues
Zostrix® may be confused with Zestril®, Zovirax®
U.S./Canadian Brand Names Capsagel® [US-OTC]; Capzasin-HP® [US-OTC]; Capzasin-P® [US-OTC]; Zostrix® [US-OTC/Can]; Zostrix®-HP [US-OTC/Can]
Therapeutic Category Analgesic, Topical
Use Topical treatment of pain associated with postherpetic neuralgia, rheumatoid arthritis, osteoarthritis, diabetic neuropathy; postsurgical pain
Usual Dosage Topical: Children ≥2 years and Adults: Apply to affected area at least 3-4 times/day; application frequency less than 3-4 times/day prevents the total depletion, inhibition of synthesis, and transport of substance P resulting in decreased clinical efficacy and increased local discomfort
Dosage Forms
Cream, topical: 0.025% (60 g); 0.075% (60 g)
Capzasin-P® [OTC]: 0.025% (45 g)
Capzasin-HP® [OTC]: 0.075% (45 g)
Zostrix® [OTC]: 0.025% (60 g)
Zostrix®-HP [OTC]: 0.075% (60 g)
Gel, topical:
Capsagel® [OTC]: 0.025% (60 g); 0.05% (60 g); 0.075% (30 g)

captopril (KAP toe pril)
Sound-Alike/Look-Alike Issues
captopril may be confused with Capitrol®, carvedilol
Synonyms ACE
U.S./Canadian Brand Names Alti-Captopril [Can]; Apo-Capto® [Can]; Capoten® [US/Can]; Gen-Captopril [Can]; Novo-Captopril [Can]; Nu-Capto [Can]; PMS-Captopril [Can]
Therapeutic Category Angiotensin-Converting Enzyme (ACE) Inhibitor
Use Management of hypertension; treatment of congestive heart failure, left ventricular dysfunction after myocardial infarction, diabetic nephropathy
Usual Dosage Note: Titrate dose according to patient's response; use lowest effective dose. Oral:
Infants: Initial: 0.15-0.3 mg/kg/dose; titrate dose upward to maximum of 6 mg/kg/day in 1-4 divided doses; usual required dose: 2.5-6 mg/kg/day
(Continued)

captopril *(Continued)*

Children: Initial: 0.5 mg/kg/dose; titrate upward to maximum of 6 mg/kg/day in 2-4 divided doses

Older Children: Initial: 6.25-12.5 mg/dose every 12-24 hours; titrate upward to maximum of 6 mg/kg/day

Adolescents: Initial: 12.5-25 mg/dose given every 8-12 hours; increase by 25 mg/dose to maximum of 450 mg/day

Adults:

Acute hypertension (urgency/emergency): 12.5-25 mg, may repeat as needed (may be given sublingually, but no therapeutic advantage demonstrated)

Hypertension:

Initial dose: 12.5-25 mg 2-3 times/day; may increase by 12.5-25 mg/dose at 1- to 2-week intervals up to 50 mg 3 times/day; maximum dose: 150 mg 3 times/day; add diuretic before further dosage increases

Usual dose range (JNC 7): 25-100 mg/day in 2 divided doses

Congestive heart failure:

Initial dose: 6.25-12.5 mg 3 times/day in conjunction with cardiac glycoside and diuretic therapy; initial dose depends upon patient's fluid/electrolyte status

Target dose: 50 mg 3 times/day

LVD after MI: Initial dose: 6.25 mg followed by 12.5 mg 3 times/day; then increase to 25 mg 3 times/day during next several days and then over next several weeks to target dose of 50 mg 3 times/day

Diabetic nephropathy: 25 mg 3 times/day; other antihypertensives often given concurrently

Dosage Forms

Tablet: 12.5 mg, 25 mg, 50 mg, 100 mg

Capoten®: 12.5 mg, 25 mg, 50 mg, 100 mg

captopril and hydrochlorothiazide (KAP toe pril & hye droe klor oh THYE a zide)

Synonyms hydrochlorothiazide and captopril

U.S./Canadian Brand Names Capozide® [US/Can]

Therapeutic Category Antihypertensive Agent, Combination

Use Management of hypertension and treatment of congestive heart failure

Usual Dosage Oral: Adults: Hypertension, CHF: May be substituted for previously titrated dosages of the individual components; alternatively, may initiate as follows:

Initial: Single tablet (captopril 25 mg/hydrochlorothiazide 15 mg) taken once daily; daily dose of captopril should not exceed 150 mg; daily dose of hydrochlorothiazide should not exceed 50 mg

Dosage Forms

Tablet:

Generics:

25/15: Captopril 25 mg and hydrochlorothiazide 15 mg

25/25: Captopril 25 mg and hydrochlorothiazide 25 mg

50/15: Captopril 50 mg and hydrochlorothiazide 15 mg

50/25: Captopril 50 mg and hydrochlorothiazide 25 mg

Brands:

Capozide®:

25/15: Captopril 25 mg and hydrochlorothiazide 15 mg

25/25: Captopril 25 mg and hydrochlorothiazide 25 mg

50/15: Captopril 50 mg and hydrochlorothiazide 15 mg

50/25: Captopril 50 mg and hydrochlorothiazide 25 mg

Capzasin-HP® [US-OTC] see capsaicin on previous page

Capzasin-P® [US-OTC] see capsaicin on previous page

Carac™ [US] see fluorouracil on page 363

Carafate® [US] see sucralfate on page 808

Carapres® [Can] see clonidine on page 204

carbachol (KAR ba kole)

Sound-Alike/Look-Alike Issues

Isopto® Carbachol may be confused with Isopto® Carpine

Synonyms carbacholine; carbamylcholine chloride

U.S./Canadian Brand Names Isopto® Carbachol [US/Can]; Miostat® [US/Can]

Therapeutic Category Cholinergic Agent

Use Lowers intraocular pressure in the treatment of glaucoma; cause miosis during surgery

Usual Dosage Adults:

Ophthalmic: Instill 1-2 drops up to 3 times/day

Intraocular: 0.5 mL instilled into anterior chamber before or after securing sutures

Dosage Forms
  Solution, intraocular:
  Miostat® [OTC]: 0.01% (1.5 mL)
  Solution, ophthalmic:
  Isopto® Carbachol [OTC]: 1.5% (15 mL); 3% (15 mL)

carbacholine *see* carbachol *on previous page*

carbamazepine (kar ba MAZ e peen)

Sound-Alike/Look-Alike Issues
  Carbatrol® may be confused with Cartrol®
  Epitol® may be confused with Epinal®
  Tegretol®, Tegretol®-XR may be confused with Mebaral®, Tegrin®, Toprol-XL®, Toradol®, Trental®
Synonyms CBZ; SPD417
U.S./Canadian Brand Names Apo-Carbamazepine® [Can]; Carbatrol® [US]; Epitol® [US]; Equetro™ [US]; Gen-Carbamazepine CR [Can]; Mapezine® [Can]; Novo-Carbamaz [Can]; Nu-Carbamazepine [Can]; PMS-Carbamazepine [Can]; Taro-Carbamazepine Chewable [Can]; Tegretol® [US/Can]; Tegretol®-XR [US]
Therapeutic Category Anticonvulsant
Use
  Carbatrol®, Tegretol®, Tegretol®-XR: Partial seizures with complex symptomatology (psychomotor, temporal lobe), generalized tonic-clonic seizures (grand mal), mixed seizure patterns, trigeminal neuralgia
  Equetro™: Acute manic and mixed episodes associated with bipolar 1 disorder
Usual Dosage Dosage must be adjusted according to patient's response and serum concentrations. Administer tablets (chewable or conventional) in 2-3 divided doses daily and suspension in 4 divided doses daily.
  Oral:
  Epilepsy:
  Children:
    <6 years: Initial: 10-20 mg/kg/day divided twice or 3 times daily as tablets or 4 times/day as suspension; increase dose every week until optimal response and therapeutic levels are achieved
      Maintenance dose: Divide into 3-4 doses daily (tablets or suspension); maximum recommended dose: 35 mg/kg/day
    6-12 years: Initial: 100 mg twice daily (tablets or extended release tablets) or 50 mg of suspension 4 times/day (200 mg/day); increase by up to 100 mg/day at weekly intervals using a twice daily regimen of extended release tablets or 3-4 times daily regimen of other formulations until optimal response and therapeutic levels are achieved
      Maintenance: Usual: 400-800 mg/day; maximum recommended dose: 1000 mg/day
      Note: Children <12 years who receive ≥400 mg/day of carbamazepine may be converted to extended release capsules (Carbatrol®) using the same total daily dosage divided twice daily
    Children >12 years and Adults: Initial: 200 mg twice daily (tablets, extended release tablets, or extended release capsules) or 100 mg of suspension 4 times/day (400 mg daily); increase by up to 200 mg/day at weekly intervals using a twice daily regimen of extended release tablets or capsules, or a 3-4 times/day regimen of other formulations until optimal response and therapeutic levels are achieved; usual dose: 800-1200 mg/day
    Maximum recommended doses:
      Children 12-15 years: 1000 mg/day
      Children >15 years: 1200 mg/day
      Adults: 1600 mg/day; however, some patients have required up to 1.6-2.4 g/day
  Trigeminal or glossopharyngeal neuralgia: Adults: Initial: 100 mg twice daily with food, gradually increasing in increments of 100 mg twice daily as needed
      Maintenance: Usual: 400-800 mg daily in 2 divided doses; maximum dose: 1200 mg/day
  Bipolar disorder: Adults: Initial: 400 mg/day in divided doses, twice daily; may adjust by 200 mg daily increments; maximum dose: 1600 mg/day.
      Note: Equetro™ is the only formulation specifically approved by the FDA for the managment of bipolar disorder.
Dosage Forms
  Capsule, extended release:
  Carbatrol®, Equetro™: 100 mg, 200 mg, 300 mg
  Suspension, oral: 100 mg/5 mL
  Tegretol®: 100 mg/5 mL
  Tablet: 200 mg
  Epitol®, Tegretol®: 200 mg
  Tablet, chewable: 100 mg
  Tegretol®: 100 mg
  Tablet, extended release:
  Tegretol®-XR: 100 mg, 200 mg, 400 mg

carbamide *see* urea *on page 877*

carbamide peroxide (KAR ba mide per OKS ide)

Synonyms urea peroxide

U.S./Canadian Brand Names Cankaid® [US-OTC]; Debrox® [US-OTC]; Dent's Ear Wax [US-OTC]; E•R•O [US-OTC]; Gly-Oxide® [US-OTC]; Murine® Ear Wax Removal System [US-OTC]; Orajel® Perioseptic® Spot Treatment [US-OTC]

Therapeutic Category Antiinfective Agent, Oral; Otic Agent, Ceruminolytic

Use Relief of minor inflammation of gums, oral mucosal surfaces, and lips including canker sores and dental irritation; emulsify and disperse ear wax

Usual Dosage Children and Adults:

Oral: Inflammation/dental irritation: Solution (should not be used for >7 days): Oral preparation should not be used in children <2 years of age; apply several drops undiluted on affected area 4 times/day after meals and at bedtime; expectorate after 2-3 minutes **or** place 10 drops onto tongue, mix with saliva, swish for several minutes, expectorate

Otic:

Children <12 years: Tilt head sideways and individualize the dose according to patient size; 3 drops (range: 1-5 drops) twice daily for up to 4 days, tip of applicator should not enter ear canal; keep drops in ear for several minutes by keeping head tilted and placing cotton in ear

Children ≥12 years and Adults: Tilt head sideways and instill 5-10 drops twice daily up to 4 days, tip of applicator should not enter ear canal; keep drops in ear for several minutes by keeping head tilted and placing cotton in ear

Dosage Forms

Liquid, oral: 10% (60 mL)

Cankaid®: 10% (22 mL)

Gly-Oxide®: 10% (15 mL, 60 mL)

Solution, otic [drops]: 6.5% (15 mL)

Auraphene® B [OTC]: 6.5% (15 mL)

Auro® [OTC]: 6.5% (22.2 mL)

Debrox® [OTC]: 6.5% (15 mL, 30 mL)

E•R•O [OTC], Murine® Ear Wax Removal System [OTC], Otix® [OTC]: 6.5% (15 mL)

carbamylcholine chloride *see* carbachol *on page 146*

Carbaphen 12® [US] *see* carbetapentane, phenylephrine, and chlorpheniramine *on page 150*

Carbaphen 12 Ped® [US] *see* carbetapentane, phenylephrine, and chlorpheniramine *on page 150*

Carbastat® *(Discontinued)* *see* carbachol *on page 146*

Carbatrol® [US] *see* carbamazepine *on previous page*

Carbaxefed DM RF *(Discontinued)* *see* carbinoxamine, pseudoephedrine, and dextromethorphan *on page 152*

Carbaxefed RF *(Discontinued)* *see* carbinoxamine and pseudoephedrine *on page 151*

carbenicillin (kar ben i SIL in)

Synonyms carbenicillin indanyl sodium; carindacillin

U.S./Canadian Brand Names Geocillin® [US]

Therapeutic Category Penicillin

Use Treatment of serious urinary tract infections and prostatitis caused by susceptible gram-negative aerobic bacilli

Usual Dosage

Usual dosage range:

Children: Oral: 30-50 mg/kg/day divided every 6 hours (maximum dose: 2-3 g/day)

Adults: Oral: 1-2 tablets every 6 hours

Indication-specific dosing:

Adults: Oral:

Prostatitis: 2 tablets every 6 hours

Urinary tract infections: 1-2 tablets every 6 hours

Dosage Forms

Tablet:

Geocillin®: 382 mg

carbenicillin indanyl sodium *see* carbenicillin *on this page*

carbetapentane and chlorpheniramine (kar bay ta PEN tane & klor fen IR a meen)

Synonyms carbetapentane tannate and chlorpheniramine tannate; chlorpheniramine and carbetapentane

U.S./Canadian Brand Names Tannate 12 S [US]; Tannic-12 S [US]; Tannic-12 [US]; Tannihist-12 RF [US]; Tussi-12 S™ [US]; Tussi-12® [US]; Tussizone-12 RF™ [US]

Therapeutic Category Antihistamine/Antitussive

Use Symptomatic relief of cough associated with upper respiratory tract conditions, such as the common cold, bronchitis, bronchial asthma

Usual Dosage Oral:

Children: Based on carbetapentane 30 mg and chlorpheniramine 4 mg per 5 mL suspension:

2-6 years: 2.5-5 mL every 12 hours

>6 years: 5-10 mL every 12 hours

Adults: Based on carbetapentane 60 mg and chlorpheniramine 5 mg per tablet: 1-2 tablets every 12 hours

Dosage Forms

Suspension:

C-Tanna 12, Tannate 12 S, Tannic-12 S, Trionate®, Tussi-12 S™, Tustan 12S™: Carbetapentane 30 mg and chlorpheniramine 4 mg per 5 mL

Tablet:

Trionate®, Tussi-12®, Tussizone-12 RF™: Carbetapentane 60 mg and chlorpheniramine 5 mg

carbetapentane and phenylephrine (kar bay ta PEN tane & fen il EF rin)

Synonyms phenylephrine tannate and carbetapentane tannate

U.S./Canadian Brand Names L-All 12 [US]

Therapeutic Category Antitussive; Antitussive/Decongestant; Sympathomimetic

Use Symptomatic relief of upper respiratory tract conditions such as the common cold, bronchial asthma, and bronchitis (acute and chronic)

Usual Dosage Oral:

Children:

2-6 years: 2.5 mL every 12 hours, not to exceed 5 mL/24 hours

6-12 years: 5 mL every 12 hours, not to exceed 10 mL/24 hours

Children >12 years and Adults: 5-10 mL every 12 hours, not to exceed 20 mL/24 hours

carbetapentane and pseudoephedrine (kar bay ta PEN tane & soo doe e FED rin)

Synonyms carbetapentane tannate and pseudoephedrine tannate; pseudoephedrine and carbetapentane

U.S./Canadian Brand Names Respi-Tann™ [US]

Therapeutic Category Antitussive/Decongestant

Use Relief of cough and congestion due to the common cold, influenza, sinusitis, or bronchitis

Usual Dosage Relief of cough and congestion: Oral:

Children:

2-6 years: ½ tablet or 2.5 mL suspension every 12 hours (maximum: 4 doses/24 hours)

6-12 years: 1 tablet or 5 mL suspension every 12 hours (maximum: 4 doses/24 hours)

Children >12 years and Adults: 2 tablets or 10 mL suspension every 12 hours (maximum: 4 doses/24 hours)

Dosage Forms

Suspension: Carbetapentane 25 mg and pseudoephedrine 75 mg per 5 mL

Respi-Tann™: Carbetapentane 25 mg and pseudoephedrine 75 mg per 5 mL

Tablet, chewable:

Respi-Tann™: Carbetapentane 25 mg and pseudoephedrine 75 mg

carbetapentane, ephedrine, phenylephrine, and chlorpheniramine *see* chlorpheniramine, ephedrine, phenylephrine, and carbetapentane *on page 179*

carbetapentane, guaifenesin, and phenylephrine

(kar bay ta PEN tane, gwye FEN e sin, & fen il EF rin)

Synonyms guaifenesin, carbetapentane citrate, and phenylephrine hydrochloride; phenylephrine hydrochloride, carbetapentane citrate, and guaifenesin

U.S./Canadian Brand Names Carbetaplex [US]; Gentex LQ [US]; Levall™ [US]; Phencarb GG [US]

Therapeutic Category Antitussive; Expectorant; Expectorant/Decongestant/Antitussive; Sympathomimetic

Use Relief of nonproductive cough accompanying respiratory tract congestion associated with the common cold, influenza, sinusitis, and bronchitis

Usual Dosage Oral:

Children 2-6 years:

Gentex LQ: 2.5 mL every 4-6 hours

Levall™: 1.25 mL every 4-6 hours; maximum dose of phenylephrine: 15 mg/24 hours

Children 6-12 years:

Gentex LQ: 5 mL every 4-6 hours

(Continued)

149

carbetapentane, guaifenesin, and phenylephrine *(Continued)*

Levall™: 2.5 mL every 4-6 hours; maximum dose of phenylephrine: 30 mg/24 hours
Children ≥12 years and Adults:
Gentex LQ: 5-10 mL every 4-6 hours
Levall™: 5 mL every 4-6 hours; maximum dose of phenylephrine: 60 mg/24 hours

Dosage Forms
Liquid:
Carbetaplex: Carbetapentane 20 mg, guaifenesin 100 mg, and phenylephrine 15 mg per 5 mL
Gentex LQ: Carbetapentane 20 mg, guaifenesin 100 mg, and phenylephrine 10 mg per 5 mL
Levall™: Carbetapentane 15 mg, guaifenesin 100 mg, and phenylephrine 5 mg per 5 mL
Phencarb GG: Carbetapentane 20 mg, guaifenesin 100 mg, and phenylephrine 10 mg per 5 mL

carbetapentane, phenylephrine, and chlorpheniramine

(kar bay ta PEN tane, fen il EF rin, & klor fen IR a meen)

Synonyms chlorpheniramine, carbetapentane, and phenylephrine; phenylephrine, chlorpheniramine, and carbetapentane

U.S./Canadian Brand Names Carbaphen 12 Ped® [US]; Carbaphen 12® [US]

Therapeutic Category Antihistamine/Decongestant/Antitussive; Antitussive; Sympathomimetic

Use Symptomatic relief of cough, nasal congestion, and discharge associated with the common cold, bronchial asthma, acute and chronic bronchitis, and other respiratory tract conditions

Usual Dosage Oral: Relief of cough, congestion:
Children 2-6 years:
Carbaphen 12 Ped®: 1-2 mL every 12 hours
XiraTuss suspension: 2.5-5 mL every 12 hours
Children 6-12 years:
Carbaphen 12 Ped®: 2-4 mL every 12 hours
XiraTuss suspension: 5-10 mL every 12 hours
Children >12 years and Adults:
Carbaphen 12®: 5-10 mL every 12 hours
XiraTuss tablet: 1-2 tablets every 12 hours

Dosage Forms
Suspension:
Carbaphen 12®: Carbetapentane 60 mg, phenylephrine 20 mg, and chlorpheniramine 8 mg per 5 mL
Carbaphen 12 Ped®: Carbetapentane 15 mg, phenylephrine 2.5 mg, and chlorpheniramine 2 mg per 1 mL

carbetapentane, phenylephrine, and pyrilamine

(kar bay ta PEN tane, fen il EF rin, & peer Il a meen)

Synonyms phenylephrine tannate, carbetapentane tannate, and pyrilamine tannate; pyrilamine, phenylephrine, and carbetapentane

U.S./Canadian Brand Names C-Tanna 12D [US]; Tussi-12® D [US]; Tussi-12® DS [US]

Therapeutic Category Antihistamine; Antihistamine/Decongestant/Antitussive; Antitussive; Decongestant

Use Symptomatic relief of cough associated with respiratory tract conditions such as the common cold, bronchial asthma, acute and chronic bronchitis

Usual Dosage Oral: Relief of cough:
Children:
2-6 years (Tussi-12® DS): 2.5-5 mL every 12 hours
6-11 years:
Tussi-12® D: ¹/₂ to 1 tablet every 12 hours
Tussi-12® DS: 5-10 mL every 12 hours
Children ≥12 years and Adults (Tussi-12® D): 1-2 tablets every 12 hours

Dosage Forms
Suspension:
C-Tanna 12D: Carbetapentane 30 mg, pyrilamine 30 mg, and phenylephrine 5 mg per 5 mL
Tussi-12® DS: Carbetapentane 30 mg, pyrilamine 30 mg, and phenylephrine 5 mg per 5 mL
Tablet:
C-Tanna 12D, Tussi-12® D: Carbetapentane 60 mg, pyrilamine 40 mg, and phenylephrine 10 mg

carbetapentane tannate and chlorpheniramine tannate *see* carbetapentane and chlorpheniramine *on previous page*

carbetapentane tannate and pseudoephedrine tannate *see* carbetapentane and pseudoephedrine *on previous page*

Carbetaplex [US] *see* carbetapentane, guaifenesin, and phenylephrine *on previous page*

carbetocin *(Canada only)* (kar BE toe sin)
U.S./Canadian Brand Names Duratocin™ [Can]
Therapeutic Category Uteronic Agent
Use For the prevention of uterine atony and postpartum hemorrhage following elective cesarean section under epidural or spinal anesthesia.
Usual Dosage A single I.V. dose of 100 mcg (1 mL) is administered by bolus injection, over 1 minute, only when delivery of the infant has been completed by cesarean section under epidural anesthetic. Carbetocin can be administered either before or after delivery of the placenta
Dosage Forms Injection: 1 mcg/mL (1 mL)

carbidopa (kar bi DOE pa)
U.S./Canadian Brand Names Lodosyn® [US]
Therapeutic Category Anti-Parkinson Agent (Dopamine Agonist)
Use Given with levodopa in the treatment of parkinsonism to enable a lower dosage of levodopa to be used and a more rapid response to be obtained and to decrease side effects; for details of administration and dosage, see levodopa; has no effect without levodopa
Usual Dosage Oral: Adults: 70-100 mg/day; maximum daily dose: 200 mg
Dosage Forms
Tablet:
Lodosyn®: 25 mg

carbidopa and levodopa *see* levodopa and carbidopa *on page 500*

carbidopa, levodopa, and entacapone *see* levodopa, carbidopa, and entacapone *on page 500*

Carbihist *(Discontinued) see* carbinoxamine *on this page*

carbinoxamine (kar bi NOKS a meen)
Synonyms carbinoxamine maleate
U.S./Canadian Brand Names Palgic® [US]
Therapeutic Category Antihistamine
Use Seasonal and perennial allergic rhinitis; vasomotor rhinitis; urticaria; decrease severity of other allergic reactions
Usual Dosage Oral (Palgic®):
Children:
  >3-6 years: 2-5 mg 3-4 times/day
  >6 years: 4-6 mg 3-4 times/day
Adults: 4-8 mg 3-4 times/day
Dosage Forms
Solution:
Palgic®: 4 mg/5 mL
Tablet [scored]:
Palgic®: 4 mg

carbinoxamine and pseudoephedrine (kar bi NOKS a meen & soo doe e FED rin)
Synonyms pseudoephedrine and carbinoxamine
U.S./Canadian Brand Names Hydro-Tussin™-CBX [US]
Therapeutic Category Antihistamine/Decongestant Combination
Use Seasonal and perennial allergic rhinitis; vasomotor rhinitis
Usual Dosage Oral:
Children:
  Drops (Andehist NR, Carbaxefed RF, Sildec):
  1-3 months: 0.25 mL 4 times/day
  3-6 months: 0.5 mL 4 times/day
  6-12 months: 0.75 mL 4 times/day
  12-24 months: 1 mL 4 times/day
  Liquid (Pediatex™-D):
  1-3 months: 1.25 mL up to 4 times/day
  3-6 months: 2.5 mL up to 4 times/day
  6-9 months: 3.75 mL up to 4 times/day
  9-18 months: 3.75-5 mL up to 4 times/day
  18 months to 6 years: 5 mL 3-4 times/day
  >6 years: Refer to adult dosing
  Syrup (Hydro-Tussin™-CBX, Palgic®-DS):
  1-3 months: 1.25 mL up to 4 times/day
(Continued)

carbinoxamine and pseudoephedrine *(Continued)*

3-6 months: 2.5 mL up to 4 times/day
6-9 months: 3.75 mL up to 4 times/day
9-18 months: 3.75-5 mL up to 4 times/day
18 months to 6 years: 5 mL 3-4 times/day
>6 years: Refer to adult dosing
Tablet, timed release:
  6-12 years (Palgic®-D): One-half tablet every 12 hours
  ≥12 years (Palgic®-D): Refer to adult dosing
Adults:
  Liquid (Pediatex™-D): 10 mL 4 times/day
  Syrup (Hydro-Tussin™-CBX, Palgic®-DS): 10 mL 4 times/day
  Tablet, timed release (Palgic®-D): 1 tablet every 12 hours

Dosage Forms
  Syrup: Carbinoxamine 2 mg and pseudoephedrine 25 mg per 5 mL
  Hydro-Tussin™-CBX: Carbinoxamine 2 mg and pseudoephedrine 25 mg per 5 mL

carbinoxamine, dextromethorphan, and pseudoephedrine *see* carbinoxamine, pseudoephedrine, and dextromethorphan *on this page*

carbinoxamine maleate *see* carbinoxamine *on previous page*

Carbinoxamine PD *(Discontinued)* *see* carbinoxamine *on previous page*

carbinoxamine, pseudoephedrine, and dextromethorphan

(kar bi NOKS a meen, soo doe e FED rin, & deks troe meth OR fan)

Sound-Alike/Look-Alike Issues
  Tussafed® may be confused with Tussafin®

Synonyms carbinoxamine, dextromethorphan, and pseudoephedrine; dextromethorphan, carbinoxamine, and pseudoephedrine; dextromethorphan, pseudoephedrine, and carbinoxamine; pseudoephedrine, carbinoxamine, and dextromethorphan; pseudoephedrine, dextromethorphan, and carbinoxamine

Therapeutic Category Antihistamine/Decongestant/Antitussive

Use Relief of coughs and upper respiratory symptoms, including nasal congestion, associated with allergy or the common cold

Usual Dosage Oral:
  Drops: Infants and Children:
    1-3 months: 1/4 mL 4 times/day
    3-6 months: 1/2 mL 4 times/day
    6-12 months: 3/4 mL 4 times/day
    12-24 months: 1 mL 4 times/day
  Liquid (Pediatex™ DM):
    Children 18 months to 6 years: 2.5 mL 4 times/day
    Children 6-12 years: 5 mL 4 times/day
    Children ≥12 years and Adults: 10 mL 4 times/day
  Syrup (Tussafed®):
    Children 18 months to 6 years: 2.5 mL 4 times/day
    Children >6 years and Adults: 5 mL 4 times/day

carbinoxamine, pseudoephedrine, and hydrocodone *see* hydrocodone, carbinoxamine, and pseudoephedrine *on page 430*

Carbiset® Tablet *(Discontinued)* *see* carbinoxamine and pseudoephedrine *on previous page*

Carbiset-TR® Tablet *(Discontinued)* *see* carbinoxamine and pseudoephedrine *on previous page*

Carbocaine® [US/Can] *see* mepivacaine *on page 543*

Carbocaine® 2% with Neo-Cobefrin® [US] *see* mepivacaine and levonordefrin *on page 544*

Carbodec® Syrup *(Discontinued)* *see* carbinoxamine and pseudoephedrine *on previous page*

Carbodec® Tablet *(Discontinued)* *see* carbinoxamine and pseudoephedrine *on previous page*

Carbodec® TR Tablet *(Discontinued)* *see* carbinoxamine and pseudoephedrine *on previous page*

Carbofed DM [US] *see* brompheniramine, pseudoephedrine, and dextromethorphan *on page 122*

carbolic acid *see* phenol *on page 673*

Carbolith™ [Can] *see* lithium *on page 513*

carboplatin (KAR boe pla tin)
Sound-Alike/Look-Alike Issues
carboplatin may be confused with cisplatin, oxaliplatin
Paraplatin® may be confused with Platinol®
Synonyms CBDCA; NSC-241240
U.S./Canadian Brand Names Paraplatin-AQ [Can]
Therapeutic Category Antineoplastic Agent
Use Treatment of ovarian cancer
Usual Dosage Refer to individual protocols: **Note:** Doses for adults are usually determined by the AUC using the Calvert formula.

IVPB, I.V. infusion: Adults:
Ovarian cancer: 300-360 mg/m^2 every 4 weeks
In adults, dosing is commonly calculated using the Calvert formula:
Total dose (mg) = Target AUC x (GFR+ 25)
Usual target AUCs:
Previously untreated patients: 6-8
Previously treated patients: 4-6
Dosage Forms
Injection, powder for reconstitution: 50 mg, 150 mg, 450 mg
Injection, solution: 10 mg/mL (5 mL, 15 mL, 45 mL, 60 mL)

carboprost *see* carboprost tromethamine *on this page*

carboprost tromethamine (KAR boe prost tro METH a meen)
Synonyms carboprost; prostaglandin F$_2$
U.S./Canadian Brand Names Hemabate® [US/Can]
Therapeutic Category Prostaglandin
Use Termination of pregnancy; treatment of refractory postpartum uterine bleeding
Usual Dosage I.M.: Adults:
Abortion: Initial: 250 mcg, then 250 mcg at 1.5- to 3.5-hour intervals, depending on uterine response; a 500 mcg dose may be given if uterine response is not adequate after several 250 mcg doses; do not exceed 12 mg total dose or continuous administration for >2 days
Refractory postpartum uterine bleeding: Initial: 250 mcg; if needed, may repeat at 15- to 90-minute intervals; maximum total dose: 2 mg (8 doses)
Dosage Forms
Injection, solution:
Hemabate®: Carboprost 250 mcg and tromethamine 83 mcg per mL (1 mL)

carbose D *see* carboxymethylcellulose *on this page*

Carboxine *(Discontinued) see* carbinoxamine *on page 151*

Carboxine-PSE *(Discontinued) see* carbinoxamine and pseudoephedrine *on page 151*

carboxymethylcellulose (kar boks ee meth il SEL yoo lose)
Synonyms carbose D; carboxymethylcellulose sodium
U.S./Canadian Brand Names Celluvisc™ [Can]; Refresh Liquigel™ [US-OTC]; Refresh Plus® [US-OTC/Can]; Refresh Tears® [US-OTC/Can]; Tears Again® Gel Drops™ [US-OTC]; Tears Again® Night and Day™ [US-OTC]; Theratears® [US]
Therapeutic Category Ophthalmic Agent, Miscellaneous
Use Artificial tear substitute
Usual Dosage Ophthalmic: Adults: Instill 1-2 drops into eye(s) 3-4 times/day
Dosage Forms
Gel, ophthalmic: 1.5% (3.5 g)
Tears Again® Night and Day™ [OTC]: 1.5% (3.5 g)
Solution ophthalmic: 0.25% (0.6 mL, 15 mL); 0.5% (0.4 mL, 15 mL); 0.7% (15 mL); 1% (15 mL)
Refresh Liquigel™ [OTC]: 1% (15 mL)
Refresh Plus® [OTC] [preservative free]: 0.5% (0.4 mL)
Refresh Tears® [OTC]: 0.5% (15 mL)
Tears Again® Gel Drops™ [OTC]: 0.7% (15 mL)
Theratears®: 0.25% (0.6 mL [preservative free], 15 mL)

carboxymethylcellulose sodium *see* carboxymethylcellulose *on this page*

Cardene® [US] *see* nicardipine *on page 603*

Cardene® I.V. [US] *see* nicardipine *on page 603*

Cardene® **SR [US]** *see* nicardipine *on page 603*

Cardio-Green® *(Discontinued) see* indocyanine green *on page 453*

Cardioquin® *(Discontinued) see* quinidine *on page 740*

Cardizem® **[US/Can]** *see* diltiazem *on page 261*

Cardizem® **CD [US/Can]** *see* diltiazem *on page 261*

Cardizem® **Injection** *(Discontinued) see* diltiazem *on page 261*

Cardizem® **LA [US]** *see* diltiazem *on page 261*

Cardizem® **SR [Can]** *see* diltiazem *on page 261*

Cardizem® **SR** *(Discontinued) see* diltiazem *on page 261*

Cardura® **[US]** *see* doxazosin *on page 278*

Cardura-1™ **[Can]** *see* doxazosin *on page 278*

Cardura-2™ **[Can]** *see* doxazosin *on page 278*

Cardura-4™ **[Can]** *see* doxazosin *on page 278*

Cardura® **XL [US]** *see* doxazosin *on page 278*

CareNatal™ **DHA [US]** *see* vitamins (multiple/prenatal) *on page 896*

Carimune™ *(Discontinued) see* immune globulin (intravenous) *on page 451*

Carimune™ **NF [US]** *see* immune globulin (intravenous) *on page 451*

carindacillin *see* carbenicillin *on page 148*

carisoprodate *see* carisoprodol *on this page*

carisoprodol (kar eye soe PROE dole)

Synonyms carisoprodate; isobamate
U.S./Canadian Brand Names Soma® [US/Can]
Therapeutic Category Skeletal Muscle Relaxant
Use Short-term (2-3 weeks) relief of skeletal muscle pain
Usual Dosage Oral: Children ≥12 years and Adults: 350 mg 3-4 times/day; take last dose at bedtime
Dosage Forms
  Tablet: 350 mg
  Soma®: 250 mg, 350 mg

carisoprodol and aspirin (kar eye soe PROE dole & AS pir in)

Synonyms aspirin and carisoprodol
U.S./Canadian Brand Names Soma® Compound [US]
Therapeutic Category Skeletal Muscle Relaxant
Use Skeletal muscle relaxant
Usual Dosage Oral: Adults: 1-2 tablets 4 times/day
Dosage Forms
  Tablet: Carisoprodol 200 mg and aspirin 325 mg
  Soma® Compound: Carisoprodol 200 mg and aspirin 325 mg

carisoprodol, aspirin, and codeine (kar eye soe PROE dole, AS pir in, and KOE deen)

Synonyms aspirin, carisoprodol, and codeine; codeine, aspirin, and carisoprodol
U.S./Canadian Brand Names Soma® Compound w/Codeine [US]
Therapeutic Category Skeletal Muscle Relaxant
Controlled Substance C-III
Use Skeletal muscle relaxant
Usual Dosage Oral: Adults: 1 or 2 tablets 4 times/day
Dosage Forms
  Tablet: Carisoprodol 200 mg, aspirin 325 mg, and codeine 16 mg
  Soma® Compound w/Codeine: Carisoprodol 200 mg, aspirin 325 mg, and codeine 16 mg

Carmol® **10 [US-OTC]** *see* urea *on page 877*

Carmol® **20 [US-OTC]** *see* urea *on page 877*

Carmol® **40 [US]** *see* urea *on page 877*

Carmol® **Deep Cleaning [US]** *see* urea *on page 877*

Carmol-HC® **[US]** *see* urea and hydrocortisone *on page 878*

Carmol® Scalp [US] *see* sulfacetamide *on page 810*

carmustine (kar MUS teen)
Sound-Alike/Look-Alike Issues
carmustine may be confused with lomustine
Synonyms BCNU; bis-chloronitrosourea; carmustinum; NSC-409962; WR-139021
U.S./Canadian Brand Names BiCNU® [US/Can]; Gliadel Wafer® [Can]; Gliadel® [US]
Therapeutic Category Antineoplastic Agent
Use
Injection: Treatment of brain tumors (glioblastoma, brainstem glioma, medulloblastoma, astrocytoma, ependymoma, and metastatic brain tumors), multiple myeloma, Hodgkin disease (relapsed or refractory), non-Hodgkin lymphomas (relapsed or refractory),
Wafer (implant): Adjunct to surgery in patients with recurrent glioblastoma multiforme; adjunct to surgery and radiation in patients with high-grade malignant glioma
Usual Dosage I.V. (refer to individual protocols): Adults:
Usual dosage (per manufacturer labeling): 150-200 mg/m^2 every 6 weeks **or** 75-100 mg/m^2/day for 2 days every 6 weeks
Primary brain cancer:
150-200 mg/m^2 every 6-8 weeks as a single dose **or**
75-120 mg/m^2 days 1 and 2 every 6-8 weeks **or**
20-65 mg/m^2 every 4-6 weeks **or**
0.5-1 mg/kg every 4-6 weeks **or**
40-80 mg/m^2/day for 3 days every 6-8 weeks
Autologous BMT: ALL OF THE FOLLOWING DOSES ARE FATAL WITHOUT BMT
Combination therapy: Up to 300-900 mg/m^2
Single-agent therapy: Up to 1200 mg/m^2 (fatal necrosis is associated with doses >2 g/m^2)
Implantation (wafer): Recurrent glioblastoma multiforme, malignant glioma: Up to 8 wafers may be placed in the resection cavity (total dose 62.6 mg); should the size and shape not accommodate 8 wafers, the maximum number of wafers allowed should be placed
Dosage Forms
Injection, powder for reconstitution:
BiCNU®: 100 mg
Implant:
Gliadel®: 7.7 mg (8s)

carmustinum *see* carmustine *on this page*
Carnation Instant Breakfast® [US-OTC] *see* nutritional formula, enteral/oral *on page 622*
Carnitor® [US/Can] *see* levocarnitine *on page 499*
Carnitor® SF [US] *see* levocarnitine *on page 499*
Carrington Antifungal [US-OTC] *see* miconazole *on page 566*

carteolol (KAR tee oh lole)
Sound-Alike/Look-Alike Issues
carteolol may be confused with carvedilol
Synonyms carteolol hydrochloride
U.S./Canadian Brand Names Ocupress® Ophthalmic [Can]
Therapeutic Category Beta-Adrenergic Blocker
Use Treatment of chronic open-angle glaucoma and intraocular hypertension
Usual Dosage Ophthalmic: Adults: Instill 1 drop in affected eye(s) twice daily.
Dosage Forms
Solution, ophthalmic, as hydrochloride: 1% (5 mL, 10 mL, 15 mL)

carteolol hydrochloride *see* carteolol *on this page*
Carter's Little Pills® [Can] *see* bisacodyl *on page 112*
Carter's Little Pills® (Discontinued) *see* bisacodyl *on page 112*
Cartia XT™ [US] *see* diltiazem *on page 261*

carvedilol (KAR ve dil ole)
Sound-Alike/Look-Alike Issues
carvedilol may be confused with captopril, carteolol
U.S./Canadian Brand Names Apo-Carvedilol® [Can]; Coreg CR™ [US]; Coreg® [US/Can]; Novo-Carvedilol [Can]; PMS-Carvedilol [Can]; RAN™-Carvedilol [Can]; ratio-Carvedilol [Can]
(Continued)

carvedilol *(Continued)*

Therapeutic Category Beta-Adrenergic Blocker

Use Mild-to-severe heart failure of ischemic or cardiomyopathic origin (usually in addition to standardized therapy); left ventricular dysfunction following myocardial infarction (MI) (clinically stable with LVEF ≤40%); management of hypertension

Usual Dosage Oral: Adults: Reduce dosage if heart rate drops to <55 beats/minute.

Hypertension:

Immediate release: 6.25 mg twice daily; if tolerated, dose should be maintained for 1-2 weeks, then increased to 12.5 mg twice daily. Dosage may be increased to a maximum of 25 mg twice daily after 1-2 weeks; maximum dose: 50 mg/day.

Extended release: Initial: 20 mg once daily, if tolerated, dose should be maintained for 1-2 weeks then increased to 40 mg once daily if necessary; maximum dose: 80 mg once daily

Congestive heart failure:

Immediate release: 3.125 mg twice daily for 2 weeks; if this dose is tolerated, may increase to 6.25 mg twice daily. Double the dose every 2 weeks to the highest dose tolerated by patient. (Prior to initiating therapy, other heart failure medications should be stabilized and fluid retention minimized.)

Maximum recommended dose:

Mild-to-moderate heart failure:

<85 kg: 25 mg twice daily

>85 kg: 50 mg twice daily

Severe heart failure: 25 mg twice daily

Extended release: Initial: 10 mg once daily for 2 weeks; if the dose is tolerated, increase dose to 20 mg, 40 mg, and 80 mg over successive intervals of at least 2 weeks. Maintain on lower dose if higher dose is not tolerated.

Left ventricular dysfunction following MI: **Note:** Should be initiated only after patient is hemodynamically stable and fluid retention has been minimized.

Immediate release: Initial 3.125-6.25 mg twice daily; increase dosage incrementally (ie, from 6.25-12.5 mg twice daily) at intervals of 3-10 days, based on tolerance, to a target dose of 25 mg twice daily.

Extended release: Initial: 20 mg once daily; increase dosage incrementally at intervals of 3-10 days. Target dose: 80 mg once daily.

Conversion from immediate release to extended release (Coreg CR™):

Current dose immediate release tablets 3.125 mg twice daily: Convert to extended release capsules 10 mg once daily

Current dose immediate release tablets 6.25 mg twice daily: Convert to extended release capsules 20 mg once daily

Current dose immediate release tablets 12.5 mg twice daily: Convert to extended release capsules 40 mg once daily

Current dose immediate release tablets 25 mg twice daily: Convert to extended release capsules 80 mg once daily

Dosage Forms

Capsule, extended release:

Coreg CR™: 10 mg, 20 mg, 40 mg, 80 mg

Tablet: 3.125 mg, 6.25 mg, 12.5 mg, 25 mg

Coreg®: 3.125 mg, 6.25 mg, 12.5 mg, 25 mg

Casodex® **[US/Can]** *see* bicalutamide *on page 111*

caspofungin *(kas poe FUN jin)*

Synonyms caspofungin acetate

U.S./Canadian Brand Names Cancidas® [US/Can]

Therapeutic Category Antifungal Agent, Systemic

Use Treatment of invasive *Aspergillus* infections in patients who are refractory or intolerant of other therapy; treatment of candidemia and other *Candida* infections (intra-abdominal abscesses, esophageal, peritonitis, pleural space); empirical treatment for presumed fungal infections in febrile neutropenic patient

Usual Dosage I.V.: Adults: **Note:** Duration of caspofungin treatment should be determined by patient status and clinical response. Empiric therapy should be given until neutropenia resolves. In patients with positive cultures, treatment should continue until 14 days after last positive culture. In neutropenic patients, treatment should be given at least 7 days after both signs and symptoms of infection **and** neutropenia resolve.

Empiric therapy: Initial dose: 70 mg on day 1; subsequent dosing: 50 mg/day; may increase up to 70 mg/day if tolerated, but clinical response is inadequate

Invasive *Aspergillus*, candidiasis: Initial dose: 70 mg on day 1; subsequent dosing: 50 mg/day

Esophageal candidiasis: 50 mg/day; **Note:** The majority of patients studied for this indication also had oropharyngeal involvement.

Concomitant use of an enzyme inducer:

Patients receiving rifampin: 70 mg caspofungin daily

Patients receiving carbamazepine, dexamethasone, efavirenz, nevirapine, **or** phenytoin (and possibly other enzyme inducers) may require an increased daily dose of caspofungin (70 mg/day).

Dosage Forms
Injection, powder for reconstitution:
Cancidas®: 50 mg, 70 mg

caspofungin acetate *see* caspofungin *on previous page*
Castellani Paint Modified [US-OTC] *see* phenol *on page 673*

castor oil (KAS tor oyl)
Synonyms oleum ricini
Therapeutic Category Laxative
Use Preparation for rectal or bowel examination or surgery; rarely used to relieve constipation; also applied to skin as emollient and protectant
Usual Dosage Oral: Oil:
Children 2-11 years: 5-15 mL as a single dose
Children ≥12 years and Adults: 15-60 mL as a single dose
Dosage Forms
Oil, oral: 100%

castor oil, trypsin, and balsam peru *see* trypsin, balsam peru, and castor oil *on page 872*

Cataflam® [US/Can] *see* diclofenac *on page 253*

Catapres® [US] *see* clonidine *on page 204*

Catapres-TTS® [US] *see* clonidine *on page 204*

catechins *see* sinecatechins *on page 788*

Cathflo® Activase® [US/Can] *see* alteplase *on page 34*

Caverject® [US/Can] *see* alprostadil *on page 33*

Caverject Impulse® [US] *see* alprostadil *on page 33*

CaviRinse™ [US] *see* fluoride *on page 361*

CB-1348 *see* chlorambucil *on page 172*

CBDCA *see* carboplatin *on page 153*

CBZ *see* carbamazepine *on page 147*

CC-5013 *see* lenalidomide *on page 495*

CCI-779 *see* temsirolimus *on page 824*

CCNU *see* lomustine *on page 515*

C-Crystals® *(Discontinued)* *see* ascorbic acid *on page 76*

2-CdA *see* cladribine *on page 196*

CDDP *see* cisplatin *on page 194*

CDX *see* bicalutamide *on page 111*

Cebid® *(Discontinued)* *see* ascorbic acid *on page 76*

Ceclor® [Can] *see* cefaclor *on this page*

Ceclor® *(Discontinued)* *see* cefaclor *on this page*

Cecon® [US-OTC] *see* ascorbic acid *on page 76*

Cedax® [US] *see* ceftibuten *on page 163*

Cedocard®-SR [Can] *see* isosorbide dinitrate *on page 476*

CEE *see* estrogens (conjugated/equine) *on page 318*

CeeNU® [US/Can] *see* lomustine *on page 515*

Ceepryn® *(Discontinued)* *see* cetylpyridinium *on page 170*

cefaclor (SEF a klor)
Sound-Alike/Look-Alike Issues
cefaclor may be confused with cephalexin
U.S./Canadian Brand Names Apo-Cefaclor® [Can]; Ceclor® [Can]; Novo-Cefaclor [Can]; Nu-Cefaclor [Can]; PMS-Cefaclor [Can]; Raniclor™ [US]
(Continued)

cefaclor *(Continued)*

Therapeutic Category Cephalosporin (Second Generation)

Use Treatment of susceptible bacterial infections including otitis media, lower respiratory tract infections, acute exacerbations of chronic bronchitis, pharyngitis and tonsillitis, urinary tract infections, skin and skin structure infections

Usual Dosage

Usual dosage range:

Children >1 month: Oral: 20-40 mg/kg/day divided every 8-12 hours (maximum dose: 1 g/day)

Adults: Oral: 250-500 mg every 8 hours

Indication-specific dosing:

Children: Oral:

Otitis media: 40 mg/kg/day divided every 12 hours

Pharyngitis: 20 mg/kg/day divided every 12 hours

Dosage Forms

Capsule: 250 mg, 500 mg

Powder for oral suspension: 125 mg/5 mL, 250 mg/5 mL, 375 mg/5 mL

Tablet, chewable:

Raniclor™: 250 mg, 375 mg

Tablet, extended release: 500 mg

cefadroxil (sef a DROKS il)

Synonyms cefadroxil monohydrate

U.S./Canadian Brand Names Apo-Cefadroxil® [Can]; Duricef® [US/Can]; Novo-Cefadroxil [Can]

Therapeutic Category Cephalosporin (First Generation)

Use Treatment of susceptible bacterial infections, including those caused by group A beta-hemolytic *Streptococcus*; prophylaxis against infective endocarditis in patients who are allergic to penicillin and undergoing surgical or dental procedures

Usual Dosage

Usual dosage range: Oral:

Children: 30 mg/kg/day divided twice daily up to a maximum of 2 g/day

Adults: 1-2 g/day in 2 divided doses

Indication-specific dosing:

Prophylaxis against bacterial endocarditis:

Children: Oral: 50 mg/kg 1 hour prior to the procedure

Adults: Oral: 2 g 1 hour prior to the procedure

Dosage Forms

Capsule: 500 mg

Powder for oral suspension: 250 mg/5 mL, 500 mg/5 mL

Duricef®: 250 mg/5 mL, 500 mg/5 mL

Tablet: 1 g

cefadroxil monohydrate *see* cefadroxil *on this page*

Cefanex® *(Discontinued)* *see* cephalexin *on page 167*

cefazolin (sef A zoe lin)

Sound-Alike/Look-Alike Issues

cefazolin may be confused with cefprozil, cephalexin, cephalothin

Kefzol® may be confused with Cefzil®

Synonyms cefazolin sodium

Therapeutic Category Cephalosporin (First Generation)

Use Treatment of respiratory tract, skin and skin structure, genital, urinary tract, biliary tract, bone and joint infections, and septicemia due to susceptible gram-positive cocci (except enterococcus); some gram-negative bacilli including *E. coli*, *Proteus*, and *Klebsiella* may be susceptible; perioperative prophylaxis

Usual Dosage

Usual dosage range: I.M., I.V.:

Children >1 month: 25-100 mg/kg/day divided every 6-8 hours; maximum: 6 g/day

Adults: 250 mg to 2 g every 6-12 (usually 8) hours, depending on severity of infection; maximum dose: 12 g/day

Indication-specific dosing:

Prophylaxis in total joint replacement patient: Adults: I.M., I.V.: 1 g 1 hour prior to the procedure

Mild-to-moderate infections: Adults: 500 mg to 1 g every 6-8 hours

Mild infection with gram-positive cocci: Adults: 250-500 mg every 8 hours

Perioperative prophylaxis: Adults: 1 g given 30 minutes prior to surgery (repeat with 500 mg to 1 g during prolonged surgery); followed by 500 mg to 1 g every 6-9 hours for 24 hours postop

Pneumococcal pneumonia: Adults: 500 mg every 12 hours
Severe infection: Adults: 1-2 g every 6 hours
UTI (uncomplicated): Adults: 1 g every 12 hours
Dosage Forms
Infusion [premixed in D$_5$W]: 1 g (50 mL)
Injection, powder for reconstitution: 500 mg, 1 g, 10 g, 20 g

cefazolin sodium *see* cefazolin *on previous page*

cefdinir (SEF di ner)
Synonyms CFDN
U.S./Canadian Brand Names Omnicef® [US/Can]
Therapeutic Category Cephalosporin (Third Generation)
Use Treatment of community-acquired pneumonia, acute exacerbations of chronic bronchitis, acute bacterial otitis media, acute maxillary sinusitis, pharyngitis/tonsillitis, and uncomplicated skin and skin structure infections.
Usual Dosage
Usual dosage range:
Children 6 months to 12 years: Oral: 7 mg/kg/dose twice daily or 14 mg/kg/dose once daily (maximum: 600 mg/day)
Adolescents and Adults: Oral: 300 mg twice daily or 600 mg once daily
Indication-specific dosing:
Children 6 months to 12 years: Oral:
Acute bacterial otitis media, pharyngitis/tonsillitis: 7 mg/kg/dose twice daily for 5-10 days **or** 14 mg/kg/dose once daily for 10 days (maximum: 600 mg/day)
Acute maxillary sinusitis: 7 mg/kg/dose twice daily **or** 14 mg/kg/dose once daily for 10 days (maximum: 600 mg/day)
Uncomplicated skin and skin structure infections: 7 mg/kg/dose twice daily for 10 days (maximum: 600 mg/day)
Adolescents and Adults:
Acute exacerbations of chronic bronchitis, pharyngitis/tonsillitis: 300 mg twice daily for 5-10 days **or** 600 mg once daily for 10 days
Acute maxillary sinusitis: 300 mg twice daily **or** 600 mg once daily for 10 days
Community-acquired pneumonia, uncomplicated skin and skin structure infections: 300 mg twice daily for 10 days
Dosage Forms
Capsule: 300 mg
Omnicef®: 300 mg
Powder for oral suspension: 125 mg/5 mL; 250 mg/5 mL
Omnicef®: 125 mg/5 mL (60 mL, 100 mL), 250 mg/5 mL (60 mL, 100 mL)

cefditoren (sef de TOR en)
Synonyms cefditoren pivoxil
U.S./Canadian Brand Names Spectracef™ [US]
Therapeutic Category Antibiotic, Cephalosporin
Use Treatment of acute bacterial exacerbation of chronic bronchitis or community-acquired pneumonia (due to susceptible organisms including *Haemophilus influenzae, Haemophilus parainfluenzae, Streptococcus pneumoniae*-penicillin susceptible only, *Moraxella catarrhalis*); pharyngitis or tonsillitis (*Streptococcus pyogenes*); and uncomplicated skin and skin-structure infections (*Staphylococcus aureus* - not MRSA, *Streptococcus pyogenes*)
Usual Dosage
Usual dosage range:
Children ≥12 years and Adults: Oral: 200-400 mg twice daily
Indication-specific dosing:
Children ≥12 years and Adults: Oral:
Acute bacterial exacerbation of chronic bronchitis: 400 mg twice daily for 10 days
Community-acquired pneumonia: 400 mg twice daily for 14 days
Pharyngitis, tonsillitis, uncomplicated skin and skin structure infections: 200 mg twice daily for 10 days
Dosage Forms
Tablet:
Spectracef®: 200 mg

cefditoren pivoxil *see* cefditoren *on this page*

cefepime (SEF e pim)

Synonyms cefepime hydrochloride
U.S./Canadian Brand Names Maxipime® [US/Can]
Therapeutic Category Cephalosporin (Fourth Generation)
Use Treatment of uncomplicated and complicated urinary tract infections, including pyelonephritis caused by typical urinary tract pathogens; monotherapy for febrile neutropenia; uncomplicated skin and skin structure infections caused by *Streptococcus pyogenes*; moderate-to-severe pneumonia caused by pneumococcus, *Pseudomonas aeruginosa*, and other gram-negative organisms; complicated intra-abdominal infections (in combination with metronidazole). Also active against methicillin-susceptible staphylococci, *Enterobacter* sp, and many other gram-negative bacilli.

Children 2 months to 16 years: Empiric therapy of febrile neutropenia patients, uncomplicated skin/soft tissue infections, pneumonia, and uncomplicated/complicated urinary tract infections.

Usual Dosage
Usual dosage range:
Children: I.V.: 50 mg/kg every 8-12 hours
Adults: I.V.: 1-2 g every 6-12 hours
Indication-specific dosing:
Children >2 months: I.V.:
Febrile neutropenia: 50 mg/kg every 8 hours for 7-10 days
Uncomplicated skin/soft tissue infections, pneumonia, complicated/uncomplicated UTI: 50 mg/kg twice daily
Adults:
Brain abscess *(Pseudomonas)*, meningitis (postsurgical): I.V.: 2 g every 8 hours
Hospital-acquired pneumonia (HAP): I.V.: 1-2 g every 8-12 hours (American Thoracic Society/ATS guidelines)
Monotherapy for febrile neutropenic patients: I.V: 2 g every 8 hours for 7 days or until the neutropenia resolves
Otitis externa (malignant), pneumonia: I.V.: 2 g every 12 hours
Peritonitis (spontaneous): I.V.: 2 g every 12 hours with metronidazole
Septic lateral/cavernous sinus thrombosis: I.V.: 2 g every 8-12 hours; with metronidazole for lateral
Urinary tract infections (mild to moderate) I.M., I.V.: 500-1000 mg every 12 hours
Dosage Forms
Injection, powder for reconstitution: 1 g, 2 g
Maxipime®: 500 mg, 1 g, 2 g

cefepime hydrochloride *see* cefepime *on this page*

Cefizox® [US/Can] *see* ceftizoxime *on page 164*

Cefotan® *(Discontinued)*

cefotaxime (sef oh TAKS eem)

Sound-Alike/Look-Alike Issues
cefotaxime may be confused with cefoxitin, ceftizoxime, cefuroxime
Synonyms cefotaxime sodium
U.S./Canadian Brand Names Claforan® [US/Can]
Therapeutic Category Cephalosporin (Third Generation)
Use Treatment of susceptible infection in respiratory tract, skin and skin structure, bone and joint, urinary tract, gynecologic as well as septicemia, and documented or suspected meningitis. Active against most gram-negative bacilli (not *Pseudomonas*) and gram-positive cocci (not enterococcus). Active against many penicillin-resistant pneumococci.
Usual Dosage
Usual dosage range:
Infants and Children 1 month to 12 years <50 kg: I.M., I.V.: 50-200 mg/kg/day in divided doses every 6-8 hours
Children >12 years and Adults: I.M., I.V.: 1-2 g every 4-12 hours
Indication-specific dosing:
Infants and Children 1 month to 12 years:
Epiglottitis: I.M., I.V.: 150-200 mg/kg/day in 4 divided doses with clindamycin for 7-10 days
Meningitis: I.M., I.V.: 200 mg/kg/day in divided doses every 6 hours
Pneumonia: I.V.: 200 mg/kg/day divided every 8 hours
Sepsis: I.V.: 150 mg/kg/day divided every 8 hours
Typhoid fever: I.M., I.V.: 150-200 mg/kg/day in 3-4 divided doses (maximum: 12 g/day); fluoroquinolone resistant: 80 mg/kg/day in 3-4 divided doses (maximum: 12 g/day)
Children >12 years and Adults:
Arthritis (septic): I.V.: 1 g every 8 hours

Brain abscess, meningitis: I.V.: 2 g every 4-6 hours

Caesarean section: I.M., I.V.: 1 g as soon as the umbilical cord is clamped, then 1 g at 6- and 12-hour intervals

Epiglottitis: I.V.: 2 g every 4-8 hours

Gonorrhea: I.M.: 1 g as a single dose
Disseminated: I.V.: 1 g every 8 hours

Life-threatening infections: I.V.: 2 g every 4 hours

Liver abscess: I.V.: 1-2 g every 6 hours

Lyme disease:
Cardiac manifestations: I.V.: 2 g every 4 hours
CNS manifestations: I.V.: 2 g every 8 hours for 14-28 days

Moderate-to-severe infections: I.M., I.V.: 1-2 g every 8 hours

Orbital cellulitis: I.V.: 2 g every 4 hours

Peritonitis (spontaneous): I.V.: 2 g every 8 hours, unless life-threatening then 2 g every 4 hours

Septicemia: I.V.: 2 g every 6-8 hours

Skin and soft tissue:
Mixed, necrotizing: I.V.: 2 g every 6 hours, with metronidazole or clindamycin
Bite wounds (animal): I.V.: 2 g every 6 hours

Surgical prophylaxis: I.M., I.V.: 1 g 30-90 minutes before surgery

Uncomplicated infections: I.M., I.V.: 1 g every 12 hours

Dosage Forms
Infusion, as sodium [premixed iso-osmotic solution]:
Claforan®: 1 g (50 mL); 2 g (50 mL)

Injection, powder for reconstitution: 500 mg, 1 g, 2 g, 10 g, 20 g
Claforan®: 500 mg, 1 g, 2 g, 10 g

cefotaxime sodium *see* cefotaxime *on previous page*

cefoxitin (se FOKS i tin)

Sound-Alike/Look-Alike Issues
cefoxitin may be confused with cefotaxime, cefotetan, Cytoxan®
Mefoxin® may be confused with Lanoxin®

Synonyms cefoxitin sodium

U.S./Canadian Brand Names Apo-Cefoxitin® [Can]; Mefoxin® [US]

Therapeutic Category Cephalosporin (Second Generation)

Use Less active against staphylococci and streptococci than first generation cephalosporins, but active against anaerobes including *Bacteroides fragilis*; active against gram-negative enteric bacilli including *E. coli, Klebsiella*, and *Proteus*; used predominantly for respiratory tract, skin and skin structure, bone and joint, urinary tract and gynecologic as well as septicemia; surgical prophylaxis; intraabdominal infections and other mixed infections; indicated for bacterial *Eikenella corrodens* infections

Usual Dosage
Usual dosage range:
Infants >3 months and Children: I.M., I.V.: 80-160 mg/kg/day in divided doses every 4-6 hours (maximum dose: 12 g/day)
Adults: I.M., I.V.: 1-2 g every 6-8 hours (maximum dose: 12 g/day)
Note: I.M. injection is painful

Indication-specific dosing:
Infants >3 months and Children:
Mild-to-moderate infection: I.M., I.V.: 80-100 mg/kg/day in divided doses every 4-6 hours
Perioperative prophylaxis: I.V.: 30-40 mg/kg 30-60 minutes prior to surgery followed by 30-40 mg/kg/dose every 6 hours for no more than 24 hours after surgery depending on the procedure
Severe infection: I.M., I.V.: 100-160 mg/kg/day in divided doses every 4-6 hours
Adolescents and Adults:
Perioperative prophylaxis: I.M., I.V.: 1-2 g 30-60 minutes prior to surgery followed by 1-2 g every 6-8 hours for no more than 24 hours after surgery depending on the procedure
Adults:
Amnionitis, endomyometritis: I.M., I.V.: 2 g every 6-8 hours
Aspiration pneumonia, empyema, orbital cellulitis, parapharyngeal space, human bites: I.M., I.V.: 2 g every 8 hours
Liver abscess: I.V.: 1 g every 4 hours
Mycobacterium species, not MTB or MAI: I.V.: 12 g/day with amikacin
Pelvic inflammatory disease:
Inpatients: I.V.: 2 g every 6 hours **plus** doxycycline 100 mg I.V. or 100 mg orally every 12 hours until improved, followed by doxycycline 100 mg orally twice daily to complete 14 days
Outpatients: I.M.: 2 g **plus** probenecid 1 g orally as a single dose, followed by doxycycline 100 mg orally twice daily for 14 days

(Continued)

cefoxitin *(Continued)*

Dosage Forms
Infusion [premixed iso-osmotic solution]:
Mefoxin®: 1 g (50 mL); 2 g (50 mL)
Injection, powder for reconstitution: 1 g, 2 g, 10 g
Mefoxin®: 1 g, 2 g, 10 g

cefoxitin sodium *see* cefoxitin *on previous page*

cefpodoxime (sef pode OKS eem)

Sound-Alike/Look-Alike Issues
Vantin® may be confused with Ventolin®
Synonyms cefpodoxime proxetil
U.S./Canadian Brand Names Vantin® [US/Can]
Therapeutic Category Cephalosporin (Second Generation)
Use Treatment of susceptible acute, community-acquired pneumonia caused by *S. pneumoniae* or nonbeta-lactamase producing *H. influenzae*; acute uncomplicated gonorrhea caused by *N. gonorrhoeae*; uncomplicated skin and skin structure infections caused by *S. aureus* or *S. pyogenes*; acute otitis media caused by *S. pneumoniae, H. influenzae,* or *M. catarrhalis*; pharyngitis or tonsillitis; and uncomplicated urinary tract infections caused by *E. coli, Klebsiella,* and *Proteus*
Usual Dosage
Usual dosage range:
Children 2 months to 12 years: Oral: 10 mg/kg/day divided every 12 hours (maximum dose: 400 mg/day)
Children ≥12 years and Adults: Oral: 100-400 mg every 12 hours
Indication-specific dosing:
Children 2 months to 12 years: Oral:
Acute maxillary sinusitis: 10 mg/kg/day divided every 12 hours for 10 days (maximum: 200 mg/dose)
Acute otitis media: 10 mg/kg/day divided every 12 hours (400 mg/day) for 5 days (maximum: 200 mg/dose)
Pharyngitis/tonsillitis: 10 mg/kg/day in 2 divided doses for 5-10 days (maximum: 100 mg/dose)
Children ≥12 years and Adults: Oral:
Acute community-acquired pneumonia and bacterial exacerbations of chronic bronchitis: 200 mg every 12 hours for 14 days and 10 days, respectively
Acute maxillary sinusitis: 200 mg every 12 hours for 10 days
Pharyngitis/tonsillitis: 100 mg every 12 hours for 5-10 days
Skin and skin structure: 400 mg every 12 hours for 7-14 days
Uncomplicated gonorrhea (male and female) and rectal gonococcal infections (female): 200 mg as a single dose
Uncomplicated urinary tract infection: 100 mg every 12 hours for 7 days
Dosage Forms
Granules for oral suspension:
Vantin®: 50 mg/5 mL, 100 mg/5 mL
Tablet: 100 mg, 200 mg
Vantin®: 100 mg, 200 mg

cefpodoxime proxetil *see* cefpodoxime *on this page*

cefprozil (sef PROE zil)

Sound-Alike/Look-Alike Issues
cefprozil may be confused with cefazolin, cefuroxime
Cefzil® may be confused with Cefol®, Ceftin®, Kefzol®
U.S./Canadian Brand Names Apo-Cefprozil® [Can]; Cefzil® [US/Can]
Therapeutic Category Cephalosporin (Second Generation)
Use Treatment of otitis media and infections involving the respiratory tract and skin and skin structure; active against methicillin-sensitive staphylococci, many streptococci, and various gram-negative bacilli including *E. coli*, some *Klebsiella, P. mirabilis, H. influenzae,* and *Moraxella*.
Usual Dosage
Usual dosage range:
Infants and Children >6 months to 12 years: Oral: 7.5-15 mg/kg/day divided every 12 hours
Children >12 years and Adults: Oral: 250-500 mg every 12 hours or 500 mg every 24 hours
Indication-specific dosing:
Infants and Children >6 months to 12 years: Oral:
Otitis media: 15 mg/kg every 12 hours for 10 days

Children 2-12 years: Oral:
Pharyngitis/tonsillitis: 7.5-15 mg/kg/day divided every 12 hours for 10 days (administer for >10 days if due to *S. pyogenes*); maximum: 1 g/day
Uncomplicated skin and skin structure infections: 20 mg/kg every 24 hours for 10 days; maximum: 1 g/day
Children >12 years and Adults: Oral:
Pharyngitis/tonsillitis: 500 mg every 24 hours for 10 days
Secondary bacterial infection of acute bronchitis or acute bacterial exacerbation of chronic bronchitis: 500 mg every 12 hours for 10 days
Uncomplicated skin and skin structure infections: 250 mg every 12 hours or 500 mg every 12-24 hours for 10 days
Dosage Forms
Powder for oral suspension: 125 mg/5 mL, 250 mg/5 mL
Cefzil®: 125 mg/5 mL, 250 mg/5 mL
Tablet: 250 mg, 500 mg
Cefzil®: 250 mg, 500 mg

ceftazidime (SEF tay zi deem)

Sound-Alike/Look-Alike Issues
ceftazidime may be confused with ceftizoxime
Ceptaz® may be confused with Septra®
Tazicef® may be confused with Tazidime®
Tazidime® may be confused with Tazicef®
U.S./Canadian Brand Names Fortaz® [US/Can]; Tazicef® [US]
Therapeutic Category Cephalosporin (Third Generation)
Use Treatment of documented susceptible *Pseudomonas aeruginosa* infection and infections due to other susceptible aerobic gram-negative organisms; empiric therapy of a febrile, granulocytopenic patient
Usual Dosage
Usual dosage range:
Infants and Children 1 month to 12 years: I.V.: 30-50 mg/kg/dose every 8 hours (maximum dose: 6 g/day)
Adults: I.M., I.V.: 500 mg to 2 g every 8-12 hours
Indication-specific dosing:
Bacterial arthritis (gram-negative bacilli): I.V.: 1-2 g every 8 hours
Cystic fibrosis: I.V.: 30-50 mg/kg every 8 hours (maximum: 6 g/day)
Melioidosis: I.V.: 40 mg/kg every 8 hours for 10 days, followed by oral therapy with doxycycline or TMP/SMX
Otitis externa: I.V.: 2 g every 8 hours
Peritonitis (CAPD):
Anuric, intermittent: 1000-1500 mg/day
Anuric, continuous (per liter exchange): Loading dose: 250 mg; maintenance dose: 125 mg
Severe infections, including meningitis, complicated pneumonia, endophthalmitis, CNS infection, osteomyelitis, intra-abdominal and gynecological, skin and soft tissue: I.V.: 2 g every 8 hours
Dosage Forms
Infusion [premixed iso-osmotic solution]:
Fortaz®: 1 g (50 mL); 2 g (50 mL)
Injection, powder for reconstitution:
Fortaz®: 500 mg, 1 g, 2 g, 6 g
Tazicef®: 1 g, 2 g, 6 g

ceftibuten (sef TYE byoo ten)

U.S./Canadian Brand Names Cedax® [US]
Therapeutic Category Cephalosporin (Third Generation)
Use Oral cephalosporin for treatment of bronchitis, otitis media, and pharyngitis/tonsillitis due to *H. influenzae* and *M. catarrhalis*, both beta-lactamase-producing and nonproducing strains, as well as *S. pneumoniae* (weak) and *S. pyogenes*
Usual Dosage Oral:
Children <12 years: 9 mg/kg/day for 10 days (maximum dose: 400 mg/day)
Children ≥12 years and Adults: 400 mg once daily for 10 days (maximum dose: 400 mg/day)
Dosage Forms
Capsule:
Cedax®: 400 mg
Powder for oral suspension:
Cedax®: 90 mg/5 mL

Ceftin® [US/Can] *see* cefuroxime *on page 165*

Ceftin® **Tablet 125 mg** *(Discontinued)* *see* cefuroxime *on next page*

ceftizoxime (sef ti ZOKS eem)
Sound-Alike/Look-Alike Issues
   ceftizoxime may be confused with cefotaxime, ceftazidime, cefuroxime
Synonyms ceftizoxime sodium
U.S./Canadian Brand Names Cefizox® [US/Can]
Therapeutic Category Cephalosporin (Third Generation)
Use Treatment of susceptible bacterial infections, mainly respiratory tract, skin and skin structure, bone and joint, urinary tract and gynecologic, as well as septicemia; active against many gram-negative bacilli (not *Pseudomonas*), some gram-positive cocci (not *Enterococcus*), and some anaerobes
Usual Dosage
   Usual dosage range:
      Children ≥6 months: I.M., I.V.: 150-200 mg/kg/day divided every 6-8 hours (maximum: 12 g/24 hours)
      Adults: I.M., I.V.: 1-4 g every 8-12 hours
   Indication-specific dosing:
      Adults:
      Gonococcal:
         Disseminated infection: I.M., I.V.: 1 g every 8 hours
         Uncomplicated: I.M.: 1 g as single dose
      Life-threatening infections: I.V.: 2 g every 4 hours or 4 g every 8 hours
Dosage Forms
   Infusion [premixed iso-osmotic solution]:
      Cefizox®: 1 g (50 mL); 2 g (50 mL)

ceftizoxime sodium *see* ceftizoxime *on this page*

ceftriaxone (sef trye AKS one)
Sound-Alike/Look-Alike Issues
   Rocephin® may be confused with Roferon®
Synonyms ceftriaxone sodium
U.S./Canadian Brand Names Rocephin® [US/Can]
Therapeutic Category Cephalosporin (Third Generation)
Use Treatment of lower respiratory tract infections, acute bacterial otitis media, skin and skin structure infections, bone and joint infections, intraabdominal and urinary tract infections, pelvic inflammatory disease (PID), uncomplicated gonorrhea, bacterial septicemia, and meningitis; used in surgical prophylaxis
Usual Dosage
   Usual dosage range:
      Infants and Children: I.M., I.V.: 50-100 mg/kg/day in 1-2 divided doses (maximum: 4 g/day)
      Adults: I.M., I.V.: 1-2 g every 12-24 hours
   Indication-specific dosing:
      Infants and Children:
      Epiglottitis: I.M., I.V.: 50-100 mg/kg once daily for 7-10 days with clindamycin
      Mild-to-moderate infections: I.M., I.V.: 50-75 mg/kg/day in 1-2 divided doses every 12-24 hours (maximum: 2 g/day); continue until at least 2 days after signs and symptoms of infection have resolved
      Meningitis:
      Gonococcal, complicated:
         <45 kg: I.V.: 50 mg/kg/day given every 12 hours (maximum: 2 g/day); usual duration of treatment is 10-14 days
         >45 kg: I.V.: 1-2 g every 12 hours; usual duration of treatment is 10-14 days
      Uncomplicated: I.M., I.V.: Loading dose of 100 mg/kg (maximum: 4 g), followed by 100 mg/kg/day divided every 12-24 hours (maximum: 4 g/day); usual duration of treatment is 7-14 days
      Otitis media: *Acute:* I.M., I.V.: 50 mg/kg in a single dose (maximum: 1 g)
      Pneumonia: I.V.: 50-75 mg/kg once daily
      Prophylaxis against infective endocarditis: I.M., I.V.: 50 mg/kg 30-60 minutes before procedure; maximum dose: 1 g
      Serious infections: I.V.: 80-100 mg/kg/day in 1-2 divided doses (maximum: 4 g/day)
      Typhoid fever: I.V.: 100 mg/kg once daily (maximum 4 g)
      Adults:
      Arthritis (septic): I.V.: 1-2 g once daily
      Brain abscess and necrotizing fasciitis: I.V.: 2 g every 12 hours
      Cavernous sinus thrombosis: I.V.: 1 g every 12 hours with vancomycin or linezolid
      Endocarditis, acute native valve: I.V.: 2 g once daily for 2-4 weeks
      Lyme disease: I.V.: 2 g once daily for 14-28 days
      Mastoiditis (hospitalized): I.V.: 2 g once daily; >60 years old: 1 g once daily

Meningitis: I.V.: 2 g every 12 hours for 7-14 days (longer courses may be necessary for selected organisms)

Pelvic inflammatory disease: I.M.: 250 mg in a single dose

Pneumonia, community-acquired: I.V.: 2 g once daily; >65 years of age: 1 g once daily

Prophylaxis against infective endocarditis: I.M., I.V.: 1 g 30-60 minutes before procedure. **Note:** Intramuscular injections should be avoided in patients who are receiving anticoagulant therapy. In these circumstances, orally administered regimens should be given whenever possible. Intravenously administered antibiotics should be used for patients who are unable to tolerate or absorb oral medications.

Septic/toxic shock: I.V.: 2 g once daily; with clindamycin for toxic shock

Surgical prophylaxis: I.V.: 1 g 30 minutes to 2 hours before surgery

Syphilis: I.M., I.V.: 1 g once daily for 8-10 days

Typhoid fever: I.V.: 2-3 g once daily for 7-14 days

Dosage Forms

Infusion [premixed in dextrose]: 1 g (50 mL); 2 g (50 mL)

Injection, powder for reconstitution: 250 mg, 500 mg, 1 g, 2 g, 10 g

Rocephin®: 250 mg, 500 mg, 1 g, 2 g, 10 g

ceftriaxone sodium see ceftriaxone *on previous page*

cefuroxime (se fyoor OKS eem)

Sound-Alike/Look-Alike Issues

cefuroxime may be confused with cefotaxime, cefprozil, ceftizoxime, deferoxamine

Ceftin® may be confused with Cefotan®, cefotetan, Cefzil®, Cipro®

Zinacef® may be confused with Zithromax®

Synonyms cefuroxime axetil; cefuroxime sodium

U.S./Canadian Brand Names Apo-Cefuroxime® [Can]; Ceftin® [US/Can]; ratio-Cefuroxime [Can]; Zinacef® [US/Can]

Therapeutic Category Cephalosporin (Second Generation)

Use Treatment of infections caused by staphylococci, group B streptococci, *H. influenzae* (type A and B), *E. coli*, *Enterobacter*, *Salmonella*, and *Klebsiella*; treatment of susceptible infections of the upper and lower respiratory tract, otitis media, urinary tract, uncomplicated skin and soft tissue, bone and joint, sepsis, uncomplicated gonorrhea, and early Lyme disease; preoperative prophylaxis of susceptible infections

Usual Dosage Note: Cefuroxime axetil film-coated tablets and oral suspension are not bioequivalent and are not substitutable on a mg/mg basis

Usual dosage range:

Neonates: I.M., I.V.: 50-100 mg/kg/day divided every 12 hours

Children <13 years:

Oral: 20-30 mg/kg/day in 2 divided doses

I.M., I.V.: 75-150 mg/kg/day divided every 8 hours (maximum dose: 6 g/day)

Children ≥13 years and Adults:

Oral: 250-500 mg twice daily

I.M., I.V.: 750 mg to 1.5 g every 6-8 hours or 100-150 mg/kg/day in divided doses every 6-8 hours (maximum: 6 g/day)

Indication-specific dosing:

Children ≥3 months to 12 years:

Acute bacterial maxillary sinusitis, acute otitis media, and impetigo:

Oral: Suspension: 30 mg/kg/day in 2 divided doses for 10 days (maximum dose: 1 g/day); tablet: 250 mg twice daily for 10 days

I.M., I.V.: 75-150 mg/kg/day divided every 8 hours (maximum dose: 6 g/day)

Epiglottitis: Oral: 150 mg/kg/day in 3 divided doses for 7-10 days

Pharyngitis/tonsillitis:

Oral: Suspension: 20 mg/kg/day (maximum: 500 mg/day) in 2 divided doses for 10 days; tablet: 125 mg every 12 hours for 10 days

I.M., I.V.: 75-150 mg/kg day divided every 8 hours (maximum: 6 g/day)

Children ≥13 years and Adults:

Bronchitis (acute and exacerbations of chronic bronchitis):

Oral: 250-500 mg every 12 hours for 10 days

I.V.: 500-750 mg every 8 hours (complete therapy with oral dosing)

Cellulitis:

Oral: 500 mg every 12 hours

Orbital: I.V.: 1.5 g every 8 hours

Gonorrhea:

Disseminated: I.M., I.V.: 750 mg every 8 hours

Uncomplicated:

Oral: 1 g as a single dose

(Continued)

cefuroxime *(Continued)*

I.M.: 1.5 g as single dose (administer in 2 different sites with probenecid)

Lyme disease (early): Oral: 500 mg twice daily for 20 days

Pharyngitis/tonsillitis and sinusitis: Oral: 250 mg twice daily for 10 days

Pneumonia (uncomplicated): I.V.: 750 mg every 8 hours

Severe or complicated infections: I.M., I.V.: 1.5 g every 8 hours (up to 1.5 g every 6 hours in life-threatening infections)

Skin/skin structure infection (uncomplicated):

Oral: 250-500 mg every 12 hours for 10 days

I.M., I.V.: 750 mg every 8 hours

Surgical prophylaxis:

I.V.: 1.5 g 30 minutes to 1 hour prior to procedure (if procedure is prolonged can give 750 mg every 8 hours I.M.)

Open heart: I.V.: 1.5 g every 12 hours to a total of 6 g

Urinary tract infection (uncomplicated):

Oral: 125-250 mg every 12 hours for 7-10 days

I.M., I.V.: 750 mg every 8 hours

Dosage Forms Note: Strength expressed as base

Infusion [premixed]: 750 mg (50 mL); 1.5 g (50 mL)

Zinacef®: 750 mg (50 mL); 1.5 g (50 mL)

Injection, powder for reconstitution: 750 mg, 1.5 g, 7.5 g

Zinacef®: 750 mg, 1.5 g, 7.5 g

Powder for oral suspension:

Ceftin®: 125 mg/5 mL, 250 mg/5 mL

Tablet: 250 mg, 500 mg

Ceftin®: 250 mg, 500 mg

cefuroxime axetil *see* cefuroxime *on previous page*

cefuroxime sodium *see* cefuroxime *on previous page*

Cefzil® [US/Can] *see* cefprozil *on page 162*

Celebrex® [US/Can] *see* celecoxib *on this page*

celecoxib (se le KOKS ib)

Sound-Alike/Look-Alike Issues

Celebrex® may be confused with Celexa®, cerebra, Cerebyx®

U.S./Canadian Brand Names Celebrex® [US/Can]; GD-Celecoxib [Can]

Therapeutic Category Nonsteroidal Antiinflammatory Drug (NSAID), COX-2 Selective

Use Relief of the signs and symptoms of osteoarthritis, ankylosing spondylitis, juvenile rheumatoid arthritis (JRA), and rheumatoid arthritis; management of acute pain; treatment of primary dysmenorrhea; decreasing intestinal polyps in familial adenomatous polyposis (FAP).

Canadian note: Celecoxib is only indicated for relief of symptoms of rheumatoid arthritis, osteoarthritis, and relief of acute pain in adults

Usual Dosage Note: Use the lowest effective dose for the shortest duration of time, consistent with individual patient goals. Oral:

Children ≥2 years: JRA

≥10 kg to ≤25 kg: 50 mg twice daily

>25 kg: 100 mg twice daily

Adults:

Acute pain or primary dysmenorrhea: Initial dose: 400 mg, followed by an additional 200 mg if needed on day 1; maintenance dose: 200 mg twice daily as needed

Ankylosing spondylitis: 200 mg/day as a single dose or in divided doses twice daily; if no effect after 6 weeks, may increase to 400 mg/day. If no response following 6 weeks of treatment with 400 mg/day, consider discontinuation and alternative treatment.

Familial adenomatous polyposis: 400 mg twice daily

Osteoarthritis: 200 mg/day as a single dose or in divided dose twice daily

Rheumatoid arthritis: 100-200 mg twice daily

Dosage Forms

Capsule:

Celebrex®: 50 mg, 100 mg, 200 mg, 400 mg

Celestone® [US] *see* betamethasone (systemic) *on page 108*

Celestone® Soluspan® [US/Can] *see* betamethasone (systemic) *on page 108*

Celexa® [US/Can] *see* citalopram *on page 194*

CellCept® **[US/Can]** *see* mycophenolate *on page 584*

Cellugel® **[US]** *see* hydroxypropyl methylcellulose *on page 439*

cellulose, oxidized regenerated (SEL yoo lose, OKS i dyzed re JEN er aye ted)

Sound-Alike/Look-Alike Issues
Surgicel® may be confused with Serentil®
Synonyms absorbable cotton; oxidized regenerated cellulose
U.S./Canadian Brand Names Surgicel® Fibrillar [US]; Surgicel® NuKnit [US]; Surgicel® [US]
Therapeutic Category Hemostatic Agent
Use Hemostatic; temporary packing for the control of capillary, venous, or small arterial hemorrhage
Usual Dosage Minimal amounts of the fabric strip are laid on the bleeding site or held firmly against the tissues until hemostasis occurs; remove excess material
Dosage Forms
  Fabric, fibrous:
    Surgicel® Fibrillar:
      1" x 2" (10s)
      2" x 4" (10s)
      4" x 4" (10s)
  Fabric, knitted:
    Surgicel® NuKnit:
      1" x 1" (24s)
      1" x 3½"(10s)
      3" x 4" (24s)
      6" x 9" (10s)
  Fabric, sheer weave:
    Surgicel®:
      ½"x 2" (24s)
      2" x 3" (24s)
      2" x 14" (24s)
      4" x 8" (24s)

Celluvisc™ **[Can]** *see* carboxymethylcellulose *on page 153*

Celontin® **[US/Can]** *see* methsuximide *on page 556*

Cemill [US-OTC] *see* ascorbic acid *on page 76*

Cena-K® *(Discontinued)* *see* potassium chloride *on page 700*

Cenestin® **[US/Can]** *see* estrogens (conjugated A/synthetic) *on page 317*

Cenolate® **[US]** *see* ascorbic acid *on page 76*

Centamin [US-OTC] *see* vitamins (multiple/oral) *on page 895*

Centany™ **[US]** *see* mupirocin *on page 582*

Centrum® **[US-OTC]** *see* vitamins (multiple/oral) *on page 895*

Centrum Kids® Complete [US-OTC] *see* vitamins (multiple/pediatric) *on page 896*

Centrum Kids® Dora the Explorer™ Complete [US-OTC] *see* vitamins (multiple/pediatric) *on page 896*

Centrum Kids® Rugrats® Complete [US-OTC] *see* vitamins (multiple/pediatric) *on page 896*

Centrum Kids® SpongeBob™ SquarePants Complete [US-OTC] *see* vitamins (multiple/pediatric) *on page 896*

Centrum® Performance™ [US-OTC] *see* vitamins (multiple/oral) *on page 895*

Centrum® Silver® [US-OTC] *see* vitamins (multiple/oral) *on page 895*

Cepacol® Antibacterial Mouthwash [US-OTC] *see* cetylpyridinium *on page 170*

Cepacol® Antibacterial Mouthwash Gold [US-OTC] *see* cetylpyridinium *on page 170*

Cepacol® Sore Throat [US-OTC] *see* benzocaine *on page 101*

Cephadyn [US] *see* butalbital and acetaminophen *on page 131*

cephalexin (sef a LEKS in)

Sound-Alike/Look-Alike Issues
cephalexin may be confused with cefaclor, cefazolin, cephalothin, ciprofloxacin
Synonyms cephalexin monohydrate
U.S./Canadian Brand Names Apo-Cephalex® [Can]; Keflex® [US]; Keftab® [Can]; Novo-Lexin [Can]; Nu-Cephalex [Can]
(Continued)

167

cephalexin (Continued)

Therapeutic Category Cephalosporin (First Generation)

Use Treatment of susceptible bacterial infections including respiratory tract infections, otitis media, skin and skin structure infections, bone infections, and genitourinary tract infections, including acute prostatitis; alternative therapy for acute infective endocarditis prophylaxis

Usual Dosage

Usual dosage range:

Children >1 year: Oral: 25-100 mg/kg/day every 6-8 hours (maximum: 4 g/day)

Adults: Oral: 250-1000 mg every 6 hours; maximum: 4 g/day

Indication-specific dosing:

Children >1 year: Oral:

Furunculosis: 25-50 mg/kg/day in 4 divided doses

Impetigo: 25 mg/kg/day in 4 divided doses

Otitis media: 75-100 mg/kg/day in 4 divided doses

Prophylaxis of infective endocarditis (dental, oral, respiratory tract, or esophageal procedures): 50 mg/kg 30-60 minutes prior to procedure (maximum: 2 g)

Severe infections: 50-100 mg/kg/day in divided doses every 6-8 hours

Skin abscess: 50 mg/kg/day in 4 divided doses (maximum: 4 g)

Streptococcal pharyngitis, skin and skin structure infections: 25-50 mg/kg/day divided every 12 hours

Children >15 years and Adults: Oral:

Cellulitis and mastitis: 500 mg every 6 hours

Furunculosis/skin abscess: 250 mg 4 times/day

Prophylaxis of infective endocarditis (dental, oral, respiratory tract, or esophageal procedures): 2 g 30-60 minutes prior to procedure

Prophylaxis in total joint replacement patients undergoing dental procedures which produce bacteremia: 2 g 1 hour prior to procedure

Streptococcal pharyngitis, skin and skin structure infections: 500 mg every 12 hours

Uncomplicated cystitis: 500 mg every 12 hours for 7-14 days

Dosage Forms

Capsule: 250 mg, 500 mg

Keflex®: 250 mg, 500 mg, 750 mg

Powder for oral suspension: 125 mg/5 mL, 250 mg/5 mL

Keflex®: 125 mg/5 mL, 250 mg/5 mL

Tablet: 250 mg, 500 mg

cephalexin monohydrate see cephalexin on previous page

cephalothin *(Discontinued)*

Cephulac® *(Discontinued)* see lactulose on page 489

Ceprotin [US] see protein C concentrate (human) on page 726

Ceptaz® *(Discontinued)* see ceftazidime on page 163

Cerebyx® [US/Can] see fosphenytoin on page 376

Ceredase® [US] see alglucerase on page 28

Cerezyme® [US/Can] see imiglucerase on page 448

Ceron [US] see chlorpheniramine and phenylephrine on page 177

Ceron-DM [US] see chlorpheniramine, phenylephrine, and dextromethorphan on page 180

Cerovel™ [US] see urea on page 877

Certain Dri® [US-OTC] see aluminum chloride hexahydrate on page 36

Certuss-D® [US] see guaifenesin, dextromethorphan, and phenylephrine on page 407

Cerubidine® [US/Can] see daunorubicin hydrochloride on page 233

Cerumenex® *(Discontinued)*

Cervidil® [US/Can] see dinoprostone on page 264

C.E.S.® [Can] see estrogens (conjugated/equine) on page 318

Cesia™ [US] see ethinyl estradiol and desogestrel on page 322

Cetacaine® [US] see benzocaine, butamben, and tetracaine on page 103

Cetacort® [US] see hydrocortisone (topical) on page 434

Cetafen® [US-OTC] see acetaminophen on page 5

Cetafen Extra® [US-OTC] see acetaminophen on page 5

Cetamide™ [Can] see sulfacetamide on page 810

Cetapred® Ophthalmic *(Discontinued)* *see* sulfacetamide and prednisolone *on page 811*

cetirizine (se TI ra zeen)
Sound-Alike/Look-Alike Issues
Zyrtec® may be confused with Serax®, Xanax®, Zantac®, Zyprexa®
Synonyms cetirizine hydrochloride; P-071; UCB-P071
U.S./Canadian Brand Names Apo-Cetirizine® [Can]; Reactine™ [Can]; Zyrtec® [US]
Therapeutic Category Antihistamine
Use Perennial and seasonal allergic rhinitis and other allergic symptoms including urticaria; chronic idiopathic urticaria
Usual Dosage Oral:
Children:
6-12 months: Chronic urticaria, perennial allergic rhinitis: 2.5 mg once daily
12 months to <2 years: Chronic urticaria, perennial allergic rhinitis: 2.5 mg once daily; may increase to 2.5 mg every 12 hours if needed
2-5 years: Chronic urticaria, perennial or seasonal allergic rhinitis: Initial: 2.5 mg once daily; may be increased to 2.5 mg every 12 hours **or** 5 mg once daily
Children ≥6 years and Adults: Chronic urticaria, perennial or seasonal allergic rhinitis: 5-10 mg once daily, depending upon symptom severity
Dosage Forms
Syrup:
Zyrtec®: 5 mg/5 mL
Tablet:
Zyrtec®: 5 mg, 10 mg
Tablet, chewable:
Zyrtec®: 5 mg, 10 mg

cetirizine and pseudoephedrine (se TI ra zeen & soo doe e FED rin)
Sound-Alike/Look-Alike Issues
Zyrtec® may be confused with Serax®, Xanax®, Zantac®, Zyprexa®
Synonyms cetirizine hydrochloride and pseudoephedrine hydrochloride; pseudoephedrine hydrochloride and cetirizine hydrochloride
U.S./Canadian Brand Names Reactine® Allergy and Sinus [Can]; Zyrtec-D 12 Hour® [US]
Therapeutic Category Antihistamine/Decongestant Combination
Use Treatment of symptoms of seasonal or perennial allergic rhinitis
Usual Dosage Oral: Children ≥12 years and Adults: Seasonal/perennial allergic rhinitis: 1 tablet twice daily
Dosage Forms
Tablet, extended release:
Zyrtec-D 12 Hour®: Cetirizine 5 mg and pseudoephedrine 120 mg

cetirizine hydrochloride *see* cetirizine *on this page*

cetirizine hydrochloride and pseudoephedrine hydrochloride *see* cetirizine and pseudoephedrine *on this page*

cetrorelix (set roe REL iks)
Synonyms cetrorelix acetate
U.S./Canadian Brand Names Cetrotide® [US/Can]
Therapeutic Category Antigonadotropic Agent
Use Inhibits premature luteinizing hormone (LH) surges in women undergoing controlled ovarian stimulation
Usual Dosage SubQ: Adults: Female: Used in conjunction with controlled ovarian stimulation therapy using gonadotropins (FSH, HMG):
Single-dose regimen: 3 mg given when serum estradiol levels show appropriate stimulation response, usually stimulation day 7 (range days 5-9). If hCG is not administered within 4 days, continue cetrorelix at 0.25 mg/day until hCG is administered.
Multiple-dose regimen: 0.25 mg morning or evening of stimulation day 5, or morning of stimulation day 6; continue until hCG is administered.
Dosage Forms
Injection, powder for reconstitution:
Cetrotide®: 0.25 mg, 3 mg

cetrorelix acetate *see* cetrorelix *on this page*

Cetrotide® [US/Can] *see* cetrorelix *on this page*

cetuximab (se TUK see mab)
Sound-Alike/Look-Alike Issues
cetuximab may be confused with bevacizumab
Synonyms C225; IMC-C225; NSC-714692
U.S./Canadian Brand Names Erbitux® [US/Can]
Therapeutic Category Antineoplastic Agent, Monoclonal Antibody; Epidermal Growth Factor Receptor (EGFR) Inhibitor
Use Treatment of metastatic colorectal cancer; treatment of squamous cell cancer of the head and neck
Usual Dosage I.V.: Adults:
Colorectal cancer:
Initial loading dose: 400 mg/m^2 infused over 120 minutes
Maintenance dose: 250 mg/m^2 infused over 60 minutes weekly
Head and neck cancer:
Initial loading dose: 400 mg/m^2 infused over 120 minutes
Maintenance dose: 250 mg/m^2 infused over 60 minutes weekly
Note: If given in combination with radiation therapy, administer loading dose 1 week prior to initiation of radiation course. Administer weekly maintenance dose 1 hour prior to radiation for the duration of radiation therapy (6-7 weeks).
Dosage Forms
Injection, solution [preservative free]:
Erbitux®: 2 mg/mL (50 mL)

cetylpyridinium (SEE til peer i DI nee um)
Synonyms cetylpyridinium chloride; CPC
U.S./Canadian Brand Names Cepacol® Antibacterial Mouthwash Gold [US-OTC]; Cepacol® Antibacterial Mouthwash [US-OTC]; DiabetAid Gingivitis Mouth Rinse [US-OTC]
Therapeutic Category Local Anesthetic
Use Antiseptic to aid in the prevention and reduction of plaque and gingivitis, and to freshen breath
Usual Dosage Oral (OTC labeling): Children ≥6 years and Adults: Rinse or gargle to freshen mouth; may be used before or after brushing
Dosage Forms
Liquid, oral [mouthwash/gargle]:
Cepacol® Antibacterial Mouthwash Gold [OTC]: 0.05%
DiabetAid Gingivitis Mouth Rinse [OTC]: 0.1%

cetylpyridinium chloride *see* cetylpyridinium *on this page*

Cevalin® *(Discontinued)* *see* ascorbic acid *on page 76*

cevimeline (se vi ME leen)
Sound-Alike/Look-Alike Issues
Evoxac® may be confused with Eurax®
Synonyms cevimeline hydrochloride
U.S./Canadian Brand Names Evoxac® [US/Can]
Therapeutic Category Cholinergic Agent
Use Treatment of symptoms of dry mouth in patients with Sjögren syndrome
Usual Dosage Oral: Adults: 30 mg 3 times/day
Dosage Forms
Capsule:
Evoxac®: 30 mg

cevimeline hydrochloride *see* cevimeline *on this page*

CFDN *see* cefdinir *on page 159*

CG *see* chorionic gonadotropin (human) *on page 187*

C-Gel [US-OTC] *see* ascorbic acid *on page 76*

CGP-42446 *see* zoledronic acid *on page 907*

CGP-57148B *see* imatinib *on page 448*

C-Gram [US-OTC] *see* ascorbic acid *on page 76*

CGS-20267 *see* letrozole *on page 496*

Champix® [Can] *see* varenicline *on page 884*

Chantix™ [US] *see* varenicline *on page 884*

Charcadole® [Can] *see* charcoal *on next page*

Charcadole®, Aqueous [Can] *see* charcoal *on this page*

Charcadole® TFS [Can] *see* charcoal *on this page*

Char-Caps [US-OTC] *see* charcoal *on this page*

CharcoAid® *(Discontinued)* *see* charcoal *on this page*

CharcoAid G® *(Discontinued)* *see* charcoal *on this page*

charcoal (CHAR kole)

Sound-Alike/Look-Alike Issues
Actidose® may be confused with Actos®

Synonyms activated carbon; activated charcoal; adsorbent charcoal; liquid antidote; medicinal carbon; medicinal charcoal

U.S./Canadian Brand Names Actidose-Aqua® [US-OTC]; Actidose® with Sorbitol [US-OTC]; Char-Caps [US-OTC]; Charcadole® TFS [Can]; Charcadole® [Can]; Charcadole®, Aqueous [Can]; Charcoal Plus® DS [US-OTC]; Charcocaps® [US-OTC]; EZ-Char™ [US-OTC]; Kerr Insta-Char® [US-OTC]

Therapeutic Category Antidote

Use Emergency treatment in poisoning by drugs and chemicals; aids the elimination of certain drugs and improves decontamination of excessive ingestions of sustained-release products or in the presence of bezoars; repetitive doses have proven useful to enhance the elimination of certain drugs (eg, carbamazepine, dapsone, phenobarbital, quinine, or theophylline); repetitive doses for gastric dialysis in uremia to adsorb various waste products; dietary supplement (digestive aid)

Usual Dosage Oral:
Acute poisoning: **Note:** ~10 g of activated charcoal for each 1 g of toxin is considered adequate; this may require multiple doses. If sorbitol is also used, sorbitol dose should not exceed 1.5 g/kg. When using multiple doses of charcoal, sorbitol should be given with every other dose (not to exceed 2 doses/day).
Children: 1 g/kg as a single dose; if multiple doses are needed, additional doses can be given as 0.25 g/kg every hour or equivalent (ie, 0.5 g/kg every 2 hours) **or**
>1 year-12 years: 25-50 g as a single dose; smaller doses (10-25 g) may be used in children 1-5 years due to smaller gut lumen capacity
Children >12 years and Adults: 25-100 g as a single dose; if multiple doses are needed, additional doses may be given as 12.5 g/hour or equivalent (ie, 25 g every 2 hours)
Dietary supplement: Adult: 500-520 mg after meals; may repeat in 2 hours if needed (maximum 10 g/day)

Dosage Forms
Capsule:
Char-Caps [OTC], Charcocaps® [OTC]: 260 mg
Liquid:
Actidose-Aqua® [OTC]: 15 g, 25 g, 50 g
Kerr Insta-Char® [OTC]: 25 g, 50 g
Liquid [with sorbitol]:
Actidose® with Sorbitol [OTC], Kerr Insta-Char® [OTC]: 25 g, 50 g
Pellet:
EZ-Char™ [OTC]: 25 g
Powder for suspension: 30 g, 240 g
Tablet:
Charcoal Plus® DS [OTC]: 250 mg

Charcoal Plus® DS [US-OTC] *see* charcoal *on this page*

Charcocaps® [US-OTC] *see* charcoal *on this page*

Chealamide® *(Discontinued)* *see* edetate disodium *on page 291*

CheeTah® [US] *see* barium *on page 94*

Chemet® [US/Can] *see* succimer *on page 808*

Cheracol® [US] *see* guaifenesin and codeine *on page 402*

Cheracol® [US-OTC] *see* phenol *on page 673*

Cheracol® D [US-OTC] *see* guaifenesin and dextromethorphan *on page 402*

Cheracol® Plus [US-OTC] *see* guaifenesin and dextromethorphan *on page 402*

Chew-C [US-OTC] *see* ascorbic acid *on page 76*

Chew-Cal [US-OTC] *see* calcium and vitamin D *on page 137*

CHG *see* chlorhexidine gluconate *on page 174*

Chibroxin® *(Discontinued)* *see* norfloxacin *on page 612*

chicken pox vaccine *see* varicella virus vaccine *on page 885*

Chiggerex® [US-OTC] *see* benzocaine *on page 101*

Chiggertox® [US-OTC] *see* benzocaine *on page 101*

Children's Advil® Cold [Can] *see* pseudoephedrine and ibuprofen *on page 729*

Children's Dimetapp® Elixir Cold & Allergy *(Discontinued)* *see* brompheniramine and pseudoephedrine *on page 120*

Children's Hold® *(Discontinued)* *see* dextromethorphan *on page 247*

Children's Kaopectate® *(Discontinued)*

Children's Motion Sickness Liquid [Can] *see* dimenhydrinate *on page 262*

Children's Pepto [US-OTC] *see* calcium carbonate *on page 138*

children's vitamins *see* vitamins (multiple/pediatric) *on page 896*

ChiRhoStim® [US] *see* secretin *on page 780*

Chirocaine® *(Discontinued)*

Chlo-Amine® Oral *(Discontinued)* *see* chlorpheniramine *on page 177*

Chlorafed® Liquid *(Discontinued)* *see* chlorpheniramine and pseudoephedrine *on page 178*

chloral *see* chloral hydrate *on this page*

chloral hydrate (KLOR al HYE drate)

Synonyms chloral; hydrated chloral; trichloroacetaldehyde monohydrate
U.S./Canadian Brand Names Aquachloral® Supprettes® [US]; PMS-Chloral Hydrate [Can]; Somnote™ [US]
Therapeutic Category Hypnotic, Nonbarbiturate
Controlled Substance C-IV
Use Short-term sedative and hypnotic (<2 weeks); sedative/hypnotic for diagnostic procedures; sedative prior to EEG evaluations
Usual Dosage
Children:
Sedation or anxiety: Oral, rectal: 5-15 mg/kg/dose every 8 hours (maximum: 500 mg/dose)
Prior to EEG: Oral, rectal: 20-25 mg/kg/dose, 30-60 minutes prior to EEG; may repeat in 30 minutes to maximum of 100 mg/kg or 2 g total
Hypnotic: Oral, rectal: 20-40 mg/kg/dose up to a maximum of 50 mg/kg/24 hours or 1 g/dose or 2 g/24 hours
Conscious sedation: Oral: 50-75 mg/kg/dose 30-60 minutes prior to procedure; may repeat 30 minutes after initial dose if needed, to a total maximum dose of 120 mg/kg or 1 g total
Adults: Oral, rectal:
Sedation, anxiety: 250 mg 3 times/day
Hypnotic: 500-1000 mg at bedtime or 30 minutes prior to procedure, not to exceed 2 g/24 hours
Dosage Forms
Capsule:
Somnote®: 500 mg
Suppository, rectal: 500 mg
Aquachloral® Supprettes®: 325 mg
Syrup: 500 mg/5 mL

chlorambucil (klor AM byoo sil)

Sound-Alike/Look-Alike Issues
chlorambucil may be confused with Chloromycetin®
Leukeran® may be confused with Alkeran®, leucovorin, Leukine®, Myleran®
Synonyms CB-1348; chlorambucilum; chloraminophene; chlorbutinum; NSC-3088; WR-139013
U.S./Canadian Brand Names Leukeran® [US/Can]
Therapeutic Category Antineoplastic Agent
Use Management of chronic lymphocytic leukemia, Hodgkin and non-Hodgkin lymphoma; breast and ovarian carcinoma; Waldenström macroglobulinemia, testicular carcinoma, thrombocythemia, choriocarcinoma
Usual Dosage Oral (refer to individual protocols): Adults:
CLL, NHL: 0.1 mg/kg/day for 3-6 weeks **or** 0.4 mg/kg (increased by 0.1 mg/kg/dose until response/toxicity observed) biweekly **or** 0.4 mg/kg (increased by 0.1 mg/kg/dose until response/toxicity observed) monthly **or** 0.03-0.1 mg/kg/day continuously
Hodgkin lymphoma: 0.2 mg/kg/day for 3-6 weeks **or** 0.4 mg/kg (increased by 0.1 mg/kg/dose until response/toxicity observed) biweekly **or** 0.4 mg/kg (increased by 0.1 mg/kg/dose until response/toxicity observed) monthly **or** 0.03-0.1 mg/kg/day continuously
Dosage Forms
Tablet:
Leukeran®: 2 mg

chlorambucilum *see* chlorambucil *on previous page*

chloraminophene *see* chlorambucil *on previous page*

chloramphenicol (klor am FEN i kole)
Sound-Alike/Look-Alike Issues
Chloromycetin® may be confused with chlorambucil, Chlor-Trimeton®
U.S./Canadian Brand Names Chloromycetin® Sodium Succinate [US]; Chloromycetin® Succinate [Can]; Chloromycetin® [Can]; Diochloram® [Can]; Pentamycetin® [Can]
Therapeutic Category Antibiotic, Miscellaneous; Antibiotic, Ophthalmic; Antibiotic, Otic
Use Treatment of serious infections due to organisms resistant to other less toxic antibiotics or when its penetrability into the site of infection is clinically superior to other antibiotics to which the organism is sensitive; useful in infections caused by *Bacteroides*, *H. influenzae*, *Neisseria meningitidis*, *Salmonella*, and *Rickettsia*; active against many vancomycin-resistant enterococci
Usual Dosage
Meningitis: I.V.: Infants >30 days and Children: 50-100 mg/kg/day divided every 6 hours
Other infections: I.V.:
Infants >30 days and Children: 50-75 mg/kg/day divided every 6 hours; maximum daily dose: 4 g/day
Adults: 50-100 mg/kg/day in divided doses every 6 hours; maximum daily dose: 4 g/day
Dosage Forms
Injection, powder for reconstitution: 1 g

ChloraPrep® [US-OTC] *see* chlorhexidine gluconate *on next page*

Chloraseptic® Gargle [US-OTC] *see* phenol *on page 673*

Chloraseptic® Mouth Pain [US-OTC] *see* phenol *on page 673*

Chloraseptic® Pocket Pump [US-OTC] *see* phenol *on page 673*

Chloraseptic® Spray [US-OTC] *see* phenol *on page 673*

Chloraseptic® Spray for Kids [US-OTC] *see* phenol *on page 673*

Chlorate® Oral (Discontinued) *see* chlorpheniramine *on page 177*

chlorbutinum *see* chlorambucil *on previous page*

Chlordex GP [US] *see* dextromethorphan, chlorpheniramine, phenylephrine, and guaifenesin *on page 248*

chlordiazepoxide (klor dye az e POKS ide)
Sound-Alike/Look-Alike Issues
Librium® may be confused with Librax®
Synonyms methaminodiazepoxide hydrochloride
U.S./Canadian Brand Names Apo-Chlordiazepoxide® [Can]; Librium® [US]
Therapeutic Category Benzodiazepine
Controlled Substance C-IV
Use Management of anxiety disorder or for the short-term relief of symptoms of anxiety; withdrawal symptoms of acute alcoholism; preoperative apprehension and anxiety
Usual Dosage
Children >6 years: Anxiety: Oral, I.M.: 0.5 mg/kg/24 hours divided every 6-8 hours
Adults:
Anxiety:
Oral: 15-100 mg divided 3-4 times/day
I.M., I.V.: Initial: 50-100 mg followed by 25-50 mg 3-4 times/day as needed
Preoperative anxiety: I.M.: 50-100 mg prior to surgery
Ethanol withdrawal symptoms: Oral, I.V.: 50-100 mg to start, dose may be repeated in 2-4 hours as necessary to a maximum of 300 mg/24 hours
Note: Up to 300 mg may be given I.M. or I.V. during a 6-hour period, but not more than this in any 24-hour period.
Dosage Forms
Capsule: 5 mg, 10 mg, 25 mg
Librium®: 5 mg, 10 mg, 25 mg
Injection, powder for reconstitution:
Librium®: 100 mg

chlordiazepoxide and amitriptyline hydrochloride *see* amitriptyline and chlordiazepoxide *on page 44*

chlordiazepoxide and clidinium *see* clidinium and chlordiazepoxide *on page 198*

chlorethazine *see* mechlorethamine *on page 535*

chlorethazine mustard *see* mechlorethamine *on page 535*

chlorhexidine gluconate (klor HEKS i deen GLOO koe nate)
Sound-Alike/Look-Alike Issues
Peridex® may be confused with Precedex™
Synonyms CHG
U.S./Canadian Brand Names Avagard™ [US-OTC]; BactoShield® CHG [US-OTC]; Betasept® [US-OTC]; ChloraPrep® [US-OTC]; Dyna-Hex® [US-OTC]; Hibiclens® [US-OTC]; Hibidil® 1:2000 [Can]; Hibistat® [US-OTC]; Operand® Chlorhexidine Gluconate [US-OTC]; ORO-Clense [Can]; Peridex® [US]; PerioChip® [US]; PerioGard® [US]
Therapeutic Category Antibiotic, Oral Rinse; Antibiotic, Topical
Use Skin cleanser for surgical scrub, cleanser for skin wounds, preoperative skin preparation, germicidal hand rinse, and as antibacterial dental rinse. Chlorhexidine is active against gram-positive and gram-negative organisms, facultative anaerobes, aerobes, and yeast.
Orphan drug: Peridex®: Oral mucositis with cytoreductive therapy when used for patients undergoing bone marrow transplant
Usual Dosage Adults:
Oral rinse (Peridex®, PerioGard®):
Floss and brush teeth, completely rinse toothpaste from mouth and swish 15 mL (one capful) undiluted oral rinse around in mouth for 30 seconds, then expectorate. Caution patient not to swallow the medicine and instruct not to eat for 2-3 hours after treatment. (Cap on bottle measures 15 mL.)
Treatment of gingivitis: Oral prophylaxis: Swish for 30 seconds with 15 mL chlorhexidine, then expectorate; repeat twice daily (morning and evening). Patient should have a reevaluation followed by a dental prophylaxis every 6 months.
Periodontal chip: One chip is inserted into a periodontal pocket with a probing pocket depth ≥5 mm. Up to 8 chips may be inserted in a single visit. Treatment is recommended every 3 months in pockets with a remaining depth ≥5 mm. If dislodgment occurs 7 days or more after placement, the subject is considered to have had the full course of treatment. If dislodgment occurs within 48 hours, a new chip should be inserted. The chip biodegrades completely and does not need to be removed. Patients should avoid dental floss at the site of PerioChip® insertion for 10 days after placement because flossing might dislodge the chip.
Insertion of periodontal chip: Pocket should be isolated and surrounding area dried prior to chip insertion. The chip should be grasped using forceps with the rounded edges away from the forceps. The chip should be inserted into the periodontal pocket to its maximum depth. It may be maneuvered into position using the tips of the forceps or a flat instrument.
Cleanser:
Surgical scrub: Scrub 3 minutes and rinse thoroughly, wash for an additional 3 minutes
Hand sanitizer (Avagard™): Dispense 1 pumpful in palm of one hand; dip fingertips of opposite hand into solution and work it under nails. Spread remainder evenly over hand and just above elbow, covering all surfaces. Repeat on other hand. Dispense another pumpful in each hand and reapply to each hand up to the wrist. Allow to dry before gloving.
Hand wash: Wash for 15 seconds and rinse
Hand rinse: Rub 15 seconds and rinse
Dosage Forms
Chip, for periodontal pocket insertion:
PerioChip®: 2.5 mg
Liquid, topical [surgical scrub]:
Avagard™ [OTC]: 1% (500 mL)
BactoShield® CHG [OTC]: 2% (120 mL, 480 mL, 750 mL, 1000 mL, 3800 mL); 4% (120 mL, 480 mL, 750 mL, 1000 mL, 3800 mL)
Betasept® [OTC]: 4% 120 mL, 240 mL, 480 mL, 960 mL, 3840 mL)
ChloraPrep® [OTC]: 2% (0.67 mL, 1.5 mL, 3 mL, 10.5 mL)
Dyna-Hex® [OTC]: 2% (120 mL, 960 mL, 3840 mL); 4% (120 mL, 960 mL, 3840 mL)
Hibiclens® [OTC]: 4% (15 mL, 120 mL, 240 mL, 480 mL, 960 mL, 3840 mL)
Operand® Chlorhexidine Gluconate [OTC]: 2% (120 mL); 4% (120 mL, 240 mL, 480 mL, 960 mL, 3840 mL)
Liquid, oral rinse: 0.12%
Peridex®, PerioGard®: 0.12%
Pad [prep pad]:
Hibistat® [OTC]: 0.5% (50s)
Sponge/Brush:
BactoShield® CHG [OTC]: 4% per sponge/brush

chlormeprazine *see* prochlorperazine *on page 716*

Chlor-Mes-D [US] *see* chlorpheniramine, phenylephrine, and methscopolamine *on page 181*

2-chlorodeoxyadenosine *see* cladribine *on page 196*

chloroethane *see* ethyl chloride *on page 334*

Chloromag® **[US]** *see* magnesium chloride *on page 524*

Chloromycetin® **[Can]** *see* chloramphenicol *on page 173*

Chloromycetin® **Sodium Succinate [US]** *see* chloramphenicol *on page 173*

Chloromycetin® **Succinate [Can]** *see* chloramphenicol *on page 173*

chlorophyll (KLOR oh fil)
Synonyms chlorophyllin
U.S./Canadian Brand Names Nullo® [US-OTC]
Therapeutic Category Gastrointestinal Agent, Miscellaneous
Use Control fecal odors in colostomy or ileostomy
Usual Dosage
Oral: Children >12 years and Adults: 100-200 mg/day in divided doses; may increase to 300 mg/day if odor is not controlled (maximum: 300 mg/day)
Ostomy: Tablet: May also place 1-2 tablets in empty pouch each time it is reused or changed.
Dosage Forms
Caplet:
Nullo® [OTC]: Chlorophyllin copper complex 100 mg

chlorophyllin *see* chlorophyll *on this page*

chlorophyllin copper complex sodium, papain, and urea *see* chlorophyllin, papain, and urea *on this page*

chlorophyllin, papain, and urea (KLOR oh fil in, pa PAY in, & yoor EE a)
Sound-Alike/Look-Alike Issues
Ziox™ may be confused with Zyvox®
Synonyms chlorophyllin copper complex sodium, papain, and urea; papain, urea, and chlorophyllin; urea, chlorophyllin, and papain
U.S./Canadian Brand Names Allanfil 405 [US]; Allanfil Spray [US]; Panafil® SE [US]; Panafil® [US]; Ziox 405™ [US]; Ziox™ [US]
Therapeutic Category Enzyme, Topical Debridement
Use Treatment of acute and chronic lesions, such as varicose, diabetic decubitus ulcers, burns, postoperative wounds, pilonidal cyst wounds, carbuncles, and miscellaneous traumatic or infected wounds
Usual Dosage Topical: Adults: Apply with each dressing change; daily or twice daily dressing changes are preferred, but may be every 2-3 days. Cover with dressing following application.
Ointment: Apply $1/_8$" thickness over the wound with clean applicator.
Spray: Completely cover the wound site so that the wound is not visible.
Dosage Forms
Emulsion [spray]:
Panafil® SE: Copper chlorophyllin complex sodium 0.5%, papain ≥521,700 USP units/g, and urea 10% (34 mL)
Ointment:
Allanfil 405, Panafil®: Chlorophyllin copper complex sodium 0.5%, papain ≥521,700 USP units/g, and urea 10% (6 g, 30 g)
Ziox™: Chlorophyllin copper complex sodium 0.5%, papain ≥521,700 USP units/g, and urea 10% (30 g)
Ziox 405™: Copper chlorophyllin complex sodium 0.5%, papain ≥521,700 USP units/g, and urea 10% (3.5 g, 30 g)
Solution [spray]:
Allanfil: Copper chlorophyllin complex sodium 0.5%, papain ≥521,700 USP units/g, and urea 10% (33 mL)

chloroprocaine (klor oh PROE kane)
Sound-Alike/Look-Alike Issues
Nesacaine® may be confused with Neptazane®
Synonyms chloroprocaine hydrochloride
U.S./Canadian Brand Names Nesacaine® [US]; Nesacaine®-CE [Can]; Nesacaine®-MPF [US]
Therapeutic Category Local Anesthetic
Use Infiltration anesthesia and peripheral and epidural anesthesia
Usual Dosage Dosage varies with anesthetic procedure, the area to be anesthetized, the vascularity of the tissues, depth of anesthesia required, degree of muscle relaxation required, and duration of anesthesia; range.
Children >3 years (normally developed): Maximum dose (without epinephrine): 11 mg/kg; for infiltration, concentrations of 0.5% to 1% are recommended; for nerve block, concentrations of 1% to 1.5% are recommended
(Continued)

chloroprocaine *(Continued)*

Adults:
Maximum single dose (without epinephrine): 11 mg/kg; maximum dose: 800 mg
Maximum single dose (with epinephrine): 14 mg/kg; maximum dose: 1000 mg
Infiltration and peripheral nerve block:
  Mandibular: 2%: 2-3 mL; total dose 40-60 mg
  Infraorbital: 2%: 0.5-1 mL; total dose 10-20 mg
  Brachial plexus: 2%; 30-40 mL; total dose 600-800 mg
  Digital (without epinephrine): 1%; 3-4 mL; total dose: 30-40 mg
  Pudendal: 2%; 10 mL each side; total dose: 400 mg
  Paracervical: 1%; 3 mL per each of four sites
  Caudal block: Preservative-free: 2% or 3%: 15-25 mL; may repeat at 40-60 minute intervals
  Lumbar epidural block: Preservative-free: 2% or 3%: 2-2.5 mL per segment; usual total volume: 15-25 mL; may repeat with doses that are 2-6 mL less than initial dose every 40-50 minutes.

Dosage Forms
Injection, solution: 1% (30 mL); 2% (30 mL)
  Nesacaine®: 1% (30 mL); 2% (30 mL)
Injection, solution [preservative free]: 2% (20 mL); 3% (20 mL)
  Nesacaine®-MPF: 2% (20 mL); 3% (20 mL)

chloroprocaine hydrochloride *see* chloroprocaine *on previous page*

Chloroptic® Ophthalmic Solution *(Discontinued)* *see* chloramphenicol *on page 173*

Chloroptic® SOP *(Discontinued)* *see* chloramphenicol *on page 173*

chloroquine *(KLOR oh kwin)*

Synonyms chloroquine phosphate
U.S./Canadian Brand Names Aralen® [US/Can]; Novo-Chloroquine [Can]
Therapeutic Category Aminoquinoline (Antimalarial)
Use Suppression or chemoprophylaxis of malaria; treatment of uncomplicated or mild-to-moderate malaria; extraintestinal amebiasis
Usual Dosage Oral:
Suppression or prophylaxis of malaria:
  Children: Administer 5 mg base/kg/week on the same day each week (not to exceed 300 mg base/dose); begin 1-2 weeks prior to exposure; continue for 4-6 weeks after leaving endemic area; if suppressive therapy is not begun prior to exposure, double the initial loading dose to 10 mg base/kg and administer in 2 divided doses 6 hours apart, followed by the usual dosage regimen
  Adults: 500 mg/week (300 mg base) on the same day each week; begin 1-2 weeks prior to exposure; continue for 4-6 weeks after leaving endemic area; if suppressive therapy is not begun prior to exposure, double the initial loading dose to 1 g (600 mg base) and administer in 2 divided doses 6 hours apart, followed by the usual dosage regimen
Acute attack:
  Children: 10 mg/kg (base) on day 1, followed by 5 mg/kg (base) 6 hours later and 5 mg/kg (base) on days 2 and 3
  Adults: 1 g (600 mg base) on day 1, followed by 500 mg (300 mg base) 6 hours later, followed by 500 mg (300 mg base) on days 2 and 3
Extraintestinal amebiasis:
  Children: 10 mg/kg (base) once daily for 2-3 weeks (up to 300 mg base/day)
  Adults: 1 g/day (600 mg base) for 2 days followed by 500 mg/day (300 mg base) for at least 2-3 weeks
Dosage Forms
Tablet: 250 mg, 500 mg
  Aralen®: 500 mg

chloroquine phosphate *see* chloroquine *on this page*

chlorothiazide *(klor oh THYE a zide)*

U.S./Canadian Brand Names Diuril® [US/Can]
Therapeutic Category Diuretic, Thiazide
Use Management of mild-to-moderate hypertension; adjunctive treatment of edema
Usual Dosage Note: The manufacturer states that I.V. and oral dosing are equivalent. Some clinicians may use lower I.V. doses, however, because of chlorothiazide's poor oral absorption. I.V. dosing in infants and children has not been well established.

Infants <6 months: Oral: 20-40 mg/kg/day in 2 divided doses (maximum dose: 375 mg/day)
Infants >6 months and Children: Oral: 10-20 mg/kg/day in 2 divided doses (maximum dose: 375 mg/day in children <2 years or 1 g/day in children 2-12 years)

Adults:
Hypertension: Oral: 500-2000 mg/day divided in 1-2 doses (manufacturer labeling); doses of 125-500 mg/day have also been recommended

Edema: Oral, I.V.: 250-1000 mg once or twice daily; intermittent treatment (eg, therapy on alternative days) may be appropriate for some patients. Maximum daily dose: 1000 mg (ACC/AHA 2005 Heart Failure Guidelines)

Dosage Forms
Injection, powder for reconstitution:
Sodium Diuril®: 500 mg
Suspension, oral:
Diuril®: 250 mg/5 mL
Tablet: 250 mg, 500 mg

Chlorphed® (Discontinued) see brompheniramine on page 120

Chlorphed®-LA Nasal Solution (Discontinued) see oxymetazoline on page 643

Chlorphen [US-OTC] see chlorpheniramine on this page

chlorpheniramine (klor fen IR a meen)

Sound-Alike/Look-Alike Issues
Chlor-Trimeton® may be confused with Chloromycetin®

Synonyms chlorpheniramine maleate; CTM

U.S./Canadian Brand Names Ahist™ [US]; Aller-Chlor® [US-OTC]; Chlor-Trimeton® [US-OTC]; Chlor-Tripolon® [Can]; Chlorphen [US-OTC]; Diabetic Tussin® Allergy Relief [US-OTC]; Novo-Pheniram [Can]; PediaTan™ [US]; QDALL® AR [US]; Teldrin® HBP [US-OTC]

Therapeutic Category Antihistamine

Use Perennial and seasonal allergic rhinitis and other allergic symptoms including urticaria

Usual Dosage Oral:
Children: 0.35 mg/kg/day in divided doses every 4-6 hours
2-6 years: 1 mg every 4-6 hours, not to exceed 6 mg in 24 hours
6-12 years: 2 mg every 4-6 hours, not to exceed 12 mg/day or sustained release 8 mg at bedtime
Children >12 years and Adults: 4 mg every 4-6 hours, not to exceed 24 mg/day or sustained release 8-12 mg every 8-12 hours, not to exceed 24 mg/day

Dosage Forms
Capsule, variable release:
QDALL® AR: Chlorpheniramine 12 mg [immediate release and sustained release]
Suspension:
PediaTan™: 8 mg/5 mL
Syrup:
Aller-Chlor® [OTC], Diabetic Tussin® Allergy Relief [OTC]: 2 mg/5 mL
Tablet: 4 mg
Aller-Chlor® [OTC], Chlor-Trimeton® [OTC], Chlorphen [OTC], Teldrin® HBP [OTC]: 4 mg
Tablet, extended release:
Chlor-Trimeton® [OTC]: 12 mg
Tablet, long acting [scored]:
Ahist™: 12 mg

chlorpheniramine, acetaminophen, and pseudoephedrine see acetaminophen, chlorpheniramine, and pseudoephedrine on page 10

chlorpheniramine and acetaminophen (klor fen IR a meen & a seet a MIN oh fen)

Synonyms acetaminophen and chlorpheniramine

U.S./Canadian Brand Names Coricidin HBP® Cold and Flu [US-OTC]

Therapeutic Category Antihistamine/Analgesic

Use Symptomatic relief of congestion, headache, aches and pains of colds and flu

Usual Dosage Oral: Adults: 2 tablets every 4 hours

Dosage Forms
Tablet:
Coricidin HBP® Cold and Flu [OTC]: Chlorpheniramine 2 mg and acetaminophen 325 mg

chlorpheniramine and carbetapentane see carbetapentane and chlorpheniramine on page 149

chlorpheniramine and phenylephrine (klor fen IR a meen & fen il EF rin)

Sound-Alike/Look-Alike Issues
Rynatan® may be confused with Rynatuss®
(Continued)

177

chlorpheniramine and phenylephrine *(Continued)*

Synonyms chlorpheniramine maleate and phenylephrine hydrochloride; chlorpheniramine tannate and phenylephrine tannate; phenylephrine and chlorpheniramine

U.S./Canadian Brand Names Actifed® Cold and Allergy [US-OTC] *[reformulation]*; AllanTan Pediatric [US]; Allerx™ Suspension [US]; C-Phen [US]; Ceron [US]; Dallergy-JR® [US]; Dec-Chlorphen [US]; Ed A-Hist® [US]; NoHist [US]; PD-Hist-D [US]; PediaTan™D [US]; Phenabid® [US]; R-Tanna [US]; Relera [US]; Rescon-Jr [US]; Rondec® [US]; Rynatan® Pediatric Suspension [US]; Rynatan® [US]; Sildec PE [US]

Therapeutic Category Antihistamine/Decongestant Combination

Use Temporary relief of upper respiratory conditions such as nasal congestion, runny nose, and sneezing due to the common cold, hay fever, or allergic or vasomotor rhinitis

Usual Dosage Antihistamine/decongestant: Oral:
Children:
  6-12 months: Rondec® Drops: 0.75 mL 4 times/day
  1-2 years: Rondec® Drops: 1 mL 4 times/day
  2-6 years:
   Allerx™: 1.25 -2.5 mL every 12 hours
   Dallergy-JR® suspension: 2.5 mL every 12 hours
   Rondec® Syrup: 1.25 mL every 4-6 hours; maximum 7.5 mL/24 hours
   Rynatan® Suspension: 2.5 -5 mL every 12 hours
  6-12 years:
   Allerx™: 2.5-5 mL every 12 hours
   Dallergy-JR®: One capsule every 12 hours; maximum 2 capsules/24 hours
   Dallergy-JR® suspension: 5 mL every 12 hours
   Ed A-Hist™: One-half caplet every 12 hours
   Rondec® Syrup: 2.5 mL every 4-6 hours; maximum 15 mL/24 hours
   Rynatan® Suspension: 5-10 mL every 12 hours
  ≥12 years: Refer to adult dosing.
Adults:
  Allerx™: 15 mL every 12 hours
  Dallergy-JR®: Two capsules every 12 hours; maximum 4 capsules/24 hours
  Dallergy-JR® suspension: 10 mL every 12 hours
  Ed A-Hist™: One caplet every 12 hours
  R-Tanna: 1-2 tablets every 12 hours
  Rondec® Syrup: 5 mL every 4-6 hours; maximum 30 mL/24 hours
  Rynatan® Tablet: 1-2 tablets every 12 hours

Dosage Forms
  Caplet, prolonged release:
  Ed A-Hist®, NoHist, Relera: Chlorpheniramine 8 mg and phenylephrine 20 mg
  Capsule, extended release:
  Dallergy-JR®: Chlorpheniramine 4 mg and phenylephrine 20 mg
  Capsule, timed release:
  Phenabid®: Chlorpheniramine 8 mg and phenylephrine 20 mg
  Liquid:
  Ed A-Hist®: Chlorpheniramine 4 mg and phenylephrine 10 mg per 5 mL
  Liquid, oral drops:
  Ceron, C-Phen, Dec-Chlorphen, PD-Hist-D, Rondec®, Sildec PE: Chlorpheniramine 1 mg and phenylephrine 3.5 mg per mL
  Suspension, oral: Chlorpheniramine 4.5 mg and phenylephrine 5 mg per 5 mL
  AllanTan Pediatric, Rinate™ Pediatric, Rynatan® Pediatric Suspension: Chlorpheniramine tannate 4.5 mg and phenylephrine tannate 5 mg per 5 mL
  AlleRx™: Chlorpheniramine 3 mg and phenylephrine 7.5 per 5 mL
  Dallergy-JR®: Chlorpheniramine tannate 4 mg and phenylephrine tannate 20 mg per 5 mL
  PediaTan™D: Chlorpheniramine tannate 8 mg and phenylephrine tannate 10 mg per 5 mL
  Syrup:
  Ceron, C-Phen, Dec-Chlorphen, PD-Hist-D, Rondec®, Sildec PE: Chlorpheniramine 4 mg and phenylephrine 12. 5 mg per 5 mL
  Tablet:
  Actifed® Cold and Allergy, Sudafed PE® Sinus and Allergy: Chlorpheniramine 4 mg and phenylephrine 10 mg
  R-Tanna, Rynatan®: Chlorpheniramine 9 mg and phenylephrine 25 mg
  Tablet, sustained release:
  Rescon-Jr: Chlorpheniramine 4 mg and phenylephrine 20 mg

chlorpheniramine and pseudoephedrine (klor fen IR a meen & soo doe e FED rin)
Sound-Alike/Look-Alike Issues
  Allerest® may be confused with Sinarest®

Chlor-Trimeton® may be confused with Chloromycetin®

Sudafed® may be confused with Sufenta®

Synonyms chlorpheniramine maleate and pseudoephedrine hydrochloride; chlorpheniramine tannate and pseudoephedrine tannate; pseudoephedrine and chlorpheniramine

U.S./Canadian Brand Names A.R.M® [US-OTC]; Allerest® Maximum Strength Allergy and Hay Fever [US-OTC]; Deconamine® SR [US]; Deconamine® [US]; Dicel™ [US]; Dynahist-ER Pediatric® [US]; Histex™ [US]; Kronofed-A® [US]; Kronofed-A®-Jr [US]; LoHist-D [US]; QDALL® [US]; Sudafed® Sinus & Allergy [US-OTC]; Sudal® 12 [US]; Triaminic® Cold and Allergy [Can]

Therapeutic Category Antihistamine/Decongestant Combination

Use Relief of nasal congestion associated with the common cold, hay fever, and other allergies, sinusitis, eustachian tube blockage, and vasomotor and allergic rhinitis

Usual Dosage General dosing guidelines; consult specific product labeling. Rhinitis/decongestant: Oral:

Children:

2-6 years:

Chlorpheniramine maleate 1 mg and pseudoephedrine hydrochloride 15 mg every 4-6 hours

Chlorpheniramine tannate 4.5 mg and pseudoephedrine tannate 75 mg: 2.5-5 mL every 12 hours (maximum: 10 mL/24 hours)

6-12 years: Chlorpheniramine maleate 2 mg and pseudoephedrine hydrochloride 30 mg every 4-6 hours (immediate release products)

Children ≥12 years and Adults:

Chlorpheniramine maleate 4 mg and pseudoephedrine hydrochloride 60 mg every 4-6 hours (immediate release products)

Chlorpheniramine tannate 4.5 mg and pseudoephedrine tannate 75 mg: 10-20 mL every 12 hours (maximum: 40 mL/24 hours)

Deconamine® SR, Kronofed-A®: Chlorpheniramine maleate 8 mg and pseudoephedrine hydrochloride 120 mg every 12 hours

Dosage Forms

Capsule, extended release: Chlorpheniramine 8 mg and pseudoephedrine 120 mg

Dynahist-ER Pediatric®: Chlorpheniramine 4 mg and pseudoephedrine 60 mg

Capsule, sustained release: Chlorpheniramine 8 mg and pseudoephedrine 120 mg

Deconamine® SR: Chlorpheniramine 8 mg and pseudoephedrine 120 mg

Liquid:

Histex™, LoHist-D: Chlorpheniramine 2 mg and pseudoephedrine 30 mg per 5 mL

Suspension:

Dicel™: Chlorpheniramine tannate 5 mg and pseudoephedrine tannate 75 mg per 5 mL

Syrup: Chlorpheniramine 2 mg and pseudoephedrine 30 mg per 5 mL

Tablet: Chlorpheniramine 4 mg and pseudoephedrine 60 mg

Allerest® Maximum Strength Allergy and Hay Fever [OTC]: Chlorpheniramine 2 mg and pseudoephedrine 30 mg

Sudafed® Sinus & Allergy [OTC]: Chlorpheniramine 4 mg and pseudoephedrine 60 mg

Tablet, chewable:

Sudal® 12: Chlorpheniramine 4 mg and pseudoephedrine 30 mg

chlorpheniramine, carbetapentane, and phenylephrine *see* carbetapentane, phenylephrine, and chlorpheniramine *on page 150*

chlorpheniramine, dextromethorphan, phenylephrine, and guaifenesin *see* dextromethorphan, chlorpheniramine, phenylephrine, and guaifenesin *on page 248*

chlorpheniramine, ephedrine, phenylephrine, and carbetapentane

(klor fen IR a meen, e FED rin, fen il EF rin, & kar bay ta PEN tane)

Sound-Alike/Look-Alike Issues

Rynatuss® may be confused with Rynatan®

Synonyms carbetapentane, ephedrine, phenylephrine, and chlorpheniramine; ephedrine, chlorpheniramine, phenylephrine, and carbetapentane; phenylephrine, ephedrine, chlorpheniramine, and carbetapentane

U.S./Canadian Brand Names Rynatuss® [US]; Tetra Tannate Pediatric [US]

Therapeutic Category Antihistamine/Decongestant/Antitussive

Use Symptomatic relief of cough with a decongestant and an antihistamine

Usual Dosage Oral:

Children:

<2 years: Titrate dose individually

2-6 years: 2.5-5 mL every 12 hours

>6 years: 5-10 mL every 12 hours

Adults: 1-2 tablets every 12 hours

(Continued)

chlorpheniramine, ephedrine, phenylephrine, and carbetapentane *(Continued)*

Dosage Forms
Suspension:
Quad Tann® Pediatric, Tetra Tannate Pediatric: Chlorpheniramine 4 mg, ephedrine 5 mg, phenylephrine 5 mg, and carbetapentane 30 mg per 5 mL
Tablet:
Rynatuss®: Chlorpheniramine 5 mg, ephedrine 10 mg, phenylephrine 10 mg, and carbetapentane 50 mg
Tablet, long acting:
Quad Tann®: Chlorpheniramine 5 mg, ephedrine 10 mg, phenylephrine 10 mg, and carbetapentane 60 mg

chlorpheniramine, hydrocodone, phenylephrine, acetaminophen, and caffeine *see* hydrocodone, chlorpheniramine, phenylephrine, acetaminophen, and caffeine *on page 431*

chlorpheniramine maleate *see* chlorpheniramine *on page 177*

chlorpheniramine maleate and hydrocodone bitartrate *see* hydrocodone and chlorpheniramine *on page 428*

chlorpheniramine maleate and phenylephrine hydrochloride *see* chlorpheniramine and phenylephrine *on page 177*

chlorpheniramine maleate and pseudoephedrine hydrochloride *see* chlorpheniramine and pseudoephedrine *on page 178*

chlorpheniramine maleate, dihydrocodeine bitartrate, and phenylephrine hydrochloride *see* dihydrocodeine, chlorpheniramine, and phenylephrine *on page 259*

chlorpheniramine maleate, ibuprofen, and pseudoephedrine *see* ibuprofen, pseudoephedrine, and chlorpheniramine *on page 445*

chlorpheniramine maleate, phenylephrine hydrochloride, and guaifenesin *see* chlorpheniramine, phenylephrine, and guaifenesin *on next page*

chlorpheniramine maleate, pseudoephedrine hydrochloride, and dextromethorphan hydrobromide *see* chlorpheniramine, pseudoephedrine, and dextromethorphan *on page 183*

chlorpheniramine, phenylephrine, and dextromethorphan
(klor fen IR a meen, fen il EF rin, & deks troe meth OR fan)
Synonyms dextromethorphan, chlorpheniramine, and phenylephrine; phenylephrine, chlorpheniramine, and dextromethorphan
U.S./Canadian Brand Names C-Phen DM [US]; Ceron-DM [US]; Corfen DM [US]; De-Chlor DM [US]; De-Chlor DR [US]; Dec-Chlorphen DM [US]; Dex PC [US]; Ed A-Hist DM [US]; Neo DM [US]; PD-Cof [US]; Phenabid DM® [US]; Rondec®-DM [US]; Sildec PE-DM [US]; Statuss™ DM [US]; Tri-Vent™ DPC [US]
Therapeutic Category Antihistamine/Decongestant/Antitussive
Use Temporary relief of cough and upper respiratory symptoms associated with allergies or the common cold
Usual Dosage Oral: Relief of cough and cold symptoms:
Children:
6-12 months (Rondec®-DM drops): 0.75 mL 4 times/day
1-2 years (Rondec®-DM drops): 1 mL 4 times/day
2-6 years:
Rondec®-DM syrup: 1.25 mL every 4-6 hours (maximum: 7.5 mL/24 hours)
Tri-Vent™ DPC: 2.5 mL every 6 hours (maximum: 10 mL/24 hours)
6-12 years:
Rondec®-DM syrup: 2.5 mL every 4-6 hours (maximum: 15 mL/24 hours)
Tri-Vent™ DPC: 5 mL every 6 hours (maximum: 20 mL/24 hours)
Children ≥12 years and Adults:
Rondec®-DM syrup: 5 mL every 4-6 hours (maximum: 30 mL/24 hours)
Tri-Vent™ DPC: 10 mL every 6 hours (maximum: 40 mL/24 hours)
Dosage Forms
Liquid:
Corfen DM: Chlorpheniramine 4 mg, phenylephrine 10 mg, and dextromethorphan 15 mg per 5 mL
De-Chlor DM: Chlorpheniramine 2 mg, phenylephrine 10 mg, and dextromethorphan 15 mg per 5 mL
De-Chlor DR: Chlorpheniramine 2 mg, phenylephrine 6 mg, and dextromethorphan 15 mg per 5 mL
Liquid, oral [drops]:
Ceron-DM, C-Phen DM, PD-Cof, Dec-Chlorphen DM, Rondec® DM, Sildec PE-DM: Chlorpheniramine 1 mg, phenylephrine 3.5 mg, and dextromethorphan 3 mg per 1 mL
Neo DM: Chlorpheniramine 0.75 mg, phenylephrine 1.75 mg, and dextromethorphan 2.75 mg per 1 mL
Syrup:
Ceron-DM, C-Phen DM, Dec-Chlorphen DM, Rondec®-DM, Sildec PE-DM: Chlorpheniramine 4 mg, phenylephrine 12.5 mg, and dextromethorphan 15 mg per 5 mL

Dex PC, Tri-Vent™ DPC: Chlorpheniramine 2 mg, phenylephrine 6 mg, and dextromethorphan 15 mg per 5 mL

Ed A-Hist DM: Chlorpheniramine 4 mg, phenylephrine 10 mg, and dextromethorphan 15 mg per 5 mL

Robitussin® Cough and Allergy: Chlorpheniramine 2 mg, phenylephrine 5 mg, and dextromethorphan 10 mg per 5 mL

Robitussin® Cough and Cold Nighttime: Chlorpheniramine 1 mg, phenylephrine 2.5 mg, and dextromethorphan 5 mg per 5 mL

Robitussin® Pediatric Cough and Cold Nighttime: Chlorpheniramine 4 mg, phenylephrine 12.5 mg, and dextromethorphan 15 mg per 5 mL

Statuss™: DM: Chlorpheniramine 2 mg, phenylephrine 10 mg, and dextromethorphan 15 mg per 5 mL

Tablet, timed release:

Phenabid DM®: Chlorpheniramine 8 mg, phenylephrine 20 mg, and dextromethorphan 30 mg

chlorpheniramine, phenylephrine, and guaifenesin

(klor fen IR a meen, fen il EF rin, & gwye FEN e sin)

Synonyms chlorpheniramine maleate, phenylephrine hydrochloride, and guaifenesin; chlorpheniramine tannate, phenylephrine tannate, and guaifenesin; guaifenesin, phenylephrine, and chlorpheniramine; phenylephrine, chlorpheniramine, and guaifenesin

U.S./Canadian Brand Names P Chlor GG [US]

Therapeutic Category Cough and Cold Combination

Use Symptomatic relief of upper respiratory symptoms associated with infections such as the common cold or allergies

Usual Dosage General dosing guidelines; consult specific product labeling.

Antihistamine/decongestant/expectorant: Oral:

Children <3 months: 2-3 drops per month of age every 4-6 hours as needed; not to exceed 4 doses/24 hours

Children 3-6 months: 0.3-0.6 mL every 4-6 hours as needed; not to exceed 4 doses/24 hours

Children 6 months to 1 year: 0.6-1 mL every 4-6 hours as needed; not to exceed 4 doses/24 hours

Children 1-2 years: 1-2 mL every 4-6 hours as needed; not to exceed 4 doses/24 hours

Dosage Forms

Liquid:

P Chlor GG [drops]: Chlorpheniramine 1 mg, phenylephrine 2 mg, and guaifenesin 20 mg per 1 mL

chlorpheniramine, phenylephrine, and hydrocodone *see* phenylephrine, hydrocodone, and chlorpheniramine *on page 678*

chlorpheniramine, phenylephrine, and methscopolamine

(klor fen IR a meen, fen il EF rin, & meth skoe POL a meen)

Synonyms methscopolamine nitrate, chlorpheniramine maleate, and phenylephrine hydrochloride; phenylephrine tannate, chlorpheniramine tannate, and methscopolamine nitrate

U.S./Canadian Brand Names aerohist plus™ [US]; aeroKid™ [US]; AH-Chew® II [US]; AH-Chew® [US]; Chlor-Mes-D [US]; Dallergy® [US]; Dehistine [US]; Duradyl® [US]; Durahist™ PE [US]; Extendryl® JR [US]; Extendryl® SR [US]; Extendryl® [US]; Hista-Vent® DA [US]; OMNIhist® II L.A. [US]; PCM Allergy [US]; PCM [US]; Phenylephrine CM [US]; Ralix [US]; Rescon® MX [US]; Rescon® [US]

Therapeutic Category Antihistamine/Decongestant/Anticholinergic

Use Treatment of upper respiratory symptoms such as respiratory congestion, allergic rhinitis, vasomotor rhinitis, sinusitis, and allergic skin reactions of urticaria and angioedema

Usual Dosage

Children 6-11 years: Relief of respiratory symptoms: Oral:

aeroKid™: 2.5-5 mL every 4 hours

Ah-Chew® suspension: 2.5-5 mL every 12 hours

Dallergy®, Durahist™ PE, OMNIhist® II L.A., Rescon® MX: One-half caplet/tablet every 12 hours

Duradryl® syrup, Extendryl syrup: 2.5-5 mL, may repeat up to every 4 hours depending on age and body weight

Extendryl® chewable tablet: One tablet every 4 hours; do not exceed 4 doses in 24 hours

Extendryl® JR: One tablet every 12 hours

Children ≥12 years and Adults: Relief of respiratory symptoms: Oral: **Note:** If disturbances in urination occur in patients without renal impairment, medication should be discontinued for 1-2 days and should then be restarted at a lower dose

aeroKid™: 5-10 mL every 3-4 hours

Ah-Chew® suspension: 5-10 mL every 12 hours

Dallergy®, Durahist™ PE, Extendryl SR, OMNIhist® II L.A., Rescon® MX: One capsule/tablet every 12 hours

Duradryl® syrup, Extendryl syrup: 5-10 mL every 3-4 hours (4 times/day)

Extendryl®: 1-2 chewable tablets every 4 hours

(Continued)

chlorpheniramine, phenylephrine, and methscopolamine *(Continued)*

Dosage Forms
Caplet, extended release:
aerohist plus™ [OTC]: Chlorpheniramine 8 mg, phenylephrine 20 mg, and methscopolamine 2.5 mg
Dallergy® [OTC]: Chlorpheniramine 12 mg, phenylephrine 20 mg, and methscopolamine 2.5 mg
Liquid:
Chlor-Mes-D [OTC]: Chlorpheniramine 2 mg, phenylephrine 10 mg, and methscopolamine 0.625 mg per 5 mL
Suspension:
Ah-Chew® [OTC]: Chlorpheniramine, phenylephrine, and methscopalamine 1.5 mg per 5 mL
Syrup:
aeroKid™ [OTC]: Chlorpheniramine 4 mg, phenylephrine 1 mg, and methscopolamine 1.25 mg per 5 mL
Dallergy [OTC]: Chlorpheniramine 2 mg, phenylephrine 8 mg, and methscopolamine 0.75 mg per 5 mL
Dehistine [OTC], Duradryl® [OTC]: Chlorpheniramine 2 mg, phenylephrine 10 mg, and methscopolamine 1.25 mg per 5 mL
Extendryl® [OTC]: Dexchlorpheniramine 1 mg, phenylephrine 10 mg, and methscopolamine 1.25 mg per 5 mL
Tablet [scored]:
Dallergy® [OTC]: Chlorpheniramine 4 mg, phenylephrine 10 mg, and methscopolamine 1.25 mg
Tablet, chewable:
AH-Chew II [OTC]: Chlorpheniramine 2 mg, phenylephrine 15 mg, and methscopolamine 1.25 mg
Extendryl [OTC], PCM [OTC]: Chlorpheniramine 2 mg, phenylephrine 10 mg, and methscopolamine 1.25 mg
Tablet, extended release: Chlorpheniramine 8 mg, phenylephrine 20 mg, and methscopolamine 1.25 mg; chlorpheniramine 12 mg, phenylephrine 20 mg, and methscopolamine 2.5 mg
Durahist™ PE [OTC]: Chlorpheniramine 8 mg, phenylephrine 20 mg, and methscopolamine 1.25 mg [scored]
Extendryl SR [OTC]: Chlorpheniramine 8 mg, phenylephrine 20 mg, and methscopolamine 2.5 mg
Extendryl® JR [OTC]: Chlorpheniramine 4 mg, phenylephrine 10 mg, and methscopolamine 1.25 mg
Hista-Vent® DA [OTC]: Chlorpheniramine 8 mg, phenylephrine 20 mg, and methscopolamine 2.5 mg [scored]
PCM Allergy [OTC]: Chlorpheniramine 12 mg, phenylephrine 20 mg, and methscopolamine 2.5 mg
Tablet, long acting [scored]:
OMNIhist® II L.A. [OTC]: Chlorpheniramine 8 mg, phenylephrine 25 mg, and methscopolamine 2.5 mg
Rescon® MX [OTC]: Chlorpheniramine 8 mg, phenylephrine 40 mg, and methscopolamine 2.5 mg
Tablet, sustained release:
Ralix [OTC]: Chlorpheniramine 8 mg, phenylephrine 40 mg, and methscopolamine 2 mg
Tablet, timed release:
Phenylephrine CM [OTC]: Chlorpheniramine 8 mg, phenylephrine 40 mg, and methscopolamine 2.5 mg
Tablet, variable release:
Rescon® [OTC]: Chlorpheniramine 12 mg and phenylephrine 40 mg [sustained release] and methscopolamine 2 mg [immediate release] [MaxRelent release]

chlorpheniramine, phenylephrine, and phenyltoloxamine
(klor fen IR a meen, fen il EF rin, & fen il tole LOKS a meen)
Synonyms phenylephrine, chlorpheniramine, and phenyltoloxamine; phenyltoloxamine, chlorpheniramine, and phenylephrine
U.S./Canadian Brand Names Comhist® [US]; Nalex®-A [US]
Therapeutic Category Antihistamine/Decongestant Combination
Use Symptomatic relief of rhinitis and nasal congestion due to colds or allergy
Usual Dosage Oral:
Children:
2-6 years: Nalex®-A liquid: 1.25-2.5 mL every 4-6 hours
6-12 years:
Nalex®-A liquid: 5 mL every 4-6 hours
Nalex®-A tablet: 1/2 tablet 2-3 times/day
Children >12 years and Adults:
Nalex®-A liquid: 10 mL every 4-6 hours
Nalex®-A tablet: 1 tablet 2-3 times/day
Dosage Forms
Liquid: Chlorpheniramine 2.5 mg, phenylephrine 5 mg, and phenyltoloxamine 7.5 mg per 5 mL
Nalex®-A, NoHist-A, Rhinacon A: Chlorpheniramine 2.5 mg, phenylephrine 5 mg, and phenyltoloxamine 7.5 mg per 5 mL
Tablet, extended release:
Rhinacon A: Chlorpheniramine 4 mg, phenylephrine 20 mg, and phenyltoloxamine 40 mg
Tablet, prolonged release:
Nalex®-A: Chlorpheniramine 4 mg, phenylephrine 20 mg, and phenyltoloxamine 40 mg

Tablet, sustained release:
Chlorex-A: Chlorpheniramine 4 mg, phenylephrine 20 mg, and phenyltoloxamine 40 mg

chlorpheniramine, phenylephrine, codeine, and potassium iodide
(klor fen IR a meen, fen il EF rin, KOE deen, & poe TASS ee um EYE oh dide)
Synonyms codeine, chlorpheniramine, phenylephrine, and potassium iodide; phenylephrine, chlorpheniramine, codeine, and potassium iodide; potassium iodide, chlorpheniramine, phenylephrine, and codeine
Therapeutic Category Antihistamine/Decongestant/Antitussive
Controlled Substance C-V
Use Symptomatic relief of rhinitis, nasal congestion and cough due to colds or allergy
Usual Dosage Children 6 months to 12 years: 1.25-10 mL every 4-6 hours

chlorpheniramine, pseudoephedrine, and acetaminophen *see* acetaminophen, chlorpheniramine, and pseudoephedrine *on page 10*

chlorpheniramine, pseudoephedrine, and codeine
(klor fen IR a meen, soo doe e FED rin, & KOE deen)
Synonyms codeine, chlorpheniramine, and pseudoephedrine; pseudoephedrine, chlorpheniramine, and codeine
Therapeutic Category Antihistamine/Decongestant/Antitussive
Controlled Substance C-V
Use Temporary relief of cough associated with minor throat or bronchial irritation or nasal congestion due to common cold, allergic rhinitis, or sinusitis
Usual Dosage Oral:
Children:
25-50 lb: 1.25-2.5 mL every 4-6 hours, up to 4 doses in 24-hour period
50-90 lb: 2.5-5 mL every 4-6 hours, up to 4 doses in 24-hour period
Adults: 10 mL every 4-6 hours, up to 4 doses in 24-hour period

chlorpheniramine, pseudoephedrine, and dextromethorphan
(klor fen IR a meen, soo doe e FED rin, & deks troe meth OR fan)
Synonyms chlorpheniramine maleate, pseudoephedrine hydrochloride, and dextromethorphan hydrobromide; chlorpheniramine tannate, pseudoephedrine tannate, and dextromethorphan tannate; dexchlorpheniramine tannate, pseudoephedrine tannate, and dextromethorphan tannate; dextromethorphan, chlorpheniramine, and pseudoephedrine; pseudoephedrine, chlorpheniramine, and dextromethorphan
U.S./Canadian Brand Names Dicel™ DM [US]; DuraTan™ Forte [US]; Kidkare Cough and Cold [US-OTC]; Rescon DM [US-OTC]; Tanafed DMX™ [US]
Therapeutic Category Antihistamine/Decongestant/Antitussive
Use Temporarily relieves nasal congestion, runny nose, cough, and sneezing due to the common cold, hay fever, or allergic rhinitis
Usual Dosage General dosing guidelines; consult specific product labeling. Relief of cold symptoms: Oral:
Children:
2-6 years:
Dexchlorpheniramine tannate 2.5 mg, pseudoephedrine tannate 75 mg, and dextromethorphan tannate 25 mg (Tanafed DMX™): 2.5-5 mL every 12 hours (maximum: 10 mL/24 hours)
Dexchlorpheniramine tannate 3.5 mg, pseudoephedrine tannate 45 mg, and dextromethorphan tannate 30 mg (DuraTan™ Forte): 1.25-2.5 mL every 12 hours (maximum: 5 mL/24 hours)
6-12 years:
Chlorpheniramine maleate 1 mg, pseudoephedrine 15 mg, and dextromethorphan hydrobromide 7.5 mg per 5 mL: 10 mL every 6 hours
Chlorpheniramine maleate 1 mg, pseudoephedrine 15 mg, and dextromethorphan hydrobromide 5 mg per tablet or 5 mL: 2 tablets or 10 mL every 4-6 hours (maximum: 4 doses/24 hours)
Chlorpheniramine maleate 2 mg, pseudoephedrine 30 mg, and dextromethorphan hydrobromide 10 mg per tablet or 5 mL (Rescon DM): 5 mL every 4-6 hours (maximum: 4 doses/24 hours)
Dexchlorpheniramine tannate 2.5 mg, pseudoephedrine tannate 75 mg, and dextromethorphan tannate 25 mg (Tanafed DMX™): 5-10 mL every 12 hours (maximum: 20 mL/24 hours)
Dexchlorpheniramine tannate 3.5 mg, pseudoephedrine tannate 45 mg, and dextromethorphan tannate 30 mg (DuraTan™ Forte): 2.5-5 mL every 12 hours (maximum: 10 mL/24 hours)
>12 years: Refer to adult dosing
Adults:
Chlorpheniramine maleate 1 mg, pseudoephedrine 15 mg, and dextromethorphan hydrobromide 7.5 mg per 5 mL: 20 mL every 6 hours
Chlorpheniramine maleate 2 mg, pseudoephedrine 30 mg, and dextromethorphan hydrobromide 10 mg per tablet or 5 mL (Rescon DM): 10 mL every 4-6 hours (maximum: 4 doses/24 hours)
(Continued)

chlorpheniramine, pseudoephedrine, and dextromethorphan *(Continued)*

Dexchlorpheniramine tannate 2.5 mg, pseudoephedrine tannate 75 mg, and dextromethorphan tannate 25 mg (Tanafed DMX™): 10-20 mL every 12 hours (maximum: 40 mL/24 hours)

Dexchlorpheniramine tannate 3.5 mg, pseudoephedrine tannate 45 mg, and dextromethorphan tannate 30 mg (DuraTan™ Forte): 5-15 mL every 12 hours (maximum: 30 mL/24 hours)

Dosage Forms

Liquid: Chlorpheniramine 1 mg, pseudoephedrine 15 mg, and dextromethorphan 5 mg per 5 mL

Kidkare Cough and Cold [OTC]: Chlorpheniramine 1 mg, pseudoephedrine 15 mg, and dextromethorphan 5 mg per 5 mL

Rescon DM [OTC]: Chlorpheniramine 2 mg, pseudoephedrine 30 mg, and dextromethorphan 10 mg per 5 mL

Suspension:

Dicel™ DM: Chlorpheniramine 5 mg, pseudoephedrine 75 mg, and dextromethorphan 25 mg per 5 mL

DuraTan™ Forte: Dexchlorpheniramine tannate 3.5 mg, pseudoephedrine tannate 45 mg, and dextromethorphan tannate 30 mg per 5 mL

Tanafed DMX™: Dexchlorpheniramine 2.5 mg, pseudoephedrine 75 mg, and dextromethorphan 25 mg

chlorpheniramine, pseudoephedrine, and dihydrocodeine *see* pseudoephedrine, dihydrocodeine, and chlorpheniramine *on page 730*

chlorpheniramine, pseudoephedrine, and hydrocodone *see* pseudoephedrine, hydrocodone, and chlorpheniramine *on page 731*

chlorpheniramine, pseudoephedrine, and methscopolamine

(klor fen IR a meen, soo doe e FED rin, & meth skoe POL a meen)

Synonyms methscopolamine, chlorpheniramine, and pseudoephedrine; methscopolamine, pseudoephedrine, and chlorpheniramine; pseudoephedrine hydrochloride, methscopolamine nitrate, and chlorpheniramine maleate; pseudoephedrine, methscopolamine, and chlorpheniramine

U.S./Canadian Brand Names AlleRx™ Dose Pack [US]; Durahist™ [US]; Hista-Vent® PSE [US]

Therapeutic Category Antihistamine/Decongestant/Anticholinergic

Use Relief of symptoms of allergic rhinitis, vasomotor rhinitis, sinusitis, and the common cold

Usual Dosage Oral:

Children 6-11 years: Durahist™, Hista-Vent® PSE: One-half tablet every 12 hours (maximum dose: 1 tablet/24 hours)

Children ≥12 years and Adults:

AllerRx™: One yellow AM tablet in the morning and one blue PM tablet in the evening

Durahist™, Hista-Vent® PSE: One tablet every 12 hours (maximum dose: 2 tablets/24 hours).

Dosage Forms

Combination package:

AlleRx™:

Tablet, controlled release: Pseudoephedrine hydrochloride 120 mg and methscopolamine nitrate 2.5 mg [yellow AM tablet]

Tablet, controlled release: Chlorpheniramine maleate 8 mg and methscopolamine nitrate 2.5 mg [blue PM tablet]

Tablet, sustained release: Chlorpheniramine maleate 8 mg, pseudoephedrine hydrochloride 60 mg, and methscopolamine nitrate 1.25 mg; chlorpheniramine maleate 8 mg, pseudoephedrine hydrochloride 90 mg, and methscopolamine nitrate 2.5 mg; chlorpheniramine maleate 8 mg, pseudoephedrine hydrochloride 120 mg, and methscopolamine nitrate 2.5 mg

Durahist™: Chlorpheniramine maleate 8 mg, pseudoephedrine hydrochloride 60 mg, and methscopolamine nitrate 1.25 mg [scored]

Hista-Vent® PSE: Chlorpheniramine maleate 8 mg, pseudoephedrine hydrochloride 120 mg, and methscopolamine nitrate 2.5 mg [dye free; scored]

chlorpheniramine tannate and phenylephrine tannate *see* chlorpheniramine and phenylephrine *on page 177*

chlorpheniramine tannate and pseudoephedrine tannate *see* chlorpheniramine and pseudoephedrine *on page 178*

chlorpheniramine tannate, phenylephrine tannate, and guaifenesin *see* chlorpheniramine, phenylephrine, and guaifenesin *on page 181*

chlorpheniramine tannate, pseudoephedrine tannate, and dextromethorphan tannate *see* chlorpheniramine, pseudoephedrine, and dextromethorphan *on previous page*

Chlor-Pro® Injection *(Discontinued)* *see* chlorpheniramine *on page 177*

chlorpromazine (klor PROE ma zeen)
Sound-Alike/Look-Alike Issues
chlorproMAZINE may be confused with chlorproPAMIDE, clomiPRAMINE, prochlorperazine, promethazine
Thorazine® may be confused with thiamine, thioridazine

Synonyms chlorpromazine hydrochloride; CPZ

Tall-Man chlorpro**MAZINE**

U.S./Canadian Brand Names Largactil® [Can]; Novo-Chlorpromazine [Can]

Therapeutic Category Phenothiazine Derivative

Use Control of mania; treatment of schizophrenia; control of nausea and vomiting; relief of restlessness and apprehension before surgery; acute intermittent porphyria; adjunct in the treatment of tetanus; intractable hiccups; combativeness and/or explosive hyperexcitable behavior in children 1-12 years of age and in short-term treatment of hyperactive children

Usual Dosage
Children ≥6 months:
Schizophrenia/psychoses:
Oral: 0.5-1 mg/kg/dose every 4-6 hours; older children may require 200 mg/day or higher
I.M., I.V.: 0.5-1 mg/kg/dose every 6-8 hours
<5 years (22.7 kg): Maximum: 40 mg/day
5-12 years (22.7-45.5 kg): Maximum: 75 mg/day
Nausea and vomiting:
Oral: 0.5-1 mg/kg/dose every 4-6 hours as needed
I.M., I.V.: 0.5-1 mg/kg/dose every 6-8 hours
<5 years (22.7 kg): Maximum: 40 mg/day
5-12 years (22.7-45.5 kg): Maximum: 75 mg/day
Adults:
Schizophrenia/psychoses:
Oral: Range: 30-2000 mg/day in 1-4 divided doses, initiate at lower doses and titrate as needed; usual dose: 400-600 mg/day; some patients may require 1-2 g/day
I.M., I.V.: Initial: 25 mg, may repeat (25-50 mg) in 1-4 hours, gradually increase to a maximum of 400 mg/dose every 4-6 hours until patient is controlled; usual dose: 300-800 mg/day
Intractable hiccups: Oral, I.M.: 25-50 mg 3-4 times/day
Nausea and vomiting:
Oral: 10-25 mg every 4-6 hours
I.M., I.V.: 25-50 mg every 4-6 hours

Dosage Forms
Injection, solution: 25 mg/mL (1 mL, 2 mL)
Tablet: 10 mg, 25 mg, 50 mg, 100 mg, 200 mg

chlorpromazine hydrochloride *see* chlorpromazine *on this page*

chlorpropamide (klor PROE pa mide)
Sound-Alike/Look-Alike Issues
chlorproPAMIDE may be confused with chlorproMAZINE
Diabinese® may be confused with DiaBeta®, Dialume®, Diamox®

Tall-Man chlorpro**PAMIDE**

U.S./Canadian Brand Names Apo-Chlorpropamide® [Can]; Diabinese® [US]; Novo-Propamide [Can]

Therapeutic Category Antidiabetic Agent, Oral

Use Management of blood sugar in type 2 diabetes mellitus (noninsulin dependent, NIDDM)

Usual Dosage Oral: The dosage of chlorpropamide is variable and should be individualized based upon the patient's response
Initial dose: Adults: 250 mg/day in mild-to-moderate diabetes in middle-aged, stable diabetic
Subsequent dosages may be increased or decreased by 50-125 mg/day at 3- to 5-day intervals
Maintenance dose: 100-250 mg/day; severe diabetics may require 500 mg/day; avoid doses >750 mg/day

Dosage Forms
Tablet: 100 mg, 250 mg
Diabinese®: 100 mg, 250 mg

chlorthalidone (klor THAL i done)
U.S./Canadian Brand Names Apo-Chlorthalidone® [Can]; Thalitone® [US]

Therapeutic Category Diuretic, Miscellaneous

Use Management of mild-to-moderate hypertension when used alone or in combination with other agents; treatment of edema associated with congestive heart failure or nephrotic syndrome. Recent studies have found chlorthalidone effective in the treatment of isolated systolic hypertension in the elderly.
(Continued)

chlorthalidone (Continued)

Usual Dosage Oral: Adults:
Hypertension: 25-100 mg/day or 100 mg 3 times/week; usual dosage range (JNC 7): 12.5-25 mg/day
Edema: Initial: 50-100 mg/day or 100 mg on alternate days; maximum dose: 200 mg/day
Heart failure-associated edema: 12.5-25 mg once daily; maximum daily dose: 100 mg (ACC/AHA 2005 Heart Failure Guidelines)

Dosage Forms
Tablet: 25 mg, 50 mg, 100 mg
Thalitone®: 15 mg

chlorthalidone and atenolol see atenolol and chlorthalidone on page 81

chlorthalidone and clonidine see clonidine and chlorthalidone on page 205

Chlor-Trimeton® [US-OTC] see chlorpheniramine on page 177

Chlor-Trimeton® Allergy D (Discontinued) see chlorpheniramine and pseudoephedrine on page 178

Chlor-Trimeton® Syrup (Discontinued) see chlorpheniramine on page 177

Chlor-Tripolon® [Can] see chlorpheniramine on page 177

Chlor-Tripolon ND® [Can] see loratadine and pseudoephedrine on page 518

chlorzoxazone (klor ZOKS a zone)

Sound-Alike/Look-Alike Issues
Parafon Forte® may be confused with Fam-Pren Forte

U.S./Canadian Brand Names Parafon Forte® DSC [US]; Parafon Forte® [Can]; Strifon Forte® [Can]
Therapeutic Category Skeletal Muscle Relaxant
Use Symptomatic treatment of muscle spasm and pain associated with acute musculoskeletal conditions
Usual Dosage Oral:
Children: 20 mg/kg/day or 600 mg/m^2/day in 3-4 divided doses
Adults: 250-500 mg 3-4 times/day up to 750 mg 3-4 times/day

Dosage Forms
Caplet: 500 mg
Parafon Forte® DSC: 500 mg
Tablet: 250 mg, 500 mg

cholecalciferol (kole e kal SI fer ole)

Synonyms D$_3$
U.S./Canadian Brand Names D-Vi-Sol® [Can]; Delta-D® [US]
Therapeutic Category Vitamin D Analog
Use Dietary supplement, treatment of vitamin D deficiency, or prophylaxis of deficiency
Usual Dosage Oral: Adults: 400-1000 units/day

Dosage Forms
Tablet: 1000 int. units
Delta-D®: 400 int. units

cholecalciferol and alendronate see alendronate and cholecalciferol on page 27

cholera and traveler's diarrhea vaccine see traveler's diarrhea and cholera vaccine (Canada only) on page 858

cholestyramine resin (koe LES teer a meen REZ in)

U.S./Canadian Brand Names Novo-Cholamine Light [Can]; Novo-Cholamine [Can]; PMS-Cholestyramine [Can]; Prevalite® [US]; Questran® Light Sugar Free [Can]; Questran® Light [US]; Questran® [US/Can]
Therapeutic Category Bile Acid Sequestrant
Use Adjunct in the management of primary hypercholesterolemia; pruritus associated with elevated levels of bile acids; diarrhea associated with excess fecal bile acids; binding toxicologic agents; pseudomembraneous colitis
Usual Dosage Oral (dosages are expressed in terms of anhydrous resin):
Children: 240 mg/kg/day in 3 divided doses; need to titrate dose depending on indication
Adults: 4 g 1-2 times/day to a maximum of 24 g/day and 6 doses/day

Dosage Forms
Powder for oral suspension: 4 g of resin/5 g of powder, 4 g of resin/5.7 g of powder, 4 g of resin/9 g of powder
Prevalite®: 4 g of resin/5.5 g of powder
Questran®: 4 g of resin/9 g of powder
Questran® Light: 4 g of resin/6.4 g of powder

choline magnesium trisalicylate (KOE leen mag NEE zhum trye sa LIS i late)

Synonyms tricosal
Therapeutic Category Analgesic, Nonnarcotic; Nonsteroidal Antiinflammatory Drug (NSAID)
Use Management of osteoarthritis, rheumatoid arthritis, and other arthritis; acute painful shoulder
Usual Dosage Oral (based on total salicylate content):
Children <37 kg: 50 mg/kg/day given in 2 divided doses; 2250 mg/day for heavier children
Adults: 500 mg to 1.5 g 2-3 times/day **or** 3 g at bedtime; usual maintenance dose: 1-4.5 g/day
Dosage Forms
Liquid: 500 mg/5 mL
Tablet: 500 mg, 750 mg, 1000 mg

Cholografin® Meglumine [US] *see* iodipamide meglumine *on page 466*

chondroitin sulfate and sodium hyaluronate *see* sodium chondroitin sulfate and sodium hyaluronate *on page 794*

Chooz® [US-OTC] *see* calcium carbonate *on page 138*

choriogonadotropin alfa *see* chorionic gonadotropin (recombinant) *on this page*

chorionic gonadotropin (human) (kor ee ON ik goe NAD oh troe pin, HYU man)

Synonyms CG; hCG
U.S./Canadian Brand Names Humegon® [Can]; Novarel® [US]; Pregnyl® [US/Can]; Profasi® HP [Can]
Therapeutic Category Gonadotropin
Use Induces ovulation and pregnancy in anovulatory, infertile females; treatment of hypogonadotropic hypogonadism, prepubertal cryptorchidism; spermatogenesis induction with follitropin alfa
Usual Dosage I.M.:
Children: Various regimens:
Prepubertal cryptorchidism:
4000 units 3 times/week for 3 weeks **or**
5000 units every second day for 4 injections **or**
500 units 3 times/week for 4-6 weeks **or**
15 injections of 500-1000 units given over 6 weeks

Hypogonadotropic hypogonadism: Male:
500-1000 units 3 times/week for 3 weeks, followed by the same dose twice weekly for 3 weeks **or**
4000 units 3 times/week for 6-9 months, then reduce dosage to 2000 units 3 times/week for additional 3 months
Adults:
Induction of ovulation: Female: 5000-10,000 units one day following last dose of menotropins
Spermatogenesis induction associated with hypogonadotropic hypogonadism: Male: Treatment regimens vary (range: 1000-2000 units 2-3 times a week). Administer hCG until serum testosterone levels are normal (may require 2-3 months of therapy), then may add follitropin alfa or menopausal gonadotropin if needed to induce spermatogenesis; continue hCG at the dose required to maintain testosterone levels.
Dosage Forms
Injection, powder for reconstitution: 10,000 units
Novarel®, Pregnyl®: 10,000 units

chorionic gonadotropin (recombinant) (kor ee ON ik goe NAD oh troe pin ree KOM be nant)

Synonyms choriogonadotropin alfa; r-hCG
U.S./Canadian Brand Names Ovidrel® [US/Can]
Therapeutic Category Gonadotropin; Ovulation Stimulator
Use As part of an assisted reproductive technology (ART) program, induces ovulation in infertile females who have been pretreated with follicle-stimulating hormones (FSH); induces ovulation and pregnancy in infertile females when the cause of infertility is functional
Usual Dosage SubQ: Adults: Female: Assisted reproductive technologies (ART) and ovulation induction: 250 mcg given 1 day following the last dose of follicle-stimulating agent. Use only after adequate follicular development has been determined. Hold treatment when there is an excessive ovarian response.
Dosage Forms
Injection, solution:
Ovidrel®: 257.5 mcg/0.515 mL (0.515 mL)

Choron® *(Discontinued)* *see* chorionic gonadotropin (human) *on this page*

chromium *see* trace metals *on page 855*

Chronovera® [Can] *see* verapamil *on page 887*

Chronulac® *(Discontinued)* *see* lactulose *on page 489*

Cl-1008 *see* pregabalin *on page 712*

Cialis® **[US/Can]** *see* tadalafil *on page 819*

Cibacalcin® *(Discontinued)* *see* calcitonin *on page 135*

ciclesonide (sye KLES oh nide)

U.S./Canadian Brand Names Alvesco® [Can]; Omnaris™ [US]

Therapeutic Category Corticosteroid, Inhalant (Oral); Corticosteroid, Nasal

Use

Intranasal: Management of seasonal and perennial allergic rhinitis

Oral inhalation: Prophylactic management of bronchial asthma

Usual Dosage

Intranasal (Omnaris™): Children ≥12 years and Adults: Rhinitis: 2 sprays (50 mcg/spray) per nostril once daily; maximum: 200 mcg/day

Oral inhalation (Alvesco®): Adults: Asthma: Initial: 400 mcg once daily; maintenance: 100-800 mcg/day (1-2 puffs once or twice daily). **Note:** Titrate to the lowest effective dose once asthma stability is achieved.

Conversion from oral to inhaled steroid: Initiation of oral inhalation therapy should begin in patients who have previously been stabilized on oral corticosteroids (OCS). A gradual dose reduction of OCS should begin ~10 days after starting inhaled therapy. Decrease daily dose by 1 mg of prednisone (or equivalent of other OCS) every 7 days in closely monitored patients, and every 10 days in patients whom close monitoring is not possible. In the presence of withdrawal symptoms, resume previous OCS dose for 1 week before attempting further dose reductions.

Dosage Forms [CAN] = Canadian brand name

Aerosol for oral inhalation:

Alvesco® [CAN]: 100 mcg/inhalation, 200 mcg/inhalation [not available in the U.S.]

Suspension, intranasal [spray]:

Omnaris™: 50 mcg/inhalation (12.5 g)

ciclopirox (sye kloe PEER oks)

Sound-Alike/Look-Alike Issues

Loprox® may be confused with Lonox®

Synonyms ciclopirox olamine

U.S./Canadian Brand Names Loprox® [US/Can]; Penlac® [US/Can]; Stieprox® [Can]

Therapeutic Category Antifungal Agent

Use

Cream/suspension: Treatment of tinea pedis (athlete's foot), tinea cruris (jock itch), tinea corporis (ringworm), cutaneous candidiasis, and tinea versicolor (pityriasis)

Gel: Treatment of tinea pedis (athlete's foot), tinea corporis (ringworm); seborrheic dermatitis of the scalp

Lacquer (solution): Topical treatment of mild-to-moderate onychomycosis of the fingernails and toenails due to *Trichophyton rubrum* (not involving the lunula) and the immediately-adjacent skin

Shampoo: Treatment of seborrheic dermatitis of the scalp

Usual Dosage Topical:

Children >10 years and Adults: Tinea pedis, tinea cruris, tinea corporis, cutaneous candidiasis, and tinea versicolor: Cream/suspension: Apply twice daily, gently massage into affected areas; if no improvement after 4 weeks of treatment, re-evaluate the diagnosis.

Children ≥12 years and Adults: Onychomycosis of the fingernails and toenails: Lacquer (solution): Apply to adjacent skin and affected nails daily (as a part of a comprehensive management program for onychomycosis). Remove with alcohol every 7 days.

Children >16 years and Adults:

Tinea pedis, tinea corporis: Gel: Apply twice daily, gently massage into affected areas and surrounding skin; if no improvement after 4 weeks of treatment, reevaluate diagnosis

Seborrheic dermatitis of the scalp:

Gel: Apply twice daily, gently massage into affected areas and surrounding skin; if no improvement after 4 weeks of treatment, reevaluate diagnosis.

Shampoo: Apply ~5 mL (1 teaspoonful) to wet hair; lather, and leave in place ~3 minutes; rinse. May use up to 10 mL for longer hair. Repeat twice weekly for 4 weeks; allow a minimum of 3 days between applications.

Dosage Forms

Cream: 0.77% (15 g, 30 g, 90 g)

Loprox®: 0.77% (15 g, 30 g, 90 g)

Gel:

Loprox®: 0.77% (30 g, 45 g, 100 g)

Shampoo:

Loprox®: 1% (120 mL)

Solution, topical [nail lacquer]:
Penlac®: 8% (6.6 mL)
Suspension, topical: 0.77% (30 mL, 60 mL)
Loprox®: 0.77% (30 mL, 60 mL)

ciclopirox olamine *see* ciclopirox *on previous page*

cidecin *see* daptomycin *on page 231*

cidofovir (si DOF o veer)
U.S./Canadian Brand Names Vistide® [US]
Therapeutic Category Antiviral Agent
Use Treatment of cytomegalovirus (CMV) retinitis in patients with acquired immunodeficiency syndrome (AIDS). **Note:** Should be administered with probenecid.
Usual Dosage Adults:
Induction: 5 mg/kg I.V. over 1 hour once weekly for 2 consecutive weeks
Maintenance: 5 mg/kg over 1 hour once every other week
Note: Administer with probenecid 2 g orally 3 hours prior to each cidofovir dose and 1 g at 2 hours and 8 hours after completion of the infusion (total: 4 g)
Hydrate with 1 L of 0.9% NS I.V. prior to cidofovir infusion; a second liter may be administered over a 1- to 3-hour period immediately following infusion, if tolerated
Dosage Forms
Injection, solution [preservative free]:
Vistide®: 75 mg/mL (5 mL)

cilazapril *(Canada only)* (sye LAY za pril)
Synonyms cilazapril monohydrate
U.S./Canadian Brand Names Apo-Cilazapril® [Can]; Inhibace® [Can]; Novo-Cilazapril [Can]
Therapeutic Category Angiotensin-Converting Enzyme (ACE) Inhibitor
Use Management of hypertension; treatment of congestive heart failure
Usual Dosage Oral:
Hypertension: 2.5-5 mg once daily (maximum dose: 10 mg/day)
Congestive heart failure: Initial: 0.5 mg once daily; if tolerated, after 5 days increase to 1 mg/day (lowest maintenance dose); may increase to maximum of 2.5 mg once daily
Dosage Forms [CAN] = Canadian brand name
Tablet:
Inhibace® [CAN], Novo-Cilazapril [CAN]: 1 mg, 2.5 mg, 5 mg [not available in the U.S.]

cilazapril monohydrate *see* cilazapril *(Canada only) on this page*

cilostazol (sil OH sta zol)
Sound-Alike/Look-Alike Issues
Pletal® may be confused with Plendil®
Synonyms OPC-13013
U.S./Canadian Brand Names Pletal® [US/Can]
Therapeutic Category Platelet Aggregation Inhibitor
Use Symptomatic management of peripheral vascular disease, primarily intermittent claudication
Usual Dosage Oral: Adults: 100 mg twice daily taken at least one-half hour before or 2 hours after breakfast and dinner; dosage should be reduced to 50 mg twice daily during concurrent therapy with inhibitors of CYP3A4 or CYP2C19
Dosage Forms
Tablet: 50 mg, 100 mg
Pletal®: 50 mg, 100 mg

Ciloxan® [US/Can] *see* ciprofloxacin *on next page*

cimetidine (sye MET i deen)
Sound-Alike/Look-Alike Issues
cimetidine may be confused with simethicone
U.S./Canadian Brand Names Apo-Cimetidine® [Can]; Gen-Cimetidine [Can]; Novo-Cimetidine [Can]; Nu-Cimet [Can]; PMS-Cimetidine [Can]; Tagamet® HB 200 [US-OTC]; Tagamet® HB [Can]
Therapeutic Category Histamine H$_2$ Antagonist
Use Short-term treatment of active duodenal ulcers and benign gastric ulcers; long-term prophylaxis of duodenal ulcer; gastric hypersecretory states; gastroesophageal reflux; prevention of upper GI bleeding in
(Continued)

cimetidine *(Continued)*

critically-ill patients; labeled for OTC use for prevention or relief of heartburn, acid indigestion, or sour stomach

Usual Dosage

Children: Oral, I.M., I.V.: 20-40 mg/kg/day in divided doses every 6 hours

Children ≥12 years and Adults: Oral: Heartburn, acid indigestion, sour stomach (OTC labeling): 200 mg up to twice daily; may take 30 minutes prior to eating foods or beverages expected to cause heartburn or indigestion

Adults:

Short-term treatment of active ulcers:

Oral: 300 mg 4 times/day or 800 mg at bedtime or 400 mg twice daily for up to 8 weeks

Note: Higher doses of 1600 mg at bedtime for 4 weeks may be beneficial for a subpopulation of patients with larger duodenal ulcers (>1 cm defined endoscopically) who are also heavy smokers (≥1 pack/day).

I.M., I.V.: 300 mg every 6 hours or 37.5 mg/hour by continuous infusion; I.V. dosage should be adjusted to maintain an intragastric pH ≥5

Prevention of upper GI bleed in critically-ill patients: 50 mg/hour by continuous infusion; I.V. dosage should be adjusted to maintain an intragastric pH ≥5

Note: Reduce dose by 50% if Cl_{cr} <30 mL/minute; treatment >7 days has not been evaluated.

Duodenal ulcer prophylaxis: Oral: 400 mg at bedtime

Gastric hypersecretory conditions: Oral, I.M., I.V.: 300-600 mg every 6 hours; dosage not to exceed 2.4 g/day

Gastroesophageal reflux disease: Oral: 400 mg 4 times/day or 800 mg twice daily for 12 weeks

Dosage Forms

Infusion [premixed in NS]: 300 mg (50 mL)

Injection, solution: 150 mg/mL (2 mL, 8 mL)

Liquid, oral: 300 mg/5 mL

Tablet: 200 mg [OTC], 300 mg, 400 mg, 800 mg

Tagamet® HB 200 [OTC]: 200 mg

cinacalcet *(sin a KAL cet)*

Synonyms AMG 073; cinacalcet hydrochloride

U.S./Canadian Brand Names Sensipar™ [US]

Therapeutic Category Calcimimetic

Use Treatment of secondary hyperparathyroidism in dialysis patients; treatment of hypercalcemia in patients with parathyroid carcinoma

Usual Dosage Oral: Adults: **Do not titrate dose more frequently than every 2-4 weeks.**

Secondary hyperparathyroidism: Initial: 30 mg once daily (maximum daily dose: 180 mg); increase dose incrementally (60 mg, 90 mg, 120 mg, 180 mg once daily) as necessary to maintain iPTH level between 150-300 pg/mL.

Parathyroid carcinoma: Initial: 30 mg twice daily (maximum daily dose: 360 mg daily as 90 mg 4 times/day); increase dose incrementally (60 mg twice daily, 90 mg twice daily, 90 mg 4 times/day) as necessary to normalize serum calcium levels.

Dosage Forms

Tablet:

Sensipar™: 30 mg, 60 mg, 90 mg

cinacalcet hydrochloride *see* cinacalcet *on this page*

Cipralex® [Can] *see* escitalopram *on page 311*

Cipro® [US/Can] *see* ciprofloxacin *on this page*

Cipro® XL [Can] *see* ciprofloxacin *on this page*

Ciprodex® [US/Can] *see* ciprofloxacin and dexamethasone *on page 193*

ciprofloxacin *(sip roe FLOKS a sin)*

Sound-Alike/Look-Alike Issues

ciprofloxacin may be confused with cephalexin

Ciloxan® may be confused with cinoxacin, Cytoxan®

Cipro® may be confused with Ceftin®

Synonyms ciprofloxacin hydrochloride

U.S./Canadian Brand Names Apo-Ciproflox® [Can]; Ciloxan® [US/Can]; Cipro® XL [Can]; Cipro® XR [US]; Cipro® [US/Can]; CO Ciprofloxacin [Can]; Gen-Ciprofloxacin [Can]; Novo-Ciprofloxacin [Can]; PMS-Ciprofloxacin [Can]; Proquin® XR [US]; RAN™-Ciprofloxacin [Can]; ratio-Ciprofloxacin [Can]; Rhoxal-ciprofloxacin [Can]; Sandoz-Ciprofloxacin [Can]; Taro-Ciprofloxacin [Can]

Therapeutic Category Antibiotic, Ophthalmic; Quinolone

Use

Children: Complicated urinary tract infections and pyelonephritis due to *E. coli.* **Note:** Although effective, ciprofloxacin is not the drug of first choice in children.

Children and adults: To reduce incidence or progression of disease following exposure to aerolized *Bacillus anthracis.* Ophthalmologically, for superficial ocular infections (corneal ulcers, conjunctivitis) due to suscep-tible strains

Adults: Treatment of the following infections when caused by susceptible bacteria: Urinary tract infections; acute uncomplicated cystitis in females; chronic bacterial prostatitis; lower respiratory tract infections (including acute exacerbations of chronic bronchitis); acute sinusitis; skin and skin structure infections; bone and joint infections; complicated intra-abdominal infections (in combination with metronidazole); infectious diarrhea; typhoid fever due to *Salmonella typhi* (eradication of chronic typhoid carrier state has not been proven); uncomplicated cervical and urethra gonorrhea (due to *N. gonorrhoeae*); nosocomial pneumonia; empirical therapy for febrile neutropenic patients (in combination with piperacillin)

Note: As of April 2007, the CDC no longer recommends the use of fluoroquinolones for the treatment of gonococcal disease.

Usual Dosage Note: Extended release tablets and immediate release formulations are not interchangeable. Unless otherwise specified, oral dosing reflects the use of immediate release formulations.

Usual dosage ranges:

Children:
Oral: 20-30 mg/kg/day in 2 divided doses; maximum dose: 1.5 g/day
I.V.: 20-30 mg/kg/day divided every 12 hours; maximum dose: 800 mg/day

Adults:
Oral: 250-750 mg every 12 hours
I.V.: 200-400 mg every 12 hours

Indication-specific dosing:

Children:

Anthrax:

Inhalational (postexposure prophylaxis):
Oral: 15 mg/kg/dose every 12 hours for 60 days; maximum: 500 mg/dose
I.V.: 10 mg/kg/dose every 12 hours for 60 days; do **not** exceed 400 mg/dose (800 mg/day)

Cutaneous (treatment, CDC guidelines): Oral: 10-15 mg/kg every 12 hours for 60 days (maximum: 1 g/day); amoxicillin 80 mg/kg/day divided every 8 hours is an option for completion of treatment after clinical improvement. **Note:** In the presence of systemic involvement, extensive edema, lesions on head/neck, refer to I.V. dosing for treatment of inhalational/gastrointestinal/oropharyngeal anthrax.

Inhalational/gastrointestinal/oropharyngeal (treatment, CDC guidelines): I.V.: Initial: 10-15 mg/kg every 12 hours for 60 days (maximum: 500 mg/dose); switch to oral therapy when clinically appropriate; refer to adult dosing for notes on combined therapy and duration

Bacterial conjunctivitis: See adult dosing

Corneal ulcer: See adult dosing

Urinary tract infection (complicated) or pyelonephritis:
Oral: 20-30 mg/kg/day in 2 divided doses (every 12 hours) for 10-21 days; maximum: 1.5 g/day
I.V.: 6-10 mg/kg every 8 hours for 10-21 days (maximum: 400 mg/dose)

Adults:

Anthrax:

Inhalational (postexposure prophylaxis):
Oral: 500 mg every 12 hours for 60 days
I.V.: 400 mg every 12 hours for 60 days

Cutaneous (treatment, CDC guidelines): Oral: Immediate release formulation: 500 mg every 12 hours for 60 days. **Note:** In the presence of systemic involvement, extensive edema, lesions on head/neck, refer to I.V. dosing for treatment of inhalational/gastrointestinal/oropharyngeal anthrax

Inhalational/gastrointestinal/oropharyngeal (treatment, CDC guidelines): I.V.: 400 mg every 12 hours. **Note:** Initial treatment should include two or more agents predicted to be effective (per CDC recommen-dations). Continue combined therapy for 60 days.

Bacterial conjunctivitis:
Ophthalmic solution: Instill 1-2 drops in eye(s) every 2 hours while awake for 2 days and 1-2 drops every 4 hours while awake for the next 5 days
Ophthalmic ointment: Apply a 1/2" ribbon into the conjunctival sac 3 times/day for the first 2 days, followed by a 1/2" ribbon applied twice daily for the next 5 days

Bone/joint infections:
Oral: 500-750 mg twice daily for 4-6 weeks
I.V.: Mild to moderate: 400 mg every 12 hours for 4-6 weeks; Severe/complicated: 400 mg every 8 hours for 4-6 weeks

Chancroid (CDC guidelines): Oral: 500 mg twice daily for 3 days

Corneal ulcer: Ophthalmic solution: Instill 2 drops into affected eye every 15 minutes for the first 6 hours, then 2 drops into the affected eye every 30 minutes for the remainder of the first day. On day 2, instill 2

(Continued)

ciprofloxacin *(Continued)*

drops into the affected eye hourly. On days 3-14, instill 2 drops into affected eye every 4 hours. Treatment may continue after day 14 if reepithelialization has not occurred.

Febrile neutropenia*: I.V.: 400 mg every 8 hours for 7-14 days

Gonococcal infections:

Urethral/cervical gonococcal infections: Oral: 250-500 mg as a single dose (CDC recommends concomitant doxycycline or azithromycin due to possible coinfection with *Chlamydia*; **Note:** As of April 2007, the CDC no longer recommends the use of fluoroquinolones for the treatment of uncomplicated gonococcal disease.

Disseminated gonococcal infection (CDC guidelines): Oral: 500 mg twice daily to complete 7 days of therapy (initial treatment with ceftriaxone 1 g I.M./I.V. daily for 24-48 hours after improvement begins); **Note:** As of April 2007, the CDC no longer recommends the use of fluoroquinolones for the treatment of more serious gonococcal disease, unless no other options exist and susceptibility can be confirmed via culture.

Infectious diarrhea: Oral:

Salmonella: 500 mg twice daily for 5-7 days

Shigella: 500 mg twice daily for 3 days

Traveler's diarrhea: Mild: 750 mg for one dose; Severe: 500 mg twice daily for 3 days

Vibrio cholerae: 1 g for one dose

Intra-abdominal*:

Oral: 500 mg every 12 hours for 7-14 days

I.V.: 400 mg every 12 hours for 7-14 days

Lower respiratory tract, skin/skin structure infections:

Oral: 500-750 mg twice daily for 7-14 days

I.V.: Mild to moderate: 400 mg every 12 hours for 7-14 days; Severe/complicated: 400 mg every 8 hours for 7-14 days

Nosocomial pneumonia: I.V.: 400 mg every 8 hours for 10-14 days

Prostatitis (chronic, bacterial): Oral: 500 mg every 12 hours for 28 days

Sinusitis (acute): Oral: 500 mg every 12 hours for 10 days

Typhoid fever: Oral: 500 mg every 12 hours for 10 days

Urinary tract infection:

Acute uncomplicated, cystitis:

Oral:

Immediate release formulation: 250 mg every 12 hours for 3 days

Extended release formulation (Cipro® XR, Proquin® XR): 500 mg every 24 hours for 3 days

I.V.: 200 mg every 12 hours for 7-14 days

Complicated (including pyelonephritis):

Oral:

Immediate release formulation: 500 mg every 12 hours for 7-14 days

Extended release formulation (Cipro® XR): 1000 mg every 24 hours for 7-14 days

I.V.: 400 mg every 12 hours for 7-14 days

*Combination therapy generally recommended.

Dosage Forms

Infusion [premixed in D₅W]:

Cipro®: 200 mg (100 mL); 400 mg (200 mL)

Injection, solution: 10 mg/mL (20 mL, 40 mL)

Cipro®: 10 mg/mL (20 mL, 40 mL)

Microcapsules for suspension, oral:

Cipro®: 250 mg/5 mL, 500 mg/5 mL

Ointment, ophthalmic:

Ciloxan®: 3.33 mg/g [0.3% base] (3.5 g)

Solution, ophthalmic: 3.5 mg/mL (2.5 mL, 5mL, 10 mL) [0.3% base]

Ciloxan®: 3.5 mg/mL (2.5 mL, 5 mL, 10 mL) [0.3% base]

Tablet: 250 mg, 500 mg, 750 mg

Cipro®: 100 mg, 250 mg, 500 mg, 750 mg

Tablet, extended release: 500 mg, 1000 mg

Cipro® XR: 500 mg, 1000 mg

Proquin® XR: 500 mg

Tablet, extended release [dose pack]:

Proquin® XR: 500 mg (3s)

ciprofloxacin and dexamethasone (sip roe FLOKS a sin & deks a METH a sone)
Synonyms ciprofloxacin hydrochloride and dexamethasone; dexamethasone and ciprofloxacin
U.S./Canadian Brand Names Ciprodex® [US/Can]
Therapeutic Category Antibiotic/Corticosteroid, Otic
Use Treatment of acute otitis media in pediatric patients with tympanostomy tubes or acute otitis externa in children and adults
Usual Dosage Otic:
  Children: Acute otitis media in patients with tympanostomy tubes or acute otitis externa: Instill 4 drops into affected ear(s) twice daily for 7 days
  Adults: Acute otitis externa: Instill 4 drops into affected ear(s) twice daily for 7 days
Dosage Forms
  Suspension, otic:
  Ciprodex®: Ciprofloxacin 0.3% and dexamethasone 0.1% (7.5 mL)

ciprofloxacin and hydrocortisone (sip roe FLOKS a sin & hye droe KOR ti sone)
Synonyms ciprofloxacin hydrochloride and hydrocortisone; hydrocortisone and ciprofloxacin
U.S./Canadian Brand Names Cipro® HC [US/Can]
Therapeutic Category Antibiotic/Corticosteroid, Otic
Use Treatment of acute otitis externa, sometimes known as "swimmer's ear"
Usual Dosage Otic: Children >1 year of age and Adults: The recommended dosage for all patients is three drops of the suspension in the affected ear twice daily for 7 days; twice-daily dosing schedule is more convenient for patients than that of existing treatments with hydrocortisone, which are typically administered three or four times a day; a twice-daily dosage schedule may be especially helpful for parents and caregivers of young children
Dosage Forms
  Suspension, otic:
  Cipro® HC: Ciprofloxacin 0.2% and hydrocortisone 1% (10 mL)

ciprofloxacin hydrochloride see ciprofloxacin on page 190

ciprofloxacin hydrochloride and dexamethasone see ciprofloxacin and dexamethasone on this page

ciprofloxacin hydrochloride and hydrocortisone see ciprofloxacin and hydrocortisone on this page

Cipro® HC [US/Can] see ciprofloxacin and hydrocortisone on this page

Cipro® XR [US] see ciprofloxacin on page 190

cisapride (SIS a pride)
Sound-Alike/Look-Alike Issues
  Propulsid® may be confused with propranolol
U.S./Canadian Brand Names Propulsid® [US]
Therapeutic Category Gastrointestinal Agent, Prokinetic
Use Treatment of nocturnal symptoms of gastroesophageal reflux disease (GERD); has demonstrated effectiveness for gastroparesis, refractory constipation, and nonulcer dyspepsia
Usual Dosage Oral:
  Children: 0.15-0.3 mg/kg/dose 3-4 times/day; maximum: 10 mg/dose
  Adults: Initial: 10 mg 4 times/day at least 15 minutes before meals and at bedtime; in some patients the dosage will need to be increased to 20 mg to obtain a satisfactory result

cisatracurium (sis a tra KYOO ree um)
Sound-Alike/Look-Alike Issues
  Nimbex® may be confused with Revex®
Synonyms cisatracurium besylate
U.S./Canadian Brand Names Nimbex® [US/Can]
Therapeutic Category Skeletal Muscle Relaxant
Use Adjunct to general anesthesia to facilitate endotracheal intubation and to relax skeletal muscles during surgery; to facilitate mechanical ventilation in ICU patients; does not relieve pain or produce sedation
Usual Dosage I.V. (not to be used I.M.):
  Operating room administration:
  Infants 1-23 months: 0.15 mg/kg over 5-10 seconds during either halothane or opioid anesthesia
  Children 2-12 years: Intubating doses: 0.1-0.15 mg/kg over 5-15 seconds during either halothane or opioid anesthesia. (**Note:** When given during stable opioid/nitrous oxide/oxygen anesthesia, 0.1 mg/kg produces maximum neuromuscular block in an average of 2.8 minutes and clinically effective block for 28 minutes.)
  (Continued)

cisatracurium *(Continued)*

Adults: Intubating doses: 0.15-0.2 mg/kg as component of propofol/nitrous oxide/oxygen induction-intubation technique. (**Note:** May produce generally good or excellent conditions for tracheal intubation in 1.5-2 minutes with clinically effective duration of action during propofol anesthesia of 55-61 minutes.); initial dose after succinylcholine for intubation: 0.1 mg/kg; maintenance dose: 0.03 mg/kg 40-60 minutes after initial dose, then at ~20-minute intervals based on clinical criteria

Children ≥2 years and Adults: Continuous infusion: After an initial bolus, a diluted solution can be given by continuous infusion for maintenance of neuromuscular blockade during extended surgery; adjust the rate of administration according to the patient's response as determined by peripheral nerve stimulation. An initial infusion rate of 3 mcg/kg/minute may be required to rapidly counteract the spontaneous recovery of neuromuscular function; thereafter, a rate of 1-2 mcg/kg/minute should be adequate to maintain continuous neuromuscular block in the 89% to 99% range in most pediatric and adult patients. Consider reduction of the infusion rate by 30% to 40% when administering during stable isoflurane, enflurane, sevoflurane, or desflurane anesthesia. Spontaneous recovery from neuromuscular blockade following discontinuation of infusion of cisatracurium may be expected to proceed at a rate comparable to that following single bolus administration.

Intensive care unit administration: Follow the principles for infusion in the operating room. At initial signs of recovery from bolus dose, begin the infusion at a dose of 3 mcg/kg/minute and adjust rates accordingly; dosage ranges of 0.5-10 mcg/kg/minute have been reported. If patient is allowed to recover from neuromuscular blockade, readministration of a bolus dose may be necessary to quickly reestablish neuromuscular block prior to reinstituting the infusion.

Dosage Forms
Injection, solution:
Nimbex®: 2 mg/mL (5 mL, 10 mL); 10 mg/mL (20 mL)

cisatracurium besylate *see* cisatracurium *on previous page*

cisplatin (SIS pla tin)

Sound-Alike/Look-Alike Issues
cisplatin may be confused with carboplatin
Platinol®-AQ may be confused with Paraplatin®, Patanol®, Plaquenil®

Synonyms CDDP

Therapeutic Category Antineoplastic Agent

Use Treatment of head and neck, breast, testicular, and ovarian cancer; Hodgkin and non-Hodgkin lymphoma; neuroblastoma; sarcomas, bladder, gastric, lung, esophageal, cervical, and prostate cancer; myeloma, melanoma, mesothelioma, small cell lung cancer, and osteosarcoma

Usual Dosage Refer to individual protocols. **VERIFY ANY CISPLATIN DOSE EXCEEDING 100 mg/m^2 PER COURSE.**
Adults:
Advanced bladder cancer: 50-70 mg/m^2 every 3-4 weeks
Malignant pleural mesothelioma in combination with pemetrexed: 75 mg/m^2 on day 1 of each 21-day cycle; see pemetrexed monograph for additional details
Metastatic ovarian cancer: 75-100 mg/m^2 every 3-4 weeks
Intraperitoneal: Cisplatin has been administered intraperitoneal with systemic sodium thiosulfate for ovarian cancer; doses up to 90-270 mg/m^2 have been administered and retained for 4 hours before draining
Testicular cancer: 10-20 mg/m^2/day for 5 days repeated every 3-4 weeks

Dosage Forms
Injection, solution [preservative free]: 1 mg/mL (50 mL, 100 mL, 200 mL)

13-*cis*-retinoic acid *see* isotretinoin *on page 477*

citalopram (sye TAL oh pram)

Sound-Alike/Look-Alike Issues
Celexa® may be confused with Celebrex®, Cerebra®, Cerebyx®, Ranexa™, Zyprexa®

Synonyms citalopram hydrobromide; nitalapram

U.S./Canadian Brand Names Apo-Citalopram® [Can]; Celexa® [US/Can]; CO Citalopram [Can]; Dom-Citalopram [Can]; Gen-Citalopram [Can]; Novo-Citalopram [Can]; PHL-Citalopram [Can]; PMS-Citalopram [Can]; RAN™-Citalopram [Can]; ratio-Citalopram [Can]; Rhoxal-citalopram [Can]; Sandoz-Citalopram [Can]

Therapeutic Category Antidepressant

Use Treatment of depression

Usual Dosage Oral: Adults: Depression: Initial: 20 mg/day, generally with an increase to 40 mg/day; doses of more than 40 mg are not usually necessary. Should a dose increase be necessary, it should occur in 20 mg increments at intervals of no less than 1 week. Maximum dose: 60 mg/day

Dosage Forms
Solution, oral: 10 mg/5 mL
Celexa®: 10 mg/5 mL

Tablet: 10 mg, 20 mg, 40 mg
Celexa®: 10 mg, 20 mg, 40 mg

citalopram hydrobromide *see* citalopram *on previous page*

Citanest® Plain [US/Can] *see* prilocaine *on page 713*

Citracal® [US-OTC] *see* calcium citrate *on page 140*

Citracal® Prenatal 90+DHA [US] *see* vitamins (multiple/prenatal) *on page 896*

Citracal® Prenatal +DHA [US] *see* vitamins (multiple/prenatal) *on page 896*

citrate of magnesia *see* magnesium citrate *on page 525*

citric acid and D-gluconic acid irrigant *see* citric acid, magnesium carbonate, and glucono-delta-lactone *on this page*

citric acid and potassium citrate *see* potassium citrate and citric acid *on page 701*

citric acid bladder mixture *see* citric acid, magnesium carbonate, and glucono-delta-lactone *on this page*

citric acid, magnesium carbonate, and glucono-delta-lactone
(SI trik AS id, mag NEE see um KAR bo nate, and GLOO kon o DEL ta LAK tone)
Sound-Alike/Look-Alike Issues
Renacidin® may be confused with Remicade®
Synonyms citric acid and D-gluconic acid irrigant; citric acid bladder mixture; citric acid, magnesium hydroxycarbonate, D-gluconic acid, magnesium acid citrate, and calcium carbonate; hemiacidrin
U.S./Canadian Brand Names Renacidin® [US]
Therapeutic Category Irrigating Solution
Use Prevention of formation of calcifications of indwelling urinary tract catheters; treatment of renal and bladder calculi of the apatite or struvite type
Usual Dosage Adults:
Dissolution or prevention of calcifications: Irrigation (indwelling urethral catheters): 30-60 mL 2-3 times/day by means of a rubber syringe
Renal calculi: Irrigation: Infuse NS at 60 mL/hour and increase until pain, elevated pressure, or maximum flow rate of 120 mL/hour is reached. Begin flow of solution at maximum rate achieved with NS.
Bladder calculi: 30 mL instilled through urinary catheter; clamp for 30-60 minutes, then release and drain; repeat 4-6 times/day
Dosage Forms
Solution, irrigation:
Renacidin®: Citric acid 6.602 g, magnesium carbonate 3.177 g, glucono-delta-lactone 0.198 g per 100 mL (500 mL)

citric acid, magnesium hydroxycarbonate, D-gluconic acid, magnesium acid citrate, and calcium carbonate *see* citric acid, magnesium carbonate, and glucono-delta-lactone *on this page*

citric acid, sodium citrate, and potassium citrate
(SIT rik AS id, SOW dee um SIT rate, & poe TASS ee um SIT rate)
Synonyms potassium citrate, citric acid, and sodium citrate; sodium citrate, citric acid, and potassium citrate
U.S./Canadian Brand Names Cytra-3 [US]; Polycitra® [US]; Polycitra®-LC [US]
Therapeutic Category Alkalinizing Agent
Use Conditions where long-term maintenance of an alkaline urine is desirable as in control and dissolution of uric acid and cystine calculi of the urinary tract
Usual Dosage Oral:
Children: 5-15 mL diluted in water after meals and at bedtime
Adults: 15-30 mL diluted in water after meals and at bedtime
Dosage Forms
Solution, oral:
Cytra-3, Polycitra®-LC: Citric acid 334 mg, sodium citrate 500 mg, and potassium citrate 550 mg per 5 mL
Syrup, oral: Citric acid 334 mg, sodium citrate 500 mg, and potassium citrate 550 mg per 5 mL
Polycitra®: Citric acid 334 mg, sodium citrate 500 mg, and potassium citrate 550 mg per 5 mL

Citroma® [US-OTC] *see* magnesium citrate *on page 525*

Citro-Mag® [Can] *see* magnesium citrate *on page 525*

Citrotein® [US-OTC] *see* nutritional formula, enteral/oral *on page 622*

citrovorum factor *see* leucovorin *on page 496*

Citrucel® **[US-OTC]** *see* methylcellulose *on page 557*

Citrucel® **Fiber Shake [US-OTC]** *see* methylcellulose *on page 557*

Citrucel® **Fiber Smoothie [US-OTC]** *see* methylcellulose *on page 557*

CL-118,532 *see* triptorelin *on page 870*

CI-719 *see* gemfibrozil *on page 387*

CL-825 *see* pentostatin *on page 667*

CL-184116 *see* porfimer *on page 698*

cladribine (KLA dri been)
Sound-Alike/Look-Alike Issues
cladribine may be confused with clofarabine
Leustatin® may be confused with lovastatin
Synonyms 2-CdA; 2-chlorodeoxyadenosine; NSC-105014
U.S./Canadian Brand Names Leustatin® [US/Can]
Therapeutic Category Antineoplastic Agent
Use Treatment of hairy cell leukemia
Usual Dosage I.V. (refer to individual protocols): Adults: Hairy cell leukemia: Continuous infusion: 0.09 mg/kg/day days 1-7; may be repeated every 28-35 days
Dosage Forms
  Injection, solution [preservative free]: 1 mg/mL (10 mL)
    Leustatin®: 1 mg/mL (10 mL)

Claforan® **[US/Can]** *see* cefotaxime *on page 160*

Claravis™ **[US]** *see* isotretinoin *on page 477*

Clarinex® **[US]** *see* desloratadine *on page 238*

Clarinex-D® **12 Hour [US]** *see* desloratadine and pseudoephedrine *on page 239*

Clarinex-D® **24 Hour [US]** *see* desloratadine and pseudoephedrine *on page 239*

Claripel™ **[US]** *see* hydroquinone *on page 437*

clarithromycin (kla RITH roe mye sin)
Sound-Alike/Look-Alike Issues
clarithromycin may be confused with erythromycin
U.S./Canadian Brand Names Biaxin® XL [US/Can]; Biaxin® [US/Can]; ratio-Clarithromycin [Can]
Therapeutic Category Macrolide (Antibiotic)
Use
  Children:
    Acute otitis media (*H. influenzae, M. catarrhalis,* or *S. pneumoniae*)
    Community-acquired pneumonia due to susceptible *Mycoplasma pneumoniae, S. pneumoniae,* or *Chlamydia pneumoniae* (TWAR)
    Pharyngitis/tonsillitis, acute maxillary sinusitis, uncomplicated skin/skin structure infections, and mycobacterial infections
    Prevention of disseminated mycobacterial infections due to MAC disease in patients with advanced HIV infection
  Adults:
    Pharyngitis/tonsillitis due to susceptible *S. pyogenes*
    Acute maxillary sinusitis and acute exacerbation of chronic bronchitis due to susceptible *H. influenzae, M. catarrhalis,* or *S. pneumoniae*
    Community-acquired pneumonia due to susceptible *H. influenzae, H. parainfluenzae, Mycoplasma pneumoniae, S. pneumoniae,* or *Chlamydia pneumoniae* (TWAR)
    Uncomplicated skin/skin structure infections due to susceptible *S. aureus, S. pyogenes*
    Disseminated mycobacterial infections due to *M. avium* or *M. intracellulare*
    Prevention of disseminated mycobacterial infections due to *M. avium* complex (MAC) disease (eg, patients with advanced HIV infection)
    Duodenal ulcer disease due to *H. pylori* in regimens with other drugs including amoxicillin and lansoprazole or omeprazole, ranitidine bismuth citrate, bismuth subsalicylate, tetracycline, and/or an H_2 antagonist
Usual Dosage
  Usual dosage range:
    Children ≥6 months: Oral: 7.5 mg/kg every 12 hours (maximum: 500 mg/dose)
    Adults: Oral: 250-500 mg every 12 hours **or** 1000 mg (two 500 mg extended release tablets) once daily for 7-14 days

Indication-specific dosing:
Children: Oral:
Community-acquired pneumonia, sinusitis, bronchitis, skin infections: 15 mg/kg/day divided every 12 hours for 10 days
Prophylaxis for infective endocarditis: 15 mg/kg 30-60 minutes before procedure
Mycobacterial infection (prevention and treatment): 7.5 mg/kg (up to 500 mg) twice daily. **Note:** Safety of clarithromycin for MAC not studied in children <20 months.
Adults: Oral:
Acute exacerbation of chronic bronchitis:
M. catarrhalis and *S. pneumoniae*: 250 mg every 12 hours for 7-14 days **or** 1000 mg (two 500 mg extended release tablets) once daily for 7 days
H. influenzae: 500 mg every 12 hours for 7-14 days or 1000 mg (two 500 mg extended release tablets) once daily for 7 days
H. parainfluenzae: 500 mg every 12 hours for 7 days or 1000 mg (two 500 mg extended release tablets) once daily for 7 days
Acute maxillary sinusitis: 500 mg every 12 hours **or** 1000 mg (two 500 mg extended release tablets) once daily for 14 days
Prophylaxis for infective endocarditis: 500 mg 30-60 minutes prior to procedure
Mycobacterial infection (prevention and treatment): 500 mg twice daily (use with other antimycobacterial drugs, eg, ethambutol or rifampin)
Peptic ulcer disease: Eradication of *Helicobacter pylori*: Dual or triple combination regimens with bismuth subsalicylate, amoxicillin, an H_2-receptor antagonist, or proton-pump inhibitor: 500 mg every 8-12 hours for 10-14 days
Pharyngitis, tonsillitis: 250 mg every 12 hours for 10 days
Pneumonia:
C. pneumoniae, *M. pneumoniae*, and *S. pneumoniae*: 250 mg every 12 hours for 7-14 days **or** 1000 mg (two 500 mg extended release tablets) once daily for 7 days
H. influenzae: 250 mg every 12 hours for 7 days **or** 1000 mg (two 500 mg extended release tablets) once daily for 7 days
Skin and skin structure infection, uncomplicated: 250 mg every 12 hours for 7-14 days
Dosage Forms
Granules for oral suspension: 125 mg/5 mL (50 mL, 100 mL); 250 mg/5 mL (50 mL, 100 mL)
Biaxin®: 125 mg/5 mL, 250 mg/5 mL
Tablet: 250 mg, 500 mg
Biaxin®: 250 mg, 500 mg
Tablet, extended release: 500 mg
Biaxin® XL: 500 mg

clarithromycin, lansoprazole, and amoxicillin *see* lansoprazole, amoxicillin, and clarithromycin *on page 493*

Claritin® [Can] *see* loratadine *on page 517*

Claritin® 24 Hour Allergy [US-OTC] *see* loratadine *on page 517*

Claritin-D® 12-Hour [US-OTC] *see* loratadine and pseudoephedrine *on page 518*

Claritin-D® 24-Hour [US-OTC] *see* loratadine and pseudoephedrine *on page 518*

Claritin® Allergic Decongestant [Can] *see* oxymetazoline *on page 643*

Claritin® Extra [Can] *see* loratadine and pseudoephedrine *on page 518*

Claritin® Hives Relief [US-OTC] *see* loratadine *on page 517*

Claritin® Kids [Can] *see* loratadine *on page 517*

Claritin® Liberator [Can] *see* loratadine and pseudoephedrine *on page 518*

Clarus™ [Can] *see* isotretinoin *on page 477*

Clasteon® [Can] *see* clodronate *(Canada only) on page 202*

clavulanic acid and amoxicillin *see* amoxicillin and clavulanate potassium *on page 49*

Clavulin® [Can] *see* amoxicillin and clavulanate potassium *on page 49*

Clear Away® Disc *(Discontinued)* *see* salicylic acid *on page 772*

Clear By Design® Gel *(Discontinued)* *see* benzoyl peroxide *on page 103*

Clear eyes® for Dry Eyes and ACR Relief [US-OTC] *see* naphazoline *on page 590*

Clear eyes® for Dry Eyes and Redness Relief [US-OTC] *see* naphazoline *on page 590*

Clear eyes® Redness Relief [US-OTC] *see* naphazoline *on page 590*

Clear eyes® Seasonal Relief [US-OTC] *see* naphazoline *on page 590*

Clearplex [US-OTC] *see* benzoyl peroxide *on page 103*

Clearsil® Maximum Strength *(Discontinued)* *see* benzoyl peroxide *on page 103*

Clear Tussin® 30 *(Discontinued)* *see* guaifenesin and dextromethorphan *on page 402*

clemastine (KLEM as teen)

Synonyms clemastine fumarate
U.S./Canadian Brand Names Dayhist® Allergy [US-OTC]; Tavist® Allergy [US-OTC]
Therapeutic Category Antihistamine
Use Perennial and seasonal allergic rhinitis and other allergic symptoms including urticaria
Usual Dosage Oral:
Infants and Children <6 years: 0.05 mg/kg/day as **clemastine base** or 0.335-0.67 mg/day clemastine fumarate (0.25-0.5 mg base/day) divided into 2 or 3 doses; maximum daily dosage: 1.34 mg (1 mg base)
Children 6-12 years: 0.67-1.34 mg clemastine fumarate (0.5-1 mg base) twice daily; do not exceed 4.02 mg/day (3 mg/day base)
Children ≥12 years and Adults:
1.34 mg clemastine fumarate (1 mg base) twice daily to 2.68 mg (2 mg base) 3 times/day; do not exceed 8.04 mg/day (6 mg base)
OTC labeling: 1.34 mg clemastine fumarate (1 mg base) twice daily; do not exceed 2 mg base/24 hours
Dosage Forms
Syrup: 0.67 mg/5 mL [0.5 mg base/5 mL; prescription formulation]
Tablet: 1.34 mg [1 mg base; OTC], 2.68 mg [2 mg base; prescription formulation]
Dayhist® Allergy [OTC], Tavist® Allergy [OTC]: 1.34 mg [1 mg base]

clemastine fumarate *see* clemastine *on this page*

Clenia™ [US] *see* sulfur and sulfacetamide *on page 815*

Cleocin® [US] *see* clindamycin *on this page*

Cleocin HCl® [US] *see* clindamycin *on this page*

Cleocin Pediatric® [US] *see* clindamycin *on this page*

Cleocin Phosphate® [US] *see* clindamycin *on this page*

Cleocin T® [US] *see* clindamycin *on this page*

Cleocin® Vaginal Ovule [US] *see* clindamycin *on this page*

clidinium and chlordiazepoxide (kli DI nee um & klor dye az e POKS ide)

Sound-Alike/Look-Alike Issues
Librax® may be confused with Librium®
Synonyms chlordiazepoxide and clidinium
U.S./Canadian Brand Names Apo-Chlorax® [Can]; Librax® [US/Can]
Therapeutic Category Anticholinergic Agent
Use Adjunct treatment of peptic ulcer; treatment of irritable bowel syndrome
Usual Dosage Oral: 1-2 capsules 3-4 times/day, before meals or food and at bedtime
Dosage Forms
Capsule: Clidinium 2.5 mg and chlordiazepoxide 5 mg
Librax® [original formulation]: Clidinium 2.5 mg and chlordiazepoxide 5 mg

Climara® [US/Can] *see* estradiol *on page 313*

ClimaraPro® [US] *see* estradiol and levonorgestrel *on page 315*

Clinac™ BPO [US] *see* benzoyl peroxide *on page 103*

Clindagel® [US] *see* clindamycin *on this page*

ClindaMax™ [US] *see* clindamycin *on this page*

clindamycin (klin da MYE sin)

Sound-Alike/Look-Alike Issues
Cleocin® may be confused with bleomycin, Clinoril®, Lincocin®
Synonyms clindamycin hydrochloride; clindamycin palmitate; clindamycin phosphate
U.S./Canadian Brand Names Alti-Clindamycin [Can]; Apo-Clindamycin® [Can]; Cleocin HCl® [US]; Cleocin Pediatric® [US]; Cleocin Phosphate® [US]; Cleocin T® [US]; Cleocin® Vaginal Ovule [US]; Cleocin® [US]; Clindagel® [US]; ClindaMax™ [US]; Clindamycin Injection, USP [Can]; Clindesse™ [US]; Clindoxyl® [Can]; Dalacin® C [Can]; Dalacin® T [Can]; Dalacin® Vaginal [Can]; Evoclin™ [US]; Novo-Clindamycin [Can]; Riva-Clindamycin [Can]; Taro-Clindamycin [Can]

Therapeutic Category Acne Products; Antibiotic, Miscellaneous

Use Treatment against aerobic and anaerobic streptococci (except enterococci), most staphylococci, *Bacteroides* sp and *Actinomyces*; bacterial vaginosis (vaginal cream, vaginal suppository); pelvic inflammatory disease (I.V.); topically in treatment of severe acne; vaginally for *Gardnerella vaginalis*

Usual Dosage

Usual dosage ranges:

Infants and Children:

Oral: 8-20 mg/kg/day as hydrochloride; 8-25 mg/kg/day as palmitate in 3-4 divided doses (minimum dose of palmitate: 37.5 mg 3 times/day)

I.M., I.V.:

<1 month: 15-20 mg/kg/day

>1 month: 20-40 mg/kg/day in 3-4 divided doses

Adults:

Oral: 150-450 mg/dose every 6-8 hours; maximum dose: 1.8 g/day

I.M., I.V.: 1.2-1.8 g/day in 2-4 divided doses; maximum dose: 4.8 g/day

Indication-specific dosing:

Children:

Anthrax: I.V.: 7.5 mg/kg every 6 hours

Babesiosis: Oral: 20-40 mg/kg/day divided every 8 hours for 7 days plus quinine

Orofacial infections: 8-25 mg/kg in 3-4 equally divided doses

Prophylaxis of infective endocarditis:

Oral: 20 mg/kg 30-60 minutes before procedure

I.V.: 20 mg/kg 30-60 minutes before procedure. **Note:** Intramuscular injections should be avoided in patients who are receiving anticoagulant therapy. In these circumstances, orally administered regimens should be given whenever possible. Intravenously administered antibiotics should be used for patients who are unable to tolerate or absorb oral medications.

Children ≥12 years and Adults:

Acne vulgaris: Topical:

Gel, pledget, lotion, solution: Apply a thin film twice daily

Foam (Evoclin™): Apply once daily

Adults:

Amnionitis: I.V.: 450-900 mg every 8 hours

Anthrax: I.V.: 900 mg every 8 hours with ciprofloxacin or doxycycline

Babesiosis:

Oral: 600 mg 3 times/day for 7 days with quinine

I.V.: 1.2 g twice daily

Bacterial vaginosis: Intravaginal:

Suppositories: Insert one ovule (100 mg clindamycin) daily into vagina at bedtime for 3 days

Cream:

Cleocin®: One full applicator inserted intravaginally once daily before bedtime for 3 or 7 consecutive days in nonpregnant patients or for 7 consecutive days in pregnant patients

Clindesse™: One full applicator inserted intravaginally as a single dose at anytime during the day in nonpregnant patients

Bite wounds (canine): Oral: 300 mg 4 times/day with a fluoroquinolone

Gangrenous myositis: I.V.: 900 mg every 8 hours with penicillin G

Group B streptococcus (neonatal prophylaxis): I.V.: 900 mg every 8 hours until delivery

Orofacial/parapharyngeal space infections:

Oral: 150-450 mg every 6 hours for 7 days, maximum 1.8 g/day

I.V.: 600-900 mg every 8 hours

Pelvic inflammatory disease: I.V.: 900 mg every 8 hours with gentamicin 2 mg/kg, then 1.5 mg/kg every 8 hours; continue after discharge with doxycycline 100 mg twice daily to complete 14 days of total therapy

Prophylaxis of infective endocarditis:

Oral: 600 mg 30-60 minutes before procedure

I.V.: 600 mg 30-60 minutes before procedure. **Note:** Intramuscular injections should be avoided in patients who are receiving anticoagulant therapy. In these circumstances, orally administered regimens should be given whenever possible. Intravenously administered antibiotics should be used for patients who are unable to tolerate or absorb oral medications.

Prophylaxis in total joint replacement patients undergoing dental procedures which produce bacteremia:

Oral: 600 mg 1 hour prior to procedure

I.V.: 600 mg 1 hour prior to procedure (for patients unable to take oral medication)

Toxic shock syndrome: I.V.: 900 mg every 8 hours with penicillin G or ceftriaxone

Dosage Forms

Capsule: 150 mg, 300 mg

Cleocin HCl®: 75 mg, 150 mg, 300 mg

(Continued)

clindamycin *(Continued)*

Cream, vaginal:
Cleocin®: 2% (40 g)
Clindesse™: 2% (5 g)
Foam, topical:
Evoclin™: 1% (50 g, 100 g)
Gel, topical: 1% (30 g, 60 g)
Cleocin T®: 1% (30 g, 60 g)
Clindagel®: 1% (40 mL, 75 mL)
ClindaMax™: 1% (30 g, 60 g)
Granules for oral solution:
Cleocin Pediatric®: 75 mg/5 mL
Infusion [premixed in D_5W]:
Cleocin Phosphate®: 300 mg (50 mL); 600 mg (50 mL); 900 mg (50 mL)
Injection, solution: 150 mg/mL (2 mL, 4 mL, 6 mL, 60 mL)
Cleocin Phosphate®: 150 mg/mL (2 mL, 4 mL, 6 mL, 60 mL)
Lotion: 1% (60 mL)
Cleocin T®, ClindaMax™: 1% (60 mL)
Pledgets, topical: 1% (60s)
Cleocin T®: 1% (60s)
Solution, topical: 1% (30 mL, 60 mL)
Cleocin T®: 1% (30 mL, 60 mL)
Suppository, vaginal:
Cleocin® Vaginal Ovule: 100 mg (3s)

clindamycin and benzoyl peroxide (klin da MYE sin & BEN zoe il peer OKS ide)

Synonyms benzoyl peroxide and clindamycin; clindamycin phosphate and benzoyl peroxide
U.S./Canadian Brand Names BenzaClin® [US/Can]; Duac™ [US]
Therapeutic Category Topical Skin Product; Topical Skin Product, Acne
Use Topical treatment of acne vulgaris
Usual Dosage Topical: Children ≥12 years and Adults: Apply to affected areas after skin has been cleansed and dried
BenzaClin®: Acne: Apply twice daily (morning and evening)
Duac™: Inflammatory acne: Apply once daily in the evening
Dosage Forms
Gel, topical:
BenzaClin®: Clindamycin 1% and benzoyl peroxide 5% (25 g, 50 g)
Duac™: Clindamycin 1% and benzoyl peroxide 5% (45 g)

clindamycin and tretinoin (klin da MYE sin & TRET i noyn)

Synonyms clindamycin phosphate and tretinoin; tretinoin and clindamycin
U.S./Canadian Brand Names Ziana™ [US]
Therapeutic Category Acne Products; Retinoic Acid Derivative; Topical Skin Product; Topical Skin Product, Acne
Use Treatment of acne vulgaris
Usual Dosage Topical: Children ≥12 years and Adults: Apply pea-size amount to entire face once daily at bedtime

clindamycin hydrochloride *see* clindamycin *on page 198*

Clindamycin Injection, USP [Can] *see* clindamycin *on page 198*

clindamycin palmitate *see* clindamycin *on page 198*

clindamycin phosphate *see* clindamycin *on page 198*

clindamycin phosphate and benzoyl peroxide *see* clindamycin and benzoyl peroxide *on this page*

clindamycin phosphate and tretinoin *see* clindamycin and tretinoin *on this page*

Clindesse™ [US] *see* clindamycin *on page 198*

Clindets® *(Discontinued)* *see* clindamycin *on page 198*

Clindex® *(Discontinued)* *see* clidinium and chlordiazepoxide *on page 198*

Clindoxyl® [Can] *see* clindamycin *on page 198*

Clinoril® [US] *see* sulindac *on page 815*

clioquinol and flumethasone *(Canada only)* (klye ok KWIN ole & floo METH a sone)

Synonyms flumethasone and clioquinol; iodochlorhydroxyquin and flumethasone

U.S./Canadian Brand Names Locacorten® Vioform® [Can]

Therapeutic Category Antibiotic, Topical; Corticosteroid, Topical

Use Treatment of corticosteroid-responsive dermatoses complicated by infection with bacterial and/or fungal agents

Usual Dosage Children >2 years and Adults:

Otic solution (drops): Instill 2-3 drops into affected ear(s) 2 times/day; generally limit duration to 10 days

Topical: Apply in a thin layer to affected area 2-3 times/day; generally limit duration to 7 days

Dosage Forms [CAN] = Canadian brand name

Cream, topical:

Locacorten® Vioform® [CAN]: Clioquinol 3% and flumethasone 0.02% (15 g, 50 g) [not available in the U.S.]

Solution, otic:

Locacorten® Vioform® [CAN]: Clioquinol 1% and flumethasone 0.02% (10 mL) [not available in the U.S.]

Clobazam-10 [Can] *see* clobazam *(Canada only)* on this page

clobazam *(Canada only)* (KLOE ba zam)

U.S./Canadian Brand Names Alti-Clobazam [Can]; Apo-Clobazam® [Can]; Clobazam-10 [Can]; Dom-Clobazam [Can]; Frisium® [Can]; Novo-Clobazam [Can]; PMS-Clobazam [Can]; ratio-Clobazam [Can]

Therapeutic Category Anticonvulsant; Antidepressant

Use Adjunctive treatment of epilepsy

Usual Dosage Oral:

Children:

<2 years: Initial 0.5-1 mg/kg/day

2-16 years: Initial: 5 mg/day; may be increased (no more frequently than every 5 days) to a maximum of 40 mg/day

Adults: Initial: 5-15 mg/day; dosage may be gradually adjusted (based on tolerance and seizure control) to a maximum of 80 mg/day

Note: Daily doses of up to 30 mg may be taken as a single dose at bedtime; higher doses should be divided.

Dosage Forms [CAN] = Canadian brand name

Tablet: 10 mg [not available in the U.S.]

Alti-Clobazam [CAN], Apo-Clobazam® [CAN], Clobazam-10 [CAN], Dom-Clobazam [CAN], Frisium® [CAN], Novo-Clobazam [CAN], PMS-Clobazam [CAN], ration-Clobazam [CAN]: 10 mg [not available in the U.S.]

clobetasol (kloe BAY ta sol)

Synonyms clobetasol propionate

U.S./Canadian Brand Names Clobevate® [US]; Clobex® [US/Can]; Cormax® [US]; Dermovate® [Can]; Gen-Clobetasol [Can]; Novo-Clobetasol [Can]; Olux-E™ [US]; Olux® [US]; Taro-Clobetasol [Can]; Temovate E® [US]; Temovate® [US]

Therapeutic Category Corticosteroid, Topical

Use Short-term relief of inflammation of moderate-to-severe corticosteroid-responsive dermatoses (very high potency topical corticosteroid)

Usual Dosage Topical: Discontinue when control achieved; if improvement not seen within 2 weeks, reassessment of diagnosis may be necessary.

Children ≥12 years and Adults:

Steroid-responsive dermatoses:

Cream, emollient cream, gel, ointment: Apply twice daily for up to 2 weeks (maximum dose: 50 g/week)

Foam (Olux-E™): Apply to affected area twice daily for up to 2 weeks (maximum dose: 50 g/week); do not apply to face or intertriginous areas

Steroid-responsive dermatoses: Foam (Olux®), solution: Apply to affected scalp twice daily for up to 2 weeks (maximum dose: 50 g/week or 50 mL/week)

Mild-to-moderate plaque-type psoriasis of nonscalp areas: Foam (Olux®): Apply to affected area twice daily for up to 2 weeks (maximum dose: 50 g/week); do not apply to face or intertriginous areas

Children ≥16 years and Adults: Moderate-to-severe plaque-type psoriasis: Emollient cream, lotion: Apply twice daily for up to 2 weeks, has been used for up to 4 weeks when application is <10% of body surface area; use with caution (maximum dose: 50 g/week)

Children ≥18 years and Adults:

Moderate-to-severe plaque-type psoriasis: Spray: Apply by spraying directly onto affected area twice daily; should be gently rubbed into skin. Should be used for not longer than 4 weeks; treatment beyond 2 weeks should be limited to localized lesions which have not improved sufficiently. Total dose should not exceed 50 g/week or 59 mL/week.

Scalp psoriasis: Shampoo: Apply thin film to dry scalp once daily; leave in place for 15 minutes, then add water, lather; rinse thoroughly

Steroid-responsive dermatoses: Lotion: Apply twice daily for up to 2 weeks (maximum dose: 50 g/week)

(Continued)

clobetasol *(Continued)*

Dosage Forms
Cream: 0.05% (15 g, 30 g, 45 g, 60 g)
Cormax®: 0.05% (30 g)
Temovate®: 0.05% (30 g, 60 g)
Cream [in emollient base]: 0.05% (15 g, 30 g, 60 g)
Temovate E®: 0.05% (60 g)
Foam, topical:
Olux®, Olux-E™: 0.05% (50 g, 100 g)
Gel: 0.05% (15 g, 30 g, 60 g)
Clobevate®: 0.05% (15 g, 30 g, 60 g)
Temovate®: 0.05% (60 g)
Lotion: 0.05% (30 mL, 59 mL)
Clobex®: 0.05% (30 mL, 59 mL)
Ointment: 0.05% (15 g, 30 g, 45 g, 60 g)
Cormax®: 0.05% (15 g, 45 g)
Temovate®: 0.05% (15 g, 30 g)
Shampoo: 0.05% (120 mL)
Clobex®: 0.05% (120 mL)
Solution, topical [for scalp application]: 0.05% (25 mL, 50 mL)
Cormax®: 0.05% (25 mL, 50 mL)
Temovate®: 0.05% (50 mL) [contains isopropyl alcohol 40%]
Spray, topical [spray]: 0.05% (60 mL)
Clobex®: 0.05% (60 mL, 125 mL)

clobetasol propionate *see* clobetasol *on previous page*

Clobevate® [US] *see* clobetasol *on previous page*

Clobex® [US/Can] *see* clobetasol *on previous page*

clocortolone (kloe KOR toe lone)

Sound-Alike/Look-Alike Issues
Cloderm® may be confused with Clocort®
Synonyms clocortolone pivalate
U.S./Canadian Brand Names Cloderm® [US/Can]
Therapeutic Category Corticosteroid, Topical
Use Inflammation of corticosteroid-responsive dermatoses (intermediate-potency topical corticosteroid)
Usual Dosage Adults: Apply sparingly and gently; rub into affected area from 1-4 times/day. Therapy should be discontinued when control is achieved; if no improvement is seen, reassessment of diagnosis may be necessary.
Dosage Forms
Cream:
Cloderm®: 0.1% (45 g, 90 g)

clocortolone pivalate *see* clocortolone *on this page*

Cloderm® [US/Can] *see* clocortolone *on this page*

clodronate *(Canada only)* (KLOE droh nate)

Synonyms clodronate disodium
U.S./Canadian Brand Names Bonefos® [Can]; Clasteon® [Can]; Ostac® [Can]
Therapeutic Category Bisphosphonate Derivative
Use Management of hypercalcemia of malignancy
Usual Dosage
I.V.:
Multiple infusions: 300 mg/day; should not be prolonged beyond 10 days.
Single infusion: 1500 mg as a single dose
Oral: Recommended daily maintenance dose following I.V. therapy: Range: 1600 mg (4 capsules) to 2400 mg (6 capsules) given in single or 2 divided doses; maximum recommended daily dose: 3200 mg (8 capsules). Should be taken at least 1 hour before or after food, because food may decrease the amount of clodronate absorbed by the body.
Dosage Forms [CAN] = Canadian brand name
Injection:
Bonefos® [CAN]: 30 mg/mL (10 mL); 60 mg/mL (5 mL) [not available in the U.S.]
Capsule:
Bonefos® [CAN], Clasteon [CAN]: 400 mg [not available in the U.S.]

clodronate disodium *see* clodronate *(Canada only) on previous page*

clofarabine (klo FARE a been)
Synonyms Clofarex; NSC606869
U.S./Canadian Brand Names Clolar™ [US]
Therapeutic Category Antineoplastic Agent, Antimetabolite (Purine Antagonist)
Use Treatment of relapsed or refractory acute lymphoblastic leukemia
Usual Dosage I.V.: Children and Adults 1-21 years: ALL: 52 mg/m^2/day days 1 through 5; repeat every 2-6 weeks
Dosage Forms
Injection, solution [preservative free]:
Clolar™: 1 mg/mL (20 mL)

Clofarex *see* clofarabine *on this page*

Clolar™ [US] *see* clofarabine *on this page*

Clomid® [US/Can] *see* clomiphene *on this page*

clomiphene (KLOE mi feen)
Sound-Alike/Look-Alike Issues
clomiPHENE may be confused with clomiPRAMINE, clonidine
Clomid® may be confused with clonidine
Serophene® may be confused with Sarafem®
Synonyms clomiphene citrate
Tall-Man clomiPHENE
U.S./Canadian Brand Names Clomid® [US/Can]; Milophene® [Can]; Serophene® [US/Can]
Therapeutic Category Ovulation Stimulator
Use Treatment of ovulatory failure in patients desiring pregnancy
Usual Dosage Oral: Adults:
Male (infertility): 25 mg/day for 25 days with 5 days rest, or 100 mg every Monday, Wednesday, Friday
Female (ovulatory failure): 50 mg/day for 5 days (first course); start the regimen on or about the fifth day of cycle. The dose should be increased only in those patients who do not ovulate in response to cyclic 50 mg Clomid®. A low dosage or duration of treatment course is particularly recommended if unusual sensitivity to pituitary gonadotropin is suspected, such as in patients with polycystic ovary syndrome.

If ovulation does not appear to occur after the first course of therapy, a second course of 100 mg/day (two 50 mg tablets given as a single daily dose) for 5 days should be given. This course may be started as early as 30 days after the previous one after precautions are taken to exclude the presence of pregnancy. Increasing the dosage or duration of therapy beyond 100 mg/day for 5 days is not recommended. The majority of patients who are going to ovulate will do so after the first course of therapy. If ovulation does not occur after 3 courses of therapy, further treatment is not recommended and the patient should be reevaluated. If 3 ovulatory responses occur, but pregnancy has not been achieved, further treatment is not recommended. If menses does not occur after an ovulatory response, the patient should be reevaluated. Long-term cyclic therapy is not recommended beyond a total of about 6 cycles.
Dosage Forms
Tablet [scored]: 50 mg
Clomid®, Serophene®: 50 mg

clomiphene citrate *see* clomiphene *on this page*

clomipramine (kloe MI pra meen)
Sound-Alike/Look-Alike Issues
clomiPRAMINE may be confused with chlorproMAZINE, clomiPHENE, desipramine, Norpramin®
Anafranil® may be confused with alfentanil, enalapril, nafarelin
Synonyms clomipramine hydrochloride
Tall-Man clomiPRAMINE
U.S./Canadian Brand Names Anafranil® [US/Can]; Apo-Clomipramine® [Can]; CO Clomipramine [Can]; Gen-Clomipramine [Can]
Therapeutic Category Antidepressant, Tricyclic (Tertiary Amine)
Use Treatment of obsessive-compulsive disorder (OCD)
Usual Dosage Oral: Initial:
Children:
<10 years: Safety and efficacy have not been established.
≥10 years: OCD: 25 mg/day; gradually increase, as tolerated, to a maximum of 3 mg/kg/day or 200 mg/day (whichever is smaller)
(Continued)

clomipramine *(Continued)*

Adults: OCD: 25 mg/day and gradually increase, as tolerated, to 100 mg/day the first 2 weeks, may then be increased to a total of 250 mg/day maximum

Dosage Forms
Capsule: 25 mg, 50 mg, 75 mg
Anafranil®: 25 mg, 50 mg, 75 mg

clomipramine hydrochloride *see* clomipramine *on previous page*

Clonapam [Can] *see* clonazepam *on this page*

clonazepam (kloe NA ze pam)

Sound-Alike/Look-Alike Issues
clonazepam may be confused with clofazimine, clonidine, clorazepate, clozapine, lorazepam
Klonopin® may be confused with clofazimine, clonidine, clorazepate, clozapine, lorazepam
U.S./Canadian Brand Names Alti-Clonazepam [Can]; Apo-Clonazepam® [Can]; Clonapam [Can]; CO Clonazepam [Can]; Gen-Clonazepam [Can]; Klonopin® [US/Can]; Novo-Clonazepam [Can]; Nu-Clonazepam [Can]; PMS-Clonazepam [Can]; Rho®-Clonazepam [Can]; Rivotril® [Can]; Sandoz-Clonazepam [Can]
Therapeutic Category Benzodiazepine
Controlled Substance C-IV
Use Alone or as an adjunct in the treatment of petit mal variant (Lennox-Gastaut), akinetic, and myoclonic seizures; petit mal (absence) seizures unresponsive to succimides; panic disorder with or without agoraphobia
Usual Dosage Oral:
Children <10 years or 30 kg: Seizure disorders:
Initial daily dose: 0.01-0.03 mg/kg/day (maximum: 0.05 mg/kg/day) given in 2-3 divided doses; increase by no more than 0.5 mg every third day until seizures are controlled or adverse effects seen
Usual maintenance dose: 0.1-0.2 mg/kg/day divided 3 times/day, not to exceed 0.2 mg/kg/day
Adults:
Burning mouth syndrome (dental use): 0.25-3 mg/day in 2 divided doses, in morning and evening
Seizure disorders:
Initial daily dose not to exceed 1.5 mg given in 3 divided doses; may increase by 0.5-1 mg every third day until seizures are controlled or adverse effects seen (maximum: 20 mg/day)
Usual maintenance dose: 0.05-0.2 mg/kg; do not exceed 20 mg/day
Panic disorder: 0.25 mg twice daily; increase in increments of 0.125-0.25 mg twice daily every 3 days; target dose: 1 mg/day (maximum: 4 mg/day)
Discontinuation of treatment: To discontinue, treatment should be withdrawn gradually. Decrease dose by 0.125 mg twice daily every 3 days until medication is completely withdrawn.
Dosage Forms
Tablet: 0.5 mg, 1 mg, 2 mg
Klonopin®: 0.5 mg, 1 mg, 2 mg
Tablet, orally disintegrating [wafer]: 0.125 mg, 0.25 mg, 0.5 mg, 1 mg, 2 mg
Klonopin®: 0.125 mg, 0.25 mg, 0.5 mg, 1 mg, 2 mg

clonidine (KLON i deen)

Sound-Alike/Look-Alike Issues
clonidine may be confused with Clomid®, clomiPHENE, clonazepam, clozapine, Klonopin®, quinidine
Catapres® may be confused with Cataflam®, Cetapred®, Combipres®
Synonyms clonidine hydrochloride
U.S./Canadian Brand Names Apo-Clonidine® [Can]; Carapres® [Can]; Catapres-TTS® [US]; Catapres® [US]; Dixarit® [Can]; Duraclon™ [US]; Novo-Clonidine [Can]; Nu-Clonidine [Can]
Therapeutic Category Alpha-Adrenergic Agonist
Use Management of mild-to-moderate hypertension; either used alone or in combination with other antihypertensives
Orphan drug: Duraclon™: For continuous epidural administration as adjunctive therapy with intraspinal opiates for treatment of cancer pain in patients tolerant to or unresponsive to intraspinal opiates
Usual Dosage
Children:
Oral:
Hypertension: Children ≥12 years: Initial: 0.2 mg/day in 2 divided doses; increase gradually at 5- to 7-day intervals; maximum: 2.4 mg/day
Clonidine tolerance test (test of growth hormone release from pituitary): 0.15 mg/m^2 or 4 mcg/kg as single dose

Epidural infusion: Pain management: Reserved for patients with severe intractable pain, unresponsive to other analgesics or epidural or spinal opiates: Initial: 0.5 mcg/kg/hour; adjust with caution, based on clinical effect

Adults:

Oral:

Acute hypertension (urgency): Initial 0.1-0.2 mg; may be followed by additional doses of 0.1 mg every hour, if necessary, to a maximum total dose of 0.6 mg.

Hypertension: Initial dose: 0.1 mg twice daily (maximum recommended dose: 2.4 mg/day); usual dose range (JNC 7): 0.1-0.8 mg/day in 2 divided doses

Nicotine withdrawal symptoms: 0.1 mg twice daily to maximum of 0.4 mg/day for 3-4 weeks

Transdermal: Hypertension: Apply once every 7 days; for initial therapy start with 0.1 mg and increase by 0.1 mg at 1- to 2-week intervals (dosages >0.6 mg do not improve efficacy); usual dose range (JNC 7): 0.1-0.3 mg once weekly

Note: If transitioning from oral to transdermal therapy, overlap oral regimen for 1-2 days; transdermal route takes 2-3 days to achieve therapeutic effects.

Conversion from oral to transdermal:

Day 1: Place Catapres-TTS® 1; administer 100% of oral dose.

Day 2: Administer 50% of oral dose.

Day 3: Administer 25% of oral dose.

Day 4: Patch remains, no further oral supplement necessary.

Epidural infusion: Pain management: Starting dose: 30 mcg/hour; titrate as required for relief of pain or presence of side effects; minimal experience with doses >40 mcg/hour; should be considered an adjunct to intraspinal opiate therapy

Dosage Forms

Injection, epidural solution [preservative free]:

Duraclon™: 100 mcg/mL (10 mL); 500 mcg/mL (10 mL)

Patch, transdermal [once-weekly patch]:

Catapres-TTS®-1: 0.1 mg/24 hours (4s)

Catapres-TTS®-2: 0.2 mg/24 hours (4s)

Catapres-TTS®-3: 0.3 mg/24 hours (4s)

Tablet: 0.1 mg, 0.2 mg, 0.3 mg

Catapres®: 0.1 mg, 0.2 mg, 0.3 mg

clonidine and chlorthalidone (KLON i deen & klor THAL i done)

Sound-Alike/Look-Alike Issues

Combipres® may be confused with Catapres®

Synonyms chlorthalidone and clonidine

U.S./Canadian Brand Names Clorpres® [US]

Therapeutic Category Antihypertensive Agent, Combination

Use Management of mild-to-moderate hypertension

Usual Dosage Oral: 1 tablet 1-2 times/day; maximum: 0.6 mg clonidine and 30 mg chlorthalidone

Dosage Forms

Tablet:

Clorpres®: 0.1: Clonidine 0.1 mg and chlorthalidone 15 mg; 0.2: Clonidine 0.2 mg and chlorthalidone 15 mg; 0.3: Clonidine 0.3 mg and chlorthalidone 15 mg

clonidine hydrochloride *see* clonidine *on previous page*

clopidogrel (kloh PID oh grel)

Sound-Alike/Look-Alike Issues

Plavix® may be confused with Elavil®, Paxil®

Synonyms clopidogrel bisulfate

U.S./Canadian Brand Names Plavix® [US/Can]

Therapeutic Category Antiplatelet Agent

Use Reduces rate of atherothrombotic events (myocardial infarction, stroke, vascular deaths) in patients with recent MI or stroke, or established peripheral arterial disease; reduces rate of atherothrombotic events in patients with unstable angina or non-ST-segment elevation acute coronary syndromes (unstable angina and non-ST-segment elevation MI) managed medically or through PCI (with or without stent) or CABG; reduces rate of death and atherothrombotic events in patients with ST-segment elevation MI (STEMI) managed medically

Usual Dosage Oral: Adults:

Recent MI, recent stroke, or established arterial disease: 75 mg once daily

Non-ST-segment elevation acute coronary syndrome: Initial: 300 mg loading dose, followed by 75 mg once daily (in combination with aspirin 75-325 mg once daily). **Note:** A loading dose of 600 mg has been used in some investigations; limited research exists comparing the two doses.

(Continued)

clopidogrel (Continued)

Note: Drug-eluting stents: Duration of clopidogrel (in combination with aspirin): Ideally 12 months following drug-eluting stent placement in patients not at high risk for bleeding; at a minimum, 1-, 3-, and 6 months for bare metal, sirolimus, and paclitaxel stents, respectively, for uninterrupted therapy.
ST-segment elevation MI: 75 mg once daily (in combination with aspirin 75-162 mg/day). CLARITY used a 300 mg loading dose of clopidogrel. The duration of therapy was <28 days (usually until hospital discharge).

Dosage Forms
  Tablet:
  Plavix®: 75 mg

clopidogrel bisulfate see clopidogrel on previous page

Clopixol® [Can] see zuclopenthixol (Canada only) on page 909

Clopixol-Acuphase® [Can] see zuclopenthixol (Canada only) on page 909

Clopixol® Depot [Can] see zuclopenthixol (Canada only) on page 909

clorazepate (klor AZ e pate)

Sound-Alike/Look-Alike Issues
  clorazepate may be confused with clofibrate, clonazepam
Synonyms clorazepate dipotassium
U.S./Canadian Brand Names Apo-Clorazepate® [Can]; Novo-Clopate [Can]; Tranxene® SD™ [US]; Tranxene® SD™-Half Strength [US]; Tranxene® T-Tab® [US]
Therapeutic Category Anticonvulsant; Benzodiazepine
Controlled Substance C-IV
Use Treatment of generalized anxiety disorder; management of ethanol withdrawal; adjunct anticonvulsant in management of partial seizures
Usual Dosage Oral:
  Children 9-12 years: Anticonvulsant: Initial: 3.75-7.5 mg/dose twice daily; increase dose by 3.75 mg at weekly intervals, not to exceed 60 mg/day in 2-3 divided doses
  Children >12 years and Adults: Anticonvulsant: Initial: Up to 7.5 mg/dose 2-3 times/day; increase dose by 7.5 mg at weekly intervals, not to exceed 90 mg/day
  Adults:
  Anxiety:
    Regular release tablets (Tranxene® T-Tab®): 7.5-15 mg 2-4 times/day
    Sustained release (Tranxene® SD): 11.25 or 22.5 mg once daily at bedtime
  Ethanol withdrawal: Initial: 30 mg, then 15 mg 2-4 times/day on first day; maximum daily dose: 90 mg; gradually decrease dose over subsequent days
Dosage Forms
  Tablet: 3.75 mg, 7.5 mg, 15 mg
  Tranxene® SD™: 22.5 mg
  Tranxene® SD™-Half Strength: 11.25 mg
  Tranxene® T-Tab®: 3.75 mg, 7.5 mg, 15 mg

clorazepate dipotassium see clorazepate on this page

Clorpactin® WCS-90 [US-OTC] see oxychlorosene on page 640

Clorpres® [US] see clonidine and chlorthalidone on previous page

Clotrimaderm [Can] see clotrimazole on this page

clotrimazole (kloe TRIM a zole)

Sound-Alike/Look-Alike Issues
  clotrimazole may be confused with co-trimoxazole
  Lotrimin® may be confused with Lotrisone®, Otrivin®
  Mycelex® may be confused with Myoflex®
U.S./Canadian Brand Names Canesten® Topical [Can]; Canesten® Vaginal [Can]; Clotrimaderm [Can]; Cruex® Cream [US-OTC]; Gyne-Lotrimin® 3 [US-OTC]; Lotrimin® AF Athlete's Foot Cream [US-OTC]; Lotrimin® AF Athlete's Foot Solution [US-OTC]; Lotrimin® AF Jock Itch Cream [US-OTC]; Mycelex® Twin Pack [US-OTC]; Mycelex® [US]; Mycelex®-7 [US-OTC]; Trivagizole-3® [Can]
Therapeutic Category Antifungal Agent
Use Treatment of susceptible fungal infections, including oropharyngeal candidiasis, dermatophytoses, superficial mycoses, and cutaneous candidiasis, as well as vulvovaginal candidiasis; limited data suggest that clotrimazole troches may be effective for prophylaxis against oropharyngeal candidiasis in neutropenic patients

Usual Dosage
Children >3 years and Adults:
Oral:
Prophylaxis: 10 mg troche dissolved 3 times/day for the duration of chemotherapy or until steroids are reduced to maintenance levels
Treatment: 10 mg troche dissolved slowly 5 times/day for 14 consecutive days
Topical (cream, solution): Apply twice daily; if no improvement occurs after 4 weeks of therapy, re-evaluate diagnosis
Children >12 years and Adults:
Vaginal:
Cream:
1%: Insert 1 applicatorful vaginal cream daily (preferably at bedtime) for 7 consecutive days
2%: Insert 1 applicatorful vaginal cream daily (preferably at bedtime) for 3 consecutive days
Tablet: Insert 100 mg/day for 7 days or 500 mg single dose
Topical (cream, solution): Apply to affected area twice daily (morning and evening) for 7 consecutive days

Dosage Forms
Combination pack:
Mycelex®-7 [OTC]: Vaginal tablet 100 mg (7s) and vaginal cream 1% (7 g)
Cream, topical: 1% (15 g, 30 g, 45 g)
Cruex® [OTC]: 1% (15 g)
Lotrimin® AF Athlete's Foot [OTC]: 1% (12 g, 24 g)
Lotrimin® AF Jock Itch [OTC]: 1% (12 g)
Cream, vaginal: 2% (21 g)
Mycelex®-7 [OTC]: 1% (45 g)
Solution, topical: 1% (10 mL, 30 mL)
Lotrimin® AF Athlete's Foot [OTC]: 1% (10 mL)
Tablet, vaginal:
Gyne-Lotrimin® 3: 200 mg (3s)
Troche: 10 mg
Mycelex®: 10 mg

clotrimazole and betamethasone *see* betamethasone and clotrimazole *on page 108*

cloxacillin (kloks a SIL in)
Synonyms cloxacillin sodium
U.S./Canadian Brand Names Apo-Cloxi® [Can]; Novo-Cloxin [Can]; Nu-Cloxi [Can]; Riva-Cloxacillin [Can]
Therapeutic Category Penicillin
Use Treatment of susceptible bacterial infections, notably penicillinase-producing staphylococci causing respiratory tract, skin and skin structure, bone and joint, urinary tract infections
Usual Dosage Oral:
Children >1 month and <20 kg: 50-100 mg/kg/day in divided doses every 6 hours; (maximum: 4 g/day)
Children >20 kg and Adults: 250-500 mg every 6 hours
Dosage Forms [CAN] = Canadian brand name
Capsule: 250 mg, 500 mg [not available in the U.S.]
Apo-Cloxi® [CAN], Novo-Cloxin [CAN], Nu-Cloxi [CAN]: 250 mg, 500 mg [not available in the U.S.]
Powder for oral suspension: 125 mg/5 mL [not available in the U.S.]
Apo-Cloxi® [CAN], Novo-Cloxin [CAN], Nu-Cloxi [CAN]: 125 mg/5 mL [not available in the U.S.]

cloxacillin sodium *see* cloxacillin *on this page*

Cloxapen® *(Discontinued)* *see* cloxacillin *on this page*

clozapine (KLOE za peen)
Sound-Alike/Look-Alike Issues
clozapine may be confused with clofazimine, clonidine, Klonopin®
Clozaril® may be confused with Clinoril®, Colazal®
U.S./Canadian Brand Names Apo-Clozapine® [Can]; Clozaril® [US/Can]; FazaClo® [US]; Gen-Clozapine [Can]
Therapeutic Category Antipsychotic Agent, Dibenzodiazepine
Use Treatment-refractory schizophrenia; to reduce risk of recurrent suicidal behavior in schizophrenia or schizoaffective disorder
Usual Dosage Oral: Adults:
Schizophrenia: Initial: 12.5 mg once or twice daily; increased, as tolerated, in increments of 25-50 mg/day to a target dose of 300-450 mg/day after 2-4 weeks, may require doses as high as 600-900 mg/day
(Continued)

clozapine *(Continued)*

Reduce risk of suicidal behavior: Initial: 12.5 mg once or twice daily; increased, as tolerated, in increments of 25-50 mg/day to a target dose of 300-450 mg/day after 2-4 weeks; median dose is ~300 mg/day (range: 12.5-900 mg)

Termination of therapy: If dosing is interrupted for ≥48 hours, therapy must be reinitiated at 12.5-25 mg/day; may be increased more rapidly than with initial titration, unless cardiopulmonary arrest occurred during initial titration.

In the event of planned termination of clozapine, gradual reduction in dose over a 1- to 2-week period is recommended. If conditions warrant abrupt discontinuation (leukopenia), monitor patient for psychosis and cholinergic rebound (headache, nausea, vomiting, diarrhea).

Patients discontinued on clozapine therapy due to WBC <2000/mm^3 or ANC <1000/mm^3 should not be restarted on clozapine.

Dosage Forms

Tablet: 12.5 mg, 25 mg, 50 mg, 100 mg, 200 mg
Clozaril®: 25 mg, 100 mg

Tablet, orally disintegrating:
FazaClo®: 25 mg, 100 mg

Clozaril® [US/Can] *see* clozapine *on previous page*

Clysodrast® *(Discontinued)* *see* bisacodyl *on page 112*

CMA-676 *see* gemtuzumab ozogamicin *on page 388*

CMV-IGIV *see* cytomegalovirus immune globulin (intravenous-human) *on page 227*

CNJ-016™ [US] *see* vaccinia immune globulin (intravenous) *on page 879*

CoActifed® [Can] *see* triprolidine, pseudoephedrine, and codeine *(Canada only)* *on page 869*

coagulant complex inhibitor *see* antiinhibitor coagulant complex *on page 61*

coagulation factor VIIa *see* factor VIIa (recombinant) *on page 339*

CO Alendronate [Can] *see* alendronate *on page 27*

coal tar *(KOLE tar)*

Sound-Alike/Look-Alike Issues

Pentrax® may be confused with Permax®
Tegrin® may be confused with Tegretol®

Synonyms crude coal tar; LCD; pix carbonis

U.S./Canadian Brand Names Balnetar® [US-OTC/Can]; Betatar® Gel [US-OTC]; Cutar® [US-OTC]; Denorex® Original Therapeutic Strength [US-OTC]; DHS™ Tar [US-OTC]; DHS™ Targel [US-OTC]; Doak® Tar [US-OTC]; Estar® [Can]; Exorex® [US]; Fototar® [US-OTC]; Ionil T® Plus [US-OTC]; Ionil T® [US-OTC]; MG 217® Medicated Tar [US-OTC]; MG 217® [US-OTC]; Neutrogena® T/Gel Extra Strength [US-OTC]; Neutrogena® T/Gel Stubborn Itch Control [US-OTC]; Neutrogena® T/Gel [US-OTC]; Oxipor® VHC [US-OTC]; Polytar® [US-OTC]; Reme-T™ [Can]; Targel® [Can]; Tera-Gel™ [US-OTC]; Zetar® [US-OTC]

Therapeutic Category Antipsoriatic Agent; Antiseborrheic Agent, Topical

Use Topically for controlling dandruff, seborrheic dermatitis, or psoriasis

Usual Dosage Topical:

Bath: Add appropriate amount to bath water; for adults usually 60-90 mL of a 5% to 20% solution or 15-25 mL of 30% lotion; soak 5-20 minutes, then pat dry; use once daily to 3 days

Shampoo: Rub shampoo onto wet hair and scalp, rinse thoroughly; repeat; leave on 5 minutes; rinse thoroughly; apply twice weekly for the first 2 weeks then once weekly or more often if needed

Soap: Use on affected areas in place of regular soap. Work into a lather using warm water; massage into skin; rinse.

Skin: Apply to the affected area 1-4 times/day; decrease frequency to 2-3 times/week once condition has been controlled

Scalp psoriasis: Tar oil bath or coal tar solution may be painted sparingly to the lesions 3-12 hours before each shampoo

Psoriasis of the body, arms, legs: Apply at bedtime; if thick scales are present, use product with salicylic acid and apply several times during the day

Dosage Forms

Cream:
Fototar®: Coal tar 2% (85 g, 454 g)

Emulsion, topical:
Cutar® [OTC]: Coal tar solution 7.5% (180 mL, 3840 mL)
Exorex®: Coal tar 1% (240 mL)

Gel, shampoo:
DHS™ Targel [OTC]: Coal tar solution 2.9% (240 mL)

Liquid:
Doak® Tar Distillate: Coal tar 40% (60 mL)
Lotion, topical:
Doak® Tar [OTC]: Coal tar distillate 5% (240 mL)
Exorex®: Coal tar 1% (240 mL)
MG 217® [OTC]: Coal tar solution 5% (120 mL)
Oxipor® VHC [OTC]: Coal tar solution 25% (60 mL, 120 mL)
Oil, topical:
Balnetar®: Coal tar 2.5% (225 mL) [for use in bath]
Doak® Tar [OTC]: Coal tar distillate 2% (240 mL)
Ointment, topical:
MG 217® [OTC]: Coal tar solution 10% (107 g, 430 g)
Shampoo:
Betatar Gel® [OTC]: Coal tar solution 5% (240 mL)
Denorex® Original Therapeutic Strength [OTC]: Coal tar solution 12.5% (120 mL, 240 mL, 360 mL)
DHS™ Tar [OTC]: Coal tar solution 2.9% (120 mL, 240 mL, 480 mL)
Doak® Tar [OTC]: Coal tar distillate 3% (240 mL)
Ionil T® Plus [OTC]: Coal tar 2% (240 mL)
MG 217® Medicated Tar [OTC]: Coal tar solution 15% (120 mL, 240 mL)
Neutrogena® T/Gel [OTC]: Coal tar 0.5% (132 mL, 480 mL)
Neutrogena® T/Gel Extra Strength [OTC]: Coal tar extract 4% (132 mL)
Neutrogena® T/Gel Stubborn Itch Control [OTC]: Coal tar extract 2% (132 mL)
Polytar® [OTC]: Coal tar 0.5% (177 mL)
Reme-T™ [OTC]: Coal tar 5% (236 mL)
Tera-Gel™ [OTC]: Solubilized coal tar 0.5% (120 mL, 240 mL)
Zetar® [OTC]: Coal tar 1% (180 mL)
Soap:
Polytar® [OTC]: Coal tar 0.5% (113 g)

coal tar and salicylic acid (KOLE tar & sal i SIL ik AS id)

Synonyms salicylic acid and coal tar
U.S./Canadian Brand Names Sebcur/T® [Can]; Tarsum® [US-OTC]; X-Seb T® Pearl [US-OTC]; X-Seb T® Plus [US-OTC]
Therapeutic Category Antipsoriatic Agent; Antiseborrheic Agent, Topical
Use Seborrheal dermatitis, dandruff, psoriasis
Usual Dosage Psoriasis: Scalp:
Gel: Apply directly to plaques; may leave in place for up to 1 hour. Apply water and work into a lather; rinse.
Shampoo: Apply to wet hair; massage into scalp; rinse.
Dosage Forms
Gel [shampoo]: Coal tar solution 10% [equivalent to coal tar 2%] and salicylic acid (120 mL, 240 mL)
Tarsum® [OTC]: Coal tar solution 10% [equivalent to coal tar 2%] and salicylic acid (120 mL, 240 mL)
Shampoo, topical: Coal tar solution 10% [equivalent to coal tar 2%] and salicylic acid (120 mL, 240 mL)
X-Seb T® Pearl [OTC], X-Seb T® Plus [OTC]: Coal tar solution 10% [equivalent to coal tar 2%] and salicylic acid (120 mL, 240 mL)

CO Azithromycin [Can] *see azithromycin on page 88*

Cobex® *(Discontinued) see cyanocobalamin on page 220*

CO Bicalutamide [Can] *see bicalutamide on page 111*

cocaine (koe KANE)

Synonyms cocaine hydrochloride
Therapeutic Category Local Anesthetic
Controlled Substance C-II
Use Topical anesthesia for mucous membranes
Usual Dosage Topical application (ear, nose, throat, bronchoscopy): Dosage depends on the area to be anesthetized, tissue vascularity, technique of anesthesia, and individual patient tolerance; the lowest dose necessary to produce adequate anesthesia should be used; concentrations of 1% to 10% are used (not to exceed 1 mg/kg). Use reduced dosages for children, elderly, or debilitated patients.
Dosage Forms
Powder, for prescription compounding: 1 g, 5 g, 25 g
Solution, topical: 4% (4 mL, 10 mL); 10% (4 mL, 10 mL)

cocaine hydrochloride *see cocaine on this page*

CO Ciprofloxacin [Can] *see ciprofloxacin on page 190*

CO Citalopram [Can] *see* citalopram *on page 194*

CO Clomipramine [Can] *see* clomipramine *on page 203*

CO Clonazepam [Can] *see* clonazepam *on page 204*

Codal-DM [US-OTC] *see* phenylephrine, pyrilamine, and dextromethorphan *on page 679*

Codamine® *(Discontinued)*

Codamine® Pediatric *(Discontinued)*

Codehist® DH *(Discontinued)* *see* chlorpheniramine, pseudoephedrine, and codeine *on page 183*

codeine (KOE deen)

Sound-Alike/Look-Alike Issues
codeine may be confused with Cardene®, Cophene®, Cordran®, iodine, Lodine®

Synonyms codeine phosphate; codeine sulfate; methylmorphine

U.S./Canadian Brand Names Codeine Contin® [Can]

Therapeutic Category Analgesic, Narcotic; Antitussive

Controlled Substance C-II

Use Treatment of mild-to-moderate pain; antitussive in lower doses; dextromethorphan has equivalent antitussive activity but has much lower toxicity in accidental overdose

Usual Dosage Note: These are guidelines and do not represent the maximum doses that may be required in all patients. Doses should be titrated to pain relief/prevention. Doses >1.5 mg/kg body weight are not recommended.

Analgesic:

Children: Oral, I.M., SubQ: 0.5-1 mg/kg/dose every 4-6 hours as needed; maximum: 60 mg/dose

Adults:

Oral: 30 mg every 4-6 hours as needed; patients with prior opiate exposure may require higher initial doses. Usual range: 15-120 mg every 4-6 hours as needed

Oral, controlled release formulation (Codeine Contin®, not available in U.S.): 50-300 mg every 12 hours. **Note:** A patient's codeine requirement should be established using prompt release formulations; conversion to long-acting products may be considered when chronic, continuous treatment is required. Higher dosages should be reserved for use only in opioid-tolerant patients.

I.M., SubQ: 30 mg every 4-6 hours as needed; patients with prior opiate exposure may require higher initial doses. Usual range: 15-120 mg every 4-6 hours as needed; more frequent dosing may be needed

Antitussive: Oral (for nonproductive cough):

Children: 1-1.5 mg/kg/day in divided doses every 4-6 hours as needed: Alternative dose according to age:

2-6 years: 2.5-5 mg every 4-6 hours as needed; maximum: 30 mg/day

6-12 years: 5-10 mg every 4-6 hours as needed; maximum: 60 mg/day

Adults: 10-20 mg/dose every 4-6 hours as needed; maximum: 120 mg/day

Dosage Forms [CAN] = Canadian brand name

Injection: 15 mg/mL (2 mL); 30 mg/mL (2 mL)

Powder, for prescription compounding: 10 g, 25 g

Tablet: 15 mg, 30 mg, 60 mg

Tablet, controlled release: 50 mg, 100 mg, 150 mg, 200 mg

Codeine Contin® [CAN]: 50 mg, 100 mg, 150 mg, 200 mg [not available in the U.S.]

codeine, acetaminophen, butalbital, and caffeine *see* butalbital, acetaminophen, caffeine, and codeine *on page 130*

codeine and acetaminophen *see* acetaminophen and codeine *on page 6*

codeine and butalbital compound *see* butalbital, aspirin, caffeine, and codeine *on page 131*

codeine and guaifenesin *see* guaifenesin and codeine *on page 402*

codeine and promethazine *see* promethazine and codeine *on page 719*

codeine, aspirin, and carisoprodol *see* carisoprodol, aspirin, and codeine *on page 154*

codeine, butalbital, aspirin, and caffeine *see* butalbital, aspirin, caffeine, and codeine *on page 131*

codeine, chlorpheniramine, and pseudoephedrine *see* chlorpheniramine, pseudoephedrine, and codeine *on page 183*

codeine, chlorpheniramine, phenylephrine, and potassium iodide *see* chlorpheniramine, phenylephrine, codeine, and potassium iodide *on page 183*

Codeine Contin® [Can] *see* codeine *on this page*

codeine, doxylamine, and acetaminophen *see* acetaminophen, codeine, and doxylamine *(Canada only) on page 11*

codeine, guaifenesin, and pseudoephedrine *see* guaifenesin, pseudoephedrine, and codeine *on page 408*

codeine phosphate *see* codeine *on previous page*

codeine, promethazine, and phenylephrine *see* promethazine, phenylephrine, and codeine *on page 720*

codeine, pseudoephedrine, and triprolidine *see* triprolidine, pseudoephedrine, and codeine *(Canada only) on page 869*

codeine sulfate *see* codeine *on previous page*

codeine, triprolidine, and pseudoephedrine *see* triprolidine, pseudoephedrine, and codeine *(Canada only) on page 869*

Codiclear® DH [US] *see* hydrocodone and guaifenesin *on page 429*

codimal® DM [US-OTC] *see* phenylephrine, pyrilamine, and dextromethorphan *on page 679*

Codituss DM [US-OTC] *see* phenylephrine, pyrilamine, and dextromethorphan *on page 679*

cod liver oil *see* vitamin A and vitamin D *on page 893*

CO Fluoxetine [Can] *see* fluoxetine *on page 364*

Cogentin® [US] *see* benztropine *on page 105*

Co-Gesic® [US] *see* hydrocodone and acetaminophen *on page 427*

CO Glimepiride [Can] *see* glimepiride *on page 393*

Cognex® [US] *see* tacrine *on page 818*

CO Ipra-Sal [Can] *see* ipratropium and albuterol *on page 471*

Colace® [US-OTC/Can] *see* docusate *on page 273*

Colace® Adult/Children Suppositories [US-OTC] *see* glycerin *on page 397*

Colace® Infant/Children Suppositories [US-OTC] *see* glycerin *on page 397*

Colax-C® [Can] *see* docusate *on page 273*

Colazal® [US] *see* balsalazide *on page 93*

ColBenemid® *(Discontinued)* *see* colchicine and probenecid *on this page*

colchicine (KOL chi seen)
Therapeutic Category Antigout Agent
Use Treatment of acute gouty arthritis attacks and prevention of recurrences of such attacks
Usual Dosage
Gouty arthritis: Adults:
Prophylaxis of acute attacks: Oral: 0.6 mg twice daily; initial and/or subsequent dosage may be decreased (ie, 0.6 mg once daily) in patients at risk of toxicity or in those who are intolerant (including weakness, loose stools, or diarrhea); range: 0.6 mg every other day to 0.6 mg 3 times/day
Acute attacks:
Oral: Initial: 0.6-1.2 mg, followed by 0.6 every 1-2 hours; some clinicians recommend a maximum of 3 doses; more aggressive approaches have recommended a maximum dose of up to 6 mg. Wait at least 3 days before initiating another course of therapy
I.V.: Initial: 1-2 mg, then 0.5 mg every 6 hours until response, not to exceed total dose of 4 mg. If pain recurs, it may be necessary to administer additional daily doses. The amount of colchicine administered intravenously in an acute treatment period (generally ~1 week) should not exceed a total dose of 4 mg. Do not administer more colchicine by any route for at least 7 days after a full course of I.V. therapy.
Note: Many experts would avoid use because of potential for serious, life-threatening complications. Should not be administered to patients with renal insufficiency, hepatobiliary obstruction, patients >70 years of age, or recent oral colchicine use. Should be reserved for hospitalized patients who are under the care of a physician experienced in the use of intravenous colchicine.
Surgery: Gouty arthritis, prophylaxis of recurrent attacks: Adults: Oral: 0.6 mg/day or every other day; patients who are to undergo surgical procedures may receive 0.6 mg 3 times/day for 3 days before and 3 days after surgery
Dosage Forms
Injection, solution: 0.5 mg/mL (2 mL)
Tablet: 0.6 mg

colchicine and probenecid (KOL chi seen & proe BEN e sid)
Synonyms probenecid and colchicine
Therapeutic Category Antigout Agent
Use Treatment of chronic gouty arthritis when complicated by frequent, recurrent acute attacks of gout
(Continued)

colchicine and probenecid *(Continued)*
Usual Dosage Oral: Adults: 1 tablet daily for 1 week, then 1 tablet twice daily thereafter
Dosage Forms
  Tablet: Colchicine 0.5 mg and probenecid 0.5 g

Coldcough [US] *see* pseudoephedrine, dihydrocodeine, and chlorpheniramine *on page 730*

Coldcough HC [US] *see* pseudoephedrine, hydrocodone, and chlorpheniramine *on page 731*

Coldcough PD [US] *see* dihydrocodeine, chlorpheniramine, and phenylephrine *on page 259*

Coldlac-LA® *(Discontinued)*

Coldloc® *(Discontinued)*

Coldmist DM [US] *see* guaifenesin, pseudoephedrine, and dextromethorphan *on page 408*

Coldtuss DR *(Discontinued) see* chlorpheniramine, phenylephrine, and dextromethorphan *on page 180*

colesevelam *(koh le SEV a lam)*
U.S./Canadian Brand Names WelChol® [US/Can]
Therapeutic Category Antihyperlipidemic Agent, Miscellaneous; Bile Acid Sequestrant
Use Adjunctive therapy to diet and exercise in the management of elevated LDL in primary hypercholesterolemia (Fredrickson type IIa) when used alone or in combination with an HMG-CoA reductase inhibitor
Usual Dosage Oral: Adults:
  Monotherapy: 3 tablets twice daily with meals or 6 tablets once daily with a meal; maximum dose: 7 tablets/day
  Combination therapy with an HMG-CoA reductase inhibitor: 4-6 tablets daily; maximum dose: 6 tablets/day
Dosage Forms
  Tablet:
  WelChol®: 625 mg

Colestid® **[US/Can]** *see* colestipol *on this page*

colestipol *(koe LES ti pole)*
Synonyms colestipol hydrochloride
U.S./Canadian Brand Names Colestid® [US/Can]
Therapeutic Category Antihyperlipidemic Agent, Miscellaneous
Use Adjunct in management of primary hypercholesterolemia; regression of arteriolosclerosis; relief of pruritus associated with elevated levels of bile acids; possibly used to decrease plasma half-life of digoxin in toxicity
Usual Dosage Oral: Adults:
  Granules: 5-30 g/day given once or in divided doses 2-4 times/day; initial dose: 5 g 1-2 times/day; increase by 5 g at 1- to 2-month intervals
  Tablets: 2-16 g/day; initial dose: 2 g 1-2 times/day; increase by 2 g at 1- to 2-month intervals
Dosage Forms
  Granules:
  Colestid®: 5 g/7.5 g (300 g, 450 g, 500 g); 5 g/7.5 g packet (30s, 60s, 90s)
  Tablet:
  Colestid®: 1 g

colestipol hydrochloride *see* colestipol *on this page*

CO Levetiracetam [Can] *see* levetiracetam *on page 498*

colistimethate *(koe lis ti METH ate)*
Synonyms colistimethate sodium; colistin methanesulfonate; colistin sulfomethate; pentasodium colistin methanesulfonate
U.S./Canadian Brand Names Coly-Mycin® M [US/Can]
Therapeutic Category Antibiotic, Miscellaneous
Use Treatment of infections due to sensitive strains of certain gram-negative bacilli which are resistant to other antibacterials or in patients allergic to other antibacterials
Usual Dosage Note: Doses should be based on ideal body weight in obese patients; dosage expressed in terms of colistin.
  Children and Adults: Susceptible infections: I.M., I.V.: 2.5-5 mg/kg/day in 2-4 divided doses
Dosage Forms
  Injection, powder for reconstitution, as colistin base: 150 mg
  Coly-Mycin® M: 150 mg

colistimethate sodium *see* colistimethate *on previous page*

colistin methanesulfonate *see* colistimethate *on previous page*

colistin, neomycin, hydrocortisone, and thonzonium *see* neomycin, colistin, hydrocortisone, and thonzonium *on page 597*

colistin sulfomethate *see* colistimethate *on previous page*

collagen *see* collagen hemostat *on this page*

collagen absorbable hemostat *see* collagen hemostat *on this page*

collagenase (KOL la je nase)
U.S./Canadian Brand Names Santyl® [US]
Therapeutic Category Enzyme
Use Promotes debridement of necrotic tissue in dermal ulcers and severe burns
  Orphan drug: Injection: Treatment of Peyronie disease; treatment of Dupuytren disease
Usual Dosage Topical: Apply once daily (or more frequently if the dressing becomes soiled)
Dosage Forms
  Ointment:
  Santyl®: 250 units/g (15 g, 30 g)

collagen hemostat (KOL la jen HEE moe stat)
Sound-Alike/Look-Alike Issues
  Avitene® may be confused with Ativan®
Synonyms collagen; collagen absorbable hemostat; MCH; microfibrillar collagen hemostat
U.S./Canadian Brand Names Avitene® Flour [US]; Avitene® Ultrafoam [US]; Avitene® UltraWrap™ [US]; Avitene® [US]; EndoAvitene® [US]; Helistat® [US]; Helitene® [US]; Instat™ MCH [US]; Instat™ [US]; SyringeAvitene™ [US]
Therapeutic Category Hemostatic Agent
Use Adjunct to hemostasis when control of bleeding by ligature is ineffective or impractical
Usual Dosage Apply dry directly to source of bleeding; remove excess material after ~10-15 minutes
Dosage Forms
  Pad:
  Instat™: 1 inch x 2 inch (24s); 3 inch x 4 inch (24s)
  Powder:
  Avitene® Flour [microfibrillar product]: 0.5 g, 1 g, 5 g
  Helitene®: 0.5 g, 1 g
  Instat™ MCH [microfibrillar product]: 0.5 g, 1 g
  SyringeAvitene™ [microfibrillar product, prefilled syringe]: 1 g
  Sheet:
  Avitene® [microfibrillar product, nonwoven web]: 35 mm x 35 mm (1s); 70 mm x 35 mm (6s, 12s); 70 mm x 70 mm (6s, 12s)
  EndoAvitene® [microfibrillar product, preloaded applicator]: 5 mm diameter (6s); 10 mm diameter (6s)
  Sponge:
  Avitene® Ultrafoam [microfibrillar product]: 2 cm x 6.25 cm x 7 mm (12s); 8 cm x 6.25 cm x 1 cm (6s); 8 cm x 12.5 cm x 1 cm (6s); 8 cm x 12.5 cm x 3 mm (6s)
  Avitene® UltraWrap™ [microfibrillar product]: 8 cm x 12.5 cm (6s)
  Helistat®: 0.5 inch x 1 inch x 7 mm (18s); 3 inch x 4 inch x 5 inch (10s)

Colocort® [US] *see* hydrocortisone (rectal) *on page 433*

CO Lovastatin [Can] *see* lovastatin *on page 520*

Coly-Mycin® M [US/Can] *see* colistimethate *on previous page*

Coly-Mycin® S [US] *see* neomycin, colistin, hydrocortisone, and thonzonium *on page 597*

Colyte® [US/Can] *see* polyethylene glycol-electrolyte solution *on page 695*

Combantrin™ [Can] *see* pyrantel pamoate *on page 733*

Combigan® [Can] *see* brimonidine and timolol *(Canada only)* *on page 118*

CombiPatch® [US] *see* estradiol and norethindrone *on page 316*

Combipres® *(Discontinued)* *see* clonidine and chlorthalidone *on page 205*

Combivent® [US/Can] *see* ipratropium and albuterol *on page 471*

Combivir® [US/Can] *see* zidovudine and lamivudine *on page 904*

Combunox™ [US] *see* oxycodone and ibuprofen *on page 642*

CO Meloxicam [Can] *see* meloxicam *on page 539*

Comfort® **Ophthalmic** *(Discontinued)* see naphazoline *on page 590*

Comfort® **Tears Solution** *(Discontinued)* see artificial tears *on page 75*

Comhist® **[US]** see chlorpheniramine, phenylephrine, and phenyltoloxamine *on page 182*

CO Mirtazapine [Can] see mirtazapine *on page 572*

Commit® **[US-OTC]** see nicotine *on page 604*

Compazine® **[Can]** see prochlorperazine *on page 716*

Compazine® *(Discontinued)* see prochlorperazine *on page 716*

Compound 347™ **[US]** see enflurane *on page 297*

compound E see cortisone acetate *on page 217*

compound F see hydrocortisone (systemic) *on page 433*

compound S see zidovudine *on page 904*

compound S, abacavir, and lamivudine see abacavir, lamivudine, and zidovudine *on page 2*

Compound W® **[US-OTC]** see salicylic acid *on page 772*

Compound W® **One Step Wart Remover [US-OTC]** see salicylic acid *on page 772*

Compoz® **Nighttime Sleep Aid [US-OTC]** see diphenhydramine *on page 265*

Compro™ **[US]** see prochlorperazine *on page 716*

Comtan® **[US/Can]** see entacapone *on page 299*

Comtrex® **Flu Therapy Nighttime [US-OTC]** see acetaminophen, chlorpheniramine, and pseudoephedrine *on page 10*

Comtrex® **Maximum Strength Sinus and Nasal Decongestant** *(Discontinued)* see acetaminophen, chlorpheniramine, and pseudoephedrine *on page 10*

Comtrex® **Non-Drowsy Cold and Cough Relief** *(Discontinued)* see acetaminophen, dextromethorphan, and pseudoephedrine *on page 12*

Comtrex® **Sore Throat Maximum Strength [US-OTC]** see acetaminophen *on page 5*

Comvax® **[US]** see *Haemophilus* B conjugate and hepatitis B vaccine *on page 411*

Conceptrol® **[US-OTC]** see nonoxynol 9 *on page 610*

Concerta® **[US/Can]** see methylphenidate *on page 558*

Condyline™ **[Can]** see podofilox *on page 693*

Condylox® **[US]** see podofilox *on page 693*

Conex® *(Discontinued)*

Congess® **Jr** *(Discontinued)* see guaifenesin and pseudoephedrine *on page 406*

Congess® **Sr** *(Discontinued)* see guaifenesin and pseudoephedrine *on page 406*

Congestac® **[US-OTC]** see guaifenesin and pseudoephedrine *on page 406*

conivaptan (koe NYE vap tan)
Synonyms conivaptan hydrochloride; YM087
U.S./Canadian Brand Names Vaprisol® [US]
Therapeutic Category Vasopressin Antagonist
Use Treatment of euvolemic and hypervolemic hyponatremia in hospitalized patients
Usual Dosage I.V.: Adults:
Loading dose: 20 mg infused over 30 minutes, followed by continuous infusion of 20 mg over 24 hours
Maintenance: 20 mg/day as continuous infusion over 24 hours; may titrate to maximum of 40 mg/day if serum sodium not rising sufficiently; total duration of therapy not to exceed 4 days
Dosage Forms
Injection, solution:
Vaprisol®: 5 mg/mL (4 mL)

conivaptan hydrochloride see conivaptan *on this page*

conjugated estrogen and methyltestosterone see estrogens (esterified) and methyltestosterone *on page 320*

CO Norfloxacin [Can] see norfloxacin *on page 612*

Conray® **[US]** see iothalamate meglumine *on page 469*

Conray® **30 [US]** see iothalamate meglumine *on page 469*

Conray® **43 [US]** see iothalamate meglumine *on page 469*

Conray® 400 [US] *see* iothalamate sodium *on page 469*

Constulose [US] *see* lactulose *on page 489*

Contac® Cold 12 Hour Relief Non Drowsy [Can] *see* pseudoephedrine *on page 727*

Contac® Cold 12 Hour Relief Non Drowsy *(Discontinued)* *see* pseudoephedrine *on page 727*

Contac® Cold and Sore Throat, Non Drowsy, Extra Strength [Can] *see* acetaminophen and pseudoephedrine *on page 8*

Contac® Cold-Chest Congestion, Non Drowsy, Regular Strength [Can] *see* guaifenesin and pseudoephedrine *on page 406*

Contac® Cold *(Discontinued)* *see* pseudoephedrine *on page 727*

Contac® Complete [Can] *see* acetaminophen, dextromethorphan, and pseudoephedrine *on page 12*

Contac® Cough, Cold and Flu Day & Night™ [Can] *see* acetaminophen, dextromethorphan, and pseudoephedrine *on page 12*

Contac® Cough Formula Liquid *(Discontinued)* *see* guaifenesin and dextromethorphan *on page 402*

ControlRx® [US] *see* fluoride *on page 361*

Contuss® *(Discontinued)*

Contuss® XT *(Discontinued)*

CO Paroxetine [Can] *see* paroxetine *on page 654*

Copaxone® [US/Can] *see* glatiramer acetate *on page 392*

COPD [US] *see* dyphylline and guaifenesin *on page 288*

Copegus® [US] *see* ribavirin *on page 755*

Cophene-B® *(Discontinued)* *see* brompheniramine *on page 120*

Cophene XP® *(Discontinued)* *see* hydrocodone, pseudoephedrine, and guaifenesin *on page 432*

copolymer-1 *see* glatiramer acetate *on page 392*

copper *see* trace metals *on page 855*

CO Pravastatin [Can] *see* pravastatin *on page 707*

Co-Pyronil® 2 Pulvules® *(Discontinued)* *see* chlorpheniramine and pseudoephedrine *on page 178*

CO Ranitidine [Can] *see* ranitidine *on page 744*

Cordarone® [US/Can] *see* amiodarone *on page 43*

Cordran® [US/Can] *see* flurandrenolide *on page 366*

Cordran® SP [US] *see* flurandrenolide *on page 366*

Cordron-D NR *(Discontinued)* *see* carbinoxamine and pseudoephedrine *on page 151*

Cordron-DM NR *(Discontinued)* *see* carbinoxamine, pseudoephedrine, and dextromethorphan *on page 152*

Cordron-HC *(Discontinued)* *see* pseudoephedrine, hydrocodone, and chlorpheniramine *on page 731*

Cordron-HC NR [US] *see* pseudoephedrine, hydrocodone, and chlorpheniramine *on page 731*

Coreg® [US/Can] *see* carvedilol *on page 155*

Coreg CR™ [US] *see* carvedilol *on page 155*

Corfen DM [US] *see* chlorpheniramine, phenylephrine, and dextromethorphan *on page 180*

Corgard® [US/Can] *see* nadolol *on page 586*

Coricidin HBP® Chest Congestion and Cough [US-OTC] *see* guaifenesin and dextromethorphan *on page 402*

Coricidin HBP® Cold and Flu [US-OTC] *see* chlorpheniramine and acetaminophen *on page 177*

Corlopam® [US/Can] *see* fenoldopam *on page 345*

Cormax® [US] *see* clobetasol *on page 201*

Coronex® [Can] *see* isosorbide dinitrate *on page 476*

Correctol® Tablets [US-OTC] *see* bisacodyl *on page 112*

Cortaid® Intensive Therapy [US-OTC] *see* hydrocortisone (topical) *on page 434*

Cortaid® Maximum Strength [US-OTC] *see* hydrocortisone (topical) *on page 434*

Cortaid® Sensitive Skin [US-OTC] *see* hydrocortisone (topical) *on page 434*

Cortamed® **[Can]** *see* hydrocortisone (topical) *on page 434*

Cortatrigen® **Otic** *(Discontinued)* *see* neomycin, polymyxin B, and hydrocortisone *on page 597*

Cortef® **[US/Can]** *see* hydrocortisone (systemic) *on page 433*

Cortenema® **[Can]** *see* hydrocortisone (rectal) *on page 433*

Corticool® **[US-OTC]** *see* hydrocortisone (topical) *on page 434*

corticorelin (kor ti koe REL in)
Sound-Alike/Look-Alike Issues
corticorelin may be confused with corticotropin
Acthrel® may be confused with Acthar®
Synonyms corticorelin ovine triflutate; human corticotrophin-releasing hormone, analogue; ovine corticotrophin-releasing hormone
U.S./Canadian Brand Names Acthrel® [US]
Therapeutic Category Diagnostic Agent, ACTH-Dependent Hypercortisolism
Use Diagnostic test used in adrenocorticotropic hormone (ACTH)-dependent Cushing syndrome to differentiate between pituitary and ectopic production of ACTH
Usual Dosage I.V.: Adults: Testing pituitary corticotrophin function: 1 mcg/kg; dosages >100 mcg have been associated with an increase in adverse effects

Note: Venous blood samples should be drawn 15 minutes before and immediately prior to corticorelin administration to determine baseline ACTH and cortisol. At 15-, 30-, and 60 minutes after administration, venous blood samples should be drawn again to determine response. **Basal and peak responses differ depending on AM or PM administration; therefore, any repeat evaluations are recommended to be done at the same time of day as initial testing.**
Dosage Forms
Injection, powder for reconstitution:
Acthrel®: 100 mcg

corticorelin ovine triflutate *see* corticorelin *on this page*

corticotropin (kor ti koe TROE pin)
Sound-Alike/Look-Alike Issues
corticotropin may be confused with corticorelin
Synonyms ACTH; adrenocorticotropic hormone; corticotropin, repository
U.S./Canadian Brand Names H.P. Acthar® Gel [US]
Therapeutic Category Adrenal Corticosteroid
Use Acute exacerbations of multiple sclerosis; diagnostic aid in adrenocortical insufficiency, severe muscle weakness in myasthenia gravis

Cosyntropin is preferred over corticotropin for diagnostic test of adrenocortical insufficiency (cosyntropin is less allergenic and test is shorter in duration)
Usual Dosage
Children:
Antiinflammatory/immunosuppressant: I.M.: 0.8 units/kg/day or 25 units/m^2/day divided every 12-24 hours
Infantile spasms: Various regimens have been used. Some neurologists recommend low-dose ACTH (5-40 units/day) for short periods (1-6 weeks), while others recommend larger doses of ACTH (40-160 units/day) for long periods of treatment (3-12 months). Well designed comparative dosing studies are needed. Example of low dose regimen:
Initial: I.M.: 20 units/day for 2 weeks, if patient responds, taper and discontinue; if patient does not respond, increase dose to 30 units/day for 4 weeks then taper and discontinue
I.M. usual dose: 20-40 units/day or 5-8 units/kg/day in 1-2 divided doses; range: 5-160 units/day
Oral prednisone (2 mg/kg/day) was as effective as I.M. ACTH gel (20 units/day) in controlling infantile spasms
Adults: Acute exacerbation of multiple sclerosis: I.M.: 80-120 units/day for 2-3 weeks
Repository injection: I.M., SubQ: 40-80 units every 24-72 hours
Dosage Forms
Injection, gelatin:
H.P. Acthar® Gel: 80 units/mL (5 mL)

corticotropin, repository *see* corticotropin *on this page*

Cortifoam® **[US/Can]** *see* hydrocortisone (rectal) *on page 433*

Cortimyxin® **[Can]** *see* neomycin, polymyxin B, and hydrocortisone *on page 597*

cortisol *see* hydrocortisone (systemic) *on page 433*

cortisone acetate (KOR ti sone AS e tate)
Sound-Alike/Look-Alike Issues
cortisone may be confused with Cortizone®
Synonyms compound E
Therapeutic Category Adrenal Corticosteroid
Use Management of adrenocortical insufficiency
Usual Dosage If possible, administer glucocorticoids before 9 AM to minimize adrenocortical suppression; dosing depends upon the condition being treated and the response of the patient; **Note:** Supplemental doses may be warranted during times of stress in the course of withdrawing therapy
Children:
Antiinflammatory or immunosuppressive: Oral: 2.5-10 mg/kg/day **or** 20-300 mg/m^2/day in divided doses every 6-8 hours
Physiologic replacement: Oral: 0.5-0.75 mg/kg/day **or** 20-25 mg/m^2/day in divided doses every 8 hours
Adults:
Antiinflammatory or immunosuppressive: Oral: 25-300 mg/day in divided doses every 12-24 hours
Physiologic replacement: Oral: 25-35 mg/day
Dosage Forms
Tablet: 25 mg

Cortisporin® Cream [US] *see* neomycin, polymyxin B, and hydrocortisone *on page 597*

Cortisporin® Ointment [US] *see* bacitracin, neomycin, polymyxin B, and hydrocortisone *on page 92*

Cortisporin® Ophthalmic [US] *see* neomycin, polymyxin B, and hydrocortisone *on page 597*

Cortisporin® Otic [US/Can] *see* neomycin, polymyxin B, and hydrocortisone *on page 597*

Cortisporin®-TC [US] *see* neomycin, colistin, hydrocortisone, and thonzonium *on page 597*

Cortisporin® Topical Cream *(Discontinued)* *see* neomycin, polymyxin B, and hydrocortisone *on page 597*

Cortisporin® Topical Ointment [Can] *see* bacitracin, neomycin, polymyxin B, and hydrocortisone *on page 92*

Cortizone®-10 Maximum Strength [US-OTC] *see* hydrocortisone (topical) *on page 434*

Cortizone®-10 Plus Maximum Strength [US-OTC] *see* hydrocortisone (topical) *on page 434*

Cortizone®-10 Quick Shot [US-OTC] *see* hydrocortisone (topical) *on page 434*

Cortone® *(Discontinued)*

Cortrosyn® [US/Can] *see* cosyntropin *on this page*

Corvert® [US] *see* ibutilide *on page 445*

Corzide® [US] *see* nadolol and bendroflumethiazide *on page 586*

CO Simvastatin [Can] *see* simvastatin *on page 787*

Cosmegen® [US/Can] *see* dactinomycin *on page 228*

Cosopt® [US/Can] *see* dorzolamide and timolol *on page 277*

CO Sotalol [Can] *see* sotalol *on page 802*

CO Sumatriptan [Can] *see* sumatriptan *on page 815*

cosyntropin (koe sin TROE pin)
Sound-Alike/Look-Alike Issues
Cortrosyn® may be confused with Cotazym®
Synonyms synacthen; tetracosactide
U.S./Canadian Brand Names Cortrosyn® [US/Can]
Therapeutic Category Diagnostic Agent
Use Diagnostic test to differentiate primary adrenal from secondary (pituitary) adrenocortical insufficiency
Usual Dosage Adrenocortical insufficiency: I.M., I.V. (over 2 minutes): Peak plasma cortisol concentrations usually occur 45-60 minutes after cosyntropin administration
Children <2 years: 0.125 mg
Children >2 years and Adults: 0.25-0.75 mg
When greater cortisol stimulation is needed, an I.V. infusion may be used:
Children >2 years and Adults: 0.25 mg administered at 0.04 mg/hour over 6 hours
Dosage Forms
Injection, powder for reconstitution:
Cortrosyn®: 0.25 mg

Cotazym® **[Can]** *see* pancrelipase *on page 648*

Cotazym® *(Discontinued)* *see* pancrelipase *on page 648*

Cotazym-S® *(Discontinued)* *see* pancrelipase *on page 648*

CO Temazepam **[Can]** *see* temazepam *on page 823*

co-trimoxazole *see* sulfamethoxazole and trimethoprim *on page 813*

Coughcold HCM **[US]** *see* hydrocodone and pseudoephedrine *on page 430*

Coughtuss **[US]** *see* phenylephrine, hydrocodone, and chlorpheniramine *on page 678*

Coumadin® **[US/Can]** *see* warfarin *on page 899*

Covan® **[Can]** *see* triprolidine, pseudoephedrine, and codeine *(Canada only)* *on page 869*

Covera® **[Can]** *see* verapamil *on page 887*

Covera-HS® **[US/Can]** *see* verapamil *on page 887*

Coversyl® **[Can]** *see* perindopril erbumine *on page 669*

Coversyl® **Plus [Can]** *see* perindopril erbumine and indapamide *(Canada only)* *on page 669*

co-vidarabine *see* pentostatin *on page 667*

coviracil *see* emtricitabine *on page 295*

Cozaar® **[US/Can]** *see* losartan *on page 519*

CO Zopiclone **[Can]** *see* zopiclone *(Canada only)* *on page 909*

CP358774 *see* erlotinib *on page 307*

CPC *see* cetylpyridinium *on page 170*

C-Phen **[US]** *see* chlorpheniramine and phenylephrine *on page 177*

C-Phen DM **[US]** *see* chlorpheniramine, phenylephrine, and dextromethorphan *on page 180*

CPM *see* cyclophosphamide *on page 222*

CPT-11 *see* irinotecan *on page 472*

CPZ *see* chlorpromazine *on page 185*

Crantex HC **[US]** *see* hydrocodone, phenylephrine, and guaifenesin *on page 431*

Crantex LA **[US]** *see* guaifenesin and phenylephrine *on page 404*

Creomulsion® **Cough [US-OTC]** *see* dextromethorphan *on page 247*

Creomulsion® **for Children [US-OTC]** *see* dextromethorphan *on page 247*

Creon® **[US/Can]** *see* pancrelipase *on page 648*

Creo-Terpin® **[US-OTC]** *see* dextromethorphan *on page 247*

Crestor® **[US/Can]** *see* rosuvastatin *on page 768*

Cresylate® **[US]** *see* m-cresyl acetate *on page 532*

Crinone® **[US/Can]** *see* progesterone *on page 718*

Critic-Aid Skin Care® **[US-OTC]** *see* zinc oxide *on page 906*

Criticare HN® **[US-OTC]** *see* nutritional formula, enteral/oral *on page 622*

Crixivan® **[US/Can]** *see* indinavir *on page 453*

CroFab™ **[Ovine] [US]** *see* antivenin *(Crotalidae)* polyvalent *on page 63*

Crolom® **[US]** *see* cromolyn sodium *on this page*

cromoglycic acid *see* cromolyn sodium *on this page*

cromolyn sodium (KROE moe lin SOW dee um)

Sound-Alike/Look-Alike Issues
Intal® may be confused with Endal®
NasalCrom® may be confused with Nasacort®, Nasalide®
Synonyms cromoglycic acid; disodium cromoglycate; DSCG
U.S./Canadian Brand Names Apo-Cromolyn® [Can]; Crolom® [US]; Gastrocrom® [US]; Intal® [US/Can];
Nalcrom® [Can]; NasalCrom® [US-OTC]; Nu-Cromolyn [Can]; Opticrom® [US/Can]
Therapeutic Category Mast Cell Stabilizer
Use
Inhalation: May be used as an adjunct in the prophylaxis of allergic disorders, including asthma; prevention of
exercise-induced bronchospasm
Nasal: Prevention and treatment of seasonal and perennial allergic rhinitis

Oral: Systemic mastocytosis

Ophthalmic: Treatment of vernal keratoconjunctivitis, vernal conjunctivitis, and vernal keratitis

Usual Dosage

Oral:

Systemic mastocytosis:

Children 2-12 years: 100 mg 4 times/day; not to exceed 40 mg/kg/day; given $1/2$ hour prior to meals and at bedtime

Children >12 years and Adults: 200 mg 4 times/day; given $1/2$ hour prior to meals and at bedtime; if control of symptoms is not seen within 2-3 weeks, dose may be increased to a maximum 40 mg/kg/day

Inhalation:

For chronic control of asthma, taper frequency to the lowest effective dose (ie, 4 times/day to 3 times/day to twice daily): **Note:** Not effective for immediate relief of symptoms in acute asthmatic attacks; must be used at regular intervals for 2-4 weeks to be effective.

Nebulization solution: Children >2 years and Adults: Initial: 20 mg 4 times/day; usual dose: 20 mg 3-4 times/day

Metered spray:

Children 5-12 years: Initial: 2 inhalations 4 times/day; usual dose: 1-2 inhalations 3-4 times/day

Children ≥12 years and Adults: Initial: 2 inhalations 4 times/day; usual dose: 2-4 inhalations 3-4 times/day

Prevention of allergen- or exercise-induced bronchospasm: Administer 10-15 minutes prior to exercise or allergen exposure but no longer than 1 hour before:

Nebulization solution: Children >2 years and Adults: Single dose of 20 mg

Metered spray: Children >5 years and Adults: Single dose of 2 inhalations

Ophthalmic: Children >4 years and Adults: 1-2 drops in each eye 4-6 times/day

Nasal: Allergic rhinitis (treatment and prophylaxis): Children ≥2 years and Adults: 1 spray into each nostril 3-4 times/day; may be increased to 6 times/day (symptomatic relief may require 2-4 weeks)

Dosage Forms

Aerosol, for oral inhalation:

Intal®: 800 mcg/inhalation (8.1 g, 14.2 g)

Solution for nebulization: 20 mg/2 mL (60s, 120s)

Intal®: 20 mg/2 mL (60s, 120s)

Solution, intranasal [spray]:

NasalCrom® [OTC]: 40 mg/mL (13 mL, 26 mL)

Solution, ophthalmic: 4% (10 mL)

Crolom®: 4% (10 mL)

Solution, oral [concentrate]:

Gastrocrom®: 100 mg/5 mL

Crosseal™ *(Discontinued)* see fibrin sealant kit on page 351

crotalidae antivenin see antivenin *(Crotalidae)* polyvalent on page 63

crotaline antivenin, polyvalent see antivenin *(Crotalidae)* polyvalent on page 63

crotamiton (kroe TAM i tonn)

Sound-Alike/Look-Alike Issues

Eurax® may be confused with Efudex®, Eulexin®, Evoxac™, Serax®, Urex®

U.S./Canadian Brand Names Eurax® [US]

Therapeutic Category Scabicides/Pediculicides

Use Treatment of scabies (*Sarcoptes scabiei*) and symptomatic treatment of pruritus

Usual Dosage Topical:

Scabicide: Children and Adults: Wash thoroughly and scrub away loose scales, then towel dry; apply a thin layer and massage drug onto skin of the entire body from the neck to the toes (with special attention to skin folds, creases, and interdigital spaces). Repeat application in 24 hours. Take a cleansing bath 48 hours after the final application. Treatment may be repeated after 7-10 days if live mites are still present.

Pruritus: Massage into affected areas until medication is completely absorbed; repeat as necessary

Dosage Forms

Cream:

Eurax®: 10% (60 g)

Lotion:

Eurax®: 10% (60 mL, 480 mL)

crude coal tar see coal tar on page 208

Cruex® Cream [US-OTC] see clotrimazole on page 206

Cryselle™ [US] see ethinyl estradiol and norgestrel on page 332

crystalline penicillin see penicillin G (parenteral/aqueous) on page 662

Crystamine® *(Discontinued)* see cyanocobalamin on next page

Crysti 1000® *(Discontinued)* *see* cyanocobalamin *on this page*

CsA *see* cyclosporine *on page 223*

C-Tanna 12D [US] *see* carbetapentane, phenylephrine, and pyrilamine *on page 150*

C-Time [US-OTC] *see* ascorbic acid *on page 76*

CTLA-4Ig *see* abatacept *on page 3*

CTM *see* chlorpheniramine *on page 177*

CTX *see* cyclophosphamide *on page 222*

Cubicin® **[US]** *see* daptomycin *on page 231*

Culturelle® **[US-OTC]** *see* Lactobacillus *on page 488*

Cuprimine® **[US/Can]** *see* penicillamine *on page 661*

Curasore [US-OTC] *see* pramoxine *on page 706*

Curosurf® **[US/Can]** *see* poractant alfa *on page 697*

Cutar® **[US-OTC]** *see* coal tar *on page 208*

Cutivate® **[US/Can]** *see* fluticasone (topical) *on page 369*

CyA *see* cyclosporine *on page 223*

cyanide antidote kit *see* sodium nitrite, sodium thiosulfate, and amyl nitrite *on page 794*

Cyanide Antidote Package [US] *see* sodium nitrite, sodium thiosulfate, and amyl nitrite *on page 794*

cyanocobalamin (sye an oh koe BAL a min)

Synonyms vitamin B_{12}
U.S./Canadian Brand Names Nascobal® [US]; Twelve Resin-K [US]
Therapeutic Category Vitamin, Water Soluble
Use Treatment of pernicious anemia; vitamin B_{12} deficiency due to dietary deficiencies or malabsorption diseases, inadequate secretion of intrinsic factor, and inadequate utilization of B_{12} (eg, during neoplastic treatment); increased B_{12} requirements due to pregnancy, thyrotoxicosis, hemorrhage, malignancy, liver or kidney disease
Usual Dosage
  Adequate intake:
  Children:
    0-6 months: 0.4 mcg/day
    7-12 months: 0.5 mcg/day
  Recommended intake:
  Children:
    1-3 years: 0.9 mcg/day
    4-8 years: 1.2 mcg/day
    9-13 years: 1.8 mcg/day
    Children >14 years and Adults: 2.4 mcg/day
    Pregnancy: 2.6 mcg/day
    Lactation: 2.8 mcg/day
  Vitamin B_{12} deficiency:
  I.M., deep SubQ:
    Children (dosage not well established): 0.2 mcg/kg for 2 days, followed by 1000 mcg/day for 2-7 days, followed by 100 mcg/week for one month; for malabsorptive causes of B_{12} deficiency, monthly maintenance doses of 100 mcg have been recommended **or** as an alternative 100 mcg/day for 10-15 days, then once or twice weekly for several months
    Adults: Initial: 30 mcg/day for 5-10 days; maintenance: 100-200 mcg/month
    Intranasal: Adults: 500 mcg in one nostril once weekly
    Oral: Adults: 250 mcg/day
  Pernicious anemia: I.M., deep SubQ (administer concomitantly with folic acid if needed, 1 mg/day for 1 month):
    Children: 30-50 mcg/day for 2 or more weeks (to a total dose of 1000-5000 mcg), then follow with 100 mcg/month as maintenance dosage
    Adults: 100 mcg/day for 6-7 days; if improvement, administer same dose on alternate days for 7 doses, then every 3-4 days for 2-3 weeks; once hematologic values have returned to normal, maintenance dosage: 100 mcg/month. **Note:** Alternative dosing of 1000 mcg/day for 5 days (followed by 500-1000 mcg/month) has been used.
    Hematologic remission (without evidence of nervous system involvement): Adults:
    Intranasal: 500 mcg in one nostril once weekly
    Oral: 1000-2000 mcg/day

I.M., SubQ: 100-1000 mcg/month
Schilling test: Adults: I.M.: 1000 mcg
Dosage Forms
  Injection, solution: 1000 mcg/mL (1 mL, 10 mL, 30 mL)
  Lozenge [OTC]: 100 mcg, 250 mcg, 500 mcg
  Solution, intranasal spray: 500 mcg/0.1 mL actuation (2.3 mL)
   Nascobal®: 500 mcg/0.1 mL actuation (2.3 mL)
  Tablet [OTC]: 50 mcg, 100 mcg, 250 mcg, 500 mcg, 1000 mcg, 5000 mcg
   Twelve Resin-K: 1000 mcg
  Tablet, extended release [OTC]: 1000 mcg, 1500 mcg
  Tablet, sublingual [OTC]: 2500 mcg

cyanocobalamin, folic acid, and pyridoxine *see* folic acid, cyanocobalamin, and pyridoxine *on page 371*

Cyanoject® *(Discontinued)* *see* cyanocobalamin *on previous page*

Cyclen® [Can] *see* ethinyl estradiol and norgestimate *on page 331*

Cyclessa® [US/Can] *see* ethinyl estradiol and desogestrel *on page 322*

cyclobenzaprine (sye kloe BEN za preen)
Sound-Alike/Look-Alike Issues
  cyclobenzaprine may be confused with cycloSERINE, cyproheptadine
  Flexeril® may be confused with Floxin®
Synonyms cyclobenzaprine hydrochloride
U.S./Canadian Brand Names Apo-Cyclobenzaprine® [Can]; Fexmid™ [US]; Flexeril® [US/Can]; Flexitec [Can]; Gen-Cyclobenzaprine [Can]; Novo-Cycloprine [Can]; Nu-Cyclobenzaprine [Can]
Therapeutic Category Skeletal Muscle Relaxant
Use Treatment of muscle spasm associated with acute painful musculoskeletal conditions
Usual Dosage Oral: **Note:** Do not use longer than 2-3 weeks. Children ≥15 years and Adults: Initial: 5 mg 3 times/day; may increase to 7.5-10 mg 3 times/day if needed
Dosage Forms
  Tablet: 5 mg, 10 mg
   Fexmid™: 7.5 mg
   Flexeril®: 5 mg, 10 mg

cyclobenzaprine hydrochloride *see* cyclobenzaprine *on this page*

Cyclocort® [Can] *see* amcinonide *on page 39*

Cyclocort® *(Discontinued)* *see* amcinonide *on page 39*

Cyclogyl® [US/Can] *see* cyclopentolate *on this page*

Cyclomen® [Can] *see* danazol *on page 230*

Cyclomydril® [US] *see* cyclopentolate and phenylephrine *on this page*

cyclopentolate (sye kloe PEN toe late)
Synonyms cyclopentolate hydrochloride
U.S./Canadian Brand Names Cyclogyl® [US/Can]; Cylate® [US]; Diopentolate® [Can]
Therapeutic Category Anticholinergic Agent
Use Diagnostic procedures requiring mydriasis and cycloplegia
Usual Dosage Ophthalmic:
  Neonates and Infants: **Note:** Cyclopentolate and phenylephrine combination formulation is the preferred agent for use in neonates and infants due to lower cyclopentolate concentration and reduced risk for systemic reactions
  Children: Instill 1 drop of 0.5%, 1%, or 2% in eye followed by 1 drop of 0.5% or 1% in 5 minutes, if necessary
  Adults: Instill 1 drop of 1% followed by another drop in 5 minutes; 2% solution in heavily pigmented iris
Dosage Forms
  Solution, ophthalmic: 1% (2 mL, 15 mL)
   Cylate®: 1% (2 mL, 15 mL)
   Cyclogyl®: 0.5% (15 mL); 1% (2 mL, 5 mL, 15 mL); 2% (2 mL, 5 mL, 15 mL)

cyclopentolate and phenylephrine (sye kloe PEN toe late & fen il EF rin)
Synonyms phenylephrine and cyclopentolate
U.S./Canadian Brand Names Cyclomydril® [US]
Therapeutic Category Anticholinergic/Adrenergic Agonist
Use Induce mydriasis greater than that produced with cyclopentolate HCl alone
  (Continued)

221

cyclopentolate and phenylephrine *(Continued)*

Usual Dosage Ophthalmic: Neonates, Infants, Children, and Adults: Instill 1 drop into the eye every 5-10 minutes, for up to 3 doses, approximately 40-50 minutes before the examination

Dosage Forms
Solution, ophthalmic:
Cyclomydril®: Cyclopentolate 0.2% and phenylephrine 1% (2 mL, 5 mL)

cyclopentolate hydrochloride *see* cyclopentolate *on previous page*

cyclophosphamide (sye kloe FOS fa mide)

Sound-Alike/Look-Alike Issues
cyclophosphamide may be confused with cycloSPORINE, ifosfamide
Cytoxan® may be confused with cefoxitin, Centoxin®, Ciloxan®, cytarabine, CytoGam®, Cytosar®, Cytosar-U®, Cytotec®

Synonyms CPM; CTX; CYT; NSC-26271

U.S./Canadian Brand Names Cytoxan® [US/Can]; Procytox® [Can]

Therapeutic Category Antineoplastic Agent

Use
Oncologic: Treatment of Hodgkin and non-Hodgkin lymphoma, Burkitt lymphoma, chronic lymphocytic leukemia (CLL), chronic myelocytic leukemia (CML), acute myelocytic leukemia (AML), acute lymphocytic leukemia (ALL), mycosis fungoides, multiple myeloma, neuroblastoma, retinoblastoma, rhabdomyosarcoma, Ewing sarcoma; breast, testicular, endometrial, ovarian, and lung cancers, and in conditioning regimens for bone marrow transplantation

Nononcologic: Prophylaxis of rejection for kidney, heart, liver, and bone marrow transplants, severe rheumatoid disorders, nephrotic syndrome, Wegener granulomatosis, idiopathic pulmonary hemosideroses, myasthenia gravis, multiple sclerosis, systemic lupus erythematosus, lupus nephritis, autoimmune hemolytic anemia, idiopathic thrombocytic purpura (ITP), macroglobulinemia, and antibody-induced pure red cell aplasia

Usual Dosage Refer to individual protocols
Children:
SLE: I.V.: 500-750 mg/m^2 every month; maximum dose: 1 g/m^2
JRA/vasculitis: I.V.: 10 mg/kg every 2 weeks
Children and Adults:
Oral: 50-100 mg/m^2/day as continuous therapy or 400-1000 mg/m^2 in divided doses over 4-5 days as intermittent therapy
I.V.:
Single doses: 400-1800 mg/m^2 (30-50 mg/kg) per treatment course (1-5 days) which can be repeated at 2-4 week intervals
Continuous daily doses: 60-120 mg/m^2 (1-2.5 mg/kg) per day
Autologous BMT: IVPB: 50 mg/kg/dose x 4 days or 60 mg/kg/dose for 2 days; total dose is usually divided over 2-4 days
Nephrotic syndrome: Oral: 2-3 mg/kg/day every day for up to 12 weeks when corticosteroids are unsuccessful

Dosage Forms
Injection, powder for reconstitution:
Cytoxan®: 500 mg, 1 g, 2 g
Tablet: 25 mg, 50 mg
Cytoxan®: 25 mg, 50 mg

cycloserine (sye kloe SER een)

Sound-Alike/Look-Alike Issues
cycloSERINE may be confused with cyclobenzaprine, cycloSPORINE

Tall-Man cycloSERINE

U.S./Canadian Brand Names Seromycin® [US]

Therapeutic Category Antibiotic, Miscellaneous

Use Adjunctive treatment in pulmonary or extrapulmonary tuberculosis

Usual Dosage Some neurotoxic effects may be relieved or prevented by concomitant administration of pyridoxine

Tuberculosis: Oral:
Children: 10-20 mg/kg/day in 2 divided doses up to 1000 mg/day for 18-24 months
Adults: Initial: 250 mg every 12 hours for 14 days, then administer 500 mg to 1 g/day in 2 divided doses for 18-24 months (maximum daily dose: 1 g)

Dosage Forms
Capsule:
Seromycin®: 250 mg

cyclosporin A *see* cyclosporine *on this page*

cyclosporine (SYE kloe spor een)
Sound-Alike/Look-Alike Issues
cycloSPORINE may be confused with cyclophosphamide, Cyklokapron®, cycloSERINE
Gengraf® may be confused with Prograf®
Neoral® may be confused with Neurontin®, Nizoral®
Sandimmune® may be confused with Sandostatin®

Synonyms CsA; CyA; cyclosporin A
Tall-Man cycloSPORINE
U.S./Canadian Brand Names Gengraf® [US]; Neoral® [US/Can]; Restasis® [US]; Rhoxal-cyclosporine [Can]; Sandimmune® I.V. [Can]; Sandimmune® [US]; Sandoz-Cyclosporine [Can]
Therapeutic Category Immunosuppressant Agent
Use Prophylaxis of organ rejection in kidney, liver, and heart transplants, has been used with azathioprine and/or corticosteroids; severe, active rheumatoid arthritis (RA) not responsive to methotrexate alone; severe, recalcitrant plaque psoriasis in nonimmunocompromised adults unresponsive to or unable to tolerate other systemic therapy

Ophthalmic emulsion (Restasis®): Increase tear production when suppressed tear production is presumed to be due to keratoconjunctivitis sicca-associated ocular inflammation (in patients not already using topical anti-inflammatory drugs or punctal plugs)
Usual Dosage Neoral®/Genraf® and Sandimmune® are not bioequivalent and cannot be used interchangeably.
Children: Transplant: Refer to adult dosing; children may require, and are able to tolerate, larger doses than adults.
Adults:
Newly-transplanted patients: Adjunct therapy with corticosteroids is recommended. Initial dose should be given 4-12 hours prior to transplant or may be given postoperatively; adjust initial dose to achieve desired plasma concentration
Oral: Dose is dependent upon type of transplant and formulation:
Cyclosporine (modified):
Renal: 9 ± 3 mg/kg/day, divided twice daily
Liver: 8 ± 4 mg/kg/day, divided twice daily
Heart: 7 ± 3 mg/kg/day, divided twice daily
Cyclosporine (nonmodified): Initial dose: 15 mg/kg/day as a single dose (range 14-18 mg/kg); lower doses of 10-14 mg/kg/day have been used for renal transplants. Continue initial dose daily for 1-2 weeks; taper by 5% per week to a maintenance dose of 5-10 mg/kg/day; some renal transplant patients may be dosed as low as 3 mg/kg/day
Note: When using the non-modified formulation, cyclosporine levels may increase in liver transplant patients when the T-tube is closed; dose may need decreased
I.V.: Cyclosporine (nonmodified): Manufacturer's labeling: Initial dose: 5-6 mg/kg/day as a single dose (1/3 the oral dose), infused over 2-6 hours; use should be limited to patients unable to take capsules or oral solution; patients should be switched to an oral dosage form as soon as possible
Note: Many transplant centers administer cyclosporine as "divided dose" infusions (in 2-3 doses/day) or as a continuous (24-hour) infusion; dosages range from 3-7.5 mg/kg/day. Specific institutional protocols should be consulted.
Conversion to cyclosporine (modified) from cyclosporine (nonmodified): Start with daily dose previously used and adjust to obtain preconversion cyclosporine trough concentration. Plasma concentrations should be monitored every 4-7 days and dose adjusted as necessary, until desired trough level is obtained. When transferring patients with previously poor absorption of cyclosporine (nonmodified), monitor trough levels at least twice weekly (especially if initial dose exceeds 10 mg/kg/day); high plasma levels are likely to occur.
Rheumatoid arthritis: Oral: Cyclosporine (modified): Initial dose: 2.5 mg/kg/day, divided twice daily; salicylates, NSAIDs, and oral glucocorticoids may be continued; dose may be increased by 0.5-0.75 mg/kg/day if insufficient response is seen after 8 weeks of treatment; additional dosage increases may be made again at 12 weeks (maximum dose: 4 mg/kg/day). Discontinue if no benefit is seen by 16 weeks of therapy.
Note: Increase the frequency of blood pressure monitoring after each alteration in dosage of cyclosporine. Cyclosporine dosage should be decreased by 25% to 50% in patients with no history of hypertension who develop sustained hypertension during therapy and, if hypertension persists, treatment with cyclosporine should be discontinued.
Psoriasis: Oral: Cyclosporine (modified): Initial dose: 2.5 mg/kg/day, divided twice daily; dose may be increased by 0.5 mg/kg/day if insufficient response is seen after 4 weeks of treatment. Additional dosage increases may be made every 2 weeks if needed (maximum dose: 4 mg/kg/day). Discontinue if no benefit is seen by 6 weeks of therapy. Once patients are adequately controlled, the dose should be decreased to the lowest effective dose. Doses lower than 2.5 mg/kg/day may be effective. Treatment longer than 1 year is not recommended.
(Continued)

cyclosporine *(Continued)*

Note: Increase the frequency of blood pressure monitoring after each alteration in dosage of cyclosporine. Cyclosporine dosage should be decreased by 25% to 50% in patients with no history of hypertension who develop sustained hypertension during therapy and, if hypertension persists, treatment with cyclosporine should be discontinued.

Keratoconjunctivitis sicca: Ophthalmic (Restasis®): Children ≥16 years and Adults: Instill 1 drop in each eye every 12 hours

Dosage Forms

Capsule, soft gel, modified: 25 mg, 100 mg
Gengraf®, Neoral®: 25 mg, 100 mg
Capsule, soft gel, non-modified: 25 mg, 100 mg
Sandimmune®: 25 mg, 100 mg
Emulsion, ophthalmic [preservative free, single-use vial]: 0.05% (0.4 mL)
Restasis®: 0.05% (0.4 mL)
Injection, solution, non-modified: 50 mg/mL (5 mL)
Sandimmune®: 50 mg/mL (5 mL)
Solution, oral, modified: 100 mg/mL
Gengraf®, Neoral®: 100 mg/mL
Solution, oral, non-modified: 100 mg/mL
Sandimmune®: 100 mg/mL

Cycofed® Pediatric *(Discontinued)* *see* guaifenesin, pseudoephedrine, and codeine *on page 408*

Cyestra-35 [Can] *see* cyproterone *(Canada only) on next page*

Cyklokapron® [US/Can] *see* tranexamic acid *on page 857*

Cylate® [US] *see* cyclopentolate *on page 221*

Cylex® [US-OTC] *see* benzocaine *on page 101*

Cymbalta® [US] *see* duloxetine *on page 286*

Cyomin® *(Discontinued)* *see* cyanocobalamin *on page 220*

cyproheptadine (si proe HEP ta deen)

Sound-Alike/Look-Alike Issues
cyproheptadine may be confused with cyclobenzaprine
Periactin® may be confused with Perative®, Percodan®, Persantine®

Synonyms cyproheptadine hydrochloride

Therapeutic Category Antihistamine

Use Perennial and seasonal allergic rhinitis and other allergic symptoms including urticaria

Usual Dosage Oral:

Children:
Allergic conditions: 0.25 mg/kg/day or 8 mg/m²/day in 2-3 divided doses **or**
2-6 years: 2 mg every 8-12 hours (not to exceed 12 mg/day)
7-14 years: 4 mg every 8-12 hours (not to exceed 16 mg/day)
Migraine headaches: 4 mg 2-3 times/day

Children ≥12 years and Adults: Spasticity associated with spinal cord damage: 4 mg at bedtime; increase by a 4 mg dose every 3-4 days; average daily dose: 16 mg in divided doses; not to exceed 36 mg/day

Children >13 years and Adults: Appetite stimulation (anorexia nervosa): 2 mg 4 times/day; may be increased gradually over a 3-week period to 8 mg 4 times/day

Adults:
Allergic conditions: 4-20 mg/day divided every 8 hours (not to exceed 0.5 mg/kg/day)
Cluster headaches: 4 mg 4 times/day
Migraine headaches: 4-8 mg 3 times/day

Dosage Forms
Syrup: 2 mg/5 mL
Tablet: 4 mg

cyproheptadine hydrochloride *see* cyproheptadine *on this page*

cyproterone acetate *see* cyproterone *(Canada only) on next page*

cyproterone and ethinyl estradiol *(Canada only)*
(sye PROE ter one & ETH in il es tra DYE ole)

Synonyms ethinyl estradiol and cyproterone acetate

U.S./Canadian Brand Names Diane-35 [Can]

Therapeutic Category Acne Products; Estrogen and Androgen Combination

Use Treatment of females with severe acne, unresponsive to other therapies, with associated symptoms of androgenization (including mild hirsutism or seborrhea). **Should not be used solely for contraception;** however, will provide reliable contraception if taken as recommended for approved indications.

Usual Dosage Oral: Adults: Female: Acne: One tablet daily for 21 days, followed by 7 days off; first cycle should begin on the first day of menstrual flow. Discontinue therapy 3-4 cycles after symptoms have resolved.

Dosage Forms CAN = [Canadian brand name]

Tablet:
Diane-35 [CAN]: Cyproterone 2 mg and ethinyl estradiol 0.35 mg (21s) [not available in the U.S.]

cyproterone *(Canada only)* (sye PROE ter one)

Synonyms cyproterone acetate

U.S./Canadian Brand Names Androcur® Depot [Can]; Androcur® [Can]; Apo-Cyproterone® [Can]; Cyestra-35 [Can]; Gen-Cyproterone [Can]; Novo-Cyproterone [Can]

Therapeutic Category Antiandrogen; Progestin

Use Palliative treatment of advanced prostate carcinoma

Usual Dosage Adults: Males: Prostatic carcinoma (palliative treatment):
Oral: 200-300 mg/day in 2-3 divided doses; following orchiectomy, reduce dose to 100-200 mg/day; should be taken with meals
I.M. (depot): 300 mg (3 mL) once weekly; reduce dose in orchiectomized patients to 300 mg every 2 weeks

Dosage Forms [CAN] = Canadian brand name:

Injection, solution: 100 mg/mL (3 mL) [not available in the U.S.]
Androcur® Depot [CAN]: 100 mg/mL (3 mL) [not available in the U.S.]
Tablet: 50 mg [not available in the U.S.]
Androcur® [CAN], Apo-Cyproterone® [CAN], Gen-Cyproterone [CAN]: 50 mg [not available in the U.S.]

Cystadane® [US/Can] *see* betaine *on page 107*

Cystagon® [US] *see* cysteamine *on this page*

cysteamine (sis TEE a meen)

Synonyms cysteamine bitartrate

U.S./Canadian Brand Names Cystagon® [US]

Therapeutic Category Urinary Tract Product

Use Treatment of nephropathic cystinosis

Usual Dosage Oral: Initiate therapy with $1/4$ to $1/6$ of maintenance dose; titrate slowly upward over 4-6 weeks.
Note: Dosage may be increased if cystine levels are <1 nmol/$1/2$ cystine/mg protein, although intolerance and incidence of adverse events may be increased.
Children <12 years: Maintenance: 1.3 g/m^2/day or 60 mg/kg/day divided into 4 doses (maximum dose: 1.95 g/m^2/day or 90 mg/kg/day)
Children >12 years and Adults (>110 lb): 2 g/day in 4 divided doses; maximum dose: 1.95 g/m^2/day or 90 mg/kg/day

Dosage Forms
Capsule:
Cystagon®: 50 mg, 150 mg

cysteamine bitartrate *see* cysteamine *on this page*

cysteine (SIS te een)

Synonyms cysteine hydrochloride

Therapeutic Category Nutritional Supplement

Use Supplement to crystalline amino acid solutions, in particular the specialized pediatric formulas (eg, Aminosyn® PF, TrophAmine®) to meet the intravenous amino acid nutritional requirements of infants receiving parenteral nutrition (PN)

Usual Dosage I.V.: Neonates and Infants: Added as a fixed ratio to crystalline amino acid solution: 40 mg cysteine per g of amino acids; dosage will vary with the daily amino acid dosage (eg, 0.5-2.5 g/kg/day amino acids would result in 20-100 mg/kg/day cysteine); individual doses of cysteine of 0.8-1 mmol/kg/day have also been added directly to the daily PN solution; the duration of treatment relates to the need for PN; patients on chronic PN therapy have received cysteine until 6 months of age and in some cases until 2 years of age

Dosage Forms
Injection, solution: 50 mg/mL (10 mL, 50 mL)

cysteine hydrochloride *see* cysteine *on previous page*

Cystistat® **[Can]** *see* hyaluronate and derivatives *on page 423*

Cysto-Conray® **II [US]** *see* iothalamate meglumine *on page 469*

Cystografin® **[US]** *see* diatrizoate meglumine *on page 249*

Cystografin® Dilute [US] *see* diatrizoate meglumine *on page 249*

Cystospaz® **[US/Can]** *see* hyoscyamine *on page 441*

Cystospaz-M® *(Discontinued)* *see* hyoscyamine *on page 441*

CYT *see* cyclophosphamide *on page 222*

Cytadren® **[US]** *see* aminoglutethimide *on page 42*

cytarabine (sye TARE a been)

Sound-Alike/Look-Alike Issues
cytarabine may be confused with Cytadren®, Cytosar®, Cytoxan®, vidarabine
Cytosar-U® may be confused with cytarabine, Cytovene®, Cytoxan®, Neosar®
Synonyms arabinosylcytosine; ara-C; cytarabine hydrochloride; cytosine arabinosine hydrochloride; NSC-63878
U.S./Canadian Brand Names Cytosar-U® [US]; Cytosar® [Can]
Therapeutic Category Antineoplastic Agent
Use Treatment of acute myeloid leukemia (AML), acute lymphocytic leukemia (ALL), chronic myelocytic leukemia (CML; blast phase), and lymphomas; prophylaxis and treatment of meningeal leukemia
Usual Dosage Refer to individual protocols. Children and Adults:
Remission induction:
I.V.: 100-200 mg/m^2/day for 5-10 days; a second course, beginning 2-4 weeks after the initial therapy, may be required in some patients.
or 100 mg/m^2 every 12 hours for 7 days
I.T.: 5-75 mg/m^2 every 2-7 days until CNS findings normalize; or age-based dosing:
<1 year of age: 20 mg
1-2 years of age: 30 mg
2-3 years of age: 50 mg
>3 years of age: 75 mg
Remission maintenance:
I.V.: 70-200 mg/m^2/day for 2-5 days at monthly intervals
I.M., SubQ: 1-1.5 mg/kg single dose for maintenance at 1- to 4-week intervals
High-dose therapies:
Doses as high as 1-3 g/m^2 have been used for refractory or secondary leukemias or refractory non-Hodgkin lymphoma.
Doses of 1-3 g/m^2 every 12 hours for up to 12 doses have been used for leukemia
Bone marrow transplant: 1.5 g/m^2 continuous infusion over 48 hours
Dosage Forms
Injection, powder for reconstitution: 100 mg, 500 mg, 1 g, 2 g
Cytosar-U®: 100 mg, 500 mg, 1 g, 2 g
Injection, solution: 20 mg/mL (5 mL, 25 mL, 50 mL); 100 mg/mL (20 mL)
Cytosar-U®L 20 mg/mL (5 mL, 25 mL, 50 mL); 100 mg/mL (20 mL)

cytarabine hydrochloride *see* cytarabine *on this page*

cytarabine (liposomal) (sye TARE a been lip po SOE mal)

Sound-Alike/Look-Alike Issues
cytarabine may be confused with Cytadren®, Cytosar®, Cytoxan®, vidarabine
DepoCyt® may be confused with Depoject®
U.S./Canadian Brand Names DepoCyt® [US/Can]
Therapeutic Category Antineoplastic Agent, Antimetabolite (Purine)
Use Treatment of lymphomatous meningitis
Usual Dosage Note: Patients should be started on dexamethasone 4 mg twice daily (oral or I.V.) for 5 days, beginning on the day of cytarabine liposomal injection.

Intrathecal: Adults:
Induction: 50 mg every 14 days for a total of 2 doses (weeks 1 and 3)
Consolidation: 50 mg every 14 days for 3 doses (weeks 5, 7, and 9), followed by an additional dose at week 13
Maintenance: 50 mg every 28 days for 4 doses (weeks 17, 21, 25, and 29)

Dosage reduction for toxicity: If drug-related neurotoxicity develops, reduce dose to 25 mg. If toxicity persists, discontinue treatment.

Dosage Forms
Injection, suspension [preservative free]:
Depocyt®: 10 mg/mL (5 mL)

CytoGam® [US/Can] *see* cytomegalovirus immune globulin (intravenous-human) *on this page*

cytomegalovirus immune globulin (intravenous-human)
(sye toe meg a low VYE rus i MYUN GLOB yoo lin in tra VEE nus HYU man)
Sound-Alike/Look-Alike Issues
CytoGam® may be confused with Cytoxan®, Gamimune® N
Synonyms CMV-IGIV
U.S./Canadian Brand Names CytoGam® [US/Can]
Therapeutic Category Immune Globulin
Use Prophylaxis of cytomegalovirus (CMV) disease associated with kidney, lung, liver, pancreas, and heart transplants; concomitant use with ganciclovir should be considered in organ transplants (other than kidney) from CMV seropositive donors to CMV seronegative recipients
Usual Dosage I.V.: Adults:
Kidney transplant:
  Initial dose (within 72 hours of transplant): 150 mg/kg/dose
  2-, 4-, 6-, and 8 weeks after transplant: 100 mg/kg/dose
  12 and 16 weeks after transplant: 50 mg/kg/dose
Liver, lung, pancreas, or heart transplant:
  Initial dose (within 72 hours of transplant): 150 mg/kg/dose
  2-, 4-, 6-, and 8 weeks after transplant: 150 mg/kg/dose
  12 and 16 weeks after transplant: 100 mg/kg/dose
Dosage Forms
Injection, solution [preservative free]:
CytoGam®: 50 mg ± 10 mg/mL (50 mL)

Cytomel® [US/Can] *see* liothyronine *on page 510*

Cytosar® [Can] *see* cytarabine *on previous page*

Cytosar-U® [US] *see* cytarabine *on previous page*

cytosine arabinosine hydrochloride *see* cytarabine *on previous page*

Cytotec® [US] *see* misoprostol *on page 573*

Cytovene® [US/Can] *see* ganciclovir *on page 383*

Cytoxan® [US/Can] *see* cyclophosphamide *on page 222*

Cytra-3 [US] *see* citric acid, sodium citrate, and potassium citrate *on page 195*

Cytra-K [US] *see* potassium citrate and citric acid *on page 701*

Cytuss HC [US] *see* phenylephrine, hydrocodone, and chlorpheniramine *on page 678*

Cēpacol® Dual Action Maximum Strength [US-OTC] *see* dyclonine *on page 287*

Cēpastat® [US-OTC] *see* phenol *on page 673*

Cēpastat® Extra Strength [US-OTC] *see* phenol *on page 673*

D2E7 *see* adalimumab *on page 18*

D$_3$ *see* cholecalciferol *on page 186*

d4T *see* stavudine *on page 805*

DAB$_{389}$IL-2 *see* denileukin diftitox *on page 236*

dacarbazine (da KAR ba zeen)
Sound-Alike/Look-Alike Issues
dacarbazine may be confused with Dicarbosil®, procarbazine
Synonyms DIC; dimethyl triazeno imidazole carboxamide; DTIC; imidazole carboxamide; imidazole carboxamide dimethyltriazene; WR-139007
U.S./Canadian Brand Names DTIC-Dome® [US]; DTIC® [Can]
Therapeutic Category Antineoplastic Agent
Use Treatment of malignant melanoma, Hodgkin disease, soft-tissue sarcomas, fibrosarcomas, rhabdomyosarcoma, islet cell carcinoma, medullary carcinoma of the thyroid, and neuroblastoma
Usual Dosage Refer to individual protocols. Some dosage regimens include:
Intra-arterial: 50-400 mg/m^2 for 5-10 days
I.V.:
  Hodgkin disease, ABVD: 375 mg/m^2 days 1 and 15 every 4 weeks **or** 100 mg/m^2/day for 5 days
(Continued)

dacarbazine *(Continued)*

Metastatic melanoma (alone or in combination with other agents): 150-250 mg/m² days 1-5 every 3-4 weeks
Metastatic melanoma: 850 mg/m² every 3 weeks
High dose: Bone marrow/blood cell transplantation: I.V.: 1-3 g/m²; maximum dose as a single agent: 3.38 g/m²; generally combined with other high-dose chemotherapeutic drugs

Dosage Forms
Injection, powder for reconstitution: 100 mg, 200 mg, 500 mg
DTIC-Dome®: 200 mg

Dacex-DM [US] *see* guaifenesin, dextromethorphan, and phenylephrine *on page 407*

daclizumab *(dac KLYE zue mab)*

U.S./Canadian Brand Names Zenapax® [US/Can]
Therapeutic Category Immunosuppressant Agent
Use Part of an immunosuppressive regimen (including cyclosporine and corticosteroids) for the prophylaxis of acute organ rejection in patients receiving renal transplant
Usual Dosage Daclizumab is used adjunctively with other immunosuppressants (eg, cyclosporine, corticosteroids, mycophenolate mofetil, and azathioprine): I.V.:
Children: Use same weight-based dose as adults
Adults: Immunoprophylaxis against acute renal allograft rejection: 1 mg/kg infused over 15 minutes within 24 hours before transplantation (day 0), then every 14 days for 4 additional doses

Dosage Forms
Injection, solution [preservative free]:
Zenapax®: 5 mg/mL (5 mL)

Dacodyl™ [US-OTC] *see* bisacodyl *on page 112*

Dacogen™ [US] *see* decitabine *on page 234*

DACT *see* dactinomycin *on this page*

dactinomycin *(dak ti noe MYE sin)*

Sound-Alike/Look-Alike Issues
dactinomycin may be confused with daptomycin, DAUNOrubicin
actinomycin may be confused with Achromycin
Synonyms ACT; Act-D; actinomycin; actinomycin Cl; actinomycin D; DACT; NSC-3053
U.S./Canadian Brand Names Cosmegen® [US/Can]
Therapeutic Category Antineoplastic Agent
Use Treatment of testicular tumors, melanoma, gestational trophoblastic neoplasm, Wilms tumor, neuroblastoma, retinoblastoma, rhabdomyosarcoma, uterine sarcomas, Ewing sarcoma, Kaposi sarcoma, sarcoma botryoides, and soft tissue sarcoma
Usual Dosage Refer to individual protocols:
Note: Medication orders for dactinomycin are commonly written in MICROgrams (eg, 150 mcg) although many regimens list the dose in MILLIgrams (eg, mg/kg or mg/m²). One-time doses for >1000 mcg, or multiple-day doses for >500 mcg/day are not common. The dose intensity per 2-week cycle for adults and children should not exceed 15 mcg/kg/day for 5 days or 400-600 mcg/m²/day for 5 days. Some practitioners recommend calculation of the dosage for obese or edematous adult patients on the basis of body surface area in an effort to relate dosage to lean body mass.
Children >6 months: I.V.: Usual dose: 15 mcg/kg/day **or** 400-600 mcg/m²/day for 5 days every 3-6 weeks
Wilms tumor, rhabdomyosarcoma, Ewing sarcoma: 15 mcg/kg/day for 5 days (in various combination regimens and schedules)
Adults: I.V.:
Usual doses:
2.5 mg/m² in divided doses over 1 week, repeated every 2 weeks **or**
0.75-2 mg/m² every 1-4 weeks **or**
400-600 mcg/m²/day for 5 days, repeated every 3-6 weeks
Testicular cancer: 1000 mcg/m² on day 1 (as part of a combination chemotherapy regimen)
Gestational trophoblastic neoplasm: 12 mcg/kg/day for 5 days **or** 500 mcg days 1 and 2 (as part of a combination chemotherapy regimen)
Wilms tumor, Ewing sarcoma: 15 mcg/kg/day for 5 days (in various combination regimens and schedules)
Dosage Forms
Injection, powder for reconstitution:
Cosmegen®: 0.5 mg

DAD *see* mitoxantrone *on page 573*

Daily Prenatal [US] *see* vitamins (multiple/prenatal) *on page 896*

Dairyaid® [Can] *see* lactase *on page 487*

Dakin's Solution [US] *see* sodium hypochlorite solution *on page 794*

Dakrina® Ophthalmic Solution *(Discontinued)* *see* artificial tears *on page 75*

Dalacin® C [Can] *see* clindamycin *on page 198*

Dalacin® T [Can] *see* clindamycin *on page 198*

Dalacin® Vaginal [Can] *see* clindamycin *on page 198*

Dallergy® [US] *see* chlorpheniramine, phenylephrine, and methscopolamine *on page 181*

Dallergy-D® Syrup *(Discontinued)* *see* chlorpheniramine and phenylephrine *on page 177*

Dallergy-JR® [US] *see* chlorpheniramine and phenylephrine *on page 177*

Dalmane® [US/Can] *see* flurazepam *on page 366*

d-Alpha-Gems™ [US-OTC] *see* vitamin E *on page 894*

d-alpha tocopherol *see* vitamin E *on page 894*

dalteparin (dal TE pa rin)

Synonyms dalteparin sodium; NSC-714371
U.S./Canadian Brand Names Fragmin® [US/Can]
Therapeutic Category Anticoagulant (Other)
Use Prevention of deep vein thrombosis which may lead to pulmonary embolism, in patients requiring abdominal surgery who are at risk for thromboembolism complications (eg, patients >40 years of age, obesity, patients with malignancy, history of deep vein thrombosis or pulmonary embolism, and surgical procedures requiring general anesthesia and lasting >30 minutes); prevention of DVT in patients undergoing hip-replacement surgery; patients immobile during an acute illness; acute treatment of unstable angina or non-Q-wave myocardial infarction; prevention of ischemic complications in patients on concurrent aspirin therapy; in patients with cancer, extended treatment (6 months) of acute symptomatic venous thromboembolism (DVT and/or PE) to reduce the recurrence of venous thromboembolism
Usual Dosage Adults: SubQ:
Abdominal surgery:
Low-to-moderate DVT risk: 2500 int. units 1-2 hours prior to surgery, then once daily for 5-10 days postoperatively
High DVT risk: 5000 int. units the evening prior to surgery and then once daily for 5-10 days postoperatively. Alternatively in patients with malignancy: 2500 int. units 1-2 hours prior to surgery, 2500 int. units 12 hours later, then 5000 int. units once daily for 5-10 days postoperatively.
Patients undergoing total hip surgery: **Note:** Three treatment options are currently available. Dose is given for 5-10 days, although up to 14 days of treatment have been tolerated in clinical trials:
Postoperative start:
Initial: 2500 int. units 4-8 hours* after surgery
Maintenance: 5000 int. units once daily; start at least 6 hours after postsurgical dose
Preoperative (starting day of surgery):
Initial: 2500 int. units within 2 hours before surgery
Adjustment: 2500 int. units 4-8 hours* after surgery
Maintenance: 5000 int. units once daily; start at least 6 hours after postsurgical dose
Preoperative (starting evening prior to surgery):
Initial: 5000 int. units 10-14 hours before surgery
Adjustment: 5000 int. units 4-8 hours* after surgery
Maintenance: 5000 int. units once daily, allowing 24 hours between doses.
*Dose may be delayed if hemostasis is not yet achieved.
Unstable angina or non-Q-wave myocardial infarction: 120 int. units/kg body weight (maximum dose: 10,000 int. units) every 12 hours for 5-8 days with concurrent aspirin therapy. Discontinue dalteparin once patient is clinically stable.
Venous thromboembolism: Cancer patients:
Initial (month 1): 200 int. units/kg (maximum dose: 18,000 int. units) once daily for 30 days
Maintenance (months 2-6): ~150 int. units/kg (maximum dose: 18,000 int. units) once daily. If platelet count between 50,000-100,000/mm^3, reduce dose by 2,500 int. units until platelet count recovers to ≥100,000/mm^3. If platelet count <50,000/mm^3, discontinue dalteparin until platelet count recover to >50,000/mm^3.
Immobility during acute illness: 5000 int. units once daily
Dosage Forms
Injection, solution [multidose vial]:
Fragmin®: Antifactor Xa 10,000 int. units per 1 mL (9.5 mL); antifactor Xa 25,000 units per 1 mL (3.8 mL)
Injection, solution [preservative free; prefilled syringe]:
Fragmin®: Antifactor Xa 2500 int. units per 0.2 mL (0.2 mL); antifactor Xa 5000 int. units per 0.2 mL (0.2 mL); antifactor Xa 7500 int. units per 0.3 mL (0.3 mL); antifactor Xa 12,500 int. units per 0.5 mL (0.5 mL); antifactor Xa 15,000 int. units per 0.6 mL (0.6 mL); antifactor Xa 18,000 int. units per 0.72 mL (0.72 mL)
Injection, solution [preservative free; graduated prefilled syringe]: Antifactor Xa 10,000 int. units/1 mL (1 mL)

dalteparin sodium *see* dalteparin *on previous page*

Damason-P® **[US]** *see* hydrocodone and aspirin *on page 428*

danaparoid *(Canada only)* (da NAP a roid)
Synonyms danaparoid sodium
U.S./Canadian Brand Names Orgaran® [Can]
Therapeutic Category Anticoagulant (Other)
Use Prevention of postoperative deep vein thrombosis following elective hip replacement surgery
Usual Dosage SubQ: Adults: Prevention of DVT following hip replacement: 750 anti-Xa units twice daily; beginning 1-4 hours before surgery and then not sooner than 2 hours after surgery and every 12 hours until the risk of DVT has diminished. The average duration of therapy is 7-10 days.
Dosage Forms [CAN] = Canadian brand name
Injection, solution:
Orgaran® [CAN]: 750 anti-Xa units/0.6 mL (0.6 mL) [not available in the U.S.]

danaparoid sodium *see* danaparoid *(Canada only) on this page*

danazol (DA na zole)
Sound-Alike/Look-Alike Issues
danazol may be confused with Dantrium®
Danocrine® may be confused with Dacriose®
U.S./Canadian Brand Names Cyclomen® [Can]; Danocrine® [Can]
Therapeutic Category Androgen
Use Treatment of endometriosis, fibrocystic breast disease, and hereditary angioedema
Usual Dosage Oral: Adults:
Female: Endometriosis: Initial: 200-400 mg/day in 2 divided doses for mild disease; individualize dosage. Usual maintenance dose: 800 mg/day in 2 divided doses to achieve amenorrhea and rapid response to painful symptoms. Continue therapy uninterrupted for 3-6 months (up to 9 months).
Female: Fibrocystic breast disease: Range: 100-400 mg/day in 2 divided doses
Male/Female: Hereditary angioedema: Initial: 200 mg 2-3 times/day; after favorable response, decrease the dosage by 50% or less at intervals of 1-3 months or longer if the frequency of attacks dictates. If an attack occurs, increase the dosage by up to 200 mg/day.
Dosage Forms
Capsule: 50 mg, 100 mg, 200 mg

Danocrine® **[Can]** *see* danazol *on this page*

Danocrine® *(Discontinued)* *see* danazol *on this page*

Dantrium® **[US/Can]** *see* dantrolene *on this page*

dantrolene (DAN troe leen)
Sound-Alike/Look-Alike Issues
Dantrium® may be confused with danazol, Daraprim®
Synonyms dantrolene sodium
U.S./Canadian Brand Names Dantrium® [US/Can]
Therapeutic Category Skeletal Muscle Relaxant
Use Treatment of spasticity associated with spinal cord injury, stroke, cerebral palsy, or multiple sclerosis; treatment of malignant hyperthermia
Usual Dosage
Spasticity: Oral:
Children: Initial: 0.5 mg/kg/dose twice daily, increase frequency to 3-4 times/day at 4- to 7-day intervals, then increase dose by 0.5 mg/kg to a maximum of 3 mg/kg/dose 2-4 times/day up to 400 mg/day
Adults: 25 mg/day to start, increase frequency to 2-4 times/day, then increase dose by 25 mg every 4-7 days to a maximum of 100 mg 2-4 times/day or 400 mg/day

Malignant hyperthermia: Children and Adults:
Preoperative prophylaxis:
Oral: 4-8 mg/kg/day in 4 divided doses, begin 1-2 days prior to surgery with last dose 3-4 hours prior to surgery
I.V.: 2.5 mg/kg ~1$\frac{1}{4}$ hours prior to anesthesia and infused over 1 hour with additional doses as needed and individualized

Crisis: I.V.: 2.5 mg/kg; may repeat dose up to cumulative dose of 10 mg/kg; if physiologic and metabolic abnormalities reappear, repeat regimen

Postcrisis follow-up: Oral: 4-8 mg/kg/day in 4 divided doses for 1-3 days; I.V. dantrolene may be used when oral therapy is not practical; individualize dosage beginning with 1 mg/kg or more as the clinical situation dictates

Dosage Forms
Capsule: 25 mg, 50 mg, 100 mg
Dantrium®: 25 mg, 50 mg, 100 mg
Injection, powder for reconstitution:
Dantrium®: 20 mg

dantrolene sodium *see* dantrolene *on previous page*

dapcin *see* daptomycin *on this page*

dapiprazole (DA pi pray zole)

Synonyms dapiprazole hydrochloride
U.S./Canadian Brand Names Rēv-Eyes™ [US]
Therapeutic Category Alpha-Adrenergic Blocking Agent
Use Reverse dilation due to drugs (adrenergic or parasympathomimetic) after eye exams
Usual Dosage Ophthalmic: Adults: Instill 2 drops followed 5 minutes later by an additional 2 drops into the conjunctiva of each eye; should not be used more frequently than once a week in the same patient
Dosage Forms
Powder, ophthalmic:
Rēv-Eyes™: 25 mg

dapiprazole hydrochloride *see* dapiprazole *on this page*

dapsone (DAP sone)

Sound-Alike/Look-Alike Issues
dapsone may be confused with Diprosone®
Synonyms diaminodiphenylsulfone
U.S./Canadian Brand Names Aczone™ [US]
Therapeutic Category Sulfone
Use Treatment of leprosy and dermatitis herpetiformis (infections caused by *Mycobacterium leprae*); treatment of acne vulgaris
Usual Dosage Oral:
Leprosy:
Children: 1-2 mg/kg/24 hours, up to a maximum of 100 mg/day
Adults: 50-100 mg/day for 3-10 years
Dermatitis herpetiformis: Adults: Start at 50 mg/day, increase to 300 mg/day, or higher to achieve full control, reduce dosage to minimum level as soon as possible
Topical: Acne vulgaris: Children ≥12 years and Adults: Apply pea-sized amount twice daily
Dosage Forms
Gel, topical:
Aczone™: 5% (30 g)
Tablet: 25 mg, 100 mg

Daptacel® [US] *see* diphtheria, tetanus toxoids, and acellular pertussis vaccine *on page 269*

daptomycin (DAP toe mye sin)

Sound-Alike/Look-Alike Issues
daptomycin may be confused with dactinomycin
Synonyms cidecin; dapcin; LY146032
U.S./Canadian Brand Names Cubicin® [US]
Therapeutic Category Antibiotic, Cyclic Lipopeptide
Use Treatment of complicated skin and skin structure infections caused by susceptible aerobic Gram-positive organisms; *Staphylococcus aureus* bacteremia, including right-sided infective endocarditis caused by MSSA or MRSA
Usual Dosage I.V.: Adults:
Skin and soft tissue: 4 mg/kg once daily for 7-14 days
Bacteremia, right-sided endocarditis caused by MSSA or MRSA: 6 mg/kg once daily for 2-6 weeks
Dosage Forms
Injection, powder for reconstitution:
Cubicin®: 500 mg

Daranide® **[US/Can]** *see* dichlorphenamide *on page 253*

Daraprim® **[US/Can]** *see* pyrimethamine *on page 736*

darbepoetin alfa (dar be POE e tin AL fa)
Sound-Alike/Look-Alike Issues
darbepoetin alfa may be confused with epoetin alfa
Synonyms erythropoiesis-stimulating agent (ESA); erythropoiesis-stimulating protein; NSC-729969
U.S./Canadian Brand Names Aranesp® [US/Can]
Therapeutic Category Colony-Stimulating Factor; Growth Factor; Recombinant Human Erythropoietin
Use Treatment of anemia associated with chronic renal failure (CRF), including patients on dialysis (ESRD) and patients not on dialysis; anemia associated with concurrent chemotherapy for nonmyeloid malignancies
Usual Dosage Adults:
Anemia associated with CRF: I.V., SubQ: Initial: 0.45 mcg/kg once weekly; titrate to response; some patients may respond to doses given once every 2 weeks
Anemia associated with chemotherapy: SubQ: Initial: 2.25 mcg/kg once weekly; with inadequate response after 6 weeks: 4.5 mcg/kg once weekly
or
500 mcg once every 3 weeks
Dosage Forms
Injection, solution [preservative free]:
Aranesp®: 25 mcg/0.42 mL (0.42 mL); 40 mcg/ 0.4 mL (0.4 mL); 60 mcg/0.3 mL (0.3 mL); 100 mcg/0.5 mL (0.5 mL); 150 mcg/0.3 mL (0.3 mL); 200 mcg/0.4 mL (0.4 mL); 300 mcg/0.6 mL (0.6 mL); 500 mcg/mL (1 mL) [contains polysorbate 80; prefilled syringe; needle cover contains latex]
Aranesp®: 25 mcg/mL (1 mL); 40 mcg/mL (1 mL); 60 mcg/mL (1 mL); 100 mcg/mL (1 mL); 150 mcg/0.75 mL (0.75 mL); 200 mcg/mL (1 mL); 300 mcg/mL (1 mL) [contains polysorbate 80; single-dose vial]

darifenacin (dar i FEN a sin)
Synonyms darifenacin hydrobromide; UK-88,525
U.S./Canadian Brand Names Enablex® [US/Can]
Therapeutic Category Anticholinergic Agent
Use Management of symptoms of bladder overactivity (urge incontinence, urgency, and frequency)
Usual Dosage Oral: Adults: Initial: 7.5 mg once daily. If response is not adequate after a minimum of 2 weeks, dosage may be increased to 15 mg once daily.
Dosage Forms
Tablet, extended release:
Enablex®: 7.5 mg, 15 mg

darifenacin hydrobromide *see* darifenacin *on this page*

darunavir (dar OO na veer)
Synonyms darunavir ethanolate; TMC-114
U.S./Canadian Brand Names Prezista™ [US]
Therapeutic Category Antiretroviral Agent, Protease Inhibitor
Use Treatment of HIV-1 infections in combination with ritonavir and other antiretroviral agents; limited to highly treatment-experienced or multiprotease inhibitor-resistant patients
Usual Dosage Oral: Adults: 600 mg twice daily with meals
Note: Coadministration with ritonavir (100 mg twice daily) is required.
Dosage Forms
Tablet:
Prezista™: 300 mg

darunavir ethanolate *see* darunavir *on this page*

Darvocet A500™ **[US]** *see* propoxyphene and acetaminophen *on page 723*

Darvocet-N® **50 [US/Can]** *see* propoxyphene and acetaminophen *on page 723*

Darvocet-N® **100 [US/Can]** *see* propoxyphene and acetaminophen *on page 723*

Darvon® **[US]** *see* propoxyphene *on page 723*

Darvon® **Compound** *(Discontinued)* *see* propoxyphene, aspirin, and caffeine *on page 723*

Darvon-N® **[US/Can]** *see* propoxyphene *on page 723*

dasatinib (da SA ti nib)
Synonyms BMS-354825; NSC-732517
U.S./Canadian Brand Names Sprycel™ [US/Can]
Therapeutic Category Antineoplastic Agent, Tyrosine Kinase Inhibitor
Use Treatment of chronic myelogenous leukemia (CML); treatment of Philadelphia chromosome-positive (Ph+) acute lymphoblastic leukemia (ALL)
Usual Dosage Oral: Adults: CML, Ph+ ALL: 70 mg twice daily
Dosage Forms
Tablet:
Sprycel™: 20 mg, 50 mg, 70 mg

daunomycin *see* daunorubicin hydrochloride *on this page*

daunorubicin citrate (liposomal) (daw noe ROO bi sin SI trate lip po SOE mal)
Sound-Alike/Look-Alike Issues
DAUNOrubicin may be confused with dactinomycin, DOXOrubicin, epirubicin, idarubicin
DAUNOrubicin liposomal may be confused with DOXOrubicin liposomal
Liposomal formulations (DaunoXome®) may be confused with conventional formulations (Adriamycin PFS®, Adriamycin RDF®, Cerubidine®, Rubex®)
Synonyms DAUNOrubicin liposomal; liposomal DAUNOrubicin; NSC-697732
Tall-Man DAUNOrubicin citrate (liposomal)
U.S./Canadian Brand Names DaunoXome® [US]
Therapeutic Category Antineoplastic Agent
Use First-line treatment of advanced HIV-associated Kaposi sarcoma (KS)
Usual Dosage I.V. (refer to individual protocols): Adults: HIV-associated KS: 40 mg/m^2 every 2 weeks
Dosage Forms
Injection, solution [preservative free]:
DaunoXome®: 2 mg/mL (25 mL)

daunorubicin hydrochloride (daw noe ROO bi sin hye droe KLOR ide)
Sound-Alike/Look-Alike Issues
DAUNOrubicin may be confused with dactinomycin, DOXOrubicin, epirubicin, idarubicin
Conventional formulations (Cerubidine®) may be confused with liposomal formulations (DaunoXome®, Doxil®)
Synonyms daunomycin; DNR; NSC-82151; rubidomycin hydrochloride
Tall-Man DAUNOrubicin hydrochloride
U.S./Canadian Brand Names Cerubidine® [US/Can]
Therapeutic Category Antineoplastic Agent
Use Treatment of acute lymphocytic (ALL) and nonlymphocytic (ANLL) leukemias
Usual Dosage I.V. (refer to individual protocols):
Children: **Note:** Cumulative dose should not exceed 300 mg/m^2 in children >2 years; maximum cumulative doses for younger children are unknown.
ALL combination therapy: Remission induction: 25-45 mg/m^2 on day 1 every week for 4 cycles **or** 30-45 mg/m^2/day for 3 days
AML combination therapy: Induction: I.V. continuous infusion: 30-60 mg/m^2/day on days 1-3 of cycle
Note: In children <2 years or <0.5 m^2, daunorubicin should be based on weight - mg/kg: 1 mg/kg per protocol with frequency dependent on regimen employed
Adults: **Note:** Cumulative dose should not exceed 550 mg/m^2 in adults without risk factors for cardiotoxicity and should not exceed 400 mg/m^2 in adults receiving chest irradiation.
Range: 30-60 mg/m^2/day for 3-5 days, repeat dose in 3-4 weeks
AML: Single agent induction: 60 mg/m^2/day for 3 days; repeat every 3-4 weeks
AML: Combination therapy induction: 45 mg/m^2/day for 3 days of the first course of induction therapy; subsequent courses: Every day for 2 days
ALL combination therapy: 45 mg/m^2/day for 3 days
Dosage Forms
Injection, powder for reconstitution: 20 mg, 50 mg
Cerubidine®: 20 mg
Injection, solution: 5 mg/mL (4 mL, 10 mL)

DAUNOrubicin liposomal *see* daunorubicin citrate (liposomal) *on this page*

DaunoXome® [US] *see* daunorubicin citrate (liposomal) *on this page*

1-Day™ [US-OTC] *see* tioconazole *on page 845*

Dayhist® Allergy [US-OTC] *see* clemastine *on page 198*

Daypro® [US/Can] *see* oxaprozin *on page 637*

Dayto Himbin® (Discontinued) *see* yohimbine *on page 901*

Daytrana™ [US] *see* methylphenidate *on page 558*

DC 240® Softgel® (Discontinued) *see* docusate *on page 273*

dCF *see* pentostatin *on page 667*

DDAVP® [US/Can] *see* desmopressin acetate *on page 239*

ddI *see* didanosine *on page 255*

1-deamino-8-D-arginine vasopressin *see* desmopressin acetate *on page 239*

Debrox® [US-OTC] *see* carbamide peroxide *on page 148*

Decadron® [US] *see* dexamethasone (systemic) *on page 241*

Decadron® Phosphate (Discontinued) *see* dexamethasone (systemic) *on page 241*

Deca-Durabolin® [Can] *see* nandrolone *on page 590*

Deca-Durabolin® (Discontinued) *see* nandrolone *on page 590*

Decahist-DM (Discontinued) *see* carbinoxamine, pseudoephedrine, and dextromethorphan *on page 152*

Decavac™ [US] *see* diphtheria and tetanus toxoid *on page 267*

Dec-Chlorphen [US] *see* chlorpheniramine and phenylephrine *on page 177*

Dec-Chlorphen DM [US] *see* chlorpheniramine, phenylephrine, and dextromethorphan *on page 180*

De-Chlor DM [US] *see* chlorpheniramine, phenylephrine, and dextromethorphan *on page 180*

De-Chlor DR [US] *see* chlorpheniramine, phenylephrine, and dextromethorphan *on page 180*

De-Chlor G [US] *see* hydrocodone, phenylephrine, and guaifenesin *on page 431*

De-Chlor HC [US] *see* phenylephrine, hydrocodone, and chlorpheniramine *on page 678*

De-Chlor HD [US] *see* phenylephrine, hydrocodone, and chlorpheniramine *on page 678*

decitabine (de SYE ta been)
Synonyms 5-aza-2'-deoxycytidine; 5-azaC; NSC-127716
U.S./Canadian Brand Names Dacogen™ [US]
Therapeutic Category Antineoplastic Agent, Antimetabolite (Pyrimidine)
Use Treatment of myelodysplastic syndrome (MDS)
Usual Dosage I.V.: Adults: MDS: 15 mg/m^2 over 3 hours every 8 hours (45 mg/m^2/day) for 3 days (135 mg/m^2/cycle) every 6 weeks. Treatment is recommended for at least 4 cycles and may continue until the patient no longer continues to benefit.
Dosage Forms
Injection, powder for reconstitution:
Dacogen™: 50 mg

Declomycin® [US/Can] *see* demeclocycline *on page 236*

Deconamine® [US] *see* chlorpheniramine and pseudoephedrine *on page 178*

Deconamine® SR [US] *see* chlorpheniramine and pseudoephedrine *on page 178*

Deconsal® II [US] *see* guaifenesin and phenylephrine *on page 404*

Deconsal® CT [US] *see* phenylephrine and pyrilamine *on page 677*

Deep Sea [US-OTC] *see* sodium chloride *on page 792*

Defen-LA® (Discontinued) *see* guaifenesin and pseudoephedrine *on page 406*

deferasirox (de FER a sir ox)
Sound-Alike/Look-Alike Issues
deferasirox may be confused with deferoxamine
Synonyms ICL670
U.S./Canadian Brand Names Exjade® [US/Can]
Therapeutic Category Antidote; Chelating Agent
Use Treatment of chronic iron overload due to blood transfusions
Usual Dosage Oral: Children ≥2 years and Adults:
Initial: 20 mg/kg daily (calculate dose to nearest whole tablet)
Maintenance: Adjust dose every 3-6 months based on serum ferritin levels; increase by 5-10 mg/kg/day (calculate dose to nearest whole tablet); titrate. Maximum dose: 30 mg/kg/day; consider interrupting therapy

for serum ferritin <500 mcg/L. **Note:** Consider dose reduction or interruption for hearing loss or visual disturbances.

Dosage Forms
Tablet, for oral suspension:
Exjade®: 125 mg, 250 mg, 500 mg

deferoxamine (de fer OKS a meen)
Sound-Alike/Look-Alike Issues
deferoxamine may be confused with cefuroxime, deferasirox
Desferal® may be confused with desflurane, Dexferrum®, Disophrol®
Synonyms deferoxamine mesylate; desferrioxamine; NSC-644468
U.S./Canadian Brand Names Desferal® [US/Can]; PMS-Deferoxamine [Can]
Therapeutic Category Antidote
Use Acute iron intoxication or when clinical signs of significant iron toxicity exist; chronic iron overload secondary to multiple transfusions
Usual Dosage
Acute iron toxicity: **Note:** I.V. route is used when severe toxicity is evidenced by systemic symptoms (coma, shock, metabolic acidosis, or severe gastrointestinal bleeding) or potentially severe intoxications (serum iron level >500 mcg/dL). When severe symptoms are not present, the I.M. route may be preferred (per manufacturer); however, the use of deferoxamine in situations where the serum iron concentration is <500 mcg/dL or when severe toxicity is not evident is a subject of some clinical debate.
Children ≥3 years:
I.M.: 90 mg/kg/dose every 8 hours (maximum: 6 g/24 hours)
I.V.: 15 mg/kg/hour (maximum: 6 g/24 hours)
Adults: I.M., I.V.: Initial: 1000 mg, may be followed by 500 mg every 4 hours for up to 2 doses; subsequent doses of 500 mg have been administered every 4-12 hours
Maximum recommended dose: 6 g/day (per manufacturer, however, higher doses have been administered)
Chronic iron overload:
Children ≥3 years:
I.V.: 15 mg/kg/hour (maximum: 12 g/24 hours)
SubQ: 20-40 mg/kg/day over 8-12 hours (maximum: 1000-2000 mg/day)
Adults:
I.M., I.V.: 500-1000 mg/day I.M.; in addition, 2000 mg should be given I.V. with each unit of blood transfused (administer separately from blood); maximum: 1 g/day in absence of transfusions; 6 g/day if patient received transfusions
SubQ: 1-2 g every day or 20-40 mg/kg/day over 8-24 hours
Dosage Forms
Injection, powder for reconstitution: 500 mg, 2 g
Desferal®: 500 mg, 2 g

deferoxamine mesylate see deferoxamine on this page

Deficol® *(Discontinued)* see bisacodyl on page 112

Definity® [US/Can] see perflutren lipid microspheres on page 668

Degest® 2 Ophthalmic *(Discontinued)* see naphazoline on page 590

Dehistine [US] see chlorpheniramine, phenylephrine, and methscopolamine on page 181

Dehydral® [Can] see methenamine on page 551

dehydrobenzperidol see droperidol on page 284

Del Aqua® [US] see benzoyl peroxide on page 103

Delatest® Injection *(Discontinued)* see testosterone on page 828

Delatestryl® [US/Can] see testosterone on page 828

delavirdine (de la VIR deen)
Synonyms U-90152S
U.S./Canadian Brand Names Rescriptor® [US/Can]
Therapeutic Category Antiviral Agent
Use Treatment of HIV-1 infection in combination with at least two additional antiretroviral agents
Usual Dosage Oral: Adolescents ≥16 years and Adults: 400 mg 3 times/day
Dosage Forms
Tablet:
Rescriptor®: 100 mg, 200 mg

Delestrogen® [US] see estradiol on page 313

Delfen® **[US-OTC]** *see* nonoxynol 9 *on page 610*

Delsym® **[US-OTC]** *see* dextromethorphan *on page 247*

delta-9-tetrahydro-cannabinol *see* dronabinol *on page 284*

delta-9-tetrahydrocannabinol and cannabinol *see* tetrahydrocannabinol and cannabidiol *(Canada only) on page 832*

delta-9 THC *see* dronabinol *on page 284*

Delta-D® **[US]** *see* cholecalciferol *on page 186*

deltacortisone *see* prednisone *on page 710*

deltadehydrocortisone *see* prednisone *on page 710*

deltahydrocortisone *see* prednisolone (systemic) *on page 710*

Del-Vi-A® **(Discontinued)** *see* vitamin A *on page 892*

Demadex® **[US]** *see* torsemide *on page 852*

demeclocycline (dem e kloe SYE kleen)

Synonyms demeclocycline hydrochloride; demethylchlortetracycline
U.S./Canadian Brand Names Declomycin® [US/Can]
Therapeutic Category Tetracycline Derivative
Use Treatment of susceptible bacterial infections (acne, gonorrhea, pertussis, and urinary tract infections) caused by both gram-negative and gram-positive organisms
Usual Dosage Oral:
Children ≥8 years: 8-12 mg/kg/day divided every 6-12 hours
Adults: 150 mg 4 times/day or 300 mg twice daily
Dosage Forms
Tablet: 150 mg, 300 mg
Declomycin®: 150 mg, 300 mg

demeclocycline hydrochloride *see* demeclocycline *on this page*

Demerol® **[US/Can]** *see* meperidine *on page 542*

4-demethoxydaunorubicin *see* idarubicin *on page 446*

demethylchlortetracycline *see* demeclocycline *on this page*

Demser® **[US/Can]** *see* metyrosine *on page 565*

Demulen® **30 [Can]** *see* ethinyl estradiol and ethynodiol diacetate *on page 324*

Demulen® **(Discontinued)** *see* ethinyl estradiol and ethynodiol diacetate *on page 324*

Denavir® **[US]** *see* penciclovir *on page 660*

denileukin diftitox (de ni LOO kin DIF ti toks)

Synonyms DAB$_{389}$IL-2; NSC-714744
U.S./Canadian Brand Names ONTAK® [US]
Therapeutic Category Antineoplastic Agent, Miscellaneous
Use Treatment of persistent or recurrent cutaneous T-cell lymphoma whose malignant cells express the CD25 component of the IL-2 receptor
Usual Dosage I.V.: Adults: 9 or 18 mcg/kg/day days 1 through 5 every 21 days
Dosage Forms
Injection, solution [frozen]:
ONTAK®: 150 mcg/mL (2 mL)

Denorex® **Original Therapeutic Strength [US-OTC]** *see* coal tar *on page 208*

Denta 5000 Plus [US] *see* fluoride *on page 361*

DentaGel [US] *see* fluoride *on page 361*

Dentapaine [US-OTC] *see* benzocaine *on page 101*

Dent's Ear Wax [US-OTC] *see* carbamide peroxide *on page 148*

Dent's Extra Strength Toothache [US-OTC] *see* benzocaine *on page 101*

Dent's Maxi-Strength Toothache [US-OTC] *see* benzocaine *on page 101*

deoxycoformycin *see* pentostatin *on page 667*

2′-deoxycoformycin *see* pentostatin *on page 667*

Depacon® **[US]** *see* valproic acid and derivatives *on page 881*

Depade® [US] *see* naltrexone *on page 590*

Depakene® [US/Can] *see* valproic acid and derivatives *on page 881*

Depakote® [US] *see* valproic acid and derivatives *on page 881*

Depakote® ER [US] *see* valproic acid and derivatives *on page 881*

Depakote® Sprinkle [US] *see* valproic acid and derivatives *on page 881*

depAndro® Injection *(Discontinued)* *see* testosterone *on page 828*

Depen® [US/Can] *see* penicillamine *on page 661*

depGynogen® Injection *(Discontinued)* *see* estradiol *on page 313*

depMedalone® Injection *(Discontinued)* *see* methylprednisolone *on page 559*

DepoCyt® [US/Can] *see* cytarabine (liposomal) *on page 226*

DepoDur™ [US] *see* morphine sulfate *on page 578*

Depo®-Estradiol [US/Can] *see* estradiol *on page 313*

Depoject® Injection *(Discontinued)* *see* methylprednisolone *on page 559*

Depo-Medrol® [US/Can] *see* methylprednisolone *on page 559*

Deponit® Patch *(Discontinued)* *see* nitroglycerin *on page 608*

Depo-Prevera® [Can] *see* medroxyprogesterone *on page 537*

Depo-Provera® [US/Can] *see* medroxyprogesterone *on page 537*

Depo-Provera® Contraceptive [US] *see* medroxyprogesterone *on page 537*

depo-subQ provera 104™ [US] *see* medroxyprogesterone *on page 537*

Depotest® 100 [Can] *see* testosterone *on page 828*

Depotest® Injection *(Discontinued)* *see* testosterone *on page 828*

Depo®-Testosterone [US] *see* testosterone *on page 828*

deprenyl *see* selegiline *on page 780*

Dequadin® [Can] *see* dequalinium *(Canada only) on this page*

dequalinium *(Canada only)* (de kwal LI ne um)
U.S./Canadian Brand Names Dequadin® [Can]
Therapeutic Category Antibacterial, Topical; Antifungal Agent, Topical
Use Treatment of mouth and throat infections
Usual Dosage Adults:
  Lozenge: One lozenge sucked slowly every 2-3 hours
  Oral paint: Apply freely to infected area, every 2-3 hours, or as directed by physician
Dosage Forms
  Lozenge, as chloride: 0.25 mg (20s)
  Oral paint, as chloride: 0.5% (25 mL)

Dermaflex® Gel *(Discontinued)* *see* lidocaine *on page 504*

DermaFungal [US-OTC] *see* miconazole *on page 566*

Dermagran® [US-OTC] *see* aluminum hydroxide *on page 36*

Dermagran® AF [US-OTC] *see* miconazole *on page 566*

Dermamycin® [US-OTC] *see* diphenhydramine *on page 265*

Dermarest Dricort® [US-OTC] *see* hydrocortisone (topical) *on page 434*

Dermarest® Skin Correction Cream Plus [US-OTC] *see* hydroquinone *on page 437*

Derma-Smoothe/FS® [US/Can] *see* fluocinolone *on page 359*

Dermatop® [US/Can] *see* prednicarbate *on page 709*

Dermatophytin-O *(Discontinued)*

Dermazene® [US] *see* iodoquinol and hydrocortisone *on page 467*

DermaZinc™ [US-OTC] *see* pyrithione zinc *on page 737*

Dermazole [Can] *see* miconazole *on page 566*

Dermoplast® Antibacterial [US-OTC] *see* benzocaine *on page 101*

Dermoplast® Pain Relieving [US-OTC] *see* benzocaine *on page 101*

Dermovate® [Can] *see* clobetasol *on page 201*

Dermtex® **HC [US-OTC]** *see* hydrocortisone (topical) *on page 434*

Desferal® **[US/Can]** *see* deferoxamine *on page 235*

desferrioxamine *see* deferoxamine *on page 235*

desflurane (DES flure ane)

Sound-Alike/Look-Alike Issues
desflurane may be confused with Desferal®

U.S./Canadian Brand Names Suprane® [US/Can]

Therapeutic Category General Anesthetic

Use Induction and maintenance of general anesthesia (adults); maintenance of anesthesia (intubated children)

Usual Dosage
Note: Concurrent use with benzodiazepines, nitrous oxide, or opioids decreases the desflurane dose.

Children (intubated): Maintenance: Surgical levels of anesthesia range between 5.2% to 10%

Adults: The minimum alveolar concentration (MAC), the concentration at which 50% of patients do not respond to surgical incision, ranges from 6.0% (45 years of age) to 7.3% (25 years of age). The concentration at which amnesia and loss of awareness occur (MAC - awake) is 2.4%. Surgical levels of anesthesia are achieved with concentrations between 2.5% to 8.5%.

Note: Because of the higher vapor pressure of desflurane, its vaporizer is heated in order to deliver a constant concentration

Dosage Forms
Liquid, for inhalation:
Suprane®: 240 mL

desiccated thyroid *see* thyroid *on page 839*

desipramine (des IP ra meen)

Sound-Alike/Look-Alike Issues
desipramine may be confused with clomiPRAMINE, deserpidine, diphenhydrAMINE, disopyramide, imipramine, nortriptyline

Norpramin® may be confused with clomiPRAMINE, imipramine, Norpace®, nortriptyline, Tenormin®

Synonyms desipramine hydrochloride; desmethylimipramine hydrochloride

U.S./Canadian Brand Names Alti-Desipramine [Can]; Apo-Desipramine® [Can]; Norpramin® [US/Can]; Nu-Desipramine [Can]; PMS-Desipramine [Can]

Therapeutic Category Antidepressant, Tricyclic (Secondary Amine)

Use Treatment of depression

Usual Dosage Oral (dose is generally administered at bedtime): Depression:
Adolescents: Initial: 25-50 mg/day; gradually increase to 100 mg/day in single or divided doses (maximum: 150 mg/day)
Adults: Initial: 75 mg/day in divided doses; increase gradually to 150-200 mg/day in divided or single dose (maximum: 300 mg/day)

Dosage Forms
Tablet: 10 mg, 25 mg, 50 mg, 75 mg, 100 mg, 150 mg
Norpramin®: 10 mg, 25 mg, 50 mg, 75 mg, 100 mg, 150 mg

desipramine hydrochloride *see* desipramine *on this page*

Desitin® **[US-OTC]** *see* zinc oxide *on page 906*

Desitin® **Creamy [US-OTC]** *see* zinc oxide *on page 906*

desloratadine (des lor AT a deen)

U.S./Canadian Brand Names Aerius® [Can]; Clarinex® [US]

Therapeutic Category Antihistamine, Nonsedating

Use Relief of nasal and non-nasal symptoms of seasonal allergic rhinitis (SAR) and perennial allergic rhinitis (PAR); treatment of chronic idiopathic urticaria (CIU)

Usual Dosage Oral:
Children:
6-11 months: 1 mg once daily
12 months to 5 years: 1.25 mg once daily
6-11 years: 2.5 mg once daily
Children ≥12 years and Adults: 5 mg once daily

Dosage Forms
Syrup:
Clarinex®: 0.5 mg/mL

Tablet:
Clarinex®: 5 mg
Tablet, orally disintegrating:
Clarinex® RediTabs®: 2.5 mg, 5 mg

desloratadine and pseudoephedrine (des lor AT a deen & soo doe e FED rin)
Synonyms pseudoephedrine and desloratadine
U.S./Canadian Brand Names Clarinex-D® 12 Hour [US]; Clarinex-D® 24 Hour [US]
Therapeutic Category Antihistamine/Decongestant Combination, Nonsedating
Use Relief of symptoms of seasonal allergic rhinitis, in children ≥12 years of age and adults
Usual Dosage Oral: Children ≥12 years and Adults:
Clarinex-D® 12 Hour: One tablet twice daily
Clarinex-D® 24 Hour: One tablet daily
Dosage Forms
Tablet, variable release:
Clarinex-D® 12 Hour: Desloratadine 2.5 mg [immediate release] and pseudoephedrine 120 mg [extended release]
Clarinex-D® 24 Hour: Desloratadine 5 mg [immediate release] and pseudoephedrine 240 mg [extended release]

desmethylimipramine hydrochloride *see* desipramine *on previous page*

desmopressin acetate (des moe PRES in AS e tate)
Synonyms 1-deamino-8-D-arginine vasopressin
U.S./Canadian Brand Names Apo-Desmopressin® [Can]; DDAVP® [US/Can]; Minirin® [Can]; Nove-Desmopressin® [Can]; Octostim® [Can]; Stimate™ [US]
Therapeutic Category Vasopressin Analog, Synthetic
Use
Injection: Treatment of diabetes insipidus; control of bleeding in hemophilia A, and mild-to-moderate classic von Willebrand disease (type I)
Tablet, nasal solution: Treatment of diabetes insipidus; primary nocturnal enuresis
Usual Dosage
Children:
Diabetes insipidus:
Intranasal (using 100 mcg/mL nasal solution): 3 months to 12 years: Initial: 5 mcg/day (0.05 mL/day) divided 1-2 times/day; range: 5-30 mcg/day (0.05-0.3 mL/day) divided 1-2 times/day; adjust morning and evening doses separately for an adequate diurnal rhythm of water turnover; doses <10 mcg should be administered using the rhinal tube system
Oral: ≥4 years: Initial: 0.05 mg twice daily; total daily dose should be increased or decreased as needed to obtain adequate antidiuresis (range: 0.1-1.2 mg divided 2-3 times/day)
Hemophilia A and von Willebrand disease (type I):
I.V.: >3 months: 0.3 mcg/kg by slow infusion; may repeat dose if needed; begin 30 minutes before procedure
Intranasal: ≥11 months: Refer to adult dosing.
Nocturnal enuresis:
Intranasal (using 100 mcg/mL nasal solution): ≥6 years: Initial: 20 mcg (0.2 mL) at bedtime; range: 10-40 mcg; it is recommended that 1/2 of the dose be given in each nostril. **Note:** The nasal spray pump can only deliver doses of 10 mcg (0.1 mL) or multiples of 10 mcg (0.1 mL); if doses other than this are needed, the rhinal tube delivery system is preferred. For 10 mcg dose, administer in one nostril.
Oral: 0.2 mg at bedtime; dose may be titrated up to 0.6 mg to achieve desired response. Patients previously on intranasal therapy can begin oral tablets 24 hours after the last intranasal dose.
Children ≥12 years and Adults:
Diabetes insipidus:
I.V., SubQ: 2-4 mcg/day (0.5-1 mL) in 2 divided doses or 1/10 of the maintenance intranasal dose
Intranasal (using 100 mcg/mL nasal solution): 10-40 mcg/day (0.1-0.4 mL) divided 1-3 times/day; adjust morning and evening doses separately for an adequate diurnal rhythm of water turnover. **Note:** The nasal spray pump can only deliver doses of 10 mcg (0.1 mL) or multiples of 10 mcg (0.1 mL); if doses other than this are needed, the rhinal tube delivery system is preferred.
Oral: Initial: 0.05 mg twice daily; total daily dose should be increased or decreased as needed to obtain adequate antidiuresis (range: 0.1-1.2 mg divided 2-3 times/day)
Hemophilia A and mild to moderate von Willebrand disease (type I):
I.V.: 0.3 mcg/kg by slow infusion, begin 30 minutes before procedure
Intranasal: Using high concentration spray (1.5 mg/mL): <50 kg: 150 mcg (1 spray); >50 kg: 300 mcg (1 spray each nostril); repeat use is determined by the patient's clinical condition and laboratory work; if using preoperatively, administer 2 hours before surgery
(Continued)

desmopressin acetate *(Continued)*

Dosage Forms
Injection, solution: 4 mcg/mL (1 mL, 10 mL)
DDAVP®: 4 mcg/mL (1 mL, 10 mL)
Solution, intranasal: 100 mcg/mL (2.5 mL)
DDAVP®: 100 mcg/mL (2.5 mL)
Solution, intranasal [spray]: 100 mcg/mL (5 mL)
DDAVP®: 100 mcg/mL (5 mL)
Stimate™: 1.5 mg/mL (2.5 mL)
Tablet: 0.1 mg, 0.2 mg
DDAVP®: 0.1 mg, 0.2 mg

Desocort® [Can] *see* desonide *on this page*

Desogen® [US] *see* ethinyl estradiol and desogestrel *on page 322*

desogestrel and ethinyl estradiol *see* ethinyl estradiol and desogestrel *on page 322*

Desonate™ [US] *see* desonide *on this page*

desonide (DES oh nide)

U.S./Canadian Brand Names Desocort® [Can]; Desonate™ [US]; DesOwen® [US]; LoKara™ [US]; PMS-Desonide [Can]; Verdeso™ [US]
Therapeutic Category Corticosteroid, Topical
Use Adjunctive therapy for inflammation in acute and chronic corticosteroid responsive dermatosis (low potency corticosteroid); mild-to-moderate atopic dermatitis
Usual Dosage Topical:
Corticosteroid responsive dermatoses: Children and Adults: Therapy should be discontinued when control is achieved. If no improvement is seen within 2 weeks, reassessment of diagnosis may be necessary.
Cream, ointment: Apply 2-4 times/day sparingly
Lotion: Apply 2-3 times/day sparingly
Atopic dermatitis: Children ≥3 months and Adults: Aerosol, gel: Apply 2 times/day sparingly. Therapy should be discontinued when control is achieved. If no improvement is seen within 4 weeks, reassessment of diagnosis may be necessary.
Dosage Forms
Aerosol, topical [foam]:
Verdeso®: 0.05% (50 g, 100 g)
Cream, topical: 0.05% (15 g, 60 g)
DesOwen®: 0.05% (15 g, 60 g, 90 g)
Gel, topical [aqueous]:
Desonate™: 0.05% (15 g, 30 g, 60g)
Lotion, topical: 0.05% (60 mL, 120 mL)
DesOwen®, LoKara™: 0.05% (60 mL, 120 mL)
Ointment, topical: 0.05% (15 g, 60 g)
DesOwen®: 0.05% (15 g, 60 g)

DesOwen® [US] *see* desonide *on this page*

desoximetasone (des oks i MET a sone)

Sound-Alike/Look-Alike Issues
desoximetasone may be confused with dexamethasone
Topicort® may be confused with Topic®
U.S./Canadian Brand Names Taro-Desoximetasone [Can]; Topicort® [US/Can]; Topicort®-LP [US]
Therapeutic Category Corticosteroid, Topical
Use Relieves inflammation and pruritic symptoms of corticosteroid-responsive dermatosis (intermediate- to high-potency topical corticosteroid)
Usual Dosage Desoximetasone is a potent fluorinated topical corticosteroid. Therapy should be discontinued when control is achieved; if no improvement is seen, reassessment of diagnosis may be necessary.

Cream, gel: Children and Adults: Apply a thin film to affected area twice daily
Ointment: Children ≥10 years and Adults: Apply a thin film to affected area twice daily
Dosage Forms
Cream, topical: 0.25% (15 g, 60 g); 0.05% (15 g, 60 g)
Topicort®: 0.25% (15 g, 60 g)
Topicort®-LP: 0.05% (15 g, 60 g)
Gel, topical: 0.05% (15 g, 60 g)
Topicort®: 0.05% (15 g, 60 g)

Ointment, topical: 0.25% (15 g, 60 g)
Topicort®: 0.25% (15 g, 60 g)

desoxyephedrine hydrochloride *see* methamphetamine *on page 551*

Desoxyn® [US/Can] *see* methamphetamine *on page 551*

desoxyphenobarbital *see* primidone *on page 714*

Desquam-X® [US/Can] *see* benzoyl peroxide *on page 103*

Desquam-X® Wash (Discontinued) *see* benzoyl peroxide *on page 103*

Desquam-E™ [US] *see* benzoyl peroxide *on page 103*

Desyrel® [Can] *see* trazodone *on page 859*

Desyrel® (Discontinued) *see* trazodone *on page 859*

Detane® [US-OTC] *see* benzocaine *on page 101*

detemir insulin *see* insulin detemir *on page 457*

Detrol® [US/Can] *see* tolterodine *on page 850*

Detrol® LA [US/Can] *see* tolterodine *on page 850*

Detuss [US] *see* pseudoephedrine, hydrocodone, and chlorpheniramine *on page 731*

Detussin® Expectorant (Discontinued) *see* hydrocodone, pseudoephedrine, and guaifenesin *on page 432*

Dex4 Glucose [US-OTC] *see* glucose (instant) *on page 395*

Dexacidin® (Discontinued) *see* neomycin, polymyxin B, and dexamethasone *on page 597*

Dexacine™ (Discontinued) *see* neomycin, polymyxin B, and dexamethasone *on page 597*

dexamethasone and ciprofloxacin *see* ciprofloxacin and dexamethasone *on page 193*

dexamethasone and tobramycin *see* tobramycin and dexamethasone *on page 848*

Dexamethasone Intensol® [US] *see* dexamethasone (systemic) *on this page*

dexamethasone, neomycin, and polymyxin B *see* neomycin, polymyxin B, and dexamethasone *on page 597*

dexamethasone (ophthalmic) (deks a METH a sone op THAL mik)
Sound-Alike/Look-Alike Issues
dexamethasone may be confused with desoximetasone
Maxidex® may be confused with Maxzide®
Synonyms dexamethasone sodium phosphate
U.S./Canadian Brand Names Maxidex® [US/Can]
Therapeutic Category Adrenal Corticosteroid
Use Inflammatory or allergic conjunctivitis
Usual Dosage Ophthalmic: Adults:
Ointment: Apply thin coating into conjunctival sac 3-4 times/day; gradually taper dose to discontinue
Suspension: Instill 2 drops into conjunctival sac every hour during the day and every other hour during the night; gradually reduce dose to every 3-4 hours, then to 3-4 times/day
Dosage Forms
Solution, ophthalmic: 0.1% (5 mL)
Suspension, ophthalmic:
Maxidex®: 0.1% (5 mL)

dexamethasone sodium phosphate *see* dexamethasone (ophthalmic) *on this page*

dexamethasone sodium phosphate *see* dexamethasone (systemic) *on this page*

dexamethasone (systemic) (deks a METH a sone sis TEM ik)
Sound-Alike/Look-Alike Issues
dexamethasone may be confused with desoximetasone
Decadron® may be confused with Percodan®
Synonyms dexamethasone sodium phosphate
U.S./Canadian Brand Names Apo-Dexamethasone® [Can]; Decadron® [US]; Dexamethasone Intensol® [US]; Dexasone® [Can]; DexPak® TaperPak® [US]; Diodex® [Can]; PMS-Dexamethasone [Can]
Therapeutic Category Adrenal Corticosteroid
Use Systemically and locally for chronic swelling; allergic, hematologic, neoplastic, and autoimmune diseases; may be used in management of cerebral edema, septic shock, as a diagnostic agent, antiemetic
(Continued)

dexamethasone (systemic) *(Continued)*

Usual Dosage

Children:

Antiemetic (prior to chemotherapy): I.V. (should be given as sodium phosphate): 5-20 mg given 15-30 minutes before treatment

Antiinflammatory immunosuppressant: Oral, I.M., I.V. (injections should be given as sodium phosphate): 0.08-0.3 mg/kg/day **or** 2.5-10 mg/m^2/day in divided doses every 6-12 hours

Extubation or airway edema: Oral, I.M., I.V. (injections should be given as sodium phosphate): 0.5-2 mg/kg/day in divided doses every 6 hours beginning 24 hours prior to extubation and continuing for 4-6 doses afterwards

Cerebral edema: I.V. (should be given as sodium phosphate): Loading dose: 1-2 mg/kg/dose as a single dose; maintenance: 1-1.5 mg/kg/day (maximum: 16 mg/day) in divided doses every 4-6 hours for 5 days then taper for 5 days, then discontinue

Bacterial meningitis in infants and children >2 months: I.V. (should be given as sodium phosphate): 0.6 mg/kg/day in 4 divided doses every 6 hours for the first 4 days of antibiotic treatment; start dexamethasone at the time of the first dose of antibiotic

Physiologic replacement: Oral, I.M., I.V.: 0.03-0.15 mg/kg/day **or** 0.6-0.75 mg/m^2/day in divided doses every 6-12 hours

Adults:

Antiemetic:

Prophylaxis: Oral, I.V.: 10-20 mg 15-30 minutes before treatment on each treatment day

Continuous infusion regimen: Oral or I.V.: 10 mg every 12 hours on each treatment day

Mildly emetogenic therapy: Oral, I.M., I.V.: 4 mg every 4-6 hours

Delayed nausea/vomiting: Oral: 4-10 mg 1-2 times/day for 2-4 days **or**

8 mg every 12 hours for 2 days; then

4 mg every 12 hours for 2 days **or**

20 mg 1 hour before chemotherapy; then

10 mg 12 hours after chemotherapy; then

8 mg every 12 hours for 4 doses; then

4 mg every 12 hours for 4 doses

Antiinflammatory:

Oral, I.M., I.V. (injections should be given as sodium phosphate): 0.75-9 mg/day in divided doses every 6-12 hours

Intra-articular, intralesional, or soft tissue (as sodium phosphate): 0.4-6 mg/day

Chemotherapy: Oral, I.V.: 40 mg every day for 4 days, repeated every 4 weeks (VAD regimen)

Cerebral edema: I.V. 10 mg stat, 4 mg I.M./I.V. (should be given as sodium phosphate) every 6 hours until response is maximized, then switch to oral regimen, then taper off if appropriate; dosage may be reduced after 24 days and gradually discontinued over 5-7 days

Cushing syndrome, diagnostic: Oral: 1 mg at 11 PM, draw blood at 8 AM; greater accuracy for Cushing syndrome may be achieved by the following:

Dexamethasone 0.5 mg by mouth every 6 hours for 48 hours (with 24-hour urine collection for 17-hydroxycorticosteroid excretion)

Differentiation of Cushing syndrome due to ACTH excess from Cushing due to other causes: Oral: Dexamethasone 2 mg every 6 hours for 48 hours (with 24-hour urine collection for 17-hydroxycorticosteroid excretion)

Multiple sclerosis (acute exacerbation): 30 mg/day for 1 week, followed by 4-12 mg/day for 1 month

Physiological replacement: Oral, I.M., I.V. (should be given as sodium phosphate): 0.03-0.15 mg/kg/day **or** 0.6-0.75 mg/m^2/day in divided doses every 6-12 hours

Treatment of shock:

Addisonian crisis/shock (ie, adrenal insufficiency/responsive to steroid therapy): I.V. (given as sodium phosphate): 4-10 mg as a single dose, which may be repeated if necessary

Unresponsive shock (ie, unresponsive to steroid therapy): I.V. (given as sodium phosphate): 1-6 mg/kg as a single I.V. dose or up to 40 mg initially followed by repeat doses every 2-6 hours while shock persists

Hemodialysis: Supplemental dose is not necessary

Peritoneal dialysis: Supplemental dose is not necessary

Dosage Forms

Elixir: 0.5 mg/5 mL

Injection, solution: 4 mg/mL (1 mL, 5 mL, 10 mL, 25 mL, 30 mL); 10 mg/mL (1 mL, 10 mL)

Injection, solution [preservative free]: 10 mg/mL (1 mL)

Solution, oral: 0.5 mg/5 mL

Solution, oral concentrate:

Dexamethasone Intensol®: 1 mg/mL

Tablet: 0.5 mg, 0.75 mg, 1 mg, 1.5 mg, 2 mg, 4 mg, 6 mg

DexPak® TaperPak®: 1.5 mg

Dexasone® **[Can]** *see* dexamethasone (systemic) *on previous page*

dexbrompheniramine and pseudoephedrine
(deks brom fen EER a meen & soo doe e FED rin)

Synonyms pseudoephedrine and dexbrompheniramine

U.S./Canadian Brand Names Drixoral® Cold & Allergy [US-OTC]; Drixoral® [Can]

Therapeutic Category Antihistamine/Decongestant Combination

Use Relief of symptoms of upper respiratory mucosal congestion in seasonal and perennial nasal allergies, acute rhinitis, rhinosinusitis, and eustachian tube blockage

Usual Dosage Oral: Children >12 years and Adults: 1 timed release tablet every 12 hours, may require 1 tablet every 8 hours

Dosage Forms
Tablet, sustained action: Dexbrompheniramine 6 mg and pseudoephedrine 120 mg
Drixoral® Cold & Allergy [OTC]: Dexbrompheniramine 6 mg and pseudoephedrine 120 mg

Dexchlor® *(Discontinued)* see dexchlorpheniramine on this page

dexchlorpheniramine (deks klor fen EER a meen)

Synonyms dexchlorpheniramine maleate

Therapeutic Category Antihistamine

Use Perennial and seasonal allergic rhinitis and other allergic symptoms including urticaria

Usual Dosage Oral:
Children:
2-5 years: 0.5 mg every 4-6 hours (do not use timed release)
6-11 years: 1 mg every 4-6 hours or 4 mg timed release at bedtime
Adults: 2 mg every 4-6 hours or 4-6 mg timed release at bedtime or every 8-10 hours

Dosage Forms
Syrup: 2 mg/5 mL
Tablet, sustained action: 4 mg, 6 mg

dexchlorpheniramine and pseudoephedrine
(deks klor fen EER a meen & soo doe e FED rin)

Synonyms pseudoephedrine tannate and dexchlorpheniramine tannate

U.S./Canadian Brand Names Duotan PD [US]; Tanafed DP™ [US]

Therapeutic Category Alpha/Beta Agonist; Antihistamine

Use Relief of nasal congestion associated with the common cold, hay fever, and other allergies, sinusitis, and vasomotor and allergic rhinitis

Usual Dosage Oral: Rhinitis/decongestant: Dexchlorpheniramine tannate 2.5 mg and pseudoephedrine tannate 75 mg per 5 mL:

Children:
2-6 years: 2.5-5 mL every 12 hours (maximum: 10 mL/24 hours)
6-12 years: 5-10 mL every 12 hours (maximum: 20 mL/24 hours)
Children ≥12 years and Adults: 10-20 mL every 12 hours (maximum: 40 mL/24 hours)

Dosage Forms
Suspension:
Duotan PD, Tanafed DP™: Dexchlorpheniramine 2.5 mg and pseudoephedrine 75 mg per 5 mL

dexchlorpheniramine maleate see dexchlorpheniramine on this page

dexchlorpheniramine tannate, pseudoephedrine tannate, and dextromethorphan tannate see chlorpheniramine, pseudoephedrine, and dextromethorphan on page 183

Dexcon-DM *(Discontinued)* see guaifenesin, dextromethorphan, and phenylephrine on page 407

Dexcon-PE [US] see guaifenesin, dextromethorphan, and phenylephrine on page 407

Dexedrine® [US/Can] see dextroamphetamine on page 246

Dexferrum® [US] see iron dextran complex on page 473

DexFol™ [US] see vitamin B complex combinations on page 894

Dexiron™ [Can] see iron dextran complex on page 473

dexmedetomidine (deks MED e toe mi deen)
Sound-Alike/Look-Alike Issues
Precedex™ may be confused with Peridex®
(Continued)

dexmedetomidine *(Continued)*

Synonyms dexmedetomidine hydrochloride

U.S./Canadian Brand Names Precedex™ [US/Can]

Therapeutic Category Alpha-Adrenergic Agonist - Central-Acting (Alpha$_2$-Agonists); Sedative

Use Sedation of initially intubated and mechanically ventilated patients during treatment in an intensive care setting; duration of infusion should not exceed 24 hours

Usual Dosage Individualized and titrated to desired clinical effect

Adults: I.V.: Solution must be diluted prior to administration. Initial: Loading infusion of 1 mcg/kg over 10 minutes, followed by a maintenance infusion of 0.2-0.7 mcg/kg/hour; not indicated for infusions lasting >24 hours

Dosage Forms

Injection, solution [preservative free]:

Precedex™: 100 mcg/mL (2 mL)

dexmedetomidine hydrochloride *see* dexmedetomidine *on previous page*

dexmethylphenidate (dex meth il FEN i date)

Synonyms dexmethylphenidate hydrochloride

U.S./Canadian Brand Names Focalin® XR [US]; Focalin® [US]

Therapeutic Category Central Nervous System Stimulant, Nonamphetamine

Controlled Substance C-II

Use Treatment of attention-deficit/hyperactivity disorder (ADHD)

Usual Dosage Treatment of ADHD: Oral:

Children ≥6 years: Patients not currently taking methylphenidate:

Tablet: Initial: 2.5 mg twice daily; dosage may be adjusted in increments of 2.5-5 mg at weekly intervals (maximum dose: 20 mg/day); doses should be taken at least 4 hours apart

Capsule: Initial: 5 mg/day; dosage may be adjusted in increments of 5 mg/day at weekly intervals (maximum dose: 20 mg/day)

Adults: Patients not currently taking methylphenidate:

Tablet: Initial: 2.5 mg twice daily; dosage may be adjusted in increments of 2.5-5 mg at weekly intervals (maximum dose: 20 mg/day); doses should be taken at least 4 hours apart

Capsule: Initial: 10 mg/day; dosage may be adjusted in increments of 10 mg/day at weekly intervals (maximum dose: 20 mg/day)

Conversion to dexmethylphenidate from methylphenidate: Tablet, capsule: Initial: Half the total daily dose of racemic methylphenidate (maximum dexmethylphenidate dose: 20 mg/day)

Conversion from dexmethylphenidate immediate release to dexmethylphenidate extended release: When changing from Focalin® tablets to Focalin® XR capsules, patients may be switched to the same daily dose using Focalin® XR (maximum dose: 20 mg/day)

Dose reductions and discontinuation: Reduce dose or discontinue in patients with paradoxical aggravation of symptoms. Discontinue if no improvement is seen after one month of treatment.

Dosage Forms

Capsule, extended release:

Focalin® XR: 5 mg, 10 mg, 15 mg, 20 mg

Tablet: 2.5 mg, 5 mg, 10 mg

Focalin®: 2.5 mg, 5 mg, 10 mg

dexmethylphenidate hydrochloride *see* dexmethylphenidate *on this page*

DexPak® TaperPak® [US] *see* dexamethasone (systemic) *on page 241*

dexpanthenol (deks PAN the nole)

Synonyms pantothenyl alcohol

U.S./Canadian Brand Names Panthoderm® [US-OTC]

Therapeutic Category Gastrointestinal Agent, Stimulant

Use Prophylactic use to minimize paralytic ileus; treatment of postoperative distention; topical to relieve itching and to aid healing of minor dermatoses

Usual Dosage

Children and Adults: Relief of itching and aid in skin healing: Topical: Apply to affected area 1-2 times/day

Adults:

Prevention of postoperative ileus: I.M.: 250-500 mg stat, repeat in 2 hours, followed by doses every 6 hours until danger passes

Paralytic ileus: I.M.: 500 mg stat, repeat in 2 hours, followed by doses every 6 hours, if needed

Dosage Forms

Cream, topical:

Panthoderm® [OTC]: 2% (30 g, 60 g)

Injection, solution: 250 mg/mL (2 mL)

Dex PC [US] *see* chlorpheniramine, phenylephrine, and dextromethorphan *on page 180*

dexrazoxane (deks ray ZOKS ane)
Sound-Alike/Look-Alike Issues
Zinecard® may be confused with Gemzar®
Synonyms ICRF-187; NSC-169780
U.S./Canadian Brand Names Zinecard® [US/Can]
Therapeutic Category Cardiovascular Agent, Other
Use
Zinecard®: Reduction of the incidence and severity of cardiomyopathy associated with doxorubicin adminis-tration in women with metastatic breast cancer who have received a cumulative doxorubicin dose of 300 mg/m^2 and who would benefit from continuing therapy with doxorubicin. (It is not recommended for use with initial doxorubicin therapy.)
Totect™: Treatment of anthracycline-induced extravasation.
Usual Dosage I.V.: Adults: Prevention of doxorubicin cardiomyopathy: A 10:1 ratio of dexrazoxane: doxorubicin (500 mg/m^2 dexrazoxane: 50 mg/m^2 doxorubicin)
Dosage Forms
Injection, powder for reconstitution: 250 mg, 500 mg
Totect™: 500 mg
Zinecard®: 250 mg, 500 mg

dextran (DEKS tran)
Sound-Alike/Look-Alike Issues
dextran may be confused with Dexatrim®, Dexedrine®
Synonyms dextran 40; dextran 70; dextran, high molecular weight; dextran, low molecular weight
U.S./Canadian Brand Names Gentran® [US/Can]; LMD® [US]
Therapeutic Category Plasma Volume Expander
Use Blood volume expander used in treatment of shock or impending shock when blood or blood products are not available; dextran 40 is also used as a priming fluid in cardiopulmonary bypass and for prophylaxis of venous thrombosis and pulmonary embolism in surgical procedures associated with a high risk of thrombo-embolic complications
Usual Dosage I.V. (requires an infusion pump): Dose and infusion rate are dependent upon the patient's fluid status and must be individualized:
Volume expansion/shock:
Children (Dextran 40 or 70): Total dose should not exceed 20 mL/kg during first 24 hours
Adults:
Dextran 40: 500-1000 mL at a rate of 20-40 mL/minute (maximum: 20 mL/kg/day for first 24 hours); 10 mL/kg/day thereafter; therapy should not be continued beyond 5 days
Dextran 70: 500-1000 mL at a rate of 20-40 mL/minute (maximum: 20 mL/kg/day for first 24 hours)
Pump prime (Dextran 40): Varies with the volume of the pump oxygenator; generally, the 10% solution is added in a dose of 1-2 g/kg
Prophylaxis of venous thrombosis/pulmonary embolism (Dextran 40): Begin during surgical procedure and give 50-100 g on the day of surgery; an additional 50 g (500 mL) should be administered every 2-3 days during the period of risk (up to 2 weeks postoperatively); usual maximum infusion rate for nonemergency use: 4 mL/minute
Dosage Forms
Infusion [premixed in D_5W; high molecular weight]: 6% Dextran 70 (500 mL)
Infusion [premixed in D_5W; low molecular weight]: 10% Dextran 40 (500 mL)
Gentran®, LMD®: 10% Dextran 40 (500 mL)
Infusion [premixed in $D_{10}W$; high molecular weight]: 32% Dextran 70 (500 mL)
Infusion [premixed in NS; high molecular weight]: 6% Dextran 70 (500 mL)
Gentran®: 6% Dextran 70 (500 mL)
Infusion [premixed in NS; low molecular weight]: 10% Dextran (500 mL)
Gentran®, LMD®: 10% Dextran (500 mL)

dextran 40 *see* dextran *on this page*

dextran 70 *see* dextran *on this page*

dextran 1 (DEKS tran won)
Sound-Alike/Look-Alike Issues
dextran may be confused with Dexatrim®, Dexedrine®
Therapeutic Category Plasma Volume Expander
Use Prophylaxis of serious anaphylactic reactions to I.V. infusion of dextran
(Continued)

dextran 1 *(Continued)*

Usual Dosage I.V. (time between dextran 1 and dextran solution should not exceed 15 minutes):
Children: 0.3 mL/kg 1-2 minutes before I.V. infusion of dextran
Adults: 20 mL 1-2 minutes before I.V. infusion of dextran

dextran, high molecular weight *see* dextran *on previous page*

dextran, low molecular weight *see* dextran *on previous page*

dextroamphetamine (deks troe am FET a meen)

Sound-Alike/Look-Alike Issues
Dexedrine® may be confused with dextran, Excedrin®
Synonyms dextroamphetamine sulfate
U.S./Canadian Brand Names Dexedrine® [US/Can]; Dextrostat® [US]
Therapeutic Category Amphetamine
Controlled Substance C-II
Use Narcolepsy; attention deficit/hyperactivity disorder (ADHD)
Usual Dosage Oral:
Children:
Narcolepsy: 6-12 years: Initial: 5 mg/day; may increase at 5 mg increments in weekly intervals until side effects appear (maximum dose: 60 mg/day)
ADHD:
3-5 years: Initial: 2.5 mg/day given every morning; increase by 2.5 mg/day in weekly intervals until optimal response is obtained; usual range: 0.1-0.5 mg/kg/dose every morning with maximum of 40 mg/day
≥6 years: 5 mg once or twice daily; increase in increments of 5 mg/day at weekly intervals until optimal response is obtained; usual range: 0.1-0.5 mg/kg/dose every morning (5-20 mg/day) with maximum of 40 mg/day
Children >12 years and Adults: Narcolepsy: Initial: 10 mg/day, may increase at 10 mg increments in weekly intervals until side effects appear; maximum: 60 mg/day
Dosage Forms
Capsule, sustained release: 5 mg, 10 mg, 15 mg
Dexedrine® Spansule®: 5 mg, 10 mg, 15 mg
Tablet: 5 mg, 10 mg
Dextrostat®: 5 mg, 10 mg

dextroamphetamine and amphetamine (deks troe am FET a meen & am FET a meen)

Sound-Alike/Look-Alike Issues
Adderall® may be confused with Inderal®
Synonyms amphetamine and dextroamphetamine
U.S./Canadian Brand Names Adderall XR® [US/Can]; Adderall® [US]
Therapeutic Category Amphetamine
Controlled Substance C-II
Use Attention deficit/hyperactivity disorder (ADHD); narcolepsy
Usual Dosage Oral: **Note:** Use lowest effective individualized dose; administer first dose as soon as awake
ADHD:
Children 3-5 years (Adderall®): Initial 2.5 mg/day given every morning; increase daily dose in 2.5 mg increments at weekly intervals until optimal response is obtained (maximum dose: 40 mg/day given in 1-3 divided doses); use intervals of 4-6 hours between additional doses
Children ≥6 years:
Adderall®: Initial: 5 mg 1-2 times/day; increase daily dose in 5 mg increments at weekly intervals until optimal response is obtained (usual maximum dose: 40 mg/day given in 1-3 divided doses); use intervals of 4-6 hours between additional doses
Adderall XR®: 5-10 mg once daily in the morning; if needed, may increase daily dose in 5-10 mg increments at weekly intervals (maximum dose: 30 mg/day)
Adolescents 13-17 years (Adderall XR®): 10 mg once daily in the morning; may be increased to 20 mg/day after 1 week if symptoms are not controlled; higher doses (up to 60 mg)/day have been evaluated; however, there is not adequate evidence that higher doses afforded additional benefit
Adults (Adderall XR®): Initial: 20 mg once daily in the morning; higher doses (up to 60 mg once daily) have been evaluated; however, there is not adequate evidence that higher doses afforded additional benefit
Narcolepsy (Adderall®):
Children 6-12 years: Initial: 5 mg/day; increase daily dose in 5 mg at weekly intervals until optimal response is obtained (maximum dose: 60 mg/day given in 1-3 divided doses with intervals of 4-6 hours between doses)

Children >12 years and Adults: Initial: 10 mg/day; increase daily dose in 10 mg increments at weekly intervals until optimal response is obtained (maximum dose: 60 mg/day given in 1-3 divided doses with intervals of 4-6 hours between doses)

Dosage Forms
Capsule, extended release:
Adderall XR®:
5 mg [dextroamphetamine 1.25 mg, dextroamphetamine saccharate 1.25 mg, amphetamine aspartate monohydrate 1.25 mg, amphetamine sulfate 1.25 mg]
10 mg [dextroamphetamine sulfate 2.5 mg, dextroamphetamine saccharate 2.5 mg, amphetamine aspartate monohydrate 2.5 mg, amphetamine sulfate 2.5 mg]
15 mg [dextroamphetamine sulfate 3.75 mg, dextroamphetamine saccharate 3.75 mg, amphetamine aspartate monohydrate 3.75 mg, amphetamine sulfate 3.75 mg]
20 mg [dextroamphetamine sulfate 5 mg, dextroamphetamine saccharate 5 mg, amphetamine aspartate monohydrate 5 mg, amphetamine sulfate 5 mg]
25 mg [dextroamphetamine sulfate 6.25 mg, dextroamphetamine saccharate 6.25 mg, amphetamine aspartate monohydrate 6.25 mg, amphetamine sulfate 6.25 mg]
30 mg [dextroamphetamine sulfate 7.5 mg, dextroamphetamine saccharate 7.5 mg, amphetamine aspartate monohydrate 7.5 mg, amphetamine sulfate 7.5 mg]
Tablet: 5 mg, 7.5 mg, 10 mg, 12.5 mg, 15 mg, 20 mg, 30 mg
Adderall®:
5 mg [dextroamphetamine sulfate 1.25 mg, dextroamphetamine saccharate 1.25 mg, amphetamine aspartate 1.25 mg, amphetamine sulfate 1.25 mg]
7.5 mg [dextroamphetamine 1.875 mg, dextroamphetamine saccharate 1.875 mg, amphetamine aspartate 1.875 mg, amphetamine sulfate 1.875 mg]
10 mg [dextroamphetamine sulfate 2.5 mg, dextroamphetamine saccharate 2.5 mg, amphetamine aspartate 2.5 mg, amphetamine sulfate 2.5 mg]
12.5 mg [dextroamphetamine sulfate 3.125 mg, dextroamphetamine saccharate 3.125 mg, amphetamine aspartate 3.125 mg, amphetamine sulfate 3.125 mg]
15 mg [dextroamphetamine sulfate 3.75 mg, dextroamphetamine saccharate 3.75 mg, amphetamine aspartate 3.75 mg, amphetamine sulfate 3.75 mg]
20 mg [dextroamphetamine sulfate 5 mg, dextroamphetamine saccharate 5 mg, amphetamine aspartate 5 mg, amphetamine sulfate 5 mg]
30 mg [dextroamphetamine sulfate 7.5 mg, dextroamphetamine saccharate 7.5 mg, amphetamine aspartate 7.5 mg, amphetamine sulfate 7.5 mg]

dextroamphetamine sulfate *see* dextroamphetamine *on previous page*

dextromethorphan (deks troe meth OR fan)
Sound-Alike/Look-Alike Issues
Benylin® may be confused with Benadryl®, Ventolin®
Delsym® may be confused with Delfen®, Desyrel®
U.S./Canadian Brand Names Babee® Cof Syrup [US-OTC]; Creo-Terpin® [US-OTC]; Creomulsion® Cough [US-OTC]; Creomulsion® for Children [US-OTC]; Delsym® [US-OTC]; ElixSure© Cough [US-OTC]; Hold® DM [US-OTC]; PediaCare® Infants' Long-Acting Cough [US-OTC]; Robitussin® CoughGels™ [US-OTC]; Robitussin® Maximum Strength Cough [US-OTC]; Robitussin® Pediatric Cough [US-OTC]; Scot-Tussin DM® Cough Chasers [US-OTC]; Silphen DM® [US-OTC]; Triaminic® Thin Strips™ Long Acting Cough [US-OTC]; Vicks® 44® Cough Relief [US-OTC]
Therapeutic Category Antitussive
Use Symptomatic relief of coughs caused by minor viral upper respiratory tract infections or inhaled irritants; most effective for a chronic nonproductive cough
Usual Dosage Oral:
Children:
<2 years: Use only as directed by a physician
2-6 years (syrup): 2.5-7.5 mg every 4-8 hours; extended release is 15 mg twice daily (maximum: 30 mg/24 hours)
6-12 years: 5-10 mg every 4 hours or 15 mg every 6-8 hours; extended release is 30 mg twice daily (maximum: 60 mg/24 hours)
Children >12 years and Adults: 10-20 mg every 4 hours or 30 mg every 6-8 hours; extended release: 60 mg twice daily; maximum: 120 mg/day
Dosage Forms
Gelcap: 15 mg, 30 mg
Robitussin® CoughGels™ [OTC]: 15 mg
Liquid, oral: 5 mg/5 mL, 10 mg/15 mL
Creo-Terpin® [OTC], Vicks® 44® Cough Relief [OTC]: 10 mg/15 mL
Lozenge: 5 mg (10s, 20s)
Hold® DM [OTC]: 5 mg (10s)
(Continued)

dextromethorphan *(Continued)*

Scot-Tussin DM® Cough Chasers [OTC]: 5 mg (20s)
Strips, oral:
Triaminic® Thin Strips™ Long Acting Cough [OTC]: 7.5 mg
Suspension, extended release: 30 mg/5 mL (89 mL, 148 mL)
Delsym® [OTC]: 30 mg/5 mL (89 mL, 148 mL)
Syrup: 5 mg/5 mL, 7.5 mg/5 mL, 10 mg/5 mL, 15 mg/5 mL, 20 mg/15 mL
Babee® Cof Syrup [OTC], ElixSure® Cough [OTC], Robitussin® Pediatric Cough [OTC]: 7.5 mg/5 mL
Creomulsion® Cough [OTC]: 20 mg/15 mL
Creomulsion® for Children [OTC]: 5 mg/5 mL
Robitussin® Maximum Strength Cough [OTC]: 15 mg/5 mL
Silphen DM® [OTC]: 10 mg/5 mL

dextromethorphan, acetaminophen, and pseudoephedrine *see* acetaminophen, dextromethorphan, and pseudoephedrine *on page 12*

dextromethorphan and guaifenesin *see* guaifenesin and dextromethorphan *on page 402*

dextromethorphan and promethazine *see* promethazine and dextromethorphan *on page 719*

dextromethorphan and pseudoephedrine *see* pseudoephedrine and dextromethorphan *on page 728*

dextromethorphan, carbinoxamine, and pseudoephedrine *see* carbinoxamine, pseudoephedrine, and dextromethorphan *on page 152*

dextromethorphan, chlorpheniramine, and phenylephrine *see* chlorpheniramine, phenylephrine, and dextromethorphan *on page 180*

dextromethorphan, chlorpheniramine, and pseudoephedrine *see* chlorpheniramine, pseudoephedrine, and dextromethorphan *on page 183*

dextromethorphan, chlorpheniramine, phenylephrine, and guaifenesin

(deks troe meth OR fan, klor fen IR a meen, fen il EF rin, & gwye FEN e sin)
Synonyms chlorpheniramine, dextromethorphan, phenylephrine, and guaifenesin; guaifenesin, chlorpheniramine, phenylephrine, and dextromethorphan; phenylephrine hydrochloride, chlorpheniramine maleate, dextromethorphan hydrobromide, and guaifenesin
U.S./Canadian Brand Names Chlordex GP [US]; Donatussin [US]
Therapeutic Category Antihistamine/Decongestant/Antitussive/Expectorant
Use Symptomatic relief of dry, nonproductive cough and upper respiratory symptoms associated with infections such as the common cold, bronchitis, or sinusitis
Usual Dosage General dosing guidelines; consult specific product labeling.
Antitussive/antihistamine/decongestant/expectorant: Oral (Donatussin®):
Children:
2-6 years: 2.5 mL every 6 hours as needed (maximum: 10 mL/24 hours)
6-12 years: 5 mL every 6 hours as needed (maximum: 20 mL/24 hours)
Children ≥12 years and Adults: 10 mL every 6 hours as needed (maximum: 40 mL/24 hours)
Dosage Forms
Liquid:
Chlordex GP®: Dextromethorphan 7.5 mg, chlorpheniramine 2 mg, phenylephrine 10 mg, and guaifenesin 100 mg per 5 mL (480 mL)
Syrup:
Donatussin®: Dextromethorphan 15 mg, chlorpheniramine 2 mg, phenylephrine 10 mg, and guaifenesin 100 mg per 5 mL (480 mL)

dextromethorphan, guaifenesin, and pseudoephedrine *see* guaifenesin, pseudoephedrine, and dextromethorphan *on page 408*

dextromethorphan hydrobromide, acetaminophen, and phenylephrine hydrochloride *see* acetaminophen, dextromethorphan, and phenylephrine *on page 11*

dextromethorphan hydrobromide, brompheniramine maleate, and pseudoephedrine hydrochloride *see* brompheniramine, pseudoephedrine, and dextromethorphan *on page 122*

dextromethorphan, pseudoephedrine, and carbinoxamine *see* carbinoxamine, pseudoephedrine, and dextromethorphan *on page 152*

dextromethorphan tannate, pyrilamine tannate, and phenylephrine tannate *see* phenylephrine, pyrilamine, and dextromethorphan *on page 679*

dextropropoxyphene *see* propoxyphene *on page 723*

dextrose, levulose and phosphoric acid *see* fructose, dextrose, and phosphoric acid *on page 378*

Dextrostat® **[US]** *see* dextroamphetamine *on page 246*

Dey-Dose® **Isoproterenol** *(Discontinued)* *see* isoproterenol *on page 475*

Dey-Dose® **Metaproterenol** *(Discontinued)*

DFMO *see* eflornithine *on page 293*

DHAD *see* mitoxantrone *on page 573*

DHAQ *see* mitoxantrone *on page 573*

DHC® *(Discontinued)* *see* hydrocodone and acetaminophen *on page 427*

DHC Plus® *(Discontinued)*

DHE *see* dihydroergotamine *on page 260*

D.H.E. 45® **[US]** *see* dihydroergotamine *on page 260*

DHPG sodium *see* ganciclovir *on page 383*

DHS™ **Sal [US-OTC]** *see* salicylic acid *on page 772*

DHS™ **Tar [US-OTC]** *see* coal tar *on page 208*

DHS™ **Targel [US-OTC]** *see* coal tar *on page 208*

DHS™ **Zinc [US-OTC]** *see* pyrithione zinc *on page 737*

DHT™ *(Discontinued)*

DHT™ **Intensol**™ *(Discontinued)*

DiabetAid™ **Antifungal Foot Bath [US-OTC]** *see* miconazole *on page 566*

DiabetAid Gingivitis Mouth Rinse [US-OTC] *see* cetylpyridinium *on page 170*

Diabetic Tussin C® **[US]** *see* guaifenesin and codeine *on page 402*

Diabetic Tussin® **Allergy Relief [US-OTC]** *see* chlorpheniramine *on page 177*

Diabetic Tussin® **DM [US-OTC]** *see* guaifenesin and dextromethorphan *on page 402*

Diabetic Tussin® **DM Maximum Strength [US-OTC]** *see* guaifenesin and dextromethorphan *on page 402*

Diabetic Tussin® **EX [US-OTC]** *see* guaifenesin *on page 401*

Diabinese® **[US]** *see* chlorpropamide *on page 185*

Diaβeta® **[US/Can]** *see* glyburide *on page 396*

Dialose® **Tablet** *(Discontinued)* *see* docusate *on page 273*

Dialume® *(Discontinued)* *see* aluminum hydroxide *on page 36*

Diamicron® **[Can]** *see* gliclazide *(Canada only)* *on page 393*

Diamicron® **MR [Can]** *see* gliclazide *(Canada only)* *on page 393*

Diamine T.D.® *(Discontinued)* *see* brompheniramine *on page 120*

diaminocyclohexane oxalatoplatinum *see* oxaliplatin *on page 636*

diaminodiphenylsulfone *see* dapsone *on page 231*

Diamode [US-OTC] *see* loperamide *on page 515*

Diamox® **[Can]** *see* acetazolamide *on page 13*

Diamox® **250 mg Tablet** *(Discontinued)* *see* acetazolamide *on page 13*

Diamox® **Sequels**® **[US]** *see* acetazolamide *on page 13*

Diane-35 [Can] *see* cyproterone and ethinyl estradiol *(Canada only)* *on page 225*

Diar-aid® *(Discontinued)* *see* loperamide *on page 515*

Diarr-Eze [Can] *see* loperamide *on page 515*

Diastat® **[US/Can]** *see* diazepam *on page 251*

Diastat® **AcuDial**™ **[US]** *see* diazepam *on page 251*

Diastat® **Rectal Delivery System [Can]** *see* diazepam *on page 251*

diatrizoate meglumine (dye a tri ZOE ate MEG loo meen)
U.S./Canadian Brand Names Cystografin® Dilute [US]; Cystografin® [US]; Hypaque™ Meglumine [US]; Reno-30® [US]; Reno-60® [US]; Reno-Dip® [US]
Therapeutic Category Iodinated Contrast Media; Radiological/Contrast Media, Ionic
Use
Solution for instillation: Retrograde cystourethrography; retrograde or ascending pyelography
(Continued)

diatrizoate meglumine *(Continued)*

Solution for injection: Arthrography, cerebral angiography, direct cholangiography, discography, drip infusion pyelography, excretory urography, peripheral arteriography, splenoportography, venography; contrast enhancement of computed tomographic head and body imaging

Usual Dosage Dosing is based upon route of administration, type of examination, age of patient, and product used. Consult specific product information for detailed dosing.

Dosage Forms

Solution, for instillation:
Cystografin®: Diatrizoate meglumine 30% (100 mL, 300 mL)
Cystografin® Dilute: Diatrizoate meglumine 18% (300 mL)
Reno-30®: Diatrizoate meglumine 30% (50 mL)

Solution, injection:
Hypaque™ Meglumine: Diatrizoate meglumine 60% (150 mL)
Reno-60®: Diatrizoate meglumine 60% (50 mL)
Reno-Dip®: Diatrizoate meglumine 30% (300 mL)

diatrizoate meglumine and diatrizoate sodium

(dye a tri ZOE ate MEG loo meen & dye a tri ZOE ate SOW dee um)

Synonyms diatrizoate sodium and diatrizoate meglumine

U.S./Canadian Brand Names Gastrografin® [US]; Hypaque™-76 [US]; MD-76®R [US]; MD-Gastroview® [US]; RenoCal-76® [US]; Renografin®-60 [US]

Therapeutic Category Iodinated Contrast Media; Radiological/Contrast Media, Ionic

Use

Oral/rectal: Examination of GI tract; adjunct to contrast enhancement in computed tomography of the torso
Injection: Angiocardiography, aortography, central venography, cerebral angiography, cholangiography, digital arteriography, excretory urography, nephrotomography, peripheral angiography, peripheral arteriography, renal arteriography, renal venography, splenoportography, visceral arteriography; contrast enhancement of computed tomographic imaging

Usual Dosage

Radiographic exam of GI tract segments:
Oral:
Children <5 years: 30 mL, dilute 1:1 (if <10 kg or debilitated, dilute 1:3)
Children 5-10 years: 60 mL, dilute 1:1 (if <10 kg or debilitated, dilute 1:3)
Adults: 30-90 mL
Rectal enema:
Children <5 years: Dilute 1:5 in tap water
Children >5 years: Dilute 90 mL in 500 mL tap water
Adults: Dilute 240 mL in 1000 mL tap water
Tomography: Adults: Oral: 25-77 mL in 1000 mL tap water 15-30 minutes prior to imaging

Dosage Forms

Solution, injection:
Hypaque™-76: Diatrizoate meglumine 66% and diatrizoate sodium 10% (50 mL, 200 mL)
MD-76®R: Diatrizoate meglumine 66% and diatrizoate sodium 10% (50 mL, 100 mL, 150 mL, 200 mL)
RenoCal-76®: Diatrizoate meglumine 66% and diatrizoate sodium 10% (50 mL)
Renografin®-60: Diatrizoate meglumine 520 mg and diatrizoate sodium 80 mg per mL (10 mL, 50 mL, 100 mL)

Solution, oral/rectal:
Gastrografin®: Diatrizoate meglumine 660 mg and diatrizoate sodium 100 mg per mL
MD-Gastroview®: Diatrizoate meglumine 660 mg and diatrizoate sodium 100 mg per mL

diatrizoate meglumine and iodipamide meglumine

(dye a tri ZOE ate MEG loo meen & eye oh DI pa mide MEG loo meen)

Synonyms iodipamide meglumine and diatrizoate meglumine

U.S./Canadian Brand Names Sinografin® [US]

Therapeutic Category Iodinated Contrast Media; Radiological/Contrast Media, Ionic

Use Hysterosalpingography

Dosage Forms

Injection, solution [for cervical instillation]:
Sinografin®: Diatrizoate meglumine 524 mg and iodipamide meglumine 268 mg per mL (10 mL)

diatrizoate sodium (dye a tri ZOE ate SOW dee um)

U.S./Canadian Brand Names Hypaque™ Sodium [US]

Therapeutic Category Iodinated Contrast Media; Radiological/Contrast Media, Ionic

Use Radiographic examination of GI tract

Usual Dosage
Oral:
Infants and Children: 20% to 40% solution: 30-75 mL
Adults: 25% to 40% solution: 90-180 mL
Rectal: Enema:
Infants and Children: 10% to 15% solution: 100-500 mL depending on weight of patient
Adults: 15% to 25% solution: 500-1000 mL
Dosage Forms
Powder for solution, oral/rectal:
Hypaque™ Sodium: Diatrizoate sodium (250 g)

diatrizoate sodium and diatrizoate meglumine *see* diatrizoate meglumine and diatrizoate sodium *on previous page*

Diatx®Zn [US] *see* vitamins (multiple/oral) *on page 895*

Diazemuls® [Can] *see* diazepam *on this page*

Diazemuls® Injection (Discontinued) *see* diazepam *on this page*

diazepam (dye AZ e pam)
Sound-Alike/Look-Alike Issues
diazepam may be confused with diazoxide, Ditropan®, lorazepam
Valium® may be confused with Valcyte™
U.S./Canadian Brand Names Apo-Diazepam® [Can]; Diastat® AcuDial™ [US]; Diastat® Rectal Delivery System [Can]; Diastat® [US/Can]; Diazemuls® [Can]; Diazepam Intensol® [US]; Novo-Dipam [Can]; Valium® [US/Can]
Therapeutic Category Benzodiazepine
Controlled Substance C-IV
Use Management of anxiety disorders, ethanol withdrawal symptoms; skeletal muscle relaxant; treatment of convulsive disorders
Rectal gel: Management of selected, refractory epilepsy patients on stable regimens of antiepileptic drugs (AEDs) requiring intermittent use of diazepam to control episodes of increased seizure activity
Usual Dosage Oral absorption is more reliable than I.M.
Children:
Conscious sedation for procedures: Oral: 0.2-0.3 mg/kg (maximum: 10 mg) 45-60 minutes prior to procedure
Sedation/muscle relaxant/anxiety:
Oral: 0.12-0.8 mg/kg/day in divided doses every 6-8 hours
I.M., I.V.: 0.04-0.3 mg/kg/dose every 2-4 hours to a maximum of 0.6 mg/kg within an 8-hour period if needed
Status epilepticus:
Infants 30 days to 5 years: I.V.: 0.05-0.3 mg/kg/dose given over 2-3 minutes, every 15-30 minutes to a maximum total dose of 5 mg; repeat in 2-4 hours as needed **or** 0.2-0.5 mg/dose every 2-5 minutes to a maximum total dose of 5 mg
>5 years: I.V.: 0.05-0.3 mg/kg/dose given over 2-3 minutes every 15-30 minutes to a maximum total dose of 10 mg; repeat in 2-4 hours as needed **or** 1 mg/dose given over 2-3 minutes, every 2-5 minutes to a maximum total dose of 10 mg
Rectal: 0.5 mg/kg, then 0.25 mg/kg in 10 minutes if needed (prepare dose using parenteral formulation)
Anticonvulsant (acute treatment): Rectal gel:
Children <2 years: Safety and efficacy have not been studied
Children 2-5 years: 0.5 mg/kg
Children 6-11 years: 0.3 mg/kg
Children ≥12 years: 0.2 mg/kg
Note: Dosage should be rounded upward to the next available dose, 2.5, 5, 7.5, 10, 12.5, 15, 17.5, and 20 mg/dose; dose may be repeated in 4-12 hours if needed; do not use for more than 5 episodes per month or more than one episode every 5 days
Adolescents: Conscious sedation for procedures:
Oral: 10 mg
I.V.: 5 mg, may repeat with ¹/₂ dose if needed
Adults:
Anticonvulsant (acute treatment): Rectal gel: 0.2 mg/kg
Note: Dosage should be rounded upward to the next available dose, 2.5, 5, 7.5, 10, 12.5, 15, 17.5, and 20 mg/dose; dose may be repeated in 4-12 hours if needed; do not use for more than 5 episodes per month or more than one episode every 5 days.
Anxiety/sedation/skeletal muscle relaxant:
Oral: 2-10 mg 2-4 times/day
I.M., I.V.: 2-10 mg, may repeat in 3-4 hours if needed
Sedation in the ICU patient: I.V.: 0.03-0.1 mg/kg every 30 minutes to 6 hours
(Continued)

diazepam *(Continued)*

Status epilepticus: I.V.: 5-10 mg every 10-20 minutes, up to 30 mg in an 8-hour period; may repeat in 2-4 hours if necessary

Rapid tranquilization of agitated patient (administer every 30-60 minutes): Oral: 5-10 mg; average total dose for tranquilization: 20-60 mg

Dosage Forms
Gel, rectal:
Diastat®: Pediatric rectal tip [4.4 cm]: 5 mg/mL (2.5 mg, 5 mg)
Diastat® AcuDial™ delivery system:
10 mg: Pediatric/adult rectal tip [4.4 cm]: 5 mg/mL (delivers set doses of 5 mg, 7.5 mg, and 10 mg)
20 mg: Adult rectal tip [6 cm]: 5 mg/mL (delivers set doses of 10 mg, 12.5 mg, 15 mg, 17.5 mg, and 20 mg)
Injection, solution: 5 mg/mL (2 mL, 10 mL)
Solution, oral: 5 mg/5 mL
Solution, oral concentrate: 5 mg/mL
Diazepam Intensol®: 5 mg/mL
Tablet: 2 mg, 5 mg, 10 mg
Valium®: 2 mg, 5 mg, 10 mg

Diazepam Intensol® [US] *see* diazepam *on previous page*

diazoxide *(dye az OKS ide)*
Sound-Alike/Look-Alike Issues
diazoxide may be confused with diazepam, Dyazide®
Hyperstat® may be confused with Nitrostat®
U.S./Canadian Brand Names Proglycem® [US/Can]
Therapeutic Category Antihypertensive Agent; Antihypoglycemic Agent
Use
Oral: Hypoglycemia related to islet cell adenoma, carcinoma, hyperplasia, or adenomatosis, nesidioblastosis, leucine sensitivity, or extrapancreatic malignancy
I.V.: Severe hypertension
Usual Dosage
Hypertension: Children and Adults: I.V.: 1-3 mg/kg up to a maximum of 150 mg in a single injection; repeat dose in 5-15 minutes until blood pressure adequately reduced; repeat administration at intervals of 4-24 hours; monitor the blood pressure closely; do not use longer than 10 days
Hyperinsulinemic hypoglycemia: Oral: **Note:** Use lower dose listed as initial dose
Newborns and Infants: 8-15 mg/kg/day in divided doses every 8-12 hours
Children and Adults: 3-8 mg/kg/day in divided doses every 8-12 hours
Dosage Forms [CAN] = Canadian brand name
Capsule:
Proglycem® [CAN]: 50 mg [not available in the U.S.]
Suspension, oral:
Proglycem®: 50 mg/mL

Dibent® Injection *(Discontinued)* *see* dicyclomine *on page 255*

Dibenzyline® [US/Can] *see* phenoxybenzamine *on page 674*

dibucaine *(DYE byoo kane)*
U.S./Canadian Brand Names Nupercainal® [US-OTC]
Therapeutic Category Local Anesthetic
Use Fast, temporary relief of pain and itching due to hemorrhoids, minor burns
Usual Dosage Topical: Children and Adults: Apply gently to the affected areas; no more than 30 g for adults or 7.5 g for children should be used in any 24-hour period
Dosage Forms
Ointment: 1% (30 g, 454 g)
Nupercainal® [OTC]: 1% (30 g, 60g)

DIC *see* dacarbazine *on page 227*

Dicarbosil® *(Discontinued)* *see* calcium carbonate *on page 138*

Dicel™ [US] *see* chlorpheniramine and pseudoephedrine *on page 178*

Dicel™ DM [US] *see* chlorpheniramine, pseudoephedrine, and dextromethorphan *on page 183*

Dicetel® [Can] *see* pinaverium *(Canada only) on page 683*

dichloralphenazone, acetaminophen, and isometheptene *see* acetaminophen, isometheptene, and dichloralphenazone *on page 13*

dichloralphenazone, isometheptene, and acetaminophen *see* acetaminophen, isometheptene, and dichloralphenazone *on page 13*

6,7-dichloro-1,5-dihydroimidazo [2,1b] quinazolin-2(3H)-one monohydrochloride *see* anagrelide *on page 55*

dichlorodifluoromethane and trichloromonofluoromethane
(dye klor oh dye flor oh METH ane & tri klor oh mon oh flor oh METH ane)
Synonyms trichloromonofluoromethane and dichlorodifluoromethane
U.S./Canadian Brand Names Fluori-Methane® [US]
Therapeutic Category Analgesic, Topical
Use Management of pain associated with injections
Usual Dosage Invert bottle over treatment area approximately 12" away from site of application; open dispenseal spring valve completely, allowing liquid to flow in a stream from the bottle. The rate of spraying is approximately 10 cm/second and should be continued until entire muscle has been covered.
Dosage Forms
 Aerosol, topical:
  Fluori-Methane®: Dichlorodifluoromethane 15% and trichloromonofluoromethane 85% (103 mL)

dichlorotetrafluoroethane and ethyl chloride *see* ethyl chloride and dichlorotetrafluoroethane *on page 334*

dichlorphenamide (dye klor FEN a mide)
Sound-Alike/Look-Alike Issues
 Daranide® may be confused with Daraprim®
Synonyms diclofenamide
U.S./Canadian Brand Names Daranide® [US/Can]
Therapeutic Category Carbonic Anhydrase Inhibitor; Diuretic, Carbonic Anhydrase Inhibitor; Ophthalmic Agent, Antiglaucoma
Use Adjunct in treatment of open-angle glaucoma and perioperative treatment for angle-closure glaucoma
Usual Dosage Oral: Adults: 100-200 mg to start followed by 100 mg every 12 hours until desired response is obtained; maintenance dose: 25-50 mg 1-3 times/day
Dosage Forms
 Tablet:
  Daranide®: 50 mg

Dickinson's® Witch Hazel [US-OTC] *see* witch hazel *on page 900*

Diclectin® [Can] *see* doxylamine and pyridoxine *(Canada only) on page 283*

diclofenac (dye KLOE fen ak)
Sound-Alike/Look-Alike Issues
 diclofenac may be confused with Diflucan®, Duphalac®
 Cataflam® may be confused with Catapres®
 Voltaren® may be confused with tramadol, Ultram®, Verelan®
Synonyms diclofenac potassium; diclofenac sodium
U.S./Canadian Brand Names Apo-Diclo Rapide® [Can]; Apo-Diclo SR® [Can]; Apo-Diclo® [Can]; Cataflam® [US/Can]; Novo-Difenac K [Can]; Novo-Difenac [Can]; Novo-Difenac-SR [Can]; Nu-Diclo [Can]; Nu-Diclo-SR [Can]; Pennsaid® [Can]; PMS-Diclofenac SR [Can]; PMS-Diclofenac [Can]; Riva-Diclofenac [Can]; Riva-Diclofenac-K [Can]; Solaraze® [US]; Voltaren Ophthalmic® [US]; Voltaren Ophtha® [Can]; Voltaren Rapide® [Can]; Voltaren® [US/Can]; Voltaren®-XR [US]
Therapeutic Category Analgesic, Nonnarcotic; Nonsteroidal Antiinflammatory Drug (NSAID)
Use
 Immediate release: Ankylosing spondylitis; primary dysmenorrhea; acute and chronic treatment of rheumatoid arthritis, osteoarthritis
 Delayed-release tablets: Acute and chronic treatment of rheumatoid arthritis, osteoarthritis, ankylosing spondylitis
 Extended-release tablets: Chronic treatment of osteoarthritis, rheumatoid arthritis
 Ophthalmic solution: Postoperative inflammation following cataract extraction; temporary relief of pain and photophobia in patients undergoing corneal refractive surgery
 Topical gel: Actinic keratosis (AK) in conjunction with sun avoidance
Usual Dosage Adults:
 Oral:
  Analgesia/primary dysmenorrhea: Starting dose: 50 mg 3 times/day; maximum dose: 150 mg/day
  Rheumatoid arthritis: 150-200 mg/day in 2-4 divided doses (100 mg/day of sustained release product)
  Osteoarthritis: 100-150 mg/day in 2-3 divided doses (100-200 mg/day of sustained release product)
(Continued)

253

diclofenac *(Continued)*

Ankylosing spondylitis: 100-125 mg/day in 4-5 divided doses
Ophthalmic:
Cataract surgery: Instill 1 drop into affected eye 4 times/day beginning 24 hours after cataract surgery and continuing for 2 weeks
Corneal refractive surgery: Instill 1-2 drops into affected eye within the hour prior to surgery, within 15 minutes following surgery, and then continue for 4 times/day, up to 3 days
Topical: Apply gel to lesion area twice daily for 60-90 days

Dosage Forms
Gel:
Solaraze®: 30 mg/g (50 g)
Solution, ophthalmic:
Voltaren Ophthalmic®: 0.1% (2.5 mL, 5 mL)
Tablet: 50 mg
Cataflam®: 50 mg
Tablet, delayed release, enteric coated: 50 mg, 75 mg
Voltaren®: 75 mg
Tablet, extended release: 100 mg
Voltaren®-XR: 100 mg

diclofenac and misoprostol (dye KLOE fen ak & mye soe PROST ole)

Synonyms misoprostol and diclofenac
U.S./Canadian Brand Names Arthrotec® [US/Can]
Therapeutic Category Analgesic, Nonnarcotic; Prostaglandin
Use The diclofenac component is indicated for the treatment of osteoarthritis and rheumatoid arthritis; the misoprostol component is indicated for the prophylaxis of NSAID-induced gastric and duodenal ulceration
Usual Dosage Oral: Adults:
Arthrotec® 50:
Osteoarthritis: 1 tablet 2-3 times/day
Rheumatoid arthritis: 1 tablet 3-4 times/day
For both regimens, if not tolerated by patient, the dose may be reduced to 1 tablet twice daily
Arthrotec® 75:
Patients who cannot tolerate full daily Arthrotec® 50 regimens: 1 tablet twice daily
Note: The use of these tablets may not be as effective at preventing GI ulceration

Dosage Forms
Tablet:
Arthrotec®: Diclofenac 50 mg and misoprostol 200 mcg; diclofenac 75 mg and misoprostol 200 mcg

diclofenac potassium *see* diclofenac *on previous page*

diclofenac sodium *see* diclofenac *on previous page*

diclofenamide *see* dichlorphenamide *on previous page*

dicloxacillin (dye kloks a SIL in)

Synonyms dicloxacillin sodium
U.S./Canadian Brand Names Dycill® [Can]; Pathocil® [Can]
Therapeutic Category Penicillin
Use Treatment of systemic infections such as pneumonia, skin and soft tissue infections, and osteomyelitis caused by penicillinase-producing staphylococci
Usual Dosage
Usual dosage range:
Children <40 kg: Oral: 12.5-100 mg/kg/day divided every 6 hours
Children >40 kg: Oral: 125-250 mg every 6 hours
Adults: Oral: 125-1000 mg every 6 hours
Indication-specific dosing:
Children: Oral:
Furunculosis: 25-50 mg/kg/day divided every 6 hours
Osteomyelitis: 50-100 mg/kg/day in divided doses every 6 hours
Adults: Oral:
Erysipelas, furunculosis, mastitis, otitis externa, septic bursitis, skin abscess: 500 mg every 6 hours
Impetigo: 250 mg every 6 hours
Prosthetic joint (long-term suppression therapy): 250 mg twice daily
Staphylococcus aureus, **methicillin susceptible infection if no I.V. access:** 500-1000 mg every 6-8 hours

Dosage Forms
Capsule: 250 mg, 500 mg

dicloxacillin sodium *see* dicloxacillin *on previous page*

dicyclomine (dye SYE kloe meen)

Sound-Alike/Look-Alike Issues
dicyclomine may be confused with diphenhydrAMINE, doxycycline, dyclonine
Bentyl® may be confused with Aventyl®, Benadryl®, Bontril®, Cantil®, Proventil®, Trental®
Synonyms dicyclomine hydrochloride; dicycloverine hydrochloride
U.S./Canadian Brand Names Bentylol® [Can]; Bentyl® [US]; Formulex® [Can]; Lomine [Can]; Riva-Dicyclomine [Can]
Therapeutic Category Anticholinergic Agent
Use Treatment of functional bowel/irritable bowel syndrome
Usual Dosage Adults:
Oral: Initiate with 80 mg/day in 4 equally divided doses, then increase up to 160 mg/day. Duration: Safety data not available for duration >2 weeks.
I.M. (**should not be used I.V.**): 80 mg/day in 4 divided doses (20 mg/dose)
Dosage Forms
Capsule: 10 mg
Bentyl®: 10 mg
Injection, solution: 10 mg/mL (2 mL)
Bentyl®: 10 mg/mL (2 mL)
Syrup:
Bentyl®: 10 mg/5 mL
Tablet: 20 mg
Bentyl®: 20 mg

dicyclomine hydrochloride *see* dicyclomine *on this page*

dicycloverine hydrochloride *see* dicyclomine *on this page*

Di-Dak-Sol [US] *see* sodium hypochlorite solution *on page 794*

didanosine (dye DAN oh seen)

Sound-Alike/Look-Alike Issues
Videx® may be confused with Lidex®
Synonyms ddI; dideoxyinosine
U.S./Canadian Brand Names Videx® EC [US/Can]; Videx® [US/Can]
Therapeutic Category Antiviral Agent
Use Treatment of HIV infection; always to be used in combination with at least two other antiretroviral agents
Usual Dosage Treatment of HIV infection: Oral (administer on an empty stomach):
Children: Pediatric powder for oral solution (Videx®):
2 weeks to 8 months: 100 mg/m^2 twice daily is recommended by the manufacturer; 50 mg/m^2 may be considered in infants 2 weeks to 4 months
>8 months: 120 mg/m^2 twice daily; dosing range: 90-150 mg/m^2 twice daily; patients with CNS disease may require higher dose
Adolescents and Adults: Dosing based on patient weight:
Pediatric powder for oral solution (Videx®):
<60 kg: 125 mg twice daily or 250 mg once daily
≥60 kg: 200 mg twice daily or 400 mg once daily
Delayed release capsule (Videx® EC):
<60 kg: 250 mg once daily
≥60 kg; 400 mg once daily
Dosage Forms
Capsule, delayed release, enteric coated pellets: 200 mg, 250 mg, 400 mg
Capsule, delayed release, enteric coated beadlets:
Videx® EC: 125 mg, 200 mg, 250 mg, 400 mg
Powder for oral solution, pediatric:
Videx®: 2 g, 4 g

dideoxyinosine *see* didanosine *on this page*

Didrex® [US/Can] *see* benzphetamine *on page 105*

Didrocal™ [Can] *see* etidronate and calcium *on page 334*

Didronel® [US/Can] *see* etidronate disodium *on page 335*

dietary supplements *see* nutritional formula, enteral/oral *on page 622*

diethylene triamine penta-acetic acid (dye ETH i leen TRYE a meen PEN ta a SEE tik AS id)

Synonyms Ca-DTPA; diethylenetriamine pentaacetic acid; DTPA; pentetate calcium trisodium; pentetate zinc trisodium; trisodium calcium diethylenetriaminepentaacetate (Ca-DTPA); zinc diethylenetriaminepentaacetate (Zn-DTPA); Zn-DTPA

Therapeutic Category Antidote

Use Treatment of known or suspected internal contamination with plutonium, americium, or curium

Usual Dosage Internal contamination with plutonium, americium, or curium: Ca-DTPA is the preferred initial agent; sequential administration of Ca-DTPA then Zn-DTPA is recommended. I.V.:

Children <12 years:
  Initial: Ca-DTPA: 14 mg/kg/day (maximum dose: 1 g/day)
  Maintenance: Zn-DTPA: 14 mg/kg/day (maximum: 1 g/day); length of therapy depends on patient response and degree of contamination. **Note:** An equivalent dose of Ca-DTPA should be used for maintenance therapy only if Zn-DTPA is not available.

Children ≥12 years and Adults:
  Initial: Ca-DTPA: 1 g/day
  Pregnancy: Zn-DTPA 1 g/day should be used for the initial dose in pregnant women **except** in cases of high internal contamination
  Maintenance: Zn-DTPA: 1 g/day; length of therapy depends on patient response and degree of contamination. **Note:** An equivalent dose of Ca-DTPA should be used for maintenance therapy only if Zn-DTPA is not available.

Dosage Forms
Injection, solution:
  Ca-DTPA: 200 mg/mL (5 mL)
  Zn-DTPA: 200 mg/mL (5 mL)

diethylenetriamine pentaacetic acid *see* diethylene triamine penta-acetic acid *on this page*

diethylpropion (dye eth il PROE pee on)

Synonyms amfepramone; diethylpropion hydrochloride

U.S./Canadian Brand Names Tenuate® Dospan® [Can]; Tenuate® [Can]

Therapeutic Category Anorexiant

Controlled Substance C-IV

Use Short-term (few weeks) adjunct in the management of exogenous obesity

Usual Dosage Oral: Children >16 years and Adults:
  Tablet: 25 mg 3 times/day before meals or food
  Tablet, controlled release: 75 mg at midmorning

Dosage Forms
Tablet: 25 mg
Tablet, controlled release: 75 mg

diethylpropion hydrochloride *see* diethylpropion *on this page*

difenoxin and atropine (dye fen OKS in & A troe peen)

Synonyms atropine and difenoxin

U.S./Canadian Brand Names Motofen® [US]

Therapeutic Category Antidiarrheal

Controlled Substance C-IV

Use Treatment of diarrhea

Usual Dosage Oral: Adults: Initial: 2 tablets (each tablet contains difenoxin hydrochloride 1 mg and atropine sulfate 0.025 mg), then 1 tablet after each loose stool; 1 tablet every 3-4 hours, up to 8 tablets in a 24-hour period; if no improvement after 48 hours, continued administration is not indicated

Dosage Forms
Tablet:
  Motofen®: Difenoxin 1 mg and atropine 0.025 mg

Differin® [US/Can] *see* adapalene *on page 18*

Differin® XP [Can] *see* adapalene *on page 18*

Difil-G [US] *see* dyphylline and guaifenesin *on page 288*

Difil®-G Forte [US] *see* dyphylline and guaifenesin *on page 288*

diflorasone (dye FLOR a sone)
Sound-Alike/Look-Alike Issues
Psorcon® may be confused with Proscar®, ProSom®, Psorion®
Synonyms diflorasone diacetate
U.S./Canadian Brand Names ApexiCon™ E [US]; ApexiCon™ [US]; Florone® [US/Can]; Psorcon® [Can]
Therapeutic Category Corticosteroid, Topical
Use Relieves inflammation and pruritic symptoms of corticosteroid-responsive dermatosis (high to very high potency topical corticosteroid)

Maxiflor®: High potency topical corticosteroid
Psorcon®: Very high potency topical corticosteroid
Usual Dosage Topical: Apply ointment sparingly 1-3 times/day; apply cream sparingly 2-4 times/day. Therapy should be discontinued when control is achieved; if no improvement is seen, reassessment of diagnosis may be necessary.
Dosage Forms
Cream: 0.05% (15 g, 30 g, 60 g)
ApexiCon™ E, Florone®: 0.05% (30 g, 60 g)
Ointment: 0.05% (15 g, 30 g, 60 g)
ApexiCon™: 0.05% (30 g, 60 g)

diflorasone diacetate *see* diflorasone *on this page*

Diflucan® [US/Can] *see* fluconazole *on page 356*

diflunisal (dye FLOO ni sal)
Sound-Alike/Look-Alike Issues
Dolobid® may be confused with Slo-Bid®
U.S./Canadian Brand Names Apo-Diflunisal® [Can]; Novo-Diflunisal [Can]; Nu-Diflunisal [Can]
Therapeutic Category Analgesic, Nonnarcotic; Nonsteroidal Antiinflammatory Drug (NSAID)
Use Management of inflammatory disorders usually including rheumatoid arthritis and osteoarthritis; can be used as an analgesic for treatment of mild to moderate pain
Usual Dosage Oral: Adults:
Mild-to-moderate pain: Initial: 500-1000 mg followed by 250-500 mg every 8-12 hours; maximum daily dose: 1.5 g
Arthritis: 500-1000 mg/day in 2 divided doses; maximum daily dose: 1.5 g
Dosage Forms
Tablet: 500 mg

Digibind® [US/Can] *see* digoxin immune Fab *on next page*

DigiFab™ [US] *see* digoxin immune Fab *on next page*

Digitek® [US] *see* digoxin *on this page*

digoxin (di JOKS in)
Sound-Alike/Look-Alike Issues
digoxin may be confused with Desoxyn®, doxepin
Lanoxin® may be confused with Lasix®, Levoxyl®, Levsinex®, Lomotil®, Lonox®, Mefoxin®, Xanax®
U.S./Canadian Brand Names Apo-Digoxin® [Can]; Digitek® [US]; Digoxin CSD [Can]; Lanoxicaps® [US/Can]; Lanoxin® [US/Can]; Novo-Digoxin [Can]; Pediatric Digoxin CSD [Can]
Therapeutic Category Antiarrhythmic Agent, Miscellaneous; Cardiac Glycoside
Use Treatment of congestive heart failure and to slow the ventricular rate in tachyarrhythmias such as atrial fibrillation, atrial flutter, and supraventricular tachycardia (paroxysmal atrial tachycardia); cardiogenic shock
Usual Dosage When changing from oral (tablets or liquid) or I.M. to I.V. therapy, dosage should be reduced by 20% to 25%. Refer to the following:

Preterm infant[1]:
Total digitalizing dose[2]:
Oral: 20-30 mcg/kg[1]
I.V. or I.M.: 15-25 mcg/kg[1]
Daily maintenance dose[3]:
Oral: 5-7.5 mcg/kg[1]
I.V. or I.M.: 4-6 mcg/kg[1]
Full-term infant[1]:
Total digitalizing dose[2]:
Oral: 25-35 mcg/kg[1]
I.V. or I.M.: 20-30 mcg/kg[1]
(Continued)

digoxin *(Continued)*

Daily maintenance dose[3]:
Oral: 6-10 mcg/kg[1]
I.V. or I.M.: 5-8 mcg/kg[1]
1 month to 2 years[1]:
Total digitalizing dose[2]:
Oral: 35-60 mcg/kg[1]
I.V. or I.M.: 30-50 mcg/kg[1]
Daily maintenance dose[3]:
Oral: 10-15 mcg/kg[1]
I.V. or I.M.: 7.5-12 mcg/kg[1]
2-5 years[1]:
Total digitalizing dose[2]:
Oral: 30-40 mcg/kg[1]
I.V. or I.M.: 25-35 mcg/kg[1]
Daily maintenance dose[3]:
Oral: 7.5-10 mcg/kg[1]
I.V. or I.M.: 6-9 mcg/kg[1]
5-10 years[1]:
Total digitalizing dose[2]:
Oral: 20-35 mcg/kg[1]
I.V. or I.M.: 15-30 mcg/kg[1]
Daily maintenance dose[3]:
Oral: 5-10 mcg/kg[1]
I.V. or I.M.: 4-8 mcg/kg[1]
>10 years[1]:
Total digitalizing dose[2]:
Oral: 10-15 mcg/kg[1]
I.V. or I.M.: 8-12 mcg/kg[1]
Daily maintenance dose[3]:
Oral: 2.5-5 mcg/kg[1]
I.V. or I.M.: 2-3 mcg/kg[1]
Adults:
Total digitalizing dose[2]:
Oral: 0.75-1.5 mg
I.V. or I.M.: 0.5-1 mg
Daily maintenance dose[3]:
Oral: 0.125-0.5 mg
I.V. or I.M.: 0.1-0.4 mg

[1]Based on lean body weight and normal renal function for age. Decrease dose in patients with decreased renal function; digitalizing dose often not recommended in infants and children.

[2]Give one-half of the total digitalizing dose (TDD) in the initial dose, then give one-quarter of the TDD in each of two subsequent doses at 8- to 12-hour intervals. Obtain EKG 6 hours after each dose to assess potential toxicity.

[3]Divided every 12 hours in infants and children <10 years of age. Give once daily to children >10 years of age and adults.

Dosage Forms
Capsule:
Lanoxicaps®: 100 mcg, 200 mcg
Injection: 250 mcg/mL (1 mL, 2 mL)
Lanoxin®: 250 mcg/mL (2 mL)
Injection, pediatric: 100 mcg/mL (1 mL)
Solution, oral: 50 mcg/mL (2.5 mL, 5 mL, 60 mL)
Tablet: 125 mcg, 250 mcg
Digitek®, Lanoxin®: 125 mcg, 250 mcg

Digoxin CSD [Can] *see* digoxin *on previous page*

digoxin immune Fab (di JOKS in i MYUN fab)

Synonyms antidigoxin fab fragments, ovine
U.S./Canadian Brand Names Digibind® [US/Can]; DigiFab™ [US]
Therapeutic Category Antidote
Use Treatment of life-threatening or potentially life-threatening digoxin intoxication, including:
• acute digoxin ingestion (ie, >10 mg in adults or >4 mg in children)
• chronic ingestions leading to steady-state digoxin concentrations >6 ng/mL in adults or >4 ng/mL in children

- manifestations of digoxin toxicity due to overdose (life-threatening ventricular arrhythmias, progressive bradycardia, second- or third-degree heart block not responsive to atropine, serum potassium >5 mEq/L in adults or >6 mEq in children)

Usual Dosage Each vial of Digibind® 38 mg or DigiFab™ 40 mg will bind ~0.5 mg of digoxin or digitoxin.

Estimation of the dose is based on the body burden of digitalis. This may be calculated if the amount ingested is known or the postdistribution serum drug level is known (round dose to the nearest whole vial). Fab dose (in vials) based on number of tablets (0.25 mg) ingested.

5 tablets ingested: 2 vials
10 tablets ingested: 4 vials
25 tablets ingested: 10 vials
50 tablets ingested: 20 vials
75 tablets ingested: 30 vials
100 tablets ingested: 40 vials
150 tablets ingested: 60 vials
200 tablets ingested: 80 vials

Fab dose based on serum drug level postdistribution:
Digoxin: No. of vials = level (ng/mL) x body weight (kg) divided by 100
Digitoxin: No. of vials = digitoxin (ng/mL) x body weight (kg) divided by 1000
If neither amount ingested nor drug level are known, dose empirically as follows:
For acute toxicity: 20 vials, administered in 2 divided doses to decrease the possibility of a febrile reaction, and to avoid fluid overload in small children.
For chronic toxicity: 6 vials; for infants and small children (≤20kg), a single vial may be sufficient

Dosage Forms
Injection, powder for reconstitution:
Digibind®: 38 mg
DigiFab™: 40 mg

dihematoporphyrin ether *see* porfimer *on page 698*

Dihistine® DH *(Discontinued)* *see* chlorpheniramine, pseudoephedrine, and codeine *on page 183*

dihydrocodeine, aspirin, and caffeine (dye hye droe KOE deen, AS pir in, & KAF een)
Sound-Alike/Look-Alike Issues
Synalgos®-DC may be confused with Synagis®
Synonyms dihydrocodeine compound
U.S./Canadian Brand Names Synalgos®-DC [US]
Therapeutic Category Analgesic, Narcotic
Controlled Substance C-III
Use Management of mild to moderate pain that requires relaxation
Usual Dosage Oral: Adults: 1-2 capsules every 4-6 hours as needed for pain
Dosage Forms
Capsule:
Synalgos®-DC: Dihydrocodeine 16 mg, aspirin 356.4 mg, and caffeine 30 mg

dihydrocodeine bitartrate, acetaminophen, and caffeine *see* acetaminophen, caffeine, and dihydrocodeine *on page 10*

dihydrocodeine bitartrate, phenylephrine hydrochloride, and chlorpheniramine maleate *see* phenylephrine, hydrocodone, and chlorpheniramine *on page 678*

dihydrocodeine bitartrate, pseudoephedrine hydrochloride, and chlorpheniramine maleate *see* pseudoephedrine, dihydrocodeine, and chlorpheniramine *on page 730*

dihydrocodeine, chlorpheniramine, and phenylephrine
(dye hye droe KOE deen, klor fen IR a meen, & fen il EF rin)
Synonyms chlorpheniramine maleate, dihydrocodeine bitartrate, and phenylephrine hydrochloride; phenylephrine, chlorpheniramine, and dihydrocodeine
U.S./Canadian Brand Names Baltussin [US]; Coldcough PD [US]; Pancof®-PD [US]
Therapeutic Category Antihistamine; Antihistamine/Decongestant/Antitussive; Antitussive; Decongestant
Controlled Substance C-III/C-V
Use Symptomatic relief of cough and congestion associated with the upper respiratory tract
Usual Dosage Cough and congestion: Oral:
Children 2-6 years (Pancof®-PD): 1.25-2.5 mL every 4-6 hours as needed (maximum: 10 mL/24 hours)
Children 6-12 years:
Baltussin: 2.5 mL every 4-6 hours as needed
(Continued)

dihydrocodeine, chlorpheniramine, and phenylephrine *(Continued)*

Pancof®-PD: 2.5-5 mL every 4-6 hours as needed (maximum: 20 mL/24 hours)
Children ≥12 years and adults:
Baltussin: 5 mL every 4-6 hours as needed
Pancof®-PD: 5-10 mL every 4-6 hours as needed (maximum: 40 mL/24 hours)
Dosage Forms
Liquid: Dihydrocodeine 3 mg, chlorpheniramine 2 mg, and phenylephrine 7.5 mg per 5 mL
Pancof®-PD: Dihydrocodeine 3 mg, chlorpheniramine 2 mg, and phenylephrine 7.5 mg per 5 m
Syrup:
Baltussin: Dihydrocodeine 3 mg, chlorpheniramine 5 mg, and phenylephrine 20 mg per 5 mL
Coldcough PD: Dihydrocodeine 3 mg, chlorpheniramine 2 mg, and phenylephrine 7.5 mg per 5 mL

dihydrocodeine compound *see* dihydrocodeine, aspirin, and caffeine *on previous page*

dihydrocodeine, pseudoephedrine, and guaifenesin

(dye hye droe KOE deen, soo doe e FED rin, & gwye FEN e sin)
Synonyms guaifenesin, dihydrocodeine, and pseudoephedrine; pseudoephedrine hydrochloride, guaifenesin, and dihydrocodeine bitartrate
U.S./Canadian Brand Names DiHydro-GP [US]; Hydro-Tussin™ EXP [US]; Pancof®-EXP [US]
Therapeutic Category Antitussive/Decongestant/Expectorant
Use Temporary relief of cough and congestion associated with upper respiratory tract infections and allergies
Usual Dosage Oral: Cough/congestion (Hydro-Tussin™ EXP, Pancof®-EXP):
Children:
2-6 years: 1.25-2.5 mL every 4-6 hours as needed
6-12 years: 2.5-5 mL every 4-6 hours as needed
Children ≥12 years and Adults: 5-10 mL every 4-6 hours as needed
Dosage Forms
Syrup:
DiHydro-GP, Hydro-Tussin™ EXP, Pancof®-EXP: Dihydrocodeine 7.5 mg, pseudoephedrine 15 mg, and guaifenesin 100 mg per 5 mL

DiHydro-CP [US] *see* pseudoephedrine, dihydrocodeine, and chlorpheniramine *on page 730*

dihydroergotamine (dye hye droe er GOT a meen)

Synonyms DHE; dihydroergotamine mesylate
U.S./Canadian Brand Names D.H.E. 45® [US]; Migranal® [US/Can]
Therapeutic Category Ergot Alkaloid and Derivative
Use Treatment of migraine headache with or without aura; injection also indicated for treatment of cluster headaches
Usual Dosage Adults:
I.M., SubQ: 1 mg at first sign of headache; repeat hourly to a maximum dose of 3 mg total; maximum dose: 6 mg/week
I.V.: 1 mg at first sign of headache; repeat hourly up to a maximum dose of 2 mg total; maximum dose: 6 mg/week
Intranasal: 1 spray (0.5 mg) of nasal spray should be administered into each nostril; if needed, repeat after 15 minutes, up to a total of 4 sprays. **Note:** Do not exceed 3 mg (6 sprays) in a 24-hour period and no more than 8 sprays in a week.
Dosage Forms
Injection, solution: 1 mg/mL (1 mL)
D.H.E. 45®: 1 mg/mL (1 mL)
Solution, intranasal spray:
Migranal®: 4 mg/mL [0.5 mg/spray] (1 mL)

dihydroergotamine mesylate *see* dihydroergotamine *on this page*

dihydroergotoxine *see* ergoloid mesylates *on page 306*

dihydrogenated ergot alkaloids *see* ergoloid mesylates *on page 306*

DiHydro-GP [US] *see* dihydrocodeine, pseudoephedrine, and guaifenesin *on this page*

dihydrohydroxycodeinone *see* oxycodone *on page 640*

dihydromorphinone *see* hydromorphone *on page 435*

dihydroxyanthracenedione dihydrochloride *see* mitoxantrone *on page 573*

1,25 dihydroxycholecalciferol *see* calcitriol *on page 135*

dihydroxydeoxynorvinkaleukoblastine *see* vinorelbine *on page 891*

dihydroxypropyl theophylline *see* dyphylline *on page 288*

Dihyrex® **Injection** *(Discontinued) see* diphenhydramine *on page 265*

diiodohydroxyquin *see* iodoquinol *on page 467*

Dilacor® **XR [US]** *see* diltiazem *on this page*

Dilantin® **[US/Can]** *see* phenytoin *on page 680*

Dilatrate®**-SR [US]** *see* isosorbide dinitrate *on page 476*

Dilaudid® **[US/Can]** *see* hydromorphone *on page 435*

Dilaudid® **Cough Syrup** *(Discontinued) see* hydromorphone *on page 435*

Dilaudid-HP® **[US/Can]** *see* hydromorphone *on page 435*

Dilaudid-HP-Plus® **[Can]** *see* hydromorphone *on page 435*

Dilaudid® **Sterile Powder [Can]** *see* hydromorphone *on page 435*

Dilaudid-XP® **[Can]** *see* hydromorphone *on page 435*

Dilex-G [US] *see* dyphylline and guaifenesin *on page 288*

Dilocaine® **Injection** *(Discontinued) see* lidocaine *on page 504*

Dilomine® **Injection** *(Discontinued) see* dicyclomine *on page 255*

Dilor® **[Can]** *see* dyphylline *on page 288*

Dilor-G® **[US]** *see* dyphylline and guaifenesin *on page 288*

Diltia XT® **[US]** *see* diltiazem *on this page*

diltiazem (dil TYE a zem)

Sound-Alike/Look-Alike Issues
diltiazem may be confused with Dilantin®
Cardizem® may be confused with Cardene®, Cardene SR®, Cardizem CD®, Cardizem SR®, cardiem
Cartia XT™ may be confused with Procardia XL®
Tiazac® may be confused with Tigan®, Ziac®

Synonyms diltiazem hydrochloride

U.S./Canadian Brand Names Alti-Diltiazem CD [Can]; Apo-Diltiaz CD® [Can]; Apo-Diltiaz SR® [Can]; Apo-Diltiaz TZ® [Can]; Apo-Diltiaz® Injectable [Can]; Apo-Diltiaz® [Can]; Cardizem® CD [US/Can]; Cardizem® LA [US]; Cardizem® SR [Can]; Cardizem® [US/Can]; Cartia XT™ [US]; Dilacor® XR [US]; Dilt-XR [US]; Diltia XT® [US]; Diltiazem HCl ER® [Can]; Diltiazem Hydrochloride Injection [Can]; Gen-Diltiazem CD [Can]; Gen-Diltiazem [Can]; Med-Diltiazem [Can]; Novo-Diltazem [Can]; Novo-Diltazem-CD [Can]; Novo-Diltazem HCl ER [Can]; Nu-Diltiaz [Can]; Nu-Diltiaz-CD [Can]; ratio-Diltiazem CD [Can]; Rhoxal-diltiazem CD [Can]; Rhoxal-diltiazem SR [Can]; Rhoxal-diltiazem T [Can]; Sandoz-Diltiazem CD [Can]; Sandoz-Diltiazem T [Can]; Syn-Diltiazem® [Can]; Taztia XT™ [US]; Tiazac® XC [Can]; Tiazac® [US/Can]

Therapeutic Category Calcium Channel Blocker

Use
Oral: Essential hypertension; chronic stable angina or angina from coronary artery spasm
Injection: Atrial fibrillation or atrial flutter; paroxysmal supraventricular tachycardia (PSVT)

Usual Dosage Adults:
Oral:
Angina:
Capsule, extended release (Cardizem® CD, Cartia XT™, Dilacor® XR, Diltia XT®, Tiazac®): Initial: 120-180 mg once daily (maximum dose: 480 mg/day)
Tablet, extended release (Cardizem® LA): 180 mg once daily; may increase at 7- to 14-day intervals (maximum recommended dose: 360 mg/day)
Tablet, immediate release (Cardizem®): Usual starting dose: 30 mg 4 times/day; usual range: 180-360 mg/day
Hypertension:
Capsule, extended release (Cardizem® CD, Cartia XT™, Dilacor® XR, Diltia XT®, Tiazac®): Initial: 180-240 mg once daily; dose adjustment may be made after 14 days; usual dose range (JNC 7): 180-420 mg/day; Tiazac®: usual dose range: 120-540 mg/day
Capsule, sustained release: Initial: 60-120 mg twice daily; dose adjustment may be made after 14 days; usual range: 240-360 mg/day
Tablet, extended release (Cardizem® LA): Initial: 180-240 mg once daily; dose adjustment may be made after 14 days; usual dose range (JNC 7): 120-540 mg/day
I.V.: Atrial fibrillation, atrial flutter, PSVT:
Initial bolus dose: 0.25 mg/kg actual body weight over 2 minutes (average adult dose: 20 mg)
Repeat bolus dose (may be administered after 15 minutes if the response is inadequate.): 0.35 mg/kg actual body weight over 2 minutes (average adult dose: 25 mg)
(Continued)

diltiazem *(Continued)*

Continuous infusion (requires an infusion pump; infusions >24 hours or infusion rates >15 mg/hour are not recommended.): Initial infusion rate of 10 mg/hour; rate may be increased in 5 mg/hour increments up to 15 mg/hour as needed; some patients may respond to an initial rate of 5 mg/hour.

If diltiazem injection is administered by continuous infusion for >24 hours, the possibility of decreased diltiazem clearance, prolonged elimination half-life, and increased diltiazem and/or diltiazem metabolite plasma concentrations should be considered.

Conversion from I.V. diltiazem to oral diltiazem: Start oral approximately 3 hours after bolus dose.

Oral dose (mg/day) is approximately equal to [rate (mg/hour) x 3 + 3] x 10.

3 mg/hour = 120 mg/day
5 mg/hour = 180 mg/day
7 mg/hour = 240 mg/day
11 mg/hour = 360 mg/day

Dosage Forms

Capsule, extended release [once-daily dosing]: 120 mg, 180 mg, 240 mg, 300 mg, 360 mg, 420 mg
Cardizem® CD, Taztia XT™: 120 mg, 180 mg, 240 mg, 300 mg, 360 mg
Cartia XT™: 120 mg, 180 mg, 240 mg, 300 mg
Dilacor® XR, Diltia XT®: 120 mg, 180 mg, 240 mg
Tiazac®: 120 mg, 180 mg, 240 mg, 300 mg, 360 mg, 420 mg
Capsule, sustained release [twice-daily dosing]: 60 mg, 90 mg, 120 mg
Injection, solution: 5 mg/mL (5 mL, 10 mL, 25 mL)
Injection, powder for reconstitution:
Cardizem®: 25 mg
Tablet: 30 mg, 60 mg, 90 mg, 120 mg
Cardizem®: 30 mg, 60 mg, 90 mg, 120 mg
Tablet, extended release:
Cardizem® LA: 120 mg, 180 mg, 240 mg, 300 mg, 360 mg, 420 mg

Diltiazem HCl ER® [Can] *see* diltiazem *on previous page*

diltiazem hydrochloride *see* diltiazem *on previous page*

Diltiazem Hydrochloride Injection [Can] *see* diltiazem *on previous page*

Dilt-XR [US] *see* diltiazem *on previous page*

Dimaphen [US-OTC] *see* brompheniramine and pseudoephedrine *on page 120*

Dimaphen DM *(Discontinued)* *see* brompheniramine, pseudoephedrine, and dextromethorphan *on page 122*

dimenhydrinate *(dye men HYE dri nate)*

Sound-Alike/Look-Alike Issues
dimenhyDRINATE may be confused with diphenhydrAMINE
Tall-Man dimenhy**DRINATE**
U.S./Canadian Brand Names Apo-Dimenhydrinate® [Can]; Children's Motion Sickness Liquid [Can]; Dinate® [Can]; Dramamine® [US-OTC]; Gravol® [Can]; Jamp® Travel Tablet [Can]; Nauseatol [Can]; Novo-Dimenate [Can]; SAB-Dimenhydrinate [Can]
Therapeutic Category Antihistamine
Use Treatment and prevention of nausea, vertigo, and vomiting associated with motion sickness
Dosage forms available in Canada (not available in the U.S.), including parenteral formulations and suppositories, are also approved for the treatment of postoperative nausea and vomiting and treatment of radiation sickness.
Usual Dosage Oral:
Children:
2-5 years: 12.5-25 mg every 6-8 hours, maximum: 75 mg/day
6-12 years: 25-50 mg every 6-8 hours, maximum: 150 mg/day
Adults: 50-100 mg every 4-6 hours, not to exceed 400 mg/day
Gravol® L/A (not available in the U.S.): 75-150 mg every 8-12 hours, up to a maximum of five 75 mg caplets or three 100 mg caplets in 24 hours

Additional formulations/uses (approved in Canada) for parenteral/suppository formulations (not available in U.S.):
I.M., I.V., rectal: Adults:
Postoperative nausea and vomiting: 50-100 mg administered 30-60 minutes prior to radiation therapy; may be repeated as needed up to a maximum of 400 mg in 24 hours
Radiation sickness: 50-100 mg administered 30-60 minutes prior to radiation therapy. May be repeated as needed up to a maximum of 400 mg in 24 hours

Dosage Forms [CAN] = Canadian brand name
  Capsule, softgel: 50 mg [not available in the U.S.]
    Gravol® [CAN]: 50 mg [not available in the U.S.]
  Capsule, long-acting: 75 mg, 100 mg [not available in the U.S.]
    Gravol® L/A [CAN]: 75 mg, 100 mg [not available in the U.S.]
  Injection, solution: 10 mg/mL (5 mL); 50 mg/mL (1 mL, 5 mL) [not available in the U.S.]
    Gravol® I.M. [CAN]: 50 mg/mL (1 mL, 5 mL) [not available in the U.S.]
    Gravol® I.V. [CAN]: 10 mg/mL (5 mL) [not available in the U.S.]
  Solution, oral: 3 mg/mL [not available in the U.S.]
    Gravol® [CAN], Children's Motion Sickness [CAN]: 3 mg/mL [not available in the U.S.]
  Suppository, rectal: 75 mg, 100 mg [not available in the U.S.]
    Gravol® [CAN], Sab-Dimenhydrinate [CAN]: 75 mg, 100 mg [not available in the U.S.]
  Tablet: 50 mg
    Dinate® [CAN], Dramamine® [OTC], Jamp® Travel Tablet [CAN], Nauseatol® [CAN]: 50 mg
    Gravol® Filmkote Jr [CAN]: 25 mg [not available in the U.S.]
    Gravol® Filmkote [CAN]: 50 mg [not available in the U.S.]
  Tablet, chewable: 50 mg
    Dramamine® [OTC]: 50 mg
    Gravol® Chewable for Children [CAN]: 25 mg [not available in the U.S.]
    Gravol® Chewable for Adults [CAN]: 50 mg [not available in the U.S.]

dimercaprol (dye mer KAP role)
  Synonyms BAL; British anti-lewisite; dithioglycerol
  U.S./Canadian Brand Names BAL in Oil® [US]
  Therapeutic Category Chelating Agent
  Use Antidote to gold, arsenic (except arsine), or acute mercury poisoning (except nonalkyl mercury); adjunct to edetate calcium disodium in lead poisoning
  Usual Dosage Note: Premedication with an antihistamine is recommended.
    Children and Adults: Deep I.M.:
      Mild arsenic or gold poisoning: 2.5 mg/kg every 6 hours for 2 days, then every 12 hours for 1 day, followed by once daily for 10 days
      Severe arsenic or gold poisoning: 3 mg/kg every 4 hours for 2 days, then every 6 hours for 1 day, followed every 12 hours for 10 days
      Mercury poisoning: 5 mg/kg initially, followed by 2.5 mg/kg 1-2 times/day for 10 days
      Lead poisoning:
        Acute encephalopathy or blood lead levels >70 mcg/dL (in conjunction with calcium EDTA): 4 mg/kg loading dose, followed by 4 mg/kg every 4 hours for 2-7 days (calcium EDTA is not administered with the loading dose; begin calcium EDTA with the second dose)
        Mild (in conjunction with calcium EDTA): 4 mg/kg/dose loading dose, followed by 3 mg/kg/dose every 4 hours for 2-7 days (calcium EDTA is not administered with the loading dose; begin calcium EDTA with the second dose)
  Dosage Forms
  Injection, oil:
    BAL in Oil®: 100 mg/mL (3 mL)

Dimetabs® Oral *(Discontinued)* see dimenhydrinate on previous page

Dimetapp® 12-Hour Non-Drowsy Extentabs® *(Discontinued)* see pseudoephedrine on page 727

Dimetapp® Children's ND *(Discontinued)* see loratadine on page 517

Dimetapp® Decongestant Infant *(Discontinued)* see pseudoephedrine on page 727

Dimetapp® DM Children's Cold and Cough *(Discontinued)* see brompheniramine, pseudoephedrine, and dextromethorphan on page 122

Dimetapp® Infant Decongestant Plus Cough *(Discontinued)* see pseudoephedrine and dextromethorphan on page 728

Dimetapp® Sinus Caplets *(Discontinued)* see pseudoephedrine and ibuprofen on page 729

Dimetapp® Toddler's [US-OTC] see phenylephrine on page 675

dimethyl sulfoxide (dye meth il sul FOKS ide)
  Synonyms DMSO
  U.S./Canadian Brand Names Dimethyl Sulfoxide Irrigation, USP [Can]; Kemsol® [Can]; Rimso®-50 [US/Can]
  Therapeutic Category Urinary Tract Product
  Use Symptomatic relief of interstitial cystitis
    (Continued)

dimethyl sulfoxide *(Continued)*

Usual Dosage Instill 50 mL directly into bladder and allow to remain for 15 minutes; repeat every 2 weeks until maximum symptomatic relief is obtained

Dosage Forms
Solution, intravesical: 50% [500 mg/mL] (50 mL)
Rimso®-50: 50% [500 mg/mL] (50 mL)

Dimethyl Sulfoxide Irrigation, USP [Can] see dimethyl sulfoxide *on previous page*

dimethyl triazeno imidazole carboxamide see dacarbazine *on page 227*

Dinate® [Can] see dimenhydrinate *on page 262*

Dinate® Injection *(Discontinued)* see dimenhydrinate *on page 262*

dinoprostone (dye noe PROST one)

Sound-Alike/Look-Alike Issues
Prepidil® may be confused with Bepridil®
Synonyms PGE$_2$; prostaglandin E$_2$
U.S./Canadian Brand Names Cervidil® [US/Can]; Prepidil® [US/Can]; Prostin E$_2$® [US/Can]
Therapeutic Category Prostaglandin
Use
Gel: Promote cervical ripening in patients at or near term in whom there is a medical or obstetrical indication for the induction of labor
Suppositories: Terminate pregnancy from 12th through 20th week of gestation; evacuate uterus in cases of missed abortion or intrauterine fetal death up to 28 weeks of gestation; manage benign hydatidiform mole (nonmetastatic gestational trophoblastic disease)
Vaginal insert: Initiation and/or continuation of cervical ripening in patients at or near term in whom there is a medical or obstetrical indication for the induction of labor
Usual Dosage Females of reproductive age:
Abortifacient: Vaginal suppository: Insert 20 mg (1 suppository) high in vagina, repeat at 3- to 5-hour intervals until abortion occurs; continued administration for longer than 2 days is not advisable
Cervical ripening:
Endocervical gel: Using catheter supplied with gel, insert 0.5 mg into the cervical canal. May repeat every 6 hours if needed. Maximum cumulative dose: 1.5 mg/24 hours
Vaginal insert: Insert 10 mg transversely into the posterior fornix of the vagina (to be removed at the onset of active labor or after 12 hours)
Dosage Forms
Gel, endocervical:
Prepidil®: 0.5 mg/3 g syringe
Insert, vaginal:
Cervidil®: 10 mg
Suppository, vaginal:
Prostin E$_2$®: 20 mg

Diocaine® [Can] see proparacaine *on page 721*

Diocarpine [Can] see pilocarpine *on page 682*

Diochloram® [Can] see chloramphenicol *on page 173*

Diocto® [US-OTC] see docusate *on page 273*

Diocto C® *(Discontinued)*

Diocto-K® *(Discontinued)* see docusate *on page 273*

Diocto-K Plus® *(Discontinued)* see docusate *on page 273*

dioctyl calcium sulfosuccinate see docusate *on page 273*

dioctyl sodium sulfosuccinate see docusate *on page 273*

Diodex® [Can] see dexamethasone (systemic) *on page 241*

Diodoquin® [Can] see iodoquinol *on page 467*

Diogent® [Can] see gentamicin *on page 390*

Diomycin® [Can] see erythromycin *on page 309*

Dionephrine® [Can] see phenylephrine *on page 675*

Diopentolate® [Can] see cyclopentolate *on page 221*

Diopred® [Can] see prednisolone (systemic) *on page 710*

Dioptic's Atropine Solution [Can] see atropine *on page 83*

Dioptimyd® **[Can]** *see* sulfacetamide and prednisolone *on page 811*

Dioptrol® **[Can]** *see* neomycin, polymyxin B, and dexamethasone *on page 597*

Diosulf™ **[Can]** *see* sulfacetamide *on page 810*

Diotame® **[US-OTC]** *see* bismuth *on page 113*

Diotrope® **[Can]** *see* tropicamide *on page 871*

Dioval® **Injection** *(Discontinued)* *see* estradiol *on page 313*

Diovan® **[US/Can]** *see* valsartan *on page 882*

Diovan HCT® **[US/Can]** *see* valsartan and hydrochlorothiazide *on page 882*

Diovol® **[Can]** *see* aluminum hydroxide and magnesium hydroxide *on page 37*

Diovol® **Ex [Can]** *see* aluminum hydroxide and magnesium hydroxide *on page 37*

Diovol Plus® **[Can]** *see* aluminum hydroxide, magnesium hydroxide, and simethicone *on page 37*

Dipentum® **[US/Can]** *see* olsalazine *on page 628*

Diphen® **[US-OTC]** *see* diphenhydramine *on this page*

Diphenacen 50® **Injection** *(Discontinued)* *see* diphenhydramine *on this page*

Diphen® **AF [US-OTC]** *see* diphenhydramine *on this page*

Diphenatol® *(Discontinued)* *see* diphenoxylate and atropine *on page 267*

Diphenhist [US-OTC] *see* diphenhydramine *on this page*

diphenhydramine (dye fen HYE dra meen)

Sound-Alike/Look-Alike Issues
diphenhydrAMINE may be confused with desipramine, dicyclomine, dimenhyDRINATE
Benadryl® may be confused with benazepril, Bentyl®, Benylin®, Caladryl®

Synonyms diphenhydramine citrate; diphenhydramine hydrochloride; diphenhydramine tannate

Tall-Man diphenhydr**AMINE**

U.S./Canadian Brand Names Aler-Cap [US-OTC]; Aler-Dryl [US-OTC]; Aler-Tab [US-OTC]; Allerdryl® [Can]; AllerMax® [US-OTC]; Allernix [Can]; Altaryl® [US-OTC]; Banophen® Anti-Itch [US-OTC]; Banophen® [US-OTC]; Ben-Tann [US]; Benadryl® Allergy [US-OTC]; Benadryl® Children's Allergy Fastmelt® [US-OTC]; Benadryl® Children's Allergy [US-OTC]; Benadryl® Children's Dye-Free Allergy [US-OTC]; Benadryl® Injection [US]; Benadryl® Itch Stopping Extra Strength [US-OTC]; Benadryl® Itch Stopping [US-OTC]; Benadryl® [Can]; Compoz® Nighttime Sleep Aid [US-OTC]; Dermamycin® [US-OTC]; Diphenhist [US-OTC]; Diphen® AF [US-OTC]; Diphen® [US-OTC]; Dytan™ [US]; Genahist® [US-OTC]; Hydramine® [US-OTC]; Nytol® Extra Strength [Can]; Nytol® Quick Caps [US-OTC]; Nytol® Quick Gels [US-OTC]; Nytol® [Can]; PMS-Diphenhydramine [Can]; Siladryl® Allergy [US-OTC]; Silphen® [US-OTC]; Simply Sleep® [US-OTC/Can]; Sleep-ettes D [US-OTC]; Sleepinal® [US-OTC]; Sominex® Maximum Strength [US-OTC]; Sominex® [US-OTC]; Triaminic® Thin Strips™ Cough and Runny Nose [US-OTC]; Twilite® [US-OTC]; Unisom® Maximum Strength SleepGels® [US-OTC]

Therapeutic Category Antihistamine

Use Symptomatic relief of allergic symptoms caused by histamine release including nasal allergies and allergic dermatosis; adjunct to epinephrine in the treatment of anaphylaxis; nighttime sleep aid; prevention or treatment of motion sickness; antitussive; management of parkinsonian syndrome including drug-induced extrapyramidal symptoms; topically for relief of pain and itching associated with insect bites, minor cuts and burns, or rashes due to poison ivy, poison oak, and poison sumac

Usual Dosage Note: Dosages are expressed as the hydrochloride salt.
Children:
Allergic reactions or motion sickness: Oral, I.M., I.V.: 5 mg/kg/day or 150 mg/m²/day in divided doses every 6-8 hours, not to exceed 300 mg/day
Alternate dosing by age: Oral:
2 to <6 years: 6.25 mg every 4-6 hours; maximum: 37.5 mg/day
6 to <12 years: 12.5-25 mg every 4-6 hours; maximum: 150 mg/day
≥12 years: 25-50 mg every 4-6 hours; maximum: 300 mg/day
Night-time sleep aid: Oral: Children ≥12 years: 50 mg at bedtime
Antitussive: Oral:
2 to <6 years: 6.25 mg every 4 hours; maximum 37.5 mg/day
6 to <12 years: 12.5 mg every 4 hours; maximum 75 mg/day
≥12 years: 25 mg every 4 hours; maximum 150 mg/day
Treatment of dystonic reactions: I.M., I.V.: 0.5-1 mg/kg/dose
Relief of pain and itching: Topical: Children ≥2 years: Apply 1% or 2% to affected area up to 3-4 times/day
Adults:
Allergic reactions or motion sickness: Oral: 25-50 mg every 6-8 hours
Antitussive: Oral: 25 mg every 4 hours; maximum 150 mg/24 hours
(Continued)

diphenhydramine *(Continued)*

Nighttime sleep aid: Oral: 50 mg at bedtime

Allergic reactions or motion sickness: I.M., I.V.: 10-50 mg per dose; single doses up to 100 mg may be used if needed; not to exceed 400 mg/day

Dystonic reaction: I.M., I.V.: 50 mg in a single dose; may repeat in 20-30 minutes if necessary

Relief of pain and itching: Topical: Apply 1% or 2% to affected area up to 3-4 times/day

Dosage Forms

Caplet: 25 mg, 50 mg

Aler-Dryl [OTC], AllerMax® [OTC], Compoz® Nighttime Sleep Aid [OTC], Sleep-ettes D [OTC], Sominex® Maximum Strength [OTC], Twilite® [OTC]: 50 mg

Nytol® Quick Caps [OTC], Simply Sleep® [OTC]: 25 mg

Capsule: 25 mg, 50 mg

Aler-Cap [OTC], Banophen® [OTC], Benadryl® Allergy [OTC], Diphen® [OTC], Diphenhist [OTC], Genahist® [OTC]: 25 mg

Sleepinal® [OTC]: 50 mg

Capsule, softgel: 50 mg

Benadryl® Dye-Free Allergy [OTC]: 25 mg

Compoz® Nighttime Sleep Aid [OTC], Nytol® Quick Gels [OTC], Sleepinal® [OTC], Unisom® Maximum Strength SleepGels® [OTC]: 50 mg

Captab: 25 mg

Diphenhist® [OTC]: 25 mg

Cream: 2% (30 g)

Banophen® Anti-Itch [OTC], Benadryl® Itch Stopping Extra Strength [OTC], Diphenhist® [OTC]: 2% (30 g)

Benadryl® Itch Stopping [OTC]: 1% (30 g)

Elixir:

Altaryl [OTC], Banophen® [OTC], Diphen AF [OTC]: 12.5 mg/5 mL

Gel, topical: 2% (120 mL, 28 g, 42 g)

Benadryl® Itch Stopping Extra Strength [OTC]: 2% (120 mL)

Injection, solution: 50 mg/mL (1 mL, 10 mL)

Liquid, as hydrochloride:

AllerMax® [OTC], Benadryl® Allergy [OTC], Benadryl® Children's Dye-Free Allergy [OTC], Genahist® [OTC], Hydramine® [OTC], Siladryl® Allergy [OTC]: 12.5 mg/5 mL

Liquid, topical [stick]:

Benadryl® Itch Stopping Extra Strength [OTC]: 2% (14 mL)

Solution, oral:

Diphenhis [OTC]: 12.5 mg/5mL

Solution, topical [spray]: 2% (60 mL)

Benadryl® Itch Stopping Extra Strength [OTC], Dermamycin® [OTC]: 2% (60 mL)

Strips, oral:

Benadryl® Allergy [OTC]: 25 mg (10s)

Benadryl® Children's Allergy [OTC]: 12. 5 mg (10s)

Triaminic® Thin Strips™ Cough and Runny Nose [OTC]: 12. 5 mg (16s)

Suspension:

Ben-Tann, Dytan™: 25 mg/5 mL

Syrup: 12.5 mg/5 mL

Silphen® Cough [OTC]: 12.5 mg/5 mL

Tablet: 25 mg, 50 mg

Aler-Tab [OTC], Benadryl® Allergy [OTC], Genahist® [OTC], Sominex® [OTC]: 25 mg

Tablet, chewable:

Benadryl® Children's Allergy [OTC]: 12.5 mg

Dytan™: 25 mg

Tablet, orally disintegrating:

Benadryl® Children's Allergy Fastmelt® [OTC]: 19 mg

diphenhydramine and acetaminophen *see* acetaminophen and diphenhydramine *on page 7*

diphenhydramine and pseudoephedrine (dye fen HYE dra meen & soo doe e FED rin)

Sound-Alike/Look-Alike Issues

Benadryl® may be confused with benazepril, Bentyl®, Benylin®, Caladryl®

Synonyms pseudoephedrine and diphenhydramine

U.S./Canadian Brand Names Benadryl-D™ Allergy and Sinus Fastmelt™ [US-OTC]; Benadryl-D™ Children's Allergy and Sinus [US-OTC]; Benadryl® Children's Allergy and Cold Fastmelt™ [US-OTC]

Therapeutic Category Antihistamine/Decongestant Combination

Use Relief of symptoms of upper respiratory mucosal congestion in seasonal and perennial nasal allergies, acute rhinitis, rhinosinusitis, and eustachian tube blockage

Usual Dosage Oral: Adults: Based on **pseudoephedrine** component: 60 mg every 4-6 hours, maximum: 240 mg/day

Dosage Forms

Liquid:

Benadryl-D™ Children's Allergy and Sinus [OTC]: Diphenhydramine 12.5 mg and pseudoephedrine 30 mg per 5 mL

Tablet, quick dissolving:

Benadryl® Children's Allergy and Cold Fastmelt™ [OTC], Benadryl-D™ Allergy and Sinus Fastmelt™ [OTC]: Diphenhydramine 19 mg and pseudoephedrine 30 mg

diphenhydramine citrate *see* diphenhydramine *on page 265*

diphenhydramine hydrochloride *see* diphenhydramine *on page 265*

diphenhydramine, hydrocodone, and phenylephrine *see* hydrocodone, phenylephrine, and diphenhydramine *on page 431*

diphenhydramine tannate *see* diphenhydramine *on page 265*

diphenoxylate and atropine (dye fen OKS i late & A troe peen)

Sound-Alike/Look-Alike Issues

Lomotil® may be confused with Lamictal®, Lamisil®, lamotrigine, Lanoxin®, Lasix®, ludiomil

Lonox® may be confused with Lanoxin®, Loprox®

Synonyms atropine and diphenoxylate

U.S./Canadian Brand Names Lomotil® [US/Can]; Lonox® [US]

Therapeutic Category Antidiarrheal

Controlled Substance C-V

Use Treatment of diarrhea

Usual Dosage Oral:

Children 2-12 years (use with caution in young children due to variable responses): Liquid: Diphenoxylate 0.3-0.4 mg/kg/day in 4 divided doses until control achieved (maximum: 10 mg/day), then reduce dose as needed; some patients may be controlled on doses as low as 25% of the initial daily dose

Adults: Diphenoxylate 5 mg 4 times/day until control achieved (maximum: 20 mg/day), then reduce dose as needed; some patients may be controlled on doses of 5 mg/day

Dosage Forms

Solution, oral: Diphenoxylate 2.5 mg and atropine 0.025 mg per 5 mL

Lomotil®: Diphenoxylate 2.5 mg and atropine 0.025 mg per 5 mL

Tablet: Diphenoxylate 2.5 mg and atropine 0.025 mg

Lomotil®, Lonox®: Diphenoxylate 2.5 mg and atropine 0.025 mg

Diphenylan Sodium® *(Discontinued)* *see* phenytoin *on page 680*

diphenylhydantoin *see* phenytoin *on page 680*

diphtheria and tetanus toxoid (dif THEER ee a & TET a nus TOKS oyd)

Synonyms DT; Td; tetanus and diphtheria toxoid

U.S./Canadian Brand Names Decavac™ [US]; Td Adsorbed [Can]

Therapeutic Category Toxoid

Use

Diphtheria and tetanus toxoids adsorbed for pediatric use (DT): Infants and children through 6 years of age: Active immunity against diphtheria and tetanus when pertussis vaccine is contraindicated

Tetanus and diphtheria toxoids adsorbed for adult use (Td) (Decavac™): Children ≥7 years of age and Adults: Active immunity against diphtheria and tetanus; tetanus prophylaxis in wound management

Usual Dosage I.M.:

Infants and Children ≤6 years (DT): Primary immunization:

6 weeks to 1 year: Three 0.5 mL doses at least 4 weeks apart; administer a reinforcing dose 6-12 months after the third injection

1-6 years: Two 0.5 mL doses at least 4 weeks apart; reinforcing dose 6-12 months after second injection; if final dose is given after seventh birthday, use adult preparation

4-6 years (booster immunization): 0.5 mL; not necessary if the fourth dose was given after fourth birthday; routinely administer booster doses at 10-year intervals with the adult preparation

Children ≥7 years and Adults (Td):

Primary immunization: Patients previously not immunized should receive 2 primary doses of 0.5 mL each, given at an interval of 4-6 weeks; third (reinforcing) dose of 0.5 mL 6-12 months later

Booster immunization: 0.5 mL every 10 years; to be given to children 11-12 years of age if at least 5 years have elapsed since last dose of toxoid containing vaccine. Subsequent routine doses are not recommended more often than every 10 years. The ACIP prefers Tdap for use in adolescents 11-18 years; refer to diphtheria, tetanus toxoids, and acellular pertussis vaccine monograph for additional information.

(Continued)

diphtheria and tetanus toxoid *(Continued)*

Tetanus prophylaxis in wound management; use of tetanus toxoid (Td) and/or tetanus immune globulin (TIG) depends upon the number of prior tetanus toxoid doses and type of wound.

Clean, minor wounds:
- Prior number of tetanus toxoid doses is unknown or <3: Td[1]
- Prior number of tetanus toxoid doses is ≥3: Td[1] only if >10 years since last dose
- If only three doses of fluid tetanus toxoid have been received, a fourth dose of toxoid, preferably an adsorbed toxoid, should be given

All other wounds:
- Prior number of tetanus toxoid doses is unknown or <3: Td[1] and TIG
- Prior number of tetanus toxoid doses is ≥3: Td[1] only if >5 years since last dose

[1]Adult tetanus and diphtheria toxoids; use pediatric preparations (DT or DTP) if the patient is <7 years old. Adapted from Report of the Committee on Infectious Diseases, American Academy of Pediatrics, Elk Grove Village, IL: American Academy of Pediatrics, 1986.

Dosage Forms
Injection, suspension, adult:
Decavac™: Diphtheria 2 Lf units and tetanus 5 Lf units per 0.5 mL (0.5 mL)
Injection, suspension, pediatric [preservative free]: Diphtheria 6.7 Lf units and tetanus 5 Lf units per 0.5 mL (0.5 mL)

diphtheria and tetanus toxoids and acellular pertussis adsorbed, hepatitis B (recombinant) and inactivated poliovirus vaccine combined *see* diphtheria, tetanus toxoids, acellular pertussis, hepatitis B (recombinant), and poliovirus (inactivated) vaccine *on this page*

diphtheria antitoxin (dif THEER ee a an tee TOKS in)
Therapeutic Category Antitoxin
Use Treatment of diphtheria (neutralizes unbound toxin, available from CDC)
Usual Dosage I.M. or slow I.V. infusion: Dosage varies; range: 20,000-120,000 units
Dosage Forms
Injection:
≥500 units/mL (40 mL)

diphtheria CRM$_{197}$ protein *see* pneumococcal conjugate vaccine (7-valent) *on page 691*

diphtheria CRM$_{197}$ protein conjugate *see* Haemophilus B conjugate vaccine *on page 411*

diphtheria, tetanus toxoids, acellular pertussis, hepatitis B (recombinant), and poliovirus (inactivated) vaccine
(dif THEER ee a, TET a nus TOKS oyds, ay CEL yoo lar per TUS sis, hep a TYE tis bee ree KOM be nant, & POE lee oh VYE rus, in ak ti VAY ted vak SEEN)
Synonyms diphtheria and tetanus toxoids and acellular pertussis adsorbed, hepatitis B (recombinant) and inactivated poliovirus vaccine combined
U.S./Canadian Brand Names Pediarix® [US/Can]
Therapeutic Category Vaccine
Use Combination vaccine for the active immunization against diphtheria, tetanus, pertussis, hepatitis B virus (all known subtypes), and poliomyelitis (caused by poliovirus types 1, 2, and 3)
Usual Dosage I.M.: Children 6 weeks to <7 years:
Immunization: 0.5 mL; repeat in 6-8 week intervals (preferably 8-week intervals) for a total of 3 doses. Vaccination usually begins at 2 months, but may be started as early as 6 weeks of age.
Use in children previously vaccinated with one or more component, and who are also scheduled to receive all vaccine components:
Hepatitis B vaccine: Infants born of HB$_s$Ag-negative mothers who received 1 dose of hepatitis B vaccine at birth may be given Pediarix® (safety data limited); use in infants who received more than 1 dose of hepatitis B vaccine has not been established. Infants who received 1 or more doses of hepatitis B vaccine (recombinant) may be given Pediarix® to complete the hepatitis B series (safety and efficacy not established).
Diphtheria and tetanus toxoids, and acellular pertussis vaccine (DTaP): Infants previously vaccinated with 1 or 2 doses of Infanrix® may use Pediarix® to complete the first 3 doses of the series (safety and efficacy not established); use of Pediarix® to complete DTaP vaccination started with products other than Infanrix® is not recommended.
Inactivated polio vaccine (IPV): Infants previously vaccinated with 1 or 2 doses of IPV may use Pediarix® to complete the first 3 doses of the series (safety and efficacy not established).
Dosage Forms
Injection, suspension [preservative free]:
Pediarix®: Diphtheria toxoid 25 Lf, tetanus toxoid 10 Lf, inactivated PT 25 mcg, FHA 25 mcg, pertactin 8 mcg, HB$_s$Ag 10 mcg, poliovirus type 1 40 DU, poliovirus type 2 8 DU, and poliovirus type 3 32 DU per 0.5 mL

diphtheria, tetanus toxoids, and acellular pertussis vaccine
(dif THEER ee a, TET a nus TOKS oyds & ay CEL yoo lar per TUS sis vak SEEN)

Synonyms DTaP; dTpa; Tdap; tetanus toxoid, reduced diphtheria toxoid, and acellular pertussis, adsorbed

U.S./Canadian Brand Names Adacel™ [US/Can]; Boostrix® [US]; Daptacel® [US]; Infanrix® [US]; Tripedia® [US]

Therapeutic Category Toxoid

Use

Daptacel®, Infanrix®, Tripedia® (DTaP): Active immunization against diphtheria, tetanus, and pertussis from age 6 weeks through 6 years of age (prior to seventh birthday)

Adacel™, Boostrix® (Tdap): Active booster immunization against diphtheria, tetanus, and pertussis

Usual Dosage

Primary immunization: Children 6 weeks to <7 years: I.M.: **Note:** Whenever possible, the same product should be used for all doses. Interruption of recommended schedule does not require starting the series over; a delay between doses should not interfere with final immunity.

Daptacel®: 0.5 mL per dose, total of 4 doses administered as follows (data insufficient to recommend a fifth dose):

Three doses, usually given at 2-, 4-, and 6 months of age; may be given as early as 6 weeks of age and repeated every 6-8 weeks

Fourth dose: Given at ~15-20 months of age, but at least 6 months after third dose

Infanrix®, Tripedia®: 0.5 mL per dose, total of 5 doses administered as follows:

Three doses, usually given at 2-, 4-, and 6 months of age; may be given as early as 6 weeks of age and repeated every 4-8 weeks

Fourth dose: Given at ~15-20 months of age, but at least 6 months after third dose

Fifth dose: Given at 5-6 years of age, prior to starting school or kindergarten; if the fourth dose is given at ≥4 years of age, the fifth dose may be omitted

Booster immunization:

ACIP recommendations:

Adolescents 11-18 years: I.M.: 0.5 mL. A single dose of Tdap should be given instead of Td in adolescents who have completed the recommended childhood DTP/DTaP series and have not received Td or Tdap; preferred age of vaccination with Tdap is 11-12 years. Adolescents who received Td but not Tdap and who have completed the recommended childhood DTP/DTaP series are encouraged to receive Tdap; an interval of at least 5 years between Td and Tdap is recommended, but lesser intervals may be used if the benefit outweighs the risk.

Adults 19-64 years (Adacel™): I.M.: 0.5 mL. A single dose should be given instead of Td in adults if they received their last dose of Td ≥10 years previous. Shorter intervals (as short as 2 years) may used among healthcare providers, adults in contact with infants, or others in settings with increased risk for pertussis, including during pertussis outbreaks. Adacel™ should only be used to replace a single booster dose of Td.

Manufacturer's labeling:

Children 10-18 years (Boostrix®): I.M.: 0.5 mL as a single dose, administered 5 years after last dose of DTwP or DTaP vaccine.

Children ≥11 years and Adults ≤64 years (Adacel™): I.M.: 0.5 mL as a single dose, administered 5 years after last dose of DTwP or DTaP vaccine.

Wound management: Adacel™ (in patients 11-64 years of age) or Boostrix® (in patients 10-18 years of age) may be used as an alternative to Td vaccine when a tetanus toxoid-containing vaccine is needed for wound management, and in whom the pertussis component is also indicated. Td vaccine is the preferred agent in children ≥7 years and adults.

ACIP recommendations: ACIP prefers Tdap for adolescents 11-18 years requiring a tetanus toxoid product and who were vaccinated against tetanus ≥5 years earlier. Adolescents who completed the primary 3 dose series containing tetanus toxoid <5 years earlier are protected against tetanus and do not need a tetanus toxoid vaccine as part of wound management. The ACIP prefers Adacel™ for use in adults <65 years requiring a tetanus toxoid product and who were vaccinated against tetanus ≥5 years earlier if they have not previously received Tdap.

Dosage Forms

Injection, suspension:

Adacel™: Diphtheria 2 Lf units, tetanus 5 Lf units, and acellular pertussis 2.5 mcg per 0.5 mL (0.5 mL)

Boostrix®: Diphtheria 2.5 Lf units, tetanus 5 Lf units, and acellular pertussis 8 mcg per 0.5 mL (0.5 mL)

Daptacel®: Diphtheria 15 Lf units, tetanus 5 Lf units, and acellular pertussis 10 mcg per 0.5 mL (0.5 mL)

Infanrix®: Diphtheria 25 Lf units, tetanus 10 Lf units, and acellular pertussis 25 mcg per 0.5 mL (0.5 mL)

Tripedia®: Diphtheria 6.7 Lf units, tetanus 5 Lf units, and acellular pertussis 46.8 mcg per 0.5 mL (7.5 mL)

Note: Tripedia® vaccine is also used to reconstitute ActHIB® to prepare TriHIBit® vaccine (diphtheria, tetanus toxoids, and acellular pertussis and *Haemophilus influenzae* b conjugate vaccine combination)

diphtheria, tetanus toxoids, and acellular pertussis vaccine and *Haemophilus influenzae* b conjugate vaccine

(dif THEER ee a, TET a nus TOKS oyds & ay CEL yoo lar per TUS sis vak SEEN & hem OF fi lus in floo EN za bee KON joo gate vak SEEN)

Synonyms *Haemophilus influenzae* b conjugate vaccine and diphtheria, tetanus toxoids, and acellular pertussis vaccine

U.S./Canadian Brand Names TriHIBit® [US]

Therapeutic Category Toxoid; Vaccine, Inactivated Bacteria

Use Active immunization of children 15-18 months of age for prevention of diphtheria, tetanus, pertussis, and invasive disease caused by *H. influenzae* type b

Usual Dosage I.M.: Children >15 months of age: 0.5 mL (as part of a general vaccination schedule; see individual vaccines). Vaccine should be used within 30 minutes of reconstitution.

Dosage Forms

Injection, suspension:

TriHIBit®: 5 Lf units tetanus toxoid, 6.7 Lf units diphtheria toxoid, 46.8 mcg pertussis antigens, and 10 mcg *H. influenzae* type b purified capsular polysaccharide per 0.5 mL (0.5 mL)

diphtheria toxoid conjugate *see Haemophilus* B conjugate vaccine *on page 411*

dipivalyl epinephrine *see dipivefrin on this page*

dipivefrin (dye PI ve frin)

Synonyms dipivalyl epinephrine; dipivefrin hydrochloride; DPE

U.S./Canadian Brand Names Ophtho-Dipivefrin™ [Can]; PMS-Dipivefrin [Can]; Propine® [US/Can]

Therapeutic Category Adrenergic Agonist Agent

Use Reduces elevated intraocular pressure in chronic open-angle glaucoma; also used to treat ocular hypertension, low tension, and secondary glaucomas

Usual Dosage Ophthalmic: Adults: Instill 1 drop every 12 hours into the eyes

Dosage Forms

Solution, ophthalmic: 0.1% (5 mL, 10 mL, 15 mL)

Propine®: 0.1% (10 mL, 15 mL)

dipivefrin hydrochloride *see dipivefrin on this page*

Diprivan® [US/Can] *see propofol on page 722*

Diprolene® [US] *see betamethasone (topical) on page 109*

Diprolene® AF [US] *see betamethasone (topical) on page 109*

Diprolene® Glycol [Can] *see betamethasone (topical) on page 109*

dipropylacetic acid *see valproic acid and derivatives on page 881*

Diprosone® [Can] *see betamethasone (topical) on page 109*

dipyridamole (dye peer ID a mole)

Sound-Alike/Look-Alike Issues

dipyridamole may be confused with disopyramide

Persantine® may be confused with Periactin®, Permitil®

U.S./Canadian Brand Names Apo-Dipyridamole FC® [Can]; Persantine® [US/Can]

Therapeutic Category Antiplatelet Agent; Vasodilator

Use

Oral: Used with warfarin to decrease thrombosis in patients after artificial heart valve replacement

I.V.: Diagnostic agent in CAD

Usual Dosage

Oral: Children ≥12 years and Adults: Adjunctive therapy for prophylaxis of thromboembolism with cardiac valve replacement: 75-100 mg 4 times/day

I.V.: Adults: Evaluation of coronary artery disease: 0.14 mg/kg/minute for 4 minutes; maximum dose: 60 mg

Dosage Forms

Injection, solution: 5 mg/mL (2 mL, 10 mL)

Tablet: 25 mg, 50 mg, 75 mg

Persantine®: 25 mg, 50 mg, 75 mg

dipyridamole and aspirin *see aspirin and dipyridamole on page 79*

Disalcid® (Discontinued) *see salsalate on page 775*

disalicylic acid *see salsalate on page 775*

DisCoVisc™ **[US]** *see* sodium chondroitin sulfate and sodium hyaluronate *on page 794*

Disobrom® *(Discontinued) see* dexbrompheniramine and pseudoephedrine *on page 243*

disodium cromoglycate *see* cromolyn sodium *on page 218*

disodium thiosulfate pentahydrate *see* sodium thiosulfate *on page 798*

***d*-isoephedrine hydrochloride** *see* pseudoephedrine *on page 727*

Disonate® *(Discontinued) see* docusate *on page 273*

disopyramide (dye soe PEER a mide)

Sound-Alike/Look-Alike Issues
disopyramide may be confused with desipramine, dipyridamole
Norpace® may be confused with Norpramin®

Synonyms disopyramide phosphate

U.S./Canadian Brand Names Norpace® CR [US]; Norpace® [US/Can]; Rythmodan® [Can]; Rythmodan®-LA [Can]

Therapeutic Category Antiarrhythmic Agent, Class I-A

Use Suppression and prevention of unifocal and multifocal atrial and premature, ventricular premature complexes, coupled ventricular tachycardia; effective in the conversion of atrial fibrillation, atrial flutter, and paroxysmal atrial tachycardia to normal sinus rhythm and prevention of the recurrence of these arrhythmias after conversion by other methods

Usual Dosage Oral:
Children:
<1 year: 10-30 mg/kg/24 hours in 4 divided doses
1-4 years: 10-20 mg/kg/24 hours in 4 divided doses
4-12 years: 10-15 mg/kg/24 hours in 4 divided doses
12-18 years: 6-15 mg/kg/24 hours in 4 divided doses
Adults:
<50 kg: 100 mg every 6 hours or 200 mg every 12 hours (controlled release)
>50 kg: 150 mg every 6 hours or 300 mg every 12 hours (controlled release); if no response, increase to 200 mg every 6 hours. Maximum dose required for patients with severe refractory ventricular tachycardia is 400 mg every 6 hours.

Dosage Forms
Capsule: 100 mg, 150 mg
Norpace®: 100 mg, 150 mg
Capsule, controlled release: 100 mg, 150 mg
Norpace® CR: 100 mg, 150 mg

disopyramide phosphate *see* disopyramide *on this page*

Disotate® *(Discontinued) see* edetate disodium *on page 291*

Di-Spaz® **Injection** *(Discontinued) see* dicyclomine *on page 255*

Di-Spaz® **Oral** *(Discontinued) see* dicyclomine *on page 255*

DisperMox™ *(Discontinued) see* amoxicillin *on page 48*

disulfiram (dye SUL fi ram)

Sound-Alike/Look-Alike Issues
disulfiram may be confused with Diflucan®
Antabuse® may be confused with Anturane®

U.S./Canadian Brand Names Antabuse® [US]

Therapeutic Category Aldehyde Dehydrogenase Inhibitor Agent

Use Management of chronic alcoholism

Usual Dosage Adults: Oral: Do not administer until the patient has abstained from ethanol for at least 12 hours

Initial: 500 mg/day as a single dose for 1-2 weeks; maximum daily dose is 500 mg
Average maintenance dose: 250 mg/day; range: 125-500 mg; duration of therapy is to continue until the patient is fully recovered socially and a basis for permanent self control has been established; maintenance therapy may be required for months or even years

Dosage Forms
Tablet:
Antabuse®: 250 mg, 500 mg

Dital® *(Discontinued) see* phendimetrazine *on page 671*

dithioglycerol *see* dimercaprol *on page 263*

dithranol *see* anthralin *on page 57*

Ditropan® **[US/Can]** *see* oxybutynin *on page 639*

Ditropan® **XL [US/Can]** *see* oxybutynin *on page 639*

Diurigen® *(Discontinued) see* chlorothiazide *on page 176*

Diuril® **[US/Can]** *see* chlorothiazide *on page 176*

divalproex sodium *see* valproic acid and derivatives *on page 881*

Divigel® **[US]** *see* estradiol *on page 313*

Dixarit® **[Can]** *see* clonidine *on page 204*

Dizac® **Injectable Emulsion** *(Discontinued) see* diazepam *on page 251*

Dizmiss® *(Discontinued) see* meclizine *on page 535*

5071-1DL(6) *see* megestrol *on page 538*

***dl*-alpha tocopherol** *see* vitamin E *on page 894*

4-DMDR *see* idarubicin *on page 446*

***D*-mannitol** *see* mannitol *on page 530*

D-Med® **Injection** *(Discontinued) see* methylprednisolone *on page 559*

D-3-mercaptovaline *see* penicillamine *on page 661*

DMSA *see* succimer *on page 808*

DMSO *see* dimethyl sulfoxide *on page 263*

DNA-derived humanized monoclonal antibody *see* alemtuzumab *on page 27*

DNR *see* daunorubicin hydrochloride *on page 233*

Doak® **Tar [US-OTC]** *see* coal tar *on page 208*

Doan's® **Extra Strength [US-OTC]** *see* magnesium salicylate *on page 528*

dobutamine (doe BYOO ta meen)
Sound-Alike/Look-Alike Issues
DOBUTamine may be confused with DOPamine
Synonyms dobutamine hydrochloride
Tall-Man DOBUTamine
U.S./Canadian Brand Names Dobutamine Injection, USP [Can]; Dobutrex® [Can]
Therapeutic Category Adrenergic Agonist Agent
Use Short-term management of patients with cardiac decompensation
Usual Dosage Administration requires the use of an infusion pump; I.V. infusion:
Neonates: 2-15 mcg/kg/minute, titrate to desired response
Children and Adults: 2.5-20 mcg/kg/minute; maximum: 40 mcg/kg/minute, titrate to desired response.
Dosage Forms
Infusion [premixed in dextrose]: 1 mg/mL (250 mL, 500 mL); 2 mg/mL (250 mL); 4 mg/mL (250 mL)
Injection, solution: 12.5 mg/mL (20 mL, 40 mL, 100 mL)

dobutamine hydrochloride *see* dobutamine *on this page*

Dobutamine Injection, USP [Can] *see* dobutamine *on this page*

Dobutrex® **[Can]** *see* dobutamine *on this page*

docetaxel (doe se TAKS el)
Sound-Alike/Look-Alike Issues
Taxotere® may be confused with Taxol®
Synonyms NSC-628503; RP-6976
U.S./Canadian Brand Names Taxotere® [US/Can]
Therapeutic Category Antineoplastic Agent
Use Treatment of breast cancer; locally-advanced or metastatic nonsmall cell lung cancer (NSCLC); hormone refractory, metastatic prostate cancer; advanced gastric adenocarcinoma; locally-advanced squamous cell head and neck cancer
Usual Dosage I.V. infusion (refer to individual protocols): Children ≥16 years and Adults:
Breast cancer:
Locally-advanced or metastatic: 60-100 mg/m^2 every 3 weeks; patients initially started at 60 mg/m^2 who do not develop toxicity may tolerate higher doses
Operable, node-positive (adjuvant treatment): 75 mg/m^2 every 3 weeks for 6 courses
Nonsmall cell lung cancer: 75 mg/m^2 every 3 weeks
Prostate cancer: 75 mg/m^2 every 3 weeks; prednisone (5 mg twice daily) is administered continuously

Gastric adenocarcinoma: 75 mg/m^2 every 3 weeks (in combination with cisplatin and fluorouracil)

Head and neck cancer: 75 mg/m^2 every 3 weeks (in combination with cisplatin and fluorouracil) for 4 cycles, followed by radiation therapy

Dosage Forms

Injection, solution [concentrate]:

Taxotere®: 20 mg/0.5 mL (0.5 mL, 2 mL)

docosanol (doe KOE san ole)

Synonyms behenyl alcohol; *n*-docosanol

U.S./Canadian Brand Names Abreva® [US-OTC]

Therapeutic Category Antiviral Agent, Topical

Use Treatment of herpes simplex of the face or lips

Usual Dosage Topical: Children ≥12 years and Adults: Apply 5 times/day to affected area of face or lips. Start at first sign of cold sore or fever blister and continue until healed.

Dosage Forms

Cream:

Abreva® [OTC]: 10% (2 g)

docusate (DOK yoo sate)

Sound-Alike/Look-Alike Issues

docusate may be confused with Doxinate®

Colace® may be confused with Calan®

Surfak® may be confused with Surbex®

Synonyms dioctyl calcium sulfosuccinate; dioctyl sodium sulfosuccinate; docusate calcium; docusate potassium; docusate sodium; DOSS; DSS

U.S./Canadian Brand Names Apo-Docusate-Sodium® [Can]; Colace® [US-OTC/Can]; Colax-C® [Can]; D-S-S® [US-OTC]; Diocto® [US-OTC]; Docusoft-S™ [US-OTC]; DOK™ [US-OTC]; DOS® [US-OTC]; Dulcolax® Stool Softener [US-OTC]; Enemeez® [US-OTC]; Fleet® Sof-Lax® [US-OTC]; Genasoft® [US-OTC]; Novo-Docusate Calcium [Can]; Novo-Docusate Sodium [Can]; Phillips'® Stool Softener Laxative [US-OTC]; PMS-Docusate Calcium [Can]; PMS-Docusate Sodium [Can]; Regulex® [Can]; Selax® [Can]; Silace [US-OTC]; Soflax™ [Can]; Surfak® [US-OTC]

Therapeutic Category Stool Softener

Use Stool softener in patients who should avoid straining during defecation and constipation associated with hard, dry stools; prophylaxis for straining (Valsalva) following myocardial infarction. A safe agent to be used in elderly; some evidence that doses <200 mg are ineffective; stool softeners are unnecessary if stool is well hydrated or "mushy" and soft; shown to be ineffective used long-term.

Usual Dosage Docusate salts are interchangeable; the amount of sodium or calcium per dosage unit is clinically insignificant

Infants and Children <3 years: Oral: 10-40 mg/day in 1-4 divided doses

Children: Oral:

3-6 years: 20-60 mg/day in 1-4 divided doses

6-12 years: 40-150 mg/day in 1-4 divided doses

Adolescents and Adults: Oral: 50-500 mg/day in 1-4 divided doses

Older Children and Adults: Rectal: Add 50-100 mg of docusate liquid to enema fluid (saline or water); administer as retention or flushing enema

Dosage Forms

Capsule: 100 mg, 240 mg, 250 mg

Colace® [OTC]: 50 mg, 100 mg

Docusoft-S™ [OTC], DOK™ [OTC], Genasoft® [OTC], Dulcolax® Stool Softener [OTC]:, Phillips'® Stool Softener Laxative [OTC] 100 mg

DOS® [OTC], D-S-S® [OTC]: 100 mg, 250 mg

Surfak® [OTC]: 240 mg

Enema, rectal: 283 mg/5 mL (5 mL)

Enemeez® [OTC]: 283 mg/5 mL 5 mL

Gelcap:

Fleet® Sof-Lax® [OTC]: 100 mg

Liquid: 150 mg/15 mL

Colace® [OTC], Diocto® [OTC], Silace [OTC]: 150 mg/15 mL

Syrup: 20 mg/5 mL, 60 mg/15 mL

Colace® [OTC], Diocto® [OTC]: 60 mg/15 mL

Silace [OTC]: 20 mg/5 mL

docusate and senna (DOK yoo sate & SEN na)

Sound-Alike/Look-Alike Issues
Senokot® may be confused with Depakote®
Synonyms senna and docusate; senna-S
U.S./Canadian Brand Names Peri-Colace® [US-OTC]; Senokot-S® [US-OTC]; SenoSol™-SS [US-OTC]
Therapeutic Category Laxative, Stimulant; Stool Softener
Use Short-term treatment of constipation
Usual Dosage Oral: Constipation: OTC ranges:
Children:
2-6 years: Initial: 4.3 mg sennosides plus 25 mg docusate ($\frac{1}{2}$ tablet) once daily (maximum: 1 tablet twice daily)
6-12 years: Initial: 8.6 sennosides plus 50 mg docusate (1 tablet) once daily (maximum: 2 tablets twice daily)
Children ≥12 years and Adults: Initial: 2 tablets (17.2 mg sennosides plus 100 mg docusate) once daily (maximum: 4 tablets twice daily)
Dosage Forms
Tablet: Docusate 50 mg and sennosides 8.6 mg
Peri-Colace® [OTC], Senokot-S® [OTC], SenoSol™-SS: Docusate 50 mg and sennosides 8.6 mg

docusate calcium *see* docusate *on previous page*

docusate potassium *see* docusate *on previous page*

docusate sodium *see* docusate *on previous page*

Docusoft Plus™ *(Discontinued)*

Docusoft-S™ [US-OTC] *see* docusate *on previous page*

dofetilide (doe FET il ide)

U.S./Canadian Brand Names Tikosyn® [US/Can]
Therapeutic Category Antiarrhythmic Agent, Class III
Use Maintenance of normal sinus rhythm in patients with chronic atrial fibrillation/atrial flutter of longer than 1-week duration who have been converted to normal sinus rhythm; conversion of atrial fibrillation and atrial flutter to normal sinus rhythm
Usual Dosage Oral: Adults:
Note: QT or QT_c must be determined prior to first dose. If QT_c >440 msec (>500 msec in patients with ventricular conduction abnormalities), dofetilide is contraindicated.
Initial: 500 mcg orally twice daily. Initial dosage must be adjusted in patients with estimated Cl_{cr} <60 mL/minute. Dofetilide may be initiated at lower doses than recommended based on physician discretion.
Modification of dosage in response to initial dose: QT_c interval should be measured 2-3 hours after the initial dose. If the QT_c >15% of baseline, or if the QT_c is >500 msec (550 msec in patients with ventricular conduction abnormalities) dofetilide should be adjusted. If the starting dose is 500 mcg twice daily, then adjust to 250 mcg twice daily. If the starting dose was 250 mcg twice daily, then adjust to 125 mcg twice daily. If the starting dose was 125 mcg twice daily then adjust to 125 mcg every day.
Continued monitoring for doses 2-5: QT_c interval must be determined 2-3 hours after each subsequent dose of dofetilide for in-hospital doses 2-5. If the measured QT_c is >500 msec (550 msec in patients with ventricular conduction abnormalities) at any time, dofetilide should be discontinued.
Chronic therapy (following the 5th dose):
QT or QT_c and creatinine clearance should be evaluated every 3 months. If QT_c >500 msec (>550 msec in patients with ventricular conduction abnormalities), dofetilide should be discontinued.
Dosage Forms
Capsule:
Tikosyn®: 125 mcg, 250 mcg, 500 mcg

Dofus [US-OTC] *see* Lactobacillus *on page 488*

DOK™ [US-OTC] *see* docusate *on previous page*

Doktors® Nasal Solution *(Discontinued)* *see* phenylephrine *on page 675*

Dolacet® Forte *(Discontinued)* *see* hydrocodone and acetaminophen *on page 427*

dolasetron (dol A se tron)

Sound-Alike/Look-Alike Issues
dolasetron may be confused with granisetron, ondansetron, palonosetron
Anzemet® may be confused with Aldomet® and Avandamet™

Synonyms dolasetron mesylate; MDL 73,147EF

U.S./Canadian Brand Names Anzemet® [US/Can]

Therapeutic Category Selective 5-HT$_3$ Receptor Antagonist

Use Prevention of nausea and vomiting associated with emetogenic cancer chemotherapy; prevention of postoperative nausea and vomiting; treatment of postoperative nausea and vomiting (injectable form only).

Note: In Canada, the use of dolasetron is contraindicated for all uses in children <18 years of age or in the treatment of postoperative nausea and vomiting in adults. These are not labeled contraindications in the U.S.

Usual Dosage Note: In Canada, the use of dolasetron is contraindicated in children <18 years of age or in the treatment of postoperative nausea and vomiting in adults. These are not labeled contraindications in the U.S.

Prevention of chemotherapy-associated nausea and vomiting (including initial and repeat courses):
Children 2-16 years:
Oral: 1.8 mg/kg within 1 hour before chemotherapy; maximum: 100 mg/dose
I.V.: 1.8 mg/kg ~30 minutes before chemotherapy; maximum: 100 mg/dose
Adults:
Oral:100 mg single dose 1 hour prior to chemotherapy
I.V.: 1.8 mg/kg or 100 mg 30 minutes prior to chemotherapy
Prevention of postoperative nausea and vomiting:
Children 2-16 years:
Oral: 1.2 mg/kg within 2 hours before surgery; maximum: 100 mg/dose
I.V.: 0.35 mg/kg (maximum: 12.5 mg) ~15 minutes before stopping anesthesia
Adults:
Oral: 100 mg within 2 hours before surgery
I.V.: 12.5 mg ~15 minutes before stopping anesthesia
Treatment of postoperative nausea and vomiting: I.V. (only):
Children: 0.35 mg/kg (maximum: 12.5 mg) as soon as needed
Adults: 12.5 mg as soon as needed

Dosage Forms
Injection, solution:
Anzemet®: 20 mg/mL (0.625 mL) [single-use Carpuject® or vial; contains mannitol 38.2 mg/mL]; 20 mg/mL (5 mL) [single-use vial; contains mannitol 38.2 mg/mL]; 20 mg/mL (25 mL) [multidose vial; contains mannitol 29 mg/mL]
Tablet:
Anzemet®: 50 mg, 100 mg

dolasetron mesylate *see* dolasetron *on previous page*

Dolene® *(Discontinued)* *see* propoxyphene *on page 723*

Dolgic® LQ [US] *see* butalbital, acetaminophen, and caffeine *on page 130*

Dolgic® Plus [US] *see* butalbital, acetaminophen, and caffeine *on page 130*

Dolobid® *(Discontinued)* *see* diflunisal *on page 257*

Dologesic® [US] *see* acetaminophen and phenyltoloxamine *on page 8*

Dolophine® [US] *see* methadone *on page 550*

Dolorac™ *(Discontinued)* *see* capsaicin *on page 145*

Dolorex® *(Discontinued)* *see* capsaicin *on page 145*

Dom-Azithromycin [Can] *see* azithromycin *on page 88*

Dom-Benzydamine [Can] *see* benzydamine *(Canada only) on page 105*

Dom-Citalopram [Can] *see* citalopram *on page 194*

Dom-Clobazam [Can] *see* clobazam *(Canada only) on page 201*

Dom-Domperidone [Can] *see* domperidone *(Canada only) on next page*

Domeboro® [US-OTC] *see* aluminum sulfate and calcium acetate *on page 38*

dome paste bandage *see* zinc gelatin *on page 905*

Dom-Fenofibrate Supra [Can] *see* fenofibrate *on page 345*

Dom-Mefenamic Acid [Can] *see* mefenamic acid *on page 537*

Dom-Methimazole [Can] *see* methimazole *on page 552*

Dom-Moclobemide [Can] *see* moclobemide *(Canada only) on page 575*

domperidone *(Canada only)* (dom PE ri done)

Synonyms domperidone maleate

U.S./Canadian Brand Names Alti-Domperidone [Can]; Apo-Domperidone® [Can]; Dom-Domperidone [Can]; FTP-Domperidone Maleate [Can]; Motilium® [Can]; Novo-Domperidone [Can]; Nu-Domperidone [Can]; PHL-Domperidone [Can]; PMS-Domperidone [Can]; RAN™-Domperidone [Can]; ratio-Domperidone [Can]

Therapeutic Category Dopamine Antagonist

Use Symptomatic management of upper GI motility disorders associated with chronic and subacute gastritis and diabetic gastroparesis; prevention of GI symptoms associated with use of dopamine-agonist anti-Parkinson agents

Usual Dosage Oral: Adults:

GI motility disorders: 10 mg 3-4 times/day, 15-30 minutes before meals; severe/resistant cases: 20 mg 3-4 times/day, 15-30 minutes before meals

Nausea/vomiting associated with dopamine-agonist anti-Parkinson agents: 20 mg 3-4 times/day

Dosage Forms [CAN] = Canadian brand name

Tablet: 10 mg [not available in the U.S.]

Alti-Domperidone [CAN], Apo-Domperidone® [CAN], Dom-Domperidone [CAN], Novo-Domperidone [CAN], Nu-Domperidone [CAN], PHL-Domperidone [CAN], PMS-Domperidone [CAN], ratio-Domperidone [CAN]: 10 mg [not available in the U.S.]

domperidone maleate *see* domperidone *(Canada only) on this page*

Dom-Sumatriptan [Can] *see* sumatriptan *on page 815*

Dom-Tiaprofenic® [Can] *see* tiaprofenic acid *(Canada only) on page 840*

Dom-Topiramate [Can] *see* topiramate *on page 851*

Dom-Zopiclone [Can] *see* zopiclone *(Canada only) on page 909*

Donatussin [US] *see* dextromethorphan, chlorpheniramine, phenylephrine, and guaifenesin *on page 248*

Donatussin [US] *see* guaifenesin and phenylephrine *on page 404*

Donatussin DC [US] *see* hydrocodone, phenylephrine, and guaifenesin *on page 431*

donepezil (doh NEP e zil)

Sound-Alike/Look-Alike Issues

Aricept® may be confused with AcipHex®, Ascriptin®, and Azilect®

Synonyms E2020

U.S./Canadian Brand Names Aricept® ODT [US]; Aricept® RDT [Can]; Aricept® [US/Can]

Therapeutic Category Acetylcholinesterase Inhibitor; Cholinergic Agent

Use Treatment of mild, moderate, or severe dementia of the Alzheimer type

Usual Dosage Oral: Adults: Dementia of Alzheimer type: Initial: 5 mg/day at bedtime; may increase to 10 mg/day at bedtime after 4-6 weeks

Dosage Forms

Tablet:

Aricept®: 5 mg, 10 mg

Tablet, orally disintegrating:

Aricept® ODT: 5 mg, 10 mg

Donnamar® *(Discontinued)* *see* hyoscyamine *on page 441*

Donnapine® *(Discontinued)* *see* hyoscyamine, atropine, scopolamine, and phenobarbital *on page 442*

Donnatal® [US] *see* hyoscyamine, atropine, scopolamine, and phenobarbital *on page 442*

Donnatal Extentabs® [US] *see* hyoscyamine, atropine, scopolamine, and phenobarbital *on page 442*

dopamine (DOE pa meen)

Sound-Alike/Look-Alike Issues

DOPamine may be confused with DOBUTamine, Dopram®

Synonyms dopamine hydrochloride

Tall-Man DOPamine

Therapeutic Category Adrenergic Agonist Agent

Use Adjunct in the treatment of shock (eg, MI, open heart surgery, renal failure, cardiac decompensation) which persists after adequate fluid volume replacement

Usual Dosage I.V. infusion (administration requires the use of an infusion pump):

Neonates: 1-20 mcg/kg/minute continuous infusion, titrate to desired response.

Children: 1-20 mcg/kg/minute, maximum: 50 mcg/kg/minute continuous infusion, titrate to desired response.

Adults: 1-5 mcg/kg/minute up to 20 mcg/kg/minute, titrate to desired response (maximum: 50 mcg/kg/minute). Infusion may be increased by 1-4 mcg/kg/minute at 10- to 30-minute intervals until optimal response is obtained.

If dosages >20-30 mcg/kg/minute are needed, a more direct-acting pressor may be more beneficial (ie, epinephrine, norepinephrine).

Dosage Forms
Infusion [premixed in D$_5$W]: 0.8 mg/mL (250 mL, 500 mL); 1.6 mg/mL (250 mL, 500 mL); 3.2 mg/mL (250 mL)
Injection, solution: 40 mg/mL (5 mL, 10 mL); 80 mg/mL (5 mL); 160 mg/mL (5 mL)

dopamine hydrochloride *see* dopamine *on previous page*

Dopram® [US] *see* doxapram *on next page*

Doral® [US/Can] *see* quazepam *on page 738*

Dormarex® 2 Oral *(Discontinued)* *see* diphenhydramine *on page 265*

dornase alfa (DOOR nase AL fa)
Synonyms recombinant human deoxyribonuclease; rhDNase
U.S./Canadian Brand Names Pulmozyme® [US/Can]
Therapeutic Category Enzyme
Use Management of cystic fibrosis patients to reduce the frequency of respiratory infections that require parenteral antibiotics in patients with FVC ≥40% of predicted; to improve pulmonary function in patients with cystic fibrosis
Usual Dosage Inhalation:
Children ≥3 months to Adults: 2.5 mg once daily through selected nebulizers; experience in children <5 years is limited
Patients unable to inhale or exhale orally throughout the entire treatment period may use Pari-Baby™ nebulizer. Some patients may benefit from twice daily administration.
Dosage Forms
Solution for nebulization [preservative free]:
Pulmozyme®: 1 mg/mL (2.5 mL)

Doryx® [US] *see* doxycycline *on page 281*

dorzolamide (dor ZOLE a mide)
Synonyms dorzolamide hydrochloride
U.S./Canadian Brand Names Trusopt® [US/Can]
Therapeutic Category Carbonic Anhydrase Inhibitor
Use Lowers intraocular pressure in patients with ocular hypertension or open-angle glaucoma
Usual Dosage Children and Adults: Reduction of intraocular pressure: Instill 1 drop in the affected eye(s) 3 times/day
Dosage Forms
Solution, ophthalmic:
Trusopt®: 2% (10 mL)

dorzolamide and timolol (dor ZOLE a mide & TYE moe lole)
Synonyms timolol and dorzolamide
U.S./Canadian Brand Names Cosopt® [US/Can]; Preservative-Free Cosopt® [Can]
Therapeutic Category Beta-Adrenergic Blocker; Carbonic Anhydrase Inhibitor
Use Reduction of intraocular pressure in patients with ocular hypertension or open-angle glaucoma
Usual Dosage Ophthalmic: Children ≥2 years and Adults: Instill 1 drop in affected eye(s) twice daily
Dosage Forms
Solution, ophthalmic:
Cosopt®: Dorzolamide 2% and timolol 0.5% (10 mL)

dorzolamide hydrochloride *see* dorzolamide *on this page*

DOS® [US-OTC] *see* docusate *on page 273*

DOSS *see* docusate *on page 273*

Dostinex® [US/Can] *see* cabergoline *on page 133*

Dovobet® [Can] *see* calcipotriene and betamethasone *on page 135*

Dovonex® [US] *see* calcipotriene *on page 135*

doxacurium (doks a KYOO ri um)

Sound-Alike/Look-Alike Issues
doxacurium may be confused with doxapram, DOXOrubicin

Synonyms doxacurium chloride

U.S./Canadian Brand Names Nuromax® [US]

Therapeutic Category Skeletal Muscle Relaxant

Use Adjunct to general anesthesia to facilitate endotracheal intubation and to relax skeletal muscles during surgery; to facilitate mechanical ventilation in ICU patients; does not relieve pain or produce sedation; the characteristics of this agent make it especially useful in procedures requiring careful maintenance of hemodynamic stability for prolonged periods

Usual Dosage Administer I.V.; dose to effect; doses will vary due to interpatient variability; use ideal body weight for obese patients

Surgery:
Children >2 years: Initial: 0.03-0.05 mg/kg followed by maintenance doses of 0.005-0.01 mg/kg after 30-45 minutes

Adults: 0.05-0.08 mg/kg with thiopental/narcotic or 0.025 mg/kg after initial dose of succinylcholine for intubation; initial maintenance dose of 0.005-0.01 mg/kg after 100-160 minutes followed by repeat doses every 30-45 minutes

Pretreatment/priming: 10% of intubating dose given 3-5 minutes before initial dose

ICU: 0.05 mg/kg bolus followed by 0.025 mg/kg every 2-3 hours or 0.25-0.75 mcg/kg/minute once initial recovery from bolus dose observed

Dosage Forms
Injection, solution:
Nuromax®: 1 mg/mL (5 mL)

doxacurium chloride see doxacurium on this page

doxapram (DOKS a pram)

Sound-Alike/Look-Alike Issues
doxapram may be confused with doxacurium, doxazosin, doxepin, Doxinate®, DOXOrubicin
Dopram® may be confused with DOPamine

Synonyms doxapram hydrochloride

U.S./Canadian Brand Names Dopram® [US]

Therapeutic Category Respiratory Stimulant

Use Respiratory and CNS stimulant for respiratory depression secondary to anesthesia, drug-induced CNS depression; acute hypercapnia secondary to COPD

Usual Dosage
Respiratory depression following anesthesia:
Intermittent injection: Initial: 0.5-1 mg/kg; may repeat at 5-minute intervals (only in patients who demonstrate initial response); maximum total dose: 2 mg/kg

I.V. infusion: Initial: 5 mg/minute until adequate response or adverse effects seen; decrease to 1-3 mg/minute; maximum total dose: 4 mg/kg

Drug-induced CNS depression:
Intermittent injection: Initial: Priming dose of 1-2 mg/kg, repeat after 5 minutes; may repeat at 1-2 hour intervals (until sustained consciousness); maximum: 3 g/day. May repeat in 24 hours if necessary.

I.V. infusion: Initial: Priming dose of 1-2 mg/kg, repeat after 5 minutes. If no response, wait 1-2 hours and repeat. If some stimulation is noted, initiate infusion at 1-3 mg/minute (depending on size of patient/depth of CNS depression); suspend infusion if patient begins to awaken. Infusion should not be continued for >2 hours. May reinstitute infusion as described above, including bolus, after rest interval of 30 minutes to 2 hours; maximum: 3 g/day

Acute hypercapnia secondary to COPD: I.V. infusion: Initial: Initiate infusion at 1-2 mg/minute (depending on size of patient/depth of CNS depression); may increase to maximum rate of 3 mg/minute; infusion should not be continued for >2 hours. Monitor arterial blood gases prior to initiation of infusion and at 30-minute intervals during the infusion (to identify possible development of acidosis/CO_2 retention). Additional infusions are not recommended (per manufacturer).

Dosage Forms
Injection, solution: 20 mg/mL (20 mL)
Dopram®: 20 mg/mL (20 mL)

doxapram hydrochloride see doxapram on this page

doxazosin (doks AY zoe sin)

Sound-Alike/Look-Alike Issues
doxazosin may be confused with doxapram, doxepin, DOXOrubicin
Cardura® may be confused with Cardene®, Cordarone®, Cordran®, Coumadin®, K-Dur®, Ridaura®

Synonyms doxazosin mesylate

U.S./Canadian Brand Names Alti-Doxazosin [Can]; Apo-Doxazosin® [Can]; Cardura-1™ [Can]; Cardura-2™ [Can]; Cardura-4™ [Can]; Cardura® XL [US]; Cardura® [US]; Gen-Doxazosin [Can]; Novo-Doxazosin [Can]

Therapeutic Category Alpha-Adrenergic Blocking Agent

Use Treatment of hypertension alone or in conjunction with diuretics, ACE inhibitors, beta-blockers, or calcium antagonists; treatment of urinary outflow obstruction and/or obstructive and irritative symptoms associated with benign prostatic hyperplasia (BPH), particularly useful in patients with troublesome symptoms who are unable or unwilling to undergo invasive procedures, but who require rapid symptomatic relief; can be used in combination with finasteride

Usual Dosage Oral: Adults:

Immediate release: 1 mg once daily in morning or evening; may be increased to 2 mg once daily. Thereafter titrate upwards, if needed, over several weeks, balancing therapeutic benefit with doxazosin-induced postural hypotension.

Hypertension: Maximum dose: 16 mg/day

BPH: Goal: 4-8 mg/day; maximum dose: 8 mg/day

Extended release: BPH: 4 mg once daily with breakfast; titrate based on response and tolerability every 3-4 weeks to maximum recommended dose of 8 mg/day

Reinitiation of therapy: If therapy is discontinued for several days, restart at 4 mg dose and titrate as before.

Conversion to extended release from immediate release: Initiate with 4 mg once daily; omit final evening dose of immediate release prior to starting morning dosing with extended release product.

Dosage Forms

Tablet: 1 mg, 2 mg, 4 mg, 8 mg

Cardura®: 1 mg, 2 mg, 4 mg, 8 mg

Tablet, extended release:

Cardura® XL: 4 mg, 8 mg

doxazosin mesylate see doxazosin *on previous page*

doxepin (DOKS e pin)

Sound-Alike/Look-Alike Issues

doxepin may be confused with digoxin, doxapram, doxazosin, Doxidan®, doxycycline

Sinequan® may be confused with saquinavir, Serentil®, Seroquel®, Singulair®

Zonalon® may be confused with Zone-A Forte®

Synonyms doxepin hydrochloride

U.S./Canadian Brand Names Apo-Doxepin® [Can]; Novo-Doxepin [Can]; Prudoxin™ [US]; Sinequan® [Can]; Zonalon® [US/Can]

Therapeutic Category Antidepressant, Tricyclic (Tertiary Amine); Topical Skin Product

Use

Oral: Depression

Topical: Short-term (<8 days) management of moderate pruritus in adults with atopic dermatitis or lichen simplex chronicus

Usual Dosage

Oral: Topical: Burning mouth syndrome (dental use): Cream: Apply 3-4 times daily

Oral (entire daily dose may be given at bedtime):

Depression or anxiety:

Adolescents: Initial: 25-50 mg/day in single or divided doses; gradually increase to 100 mg/day

Adults: Initial: 25-150 mg/day at bedtime or in 2-3 divided doses; may gradually increase up to 300 mg/day; single dose should not exceed 150 mg; select patients may respond to 25-50 mg/day

Chronic urticaria, angioedema, nocturnal pruritus: Adults: 10-30 mg/day

Topical: Pruritus: Adults: Apply a thin film 4 times/day with at least 3- to 4-hour interval between applications; not recommended for use >8 days. **Note:** Low-dose (25-50 mg) oral administration has also been used to treat pruritus, but systemic effects are increased.

Dosage Forms

Capsule: 10 mg, 25 mg, 50 mg, 75 mg, 100 mg, 150 mg

Cream:

Prudoxin™: 5% (45 g)

Zonalon®: 5% (30 g, 45 g)

Solution, oral concentrate: 10 mg/mL

doxepin hydrochloride see doxepin *on this page*

doxercalciferol (doks er kal si fe FEER ole)

Synonyms 1α-hydroxyergocalciferol
U.S./Canadian Brand Names Hectorol® [US/Can]
Therapeutic Category Vitamin D Analog
Use Treatment of secondary hyperparathyroidism in patients with chronic kidney disease
Usual Dosage
Oral:
Dialysis patients: Dose should be titrated to lower iPTH to 150-300 pg/mL; dose is adjusted at 8-week intervals (maximum dose: 20 mcg 3 times/week)
Initial dose: iPTH >400 pg/mL: 10 mcg 3 times/week at dialysis
Dose titration:
iPTH level decreased by 50% and >300 pg/mL: Dose can be increased to 12.5 mcg 3 times/week for 8 more weeks; this titration process can continue at 8-week intervals; each increase should be by 2.5 mcg/dose
iPTH level 150-300 pg/mL: Maintain current dose
iPTH level <100 pg/mL: Suspend doxercalciferol for 1 week; resume at a reduced dose; decrease each dose (not weekly dose) by at least 2.5 mcg
Predialysis patients: Dose should be titrated to lower iPTH to 35-70 pg/mL with stage 3 disease or to 70-110 pg/mL with stage 4 disease: Dose may be adjusted at 2-week intervals (maximum dose: 3.5 mcg/day)
Initial dose: 1 mcg/day
Dose titration:
iPTH level >70 pg/mL with stage 3 disease or >110 pg/mL with stage 4 disease: Increase dose by 0.5 mcg every 2 weeks as necessary
iPTH level 35-70 pg/mL with stage 3 disease or 70-110 pg/mL with stage 4 disease: Maintain current dose
iPTH level is <35 pg/mL with stage 3 disease or <70 pg/mL with stage 4 disease: Suspend doxercalciferol for 1 week, then resume at a reduced dose (at least 0.5 mcg lower)
I.V.:
Dialysis patients: Dose should be titrated to lower iPTH to 150-300 pg/mL; dose is adjusted at 8-week intervals (maximum dose: 18 mcg/week)
Initial dose: iPTH level >400 pg/mL: 4 mcg 3 times/week after dialysis, administered as a bolus dose
Dose titration:
iPTH level decreased by <50% and >300 pg/mL: Dose can be increased by 1-2 mcg at 8-week intervals, as necessary
iPTH level decreased by >50% and >300 pg/mL: Maintain current dose
iPTH level 150-300 pg/mL: Maintain the current dose
iPTH level <100 pg/mL: Suspend doxercalciferol for 1 week; resume at a reduced dose (at least 1 mcg lower)
Dosage Forms
Capsule:
Hectorol®: 0.5 mcg, 2.5 mcg
Injection, solution:
Hectorol®: 2 mcg/mL (2 mL)

Doxidan® [US-OTC] see bisacodyl on page 112

Doxil® [US] see doxorubicin (liposomal) on next page

doxorubicin (doks oh ROO bi sin)

Sound-Alike/Look-Alike Issues
DOXOrubicin may be confused with dactinomycin, DAUNOrubicin, doxacurium, doxapram, doxazosin, epirubicin, idarubicin
Adriamycin PFS® may be confused with achromycin, Aredia®, Idamycin®
Rubex® may be confused with Robaxin®
ADR is an error-prone abbreviation
conventional formulations (Adriamycin PFS®, Adriamycin RDF®, Rubex®) may be confused with liposomal formulations (DaunoXome®, Doxil®)
Synonyms adria; doxorubicin hydrochloride; hydroxydaunomycin hydrochloride; hydroxyldaunorubicin hydrochloride; NSC-123127
Tall-Man DOXOrubicin
U.S./Canadian Brand Names Adriamycin® [US/Can]
Therapeutic Category Antineoplastic Agent
Use Treatment of leukemias, lymphomas, multiple myeloma, osseous and nonosseous sarcomas, mesotheliomas, germ cell tumors of the ovary or testis, and carcinomas of the head and neck, thyroid, lung, breast, stomach, pancreas, liver, ovary, bladder, prostate, uterus, neuroblastoma and Wilms tumor.
Usual Dosage Refer to individual protocols. I.V.:
Children:
35-75 mg/m² as a single dose, repeat every 21 days **or**

20-30 mg/m² once weekly **or**
60-90 mg/m² given as a continuous infusion over 96 hours every 3-4 weeks
Adults: Usual or typical dose: 60-75 mg/m² as a single dose, repeat every 21 days **or** other dosage regimens like 20-30 mg/m²/day for 2-3 days, repeat in 4 weeks **or** 20 mg/m² once weekly

Dosage Forms
Injection, powder for reconstitution: 10 mg, 50 mg
Adriamycin®: 10 mg, 20 mg, 50 mg
Injection, solution: 2 mg/mL (5 mL, 10 mL, 25 mL, 100 mL)
Adriamycin®: 2 mg/mL (5 mL, 10 mL, 25 mL, 100 mL)

doxorubicin hydrochloride *see* doxorubicin *on previous page*

DOXOrubicin hydrochloride (liposomal) *see* doxorubicin (liposomal) *on this page*

doxorubicin (liposomal) (doks oh ROO bi sin lip pah SOW mal)

Sound-Alike/Look-Alike Issues
DOXOrubicin may be confused with dactinomycin, DAUNOrubicin, doxacurium, doxapram, doxazosin, epirubicin, idarubicin
DOXOrubicin liposomal may be confused with DAUNOrubicin liposomal
Doxil® may be confused with Doxy®, Paxil®
liposomal formulations (Doxil®) may be confused with conventional formulations (Adriamycin PFS®, Adriamycin RDF®, Cerubidine®, Rubex®).

Synonyms DOXOrubicin hydrochloride (liposomal); liposomal DOXOrubicin; NSC-712227; pegylated liposomal DOXOrubicin

Tall-Man DOXOrubicin (liposomal)

U.S./Canadian Brand Names Caelyx® [Can]; Doxil® [US]

Therapeutic Category Antineoplastic Agent

Use Treatment of ovarian cancer, multiple myeloma, and AIDS-related Kaposi sarcoma

Usual Dosage Refer to individual protocols. **Liposomal formulations of doxorubicin should NOT be substituted for conventional doxorubicin hydrochloride on a mg-per-mg basis.**
AIDS-related Kaposi sarcoma: I.V.: 20 mg/m²/dose once every 3 weeks
Multiple myeloma: I.V.: 30 mg/m²/dose every 3 weeks (in combination with bortezomib)
Ovarian cancer: I.V.: 50 mg/m²/dose every 4 weeks

Dosage Forms
Injection, solution:
Doxil®: 2 mg/mL (10 mL, 25 mL)

Doxy-100® [US] *see* doxycycline *on this page*

Doxycin [Can] *see* doxycycline *on this page*

doxycycline (doks i SYE kleen)

Sound-Alike/Look-Alike Issues
doxycycline may be confused with dicyclomine, doxepin, doxylamine
Doxy-100® may be confused with Doxil®
Monodox® may be confused with Maalox®

Synonyms doxycycline calcium; doxycycline hyclate; doxycycline monohydrate

U.S./Canadian Brand Names Adoxa® [US]; Apo-Doxy Tabs® [Can]; Apo-Doxy® [Can]; Doryx® [US]; Doxy-100® [US]; Doxycin [Can]; Doxytec [Can]; Monodox® [US]; Novo-Doxylin [Can]; Nu-Doxycycline [Can]; Oracea™ [US]; Periostat® [US/Can]; Vibra-Tabs® [US/Can]; Vibramycin® [US]

Therapeutic Category Tetracycline Derivative

Use Principally in the treatment of infections caused by susceptible *Rickettsia*, *Chlamydia*, and *Mycoplasma*; alternative to mefloquine for malaria prophylaxis; treatment for syphilis, uncomplicated *Neisseria gonorrhoeae*, *Listeria*, *Actinomyces israelii*, and *Clostridium* infections in penicillin-allergic patients; used for community-acquired pneumonia and other common infections due to susceptible organisms; anthrax due to *Bacillus anthracis,* including inhalational anthrax (postexposure); treatment of infections caused by uncommon susceptible gram-negative and gram-positive organisms including *Borrelia recurrentis, Ureaplasma urealyticum, Haemophilus ducreyi, Yersinia pestis, Francisella tularensis, Vibrio cholerae, Campylobacter fetus, Brucella* spp, *Bartonella bacilliformis*, and *Calymmatobacterium granulomatis,* Q fever, Lyme disease; treatment of inflammatory lesions associated with rosacea

Usual Dosage
Usual dosage range:
Children >8 years (<45 kg): Oral, I.V.: 2-5 mg/kg/day in 1-2 divided doses, not to exceed 200 mg/day
Children >8 years (>45 kg) and Adults: Oral, I.V.: 100-200 mg/day in 1-2 divided doses
(Continued)

doxycycline *(Continued)*

Indication-specific dosing:

Children:

Anthrax: Doxycycline should be used in children if antibiotic susceptibility testing, exhaustion of drug supplies, or allergic reaction preclude use of penicillin or ciprofloxacin. For treatment, the consensus recommendation does not include a loading dose for doxycycline.

Inhalational (postexposure prophylaxis) (MMWR, 2001, 50:889-893): Oral, I.V. (use oral route when possible):

≤8 years: 2.2 mg/kg every 12 hours for 60 days

>8 years and ≤45 kg: 2.2 mg/kg every 12 hours for 60 days

>8 years and >45 kg: 100 mg every 12 hours for 60 days

Cutaneous (treatment): Oral: See dosing for "Inhalational (postexposure prophylaxis)"

Note: In the presence of systemic involvement, extensive edema, and/or lesions on head/neck, doxycycline should initially be administered I.V.

Inhalational/gastrointestinal/oropharyngeal (treatment): I.V.: Refer to dosing for inhalational anthrax (postexposure prophylaxis); switch to oral therapy when clinically appropriate

Note: Initial treatment should include two or more agents predicted to be effective (per CDC recommendations). Agents suggested for use in conjunction with doxycycline or ciprofloxacin include rifampin, vancomycin, imipenem, penicillin, ampicillin, chloramphenicol, clindamycin, and clarithromycin. May switch to oral antimicrobial therapy when clinically appropriate. Continue combined therapy for 60 days

Children ≥8 years:

Malaria prophylaxis: Oral: 2 mg/kg/day (maximum 100 mg/day). Start 1-2 days prior to travel to endemic area; continue daily during travel and for 4 weeks after leaving endemic area

Children ≥8 years (and >45 kg) and Adults:

Chlamydial infections, uncomplicated: Oral: 100 mg twice daily for ≥7 days

Lyme disease, Q fever, or tularemia: Oral: 100 mg twice daily for 14-21 days

Rickettsial disease or ehrlichiosis: Oral, I.V.: 100 mg twice daily for 7-14 days

Adults:

Anthrax:

Inhalational (postexposure prophylaxis): Oral, I.V. (use oral route when possible): 100 mg every 12 hours for 60 days (*MMWR*, 2001, 50:889-93); **Note:** Preliminary recommendation, FDA review and update is anticipated.

Cutaneous (treatment): Oral: 100 mg every 12 hours for 60 days. **Note:** In the presence of systemic involvement, extensive edema, lesions on head/neck, refer to I.V. dosing for treatment of inhalational/gastrointestinal/oropharyngeal anthrax

Inhalational/gastrointestinal/oropharyngeal (treatment): I.V.: Initial: 100 mg every 12 hours; switch to oral therapy when clinically appropriate; some recommend initial loading dose of 200 mg, followed by 100 mg every 8-12 hours (*JAMA*, 1997, 278:399-411). **Note:** Initial treatment should include two or more agents predicted to be effective (per CDC recommendations). Agents suggested for use in conjunction with doxycycline or ciprofloxacin include rifampin, vancomycin, imipenem, penicillin, ampicillin, chloramphenicol, clindamycin, and clarithromycin. May switch to oral antimicrobial therapy when clinically appropriate. Continue combined therapy for 60 days

Brucellosis: Oral: 100 mg twice daily for 6 weeks with rifampin or streptomycin

Community-acquired pneumonia, bronchitis: Oral, I.V.: 100 mg twice daily

Endometritis, salpingitis, parametritis, or peritonitis: I.V.: 100 mg twice daily with cefoxitin 2 g every 6 hours for 4 days and for ≥48 hours after patient improves; then continue with oral therapy 100 mg twice daily to complete a 10- to 14-day course of therapy

Gonococcal infection, acute (PID) in combination with another antibiotic: I.V.: 100 mg every 12 hours until improved, followed by 100 mg orally twice daily to complete 14 days

Malaria prophylaxis: 100 mg/day. Start 1-2 days prior to travel to endemic area; continue daily during travel and for 4 weeks after leaving endemic area

Nongonococcal urethritis: Oral: 100 mg twice daily for 7 days

Periodontitis: Oral (Periostat®): 20 mg twice daily as an adjunct following scaling and root planing; may be administered for up to 9 months. Safety beyond 12 months of treatment and efficacy beyond 9 months of treatment have not been established.

Rosacea: (Oracea™): Oral: 40 mg once daily in the morning

Syphilis:

Early syphilis: Oral, I.V.: 200 mg/day in divided doses for 14 days

Late syphilis: Oral, I.V.: 200 mg/day in divided doses for 28 days

***Yersinia pestis* (plague):** Oral: 100 mg twice daily for 7 days

Vibrio cholerae: Oral: 300 mg as a single dose

Dosage Forms

Capsule: 50 mg, 100 mg

Vibramycin®: 100 mg

Monodox®: 50 mg, 100 mg

Capsule, variable release:
Oracea™: 40 mg [30 mg (immediate-release) and 10 mg (delayed-release)]
Injection, powder for reconstitution: 100 mg
Doxy-100®: 100 mg
Powder for oral suspension:
Vibramycin®: 25 mg/5 mL
Syrup:
Vibramycin®: 50 mg/5 mL
Tablet: 20 mg, 50 mg, 75 mg, 100 mg, 150 mg
Adoxa®: 50 mg, 75 mg, 100 mg
Adoxa® Pak™ 1/75 [unit-dose pack]: 75 mg (31s)
Adoxa® Pak™ 1/100 [unit-dose pack]: 100 mg (31s)
Adoxa® Pak™ 1/150 [unit-dose pack]: 150 mg (30s)
Adoxa® Pak™ 2/100 [unit-dose pack]: 100 mg (60s)
Periostat®: 20 mg
Vibra-Tabs®: 100 mg
Tablet, delayed-release coated pellets:
Doryx®: 75 mg, 100 mg

doxycycline calcium *see* doxycycline *on page 281*

doxycycline hyclate *see* doxycycline *on page 281*

doxycycline monohydrate *see* doxycycline *on page 281*

doxylamine (dox IL a meen)
Sound-Alike/Look-Alike Issues
doxylamine may be confused with doxycycline
Synonyms doxylamine succinate
U.S./Canadian Brand Names Good Sense Sleep Aid [US-OTC]; Unisom® SleepTabs® [US-OTC]; Unisom®-2 [Can]
Therapeutic Category Antihistamine
Use Sleep aid; antihistamine for hypersensitivity reactions and antiemetic
Usual Dosage Oral: Adults: One tablet 30 minutes before bedtime; once daily or as instructed by healthcare professional
Dosage Forms
Tablet:
Good Sense Sleep Aid [OTC], Unisom® SleepTabs® [OTC]: 25 mg

doxylamine and pyridoxine *(Canada only)* (dox IL a meen & peer i DOX een)
Sound-Alike/Look-Alike Issues
doxylamine may be confused with doxycycline
Synonyms doxylamine succinate and pyridoxine hydrochloride; pyridoxine and doxylamine
U.S./Canadian Brand Names Diclectin® [Can]
Therapeutic Category Antihistamine; Vitamin
Use Treatment of pregnancy-associated nausea and vomiting
Usual Dosage Oral: Adults: Two delayed release tablets (a total of doxylamine 20 mg and pyridoxine 20 mg) at bedtime; in severe cases or in cases with nausea/vomiting during the day, dosage may be increased by 1 tablet in the morning and/or afternoon
Dosage Forms [CAN] = Canadian brand name
Tablet, delayed release:
Diclectin® [CAN]: Doxylamine 10 mg and pyridoxine 10 mg [not available in the U.S.]

doxylamine succinate *see* doxylamine *on this page*

doxylamine succinate and pyridoxine hydrochloride *see* doxylamine and pyridoxine *(Canada only) on this page*

doxylamine succinate, codeine phosphate, and acetaminophen *see* acetaminophen, codeine, and doxylamine *(Canada only) on page 11*

Doxytec [Can] *see* doxycycline *on page 281*

DPA *see* valproic acid and derivatives *on page 881*

D-Pan® *(Discontinued)* *see* dexpanthenol *on page 244*

DPE *see* dipivefrin *on page 270*

D-penicillamine *see* penicillamine *on page 661*

DPH *see* phenytoin *on page 680*

DPM™ **[US-OTC]** *see* urea *on page 877*

Dramamine® **[US-OTC]** *see* dimenhydrinate *on page 262*

Dramamine® **Less Drowsy Formula [US-OTC]** *see* meclizine *on page 535*

Dramilin® **Injection** *(Discontinued) see* dimenhydrinate *on page 262*

dried smallpox vaccine *see* smallpox vaccine *on page 790*

Drinex [US-OTC] *see* acetaminophen, chlorpheniramine, and pseudoephedrine *on page 10*

Drinkables® **MultiVitamins [US-OTC]** *see* vitamins (multiple/oral) *on page 895*

Drisdol® **[US/Can]** *see* ergocalciferol *on page 305*

Dristan™ **12-Hour [US-OTC]** *see* oxymetazoline *on page 643*

Dristan® **Long Lasting Nasal [Can]** *see* oxymetazoline *on page 643*

Dristan® **Long Lasting Nasal Solution** *(Discontinued) see* oxymetazoline *on page 643*

Dristan® **N.D. [Can]** *see* acetaminophen and pseudoephedrine *on page 8*

Dristan® **N.D., Extra Strength [Can]** *see* acetaminophen and pseudoephedrine *on page 8*

Dristan® **Saline Spray** *(Discontinued) see* sodium chloride *on page 792*

Drithocreme® **HP 1%** *(Discontinued) see* anthralin *on page 57*

Dritho-Scalp® **[US]** *see* anthralin *on page 57*

Drixoral® **[Can]** *see* dexbrompheniramine and pseudoephedrine *on page 243*

Drixoral® **Cold & Allergy [US-OTC]** *see* dexbrompheniramine and pseudoephedrine *on page 243*

Drixoral® **Cough & Congestion Liquid Caps** *(Discontinued) see* pseudoephedrine and dextro-methorphan *on page 728*

Drixoral® **Cough Liquid Caps** *(Discontinued) see* dextromethorphan *on page 247*

Drixoral® **Nasal [Can]** *see* oxymetazoline *on page 643*

Drixoral® **ND [Can]** *see* pseudoephedrine *on page 727*

Drixoral® **Non-Drowsy** *(Discontinued) see* pseudoephedrine *on page 727*

Drize®**-R** *(Discontinued) see* chlorpheniramine, phenylephrine, and methscopolamine *on page 181*

dronabinol (droe NAB i nol)

Sound-Alike/Look-Alike Issues
dronabinol may be confused with droperidol
Synonyms delta-9-tetrahydro-cannabinol; delta-9 THC; tetrahydrocannabinol; THC
U.S./Canadian Brand Names Marinol® [US/Can]
Therapeutic Category Antiemetic
Controlled Substance C-III
Use Chemotherapy-associated nausea and vomiting refractory to other antiemetic(s); AIDS-related anorexia
Usual Dosage Refer to individual protocols. Oral:
Antiemetic: Children and Adults: 5 mg/m² 1-3 hours before chemotherapy, then 5 mg/m²/dose every 2-4 hours after chemotherapy for a total of 4-6 doses/day; increase doses in increments of 2.5 mg/m² to a maximum of 15 mg/m²/dose.
Appetite stimulant: Adults: Initial: 2.5 mg twice daily (before lunch and dinner); titrate up to a maximum of 20 mg/day.
Dosage Forms
Capsule, gelatin:
Marinol®: 2.5 mg, 5 mg, 10 mg

droperidol (droe PER i dole)

Sound-Alike/Look-Alike Issues
droperidol may be confused with dronabinol
Inapsine® may be confused with Nebcin®
Synonyms dehydrobenzperidol
U.S./Canadian Brand Names Droperidol Injection, USP [Can]; Inapsine® [US]
Therapeutic Category Antiemetic; Antipsychotic Agent, Butyrophenone
Use Antiemetic in surgical and diagnostic procedures; preoperative medication in patients when other treatments are ineffective or inappropriate
Usual Dosage Titrate carefully to desired effect
Children 2-12 years: Nausea and vomiting: I.M., I.V.: 0.05-0.06 mg/kg (maximum initial dose: 0.1 mg/kg); additional doses may be repeated to achieve effect; administer additional doses with caution

Adults: Nausea and vomiting: I.M., I.V.: Initial: 2.5 mg; additional doses of 1.25 mg may be administered to achieve desired effect; administer additional doses with caution

Dosage Forms
Injection, solution: 2.5 mg/mL (1 mL, 2 mL)
Inapsine®: 2.5 mg/mL (1 mL, 2 mL)

Droperidol Injection, USP [Can] *see* droperidol *on previous page*

drospirenone and estradiol (droh SPYE re none & es tra DYE ole)
Synonyms E2 and DRSP; estradiol and drospirenone
U.S./Canadian Brand Names Angeliq® [US/Can]
Therapeutic Category Estrogen and Progestin Combination
Use Treatment of moderate-to-severe vasomotor symptoms associated with menopause; treatment of vulvar and vaginal atrophy associated with menopause
Usual Dosage Oral: Adults:
Moderate-to-severe vasomotor symptoms associated with menopause: One tablet daily; reevaluate patients at 3- and 6-month intervals to determine if treatment is still necessary.
Atrophic vaginitis in females with an intact uterus: One tablet daily; reevaluate patients at 3- and 6-month intervals to determine if treatment is still necessary.
Note: The lowest dose of estrogen/progestin that will control symptoms should be used; medication should be discontinued as soon as possible.
Dosage Forms
Tablet:
Angeliq®: Drospirenone 0.5 mg and estradiol 1 mg

drospirenone and ethinyl estradiol *see* ethinyl estradiol and drospirenone *on page 323*

drotrecogin alfa (dro TRE coe jin AL fa)
Synonyms activated protein C, human, recombinant; drotrecogin alfa, activated; protein C (activated), human, recombinant
U.S./Canadian Brand Names Xigris® [US/Can]
Therapeutic Category Protein C (Activated)
Use Reduction of mortality from severe sepsis (associated with organ dysfunction) in adults at high risk of death (eg, APACHE II score ≥25)
Usual Dosage I.V.: Adults: Sepsis: 24 mcg/kg/hour for a total of 96 hours; stop infusion **immediately** if clinically-important bleeding is identified
Dosage Forms
Injection, powder for reconstitution [preservative free]:
Xigris®: 5 mg, 20 mg

drotrecogin alfa, activated *see* drotrecogin alfa *on this page*

DroTuss-CP [US] *see* phenylephrine, hydrocodone, and chlorpheniramine *on page 678*

Droxia® [US] *see* hydroxyurea *on page 439*

Dr. Scholl's® Callus Remover [US-OTC] *see* salicylic acid *on page 772*

Dr. Scholl's® Clear Away [US-OTC] *see* salicylic acid *on page 772*

Dry Eye® Therapy Solution *(Discontinued)* *see* artificial tears *on page 75*

Dryox® Gel *(Discontinued)* *see* benzoyl peroxide *on page 103*

Dryox® Wash *(Discontinued)* *see* benzoyl peroxide *on page 103*

Drysol™ [US] *see* aluminum chloride hexahydrate *on page 36*

Dryvax® [US] *see* smallpox vaccine *on page 790*

DSCG *see* cromolyn sodium *on page 218*

D-ser(bu^t)^6,Azgly^10-LHRH *see* goserelin *on page 399*

D-S-S® [US-OTC] *see* docusate *on page 273*

DSS *see* docusate *on page 273*

DT *see* diphtheria and tetanus toxoid *on page 267*

D-Tann HC [US] *see* hydrocodone, phenylephrine, and diphenhydramine *on page 431*

DTaP *see* diphtheria, tetanus toxoids, and acellular pertussis vaccine *on page 269*

DTIC® [Can] *see* dacarbazine *on page 227*

DTIC *see* dacarbazine *on page 227*

DTIC-Dome® **[US]** *see* dacarbazine *on page 227*

DTPA *see* diethylene triamine penta-acetic acid *on page 256*

dTpa *see* diphtheria, tetanus toxoids, and acellular pertussis vaccine *on page 269*

D-Trp(6)-LHRH *see* triptorelin *on page 870*

Duac™ **[US]** *see* clindamycin and benzoyl peroxide *on page 200*

Duet® **[US]** *see* vitamins (multiple/prenatal) *on page 896*

Duetact™ **[US]** *see* pioglitazone and glimepiride *on page 684*

Duet™ **DHA [US]** *see* vitamins (multiple/prenatal) *on page 896*

Dukoral™ **[Can]** *see* traveler's diarrhea and cholera vaccine *(Canada only) on page 858*

Dulcolax® **[US-OTC/Can]** *see* bisacodyl *on page 112*

Dulcolax® **Stool Softener [US-OTC]** *see* docusate *on page 273*

Dull-C® **[US-OTC]** *see* ascorbic acid *on page 76*

duloxetine (doo LOX e teen)

Sound-Alike/Look-Alike Issues
duloxetine may be confused with fluoxetine

Synonyms duloxetine hydrochloride; LY248686; (+)-(S)-N-methyl-γ-(1-naphthyloxy)-2-thiophenepropylamine hydrochloride

U.S./Canadian Brand Names Cymbalta® [US]

Therapeutic Category Antidepressant, Serotonin/Norepinephrine Reuptake Inhibitor

Use Treatment of major depressive disorder (MDD); management of pain associated with diabetic neuropathy; treatment of generalized anxiety disorder (GAD)

Usual Dosage Oral: Adults:
MDD: Initial: 40-60 mg/day; dose may be divided (ie, 20 or 30 mg twice daily) or given as a single daily dose of 60 mg; maximum dose: 60 mg/day

Diabetic neuropathy: 60 mg once daily; lower initial doses may be considered in patients where tolerability is a concern and/or renal impairment is present

GAD: Initial: 30-60 mg/day as a single daily dose; patients initiated at 30 mg/day should be titrated to 60 mg/day after 1 week; maximum dose: 120 mg/day. **Note:** Doses >60 mg/day have not been demonstrated to be more effective than 60 mg/day.

Dosage Forms
Capsule, enteric coated pellets:
Cymbalta®: 20 mg, 30 mg, 60 mg

duloxetine hydrochloride *see* duloxetine *on this page*

Duocaine™ **[US]** *see* lidocaine and bupivacaine *on page 506*

DuoCet™ *(Discontinued)* *see* hydrocodone and acetaminophen *on page 427*

Duodote™ **[US]** *see* atropine and pralidoxime *on page 84*

DuoFilm® **[US-OTC/Can]** *see* salicylic acid *on page 772*

Duoforte® **27 [Can]** *see* salicylic acid *on page 772*

Duomax [US] *see* guaifenesin and phenylephrine *on page 404*

DuoNeb™ **[US]** *see* ipratropium and albuterol *on page 471*

DuoPlant® *(Discontinued)* *see* salicylic acid *on page 772*

Duotan PD [US] *see* dexchlorpheniramine and pseudoephedrine *on page 243*

Duo-Trach® **Injection** *(Discontinued)* *see* lidocaine *on page 504*

DuP 753 *see* losartan *on page 519*

Duphalac® *(Discontinued)* *see* lactulose *on page 489*

Durabolin® **[Can]** *see* nandrolone *on page 590*

Duraclon™ **[US]** *see* clonidine *on page 204*

Duradrin® *(Discontinued)* *see* acetaminophen, isometheptene, and dichloralphenazone *on page 13*

Duradyl® **[US]** *see* chlorpheniramine, phenylephrine, and methscopolamine *on page 181*

Duradyne DHC® *(Discontinued)* *see* hydrocodone and acetaminophen *on page 427*

Duragesic® **[US/Can]** *see* fentanyl *on page 346*

Dura-Gest® *(Discontinued)*

Durahist™ **[US]** *see* chlorpheniramine, pseudoephedrine, and methscopolamine *on page 184*

Durahist™ PE [US] *see* chlorpheniramine, phenylephrine, and methscopolamine *on page 181*

Duralith® [Can] *see* lithium *on page 513*

Duralone® Injection *(Discontinued)* *see* methylprednisolone *on page 559*

Duramist® Plus [US-OTC] *see* oxymetazoline *on page 643*

Duramorph® [US] *see* morphine sulfate *on page 578*

Duraphen™ II DM [US] *see* guaifenesin, dextromethorphan, and phenylephrine *on page 407*

Duraphen™ DM [US] *see* guaifenesin, dextromethorphan, and phenylephrine *on page 407*

Duraphen™ Forte [US] *see* guaifenesin, dextromethorphan, and phenylephrine *on page 407*

DuraTan™ Forte [US] *see* chlorpheniramine, pseudoephedrine, and dextromethorphan *on page 183*

Duratest® Injection *(Discontinued)* *see* testosterone *on page 828*

Durathate® Injection *(Discontinued)* *see* testosterone *on page 828*

Duration® [US-OTC] *see* oxymetazoline *on page 643*

Duratocin™ [Can] *see* carbetocin *(Canada only) on page 151*

Duratuss® [US] *see* guaifenesin and phenylephrine *on page 404*

Duratuss® DM [US] *see* guaifenesin and dextromethorphan *on page 402*

Duratuss GP® [US] *see* guaifenesin and phenylephrine *on page 404*

Duratuss® HD [US] *see* hydrocodone, phenylephrine, and guaifenesin *on page 431*

Dura-Vent®/DA *(Discontinued)* *see* chlorpheniramine, phenylephrine, and methscopolamine *on page 181*

Dura-Vent® *(Discontinued)*

Duricef® [US/Can] *see* cefadroxil *on page 158*

Duricef® Oral Suspension 125 mg/5 mL *(Discontinued)* *see* cefadroxil *on page 158*

Durolane® [Can] *see* hyaluronate and derivatives *on page 423*

Durrax® Oral *(Discontinued)* *see* hydroxyzine *on page 440*

dutasteride (doo TAS teer ide)
    U.S./Canadian Brand Names Avodart™ [US/Can]
    Therapeutic Category Antineoplastic Agent, Anthracenedione
    Use Treatment of symptomatic benign prostatic hyperplasia (BPH)
    Usual Dosage Oral: Adults: Male: 0.5 mg once daily
    Dosage Forms
      Capsule, softgel:
        Avodart™: 0.5 mg

Duvoid® [Can] *see* bethanechol *on page 110*

Duvoid® *(Discontinued)* *see* bethanechol *on page 110*

D-Vi-Sol® [Can] *see* cholecalciferol *on page 186*

DW286 *see* gemifloxacin *on page 387*

Dwelle® Ophthalmic Solution *(Discontinued)* *see* artificial tears *on page 75*

Dyazide® [US] *see* hydrochlorothiazide and triamterene *on page 427*

Dycill® [Can] *see* dicloxacillin *on page 254*

Dycill® *(Discontinued)* *see* dicloxacillin *on page 254*

Dyclone® *(Discontinued)* *see* dyclonine *on this page*

dyclonine (DYE kloe neen)
    Sound-Alike/Look-Alike Issues
      dyclonine may be confused with dicyclomine
    Synonyms dyclonine hydrochloride
    U.S./Canadian Brand Names Cēpacol® Dual Action Maximum Strength [US-OTC]; Sucrets® [US-OTC]
    Therapeutic Category Local Anesthetic
    Use Temporary relief of pain associated with oral mucosa
    Usual Dosage Oral:
      Lozenge: Children ≥2 years and Adults: One lozenge every 2 hours as needed (maximum: 10 lozenges/day)
      Spray:
        Children ≥3-12 years: 1-3 sprays, up to 4 times a day
    (Continued)

dyclonine *(Continued)*

Children ≥12 years and Adults: 1-4 sprays, up to 4 times a day
Dosage Forms
Lozenge:
Sucrets® [OTC]: 1.2 mg, 2 mg, 3 mg
Spray, oral:
Cēpacol® Dual Action Maximum Strength [OTC]: 0.1%

dyclonine hydrochloride *see* dyclonine *on previous page*

Dygase [US] *see* pancreatin *on page 648*

Dylix [US] *see* dyphylline *on this page*

Dymenate® Injection *(Discontinued)* *see* dimenhydrinate *on page 262*

Dynabac® *(Discontinued)*

Dynacin® [US] *see* minocycline *on page 571*

DynaCirc® [Can] *see* isradipine *on page 477*

DynaCirc® CR [US] *see* isradipine *on page 477*

DynaCirc® *(Discontinued)* *see* isradipine *on page 477*

Dyna-Hex® [US-OTC] *see* chlorhexidine gluconate *on page 174*

Dynahist-ER Pediatric® [US] *see* chlorpheniramine and pseudoephedrine *on page 178*

Dynapen® *(Discontinued)* *see* dicloxacillin *on page 254*

Dynatuss-EX [US] *see* guaifenesin, dextromethorphan, and phenylephrine *on page 407*

Dynex *(Discontinued)* *see* guaifenesin and pseudoephedrine *on page 406*

dyphylline *(DYE fi lin)*

Synonyms dihydroxypropyl theophylline
U.S./Canadian Brand Names Dilor® [Can]; Dylix [US]; Lufyllin® [US/Can]
Therapeutic Category Theophylline Derivative
Use Bronchodilator in reversible airway obstruction due to asthma, chronic bronchitis, or emphysema
Usual Dosage Oral: Adults: Up to 15 mg/kg 4 times/day, individualize dosage
Dosage Forms
Elixir:
Dylix: 100 mg/15 mL
Tablet:
Lufyllin®: 200 mg, 400 mg

dyphylline and guaifenesin *(DYE fi lin & gwye FEN e sin)*

Synonyms guaifenesin and dyphylline
U.S./Canadian Brand Names COPD [US]; Difil-G [US]; Difil®-G Forte [US]; Dilex-G [US]; Dilor-G® [US]; Lufyllin®-GG [US]
Therapeutic Category Expectorant; Theophylline Derivative
Use Treatment of bronchial asthma and reversible bronchospasm associated with chronic bronchitis and emphysema
Usual Dosage Oral:
Children 6-12 years:
Elixir: Lufyllin®-GG: 15-30 mL 3 or 4 times/day
Syrup: Dilex-G:
18-27 kg: 1.25-1.6 mL 4 times/day
27-36 kg: 2.5-3.3 mL 4 times/day
36.5-45 kg: 3.3-3.7 mL 4 times/day
Tablet: Lufyllin®-GG: 1/2 -1 tablet 3 or 4 times/day
Children >12 years and Adults:
Elixir: Lufyllin®-GG: 30 mL 4 times/day
Syrup:
Dilex-G: 5-10 mL 4 times/day
Difil®-G Forte: 5-10 mL 3 or 4 times/day; may double or triple (in severe cases) according to patient response
Tablet: Difil-G, Dilex-G, Lufyllin®-GG: One tablet 3 or 4 times/day
Dosage Forms
Elixir: Dyphylline 100 mg and guaifenesin 100 mg per 15 mL
Lufyllin®-GG: Dyphylline 100 mg and guaifenesin 100 mg per 15 mL

Liquid: Dyphylline 100 mg and guaifenesin 100 mg per 5 mL
  Difil®-G Forte: Dyphylline 100 mg and guaifenesin 100 mg per 5 mL
Syrup:
  Dilex-G: Dyphylline 100 mg and guaifenesin 200 mg per 5 mL
Tablet: Dyphylline 200 mg and guaifenesin 200 mg
  COPD, Lufyllin®-GG: Dyphylline 200 mg and guaifenesin 200 mg
  Difil-G: Dyphylline 200 mg and guaifenesin 300 mg
  Dilex-G: Dyphylline 200 mg and guaifenesin 400 mg

Dyrenium® [US] *see* triamterene *on page 863*

Dyrexan-OD® *(Discontinued) see* phendimetrazine *on page 671*

Dytan™ [US] *see* diphenhydramine *on page 265*

E2 and DRSP *see* drospirenone and estradiol *on page 285*

7E3 *see* abciximab *on page 3*

E2020 *see* donepezil *on page 276*

EarSol® HC [US] *see* hydrocortisone (topical) *on page 434*

Easprin® [US] *see* aspirin *on page 78*

Ebixa® [Can] *see* memantine *on page 539*

echothiophate iodide (ek oh THYE oh fate EYE oh dide)

Synonyms ecostigmine iodide
U.S./Canadian Brand Names Phospholine Iodide® [US]
Therapeutic Category Cholinesterase Inhibitor
Use Used as miotic in treatment of chronic, open-angle glaucoma; may be useful in specific cases of angle-closure glaucoma (postiridectomy or where surgery refused/contraindicated); postcataract surgery-related glaucoma; accommodative esotropia
Usual Dosage Ophthalmic:
  Children: Accommodative esotropia:
    Diagnosis: Instill 1 drop (0.125%) once daily into both eyes at bedtime for 2-3 weeks
    Treatment: Usual dose: Instill 1 drop of 0.06% once daily or 0.125% every other day (maximum: 0.125% daily). **Note:** Use lowest concentration and frequency which gives satisfactory response; if necessary, doses >0.125% daily may be used for short periods of time.
  Adults: Open-angle or secondary glaucoma:
    Initial: Instill 1 drop (0.03%) twice daily into eyes with 1 dose just prior to bedtime
    Maintenance: Some patients have been treated with 1 dose daily or every other day
    Conversion from other ophthalmic agents: If IOP control was unsatisfactory, patients may be expected to require higher doses of echothiophate (eg, ≥0.06%); however, patients should be initially started on the 0.03% strength for a short period to better tolerance.
Dosage Forms
  Powder for reconstitution, ophthalmic:
    Phospholine Iodide®: 6.25 mg [0.125%]

EC-Naprosyn® [US] *see* naproxen *on page 591*

***E. coli* asparaginase** *see* asparaginase *on page 77*

econazole (e KONE a zole)

Synonyms econazole nitrate
U.S./Canadian Brand Names Ecostatin® [Can]; Spectazole® [US/Can]
Therapeutic Category Antifungal Agent
Use Topical treatment of tinea pedis (athlete's foot), tinea cruris (jock itch), tinea corporis (ringworm), tinea versicolor, and cutaneous candidiasis
Usual Dosage Topical: Children and Adults:
  Tinea pedis, tinea cruris, tinea corporis, tinea versicolor: Apply sufficient amount to cover affected areas once daily
  Cutaneous candidiasis: Apply sufficient quantity twice daily (morning and evening)
  Duration of treatment: Candidal infections and tinea cruris, versicolor, and corporis should be treated for 2 weeks and tinea pedis for 1 month; occasionally, longer treatment periods may be required
Dosage Forms
  Cream, topical: 1% (15 g, 30 g, 85 g)

econazole nitrate *see* econazole *on this page*

Econopred® Plus [US] *see* prednisolone (ophthalmic) *on page 709*

Ecostatin® **[Can]** *see* econazole *on previous page*

ecostigmine iodide *see* echothiophate iodide *on previous page*

Ecotrin® **[US-OTC]** *see* aspirin *on page 78*

Ecotrin® **Low Strength [US-OTC]** *see* aspirin *on page 78*

Ecotrin® **Maximum Strength [US-OTC]** *see* aspirin *on page 78*

Ectosone [Can] *see* betamethasone (topical) *on page 109*

eculizumab (e kue LIZ oo mab)

U.S./Canadian Brand Names Soliris™ [US]

Therapeutic Category Monoclonal Antibody; Monoclonal Antibody, Complement Inhibitor

Use Treatment of paroxysmal nocturnal hemoglobinuria (PNH) to reduce hemolysis

Usual Dosage Note: Patients must receive meningococcal vaccine at least 2 weeks prior to treatment initiation; revaccinate according to current guidelines.

I.V.: Adults: PNH: 600 mg once weekly (±2 days) for 4 weeks, followed by 900 mg 1 week (±2 days) later; then maintenance: 900 mg every 2 weeks (±2 days) thereafter

Treatment should be administered at the recommended time interval, however, the administration day may be varied by ±2 days if serum LDH levels suggest increased hemolysis before the end of the dosing interval.

Dosage Forms

Injection, solution [preservative free]:

Soliris™: 10 mg/ml (30 mL)

Ed A-Hist® **[US]** *see* chlorpheniramine and phenylephrine *on page 177*

Ed A-Hist DM [US] *see* chlorpheniramine, phenylephrine, and dextromethorphan *on page 180*

edathamil disodium *see* edetate disodium *on next page*

Edecrin® **[US/Can]** *see* ethacrynic acid *on page 321*

edetate calcium disodium (ED e tate KAL see um dye SOW dee um)

Sound-Alike/Look-Alike Issues

Edetate calcium disodium (CaEDTA) may be confused with edetate disodium (Na₂EDTA). CDC recommends that edetate disodium should **never** be used for chelation therapy in children. Fatal hypocalcemia may result if edetate disodium is used for chelation therapy instead of edetate calcium disodium.

Synonyms CaEDTA; calcium disodium edetate; calcium EDTA; EDTA (calcium disodium)

U.S./Canadian Brand Names Calcium Disodium Versenate® [US]

Therapeutic Category Chelating Agent

Use Treatment of symptomatic acute and chronic lead poisoning or for symptomatic patients with high blood lead levels; used as an aid in the diagnosis of lead poisoning; possibly useful in poisoning by zinc, manganese, and certain heavy radioisotopes

Usual Dosage Several regimens have been recommended:

Diagnosis of lead poisoning: Mobilization test (not recommended by AAP guidelines): I.M., I.V.:

Children: 500 mg/m²/dose (maximum dose: 1 g) as a single dose or divided into 2 doses

Adults: 500 mg/m²/dose

Note: Urine is collected for 24 hours after first EDTA dose and analyzed for lead content; if the ratio of mcg of lead in urine to mg calcium EDTA given is >1, then test is considered positive; for convenience, an 8-hour urine collection may be done after a single 50 mg/kg I.M. (maximum dose: 1 g) or 500 mg/m² I.V. dose; a positive test occurs if the ratio of lead excretion to mg calcium EDTA >0.5-0.6.

Treatment of lead poisoning: Children and Adults (each regimen is specific for route): **Note:** Depending upon the blood lead level, additional courses may be necessary; repeat at least 2-4 days and preferably 2-4 weeks apart:

Symptoms of lead encephalopathy and/or blood lead level >70 mcg/dL: Treat 5 days; give in conjunction with dimercaprol; wait a minimum of 2 days with no treatment before considering a repeat course:

I.M.: 250 mg/m²/dose every 4 hours

I.V.: 50 mg/kg/day as 24-hour continuous I.V. infusion **or** 1-1.5 g/m² I.V. as either an 8- to 24-hour infusion or divided into 2 doses every 12 hours

*Symptomatic lead poisoning **without** encephalopathy or asymptomatic with blood lead level >70 mcg/dL:* Treat 3-5 days; treatment with dimercaprol is recommended until the blood lead level concentration <50 mcg/dL:

I.M.: 167 mg/m² every 4 hours

I.V.: 1 g/m² as an 8- to 24-hour infusion or divided every 12 hours

*Asymptomatic **children** with blood lead level 45-69 mcg/dL:* I.V.: 25 mg/kg/day for 5 days as an 8- to 24-hour infusion or divided into 2 doses every 12 hours

Lead nephropathy: Adults: An alternative dosing regimen reflecting the reduction in renal clearance is based upon the serum creatinine. Dose of Ca EDTA based on serum creatinine: **Note:** Repeat regimen monthly until lead levels are reduced to an acceptable level:

S_{cr} >2-3 mg/dL / Cl_{cr} 30-50 mL/minute: Reduce recommended dose by 50% and administer daily

S_{cr} >3-4 mg/dL / Cl_{cr} 20-30 mL/minute: Reduce recommended dose by 50% and administer every 48 hours

S_{cr} >4 mg/dL / Cl_{cr} <20 mL/minute: Reduce recommended dose by 50% and administer once weekly

Dosage Forms
Injection, solution:
Calcium Disodium Versenate®: 200 mg/mL (5 mL)

edetate disodium (ED e tate dye SOW dee um)

Sound-Alike/Look-Alike Issues
Edetate disodium (Na_2EDTA) may be confused with edetate calcium disodium (CaEDTA). CDC recommends that edetate disodium should **never** be used for chelation therapy in children. Fatal hypocalcemia may result if edetate disodium is used for chelation therapy instead of edetate calcium disodium.

Synonyms edathamil disodium; EDTA (disodium); Na2EDTA; sodium edetate
U.S./Canadian Brand Names Endrate® [US]
Therapeutic Category Chelating Agent
Use Emergency treatment of hypercalcemia; control digitalis-induced cardiac dysrhythmias (ventricular arrhythmias)
Usual Dosage Hypercalcemia: I.V.:
Children: 40-70 mg/kg/day slow infusion over 3-4 hours or more to a maximum of 3 g/24 hours; administer for 5 days and allow 5 days between courses of therapy
Adults: 50 mg/kg/day over 3 or more hours to a maximum of 3 g/24 hours; a suggested regimen of 5 days followed by 2 days without drug and repeated courses up to 15 total doses
Digitalis-induced arrhythmias: Children and Adults: 15 mg/kg/hour (maximum dose: 60 mg/kg/day) as continuous infusion
Dosage Forms
Injection, solution: 150 mg/mL (20 mL)
Endrate®: 150 mg/mL (20 mL)

Edex® [US] *see* alprostadil *on page 33*

edrophonium (ed roe FOE nee um)

Synonyms edrophonium chloride
U.S./Canadian Brand Names Enlon® [US/Can]; Reversol® [US]; Tensilon® [Can]
Therapeutic Category Cholinergic Agent
Use Diagnosis of myasthenia gravis; differentiation of cholinergic crises from myasthenia crises; reversal of nondepolarizing neuromuscular blockers; adjunct treatment of respiratory depression caused by curare overdose
Usual Dosage Usually administered I.V., however, if not possible, I.M. or SubQ may be used:
Infants:
I.M.: 0.5-1 mg
I.V.: Initial: 0.1 mg, followed by 0.4 mg if no response; total dose = 0.5 mg
Children:
Diagnosis: Initial: 0.04 mg/kg over 1 minute followed by 0.16 mg/kg if no response, to a maximum total dose of 5 mg for children <34 kg, or 10 mg for children >34 kg **or**
Alternative dosing (manufacturer's recommendation):
≤34 kg: 1 mg; if no response after 45 seconds, repeat dosage in 1 mg increments every 30-45 seconds, up to a total of 5 mg
>34 kg: 2 mg; if no response after 45 seconds, repeat dosage in 1 mg increments every 30-45 seconds, up to a total of 10 mg
I.M.:
<34 kg: 1 mg
>34 kg: 5 mg
Titration of oral anticholinesterase therapy: 0.04 mg/kg once given 1 hour after oral intake of the drug being used in treatment; if strength improves, an increase in neostigmine or pyridostigmine dose is indicated
Adults:
Diagnosis:
I.V.: 2 mg test dose administered over 15-30 seconds; 8 mg given 45 seconds later if no response is seen; test dose may be repeated after 30 minutes
I.M.: Initial: 10 mg; if no cholinergic reaction occurs, administer 2 mg 30 minutes later to rule out false-negative reaction
Titration of oral anticholinesterase therapy: 1-2 mg given 1 hour after oral dose of anticholinesterase; if strength improves, an increase in neostigmine or pyridostigmine dose is indicated
(Continued)

edrophonium *(Continued)*

Reversal of nondepolarizing neuromuscular blocking agents (neostigmine with atropine usually preferred): I.V.: 10 mg over 30-45 seconds; may repeat every 5-10 minutes up to 40 mg

Termination of paroxysmal atrial tachycardia: I.V. rapid injection: 5-10 mg

Differentiation of cholinergic from myasthenic crisis: I.V.: 1 mg; may repeat after 1 minute. **Note:** Intubation and controlled ventilation may be required if patient has cholinergic crisis

Dosage Forms
Injection, solution:
Enlon®: 10 mg/mL (15 mL)
Reversol®: 10 mg/mL (10 mL)

edrophonium and atropine (ed roe FOE nee um & A troe peen)

Synonyms atropine sulfate and edrophonium chloride; edrophonium chloride and atropine sulfate
U.S./Canadian Brand Names Enlon-Plus™ [US]
Therapeutic Category Anticholinergic Agent; Antidote; Cholinergic Agonist
Use Reversal of nondepolarizing neuromuscular blockers; adjunct treatment of respiratory depression caused by curare overdose
Usual Dosage I.V.: Adults: Reversal of neuromuscular blockade: 0.05 mL/kg given over 45-60 seconds. The dose delivered is 0.5-1 mg/kg of edrophonium and 0.007-0.015 mg/kg of atropine. An edrophonium dose of 1 mg/kg should rarely be exceeded. **Note:** Monitor closely for bradyarrhythmias. Have atropine on hand in case needed.
Dosage Forms
Injection, solution:
Enlon-Plus™: Edrophonium 10 mg/mL and atropine 0.14 mg/mL (5 mL, 15 mL)

edrophonium chloride *see* edrophonium *on previous page*

edrophonium chloride and atropine sulfate *see* edrophonium and atropine *on this page*

ED-SPAZ® *(Discontinued) see* hyoscyamine *on page 441*

EDTA (calcium disodium) *see* edetate calcium disodium *on page 290*

EDTA (disodium) *see* edetate disodium *on previous page*

ED-TLC [US] *see* phenylephrine, hydrocodone, and chlorpheniramine *on page 678*

ED-Tuss HC [US] *see* phenylephrine, hydrocodone, and chlorpheniramine *on page 678*

E.E.S.® **[US/Can]** *see* erythromycin *on page 309*

efalizumab (e fa li ZOO mab)

Synonyms anti-CD11a; hu1124
U.S./Canadian Brand Names Raptiva® [US]
Therapeutic Category Immunosuppressant Agent; Monoclonal Antibody
Use Treatment of chronic moderate-to-severe plaque psoriasis in patients who are candidates for systemic therapy or phototherapy
Usual Dosage SubQ: Adults: Psoriasis: Initial: 0.7 mg/kg, followed by weekly dose of 1 mg/kg (maximum: 200 mg/dose)
Dosage Forms
Injection, powder for reconstitution:
Raptiva®: 150 mg

efavirenz (e FAV e renz)

U.S./Canadian Brand Names Sustiva® [US/Can]
Therapeutic Category Nonnucleoside Reverse Transcriptase Inhibitor (NNRTI)
Use Treatment of HIV-1 infections in combination with at least two other antiretroviral agents
Usual Dosage Oral: Dosing at bedtime is recommended to limit central nervous system effects; should not be used as single-agent therapy

Children ≥3 years: Dosage is based on body weight
10 kg to <15 kg: 200 mg once daily
15 kg to <20 kg: 250 mg once daily
20 kg to <25 kg: 300 mg once daily
25 kg to <32.5 kg: 350 mg once daily
32.5 kg to <40 kg: 400 mg once daily
≥40 kg: 600 mg once daily
Adults: 600 mg once daily

Dosage Forms
Capsule:
  Sustiva®: 50 mg, 100 mg, 200 mg
Tablet:
  Sustiva®: 600 mg

efavirenz, emtricitabine, and tenofovir (e FAV e renz, em trye SYE ta been, & te NOE fo veer)

Synonyms emtricitabine, efavirenz, and tenofovir; tenofovir disoproxil fumarate, efavirenz, and emtricitabine
U.S./Canadian Brand Names Atripla™ [US]
Therapeutic Category Antiretroviral Agent, Reverse Transcriptase Inhibitor (Nonnucleoside); Antiretroviral Agent, Reverse Transcriptase Inhibitor (Nucleoside); Antiretroviral Agent, Reverse Transcriptase Inhibitor (Nucleotide)
Use Treatment of HIV infection
Usual Dosage Oral: Adults: One tablet once daily to be taken on an empty stomach (at bedtime is recommended).
Dosage Forms
  Tablet:
    Atripla™: Efavirenz 600 mg, emtricitabine 200 mg, and tenofovir disoproxil fumarate 300 mg

Effer-K™ [US] see potassium bicarbonate and potassium citrate on page 699

Effer-Syllium® (Discontinued) see psyllium on page 732

Effexor® [US] see venlafaxine on page 887

Effexor® XR [US/Can] see venlafaxine on page 887

Eflone® (Discontinued) see fluorometholone on page 363

eflornithine (ee FLOR ni theen)

Sound-Alike/Look-Alike Issues
  Vaniqa™ may be confused with Viagra®
Synonyms DFMO; eflornithine hydrochloride
U.S./Canadian Brand Names Vaniqa™ [US/Can]
Therapeutic Category Antiprotozoal; Topical Skin Product
Use Cream: Females ≥12 years: Reduce unwanted hair from face and adjacent areas under the chin
  Orphan status: Injection: Treatment of meningoencephalitic stage of *Trypanosoma brucei gambiense* infection (sleeping sickness)
Usual Dosage
  Children ≥12 years and Adults: Females: Topical: Apply thin layer of cream to affected areas of face and adjacent chin twice daily, at least 8 hours apart
  Adults: I.V. infusion: 100 mg/kg/dose given every 6 hours (over at least 45 minutes) for 14 days
Dosage Forms
  Cream, topical:
    Vaniqa™: 13.9% (30 g)
  Injection, solution:
    Vaniqa™: 200 mg/mL (100 mL) [orphan drug status]

eflornithine hydrochloride see eflornithine on this page

Efodine® (Discontinued) see povidone-iodine on page 704

eformoterol and budesonide see budesonide and formoterol on page 124

Efudex® [US/Can] see fluorouracil on page 363

E-Gems® [US-OTC] see vitamin E on page 894

E-Gems Elite® [US-OTC] see vitamin E on page 894

E-Gems Plus® [US-OTC] see vitamin E on page 894

EHDP see etidronate disodium on page 335

Elaprase™ [US] see idursulfase on page 447

Elavil® (Discontinued) see amitriptyline on page 44

Eldepryl® [US] see selegiline on page 780

Eldopaque® [US-OTC/Can] see hydroquinone on page 437

Eldopaque Forte® [US] see hydroquinone on page 437

Eldoquin® [US-OTC/Can] see hydroquinone on page 437

Eldoquin Forte® [US] see hydroquinone on page 437

electrolyte lavage solution *see* polyethylene glycol-electrolyte solution *on page 695*

Elestat™ **[US]** *see* epinastine *on page 300*

Elestrin™ **[US]** *see* estradiol *on page 313*

eletriptan (el e TRIP tan)
Synonyms eletriptan hydrobromide
U.S./Canadian Brand Names Relpax® [US/Can]
Therapeutic Category Serotonin 5-HT$_{1B, 1D}$ Receptor Agonist
Use Acute treatment of migraine, with or without aura
Usual Dosage Oral: Adults: Acute migraine: 20-40 mg; if the headache improves but returns, dose may be repeated after 2 hours have elapsed since first dose; maximum 80 mg/day.
Note: If the first dose is ineffective, diagnosis needs to be reevaluated. Safety of treating >3 headaches/month has not been established.
Dosage Forms
Tablet:
Relpax®: 20 mg, 40 mg

eletriptan hydrobromide *see* eletriptan *on this page*

Elidel® **[US/Can]** *see* pimecrolimus *on page 683*

Eligard® **[US/Can]** *see* leuprolide *on page 497*

Elimite® **[US]** *see* permethrin *on page 670*

elipten *see* aminoglutethimide *on page 42*

Elitek™ **[US]** *see* rasburicase *on page 746*

Elixomin® ***(Discontinued)*** *see* theophylline *on page 834*

Elixophyllin® ***(Discontinued)*** *see* theophylline *on page 834*

Elixophyllin-GG® **[US]** *see* theophylline and guaifenesin *on page 835*

ElixSure™ **Fever/Pain** ***(Discontinued)*** *see* acetaminophen *on page 5*

ElixSure™ **IB [US-OTC]** *see* ibuprofen *on page 444*

ElixSure© **Cough [US-OTC]** *see* dextromethorphan *on page 247*

Ellence® **[US/Can]** *see* epirubicin *on page 302*

Elmiron® **[US/Can]** *see* pentosan polysulfate sodium *on page 667*

Elocom® **[Can]** *see* mometasone *on page 576*

Elocon® **[US]** *see* mometasone *on page 576*

Eloxatin® **[US]** *see* oxaliplatin *on page 636*

Elspar® **[US/Can]** *see* asparaginase *on page 77*

Eltor® **[Can]** *see* pseudoephedrine *on page 727*

Eltroxin® **[Can]** *see* levothyroxine *on page 503*

Emadine® **[US]** *see* emedastine *on this page*

Embeline™ ***(Discontinued)*** *see* clobetasol *on page 201*

Embeline™ **E** ***(Discontinued)*** *see* clobetasol *on page 201*

Emcyt® **[US/Can]** *see* estramustine *on page 317*

Emecheck® ***(Discontinued)***

emedastine (em e DAS teen)
Synonyms emedastine difumarate
U.S./Canadian Brand Names Emadine® [US]
Therapeutic Category Antihistamine, H$_1$ Blocker, Ophthalmic
Use Treatment of allergic conjunctivitis
Usual Dosage Ophthalmic: Children ≥3 years and Adults: Instill 1 drop in affected eye up to 4 times/day
Dosage Forms
Solution, ophthalmic:
Emadine®: 0.05% (5 mL)

emedastine difumarate *see* emedastine *on this page*

Emend® **[US]** *see* aprepitant *on page 71*

Emetrol® **[US-OTC]** *see* fructose, dextrose, and phosphoric acid *on page 378*

Emitrip® *(Discontinued)* *see* amitriptyline *on page 44*

Emko® *(Discontinued)* *see* nonoxynol 9 *on page 610*

EMLA® **[US/Can]** *see* lidocaine and prilocaine *on page 507*

Emo-Cort® **[Can]** *see* hydrocortisone (topical) *on page 434*

Emsam® **[US]** *see* selegiline *on page 780*

emtricitabine (em trye SYE ta been)
Synonyms BW524W91; coviracil; FTC
U.S./Canadian Brand Names Emtriva® [US/Can]
Therapeutic Category Antiretroviral Agent, Reverse Transcriptase Inhibitor (Nucleoside)
Use Treatment of HIV infection in combination with at least two other antiretroviral agents
Usual Dosage Oral:
  Children:
    0-3 months: Solution: 3 mg/kg/day
    3 months to 17 years:
      Capsule: Children >33 kg: 200 mg once daily
      Solution: 6 mg/kg once daily; maximum: 240 mg/day
  Adults:
    Capsule: 200 mg once daily
    Solution: 240 mg once daily
Dosage Forms
  Capsule:
    Emtriva®: 200 mg
  Solution:
    Emtriva®: 10 mg/mL

emtricitabine and tenofovir (em trye SYE ta been & te NOE fo veer)
Synonyms tenofovir and emtricitabine
U.S./Canadian Brand Names Truvada® [US/Can]
Therapeutic Category Antiretroviral Agent, Reverse Transcriptase Inhibitor (Nucleoside);   Antiretroviral Agent, Reverse Transcriptase Inhibitor (Nucleotide)
Use Treatment of HIV infection in combination with other antiretroviral agents
Usual Dosage Oral: Adults: One tablet (emtricitabine 200 mg and tenofovir 300 mg) once daily
Dosage Forms
  Tablet:
    Truvada®: Emtricitabine 200 mg and tenofovir 300 mg

emtricitabine, efavirenz, and tenofovir *see* efavirenz, emtricitabine, and tenofovir *on page 293*

Emtriva® **[US/Can]** *see* emtricitabine *on this page*

Emulsoil® *(Discontinued)* *see* castor oil *on page 157*

E-Mycin® *(Discontinued)*

E-Mycin-E® *(Discontinued)*

ENA 713 *see* rivastigmine *on page 763*

Enablex® **[US/Can]** *see* darifenacin *on page 232*

enalapril (e NAL a pril)
Sound-Alike/Look-Alike Issues
  enalapril may be confused with Anafranil®, Elavil®, Eldepryl®, nafarelin, ramipril
Synonyms enalaprilat; enalapril maleate
U.S./Canadian Brand Names Vasotec® [US/Can]
Therapeutic Category Angiotensin-Converting Enzyme (ACE) Inhibitor
Use Management of mild to severe hypertension; treatment of congestive heart failure, left ventricular dysfunction after myocardial infarction
Usual Dosage Use lower listed initial dose in patients with hyponatremia, hypovolemia, severe congestive heart failure, decreased renal function, or in those receiving diuretics.

  Oral: **Enalapril**: Children 1 month to 17 years: Hypertension: Initial: 0.08 mg/kg/d (up to 5 mg) in 1-2 divided doses; adjust dosage based on patient response; doses >0.58 mg/kg (40 mg) have not been evaluated in pediatric patients
  (Continued)

enalapril *(Continued)*

Adults:

Oral: **Enalapril:**

Hypertension: 2.5-5 mg/day then increase as required, usually at 1- to 2-week intervals; usual dose range (JNC 7): 2.5-40 mg/day in 1-2 divided doses. **Note:** Initiate with 2.5 mg if patient is taking a diuretic which cannot be discontinued. May add a diuretic if blood pressure cannot be controlled with enalapril alone.

Heart failure: Initial: 2.5 mg once or twice daily (usual range: 5-40 mg/day in 2 divided doses). Titrate slowly at 1- to 2-week intervals. Target dose: 10-20 mg twice daily (ACC/AHA 2005 Heart Failure Guidelines)

Asymptomatic left ventricular dysfunction: 2.5 mg twice daily, titrated as tolerated to 20 mg/day

I.V.: **Enalaprilat:**

Hypertension: 1.25 mg/dose, given over 5 minutes every 6 hours; doses as high as 5 mg/dose every 6 hours have been tolerated for up to 36 hours. **Note:** If patients are concomitantly receiving diuretic therapy, begin with 0.625 mg I.V. over 5 minutes; if the effect is not adequate after 1 hour, repeat the dose and administer 1.25 mg at 6-hour intervals thereafter; if adequate, administer 0.625 mg I.V. every 6 hours.

Heart failure: Avoid I.V. administration in patients with unstable heart failure or those suffering acute myocardial infarction.

Conversion from I.V. to oral therapy if not concurrently on diuretics: 5 mg once daily; subsequent titration as needed; if concurrently receiving diuretics and responding to 0.625 mg I.V. every 6 hours, initiate with 2.5 mg/day.

Dosage Forms

Injection, solution: 1.25 mg/mL (1 mL, 2 mL)

Tablet: 2.5 mg, 5 mg, 10 mg, 20 mg

Vasotec®: 2.5 mg, 5 mg, 10 mg, 20 mg

enalapril and felodipine *(e NAL a pril & fe LOE di peen)*

Synonyms felodipine and enalapril

U.S./Canadian Brand Names Lexxel® [US/Can]

Therapeutic Category Antihypertensive Agent, Combination

Use Treatment of hypertension, however, not indicated for initial treatment of hypertension; replacement therapy in patients receiving separate dosage forms (for patient convenience); when monotherapy with one component fails to achieve desired antihypertensive effect, or when dose-limiting adverse effects limit upward titration of monotherapy

Usual Dosage Oral: Adults: Enalapril 5-20 mg and felodipine 2.5-10 mg once daily

Dosage Forms

Tablet, extended release:

Lexxel®: Enalapril 5 mg and felodipine 2.5 mg; enalapril 5 mg and felodipine 5 mg

enalapril and hydrochlorothiazide *(e NAL a pril & hye droe klor oh THYE a zide)*

Synonyms hydrochlorothiazide and enalapril

U.S./Canadian Brand Names Vaseretic® [US/Can]

Therapeutic Category Antihypertensive Agent, Combination

Use Treatment of hypertension

Usual Dosage Oral: Adults: Enalapril 5-10 mg and hydrochlorothiazide 12.5-25 mg once daily (maximum: 20 mg/day [enalapril]; 50 mg/day [hydrochlorothiazide])

Dosage Forms

Tablet: 5-12.5: Enalapril 5 mg and hydrochlorothiazide 12.5 mg; 10-25: Enalapril 10 mg and hydrochlorothiazide 25 mg

Vaseretic®: 5-12.5: Enalapril 5 mg and hydrochlorothiazide 12.5 mg; 10-25: enalapril 10 mg and hydrochlorothiazide 25 mg

enalaprilat *see* enalapril *on previous page*

enalapril maleate *see* enalapril *on previous page*

Enbrel® [US/Can] *see* etanercept *on page 321*

Encare® [US-OTC] *see* nonoxynol 9 *on page 610*

Encort™ [US] *see* hydrocortisone (rectal) *on page 433*

EndaCof [US] *see* hydrocodone and guaifenesin *on page 429*

EndaCof-DM [US] *see* brompheniramine, pseudoephedrine, and dextromethorphan *on page 122*

EndaCof-PD [US] *see* brompheniramine, pseudoephedrine, and dextromethorphan *on page 122*

EndaCof-XP [US] *see* hydrocodone and guaifenesin *on page 429*

Endagen™-HD *(Discontinued)* *see* phenylephrine, hydrocodone, and chlorpheniramine *on page 678*

Endantadine® [Can] *see* amantadine *on page 38*

EndoAvitene® **[US]** *see* collagen hemostat *on page 213*

Endocet® **[US/Can]** *see* oxycodone and acetaminophen *on page 641*

Endocodone® *(Discontinued) see* oxycodone *on page 640*

Endodan® **[US/Can]** *see* oxycodone and aspirin *on page 642*

Endo®**-Levodopa/Carbidopa [Can]** *see* levodopa and carbidopa *on page 500*

Endolor® *(Discontinued)*

Endometrin® **[US]** *see* progesterone *on page 718*

Endrate® **[US]** *see* edetate disodium *on page 291*

Enduron® **[Can]** *see* methyclothiazide *on page 556*

Enduron® *(Discontinued) see* methyclothiazide *on page 556*

Enduronyl® **Forte** *(Discontinued)*

Enemeez® **[US-OTC]** *see* docusate *on page 273*

Ener-B® *(Discontinued) see* cyanocobalamin *on page 220*

Enerjets [US-OTC] *see* caffeine *on page 133*

enflurane (EN floo rane)

Sound-Alike/Look-Alike Issues
enflurane may be confused with isoflurane

U.S./Canadian Brand Names Compound 347™ [US]; Ethrane® [US]

Therapeutic Category General Anesthetic

Use Maintenance of general anesthesia

Usual Dosage Minimum alveolar concentration (MAC), the concentration at which 50% of patients do not respond to surgical incision, is 1.6% for enflurane. The concentration at which amnesia and loss of awareness occur (MAC - awake) is 0.4%. Surgical levels of anesthesia are achieved with concentrations between 0.5% to 3%.

Dosage Forms
Liquid, for inhalation:
Compound 347™, Ethrane®: >99.9% (250 mL)

enfuvirtide (en FYOO vir tide)

Synonyms T-20

U.S./Canadian Brand Names Fuzeon® [US/Can]

Therapeutic Category Antiretroviral Agent, Fusion Protein Inhibitor

Use Treatment of HIV-1 infection in combination with other antiretroviral agents in treatment-experienced patients with evidence of HIV-1 replication despite ongoing antiretroviral therapy

Usual Dosage SubQ:
Children 6-16 years: 2 mg/kg twice daily (maximum dose: 90 mg twice daily)
Adolescents ≥16 years and Adults: 90 mg twice daily

Dosage Forms
Injection, powder for reconstitution [preservative free]:
Fuzeon®: 108 mg

ENG *see* etonogestrel *on page 336*

Engerix-B® **[US/Can]** *see* hepatitis B vaccine *on page 418*

Engerix-B® **and Havrix**® *see* hepatitis A inactivated and hepatitis B (recombinant) vaccine *on page 416*

enhanced-potency inactivated poliovirus vaccine *see* poliovirus vaccine (inactivated) *on page 693*

Enhancer [US] *see* barium *on page 94*

Enisyl® *(Discontinued) see* l-lysine *on page 513*

Enjuvia™ **[US]** *see* estrogens (conjugated B/synthetic) *on page 317*

Enlon® **[US/Can]** *see* edrophonium *on page 291*

Enlon-Plus™ **[US]** *see* edrophonium and atropine *on page 292*

Enomine® *(Discontinued)*

Enovil® *(Discontinued) see* amitriptyline *on page 44*

enoxaparin (ee noks a PA rin)

Sound-Alike/Look-Alike Issues
Lovenox® may be confused with Lotronex®, Protonix®
Synonyms enoxaparin sodium
U.S./Canadian Brand Names Enoxaparin Injection [Can]; Lovenox® HP [Can]; Lovenox® [US/Can]
Therapeutic Category Anticoagulant (Other)
Use

Acute coronary syndromes: Unstable angina (UA), non-ST-segment elevation (NSTEMI), and ST-segment elevation myocardial infarction (STEMI)

DVT prophylaxis: Following hip or knee replacement surgery, abdominal surgery, or in medical patients with severely-restricted mobility during acute illness in patients at risk of thromboembolic complications

DVT treatment (acute): Inpatient treatment (patients with and without pulmonary embolism) and outpatient treatment (patients without pulmonary embolism)

Note: High-risk patients include those with one or more of the following risk factors: >40 years of age, obesity, general anesthesia lasting >30 minutes, malignancy, history of deep vein thrombosis or pulmonary embolism

Usual Dosage SubQ: Adults:

DVT prophylaxis:

Hip replacement surgery:

Twice-daily dosing: 30 mg twice daily, with initial dose within 12-24 hours after surgery, and every 12 hours until risk of DVT has diminished or the patient is adequately anticoagulated on warfarin.

Once-daily dosing: 40 mg once daily, with initial dose within 9-15 hours before surgery, and daily until risk of DVT has diminished or the patient is adequately anticoagulated on warfarin.

Knee replacement surgery: 30 mg twice daily, with initial dose within 12-24 hours after surgery, and every 12 hours until risk of DVT has diminished (usually 7-10 days).

Abdominal surgery: 40 mg once daily, with initial dose given 2 hours prior to surgery; continue until risk of DVT has diminished (usual 7-10 days).

Medical patients with severely-restricted mobility during acute illness: 40 mg once daily; continue until risk of DVT has diminished

DVT treatment (acute): **Note:** Start warfarin within 72 hours and continue enoxaparin until INR is between 2.0 and 3.0 (usually 7 days).

Inpatient treatment (with or without pulmonary embolism): 1 mg/kg/dose every 12 hours or 1.5 mg/kg once daily.

Outpatient treatment (without pulmonary embolism): 1 mg/kg/dose every 12 hours.

ST-segment elevation myocardial infarction (STEMI):

Patients <75 years of age: Initial: 30 mg I.V. single bolus plus 1 mg/kg (maximum 100 mg for the first 2 doses only) SubQ every 12 hours. The first SubQ dose should be administered with the I.V. bolus. Maintenance: After first 2 doses, administer 1 mg/kg SubQ every 12 hours.

Patients ≥75 years of age: Initial: SubQ: 0.75 mg/kg every 12 hours (**Note:** No I.V. bolus is administered in this population); a maximum dose of 75 mg is recommended for the first 2 doses. Maintenance: After first 2 doses, administer 0.75 mg/kg SubQ every 12 hours

Additional notes on STEMI treatment: Therapy was continued for 8 days or until hospital discharge; optimal duration not defined. Unless contraindicated, all patients received aspirin (75-325 mg daily) in clinical trials. In patients with STEMI receiving thrombolytics, initiate enoxaparin dosing between 15 minutes before and 30 minutes after fibrinolytic therapy. In patients undergoing PCI, if balloon inflation occurs <8 hours after the last SubQ enoxaparin dose, no additional dosing is needed. If balloon inflation occurs ≥8 hours after last SubQ enoxaparin dose, a single I.V. dose of 0.3 mg/kg should be administered.

Unstable angina or non-ST-segment myocardial infarction (NSTEMI): 1 mg/kg every 12 hours in conjunction with oral aspirin therapy (100-325 mg once daily); continue until clinical stabilization (a minimum of at least 2 days)

Dosage Forms

Injection, solution [graduated prefilled syringe; preservative free]:
Lovenox®: 60 mg/0.6 mL (0.6 mL); 80 mg/0.8 mL (0.8 mL); 100 mg/mL (1 mL); 120 mg/0.8 mL (0.8 mL); 150 mg/mL (1 mL)

Injection, solution [multidose vial]:
Lovenox®: 100 mg/mL (3 mL)

Injection, solution [prefilled syringe; preservative free]:
Lovenox®: 30 mg/0.3 mL (0.3 mL); 40 mg/0.4 mL (0.4 mL)

Enoxaparin Injection [Can] *see* enoxaparin *on this page*

enoxaparin sodium *see* enoxaparin *on this page*

Enpresse™ [US] *see* ethinyl estradiol and levonorgestrel *on page 325*

Ensure® [US-OTC] *see* nutritional formula, enteral/oral *on page 622*

Ensure Plus® [US-OTC] *see* nutritional formula, enteral/oral *on page 622*

entacapone (en TA ka pone)
U.S./Canadian Brand Names Comtan® [US/Can]
Therapeutic Category Anti-Parkinson Agent; Reverse COMT Inhibitor
Use Adjunct to levodopa/carbidopa therapy in patients with idiopathic Parkinson disease who experience "wearing-off" symptoms at the end of a dosing interval
Usual Dosage Oral: Adults: 200 mg with each dose of levodopa/carbidopa, up to a maximum of 8 times/day (maximum daily dose: 1600 mg/day). To optimize therapy, the dosage of levodopa may need reduced or the dosing interval may need extended. Patients taking levodopa ≥800 mg/day or who had moderate-to-severe dyskinesias prior to therapy required an average decrease of 25% in the daily levodopa dose.
Dosage Forms
Tablet:
Comtan®: 200 mg

entacapone, carbidopa, and levodopa *see* levodopa, carbidopa, and entacapone *on page 500*

entecavir (en TE ka veer)
U.S./Canadian Brand Names Baraclude® [US/Can]
Therapeutic Category Antiretroviral Agent, Reverse Transcriptase Inhibitor (Nucleoside)
Use Treatment of chronic hepatitis B infection in adults with evidence of active viral replication and either evidence of persistent transaminase elevations or histologically-active disease
Usual Dosage Oral: Adolescents ≥16 years and Adults:
Nucleoside treatment naive: 0.5 mg daily
Lamivudine-resistant viremia (or known lamivudine-resistant mutations): 1 mg daily
Dosage Forms
Oral solution:
Baraclude®: 0.05 mg/mL
Tablet:
Baraclude®: 0.5 mg, 1 mg

enterotoxigenic *Escherichia coli* **and** *Vibrio cholera* **vaccine** *see* traveler's diarrhea and cholera vaccine *(Canada only) on page 858*

Entero Vu™ [US] *see* barium *on page 94*

Entertainer's Secret® [US-OTC] *see* saliva substitute *on page 774*

Entex® *(Discontinued)* *see* guaifenesin and phenylephrine *on page 404*

Entex® ER *(Discontinued)* *see* guaifenesin and phenylephrine *on page 404*

Entex® LA [Can] *see* guaifenesin and pseudoephedrine *on page 406*

Entex® LA *(Discontinued)* *see* guaifenesin and phenylephrine *on page 404*

Entex® PSE [US] *see* guaifenesin and pseudoephedrine *on page 406*

Entocort® [Can] *see* budesonide *on page 123*

Entocort® EC [US] *see* budesonide *on page 123*

Entrobar® [US] *see* barium *on page 94*

EntroEase® [US] *see* barium *on page 94*

Entrophen® [Can] *see* aspirin *on page 78*

Entsol® [US-OTC] *see* sodium chloride *on page 792*

Entuss-D® Liquid *(Discontinued)* *see* hydrocodone and pseudoephedrine *on page 430*

Enulose [US] *see* lactulose *on page 489*

Eperbel-S [US] *see* belladonna, phenobarbital, and ergotamine *on page 98*

ephedrine (e FED rin)
Sound-Alike/Look-Alike Issues
ephedrine may be confused with Epifrin®, epinephrine
Synonyms ephedrine sulfate
U.S./Canadian Brand Names Pretz-D® [US-OTC]
Therapeutic Category Adrenergic Agonist Agent
Use Treatment of bronchial asthma, nasal congestion, acute bronchospasm, idiopathic orthostatic hypotension, hypotension induced by spinal anesthesia
Usual Dosage
Children:
Oral, SubQ: 3 mg/kg/day or 25-100 mg/m^2/day in 4-6 divided doses every 4-6 hours
(Continued)

ephedrine *(Continued)*

    I.M., slow I.V. push: 0.2-0.3 mg/kg/dose every 4-6 hours
Adults:
    Oral: 25-50 mg every 3-4 hours as needed
    I.M., SubQ: 25-50 mg, parenteral adult dose should not exceed 150 mg in 24 hours
    I.M.: Hypotension induced by anesthesia: 25 mg
    I.V.: 5-25 mg/dose slow I.V. push repeated after 5-10 minutes as needed, then every 3-4 hours not to exceed 150 mg/24 hours
    Nasal spray:
    Children 6-12 years: 1-2 sprays into each nostril, not more frequently than every 4 hours
    Children ≥12 years and Adults: 2-3 sprays into each nostril, not more frequently than every 4 hours
Dosage Forms
    Capsule: 25 mg
    Injection, solution: 50 mg/mL (1 mL, 10 mL)
    Solution, intranasal spray: 0.25% (50 mL)
    Pretz-D® [OTC]: 0.25% (50 mL)

ephedrine, chlorpheniramine, phenylephrine, and carbetapentane *see* chlorpheniramine, ephedrine, phenylephrine, and carbetapentane *on page 179*

ephedrine sulfate *see* ephedrine *on previous page*

EpiClenz™ [US-OTC] *see* alcohol (ethyl) *on page 25*

epidermal thymocyte activating factor *see* aldesleukin *on page 26*

Epifoam® [US] *see* pramoxine and hydrocortisone *on page 707*

Epifrin® *(Discontinued)* *see* epinephrine *on this page*

epinastine *(ep i NAS teen)*
Synonyms epinastine hydrochloride
U.S./Canadian Brand Names Elestat™ [US]
Therapeutic Category Antihistamine, H₁ Blocker, Ophthalmic
Use Treatment of allergic conjunctivitis
Usual Dosage Ophthalmic: Children ≥3 years and Adults: Allergic conjunctivitis: Instill 1 drop into each eye twice daily; continue throughout period of exposure, even in the absence of symptoms
Dosage Forms
    Solution, ophthalmic:
    Elestat™: 0.05% (5 mL)

epinastine hydrochloride *see* epinastine *on this page*

epinephrine *(ep i NEF rin)*
Sound-Alike/Look-Alike Issues
    epinephrine may be confused with ephedrine
    Epifrin® may be confused with ephedrine, EpiPen®
    EpiPen® may be confused with Epifrin®
Synonyms adrenaline; epinephrine bitartrate; epinephrine hydrochloride; racepinephrine
U.S./Canadian Brand Names Adrenalin® [US/Can]; EpiPen® Jr [US/Can]; EpiPen® [US/Can]; Primatene® Mist [US-OTC]; Raphon [US-OTC]; S2® [US-OTC]; Twinject™ [US/Can]
Therapeutic Category Adrenergic Agonist Agent
Use Treatment of bronchospasms, bronchial asthma, nasal congestion, viral croup, anaphylactic reactions, cardiac arrest; added to local anesthetics to decrease systemic absorption of local anesthetics and increase duration of action; decrease superficial hemorrhage
Usual Dosage
    Neonates: Cardiac arrest: I.V.: 0.01-0.03 mg/kg (0.1-0.3 mL/kg of **1:10,000** solution) every 3-5 minutes as needed. Although I.V. route is preferred, may consider administration of doses up to 0.1 mg/kg through the endotracheal tube until I.V. access established; dilute intratracheal doses to 1-2 mL with normal saline.
    Infants and Children:
        Asystole/pulseless arrest, bradycardia, VT/VF (after failed defibrillations):
        I.V., I.O.: 0.01 mg/kg (0.1 mL/kg of **1:10,000** solution) every 3-5 minutes as needed (maximum: 1 mg)
        Intratracheal: 0.1 mg/kg (0.1 mL/kg of **1:1000** solution) every 3-5 minutes (maximum: 10 mg)
        Continuous I.V. infusion: 0.1-1 mcg/kg/minute; doses <0.3 mcg/kg/minute generally produce β-adrenergic effects and higher doses generally produce α-adrenergic vasoconstriction; titrate dosage to desired effect
        Bronchodilator: SubQ: 0.01 mg/kg (0.01 mL/kg of **1:1000**) (single doses not to exceed 0.5 mg) every 20 minutes for 3 doses
        Nebulization: 1-3 inhalations up to every 3 hours using solution prepared with 10 drops of 1:100

Children <4 years: S2® (racepinephrine, OTC labeling): Croup: 0.05 mL/kg (max 0.5 mL/dose); dilute in NS 3 mL. Administer over ~15 minutes; do not administer more frequently than every 2 hours.

Inhalation: Children ≥4 years: Primatene® Mist: Refer to adult dosing.

Decongestant: Children ≥6 years: Refer to adult dosing

Hypersensitivity reaction:

SubQ, I.V.: 0.01 mg/kg every 20 minutes; larger doses or continuous infusion may be needed for some anaphylactic reactions

Self-administration following severe allergic reactions (eg, insect stings, food): **Note:** World Health Organization (WHO) and Anaphylaxis Canada recommend the availability of 1 dose for every 10-20 minutes of travel time to a medical emergency facility:

Twinject™: SubQ, I.M.:

Children 15-30 kg: 0.15 mg

Children >30 kg: 0.3 mg

Epipen® Jr: I.M.: Children <30 kg: 0.15 mg

Epipen®: I.M.: Children ≥30 kg: 0.3 mg

Adults:

Asystole/pulseless arrest, bradycardia, VT/VF:

I.V., I.O.: 1 mg every 3-5 minutes; if this approach fails, higher doses of epinephrine (up to 0.2 mg/kg) may be indicated for treatment of specific problems (eg, beta-blocker or calcium channel blocker overdose)

Intratracheal: Administer 2-2.5 mg for VF or pulseless VT if I.V./I.O. access is delayed or cannot be established; dilute in 5-10 mL NS or distilled water. **Note:** Absorption is greater with distilled water, but causes more adverse effects on PaO_2.

Bradycardia (symptomatic) or hypotension (not responsive to atropine or pacing): I.V. infusion: 2-10 mcg/minute; titrate to desired effect

Bronchodilator:

SubQ: 0.3-0.5 mg **(1:1000)** every 20 minutes for 3 doses

Nebulization: 1-3 inhalations up to every 3 hours using solution prepared with 10 drops of the **1:100** product

S2® (racepinephrine, OTC labeling): 0.5 mL (~10 drops). Dose may be repeated not more frequently than very 3-4 hours if needed. Solution should be diluted if using jet nebulizer.

Inhalation: Primatene® Mist (OTC labeling): One inhalation, wait at least 1 minute; if relieved, may use once more. Do not use again for at least 3 hours.

Decongestant: Intranasal: Apply 1:1000 locally as drops or spray or with sterile swab

Hypersensitivity reaction:

SubQ, I.M.: 0.3-0.5 mg (1:1000) every 15-20 minutes if condition requires (I.M. route is preferred)

I.V.: 0.1 mg (1:10,000) over 5 minutes. May infuse at 1-4 mcg/minute to prevent the need to repeat injections frequently.

Self-administration following severe allergic reactions (eg, insect stings, food): **Note:** The World Health Organization (WHO) and Anaphylaxis Canada recommend the availability of one dose for every 10 to 20 minutes of travel time to a medical emergency facility. More than 2 doses should only be administered under direct medical supervision.

Twinject™: SubQ, I.M.: 0.3 mg

Epipen®: I.M.: 0.3 mg

Dosage Forms

Aerosol for oral inhalation:

Primatene® Mist [OTC]: 0.22 mg/inhalation (15 mL, 22.5 mL)

Injection, solution [prefilled auto injector]:

EpiPen®: 0.3 mg/0.3 mL [1:1000] (2 mL) [available as single unit or in double-unit pack with training unit]

EpiPen® Jr: 0.15 mg/0.3 mL [1:2000] (2 mL) [available as single unit or in double-unit pack with training unit]

Twinject™: 0.15 mg/0.15 mL [1:1000] (1.1 mL) [two 0.15 mg doses per injector]; 0.3 mg/0.3 mL [1:1000] (1.1 mL) [two 0.3 mg doses per injector]

Injection, solution: 0.1 mg/mL [1:10,000] (10 mL); 1 mg/mL [1:1000] (1 mL)

Adrenalin®: 1 mg/mL [1:1000] (1 mL, 30 mL)

Solution for oral inhalation:

Adrenalin®: 1% [10 mg/mL, 1:100] (7.5 mL)

Solution for oral inhalation [racepinephrine]:

S2®: 2.25% (0.5 mL, 15 mL)

Solution, topical [racepinephrine]:

Raphon: 2.25% (15 mL)

epinephrine and articaine hydrochloride *see* articaine and epinephrine *on page 75*

epinephrine and chlorpheniramine (ep i NEF rin & klor fen IR a meen)

Synonyms insect sting kit
U.S./Canadian Brand Names Ana-Kit® [US]
Therapeutic Category Antidote
Use Anaphylaxis emergency treatment of insect bites or stings by the sensitive patient that may occur within minutes of insect sting or exposure to an allergic substance
Usual Dosage I.M. or SubQ: Children and Adults:
Epinephrine:
<2 years: 0.05-0.1 mL
2-6 years: 0.15 mL
6-12 years: 0.2 mL
>12 years : 0.3 mL
Chlorpheniramine:
<6 years: 1 tablet
6-12 years: 2 tablets
>12 years: 4 tablets
Dosage Forms
Kit:
Ana-Kit®: Epinephrine 1:1000 (1 mL), chlorpheniramine chewable tablet 2 mg (4), sterile alcohol pads (2), tourniquet (1)

epinephrine and lidocaine *see* lidocaine and epinephrine *on page 506*

epinephrine bitartrate *see* epinephrine *on page 300*

epinephrine bitartrate and bupivacaine hydrochloride *see* bupivacaine and epinephrine *on page 126*

epinephrine hydrochloride *see* epinephrine *on page 300*

EpiPen® [US/Can] *see* epinephrine *on page 300*

EpiPen® Jr [US/Can] *see* epinephrine *on page 300*

epipodophyllotoxin *see* etoposide *on page 336*

EpiQuin™ Micro [US] *see* hydroquinone *on page 437*

epirubicin (ep i ROO bi sin)

Sound-Alike/Look-Alike Issues
epirubicin may be confused with DAUNOrubicin, DOXOrubicin, idarubicin
Ellence® may be confused with Elase®
Synonyms epirubicin hydrochloride; NSC-256942; pidorubicin; pidorubicin hydrochloride
U.S./Canadian Brand Names Ellence® [US/Can]; Pharmorubicin® [Can]
Therapeutic Category Antineoplastic Agent, Anthracycline; Antineoplastic Agent, Antibiotic
Use Adjuvant therapy for primary breast cancer
Usual Dosage Adults: I.V.: 100-120 mg/m^2 once every 3-4 weeks **or** 50-60 mg/m^2 days 1 and 8 every 3-4 weeks
Breast cancer:
CEF-120: 60 mg/m^2 on days 1 and 8 every 28 days for 6 cycles
FEC-100: 100 mg/m^2 on day 1 every 21 days for 6 cycles
Note: Patients receiving 120 mg/m^2/cycle as part of combination therapy should also receive prophylactic therapy with sulfamethoxazole/trimethoprim or a fluoroquinolone.
Dosage modifications:
Delay day 1 dose until platelets are ≥100,000/mm^3, ANC ≥1500/mm^3, and nonhematologic toxicities have recovered to ≤grade 1
Reduce day 1 dose in subsequent cycles to 75% of previous day 1 dose if patient experiences nadir platelet counts <50,000/mm^3, ANC <250/mm^3, neutropenic fever, or grade 3/4 nonhematologic toxicity during the previous cycle
For divided doses (day 1 and day 8), reduce day 8 dose to 75% of day 1 dose if platelet counts are 75,000-100,000/mm^3 and ANC is 1000-1499/mm^3; omit day 8 dose if platelets are <75,000/mm^3, ANC <1000/mm^3, or grade 3/4 nonhematologic toxicity
Dosage adjustment in bone marrow dysfunction: Heavily-treated patients, patients with preexisting bone marrow depression or neoplastic bone marrow infiltration: Lower starting doses (75-90 mg/mm^2) should be considered.
Dosage Forms
Injection, powder for reconstitution, as hydrochloride, [preservative free]: 50 mg, 200 mg [contains lactose]
Injection, solution [preservative free]: 2 mg/mL (25 mL, 100 mL)
Ellence®: 2 mg/mL (25 mL, 100 mL)

epirubicin hydrochloride *see* epirubicin *on previous page*

Epitol® **[US]** *see* carbamazepine *on page 147*

Epival® **I.V. [Can]** *see* valproic acid and derivatives *on page 881*

Epivir® **[US]** *see* lamivudine *on page 489*

Epivir-HBV® **[US]** *see* lamivudine *on page 489*

eplerenone (e PLER en one)
Sound-Alike/Look-Alike Issues
Inspra™ may be confused with Spiriva®
U.S./Canadian Brand Names Inspra™ [US]
Therapeutic Category Antihypertensive Agent; Selective Aldosterone Blocker
Use Treatment of hypertension (may be used alone or in combination with other antihypertensive agents); treatment of CHF following acute MI
Usual Dosage Oral: Adults:
Hypertension: Initial: 50 mg once daily; may increase to 50 mg twice daily if response is not adequate; may take up to 4 weeks for full therapeutic response. Doses >100 mg/day are associated with increased risk of hyperkalemia and no greater therapeutic effect.
Concurrent use with moderate CYP3A4 inhibitors: Initial: 25 mg once daily
Congestive heart failure (post-MI): Initial: 25 mg once daily; dosage goal: titrate to 50 mg once daily within 4 weeks, as tolerated
Dosage adjustment per serum potassium concentrations for CHF:
<5.0 mEq/L:
Increase dose from 25 mg every other day to 25 mg daily **or**
Increase dose from 25 mg daily to 50 mg daily
5.0-5.4 mEq/L: No adjustment needed
5.5-5.9 mEq/L:
Decrease dose from 50 mg daily to 25 mg daily **or**
Decrease dose from 25 mg daily to 25 mg every other day **or**
Decrease does from 25 mg every other day to withhold medication
≥6.0 mEq/L: Withhold medication until potassium <5.5 mEq/L, then restart at 25 mg every other day
Dosage Forms
Tablet:
Inspra™: 25 mg, 50 mg

EPO *see* epoetin alfa *on this page*

epoetin alfa (e POE e tin AL fa)
Sound-Alike/Look-Alike Issues
epoetin alfa may be confused with darbepoetin alfa
Synonyms EPO; erythropoiesis-stimulating agent (ESA); erythropoietin; NSC-724223; rHuEPO-α
U.S./Canadian Brand Names Epogen® [US]; Eprex® [Can]; Procrit® [US]
Therapeutic Category Colony-Stimulating Factor
Use Treatment of anemia related to HIV (zidovudine) therapy, chronic renal failure, antineoplastic therapy (for nonmyeloid malignancies); reduction of allogeneic blood transfusion for elective, noncardiac, nonvascular surgery
Usual Dosage Note: Use the minimum effective dose that will gradually increase the hemoglobin level to a point sufficient to avoid red blood cell transfusion. Hemoglobin levels should not exceed 12 g/dL and should not rise >1 g/dL per 2-week time period.
Chronic renal failure patients: I.V., SubQ: **Note:** Target hemoglobin levels should not exceed 12 g/dL.
Children: Initial dose: 50 units/kg 3 times/week
Adults: Initial dose: 50-100 units/kg 3 times/week
Dose adjustment: Children and Adults: Reduce dose by 25% when hemoglobin approaches 12 g/dL **or** hemoglobin increases 1 g/dL in any 2-week period. Increase dose by 25% if hemoglobin does not increase by 2 g/dL after 8 weeks of therapy (with adequate iron stores, may increase dose by 25% if hemoglobin increase <1 g/dL over 4 weeks) and hemoglobin is below suggested target range. Do not increase dose more frequently than at 4-week intervals.
Maintenance dose: Individualize to target range; limit additional dosage increases to every 4 weeks (or longer)
Dialysis patients: Median dose:
Children: 167 units/kg/week (hemodialysis) **or** 76 units/kg/week (peritoneal dialysis)
Adults: 75 units/kg 3 times/week
Nondialysis patients:
Children: Dosing range: 50-250 units/kg 1-3 times/week
Adults: Median dose: 75-150 units/kg/week
(Continued)

epoetin alfa *(Continued)*

Zidovudine-treated, HIV-infected patients (patients with erythropoietin levels >500 mU/mL are **unlikely** to respond): I.V., SubQ: **Note:** Target hemoglobin levels should not exceed 12 g/dL.

Children: Initial dose: Reported dosing range: 50-400 units/kg 2-3 times/week

Adults (with serum erythropoietin levels ≤500 and zidovudine doses ≤4200 mg): 100 units/kg 3 times/week for 8 weeks. **Dose adjustment:** Increase dose by 50-100 units/kg 3 times/week if response is not satisfactory in terms of reducing transfusion requirements or increasing hemoglobin after 8 weeks of therapy. Evaluate response every 4-8 weeks thereafter and adjust the dose accordingly by 50-100 units/kg increments 3 times/week. If patient has not responded satisfactorily to a 300 unit/kg dose 3 times/week, a response to higher doses is unlikely. Withhold dose if hemoglobin exceeds 12 g/dL and resume treatment at a 25% dose reduction when hemoglobin drops below 11g/dL.

Cancer patient on chemotherapy: Treatment of patients with erythropoietin levels >200 mU/mL is **not recommended. Note:** Target hemoglobin levels should not exceed 12 g/dL.

Children: I.V.: 600 units/kg once weekly (maximum: 40,000 units)

Adults: SubQ: Initial dose: 150 units/kg 3 times/week or 40,000 units once weekly; commonly used doses range from 10,000 units 3 times/week to 40,000-60,000 units once weekly.

Dose adjustment: Children and Adults: If response is not satisfactory after a sufficient period of evaluation (8 weeks of 3 times/week and 4 weeks of once-weekly therapy), the dose may be increased every 4 weeks (or longer) up to 300 units/kg 3 times/week, **or** when dosed weekly, increased all at once to 60,000 units weekly (adults) or 900 units/kg/week; maximum 60,000 units (pediatrics). If patient does not respond, a response to higher doses is unlikely. Stop dose if hemoglobin exceeds 12 g/dL and resume treatment at a 25% dose reduction when hemoglobin drops below 11 g/dL; reduce dose by 25% if hemoglobin increases by 1 g/dL in any 2-week period, or if hemoglobin approaches 12 g/dL.

Surgery patients: Prior to initiating treatment, obtain a hemoglobin to establish that is >10 mg/dL or ≤13 mg/dL: Adults: SubQ: Initial dose: 300 units/kg/day for 10 days before surgery, on the day of surgery, and for 4 days after surgery

Alternative dose: 600 units/kg in once weekly doses (21, 14, and 7 days before surgery) plus a fourth dose on the day of surgery

Dosage Forms

Injection, solution [preservative free]:

Epogen®, Procrit®: 2000 units/mL (1 mL); 3000 units/mL (1 mL); 4000 units/mL (1 mL); 10,000 units/mL (1 mL); 40,000 units/mL (1 mL)

Injection, solution [with preservative]:

Epogen®, Procrit®: 10,000 units/mL (2 mL); 20,000 units/mL (1 mL)

Epogen® [US] *see* epoetin alfa *on previous page*

epoprostenol *(e poe PROST en ole)*

Synonyms epoprostenol sodium; PGI₂; PGX; prostacyclin

U.S./Canadian Brand Names Flolan® [US/Can]

Therapeutic Category Platelet Inhibitor

Use Treatment of idiopathic pulmonary arterial hypertension [IPAH]; pulmonary hypertension associated with the scleroderma spectrum of disease [SSD] in NYHA Class III and Class IV patients who do not respond adequately to conventional therapy

Usual Dosage I.V.: Adults: Initial: 1-2 ng/kg/minute, increase dose in increments of 1-2 ng/kg/minute every 15 minutes or longer until dose-limiting side effects are noted or tolerance limit to epoprostenol is observed

Dosage Forms

Injection, powder for reconstitution:

Flolan®: 0.5 mg, 1.5 mg

epoprostenol sodium *see* epoprostenol *on this page*

Eprex® [Can] *see* epoetin alfa *on previous page*

eprosartan *(ep roe SAR tan)*

U.S./Canadian Brand Names Teveten® [US/Can]

Therapeutic Category Angiotensin II Receptor Antagonist

Use Treatment of hypertension; may be used alone or in combination with other antihypertensives

Usual Dosage Oral: Adults: Dosage must be individualized; can administer once or twice daily with total daily doses of 400-800 mg. Usual starting dose is 600 mg once daily as monotherapy in patients who are euvolemic. Limited clinical experience with doses >800 mg.

Dosage Forms

Tablet:

Teveten®: 400 mg, 600 mg

eprosartan and hydrochlorothiazide (ep roe SAR tan & hye droe klor oh THYE a zide)

Synonyms eprosartan mesylate and hydrochlorothiazide; hydrochlorothiazide and eprosartan

U.S./Canadian Brand Names Teveten® HCT [US/Can]; Teveten® Plus [Can]

Therapeutic Category Angiotensin II Antagonist Combination; Antihypertensive Agent, Combination; Diuretic, Thiazide

Use Treatment of hypertension (not indicated for initial treatment)

Usual Dosage Oral: Adults: Dose is individualized (combination substituted for individual components)

Usual recommended dose: Eprosartan 600 mg/hydrochlorothiazide 12.5 mg once daily (maximum dose: Eprosartan 600 mg/hydrochlorothiazide 25 mg once daily)

Dosage Forms

Tablet:

Teveten® HCT: 600 mg/12.5 mg: Eprosartan 600 mg and hydrochlorothiazide 12.5 mg; 600 mg/25 mg: Eprosartan 600 mg and hydrochlorothiazide 25 mg

eprosartan mesylate and hydrochlorothiazide see eprosartan and hydrochlorothiazide on this page

epsilon aminocaproic acid see aminocaproic acid on page 42

epsom salts see magnesium sulfate on page 529

EPT see teniposide on page 825

eptacog alfa (activated) see factor VIIa (recombinant) on page 339

eptifibatide (ep TIF i ba tide)

Synonyms intrifiban

U.S./Canadian Brand Names Integrilin® [US/Can]

Therapeutic Category Antiplatelet Agent

Use Treatment of patients with acute coronary syndrome (unstable angina/non-Q wave myocardial infarction [UA/NQMI]), including patients who are to be managed medically and those undergoing percutaneous coronary intervention (PCI including angioplasty, intracoronary stenting)

Usual Dosage I.V.: Adults:

Acute coronary syndrome: Bolus of 180 mcg/kg (maximum: 22.6 mg) over 1-2 minutes, begun as soon as possible following diagnosis, followed by a continuous infusion of 2 mcg/kg/minute (maximum: 15 mg/hour) until hospital discharge or initiation of CABG surgery, up to 72 hours. Concurrent aspirin and heparin therapy (target aPTT 50-70 seconds) are recommended.

Percutaneous coronary intervention (PCI) with or without stenting: Bolus of 180 mcg/kg (maximum: 22.6 mg) administered immediately before the initiation of PCI, followed by a continuous infusion of 2 mcg/kg/minute (maximum: 15 mg/hour). A second 180 mcg/kg bolus (maximum: 22.6 mg) should be administered 10 minutes after the first bolus. Infusion should be continued until hospital discharge or for up to 18-24 hours, whichever comes first. Concurrent aspirin (160-325 mg 1-24 hours before PCI and daily thereafter) and heparin therapy (ACT 200-300 seconds during PCI) are recommended. Heparin infusion after PCI is discouraged. In patients who undergo coronary artery bypass graft surgery, discontinue infusion prior to surgery.

Dosage Forms

Injection, solution:

Integrilin®: 0.75 mg/mL (100 mL); 2 mg/mL (10 mL, 100 mL)

Epzicom™ [US] see abacavir and lamivudine on page 2

Equagesic® [US] see meprobamate and aspirin on page 544

Equalactin® [US-OTC] see polycarbophil on page 694

Equalizer Gas Relief [US-OTC] see simethicone on page 786

Equanil® (Discontinued) see meprobamate on page 544

Equetro™ [US] see carbamazepine on page 147

Equilet® (Discontinued) see calcium carbonate on page 138

Eraxis™ [US] see anidulafungin on page 57

Erbitux® [US/Can] see cetuximab on page 170

ergocalciferol (er goe kal SIF e role)

Sound-Alike/Look-Alike Issues

Calciferol™ may be confused with calcitriol

Drisdol® may be confused with Drysol™

(Continued)

ergocalciferol *(Continued)*

Synonyms activated ergosterol; viosterol; vitamin D$_2$
U.S./Canadian Brand Names Calciferol™ [US]; Drisdol® [US/Can]; Ostoforte® [Can]
Therapeutic Category Vitamin D Analog
Use Treatment of refractory rickets, hypophosphatemia, hypoparathyroidism; dietary supplement
Usual Dosage Oral: **Note:** 1 mcg = 40 int. units
  Adequate intake:
  Infants and Children: 5 mcg/day (200 int. units/day)
  Adults:
   18-50 years: 5 mcg/day (200 int. units/day)
   51-70 years: 10 mcg/day (400 int. units/day)
  Dietary supplementation: Infants, Children, and Adults: 10 mcg/day (400 int. units/day)
  Vitamin D deficiency/insufficiency in patients with CKD stages 3-4 (K/DOQI guidelines): **Note:** Dose is based on 25-hydroxyvitamin D serum level [25(OH) D]:
  Children (treatment duration should be a total of 3 months):
   Serum 25(OH)D <5 ng/mL:
    8000 int. units/day for 4 weeks, then 4000 int. units/day for 2 months **or**
    50,000 int. units/week for 4 weeks, then 50,000 int. units twice a month for 2 months
   Serum 25(OH)D 5-15 ng/mL:
    4000 int units/day **or**
    50,000 int. units every other week
   Serum 25(OH)D 16-30 ng/mL:
    2000 int. units/day **or**
    50,000 int. units every 4 weeks
  Adults (treatment duration should be a total of 6 months):
   Serum 25(OH)D <5 ng/mL:
    50,000 int. units/week for 12 weeks, then 50,000 int. units/month
   Serum 25(OH)D 5-15 ng/mL:
    50,000 int. units/week for 4 weeks, then 50,000 int. units/month
   Serum 25(OH)D 16-30 ng/mL:
    50,000 int. units/month
  Hypoparathyroidism:
  Children: 1.25-5 mg/day (50,000-200,000 int. units) and calcium supplements
  Adults: 625 mcg to 5 mg/day (25,000-200,000 int. units) and calcium supplements
  Nutritional rickets and osteomalacia:
  Children and Adults (with normal absorption): 25-125 mcg/day (1000-5000 int. units)
  Children with malabsorption: 250-625 mcg/day (10,000-25,000 int. units)
  Adults with malabsorption: 250-7500 mcg (10,000-300,000 int. units)
  Vitamin D-*dependent* rickets:
  Children: 75-125 mcg/day (3000-5000 int. units); maximum: 1500 mcg/day
  Adults: 250 mcg to 1.5 mg/day (10,000-60,000 int. units)
  Vitamin D-*resistant* rickets: Children and Adults: 12,000-500,000 int. units/day
  Familial hypophosphatemia:
  Children: 40,000-80,000 int. units plus phosphate supplements; dose may be reduced once growth is complete
  Adults: 10,000-60,000 int. units plus phosphate supplements
Dosage Forms
  Capsule:
  Drisdol®: 50,000 int. units
  Liquid, oral [drops]:
  Calciferol™, Drisdol®: 8000 int. units/mL OTC]
  Tablet: 400 int. units [OTC]

ergoloid mesylates *(ER goe loid MES i lates)*

Synonyms dihydroergotoxine; dihydrogenated ergot alkaloids
U.S./Canadian Brand Names Hydergine® [Can]
Therapeutic Category Ergot Alkaloid and Derivative
Use Treatment of cerebrovascular insufficiency in primary progressive dementia, Alzheimer dementia, and senile onset
Usual Dosage Oral: Adults: 1 mg 3 times/day up to 4.5-12 mg/day; up to 6 months of therapy may be necessary
Dosage Forms
  Tablet: 1 mg
  Tablet, sublingual: 1 mg

Ergomar® **[US]** *see ergotamine on this page*

ergometrine maleate *see ergonovine on this page*

ergonovine (er goe NOE veen)
Synonyms ergometrine maleate; ergonovine maleate
U.S./Canadian Brand Names Ergotrate® [US]
Therapeutic Category Ergot Alkaloid and Derivative
Use Prevention and treatment of postpartum and postabortion hemorrhage caused by uterine atony or subinvolution
Usual Dosage Adults:
  I.M., I.V. (I.V. should be reserved for emergency use only): 0.2 mg, may repeat dose in 2-4 hours if needed
  Oral, SL:
    Immediate post-partum: 0.2 mg (usually given I.M. or I.V)
    Late post-partum: 0.2-0.4 mg every 6-12 hours until danger of uterine atony has passed (usually ~48 hours)
Dosage Forms
  Injection:
    Ergotrate®: 0.2 mg/mL (1 mL)
  Tablet:
    Ergotrate®: 0.2 mg

ergonovine maleate *see ergonovine on this page*

ergotamine (er GOT a meen)
Synonyms ergotamine tartrate
U.S./Canadian Brand Names Ergomar® [US]
Therapeutic Category Ergot Alkaloid and Derivative
Use Abort or prevent vascular headaches, such as migraine, migraine variants, or so-called "histaminic cephalalgia"
Usual Dosage Sublingual: One tablet under tongue at first sign, then 1 tablet every 30 minutes if needed; maximum dose: 3 tablets/24 hours, 5 tablets/week
Dosage Forms
  Tablet, sublingual:
    Ergomar®: 2 mg

ergotamine and caffeine (er GOT a meen & KAF een)
Sound-Alike/Look-Alike Issues
  Cafergot® may be confused with Carafate®
Synonyms caffeine and ergotamine; ergotamine tartrate and caffeine
U.S./Canadian Brand Names Cafergor® [Can]; Cafergot® [US]; Migergot [US]
Therapeutic Category Antimigraine Agent; Ergot Derivative; Stimulant
Use Abort or prevent vascular headaches, such as migraine, migraine variants, or so-called "histaminic cephalalgia"
Usual Dosage Adults:
  Oral: Two tablets at onset of attack; then 1 tablet every 30 minutes as needed; maximum: 6 tablets per attack; do not exceed 10 tablets/week.
  Rectal: One suppository rectally at first sign of an attack; follow with second dose after 1 hour, if needed; maximum: 2 per attack; do not exceed 5/week.
Dosage Forms
  Suppository, rectal:
    Migergot: Ergotamine tartrate 2 mg and caffeine 100 mg (12s)
  Tablet: Ergotamine tartrate 1 mg and caffeine 100 mg
    Cafergot®: Ergotamine tartrate 1 mg and caffeine 100 mg

ergotamine tartrate *see ergotamine on this page*

ergotamine tartrate and caffeine *see ergotamine and caffeine on this page*

Ergotamine Tartrate and Caffeine Cafatine® *(Discontinued) see ergotamine on this page*

ergotamine tartrate, belladonna, and phenobarbital *see belladonna, phenobarbital, and ergotamine on page 98*

Ergotrate® **[US]** *see ergonovine on this page*

erlotinib (er LOE tye nib)
Sound-Alike/Look-Alike Issues
  erlotinib may be confused with gefitinib
(Continued)

erlotinib *(Continued)*

Synonyms CP358774; erlotinib hydrochloride; NSC-718781; OSI-774; R 14-15
U.S./Canadian Brand Names Tarceva® [US/Can]
Therapeutic Category Antineoplastic, Tyrosine Kinase Inhibitor
Use Treatment of refractory advanced or metastatic nonsmall cell lung cancer (NSCLC); pancreatic cancer (first-line therapy in combination with gemcitabine)
Usual Dosage Oral: Adults: **Note:** Dose adjustments are likely to be needed when erlotinib is administered concomitantly with strong CYP3A4 inducers or inhibitors.
NSCLC: 150 mg/day
Pancreatic cancer: 100 mg/day in combination with gemcitabine
Dosage Forms
Tablet:
Tarceva®: 25 mg, 100 mg, 150 mg

erlotinib hydrochloride *see* erlotinib *on previous page*
Errin™ [US] *see* norethindrone *on page 611*
Ertaczo™ [US] *see* sertaconazole *on page 783*

ertapenem *(er ta PEN em)*

Sound-Alike/Look-Alike Issues
Invanz® may be confused with Avinza™
Synonyms ertapenem sodium; L-749,345; MK0826
U.S./Canadian Brand Names Invanz® [US/Can]
Therapeutic Category Antibiotic, Carbapenem
Use Treatment of the following moderate-severe infections: Complicated intraabdominal infections, complicated skin and skin structure infections (including diabetic foot infections without osteomyelitis), complicated UTI (including pyelonephritis), acute pelvic infections, and community-acquired pneumonia. Prophylaxis of surgical site infection following elective colorectal surgery. Antibacterial coverage includes aerobic gram-positive organisms, aerobic gram-negative organisms, anaerobic organisms.

Note: Methicillin-resistant *Staphylococcus*, *Enterococcus* spp, penicillin-resistant strains of *Streptococcus pneumoniae*, beta-lactamase-positive strains of *Haemophilus influenzae* are **resistant** to ertapenem, as are most *Pseudomonas aeruginosa*.
Usual Dosage
Usual dosage ranges:
Children 3 months to 12 years: I.M., I.V.: 15 mg/kg twice daily (maximum: 1 g/day)
Children ≥13 years and Adults: I.M., I.V.: 1 g/day
Indication-specific dosing:
Children 3 months to 12 years: I.M., I.V.:
Community-acquired pneumonia, complicated urinary tract infections (including pyelonephritis): 15 mg/kg twice daily (maximum: 1 g/day); duration of total antibiotic treatment: 10-14 days (**Note:** Duration includes possible switch to appropriate oral therapy after at least 3 days of parenteral treatment, once clinical improvement demonstrated.)
Intra-abdominal infection: 15 mg/kg twice daily (maximum: 1 g/day) for 5-14 days
Pelvic infections (acute): 15 mg/kg twice daily (maximum: 1 g/day) for 3-10 days
Skin and skin structure infections: 15 mg/kg twice daily (maximum: 1 g/day) for 7-14 days
Children ≥13 years and Adults: I.M., I.V.:
Community-acquired pneumonia, complicated urinary tract infections (including pyelonephritis): 1 g/day; duration of total antibiotic treatment: 10-14 days (**Note:** Duration includes possible switch to appropriate oral therapy after at least 3 days of parenteral treatment, once clinical improvement demonstrated.)
Intra-abdominal infection: 1 g/day for 5-14 days
Pelvic infections (acute): 1 g/day for 3-10 days
Skin and skin structure infections (including diabetic foot infections): 1 g/day for 7-14 days
Adults: I.V.:
Prophylaxis of surgical site following colorectal surgery: 1 g given 1 hour preoperatively
Dosage Forms
Injection, powder for reconstitution:
Invanz®: 1 g

ertapenem sodium *see* ertapenem *on this page*
Erwinia asparaginase *see* asparaginase *on page 77*
Erybid™ [Can] *see* erythromycin *on next page*
Eryc® [Can] *see* erythromycin *on next page*
Eryc® *(Discontinued)* *see* erythromycin *on next page*

Eryderm® [US] *see* erythromycin *on this page*

Erygel® [US] *see* erythromycin *on this page*

EryPed® [US] *see* erythromycin *on this page*

Ery-Tab® [US] *see* erythromycin *on this page*

Erythrocin® [US] *see* erythromycin *on this page*

erythromycin (er ith roe MYE sin)

Sound-Alike/Look-Alike Issues

erythromycin may be confused with azithromycin, clarithromycin, Ethmozine®

Akne-Mycin® may be confused with AK-Mycin®

E.E.S.® may be confused with DES®

Eryc® may be confused with Emcyt®, Ery-Tab®

Ery-Tab® may be confused with Eryc®

Erythrocin® may be confused with Ethmozine®

Synonyms erythromycin base; erythromycin ethylsuccinate; erythromycin lactobionate; erythromycin stearate

U.S./Canadian Brand Names Akne-Mycin® [US]; Apo-Erythro Base® [Can]; Apo-Erythro E-C® [Can]; Apo-Erythro-ES® [Can]; Apo-Erythro-S® [Can]; Diomycin® [Can]; E.E.S.® [US/Can]; Ery-Tab® [US]; Erybid™ [Can]; Eryc® [Can]; Eryderm® [US]; Erygel® [US]; EryPed® [US]; Erythrocin® [US]; Novo-Rythro Estolate [Can]; Novo-Rythro Ethylsuccinate [Can]; Nu-Erythromycin-S [Can]; PCE® [US/Can]; PMS-Erythromycin [Can]; Romycin® [US]; Sans Acne® [Can]

Therapeutic Category Acne Products; Antibiotic, Ophthalmic; Antibiotic, Topical; Macrolide (Antibiotic)

Use

Systemic: Treatment of susceptible bacterial infections including *S. pyogenes*, some *S. pneumoniae*, some *S. aureus*, *M. pneumoniae*, *Legionella pneumophila*, diphtheria, pertussis, *Chlamydia*, erythrasma, *N. gonorrhoeae*, *E. histolytica*, syphilis and nongonococcal urethritis, and *Campylobacter* gastroenteritis; used in conjunction with neomycin for decontaminating the bowel

Ophthalmic: Treatment of superficial eye infections involving the conjunctiva or cornea; neonatal ophthalmia

Topical: Treatment of acne vulgaris

Usual Dosage Note: Due to differences in absorption, 400 mg erythromycin ethylsuccinate produces the same serum levels as 250 mg erythromycin base or stearate.

Usual dosage range:

Neonates: Ophthalmic: Prophylaxis of neonatal gonococcal or chlamydial conjunctivitis: 0.5-1 cm ribbon of ointment should be instilled into each conjunctival sac

Infants and Children:

Oral:

Base: 30-50 mg/kg/day in 2-4 divided doses; maximum: 2 g/day

Ethylsuccinate: 30-50 mg/kg/day in 2-4 divided doses; maximum: 3.2 g/day

Stearate: 30-50 mg/kg/day in 2-4 divided doses; maximum: 2 g/day

I.V.: Lactobionate: 15-50 mg/kg/day divided every 6 hours, not to exceed 4 g/day

Children and Adults:

Ophthalmic: Instill ½" (1.25 cm) 2-6 times/day depending on the severity of the infection

Topical: Acne: Apply over the affected area twice daily after the skin has been thoroughly washed and patted dry

Adults:

Oral:

Base: 250-500 mg every 6-12 hours; maximum 4 g/day

Ethylsuccinate: 400-800 mg every 6-12 hours; maximum: 4 g/day

I.V.: Lactobionate: 15-20 mg/kg/day divided every 6 hours or 500 mg to 1 g every 6 hours, or given as a continuous infusion over 24 hours; maximum: 4 g/24 hours

Indication-specific dosing:

Children:

Conjunctivitis, neonatal *(C. trachomatis):* Oral: 50 mg/kg/day (base or ethylsuccinate) in 4 divided doses for 14 days

Mild/moderate infection: Oral: 30-50 mg/kg/day in divided doses every 6-12 hours

Pertussis: Oral: 40-50 mg/kg/day in 4 divided doses for 14 days; maximum 2 g/day (not preferred agent for infants <1 month due to IHPS)

Pharyngitis, tonsillitis (streptococcal): Oral: 20 mg (base)/kg/day or 40 mg (ethylsuccinate)/kg/day in 2 divided doses for 10 days. **Note:** No longer preferred therapy due to increased organism resistance.

Pneumonia *(C. trachomatis):* Oral: 50 mg/kg/day (base or ethylsuccinate) in 4 divided doses for 14-21 days

Preop bowel preparation: Oral: 20 mg (base)/kg at 1, 2, and 11 PM on the day before surgery combined with mechanical cleansing of the large intestine and oral neomycin

Severe infection: I.V.: 15-50 mg/kg/day; maximum: 4 g/day

(Continued)

erythromycin *(Continued)*

Adults:

Legionnaires disease: Oral: 1.6-4 g (ethylsuccinate)/day or 1-4 g (base)/day in divided doses for 21 days. **Note:** No longer preferred therapy and only used in nonhospitalized patients.

Lymphogranuloma venereum: Oral: 500 mg (base) 4 times/day for 21 days

Nongonococcal urethritis (including coinfection with *C. trachomatis*): Oral: 500 mg (base) 4 times/day for 7 days or 800 mg (ethylsuccinate) 4 times/day for 7 days. **Note:** May use 250 mg (base) or 400 mg (ethylsuccinate) 4 times/day for 14 days if gastrointestinal intolerance.

Pelvic inflammatory disease: I.V.: 500 mg every 6 hours for 3 days, followed by 1000 mg (base)/day orally in 2-4 divided doses for 7 days. **Note:** Not recommended therapy per current treatment guidelines.

Pertussis: Oral: 500 mg (base) every 6 hours for 14 days

Syphilis, primary: Oral: 48-64 g (ethylsuccinate) or 30-40 g (base) in divided doses over 10-15 days. **Note:** Not recommended therapy per current treatment guidelines.

Dosage Forms [CAN] = Canadian brand name

Capsule, delayed release, enteric-coated pellets: 250 mg

Gel, topical: 2% (30 g, 60 g)

Erygel®: 2% (30 g, 60 g)

Granules for oral suspension:

E.E.S.®: 200 mg/5 mL

Injection, powder for reconstitution:

Erythrocin®: 500 mg, 1 g

Ointment, ophthalmic: 0.5% [5 mg/g] (1 g, 3.5 g)

Romycin®: 0.5% [5 mg/g] (3.5 g)

Ointment, topical:

Akne-Mycin®: 2% (25 g)

Powder for oral suspension:

EryPed®: 200 mg/5 mL, 400 mg/5 mL

Powder for oral suspension [drops]:

EryPed®: 100 mg/2.5 mL

Solution, topical: 2% (60 mL)

Eryderm®: 2% (60 mL)

Sans Acne® [CAN]: 2% (60 mL) [not available in the U.S.]

Suspension, oral: 200 mg/5 mL, 400 mg/5 mL

E.E.S.®: 200 mg/5 mL, 400 mg/5 mL

Tablet: 250 mg, 400 mg, 500 mg

E.E.S.®: 400 mg

Erythrocin®: 250 mg, 500 mg

Tablet, delayed release, enteric coated:

Ery-Tab®: 250 mg, 333 mg, 500 mg

Tablet [polymer-coated particles]:

PCE®: 333 mg, 500 mg

erythromycin and benzoyl peroxide (er ith roe MYE sin & BEN zoe il per OKS ide)

Synonyms benzoyl peroxide and erythromycin

U.S./Canadian Brand Names Benzamycin® Pak [US]; Benzamycin® [US]

Therapeutic Category Acne Products

Use Topical control of acne vulgaris

Usual Dosage Apply twice daily, morning and evening

Dosage Forms

Gel, topical: Erythromycin 30 mg and benzoyl peroxide 50 mg per g (23 g, 47g)

Benzamycin®: Erythromycin 30 mg and benzoyl peroxide 50 mg per g (47 g)

Benzamycin® Pak: Erythromycin 30 mg and benzoyl peroxide 50 mg per 0.8 g packet (60s)

erythromycin and sulfisoxazole (er ith roe MYE sin & sul fi SOKS a zole)

Sound-Alike/Look-Alike Issues

Pediazole® may be confused with Pediapred®

Synonyms sulfisoxazole and erythromycin

U.S./Canadian Brand Names Pediazole® [Can]

Therapeutic Category Macrolide (Antibiotic); Sulfonamide

Use Treatment of susceptible bacterial infections of the upper and lower respiratory tract, otitis media in children caused by susceptible strains of *Haemophilus influenzae*, and many other infections in patients allergic to penicillin

Usual Dosage Oral (dosage recommendation is based on the product's erythromycin content):
Children ≥2 months: 50 mg/kg/day erythromycin and 150 mg/kg/day sulfisoxazole in divided doses every 6 hours; not to exceed 2 g erythromycin/day or 6 g sulfisoxazole/day for 10 days
Adults >45 kg: 400 mg erythromycin and 1200 mg sulfisoxazole every 6 hours
Dosage Forms **Powder for oral suspension:** Erythromycin 200 mg and sulfisoxazole 600 mg per 5 mL

erythromycin base *see* erythromycin *on page 309*

erythromycin ethylsuccinate *see* erythromycin *on page 309*

erythromycin lactobionate *see* erythromycin *on page 309*

erythromycin stearate *see* erythromycin *on page 309*

erythropoiesis-stimulating agent (ESA) *see* darbepoetin alfa *on page 232*

erythropoiesis-stimulating agent (ESA) *see* epoetin alfa *on page 303*

erythropoiesis-stimulating protein *see* darbepoetin alfa *on page 232*

erythropoietin *see* epoetin alfa *on page 303*

escitalopram (es sye TAL oh pram)
Synonyms escitalopram oxalate; Lu-26-054; S-citalopram
U.S./Canadian Brand Names Cipralex® [Can]; Lexapro® [US]
Therapeutic Category Antidepressant, Selective Serotonin Reuptake Inhibitor
Use Treatment of major depressive disorder; generalized anxiety disorders (GAD)
Usual Dosage Oral: Adults: Depression, GAD: Initial: 10 mg/day; dose may be increased to 20 mg/day after at least 1 week
Dosage Forms
  Solution, oral:
  Lexapro®: 1 mg/mL
  Tablet:
  Lexapro®: 5 mg, 10 mg, 20 mg
    Note: Cipralex® [CAN] is available only in 10 mg and 20 mg strengths.

escitalopram oxalate *see* escitalopram *on this page*

Esclim® [US] *see* estradiol *on page 313*

Eserine® [Can] *see* physostigmine *on page 681*

eserine salicylate *see* physostigmine *on page 681*

Esgic® [US] *see* butalbital, acetaminophen, and caffeine *on page 130*

Esgic-Plus™ [US] *see* butalbital, acetaminophen, and caffeine *on page 130*

Esidrix Tablets *(Discontinued)* *see* hydrochlorothiazide *on page 426*

Eskalith CR® *(Discontinued)* *see* lithium *on page 513*

Eskalith® *(Discontinued)* *see* lithium *on page 513*

esmolol (ES moe lol)
Sound-Alike/Look-Alike Issues
  esmolol may be confused with Osmitrol®
  Brevibloc® may be confused with bretylium, Brevital®, Bumex®, Buprenex®
Synonyms esmolol hydrochloride
U.S./Canadian Brand Names Brevibloc® [US/Can]
Therapeutic Category Antiarrhythmic Agent, Class II; Beta-Adrenergic Blocker
Use Treatment of supraventricular tachycardia (SVT) and atrial fibrillation/flutter (control ventricular rate); treatment of tachycardia and/or hypertension (especially intraoperative or postoperative); treatment of noncompensatory sinus tachycardia
Usual Dosage **I.V. infusion requires an infusion pump** (must be adjusted to individual response and tolerance):
Adults:
  Intraoperative tachycardia and/or hypertension (immediate control): Initial bolus: 80 mg (~1 mg/kg) over 30 seconds, followed by a 150 mcg/kg/minute infusion, if necessary. Adjust infusion rate as needed to maintain desired heart rate and/or blood pressure, up to 300 mcg/kg/minute.
  For control of postoperative hypertension, as many as one-third of patients may require higher doses (250-300 mcg/kg/minute) to control blood pressure; the safety of doses >300 mcg/kg/minute has not been studied.
(Continued)

311

esmolol (Continued)

Supraventricular tachycardia or gradual control of postoperative tachycardia/hypertension: Loading dose: 500 mcg/kg over 1 minute; follow with a 50 mcg/kg/minute infusion for 4 minutes; response to this initial infusion rate may be a rough indication of the responsiveness of the ventricular rate.

Infusion may be continued at 50 mcg/kg/minute or, if the response is inadequate, titrated upward in 50 mcg/kg/minute increments (increased no more frequently than every 4 minutes) to a maximum of 200 mcg/kg/minute.

To achieve more rapid response, following the initial loading dose and 50 mcg/kg/minute infusion, rebolus with a second 500 mcg/kg loading dose over 1 minute, and increase the maintenance infusion to 100 mcg/kg/minute for 4 minutes. If necessary, a third (and final) 500 mcg/kg loading dose may be administered, prior to increasing to an infusion rate of 150 mcg/kg/minute. After 4 minutes of the 150 mcg/kg/minute infusion, the infusion rate may be increased to a maximum rate of 200 mcg/kg/minute (without a bolus dose).

Usual dosage range (SVT): 50-200 mcg/kg/minute with average dose of 100 mcg/kg/minute.

Guidelines for transfer to oral therapy (beta blocker, calcium channel blocker):
Infusion should be reduced by 50% 30 minutes following the first dose of the alternative agent
Manufacturer suggests following the second dose of the alternative drug, patient's response should be monitored and if control is adequate for the first hours, esmolol may be discontinued.

Dosage Forms

Infusion [premixed in sodium chloride; preservative free]:
Brevibloc®: 2000 mg (100 mL) [20 mg/mL; double strength]; 2500 mg (250 mL) [10 mg/mL]
Injection, solution: 10 mg/mL (10 mL)
Brevibloc®: 10 mg/mL (10 mL); 20 mg/mL (5 mL, 100 mL); 250 mg/mL (10 mL)

esmolol hydrochloride see esmolol on previous page

E-Solve-2® Topical (Discontinued)

esomeprazole (es oh ME pray zol)

Synonyms esomeprazole magnesium; esomeprazole sodium
U.S./Canadian Brand Names Nexium® [US/Can]
Therapeutic Category Proton Pump Inhibitor
Use

Oral: Short-term (4-8 weeks) treatment of erosive esophagitis; maintaining symptom resolution and healing of erosive esophagitis; treatment of symptomatic gastroesophageal reflux disease (GERD); as part of a multi-drug regimen for *Helicobacter pylori* eradication in patients with duodenal ulcer disease (active or history of within the past 5 years); prevention of gastric ulcers in patients at risk (age ≥60 years and/or history of gastric ulcer) associated with continuous NSAID therapy; long-term treatment of pathological hypersecretory conditions including Zollinger-Ellison syndrome

I.V.: Short-term (≤10 days) treatment of gastroesophageal reflux disease (GERD) when oral therapy is not possible or appropriate

Usual Dosage

Adolescents 12-17 years: Oral: GERD: 20-40 mg once daily for up to 8 weeks
Adults:

Oral:

Erosive esophagitis (healing): Initial: 20-40 mg once daily for 4-8 weeks; if incomplete healing, may continue for an additional 4-8 weeks; maintenance: 20 mg once daily
Symptomatic GERD: 20 mg once daily for 4 weeks; may continue an additional 4 weeks if symptoms persist
Helicobacter pylori eradication: 40 mg once daily for 10 days; requires combination therapy
Prevention of NSAID-induced gastric ulcers: 20-40 mg once daily for up to 6 months
Pathological hypersecretory conditions (Zollinger-Ellison syndrome): 40 mg twice daily; adjust regimen to individual patient needs; doses up to 240 mg/day have been administered

I.V.: GERD: 20 mg or 40 mg once daily for ≤10 days; change to oral therapy as soon as appropriate

Dosage Forms Note: Strength expressed as base

Capsule, delayed release:
Nexium®: 20 mg, 40 mg
Granules, for oral suspension, delayed release, as magnesium:
Nexium®: 20 mg, 40 mg
Injection, powder for reconstitution:
Nexium®: 20 mg, 40 mg

esomeprazole magnesium see esomeprazole on this page

esomeprazole sodium see esomeprazole on this page

Esopho-Cat® [US] see barium on page 94

Esoterica® Regular [US-OTC] see hydroquinone on page 437

Especol® **[US-OTC]** *see* fructose, dextrose, and phosphoric acid *on page 378*

Estalis® **[Can]** *see* estradiol and norethindrone *on page 316*

Estalis-Sequi® **[Can]** *see* estradiol and norethindrone *on page 316*

Estar® **[Can]** *see* coal tar *on page 208*

estazolam (es TA zoe lam)

Sound-Alike/Look-Alike Issues
ProSom® may be confused with PhosLo®, Proscar®, Pro-Sof® Plus, Prozac®, Psorcon®
Therapeutic Category Benzodiazepine
Controlled Substance C-IV
Use Short-term management of insomnia
Usual Dosage Oral: Adults: 1 mg at bedtime, some patients may require 2 mg; start at doses of 0.5 mg in debilitated patients
Dosage Forms
Tablet: 1 mg, 2 mg

Ester-E™ **[US-OTC]** *see* vitamin E *on page 894*

esterified estrogen and methyltestosterone *see* estrogens (esterified) and methyltestosterone *on page 320*

esterified estrogens *see* estrogens (esterified) *on page 319*

Estivin® **II Ophthalmic** *(Discontinued)* *see* naphazoline *on page 590*

Estra-L® **Injection** *(Discontinued)* *see* estradiol *on this page*

Estrace® **[US/Can]** *see* estradiol *on this page*

Estraderm® **[US/Can]** *see* estradiol *on this page*

estradiol (es tra DYE ole)

Sound-Alike/Look-Alike Issues
Alora® may be confused with Aldara™
Elestrin™ may be confused with alosetron
Estraderm® may be confused with Testoderm®
Synonyms estradiol acetate; estradiol cypionate; estradiol hemihydrate; estradiol transdermal; estradiol valerate
U.S./Canadian Brand Names Alora® [US]; Climara® [US/Can]; Delestrogen® [US]; Depo®-Estradiol [US/Can]; Divigel® [US]; Elestrin™ [US]; Esclim® [US]; Estrace® [US/Can]; Estraderm® [US/Can]; Estradot® [Can]; Estrasorb™ [US]; Estring® [US/Can]; EstroGel® [US/Can]; Evamist® [US]; Femring® [US]; Femtrace® [US]; Gynodiol® [US]; Menostar™ [US/Can]; Oesclim® [Can]; Sandoz-Estradiol Derm 100 [Can]; Sandoz-Estradiol Derm 50 [Can]; Sandoz-Estradiol Derm 75 [Can]; Vagifem® [US/Can]; Vivelle-Dot® [US]; Vivelle® [US]
Therapeutic Category Estrogen Derivative
Use Treatment of moderate-to-severe vasomotor symptoms associated with menopause; treatment of vulvar and vaginal atrophy; hypoestrogenism (due to hypogonadism, castration, or primary ovarian failure); prostatic cancer (palliation), breast cancer (palliation), osteoporosis (prophylaxis); abnormal uterine bleeding due to hormonal imbalance; postmenopausal urogenital symptoms of the lower urinary tract (urinary urgency, dysuria)
Usual Dosage All dosage needs to be adjusted based upon the patient's response
Oral:
Prostate cancer (androgen-dependent, inoperable, progressing): 10 mg 3 times/day for at least 3 months
Breast cancer (inoperable, progressing in appropriately selected patients): 10 mg 3 times/day for at least 3 months
Osteoporosis prophylaxis in postmenopausal females: 0.5 mg/day in a cyclic regimen (3 weeks on and 1 week off)
Female hypoestrogenism (due to hypogonadism, castration, or primary ovarian failure): 1-2 mg/day; titrate as necessary to control symptoms using minimal effective dose for maintenance therapy
Moderate-to-severe vasomotor symptoms associated with menopause: 1-2 mg/day, adjusted as necessary to limit symptoms; administration should be cyclic (3 weeks on, 1 week off). Patients should be re-evaluated at 3- to 6-month intervals to determine if treatment is still necessary.
I.M.:
Prostate cancer: Valerate: ≥30 mg or more every 1-2 weeks
Moderate-to-severe vasomotor symptoms associated with menopause:
Cypionate: 1-5 mg every 3-4 weeks
Valerate: 10-20 mg every 4 weeks
Female hypoestrogenism (due to hypogonadism):
Cypionate: 1.5-2 mg monthly
(Continued)

estradiol (Continued)

Valerate: 10-20 mg every 4 weeks

Topical:

Emulsion: Moderate-to-severe vasomotor symptoms associated with menopause: 3.84 g applied once daily in the morning

Gel:

Moderate-to-severe vasomotor symptoms associated with menopause:

Divigel®: 0.25 g per day; adjust dose based on patient response. Dosing range: 0.25-1 g/day

Elestrin™: 0.87g/day applied at the same time each day

EstroGel®: 1.25 g/day applied at the same time each day

Vulvar and vaginal atrophy:

Elestrin™: 0.87g/day applied at the same time each day

EstroGel®: 1.25 g/day applied at the same time each day

Transdermal: Indicated dose may be used continuously in patients without an intact uterus. May be given continuously or cyclically (3 weeks on, 1 week off) in patients with an intact uterus (exception - Menostar™, see specific dosing instructions). When changing patients from oral to transdermal therapy, start transdermal patch 1 week after discontinuing oral hormone (may begin sooner if symptoms reappear within 1 week):

Once-weekly patch:

Moderate to severe vasomotor symptoms associated with menopause (Climara®): Apply 0.025 mg/day patch once weekly. Adjust dose as necessary to control symptoms. Patients should be re-evaluated at 3- to 6-month intervals to determine if treatment is still necessary.

Osteoporosis prophylaxis in postmenopausal women:

Climara®: Apply patch once weekly; minimum effective dose 0.025 mg/day; adjust response to therapy by biochemical markers and bone mineral density

Menostar™: Apply patch once weekly. In women with a uterus, also administer a progestin for 14 days every 6-12 months

Twice-weekly patch:

Moderate-to-severe vasomotor symptoms associated with menopause, vulvar/vaginal atrophy, female hypogonadism: Titrate to lowest dose possible to control symptoms, adjusting initial dose after the first month of therapy; reevaluate therapy at 3- to 6-month intervals to taper or discontinue medication:

Alora®, Esclim®, Estraderm®, Vivelle-Dot®: Apply 0.05 mg patch twice weekly

Vivelle®: Apply 0.0375 mg patch twice weekly

Prevention of osteoporosis in postmenopausal women:

Alora®, Vivelle®, Vivelle-Dot®: Apply 0.025 mg patch twice weekly, increase dose as necessary

Estraderm®: Apply 0.05 mg patch twice weekly

Vaginal cream: Vulvar and vaginal atrophy: Insert 2-4 g/day intravaginally for 2 weeks, then gradually reduce to 1/2 the initial dose for 2 weeks, followed by a maintenance dose of 1 g 1-3 times/week

Vaginal ring:

Postmenopausal vaginal atrophy, urogenital symptoms: Estring®: 2 mg intravaginally; following insertion, ring should remain in place for 90 days

Moderate-to-severe vasomotor symptoms associated with menopause; vulvar/vaginal atrophy: Femring®: 0.05 mg intravaginally; following insertion, ring should remain in place for 3 months; dose may be increased to 0.1 mg if needed

Vaginal tablets: Atrophic vaginitis: Vagifem®: Initial: Insert 1 tablet once daily for 2 weeks; maintenance: Insert 1 tablet twice weekly; attempts to discontinue or taper medication should be made at 3- to 6-month intervals

Dosage Forms

Cream, vaginal:

Estrace®: 0.1 mg/g (12 g) [refill]; 0.1 mg/g (42.5 g) [packaged with applicator]

Emulsion, topical:

Estrasorb™: 2.5 mg/g (56s) [each pouch contains 4.35 mg estradiol hemihydrate; contents of two pouches delivers estradiol 0.05 mg/day]

Gel, topical:

Divigel®: 0.1% (0.25 g) [foil packet; delivers estradiol 0.25 mg/packet]; (0.5 g) [foil packet; delivers 0.5 mg estradiol/packet]; (1 g) [foil packet; delivers estradiol 1 mg/packet]

Elestrin™: 0.06% (144 g) [pump; delivers estradiol 0.52 mg/0.87 g; 100 actuations]

EstroGel®: 0.06% (93 g) [pump; delivers estradiol 0.75 mg/1.25 g; 64 actuations]

Injection, oil:

Delestrogen®: 10 mg/mL (5 mL); 20 mg/mL (5 mL); 40 mg/mL (5 mL)

Depo®-Estradiol: 5 mg/mL (5 mL)

Ring, vaginal:

Estring®: 2 mg [total estradiol 2 mg; releases 7.5 mcg/day over 90 days] (1s)

Femring®: 0.05 mg [total estradiol 12.4 mg; releases 0.05 mg/day over 3 months] (1s); 0.1 mg [total estradiol 24.8 mg; releases 0.1 mg/day over 3 months] (1s)

Solution, topical [spray]:
Evamist™: 1.53 mg/spray (8.1 mL)
Tablet, oral: 0.45 mg, 0.9 mg, 1.8 mg
Femtrace®: 0.45 mg, 0.9 mg, 1.8 mg
Tablet, oral, micronized: 0.5 mg, 1 mg, 2 mg
Estrace®: 0.5 mg, 1 mg, 2 mg
Gynodiol®: 0.5 mg, 1 mg, 1.5 mg, 2 mg
Tablet, vaginal:
Vagifem®: 25 mcg
Transdermal system: 0.025 mg/24 hours [once-weekly patch] (4s); 0.0375 mg/24 hours (4s) [once weekly patch]; 0.05 mg/24 hours (4s) [once-weekly patch]; 0.06 mg/24 hours (4s) [once weekly patch]; 0.075 mg/24 hours [once-weekly patch]; 0.1 mg/24 hours (4s) [once-weekly patch]

Brands:
Alora® [twice-weekly patch]:
0.025 mg/24 hours [9 cm^2, total estradiol 0.77 mg] (8s)
0.05 mg/24 hours [18 cm^2, total estradiol 1.5 mg] (8s, 24s)
0.075 mg/24 hours [27 cm^2, total estradiol 2.3 mg] (8s)
0.1 mg/24 hours [36 cm^2, total estradiol 3.1 mg] (8s)
Climara® [once-weekly patch]:
0.025 mg/24 hours [6.5 cm^2, total estradiol 2.04 mg] (4s)
0.0375 mg/24 hours [9.375 cm^2, total estradiol 2.85 mg] (4s)
0.05 mg/24 hours [12.5 cm^2, total estradiol 3.8 mg] (4s)
0.06 mg/24 hours [15 cm^2, total estradiol 4.55 mg] (4s)
0.075 mg/24 hours [18.75 cm^2, total estradiol 5.7 mg] (4s)
0.1 mg/24 hours [25 cm^2, total estradiol 7.6 mg] (4s)
Esclim® [twice-weekly patch]:
0.025 mg/day [11 cm^2, total estradiol 5 mg] (8s)
0.0375 mg/day [16.5 cm^2, total estradiol 7.5 mg] (8s)
0.05 mg/day [22 cm^2, total estradiol 10 mg] (8s)
0.075 mg/day [33 cm^2, total estradiol 15 mg] (8s)
0.1 mg/day [44 cm^2, total estradiol 20 mg] (8s)
Estraderm® [twice-weekly patch]:
0.05 mg/24 hours [10 cm^2, total estradiol 4 mg] (8s)
0.1 mg/24 hours [20 cm^2, total estradiol 8 mg] (8s)
Menostar® [once-weekly patch]: 0.014 mg/24 hours [3.25 cm^2, total estradiol 1 mg] (4s)
Vivelle® [twice-weekly patch]:
0.05 mg/24 hours [14.5 cm^2, total estradiol 4.33 mg] (8s)
0.1 mg/24 hours [29 cm^2, total estradiol 8.66 mg] (8s)
Vivelle-Dot® [twice-weekly patch]:
0.025 mg/day [2.5 cm^2, total estradiol 0.39 mg] (8s)
0.0375 mg/day [3.75 cm^2, total estradiol 0.585 mg] (8s)
0.05 mg/day [5 cm^2, total estradiol 0.78 mg] (8s)
0.075 mg/day [7.5 cm^2, total estradiol 1.17 mg] (8s)
0.1 mg/day [10 cm^2, total estradiol 1.56 mg] (8s)

estradiol acetate *see* estradiol *on page 313*

estradiol and drospirenone *see* drospirenone and estradiol *on page 285*

estradiol and levonorgestrel (es tra DYE ole & LEE voe nor jes trel)

Synonyms levonorgestrel and estradiol
U.S./Canadian Brand Names ClimaraPro® [US]
Therapeutic Category Estrogen and Progestin Combination
Use Women with an intact uterus: Treatment of moderate-to-severe vasomotor symptoms associated with menopause; prevention of postmenopausal osteoporosis
Usual Dosage Topical: Adult females with an intact uterus: Treatment of moderate-to-severe vasomotor symptoms associated with menopause or prevention of postmenopausal osteoporosis:
Estradiol 0.045 mg/levonorgestrel 0.015 mg: Apply one patch weekly
Dosage Forms
Transdermal system:
ClimaraPro®: Estradiol 0.045 mg/24 hours and levonorgestrel 0.015 mg/24 hours (4s) [once-weekly patch]

estradiol and NGM *see* estradiol and norgestimate *on next page*

estradiol and norethindrone (es tra DYE ole & nor eth IN drone)

Synonyms norethindrone and estradiol

U.S./Canadian Brand Names Activella® [US]; CombiPatch® [US]; Estalis-Sequi® [Can]; Estalis® [Can]

Therapeutic Category Estrogen and Progestin Combination

Use Women with an intact uterus:

Tablet: Treatment of moderate-to-severe vasomotor symptoms associated with menopause; treatment of vulvar and vaginal atrophy; prophylaxis for postmenopausal osteoporosis

Transdermal patch: Treatment of moderate-to-severe vasomotor symptoms associated with menopause; treatment of vulvar and vaginal atrophy; treatment of hypoestrogenism due to hypogonadism, castration, or primary ovarian failure

Usual Dosage Note: Patients should be treated with the lowest effective dose and for the shortest duration, consistent with treatment goals. Adults:

Oral (Activella®): 1 tablet daily

Transdermal patch (CombiPatch®):

Continuous combined regimen: Apply one patch twice weekly

Continuous sequential regimen: Apply estradiol-only patch for first 14 days of cycle, followed by one CombiPatch® applied twice weekly for the remaining 14 days of a 28-day cycle

Transdermal patch, combination pack (product-specific dosing for Canadian formulation):

Estalis®: Continuous combined regimen: Apply a new patch twice weekly during a 28-day cycle

Estalis-Sequi®: Continuous sequential regimen: Apply estradiol-only patch (Vivelle®) for first 14 days, followed by one Estalis® patch applied twice weekly during the last 14 days of a 28-day cycle

Note: In women previously receiving oral estrogens, initiate upon reappearance of menopausal symptoms following discontinuation of oral therapy.

Dosage Forms [CAN] = Canadian brand name

Combination pack:

Estalis-Sequi® 140/50 [CAN; not available in U.S.]:

Transdermal system (Vivelle®): Estradiol 50 mcg per day (4s) [14.5 sq cm; total estradiol 4.33 mg]

Transdermal system (Estalis®): Norethindrone 140 mcg and estradiol 50 mcg per day (4s) [9 sq cm; total norethindrone 2.7 mg, total estradiol 0.62 mg; not available in the U.S.]

Estalis-Sequi® 250/50 [CAN; not available in U.S.]:

Transdermal system (Vivelle®): Estradiol 50 mcg per day (4s) [14.5 sq cm; total estradiol 4.33 mg]

Transdermal system (Estalis®): Norethindrone250 mcg and estradiol 50 mcg per day (4s) [16 sq cm; total norethindrone 4.8 mg, total estradiol 0.51 mg; not available in the U.S.]

Tablet:

Activella® 0.5/0.1: Estradiol 0.5 mg and norethindrone acetate 0.1mg (28s)

Activella® 1/0.5: Estradiol 1 mg and norethindrone acetate 0.5 mg (28s)

Transdermal system:

CombiPatch®:

0.05/0.14: Estradiol 0.05 mg and norethindrone 0.14 mg per day (8s) [9 sq cm]

0.05/0.25: Estradiol 0.05 mg and norethindrone 0.25 mg per day (8s) [16 sq cm]

Estalis® [CAN]:

140/50: Norethindrone 140 mcg and estradiol 50 mcg per day (8s) [9 sq cm; total norethindrone 2.7 mg, total estradiol 0.62 mg; not available in the U.S.]

250/50 Norethindrone 250 mcg and estradiol 50 mcg per day (8s) [16 sq cm; total norethindrone 4.8 mg, total estradiol 0.51 mg; not available in U.S.]

estradiol and norgestimate (es tra DYE ole & nor JES ti mate)

Synonyms estradiol and NGM; norgestimate and estradiol; ortho prefest

U.S./Canadian Brand Names Prefest™ [US]

Therapeutic Category Estrogen and Progestin Combination

Use Women with an intact uterus: Treatment of moderate to severe vasomotor symptoms associated with menopause; treatment of atrophic vaginitis; prevention of osteoporosis

Usual Dosage Oral: Adults: Females with an intact uterus: Treatment of menopausal symptoms, atrophic vaginitis, prevention of osteoporosis: Treatment is cyclical and consists of the following: One tablet of estradiol 1 mg (pink tablet) once daily for 3 days, followed by 1 tablet of estradiol 1 mg and norgestimate 0.09 mg (white tablet) once daily for 3 days; repeat sequence continuously. **Note:** This dose may not be the lowest effective combination for these indications. In case of a missed tablet, restart therapy with next available tablet in sequence (taking only 1 tablet each day).

Dosage Forms

Tablet:

Prefest™: Estradiol 1 mg [15 pink tablets] and estradiol 1 mg and norgestimate 0.09 mg [15 white tablets] (supplied in blister card of 30)

estradiol cypionate *see estradiol on page 313*

estradiol hemihydrate *see estradiol on page 313*

estradiol transdermal *see estradiol on page 313*

estradiol valerate *see estradiol on page 313*

Estradot® [Can] *see estradiol on page 313*

estramustine (es tra MUS teen)
Sound-Alike/Look-Alike Issues
estramustine may be confused with exemestane
Emcyt® may be confused with Eryc®
Synonyms estramustine phosphate; estramustine phosphate sodium; NSC-89199
U.S./Canadian Brand Names Emcyt® [US/Can]
Therapeutic Category Antineoplastic Agent
Use Palliative treatment of prostatic carcinoma (progressive or metastatic)
Usual Dosage Oral (refer to individual protocols): Adults: Males: 14 mg/kg/day (range: 10-16 mg/kg/day) in 3 or 4 divided doses
Dosage Forms
Capsule:
Emcyt®: 140 mg

estramustine phosphate *see estramustine on this page*

estramustine phosphate sodium *see estramustine on this page*

Estrasorb™ [US] *see estradiol on page 313*

Estratab® [Can] *see estrogens (esterified) on page 319*

Estratab® (Discontinued) *see estrogens (esterified) on page 319*

Estratest® [US/Can] *see estrogens (esterified) and methyltestosterone on page 320*

Estratest® H.S. [US] *see estrogens (esterified) and methyltestosterone on page 320*

Estring® [US/Can] *see estradiol on page 313*

Estro-Cyp® Injection (Discontinued) *see estradiol on page 313*

EstroGel® [US/Can] *see estradiol on page 313*

estrogenic substances, conjugated *see estrogens (conjugated/equine) on next page*

estrogens (conjugated A/synthetic) (ES troe jenz, KON joo gate ed, aye, sin THET ik)
Sound-Alike/Look-Alike Issues
Cenestin® may be confused with Senexon®
U.S./Canadian Brand Names Cenestin® [US/Can]
Therapeutic Category Estrogen Derivative
Use Treatment of moderate-to-severe vasomotor symptoms of menopause; treatment of vulvar and vaginal atrophy
Usual Dosage The lowest dose that will control symptoms should be used; medication should be discontinued as soon as possible. Oral: Adults:

Moderate-to-severe vasomotor symptoms: 0.45 mg/day; may be titrated up to 1.25 mg/day. Attempts to discontinue medication should be made at 3- to 6-month intervals.
Vulvar and vaginal atrophy: 0.3 mg/day
Dosage Forms
Tablet:
Cenestin®: 0.3 mg, 0.45 mg, 0.625 mg, 0.9 mg, 1.25 mg

estrogens (conjugated B/synthetic) (ES troe jenz, KON joo gate ed, bee, sin THET ik)
U.S./Canadian Brand Names Enjuvia™ [US]
Therapeutic Category Estrogen Derivative
Use Treatment of moderate-to-severe vasomotor symptoms of menopause; treatment of vulvar and vaginal atrophy associated with menopause; treatment of moderate-to-severe vaginal dryness and pain with intercourse associated with menopause
Usual Dosage The lowest dose that will control symptoms should be used; medication should be discontinued as soon as possible. Oral:
Adults:
Moderate-to-severe vasomotor symptoms associated with menopause: 0.3 mg/day; may be titrated up to 1.25 mg/day. Attempts to discontinue medication should be made at 3- to 6-month intervals.
Vaginal dryness/vulvar and vaginal atrophy associated with menopause: 0.3 mg/day. Attempts to discontinue medication should be made at 3- to 6-month intervals.
(Continued)

estrogens (conjugated B/synthetic) *(Continued)*

Dosage Forms
Tablet:
Enjuvia™: 0.3 mg, 0.45 mg, 0.625 mg, 1.25 mg

estrogens (conjugated/equine) (ES troe jenz KON joo gate ed, EE kwine)

Sound-Alike/Look-Alike Issues
Premarin® may be confused with Primaxin®, Provera®, Remeron®

Synonyms CEE; estrogenic substances, conjugated

U.S./Canadian Brand Names C.E.S.® [Can]; Premarin® [US/Can]

Therapeutic Category Estrogen Derivative

Use Treatment of moderate-to-severe vasomotor symptoms associated with menopause; treatment of vulvar and vaginal atrophy; hypoestrogenism (due to hypogonadism, castration, or primary ovarian failure); prostatic cancer (palliation); breast cancer (palliation); osteoporosis (prophylaxis, postmenopausal women at significant risk only); abnormal uterine bleeding

Usual Dosage Adults:

Male: Androgen-dependent prostate cancer palliation: Oral: 1.25-2.5 mg 3 times/day

Female:

Prevention of postmenopausal osteoporosis: Oral: Initial: 0.3 mg/day cyclically* or daily, depending on medical assessment of patient. Dose may be adjusted based on bone mineral density and clinical response. The lowest effective dose should be used.

Moderate to severe vasomotor symptoms associated with menopause: Oral: Initial: 0.3 mg/day, cyclically* or daily, depending on medical assessment of patient. The lowest dose that will control symptoms should be used. Medication should be discontinued as soon as possible.

Vulvar and vaginal atrophy:

Oral: Initial: 0.3 mg/day; the lowest dose that will control symptoms should be used. May be given cyclically* or daily, depending on medical assessment of patient. Medication should be discontinued as soon as possible.

Vaginal cream: Intravaginal: $^1/_2$ to 2 g/day given cyclically*

Abnormal uterine bleeding:

Acute/heavy bleeding:

I.M., I.V.: 25 mg, may repeat in 6-12 hours if needed

Note: Treatment should be followed by a low-dose oral contraceptive; medroxyprogesterone acetate along with or following estrogen therapy can also be given

Female hypogonadism: Oral: 0.3-0.625 mg/day given cyclically*; dose may be titrated in 6- to 12-month intervals; progestin treatment should be added to maintain bone mineral density once skeletal maturity is achieved.

Female castration, primary ovarian failure: Oral: 1.25 mg/day given cyclically*; adjust according to severity of symptoms and patient response. For maintenance, adjust to the lowest effective dose.

***Cyclic administration:** Either 3 weeks on, 1 week off **or** 25 days on, 5 days off

Male and Female: Breast cancer palliation, metastatic disease in selected patients: Oral: 10 mg 3 times/day for at least 3 months

Dosage Forms
Cream, vaginal:
Premarin®: 0.625 mg/g (42.5 g)
Injection, powder for reconstitution:
Premarin®: 25 mg
Tablet:
Premarin®: 0.3 mg, 0.45 mg, 0.625 mg, 0.9 mg, 1.25 mg

estrogens (conjugated/equine) and medroxyprogesterone

(ES troe jenz KON joo gate ed/EE kwine & me DROKS ee proe JES te rone)

Sound-Alike/Look-Alike Issues
Premphase® may be confused with Prempro™
Prempro™ may be confused with Premphase®

Synonyms medroxyprogesterone and estrogens (conjugated); MPA and estrogens (conjugated)

U.S./Canadian Brand Names Premphase® [US/Can]; Premplus® [Can]; Prempro™ [US/Can]

Therapeutic Category Estrogen and Progestin Combination

Use Women with an intact uterus: Treatment of moderate-to-severe vasomotor symptoms associated with menopause; treatment of atrophic vaginitis; osteoporosis (prophylaxis)

Usual Dosage Oral: Adults:

Treatment of moderate-to-severe vasomotor symptoms associated with menopause or treatment of atrophic vaginitis in females with an intact uterus. (The lowest dose that will control symptoms should be used; medication should be discontinued as soon as possible):

Premphase®: One maroon conjugated estrogen 0.625 mg tablet daily on days 1 through 14 and one light blue conjugated estrogen 0.625 mg/MPA 5 mg tablet daily on days 15 through 28; reevaluate patients at 3- and 6-month intervals to determine if treatment is still necessary; monitor patients for signs of endometrial cancer; rule out malignancy if unexplained vaginal bleeding occurs

Prempro™: One conjugated estrogen 0.3 mg/MPA 1.5 mg tablet daily; re-evaluate at 3-and 6-month intervals to determine if therapy is still needed; dose may be increased to a maximum of one conjugated estrogen 0.625 mg/MPA 5 mg tablet daily in patients with bleeding or spotting, once malignancy has been ruled out

Osteoporosis prophylaxis in females with an intact uterus:

Premphase®: One maroon conjugated estrogen 0.625 tablet daily on days 1 through 14 and one light blue conjugated estrogen 0.625 mg/MPA 5 mg tablet daily on days 15 through 28; monitor patients for signs of endometrial cancer; rule out malignancy if unexplained vaginal bleeding occurs

Prempro™: One conjugated estrogen 0.3 mg/MPA 1.5 mg tablet daily; dose may be increased to one conjugated estrogen 0.625 mg/MPA 5 mg tablet daily; in patients with bleeding or spotting, once malignancy has been ruled out

Dosage Forms

Tablet:

Premphase® [therapy pack contains two separate tablet formulations]: Conjugated estrogens 0.625 mg [14 maroon tablets] and conjugated estrogen 0.625 mg/medroxyprogesterone 5 mg [14 light blue tablets] (28s)

Prempro™:

0.3/1.5: Conjugated estrogens 0.3 mg and medroxyprogesterone 1.5 mg (28s)

0.45/1.5: Conjugated estrogens 0.45 mg and medroxyprogesterone 1.5 mg (28s)

0.625/2.5: Conjugated estrogens 0.625 mg and medroxyprogesterone 2.5 mg (28s)

0.625/5: Conjugated estrogens 0.625 mg and medroxyprogesterone 5 mg (28s)

estrogens (esterified) (ES troe jenz, es TER i fied)

Sound-Alike/Look-Alike Issues

Estratab® may be confused with Estratest®, Estratest® H.S.

Synonyms esterified estrogens

U.S./Canadian Brand Names Estratab® [Can]; Menest® [US/Can]

Therapeutic Category Estrogen Derivative

Use Treatment of moderate to severe vasomotor symptoms associated with menopause; treatment of vulvar and vaginal atrophy; hypoestrogenism (due to hypogonadism, castration, or primary ovarian failure); prostatic cancer (palliation); breast cancer (palliation); osteoporosis (prophylaxis, in women at significant risk only)

Usual Dosage Oral: Adults:

Prostate cancer (palliation): 1.25-2.5 mg 3 times/day

Female hypogonadism: 2.5-7.5 mg of estrogen daily for 20 days followed by a 10-day rest period. Administer cyclically (3 weeks on and 1 week off). If bleeding does not occur by the end of the 10-day period, repeat the same dosing schedule; the number of courses is dependent upon the responsiveness of the endometrium. If bleeding occurs before the end of the 10-day period, begin an estrogen-progestin cyclic regimen of 2.5-7.5 mg esterified estrogens daily for 20 days. During the last 5 days of estrogen therapy, give an oral progestin. If bleeding occurs before regimen is concluded, discontinue therapy and resume on the fifth day of bleeding.

Moderate to severe vasomotor symptoms associated with menopause: 1.25 mg/day administered cyclically (3 weeks on and 1 week off). If patient has not menstruated within the last 2 months or more, cyclic administration is started arbitrary. If the patient is menstruating, cyclical administration is started on day 5 of the bleeding. For short-term use only and should be discontinued as soon as possible. Re-evaluate at 3- to 6-month intervals for tapering or discontinuation of therapy.

Atopic vaginitis and kraurosis vulvae: 0.3 to ≥1.25 mg/day, depending on the tissue response of the individual patient. Administer cyclically. For short-term use only and should be discontinued as soon as possible. Re-evaluate at 3- to 6-month intervals for tapering or discontinuation of therapy.

Breast cancer (palliation): 10 mg 3 times/day for at least 3 months

Osteoporosis in postmenopausal women: Initial: 0.3 mg/day and increase to a maximum daily dose of 1.25 mg/day; initiate therapy as soon as possible after menopause; cyclically or daily, depending on medical assessment of patient. Monitor patients with an intact uterus for signs of endometrial cancer; rule out malignancy if unexplained vaginal bleeding occurs

Female castration and primary ovarian failure: 1.25 mg/day, cyclically. Adjust dosage upward or downward, according to the severity of symptoms and patient response. For maintenance, adjust dosage to lowest level that will provide effective control.

Dosage Forms

Tablet:

Menest®: 0.3 mg, 0.625 mg, 1.25 mg, 2.5 mg

estrogens (esterified) and methyltestosterone
(ES troe jenz es TER i fied & meth il tes TOS te rone)

Sound-Alike/Look-Alike Issues
Estratest® may be confused with Eskalith®, Estratab®, Estratest® H.S.
Estratest® H.S. may be confused with Eskalith®, Estratab®, Estratest®

Synonyms conjugated estrogen and methyltestosterone; esterified estrogen and methyltestosterone

U.S./Canadian Brand Names Estratest® H.S. [US]; Estratest® [US/Can]; Syntest D.S. [US]; Syntest H.S. [US]

Therapeutic Category Estrogen and Androgen Combination

Use Vasomotor symptoms of menopause

Usual Dosage Oral: Adults: Female: Lowest dose that will control symptoms should be chosen, normally given 3 weeks on and 1 week off

Dosage Forms
Tablet: Esterified estrogen 0.625 mg and methyltestosterone 1.25 mg; esterified estrogen 1.25 mg and methyltestosterone 2.5 mg;
Estratest®, Syntest D.S: Esterified estrogen 1.25 mg and methyltestosterone 2.5 mg
Estratest® H.S., Syntest H.S: Esterified estrogen 0.625 mg and methyltestosterone 1.25 mg

estropipate (ES troe pih pate)

Synonyms piperazine estrone sulfate

U.S./Canadian Brand Names Ogen® [US/Can]; Ortho-Est® [US]

Therapeutic Category Estrogen Derivative

Use Treatment of moderate to severe vasomotor symptoms associated with menopause; treatment of vulvar and vaginal atrophy; hypoestrogenism (due to hypogonadism, castration, or primary ovarian failure); osteoporosis (prophylaxis, in women at significant risk only)

Usual Dosage Oral: Adults:
Moderate to severe vasomotor symptoms associated with menopause: Usual dosage range: 0.75-6 mg estropipate daily; use the lowest dose and regimen that will control symptoms, and discontinue as soon as possible. Attempt to discontinue or taper medication at 3- to 6-month intervals. If a patient with vasomotor symptoms has not menstruated within the last ≥2 months, start the cyclic administration arbitrarily. If the patient has menstruated, start cyclic administration on day 5 of bleeding.
Female hypogonadism: 1.5-9 mg estropipate daily for the first 3 weeks, followed by a rest period of 8-10 days; use the lowest dose and regimen that will control symptoms. Repeat if bleeding does not occur by the end of the rest period. The duration of therapy necessary to product the withdrawal bleeding will vary according to the responsiveness of the endometrium. If satisfactory withdrawal bleeding does not occur, give an oral progestin in addition to estrogen during the third week of the cycle.
Female castration or primary ovarian failure: 1.5-9 mg estropipate daily for the first 3 weeks of a theoretical cycle, followed by a rest period of 8-10 days; use the lowest dose and regimen that will control symptoms
Osteoporosis prophylaxis: 0.75 mg estropipate daily for 25 days of a 31-day cycle
Atrophic vaginitis or kraurosis vulvae: 0.75-6 mg estropipate daily; administer cyclically. Use the lowest dose and regimen that will control symptoms; discontinue as soon as possible.

Dosage Forms
Tablet: 0.625 mg [estropipate 0.75 mg]; 1.25 mg [estropipate 1.5 mg]; 2.5 mg [estropipate 3 mg]
Ogen®: 0.625 mg [estropipate 0.75 mg]; 1.25 mg [estropipate 1.5 mg]; 2.5 mg [estropipate 3 mg]
Ortho-Est®: 0.625 mg [estropipate 0.75 mg]; 1.25 mg [estropipate 1.5 mg]

Estrostep® 21 *(Discontinued)* see ethinyl estradiol and norethindrone *on page 328*

Estrostep® Fe [US] see ethinyl estradiol and norethindrone *on page 328*

eszopiclone (es zoe PIK lone)

Sound-Alike/Look-Alike Issues
Lunesta™ may be confused with Neulasta®

U.S./Canadian Brand Names Lunesta™ [US]

Therapeutic Category Hypnotic, Nonbenzodiazepine

Controlled Substance C-IV

Use Treatment of insomnia

Usual Dosage Oral: Adults: Insomnia: Initial: 2 mg before bedtime (maximum dose: 3 mg)
Concurrent use with strong CYP3A4 inhibitor: 1 mg before bedtime; if needed, dose may be increased to 2 mg

Dosage Forms
Tablet:
Lunesta™: 1 mg, 2 mg, 3 mg

ETAF see aldesleukin *on page 26*

etanercept (et a NER sept)

U.S./Canadian Brand Names Enbrel® [US/Can]

Therapeutic Category Antirheumatic, Disease Modifying

Use Treatment of moderately- to severely-active rheumatoid arthritis (RA); moderately- to severely-active polyarticular juvenile rheumatoid arthritis (JRA) in patients with inadequate response to at least one disease-modifying antirheumatic drug; psoriatic arthritis; active ankylosing spondylitis (AS); moderate-to-severe chronic plaque psoriasis

Usual Dosage SubQ:

Children 4-17 years: Juvenile rheumatoid arthritis:

Once-weekly dosing (patients weighing <31 kg or ≥63 kg): 0.8 mg/kg (maximum: 50 mg/dose) once weekly

Twice-weekly dosing (patients weighing 31-62 kg): 0.4 mg/kg (maximum: 25 mg/dose) twice weekly (individual doses should be separated by 72-96 hours)

Adults:

Rheumatoid arthritis, psoriatic arthritis, ankylosing spondylitis:

Once-weekly dosing: 50 mg once weekly

Twice weekly dosing: 25 mg given twice weekly (individual doses should be separated by 72-96 hours)

Plaque psoriasis:

Initial: 50 mg twice weekly, 3-4 days apart (starting doses of 25 or 50 mg once weekly have also been used successfully); maintain initial dose for 3 months

Maintenance dose: 50 mg weekly

Dosage Forms

Injection, powder for reconstitution:

Enbrel®: 25 mg

Injection, solution:

Enbrel®: 50 mg/mL (0.51 mL, 0.98 mL)

ethacrynate sodium *see ethacrynic acid on this page*

ethacrynic acid (eth a KRIN ik AS id)

Sound-Alike/Look-Alike Issues

Edecrin® may be confused with Eulexin®, Ecotrin®

Synonyms ethacrynate sodium

U.S./Canadian Brand Names Edecrin® [US/Can]

Therapeutic Category Diuretic, Loop

Use Management of edema associated with congestive heart failure; hepatic cirrhosis or renal disease; short-term management of ascites due to malignancy, idiopathic edema, and lymphedema

Usual Dosage I.V. formulation should be diluted in D_5W or NS (1 mg/mL) and infused over several minutes.

Children: Oral: 1 mg/kg/dose once daily; increase at intervals of 2-3 days as needed, to a maximum of 3 mg/kg/day.

Adults:

Oral: 50-200 mg/day in 1-2 divided doses; may increase in increments of 25-50 mg at intervals of several days; doses up to 200 mg twice daily may be required with severe, refractory edema.

I.V.: 0.5-1 mg/kg/dose (maximum: 100 mg/dose); repeat doses not routinely recommended; however, if indicated, repeat doses every 8-12 hours.

Dosage Forms

Injection, powder for reconstitution:

Edecrin®: 50 mg

Tablet:

Edecrin®: 25 mg

ethambutol (e THAM byoo tole)

Sound-Alike/Look-Alike Issues

Myambutol® may be confused with Nembutal®

Synonyms ethambutol hydrochloride

U.S./Canadian Brand Names Etibi® [Can]; Myambutol® [US]

Therapeutic Category Antimycobacterial Agent

Use Treatment of tuberculosis and other mycobacterial diseases in conjunction with other antituberculosis agents

Usual Dosage Oral:

Treatment of tuberculosis: **Note:** Used as part of a multidrug regimen. Treatment regimens consist of an initial 2 month phase, followed by a continuation phase of 4 or 7 additional months; frequency of dosing may differ depending on phase of therapy.

Children:

Daily therapy: 15-20 mg/kg/day (maximum: 1 g/day)

(Continued)

ethambutol (Continued)

Twice weekly directly observed therapy (DOT): 50 mg/kg (maximum: 4 g/dose)
Adults (suggested doses by lean body weight):
Daily therapy: 15-25 mg/kg
40-55 kg: 800 mg
56-75 kg: 1200 mg
76-90 kg: 1600 mg (maximum dose regardless of weight)
Twice weekly directly observed therapy (DOT): 50 mg/kg
40-55 kg: 2000 mg
56-75 kg: 2800 mg
76-90 kg: 4000 mg (maximum dose regardless of weight)
Three times/week DOT: 25-30 mg/kg (maximum: 2.5 g)
40-55 kg: 1200 mg
56-75 kg: 2000 mg
76-90 kg: 2400 mg (maximum dose regardless of weight)
Disseminated *Mycobacterium avium* complex (MAC) in patients with advanced HIV infection: 15 mg/kg ethambutol in combination with azithromycin 600 mg daily
Dosage Forms
Tablet: 100 mg, 400 mg
Myambutol®: 100 mg, 400 mg

ethambutol hydrochloride *see* ethambutol *on previous page*

Ethamolin® [US] *see* ethanolamine oleate *on this page*

ethanoic acid *see* acetic acid *on page 14*

ethanol *see* alcohol (ethyl) *on page 25*

ethanolamine oleate (ETH a nol a meen OH lee ate)

Sound-Alike/Look-Alike Issues
Ethamolin® may be confused with ethanol
Synonyms monoethanolamine
U.S./Canadian Brand Names Ethamolin® [US]
Therapeutic Category Sclerosing Agent
Use Orphan drug: Sclerosing agent used for bleeding esophageal varices
Usual Dosage Adults: 1.5-5 mL per varix, up to 20 mL total or 0.4 mL/kg for a 50 kg patient; doses should be decreased in patients with severe hepatic dysfunction and should receive less than recommended maximum dose
Dosage Forms
Injection, solution:
Ethamolin®: 5% [50 mg/mL] (2 mL)

EtheDent™ [US] *see* fluoride *on page 361*

Ethezyme™ [US] *see* papain and urea *on page 652*

Ethezyme™ 830 [US] *see* papain and urea *on page 652*

ethinyl estradiol and cyproterone acetate *see* cyproterone and ethinyl estradiol *(Canada only) on page 225*

ethinyl estradiol and desogestrel (ETH in il es tra DYE ole & des oh JES trel)

Sound-Alike/Look-Alike Issues
Ortho-Cept® may be confused with Ortho-Cyclen®
Synonyms desogestrel and ethinyl estradiol
U.S./Canadian Brand Names Apri® [US]; Cesia™ [US]; Cyclessa® [US/Can]; Desogen® [US]; Kariva™ [US]; Linessa® [Can]; Marvelon® [Can]; Mircette® [US]; Ortho-Cept® [US/Can]; Reclipsen™ [US]; Solia™ [US]; Velivet™ [US]
Therapeutic Category Contraceptive, Oral
Use Prevention of pregnancy
Usual Dosage Oral: Adults: Female: Contraception:
Schedule 1 (Sunday starter): Dose begins on first Sunday after onset of menstruation; if the menstrual period starts on Sunday, take first tablet that very same day. **With a Sunday start, an additional method of contraception should be used until after the first 7 days of consecutive administration.**
For 21-tablet package: Dosage is 1 tablet daily for 21 consecutive days, followed by 7 days off of the medication; a new course begins on the 8th day after the last tablet is taken.
For 28-tablet package: Dosage is 1 tablet daily without interruption.
Schedule 2 (Day 1 starter): Dose starts on first day of menstrual cycle taking 1 tablet daily.

For 21-tablet package: Dosage is 1 tablet daily for 21 consecutive days, followed by 7 days off of the medication; a new course begins on the 8th day after the last tablet is taken.

For 28-tablet package: Dosage is 1 tablet daily without interruption.

If all doses have been taken on schedule and one menstrual period is missed, continue dosing cycle. If two consecutive menstrual periods are missed, pregnancy test is required before new dosing cycle is started.

Missed doses **monophasic formulations** (refer to package insert for complete information):

One dose missed: Take as soon as remembered or take 2 tablets next day

Two consecutive doses missed in the first 2 weeks: Take 2 tablets as soon as remembered or 2 tablets next 2 days. **An additional method of contraception should be used for 7 days after missed dose.**

Two consecutive doses missed in week 3 or three consecutive doses missed at any time:

Schedule 1 (Sunday starter): Continue to take 1 tablet daily until Sunday, then discard the rest of the pack, and a new pack is started that same day.

Schedule 2 (Day 1 starter): Current pack should be discarded, and a new pack started that same day. **An additional method of contraception should be used for 7 days after missed dose.**

Missed doses **biphasic/triphasic formulations** (refer to package insert for complete information):

One dose missed: Take as soon as remembered or take 2 tablets next day

Two consecutive doses missed in week 1 or week 2 of the pack: Take 2 tablets as soon as remembered and 2 tablets the next day. Resume taking 1 tablet daily until the pack is empty. **An additional method of contraception should be used for 7 days after a missed dose.**

Two consecutive doses missed in week 3 of the pack; **an additional method of contraception must be used for 7 days after a missed dose**:

Schedule 1 (Sunday starter): Take 1 tablet every day until Sunday. Discard the remaining pack and start a new pack of pills on the same day.

Schedule 2 (Day 1 starter): Discard the remaining pack and start a new pack the same day.

Three or more consecutive doses missed; **an additional method of contraception must be used for 7 days after a missed dose**:

Schedule 1 (Sunday starter): Take 1 tablet every day until Sunday; on Sunday, discard the pack and start a new pack.

Schedule 2 (Day 1 starter): Discard the remaining pack and begin new pack of tablets starting on the same day.

Dosage Forms

Tablet, low-dose formulations:

Kariva™:

Day 1-21: Ethinyl estradiol 0.02 mg and desogestrel 0.15 mg [21 white tablets]

Day 22-23: 2 inactive light green tablets

Day 24-28: Ethinyl estradiol 0.01 mg [5 light blue tablets] (28s)

Mircette®:

Day 1-21: Ethinyl estradiol 0.02 mg and desogestrel 0.15 mg [21 white tablets]

Day 22-23: 2 inactive green tablets

Day 24-28: Ethinyl estradiol 0.01 mg [5 yellow tablets] (28s)

Tablet, monophasic formulations:

Apri® 28: Ethinyl estradiol 0.03 mg and desogestrel 0.15 mg (28s) [21 rose tablets and 7 white inactive tablets]

Desogen®, Reclipsen™, Solia™: Ethinyl estradiol 0.03 mg and desogestrel 0.15 mg (28s) [21 white tablets and 7 green inactive tablets]

Ortho-Cept® 28: Ethinyl estradiol 0.03 mg and desogestrel 0.15 mg (28s) [21 orange tablets and 7 green inactive tablets]

Tablet, triphasic formulations:

Cesia™, Cyclessa®:

Day 1-7:Ethinyl estradiol 0.025 mg and desogestrel 0.1 mg [7 light yellow tablets]

Day 8-14: Ethinyl estradiol 0.025 mg and desogestrel 0.125 mg [7 orange tablets]

Day 14-21: Ethinyl estradiol 0.025 mg and desogestrel 0.15 mg [7 red tablets]

Day 21-28: 7 green inactive tablets (28s)

Velivet™:

Day 1-7: Ethinyl estradiol 0.025 mg and desogestrel 0.1 mg [7 beige tablets]

Day 8-14: Ethinyl estradiol 0.025 mg and desogestrel 0.125 mg [7 orange tablets]

Day 14-21: Ethinyl estradiol 0.025 mg and desogestrel 0.15 mg [7 pink tablets]

Day 21-28: 7 white inactive tablets (28s)

ethinyl estradiol and drospirenone (ETH in il es tra DYE ole & droh SPYE re none)

Synonyms drospirenone and ethinyl estradiol

U.S./Canadian Brand Names Yasmin® [US/Can]; Yaz [US]

Therapeutic Category Contraceptive

Use Females: Prevention of pregnancy; treatment of premenstrual dysphoric disorder (PMDD); treatment of acne

(Continued)

ethinyl estradiol and drospirenone *(Continued)*

Usual Dosage Oral:

Children ≥14 years and Adults: Female: Acne (Yaz): Refer to dosing for contraception

Adults: Female: Contraception (Yasmin®, Yaz), PMDD (Yaz): Dosage is 1 tablet daily for 28 consecutive days. Dose should be taken at the same time each day, either after the evening meal or at bedtime. Dosing may be started on the first day of menstrual period (Day 1 starter) or on the first Sunday after the onset of the menstrual period (Sunday starter).

Day 1 starter: Dose starts on first day of menstrual cycle taking 1 tablet daily.

Sunday starter: Dose begins on first Sunday after onset of menstruation; if the menstrual period starts on Sunday, take first tablet that very same day. **With a Sunday start, an additional method of contraception should be used until after the first 7 days of consecutive administration.**

If all doses have been taken on schedule and one menstrual period is missed, continue dosing cycle. If two consecutive menstrual periods are missed, pregnancy test is required before new dosing cycle is started.

If doses have been missed during the first 3 weeks and the menstrual period is missed, pregnancy should be ruled out prior to continuing treatment.

Missed doses (monophasic formulations) (refer to package insert for complete information):

One dose missed: Take as soon as remembered or take 2 tablets next day

Two consecutive doses missed in the first 2 weeks: Take 2 tablets as soon as remembered or 2 tablets next 2 days. **An additional method of contraception should be used for 7 days after missed dose.**

Two consecutive doses missed in week 3 or three consecutive doses missed at any time: **An additional method of contraception must be used for 7 days after a missed dose.**

Day 1 starter: Current pack should be discarded, and a new pack should be started that same day.

Sunday starter: Continue dose of 1 tablet daily until Sunday, then discard the rest of the pack, and a new pack should be started that same day.

Any number of doses missed in week 4: Continue taking one pill each day until pack is empty; no back-up method of contraception is needed

Dosage Forms

Tablet:

Yasmin®: Ethinyl estradiol 0.03 mg and drospirenone 3 mg [21 yellow active tablets and 7 white inactive tablets] (28s)

Yaz: Ethinyl estradiol 0.02 mg and drospirenone 3 mg [24 light pink tablets and 4 white inactive tablets] (28s)

ethinyl estradiol and ethynodiol diacetate

(ETH in il es tra DYE ole & e thye noe DYE ole dye AS e tate)

Sound-Alike/Look-Alike Issues

Demulen® may be confused with Dalmane®, Demerol®

Synonyms ethynodiol diacetate and ethinyl estradiol

U.S./Canadian Brand Names Demulen® 30 [Can]; Kelnor™ [US]; Zovia™ [US]

Therapeutic Category Contraceptive, Oral

Use Prevention of pregnancy

Usual Dosage Oral: Adults: Female: Contraception:

Schedule 1 (Sunday starter): Dose begins on first Sunday after onset of menstruation; if the menstrual period starts on Sunday, take first tablet that very same day. **With a Sunday start, an additional method of contraception should be used until after the first 7 days of consecutive administration.**

For 21-tablet package: 1 tablet/day for 21 consecutive days, followed by 7 days off of the medication; a new course begins on the 8th day after the last tablet is taken.

For 28-tablet package: 1 tablet/day without interruption.

Schedule 2 (Day 1 starter): Dose starts on first day of menstrual cycle taking 1 tablet daily.

For 21-tablet package: 1 tablet/day for 21 consecutive days, followed by 7 days off of the medication; a new course begins on the 8th day after the last tablet is taken.

For 28-tablet package: 1 tablet/day without interruption.

If all doses have been taken on schedule and one menstrual period is missed, continue dosing cycle. If two consecutive menstrual periods are missed, pregnancy test is required before new dosing cycle is started.

Missed doses **monophasic formulations** (refer to package insert for complete information):

One dose missed: Take as soon as remembered or take 2 tablets next day

Two consecutive doses missed in the first 2 weeks: Take 2 tablets as soon as remembered or 2 tablets next 2 days. **An additional method of contraception should be used for 7 days after missed dose.**

Two consecutive doses missed in week 3 or three consecutive doses missed at any time: **An additional method of contraception should be used for 7 days after missed dose:**

Schedule 1 (Sunday starter): Continue dose of 1 tablet daily until Sunday, then discard the rest of the pack, and a new pack should be started that same day.

Schedule 2 (Day 1 starter): Current package should be discarded, and a new pack should be started that same day.

Dosage Forms
Tablet, monophasic formulations:
Kelnor™ 1/35: Ethinyl estradiol 0.035 mg and ethynodiol diacetate 1 mg [21 light yellow tablets and 7 white inactive tablets] (28s)

Zovia™ 1/35-28: Ethinyl estradiol 0.035 mg and ethynodiol diacetate 1 mg [21 light pink tablets and 7 white inactive tablets] (28s)

Zovia™ 1/50-28: Ethinyl estradiol 0.05 mg and ethynodiol diacetate 1 mg [21 pink tablets and 7 white inactive tablets] (28s)

ethinyl estradiol and etonogestrel (ETH in il es tra DYE ole & et oh noe JES trel)
Synonyms etonogestrel and ethinyl estradiol

U.S./Canadian Brand Names NuvaRing® [US/Can]

Therapeutic Category Contraceptive; Estrogen and Progestin Combination

Use Prevention of pregnancy

Usual Dosage Vaginal: Adults: Female: Contraception: One ring, inserted vaginally and left in place for 3 consecutive weeks, then removed for 1 week. A new ring is inserted 7 days after the last was removed (even if bleeding is not complete) and should be inserted at approximately the same time of day the ring was removed the previous week.

Initial treatment should begin as follows (pregnancy should always be ruled out first):
No hormonal contraceptive use in the past month: Using the first day of menstruation as "Day 1," insert the ring on or prior to "Day 5," even if bleeding is not complete. **An additional form of contraception should be used for the following 7 days.***

Switching from combination oral contraceptive: Ring can be inserted on any day within 7 days after the last **active** tablet in the cycle was taken and no later than the first day a new cycle of tablets would begin. Additional forms of contraception are not needed.

Switching from progestin-only contraceptive: **An additional form of contraception should be used for the following 7 days with any of the following.***
If previously using a progestin-only mini-pill, insert the ring on any day of the month; do not skip days between the last pill and insertion of the ring.

If previously using an implant, insert the ring on the same day of implant removal.

If previously using a progestin-containing IUD, insert the ring on day of IUD removal.

If previously using a progestin injection, insert the ring on the day the next injection would be given.

Following complete 1st trimester abortion: Insert ring within the first five days of abortion. If not inserted within five days, follow instructions for "No hormonal contraceptive use within the past month" and instruct patient to use a nonhormonal contraceptive in the interim.

Following delivery or 2nd trimester abortion: Insert ring 4 weeks postpartum (in women who are not breast-feeding) or following 2nd trimester abortion. **An additional form of contraception should be used for the following 7 days.***

If the ring is accidentally removed from the vagina at anytime during the 3-week period of use, it may be rinsed with cool or lukewarm water (not hot) and reinserted as soon as possible. If the ring is not reinserted within three hours, contraceptive effectiveness will be decreased. **An additional form of contraception should be used until the ring has been in place for 7 consecutive days.***

If the ring has been removed for longer than 1 week, pregnancy must be ruled out prior to restarting therapy. **An additional form of contraception should be used for the following 7 days.***

If the ring has been left in place for >3 weeks, a new ring should be inserted following a 1-week (ring-free) interval. Pregnancy must be ruled out prior to insertion and **an additional form of contraception should be used for the following 7 days.***

Disconnected ring: In the event the ring disconnects at the weld joint, discard and replace with a new ring.

***Note:** Diaphragms may interfere with proper ring placement, and therefore, are not recommended for use as an additional form of contraception.

Dosage Forms
Ring, vaginal:
NuvaRing®: Ethinyl estradiol 0.015 mg/day and etonogestrel 0.12 mg/day (1s) [3-week duration]

ethinyl estradiol and levonorgestrel (ETH in il es tra DYE ole & LEE voe nor jes trel)
Sound-Alike/Look-Alike Issues
Alesse® may be confused with Aleve®

Nordette® may be confused with Nicorette®

PREVEN® may be confused with Prevnar®

Seasonale® may be confused with Seasonique™

Seasonique™ may be confused with Seasonale®

Tri-Levlen® may be confused with Trilafon®

Triphasil® may be confused with Tri-Norinyl®

(Continued)

325

ethinyl estradiol and levonorgestrel *(Continued)*

Synonyms levonorgestrel and ethinyl estradiol

U.S./Canadian Brand Names Alesse® [US/Can]; Aviane™ [US]; Enpresse™ [US]; Jolessa™ [US]; Lessina™ [US]; Levlen® [US]; Levlite™ [US]; Levora® [US]; Lutera™ [US]; Lybrel™ [US]; Min-Ovral® [Can]; Nordette® [US]; Portia™ [US]; Quasense™ [US]; Seasonale® [US]; Seasonique™ [US]; Sronyx™ [US]; Triphasil® [US/Can]; Triquilar® [Can]; Trivora® [US]

Therapeutic Category Contraceptive, Oral

Use Prevention of pregnancy; postcoital contraception

Usual Dosage Oral: Adults: Female:

Contraception, 28-day cycle:

Schedule 1 (Sunday starter): Dose begins on first Sunday after onset of menstruation; if the menstrual period starts on Sunday, take first tablet that very same day. With a Sunday start, an additional method of contraception should be used until after the first 7 days of consecutive administration:

For 21-tablet package: 1 tablet/day for 21 consecutive days, followed by 7 days off of the medication; a new course begins on the 8th day after the last tablet is taken

For 28-tablet package: 1 tablet/day without interruption

Schedule 2 (Day 1 starter): Dose starts on first day of menstrual cycle taking 1 tablet/day:

For 21-tablet package: 1 tablet/day for 21 consecutive days, followed by 7 days off of the medication; a new course begins on the 8th day after the last tablet is taken

For 28-tablet package: 1 tablet/day without interruption

If all doses have been taken on schedule and one menstrual period is missed, continue dosing cycle. If two consecutive menstrual periods are missed, pregnancy test is required before new dosing cycle is started.

Missed doses **monophasic formulations** (refer to package insert for complete information):

One dose missed: Take as soon as remembered or take 2 tablets next day

Two consecutive doses missed in the first 2 weeks: Take 2 tablets as soon as remembered or 2 tablets next 2 days. An additional method of contraception should be used for 7 days after missed dose.

Two consecutive doses missed in week 3 or three consecutive doses missed at any time: An additional method of contraception must be used for 7 days after a missed dose:

Schedule 1 (Sunday starter): Continue dose of 1 tablet daily until Sunday, then discard the rest of the pack, and a new pack should be started that same day.

Schedule 2 (Day 1 starter): Current pack should be discarded, and a new pack should be started that same day.

Missed doses **biphasic/triphasic formulations** (refer to package insert for complete information):

One dose missed: Take as soon as remembered or take 2 tablets next day.

Two consecutive doses missed in week 1 or week 2 of the pack: Take 2 tablets as soon as remembered and 2 tablets the next day. Resume taking 1 tablet daily until the pack is empty. An additional method of contraception should be used for 7 days after a missed dose.

Two consecutive doses missed in week 3 of the pack: An additional method of contraception must be used for 7 days after a missed dose.

Schedule 1 (Sunday starter): Take 1 tablet every day until Sunday. Discard the remaining pack and start a new pack of pills on the same day.

Schedule 2 (Day 1 starter): Discard the remaining pack and start a new pack the same day.

Three or more consecutive doses missed: An additional method of contraception must be used for 7 days after a missed dose.

Schedule 1 (Sunday starter): Take 1 tablet every day until Sunday; on Sunday, discard the pack and start a new pack.

Schedule 2 (Day 1 starter): Discard the remaining pack and begin new pack of tablets starting on the same day.

Contraception, 91-day cycle (extended cycle regimen): Dose begins on first Sunday after onset of menstruation; if the menstrual period starts on Sunday, take first tablet that very same day. An additional method of contraception should be used until after the first 7 days of consecutive administration:

Seasonale®: One active tablet/day for 84 consecutive days, followed by 1 inactive tablet/day for 7 days; if all doses have been taken on schedule and one menstrual period is missed, pregnancy should be ruled out prior to continuing therapy.

Seasonique™: One active tablet/day for 84 consecutive days, followed by 1 low dose estrogen tablet/day for 7 days; if all doses have been taken on schedule and one menstrual period is missed, pregnancy should be ruled out prior to continuing therapy.

Missed doses:

One dose missed: Take as soon as remembered or take 2 tablets the next day

Two consecutive doses missed: Take 2 tablets as soon as remembered or 2 tablets the next 2 days. An additional nonhormonal method of contraception should be used for 7 consecutive days after the missed dose.

Three or more consecutive doses missed: Do not take the missed doses; continue taking 1 tablet/day until pack is complete. Bleeding may occur during the following week. An additional nonhormonal method of contraception should be used for 7 consecutive days after the missed dose.

Any number of pills during week 13: Throw away the missed pills and keep taking scheduled pills until the pack is finished. A back-up method of contraception is not needed

Contraception, continuous use (extended cycle regimen): Lybrel™: Take one tablet daily, at the same time each day, without a tablet-free interval. Therapy should be initiated as follows:

No previous contraception: Begin on the first day of menstrual cycle. Back-up contraception is not needed.

Previously taking a 21-day or 28-day combination hormonal contraceptive: Begin on day 1 of the withdrawal bleed (at the latest, 7 days after the last active tablet). Back-up contraception is not needed.

Previously using a progestin-only pill: Begin the day after taking a progestin only pill. Back-up contraception is needed for the first 7 days of therapy.

Previously using contraceptive implant: Begin the day of implant removal. Back-up contraception is needed for the first 7 days of therapy.

Previously using contraceptive injection: Begin when the next injection is due. Back-up contraception is needed for the first 7 days of therapy.

Missed doses:

One dose missed: Take as soon as remembered then take the next tablet at the regular time (2 tablets in 1 day). An additional nonhormonal method of contraception should also be used for 7 consecutive days.

Two consecutive doses missed: If remembered the day of the second missed tablet, take 2 tablets as soon as remembered, then 1 tablet the next day. If remembered the day after the second tablet is missed, take 2 tablets the day remembered, then 2 tablets the next day. An additional nonhormonal method of contraception should also be used for 7 consecutive days.

Three or more consecutive doses missed: Take 1 tablet daily and contact healthcare provider; do not take the missed pills. An additional nonhormonal method of contraception should also be used for 7 consecutive days.

Dosage Forms

Tablet, low-dose formulations:

Alesse® 28: Ethinyl estradiol 0.02 mg and levonorgestrel 0.1 mg (28s) [21 pink tablets and 7 light green inactive tablets]

Aviane™ 28: Ethinyl estradiol 0.02 mg and levonorgestrel 0.1 mg (28s) [21 orange tablets and 7 light green inactive tablets]

Lessina™ 28, Levlite™ 28: Ethinyl estradiol 0.02 mg and levonorgestrel 0.1 mg (28s) [21 pink tablets and 7 white inactive tablets]

Lutera™, Sronyx™: Ethinyl estradiol 0.02 mg and levonorgestrel 0.1 mg (28s) [21 white tablets and 7 peach inactive tablets]

Tablet, monophasic formulations:

Levlen® 28: Ethinyl estradiol 0.03 mg and levonorgestrel 0.15 mg (28s) [21 light orange tablets and 7 pink inactive tablets]

Levora® 28: Ethinyl estradiol 0.03 mg and levonorgestrel 0.15 mg (28s) [21 white tablets and 7 peach inactive tablets]

Nordette® 28: Ethinyl estradiol 0.03 mg and levonorgestrel 0.15 mg (28s) [21 light orange tablets and 7 pink inactive tablets]

Portia™ 28: Ethinyl estradiol 0.03 mg and levonorgestrel 0.15 mg (28s) [21 pink tablets and 7 white inactive tablets]

Tablet, monophasic formulations [extended cycle regimen]:

Jolessa™, Seasonale®: Ethinyl estradiol 0.03 mg and levonorgestrel 0.15 mg (91s) [84 pink tablets and 7 white inactive tablets]

Lybrel™: Ethinyl estradiol 0.02 mg and levonorgestrel 0.09 mg (28s) [28 yellow tablets]

Quasense™: Ethinyl estradiol 0.03 mg and levonorgestrel 0.15 mg] (91s) [84 white tablets and 7 peach inactive tablets

Seasonique™: Ethinyl estradiol 0.03 mg and levonorgestrel 0.15 mg (91s) [84 light blue-green tablets] and ethinyl estradiol 0.01 mg [7 yellow tablets]

Tablet, triphasic formulations:

Enpresse™:

Day 1-6: Ethinyl estradiol 0.03 mg and levonorgestrel 0.05 mg [6 pink tablets]

Day 7-11: Ethinyl estradiol 0.04 mg and levonorgestrel 0.075 mg [5 white tablets]

Day 12-21: Ethinyl estradiol 0.03 mg and levonorgestrel 0.125 mg [10 orange tablets]

Day 22-28: 7 light green inactive tablets (28s)

Triphasil® 28:

Day 1-6: Ethinyl estradiol 0.03 mg and levonorgestrel 0.05 mg [6 brown tablets]

Day 7-11: Ethinyl estradiol 0.04 mg and levonorgestrel 0.075 mg [5 white tablets]

Day 12-21: Ethinyl estradiol 0.03 mg and levonorgestrel 0.125 mg [10 light yellow tablets]

Day 22-28: 7 light green inactive tablets (28s)

Trivora® 28:

Day 1-6: Ethinyl estradiol 0.03 mg and levonorgestrel 0.05 mg [6 blue tablets]

Day 7-11: Ethinyl estradiol 0.04 mg and levonorgestrel 0.075 mg [5 white tablets]

Day 12-21: Ethinyl estradiol 0.03 mg and levonorgestrel 0.125 mg [10 pink tablets]

Day 22-28: 7 peach inactive tablets (28s)

ethinyl estradiol and NGM *see* ethinyl estradiol and norgestimate *on page 331*

ethinyl estradiol and norelgestromin (ETH in il es tra DYE ole & nor el JES troe min)
Synonyms norelgestromin and ethinyl estradiol
U.S./Canadian Brand Names Evra® [Can]; Ortho Evra® [US]
Therapeutic Category Contraceptive; Estrogen and Progestin Combination
Use Prevention of pregnancy
Usual Dosage Topical: Adults: Female:
  Contraception: Apply one patch each week for 3 weeks (21 total days); followed by one week that is patch-free. Each patch should be applied on the same day each week ("patch change day") and only one patch should be worn at a time. No more than 7 days should pass during the patch-free interval.
  Schedule 1 (Sunday starter): Dose begins on first Sunday after onset of menstruation; if the menstrual period starts on Sunday, apply one patch that very same day. **With a Sunday start, an additional method of contraception (nonhormonal) should be used until after the first 7 days of consecutive administration.** Each patch change will then occur on Sunday.
  Schedule 2 (Day 1 starter): Dose starts on first day of menstrual cycle, applying one patch during the first 24 hours of menstrual cycle. No back-up method of contraception is needed as long as the patch is applied on the first day of cycle. Each patch change will then occur on that same day of the week.
  Additional dosing considerations:
  No bleeding during patch-free week/missed menstrual period: If patch has been applied as directed, continue treatment on usual "patch change day". If used correctly, no bleeding during patch-free week does not necessarily indicate pregnancy. However, if no withdrawal bleeding occurs for 2 consecutive cycles, pregnancy should be ruled out. If patch has not been applied as directed, and one menstrual period is missed, pregnancy should be ruled out prior to continuing treatment.
  If a patch becomes partially or completely detached for <24 hours: Try to reapply to same place, or replace with a new patch immediately. Do not reapply if patch is no longer sticky, if it is sticking to itself or another surface, or if it has material sticking to it.
  If a patch becomes partially or completely detached for >24 hours (or time period is unknown): Apply a new patch and use this day of the week as the new "patch change day" from this point on. **An additional method of contraception (nonhormonal) should be used until after the first 7 days of consecutive administration.**
  Switching from oral contraceptives: Apply first patch on the first day of withdrawal bleeding. If there is no bleeding within 5 days of taking the last active tablet, pregnancy must first be ruled out. If patch is applied later than the first day of bleeding, **an additional method of contraception (nonhormonal) should be used until after the first 7 days of consecutive administration**
  Use after childbirth: Therapy should not be started <4 weeks after childbirth. Pregnancy should be ruled out prior to treatment if menstrual periods have not restarted. **An additional method of contraception (nonhormonal) should be used until after the first 7 days of consecutive administration.**
  Use after abortion or miscarriage: Therapy may be started immediately if abortion/miscarriage occur within the first trimester. If therapy is not started within 5 days, follow instructions for first time use. If abortion/miscarriage occur during the second trimester, therapy should not be started for at least 4 weeks. Follow directions for use after childbirth.
Dosage Forms The Canadian formulation differs from the U.S. product in both composition and manufacturing process (although delivery rates appear similar). [CAN] = Canadian brand name.
  Patch, transdermal:
    Evra® [CAN]: Ethinyl estradiol 0.6 mg and norelgestromin 6 mg [releases ethinyl estradiol 20 mcg and norelgestromin 150 mcg per day] (1s, 3s) [not available in the U.S.]
    Ortho Evra®: Ethinyl estradiol 0.75 mg and norelgestromin 6 mg [releases ethinyl estradiol 20 mcg and norelgestromin 150 mcg per day] (1s, 3s)

ethinyl estradiol and norethindrone (ETH in il es tra DYE ole & nor eth IN drone)
Sound-Alike/Look-Alike Issues
  femhrt® may be confused with Femara®
  Modicon® may be confused with Mylicon®
  Norinyl® may be confused with Nardil®
  Tri-Norinyl® may be confused with Triphasil®
Synonyms norethindrone acetate and ethinyl estradiol
U.S./Canadian Brand Names Aranelle™ [US]; Balziva™ [US]; Brevicon® 0.5/35 [Can]; Brevicon® 1/35 [Can]; Brevicon® [US]; Estrostep® Fe [US]; Femcon™ Fe [US]; femhrt® [US/Can]; Junel™ Fe [US]; Junel™ [US]; Leena™ [US]; Loestrin® 24 Fe [US]; Loestrin® Fe [US]; Loestrin® [US]; Loestrin® 1.5/30 [Can]; Microgestin™ Fe [US]; Microgestin™ [US]; Minestrin™ 1/20 [Can]; Modicon® [US]; Necon® 0.5/35 [US]; Necon® 1/35 [US];

Necon® 10/11 [US]; Necon® 7/7/7 [US]; Norinyl® 1+35 [US]; Nortrel™ 7/7/7 [US]; Nortrel™ [US]; Ortho-Novum® [US]; Ortho® 0.5/35 [Can]; Ortho® 1/35 [Can]; Ortho® 7/7/7 [Can]; Ovcon® [US]; Select™ 1/35 [Can]; Synphasic® [Can]; Tri-Norinyl® [US]; Zenchent™ [US]

Therapeutic Category Contraceptive, Oral

Use Prevention of pregnancy; treatment of acne; moderate to severe vasomotor symptoms associated with menopause; prevention of osteoporosis (in women at significant risk only)

Usual Dosage Oral:

Adolescents ≥15 years and Adults: Female: Acne: Estrostep®: Refer to dosing for contraception

Adults: Female:

Moderate-to-severe vasomotor symptoms associated with menopause: Initial: femhrt® 0.5/2.5: 1 tablet daily; patient should be reevaluated at 3- to 6-month intervals to determine if treatment is still necessary; patient should be maintained at the lowest effective dose

Prevention of osteoporosis: Initial: femhrt® 0.5/2.5: 1 tablet daily; patient should be maintained on the lowest effective dose

Contraception:

Schedule 1 (Sunday starter): Dose begins on first Sunday after onset of menstruation; if the menstrual period starts on Sunday, take first tablet that very same day. With a Sunday start, an additional method of contraception should be used until after the first 7 days of consecutive administration.

For 21-tablet package: Dosage is 1 tablet daily for 21 consecutive days, followed by 7 days off of the medication; a new course begins on the 8th day after the last tablet is taken.

For 28-tablet package: Dosage is 1 tablet daily without interruption.

Schedule 2 (Day 1 starter): Dose starts on first day of menstrual cycle taking 1 tablet daily.

For 21-tablet package: Dosage is 1 tablet daily for 21 consecutive days, followed by 7 days off of the medication; a new course begins on the 8th day after the last tablet is taken.

For 28-tablet package: Dosage is 1 tablet daily without interruption.

If all doses have been taken on schedule and one menstrual period is missed, continue dosing cycle. If two consecutive menstrual periods are missed, pregnancy test is required before new dosing cycle is started.

Missed doses **monophasic formulations** (refer to package insert for complete information):

One dose missed: Take as soon as remembered or take 2 tablets next day Two consecutive doses missed in the first 2 weeks: Take 2 tablets as soon as remembered or 2 tablets next 2 days. An additional method of contraception should be used for 7 days after missed dose.

Two consecutive doses missed in week 3 or three consecutive doses missed at any time: An additional method of contraception must be used for 7 days after a missed dose.

Schedule 1 (Sunday starter): Continue dose of 1 tablet daily until Sunday, then discard the rest of the pack, and a new pack should be started that same day.

Schedule 2 (Day 1 starter): Current pack should be discarded, and a new pack should be started that same day.

Missed doses **biphasic/triphasic formulations** (refer to package insert for complete information):

One dose missed: Take as soon as remembered or take 2 tablets next day.

Two consecutive doses missed in week 1 or week 2 of the pack: Take 2 tablets as soon as remembered and 2 tablets the next day. Resume taking 1 tablet daily until the pack is empty. An additional method of contraception should be used for 7 days after a missed dose.

Two consecutive doses missed in week 3 of the pack: An additional method of contraception must be used for 7 days after a missed dose.

Schedule 1 (Sunday Starter): Take 1 tablet every day until Sunday. Discard the remaining pack and start a new pack of pills on the same day.

Schedule 2 (Day 1 starter): Discard the remaining pack and start a new pack the same day.

Three or more consecutive doses missed: An additional method of contraception must be used for 7 days after a missed dose.

Schedule 1 (Sunday Starter): Take 1 tablet every day until Sunday; on Sunday, discard the pack and start a new pack.

Schedule 2 (Day 1 Starter): Discard the remaining pack and begin new pack of tablets starting on the same day.

Dosage Forms

Tablet:

femhrt®: 1/5: Ethinyl estradiol 5 mcg and norethindrone 1 mg [white tablets]; 0.5/2.5: Ethinyl estradiol 2.5 mcg and norethindrone 0.5 mg [white tablets]

Tablet, monophasic formulations:

Balziva™: Ethinyl estradiol 0.035 mg and norethindrone 0.4 mg (28s) [21 light peach tablets and 7 white inactive tablets]

Brevicon®: Ethinyl estradiol 0.035 mg and norethindrone 0.5 mg (28s) [21 blue tablets and 7 orange inactive tablets]

Junel™ 21 1/20: Ethinyl estradiol 0.02 mg and norethindrone 1 mg (21s) [yellow tablets]

Junel™ 21 1.5/30: Ethinyl estradiol 0.03 mg and norethindrone 1.5 mg (21s) [pink tablets]

Junel™ Fe 1/20: Ethinyl estradiol 0.02 mg and norethindrone 1 mg (28s) [21 yellow tablets] and ferrous fumarate 75 mg [7 brown tablets]

(Continued)

ethinyl estradiol and norethindrone *(Continued)*

Junel™ Fe 1.5/30: Ethinyl estradiol 0.03 mg and norethindrone 1.5 mg (28s) [21 pink tablets] and ferrous fumarate 75 mg [7 brown tablets]

Loestrin® 21 1/20, Microgestin™ 1/20: Ethinyl estradiol 0.02 mg and norethindrone 1 mg (21s) [white tablets]

Loestrin® 21 1.5/30, Microgestin™ 1.5/30: Ethinyl estradiol 0.03 mg and norethindrone 1.5 mg (21s) [green tablets]

Loestrin® 24 Fe: 1/20: Ethinyl estradiol 0.02 mg and norethindrone acetate 1 mg (28s) [24 white tablets] and ferrous fumarate 75 mg [4 brown tablets]

Loestrin® Fe 1/20, Microgestin™ Fe 1/20: Ethinyl estradiol 0.02 mg and norethindrone 1 mg (28s) [21 white tablets] and ferrous fumarate 75 mg [7 brown tablets]

Loestrin® Fe 1.5/30, Microgestin™ Fe 1.5/30: Ethinyl estradiol 0.03 mg and norethindrone 1.5 mg (28s) [21 green tablets] and ferrous fumarate 75 mg [7 brown tablets]

Modicon® 28: Ethinyl estradiol 0.035 mg and norethindrone 0.5 mg (28s) [21 white tablets and 7 green inactive tablets]

Necon® 0.5/35-28: Ethinyl estradiol 0.035 mg and norethindrone 0.5 mg (28s) [21 light yellow tablets and 7 white inactive tablets]

Necon® 1/35-28: Ethinyl estradiol 0.035 mg and norethindrone 1 mg (28s) [21 dark yellow tablets and 7 white inactive tablets]

Norinyl® 1+35: Ethinyl estradiol 0.035 mg and norethindrone 1 mg (28s) [21 yellow-green tablets and 7 orange inactive tablets]

Nortrel™ 0.5/35 mg:
  Ethinyl estradiol 0.035 mg and norethindrone 0.5 mg (21s) [light yellow tablets]
  Ethinyl estradiol 0.035 mg and norethindrone 0.5 mg (28s) [21 light yellow tablets and 7 white inactive tablets]

Nortrel™ 1/35 mg:
  Ethinyl estradiol 0.035 mg and norethindrone 1 mg (21s) [yellow tablets]
  Ethinyl estradiol 0.035 mg and norethindrone 1 mg (21s) [21 yellow tablets and 7 white inactive tablets]

Ortho-Novum® 1/35 28: Ethinyl estradiol 0.035 mg and norethindrone 1 mg (28s) [21 peach tablets and 7 green inactive tablets]

Ovcon® 35 21-day: Ethinyl estradiol 0.035 mg and norethindrone 0.4 mg (21s) [peach tablets]

Ovcon® 35 28-day: Ethinyl estradiol 0.035 mg and norethindrone 0.4 mg (28s) [21 peach tablets and 7 green inactive tablets]

Ovcon® 50: Ethinyl estradiol 0.05 mg and norethindrone 1 mg (28s) [21 yellow tablets and 7 green inactive tablets]

Zenchent™: Ethinyl estradiol 0.035 mg and norethindrone 0.4 mg (28s) [21 light peach tablets and 7 white inactive tablets]

Tablet, chewable, monophasic formulations:

Femcon™ Fe: Ethinyl estradiol 0.035 mg and norethindrone 0.4 mg (28s) [21 white tablets and 7 brown inactive tablets] [spearmint flavor]

Tablet, biphasic formulations:

Necon® 10/11-28:
  Day 1-10: Ethinyl estradiol 0.035 mg and norethindrone 0.5 mg [10 light yellow tablets]
  Day 11-21: Ethinyl estradiol 0.035 mg and norethindrone 1 mg [11 dark yellow tablets]
  Day 22-28: 7 white inactive tablets (28s)
Ortho-Novum® 10/11-28:
  Day 1-10: Ethinyl estradiol 0.035 mg and norethindrone 0.5 mg [10 white tablets]
  Day 11-21: Ethinyl estradiol 0.035 mg and norethindrone 1 mg [11 peach tablets]
  Day 22-28: 7 green inactive tablets (28s)

Tablet, triphasic formulations:

Aranelle™:
  Day 1-7: Ethinyl estradiol 0.035 mg and norethindrone 0.5 mg [7 light yellow tablets]
  Day 8-16: Ethinyl estradiol 0.035 mg and norethindrone 1 mg [9 white tablets]
  Day 17-21: Ethinyl estradiol 0.035 mg and norethindrone 0.5 mg [5 light yellow tablets]
  Day 22-28: 7 peach inactive tablets (28s)
Estrostep® Fe:
  Day 1-5: Ethinyl estradiol 0.02 mg and norethindrone 1 mg [5 white triangular tablets]
  Day 6-12: Ethinyl estradiol 0.03 mg and norethindrone 1 mg [7 white square tablets]
  Day 13-21: Ethinyl estradiol 0.035 mg and norethindrone 1 mg [9 white round tablets]
  Day 22-28: Ferrous fumarate 75 mg [7 brown tablets] (28s)
Leena™:
  Day 1-7: Ethinyl estradiol 0.035 mg and norethindrone 0.5 mg [7 light blue tablets]
  Day 8-16: Ethinyl estradiol 0.035 mg and norethindrone 1 mg [9 light yellow-green tablets]
  Day 17-21: Ethinyl estradiol 0.035 mg and norethindrone 0.5 mg [5 light blue tablets]
  Day 22-28: 7 orange inactive tablets (28s)

Necon® 7/7/7, Ortho-Novum® 7/7/7 28:
 Day 1-7: Ethinyl estradiol 0.035 mg and norethindrone 0.5 mg [7 white tablets]
 Day 8-14: Ethinyl estradiol 0.035 mg and norethindrone 0.75 mg [7 light peach tablets]
 Day 15-21: Ethinyl estradiol 0.035 mg and norethindrone 1 mg [7 peach tablets]
 Day 22-28: 7 green inactive tablets (28s)
Nortrel™ 7/7/7 28:
 Day 1-7: Ethinyl estradiol 0.035 mg and norethindrone 0.5 mg [7 light yellow tablets]
 Day 8-14: Ethinyl estradiol 0.035 mg and norethindrone 0.75 mg [7 blue tablets]
 Day 15-21: Ethinyl estradiol 0.035 mg and norethindrone 1 mg [7 peach tablets]
 Day 22-28: 7 white inactive tablets (28s)
Ortho-Novum® 7/7/7 28:
 Day 1-7: Ethinyl estradiol 0.035 mg and norethindrone 0.5 mg [7 white tablets]
 Day 8-14: Ethinyl estradiol 0.035 mg and norethindrone 0.75 mg [7 light peach tablets]
 Day 15-21: Ethinyl estradiol 0.035 mg and norethindrone 1 mg [7 peach tablets]
 Day 22-28: 7 green inactive tablets (28s)
Tri-Norinyl® 28:
 Day 1-7: Ethinyl estradiol 0.035 mg and norethindrone 0.5 mg [7 blue tablets]
 Day 8-16: Ethinyl estradiol 0.035 mg and norethindrone 1 mg [9 yellow-green tablets]
 Day 17-21: Ethinyl estradiol 0.035 mg and norethindrone 0.5 mg [5 blue tablets]
 Day 22-28: 7 orange inactive tablets (28s)

ethinyl estradiol and norgestimate (ETH in il es tra DYE ole & nor JES ti mate)
Sound-Alike/Look-Alike Issues
Ortho-Cyclen® may be confused with Ortho-Cept®
Synonyms ethinyl estradiol and NGM; norgestimate and ethinyl estradiol
U.S./Canadian Brand Names Cyclen® [Can]; MonoNessa™ [US]; Ortho Tri-Cyclen® Lo [US]; Ortho Tri-Cyclen® [US]; Ortho-Cyclen® [US]; Previfem™ [US]; Sprintec™ [US]; Tri-Cyclen® Lo [Can]; Tri-Cyclen® [Can]; Tri-Previfem™ [US]; Tri-Sprintec™ [US]; TriNessa™ [US]
Therapeutic Category Contraceptive, Oral
Use Prevention of pregnancy; treatment of acne
Usual Dosage Oral:
 Children ≥15 years and Adults: Female: Acne (Ortho Tri-Cyclen®): Refer to dosing for contraception

 Adults: Female:
 Contraception:
  Schedule 1 (Sunday starter): Dose begins on first Sunday after onset of menstruation; if the menstrual period starts on Sunday, take first tablet that very same day. **With a Sunday start, an additional method of contraception should be used until after the first 7 days of consecutive administration.**
   For 21-tablet package: Dosage is 1 tablet daily for 21 consecutive days, followed by 7 days off of the medication; a new course begins on the 8th day after the last tablet is taken.
   For 28-tablet package: Dosage is 1 tablet daily without interruption.
  Schedule 2 (Day 1 starter): Dose starts on first day of menstrual cycle taking 1 tablet daily.
   For 21-tablet package: Dosage is 1 tablet daily for 21 consecutive days, followed by 7 days off of the medication; a new course begins on the 8th day after the last tablet is taken.
   For 28-tablet package: Dosage is 1 tablet daily without interruption.
  If all doses have been taken on schedule and one menstrual period is missed, continue dosing cycle. If two consecutive menstrual periods are missed, pregnancy test is required before new dosing cycle is started.
  Missed doses **monophasic formulations** (refer to package insert for complete information):
   One dose missed: Take as soon as remembered or take 2 tablets next day
   Two consecutive doses missed in the first 2 weeks: Take 2 tablets as soon as remembered or 2 tablets next 2 days. **An additional method of contraception should be used for 7 days after missed dose.**
   Two consecutive doses missed in week 3 or three consecutive doses missed at any time: **An additional method of contraception must be used for 7 days after a missed dose:**
    Schedule 1 (Sunday starter): Continue dose of 1 tablet daily until Sunday, then discard the rest of the pack, and a new pack should be started that same day.
    Schedule 2 (Day 1 starter): Current pack should be discarded, and a new pack should be started that same day.
  Missed doses **biphasic/triphasic formulations** (refer to package insert for complete information):
   One dose missed: Take as soon as remembered or take 2 tablets next day.
   Two consecutive doses missed in week 1 or week 2 of the pack: Take 2 tablets as soon as remembered and 2 tablets the next day. Resume taking 1 tablet daily until the pack is empty. **An additional method of contraception must be used for 7 days after a missed dose.**
   Two consecutive doses missed in week 3 of the pack. **An additional method of contraception must be used for 7 days after a missed dose.**
    Schedule 1 (Sunday starter): Take 1 tablet every day until Sunday. Discard the remaining pack and start a new pack of pills on the same day.
 (Continued)

ethinyl estradiol and norgestimate *(Continued)*

Schedule 2 (Day 1 starter): Discard the remaining pack and start a new pack the same day.

Three or more consecutive doses missed. **An additional method of contraception must be used for 7 days after a missed dose.**

Schedule 1 (Sunday starter): Take 1 tablet every day until Sunday; on Sunday, discard the pack and start a new pack.

Schedule 2 (Day 1 starter): Discard the remaining pack and begin new pack of tablets starting on the same day.

Dosage Forms

Tablet, monophasic formulations:

MonoNessa™, Ortho-Cyclen®: Ethinyl estradiol 0.035 mg and norgestimate 0.25 mg [21 blue tablets and 7 green inactive tablets] (28s)

Previfem™: Ethinyl estradiol 0.035 mg and norgestimate 0.25 mg [21 blue tablets and 7 teal inactive tablets] (28s)

Sprintec™: Ethinyl estradiol 0.035 mg and norgestimate 0.25 mg [21 blue tablets and 7 white inactive tablets] (28s)

Tablet, triphasic formulations:

Ortho Tri-Cyclen®, TriNessa™:
Day 1-7: Ethinyl estradiol 0.035 mg and norgestimate 0.18 mg [7 white tablets]
Day 8-14: Ethinyl estradiol 0.035 mg and norgestimate 0.215 mg [7 light blue tablets]
Day 15-21: Ethinyl estradiol 0.035 mg and norgestimate 0.25 mg [7 blue tablets]
Day 22-28: 7 green inactive tablets (28s)

Tri-Previfem™:
Day 1-7: Ethinyl estradiol 0.035 mg and norgestimate 0.18 mg [7 white tablets]
Day 8-14: Ethinyl estradiol 0.035 mg and norgestimate 0.215 mg [7 light blue tablets]
Day 15-21: Ethinyl estradiol 0.035 mg and norgestimate 0.25 mg [7 blue tablets]
Day 22-28: 7 teal inactive tablets (28s)

Tri-Sprintec™:
Day 1-7: Ethinyl estradiol 0.035 mg and norgestimate 0.18 mg [7 gray tablets]
Day 8-14: Ethinyl estradiol 0.035 mg and norgestimate 0.215 mg [7 light blue tablets]
Day 15-21: Ethinyl estradiol 0.035 mg and norgestimate 0.25 mg [7 blue tablets]
Day 22-28: 7 white inactive tablets (28s)

Ortho Tri-Cyclen® Lo:
Day 1-7: Ethinyl estradiol 0.025 mg and norgestimate 0.18 mg [7 white tablets]
Day 8-14: Ethinyl estradiol 0.025 mg and norgestimate 0.215 mg [7 light blue tablets]
Day 15-21: Ethinyl estradiol 0.025 mg and norgestimate 0.25 mg [7 dark blue tablets]
Day 22-28: 7 green inactive tablets (28s)

ethinyl estradiol and norgestrel (ETH in il es tra DYE ole & nor JES trel)

Synonyms morning after pill; norgestrel and ethinyl estradiol

U.S./Canadian Brand Names Cryselle™ [US]; Lo/Ovral® [US]; Low-Ogestrel® [US]; Ogestrel® [US]; Ovral® [Can]

Therapeutic Category Contraceptive, Oral

Use Prevention of pregnancy; postcoital contraceptive or "morning after" pill

Usual Dosage Oral: Adults: Female:

Contraception:

Schedule 1 (Sunday starter): Dose begins on first Sunday after onset of menstruation; if the menstrual period starts on Sunday, take first tablet that very same day. **With a Sunday start, an additional method of contraception should be used until after the first 7 days of consecutive administration.**

For 21-tablet package: Dosage is 1 tablet daily for 21 consecutive days, followed by 7 days off of the medication; a new course begins on the 8th day after the last tablet is taken.

For 28-tablet package: Dosage is 1 tablet daily without interruption.

Schedule 2 (Day 1 starter): Dose starts on first day of menstrual cycle taking 1 tablet daily.

For 21-tablet package: Dosage is 1 tablet daily for 21 consecutive days, followed by 7 days off of the medication; a new course begins on the 8th day after the last tablet is taken.

For 28-tablet package: Dosage is 1 tablet daily without interruption.

If all doses have been taken on schedule and one menstrual period is missed, continue dosing cycle. If two consecutive menstrual periods are missed, pregnancy test is required before new dosing cycle is started.

Missed doses **monophasic formulations** (refer to package insert for complete information):

One dose missed: Take as soon as remembered or take 2 tablets next day

Two consecutive doses missed in the first 2 weeks: Take 2 tablets as soon as remembered or 2 tablets next 2 days. **An additional method of contraception should be used for 7 days after missed dose.**

Two consecutive doses missed in week 3 or three consecutive doses missed at any time:

Schedule 1 (Sunday starter): Continue to take 1 tablet daily until Sunday, then discard the rest of the pack, and a new pack is started that same day.

Schedule 2 (Day 1 starter): Current pack should be discarded, and a new pack started that same day. **An additional method of contraception should be used for 7 days after missed dose.**

Postcoital contraception:
Ethinyl estradiol 0.03 mg and norgestrel 0.3 mg formulation: 4 tablets within 72 hours of unprotected intercourse and 4 tablets 12 hours after first dose
Ethinyl estradiol 0.05 mg and norgestrel 0.5 mg formulation: 2 tablets within 72 hours of unprotected intercourse and 2 tablets 12 hours after first dose

Dosage Forms
Tablet, monophasic formulations:
Cryselle™: Ethinyl estradiol 0.03 mg and norgestrel 0.3 mg [21 white tablets and 7 light green inactive tablets] (28s)
Low-Ogestrel® 28: Ethinyl estradiol 0.03 mg and norgestrel 0.3 mg [21 white tablets and 7 peach inactive tablets] (28s)
Lo/Ovral® 28: Ethinyl estradiol 0.03 mg and norgestrel 0.3 mg [21 white tablets and 7 pink inactive tablets] (28s)
Ogestrel® 28: Ethinyl estradiol 0.05 mg and norgestrel 0.5 mg [21 white tablets and 7 peach inactive tablets] (28s)

ethiofos *see amifostine* *on page 40*

ethionamide (e thye on AM ide)
U.S./Canadian Brand Names Trecator® [US/Can]
Therapeutic Category Antimycobacterial Agent
Use Treatment of tuberculosis and other mycobacterial diseases, in conjunction with other antituberculosis agents, when first-line agents have failed or resistance has been demonstrated
Usual Dosage Oral:
Children: 15-20 mg/kg/day in 2-3 divided doses, not to exceed 1 g/day
Adults: 15-20 mg/kg/day; initiate dose at 250 mg/day for 1-2 days, then increase to 250 mg twice daily for 1-2 days, with gradual increases to highest tolerated dose; average adult dose: 750 mg/day (maximum: 1 g/day in 3-4 divided doses)
Dosage Forms
Tablet:
Trecator®: 250 mg

Ethmozine® [US/Can] *see moricizine* *on page 578*

ethosuximide (eth oh SUKS i mide)
Sound-Alike/Look-Alike Issues
ethosuximide may be confused with methsuximide
Zarontin® may be confused with Xalatan®, Zantac®, Zaroxolyn®
U.S./Canadian Brand Names Zarontin® [US/Can]
Therapeutic Category Anticonvulsant
Use Management of absence (petit mal) seizures
Usual Dosage Oral:
Children 3-6 years: Initial: 250 mg/day; increase every 4-7 days; usual maintenance dose: 20 mg/kg/day; maximum dose: 1.5 g/day in divided doses
Children >6 years and Adults: Initial: 500 mg/day; increase by 250 mg as needed every 4-7 days, up to 1.5 g/day in divided doses; usual maintenance dose for most pediatric patients is 20 mg/kg/day.
Dosage Forms
Capsule: 250 mg
Zarontin®: 250 mg
Syrup: 250 mg/5 mL
Zarontin®: 250 mg/5 mL

ethotoin (ETH oh toyn)
Synonyms ethylphenylhydantoin
U.S./Canadian Brand Names Peganone® [US/Can]
Therapeutic Category Hydantoin
Use Generalized tonic-clonic or complex-partial seizures
Usual Dosage Oral: **Note:** Administer in 4-6 divided doses daily; titrate over several days based on patient response
Children ≥1 year: Maximum initial dose: 750 mg/day; usual maintenance dose: 0.5-1 g/day; maximum dose: 3 g/day
Adults: Initial dose: ≤1 g/day; usual maintenance dose: 2-3 g/day
(Continued)

ethotoin *(Continued)*
Dosage Forms
Tablet:
Peganone®: 250 mg

ETH-Oxydose™ **[Can]** *see* oxycodone *on page 640*

ethoxynaphthamido penicillin sodium *see* nafcillin *on page 587*

Ethrane® **[US]** *see* enflurane *on page 297*

ethyl alcohol *see* alcohol (ethyl) *on page 25*

ethyl aminobenzoate *see* benzocaine *on page 101*

ethyl chloride (ETH il KLOR ide)
Synonyms chloroethane
U.S./Canadian Brand Names Gebauer's Ethyl Chloride® [US]
Therapeutic Category Local Anesthetic
Use Local anesthetic in minor operative procedures and to relieve pain caused by insect stings and burns, and irritation caused by myofascial and visceral pain syndromes
Usual Dosage Dosage varies with use
Dosage Forms
Aerosol:
Gebauer's Ethyl Chloride®: 100% (103 mL)

ethyl chloride and dichlorotetrafluoroethane
(ETH il KLOR ide & dye klor oh te tra floo or oh ETH ane)
Synonyms dichlorotetrafluoroethane and ethyl chloride
U.S./Canadian Brand Names Fluro-Ethyl® [US]
Therapeutic Category Local Anesthetic
Use Topical refrigerant anesthetic to control pain associated with minor surgical procedures, dermabrasion, injections, contusions, and minor strains
Usual Dosage Press gently on side of spray valve allowing the liquid to emerge as a fine mist approximately 2" to 4" from site of application
Dosage Forms
Aerosol:
Fluro-Ethyl®: Ethyl chloride 25% and dichlorotetrafluoroethane 75% (148 mL)

ethyl esters of omega-3 fatty acids *see* omega-3-acid ethyl esters *on page 629*

ethylphenylhydantoin *see* ethotoin *on previous page*

ethynodiol diacetate and ethinyl estradiol *see* ethinyl estradiol and ethynodiol diacetate *on page 324*

Ethyol® **[US/Can]** *see* amifostine *on page 40*

Etibi® **[Can]** *see* ethambutol *on page 321*

etidronate and calcium (e ti DROE nate & KAL see um)
Synonyms calcium carbonate and etidronate disodium
U.S./Canadian Brand Names Didrocal™ [Can]
Therapeutic Category Bisphosphonate Derivative; Calcium Salt
Use Treatment and prevention of postmenopausal osteoporosis; prevention of corticosteroid-induced osteoporosis
Usual Dosage **Note:** 90-day treatment regimen involves sequential administration of two products within the packaging; not to be taken concurrently. The first blister card contains white tablets containing etidronate disodium, while the remaining four blister cards contains blue, capsule-shaped tablets containing calcium carbonate.
Oral: Adults: Etidronate disodium 400 mg once daily for 14 days, followed by calcium carbonate 1250 mg (500 mg elemental calcium) once daily for 76 days
Dosage Forms [CAN] = Canadian brand name
Combination package [each package contains five blister cards (90-day supply)]:
Didrocal™ [CAN; not available in the U.S.]
Tablet, etidronate: 400 mg (14s) [first card (white tablets)]
Tablet, calcium: 1250 mg (76s) [remaining cards (blue tablets)]

etidronate disodium (e ti DROE nate dye SOW dee um)

Sound-Alike/Look-Alike Issues
etidronate may be confused with etidocaine, etomidate, etretinate

Synonyms EHDP; sodium etidronate

U.S./Canadian Brand Names Didronel® [US/Can]; Gen-Etidronate [Can]

Therapeutic Category Bisphosphonate Derivative

Use Symptomatic treatment of Paget disease and heterotopic ossification due to spinal cord injury or after total hip replacement, hypercalcemia associated with malignancy

Usual Dosage Oral: Adults:
Paget disease:
Initial: 5-10 mg/kg/day (not to exceed 6 months) or 11-20 mg/kg/day (not to exceed 3 months). Doses >20 mg/kg/day are **not** recommended.
Retreatment: Initiate only after etidronate-free period ≥90 days. Monitor patients every 3-6 months. Retreatment regimens are the same as for initial treatment.
Heterotopic ossification:
Caused by spinal cord injury: 20 mg/kg/day for 2 weeks, then 10 mg/kg/day for 10 weeks; total treatment period: 12 weeks
Complicating total hip replacement: 20 mg/kg/day for 1 month preoperatively then 20 mg/kg/day for 3 months postoperatively; total treatment period is 4 months

Dosage Forms
Tablet:
Didronel®: 200 mg, 400 mg

etodolac (ee toe DOE lak)

Sound-Alike/Look-Alike Issues
Lodine® may be confused with codeine, iodine, Iopidine®, Lopid®

Synonyms etodolic acid

U.S./Canadian Brand Names Apo-Etodolac® [Can]; Lodine® [Can]; Utradol™ [Can]

Therapeutic Category Analgesic, Nonnarcotic; Nonsteroidal Antiinflammatory Drug (NSAID)

Use Acute and long-term use in the management of signs and symptoms of osteoarthritis; rheumatoid arthritis and juvenile rheumatoid arthritis; management of acute pain

Usual Dosage Note: For chronic conditions, response is usually observed within 2 weeks.
Children 6-16 years: Oral: Juvenile rheumatoid arthritis (Lodine® XL):
20-30 kg: 400 mg once daily
31-45 kg: 600 mg once daily
46-60 kg: 800 mg once daily
>60 kg: 1000 mg once daily
Adults: Oral:
Acute pain: 200-400 mg every 6-8 hours, as needed, not to exceed total daily doses of 1000 mg
Rheumatoid arthritis, osteoarthritis: 400 mg 2 times/day **or** 300 mg 2-3 times/day **or** 500 mg 2 times/day (doses >1000 mg/day have not been evaluated)
Lodine® XL: 400-1000 mg once daily

Dosage Forms
Capsule: 200 mg, 300 mg
Tablet: 400 mg, 500 mg
Tablet, extended release: 400 mg, 500 mg, 600 mg

etodolic acid *see* etodolac *on this page*

EtOH *see* alcohol (ethyl) *on page 25*

etomidate (e TOM i date)

Sound-Alike/Look-Alike Issues
etomidate may be confused with etidronate

U.S./Canadian Brand Names Amidate® [US/Can]

Therapeutic Category General Anesthetic

Use Induction and maintenance of general anesthesia

Usual Dosage I.V.: Children >10 years and Adults: Initial: 0.2-0.6 mg/kg over 30-60 seconds for induction of anesthesia; maintenance: 5-20 mcg/kg/minute

Dosage Forms
Injection, solution: 2 mg/mL (10 mL, 20 mL)
Amidate®: 2 mg/mL (10 mL, 20 mL)

etonogestrel (e toe noe JES trel)
Synonyms ENG; 3-keto-desogestrel
U.S./Canadian Brand Names Implanon™ [US]
Therapeutic Category Contraceptive; Progestin
Use Prevention of pregnancy; for use in women who request long-acting (up to 3 years) contraception
Usual Dosage
Children: Not for use prior to menarche.
Adults: Contraception: Subdermal: Implant 1 rod in the inner side of the upper, nondominant arm. Remove no later than 3 years after the date of insertion. After ruling out pregnancy, timing of insertion is based on the patient's contraceptive history:
No hormonal contraceptives within the past month: Insert between days 1 through 5 of menstruation, even if woman is still bleeding
Switching from combination hormonal contraceptive:
Oral tablet: Insert anytime within 7 days after the last active tablet
Vaginal ring: Insert anytime during the 7-day ring-free period
Transdermal system: Insert anytime during the 7-day patch-free period
Switching from a progestin-only contraceptive:
Oral pill: Any day during the month; do not skip days between the last pill and implant insertion
Implant: Insert on same day as removal of implant
IUD: Insert on same day as removal of IUD
Injection: Insert on day next injection is due
First trimester abortion or miscarriage: Insert immediately. If not inserted within first 5 days follow directions for "no hormonal contraception within the past month"
Following delivery or second trimester abortion: May insert between 21 and 28 days (if not exclusively breast-feeding) or after 4 weeks (if exclusively breast-feeding). Patients should use a second form of contraception for the first 7 days if insertion occurs at >4 weeks.
Note: If following above insertion schedule, no back-up contraception needed. If deviating, use back-up method for 7 days postinsertion.
Dosage Forms
Rod, subdermal:
Implanon™: 68 mg

etonogestrel and ethinyl estradiol *see* ethinyl estradiol and etonogestrel *on page 325*

Etopophos® [US] *see* etoposide phosphate *on next page*

etoposide (e toe POE side)
Sound-Alike/Look-Alike Issues
etoposide may be confused with teniposide
VePesid® may be confused with Versed
Synonyms epipodophyllotoxin; VP-16; VP-16-213
U.S./Canadian Brand Names Toposar® [US]; VePesid® [US/Can]
Therapeutic Category Antineoplastic Agent
Use Treatment of lymphomas, ANLL, lung, testicular, bladder, and prostate carcinoma, hepatoma, rhabdomyosarcoma, uterine carcinoma, neuroblastoma, mycosis fungoides, Kaposi sarcoma, histiocytosis, gestational trophoblastic disease, Ewing sarcoma, Wilms tumor, and brain tumors
Usual Dosage Refer to individual protocols:
Adults:
Small cell lung cancer (in combination with other approved chemotherapeutic drugs):
Oral: Due to poor bioavailability, oral doses should be twice the I.V. dose, rounded to the nearest 50 mg given once daily
I.V.: 35 mg/m^2/day for 4 days or 50 mg/m^2/day for 5 days every 3-4 weeks
IVPB: 60-100 mg/m^2/day for 3 days (with cisplatin)
CIV: 500 mg/m^2 over 24 hours every 3 weeks
Testicular cancer (in combination with other approved chemotherapeutic drugs):
IVPB: 50-100 mg/m^2/day for 5 days repeated every 3-4 weeks
I.V.: 100 mg/m^2 every other day for 3 doses repeated every 3-4 weeks
Dosage Forms
Capsule, softgel: 50 mg
VePesid®: 50 mg
Injection, solution: 20 mg/mL (5 mL, 25 mL, 50 mL)
Toposar®: 20 mg/mL (5 mL, 25 mL, 50 mL)

etoposide phosphate (e toe POE side FOS fate)
Sound-Alike/Look-Alike Issues
  etoposide may be confused with teniposide
U.S./Canadian Brand Names Etopophos® [US]
Therapeutic Category Antineoplastic Agent
Use Treatment of refractory testicular tumors; treatment of small cell lung cancer
Usual Dosage Refer to individual protocols. Adults: **Note:** Etoposide phosphate is a prodrug of etoposide, doses should be expressed as the desired **ETOPOSIDE** dose; **not** as the etoposide phosphate dose. (eg, etoposide phosphate equivalent to _____ mg etoposide).

  Small cell lung cancer (in combination with other approved chemotherapeutic drugs): I.V.: Etoposide 35 mg/m^2/day for 4 days to 50 mg/m^2/day for 5 days. Courses are repeated at 3- to 4-week intervals after adequate recovery from any toxicity.

  Testicular cancer (in combination with other approved chemotherapeutic agents): I.V.: Etoposide 50-100 mg/m^2/day on days 1-5 to 100 mg/m^2/day on days 1, 3, and 5. Courses are repeated at 3- to 4-week intervals after adequate recovery from any toxicity.

Dosage Forms
Injection, powder for reconstitution:
  Etopophos®: 100 mg

Etrafon® [Can] *see* amitriptyline and perphenazine *on page 45*

ETS-2% Topical *(Discontinued)*

Eudal®-SR [US] *see* guaifenesin and pseudoephedrine *on page 406*

Euflex® [Can] *see* flutamide *on page 367*

Euflexxa™ [US] *see* hyaluronate and derivatives *on page 423*

Euglucon® [Can] *see* glyburide *on page 396*

Eulexin® [US/Can] *see* flutamide *on page 367*

Eurax® [US] *see* crotamiton *on page 219*

Evac-Q-Mag® *(Discontinued)* *see* magnesium citrate *on page 525*

Evac-U-Gen [US-OTC] *see* senna *on page 781*

Evalose® *(Discontinued)* *see* lactulose *on page 489*

Evamist® [US] *see* estradiol *on page 313*

Everone® 200 [Can] *see* testosterone *on page 828*

Everone® Injection *(Discontinued)* *see* testosterone *on page 828*

Evicel™ [US] *see* fibrin sealant kit *on page 351*

Evista® [US/Can] *see* raloxifene *on page 742*

Evoclin™ [US] *see* clindamycin *on page 198*

Evoxac® [US/Can] *see* cevimeline *on page 170*

Evra® [Can] *see* ethinyl estradiol and norelgestromin *on page 328*

Exactacain™ [US] *see* benzocaine, butamben, and tetracaine *on page 103*

Exact® Acne Medication [US-OTC] *see* benzoyl peroxide *on page 103*

Excedrin® Extra Strength [US-OTC] *see* acetaminophen, aspirin, and caffeine *on page 9*

Excedrin® IB *(Discontinued)* *see* ibuprofen *on page 444*

Excedrin® Migraine [US-OTC] *see* acetaminophen, aspirin, and caffeine *on page 9*

Excedrin® P.M. [US-OTC] *see* acetaminophen and diphenhydramine *on page 7*

ExeClear [US] *see* hydrocodone and guaifenesin *on page 429*

ExeCof-XP [US] *see* hydrocodone and guaifenesin *on page 429*

ExeFen-PD [US] *see* guaifenesin and phenylephrine *on page 404*

Exelderm® [US/Can] *see* sulconazole *on page 810*

Exelon® [US/Can] *see* rivastigmine *on page 763*

exemestane (ex e MES tane)
Sound-Alike/Look-Alike Issues
  exemestane may be confused with estramustine
(Continued)

exemestane *(Continued)*

U.S./Canadian Brand Names Aromasin® [US/Can]

Therapeutic Category Antineoplastic Agent, Miscellaneous

Use Treatment of advanced breast cancer in postmenopausal women whose disease has progressed following tamoxifen therapy; adjuvant treatment of postmenopausal estrogen receptor-positive early breast cancer following 2-3 years of tamoxifen (for a total of 5 years of adjuvant therapy)

Usual Dosage Oral: Adults: 25 mg once daily

Dosage Forms
Tablet:
Aromasin®: 25 mg

exenatide *(ex EN a tide)*

Synonyms AC002993; exendin-4; LY2148568

U.S./Canadian Brand Names Byetta™ [US]

Therapeutic Category Antidiabetic Agent, Incretin Mimetic

Use Management (adjunctive) of type 2 diabetes mellitus (noninsulin dependent, NIDDM) in patients receiving a sulfonylurea, thiazolidinedione, or metformin (or a combination of these agents)

Usual Dosage SubQ: Adults: Initial: 5 mcg twice daily within 60 minutes prior to a meal; after 1 month, may be increased to 10 mcg twice daily (based on response)

Dosage Forms
Injection, solution [prefilled pen]:
Byetta™: 250 mcg/mL (1.2 mL, 2.4 mL)

ezetimibe (ez ET i mibe)
Sound-Alike/Look-Alike Issues
Zetia™ may be confused with Zestril®
U.S./Canadian Brand Names Ezetrol® [Can]; Zetia™ [US]
Therapeutic Category Antilipemic Agent, 2-Azetidinone
Use Use in combination with dietary therapy for the treatment of primary hypercholesterolemia (as monotherapy or in combination with HMG-CoA reductase inhibitors); homozygous sitosterolemia; homozygous familial hypercholesterolemia (in combination with atorvastatin or simvastatin); mixed hyperlipidemia (in combination with fenofibrate)
Usual Dosage Oral:
Hyperlipidemias: Children ≥10 years and Adults: 10 mg/day
Sitosterolemia: Adults: 10 mg/day
Dosage Forms
Tablet:
Zetia™: 10 mg

ezetimibe and simvastatin (ez ET i mibe & SIM va stat in)
Sound-Alike/Look-Alike Issues
Vytorin® may be confused with Vyvanse™
U.S./Canadian Brand Names Vytorin® [US]
Therapeutic Category Antilipemic Agent, 2-Azetidinone
Use Used in combination with dietary modification for the treatment of primary hypercholesterolemia and homozygous familial hypercholesterolemia
Usual Dosage Oral: Adults:
Homozygous familial hypercholesterolemia: Ezetimibe 10 mg and simvastatin 40 mg once daily or ezetimibe 10 mg and simvastatin 80 mg once daily in the evening. Dosing range: Ezetimibe 10 mg and simvastatin 10-80 mg once daily.
Hyperlipidemias: Initial: Ezetimibe 10 mg and simvastatin 20 mg once daily in the evening
Patients who require less aggressive reduction in LDL-C: Initial: Ezetimibe 10 mg and simvastatin 10 mg once daily
Patients who require >55% reduction in LDL-C: Initial: Ezetimibe 10 mg and simvastatin 40 mg once daily
Dosage Forms
Tablet:
Vytorin®:
10/10: Ezetimibe 10 mg and simvastatin 10 mg
10/20: Ezetimibe 10 mg and simvastatin 20 mg
10/40: Ezetimibe 10 mg and simvastatin 40 mg
10/80: Ezetimibe 10 mg and simvastatin 80 mg

Ezetrol® [Can] *see* ezetimibe *on this page*

Ezide® (Discontinued) *see* hydrochlorothiazide *on page 426*

E•R•O [US-OTC] *see* carbamide peroxide *on page 148*

F₃T *see* trifluridine *on page 866*

Fabrazyme® [US/Can] *see* agalsidase beta *on page 21*

Factive® [US/Can] *see* gemifloxacin *on page 387*

factor VIIa (recombinant) (FAK ter SEV en aye ree KOM be nant)
Sound-Alike/Look-Alike Issues
NovoSeven® may be confused with Novacet®
Synonyms coagulation factor VIIa; eptacog alfa (activated); rFVIIa
U.S./Canadian Brand Names Niastase® [Can]; NovoSeven® [US]
Therapeutic Category Antihemophilic Agent; Blood Product Derivative
Use Treatment of bleeding episodes and prevention of bleeding in surgical interventions in patients with hemophilia A or B with inhibitors to factor VIII or factor IX and in patients with congenital factor VII deficiency
Usual Dosage Children and Adults: I.V. administration only: Hemophilia A or B with inhibitors:
Bleeding episodes: 90 mcg/kg every 2 hours until hemostasis is achieved or until the treatment is judged ineffective. The dose and interval may be adjusted based upon the severity of bleeding and the degree of hemostasis achieved. For patients experiencing severe bleeds, dosing should be continued at 3- to 6-hour intervals after hemostasis has been achieved and the duration of dosing should be minimized.
Surgical interventions: 90 mcg/kg immediately before surgery, repeat at 2-hour intervals for the duration of surgery. Continue every 2 hours for 48 hours, then every 2-6 hours until healed for minor surgery; continue every 2 hours for 5 days, then every 4 hours until healed for major surgery.
(Continued)

factor VIIa (recombinant) *(Continued)*

Congenital factor VII deficiency: Bleeding episodes and surgical interventions: 15-30 mcg/kg every 4-6 hours until hemostasis. Doses as low as 10 mcg/kg have been effective.

Dosage Forms

Injection, powder for reconstitution [preservative free]:
NovoSeven®: 1.2 mg, 2.4 mg, 4.8 mg

factor VIII (human) *see* antihemophilic factor (human) *on page 58*

factor VIII (human) *see* antihemophilic factor/von Willebrand factor complex (human) *on page 60*

factor VIII (recombinant) *see* antihemophilic factor (recombinant) *on page 59*

factor IX (FAK ter nyne)

U.S./Canadian Brand Names AlphaNine® SD [US]; BeneFix® [US/Can]; Immunine® VH [Can]; Mononine® [US/Can]

Therapeutic Category Antihemophilic Agent

Use Control bleeding in patients with factor IX deficiency (hemophilia B or Christmas disease)

Usual Dosage Dosage is expressed in units of factor IX activity and must be individualized. I.V. only:

Formula for units required to raise blood level %:

AlphaNine® SD, Mononine®: Children and Adults:

Number of factor IX units required = body weight (in kg) x desired factor IX level increase (% normal) x 1 unit/kg

For example, for a 100% level a patient who has an actual level of 20%: Number of factor IX units needed = 70 kg x 80% x 1 unit/kg = 5600 units

BeneFix®:

Children <15 years:

Number of factor IX units required = body weight (in kg) x desired factor IX level increase (% normal) x 1.4 units/kg

Adults:

Number of factor IX units required = body weight (in kg) x desired factor IX level increase (% normal) x 1.2 units/kg

Guidelines: As a general rule, the level of factor IX required for treatment of different conditions is listed below:

Minor spontaneous hemorrhage, prophylaxis:

Desired levels of factor IX for hemostasis: 15% to 25%

Initial loading dose to achieve desired level: 20-30 units/kg

Frequency of dosing: Every 12-24 hours if necessary

Duration of treatment: 1-2 days

Moderate hemorrhage:

Desired levels of factor IX for hemostasis: 25% to 50%

Initial loading dose to achieve desired level: 25-50 units/kg

Frequency of dosing: Every 12-24 hours

Duration of treatment: 2-7 days

Major hemorrhage:

Desired levels of factor IX for hemostasis: >50%

Initial loading dose to achieve desired level: 30-50 units/kg

Frequency of dosing: Every 12-24 hours, depending on half-life and measured factor IX levels (after 3-5 days, maintain at least 20% activity)

Duration of treatment: 7-10 days, depending upon nature of insult

Surgery:

Desired levels of factor IX for hemostasis: 50% to 100%

Initial loading dose to achieve desired level: 50-100 units/kg

Frequency of dosing: Every 12-24 hours, depending on half-life and measured factor IX levels

Duration of treatment: 7-10 days, depending upon nature of insult

Dosage Forms

Injection, powder for reconstitution (exact potency labeled on each vial):
AlphaNine® SD, BeneFix®, Mononine®

factor IX complex (human) (FAK ter nyne KOM pleks HYU man)

Synonyms prothrombin complex concentrate
U.S./Canadian Brand Names Bebulin® VH [US]; Profilnine® SD [US]
Therapeutic Category Antihemophilic Agent
Use

Control bleeding in patients with factor IX deficiency (hemophilia B or Christmas disease) **Note:** Factor IX concentrate containing **only** factor IX is also available and preferable for this indication.
Prevention/control of bleeding in hemophilia A patients with inhibitors to factor VIII.
Prevention/control of bleeding in patients with factor VII deficiency.
Emergency correction of the coagulopathy of warfarin excess in critical situations.

Usual Dosage Children and Adults: Dosage is expressed in units of factor IX activity and must be individualized. I.V. only:

Formula for units required to raise blood level %:
Total blood volume (mL blood/kg) = 70 mL/kg (adults), 80 mL/kg (children)
Plasma volume = total blood volume (mL) x [1 - Hct (in decimals)]
For example, for a 70 kg adult with a Hct = 40%: Plasma volume = [70 kg x 70 mL/kg] x [1 - 0.4] = 2940 mL
To calculate number of units needed to increase level to desired range (highly individualized and dependent on patient's condition): Number of units = desired level increase [desired level - actual level] x plasma volume (in mL)
For example, for a 100% level in the above patient who has an actual level of 20%: Number of units needed = [1 (for a 100% level) - 0.2] x 2940 mL = 2352 units
As a general rule, the level of factor IX required for treatment of different conditions is listed below:

Minor Spontaneous Hemorrhage, Prophylaxis:
Desired levels of factor IX for hemostasis: 15% to 25%
Initial loading dose to achieve desired level: <20-30 units/kg
Frequency of dosing: Once; repeated in 24 hours if necessary
Duration of treatment: Once; repeated if necessary

Major Trauma or Surgery:
Desired levels of factor IX for hemostasis: 25% to 50%
Initial loading dose to achieve desired level: <75 units/kg
Frequency of dosing: Every 18-30 hours, depending on half-life and measured factor IX levels
Duration of treatment: Up to 10 days, depending upon nature of insult

Factor VIII inhibitor patients: 75 units/kg/dose; may be given every 6-12 hours
Anticoagulant overdosage: I.V.: 15 units/kg
Dosage Forms
Injection, powder for reconstitution [single-dose vial; exact potency labeled on each vial]:
Bebulin® VH, Profilnine® SD

Factrel® [US] see gonadorelin on page 399

famciclovir (fam SYE kloe veer)

U.S./Canadian Brand Names Apo-Famciclovir [Can]; Famvir® [US/Can]; PMS-Famciclovir [Can]
Therapeutic Category Antiviral Agent
Use Treatment of acute herpes zoster (shingles); treatment and suppression of recurrent episodes of genital herpes in immunocompetent patients; treatment of herpes labialis (cold sores) in immunocompetent patients; treatment of recurrent mucocutaneous/genital herpes simplex in HIV-infected patients
Usual Dosage Oral: Adults:
Acute herpes zoster: 500 mg every 8 hours for 7 days (**Note:** Initiate therapy within 72 hours of rash onset.)
Recurrent genital herpes simplex in immunocompetent patients:
Initial: 1000 mg twice daily for 1 day (**Note:** initiate therapy within 6 hours of symptoms/lesions.)
Suppressive therapy: 250 mg twice daily for up to 1 year
Recurrent herpes labialis (cold sores): 1500 mg as a single dose; initiate therapy at first sign or symptom such as tingling, burning, or itching (initiated within 1 hour in clinical studies)
Recurrent mucocutaneous/genital herpes simplex in HIV patients: 500 mg twice daily for 7 days
Dosage Forms
Tablet:
Famvir®: 125 mg, 250 mg, 500 mg

famotidine (fa MOE ti deen)

U.S./Canadian Brand Names Apo-Famotidine® Injectable [Can]; Apo-Famotidine® [Can]; Famotidine Omega [Can]; Gen-Famotidine [Can]; Novo-Famotidine [Can]; Nu-Famotidine [Can]; Pepcid® AC [US-OTC/Can]; Pepcid® I.V. [Can]; Pepcid® [US/Can]; ratio-Famotidine [Can]; Riva-Famotidine [Can]; Ulcidine [Can]
(Continued)

famotidine *(Continued)*

Therapeutic Category Histamine H_2 Antagonist

Use Therapy and treatment of duodenal ulcer, gastric ulcer; control gastric pH in critically-ill patients; symptomatic relief in gastritis, gastroesophageal reflux, active benign ulcer, and pathological hypersecretory conditions

OTC labeling: Relief of heartburn, acid indigestion, and sour stomach

Usual Dosage
Children: Treatment duration and dose should be individualized
Peptic ulcer: 1-16 years:
Oral: 0.5 mg/kg/day at bedtime or divided twice daily (maximum dose: 40 mg/day); doses of up to 1 mg/kg/day have been used in clinical studies
I.V.: 0.25 mg/kg every 12 hours (maximum dose: 40 mg/day); doses of up to 0.5 mg/kg have been used in clinical studies
GERD: Oral:
<3 months: 0.5 mg/kg once daily
3-12 months: 0.5 mg/kg twice daily
1-16 years: 1 mg/kg/day divided twice daily (maximum dose: 40 mg twice daily); doses of up to 2 mg/kg/day have been used in clinical studies

Children ≥12 years and Adults: Heartburn, indigestion, sour stomach: OTC labeling: Oral: 10-20 mg every 12 hours; dose may be taken 15-60 minutes before eating foods known to cause heartburn

Adults:
Duodenal ulcer: Oral: Acute therapy: 40 mg/day at bedtime for 4-8 weeks; maintenance therapy: 20 mg/day at bedtime
Gastric ulcer: Oral: Acute therapy: 40 mg/day at bedtime
Hypersecretory conditions: Oral: Initial: 20 mg every 6 hours, may increase in increments up to 160 mg every 6 hours
GERD: Oral: 20 mg twice daily for 6 weeks
Esophagitis and accompanying symptoms due to GERD: Oral: 20 mg or 40 mg twice daily for up to 12 weeks
Patients unable to take oral medication: I.V.: 20 mg every 12 hours

Dosage Forms
Infusion [premixed in NS]:
Pepcid®: 20 mg (50 mL)
Injection, solution: 10 mg/mL (4 mL, 20 mL, 50 mL)
Pepcid®: 10 mg/mL (20 mL)
Injection, solution [preservative free]: 10 mg/mL (2 mL)
Pepcid®: 10 mg/mL (2 mL)
Powder for oral suspension:
Pepcid®: 40 mg/5 mL
Tablet: 10 mg [OTC], 20 mg, 40 mg
Pepcid®: 20 mg, 40 mg
Pepcid® AC [OTC]: 10 mg, 20 mg
Tablet, chewable:
Pepcid® AC [OTC]: 10 mg

famotidine, calcium carbonate, and magnesium hydroxide

(fa MOE ti deen, KAL see um KAR bun ate, & mag NEE zhum hye DROKS ide)

Synonyms calcium carbonate, magnesium hydroxide, and famotidine; magnesium hydroxide, famotidine, and calcium carbonate

U.S./Canadian Brand Names Pepcid® Complete [US-OTC/Can]

Therapeutic Category Antacid; Histamine H_2 Antagonist

Use Relief of heartburn due to acid indigestion

Usual Dosage Oral: Children ≥12 years and Adults: Relief of heartburn due to acid indigestion: Pepcid® Complete: 1 tablet as needed; no more than 2 tablets in 24 hours; do **not** swallow whole, chew tablet completely before swallowing; do not use for longer than 14 days

Dosage Forms
Tablet, chewable:
Pepcid® Complete [OTC]: Famotidine 10 mg, calcium carbonate 800 mg, and magnesium hydroxide 165 mg

Famotidine Omega [Can] *see* famotidine *on previous page*

Famvir® [US/Can] *see* famciclovir *on previous page*

Fansidar® [US] *see* sulfadoxine and pyrimethamine *on page 812*

Fareston® [US/Can] *see* toremifene *on page 852*

Faslodex® [US] *see* fulvestrant *on page 378*

Fasturtec® **[Can]** *see* rasburicase *on page 746*

fat emulsion (fat e MUL shun)

Synonyms intravenous fat emulsion

U.S./Canadian Brand Names Intralipid® [US/Can]; Liposyn® II [US/Can]; Liposyn® III [US]

Therapeutic Category Intravenous Nutritional Therapy

Use Source of calories and essential fatty acids for patients requiring parenteral nutrition of extended duration; prevention and treatment of essential fatty acid deficiency (EFAD)

Usual Dosage I.V.: **Note:** At the onset of therapy, the patient should be observed for any immediate allergic reactions.

Premature infants: Initial dose: 0.25-0.5 g/kg/day, increase by 0.25-0.5 g/kg/day to a maximum of 3 g/kg/day depending on needs/nutritional goals; limit to 1 g/kg/day if on phototherapy; should be administered over 24 hours (A.S.P.E.N. guidelines)

Infants and Children: Initial dose: 0.5-1 g/kg/day, increase by 0.5 g/kg/day to a maximum of 3 g/kg/day depending on needs/nutritional goals; may administer over 24 hours (A.S.P.E.N. guidelines)

Note: Pediatric patients: Monitor triglycerides while receiving intralipids. If serum triglyceride levels >200 mg/dL, stop infusion and restart at 0.5-1g/kg/day. Intravenous heparin (1 unit/mL of parenteral nutrition) may enhance the clearance of lipid emulsions.

Adults: Initial dose: 1 g/kg/day, increase by 0.5-1 g/kg/day to a maximum of 2.5-3 g/kg/day

Prevention of essential fatty acid deficiency (EFAD): Administer 8% to 10% of total caloric intake as fat emulsion (may be higher in stressed patients with EFAD); may be given 2-3 times weekly to meet essential fatty acid requirements

Dosage Forms

Injection, emulsion [soybean oil]:

Intralipid®: 10% [100 mg/mL] (100 mL, 250 mL, 500 mL); 20% [200 mg/mL] (50 mL, 100 mL, 250 mL, 500 mL, 1000 mL); 30% [300 mg/mL] (500 mL)

Liposyn® II: 10% (200 mL, 500 mL); 20% (200 mL, 500 mL)

Liposyn® III: 10% [100 mg/mL] (200 mL, 500 mL); 20% [200 mg/mL] (200 mL, 500 mL); 30% [300 mg/mL] (500 mL)

FazaClo® **[US]** *see* clozapine *on page 207*

5-FC *see* flucytosine *on page 357*

FC1157a *see* toremifene *on page 852*

Fedahist® **Expectorant** *(Discontinued) see* guaifenesin and pseudoephedrine *on page 406*

Fedahist® **Expectorant Pediatric** *(Discontinued) see* guaifenesin and pseudoephedrine *on page 406*

Fedahist® **Tablet** *(Discontinued) see* chlorpheniramine and pseudoephedrine *on page 178*

Feen-A-Mint® *(Discontinued) see* bisacodyl *on page 112*

Feiba VH [US] *see* antiinhibitor coagulant complex *on page 61*

Feiba VH Immuno [Can] *see* antiinhibitor coagulant complex *on page 61*

felbamate (FEL ba mate)

U.S./Canadian Brand Names Felbatol® [US]

Therapeutic Category Anticonvulsant

Use Not as a first-line antiepileptic treatment; only in those patients who respond inadequately to alternative treatments and whose epilepsy is so severe that a substantial risk of aplastic anemia and/or liver failure is deemed acceptable in light of the benefits conferred by its use. Patient must be fully advised of risk and provide signed written informed consent. Felbamate can be used as either monotherapy or adjunctive therapy in the treatment of partial seizures (with and without generalization) and in adults with epilepsy.

Orphan drug: Adjunctive therapy in the treatment of partial and generalized seizures associated with Lennox-Gastaut syndrome in children

Usual Dosage Anticonvulsant:

Monotherapy: Children >14 years and Adults:

Initial: 1200 mg/day in divided doses 3 or 4 times/day; titrate previously untreated patients under close clinical supervision, increasing the dosage in 600 mg increments every 2 weeks to 2400 mg/day based on clinical response and thereafter to 3600 mg/day as clinically indicated

Conversion to monotherapy: Initiate at 1200 mg/day in divided doses 3 or 4 times/day, reduce the dosage of the concomitant anticonvulsant(s) by 20% to 33% at the initiation of felbamate therapy; at week 2, increase the felbamate dosage to 2400 mg/day while reducing the dosage of the other anticonvulsant(s) up to an additional 33% of their original dosage; at week 3, increase the felbamate dosage up to 3600 mg/day and continue to reduce the dosage of the other anticonvulsant(s) as clinically indicated

(Continued)

felbamate *(Continued)*

Adjunctive therapy: Children with Lennox-Gastaut and ages 2-14 years:
Week 1:
  Felbamate: 15 mg/kg/day divided 3-4 times/day
  Concomitant anticonvulsant(s): Reduce original dosage by 20% to 30%
Week 2:
  Felbamate: 30 mg/kg/day divided 3-4 times/day
  Concomitant anticonvulsant(s): Reduce original dosage up to an additional 33%
Week 3:
  Felbamate: 45 mg/kg/day divided 3-4 times/day
  Concomitant anticonvulsant(s): Reduce dosage as clinically indicated
Adjunctive therapy: Children >14 years and Adults:
Week 1:
  Felbamate: 1200 mg/day initial dose
  Concomitant anticonvulsant(s): Reduce original dosage by 20% to 33%
Week 2:
  Felbamate: 2400 mg/day (therapeutic range)
  Concomitant anticonvulsant(s): Reduce original dosage by up to an additional 33%
Week 3:
  Felbamate: 3600 mg/day (therapeutic range)
  Concomitant anticonvulsant(s): Reduce original dosage as clinically indicated
Dosage Forms
  Suspension, oral:
    Felbatol®: 600 mg/5 mL
  Tablet:
    Felbatol®: 400 mg

Felbatol® [US] *see* felbamate *on previous page*

Feldene® [US] *see* piroxicam *on page 687*

felodipine (fe LOE di peen)

Sound-Alike/Look-Alike Issues
  Plendil® may be confused with Isordil®, pindolol, Pletal®, Prilosec®, Prinivil®
U.S./Canadian Brand Names Plendil® [US/Can]; Renedil® [Can]
Therapeutic Category Calcium Channel Blocker
Use Treatment of hypertension
Usual Dosage Oral: Adults: 2.5-10 mg once daily; usual initial dose: 5 mg; increase by 5 mg at 2-week intervals, as needed, to a maximum of 20 mg/day
  Usual dose range (JNC 7) for hypertension: 2.5-20 mg once daily
Dosage Forms
  Tablet, extended release:
    Plendil®: 2.5 mg, 5 mg, 10 mg

felodipine and enalapril *see* enalapril and felodipine *on page 296*

Femara® [US/Can] *see* letrozole *on page 496*

Fematrol [US-OTC] *see* bisacodyl *on page 112*

Femcet® *(Discontinued)*

Femcon™ Fe [US] *see* ethinyl estradiol and norethindrone *on page 328*

Femguard® *(Discontinued)* *see* sulfabenzamide, sulfacetamide, and sulfathiazole *on page 810*

femhrt® [US/Can] *see* ethinyl estradiol and norethindrone *on page 328*

Femilax™ [US-OTC] *see* bisacodyl *on page 112*

Femiron® [US-OTC] *see* ferrous fumarate *on page 349*

Fem-Prin® [US-OTC] *see* acetaminophen, aspirin, and caffeine *on page 9*

Femring® [US] *see* estradiol *on page 313*

Femstat® One [Can] *see* butoconazole *on page 132*

Femtrace® [US] *see* estradiol *on page 313*

fenofibrate (fen oh FYE brate)

Synonyms procetofene; proctofene

U.S./Canadian Brand Names Antara™ [US]; Apo-Feno-Micro® [Can]; Apo-Fenofibrate® [Can]; Dom-Fenofibrate Supra [Can]; Gen-Fenofibrate Micro [Can]; Lipidil EZ® [Can]; Lipidil Micro® [Can]; Lipidil Supra® [Can]; Lipofen™ [US]; Lofibra™ [US]; Novo-Fenofibrate [Can]; Novo-Fenofibrate-S [Can]; Nu-Fenofibrate [Can]; PHL-Fenofibrate Supra [Can]; PMS-Fenofibrate Micro [Can]; PMS-Fenofibrate Supra [Can]; ratio-Fenofibrate MC [Can]; Sandoz Fenofibrate S [Can]; TriCor® [US/Can]; Triglide™ [US]

Therapeutic Category Antihyperlipidemic Agent, Miscellaneous

Use Adjunct to dietary therapy for the treatment of adults with elevations of serum triglyceride levels (types IV and V hyperlipidemia); adjunct to dietary therapy for the reduction of low density lipoprotein cholesterol (LDL-C), total cholesterol (total-C), triglycerides, and apolipoprotein B (apo B) in adult patients with primary hypercholesterolemia or mixed dyslipidemia (Fredrickson types IIa and IIb)

Usual Dosage Oral:

Adults:

Hypertriglyceridemia: Initial:

Antara™: 43-130 mg/day

Lipofen™: 50-150 mg/day; maximum dose: 150 mg/day

Lofibra™: 67 mg/day with meals, up to 200 mg/day

TriCor®: 48 mg/day, up to 145 mg/day

Triglide™: 50-160 mg/day

Hypercholesterolemia or mixed hyperlipidemia:

Antara™: 130 mg/day

Lipofen™: 150 mg/day

Lofibra™: 200 mg/day with meals

TriCor®: 145 mg/day

Triglide™: 160 mg/day

Dosage Forms

Capsule:

Lipofen™: 50 mg, 100 mg, 150 mg

Capsule [micronized]: 67 mg, 134 mg, 200 mg

Antara™: 43 mg, 130 mg

Lofibra™: 67 mg, 134 mg, 200 mg

Tablet: 54 mg, 160 mg

TriCor®: 48 mg, 145 mg

Triglide™: 50 mg, 160 mg

fenoldopam (fe NOL doe pam)

Synonyms fenoldopam mesylate

U.S./Canadian Brand Names Corlopam® [US/Can]

Therapeutic Category Antihypertensive Agent

Use Treatment of severe hypertension (up to 48 hours in adults), including in patients with renal compromise; short-term (up to 4 hours) blood pressure reduction in pediatric patients

Usual Dosage I.V.: Hypertension, severe:

Children: Initial: 0.2 mcg/kg/minute; may be increased to dosages of 0.3-0.5 mcg/kg/minute every 20-30 minutes (maximum dose: 0.8 mcg/kg/minute); limited to short-term (4 hours) use

Adults: Initial: 0.1-0.3 mcg/kg/minute (lower initial doses may be associated with less reflex tachycardia); may be increased in increments of 0.05-0.1 mcg/kg/minute every 15 minutes until target blood pressure is reached; the maximal infusion rate reported in clinical studies was 1.6 mcg/kg/minute

Dosage Forms

Injection, solution: 10 mg/mL (1 mL, 2 mL)

Corlopam®: 10 mg/mL (1 mL, 2 mL)

fenoldopam mesylate see fenoldopam on this page

fenoprofen (fen oh PROE fen)

Sound-Alike/Look-Alike Issues

fenoprofen may be confused with flurbiprofen

Nalfon® may be confused with Naldecon®

Synonyms fenoprofen calcium

U.S./Canadian Brand Names Nalfon® [US/Can]

Therapeutic Category Analgesic, Nonnarcotic; Nonsteroidal Antiinflammatory Drug (NSAID)

Use Symptomatic treatment of acute and chronic rheumatoid arthritis and osteoarthritis; relief of mild to moderate pain

Usual Dosage Oral: Adults:

Rheumatoid arthritis: 300-600 mg 3-4 times/day up to 3.2 g/day

(Continued)

fenoprofen *(Continued)*

Mild to moderate pain: 200 mg every 4-6 hours as needed
Dosage Forms
Capsule:
Nalfon®: 200 mg
Tablet: 600 mg

fenoprofen calcium *see* fenoprofen *on previous page*

fenoterol *(Canada only)* (fen oh TER ole)

Synonyms fenoterol hydrobromide
U.S./Canadian Brand Names Berotec® [Can]
Therapeutic Category Beta$_2$-Adrenergic Agonist Agent
Use Treatment and prevention of symptoms of reversible obstructive pulmonary disease (including asthma and acute bronchospasm), chronic bronchitis, emphysema
Usual Dosage Inhalation: Children ≥12 years of age and Adults:
MDI:
Acute treatment: 1 puff initially; may repeat in 5 minutes; if relief is not evident, additional doses and/or other therapy may be necessary
Intermittent/long-term treatment: 1-2 puffs 3-4 times/day (maximum of 8 puffs/24 hours)
Solution: 0.5-1 mg (up to maximum of 2.5 mg)
Dosage Forms [CAN] = Canadian brand name
Aerosol for inhalation: MDI:
Berotec® [CAN]: 100 mcg/dose [not available in the U.S.]
Solution for inhalation:
Berotec® [CAN] 0.625 mg/mL (2 mL); 0.25 mg/mL (2 mL) [not available in the U.S.]

fenoterol hydrobromide *see* fenoterol *(Canada only) on this page*

fentanyl (FEN ta nil)

Sound-Alike/Look-Alike Issues
fentanyl may be confused with alfentanil, sufentanil
Synonyms fentanyl citrate; fentanyl hydrochloride; OTFC (oral transmucosal fentanyl citrate)
U.S./Canadian Brand Names Actiq® [US/Can]; Duragesic® [US/Can]; Fentanyl Citrate Injection, USP [Can]; Fentora™ [US]; Ionsys™ [US]; Sublimaze® [US]
Therapeutic Category Analgesic, Narcotic; General Anesthetic
Controlled Substance C-II
Use
Injection: Sedation, relief of pain, preoperative medication, adjunct to general or regional anesthesia
Iontophoretic transdermal system (Ionsys™): Short-term in-hospital management of acute postoperative pain
Transdermal patch (eg, Duragesic®): Management of moderate-to-severe chronic pain
Transmucosal lozenge (eg, Actiq®), buccal tablet (Fentora™): Management of breakthrough cancer pain
Usual Dosage Note: These are guidelines and do not represent the maximum doses that may be required in all patients. Doses should be titrated to pain relief/prevention. Monitor vital signs routinely. Single I.M. doses have a duration of 1-2 hours, single I.V. doses last 0.5-1 hour.
Sedation for minor procedures/analgesia:
Children 1-12 years:
Sedation for minor procedures/analgesia: I.M., I.V.: 1-2 mcg/kg/dose; may repeat at 30- to 60-minute intervals. **Note:** Children 18-36 months of age may require 2-3 mcg/kg/dose
Continuous sedation/analgesia: Initial I.V. bolus: 1-2 mcg/kg; then 1-3 mcg/kg/hour to a maximum dose of 5 mcg/kg/hour
Children >12 years and Adults: I.V.: 25-50 mcg; may repeat every 3-5 minutes to desired effect or adverse event; maximum dose of 500 mcg/4 hours; higher doses are used for major procedures
Surgery: Adults:
Premedication: I.M., slow I.V.: 25-100 mcg/dose 30-60 minutes prior to surgery
Adjunct to regional anesthesia: Slow I.V.: 25-100 mcg/dose over 1-2 minutes. **Note:** An I.V. should be in place with regional anesthesia so the I.M. route is rarely used but still maintained as an option in the package labeling.
Adjunct to general anesthesia: Slow I.V.:
Low dose: 0.5-2 mcg/kg/dose depending on the indication. For example, 0.5 mcg/kg will provide analgesia or reduce the amount of propofol needed for laryngeal mask airway insertion with minimal respiratory depression. However, to blunt the hemodynamic response to intubation 2 mcg/kg is often necessary.
Moderate dose: Initial: 2-15 mcg/kg/dose; Maintenance (bolus or infusion): 1-2 mcg/kg/hour. Discontinuing fentanyl infusion 30-60 minutes prior to the end of surgery will usually allow adequate ventilation upon

emergence from anesthesia. For "fast-tracking" and early extubation following major surgery, total fentanyl doses are limited to 10-15 mcg/kg.

High dose: **Note:** High-dose (20-50 mcg/kg/dose) fentanyl is rarely used, but is still maintained in the package labeling.

Acute pain management: Adults:

Severe: I.M, I.V.: 50-100 mcg/dose every 1-2 hours as needed; patients with prior opiate exposure may tolerate higher initial doses

Patient-controlled analgesia (PCA): I.V.: Usual concentration: 10 mcg/mL

Demand dose: Usual: 10 mcg; range: 10-50 mcg

Lockout interval: 5-8 minutes

Mechanically-ventilated patients (based on 70 kg patient): Slow I.V.: 0.35-1.5 mcg/kg every 30-60 minutes as needed; infusion: 0.7-10 mcg/kg/hour

Iontophoretic transdermal system: 40 mcg per activation on-demand (maximum: 6 doses/hour). **Note:** Patient's pain should be controlled prior to initiating system. Instruct patient how to operate system. Only the patient should initiate system. Each system operates for 24 hours or until 80 doses have been administered, whichever comes first.

Breakthrough cancer pain: For patients who are tolerant to and currently receiving opioid therapy for persistent cancer pain; dosing should be individually titrated to provide adequate analgesia with minimal side effects. Dose titration should be done if patient requires more than 1 dose/breakthrough pain episode for several consecutive episodes. Patients experiencing >4 breakthrough pain episodes/day should have the dose of their long-term opioid re-evaluated.

Children ≥16 years and Adults: Lozenge: Initial dose: 200 mcg; the second dose may be started 15 minutes after completion of the first dose. Consumption should be limited to ≤4 units/day.

Adults: Buccal tablet (Fentora™): Initial dose: 100 mcg; a second 100 mcg dose, if needed, may be started 30 minutes after the start of the first dose. **Note:** For patients previously using the transmucosal lozenge (Actiq®), the initial dose should be selected using the conversions listed below (maximum: 2 doses per breakthrough pain episode every 4 hours).

Dose titration, if required, should be done using multiples of the 100 mcg tablets. Patient can take two 100 mcg tablets (one on each side of mouth). If that dose is not successful, can use four 100 mcg tablets (two on each side of mouth). If titration requires >400 mcg/dose, then use 200 mcg tablets.

Conversion from lozenge to buccal tablet (Fentora™):

Lozenge dose 200-400 mcg, then buccal tablet 100 mcg

Lozenge dose 600-800 mcg, then buccal tablet 200 mcg

Lozenge dose 1200-1600 mcg, then buccal tablet 400 mcg

Note: Four 100 mcg buccal tablets deliver approximately 12% and 13% higher values of C_{max} and AUC, respectively, compared to one 400 mcg buccal tablet. To prevent confusion, patient should only have one strength available at a time. Using more than four buccal tablets at a time has not been studied.

Chronic pain management: Children ≥2 years and Adults (opioid-tolerant patients): Transdermal patch (eg, Duragesic®):

Initial: To convert patients from oral or parenteral opioids to transdermal patch, a 24-hour analgesic requirement should be calculated (based on prior opiate use). The initial fentanyl dosage may be approximated from the 24-hour morphine dosage and titrated to minimize adverse effects and provide analgesia. With the initial application, the absorption of transdermal fentanyl requires several hours to reach plateau; therefore transdermal fentanyl is inappropriate for management of acute pain. Change patch every 72 hours.

Conversion from continuous infusion of fentanyl: In patients who have adequate pain relief with a fentanyl infusion, fentanyl may be converted to transdermal dosing at a rate equivalent to the intravenous rate. A two-step taper of the infusion to be completed over 12 hours has been recommended after the patch is applied. The infusion is decreased to 50% of the original rate six hours after the application of the first patch, and subsequently discontinued twelve hours after application.

Titration: Short-acting agents may be required until analgesic efficacy is established and/or as supplements for "breakthrough" pain. The amount of supplemental doses should be closely monitored. Appropriate dosage increases may be based on daily supplemental dosage using the ratio of 45 mg/24 hours of oral morphine to a 12.5 mcg/hour increase in fentanyl dosage.

Frequency of adjustment: The dosage should not be titrated more frequently than every 3 days after the initial dose or every 6 days thereafter. Patients should wear a consistent fentanyl dosage through two applications (6 days) before dosage increase based on supplemental opiate dosages can be estimated.

Frequency of application: The majority of patients may be controlled on every 72-hour administration; however, a small number of patients require every 48-hour administration.

Dosage Forms

Infusion [premixed in NS]: 0.05 mg (10 mL); 1 mg (100 mL); 1.25 mg (250 mL); 2 mg (100 mL); 2.5 mg (250 mL)

Injection, solution [preservative free]: 0.05 mg/mL (2 mL, 5 mL, 10 mL, 20 mL, 30 mL, 50 mL)

Sublimaze®: 0.05 mg/mL (2 mL, 5 mL, 10 mL, 20 mL)

Lozenge, oral [transmucosal]: 200 mcg, 400 mcg, 600 mcg, 800 mcg, 1200 mcg, 1600 mcg

(Continued)

fentanyl *(Continued)*

Actiq®: 200 mcg, 400 mcg, 600 mcg, 800 mcg, 1200 mcg, 1600 mcg [mounted on a plastic radiopaque handle; contains sugar 2 g/unit; raspberry flavor]

Tablet, for buccal application:

Fentora™: 100 mcg, 200 mcg, 300 mcg, 400 mcg, 600 mcg, 800 mcg

Transdermal system, topical: 12 (5s) [delivers 12.5 mcg/hour; 3.13 cm^2]; 12 (5s) [delivers 12.5 mcg/hour; 5 cm^2]; 25 (5s) [delivers 25 mcg/hour; 10 cm^2]; 25 (5s) [delivers 25 mcg/hour; 6.25 cm^2]; 50 (5s) [delivers 50 mcg/hour; 12.5 cm^2]; 50 (5s) [delivers 50 mcg/hour; 20 cm^2]; 75 (5s) [delivers 75 mcg/hour; 18.75 cm^2]; 75 (5s) [delivers 75 mcg/hour; 30 cm^2]; 100 (5s) [delivers 100 mcg/hour; 25 cm^2]; 100 (5s) [delivers 100 mcg/hour; 40 cm^2]

Duragesic®: 12 [delivers 12.5 mcg/hour; 5 cm^2] (5s); 25 [delivers 25 mcg/hour; 10 cm^2] (5s); 50 [delivers 50 mcg/hour; 20 cm^2] (5s); 75 [delivers 75 mcg/hour; 30 cm^2] (5s); 100 [delivers 100 mcg/hour; 40 cm^2] (5s)

Transdermal iontophoretic system, topical:

Ionsys™: Fentanyl 40 mcg/dose [80 doses/patch; contains 3-volt lithium battery]

fentanyl citrate *see* fentanyl *on page 346*

Fentanyl Citrate Injection, USP [Can] *see* fentanyl *on page 346*

fentanyl hydrochloride *see* fentanyl *on page 346*

Fentanyl Oralet® *(Discontinued)* *see* fentanyl *on page 346*

Fentora™ [US] *see* fentanyl *on page 346*

Feosol® [US-OTC] *see* ferrous sulfate *on page 350*

Feosol® Elixir *(Discontinued)* *see* ferrous sulfate *on page 350*

Feostat® *(Discontinued)* *see* ferrous fumarate *on next page*

Ferancee® *(Discontinued)* *see* ferrous sulfate and ascorbic acid *on page 350*

Feratab® [US-OTC] *see* ferrous sulfate *on page 350*

Fer-Gen-Sol [US-OTC] *see* ferrous sulfate *on page 350*

Fergon® [US-OTC] *see* ferrous gluconate *on next page*

Feridex I.V.® [US] *see* ferumoxides *on page 350*

Fer-In-Sol® [US-OTC/Can] *see* ferrous sulfate *on page 350*

Fer-In-Sol® Syrup *(Discontinued)* *see* ferrous sulfate *on page 350*

Fer-Iron® [US-OTC] *see* ferrous sulfate *on page 350*

Fermalac [Can] *see* Lactobacillus *on page 488*

Ferodan™ [Can] *see* ferrous sulfate *on page 350*

Fero-Grad 500® [US-OTC] *see* ferrous sulfate and ascorbic acid *on page 350*

Fero-Gradumet® *(Discontinued)* *see* ferrous sulfate *on page 350*

Ferospace® *(Discontinued)* *see* ferrous sulfate *on page 350*

Ferralet® *(Discontinued)* *see* ferrous gluconate *on next page*

Ferralyn® Lanacaps® *(Discontinued)* *see* ferrous sulfate *on page 350*

Ferra-TD® *(Discontinued)* *see* ferrous sulfate *on page 350*

Ferretts [US-OTC] *see* ferrous fumarate *on next page*

Ferrex 150 [US-OTC] *see* polysaccharide-iron complex *on page 697*

ferric (III) hexacyanoferrate (II) *see* ferric hexacyanoferrate *on next page*

ferric gluconate *(FER ik GLOO koe nate)*

Sound-Alike/Look-Alike Issues

Ferrlecit® may be confused with Ferralet®

Synonyms sodium ferric gluconate

U.S./Canadian Brand Names Ferrlecit® [US/Can]

Therapeutic Category Iron Salt

Use Repletion of total body iron content in patients with iron-deficiency anemia who are undergoing hemodialysis in conjunction with erythropoietin therapy

Usual Dosage I.V.: Repletion of iron in hemodialysis patients:

Children ≥6 years: 1.5 mg/kg of elemental iron (maximum: 125 mg/dose) diluted in NS 25 mL, administered over 60 minutes at 8 sequential dialysis sessions

Adults: 125 mg elemental iron per 10 mL (either by I.V. infusion or slow I.V. injection). Most patients will require a cumulative dose of 1 g elemental iron over approximately 8 sequential dialysis treatments to achieve a favorable response.

Note: A test dose of 2 mL diluted in NS 50 mL administered over 60 minutes was previously recommended (not in current manufacturer labeling). Doses >125 mg are associated with increased adverse events.

Dosage Forms
Injection, solution:
Ferrlecit®: Elemental iron 12.5 mg/mL (5 mL)

ferric hexacyanoferrate (FER ik hex a SYE an oh fer ate)

Synonyms ferric (III) hexacyanoferrate (II); insoluble prussian blue; prussian blue
U.S./Canadian Brand Names Radiogardase™ [US]
Therapeutic Category Antidote
Use Treatment of known or suspected internal contamination with radioactive cesium and/or radioactive or nonradioactive thallium
Usual Dosage Oral: Internal contamination with radioactive cesium and/or radioactive or nonradioactive thallium:
Children 2-12 years: 1 g 3 times/day; treatment should begin as soon as possible following exposure, but is also effective if therapy is delayed
Children >12 years and Adults: 3 g 3 times/day; treatment should begin as soon as possible following exposure, but is also effective if therapy is delayed
Note: Cesium exposure: Once internal radioactivity is substantially decreased, dosage may be reduced to 1-2 g 3 times/day to improve gastrointestinal tolerance
Dosage Forms
Capsule:
Radiogardase™: 0.5 g

Ferrlecit® **[US/Can]** *see* ferric gluconate *on previous page*

Ferro-Sequels® **[US-OTC]** *see* ferrous fumarate *on this page*

ferrous fumarate (FER us FYOO ma rate)

Sound-Alike/Look-Alike Issues
Feostat® may be confused with Feosol®
Synonyms iron fumarate
U.S./Canadian Brand Names Femiron® [US-OTC]; Ferretts [US-OTC]; Ferro-Sequels® [US-OTC]; Hemocyte® [US-OTC]; Ircon® [US-OTC]; Nephro-Fer® [US-OTC]; Palafer® [Can]
Therapeutic Category Electrolyte Supplement, Oral
Use Prevention and treatment of iron-deficiency anemias
Usual Dosage Oral **(dose expressed in terms of elemental iron):**
Children:
Severe iron-deficiency anemia: 4-6 mg Fe/kg/day in 3 divided doses
Mild to moderate iron deficiency anemia: 3 mg Fe/kg/day in 1-2 divided doses
Prophylaxis: 1-2 mg Fe/kg/day
Adults:
Iron deficiency: 60-100 mg twice daily up to 60 mg 2 times/day
Prophylaxis: 60-100 mg/day
To avoid GI upset, start with a single daily dose and increase by 1 tablet/day each week or as tolerated until desired daily dose is achieved
Dosage Forms
Tablet: 324 mg
Femiron® [OTC]: 63 mg
Ferretts [OTC]: 325 mg
Hemocyte® [OTC]: 324 mg
Ircon® [OTC]: 200 mg
Nephro-Fer® [OTC]: 350 mg
Tablet, timed release:
Ferro-Sequels® [OTC]: 150 mg

ferrous gluconate (FER us GLOO koe nate)

Synonyms iron gluconate
U.S./Canadian Brand Names Apo-Ferrous Gluconate® [Can]; Fergon® [US-OTC]; Novo-Ferrogluc [Can]
Therapeutic Category Electrolyte Supplement, Oral
Use Prevention and treatment of iron-deficiency anemias
(Continued)

ferrous gluconate *(Continued)*

Usual Dosage Oral **(dose expressed in terms of elemental iron):**
Children:
Severe iron-deficiency anemia: 4-6 mg Fe/kg/day in 3 divided doses
Mild to moderate iron deficiency anemia: 3 mg Fe/kg/day in 1-2 divided doses
Prophylaxis: 1-2 mg Fe/kg/day
Adults:
Iron deficiency: 60 mg twice daily up to 60 mg 4 times/day
Prophylaxis: 60 mg/day
Dosage Forms
Tablet: 246 mg, 300 mg, 325 mg
Fergon® [OTC]: 240 mg

ferrous sulfate *(FER us SUL fate)*

Sound-Alike/Look-Alike Issues
Feosol® may be confused with Feostat®, Fer-In-Sol®
Fer-In-Sol® may be confused with Feosol®
Slow FE® may be confused with Slow-K®
Synonyms $FeSO_4$; iron sulfate
U.S./Canadian Brand Names Apo-Ferrous Sulfate® [Can]; Feosol® [US-OTC]; Fer-Gen-Sol [US-OTC]; Fer-In-Sol® [US-OTC/Can]; Fer-Iron® [US-OTC]; Feratab® [US-OTC]; Ferodan™ [Can]; Slow FE® [US-OTC]
Therapeutic Category Electrolyte Supplement, Oral
Use Prevention and treatment of iron-deficiency anemias
Usual Dosage Oral:
Children **(dose expressed in terms of elemental iron):**
Severe iron-deficiency anemia: 4-6 mg Fe/kg/day in 3 divided doses
Mild to moderate iron deficiency anemia: 3 mg Fe/kg/day in 1-2 divided doses
Prophylaxis: 1-2 mg Fe/kg/day up to a maximum of 15 mg/day
Adults **(dose expressed in terms of ferrous sulfate):**
Iron deficiency: 300 mg twice daily up to 300 mg 4 times/day or 250 mg (extended release) 1-2 times/day
Prophylaxis: 300 mg/day
Dosage Forms
Elixir: 220 mg/5 mL
Liquid, oral drops: 75 mg/0.6 mL
Fer-Gen-Sol [OTC], Fer-In-Sol® [OTC], Fer-Iron® [OTC]: 75 mg/0.6 mL
Tablet: 324 mg, 325 mg
Feratab® [OTC]: 300 mg
Tablet, exsiccated: 200 mg
Feosol® [OTC]: 200 mg
Tablet, exsiccated, timed release: 160 mg
Slow FE® [OTC]: 160 mg

ferrous sulfate and ascorbic acid *(FER us SUL fate & a SKOR bik AS id)*

Synonyms ascorbic acid and ferrous sulfate; iron sulfate and vitamin C
U.S./Canadian Brand Names Fero-Grad 500® [US-OTC]
Therapeutic Category Vitamin
Use Treatment of iron deficiency in nonpregnant adults; treatment and prevention of iron deficiency in pregnant adults
Usual Dosage Oral: Adults: 1 tablet daily
Dosage Forms
Tablet, controlled release:
Fero-Grad 500® [OTC]: Ferrous sulfate 525 mg and ascorbic acid 500 mg

Fertinorm® H.P. [Can] *see* urofollitropin *on page 878*

ferumoxides *(fer yoo MOX ides)*

Sound-Alike/Look-Alike Issues
Feridex I.V.® may be confused with Fertinex®
U.S./Canadian Brand Names Feridex I.V.® [US]
Therapeutic Category Radiopaque Agents
Use For I.V. administration as an adjunct to MRI (in adult patients) to enhance the T2 weighted images used in the detection and evaluation of lesions of the liver
Usual Dosage Adults: 0.56 mg of iron (0.05 mL Feridex I.V.®)/kg body weight diluted in 100 mL of 5% dextrose and infused over 30 minutes; a 5-micron filter is recommended; do not administer undiluted

Dosage Forms
Injection, solution:
Feridex I.V.®: Iron 11.2 mg/mL (5 mL)

FeSO₄ *see* ferrous sulfate *on previous page*

Fe-Tinic™ **150 (*Discontinued*)** *see* polysaccharide-iron complex *on page 697*

FeverAll® [US-OTC] *see* acetaminophen *on page 5*

Fexmid™ **[US]** *see* cyclobenzaprine *on page 221*

fexofenadine (feks oh FEN a deen)
Sound-Alike/Look-Alike Issues
Allegra® may be confused with Viagra®
Synonyms fexofenadine hydrochloride
U.S./Canadian Brand Names Allegra® [US/Can]
Therapeutic Category Antihistamine
Use Relief of symptoms associated with seasonal allergic rhinitis; treatment of chronic idiopathic urticaria
Usual Dosage Oral:
Chronic idiopathic urticaria: Children 6 months to <2 years: 15 mg twice daily
Chronic idiopathic urticaria, seasonal allergic rhinitis:
Children 2-11 years: 30 mg twice daily
Children ≥12 years and Adults: 60 mg twice daily **or** 180 mg once daily
Dosage Forms
Suspension:
Allegra®: 6 mg/mL
Tablet: 30 mg, 60 mg, 180 mg
Allegra®: 30 mg, 60 mg, 180 mg

fexofenadine and pseudoephedrine (feks oh FEN a deen & soo doe e FED rin)
Sound-Alike/Look-Alike Issues
Allegra-D® may be confused with Viagra®
Synonyms pseudoephedrine and fexofenadine
U.S./Canadian Brand Names Allegra-D® 12 Hour [US]; Allegra-D® 24 Hour [US]; Allegra-D® [Can]
Therapeutic Category Antihistamine/Decongestant Combination
Use Relief of symptoms associated with seasonal allergic rhinitis in adults and children ≥12 years of age
Usual Dosage Oral: Children ≥12 years and Adults:
Allegra-D® 12 Hour: One tablet twice daily
Allegra-D® 24 Hour: One tablet once daily
Dosage Forms
Tablet, extended release:
Allegra-D® 12 Hour: Fexofenadine 60 mg [immediate release] and pseudoephedrine 120 mg [extended release]
Allegra-D® 24 Hour: Fexofenadine 180 mg [immediate release] and pseudoephedrine 240 mg [extended release]

fexofenadine hydrochloride *see* fexofenadine *on this page*

Fiberall® [US] *see* psyllium *on page 732*

FiberCon® [US-OTC] *see* polycarbophil *on page 694*

Fiber-Lax® [US-OTC] *see* polycarbophil *on page 694*

Fiber-Tabs™ **[US-OTC]** *see* polycarbophil *on page 694*

fibrin sealant (human) *see* fibrin sealant kit *on this page*

fibrin sealant kit (FI brin SEEL ent kit)
Synonyms fibrin sealant (human); FS
U.S./Canadian Brand Names Evicel™ [US]; Tisseel® VH [US/Can]
Therapeutic Category Hemostatic Agent
Use
Evicel™: Adjunct to hemostasis in liver or vascular surgery when control of bleeding by conventional surgical techniques is ineffective or impractical
Tisseel® VH: Adjunct to hemostasis in cardiopulmonary bypass surgery and splenic injury (due to blunt or penetrating trauma to the abdomen) when the control of bleeding by conventional surgical techniques is ineffective or impractical; adjunctive sealant for closure of colostomies; hemostatic agent in heparinized patients undergoing cardiopulmonary bypass
(Continued)

fibrin sealant kit *(Continued)*

Usual Dosage Adjunct to hemostasis: Apply topically; actual dose is based on size of surface to be covered:

Evicel™: Children and Adults: Spray or drop onto surface of bleeding tissue in short bursts (0.1-0.2 mL); if hemostatic effect is not complete, apply a second layer. To cover a layer of 1 mm thickness:
Maximum area to be sealed: 20 cm^2
Required size of Evicel™ kit: 2 mL
Maximum area to be sealed: 40 cm^2
Required size of Evicel™ kit: 4 mL
Maximum area to be sealed: 100 cm^2
Required size of Evicel™ kit: 10 mL

Tisseel® VH: Adults: Apply in thin layers to avoid excess formation of granulation tissue and slow absorption of the sealant. Following application, hold the sealed parts in the desired position for 3-5 minutes. To prevent sealant from adhering to gloves or surgical instruments, wet them with saline prior to contact.
Maximum area to be sealed: 8 cm^2
Required package size of Tisseel® VH: 2 mL
Maximum area to be sealed: 16 cm^2
Required package size of Tisseel® VH: 4 mL
Maximum area to be sealed: 40 cm^2
Required package size of Tisseel® VH: 10 mL

Dosage Forms

Topical: Kit:
Evicel™ [preservative free; each 2 mL kit contains]:
Solution, topical: Fibrinogen 55-85 mg/mL (1 mL)
Solution, topical: Thrombin 800-1200 int. units/mL and calcium chloride 5.6-6.2 mg/mL (1 mL)
Evicel™ [preservative free; each 4 mL kit contains]:
Solution, topical: Fibrinogen 55-85 mg/mL (2 mL)
Solution, topical: Thrombin 800-1200 int. units/mL and calcium chloride 5.6-6.2 mg/mL (2 mL)
Evicel™ [preservative free; each 10 mL kit contains]:
Solution, topical: Fibrinogen 55-85 mg/mL (5 mL)
Solution, topical: Thrombin 800-1200 int. units/mL and calcium chloride 5.6-6.2 mg/mL (5 mL)
Tisseel® VH [each 2 mL, 4 mL, or 10 mL kit contains]:
Powder, for solution, topical: Fibrinogen 67-106 mg/mL
Powder, for solution, topical: Thrombin 400-625 int. units/mL
Solution, topical: Calcium chloride 36-44 μmol/mL
Solution, topical: Aprotinin 2250-3750 KIU/mL
Tisseel® VH [each dual-chamber 2 mL, 4 mL, or 10 mL prefilled syringe contains]:
Solution, topical:
Sealer protein chamber: Fibrinogen 67-106 mg/mL and aprotinin 2250-3750 KIU/mL
Thrombin chamber: Thrombin 400-625 int. units/mL and calcium chloride 36-44 μmol/mL

Fibro-XL [US-OTC] *see* psyllium *on page 732*

Fibro-Lax [US-OTC] *see* psyllium *on page 732*

filgrastim *(fil GRA stim)*

Sound-Alike/Look-Alike Issues
Neupogen® may be confused with Epogen®, Neumega®, Neupro®, Nutramigen®

Synonyms G-CSF; granulocyte colony stimulating factor; NSC-614629

U.S./Canadian Brand Names Neupogen® [US/Can]

Therapeutic Category Colony-Stimulating Factor

Use Stimulation of granulocyte production in chemotherapy-induced neutropenia (nonmyeloid malignancies, acute myeloid leukemia, and bone marrow transplantation); severe chronic neutropenia (SCN); patients undergoing peripheral blood progenitor cell (PBPC) collection

Usual Dosage Refer to individual protocols.

Dosing, even in morbidly obese patients, should be based on actual body weight. Rounding doses to the nearest vial size often enhances patient convenience and reduces costs without compromising clinical response.

Children and Adults:
Chemotherapy-induced neutropenia: SubQ, I.V.: 5 mcg/kg/day; doses may be increased by 5 mcg/kg according to the duration and severity of the neutropenia; continue for up to 14 days or until the ANC reaches 10,000/mm^3
Bone marrow transplantation: SubQ, I.V.: 10 mcg/kg/day; adjust the dose according to the duration and severity of neutropenia; recommended steps based on neutrophil response:
When ANC >1000/mm^3 for 3 consecutive days: Reduce filgrastim dose to 5 mcg/kg/day
If ANC remains >1000/mm^3 for 3 more consecutive days: Discontinue filgrastim

If ANC decreases to <1000/mm^3: Resume at 5 mcg/kg/day
If ANC decreases <1000/mm^3 during the 5 mcg/kg/day dose, increase filgrastim to 10 mcg/kg/day and follow the above steps
Peripheral blood progenitor cell (PBPC) collection: SubQ: 10 mcg/kg daily in donors, usually for 6-7 days. Begin at least 4 days before the first leukopheresis and continue until the last leukopheresis; consider dose adjustment for WBC >100,000/mm^3
Severe chronic neutropenia: SubQ:
  Congenital: 6 mcg/kg twice daily; adjust the dose based on ANC and clinical response
  Idiopathic/cyclic: 5 mcg/kg/day; adjust the dose based on ANC and clinical response
Dosage Forms
  Injection, solution [preservative free]:
    Neupogen®: 300 mcg/mL (1 mL, 1.6 mL) [vial]; 600 mcg/mL (0.5 mL, 0.8 mL) [prefilled Singleject® syringe]

Finacea® [US/Can] *see* azelaic acid *on page 88*

finasteride (fi NAS teer ide)
Sound-Alike/Look-Alike Issues
  Proscar® may be confused with ProSom®, Prozac®, Psorcon®
U.S./Canadian Brand Names Propecia® [US/Can]; Proscar® [US/Can]
Therapeutic Category Antiandrogen
Use
  Propecia®: Treatment of male pattern hair loss in **men only**. Safety and efficacy were demonstrated in men between 18-41 years of age.
  Proscar®: Treatment of symptomatic benign prostatic hyperplasia (BPH); can be used in combination with an alpha-blocker, doxazosin
Usual Dosage Oral: Adults: Male:
  Benign prostatic hyperplasia (Proscar®): 5 mg/day as a single dose; clinical responses occur within 12 weeks to 6 months of initiation of therapy; long-term administration is recommended for maximal response
  Male pattern baldness (Propecia®): 1 mg daily
Dosage Forms
  Tablet: 5 mg
    Propecia®: 1 mg
    Proscar®: 5 mg

Fiorgen PF® *(Discontinued)*

Fioricet® [US] *see* butalbital, acetaminophen, and caffeine *on page 130*

Fioricet® with Codeine [US] *see* butalbital, acetaminophen, caffeine, and codeine *on page 130*

Fiorinal® [US/Can] *see* butalbital, aspirin, and caffeine *on page 131*

Fiorinal®-C 1/2 [Can] *see* butalbital, aspirin, caffeine, and codeine *on page 131*

Fiorinal®-C 1/4 [Can] *see* butalbital, aspirin, caffeine, and codeine *on page 131*

Fiorinal® With Codeine [US] *see* butalbital, aspirin, caffeine, and codeine *on page 131*

First® Testosterone [US] *see* testosterone *on page 828*

First® Testosterone MC [US] *see* testosterone *on page 828*

fisalamine *see* mesalamine *on page 546*

fish oil *see* omega-3-acid ethyl esters *on page 629*

FK506 *see* tacrolimus *on page 818*

Flagyl® [US/Can] *see* metronidazole *on page 563*

Flagyl ER® [US] *see* metronidazole *on page 563*

Flagystatin® [Can] *see* metronidazole and nystatin *(Canada only) on page 564*

Flamazine® [Can] *see* silver sulfadiazine *on page 786*

Flarex® [US/Can] *see* fluorometholone *on page 363*

flavan *see* flavocoxid *on this page*

flavocoxid (fla vo KOKS id)
Synonyms flavan; flavonoid
U.S./Canadian Brand Names Limbrel™ [US]
Therapeutic Category Antiinflammatory Agent
Use Clinical dietary management of osteoarthritis, including associated inflammation
Usual Dosage Oral: 250 mg every 8-12 hours
  (Continued)

353

flavocoxid *(Continued)*

Dosage Forms
Capsule:
Limbrel™: 250 mg

flavonoid *see* flavocoxid *on previous page*

Flavorcee® *(Discontinued)* *see* ascorbic acid *on page 76*

flavoxate *(fla VOKS ate)*

Sound-Alike/Look-Alike Issues
flavoxate may be confused with fluvoxamine
Urispas® may be confused with Urised®
Synonyms flavoxate hydrochloride
U.S./Canadian Brand Names Apo-Flavoxate® [Can]; Urispas® [US/Can]
Therapeutic Category Antispasmodic Agent, Urinary
Use Antispasmodic to provide symptomatic relief of dysuria, nocturia, suprapubic pain, urgency, and incontinence due to detrusor instability and hyperreflexia in elderly with cystitis, urethritis, urethrocystitis, urethrotrigonitis, and prostatitis
Usual Dosage Oral: Children >12 years and Adults: 100-200 mg 3-4 times/day; reduce the dose when symptoms improve
Dosage Forms
Tablet: 100 mg
Urispas®: 100 mg

flavoxate hydrochloride *see* flavoxate *on this page*

Flebogamma® [US] *see* immune globulin (intravenous) *on page 451*

flecainide *(fle KAY nide)*

Sound-Alike/Look-Alike Issues
flecainide may be confused with fluconazole
Tambocor™ may be confused with tamoxifen
Synonyms flecainide acetate
U.S./Canadian Brand Names Apo-Flecainide® [Can]; Tambocor™ [US/Can]
Therapeutic Category Antiarrhythmic Agent, Class I-C
Use Prevention and suppression of documented life-threatening ventricular arrhythmias (eg, sustained ventricular tachycardia); controlling symptomatic, disabling supraventricular tachycardias in patients without structural heart disease in whom other agents fail
Usual Dosage Oral:
Children:
Initial: 3 mg/kg/day or 50-100 mg/m^2/day in 3 divided doses
Usual: 3-6 mg/kg/day or 100-150 mg/m^2/day in 3 divided doses; up to 11 mg/kg/day or 200 mg/m^2/day for uncontrolled patients with subtherapeutic levels
Adults:
Life-threatening ventricular arrhythmias:
Initial: 100 mg every 12 hours
Increase by 50-100 mg/day (given in 2 doses/day) every 4 days; maximum: 400 mg/day.
Use of higher initial doses and more rapid dosage adjustments have resulted in an increased incidence of proarrhythmic events and congestive heart failure, particularly during the first few days. Do not use a loading dose. Use very cautiously in patients with history of congestive heart failure or myocardial infarction.
Prevention of paroxysmal supraventricular arrhythmias in patients with disabling symptoms but no structural heart disease:
Initial: 50 mg every 12 hours
Increase by 50 mg twice daily at 4-day intervals; maximum: 300 mg/day.
Dosage Forms
Tablet: 50 mg, 100 mg, 150 mg
Tambocor™: 50 mg, 100 mg, 150 mg

flecainide acetate *see* flecainide *on this page*

Fleet® Accu-Prep® [US-OTC] *see* sodium phosphates *on page 796*

Fleet® Babylax® [US-OTC] *see* glycerin *on page 397*

Fleet® Bisacodyl [US-OTC] *see* bisacodyl *on page 112*

Fleet Enema® [Can] *see* sodium phosphates *on page 796*

Fleet® Flavored Castor Oil *(Discontinued)* see castor oil *on page 157*

Fleet® Glycerin Suppositories [US-OTC] see glycerin *on page 397*

Fleet® Glycerin Suppositories Maximum Strength [US-OTC] see glycerin *on page 397*

Fleet® Laxative *(Discontinued)* see bisacodyl *on page 112*

Fleet® Liquid Glycerin Suppositories [US-OTC] see glycerin *on page 397*

Fleet® Phospho-Soda® [US-OTC] see sodium phosphates *on page 796*

Fleet® Phospho-Soda® Oral Laxative [Can] see sodium phosphates *on page 796*

Fleet® Sof-Lax® [US-OTC] see docusate *on page 273*

Fleet® Stimulant Laxative [US-OTC] see bisacodyl *on page 112*

Fletcher's® [US-OTC] see senna *on page 781*

Flexaphen® *(Discontinued)* see chlorzoxazone *on page 186*

Flexbumin [US] see albumin *on page 22*

Flexeril® [US/Can] see cyclobenzaprine *on page 221*

Flexitec [Can] see cyclobenzaprine *on page 221*

Flex-Power [US-OTC] see trolamine *on page 870*

Flextra 650 [US] see acetaminophen and phenyltoloxamine *on page 8*

Flextra-DS [US] see acetaminophen and phenyltoloxamine *on page 8*

Flintstones® Complete [US-OTC] see vitamins (multiple/pediatric) *on page 896*

Flintstones™ Gummies [US-OTC] see vitamins (multiple/pediatric) *on page 896*

Flintstones™ Plus Immunity Support [US-OTC] see vitamins (multiple/pediatric) *on page 896*

Flintstones® Plus Iron [US-OTC] see vitamins (multiple/pediatric) *on page 896*

Flintstones™ Sour Gummies [US-OTC] see vitamins (multiple/pediatric) *on page 896*

floctafenina see floctafenine *(Canada only)* on this page

floctafenine *(Canada only)* (flok ta FEN een)

Synonyms floctafenina; floctafeninum
U.S./Canadian Brand Names Apo-Floctafenine® [Can]; Idarac® [Can]
Therapeutic Category Nonsteroidal Antiinflammatory Drug (NSAID), Oral
Use Short-term management of acute, mild-to-moderate pain
Usual Dosage Oral: Adults: 200-400 mg every 6-8 hours as needed, up to a maximum of 1200 mg/day
Dosage Forms [CAN] = Canadian brand name
  Tablet:
    Apo-Floctafenine® [CAN]: 200 mg, 400 mg [not available in the U.S.]

floctafeninum see floctafenine *(Canada only)* on this page

Flolan® [US/Can] see epoprostenol *on page 304*

Flomax® [US/Can] see tamsulosin *on page 820*

Flomax® CR [Can] see tamsulosin *on page 820*

Flonase® [US/Can] see fluticasone (nasal) *on page 368*

Flora-Q™ [US-OTC] see Lactobacillus *on page 488*

Florastor® [US-OTC] see *Saccharomyces boulardii* *on page 771*

Florastor® Kids [US-OTC] see *Saccharomyces boulardii* *on page 771*

Florazole® ER [Can] see metronidazole *on page 563*

Florical® [US-OTC] see calcium carbonate *on page 138*

Florinef® [Can] see fludrocortisone *on page 357*

Florinef® *(Discontinued)* see fludrocortisone *on page 357*

Florone® [US/Can] see diflorasone *on page 257*

Florone E® *(Discontinued)* see diflorasone *on page 257*

Flovent® Diskus® [Can] see fluticasone (oral inhalation) *on page 369*

Flovent® HFA [US/Can] see fluticasone (oral inhalation) *on page 369*

Floxin® [US/Can] see ofloxacin *on page 625*

floxuridine (floks YOOR i deen)

Sound-Alike/Look-Alike Issues
floxuridine may be confused with Fludara®, fludarabine
FUDR® may be confused with Fludara®

Synonyms fluorodeoxyuridine; 5-FUDR; NSC-27640

U.S./Canadian Brand Names FUDR® [US/Can]

Therapeutic Category Antineoplastic Agent

Use Management of hepatic metastases of colorectal and gastric cancers

Usual Dosage Refer to individual protocols.
Intra-arterial:
0.1-0.6 mg/kg/day
4-20 mg/day

Dosage Forms
Injection, powder for reconstitution: 500 mg
FUDR®: 500 mg

Fluanxol® [Can] *see* flupenthixol *(Canada only)* on page 365

Fluarix® [US] *see* influenza virus vaccine *on page 455*

flubenisolone *see* betamethasone (topical) *on page 109*

Flucaine® [US] *see* proparacaine and fluorescein *on page 722*

fluconazole (floo KOE na zole)

Sound-Alike/Look-Alike Issues
fluconazole may be confused with flecainide
Diflucan® may be confused with diclofenac, Diprivan®, disulfiram

U.S./Canadian Brand Names Apo-Fluconazole® [Can]; Diflucan® [US/Can]; Fluconazole Injection [Can]; Fluconazole Omega [Can]; Gen-Fluconazole [Can]; GMD-Fluconazole [Can]; Novo-Fluconazole [Can]; Riva-Fluconazole [Can]

Therapeutic Category Antifungal Agent

Use Treatment of candidiasis (vaginal, oropharyngeal, esophageal, urinary tract infections, peritonitis, pneumonia, and systemic infections); cryptococcal meningitis; antifungal prophylaxis in allogeneic bone marrow transplant recipients

Usual Dosage The daily dose of fluconazole is the same for oral and I.V. administration
Usual dosage ranges:
Neonates: First 2 weeks of life, especially premature neonates: Same dose as older children every 72 hours
Children: Loading dose: 6-12 mg/kg; maintenance: 3-12 mg/kg/day; duration and dosage depends on severity of infection
Adults: 200-800 mg/day; duration and dosage depends on severity of infection

Indication-specific dosing:
Children:
Candidiasis:
Oropharyngeal: Loading dose: 6 mg/kg; maintenance: 3 mg/kg/day for 2 weeks
Esophageal: Loading dose: 6 mg/kg; maintenance: 3-12 mg/kg/day for 21 days and at least 2 weeks following resolution of symptoms
Systemic infection: 6 mg/kg every 12 hours for 28 days
Meningitis, cryptococcal: Loading dose: 12 mg/kg; maintenance: 6-12 mg/kg/day for 10-12 weeks following negative CSF culture; relapse suppression (HIV-positive): 6 mg/kg/day
Adults:
Candidiasis:
Candidemia (neutropenic and non-neutropenic): 400-800 mg/day for 14 days after last positive blood culture and resolution of signs/symptoms
Chronic, disseminated: 400-800 mg/day for 3-6 months
Oropharyngeal (long-term suppression): 200 mg/day; chronic therapy is recommended in immunocompromised patients with history of oropharyngeal candidiasis (OPC)
Osteomyelitis: 400-800 mg/day for 6-12 months
Esophageal: 200 mg on day 1, then 100-200 mg/day for 2-3 weeks after clinical improvement
Prophylaxis in bone marrow transplant: 400 mg/day; begin 3 days before onset of neutropenia and continue for 7 days after neutrophils >1000 cells/mm^3
Urinary: 200 mg/day for 1-2 weeks
Vaginal: 150 mg as a single dose
Endophthalmitis: 400-800 mg/day for 6-12 weeks after surgical intervention.
Meningitis, cryptococcal: Amphotericin 0.7-1 mg/kg +/- 5-FC for 2 weeks then fluconazole 400 mg/day for at least 10 weeks (consider life-long in HIV-positive); maintenance (HIV-positive): 200-400 mg/day life-long

Dosage Forms
Infusion [premixed in sodium chloride or dextrose]: 200 mg (100 mL); 400 mg (200 mL)
Diflucan® [premixed in sodium chloride or dextrose]: 200 mg (100 mL); 400 mg (200 mL)
Powder for oral suspension: 10 mg/mL, 40 mg/mL
Diflucan®: 10 mg/mL, 40 mg/mL
Tablet: 50 mg, 100 mg, 150 mg, 200 mg
Diflucan®: 50 mg, 100 mg, 150 mg, 200 mg

Fluconazole Injection [Can] see fluconazole on previous page
Fluconazole Omega [Can] see fluconazole on previous page

flucytosine (floo SYE toe seen)
Sound-Alike/Look-Alike Issues
flucytosine may be confused with fluorouracil
Ancobon® may be confused with Oncovin®
Synonyms 5-FC; 5-fluorocytosine; 5-flurocytosine
U.S./Canadian Brand Names Ancobon® [US/Can]
Therapeutic Category Antifungal Agent
Use Adjunctive treatment of systemic fungal infections (eg, septicemia, endocarditis, UTI, meningitis, or pulmonary) caused by susceptible strains of *Candida* or *Cryptococcus*
Usual Dosage
Usual dosage ranges: Adults: Oral: 50-150 mg/kg/day in divided doses every 6 hours

Indication-specific dosing:
Adults: Oral:
Endocarditis: 25-37.5 mg/kg every 6 hours (with amphotericin B) for at least 6 weeks after valve replacement
Meningoencephalitis, cryptococcal: Induction: 25 mg/kg (with amphotericin B) every 6 hours for 2 weeks; if clinical improvement, may discontinue both amphotericin and flucytosine and follow with an extended course of fluconazole (400 mg/day); alternatively, may continue flucytosine for 6-10 weeks (with amphotericin B) without conversion to fluconazole treatment
Dosage Forms
Capsule:
Ancobon®: 250 mg, 500 mg

Fludara® [US/Can] see fludarabine on this page

fludarabine (floo DARE a been)
Sound-Alike/Look-Alike Issues
fludarabine may be confused with floxuridine, Flumadine®
Fludara® may be confused with FUDR®
Synonyms fludarabine phosphate; NSC-312887
U.S./Canadian Brand Names Beneflur® [Can]; Fludara® [US/Can]
Therapeutic Category Antineoplastic Agent
Use
I.V.: Treatment of chronic lymphocytic leukemia (CLL) (including refractory CLL); non-Hodgkin lymphoma in adults
Oral (formulation not available in U.S.): Approved in Canada for treatment of CLL
Usual Dosage Adults:
I.V.:
Chronic lymphocytic leukemia: 25 mg/m^2/day for 5 days every 28 days
Non-hodgkin lymphoma: Loading dose: 20 mg/m^2 followed by 30 mg/m^2/day for 48 hours
Oral: **Note:** Formulation available in Canada; not available in U.S.: CLL: 40 mg/m^2 once daily for 5 days every 28 days
Dosage Forms [CAN] = Canadian brand name
Injection, powder for reconstitution: 50 mg
Fludara®: 50 mg
Tablet: 10 mg [not available in the U.S.]
Fludara® [CAN]: 10 mg [not available in the U.S.]

fludarabine phosphate see fludarabine on this page

fludrocortisone (floo droe KOR ti sone)
Sound-Alike/Look-Alike Issues
Florinef® may be confused with Fiorinal®
(Continued)

fludrocortisone *(Continued)*

Synonyms 9α-fluorohydrocortisone acetate; fludrocortisone acetate; fluohydrisone acetate; fluohydrocortisone acetate

U.S./Canadian Brand Names Florinef® [Can]

Therapeutic Category Adrenal Corticosteroid (Mineralocorticoid)

Use Partial replacement therapy for primary and secondary adrenocortical insufficiency in Addison disease; treatment of salt-losing adrenogenital syndrome

Usual Dosage Oral:

Infants and Children: 0.05-0.1 mg/day

Adults: 0.1-0.2 mg/day with ranges of 0.1 mg 3 times/week to 0.2 mg/day

Addison disease: Initial: 0.1 mg/day; if transient hypertension develops, reduce the dose to 0.05 mg/day. Preferred administration with cortisone (10-37.5 mg/day) or hydrocortisone (10-30 mg/day).

Salt-losing adrenogenital syndrome: 0.1-0.2 mg/day

Dosage Forms

Tablet: 0.1 mg

fludrocortisone acetate *see* fludrocortisone *on previous page*

FluLaval™ [US] *see* influenza virus vaccine *on page 455*

Flumadine® [US/Can] *see* rimantadine *on page 759*

flumazenil *(FLOO may ze nil)*

U.S./Canadian Brand Names Anexate® [Can]; Flumazenil Injection [Can]; Flumazenil Injection, USP [Can]; Romazicon® [US/Can]

Therapeutic Category Antidote

Use Benzodiazepine antagonist; reverses sedative effects of benzodiazepines used in conscious sedation and general anesthesia; treatment of benzodiazepine overdose

Usual Dosage I.V.:

Children: Reversal of conscious sedation and general anesthesia:

Initial: 0.01 mg/kg over 15 seconds (maximum: 0.2 mg)

Repeat doses (maximum: 4 doses): 0.005-0.01 mg/kg (maximum: 0.2 mg) repeated at 1-minute intervals

Maximum total cumulative dose: 1 mg or 0.05 mg/kg (whichever is lower)

Adults:

Reversal of conscious sedation and general anesthesia:

Initial: 0.2 mg over 15 seconds

Repeat doses: If desired level of consciousness is not obtained, 0.2 mg may be repeated at 1-minute intervals.

Maximum total cumulative dose: 1 mg (usual dose: 0.6-1 mg). In the event of resedation: Repeat doses may be given at 20-minute intervals with maximum of 1 mg/dose and 3 mg/hour

Suspected benzodiazepine overdose:

Initial: 0.2 mg over 30 seconds; if the desired level of consciousness is not obtained, 0.3 mg can be given over 30 seconds

Repeat doses: 0.5 mg over 30 seconds repeated at 1-minute intervals

Maximum total cumulative dose: 3 mg (usual dose: 1-3 mg). Patients with a partial response at 3 mg may require additional titration up to a total dose of 5 mg. If a patient has not responded 5 minutes after cumulative dose of 5 mg, the major cause of sedation is not likely due to benzodiazepines. In the event of resedation: May repeat doses at 20-minute intervals with maximum of 1 mg/dose and 3 mg/hour.

Resedation: Repeated doses may be given at 20-minute intervals as needed; repeat treatment doses of 1 mg (at a rate of 0.5 mg/minute) should be given at any time and no more than 3 mg should be given in any hour. After intoxication with high doses of benzodiazepines, the duration of a single dose of flumazenil is not expected to exceed 1 hour; if desired, the period of wakefulness may be prolonged with repeated low intravenous doses of flumazenil, or by an infusion of 0.1-0.4 mg/hour. Most patients with benzodiazepine overdose will respond to a cumulative dose of 1-3 mg and doses >3 mg do not reliably produce additional effects. Rarely, patients with a partial response at 3 mg may require additional titration up to a total dose of 5 mg. **If a patient has not responded 5 minutes after receiving a cumulative dose of 5 mg, the major cause of sedation is not likely to be due to benzodiazepines.**

Dosage Forms

Injection, solution: 0.1 mg/mL (5 mL, 10 mL)

Romazicon®: 0.1 mg/mL (5 mL, 10 mL)

Flumazenil Injection [Can] *see* flumazenil *on this page*

Flumazenil Injection, USP [Can] *see* flumazenil *on this page*

flumethasone and clioquinol *see* clioquinol and flumethasone *(Canada only) on page 201*

fluMist® [US] *see* influenza virus vaccine *on page 455*

flunarizine *(Canada only)* (floo NAR i zeen)

Synonyms flunarizine hydrochloride

U.S./Canadian Brand Names Apo-Flunarizine® [Can]; Novo-Flunarizine [Can]; Sibelium® [Can]

Therapeutic Category Calcium-Entry Blocker (Selective)

Use Prophylaxis of classic (with aura) or common (without aura) migraine; symptomatic treatment of vestibular vertigo (due to a diagnosed functional disorder of the vestibular system)

Usual Dosage Oral:

Adults (<65 years): Usual dose: 5-10 mg/day, usually administered at bedtime

Migraine prophylaxis: Initial dose: 10 mg at bedtime

Maintenance dose (following initial control of symptoms): 10 mg at bedtime administered 5 consecutive days, followed by 2 consecutive medication-free days each week.

Duration of therapy: In nonresponders, discontinue if no response occurs within 2 months. If response is noted, discontinue after 6 months; restart if patient relapses.

Vertigo: Initial dose: 10 mg at bedtime until symptoms are controlled

Duration of therapy:

Chronic vertigo: Discontinue if no response within 1 month.

Paroxysmal vertigo: Discontinue if no response is noted within 2 months.

Dosage Forms [CAN] = Canadian brand name

Capsule:

Apo-Flunarizine® [CAN], Novo-Flunarizine [CAN], Sibelium® [CAN]: 5 mg [not available in the U.S.]

flunarizine hydrochloride *see* flunarizine *(Canada only)* on this page

flunisolide (floo NISS oh lide)

Sound-Alike/Look-Alike Issues

flunisolide may be confused with Flumadine®, fluocinonide

Nasarel® may be confused with Nizoral®

U.S./Canadian Brand Names AeroBid® [US]; AeroBid®-M [US]; Aerospan™ [US]; Alti-Flunisolide [Can]; Apo-Flunisolide® [Can]; Nasalide® [Can]; Nasarel® [US]; PMS-Flunisolide [Can]; Rhinalar® [Can]

Therapeutic Category Adrenal Corticosteroid

Use Steroid-dependent asthma; nasal solution is used for seasonal or perennial rhinitis

Usual Dosage Note: AeroBid® and Aerospan™ are not interchangeable; dosing changes when switching from one to another.

Oral Inhalation: Asthma:

AeroBid®:

Children 6-15 years: 2 inhalations twice daily (morning and evening); up to 4 inhalations/day

Children ≥16 years and Adults: 2 inhalations twice daily (morning and evening); up to 8 inhalations/day maximum

Aerospan™:

Children 6-11 years: 1 inhalation twice daily; up to 4 inhalations/day

Children ≥12 years and Adults: 2 inhalations twice daily; up to 8 inhalations/day

Intranasal: Rhinitis:

Children 6-14 years: 1 spray each nostril 3 times daily **or** 2 sprays in each nostril twice daily; not to exceed 4 sprays/day in each nostril (200 mcg/day)

Children ≥15 years and Adults: 2 sprays each nostril twice daily (morning and evening); may increase to 2 sprays 3 times daily; maximum dose: 8 sprays/day in each nostril (400 mcg/day)

Dosage Forms

Aerosol for oral inhalation:

AeroBid®, AeroBid®-M: 250 mcg/actuation (7 g)

Aerospan™: 80 mcg/actuation (5.1 g); 80 mcg/actuation (8.9 g)

Solution, intranasal [spray]: 29 mcg/actuation (25 mL)

Nasarel®: 29 mcg/actuation (25 mL)

fluocinolone (floo oh SIN oh lone)

Sound-Alike/Look-Alike Issues

fluocinolone may be confused with fluocinonide

Synonyms fluocinolone acetonide

U.S./Canadian Brand Names Capex™ [US/Can]; Derma-Smoothe/FS® [US/Can]; Retisert™ [US]; Synalar® [US/Can]

Therapeutic Category Corticosteroid, Topical

Use Relief of susceptible inflammatory dermatosis [low, medium, high potency topical corticosteroid]; psoriasis of the scalp; atopic dermatitis in children ≥2 years of age

Ocular implant (Retisert™): Treatment of chronic, noninfectious uveitis affecting the posterior segment of the eye.

(Continued)

fluocinolone (Continued)

Usual Dosage

Children ≥2 years: Topical: Atopic dermatitis (Derma-Smoothe/FS®): Moisten skin; apply to affected area twice daily; do not use for longer than 4 weeks

Children and Adults: Topical: Corticosteroid-responsive dermatoses: Cream, ointment, solution: Apply a thin layer to affected area 2-4 times/day; may use occlusive dressings to manage psoriasis or recalcitrant conditions

Adults:

Topical:

Atopic dermatitis (Derma-Smoothe/FS®): Apply thin film to affected area 3 times/day

Inflammatory and pruritic manifestations (dental use): Apply to oral lesion 4 times/day, after meals and at bedtime

Scalp psoriasis (Derma-Smoothe/FS®): Massage thoroughly into wet or dampened hair/scalp; cover with shower cap. Leave on overnight (or for at least 4 hours). Remove by washing hair with shampoo and rinsing thoroughly.

Seborrheic dermatitis of the scalp (Capex™): Apply no more than 1 ounce to scalp once daily; work into lather and allow to remain on scalp for ~5 minutes. Remove from hair and scalp by rinsing thoroughly with water.

Ocular implant: Chronic uveitis: One silicone-encased tablet (0.59 mg) surgically implanted into the posterior segment of the eye is designed to release 0.6 mcg/day, decreasing over 30 days to a steady-state release rate of 0.3-0.4 mcg/day for 30 months. Recurrence of uveitis denotes depletion of tablet, requiring reimplantation.

Dosage Forms

Cream: 0.01% (15 g, 60 g); 0.025% (15 g, 60 g)

Implant, intravitreal:

Retisert™: 0.59 mg

Oil:

Derma-Smoothe/FS® [eczema oil]: 0.01% (120 mL)

Derma-Smoothe/FS® [scalp oil]: 0.01% (120 mL)

Ointment: 0.025% (60 g)

Shampoo:

Capex™: 0.01% (120 mL)

Solution: 0.01% (60 mL)

fluocinolone acetonide see fluocinolone on previous page

fluocinolone, hydroquinone, and tretinoin

(floo oh SIN oh lone, HYE droe kwin one, & TRET i noyn)

Synonyms hydroquinone, fluocinolone acetonide, and tretinoin; tretinoin, fluocinolone acetonide, and hydroquinone

U.S./Canadian Brand Names Tri-Luma™ [US]

Therapeutic Category Corticosteroid, Topical; Depigmenting Agent; Retinoic Acid Derivative

Use Short-term treatment of moderate to severe melasma of the face

Usual Dosage Topical: Adults: Melasma: Apply a thin film once daily to hyperpigmented areas of melasma (including 1/2 inch of normal-appearing surrounding skin). Apply 30 minutes prior to bedtime; not indicated for use beyond 8 weeks. Do not use occlusive dressings.

Dosage Forms

Cream, topical:

Tri-Luma™: Hydroquinone 4%, tretinoin 0.05%, fluocinolone 0.01% (30 g)

fluocinonide (floo oh SIN oh nide)

Sound-Alike/Look-Alike Issues

fluocinonide may be confused with flunisolide, fluocinolone

Lidex® may be confused with Lasix®, Videx®, Wydase®

U.S./Canadian Brand Names Lidemol® [Can]; Lidex-E® [US]; Lidex® [US/Can]; Lyderm® [Can]; Tiamol® [Can]; Topsyn® [Can]; Vanos™ [US]

Therapeutic Category Corticosteroid, Topical

Use Anti-inflammatory, antipruritic; treatment of plaque-type psoriasis (up to 10% of body surface area) [high-potency topical corticosteroid]

Usual Dosage

Children and Adults: Pruritus and inflammation: Topical (0.5% cream): Apply thin layer to affected area 2-4 times/day depending on the severity of the condition. Therapy should be discontinued when control is achieved; if no improvement is seen, reassessment of diagnosis may be necessary.

Children ≥12 years and Adults: Plaque-type psoriasis (Vanos™): Topical (0.1% cream): Apply a thin layer once or twice daily to affected areas (limited to <10% of body surface area). **Note:** Not recommended for use >2 consecutive weeks or >60 g/week total exposure. Discontinue when control is achieved.

Dosage Forms
Cream: 0.1% (30 g, 60 g)
Vanos™: 0.1% (30 g, 60 g)
Cream, anhydrous, emollient: 0.05% (15 g, 30 g, 60 g)
Lidex®: 0.05% (15 g, 30 g, 60 g)
Cream, aqueous, emollient: 0.05% (15 g, 30 g, 60 g)
Lidex-E®: 0.05% (15 g, 30 g, 60 g)
Gel: 0.05% (15 g, 30 g, 60 g)
Lidex®: 0.05% (15 g, 30 g, 60 g)
Ointment: 0.05% (15 g, 30 g, 60 g)
Lidex®: 0.05% (15 g, 30 g, 60 g)
Solution: 0.05% (60 mL)
Lidex®: 0.05% (60 mL)

fluohydrisone acetate *see* fludrocortisone *on page 357*

fluohydrocortisone acetate *see* fludrocortisone *on page 357*

Fluonid® Topical *(Discontinued)* *see* fluocinolone *on page 359*

Fluor-I-Strip-AT® [US] *see* fluorescein *on this page*

Fluoracaine® [US] *see* proparacaine and fluorescein *on page 722*

Fluor-A-Day [US/Can] *see* fluoride *on this page*

FluorCare® Neutral *(Discontinued)* *see* fluoride *on this page*

fluorescein (FLURE e seen)
Synonyms fluorescein sodium; sodium fluorescein; soluble fluorescein
U.S./Canadian Brand Names AK-Fluor® [US]; Angiofluor™ Lite [US]; Fluor-I-Strip-AT® [US]; Fluorescite® [US/Can]; Fluorets® [US]; Ful-Glo® [US]
Therapeutic Category Diagnostic Agent
Use
Injection: Diagnostic aid in ophthalmic angiography and angioscopy
Topical: To stain the anterior segment of the eye for procedures (such as fitting contact lenses), disclosing corneal injury, and in applanation tonometry
Usual Dosage
Ophthalmic: Strips: Children and Adults: Moisten strip with sterile water, saline or ophthalmic fluid. Touch conjunctiva or fornix with tip of strip until adequately stained. For best results, patient should blink several times after application.
Injection:
Children: 3.5 mg/lb (7.7 mg/kg) injected rapidly into antecubital vein
Adults: 500-750 mg injected rapidly into antecubital vein
Note: Prior to use, an intradermal test dose of 0.05 mL may be used if an allergy is suspected. Evaluate 30-60 minutes following intradermal injection.
Oral: Adults: 1 g of injection solution has been administered orally in patients with inaccessible veins and when early phases of an angiogram are not needed.
Dosage Forms
Injection, solution, as sodium:
AK-Fluor, Angiofluor™ Lite, Fluorescite®: 10% (5 mL); 25% (2 mL)
Strip, ophthalmic, as sodium: 1 mg
Fluorets®, Fluor-I-Strip-AT®: 1 mg
Ful-Glo®: 0.6 mg

fluorescein and proparacaine *see* proparacaine and fluorescein *on page 722*

fluorescein sodium *see* fluorescein *on this page*

Fluorescite® [US/Can] *see* fluorescein *on this page*

Fluorets® [US] *see* fluorescein *on this page*

fluoride (FLOR ide)
Sound-Alike/Look-Alike Issues
Luride® may be confused with Lortab®
Phos-Flur® may be confused with PhosLo®
Thera-Flur-N® may be confused with Thera-Flu®
(Continued)

fluoride *(Continued)*

Synonyms acidulated phosphate fluoride; sodium fluoride; stannous fluoride

U.S./Canadian Brand Names ACT® Plus [US-OTC]; ACT® x2™ [US-OTC]; ACT® [US-OTC]; CaviRinse™ [US]; ControlRx® [US]; Denta 5000 Plus [US]; DentaGel [US]; EtheDent™ [US]; Fluor-A-Day [US/Can]; Fluorigard® [US-OTC]; Fluorinse® [US]; Flura-Drops® [US]; Gel-Kam® Rinse [US]; Gel-Kam® [US-OTC]; Just for Kids™ [US-OTC]; Lozi-Flur™ [US]; Luride® Lozi-Tab® [US]; Luride® [US]; NeutraCare® [US]; NeutraGard® Advanced [US]; NeutraGard® Plus [US]; NeutraGard® [US-OTC]; Omnii Gel™ [US-OTC]; PerioMed™ [US]; Pharmaflur® 1.1 [US]; Pharmaflur® [US]; Phos-Flur® Rinse [US-OTC]; Phos-Flur® [US]; PreviDent® 5000 Plus™ [US]; PreviDent® [US]; StanGard® Perio [US]; StanGard® [US]; Stop® [US]; Thera-Flur-N® [US]

Therapeutic Category Mineral, Oral

Use Prevention of dental caries

Usual Dosage Oral:

The recommended daily dose of oral fluoride supplement (mg), based on fluoride ion content (ppm) in drinking water (2.2 mg of sodium fluoride is equivalent to 1 mg of fluoride ion): Adapted from Recommeded Dosage Schedule of The American Dental Association, The American Academy of Pediatric Dentistry, and The American Academy of Pediatrics:

Less than 0.3 ppm:
Birth to 6 months: 0 mg
6 months to 3 years: 0.25 mg
3-6 years: 0.5 mg
6-16 years: 1 mg
0.3-0.6 ppm:
Birth to 3 years: 0 mg
3-6 years: 0.25 mg
6-16 years: 0.5 mg

Cream: Children ≥6 years and Adults: Brush teeth with cream once daily regardless of fluoride content of drinking water

Dental rinse or gel:
Children 6-12 years: 5-10 mL rinse or apply to teeth and spit daily after brushing
Adults: 10 mL rinse or apply to teeth and spit daily after brushing
PreviDent® rinse: Children >6 years and Adults: Once weekly, rinse 10 mL vigorously around and between teeth for 1 minute, then spit; this should be done preferably at bedtime, after thoroughly brushing teeth; for maximum benefit, do not eat, drink, or rinse mouth for at least 30 minutes after treatment; do not swallow
Fluorinse®: Children >6 years and Adults: Once weekly, vigorously swish 5-10 mL in mouth for 1 minute, then spit

Lozenge (Lozi-Flur™): Adults: One lozenge daily regardless of fluoride content of drinking water

Dosage Forms

Cream, oral [toothpaste]: 1.1% (51 g)
Denta 5000 Plus, EtheDent™: 1.1% (51g)
Gel-drops:
Thera-Flur-N®: 1.1% (24 mL)
Gel, topical: 1.1% (56 g)
DentaGel, EtheDent™: 1.1% (56 g)
Gel-Kam® [OTC]: 0.4% (129 g)
Just for Kids™ [OTC], Omnii Gel™ [OTC], StanGard®: 0.4% (122 g)
NeutraCare®, NeutraGard® Advanced, Phos-Flur®, PreviDent®: 1.1% (60 g)
Stop®: 0.4% (120 g)
Lozenge:
Lozi-Flur™: 2.21 mg
Paste, oral [toothpaste]: 1.1% (56 g)
ControlRx®: 1.1% (56 g)
Solution, oral drops: 1.1 mg/mL
Flura-Drops®: 0.55 mg/drop
Luride®: 1.1 mg/mL
Solution, oral rinse: 0.05%, 0.2%, 0.44%, 0.5%
ACT® [OTC], ACT® Plus [OCT], Fluorigard® [OTC], NeutraGard® [OTC]: 0.05%
ACT® x2™ [OTCT]: 0.5%
CaviRinse™, Fluorinse®, NeutraGard® Plus, PreviDent®: 0.2%
Phos-Flur® [OTC]: 0.44%
Solution, oral rinse concentrate: 0.63%
Gel-Kam®, PerioMed™, StanGard® Perio: 0.63%
Tablet, chewable: 0.5 mg, 1.1 mg, 2.2 mg
EtheDent™, Luride® Lozi-Tab®: 0.55 mg, 1.1 mg, 2.2 mg
Fluor-A-Day: 0.56 mg, 1.1 mg, 2.21 mg
Pharmaflur®: 2.2 mg
Pharmaflur® 1.1: 1.1 mg

Fluorigard® **[US-OTC]** *see* fluoride *on page 361*

Fluori-Methane® **[US]** *see* dichlorodifluoromethane and trichloromonofluoromethane *on page 253*

Fluorinse® **[US]** *see* fluoride *on page 361*

Fluoritab® *(Discontinued) see* fluoride *on page 361*

5-fluorocytosine *see* flucytosine *on page 357*

fluorodeoxyuridine *see* floxuridine *on page 356*

9α-fluorohydrocortisone acetate *see* fludrocortisone *on page 357*

fluorometholone (flure oh METH oh lone)
    U.S./Canadian Brand Names Flarex® [US/Can]; FML® Forte [US/Can]; FML® [US/Can]; PMS-Fluorometholone [Can]
    Therapeutic Category Adrenal Corticosteroid
    Use Treatment of steroid-responsive inflammatory conditions of the eye
    Usual Dosage Ophthalmic:
      Children >2 years and Adults: Reevaluate therapy if improvement is not seen within 2 days; use care not to discontinue prematurely; in chronic conditions, gradually decrease dosing frequency prior to discontinuing treatment
      Ointment (FML®): Apply small amount (~1/2 inch ribbon) to conjunctival sac 1-3 times/day; may increase application to every 4 hours during the initial 24-48 hours
      Suspension:
        FML®: Instill 1 drop into conjunctival sac 2-4 times/day; may instill 1 drop every 4 hours during initial 24-48 hours
        FML® Forte: Instill 1 drop into conjunctival sac 2-4 times/day
      Adults: Suspension (Flarex®): Instill 1-2 drops into conjunctival sac 4 times/day; may increase application to 2 drops every 2 hours during initial 24-48 hours. Consult prescriber if no improvement after 14 days.
    Dosage Forms
    Ointment, ophthalmic:
      FML®: 0.1% (3.5 g)
    Suspension, ophthalmic: 0.1% (5 mL, 10 mL, 15 mL)
      Flarex®: 0.1% (5 mL)
      FML®: 0.1% (5 mL, 10 mL, 15 mL)
      FML® Forte: 0.25% (2 mL, 5 mL, 10 mL, 15 mL)

fluorometholone and sulfacetamide *see* sulfacetamide sodium and fluorometholone *on page 811*

Fluor-Op® *(Discontinued) see* fluorometholone *on this page*

Fluoroplex® **[US]** *see* fluorouracil *on this page*

fluorouracil (flure oh YOOR a sil)
    Sound-Alike/Look-Alike Issues
      fluorouracil may be confused with flucytosine
      Efudex® may be confused with Efidac (Efidac 24®), Eurax®
    Synonyms 5-fluorouracil; FU; 5-FU
    U.S./Canadian Brand Names Adrucil® [US]; Carac™ [US]; Efudex® [US/Can]; Fluoroplex® [US]
    Therapeutic Category Antineoplastic Agent
    Use Treatment of carcinomas of the breast, colon, head and neck, pancreas, rectum, or stomach; topically for the management of actinic or solar keratoses and superficial basal cell carcinomas
    Usual Dosage Adults:
      Refer to individual protocols:
      I.V. bolus: 500-600 mg/m^2 every 3-4 weeks **or** 425 mg/m^2 on days 1-5 every 4 weeks
      Continuous I.V. infusion: 1000 mg/m^2/day for 4-5 days every 3-4 weeks **or**
      2300-2600 mg/m^2 on day 1 every week **or**
      300-400 mg/m^2/day **or**
      225 mg/m^2/day for 5-8 weeks (with radiation therapy)
      Actinic keratoses: Topical:
      Carac™: Apply thin film to lesions once daily for up to 4 weeks, as tolerated
      Efudex®: Apply to lesions twice daily for 2-4 weeks; complete healing may not be evident for 1-2 months following treatment
      Fluoroplex®: Apply to lesions twice daily for 2-6 weeks
      Superficial basal cell carcinoma: Topical: Efudex® 5%: Apply to affected lesions twice daily for 3-6 weeks; treatment may be continued for up to 10-12 weeks
    (Continued)

fluorouracil *(Continued)*

Dosage Forms
Cream, topical:
Carac™: 0.5% (30 g)
Efudex®: 5% (25 g, 40 g)
Fluoroplex®: 1% (30 g)
Injection, solution: 50 mg/mL (10 mL, 20 mL, 50 mL, 100 mL)
Adrucil®: 50 mg/mL (10 mL, 50 mL, 100 mL)
Solution, topical: 2% (10 mL); 5% (10 mL)
Efudex®: 2% (10 mL); 5% (10 mL)

5-fluorouracil see fluorouracil *on previous page*

Fluothane® *(Discontinued)* see halothane *on page 413*

fluoxetine (floo OKS e teen)

Sound-Alike/Look-Alike Issues
fluoxetine may be confused with duloxetine, fluvastatin, fluvoxamine
Prozac® may be confused with Prilosec®, Proscar®, ProSom®, ProStep®
Sarafem® may be confused with Serophene®
Synonyms fluoxetine hydrochloride
U.S./Canadian Brand Names Alti-Fluoxetine [Can]; Apo-Fluoxetine® [Can]; BCI-Fluoxetine [Can]; CO Fluoxetine [Can]; FXT [Can]; Gen-Fluoxetine [Can]; Novo-Fluoxetine [Can]; Nu-Fluoxetine [Can]; PMS-Fluoxetine [Can]; Prozac® Weekly™ [US]; Prozac® [US/Can]; Rhoxal-fluoxetine [Can]; Sandoz-Fluoxetine [Can]; Sarafem® [US]
Therapeutic Category Antidepressant, Selective Serotonin Reuptake Inhibitor
Use Treatment of major depressive disorder (MDD); treatment of binge-eating and vomiting in patients with moderate-to-severe bulimia nervosa; obsessive-compulsive disorder (OCD); premenstrual dysphoric disorder (PMDD); panic disorder with or without agoraphobia
Usual Dosage Oral: **Note:** Upon discontinuation of fluoxetine therapy, gradually taper dose. If intolerable symptoms occur following a dose reduction, consider resuming the previously prescribed dose and/or decrease dose at a more gradual rate.
Children:
Depression: 8-18 years: 10-20 mg/day; lower-weight children can be started at 10 mg/day, may increase to 20 mg/day after 1 week if needed
OCD: 7-18 years: Initial: 10 mg/day; in adolescents and higher-weight children, dose may be increased to 20 mg/day after 2 weeks. Range: 10-60 mg/day
Adults: 20 mg/day in the morning; may increase after several weeks by 20 mg/day increments; maximum: 80 mg/day; doses >20 mg may be given once daily or divided twice daily. **Note:** Lower doses of 5-10 mg/day have been used for initial treatment.
Usual dosage range:
Bulimia nervosa: 60-80 mg/day
Depression: 20-40 mg/day; patients maintained on Prozac® 20 mg/day may be changed to Prozac® Weekly™ 90 mg/week, starting dose 7 days after the last 20 mg/day dose
OCD: 40-80 mg/day
Panic disorder: Initial: 10 mg/day; after 1 week, increase to 20 mg/day; may increase after several weeks; doses >60 mg/day have not been evaluated
PMDD (Sarafem®): 20 mg/day continuously, **or** 20 mg/day starting 14 days prior to menstruation and through first full day of menses (repeat with each cycle)
Dosage Forms
Capsule: 10 mg, 20 mg, 40 mg
Prozac®: 10 mg, 20 mg, 40 mg
Sarafem®: 10 mg, 20 mg
Capsule, delayed release:
Prozac® Weekly™: 90 mg
Solution, oral: 20 mg/5 mL
Prozac®: 20 mg/5 mL
Tablet: 10 mg, 20 mg

fluoxetine and olanzapine see olanzapine and fluoxetine *on page 627*

fluoxetine hydrochloride see fluoxetine *on this page*

fluoxymesterone (floo oks i MES te rone)

Sound-Alike/Look-Alike Issues
Halotestin® may be confused with Haldol®, haloperidol, halothane

U.S./Canadian Brand Names Halotestin® [US]
Therapeutic Category Androgen
Controlled Substance C-III
Use Replacement of endogenous testicular hormone; in females, palliative treatment of breast cancer
Usual Dosage Adults: Oral:
  Male:
  Hypogonadism: 5-20 mg/day
  Delayed puberty: 2.5-20 mg/day for 4-6 months
  Female: Inoperable breast carcinoma: 10-40 mg/day in divided doses for 1-3 months
Dosage Forms
  Tablet: 10 mg
  Halotestin®: 2 mg, 5 mg

flupenthixol *(Canada only)* (floo pen THIKS ol)

Synonyms flupenthixol decanoate; flupenthixol dihydrochloride
U.S./Canadian Brand Names Fluanxol® [Can]
Therapeutic Category Antipsychotic Agent; Thioxanthene Derivative
Use Maintenance therapy of chronic schizophrenic patients whose main manifestations do **not** include excitement, agitation, or hyperactivity
Usual Dosage
  I.M. (depot): Flupenthixol is administered by deep I.M. injection, preferably in the gluteus maximus, **NOT for I.V. use**; maintenance dosages are given at 2- to 3-week intervals
  Patients not previously treated with long-acting depot neuroleptics should be given an initial test dose of 5-20 mg. An initial dose of 20 mg is usually well tolerated; however, a 5 mg test dose is recommended in elderly, frail, and cachectic patients, and in patients whose individual or family history suggests a predisposition to extrapyramidal reactions. In the subsequent 5-10 days, the therapeutic response and the appearance of extrapyramidal symptoms should be carefully monitored. Oral neuroleptic drugs may be continued, but dosage should be reduced during this overlapping period and eventually discontinued.
  Oral: Initial: 1 mg 3 times/day; dose must be individualized. May be increased by 1 mg every 2-3 days based on tolerance and control of symptoms. Usual maintenance dosage: 3-6 mg/day in divided doses (doses ≥12 mg/day used in some patients).
Dosage Forms [CAN] = Canadian brand name
  Injection, solution [depot]:
  Fluanxol® [CAN]: 20 mg/mL (10 mL); 100 mg/mL (2 mL) [not available in the U.S.]
  Tablet:
  Fluanxol® [CAN]: 0.5 mg, 3 mg [not available in the U.S.]

flupenthixol decanoate see flupenthixol *(Canada only)* on this page
flupenthixol dihydrochloride see flupenthixol *(Canada only)* on this page

fluphenazine (floo FEN a zeen)

Sound-Alike/Look-Alike Issues
  Prolixin® may be confused with Proloprim®
Synonyms fluphenazine decanoate
U.S./Canadian Brand Names Apo-Fluphenazine Decanoate® [Can]; Apo-Fluphenazine® [Can]; Modecate® Concentrate [Can]; Modecate® [Can]; PMS-Fluphenazine Decanoate [Can]; Prolixin Decanoate® [US]
Therapeutic Category Phenothiazine Derivative
Use Management of manifestations of psychotic disorders and schizophrenia; depot formulation may offer improved outcome in individuals with psychosis who are nonadherent with oral antipsychotics
Usual Dosage Adults: Psychoses:
  Oral: 0.5-10 mg/day in divided doses at 6- to 8-hour intervals; some patients may require up to 40 mg/day
  I.M.: 2.5-10 mg/day in divided doses at 6- to 8-hour intervals (parenteral dose is $^1/_3$ to $^1/_2$ the oral dose for the hydrochloride salts)
  I.M. (decanoate): 12.5-37.5 mg every 2 weeks
  Conversion from hydrochloride to decanoate I.M. 0.5 mL (12.5 mg) decanoate every 3 weeks is approximately equivalent to 10 mg hydrochloride/day
Dosage Forms
  Injection, oil: 25 mg/mL (5 mL)
  Prolixin Decanoate®: 25 mg/mL (5 mL)
  Injection, solution: 2.5 mg/mL (10 mL)
  Tablet: 1 mg, 2.5 mg, 5 mg, 10 mg

fluphenazine decanoate see fluphenazine on this page
Flura® *(Discontinued)* see fluoride on page 361

Flura-Drops® **[US]** *see* fluoride *on page 361*

flurandrenolide (flure an DREN oh lide)
Sound-Alike/Look-Alike Issues
Cordran® may be confused with Cardura®, codeine, Cordarone®
Synonyms flurandrenolone
U.S./Canadian Brand Names Cordran® SP [US]; Cordran® [US/Can]
Therapeutic Category Corticosteroid, Topical
Use Inflammation of corticosteroid-responsive dermatoses [medium potency topical corticosteroid]
Usual Dosage Topical: Therapy should be discontinued when control is achieved; if no improvement is seen, reassessment of diagnosis may be necessary.
Children:
Ointment, cream: Apply sparingly 1-2 times/day
Tape: Apply once daily
Adults: Cream, lotion, ointment: Apply sparingly 2-3 times/day
Dosage Forms
Cream, emulsified:
Cordran® SP: 0.025% (30 g, 60 g); 0.05% (15 g, 30 g, 60 g)
Lotion:
Cordran®: 0.05% (15 mL, 60 mL)
Ointment:
Cordran®: 0.025% (30 g, 60 g); 0.05% (15 g, 30 g, 60 g)
Tape, topical [roll]:
Cordran®: 4 mcg/cm^2 (7.5 cm x 60 cm, 7.5 cm x 200 cm)

flurandrenolone *see* flurandrenolide *on this page*

Flurate® Ophthalmic Solution *(Discontinued)* *see* fluorescein *on page 361*

flurazepam (flure AZ e pam)
Sound-Alike/Look-Alike Issues
flurazepam may be confused with temazepam
Dalmane® may be confused with Demulen®, Dialume®
Synonyms flurazepam hydrochloride
U.S./Canadian Brand Names Apo-Flurazepam® [Can]; Dalmane® [US/Can]; Som Pam [Can]
Therapeutic Category Benzodiazepine
Controlled Substance C-IV
Use Short-term treatment of insomnia
Usual Dosage Oral: Insomnia:
Children: ≥15 years: 15 mg at bedtime
Adults: 15-30 mg at bedtime
Dosage Forms
Capsule: 15 mg, 30 mg
Dalmane®: 15 mg, 30 mg

flurazepam hydrochloride *see* flurazepam *on this page*

flurbiprofen (flure BI proe fen)
Sound-Alike/Look-Alike Issues
flurbiprofen may be confused with fenoprofen
Ansaid® may be confused with Asacol®, Axid®
Ocufen® may be confused with Ocuflox®, Ocupress®
Synonyms flurbiprofen sodium
U.S./Canadian Brand Names Alti-Flurbiprofen [Can]; Ansaid® [Can]; Apo-Flurbiprofen® [Can]; Froben-SR® [Can]; Froben® [Can]; Novo-Flurprofen [Can]; Nu-Flurprofen [Can]; Ocufen® [US/Can]
Therapeutic Category Analgesic, Nonnarcotic; Nonsteroidal Antiinflammatory Drug (NSAID)
Use
Oral: Treatment of rheumatoid arthritis and osteoarthritis
Ophthalmic: Inhibition of intraoperative miosis
Usual Dosage
Oral:
Rheumatoid arthritis and osteoarthritis: 200-300 mg/day in 2-, 3-, or 4 divided doses; do not administer more than 100 mg for any single dose; maximum: 300 mg/day
Dental: Management of postoperative pain: 100 mg every 12 hours

Ophthalmic: Instill 1 drop every 30 minutes, beginning 2 hours prior to surgery (total of 4 drops in each affected eye)
Dosage Forms
  Solution, ophthalmic: 0.03% (2.5 mL)
    Ocufen®: 0.03% (2.5 mL)
  Tablet: 50 mg, 100 mg

flurbiprofen sodium *see* flurbiprofen *on previous page*

5-flurocytosine *see* flucytosine *on page 357*

Fluro-Ethyl® [US] *see* ethyl chloride and dichlorotetrafluoroethane *on page 334*

Flurosyn® Topical *(Discontinued)* *see* fluocinolone *on page 359*

FluShield® *(Discontinued)* *see* influenza virus vaccine *on page 455*

flutamide (FLOO ta mide)
Sound-Alike/Look-Alike Issues
  flutamide may be confused with Flumadine®, thalidomide
  Eulexin® may be confused with Edecrin®, Eurax®
Synonyms niftolid; NSC-147834; 4'-nitro-3'-trifluoromethylisobutyrantide; SCH 13521
U.S./Canadian Brand Names Apo-Flutamide® [Can]; Euflex® [Can]; Eulexin® [US/Can]; Novo-Flutamide [Can]
Therapeutic Category Antiandrogen
Use Treatment of metastatic prostatic carcinoma in combination therapy with LHRH agonist analogues
Usual Dosage Oral: Adults: Prostatic carcinoma: 250 mg 3 times/day
Dosage Forms
  Capsule: 125 mg
    Eulexin®: 125 mg

fluticasone and salmeterol (floo TIK a sone & sal ME te role)
Sound-Alike/Look-Alike Issues
  Advair may be confused with Advicor®
Synonyms fluticasone propionate and salmeterol xinafoate; salmeterol and fluticasone
U.S./Canadian Brand Names Advair Diskus® [US/Can]; Advair® HFA [US]
Therapeutic Category Beta$_2$-Adrenergic Agonist Agent; Corticosteroid, Inhalant
Use Maintenance treatment of asthma; maintenance treatment of COPD associated with chronic bronchitis
Usual Dosage Oral inhalation: **Note:** Do not use to transfer patients from systemic corticosteroid therapy.
  COPD: Adults: Advair Diskus®: Fluticasone 250 mcg/salmeterol 50 mcg twice daily, 12 hours apart. **Note:** This is the maximum dose.

  Asthma:
    Children 4-11 years: Advair Diskus®: Fluticasone 100 mcg/salmeterol 50 mcg twice daily, 12 hours apart. **Note:** This is the maximum dose.
    Children ≥12 and Adults:
      Advair Diskus®: One inhalation twice daily, morning and evening, 12 hours apart
       Maximum dose: Fluticasone 500 mcg/salmeterol 50 mcg per inhalation
      Advair® HFA: Two inhalations twice daily, morning and evening, 12 hours apart
       Maximum dose: Fluticasone 230 mcg/salmeterol 21 mcg per inhalation
    Note: Initial dose prescribed should be based upon previous dose of inhaled-steroid asthma therapy. Dose should be increased after 2 weeks if adequate response is not achieved. Patients should be titrated to lowest effective dose once stable. Each suggestion below specifies the product strength to use; remember to **use 1 inhalation for Diskus® and 2 inhalations for HFA.**

  Patients not currently on inhaled corticosteroids:
  Advair Diskus®: Fluticasone 100 mcg/salmeterol 50 mcg **or** fluticasone 250 mcg/salmeterol 50 mcg
  Advair® HFA: Fluticasone 45 mcg/salmeterol 21 mcg **or** fluticasone 115 mcg/salmeterol 21 mcg
  Patients currently using inhaled beclomethasone dipropionate:
    ≤160 mcg/day: Advair Diskus®: Fluticasone 100 mcg/salmeterol 50 mcg **or** Advair® HFA: Fluticasone 45 mcg/salmeterol 21 mcg
    320 mcg/day: Advair Diskus®: Fluticasone 250 mcg/salmeterol 50 mcg **or** Advair® HFA: Fluticasone 115 mcg/salmeterol 21 mcg
    640 mcg/day: Advair Diskus®: Fluticasone 500 mcg/salmeterol 50 mcg **or** Advair® HFA: Fluticasone 230 mcg/salmeterol 21 mcg
  Patients currently using inhaled budesonide:
    ≤400 mcg/day: Advair Diskus®: Fluticasone 100 mcg/salmeterol 50 mcg **or** Advair® HFA: Fluticasone 45 mcg/salmeterol 21 mcg
(Continued)

fluticasone and salmeterol *(Continued)*

800-1200 mcg/day: Advair Diskus®: Fluticasone 250 mcg/salmeterol 50 mcg **or** Advair® HFA: Fluticasone 115 mcg/salmeterol 21mcg

1600 mcg/day: Advair Diskus®: Fluticasone 500 mcg/salmeterol 50 mcg **or** Advair® HFA: Fluticasone 230 mcg/salmeterol 21 mcg

Patients currently using inhaled flunisolide CFC aerosol:

≤1000 mcg/day: Advair Diskus®: Fluticasone 100 mcg/salmeterol 50 mcg **or** Advair® HFA: Fluticasone 45 mcg/salmeterol 21 mcg

1250-2000 mcg/day: Advair Diskus®: Fluticasone 250 mcg/salmeterol 50 mcg **or** Advair® HFA: Fluticasone 115 mcg/salmeterol 21 mcg

Patients currently using inhaled fluticasone HFA aerosol:

≤176 mcg/day: Advair Diskus®: Fluticasone 100 mcg/salmeterol 50 mcg **or** Advair® HFA: Fluticasone 45 mcg/salmeterol 21 mcg

440 mcg/day: Advair Diskus®: Fluticasone 250 mcg/salmeterol 50 mcg **or** Advair® HFA: Fluticasone 115 mcg/salmeterol 21 mcg

660-880 mcg/day: Advair Diskus®: Fluticasone 500 mcg/salmeterol 50 mcg **or** Advair® HFA: Fluticasone 230 mcg/salmeterol 21 mcg

Patients currently using inhaled fluticasone propionate powder:

≤200 mcg/day: Advair Diskus®: Fluticasone 100 mcg/salmeterol 50 mcg **or** Advair® HFA: Fluticasone 45 mcg/salmeterol 21 mcg

500 mcg/day: Advair Diskus®: Fluticasone 250 mcg/salmeterol 50 mcg **or** Advair® HFA: Fluticasone 115 mcg/salmeterol 21 mcg

1000 mcg/day: Advair Diskus®: Fluticasone 500 mcg/salmeterol 50 mcg **or** Advair® HFA: Fluticasone 230 mcg/salmeterol 21 mcg

Patients currently using inhaled mometasone furoate powder:

220 mcg/day: Advair Diskus®: Fluticasone 100 mcg/salmeterol 50 mcg **or** Advair® HFA: Fluticasone 45 mcg/salmeterol 21 mcg

440 mcg/day: Advair Diskus®: Fluticasone 250 mcg/salmeterol 50 mcg **or** Advair® HFA: Fluticasone 115 mcg/salmeterol 21 mcg

880 mcg/day: Advair Diskus®: Fluticasone 500 mcg/salmeterol 50 mcg **or** Advair® HFA: Fluticasone 230 mcg/salmeterol 21 mcg

Patients currently using inhaled triamcinolone acetonide:

≤1000 mcg/day: Advair Diskus®: Fluticasone 100 mcg/salmeterol 50 mcg **or** Advair® HFA: Fluticasone 45 mcg/salmeterol 21 mcg

1100-1600 mcg/day: Advair Diskus®: Fluticasone 250 mcg/salmeterol 50 mcg **or** Advair® HFA: Fluticasone 115 mcg/salmeterol 21 mcg

Dosage Forms

Aerosol, for oral inhalation:

Advair® HFA:

45/21: Fluticasone 45 mcg and salmeterol 30.45 mcg (12 g)

115/21: Fluticasone 115 mcg and salmeterol 30.45 mcg (12 g)

230/21: Fluticasone 230 mcg and salmeterol 30.45 mcg (12 g)

Powder for oral inhalation:

Advair Diskus®:

100/50: Fluticasone 100 mcg and salmeterol 50 mcg (28s, 60s)

250/50: Fluticasone 250 mcg and salmeterol 50 mcg (28s, 60s)

500/50: Fluticasone 500 mcg and salmeterol 50 mcg (28s, 60s)

fluticasone (nasal) (floo TIK a sone NAY sal)

U.S./Canadian Brand Names Flonase® [US/Can]

Therapeutic Category Adrenal Corticosteroid

Use Intranasal: Management of seasonal and perennial allergic rhinitis and nonallergic rhinitis in patients ≥4 years of age

Usual Dosage Rhinitis: Intranasal:

Children ≥4 years and Adolescents: Initial: 1 spray (50 mcg/spray) per nostril once daily; patients not adequately responding or patients with more severe symptoms may use 2 sprays (100 mcg) per nostril. Depending on response, dosage may be reduced to 100 mcg daily. Total daily dosage should not exceed 2 sprays in each nostril (200 mcg)/day. Dosing should be at regular intervals.

Adults: Initial: 2 sprays (50 mcg/spray) per nostril once daily; may also be divided into 100 mcg twice a day. After the first few days, dosage may be reduced to 1 spray per nostril once daily for maintenance therapy. Dosing should be at regular intervals.

Dosage Forms

Suspension, intranasal, as furoate [spray]:

Veramyst™: 27.5 mcg/inhalation (10 g)

Suspension, intranasal, as propionate [spray]: 50 mcg/inhalation (16 g)

Flonase®: 50 mcg/inhalation (16 g)

fluticasone (oral inhalation) (floo TIK a sone or al in ha LAY shun)
U.S./Canadian Brand Names Flovent® Diskus® [Can]; Flovent® HFA [US/Can]

Therapeutic Category Adrenal Corticosteroid

Use Inhalation: Maintenance treatment of asthma as prophylactic therapy. It is also indicated for patients requiring oral corticosteroid therapy for asthma to assist in total discontinuation or reduction of total oral dose. NOT indicated for the relief of acute bronchospasm.

Usual Dosage Inhalation, oral: Asthma:

Flovent®, Flovent® HFA: Children ≥12 years: Refer to Adults dosing.

Flovent® Diskus® [Can]:

Children 4-16 years: Usual starting dose: 50-100 mcg twice daily; may increase to 200 mcg twice daily in patients not adequately controlled; titrate to the lowest effective dose once asthma stability is achieved

Children ≥16 years: Refer to Adults dosing.

Adults: **Note:** Titrate to the lowest effective dose once asthma stability is achieved

Flovent®, Flovent® HFA: Manufacturers labeling: Dosing based on previous therapy

Bronchodilator alone: Recommended starting dose: 88 mcg twice daily; highest recommended dose: 440 mcg twice daily

Inhaled corticosteroids: Recommended starting dose: 88-220 mcg twice daily; highest recommended dose: 440 mcg twice daily; a higher starting dose may be considered in patients previously requiring higher doses of inhaled corticosteroids

Oral corticosteroids: Recommended starting dose:

Flovent®: 880 mcg twice daily

Flovent® HFA: 440 mcg twice daily

Highest recommended dose: 880 mcg twice daily; starting dose is patient dependent. In patients on chronic oral corticosteroids therapy, reduce prednisone dose no faster than 2.5-5 mg/day on a weekly basis; begin taper after 1 week of fluticasone therapy

NIH Asthma Guidelines (administer in divided doses twice daily).

"Low" dose: 88-264 mcg/day

"Medium" dose: 264-660 mcg/day

"High" dose: >660 mcg/day

Flovent® Diskus® [CAN]:

Mild asthma: 100-250 mcg twice daily

Moderate asthma: 250-500 mcg twice da

Severe asthma: 500 mcg twice daily; may increase to 1000 mcg twice daily in very severe patients requiring high doses of corticosteroids

Dosage Forms [CAN] = Canadian brand name

Aerosol for oral inhalation [CFC free]:

Flovent® HFA: 44 mcg/inhalation (10.6 g); 110 mcg/inhalation (12 g); 220 mcg/inhalation (12 g)

Powder for oral inhalation [prefilled blister pack]:

Flovent® Diskus® [U.S.]: 50 mcg (60s)

Flovent® Diskus®) [CAN]: 50 mcg (28s, 60s); 100 mcg (28s, 60s); 250 mcg (28s, 60s); 500 mcg (28s, 60s) [not available in the U.S.]

fluticasone propionate and salmeterol xinafoate *see* fluticasone and salmeterol *on page 367*

fluticasone (topical) (floo TIK a sone TOP i kal)
Sound-Alike/Look-Alike Issues

Cutivate® may be confused with Ultravate®

U.S./Canadian Brand Names Cutivate® [US/Can]

Therapeutic Category Adrenal Corticosteroid; Corticosteroid, Topical

Use Relief of inflammation and pruritus associated with corticosteroid-responsive dermatoses; atopic dermatitis

Usual Dosage Topical:

Corticosteroid-responsive dermatoses:

Children ≥3 months: Cream: Apply sparingly to affected area twice daily. If no improvement is seen within 2 weeks, reassessment of diagnosis may be necessary

Adults: Cream, lotion, ointment: Apply sparingly to affected area twice daily. If no improvement is seen within 2 weeks, reassessment of diagnosis may be necessary.

Atopic dermatitis:

Children ≥3 months: Cream: Apply sparingly to affected area twice daily. If no improvement is seen within 2 weeks, reassessment of diagnosis may be necessary.

Children ≥1 year: Lotion: Apply sparingly to affected area twice daily

Adults: Cream, lotion: Apply sparingly to affected area once or twice daily. If no improvement is seen within 2 weeks, reassessment of diagnosis may be necessary

(Continued)

fluticasone (topical) *(Continued)*

Dosage Forms
Cream: 0.05% (15 g, 30 g, 60 g)
Cutivate®: 0.05% (30 g, 60 g)
Lotion:
Cutivate®: 0.05% (60 mL)
Ointment: 0.005% (15 g, 30 g, 60 g)
Cutivate®: 0.005% (30 g, 60 g)

fluvastatin (FLOO va sta tin)

Sound-Alike/Look-Alike Issues
fluvastatin may be confused with fluoxetine
U.S./Canadian Brand Names Lescol® XL [US/Can]; Lescol® [US/Can]
Therapeutic Category HMG-CoA Reductase Inhibitor
Use To be used as a component of multiple risk factor intervention in patients at risk for atherosclerosis vascular disease due to hypercholesterolemia

Adjunct to dietary therapy to reduce elevated total cholesterol (total-C), LDL-C, triglyceride, and apolipoprotein B (apo-B) levels and to increase HDL-C in primary hypercholesterolemia and mixed dyslipidemia (Fredrickson types IIa and IIb); to slow the progression of coronary atherosclerosis in patients with coronary heart disease; reduce risk of coronary revascularization procedures in patients with coronary heart disease

Usual Dosage
Adolescents 10-16 years: Oral: Heterozygous familial hypercholesterolemia: Initial: 20 mg once daily; may increase every 6 weeks based on tolerability and response to a maximum recommended dose of 80 mg/day, given in 2 divided doses (immediate release capsule) or as a single daily dose (extended release tablet)
Note: Indicated only for adjunctive therapy when diet alone cannot reduce LDL-C below 190 mg/dL, or 160 mg/dL (with cardiovascular risk factors). Female patients must be 1 year postmenarche.
Adults: Oral:
Patients requiring ≥25% decrease in LDL-C: 40 mg capsule once daily in the evening, 80 mg extended release tablet once daily (anytime), or 40 mg capsule twice daily
Patients requiring <25% decrease in LDL-C: Initial: 20 mg capsule once daily in the evening; may increase based on tolerability and response to a maximum recommended dose of 80 mg/day, given in 2 divided doses (immediate release capsule) or as a single daily dose (extended release tablet)

Dosage Forms
Capsule:
Lescol®: 20 mg, 40 mg
Tablet, extended release:
Lescol® XL: 80 mg

Fluviral S/F® **[Can]** *see* influenza virus vaccine *on page 455*
Fluvirin® **[US]** *see* influenza virus vaccine *on page 455*

fluvoxamine (floo VOKS a meen)

Sound-Alike/Look-Alike Issues
fluvoxamine may be confused with flavoxate, fluoxetine
Luvox® may be confused with Lasix®, Levoxyl®
U.S./Canadian Brand Names Alti-Fluvoxamine [Can]; Apo-Fluvoxamine® [Can]; Luvox® [Can]; Novo-Fluvoxamine [Can]; Nu-Fluvoxamine [Can]; PMS-Fluvoxamine [Can]; Rhoxal-fluvoxamine [Can]; Sandoz-Fluvoxamine [Can]
Therapeutic Category Antidepressant, Selective Serotonin Reuptake Inhibitor
Use Treatment of obsessive-compulsive disorder (OCD) in children ≥8 years of age and adults
Usual Dosage Oral: **Note:** When total daily dose exceeds 50 mg, the dose should be given in 2 divided doses:
Children 8-17 years: Initial: 25 mg at bedtime; adjust in 25 mg increments at 4- to 7-day intervals, as tolerated, to maximum therapeutic benefit: Range: 50-200 mg/day
Maximum: Children 8-11 years: 200 mg/day, adolescents: 300 mg/day; lower doses may be effective in female versus male patients
Adults: Initial: 50 mg at bedtime; adjust in 50 mg increments at 4- to 7-day intervals; usual dose range: 100-300 mg/day; divide total daily dose into 2 doses; administer larger portion at bedtime
Dosage Forms
Tablet: 25 mg, 50 mg, 100 mg

Fluzone® **[US]** *see* influenza virus vaccine *on page 455*
FML® **[US/Can]** *see* fluorometholone *on page 363*
FML® Forte [US/Can] *see* fluorometholone *on page 363*

FML-S® **[US]** *see* sulfacetamide sodium and fluorometholone *on page 811*

Focalin® **[US]** *see* dexmethylphenidate *on page 244*

Focalin® **XR [US]** *see* dexmethylphenidate *on page 244*

Foille® **[US-OTC]** *see* benzocaine *on page 101*

folacin *see* folic acid *on this page*

folacin, vitamin B₁₂, and vitamin B₆ *see* folic acid, cyanocobalamin, and pyridoxine *on this page*

folate *see* folic acid *on this page*

Folbee [US] *see* folic acid, cyanocobalamin, and pyridoxine *on this page*

Folex® **PFS**™ **(Discontinued)** *see* methotrexate *on page 553*

Folgard® **[US-OTC]** *see* folic acid, cyanocobalamin, and pyridoxine *on this page*

Folgard RX 2.2® **(Discontinued)** *see* folic acid, cyanocobalamin, and pyridoxine *on this page*

folic acid (FOE lik AS id)

Sound-Alike/Look-Alike Issues
folic acid may be confused with folinic acid

Synonyms folacin; folate; pteroylglutamic acid

U.S./Canadian Brand Names Apo-Folic® [Can]

Therapeutic Category Vitamin, Water Soluble

Use Treatment of megaloblastic and macrocytic anemias due to folate deficiency; dietary supplement to prevent neural tube defects

Usual Dosage
Oral, I.M., I.V., SubQ: Anemia:
Infants: 0.1 mg/day
Children <4 years: Up to 0.3 mg/day
Children >4 years and Adults: 0.4 mg/day
Pregnant and lactating women: 0.8 mg/day
Oral:
RDA: Expressed as dietary folate equivalents:
Children:
1-3 years: 150 mcg/day
4-8 years: 200 mcg/day
9-13 years: 300 mcg/day
Children ≥14 years and Adults: 400 mcg/day
Prevention of neural tube defects:
Females of childbearing potential: 400 mcg/day
Females at high risk or with family history of neural tube defects: 4 mg/day

Dosage Forms
Injection, solution: 5 mg/mL (10 mL)
Tablet: 0.4 mg, 0.8 mg, 1 mg

folic acid, cyanocobalamin, and pyridoxine

(FOE lik AS id, sye an oh koe BAL a min, & peer i DOKS een)

Synonyms cyanocobalamin, folic acid, and pyridoxine; folacin, vitamin B₁₂, and vitamin B₆; pyridoxine, folic acid, and cyanocobalamin

U.S./Canadian Brand Names AllanFol RX [US]; Folbee [US]; Folgard® [US-OTC]; Foltx® [US]; Tricardio B [US]

Therapeutic Category Vitamin

Use Nutritional supplement in end-stage renal failure, dialysis, hyperhomocysteinemia, homocystinuria, malabsorption syndromes, dietary deficiencies

Usual Dosage Oral: Adults: 1 tablet daily

Dosage Forms
Tablet: Folic acid 0.8 mg, cyanocobalamin 1000 mcg, and pyridoxine 50 mg
AllanFol RX: Folic acid 2.2 mg, cyanocobalamin 1000 mcg, and pyridoxine hydrochloride 25 mg
Folbee: Folic acid 2.5 mg, cyanocobalamin 1000 mcg, and pyridoxine 25 mg
Folgard® [OTC]: Folic acid 0.8 mg, cyanocobalamin 115 mcg, and pyridoxine 10 mg
Foltx®: Folic acid 2.5 mg, cyanocobalamin 2000 mcg, and pyridoxine 25 mg
Tricardio B: Folic acid 0.4 mg, cyanocobalamin 250 mcg, and pyridoxine 25 mg

folinic acid *see* leucovorin *on page 496*

follicle-stimulating hormone, human *see* urofollitropin *on page 878*

follicle stimulating hormone, recombinant *see* follitropin alfa *on next page*

follicle stimulating hormone, recombinant *see* follitropin beta *on this page*

Follistim® AQ [US] *see* follitropin beta *on this page*

Follistim® AQ Cartridge [US] *see* follitropin beta *on this page*

follitropin alfa (foe li TRO pin AL fa)

Synonyms follicle stimulating hormone, recombinant; rFSH-alpha; rhFSH-alpha

U.S./Canadian Brand Names Gonal-f® Pen [Can]; Gonal-f® RFF [US]; Gonal-f® [US/Can]

Therapeutic Category Ovulation Stimulator

Use

Gonal-f®: Ovulation induction in patients in whom the cause of infertility is functional and not caused by primary ovarian failure; development of multiple follicles with Assisted Reproductive Technology (ART); spermatogenesis induction

Gonal-f® RFF: Ovulation induction in patients in whom the cause of infertility is functional and not caused by primary ovarian failure; development of multiple follicles with ART

Usual Dosage Adults: **Note:** Dose should be individualized. Use the lowest dose consistent with the expectation of good results. Over the course of treatment, doses may vary depending on individual patient response.

Gonal-f®, Gonal-f® RFF: Female:

Ovulation induction: SubQ: Initial: 75 int. units/day; incremental dose adjustments of up to 37.5 int. units may be considered after 14 days; further dose increases of the same magnitude can be made, if necessary, every 7 days (maximum dose: 300 int. units/day). If response to follitropin is appropriate, hCG is given 1 day following the last dose. Withhold hCG if serum estradiol is >2000 pg/mL, if the ovaries are abnormally enlarged, or if abdominal pain occurs. In general, therapy should not exceed 35 days.

ART: SubQ: Initiate therapy with follitropin alfa in the early follicular phase (cycle day 2 or day 3) at a dose of 150 int. units/day, until sufficient follicular development is attained. In most cases, therapy should not exceed 10 days. In patients ≥35 years whose endogenous gonadotropin levels are suppressed, initiate follitropin alfa at a dose of 225 int. units/day. Continue treatment until adequate follicular development is indicated as determined by ultrasound in combination with measurement of serum estradiol levels. Consider adjustments to dose after 5 days based on the patient's response; adjust subsequent dosage every 3-5 days by ≤75-150 int. units additionally at each adjustment. Doses >450 int. units/day are not recommended. Once adequate follicular development is evident, administer hCG to induce final follicular maturation in preparation for oocyte. Withhold hCG if the ovaries are abnormally enlarged.

Gonal-f®: Male: Spermatogenesis induction: SubQ: Therapy should begin with hCG pretreatment until serum testosterone is in normal range, then 150 int. units 3 times/week with hCG 3 times/week; continue with lowest dose needed to induce spermatogenesis (maximum dose: 300 int. units 3 times/week); may be given for up to 18 months

Dosage Forms

Injection, powder for reconstitution [rDNA origin]:

Gonal-f®: 450 int. units

Gonal-f® RFF: 75 int. units

Injection, solution [rDNA origin]:

Gonal-f® RFF: 300 int. units/0.5 mL (0.5 mL); 450 int. units/0.75 mL (0.75 mL); 900 int. units/1.5 mL (1.5 mL)

follitropin beta (foe li TRO pin BAY ta)

Synonyms follicle stimulating hormone, recombinant; rFSH-beta; rhFSH-beta

U.S./Canadian Brand Names Follistim® AQ Cartridge [US]; Follistim® AQ [US]; Puregon® [Can]

Therapeutic Category Ovulation Stimulator

Use Ovulation induction in patients in whom the cause of infertility is functional and not caused by primary ovarian failure; development of multiple follicles with Assisted Reproductive Technology (ART)

Usual Dosage Adults: Female: **Note:** Dose should be individualized. Use the lowest dose consistent with the expectation of good results. Over the course of treatment, doses may vary depending on individual patient response.

Ovulation induction:

Follistim® AQ: I.M., SubQ: Stepwise approach: Initiate therapy with 75 int. units/day for up to 14 days. Increase by 37.5 int. units at weekly intervals until follicular growth or serum estradiol levels indicate an adequate response. The maximum (individualized) daily dose that has been safely used for ovulation induction in patients during clinical trials is 300 int. units. If response to follitropin is appropriate, hCG is given 1 day following the last dose. Withhold hCG if the ovaries are abnormally enlarged, or if abdominal pain occurs.

Follistim® AQ Cartridge: SubQ: Stepwise approach: Initiate therapy with 75 int. units/day for up to 7 days. Increase by 25 or 50 int. units at weekly intervals until follicular growth or serum estradiol levels indicate an adequate response. The maximum (individualized) daily dose that has been safely used for ovulation induction in patients during clinical trials is 175 int. units. If response to follitropin is appropriate, hCG is given 1 day following the last dose. Withhold hCG if the ovaries are abnormally enlarged, or if abdominal pain occurs.

ART:

Follistim® AQ: I.M., SubQ: A starting dose of 150-225 int. units is recommended for at least the first 4 days of treatment. The dose may be adjusted for the individual patient based upon their ovarian response. The usual maintenance dose was 75-300 int. units for 6-12 days; 375-600 int. units in patients who were poor responders. The maximum daily dose used in clinical studies is 600 int. units. When a sufficient number of follicles of adequate size are present, the final maturation of the follicles is induced by administering hCG. Oocyte retrieval is performed 34-36 hours later. Withhold hCG in cases where the ovaries are abnormally enlarged on the last day of follitropin beta therapy.

Follistim® AQ Cartridge: SubQ: A starting dose of 150-225 int. units is recommended for at least the first 5 days of treatment. The dose may be adjusted for the individual patient based upon their ovarian response. The maximum daily dose used in clinical studies is 450 int. units. When a sufficient number of follicles of adequate size are present, the final maturation of the follicles is induced by administering hCG. Oocyte retrieval is performed 34-36 hours later. Withhold hCG in cases where the ovaries are abnormally enlarged on the last day of follitropin beta therapy.

Dosage Forms

Injection, solution [rDNA origin]:

Follistim® AQ Cartridge: 175 int. units/0.21 mL (0.21 mL); 350 int. units/0.42 mL (0.42 mL); 650 int. units/0.78 mL (0.78 mL); 975 int. units/1.17 mL (1.17 mL)

Injection, solution [rDNA origin; single-dose]:

Follistim® AQ: 75 int. units/0.5 mL (0.5 mL); 150 int. units/0.5 mL (0.5 mL)

Foltx® [US] *see* folic acid, cyanocobalamin, and pyridoxine *on page 371*

Folvite® (Discontinued) *see* folic acid *on page 371*

fomepizole (foe ME pi zole)

Synonyms 4-methylpyrazole; 4-MP

U.S./Canadian Brand Names Antizol® [US]

Therapeutic Category Antidote

Use Treatment of methanol or ethylene glycol poisoning alone or in combination with hemodialysis

Usual Dosage I.V.: Adults: Ethylene glycol and methanol toxicity: A loading dose of 15 mg/kg should be administered, followed by doses of 10 mg/kg every 12 hours for 4 doses, then 15 mg/kg every 12 hours thereafter until ethylene glycol levels have been reduced <20 mg/dL and patient is asymptomatic with normal pH

Dosage Forms

Injection, solution [preservative free]:

Antizol®: 1 g/mL (1.5 mL)

fondaparinux (fon da PARE i nuks)

Synonyms fondaparinux sodium

U.S./Canadian Brand Names Arixtra® [US/Can]

Therapeutic Category Factor Xa Inhibitor

Use Prophylaxis of deep vein thrombosis (DVT) in patients undergoing surgery for hip replacement, knee replacement, hip fracture (including extended prophylaxis following hip fracture surgery), or abdominal surgery (in patients at risk for thromboembolic complications); treatment of acute pulmonary embolism (PE); treatment of acute DVT without PE

Note: Additional Canadian approvals (not approved in U.S.): Unstable angina or non-ST segment elevation myocardial infarction (UA/NSTEMI) for the prevention of death and subsequent MI; ST segment elevation MI (STEMI) for the prevention of death and myocardial reinfarction

Usual Dosage SubQ:

DVT prophylaxis: Adults ≥50 kg: 2.5 mg once daily. **Note:** Initiate dose after hemostasis has been established, 6-8 hours postoperatively.

Usual duration: 5-9 days (up to 10 days following abdominal surgery or up to 11 days following hip replacement or knee replacement)

Extended prophylaxis is recommended following hip fracture surgery (has been tolerated for up to 32 days).

Acute DVT/PE treatment: Adults: **Note:** Concomitant treatment with warfarin sodium should be initiated as soon as possible, usually within 72 hours:

<50 kg: 5 mg once daily

50-100 kg: 7.5 mg once daily

>100 kg: 10 mg once daily

Usual duration: 5-9 days (has been administered up to 26 days)

Dosage Forms

Injection, solution:

Arixtra®: 2.5 mg/0.5 mL (0.5 mL); 5 mg/0.4 mL (0.4 mL); 7.5 mg/0.6 mL (0.6 mL); 10 mg/0.8 mL (0.8 mL)

fondaparinux sodium *see* fondaparinux *on this page*

Foradil® **[Can]** *see* formoterol *on this page*

Foradil® **Aerolizer**™ **[US]** *see* formoterol *on this page*

Forane® **[US/Can]** *see* isoflurane *on page 474*

formoterol (for MOH te rol)

Sound-Alike/Look-Alike Issues
Foradil® may be confused with Toradol®

Synonyms formoterol fumarate

U.S./Canadian Brand Names Foradil® Aerolizer™ [US]; Foradil® [Can]; Oxeze® Turbuhaler® [Can]

Therapeutic Category Beta₂-Adrenergic Agonist Agent

Use Maintenance treatment of asthma and prevention of bronchospasm in patients ≥5 years of age with reversible obstructive airway disease, including patients with symptoms of nocturnal asthma, who require regular treatment with inhaled, short-acting beta₂-agonists; maintenance treatment of bronchoconstriction in patients with COPD; prevention of exercise-induced bronchospasm in patients ≥5 years of age

Note:
Oxeze® is also approved in Canada for acute relief of symptoms ("on demand" treatment) in patients ≥6 years of age.
Perforomist™ is only indicated for maintenance treatment of bronchoconstriction in patients with COPD.

Usual Dosage
Asthma maintenance treatment: Children ≥5 years and Adults: Inhalation: 12 mcg capsule every 12 hours
Oxeze® (CAN): **Note:** Not labeled for use in the U.S.: Children ≥6 years and Adults: Inhalation: 6 mcg or 12 mcg every 12 hours. Maximum dose: Children: 24 mcg/day; Adults: 48 mcg/day
Prevention of exercise-induced bronchospasm: Children ≥5 years and Adults: Inhalation: 12 mcg capsule at least 15 minutes before exercise on an "as needed" basis; additional doses should not be used for another 12 hours. **Note:** If already using for asthma maintenance then should not use additional doses for exercise-induced bronchospasm.
Oxeze® (CAN): **Note:** Not labeled for use in the U.S.: Children ≥6 years and Adults: Inhalation: 6 mcg or 12 mcg at least 15 minutes before exercise.
COPD maintenance treatment: Adults: Inhalation: 12 mcg capsule every 12 hours

Additional indication for Oxeze® **(approved in Canada):** Acute ("on demand") relief of bronchoconstriction: Children ≥12 years and Adults: 6 mcg or 12 mcg as a single dose (maximum dose: 72 mcg in any 24-hour period). The prolonged use of high dosages (48 mcg/day for ≥3 consecutive days) may be a sign of suboptimal control, and should prompt the re-evaluation of therapy.

Dosage Forms [CAN] = Canadian brand name
Powder for oral inhalation:
Foradil® Aerolizer™ [capsule]: 12 mcg (12s, 60s)
Oxeze® Turbuhaler® [CAN]: 6 mcg/inhalation, 12 mcg/inhalation [not available in the U.S.]
Solution for nebulization:
Perforomist™: 20 mcg/2 mL (2 mL)

formoterol fumarate *see* formoterol *on this page*

formoterol fumarate dehydrate and budesonide *see* budesonide and formoterol *on page 124*

Formula EM [US-OTC] *see* fructose, dextrose, and phosphoric acid *on page 378*

Formula Q® ***(Discontinued)*** *see* quinine *on page 740*

Formulation R™ **[US-OTC]** *see* phenylephrine *on page 675*

Formulex® **[Can]** *see* dicyclomine *on page 255*

5-formyl tetrahydrofolate *see* leucovorin *on page 496*

Fortamet® **[US]** *see* metformin *on page 548*

Fortaz® **[US/Can]** *see* ceftazidime *on page 163*

Forteo™ **[US/Can]** *see* teriparatide *on page 827*

Fortical® **[US]** *see* calcitonin *on page 135*

Fortovase® ***(Discontinued)*** *see* saquinavir *on page 776*

Fosamax® **[US/Can]** *see* alendronate *on page 27*

Fosamax Plus D™ **[US]** *see* alendronate and cholecalciferol *on page 27*

fosamprenavir (FOS am pren a veer)

Sound-Alike/Look-Alike Issues
Lexiva® may be confused with Levitra®

Synonyms fosamprenavir calcium; GW433908G
U.S./Canadian Brand Names Lexiva® [US]; Telzir® [Can]
Therapeutic Category Antiretroviral Agent, Protease Inhibitor
Use Treatment of HIV infections in combination with at least two other antiretroviral agents
Usual Dosage Oral: HIV infection:
Children:
Antiretroviral therapy-naive patients:
Children 2-5 years of age: Fosamprenavir 30 mg/kg twice daily (not to exceed adult dosage of 1400 mg twice daily)
Children ≥6 years of age:
Unboosted regimen: Fosamprenavir 30 mg/kg twice daily (not to exceed adult dosage of 1400 mg twice daily)
Ritonavir-boosted regimen: Fosamprenavir 18 mg/kg twice daily plus ritonavir 3 mg/kg twice daily (not to exceed the adult dose of 700 mg plus ritonavir 100 mg twice daily)
Protease inhibitor-experienced patients: Children ≥6 years of age: Fosamprenavir 18 mg/kg plus ritonavir 3 mg/kg twice daily (not to exceed the adult dose of 700 mg plus ritonavir 100 mg twice daily)
Notes: The adult regimen of 1400 mg twice daily may be used for pediatric patients who weigh ≥47 kg. When combined with ritonavir, fosamprenavir tablets may be administered to children who weigh ≥39 kg while ritonavir capsules may be used for pediatric patients who weigh ≥33 kg.

Adults:
Antiretroviral therapy-naive patients:
Unboosted regimen: 1400 mg twice daily (without ritonavir)
Ritonavir-boosted regimens:
Once-daily regimen: Fosamprenavir 1400 mg plus ritonavir 200 mg once daily
Twice-daily regimen: Fosamprenavir 700 mg plus ritonavir 100 mg twice daily
Protease inhibitor-experienced patients: Fosamprenavir 700 mg plus ritonavir 100 mg twice daily. **Note:** Once-daily administration is not recommended in protease inhibitor-experienced patients.
Combination therapy with efavirenz (ritonavir-boosted regimen):
Once-daily regimen: Fosamprenavir 1400 mg daily plus ritonavir 300 mg once daily
Twice-daily regimen: No dosage adjustment recommended for twice-daily regimen
Combination therapy with nevirapine (ritonavir-boosted regimen): Fosamprenavir 700 mg plus ritonavir 100 mg twice daily
Dosage Forms [CAN] = Canadian brand name
Tablet:
Lexiva®: 700 mg
Suspension, oral:
Telzir® [CAN]: 50 mg/mL [not available in the U.S.]

fosamprenavir calcium *see fosamprenavir on previous page*

Fosavance [Can] *see alendronate and cholecalciferol on page 27*

foscarnet (fos KAR net)
Synonyms PFA; phosphonoformate; phosphonoformic acid
U.S./Canadian Brand Names Foscavir® [US/Can]
Therapeutic Category Antiviral Agent
Use
Treatment of mucotaneous herpesvirus infections suspected to be caused by acyclovir-resistant (HSV, VZV) or ganciclovir-resistant (CMV) strains; this occurs almost exclusively in immunocompromised persons (eg, with advanced AIDS) who have received prolonged treatment for a herpesvirus infection
Treatment of CMV retinitis in persons with AIDS
Usual Dosage
CMV retinitis: I.V.:
Induction treatment: 60 mg/kg/dose every 8 hours **or** 90 mg/kg every 12 hours for 14-21 days
Maintenance therapy: 90-120 mg/kg/day as a single infusion
Herpes simplex infections (acyclovir-resistant): Induction: I.V.: 40 mg/kg/dose every 8-12 hours for 14-21 days
Dosage Forms
Injection, solution: 24 mg/mL (250 mL, 500 mL)
Foscavir®: 24 mg/mL (500 mL)

Foscavir® [US/Can] *see foscarnet on this page*

fosfomycin (fos foe MYE sin)
Sound-Alike/Look-Alike Issues
Monurol™ may be confused with Monopril®
(Continued)

fosfomycin (Continued)

Synonyms fosfomycin tromethamine

U.S./Canadian Brand Names Monurol™ [US/Can]

Therapeutic Category Antibiotic, Miscellaneous

Use Single oral dose in the treatment of uncomplicated urinary tract infections in women due to susceptible strains of *E. coli* and *Enterococcus*; may have an advantage over other agents since it maintains high concentration in the urine for up to 48 hours

Usual Dosage Oral: Adults: Female: Uncomplicated UTI: Single dose of 3 g in 4 oz of water

Dosage Forms
Powder:
Monurol™: 3 g

fosfomycin tromethamine *see fosfomycin on previous page*

fosinopril (foe SIN oh pril)

Sound-Alike/Look-Alike Issues
fosinopril may be confused with lisinopril
Monopril® may be confused with Accupril®, minoxidil, moexipril, Monoket®, Monurol™, ramipril

Synonyms fosinopril sodium

U.S./Canadian Brand Names Apo-Fosinopril® [Can]; Monopril® [US/Can]; Novo-Fosinopril [Can]; ratio-Fosinopril [Can]; Riva-Fosinopril [Can]

Therapeutic Category Angiotensin-Converting Enzyme (ACE) Inhibitor

Use Treatment of hypertension, either alone or in combination with other antihypertensive agents; treatment of congestive heart failure, left ventricular dysfunction after myocardial infarction

Usual Dosage Oral:
Children ≥6 years and >50 kg: Hypertension: Initial: 5-10 mg once daily (maximum: 40 mg/day)
Adults:
Hypertension: Initial: 10 mg/day; most patients are maintained on 20-40 mg/day. May need to divide the dose into two if trough effect is inadequate; discontinue the diuretic, if possible 2-3 days before initiation of therapy; resume diuretic therapy carefully, if needed.
Heart failure: Initial: 10 mg/day (5 mg if renal dysfunction present) and increase, as needed, to a maximum of 40 mg once daily over several weeks; usual dose: 20-40 mg/day. If hypotension, orthostasis, or azotemia occur during titration, consider decreasing concomitant diuretic dose, if any.

Dosage Forms
Tablet: 10 mg, 20 mg, 40 mg
Monopril®: 10 mg, 20 mg, 40 mg

fosinopril and hydrochlorothiazide (foe SIN oh pril & hye droe klor oh THYE a zide)

Sound-Alike/Look-Alike Issues
Monopril® may be confused with Accupril®, minoxidil, moexipril, Monoket®, Monurol™, ramipril

Synonyms hydrochlorothiazide and fosinopril

U.S./Canadian Brand Names Monopril-HCT® [US/Can]

Therapeutic Category Angiotensin-Converting Enzyme (ACE) Inhibitor

Use Treatment of hypertension; not indicated for first-line treatment

Usual Dosage Note: A patient whose blood pressure is not adequately controlled with fosinopril or hydrochlorothiazide monotherapy may be switched to combination therapy; **not** for initial treatment.
Adults: Oral: Hypertension: Fosinopril 10-80 mg per day, hydrochlorothiazide 12.5-50 mg per day

Dosage Forms
Tablet: 0/12.5: Fosinopril 10 mg and hydrochlorothiazide 12.5 mg; 20/12.5: Fosinopril 20 mg and hydrochlorothiazide 12.5 mg
Monopril-HCT®: 10/12.5: Fosinopril 10 mg and hydrochlorothiazide 12.5 mg; 20/12.5: Fosinopril 20 mg and hydrochlorothiazide 12.5 mg

fosinopril sodium *see fosinopril on this page*

fosphenytoin (FOS fen i toyn)

Sound-Alike/Look-Alike Issues
Cerebyx® may be confused with Celebrex®, Celexa™, Cerezyme®

Synonyms fosphenytoin sodium

U.S./Canadian Brand Names Cerebyx® [US/Can]

Therapeutic Category Hydantoin

Use Used for the control of generalized convulsive status epilepticus and prevention and treatment of seizures occurring during neurosurgery; indicated for short-term parenteral administration when other means of phenytoin administration are unavailable, inappropriate, or deemed less advantageous (the safety and effectiveness of fosphenytoin in this use has not been systematically evaluated for more than 5 days)

Usual Dosage The dose, concentration in solutions, and infusion rates for fosphenytoin are expressed as phenytoin sodium equivalents (PE); fosphenytoin should always be prescribed and dispensed in phenytoin sodium equivalents (PE)

Adults:

Status epilepticus: I.V.: Loading dose: 15-20 mg PE/kg I.V. administered at 100-150 mg PE/minute

Nonemergent loading and maintenance dosing: I.V. or I.M.:

Loading dose: 10-20 mg PE/kg I.V. or I.M. (maximum I.V. rate: 150 mg PE/minute)

Initial daily maintenance dose: 4-6 mg PE/kg/day I.V. or I.M.

I.M. or I.V. substitution for oral phenytoin therapy: May be substituted for oral phenytoin sodium at the same total daily dose; however, Dilantin® capsules are ~90% bioavailable by the oral route; phenytoin, supplied as fosphenytoin, is 100% bioavailable by both the I.M. and I.V. routes; for this reason, plasma phenytoin concentrations may increase when I.M. or I.V. fosphenytoin is substituted for oral phenytoin sodium therapy; in clinical trials I.M. fosphenytoin was administered as a single daily dose utilizing either 1 or 2 injection sites; some patients may require more frequent dosing

Dosage Forms

Injection, solution: 75 mg/mL (2 mL, 10 mL) [equivalent to phenytoin sodium 50 mg/mL]

Cerebyx®: 75 mg/mL (2 mL, 10 mL) [equivalent to phenytoin sodium 50 mg/mL]

fosphenytoin sodium *see* fosphenytoin *on previous page*

Fosrenol™ [US] *see* lanthanum *on page 494*

Fostex® 10% BPO [US-OTC] *see* benzoyl peroxide *on page 103*

Fototar® [US-OTC] *see* coal tar *on page 208*

Fragmin® [US/Can] *see* dalteparin *on page 229*

framycetin *(Canada only)* (fra mye CEE tin)

U.S./Canadian Brand Names Sofra-Tulle® [Can]

Therapeutic Category Antibiotic, Topical

Use Treatment of infected or potentially infected burns, wounds, ulcers, and graft sites

Usual Dosage A single layer to be applied directly to the wound and covered with an appropriate dressing. If exudative, dressings should be changed at least daily. In case of leg ulcers, cut dressing accurately to size of ulcer to decrease the risk of sensitization and to avoid contact with surrounding healthy skin.

Dosage Forms Gauze dressing: 1% (10 cm x 10 cm)

Fraxiparine™ [Can] *see* nadroparin *(Canada only) on page 586*

Fraxiparine™ Forte [Can] *see* nadroparin *(Canada only) on page 586*

Freedavite [US-OTC] *see* vitamins (multiple/oral) *on page 895*

Freezone® [US-OTC] *see* salicylic acid *on page 772*

Frisium® [Can] *see* clobazam *(Canada only) on page 201*

Froben® [Can] *see* flurbiprofen *on page 366*

Froben-SR® [Can] *see* flurbiprofen *on page 366*

Frova® [US] *see* frovatriptan *on this page*

frovatriptan (froe va TRIP tan)

Synonyms frovatriptan succinate

U.S./Canadian Brand Names Frova® [US]

Therapeutic Category Antimigraine Agent; Serotonin 5-HT$_{1B, 1D}$ Receptor Agonist

Use Acute treatment of migraine with or without aura in adults

Usual Dosage Oral: Adults: Migraine: 2.5 mg; if headache recurs, a second dose may be given if first dose provided some relief and at least 2 hours have elapsed since the first dose (maximum daily dose: 7.5 mg)

Dosage Forms

Tablet:

Frova®: 2.5 mg

frovatriptan succinate *see* frovatriptan *on this page*

fructose, dextrose, and phosphoric acid (FRUK tose, DEKS trose, & foss FOR ik AS id)

Sound-Alike/Look-Alike Issues
Emetrol® may be confused with emetine

Synonyms dextrose, levulose and phosphoric acid; levulose, dextrose and phosphoric acid; phosphorated carbohydrate solution; phosphoric acid, levulose and dextrose

U.S./Canadian Brand Names Emetrol® [US-OTC]; Especol® [US-OTC]; Formula EM [US-OTC]; Kalmz [US-OTC]; Nausea Relief [US-OTC]; Nausetrol® [US-OTC]

Therapeutic Category Antiemetic

Use Relief of nausea associated with upset stomach that occurs with intestinal or stomach flu, and food indiscretions

Usual Dosage Oral: Nausea:
Children 2-12 years: 5-10 mL; repeat dose every 15 minutes until distress subsides; do not take for more than 1 hour (5 doses)
Children ≥12 years and Adults: 15-30 mL; repeat dose every 15 minutes until distress subsides; do not take for more than 1 hour (5 doses)

Dosage Forms
Liquid, oral: Fructose 1.87 g, dextrose 1.87 g, and phosphoric acid 21.5 mg per 5 mL
Emetrol® [OTC], Especol® [OTC], Formula EM [OTC], Kalmz [OTC], Nausea Relief [OTC], Nausetrol® [OTC]: Fructose 1.87 g, dextrose 1.87 g, and phosphoric acid 21.5 mg per 5 mL

frusemide *see* furosemide *on next page*

FS *see* fibrin sealant kit *on page 351*

FS Shampoo® Topical *(Discontinued) see* fluocinolone *on page 359*

FTC *see* emtricitabine *on page 295*

FTP-Domperidone Maleate [Can] *see* domperidone *(Canada only) on page 276*

FU *see* fluorouracil *on page 363*

5-FU *see* fluorouracil *on page 363*

Fucidin® [Can] *see* fusidic acid *(Canada only) on next page*

Fucithalmic® [Can] *see* fusidic acid *(Canada only) on next page*

FUDR® [US/Can] *see* floxuridine *on page 356*

5-FUDR *see* floxuridine *on page 356*

Ful-Glo® [US] *see* fluorescein *on page 361*

fulvestrant (fool VES trant)

Synonyms ICI-182,780; zeneca 182,780; ZM-182,780
U.S./Canadian Brand Names Faslodex® [US]
Therapeutic Category Antineoplastic Agent, Estrogen Receptor Antagonist
Use Treatment of hormone receptor positive metastatic breast cancer in postmenopausal women with disease progression following antiestrogen therapy
Usual Dosage I.M.: Adults (postmenopausal women): 250 mg at 1-month intervals
Dosage Forms
Injection, solution [prefilled syringe]:
Faslodex®: 50 mg/mL (2.5 mL, 5 mL)

Fumasorb® *(Discontinued) see* ferrous fumarate *on page 349*

Fumerin® *(Discontinued) see* ferrous fumarate *on page 349*

Funduscein® Injection *(Discontinued) see* fluorescein *on page 361*

Fungi-Guard [US-OTC] *see* tolnaftate *on page 849*

Fungi-Nail® [US-OTC] *see* undecylenic acid and derivatives *on page 876*

Fungizone® [Can] *see* amphotericin B (conventional) *on page 51*

Fung-O® [US-OTC] *see* salicylic acid *on page 772*

Fungoid® Tincture [US-OTC] *see* miconazole *on page 566*

Furacin® Topical *(Discontinued)*

Furadantin® [US] *see* nitrofurantoin *on page 607*

Furalan® *(Discontinued) see* nitrofurantoin *on page 607*

Furan® *(Discontinued) see* nitrofurantoin *on page 607*

Furanlte® *(Discontinued) see* nitrofurantoin *on page 607*

furazosin *see* prazosin *on page 708*

furosemide (fyoor OH se mide)

Sound-Alike/Look-Alike Issues

furosemide may be confused with torsemide

Lasix® may be confused with Esidrix®, Lanoxin®, Lidex®, Lomotil®, Luvox®, Luxiq®

Synonyms frusemide

U.S./Canadian Brand Names Apo-Furosemide® [Can]; Furosemide Injection, USP [Can]; Furosemide Special [Can]; Lasix® Special [Can]; Lasix® [US/Can]; Novo-Semide [Can]

Therapeutic Category Diuretic, Loop

Use Management of edema associated with congestive heart failure and hepatic or renal disease; alone or in combination with antihypertensives in treatment of hypertension

Usual Dosage

Infants and Children:

Oral: 0.5-2 mg/kg/dose increased in increments of 1 mg/kg/dose with each succeeding dose until a satisfactory effect is achieved to a maximum of 6 mg/kg/dose no more frequently than 6 hours.

I.M., I.V.: 1 mg/kg/dose, increasing by each succeeding dose at 1 mg/kg/dose at intervals of 6-12 hours until a satisfactory response up to 6 mg/kg/dose.

Adults:

Oral: 20-80 mg/dose initially increased in increments of 20-40 mg/dose at intervals of 6-8 hours; usual maintenance dose interval is twice daily or every day; may be titrated up to 600 mg/day with severe edematous states.

Hypertension (JNC 7): 20-80 mg/day in 2 divided doses

I.M., I.V.: 20-40 mg/dose, may be repeated in 1-2 hours as needed and increased by 20 mg/dose until the desired effect has been obtained. Usual dosing interval: 6-12 hours; for acute pulmonary edema, the usual dose is 40 mg I.V. over 1-2 minutes. If not adequate, may increase dose to 80 mg. **Note:** ACC/AHA 2005 guidelines for chronic congestive heart failure recommend a maximum single dose of 160-200 mg.

Continuous I.V. infusion: Initial I.V. bolus dose 20-40 mg, followed by continuous I.V. infusion doses of 10-40 mg/hour. If urine output is <1 mL/kg/hour, double as necessary to a maximum of 80-160 mg/hour. The risk associated with higher infusion rates (80-160 mg/hour) must be weighed against alternative strategies. **Note:** ACC/AHA 2005 guidelines for chronic congestive heart failure recommend 40 mg I.V. load, then 10-40 mg/hour infusion.

Refractory heart failure: Oral, I.V.: Doses up to 8 g/day have been used.

Dosage Forms

Injection, solution: 10 mg/mL (2 mL, 4 mL, 8 mL, 10 mL)

Solution, oral: 10 mg/mL, 40 mg/5 mL

Tablet: 20 mg, 40 mg, 80 mg

Lasix®: 20 mg, 40 mg, 80 mg

Furosemide Injection, USP [Can] *see* furosemide *on this page*

Furosemide Special [Can] *see* furosemide *on this page*

fusidic acid *(Canada only)* (fyoo SI dik AS id)

Synonyms sodium fusidate

U.S./Canadian Brand Names Fucidin® [Can]; Fucithalmic® [Can]

Therapeutic Category Antifungal Agent, Systemic

Use

Systemic: Treatment of skin and soft tissue infections, or osteomyelitis, caused by susceptible organisms, including *Staphylococcus aureus* (penicillinase-producing or nonpenicillinase strains); may be used in the treatment of pneumonia, septicemia, endocarditis, burns, and cystic fibrosis caused by susceptible organisms when other antibiotics have failed

Topical: Treatment of primary and secondary skin infections caused by susceptible organisms

Ophthalmic: Treatment of superficial infections of the eye and conjunctiva caused by susceptible organisms

Usual Dosage

I.V.:

Children ≤12 years: 20 mg/kg/day in 3 divided doses

Children >12 years and Adults: 500 mg sodium fusidate 3 times/day

Ophthalmic: Children ≥2 years and Adults: Instill 1 drop in each eye every 12 hours for 7 days

Topical: Children and Adults: Apply to affected area 3-4 times/day until favorable results are achieved. If a gauze dressing is used, frequency of application may be reduced to 1-2 times/day.

Oral: Adults: 500 mg sodium fusidate 3 times/day. (**Note:** Oral dosage may be increased to 1000 mg 3 times/day in fulminating infections.)

Dosage Forms [CAN] = Canadian brand name

Cream:

Fucidin® [CAN]: 2% (15 g, 30 g) [not available in the U.S.]

(Continued)

fusidic acid *(Canada only)* *(Continued)*

Injection, powder for reconstitution:
Fucidin® [CAN]: 500 mg [not available in the U.S.]
Ointment, topical:
Fucidin® [CAN]: 2% (15 g, 30 g) [not available in the U.S.]
Suspension, ophthalmic:
Fucithalmic® [CAN]: 10 mg/g [1%] (0.2 g) [unit-dose, without preservative]; (3 g, 5 g) [multidose, contains benzalkonium chloride] [not available in the U.S.]
Tablet:
Fucidin® [CAN]: 250 mg [not available in the U.S.]

Fuzeon® [US/Can] *see* enfuvirtide *on page 297*

FVIII/vWF *see* antihemophilic factor/von Willebrand factor complex (human) *on page 60*

FXT [Can] *see* fluoxetine *on page 364*

GAA *see* alglucosidase alfa *on page 29*

gabapentin (GA ba pen tin)

Sound-Alike/Look-Alike Issues
Neurontin® may be confused with Neoral®, Noroxin®
U.S./Canadian Brand Names Apo-Gabapentin® [Can]; BCI-Gabapentin [Can]; Gen-Gabapentin [Can]; Neurontin® [US/Can]; Novo-Gabapentin [Can]; Nu-Gabapentin [Can]; PMS-Gabapentin [Can]
Therapeutic Category Anticonvulsant
Use Adjunct for treatment of partial seizures with and without secondary generalized seizures in patients >12 years of age with epilepsy; adjunct for treatment of partial seizures in pediatric patients 3-12 years of age; management of postherpetic neuralgia (PHN) in adults
Usual Dosage Oral:
Children: Anticonvulsant:
3-12 years: Initial: 10-15 mg/kg/day in 3 divided doses; titrate to effective dose over ~3 days; dosages of up to 50 mg/kg/day have been tolerated in clinical studies
3-4 years: Effective dose: 40 mg/kg/day in 3 divided doses
≥5-12 years: Effective dose: 25-35 mg/kg/day in 3 divided doses
See "Note" in Adults dosing.
Children >12 years and Adults:
Anticonvulsant: Initial: 300 mg 3 times/day; if necessary the dose may be increased up to 1800 mg/day. Doses of up to 2400 mg/day have been tolerated in long-term clinical studies; up to 3600 mg/day has been tolerated in short-term studies.
Note: If gabapentin is discontinued or if another anticonvulsant is added to therapy, it should be done slowly over a minimum of 1 week
Adults: Postherpetic neuralgia or neuropathic pain: Day 1: 300 mg, Day 2: 300 mg twice daily, Day 3: 300 mg 3 times/day; dose may be titrated as needed for pain relief (range: 1800-3600 mg/day, daily doses >1800 mg do not generally show greater benefit)
Dosage Forms
Capsule: 100 mg, 300 mg, 400 mg
Neurontin®: 100 mg, 300 mg, 400 mg
Solution, oral:
Neurontin®: 250 mg/5 mL
Tablet: 100 mg, 300 mg, 400 mg, 600 mg, 800 mg
Neurontin®: 600 mg, 800 mg

Gabitril® [US/Can] *see* tiagabine *on page 840*

gadobenate dimeglumine (gad oh BEN ate dye MEG loo meen)

Synonyms gadolinium-BOPTA; Gd-BOPTA
U.S./Canadian Brand Names Multihance® Multipak™ [US]; Multihance® [US]
Therapeutic Category Diagnostic Agent; Radiological/Contrast Media, Nonionic
Use Contrast medium for magnetic resonance imaging (MRI) to visualize CNS lesions with abnormal vascularity in the brain, spine, and associated tissues
Usual Dosage I.V.: Adults: CNS lesions: 0.1 mmol/kg (0.2 mL/kg)
Dosage Forms
Injection, solution [preservative free]:
Multihance®: 529 mg/mL (5 mL, 10 mL, 15 mL, 20 mL)
Multihance® Multipack™: 529 mg/mL (50 mL, 100 mL)

gadobutrol *(Canada only)* (gad oh BYOO trol)
Sound-Alike/Look-Alike Issues
  Gadovist® may be confused with Magnevist®, Vasovist™
Synonyms gadovist 1.0
U.S./Canadian Brand Names Gadovist® [Can]
Therapeutic Category Gadolinium-Containing Contrast Agent; Radiological/Contrast Media, Nonionic
Use Contrast medium for magnetic resonance imaging (MRI) of CNS lesions (brain, spine, and associated tissues); perfusion studies to diagnose stroke, or to detect focal cerebral ischemia or tumor perfusion; contrast-enhanced magnetic resonance angiography (CE-MRA)
Usual Dosage I.V.: Adults:
  General CNS imaging: 0.1 mmol/kg (0.1 mL/kg); if needed, a second dose of 0.1-0.2 mmol/kg (0.1-0.2 mL/kg) may be repeated once within 30 minutes of the first dose
  Exclusion of metastatic or recurrent tumors: 0. 3 mmol/kg (0.3 mL/kg)
  Perfusion studies: 0. 3 mmol/kg (0.3 mL/kg)
  CE-MRA:
   Imaging of a single field of view (FOV):
   Patient weight <75 kg: 7.5 mL
   Patient weight ≥75 kg: 10 mL
   Imaging >1 FOV:
   Patient weight <75 kg: 15 mL
   Patient weight ≥75 kg: 20 mL
Dosage Forms [CAN] = Canadian brand name
  Injection, solution [preservative free]:
  Gadovist® [CAN]: 604.72 mg/mL (15 mL) [not available in U.S.]

gadodiamide (gad oh DYE a mide)
Synonyms gadolinium-DTPA-BMA; Gd-DTPA-BMA
U.S./Canadian Brand Names Omniscan™ [US]
Therapeutic Category Radiological/Contrast Media, Nonionic
Use Contrast medium for magnetic resonance imaging (MRI) to visualize CNS lesions with abnormal vascularity in the brain, spine and associated tissues, and to visualize body lesions with abnormal vascularity within the thoracic (noncardiac), abdominal, pelvic cavities and retroperitoneal space
Usual Dosage I.V.:
  Children ≥2 years:
  Body imaging:
   Kidney: 0.05 mmol/kg (0.1 mL/kg); the safety of additional doses has not been studied
   Intrathoracic (noncardiac), intra-abdominal, pelvic cavities: 0.1 mmol/kg (0.2 mL/kg)
   CNS imaging: 0.1 mmol/kg (0.2 mL/kg); the safety of additional doses has not been studied
  Adults:
  Body imaging:
   Kidney: 0.05 mmol/kg (0.1 mL/kg); the safety of additional doses has not been studied
   Intrathoracic (noncardiac), intra-abdominal, pelvic cavities: 0.1 mmol/kg (0.2 mL/kg); the safety of additional doses has not been studied
   CNS imaging: 0.1 mmol/kg (0.2 mL/kg); if needed, a second dose of 0.2 mmol/kg (0.4 mL/kg) may be repeated once within 20 minutes of the first dose
Dosage Forms
  Injection, solution [preservative free]:
  Omniscan™: 287 mg/mL (5 mL, 10 mL, 15 mL, 20 mL, 50 mL)

gadofosveset *(Canada only)* (gad oh FOS ve set)
Sound-Alike/Look-Alike Issues
  Vasovist® may be confused with Magnevist®, Gadovist®
Synonyms gadofosveset trisodium
U.S./Canadian Brand Names Vasovist® [Can]
Therapeutic Category Gadolinium-Containing Contrast Agent; Radiological/Contrast Media, Paramagnetic Agent
Use Contrast medium used to enhance visualization of abdominal or limb vasculature in magnetic resonance angiography (MRA)
Usual Dosage I.V.: Adults: MRA: 0.03 mmol/kg (0.12 mL/kg); doses >0.03 mmol/kg are not recommended
Dosage Forms [CAN] = Canadian brand name
  Injection, solution [preservative free]:
  Vasovist® [CAN]: 0.25 mmoL/mL (10 mL, 15 mL, 20 mL) [not available in U.S.]

gadofosveset trisodium *see* gadofosveset *(Canada only) on this page*

gadolinium-DTPA *see* gadopentetate dimeglumine *on this page*

gadolinium-DTPA-BMA *see* gadodiamide *on previous page*

gadolinium-DTPA-BMEA *see* gadoversetamide *on this page*

gadolinium-HP-DO3A *see* gadoteridol *on this page*

gadolinum-BOPTA *see* gadobenate dimeglumine *on page 380*

gadopentetate dimeglumine (gad oh PEN te tate dye MEG loo meen)
Synonyms gadolinium-DTPA; Gd-DTPA
U.S./Canadian Brand Names Magnevist® [US/Can]
Therapeutic Category Radiological/Contrast Media, Paramagnetic Agent
Use Contrast medium for magnetic resonance imaging (MRI) to visualize lesions with abnormal vascularity in the brain, spine and associated tissues, head and neck, and body (excluding the heart)
Usual Dosage I.V.: Children ≥2 years and Adults: MRI: 0.2 mL/kg (0.1 mmol/kg) at ≤10 mL/15 seconds; complete imaging procedure within 1 hour of injection
Note: Dosing for patients >130 kg (286 pounds) has not been studied.
Dosage Forms
Injection, solution [preservative free]:
Magnevist®: Gadopentetate dimeglumine 469.01 mg/mL (5 mL, 10 mL, 15 mL, 20 mL, 50 mL, 100 mL)

gadoteridol (gad oh TER i dol)
Synonyms gadolinium-HP-DO3A; Gd-HP-DO3A
U.S./Canadian Brand Names ProHance® [US]
Therapeutic Category Radiological/Contrast Media, Nonionic
Use Contrast medium for magnetic resonance imaging (MRI) to visualize CNS lesions with abnormal vascularity in the brain, spine, and associated tissues and to visualize extracranial/extraspinal tissues in the head and neck
Usual Dosage I.V.:
Children ≥2 years: CNS imaging: 0.1 mmol/kg (0.2 mL/kg); the safety of additional doses has not been studied
Adults:
CNS imaging: 0.1 mmol/kg (0.2 mL/kg); if needed, a second dose of 0.2 mmol/kg (0.4 mL/kg) may be repeated once within 30 minutes of the first dose
Extracranial/extraspinal tissue: 0.1 mmol/kg (0.2 mL/kg)
Dosage Forms Injection, solution [preservative free]:
ProHance®: 279.3 mg/mL (5 mL, 10 mL, 15 mL, 17 mL, 20 mL, 50 mL) [contains calteridol calcium 0.23 mg/mL and tromethamine 1.21 mg/mL]
ProHance® Multipack™: 279.3 mg/mL (50 mL) [contains calteridol calcium 0.23 mg/mL and tromethamine 1.21 mg/mL; pharmacy bulk package]

gadoversetamide (gad oh ver SET a mide)
Synonyms gadolinium-DTPA-BMEA; Gd-DTPA-BMEA
U.S./Canadian Brand Names OptiMARK® [US]
Therapeutic Category Radiological/Contrast Media, Nonionic
Use Contrast medium for magnetic resonance imaging (MRI) to visualize lesions with abnormal vascularity in the liver or CNS (brain, spine, and associated tissues)
Usual Dosage I.V.: Adults: CNS or liver lesions: 0.1 mmol/kg (0.2 mL/kg)
Dosage Forms
Injection, solution [preservative free]:
OptiMARK®: 330.9 mg/mL (5 mL, 10 mL, 15 mL, 20 mL, 30 mL, 50 mL)

Gadovist® [Can] *see* gadobutrol *(Canada only) on previous page*

gadovist 1.0 *see* gadobutrol *(Canada only) on previous page*

galantamine (ga LAN ta meen)
Sound-Alike/Look-Alike Issues
Razadyne™ may be confused with Rozerem™
Reminyl® may be confused with Amaryl®
Synonyms galantamine hydrobromide
U.S./Canadian Brand Names Razadyne™ ER [US]; Razadyne™ [US]; Reminyl® ER [Can]; Reminyl® [Can]
Therapeutic Category Acetylcholinesterase Inhibitor (Central)
Use Treatment of mild-to-moderate dementia of Alzheimer disease

Usual Dosage Oral: Adults:

Note: Oral solution and tablet should be taken with breakfast and dinner; capsule should be taken with breakfast. If therapy is interrupted for ≥3 days, restart at the lowest dose and increase to current dose.

Immediate release tablet or solution: Mild-to-moderate dementia of Alzheimer: Initial: 4 mg twice a day for 4 weeks; if tolerated, increase to 8 mg twice daily for ≥4 weeks; if tolerated, increase to 12 mg twice daily

Range: 16-24 mg/day in 2 divided doses

Extended-release capsule: Initial: 8 mg once daily for 4 weeks; if tolerated, increase to 16 mg once daily for ≥4 weeks; if tolerated, increase to 24 mg once daily

Range: 16-24 mg once daily

Conversion to galantamine from other cholinesterase inhibitors: Patients experiencing poor tolerability with donepezil or rivastigmine should wait until side effects subside or allow a 7-day washout period prior to beginning galantamine. Patients not experiencing side effects with donepezil or rivastigmine may begin galantamine therapy the day immediately following discontinuation of previous therapy.

Dosage Forms

Capsule, extended release:
Razadyne™ ER: 8 mg, 16 mg, 24 mg
Solution, oral:
Razadyne™: 4 mg/mL
Tablet:
Razadyne™: 4 mg, 8 mg, 12 mg

galantamine hydrobromide *see galantamine on previous page*

galsulfase (gal SUL fase)

Synonyms recombinant N-acetylgalactosamine 4-sulfatase; rhASB

U.S./Canadian Brand Names Naglazyme™ [US]

Therapeutic Category Enzyme

Use Replacement therapy in mucopolysaccharidosis VI (MPS VI; Maroteaux-Lamy Syndrome) for improvement of walking and stair-climbing capacity

Usual Dosage Note: Premedicate with antihistamines with/without antipyretics 30-60 minutes prior to infusion. MPS VI: Children >5 years and Adults: I.V.: 1 mg/kg once weekly

Dosage Forms

Injection, solution [preservative free]:
Naglazyme™: 5 mg/5 mL (5 mL)

Gamimune® N [Can] *see immune globulin (intravenous) on page 451*

Gamimune® N Injection *(Discontinued)* *see immune globulin (intravenous) on page 451*

gamma benzene hexachloride *see lindane on page 509*

Gamma E-Gems® [US-OTC] *see vitamin E on page 894*

Gamma-E Plus [US-OTC] *see vitamin E on page 894*

Gammagard® Liquid [US/Can] *see immune globulin (intravenous) on page 451*

Gammagard® S/D [US/Can] *see immune globulin (intravenous) on page 451*

gamma globulin *see immune globulin (intramuscular) on page 450*

gamma hydroxybutyric acid *see sodium oxybate on page 795*

gammaphos *see amifostine on page 40*

Gammar®-P I.V. [US] *see immune globulin (intravenous) on page 451*

GammaSTAN™ S/D [US] *see immune globulin (intramuscular) on page 450*

Gamulin® Rh *(Discontinued)*

Gamunex® [US/Can] *see immune globulin (intravenous) on page 451*

ganciclovir (gan SYE kloe veer)

Sound-Alike/Look-Alike Issues
Cytovene® may be confused with Cytosar®, Cytosar-U®

Synonyms DHPG sodium; GCV sodium; nordeoxyguanosine

U.S./Canadian Brand Names Cytovene® [US/Can]; Vitrasert® [US/Can]

Therapeutic Category Antiviral Agent

Use

Parenteral: Treatment of CMV retinitis in immunocompromised individuals, including patients with acquired immunodeficiency syndrome; prophylaxis of CMV infection in transplant patients

Oral: Alternative to the I.V. formulation for maintenance treatment of CMV retinitis in immunocompromised patients, including patients with AIDS, in whom retinitis is stable following appropriate induction therapy and (Continued)

ganciclovir *(Continued)*

for whom the risk of more rapid progression is balanced by the benefit associated with avoiding daily I.V. infusions.

Implant: Treatment of CMV retinitis

Usual Dosage

CMV retinitis: Slow I.V. infusion (dosing is based on total body weight):

Children >3 months and Adults:

Induction therapy: 5 mg/kg/dose every 12 hours for 14-21 days followed by maintenance therapy

Maintenance therapy: 5 mg/kg/day as a single daily dose for 7 days/week or 6 mg/kg/day for 5 days/week

CMV retinitis: Oral: 1000 mg 3 times/day with food **or** 500 mg 6 times/day with food

Prevention of CMV disease in patients with advanced HIV infection and normal renal function: Oral: 1000 mg 3 times/day with food

Prevention of CMV disease in transplant patients: Same initial and maintenance dose as CMV retinitis except duration of initial course is 7-14 days, duration of maintenance therapy is dependent on clinical condition and degree of immunosuppression

Intravitreal implant: One implant for 5- to 8-month period; following depletion of ganciclovir, as evidenced by progression of retinitis, implant may be removed and replaced

Dosage Forms

Capsule: 250 mg, 500 mg

Implant, intravitreal:

Vitrasert®: 4.5 mg [released gradually over 5-8 months]

Injection, powder for reconstitution:

Cytovene®: 500 mg

Ganidin NR [US] *see* guaifenesin *on page 401*

ganirelix *(ga ni REL ix)*

Synonyms ganirelix acetate

U.S./Canadian Brand Names Orgalutran® [Can]

Therapeutic Category Antigonadotropic Agent

Use Inhibits premature luteinizing hormone (LH) surges in women undergoing controlled ovarian hyperstimulation in fertility clinics.

Usual Dosage SubQ: Adults: 250 mcg/day during the mid-to-late phase after initiating follicle-stimulating hormone on day 2 or 3 of cycle. Treatment should be continued daily until the day of chorionic gonadotropin administration.

Dosage Forms

Injection, solution: 250 mcg/0.5 mL

ganirelix acetate *see* ganirelix *on this page*

Gani-Tuss DM NR [US] *see* guaifenesin and dextromethorphan *on page 402*

Gani-Tuss® NR [US] *see* guaifenesin and codeine *on page 402*

Gantrisin® [US] *see* sulfisoxazole *on page 814*

GAR-936 *see* tigecycline *on page 842*

Garamycin® [Can] *see* gentamicin *on page 390*

Garamycin® *(Discontinued)* *see* gentamicin *on page 390*

Gardasil® [US] *see* papillomavirus (Types 6, 11, 16, 18) recombinant vaccine *on page 652*

Gas-X® [US-OTC] *see* simethicone *on page 786*

Gas-X® Extra Strength [US-OTC] *see* simethicone *on page 786*

Gas-X® Maximum Strength [US-OTC] *see* simethicone *on page 786*

GasAid [US-OTC] *see* simethicone *on page 786*

Gas Ban™ [US-OTC] *see* calcium carbonate and simethicone *on page 139*

Gas-Ban DS® *(Discontinued)* *see* aluminum hydroxide, magnesium hydroxide, and simethicone *on page 37*

Gastrocrom® [US] *see* cromolyn sodium *on page 218*

Gastrografin® [US] *see* diatrizoate meglumine and diatrizoate sodium *on page 250*

Gastrosed™ *(Discontinued)* *see* hyoscyamine *on page 441*

gatifloxacin (gat i FLOKS a sin)
U.S./Canadian Brand Names Tequin® [Can]; Zymar™ [US/Can]
Therapeutic Category Antibiotic, Quinolone
Use Treatment of bacterial conjunctivitis
Usual Dosage
  Usual dosage range:
    Adults: Oral, I.V.: 400 mg once daily
  Indication-specific dosing:
    Children ≥1 year and Adults:
    Bacterial conjunctivitis: Ophthalmic:
      Days 1 and 2: Instill 1 drop into affected eye(s) every 2 hours while awake (maximum: 8 times/day)
      Days 3-7: Instill 1 drop into affected eye(s) up to 4 times/day while awake
    Adults: Oral, I.V.:
    Acute bacterial exacerbation of chronic bronchitis: 400 mg every 24 hours for 5 days
    Acute sinusitis: 400 mg every 24 hours for 10 days
    Community-acquired pneumonia (including atypical organisms): 400 mg every 24 hours for 7-14 days
    Pyelonephritis (acute): 400 mg every 24 hours for 7-10 days
    Skin/skin structure infections (uncomplicated): 400 mg every 24 hours for 7-10 days
    Urinary tract infections:
      Complicated: 400 mg every 24 hours for 7-10 days
      Uncomplicated, cystitis: 400 mg single dose or 200 mg every 24 hours for 3 days
    Urethral gonorrhea in men (uncomplicated), cervical or rectal gonorrhea in women, and pharyngitis (gonococcal): 400 mg single dose
Dosage Forms
  Solution, ophthalmic:
    Zymar®: 0.3% (5 mL)

Gaviscon® Extra Strength [US-OTC] *see* aluminum hydroxide and magnesium carbonate *on page 36*

Gaviscon® Liquid [US-OTC] *see* aluminum hydroxide and magnesium carbonate *on page 36*

Gaviscon® Tablet [US-OTC] *see* aluminum hydroxide and magnesium trisilicate *on page 37*

G-CSF *see* filgrastim *on page 352*

G-CSF (PEG conjugate) *see* pegfilgrastim *on page 657*

GCV sodium *see* ganciclovir *on page 383*

Gd-BOPTA *see* gadobenate dimeglumine *on page 380*

GD-Celecoxib [Can] *see* celecoxib *on page 166*

Gd-DTPA *see* gadopentetate dimeglumine *on page 382*

Gd-DTPA-BMA *see* gadodiamide *on page 381*

Gd-DTPA-BMEA *see* gadoversetamide *on page 382*

Gd-HP-DO3A *see* gadoteridol *on page 382*

GD-Quinapril [Can] *see* quinapril *on page 739*

GD-Sildenafil [US] *see* sildenafil *on page 785*

Gebauer's Ethyl Chloride® [US] *see* ethyl chloride *on page 334*

Gee Gee® *(Discontinued)* *see* guaifenesin *on page 401*

gefitinib (ge FI tye nib)
Sound-Alike/Look-Alike Issues
  gefitinib may be confused with erlotinib
Synonyms NSC-715055; ZD1839
U.S./Canadian Brand Names IRESSA® [US]
Therapeutic Category Antineoplastic, Tyrosine Kinase Inhibitor
Use
  U.S. labeling: Treatment of locally advanced or metastatic nonsmall cell lung cancer after failure of platinum-based and docetaxel therapies. Treatment is limited to patients who are benefiting or have benefited from treatment with gefitinib.
  Note: Due to the lack of improved survival data from clinical trials of gefitinib, and in response to positive survival data with another EGFR inhibitor, physicians are advised to use other treatment options in advanced nonsmall cell lung cancer patients following one or two prior chemotherapy regimens when they are refractory/intolerant to their most recent regimen.
(Continued)

gefitinib *(Continued)*

Canada labeling: Approved indication is limited to NSCLC patients with epidermal growth factor receptor (EGFR) expression status positive or unknown.

Usual Dosage Note: In response to the lack of improved survival data from the ISEL trial, AstraZeneca has temporarily suspended promotion of this drug.

Oral: Adults: 250 mg/day; consider 500 mg/day in patients receiving effective CYP3A4 inducers (eg, rifampin, phenytoin)

Dosage Forms
Tablet:
IRESSA®: 250 mg

gelatin (absorbable) (JEL a tin, ab SORB a ble)

Synonyms absorbable gelatin sponge
U.S./Canadian Brand Names Gelfilm® [US]; Gelfoam® [US]
Therapeutic Category Hemostatic Agent
Use Adjunct to provide hemostasis in surgery; open prostatic surgery
Usual Dosage Hemostasis: Apply packs or sponges dry or saturated with sodium chloride. When applied dry, hold in place with moderate pressure. When applied wet, squeeze to remove air bubbles. The powder is applied as a paste prepared by adding approximately 4 mL of sterile saline solution to the powder.
Dosage Forms
Film, ophthalmic:
Gelfilm®: 25 mm x 50 mm (6s)
Film, topical:
Gelfilm®: 100 mm x 125 mm (1s)
Powder, topical:
Gelfoam®: 1 g
Sponge, dental:
Gelfoam®: Size 4 (12s)
Sponge, topical:
Gelfoam®:
Size 50 (4s)
Size 100 (6s)
Size 200 (6s)
Size 2 cm (1s)
Size 6 cm (6s)
Size 12-7 mm (12s)

gelatin, pectin, and methylcellulose (JEL a tin, PEK tin, & meth il SEL yoo lose)

Synonyms methylcellulose, gelatin, and pectin; pectin, gelatin, and methylcellulose
Therapeutic Category Protectant, Topical
Use Temporary relief from minor oral irritations
Usual Dosage Press small dabs into place until the involved area is coated with a thin film; do not try to spread onto area; may be used as often as needed

Gelfilm® [US] *see* gelatin (absorbable) *on this page*

Gelfoam® [US] *see* gelatin (absorbable) *on this page*

Gel-Kam® [US-OTC] *see* fluoride *on page 361*

Gel-Kam® Rinse [US] *see* fluoride *on page 361*

GelRite [US-OTC] *see* alcohol (ethyl) *on page 25*

Gel-Stat™ [US-OTC] *see* alcohol (ethyl) *on page 25*

Gel-Tin® *(Discontinued)* *see* fluoride *on page 361*

Gelucast® [US] *see* zinc gelatin *on page 905*

Gelusil® [US-OTC/Can] *see* aluminum hydroxide, magnesium hydroxide, and simethicone *on page 37*

Gelusil® Extra Strength [Can] *see* aluminum hydroxide and magnesium hydroxide *on page 37*

gemcitabine (jem SITE a been)

Sound-Alike/Look-Alike Issues
Gemzar® may be confused with Zinecard®

Synonyms gemcitabine hydrochloride; NSC-613327

U.S./Canadian Brand Names Gemzar® [US/Can]

Therapeutic Category Antineoplastic Agent

Use Treatment of metastatic breast cancer; locally-advanced or metastatic nonsmall cell lung cancer (NSCLC) or pancreatic cancer; advanced, relapsed ovarian cancer

Usual Dosage Refer to individual protocols. **Note**: Prolongation of the infusion time >60 minutes and administration more frequently than once weekly have been shown to increase toxicity. I.V.:

Pancreatic cancer: Initial: 1000 mg/m^2 weekly for up to 7 weeks followed by 1 week rest; then weekly for 3 weeks out of every 4 weeks.

Dose adjustment: Patients who complete an entire cycle of therapy may have the dose in subsequent cycles increased by 25% as long as the absolute granulocyte count (AGC) nadir is >1500 x 10^6/L, platelet nadir is >100,000 x 10^6/L, and nonhematologic toxicity is less than WHO Grade 1. If the increased dose is tolerated (with the same parameters) the dose in subsequent cycles may again be increased by 20%.

Nonsmall cell lung cancer:

1000 mg/m^2 days 1, 8, and 15; repeat cycle every 28 days

or

1250 mg/m^2 days 1 and 8; repeat cycle every 21 days

Breast cancer: 1250 mg/m^2 days 1 and 8; repeat cycle every 21 days

Ovarian cancer: 1000 mg/m^2 days 1 and 8; repeat cycle every 21 days

Dosage Forms

Injection, powder for reconstitution:

Gemzar®: 200 mg, 1 g

gemcitabine hydrochloride *see* gemcitabine *on previous page*

gemfibrozil (jem FI broe zil)

Sound-Alike/Look-Alike Issues

Lopid® may be confused with Levbid®, Lodine®, Lorabid®, Slo-bid™

Synonyms CI-719

U.S./Canadian Brand Names Apo-Gemfibrozil® [Can]; Gen-Gemfibrozil [Can]; GMD-Gemfibrozil [Can]; Lopid® [US/Can]; Novo-Gemfibrozil [Can]; Nu-Gemfibrozil [Can]; PMS-Gemfibrozil [Can]

Therapeutic Category Antihyperlipidemic Agent, Miscellaneous

Use Treatment of hypertriglyceridemia in types IV and V hyperlipidemia for patients who are at greater risk for pancreatitis and who have not responded to dietary intervention

Usual Dosage Oral: Adults: 1200 mg/day in 2 divided doses, 30 minutes before breakfast and dinner

Dosage Forms

Tablet: 600 mg

Lopid®: 600 mg

gemifloxacin (je mi FLOKS a sin)

Synonyms DW286; gemifloxacin mesylate; LA 20304a; SB-265805

U.S./Canadian Brand Names Factive® [US/Can]

Therapeutic Category Antibiotic, Quinolone

Use Treatment of acute exacerbation of chronic bronchitis; treatment of community-acquired pneumonia (CAP), including pneumonia caused by multidrug-resistant strains of *S. pneumoniae* (MDRSP)

Usual Dosage

Usual dosage range:

Adults: Oral: 320 mg once daily

Indication-specific dosing:

Adults: Oral:

Acute exacerbations of chronic bronchitis: 320 mg once daily for 5 days

Community-acquired pneumonia (mild to moderate): 320 mg once daily for 5 or 7 days (decision to use 5- or 7-day regimen should be guided by initial sputum culture; 7 days are recommended for MDRSP, *Klebsiella*, or *M. catarrhalis* infection)

Dosage Forms

Tablet:

Factive®: 320 mg

gemifloxacin mesylate *see* gemifloxacin *on this page*

gemtuzumab ozogamicin (gem TOO zoo mab oh zog a MY sin)

Synonyms CMA-676; NSC-720568

U.S./Canadian Brand Names Mylotarg® [US/Can]

Therapeutic Category Antineoplastic Agent, Natural Source (Plant) Derivative

Use Treatment of relapsed CD33 positive acute myeloid leukemia (AML) in patients ≥60 years of age who are not candidates for cytotoxic chemotherapy

Usual Dosage I.V.:

Children: **Note:** Patients should receive diphenhydramine (1 mg/kg) 1 hour prior to infusion and acetaminophen 15 mg/kg 1 hour prior to infusion and every 4 hours for 2 additional doses.

Adults: **Note:** Patients should receive diphenhydramine 50 mg orally and acetaminophen 650-1000 mg orally 1 hour prior to administration of each dose. Acetaminophen dosage should be repeated as needed every 4 hours for 2 additional doses. Pretreatment with methylprednisolone may ameliorate infusion-related symptoms.

AML: ≥60 years: 9 mg/m^2 infused over 2 hours. A full treatment course is a total of 2 doses administered with 14 days between doses. Full hematologic recovery is not necessary for administration of the second dose. There has been only limited experience with repeat courses of gemtuzumab ozogamicin.

Dosage Forms

Injection, powder for reconstitution:

Mylotarg®: 5 mg

Gemzar® [US/Can] *see* gemcitabine *on page 386*

Genabid® *(Discontinued)*

Genac® [US-OTC] *see* triprolidine and pseudoephedrine *on page 869*

Gen-Acebutolol [Can] *see* acebutolol *on page 4*

Genaced™ [US-OTC] *see* acetaminophen, aspirin, and caffeine *on page 9*

Genacote™ [US-OTC] *see* aspirin *on page 78*

Gen-Acyclovir [Can] *see* acyclovir *on page 17*

Genahist® [US-OTC] *see* diphenhydramine *on page 265*

Gen-Alendronate [Can] *see* alendronate *on page 27*

Gen-Alprazolam [Can] *see* alprazolam *on page 32*

Gen-Amilazide [Can] *see* amiloride and hydrochlorothiazide *on page 42*

Genamin® Expectorant *(Discontinued)*

Gen-Amiodarone [Can] *see* amiodarone *on page 43*

Gen-Amoxicillin [Can] *see* amoxicillin *on page 48*

Gen-Anagrelide [Can] *see* anagrelide *on page 55*

Genapap™ [US-OTC] *see* acetaminophen *on page 5*

Genapap™ Children [US-OTC] *see* acetaminophen *on page 5*

Genapap™ Extra Strength [US-OTC] *see* acetaminophen *on page 5*

Genapap™ Infant [US-OTC] *see* acetaminophen *on page 5*

Genapap™ Sinus Maximum Strength [US-OTC] *see* acetaminophen and pseudoephedrine *on page 8*

Genaphed® [US-OTC] *see* pseudoephedrine *on page 727*

Genasal [US-OTC] *see* oxymetazoline *on page 643*

Genasoft® [US-OTC] *see* docusate *on page 273*

Genasyme® [US-OTC] *see* simethicone *on page 786*

Gen-Atenolol [Can] *see* atenolol *on page 80*

Genaton™ [US-OTC] *see* aluminum hydroxide and magnesium carbonate *on page 36*

Genaton Tablet [US-OTC] *see* aluminum hydroxide and magnesium trisilicate *on page 37*

Genatuss® *(Discontinued)* *see* guaifenesin *on page 401*

Genatuss DM® [US-OTC] *see* guaifenesin and dextromethorphan *on page 402*

Gen-Azathioprine [Can] *see* azathioprine *on page 87*

Gen-Baclofen [Can] *see* baclofen *on page 92*

Gen-Beclo [Can] *see* beclomethasone *on page 97*

Gen-Bromazepam [Can] *see* bromazepam *(Canada only) on page 119*

Gen-Budesonide AQ [Can] *see* budesonide *on page 123*

Gen-Buspirone [Can] *see* buspirone *on page 129*

Gencalc® 600 *(Discontinued)* *see* calcium carbonate *on page 138*

Gen-Captopril [Can] *see* captopril *on page 145*

Gen-Carbamazepine CR [Can] *see* carbamazepine *on page 147*

Gen-Cimetidine [Can] *see* cimetidine *on page 189*

Gen-Ciprofloxacin [Can] *see* ciprofloxacin *on page 190*

Gen-Citalopram [Can] *see* citalopram *on page 194*

Gen-Clobetasol [Can] *see* clobetasol *on page 201*

Gen-Clomipramine [Can] *see* clomipramine *on page 203*

Gen-Clonazepam [Can] *see* clonazepam *on page 204*

Gen-Clozapine [Can] *see* clozapine *on page 207*

Gen-Combo Sterinebs [Can] *see* ipratropium and albuterol *on page 471*

Gen-Cyclobenzaprine [Can] *see* cyclobenzaprine *on page 221*

Gen-Cyproterone [Can] *see* cyproterone *(Canada only) on page 225*

Gen-Diltiazem [Can] *see* diltiazem *on page 261*

Gen-Diltiazem CD [Can] *see* diltiazem *on page 261*

Gen-Divalproex [Can] *see* valproic acid and derivatives *on page 881*

Gen-Doxazosin [Can] *see* doxazosin *on page 278*

Genebs [US-OTC] *see* acetaminophen *on page 5*

Genebs Extra Strength [US-OTC] *see* acetaminophen *on page 5*

Generlac [US] *see* lactulose *on page 489*

Genesec™ [US-OTC] *see* acetaminophen and phenyltoloxamine *on page 8*

Gen-Etidronate [Can] *see* etidronate disodium *on page 335*

Genexa™ LA [US] *see* guaifenesin and phenylephrine *on page 404*

Geneye® [US-OTC] *see* tetrahydrozoline *on page 832*

Gen-Famotidine [Can] *see* famotidine *on page 341*

Gen-Fenofibrate Micro [Can] *see* fenofibrate *on page 345*

Genfiber® [US-OTC] *see* psyllium *on page 732*

Gen-Fluconazole [Can] *see* fluconazole *on page 356*

Gen-Fluoxetine [Can] *see* fluoxetine *on page 364*

Gen-Gabapentin [Can] *see* gabapentin *on page 380*

Gen-Gemfibrozil [Can] *see* gemfibrozil *on page 387*

Gen-Gliclazide [Can] *see* gliclazide *(Canada only) on page 393*

Gen-Glybe [Can] *see* glyburide *on page 396*

Gengraf® [US] *see* cyclosporine *on page 223*

Gen-Hydroxychloroquine [Can] *see* hydroxychloroquine *on page 438*

Gen-Hydroxyurea [Can] *see* hydroxyurea *on page 439*

Gen-Indapamide [Can] *see* indapamide *on page 452*

Gen-Ipratropium [Can] *see* ipratropium *on page 470*

Gen-K® *(Discontinued)* *see* potassium chloride *on page 700*

Gen-Lamotrigine [Can] *see* lamotrigine *on page 490*

Gen-Levothyroxine [Can] *see* levothyroxine *on page 503*

Gen-Lovastatin [Can] *see* lovastatin *on page 520*

Gen-Medroxy [Can] *see* medroxyprogesterone *on page 537*

Gen-Meloxicam [Can] *see* meloxicam *on page 539*

Gen-Metformin [Can] *see* metformin *on page 548*

Gen-Minocycline [Can] *see* minocycline *on page 571*

Gen-Mirtazapine [Can] *see* mirtazapine *on page 572*

Gen-Nabumetone [Can] *see* nabumetone *on page 585*

Gen-Naproxen EC [Can] *see* naproxen *on page 591*

Gen-Nitro [Can] *see* nitroglycerin *on page 608*

Gen-Nizatidine [Can] *see* nizatidine *on page 610*

Gen-Nortriptyline [Can] *see* nortriptyline *on page 613*

Genoptic® *(Discontinued)* *see* gentamicin *on this page*

Genora® 0.5/35 *(Discontinued)* *see* ethinyl estradiol and norethindrone *on page 328*

Genora® 1/35 *(Discontinued)* *see* ethinyl estradiol and norethindrone *on page 328*

Genora® 1/50 *(Discontinued)* *see* mestranol and norethindrone *on page 547*

Genotropin® [US] *see* somatropin *on page 799*

Genotropin Miniquick® [US] *see* somatropin *on page 799*

Gen-Oxybutynin [Can] *see* oxybutynin *on page 639*

Gen-Paroxetine [Can] *see* paroxetine *on page 654*

Gen-Pindolol [Can] *see* pindolol *on page 683*

Gen-Piroxicam [Can] *see* piroxicam *on page 687*

Genpril® [US-OTC] *see* ibuprofen *on page 444*

Gen-Ranidine [Can] *see* ranitidine *on page 744*

Gen-Salbutamol [Can] *see* albuterol *on page 23*

Gen-Selegiline [Can] *see* selegiline *on page 780*

Gen-Sertraline [Can] *see* sertraline *on page 783*

Gen-Simvastatin [Can] *see* simvastatin *on page 787*

Gen-Sotalol [Can] *see* sotalol *on page 802*

Gen-Sumatriptan [Can] *see* sumatriptan *on page 815*

Gentacidin® *(Discontinued)* *see* gentamicin *on this page*

Gentak® [US] *see* gentamicin *on this page*

gentamicin (jen ta MYE sin)

Sound-Alike/Look-Alike Issues
gentamicin may be confused with kanamycin
Garamycin® may be confused with kanamycin, Terramycin®

Synonyms gentamicin sulfate

U.S./Canadian Brand Names Alcomicin® [Can]; Diogent® [Can]; Garamycin® [Can]; Gentak® [US]; Gentamicin Injection, USP [Can]; SAB-Gentamicin [Can]

Therapeutic Category Aminoglycoside (Antibiotic); Antibiotic, Ophthalmic; Antibiotic, Topical

Use Treatment of susceptible bacterial infections, normally gram-negative organisms including *Pseudomonas*, *Proteus*, *Serratia*, and gram-positive *Staphylococcus*; treatment of bone infections, respiratory tract infections, skin and soft tissue infections, as well as abdominal and urinary tract infections, endocarditis, and septicemia; used topically to treat superficial infections of the skin or ophthalmic infections caused by susceptible bacteria; prevention of infective endocarditis prior to dental or surgical procedures

Usual Dosage Note: Dosage Individualization is **critical** because of the low therapeutic index.

Use of ideal body weight (IBW) for determining the mg/kg/dose appears to be more accurate than dosing on the basis of total body weight (TBW). In morbid obesity, dosage requirement may best be estimated using a dosing weight of IBW + 0.4 (TBW - IBW).

Initial and periodic plasma drug levels (eg, peak and trough with conventional dosing) should be determined, particularly in critically-ill patients with serious infections or in disease states known to significantly alter aminoglycoside pharmacokinetics (eg, cystic fibrosis, burns, or major surgery).

Usual dosage ranges:
Infants and Children <5 years: I.M., I.V.: 2.5 mg/kg/dose every 8 hours*
Children ≥5 years: I.M., I.V.: 2-2.5 mg/kg/dose every 8 hours*
*Note: Higher individual doses and/or more frequent intervals (eg, every 6 hours) may be required in selected clinical situations (cystic fibrosis) or serum levels document the need
Children and Adults:
 Intrathecal: 4-8 mg/day
 Ophthalmic:
  Ointment: Instill 1/2" (1.25 cm) 2-3 times/day to every 3-4 hours
  Solution: Instill 1-2 drops every 2-4 hours, up to 2 drops every hour for severe infections
 Topical: Apply 3-4 times/day to affected area

Adults: I.M., I.V.:
Conventional: 1-2.5 mg/kg/dose every 8-12 hours; to ensure adequate peak concentrations early in therapy, higher initial dosage may be considered in selected patients when extracellular water is increased (edema, septic shock, postsurgical, or trauma)
Once daily: 4-7 mg/kg/dose once daily; some clinicians recommend this approach for all patients with normal renal function; this dose is at least as efficacious with similar, if not less, toxicity than conventional dosing

Indication-specific dosing:
Neonates: I.V.:
Meningitis:
0-7 days of age: <2000 g: 2.5 mg/kg every 18-24 hours; >2000 g: 2.5 mg/kg every 12 hours
8-28 days of age: <2000 g: 2.5 mg/kg every 8-12 hours; >2000 g: 2.5 mg/kg every 8 hours
Children and Adults: I.M., I.V.:
Brucellosis: 240 mg (I.M.) daily or 5 mg/kg (I.V.) daily for 7 days; either regimen recommended in combination with doxycycline
Cholangitis: 4-6 mg/kg once daily with ampicillin
Diverticulitis (complicated): 1.5-2 mg/kg every 8 hours (with ampicillin and metronidazole)
Endocarditis prophylaxis: Dental, oral, upper respiratory procedures, GI/GU procedures: 1.5 mg/kg with ampicillin (50 mg/kg) 30 minutes prior to procedure
Endocarditis or synergy (for Gram-positive infections): 1 mg/kg every 8 hours (with ampicillin)
Meningitis:
Enterococcus sp or *Pseudomonas aeruginosa*: Loading dose 2 mg/kg, then 1.7 mg/kg/dose every 8 hours (administered with another bacteriocidal drug)
Listeria: 5-7 mg/kg/day (with penicillin) for 1 week
Pelvic inflammatory disease: Loading dose: 2 mg/kg, then 1.5 mg/kg every 8 hours
Alternate therapy: 4.5 mg/kg once daily
Plague (*Yersinia pestis*): Treatment: 5 mg/kg/day, followed by postexposure prophylaxis with doxycycline
Pneumonia, hospital- or ventilator-associated: 7 mg/kg/day (with antipseudomonal beta-lactam or carbapenem)
Tularemia: 5 mg/kg/day divided every 8 hours for 1-2 weeks
Urinary tract infection: 1.5 mg/kg/dose every 8 hours
Dosage Forms
Cream, topical: 0.1% (15 g, 30 g)
Infusion [premixed in NS]: 40 mg (50 mL); 60 mg (50 mL, 100 mL); 70 mg (50 mL); 80 mg (50 mL, 100 mL); 90 mg (100 mL); 100 mg (50 mL, 100 mL); 120 mg (100 mL)
Injection, solution: 10 mg/mL (6 mL, 8 mL, 10 mL); 40 mg/mL (2 mL, 20 mL)
ADD-Vantage® vial: 10 mg/mL (6 mL, 8 mL, 10 mL)
Injection, solution, pediatric: 10 mg/mL (2 mL)
Injection, solution, pediatric [preservative free]: 10 mg/mL (2 mL)
Ointment, ophthalmic: 0.3% [3 mg/g] (3.5 g)
Gentak®: 0.3% [3 mg/g] (3.5 g)
Ointment, topical: 0.1% (15 g, 30 g)
Solution, ophthalmic: 0.3% (5 mL, 15 mL)
Gentak®: 0.3% (5 mL)

gentamicin and prednisolone *see* prednisolone and gentamicin *on page 709*

Gentamicin Injection, USP [Can] *see* gentamicin *on previous page*

gentamicin sulfate *see* gentamicin *on previous page*

Gen-Tamoxifen [Can] *see* tamoxifen *on page 819*

GenTeal® [US-OTC/Can] *see* hydroxypropyl methylcellulose *on page 439*

GenTeal® Mild [US-OTC] *see* hydroxypropyl methylcellulose *on page 439*

Gen-Temazepam [Can] *see* temazepam *on page 823*

Gentex HC [US] *see* hydrocodone, phenylephrine, and guaifenesin *on page 431*

Gentex LA [US] *see* guaifenesin and phenylephrine *on page 404*

Gentex LQ [US] *see* carbetapentane, guaifenesin, and phenylephrine *on page 149*

Gen-Ticlopidine [Can] *see* ticlopidine *on page 842*

Gen-Timolol [Can] *see* timolol *on page 843*

Gen-Tizanidine [Can] *see* tizanidine *on page 846*

Gentlax® [Can] *see* bisacodyl *on page 112*

Gentlax® (Discontinued) *see* bisacodyl *on page 112*

Gen-Topiramate [Can] *see* topiramate *on page 851*

Gentran® **[US/Can]** *see* dextran *on page 245*

Gentrasul® *(Discontinued) see* gentamicin *on page 390*

Gen-Trazodone [Can] *see* trazodone *on page 859*

Gen-Triazolam [Can] *see* triazolam *on page 864*

Gentuss-HC [US] *see* hydrocodone, phenylephrine, and diphenhydramine *on page 431*

Gen-Verapamil [Can] *see* verapamil *on page 887*

Gen-Verapamil SR [Can] *see* verapamil *on page 887*

Gen-Warfarin [Can] *see* warfarin *on page 899*

Gen-Zopiclone [Can] *see* zopiclone *(Canada only) on page 909*

Geocillin® **[US]** *see* carbenicillin *on page 148*

Geodon® **[US]** *see* ziprasidone *on page 907*

Geref® **Diagnostic [US]** *see* sermorelin acetate *on page 782*

Geref® *(Discontinued) see* sermorelin acetate *on page 782*

Geriation [US-OTC] *see* vitamins (multiple/oral) *on page 895*

Geridium® *(Discontinued) see* phenazopyridine *on page 671*

Geri-Freeda [US-OTC] *see* vitamins (multiple/oral) *on page 895*

Geri-Hydrolac™ **[US-OTC]** *see* lactic acid and ammonium hydroxide *on page 487*

Geri-Hydrolac™**-12 [US-OTC]** *see* lactic acid and ammonium hydroxide *on page 487*

Geritol Complete® **[US-OTC]** *see* vitamins (multiple/oral) *on page 895*

Geritol Extend® **[US-OTC]** *see* vitamins (multiple/oral) *on page 895*

Geritol® **Tonic [US-OTC]** *see* vitamins (multiple/oral) *on page 895*

German measles vaccine *see* rubella virus vaccine (live) *on page 770*

Gevrabon® **[US-OTC]** *see* vitamin B complex combinations *on page 894*

GF196960 *see* tadalafil *on page 819*

GG *see* guaifenesin *on page 401*

GG-Cen® *(Discontinued) see* guaifenesin *on page 401*

GHB *see* sodium oxybate *on page 795*

GI87084B *see* remifentanil *on page 748*

Gilphex TR® **[US]** *see* guaifenesin and phenylephrine *on page 404*

Giltuss® **[US]** *see* guaifenesin, dextromethorphan, and phenylephrine *on page 407*

Giltuss HC® **[US]** *see* hydrocodone, phenylephrine, and guaifenesin *on page 431*

Giltuss Pediatric® **[US]** *see* guaifenesin, dextromethorphan, and phenylephrine *on page 407*

Giltuss TR® **[US]** *see* guaifenesin, dextromethorphan, and phenylephrine *on page 407*

Gladase® **[US]** *see* papain and urea *on page 652*

glargine insulin *see* insulin glargine *on page 458*

glatiramer acetate (gla TIR a mer AS e tate)

Sound-Alike/Look-Alike Issues
Copaxone® may be confused with Compazine®
Synonyms copolymer-1
U.S./Canadian Brand Names Copaxone® [US/Can]
Therapeutic Category Biological, Miscellaneous
Use Management of relapsing-remitting type multiple sclerosis
Usual Dosage SubQ: Adults: 20 mg daily
Dosage Forms
 Injection, solution [preservative free]:
  Copaxone®: 20 mg/mL (1 mL)

Glaucon® *(Discontinued) see* epinephrine *on page 300*

Gleevec® **[US/Can]** *see* imatinib *on page 448*

Gliadel® **[US]** *see* carmustine *on page 155*

Gliadel Wafer® **[Can]** *see* carmustine *on page 155*

glibenclamide *see* glyburide *on page 396*

Gliclazide-80 [Can] *see* gliclazide *(Canada only) on this page*

gliclazide *(Canada only)* (GLYE kla zide)

U.S./Canadian Brand Names Apo-Gliclazide® [Can]; Diamicron® MR [Can]; Diamicron® [Can]; Gen-Gliclazide [Can]; Gliclazide-80 [Can]; Novo-Gliclazide [Can]; Sandoz-Gliclazide [Can]

Therapeutic Category Antidiabetic Agent; Hypoglycemic Agent, Oral; Sulfonylurea Agent

Use Management of type 2 diabetes mellitus (noninsulin-dependent, NIDDM)

Usual Dosage Oral: Adults:

Immediate release tablet: Initial: 80-160 mg/day; typical dose range 80-320 mg/day; dosage of ≥160 mg should be divided into 2 equal parts for twice-daily administration; maximum dose: 320 mg/day; should be taken with meals

Sustained release tablet: 30-120 mg once daily

Note: There is no fixed dosage regimen for the management of diabetes mellitus with gliclazide or any other hypoglycemic agent. Dose must be individualized based on frequent determinations of blood glucose during dose titration and throughout maintenance.

Dosage Forms [CAN] = Canadian brand name

Tablet: 80 mg [not available in the U.S.]

Diamicron® [CAN]: 80 mg [not available in the U.S.]

Tablet, sustained release:

Diamicron® MR [CAN]: 30 mg [not available in the U.S.]

glimepiride (GLYE me pye ride)

Sound-Alike/Look-Alike Issues

glimepiride may be confused with glipiZIDE

Amaryl® may be confused with Altace®, Amerge®, Reminyl®

U.S./Canadian Brand Names Amaryl® [US/Can]; CO Glimepiride [Can]; Novo-Glimepiride [Can]; ratio-Glimepiride [Can]; Rhoxal-glimepiride [Can]; Sandoz-Glimepiride [Can]

Therapeutic Category Antidiabetic Agent, Oral

Use Management of type 2 diabetes mellitus (noninsulin-dependent, NIDDM) as an adjunct to diet and exercise to lower blood glucose; may be used in combination with metformin or insulin in patients whose hyperglycemia cannot be controlled by diet and exercise in conjunction with a single oral hypoglycemic agent

Usual Dosage

Oral: Adults: Initial: 1-2 mg once daily, administered with breakfast or the first main meal; usual maintenance dose: 1-4 mg once daily; after a dose of 2 mg once daily, increase in increments of 2 mg at 1- to 2-week intervals based upon the patient's blood glucose response to a maximum of 8 mg once daily. If inadequate response to maximal dose, combination therapy with metformin may be considered.

Combination with insulin therapy (fasting glucose level for instituting combination therapy is in the range of >150 mg/dL in plasma or serum depending on the patient): initial recommended dose: 8 mg once daily with the first main meal

After starting with low-dose insulin, upward adjustments of insulin can be done approximately weekly as guided by frequent measurements of fasting blood glucose. Once stable, combination-therapy patients should monitor their capillary blood glucose on an ongoing basis, preferably daily.

Conversion from therapy with long half-life agents: Observe patient carefully for 1-2 weeks when converting from a longer half-life agent (eg, chlorpropamide) to glimepiride due to overlapping hypoglycemic effects.

Dosage Forms

Tablet: 1 mg, 2 mg, 4 mg

Amaryl®: 1 mg, 2 mg, 4 mg

glimepiride and pioglitazone *see* pioglitazone and glimepiride *on page 684*

glimepiride and pioglitazone hydrochloride *see* pioglitazone and glimepiride *on page 684*

glimepiride and rosiglitazone maleate *see* rosiglitazone and glimepiride *on page 767*

glipizide (GLIP i zide)

Sound-Alike/Look-Alike Issues

glipiZIDE may be confused with glimepiride, glyBURIDE

Glucotrol® may be confused with Glucophage®, Glucotrol® XL, glyBURIDE

Glucotrol® XL may be confused with Glucotrol®

Synonyms glydiazinamide

Tall-Man glipiZIDE

U.S./Canadian Brand Names Glucotrol® XL [US]; Glucotrol® [US]

Therapeutic Category Antidiabetic Agent, Oral

Use Management of type 2 diabetes mellitus (noninsulin-dependent, NIDDM)

(Continued)

glipizide *(Continued)*

Usual Dosage Oral (allow several days between dose titrations): Adults: Initial: 5 mg/day; adjust dosage at 2.5-5 mg daily increments as determined by blood glucose response at intervals of several days.

Immediate release tablet: Maximum recommended once-daily dose: 15 mg; maximum recommended total daily dose: 40 mg. Doses >15 mg/day should be administered in divided doses.

Extended release tablet (Glucotrol® XL): Maximum recommended dose: 20 mg

When transferring from insulin to glipizide:

Current insulin requirement ≤20 units: Discontinue insulin and initiate glipizide at usual dose

Current insulin requirement >20 units: Decrease insulin by 50% and initiate glipizide at usual dose; gradually decrease insulin dose based on patient response. Several days should elapse between dosage changes.

Dosage Forms

Tablet: 5 mg, 10 mg

Glucotrol®: 5 mg, 10 mg

Tablet, extended release:2.5 mg, 5 mg, 10 mg

Glucotrol® XL: 2.5 mg, 5 mg, 10 mg

glipizide and metformin (GLIP i zide & met FOR min)

Synonyms glipizide and metformin hydrochloride; metformin and glipizide

U.S./Canadian Brand Names Metaglip™ [US]

Therapeutic Category Antidiabetic Agent (Biguanide); Antidiabetic Agent (Sulfonylurea)

Use Initial therapy for management of type 2 diabetes mellitus (noninsulin-dependent, NIDDM) when hyperglycemia cannot be managed with diet and exercise alone. Second-line therapy for management of type 2 diabetes (NIDDM) when hyperglycemia cannot be managed with a sulfonylurea or metformin along with diet and exercise.

Usual Dosage Oral: Adults:

Type 2 diabetes, first-line therapy: Initial: Glipizide 2.5 mg/metformin 250 mg once daily with a meal. Dose adjustment: Increase dose by 1 tablet/day every 2 weeks, up to a maximum of glipizide 10 mg/metformin 1000 mg daily

Patients with fasting plasma glucose (FPG) 280-320 mg/dL: Consider glipizide 2.5 mg/metformin 500 mg twice daily. Dose adjustment: Increase dose by 1 tablet/day every 2 weeks, up to a maximum of glipizide 10 mg/metformin 2000 mg daily in divided doses

Type 2 diabetes, second-line therapy: Glipizide 2.5 mg/metformin 500 mg **or** glipizide 5 mg/metformin 500 mg twice daily with morning and evening meals; starting dose should not exceed current daily dose of glipizide (or sulfonylurea equivalent) or metformin. Dose adjustment: Titrate dose in increments of no more than glipizide 5 mg/metformin 500 mg, up to a maximum dose of glipizide 20 mg/metformin 2000 mg daily.

Dosage Forms

Tablet: 2.5/250: Glipizide 2.5 mg and metformin 250 mg; 2.5/500: Glipizide 2.5 mg and metformin 500 mg; 5/500: Glipizide 5 mg and metformin 500 mg

Metaglip™: 2.5/250: Glipizide 2.5 mg and metformin 250 mg; 2.5/500: Glipizide 2.5 mg and metformin 500 mg; 5/500: Glipizide 5 mg and metformin 500 mg

glipizide and metformin hydrochloride *see* glipizide and metformin *on this page*

glivec *see* imatinib *on page 448*

GlucaGen® [US] *see* glucagon *on this page*

GlucaGen® Diagnostic Kit [US] *see* glucagon *on this page*

GlucaGen® HypoKit™ [US] *see* glucagon *on this page*

glucagon (GLOO ka gon)

Sound-Alike/Look-Alike Issues

glucagon may be confused with Glaucon®

Synonyms glucagon hydrochloride

U.S./Canadian Brand Names GlucaGen® Diagnostic Kit [US]; GlucaGen® HypoKit™ [US]; GlucaGen® [US]; Glucagon Emergency Kit [US]

Therapeutic Category Antihypoglycemic Agent

Use Management of hypoglycemia; diagnostic aid in radiologic examinations to temporarily inhibit GI tract movement

Usual Dosage

Hypoglycemia or insulin shock therapy: I.M., I.V., SubQ:

Children <20 kg: 0.5 mg or 20-30 mcg/kg/dose; repeated in 20 minutes as needed

Children ≥20 kg and Adults: 1 mg; may repeat in 20 minutes as needed

Note: If patient fails to respond to glucagon, I.V. dextrose must be given.

Diagnostic aid: Adults: I.M., I.V.: 0.25-2 mg 10 minutes prior to procedure

Dosage Forms
  Injection, powder for reconstitution:
    GlucaGen®, GlucaGen® Diagnostic Kit, GlucaGen® HypoKit™, Glucagon®, Glucagon Emergency Kit: 1 mg

Glucagon Diagnostic Kit *(Discontinued)* see glucagon *on previous page*

Glucagon Emergency Kit [US] see glucagon *on previous page*

glucagon hydrochloride see glucagon *on previous page*

glucocerebrosidase see alglucerase *on page 28*

GlucoNorm® [Can] see repaglinide *on page 750*

Glucophage® [US/Can] see metformin *on page 548*

Glucophage® XR [US] see metformin *on page 548*

glucose (instant) (GLOO kose IN stant)
  Sound-Alike/Look-Alike Issues
    Glutose™ may be confused with Glutofac®
  U.S./Canadian Brand Names B-D™ Glucose [US-OTC]; Dex4 Glucose [US-OTC]; Glutol™ [US-OTC]; Glutose™ [US-OTC]; Insta-Glucose® [US-OTC]
  Therapeutic Category Antihypoglycemic Agent
  Use Management of hypoglycemia
  Usual Dosage Oral: Adults: 10-20 g
  Dosage Forms
    Gel, oral:
      Glutose™: 40% (15 g, 45 g)
      Insta-Glucose®: 40% (30 g)
    Solution, oral:
      Glutol™: 55% [100 g dextrose/180 mL] (180 mL)
    Tablet, chewable:
      B-D™ Glucose: 5 g
      Dex4 Glucose: 4 g

glucose polymers (GLOO kose POL i merz)
  U.S./Canadian Brand Names Moducal® [US-OTC]; Polycose® [US-OTC]
  Therapeutic Category Nutritional Supplement
  Use Supplies calories for those persons not able to meet the caloric requirement with usual food intake
  Usual Dosage Oral: Adults: Add to foods or beverages or mix in water
  Dosage Forms
    Liquid:
      Polycose® [OTC]: 43%
    Powder:
      Moducal® [OTC]: 368 g
      Polycose® [OTC]: 350 g

Glucotrol® [US] see glipizide *on page 393*

Glucotrol® XL [US] see glipizide *on page 393*

Glucovance® [US] see glyburide and metformin *on next page*

glulisine insulin see insulin glulisine *on page 458*

Glumetza™ [US/Can] see metformin *on page 548*

glutamic acid (gloo TAM ik AS id)
  Synonyms glutamic acid hydrochloride
  Therapeutic Category Gastrointestinal Agent, Miscellaneous
  Use Treatment of hypochlorhydria and achlorhydria
  Usual Dosage Oral: Adults:
    Tablet/powder: 500-1000 mg/day before meals or food
    Capsule: 1-3 capsules 3 times/day before meals
  Dosage Forms
    Capsule: 340 mg
    Tablet: 500 mg

glutamic acid hydrochloride see glutamic acid *on this page*

Glutofac®-MX [US] see vitamins (multiple/oral) *on page 895*

Glutofac®-ZX [US] *see* vitamins (multiple/oral) *on page 895*

Glutol™ [US-OTC] *see* glucose (instant) *on previous page*

Glutose™ [US-OTC] *see* glucose (instant) *on previous page*

Glyate® *(Discontinued) see* guaifenesin *on page 401*

glybenclamide *see* glyburide *on this page*

glybenzcyclamide *see* glyburide *on this page*

glyburide (GLYE byoor ide)
Sound-Alike/Look-Alike Issues
glyBURIDE may be confused with glipiZIDE, Glucotrol®
Diaβeta® may be confused with Diabinese®, Zebeta®
Micronase® may be confused with microK®, miconazole, Micronor®, Microzide™
Synonyms glibenclamide; glybenclamide; glybenzcyclamide
Tall-Man glyBURIDE
U.S./Canadian Brand Names Albert® Glyburide [Can]; Apo-Glyburide® [Can]; Diaβeta® [US/Can]; Euglucon® [Can]; Gen-Glybe [Can]; Glynase® PresTab® [US]; Micronase® [US]; Novo-Glyburide [Can]; Nu-Glyburide [Can]; PMS-Glyburide [Can]; ratio-Glyburide [Can]; Sandoz-Glyburide [Can]
Therapeutic Category Antidiabetic Agent, Oral
Use Management of type 2 diabetes mellitus (noninsulin-dependent, NIDDM)
Usual Dosage Oral: Adults:
Diaβeta®, Micronase®:
Initial: 2.5-5 mg/day, administered with breakfast or the first main meal of the day. In patients who are more sensitive to hypoglycemic drugs, start at 1.25 mg/day.
Increase in increments of no more than 2.5 mg/day at weekly intervals based on the patient's blood glucose response
Maintenance: 1.25-20 mg/day given as single or divided doses; maximum: 20 mg/day
Micronized tablets (Glynase® PresTab®): Adults:
Initial: 1.5-3 mg/day, administered with breakfast or the first main meal of the day in patients who are more sensitive to hypoglycemic drugs, start at 0.75 mg/day. Increase in increments of no more than 1.5 mg/day in weekly intervals based on the patient's blood glucose response.
Maintenance: 0.75-12 mg/day given as a single dose or in divided doses. Some patients (especially those receiving >6 mg/day) may have a more satisfactory response with twice-daily dosing. Maximum: 12 mg/day
Dosage Forms
Tablet: 1.25 mg, 2.5 mg, 5 mg
Diaβeta®, Micronase®: 1.25 mg, 2.5 mg, 5 mg
Tablet, micronized: 1.5 mg, 3 mg, 6 mg
Glynase® PresTab®: 3 mg, 6 mg

glyburide and metformin (GLYE byoor ide & met FOR min)
Sound-Alike/Look-Alike Issues
Glucovance® may be confused with Vyvanse™
Synonyms glyburide and metformin hydrochloride; metformin and glyburide
U.S./Canadian Brand Names Glucovance® [US]
Therapeutic Category Antidiabetic Agent (Sulfonylurea); Antidiabetic Agent, Oral
Use Initial therapy for management of type 2 diabetes mellitus (noninsulin-dependent, NIDDM). Second-line therapy for management of type 2 diabetes (NIDDM) when hyperglycemia cannot be managed with a sulfonylurea or metformin; combination therapy with a thiazolidinedione may be required to achieve additional control.
Usual Dosage Note: Dose must be individualized. Dosages expressed as glyburide/metformin components. Adults: Oral:
Initial therapy (no prior treatment with sulfonylurea or metformin): 1.25 mg/250 mg once daily with a meal; patients with Hb A_{1c} >9% or fasting plasma glucose (FPG) >200 mg/dL may start with 1.25 mg/250 mg twice daily
Dosage may be increased in increments of 1.25 mg/250 mg, at intervals of not less than 2 weeks; maximum daily dose: 10 mg/2000 mg (limited experience with higher doses)
Previously treated with a sulfonylurea or metformin alone: Initial: 2.5 mg/500 mg or 5 mg/500 mg twice daily; increase in increments no greater than 5 mg/500 mg; maximum daily dose: 20 mg/2000 mg
When switching patients previously on a sulfonylurea and metformin together, do not exceed the daily dose of glyburide (or glyburide equivalent) or metformin.
Note: May combine with a thiazolidinedione in patients with an inadequate response to glyburide/metformin therapy (risk of hypoglycemia may be increased).

Dosage Forms
 Tablet: Glyburide 1.25 mg and metformin 250 mg; glyburide 2.5 mg and metformin 500 mg; glyburide 5 mg and metformin 500 mg
 Glucovance®: 1.25 mg/250 mg: Glyburide 1.25 mg and metformin 250 mg; 2.5 mg/500 mg: Glyburide 2.5 mg and metformin 500 mg; 5 mg/500 mg: Glyburide 5 mg and metformin 500 mg

glyburide and metformin hydrochloride *see* glyburide and metformin *on previous page*

glycerin (GLIS er in)
Synonyms glycerol
U.S./Canadian Brand Names Bausch & Lomb® Computer Eye Drops [US-OTC]; Colace® Adult/Children Suppositories [US-OTC]; Colace® Infant/Children Suppositories [US-OTC]; Fleet® Babylax® [US-OTC]; Fleet® Glycerin Suppositories Maximum Strength [US-OTC]; Fleet® Glycerin Suppositories [US-OTC]; Fleet® Liquid Glycerin Suppositories [US-OTC]; Sani-Supp® [US-OTC]
Therapeutic Category Laxative; Ophthalmic Agent, Miscellaneous
Use Constipation; reduction of intraocular pressure; reduction of corneal edema; glycerin has been administered orally to reduce intracranial pressure
Usual Dosage
 Constipation: Rectal:
  Children <6 years: 1 infant suppository 1-2 times/day as needed or 2-5 mL as an enema
  Children >6 years and Adults: 1 adult suppository 1-2 times/day as needed or 5-15 mL as an enema
 Children and Adults:
  Reduction of intraocular pressure: Oral: 1-1.8 g/kg 1-1½ hours preoperatively; additional doses may be administered at 5-hour intervals
  Reduction of intracranial pressure: Oral: 1.5 g/kg/day divided every 4 hours; 1 g/kg/dose every 6 hours has also been used
  Reduction of corneal edema: Ophthalmic solution: Instill 1-2 drops in eye(s) prior to examination OR for lubricant effect, instill 1-2 drops in eye(s) every 3-4 hours
Dosage Forms
 Solution, ophthalmic, sterile:
  Bausch & Lomb® Computer Eye Drops [OTC]: 1% (15 mL)
 Solution, rectal:
  Fleet® Babylax® [OTC]: 2.3 g/2.3 mL (4 mL)
  Fleet® Liquid Glycerin Suppositories [OTC]: 5.6 g/5.5 mL (7.5 mL)
 Suppository, rectal: 82.5% (12s, 25s) [pediatric size]; 82.5% (12s, 24s, 25s, 50s, 100s) [adult size]
  Colace® Adult/Children [OTC]: 2.1 g (12s, 24s, 48s, 100s)
  Colace® Infant/Children [OTC]: 1.2 g (12s, 24s)
  Fleet® Glycerin Suppositories [OTC]: 1 g (12s) [pediatric size]; 2g (12s, 24s, 50s) [adult size]
  Fleet® Glycerin Suppositories Maximum Strength [OTC]: 3g (18s) [adult size]
  Sani-Supp® [OTC]: 82.5% (10s, 25s) [pediatric size]; 82.5% (10s, 25s, 50s) [adult size]

glycerol *see* glycerin *on this page*

glycerol guaiacolate *see* guaifenesin *on page 401*

Glycerol-T® *(Discontinued) see* theophylline and guaifenesin *on page 835*

glycerol triacetate *see* triacetin *on page 861*

glyceryl trinitrate *see* nitroglycerin *on page 608*

Glycofed® *(Discontinued) see* guaifenesin and pseudoephedrine *on page 406*

GlycoLax® [US] *see* polyethylene glycol 3350 *on page 694*

Glycon [Can] *see* metformin *on page 548*

glycopyrrolate (glye koe PYE roe late)
Synonyms glycopyrronium bromide
U.S./Canadian Brand Names Glycopyrrolate Injection, USP [Can]; Robinul® Forte [US]; Robinul® [US]
Therapeutic Category Anticholinergic Agent
Use Inhibit salivation and excessive secretions of the respiratory tract preoperatively; reversal of neuromuscular blockade; control of upper airway secretions; adjunct in treatment of peptic ulcer
Usual Dosage
 Children:
  Reduction of secretions (preanesthetic):
   Oral: 40-100 mcg/kg/dose 3-4 times/day
   I.M., I.V.: 4-10 mcg/kg/dose every 3-4 hours; maximum: 0.2 mg/dose or 0.8 mg/24 hours
   Intraoperative: I.V.: 4 mcg/kg not to exceed 0.1 mg; repeat at 2- to 3-minute intervals as needed
(Continued)

glycopyrrolate *(Continued)*

Preoperative: I.M.:
  <2 years: 4-9 mcg/kg 30-60 minutes before procedure
  >2 years: 4 mcg/kg 30-60 minutes before procedure
Children and Adults: Reverse neuromuscular blockade: I.V.: 0.2 mg for each 1 mg of neostigmine or 5 mg of pyridostigmine administered or 5-15 mcg/kg glycopyrrolate with 25-70 mcg/kg of neostigmine or 0.1-0.3 mg/kg of pyridostigmine (agents usually administered simultaneously, but glycopyrrolate may be administered first if bradycardia is present)
Adults:
  Reduction of secretions:
    Intraoperative: I.V.: 0.1 mg repeated as needed at 2- to 3-minute intervals
    Preoperative: I.M.: 4 mcg/kg 30-60 minutes before procedure
  Peptic ulcer:
    Oral: 1-2 mg 2-3 times/day
    I.M., I.V.: 0.1-0.2 mg 3-4 times/day

Dosage Forms
  Injection, solution: 0.2 mg/mL (1 mL, 2 mL, 5 mL, 20 mL)
  Robinul®: 0.2 mg/mL (1 mL, 2 mL, 5 mL)
  Tablet:
    Robinul®: 1 mg
    Robinul® Forte: 2 mg

Glycopyrrolate Injection, USP [Can] *see* glycopyrrolate *on previous page*

glycopyrronium bromide *see* glycopyrrolate *on previous page*

Glycotuss® *(Discontinued)* *see* guaifenesin *on page 401*

Glycotuss-dM® *(Discontinued)* *see* guaifenesin and dextromethorphan *on page 402*

glydiazinamide *see* glipizide *on page 393*

Glynase® PresTab® [US] *see* glyburide *on page 396*

Gly-Oxide® [US-OTC] *see* carbamide peroxide *on page 148*

Glyquin® [US] *see* hydroquinone *on page 437*

Glyquin-XM™ [US/Can] *see* hydroquinone *on page 437*

Glyset® [US/Can] *see* miglitol *on page 570*

GM-CSF *see* sargramostim *on page 777*

GMD-Azithromycin [Can] *see* azithromycin *on page 88*

GMD-Fluconazole [Can] *see* fluconazole *on page 356*

GMD-Gemfibrozil [Can] *see* gemfibrozil *on page 387*

GMD-Sertraline [Can] *see* sertraline *on page 783*

G-myticin® *(Discontinued)* *see* gentamicin *on page 390*

GnRH *see* gonadorelin *on next page*

Gold Bond® Antifungal *(Discontinued)* *see* tolnaftate *on page 849*

gold sodium thiomalate (gold SOW dee um thye oh MAL ate)

Synonyms sodium aurothiomalate
U.S./Canadian Brand Names Myochrysine® [US/Can]
Therapeutic Category Gold Compound
Use Treatment of progressive rheumatoid arthritis
Usual Dosage I.M.:
  Children: Initial: Test dose of 10 mg is recommended, followed by 1 mg/kg/week for 20 weeks; maintenance: 1 mg/kg/dose at 2- to 4-week intervals thereafter for as long as therapy is clinically beneficial and toxicity does not develop. Administration for 2-4 months is usually required before clinical improvement is observed.
  Adults: 10 mg first week; 25 mg second week; then 25-50 mg/week until 1 g cumulative dose has been given; if improvement occurs without adverse reactions, administer 25-50 mg every 2-3 weeks for 2-20 weeks, then every 3-4 weeks indefinitely

Dosage Forms
  Injection, solution:
    Myochrysine®: 50 mg/mL (1 mL, 10 mL)

GoLYTELY® [US] *see* polyethylene glycol-electrolyte solution *on page 695*

gonadorelin (goe nad oh RELL in)

Sound-Alike/Look-Alike Issues
gonadorelin may be confused with gonadotropin, guanadrel
Factrel® may be confused with Sectral®
gonadotropin may be confused with gonadorelin

Synonyms GnRH; gonadorelin acetate; gonadorelin hydrochloride; gonadotropin releasing hormone; LHRH; LRH; luteinizing hormone releasing hormone

U.S./Canadian Brand Names Factrel® [US]; Lutrepulse™ [Can]

Therapeutic Category Diagnostic Agent; Gonadotropin

Use Evaluation of functional capacity and response of gonadotrophic hormones; evaluate abnormal gonadotropin regulation as in precocious puberty and delayed puberty.

Orphan drug: Lutrepulse®: Induction of ovulation in females with hypothalamic amenorrhea

Usual Dosage
Diagnostic test: Children >12 years and Female Adults: I.V., SubQ hydrochloride salt: 100 mcg administered in women during early phase of menstrual cycle (day 1-7)
Primary hypothalamic amenorrhea: Female Adults: Acetate: I.V.: 5 mcg every 90 minutes via Lutrepulse® pump kit at treatment intervals of 21 days (pump will pulsate every 90 minutes for 7 days)

Dosage Forms
Injection, powder for reconstitution:
Factrel®: 100 mcg

gonadorelin acetate *see* gonadorelin *on this page*

gonadorelin hydrochloride *see* gonadorelin *on this page*

gonadotropin releasing hormone *see* gonadorelin *on this page*

Gonak™ [US-OTC] *see* hydroxypropyl methylcellulose *on page 439*

Gonal-f® [US/Can] *see* follitropin alfa *on page 372*

Gonal-f® Pen [Can] *see* follitropin alfa *on page 372*

Gonal-f® RFF [US] *see* follitropin alfa *on page 372*

gonioscopic ophthalmic solution *see* hydroxypropyl methylcellulose *on page 439*

Goniosoft™ [US] *see* hydroxypropyl methylcellulose *on page 439*

Goniosol® (Discontinued) *see* hydroxypropyl methylcellulose *on page 439*

Good Sense Sleep Aid [US-OTC] *see* doxylamine *on page 283*

Goody's® Extra Strength Headache Powder [US-OTC] *see* acetaminophen, aspirin, and caffeine *on page 9*

Goody's® Extra Strength Pain Relief [US-OTC] *see* acetaminophen, aspirin, and caffeine *on page 9*

Goody's PM® [US-OTC] *see* acetaminophen and diphenhydramine *on page 7*

Gordofilm® [US-OTC] *see* salicylic acid *on page 772*

Gordon Boro-Packs [US-OTC] *see* aluminum sulfate and calcium acetate *on page 38*

Gormel® [US-OTC] *see* urea *on page 877*

goserelin (GOE se rel in)

Synonyms D-ser(bu^t)^6,Azgly^{10}-LHRH; goserelin acetate; ICI-118630; NSC-606864

U.S./Canadian Brand Names Zoladex® LA [Can]; Zoladex® [US/Can]

Therapeutic Category Gonadotropin-Releasing Hormone Analog

Use Palliative treatment of advanced breast cancer and carcinoma of the prostate; treatment of endometriosis, including pain relief and reduction of endometriotic lesions; endometrial thinning agent as part of treatment for dysfunctional uterine bleeding

Usual Dosage SubQ: Adults:
Prostate cancer:
Monthly implant: 3.6 mg injected into upper abdomen every 28 days
3-month implant: 10.8 mg injected into the upper abdominal wall every 12 weeks
Breast cancer, endometriosis, endometrial thinning: Monthly implant: 3.6 mg injected into upper abdomen every 28 days
Note: For breast cancer, treatment may continue indefinitely; for endometriosis, it is recommended that duration of treatment not exceed 6 months. Only 1-2 doses are recommended for endometrial thinning.

Dosage Forms
Implant, subcutaneous:
Zoladex®: 3.6 mg [1-month implant packaged with 16-gauge hypodermic needle]; 10.8 mg [3-month implant packaged with 14-gauge hypodermic needle]

goserelin acetate *see* goserelin *on previous page*

GP 47680 *see* oxcarbazepine *on page 638*

GR38032R *see* ondansetron *on page 630*

gramicidin, neomycin, and polymyxin B *see* neomycin, polymyxin B, and gramicidin *on page 597*

granisetron (gra NI se tron)

Sound-Alike/Look-Alike Issues
granisetron may be confused with dolasetron, ondansetron, palonosetron

Synonyms BRL 43694

U.S./Canadian Brand Names Kytril® [US/Can]

Therapeutic Category Selective 5-HT$_3$ Receptor Antagonist

Use Prophylaxis of nausea and vomiting associated with emetogenic chemotherapy and radiation therapy, (including total body irradiation and fractionated abdominal radiation); prophylaxis and treatment of postoperative nausea and vomiting (PONV)

Generally **not** recommended for treatment of existing chemotherapy-induced emesis (CIE) or for prophylaxis of nausea from agents with a low emetogenic potential.

Usual Dosage
Oral: Adults:
Prophylaxis of chemotherapy-related emesis: 2 mg once daily up to 1 hour before chemotherapy or 1 mg twice daily; the first 1 mg dose should be given up to 1 hour before chemotherapy.
Prophylaxis of radiation therapy-associated emesis: 2 mg once daily given 1 hour before radiation therapy.
I.V.:
Children ≥2 years and Adults: Prophylaxis of chemotherapy-related emesis:
Within U.S.: 10 mcg/kg/dose (maximum: 1 mg/dose) given 30 minutes prior to chemotherapy; for some drugs (eg, carboplatin, cyclophosphamide) with a later onset of emetic action, 10 mcg/kg every 12 hours may be necessary.
Outside U.S.: 40 mcg/kg/dose (or 3 mg/dose); maximum: 9 mg/24 hours
Breakthrough: Granisetron has not been shown to be effective in teminating nausea or vomiting once it occurs and should not be used for this purpose.
Adults: PONV:
Prevention: 1 mg given undiluted over 30 seconds; administer before induction of anesthesia or immediately before reversal of anesthesia
Treatment: 1 mg given undiluted over 30 seconds

Dosage Forms
Injection, solution:
Kytril®: 1 mg/mL (1 mL, 4 mL)
Injection, solution [preservative free]:
Kytril®: 0.1 mg/mL (1 mL)
Solution, oral:
Kytril®: 2 mg/10 mL
Tablet:
Kytril®: 1 mg

Granulex® [US] *see* trypsin, balsam peru, and castor oil *on page 872*

granulocyte colony stimulating factor *see* filgrastim *on page 352*

granulocyte colony stimulating factor (PEG conjugate) *see* pegfilgrastim *on page 657*

granulocyte-macrophage colony stimulating factor *see* sargramostim *on page 777*

Gravol® [Can] *see* dimenhydrinate *on page 262*

green tea extract *see* sinecatechins *on page 788*

Grifulvin® V [US] *see* griseofulvin *on this page*

Grifulvin® V Tablet 250 mg and 500 mg (Discontinued) *see* griseofulvin *on this page*

Grisactin® Ultra (Discontinued) *see* griseofulvin *on this page*

griseofulvin (gri see oh FUL vin)

Synonyms griseofulvin microsize; griseofulvin ultramicrosize

U.S./Canadian Brand Names Grifulvin® V [US]; Gris-PEG® [US]

Therapeutic Category Antifungal Agent

Use Treatment of susceptible tinea infections of the skin, hair, and nails

Usual Dosage Oral:
Children >2 years:
Microsize: 10-20 mg/kg/day in single or 2 divided doses.

Ultramicrosize: Usual: 7.3 mg/kg/day in single dose or 2 divided doses; range: 5-15 mg/kg/day in single dose or 2 divided doses (maximum: 750 mg/day)

Adults:

Microsize: 500-1000 mg/day in single or divided doses

Ultramicrosize: 375 mg/day in single or divided doses; doses up to 750 mg/day have been used for infections more difficult to eradicate such as tinea unguium and tinea pedis

Duration of therapy depends on the site of infection:

Tinea corporis: 2-4 weeks

Tinea capitis: 4-6 weeks or longer (up to 8-12 weeks)

Tinea pedis: 4-8 weeks

Tinea unguium: 3-6 months or longer

Dosage Forms

Suspension, oral, microsize: 125 mg/5 mL

Grifulvin® V: 125 mg/5 mL

Tablet, microsize:

Grifulvin® V: 500 mg

Tablet, ultramicrosize:

Gris-PEG®: 125 mg, 250 mg

griseofulvin microsize *see* griseofulvin *on previous page*

griseofulvin ultramicrosize *see* griseofulvin *on previous page*

Gris-PEG® [US] *see* griseofulvin *on previous page*

Guaicon DM [US-OTC] *see* guaifenesin and dextromethorphan *on next page*

Guaifed® [US] *see* guaifenesin and phenylephrine *on page 404*

Guaifed-PD® [US] *see* guaifenesin and phenylephrine *on page 404*

Guaifen™ DM [US] *see* guaifenesin, dextromethorphan, and phenylephrine *on page 407*

guaifenesin (gwye FEN e sin)

Sound-Alike/Look-Alike Issues

guaifenesin may be confused with guanfacine

Mucinex® may be confused with Mucomyst®

Naldecon® may be confused with Nalfon®

Synonyms GG; glycerol guaiacolate

U.S./Canadian Brand Names Allfen Jr [US]; Balminil Expectorant [Can]; Benylin® E Extra Strength [Can]; Diabetic Tussin® EX [US-OTC]; Ganidin NR [US]; Guiatuss™ [US-OTC]; Koffex Expectorant [Can]; Mucinex® Maximum Strength [US-OTC]; Mucinex® [US-OTC]; Mucinex®, Children's Mini-Melts™ [US-OTC]; Mucinex®, Children's [US-OTC]; Mucinex®, Junior Mini-Melts™ [US-OTC]; Organidin® NR [US]; Phanasin® Diabetic Choice [US-OTC]; Phanasin® [US-OTC]; Robitussin® [US-OTC/Can]; Scot-Tussin® Expectorant [US-OTC]; Siltussin DAS [US-OTC]; Siltussin SA [US-OTC]; Vicks® Casero™ Chest Congestion Relief [US-OTC]; XPECT™ [US-OTC]

Therapeutic Category Expectorant

Use Help loosen phlegm and thin bronchial secretions to make coughs more productive

Usual Dosage Oral:

Children:

6 months to 2 years: 25-50 mg every 4 hours, not to exceed 300 mg/day

2-5 years: 50-100 mg every 4 hours, not to exceed 600 mg/day

6-11 years: 100-200 mg every 4 hours, not to exceed 1.2 g/day

Children >12 years and Adults: 200-400 mg every 4 hours to a maximum of 2.4 g/day

Extended release tablet: 600-1200 mg every 12 hours, not to exceed 2.4 g/day

Dosage Forms

Caplet:

Refenesen™ 400 [OTC]: 400 mg

Granules, oral:

Mucinex® Children's Mini-Melts™ [OTC]: 50 mg/packet (12s)

Mucinex® Junior Mini-Melts™ [OTC]: 100 mg/packet (12s)

Liquid: 100 mg/5 mL

Diabetic Tussin EX® [OTC], Ganidin NR, Mucinex® Children's [OTC], Organidin® NR, Siltussin DAS [OTC]: 100 mg/5 mL

Syrup: 100 mg/5 mL

Guiatuss™ [OTC], Phanasin® [OTC], Phanasin® Diabetic Choice [OTC], Robitussin® [OTC], Scot-Tussin® Expectorant [OTC], Siltussin SA [OTC]: 100 mg/5 mL

Vicks® Casero™ [OTC]: 100 mg/6.25 mL

Tablet: 200 mg

Allfen Jr: 400 mg

(Continued)

guaifenesin *(Continued)*
Organidin® NR: 200 mg
Refenesen™ [OTC]: 200 mg
XPECT™ [OTC]: 400 mg
Tablet, extended release:
Mucinex® [OTC]: 600 mg
Mucinex® Maximum Strength [OTC]: 1200 mg

Guaifenesin AC [US] *see* guaifenesin and codeine *on this page*

guaifenesin and codeine (gwye FEN e sin & KOE deen)
Synonyms codeine and guaifenesin
U.S./Canadian Brand Names Brontex® [US]; Cheracol® [US]; Diabetic Tussin C® [US]; Gani-Tuss® NR [US]; Guaifenesin AC [US]; Guaituss AC [US]; Kolephrin® #1 [US]; Mytussin® AC [US]; Robafen® AC [US]; Romilar® AC [US]; Tussi-Organidin® NR [US]; Tussi-Organidin® S-NR [US]
Therapeutic Category Antitussive/Expectorant
Controlled Substance C-V
Use Temporary control of cough due to minor throat and bronchial irritation
Usual Dosage Oral: **Note:** Also refer to specific product labeling:
Children:
2-6 years (Diabetic Tussin C® liquid, Tussi-Organidin® NR): Codeine 1 mg/kg/day in 4 divided doses
6-12 years (Diabetic Tussin C®, Kolephrin® #1, Romilar® AC, Tussi-Organidin® NR liquid): 5 mL every 4 hours; maximum 30 mL/24 hours
Children ≥12 years and Adults:
Brontex® tablets: 1 tablet every 4 hours; maximum 6 tablets/24 hours
Diabetic Tussin C®, Kolephrin® #1, Romilar® AC, Tussi-Organidin® NR liquid: 10 mL every 4 hours; maximum 60 mL/24 hours
Dosage Forms
Liquid:
Brontex®: Guaifenesin 75 mg and codeine 2.5 mg per 5 mL
Diabetic Tussin C®: Guaifenesin 200 mg and codeine 10 mg per 5 mL
Gani-Tuss® NR, Guaifenesin AC, Kolephrin® #1: Guaifenesin 100 mg and codeine 10 mg per 5 mL
Tussi-Organidin® NR, Tussi-Organidin® S-NR: Guaifenesin 300 mg and codeine 10 mg per 5 mL
Syrup:
Cheracol®, Guaituss AC, Mytussin® AC, Robafen® AC, Romilar® AC: Guaifenesin 100 mg and codeine 10 mg per 5 mL
Tablet: Guaifenesin 300 mg and codeine 10 mg
Brontex®: Guaifenesin 300 mg and codeine 10 mg

guaifenesin and dextromethorphan (gwye FEN e sin & deks troe meth OR fan)
Sound-Alike/Look-Alike Issues
Benylin® may be confused with Benadryl®, Ventolin®
Synonyms dextromethorphan and guaifenesin
U.S./Canadian Brand Names Allfen-DM [US]; Altarussin DM [US-OTC]; Balminil DM E [Can]; Benylin® DM-E [Can]; Cheracol® D [US-OTC]; Cheracol® Plus [US-OTC]; Coricidin HBP® Chest Congestion and Cough [US-OTC]; Diabetic Tussin® DM Maximum Strength [US-OTC]; Diabetic Tussin® DM [US-OTC]; Duratuss® DM [US]; Gani-Tuss DM NR [US]; Genatuss DM® [US-OTC]; Guaicon DM [US-OTC]; Guaifenex® DM [US]; Guia-D [US]; Guaicon DMS [US-OTC]; Guiatuss-DM® [US-OTC]; Hydro-Tussin™ DM [US]; Koffex DM-Expectorant [Can]; Kolephrin® GG/DM [US-OTC]; Mintab DM [US]; Mucinex® Children's Cough [US-OTC]; Mucinex® DM Maximum Strength [US-OTC]; Mucinex® DM [US-OTC]; Phanatuss® DM [US-OTC]; Phlemex [US]; Respa-DM® [US]; Robafen DM Clear [US-OTC]; Robafen DM [US-OTC]; Robitussin® Cough and Congestion [US-OTC]; Robitussin® DM Infant [US-OTC]; Robitussin® DM [US-OTC/Can]; Robitussin® Sugar Free Cough [US-OTC]; Safe Tussin® [US-OTC]; Scot-Tussin® Senior [US-OTC]; Silexin® [US-OTC]; Siltussin DM DAS [US-OTC]; Siltussin DM [US-OTC]; Simuc-DM [US]; Su-Tuss DM [US]; Touro® DM [US]; Tussi-Organidin® DM NR [US]; Tussi-Organidin® DM-S NR [US]; Vicks® 44E [US-OTC]; Vicks® Pediatric Formula 44E [US-OTC]; Z-Cof LA™ [US]
Therapeutic Category Antitussive/Expectorant
Use Temporary control of cough due to minor throat and bronchial irritation
Usual Dosage Oral:
Children 2-6 years:
General dosing guidelines: Guaifenesin 50-100 mg and dextromethorphan 2.5-5 mg every 4 hours (maximum dose: Guaifenesin 600 mg and dextromethorphan 30 mg per day)
Product-specific labeling:
Guaifenex® DM, Touro® DM: ½ tablet every 12 hours (maximum: 1 tablet/24 hour)

Robitussin® DM, Robitussin® DM Infant, Robitussin® Sugar Free Cough: 2.5 mL every 4 hours (maximum: 6 doses/24 hours)

Vicks® Pediatric Formula 44E: 7.5 mL every 4 hours (maximum: 6 doses/24 hours)

Children: 6-12 years:

General dosing guidelines: Guaifenesin 100-200 mg and dextromethorphan 5-10 mg every 4 hours (maximum dose: Guaifenesin 1200 mg and dextromethorphan 60 mg per day)

Product-specific labeling:

Guaifenex® DM, Touro® DM: 1 tablet every 12 hours (maximum: 2 tablets/24 hours)

Robitussin® DM, Robitussin® Sugar Free Cough: 5 mL every 4 hours (maximum: 6 doses/24 hours)

Vicks® 44E: 7.5 mL every 4 hours (maximum: 6 doses/24 hours)

Vicks® Pediatric Formula 44E: 15 mL every 4 hours (maximum: 6 doses/24 hours)

Z-Cof LA™: 1/2 tablet very 12 hours

Children ≥12 years and Adults:

General dosing guidelines: Guaifenesin 200-400 mg and dextromethorphan 10-20 mg every 4 hours (maximum dose: Guaifenesin 2400 mg and dextromethorphan 120 mg per day)

Product-specific labeling:

Guaifenex® DM, Mucinex® DM, Touro® DM: 1-2 tablets every 12 hours (maximum: 4 tablets/24 hours)

Robitussin® DM, Robitussin® Sugar Free Cough: 10 mL every 4 hours (maximum: 6 doses/24 hours)

Vicks® 44E: 15 mL every 4 hours (maximum: 6 doses/24 hours)

Vicks® Pediatric Formula 44E: 30 mL every 4 hours (maximum: 6 doses/24 hours)

Z-Cof LA™: 1 tablet every 12 hours

Dosage Forms

Caplet:

Fenesin DM IR: Guaifenesin 400 mg and dextromethorphan 15 mg

Refenesen™ DM [OTC]: Guaifenesin 400 mg and dextromethorphan 20 mg

Capsule, softgel:

Coricidin HBP® Chest Congestion and Cough [OTC]: Guaifenesin 200 mg and dextromethorphan 10 mg

Elixir:

Duratuss DM®, Simuc-DM: Guaifenesin 225 mg and dextromethorphan 25 mg per 5 mL

Su-Tuss DM: Guaifenesin 200 mg and dextromethorphan 20 mg per 5 mL

Liquid: Guaifenesin 100 mg and dextromethorphan 10 mg per 5 mL; guaifenesin 300 mg and dextromethorphan 10 mg per 5 mL

Diabetic Tussin® DM [OTC], Gani-Tuss® DM NR: Guaifenesin 100 mg and dextromethorphan 10 mg per 5 mL

Diabetic Tussin® DM Maximum Strength [OTC]: Guaifenesin 200 mg and dextromethorphan 10 mg per 5 mL

Double Tussin DM [OTC]: Guaifenesin 300 mg and dextromethorphan 200 mg per 5 mL

Hydro-Tussin™ DM: Guaifenesin 200 mg and dextromethorphan 20 mg per 5 mL

Kolephrin® GG/DM [OTC]: Guaifenesin 150 mg and dextromethorphan 10 mg per 5 mL

Mucinex® Children's Cough [OTC]: Guaifenesin 100 mg and dextromethorphan 5 mg per 5 mL

Safe Tussin® DM [OTC]: Guaifenesin 100 mg and dextromethorphan 15 mg per 5 mL

Scot-Tussin® Senior [OTC]: Guaifenesin 200 mg and dextromethorphan 15 mg per 5 mL

Tussi-Organidin® DM NR: Guaifenesin 300 mg and dextromethorphan 10 mg per 5 mL

Tussi-Organidin® DM-S NR: Guaifenesin 300 mg and dextromethorphan 10 mg per 5 mL

Vicks® 44E [OTC]: Guaifenesin 200 mg and dextromethorphan hydrobromide 20 mg per 15 mL

Vicks® Pediatric Formula 44E [OTC]: Guaifenesin 100 mg and dextromethorphan hydrobromide 10 mg per 15 mL

Syrup: Guaifenesin 100 mg and dextromethorphan 10 mg per 5 mL

Altarussin DM [OTC], Cheracol® D [OTC], Cheracol® Plus [OTC], Genatuss DM® [OTC], Guiatuss® DM [OTC], Guaicon DM [OTC], Guaicon DMS [OTC], Phanatuss® DM [OTC], Robafen® DM [OTC], Robafen DM Clear [OTC], Robitussin® Cough and Congestion [OTC], Robitussin®-DM [OTC], Robitussin® Sugar Free Cough [OTC], Silexin [OTC], Siltussin DM [OTC], Siltussin DM DAS [OTC]: Guaifenesin 100 mg and dextromethorphan 10 mg per 5 mL

Mintab DM: Guaifenesin 200 mg and dextromethorphan hydrobromide 10 mg per 5 mL

Tablet: Guaifenesin 1000 mg and dextromethorphan hydrobromide 60 mg; guaifenesin 1200 mg and dextromethorphan hydrobromide 60 mg

Silexin: Guaifenesin 100 mg and dextromethorphan hydrobromide 10 mg

Tablet, extended release:

Guaifenex® DM, Mucinex® DM [OTC], Respa-DM®: Guaifenesin 600 mg and dextromethorphan 30 mg

Mucophen® DM: Guaifenesin 1000 mg and dextromethorphan 60 mg

Mucinex® DM Maximum Strength: Guaifenesin 1200 mg and dextromethorphan 60 mg

Phlemex: Guaifenesin 1200 mg and dextromethorphan 20 mg

Touro® DM: Guaifenesin 575 mg and dextromethorphan 30 mg

Tablet, long-acting: Guaifenesin 1000 mg and dextromethorphan 60 mg

Z-Cof LA [scored]: Guaifenesin 650 mg and dextromethorphan 30 mg

Tablet, sustained release:

Allfen-DM: Guaifenesin 1000 mg and dextromethorphan 55 mg

(Continued)

guaifenesin and dextromethorphan (Continued)

Relacon LAX: Guaifenesin 835 mg and dextromethorphan 30 mg
Tussi-Bid®: Guaifenesin 1200 mg and dextromethorphan 60 mg
Tablet, timed release [scored]: Guaifenesin 1200 mg and dextromethorphan 60 mg
Guia-D: Guaifenesin 1000 mg and dextromethorphan 60 mg

guaifenesin and dyphylline see dyphylline and guaifenesin on page 288
guaifenesin and hydrocodone see hydrocodone and guaifenesin on page 429

guaifenesin and phenylephrine (gwye FEN e sin & fen il EF rin)
Sound-Alike/Look-Alike Issues
Endal® may be confused with Depen®, Intal®
Entex® may be confused with Tenex®
Entex® LA brand name represents a different product in the U.S. than it does in Canada. In the U.S., Entex® LA contains guaifenesin and phenylephrine, while in Canada the product bearing this brand name contains guaifenesin and pseudoephedrine.
Synonyms guaifenesin and phenylephrine tannate; phenylephrine hydrochloride and guaifenesin
U.S./Canadian Brand Names Aldex™ [US]; Crantex LA [US]; Deconsal® II [US]; Donatussin [US]; Duomax [US]; Duratuss GP® [US]; Duratuss® [US]; ExeFen-PD [US]; ExeTuss [US]; ExeTuss-GP [US]; Genexa™ LA [US]; Gentex LA [US]; Gilphex TR® [US]; Guaifed-PD® [US]; Guaifed® [US]; Guaiphen-D 1200 [US]; Guaiphen-D [US]; Guaiphen-PD [US]; Liquibid-D [US]; Nasex-G [US]; Nexphen PD [US]; norel® EX [US]; Pendex [US]; PhenaVent™ D [US]; PhenaVent™ LA [US]; PhenaVent™ Ped [US]; PhenaVent™ [US]; Prolex®-D [US]; Prolex®-PD [US]; Rescon GG [US]; Respa® PE [US]; Sil-Tex [US]; Simuc [US]; Sina-12X [US]; SINUvent® PE [US]; XPECT-PE™ [US]
Therapeutic Category Cold Preparation
Use Temporary relief of nasal congestion, sinusitis, rhinitis and hay fever; temporary relief of cough associated with upper respiratory tract conditions, especially when associated with dry, nonproductive cough
Usual Dosage Oral:
Children 3-6 months (Donatussin): 0.3-0.6 mL; may repeat every 4-6 hours as needed; maximum 4 doses/24 hours
Children 6 months-1 year (Donatussin): 0.6-1 mL; may repeat every 4-6 hours as needed; maximum: 4 doses/24 hours
Children 1-2 years (Donatussin): 1-2 mL; may repeat every 4-6 hours as needed; maximum: 4 doses/24 hours
Children 2-6 years:
Entex®, Rescon GG, Sil-Tex: 2.5 mL every 4-6 hours; maximum: 10 mL/24 hours
Sina-12X suspension: 2.5-5 mL every 12 hours
Children 6-12 years:
Aldex™, Crantex LA, Duomax, ExeTuss, Gentex LA, Liquibid-D®, Liquibid-D® 1200, PhenaVent™ D, Sina-12X tablet: One-half tablet every 12 hours; maximum: 1 tablet/24 hours
Deconsal® II: One capsule daily
Entex®, Rescon GG: 5 mL every 4-6 hours; maximum: 20 mL/24 hours
ExeFen PD, Prolex®-D, Prolex®-PD: One-half to 1 tablet every 12 hours
Guaifed-PD®, PhenaVent™ Ped: One capsule every 12 hours
Liquibid®-PD, SINUvent® PE: One tablet every 12 hours; maximum: 2 tablets/24 hours
Sina-12X suspension: Refer to adult dosing.
Children ≥12 years:
Aldex™, Crantex LA, Deconsal® II, Duomax, Entex®, Entex® LA, ExeFen PD, ExeTuss, ExeTuss-GP, Gentex LA, Guaifed®, Guaifed-PD®, Liquibid-D®, Liquibid®-PD, Liquibid-D® 1200, PhenaVent™, PhenaVent™ D, PhenaVent™ LA, PhenaVent™ Ped, Prolex®-D, Prolex®-PD, Rescon GG, Sil-Tex, Sina-12X, SINUvent® PE: Refer to adult dosing
Entex® ER: One capsule every 12 hours
Adults:
Aldex™, Crantex LA, Duomax, ExeTuss, ExeTuss-GP, Gentex LA, XPECT-PE™, Liquibid-D®, Liquibid-D® 1200, PhenaVent™ D: One tablet every 12 hours
Deconsal® II: 1-2 capsules every 12 hours; maximum: 3 capsules/24 hours
Entex®, Sil-Tex: 5-10 mL every 4-6 hours; maximum: 40 mL/24 hours
Entex® ER, Guaifed-PD®, PhenaVent™ Ped: 1-2 capsules every 12 hours
Entex® LA, Guaifed®, PhenaVent™, PhenaVent™ LA: One capsule every 12 hours; maximum: 2 capsules/24 hours
ExeFen PD, Prolex®-D, Prolex®-PD: 1-2 tablets every 12 hours
Liquibid®-PD, SINUvent® PE: Two tablets every 12 hours
Rescon GG: 10 mL every 4-6 hours; maximum: 40 mL/24 hours
Sina-12X suspension: 5-10 mL every 12 hours
Sina-12X tablet: 1-2 tablets every 12 hours; maximum: 4 tablets/24 hours

Dosage Forms
Caplet:
Refenesen™ PE [OTC]: Guaifenesin 400 mg and phenylephrine 10 mg
Capsule:
Nexphen PD: Guaifenesin 200 mg and phenylephrine hydrochloride 7 mg
Capsule, variable release:
Deconsal® II: Guaifenesin 375 mg [immediate release] and phenylephrine 20 mg [extended release]
Guaifed®, PhenaVent™: Guaifenesin 400 mg [immediate release] and phenylephrine 15 mg [extended release]
Guaifed-PD®, PhenaVent™ Ped: Guaifenesin 200 mg [immediate release] and phenylephrine 7.5 mg [extended release]
Genexa™ LA, PhenaVent™ LA: Guaifenesin 400 mg [immediate release] and phenylephrine 30 mg [extended release]
Liquid: Guaifenesin 100 mg and phenylephrine 7.5 mg per 5 mL
Rescon GG [OTC]: Guaifenesin 100 mg and phenylephrine 5 mg per 5 mL
Sil-Tex: Guaifenesin 100 mg and phenylephrine 7.5 mg per 5 mL
Liquid [drops]:
Donatussin: Guaifenesin 20 mg and phenylephrine hydrochloride 1.5 mg
Suspension:
Sina-12X: Guaifenesin 100 mg and phenylephrine 5 mg per 5 mL
Tablet:
Sina-12X: Guaifenesin 200 mg and phenylephrine 25 mg
Tablet, extended release: Guaifenesin 600 mg and phenylephrine 20 mg; guaifenesin 600 mg and phenylephrine 40 mg; guaifenesin 1200 mg and phenylephrine 40 mg
Aldex™: Guaifenesin 650 mg and phenylephrine 25 mg
ExeFen-PD: Guaifenesin 600 mg and phenylephrine 10 mg
Gentex LA: Guaifenesin 650 mg and phenylephrine 23.75 mg
Simuc: Guaifenesin 900 mg and phenylephrine 25 mg
SINUvent® PE: Guaifenesin 600 mg and phenylephrine 15 mg
Tablet, prolonged release:
Respa® PE: Guaifenesin 600 mg and phenylephrine 18 mg
Tablet, sustained release: Guaifenesin 600 mg and phenylephrine 30 mg
Crantex LA: Guaifenesin 600 mg and phenylephrine 30 mg
Duratuss®, ExeTuss, XPECT-PE™: Guaifenesin 1200 mg and phenylephrine 25 mg
Duratuss GP®, ExeTuss-GP: Guaifenesin 1200 mg and phenylephrine hydrochloride 25 mg
Nasex-G: Guaifenesin 835 mg and phenylephrine hydrochloride 25 mg
Pendex, Prolex®-PD: Guaifenesin 600 mg and phenylephrine hydrochloride 10 mg
Prolex™-D: Guaifenesin 600 mg and phenylephrine 20 mg
Tablet, timed release:
Gilphex TR®: Guaifenesin 600 mg and phenylephrine hydrochloride 25 mg [sugar free, dye free; scored]
Guaiphen-D: Guaifenesin 600 mg and phenylephrine hydrochloride 40 mg
Guaiphen-D 1200: Guaifenesin 1200 mg and phenylephrine hydrochloride 40 mg
Guaiphen-PD: Guaifenesin 275 mg and phenylephrine hydrochloride 25 mg
Tablet, variable release:
Liquibid-D®: Guaifenesin 400 mg and phenylephrine 10 mg [immediate release] and guaifenesin 800 mg and phenylephrine 30 mg [sustained release]
norel® EX: Guaifenesin 400 mg [immediate release] and guaifenesin 400 mg and phenylephrine hydrochloride 40 mg [extended release]

guaifenesin and phenylephrine tannate *see* guaifenesin and phenylephrine *on previous page*

guaifenesin and potassium guaiacolsulfonate
(gwye FEN e sin & poe TASS ee um gwye a kole SUL foe nate)
Synonyms potassium guaiacolsulfonate and guaifenesin
U.S./Canadian Brand Names Allfen *(reformulation)* [US]; Humibid® LA *(reformulation)* [US]
Therapeutic Category Expectorant
Use Temporary control of cough associated with respiratory tract infections and related conditions which are complicated by tenacious mucus and/or mucous plugs and congestion
Usual Dosage Oral: Relief of cough:
Children 6-12 years (Allfen): One-half tablet every 12 hours; maximum 1 tablet/24 hours
Children ≥12 years and Adults (Allfen, Humibid® LA): One tablet every 12 hours; maximum 2 tablets/24 hours
Dosage Forms
Tablet, sustained release:
Allfen (*reformulation*): Guaifenesin 1000 mg and potassium 150 mg
Humibid® LA (*reformulation*): Guaifenesin 600 mg and potassium 300 mg

guaifenesin and pseudoephedrine (gwye FEN e sin & soo doe e FED rin)

Sound-Alike/Look-Alike Issues

Entex® may be confused with Tenex®

Entex® LA brand name represents a different product in the U.S. than it does in Canada. In the U.S., Entex® LA contains guaifenesin and phenylephrine, while in Canada the product bearing this brand name contains guaifenesin and pseudoephedrine.

Profen II® may be confused with Profen II DM®, Profen Forte®, Profen Forte™ DM

Profen Forte® may be confused with Profen II®, Profen II DM®, Profen Forte™ DM

Synonyms pseudoephedrine and guaifenesin

U.S./Canadian Brand Names Ambifed-G [US]; Congestac® [US-OTC]; Contac® Cold-Chest Congestion, Non Drowsy, Regular Strength [Can]; Entex® LA [Can]; Entex® PSE [US]; Eudal®-SR [US]; Guaifenex® GP [US]; Guaifenex® PSE [US]; Guaimax-D® [US]; Levall G [US]; Maxifed-G® [US]; Maxifed® [US]; Mucinex® D Maximum Strength [US-OTC]; Mucinex®-D [US-OTC]; Nasatab® LA [US]; Novahistex® Expectorant with Decongestant [Can]; Pseudo GG TR [US]; Pseudo Max [US]; Pseudovent™ 400 [US]; Pseudovent™ [US]; Pseudovent™-Ped [US]; Refenesen Plus [US-OTC]; Respaire®-120 SR [US]; Respaire®-60 SR [US]; Respa®-1st [US]; Sinutab® Non-Drying [US-OTC]; Touro LA® [US]

Therapeutic Category Expectorant/Decongestant

Use Temporary relief of nasal congestion and to help loosen phlegm and thin bronchial secretions in the treatment of cough

Usual Dosage Oral:

Children 2-6 years:

Guaifenex® PSE 60: One-half tablet every 12 hours (maximum: 1 tablet/12 hours)

Maxifed-G®: One-third to $^1/_2$ tablet every 12 hours (maximum: 1 tablet/12 hours)

Children 6-12 years:

Ambifed-G, Dynex, Eudal®-SR, Guaimax-D®, Guaifenex® PSE 80, Guaifenex® PSE 120, Maxifed®, Nasatab® LA: One-half caplet or tablet every 12 hours (maximum: 1 tablet/24 hours)

Congestac®: One-half caplet every 4-6 hours (maximum: 2 caplets/24 hours)

Guaifenex® PSE 60, PanMist®-JR, Pseudovent™-Ped, Respaire®-60 SR: One tablet or capsule every 12 hours (maximum: 2 tablets or capsules every 24 hours)

Levall G: One capsule every 24 hours

Maxifed-G®: One-half to 1 tablet every 12 hours (maximum: 2 tablets/24 hours)

Children >12 years and Adults:

Ambifed-G, Dynex, Entex® PSE, Eudal®- SR, G-Phed, Guaifenex® GP, Guaifenex® PSE 120, Guaimax-D®, Levall G, Mucinex®-D 1200/120, Nasatab® LA, Pseudovent™, Respaire®-120 SR, Touro LA: One tablet or capsule every 12 hours (maximum: 2 tablets or capsules in 24 hours)

Congestac®: One caplet every 4-6 hours (maximum: 4 caplets in 24 hours)

Guaifenex® PSE 60, Maxifed-G®, Mucinex®-D 600/60, Pseudovent™-Ped, Respaire®-60 SR: 1-2 tablets or capsules every 12 hours (maximum: 4 tablets or capsules/24 hours)

Guaifenex® PSE 80: One tablet every twelve hours (maximum: 3 tablets/24 hours)

Guaifenex™ RX: 1-2 of the AM tablets every morning and 1-2 of the PM tablets 12 hours following morning dose

Maxifed®: One to 1$^1/_2$ tablets every 12 hours (maximum: 3 tablets/24 hours)

Sudafed® Non-Drying Sinus: Two capsules every 4 hours (maximum: 4 doses/24 hours)

Dosage Forms

Caplet:

Congestac® [OTC], Refenesen Plus [OTC]: Guaifenesin 400 mg and pseudoephedrine 60 mg

Caplet, long-acting:

Touro LA®: Guaifenesin 500 mg and pseudoephedrine 120 mg

Caplet, prolonged release:

Ambifed-G: Guaifenesin 1000 mg and pseudoephedrine 60 mg

Capsule, extended release:

Respaire®-60 SR: Guaifenesin 200 mg and pseudoephedrine 60 mg

Respaire®-120 SR: Guaifenesin 250 mg and pseudoephedrine 120 mg

Capsule, liquicap:

Sinutab® Non-Drying [OTC]: Guaifenesin 200 mg and pseudoephedrine 30 mg

Capsule, variable release:

Entex® PSE, Pseudovent™ 400: Guaifenesin 400 mg [immediate release] and pseudoephedrine 120 mg [extended release]

Levall G: Guaifenesin 400 mg [immediate release] and pseudoephedrine 90 mg [extended release]

Pseudovent™: Guaifenesin 250 mg [immediate release] and pseudoephedrine 120 mg [prolonged release]

Pseudovent™-Ped: Guaifenesin 300 mg [immediate release] and pseudoephedrine 60 mg [prolonged release]

Syrup: Guaifenesin 200 mg and pseudoephedrine 40 mg per 5 mL

Tablet, extended release:

Guaifenex® GP, Mucinex® D Maximum Strength [OTC]: Guaifenesin 1200 mg and pseudoephedrine 120 mg

Guaifenex® PSE 60: Guaifenesin 600 mg and pseudoephedrine 60 mg
Guaifenex® PSE 80: Guaifenesin 800 mg and pseudoephedrine 80 mg
Guaifenex® PSE 85: Guaifenesin 795 mg and pseudoephedrine hydrochloride 85 mg
Guaifenex® PSE 120: Guaifenesin 600 mg and pseudoephedrine hydrochloride 120 mg
Guaimax-D®: Guaifenesin 600 mg and pseudoephedrine 120 mg
Maxifed®: Guaifenesin 780 mg and pseudoephedrine 80 mg
Maxifed-G®: Guaifenesin 580 mg and pseudoephedrine 60 mg
Mucinex®-D [OTC] 600/60: Guaifenesin 600 mg and pseudoephedrine 60 mg
Pseudo Max: Guaifenesin 700 mg and pseudoephedrine 80 mg
Tablet, sustained release:
Nasatab® LA: Guaifenesin 500 mg and pseudoephedrine 120 mg
Respa®-1st: Guaifenesin 600 mg and pseudoephedrine 58 mg

guaifenesin and theophylline *see* theophylline and guaifenesin *on page 835*

guaifenesin, carbetapentane citrate, and phenylephrine hydrochloride *see* carbetapentane, guaifenesin, and phenylephrine *on page 149*

guaifenesin, chlorpheniramine, phenylephrine, and dextromethorphan *see* dextromethorphan, chlorpheniramine, phenylephrine, and guaifenesin *on page 248*

guaifenesin, dextromethorphan, and phenylephrine
(gwye FEN e sin, deks troe meth OR fan, & fen il EF rin)
Synonyms guaifenesin, dextromethorphan hydrobromide, and phenylephrine hydrochloride; phenylephrine hydrochloride, guaifenesin, and dextromethorphan hydrobromide
U.S./Canadian Brand Names Anextuss [US]; Certuss-D® [US]; Dacex-DM [US]; Dexcon-PE [US]; Duraphen™ DM [US]; Duraphen™ Forte [US]; Duraphen™ II DM [US]; Dynatuss-EX [US]; Giltuss Pediatric® [US]; Giltuss TR® [US]; Giltuss® [US]; Guaifen™ DM [US]; Maxiphen DM [US]; SINUtuss® DM [US]; TriTuss® ER [US]; TriTuss® [US]
Therapeutic Category Antitussive; Decongestant
Use Symptomatic relief of dry nonproductive coughs and upper respiratory symptoms associated with hay fever, colds, or the flu
Usual Dosage Also refer to specific product labeling.
Oral:
Children 6-12 years (Certuss-D, Duraphen™ DM, Duraphen™ Forte, Duraphen™ II DM, Maxiphen DM): One-half tablet every 12 hours, not to exceed 1 tablet/24 hours
Children ≥12 years and Adults:
Certuss-D, Duraphen™ DM, Duraphen™ Forte, Maxiphen DM: One tablet every 12 hours, not to exceed 2 tablets/24 hours
Duraphen™ II DM: 1-1$^1/_2$ tablets twice daily, not to exceed 3 tablets/24 hours
Dosage Forms
Caplet:
Dexcon-PE: Guaifenesin 550 mg, dextromethorphan 25 mg, and phenylephrine 20 mg
Caplet, extended release:
TriTuss®-ER: Guaifenesin 600 mg, dextromethorphan 30 mg, and phenylephrine 10 mg
Liquid:
Giltuss®: Guaifenesin 300 mg, dextromethorphan 15 mg, and phenylephrine 10 mg per 5 mL
Giltuss Pediatric®: Guaifenesin 50 mg, dextromethorphan 5 mg, and phenylephrine 2.5 mg per mL
Liquid, oral [drops]: Guaifenesin 50 mg, dextromethorphan 5 mg, and phenylephrine 2.5 mg per mL
Robitussin® Pediatric Cold and Cough CF: Guaifenesin 100 mg, dextromethorphan 5 mg, and phenylephrine 2.5 mg per 2.5 mL
Syrup: Guaifenesin 200 mg, dextromethorphan 30 mg, and phenylephrine 10 mg
Dacex-DM, TriTuss®: Guaifenesin 175 mg, dextromethorphan 25 mg, and phenylephrine 12.5 mg per 5 mL
Dynatuss-Ex: Guaifenesin 200 mg, dextromethorphan 30 mg, and phenylephrine 10 mg (473 mL)
Robitussin® Cold and Cough CF: Guaifenesin 100 mg, dextromethorphan 10 mg, and phenylephrine 5 mg per 5 mL
Tablet [scored]:
SINUtuss™ DM: Guaifenesin 600 mg, dextromethorphan hydrobromide 30 mg, and phenylephrine hydrochloride 15 mg
Tablet, extended release [scored]:
Duraphen™ II DM: Guaifenesin 800 mg, dextromethorphan 20 mg, and phenylephrine 20 mg
Duraphen™ Forte: Guaifenesin 1200 mg, dextromethorphan 30 mg, and phenylephrine 30 mg
Tablet, prolonged release [scored]:
Maxiphen DM: Guaifenesin 1000 mg, dextromethorphan 60 mg, and phenylephrine 40 mg
Tablet, sustained release: Guaifenesin 1200 mg, dextromethorphan 20 mg, and phenylephrine 40 mg
Anextuss: Guaifenesin 600 mg, dextromethorphan 60 mg, and phenylephrine 40 mg
Certuss-D® [scored]: Guaifenesin 600 mg, dextromethorphan 60 mg, and phenylephrine 40 mg
(Continued)

guaifenesin, dextromethorphan, and phenylephrine *(Continued)*

Duraphen™ DM [scored], Guaifen™ DM [scored]: Guaifenesin 1200 mg, dextromethorphan 20 mg, and phenylephrine 40 mg
Tablet, timed release [scored]:
Giltuss TR®: Guaifenesin 600 mg, dextromethorphan 30 mg, and phenylephrine 20 mg

guaifenesin, dextromethorphan hydrobromide, and phenylephrine hydrochloride *see* guaifenesin, dextromethorphan, and phenylephrine *on previous page*

guaifenesin, dihydrocodeine, and pseudoephedrine *see* dihydrocodeine, pseudoephedrine, and guaifenesin *on page 260*

guaifenesin, hydrocodone, and pseudoephedrine *see* hydrocodone, pseudoephedrine, and guaifenesin *on page 432*

guaifenesin, hydrocodone bitartrate, and phenylephrine hydrochloride *see* hydrocodone, phenylephrine, and guaifenesin *on page 431*

guaifenesin, phenylephrine, and chlorpheniramine *see* chlorpheniramine, phenylephrine, and guaifenesin *on page 181*

guaifenesin, pseudoephedrine, and codeine

(gwye FEN e sin, soo doe e FED rin, & KOE deen)
Synonyms codeine, guaifenesin, and pseudoephedrine; pseudoephedrine, guaifenesin, and codeine
U.S./Canadian Brand Names Benylin® 3.3 mg-D-E [Can]; Calmylin with Codeine [Can]; Guiatuss DAC [US]; Mytussin® DAC [US]
Therapeutic Category Antitussive/Decongestant/Expectorant
Controlled Substance C-III; C-V
Use Temporarily relieves nasal congestion and controls cough associated with upper respiratory infections and related conditions (common cold, sinusitis, bronchitis, influenza)
Usual Dosage Oral:
Children 2-6 years:
Nucofed® Pediatric: 2.5 mL every 6 hours (maximum 10 mL/24 hours)
Nucofed®: 1.25 mL every 6 hours (maximum 5 mL/24 hours)
Children 6-12 years:
Guaituss DAC: 5 mL every 4 hours (maximum 20 mL/24 hours)
Nucofed® Pediatric: 5 mL every 6 hours (maximum 20 mL/24 hours)
Nucofed®: 2.5 mL every 6 hours (maximum 10 mL/24hours)
Children >12 years and Adults:
Guaituss DAC: 10 mL every 4 hours (maximum 40 mL/24 hours)
Nucofed® Pediatric: 10 mL every 6 hours (maximum 40 mL/24 hours)
Nucofed®: 5 mL every 6 hours (maximum 20 mL/24 hours)
Dosage Forms
Syrup: Guaifenesin 100 mg, pseudoephedrine 30 mg, and codeine 10 mg per 5 mL; guaifenesin 200 mg, pseudoephedrine 60 mg, and codeine 20 mg per 5 mL
Guiatuss DAC, Mytussin® DAC: Guaifenesin 100 mg, pseudoephedrine 30 mg, and codeine 10 mg per 5 mL

guaifenesin, pseudoephedrine, and dextromethorphan

(gwye FEN e sin, soo doe e FED rin, & deks troe meth OR fan)
Sound-Alike/Look-Alike Issues
Profen II DM® may be confused with Profen II®, Profen Forte®, Profen Forte™ DM
Profen Forte™ DM may be confused with Profen II®, Profen II DM®, Profen Forte®
Synonyms dextromethorphan, guaifenesin, and pseudoephedrine; pseudoephedrine, dextromethorphan, and guaifenesin
U.S./Canadian Brand Names Ambifed-G DM [US]; Balminil DM + Decongestant + Expectorant [Can]; Benylin® DM-D-E [Can]; Coldmist DM [US]; Koffex DM + Decongestant + Expectorant [Can]; Maxifed DM [US]; Maxifed DMX [US]; Medent-DM [US]; Novahistex® DM Decongestant Expectorant [Can]; Novahistine® DM Decongestant Expectorant [Can]; Profen Forte™ DM [US]; Profen II DM® [US]; Pseudo Max DMX [US]; Pseudovent™ DM [US]; Relacon-DM NR [US]; Robitussin® Cough and Cold CF [US-OTC]; Robitussin® Cough and Cold Infant CF [US-OTC]; Robitussin® Cough and Cold® [US-OTC/Can]; Ru-Tuss DM [US]; Touro® CC [US]; Touro® CC-LD [US]; Tri-Vent™ DM [US]; Trikof-D® [US]; Tusnel Pediatric® [US]; Z-Cof™ DM [US]
Therapeutic Category Cold Preparation
Use Temporarily relieves nasal congestion and controls cough due to minor throat and bronchial irritation; helps loosen phlegm and thin bronchial secretions to make coughs more productive

Usual Dosage Note: Also refer to specific product labeling.

Children 2-6 years:
Maxifed DM: $1/3$ to $1/2$ tablet every 12 hours, not to exceed 1 tablet/24 hours
Tri-Vent™ DM: 2.5 mL up to 3-4 times/day, not to exceed pseudoephedrine 4 mg/kg/day
Profen II DM (syrup): 1.25-2.5 mL every 4 hours, not to exceed 15 mL/24 hours
Robitussin® Pediatric Cough and Cold Infant: 2.5 mL every 4-6 hours, not to exceed 4 doses/24 hours
Touro® CC: $1/2$ tablet every 12 hour, not to exceed 1 tablet/24 hours
Z-Cof™ DM: 2.5 mL 2-3 times/day, not to exceed 7.5 mL/24 hours

Children 6-12 years:
Ambifed-G DM, Profen Forte™ DM, Profen II DM®: $1/2$ tablet every 12 hours not to exceed 1 tablet/24 hours
Maxifed DM: $1/2$ to 1 tablet every 12 hours, not to exceed 2 tablets/24 hours
Tri-Vent™ DM: 5 mL up to 3-4 times/day, not to exceed pseudoephedrine 4 mg/kg/day
Touro® CC, Pseudovent™ DM: 1 tablet every 12 hours, not to exceed 2 tablets/24 hours
Profen II DM (syrup): 2.5-5 mL every 4 hours, not to exceed 30 mL/24 hours
Z-Cof™ DM: 5 mL 2-3 times/day, not to exceed 15 mL/24 hours

Children ≥12 years and Adults:
Ambifed-G DM, Aquatab® C, Profen Forte™ DM: 1 tablet every 12 hours not to exceed 2 tablets/24 hours
Maxifed DM, Touro® CC, Pseudovent™ DM: 1-2 tablets every 12 hours, not to exceed 4 tablets/24 hours
Tri-Vent™ DM: Up to 10 mL 3-4 times/day, not to exceed pseudoephedrine 240 mg/24 hours
Profen II DM (tablet): 1 to $1^{1}/_2$ tablets every 12 hours, not to exceed 3 tablets/24 hours
Profen II DM (syrup): 5-10 mL every 4 hours, not to exceed 60 mL/24 hours
Z-Cof™ DM: 10 mL 2-3 times/day, not to exceed 30 mL/24 hours

Dosage Forms
Caplet, prolonged release:
Ambifed-G DM: Guaifenesin 1000 mg, pseudoephedrine 60 mg, and dextromethorphan 30 mg
Caplet, sustained release:
Touro® CC: Guaifenesin 575 mg, pseudoephedrine 60 mg, and dextromethorphan 30 mg
Touro® CC-LD: Guaifenesin 575 mg, pseudoephedrine 25 mg, and dextromethorphan 30 mg
Capsule, softgel:
Robitussin® Cough and Cold [OTC]: Guaifenesin 200 mg, pseudoephedrine 30 mg, and dextromethorphan 10 mg
Liquid: Guaifenesin 100 mg, pseudoephedrine 30 mg, and dextromethorphan 10 mg per 5 mL
Profen II DM®: Guaifenesin 200 mg, pseudoephedrine 15 mg, and dextromethorphan 10 mg per 5 mL
Relacon-DM NR, Z-Cof™ DM: Guaifenesin 200 mg, pseudoephedrine 40 mg, and dextromethorphan 15 mg
Tusnel Pediatric®: Guaifenesin 50 mg, pseudoephedrine 15 mg, and dextromethorphan 5 mg per 5 mL
Liquid, oral drops:
Robitussin® Cough and Cold Infant CF [OTC]: Guaifenesin 100 mg, pseudoephedrine 15 mg, and dextromethorphan 5 mg per 2.5 mL
Syrup: Guaifenesin 100 mg, pseudoephedrine 45 mg, and dextromethorphan 15 mg per 5 mL
Robitussin® Cough and Cold CF [OTC]: Guaifenesin 100 mg, pseudoephedrine 30 mg, and dextromethorphan 10 mg per 5 mL
Ru-Tuss DM: Guaifenesin 100 mg, pseudoephedrine 45 mg, and dextromethorphan 15 mg per 5 mL
Tri-Vent™ DM: Guaifenesin 100 mg, pseudoephedrine 40 mg, and dextromethorphan 15 mg per 5 mL
Tablet, extended release: Guaifenesin 100 mg, pseudoephedrine hydrochloride 30 mg, and dextromethorphan hydrobromide 10 mg; guaifenesin 800 mg, pseudoephedrine 60 mg, and dextromethorphan 30 mg; guaifenesin 1200 mg, pseudoephedrine 60 mg, and dextromethorphan 60 mg; guaifenesin 1200 mg, pseudoephedrine 120 mg, and dextromethorphan 60 mg; guaifenesin 800 mg, pseudoephedrine 90 mg, and dextromethorphan 60 mg; guaifenesin 550 mg, pseudoephedrine 60 mg, and dextromethorphan 30 mg; guaifenesin 595 mg, pseudoephedrine 48 mg, and dextromethorphan 32 mg; guaifenesin 600 mg, pseudoephedrine 60 mg, and dextromethorphan 30 mg
Pseudovent™ DM: Guaifenesin 595 mg, pseudoephedrine 48 mg, and dextromethorphan 32 mg
Profen Forte™ DM: Guaifenesin 800 mg, pseudoephedrine 90 mg, and dextromethorphan 60 mg
Profen II DM®: Guaifenesin 800 mg, pseudoephedrine 45 mg, and dextromethorphan 30 mg
Tablet, long acting:
Medent-DM: Guaifenesin 800 mg, pseudoephedrine 60 mg, and dextromethorphan 30 mg
Tablet, sustained release:
Maxifed DM: Guaifenesin 580 mg, pseudoephedrine 60 mg, and dextromethorphan 30 mg
Maxifed DM: Guaifenesin 780 mg, pseudoephedrine 80 mg, and dextromethorphan 40 mg
Pseudo Max DMX: Guaifenesin 700 mg, pseudoephedrine 80 mg, and dextromethorphan 40 mg
Trikof-D®: Guaifenesin 600 mg, pseudoephedrine 50 mg, and dextromethorphan 30 mg

Guaifenex® *(Discontinued)*

Guaifenex® DM [US] *see* guaifenesin and dextromethorphan *on page 402*

Guaifenex® GP [US] *see* guaifenesin and pseudoephedrine *on page 406*

Guaifenex® PPA 75 *(Discontinued)*

Guaifenex® PSE [US] *see* guaifenesin and pseudoephedrine *on page 406*

Guaifenex™-Rx *(Discontinued)* *see* guaifenesin and pseudoephedrine *on page 406*

Guaifenex™-Rx DM *(Discontinued)* *see* guaifenesin, pseudoephedrine, and dextromethorphan *on page 408*

Guaimax-D® [US] *see* guaifenesin and pseudoephedrine *on page 406*

Guaipax® *(Discontinued)*

Guaiphen-D [US] *see* guaifenesin and phenylephrine *on page 404*

Guaiphen-D 1200 [US] *see* guaifenesin and phenylephrine *on page 404*

Guaiphen-PD [US] *see* guaifenesin and phenylephrine *on page 404*

Guaitab® *(Discontinued)* *see* guaifenesin and pseudoephedrine *on page 406*

Guaituss AC [US] *see* guaifenesin and codeine *on page 402*

Guaituss CF® *(Discontinued)*

Guaivent® *(Discontinued)* *see* guaifenesin and pseudoephedrine *on page 406*

guanabenz (GWAHN a benz)
Sound-Alike/Look-Alike Issues
guanabenz may be confused with guanadrel, guanfacine
Synonyms guanabenz acetate
U.S./Canadian Brand Names Wytensin® [Can]
Therapeutic Category Alpha-Adrenergic Agonist
Use Management of hypertension
Usual Dosage Oral: Adults: Initial: 4 mg twice daily; increase in increments of 4-8 mg/day every 1-2 weeks to a maximum of 32 mg twice daily.
Dosage Forms
Tablet: 4 mg, 8 mg

guanabenz acetate *see* guanabenz *on this page*

guanfacine (GWAHN fa seen)
Sound-Alike/Look-Alike Issues
guanfacine may be confused with guaifenesin, guanabenz, guanidine
Tenex® may be confused with Entex®, Ten-K®, Xanax®
Synonyms guanfacine hydrochloride
U.S./Canadian Brand Names Tenex® [US/Can]
Therapeutic Category Alpha-Adrenergic Agonist
Use Management of hypertension
Usual Dosage Oral: Adults: Hypertension: 1 mg usually at bedtime, may increase if needed at 3- to 4-week intervals; usual dose range (JNC 7): 0.5-2 mg once daily
Dosage Forms
Tablet: 1 mg, 2 mg
Tenex®: 1 mg, 2 mg

guanfacine hydrochloride *see* guanfacine *on this page*

guanidine (GWAHN i deen)
Sound-Alike/Look-Alike Issues
guanidine may be confused with guanfacine, guanethidine
Synonyms guanidine hydrochloride
Therapeutic Category Cholinergic Agent
Use Reduction of the symptoms of muscle weakness associated with the myasthenic syndrome of Eaton-Lambert, not for myasthenia gravis
Usual Dosage Oral: Adults: Eaton-Lambert syndrome: Initial: 10-15 mg/kg/day in 3-4 divided doses, gradually increase to 35 mg/kg/day or up to development of side effects
Dosage Forms
Tablet: 125 mg

guanidine hydrochloride *see* guanidine *on this page*

Guia-D [US] *see* guaifenesin and dextromethorphan *on page 402*

Guiacon DMS [US-OTC] *see* guaifenesin and dextromethorphan *on page 402*

GuiaCough® *(Discontinued)* *see* guaifenesin and dextromethorphan *on page 402*

GuiaCough® Expectorant *(Discontinued)* *see* guaifenesin *on page 401*

Guiaplex™ HC [US] *see* hydrocodone, phenylephrine, and guaifenesin *on page 431*

Guiatex® *(Discontinued)*

Guiatuss™ [US-OTC] *see* guaifenesin *on page 401*

Guiatuss DAC [US] *see* guaifenesin, pseudoephedrine, and codeine *on page 408*

Guiatuss-DM® [US-OTC] *see* guaifenesin and dextromethorphan *on page 402*

gum benjamin *see* benzoin *on page 103*

GW506U78 *see* nelarabine *on page 595*

GW-1000-02 *see* tetrahydrocannabinol and cannabidiol *(Canada only)* *on page 832*

GW433908G *see* fosamprenavir *on page 374*

GW572016 *see* lapatinib *on page 494*

G-well® *(Discontinued)* *see* lindane *on page 509*

Gynazole-1® [US/Can] *see* butoconazole *on page 132*

Gyne-Lotrimin® 3 [US-OTC] *see* clotrimazole *on page 206*

Gyne-Sulf® *(Discontinued)* *see* sulfabenzamide, sulfacetamide, and sulfathiazole *on page 810*

Gynodiol® [US] *see* estradiol *on page 313*

Gynogen L.A.® Injection *(Discontinued)* *see* estradiol *on page 313*

Gynol II® [US-OTC] *see* nonoxynol 9 *on page 610*

Gynovite® Plus [US-OTC] *see* vitamins (multiple/oral) *on page 895*

Habitrol® [Can] *see* nicotine *on page 604*

Haemophilus B conjugate and hepatitis B vaccine
(he MOF i lus bee KON joo gate & hep a TYE tis bee vak SEEN)
Sound-Alike/Look-Alike Issues
  Comvax® may be confused with Recombivax [Recombivax HB®]
Synonyms *Haemophilus* b (meningococcal protein conjugate) conjugate vaccine; hepatitis b vaccine (recombinant); Hib conjugate vaccine
U.S./Canadian Brand Names Comvax® [US]
Therapeutic Category Vaccine, Inactivated Virus
Use
  Immunization against invasive disease caused by *H. influenzae* type b and against infection caused by all known subtypes of hepatitis B virus in infants 6 weeks to 15 months of age born of hepatitis B surface antigen (HB$_s$Ag) negative mothers
  Infants born of HB$_s$Ag-positive mothers or mothers of unknown HB$_s$Ag status should receive hepatitis B immune globulin and hepatitis B vaccine (recombinant) at birth and should complete the hepatitis B vaccination series given according to a particular schedule
Usual Dosage Infants: I.M.: 0.5 mL at 2, 4, and 12-15 months of age (total of 3 doses)
  If the recommended schedule cannot be followed, the interval between the first two doses should be at least 6 weeks and the interval between the second and third dose should be as close as possible to 8-11 months. Minimum age for first dose is 6 weeks.
  Modified Schedule: Children who receive one dose of hepatitis B vaccine at or shortly after birth may receive Comvax® on a schedule of 2, 4, and 12-15 months of age
Dosage Forms
  Injection, suspension [preservative free]:
  Comvax®: *Haemophilus* b PRP 7.5 mcg and HB$_s$Ag 5 mcg per 0.5 mL (0.5 mL)

Haemophilus B conjugate vaccine (he MOF fi lus bee KON joo gate vak SEEN)
Synonyms diphtheria CRM$_{197}$ protein conjugate; diphtheria toxoid conjugate; *Haemophilus* b oligosaccharide conjugate vaccine; *Haemophilus* b polysaccharide vaccine; HbCV; HbOC; Hib polysaccharide conjugate; PRP-OMP; PRP-T
U.S./Canadian Brand Names ActHIB® [US/Can]; PedvaxHIB® [US/Can]
Therapeutic Category Vaccine, Inactivated Bacteria
Use Routine immunization of children 2 months to 5 years of age against invasive disease caused by *H. influenzae* type b

  Unimmunized children ≥5 years of age with a chronic illness known to be associated with increased risk of *Haemophilus influenzae* type b disease, specifically, persons with anatomic or functional asplenia or sickle cell anemia or those who have undergone splenectomy, should receive *Haemophilus influenzae* type b (Hib) vaccine.
(Continued)

Haemophilus B conjugate vaccine *(Continued)*

Haemophilus b conjugate vaccines are not indicated for prevention of bronchitis or other infections due to *H. influenzae* in adults; adults with specific dysfunction or certain complement deficiencies who are at especially high risk of *H. influenzae* type b infection (HIV-infected adults); patients with Hodgkin disease (vaccinated at least 2 weeks before the initiation of chemotherapy or 3 months after the end of chemotherapy)

Usual Dosage Children: I.M.: 0.5 mL as a single dose should be administered; do not inject I.V.

Dosage Forms
Injection, powder for reconstitution [preservative free]:
ActHIB®: *Haemophilus* b capsular polysaccharide 10 mcg and tetanus toxoid 24 mcg per dose
Injection, suspension:
PedvaxHIB®: *Haemophilus* b capsular polysaccharide 7.5 mcg and *Neisseria meningitidis* OMPC 125 mcg per 0.5 mL (0.5 mL)

Haemophilus b (meningococcal protein conjugate) conjugate vaccine see *Haemophilus* B conjugate and hepatitis B vaccine *on previous page*

Haemophilus b oligosaccharide conjugate vaccine see *Haemophilus* B conjugate vaccine *on previous page*

Haemophilus b polysaccharide vaccine see *Haemophilus* B conjugate vaccine *on previous page*

Haemophilus influenzae b conjugate vaccine and diphtheria, tetanus toxoids, and acellular pertussis vaccine see diphtheria, tetanus toxoids, and acellular pertussis vaccine and *Haemophilus influenzae* b conjugate vaccine *on page 270*

halcinonide (hal SIN oh nide)
Sound-Alike/Look-Alike Issues
halcinonide may be confused with Halcion®
Halog® may be confused with Haldol®, Mycolog®
U.S./Canadian Brand Names Halog® [US/Can]
Therapeutic Category Corticosteroid, Topical
Use Inflammation of corticosteroid-responsive dermatoses [high potency topical corticosteroid]
Usual Dosage Topical: Children and Adults: Steroid-responsive dermatoses: Apply sparingly 1-3 times/day, occlusive dressing may be used for severe or resistant dermatoses; a thin film is effective; do not overuse. Therapy should be discontinued when control is achieved; if no improvement is seen, reassessment of diagnosis may be necessary.
Dosage Forms
Solution, topical:
Halog®: 0.1% (20 mL, 60 mL)

Halcion® [Can] see triazolam *on page 864*

Halcion® (Discontinued) see triazolam *on page 864*

Haldol® [US] see haloperidol *on next page*

Haldol® Decanoate [US] see haloperidol *on next page*

Haley's M-O see magnesium hydroxide and mineral oil *on page 527*

HalfLytely® and Bisacodyl [US] see polyethylene glycol-electrolyte solution and bisacodyl *on page 695*

Halfprin® [US-OTC] see aspirin *on page 78*

halobetasol (hal oh BAY ta sol)
Sound-Alike/Look-Alike Issues
Ultravate® may be confused with Cutivate®
Synonyms halobetasol propionate
U.S./Canadian Brand Names Ultravate® [US/Can]
Therapeutic Category Corticosteroid, Topical
Use Relief of inflammatory and pruritic manifestations of corticosteroid-response dermatoses [super high potency topical corticosteroid]
Usual Dosage Topical: Children ≥12 years and Adults:
Inflammatory and pruritic manifestations (dental use): Cream: Apply sparingly to lesion twice daily. Treatment should not exceed 2 consecutive weeks and total dosage should not exceed 50 g/week. Therapy should be discontinued when control is achieved; if no improvement is seen, reassessment of diagnosis may be necessary.
Steroid-responsive dermatoses: Apply sparingly to skin twice daily, rub in gently and completely; treatment should not exceed 2 consecutive weeks and total dosage should not exceed 50 g/week. Therapy should be

discontinued when control is achieved; if no improvement is seen, reassessment of diagnosis may be necessary.

Dosage Forms
Cream: 0.05% (15 g, 50 g)
Ultravate®: 0.05% (15 g, 50 g)
Ointment: 0.05% (15 g, 50 g)
Ultravate®: 0.05% (15 g, 50 g)

halobetasol propionate *see* halobetasol *on previous page*

Halog® **[US/Can]** *see* halcinonide *on previous page*

Halog®-E *(Discontinued)* *see* halcinonide *on previous page*

haloperidol (ha loe PER i dole)

Sound-Alike/Look-Alike Issues
haloperidol may be confused Halotestin®
Haldol® may be confused with Halcion®, Halenol®, Halog®, Halotestin®, Stadol®

Synonyms haloperidol decanoate; haloperidol lactate

U.S./Canadian Brand Names Apo-Haloperidol LA® [Can]; Apo-Haloperidol® [Can]; Haldol® Decanoate [US]; Haldol® [US]; Haloperidol Injection, USP [Can]; Haloperidol Long Acting [Can]; Haloperidol-LA Omega [Can]; Haloperidol-LA [Can]; Novo-Peridol [Can]; Peridol [Can]; PMS-Haloperidol LA [Can]

Therapeutic Category Antipsychotic Agent, Butyrophenone

Use Management of schizophrenia; control of tics and vocal utterances of Tourette disorder in children and adults; severe behavioral problems in children

Usual Dosage
Children: 3-12 years (15-40 kg): Oral:
Initial: 0.05 mg/kg/day or 0.25-0.5 mg/day given in 2-3 divided doses; increase by 0.25-0.5 mg every 5-7 days; maximum: 0.15 mg/kg/day
Usual maintenance:
Agitation or hyperkinesia: 0.01-0.03 mg/kg/day once daily
Nonpsychotic disorders: 0.05-0.075 mg/kg/day in 2-3 divided doses
Psychotic disorders: 0.05-0.15 mg/kg/day in 2-3 divided doses
Children 6-12 years: Sedation/psychotic disorders: I.M. (as lactate): 1-3 mg/dose every 4-8 hours to a maximum of 0.15 mg/kg/day; change over to oral therapy as soon as able
Adults: Psychosis:
Oral: 0.5-5 mg 2-3 times/day; usual maximum: 30 mg/day
I.M. (as lactate): 2-5 mg every 4-8 hours as needed
I.M. (as decanoate): Initial: 10-20 times the daily oral dose administered at 4-week intervals
Maintenance dose: 10-15 times initial oral dose; used to stabilize psychiatric symptoms

Dosage Forms
Injection, oil: 50 mg/mL (1 mL, 5 mL); 100 mg/mL (1 mL, 5 mL)
Injection, solution: 5 mg/mL (1 mL, 10 mL)
Haldol®: 5 mg/mL (1 mL)
Solution, oral concentrate: 2 mg/mL
Tablet: 0.5 mg, 1 mg, 2 mg, 5 mg, 10 mg, 20 mg

haloperidol decanoate *see* haloperidol *on this page*

Haloperidol Injection, USP [Can] *see* haloperidol *on this page*

Haloperidol-LA [Can] *see* haloperidol *on this page*

haloperidol lactate *see* haloperidol *on this page*

Haloperidol-LA Omega [Can] *see* haloperidol *on this page*

Haloperidol Long Acting [Can] *see* haloperidol *on this page*

Halotestin® **[US]** *see* fluoxymesterone *on page 364*

halothane (HA loe thane)

Sound-Alike/Look-Alike Issues
halothane may be confused with Halotestin®

Therapeutic Category General Anesthetic

Use Induction and maintenance of general anesthesia

Usual Dosage Minimum alveolar concentration (MAC), the concentration at which 50% of patients do not respond to surgical incision, is 0.74% for halothane. The concentration at which amnesia and loss of awareness occur (MAC - awake) is 0.41%. Surgical levels of anesthesia are maintained with concentrations between 0.5% to 2%; inspired concentrations of up to 3% required for induction of anesthesia.
(Continued)

halothane *(Continued)*
Dosage Forms
Liquid: 250 mL

Halotussin® *(Discontinued)* *see* guaifenesin *on page 401*

Halotussin® **DM** *(Discontinued)* *see* guaifenesin and dextromethorphan *on page 402*

Halotussin® **PE** *(Discontinued)* *see* guaifenesin and pseudoephedrine *on page 406*

Haltran® *(Discontinued)* *see* ibuprofen *on page 444*

hamamelis water *see* witch hazel *on page 900*

HandClens® **[US-OTC]** *see* benzalkonium chloride *on page 100*

Havrix® **[US/Can]** *see* hepatitis A vaccine *on page 417*

Havrix® **and Engerix-B**® *see* hepatitis A inactivated and hepatitis B (recombinant) vaccine *on page 416*

HbCV *see* Haemophilus B conjugate vaccine *on page 411*

HBIG *see* hepatitis B immune globulin *on page 417*

hBNP *see* nesiritide *on page 600*

HbOC *see* Haemophilus B conjugate vaccine *on page 411*

hCG *see* chorionic gonadotropin (human) *on page 187*

HD 200® **Plus [US]** *see* barium *on page 94*

HDA® **Toothache [US-OTC]** *see* benzocaine *on page 101*

HDCV *see* rabies virus vaccine *on page 742*

Head & Shoulders® **Citrus Breeze [US-OTC]** *see* pyrithione zinc *on page 737*

Head & Shoulders® **Classic Clean [US-OTC]** *see* pyrithione zinc *on page 737*

Head & Shoulders® **Classic Clean 2-In-1 [US-OTC]** *see* pyrithione zinc *on page 737*

Head & Shoulders® **Dry Scalp Care [US-OTC]** *see* pyrithione zinc *on page 737*

Head & Shoulders® **Extra Volume [US-OTC]** *see* pyrithione zinc *on page 737*

Head & Shoulders® **Intensive Treatment [US-OTC]** *see* selenium sulfide *on page 780*

Head & Shoulders® **Leave-in Treatment [US-OTC]** *see* pyrithione zinc *on page 737*

Head & Shoulders® **Refresh [US-OTC]** *see* pyrithione zinc *on page 737*

Head & Shoulders® **Sensitive Care [US-OTC]** *see* pyrithione zinc *on page 737*

Head & Shoulders® **Smooth & Silky 2-In-1 [US-OTC]** *see* pyrithione zinc *on page 737*

Healon® **[US/Can]** *see* hyaluronate and derivatives *on page 423*

Healon®**5 [US]** *see* hyaluronate and derivatives *on page 423*

Healon GV® **[US/Can]** *see* hyaluronate and derivatives *on page 423*

Hectorol® **[US/Can]** *see* doxercalciferol *on page 280*

Helidac® **[US]** *see* bismuth, metronidazole, and tetracycline *on page 113*

Helistat® **[US]** *see* collagen hemostat *on page 213*

Helitene® **[US]** *see* collagen hemostat *on page 213*

Helixate® **FS [US/Can]** *see* antihemophilic factor (recombinant) *on page 59*

Hemabate® **[US/Can]** *see* carboprost tromethamine *on page 153*

hematin *see* hemin *on this page*

hemiacidrin *see* citric acid, magnesium carbonate, and glucono-delta-lactone *on page 195*

hemin (HEE min)
Synonyms hematin
U.S./Canadian Brand Names Panhematin® [US]
Therapeutic Category Blood Modifiers
Use Treatment of recurrent attacks of acute intermittent porphyria (AIP)
Usual Dosage I.V.: Children ≥16 years and Adults: 1-4 mg/kg/day administered over 10-15 minutes for 3-14 days; may be repeated no earlier than every 12 hours; not to exceed 6 mg/kg in any 24-hour period
Dosage Forms
Injection, powder for reconstitution [preservative free]:
Panhematin®: 313 mg

Hemocyte® [US-OTC] *see* ferrous fumarate *on page 349*

Hemocyte Plus® [US] *see* vitamins (multiple/oral) *on page 895*

Hemofil M [US/Can] *see* antihemophilic factor (human) *on page 58*

Hemril®-30 [US] *see* hydrocortisone (rectal) *on page 433*

HepaGam B™ [US/Can] *see* hepatitis B immune globulin *on page 417*

Hepalean® [Can] *see* heparin *on this page*

Hepalean® Leo [Can] *see* heparin *on this page*

Hepalean®-LOK [Can] *see* heparin *on this page*

heparin (HEP a rin)
Sound-Alike/Look-Alike Issues
heparin may be confused with Hespan®

Synonyms heparin calcium; heparin lock flush; heparin sodium

U.S./Canadian Brand Names Hep-Lock U/P [US]; Hep-Lock® [US]; Hepalean® Leo [Can]; Hepalean® [Can]; Hepalean®-LOK [Can]; HepFlush®-10 [US]

Therapeutic Category Anticoagulant (Other)

Use Prophylaxis and treatment of thromboembolic disorders

Note: Heparin lock flush solution is intended only to maintain patency of I.V. devices and is **not** to be used for anticoagulant therapy.

Usual Dosage
Children:

Intermittent I.V.: Initial: 50-100 units/kg, then 50-100 units/kg every 4 hours

I.V. infusion: Initial: 50 units/kg, then 15-25 units/kg/hour; increase dose by 2-4 units/kg/hour every 6-8 hours as required

Adults:

Prophylaxis (low-dose heparin): SubQ: 5000 units every 8-12 hours

Intermittent I.V.: Initial: 10,000 units, then 50-70 units/kg (5000-10,000 units) every 4-6 hours

I.V. infusion (weight-based dosing per institutional nomogram recommended):

Acute coronary syndromes: MI: Fibrinolytic therapy:

Full-dose alteplase, reteplase, or tenecteplase with dosing as follows: Concurrent bolus of 60 units/kg (maximum: 4000 units), then 12 units/kg/hour (maximum: 1000 units/hour) as continuous infusion. Check aPTT every 4-6 hours; adjust to target of 1.5-2 times the upper limit of control (50-70 seconds in clinical trials); usual range 10-30 units/kg/hour. Duration of heparin therapy depends on concurrent therapy and the specific patient risks for systemic or venous thromboembolism.

Combination regimen (unlabeled): Half-dose tenecteplase (15-25 mg based on weight) and abciximab 0.25 mg/kg bolus then 0.125 mcg/kg/minute (maximum 10 mcg/minute) for 12 hours with heparin dosing as follows: Concurrent bolus of 40 units/kg (maximum 3000 units), then 7 units/kg/hour (maximum: 800 units/hour) as continuous infusion. Adjust to a aPTT target of 50-70 seconds.

Streptokinase: Heparin use optional depending on concurrent therapy and specific patient risks for systemic or venous thromboembolism (anterior MI, CHF, previous embolus, atrial fibrillation, LV thrombus): If heparin is administered, start when aPTT <2 times the upper limit of control; do not use a bolus, but initiate infusion adjusted to a target aPTT of 1.5-2 times the upper limit of control (50-70 seconds in clinical trials). If heparin is not administered by infusion, 7500-12,500 units SubQ every 12 hours (when aPTT <2 times the upper limit of control) is recommended.

Percutaneous coronary intervention: Heparin bolus and infusion may be administered to an activated clotting time (ACT) of 300-350 seconds if no concurrent GPIIb/IIIa receptor antagonist is administered or 200-250 seconds if a GPIIb/IIIa receptor antagonist is administered.

Treatment of unstable angina (high-risk and some intermediate-risk patients): Initial bolus of 60-70 units/kg (maximum: 5000 units), followed by an initial infusion of 12-15 units/kg/hour (maximum: 1000 units/hour). The American College of Chest Physicians consensus conference has recommended dosage adjustments to correspond to a therapeutic range equivalent to heparin levels of 0.3-0.7 units/mL by antifactor Xa determinations.

Treatment of venous thromboembolism:

DVT/PE: I.V. push: 80 units/kg followed by continuous infusion of 18 units/kg/hour

DVT: SubQ: 17,500 units every 12 hours

Line flushing: When using daily flushes of heparin to maintain patency of single and double lumen central catheters, 10 units/mL is commonly used for younger infants (eg, <10 kg) while 100 units/mL is used for older infants, children, and adults. Capped PVC catheters and peripheral heparin locks require flushing more frequently (eg, every 6-8 hours). Volume of heparin flush is usually similar to volume of catheter (or slightly greater). Additional flushes should be given when stagnant blood is observed in catheter, after catheter is used for drug or blood administration, and after blood withdrawal from catheter.

(Continued)

heparin *(Continued)*

Addition of heparin (0.5-3 unit/mL) to peripheral and central parenteral nutrition has not been shown to decrease catheter-related thrombosis. The final concentration of heparin used for TPN solutions may need to be decreased to 0.5 units/mL in small infants receiving larger amounts of volume in order to avoid approaching therapeutic amounts. Arterial lines are heparinized with a final concentration of 1 unit/mL.

Dosage Forms

Infusion [premixed in NaCl 0.45%; porcine intestinal mucosa source]: 12,500 units (250 mL); 25,000 units (250 mL, 500 mL)

Infusion [preservative free; premixed in D_5W; porcine intestinal mucosa source]: 10,000 units (100 mL); 12,500 units (250 mL); 20,000 units (500 mL); 25,000 units (250 mL, 500 mL)

Infusion [preservative free; premixed in NaCl 0.9%; porcine intestinal mucosa source]: 1000 units (500 mL); 2000 units (1000 mL)

Injection, solution [lock flush preparation; porcine intestinal mucosa source; multidose vial]: 10 units/mL (1 mL, 10 mL, 30 mL); 100 units/mL (1 mL, 5 mL, 10 mL, 30 mL)

Hep-Lock®: 10 units/mL (1 mL, 2 mL, 10 mL, 30 mL); 100 units/mL (1 mL, 2 mL, 10 mL, 30 mL)

Injection, solution [lock flush preparation; porcine intestinal mucosa source; prefilled syringe]: 10 units/mL (1 mL, 2 mL, 3 mL, 5 mL); 100 units/mL (1 mL, 2 mL, 3 mL, 5 mL)

Injection, solution [preservative free; lock flush preparation; porcine intestinal mucosa source; prefilled syringe]: 100 units/mL (5 mL)

Injection, solution [preservative free; lock flush preparation; porcine intestinal mucosa source; vial]: 10 units/ mL (10 mL)

HepFlush®-10: 10 units/mL (10 mL)

Hep-Lock U/P: 10 units/mL (1 mL); 100 units/mL (1 mL)

Injection, solution [porcine intestinal mucosa source; multidose vial]: 1000 units/mL (1 mL, 10 mL, 30 mL); 5000 units/mL (1 mL, 10 mL); 10,000 units/mL (1 mL, 4 mL, 5 mL); 20,000 units/mL (1 mL)

Injection, solution [porcine intestinal mucosa source; prefilled syringe]: 5000 units/mL (1 mL)

Injection, solution [preservative free; porcine intestinal mucosa source; prefilled syringe]: 10,000 units/mL (0.5 mL)

Injection, solution [preservative free; porcine intestinal mucosa source; vial]: 1000 units/mL (2 mL); 2000 units/mL (5 mL); 2500 units/mL (10 mL)

heparin calcium *see* heparin *on previous page*

heparin cofactor I *see* antithrombin III *on page 62*

heparin lock flush *see* heparin *on previous page*

heparin sodium *see* heparin *on previous page*

hepatitis A inactivated and hepatitis B (recombinant) vaccine

(hep a TYE tis aye in ak ti VAY ted & hep a TYE tis bee ree KOM be nant vak SEEN)

Synonyms Engerix-B® and Havrix®; Havrix® and Engerix-B®; hepatitis B (recombinant) and hepatitis A inactivated vaccine

U.S./Canadian Brand Names Twinrix® [US/Can]

Therapeutic Category Vaccine

Use Active immunization against disease caused by hepatitis A virus and hepatitis B virus (all known subtypes) in populations desiring protection against or at high risk of exposure to these viruses.

Populations include travelers to areas of intermediate/high endemicity for **both** HAV and HBV; those at increased risk of HBV infection due to behavioral or occupational factors; patients with chronic liver disease; laboratory workers who handle live HAV and HBV; healthcare workers, police, and other personnel who render first-aid or medical assistance; workers who come in contact with sewage; employees of day care centers and correctional facilities; patients/staff of hemodialysis units; male homosexuals; patients frequently receiving blood products; military personnel; users of injectable illicit drugs; close household contacts of patients with hepatitis A and hepatitis B infection; residents of drug and alcohol treatment centers

Usual Dosage I.M.: Adults: Primary immunization: Three doses (1 mL each) given on a 0-, 1-, and 6-month schedule

Alternative regimen: Accelerated regimen (1 mL doses at day 0, 7, and 21-30, followed by a booster at 12 months) has demonstrated similar safety, tolerability, and immunogenicity to the standard regimen.

Dosage Forms

Injection, suspension [preservative free]:

Twinrix®: Inactivated hepatitis A virus 720 ELISA units and hepatitis B surface antigen 20 mcg per mL (1 mL)

hepatitis A vaccine (hep a TYE tis aye vak SEEN)

U.S./Canadian Brand Names Avaxim® [Can]; Avaxim®-Pediatric [Can]; Havrix® [US/Can]; VAQTA® [US/Can]

Therapeutic Category Vaccine, Inactivated Virus

Use

Active immunization against disease caused by hepatitis A virus in populations desiring protection against or at high risk of exposure

Populations at high risk of exposure to hepatitis A virus may include children and adolescents in selected states and regions, travelers to developing countries, household and sexual contacts of persons infected with hepatitis A, child day-care employees, patients with chronic liver disease, illicit drug users, male homosexuals, institutional workers (eg, institutions for the mentally and physically handicapped persons, prisons), patients with clotting-factor disorders, and healthcare workers who may be exposed to hepatitis A virus (eg, laboratory employees)

The CDC recommends routine vaccination of all children ≥1 year of age.

Usual Dosage I.M.: **Note:** Primary immunization should be given at least 2 weeks prior to expected exposure:

Havrix®:

Children 12 months to 18 years: 720 ELISA units (0.5 mL) with a booster dose of 720 ELISA units 6-12 months following primary immunization

Adults: 1440 ELISA units (1 mL) with a booster dose of 1440 ELISA units 6-12 months following primary immunization

VAQTA®:

Children 12 months to 18 years: 25 units (0.5 mL) with 25 units (0.5 mL) booster dose of 25 units to be given 6-18 months after primary immunization (6-12 months if initial dose was with Havrix®)

Adults: 50 units (1 mL) with 50 units (1 mL) booster dose of 50 units to be given 6-18 months after primary immunization (6-12 months if initial dose was with Havrix®)

Dosage Forms

Injection, suspension [adult formulation; preservative free]:

Havrix®: Viral antigen 1440 ELISA units/mL (1 mL)

VAQTA®: HAV antigen 50 units/mL (1 mL)

Injection, suspension [pediatric formulation; preservative free]:

Havrix®: Viral antigen 720 ELISA units/0.5 mL (0.5 mL)

Injection, suspension [pediatric/adolescent formulation; preservative free]:

VAQTA®: HAV antigen 25 units/0.5 mL (0.5 mL)

hepatitis B immune globulin (hep a TYE tis bee i MYUN GLOB yoo lin)

Synonyms HBIG

U.S./Canadian Brand Names HepaGam B™ [US/Can]; HyperHep B® [Can]; HyperHEP B™ S/D [US]; Nabi-HB® [US]

Therapeutic Category Immune Globulin

Use

Passive prophylactic immunity to hepatitis B following: Acute exposure to blood containing hepatitis B surface antigen (HBsAg); perinatal exposure of infants born to HBsAg-positive mothers; sexual exposure to HBsAg-positive persons; household exposure to persons with acute HBV infection

Prevention of hepatitis B virus recurrence after liver transplantation in HBsAg-positive transplant patients

Note: Hepatitis B immune globulin is not indicated for treatment of active hepatitis B infection and is ineffective in the treatment of chronic active hepatitis B infection.

Usual Dosage

I.M.:

Newborns: Perinatal exposure of infants born to HBsAg-positive mothers: 0.5 mL as soon after birth as possible (within 12 hours); active vaccination with hepatitis B vaccine may begin at the same time in a different site (if not contraindicated). If first dose of hepatitis B vaccine is delayed for as long as 3 months, dose may be repeated. If hepatitis B vaccine is refused, dose may be repeated at 3 and 6 months.

Infants <12 months: Household exposure prophylaxis: 0.5 mL (to be administered if mother or primary caregiver has acute HBV infection)

Children ≥12 months and Adults: Postexposure prophylaxis: 0.06 mL/kg as soon as possible after exposure (ie, within 24 hours of needlestick, ocular, or mucosal exposure or within 14 days of sexual exposure); usual dose: 3-5 mL; repeat at 28-30 days after exposure in nonresponders to hepatitis B vaccine or in patients who refuse vaccination

Note: HBIG may be administered at the same time (but at a different site) or up to 1 month preceding hepatitis B vaccination without impairing the active immune response

I.V.: Adults: Prevention of hepatitis B virus recurrence after liver transplantation (HepaGam B™): 20,000 int. units/dose according to the following schedule:

Anhepatic phase (Initial dose): One dose given with the liver transplant

Week 1 postop: One dose daily for 7 days (days 1-7)

Weeks 2-12 postop: One dose every 2 weeks starting day 14

Month 4 onward: One dose monthly starting on month 4

(Continued)

hepatitis B immune globulin *(Continued)*

Dose adjustment: Adjust dose to reach anti-HBs levels of 500 int. units/L within the first week after transplantation. In patients with surgical bleeding, abdominal fluid drainage >500 mL or those undergoing plasmapheresis, administer 10,000 int. units/dose every 6 hours until target anti-HBs levels are reached.

Dosage Forms Note: Potency expressed in international units (as compared to the WHO standard) is noted by individual lot on the vial label.

Injection, solution [preservative free]:
HyperHEP B™ S/D: 15% to 18% (0.5 mL, 1 mL, 5 mL)
Nabi-HB®: 5% (1 mL, 5 mL) [>312 int. units/mL]
HepaGam B™: 5% (1 mL, 5 mL) [>312 int. units/mL]

hepatitis B inactivated virus vaccine (recombinant DNA) *see* hepatitis B vaccine *on this page*

hepatitis B (recombinant) and hepatitis A inactivated vaccine *see* hepatitis A inactivated and hepatitis B (recombinant) vaccine *on page 416*

hepatitis B vaccine *(hep a TYE tis bee vak SEEN)*

Sound-Alike/Look-Alike Issues
Recombivax HB® may be confused with Comvax®

Synonyms hepatitis B inactivated virus vaccine (recombinant DNA)

U.S./Canadian Brand Names Engerix-B® [US/Can]; Recombivax HB® [US/Can]

Therapeutic Category Vaccine, Inactivated Virus

Use Immunization against infection caused by all known subtypes of hepatitis B virus, in individuals considered at high risk of potential exposure to hepatitis B virus or HB$_s$Ag-positive materials:

Healthcare workers[1]
Special patient groups (eg, adolescents, infants born to HB$_s$Ag-positive mothers, children born after 11/21/91, military personnel)
Hemodialysis patients[2] (see dosing recommendations), recipients of certain blood products[3]
Lifestyle factors: Homosexual and bisexual men, intravenous drug abusers, heterosexually-active persons with multiple sexual partners or recently acquired sexually-transmitted diseases
Environmental factors: Household and sexual contacts of HBV carriers; prison inmates; clients and staff of institutions for the mentally handicapped; residents, immigrants, and refugees from areas with endemic HBV infection; international travelers at increased risk of acquiring HBV infection
[1]The risk of hepatitis B virus (HBV) infection for healthcare workers varies both between hospitals and within hospitals. Hepatitis B vaccination is recommended for all healthcare workers with blood exposure.
[2]Hemodialysis patients often respond poorly to hepatitis B vaccination; higher vaccine doses or increased number of doses are required. A special formulation of one vaccine is now available for such persons (Recombivax HB®, 40 mcg/mL). The anti-HB$_s$(antibody to hepatitis B surface antigen) response of such persons should be tested after they are vaccinated, and those who have not responded should be revaccinated with 1-3 additional doses. Patients with chronic renal disease should be vaccinated as early as possible, ideally before they require hemodialysis. In addition, their anti-HB$_s$ levels should be monitored at 6- to 12-month intervals to assess the need for revaccination.
[3]Patients with hemophilia should be immunized subcutaneously, not intramuscularly.

Usual Dosage I.M.:
Immunization regimen: Regimen consists of 3 doses (0, 1, and 6 months): First dose given on the elected date, second dose given 1 month later, third dose given 6 months after the first dose.
Note: Infants born to mothers whose HB$_s$Ag status is unknown should follow the regimen for HB$_s$Ag-positive mothers, omitting the dose of HBIG.
Note: Preterm infants <2000 g and born to HB$_s$Ag-negative mothers should have the first dose delayed until 1 month after birth or hospital discharge due to decreased immune response in underweight infants.

Initial dose:
Birth (infants born of HB$_s$Ag-negative mothers) to 19 years:
Recombivax HB®: 0.5 mL (5 mcg/0.5 mL pediatric/adolescent formulation) **or**
Engerix-B®: 0.5 mL (10 mcg/0.5 mL formulation)
20 years and older:
Recombivax HB®: 1 mL (10 mcg/mL adult formulation) **or**
Engerix-B®: 1 mL (20 mcg/mL formulation)
Dialysis or immunocompromised patients (revaccinate if anti-HB$_s$ <10 mIU/mL ≥1-2 months after third dose):
Recombivax HB®: 1 mL (40 mcg/mL dialysis formulation) **or**
Engerix-B®: 2 mL (two 1 mL doses given at different sites using the 20 mcg/mL formulation)
1-month dose:
Birth (infants born of HB$_s$Ag-negative mothers) to 19 years:
Recombivax HB®: 0.5 mL (5 mcg/0.5 mL pediatric/adolescent formulation) **or**
Engerix-B®: 0.5 mL (10 mcg/0.5 mL formulation)

20 years and older:
  Recombivax HB®: 1 mL (10 mcg/mL adult formulation) **or**
  Engerix-B®: 1 mL (20 mcg/mL formulation)
  Dialysis or immunocompromised patients (revaccinate if anti-HB$_s$ <10 mIU/mL ≥1-2 months after third dose):
  Recombivax HB®: 1 mL (40 mcg/mL dialysis formulation) **or**
  Engerix-B®: 2 mL (two 1 mL doses given at different sites using the 20 mcg/mL formulation)
2-month dose:
  Dialysis or immunocompromised patients (revaccinate if anti-HB$_s$ <10 mIU/mL ≥1-2 months after third dose):
  Engerix-B®: 2 mL (two 1 mL doses given at different sites using the 20 mcg/mL formulation)
6-month dose (final dose in series should not be administered before age of 24 weeks):
  Birth (infants born of HB$_s$Ag-negative mothers) to 19 years:
  Recombivax HB®: 0.5 mL (5 mcg/0.5 mL pediatric/adolescent formulation)
  Engerix-B®: 0.5 mL (10 mcg/0.5 mL formulation)
  20 years and older:
  Recombivax HB®: 1 mL (10 mcg/mL adult formulation) **or**
  Engerix-B®: 1 mL (20 mcg/mL formulation)
  Dialysis or immunocompromised patients (revaccinate if anti-HB$_s$ <10 mIU/mL ≥1-2 months after third dose):
  Recombivax HB®: 1 mL (40 mcg/mL dialysis formulation) **or**
  Engerix-B®: 2 mL (two 1 mL doses given at different sites using the 20 mcg/mL formulation)
  Alternative dosing schedule for **Recombivax HB**®:
    Children 11-15 years (10 mcg/mL adult formulation): First dose of 1 mL given on the elected date, second dose given 4-6 months later
    Adults ≥20 years: Doses may be administered at 0, 1, and 4 months **or** at 0, 2, and 4 months
  Alternative dosing schedules for **Engerix-B**®:
    Children ≤10 years (10 mcg/0.5 mL formulation): High-risk children: 0.5 mL at 0, 1, 2, and 12 months; lower-risk children ages 5-10 who are candidates for an extended administration schedule may receive an alternative regimen of 0.5 mL at 0, 12, and 24 months. If booster dose is needed, revaccinate with 0.5 mL.
    Adolescents 11-19 years (20 mcg/mL formulation): 1 mL at 0, 1, and 6 months. High-risk adolescents: 1 mL at 0, 1, 2, and 12 months; lower-risk adolescents 11-16 years who are candidates for an extended administration schedule may receive an alternative regimen of 0.5 mL (using the 10 mcg/0.5 mL) formulation at 0, 12, and 24 months. If booster dose is needed, revaccinate with 20 mcg.
    Adults ≥20 years:
    Doses may be administered at 0, 1, and 4 months **or** at 0, 2, and 4 months
    High-risk adults (20 mcg/mL formulation): 1 mL at 0, 1, 2, and 12 months. If booster dose is needed, revaccinate with 1 mL.
Postexposure prophylaxis: **Note:** High-risk individuals may include children born of hepatitis B-infected mothers, those who have been or might be exposed or those who have traveled to high-risk areas.

Postexposure prophylaxis recommended dosage for infants born to HB$_s$Ag-positive mothers (by product / age):
Engerix-B® (pediatric formulation 10 mcg/0.5 mL):
  Give 0.5 mL at birth (≤12 hours); repeat 0.5 mL at 1 month and 6 months.
  The first dose may be given at birth at the same time as HBIG, but give in the opposite anterolateral thigh. This may better ensure vaccine absorption.
  An alternate regimen is administration of the vaccine at birth, and at 1, 2, and 12 months later.
Recombivax HB® (pediatric/adolescent formulation 5 mcg/0.5 mL):
  Give 0.5 mL at birth (≤12 hours); repeat 0.5 mL at 1 month and 6 months
  The first dose may be given at birth at the same time as HBIG, but give in the opposite anterolateral thigh. This may better ensure vaccine absorption.
Hepatitis B immune globulin: Give 0.5 mL at birth (or within 7 days of birth).
Dosage Forms
  Injection, suspension [preservative free] [recombinant DNA]:
  Engerix-B®:
    Adult: Hepatitis B surface antigen 20 mcg/mL (1 mL)
    Pediatric/adolescent: Hepatitis B surface antigen 10 mcg/0.5 mL (0.5 mL)
  Recombivax HB®:
    Adult: Hepatitis B surface antigen 10 mcg/mL (1 mL, 3 mL)
    Dialysis: Hepatitis B surface antigen 40 mcg/mL (1 mL)
    Pediatric/adolescent: Hepatitis B surface antigen 5 mcg/0.5 mL (0.5 mL)

hepatitis b vaccine (recombinant) *see Haemophilus* B conjugate and hepatitis B vaccine *on page 411*

HepFlush®-10 [US] *see* heparin *on page 415*

Hep-Lock® [US] *see* heparin *on page 415*

Hep-Lock U/P [US] *see* heparin *on page 415*

Hepsera™ [US/Can] *see* adefovir *on page 19*

Heptalac® *(Discontinued)* see lactulose *on page 489*

Heptovir® [Can] see lamivudine *on page 489*

Herceptin® [US/Can] see trastuzumab *on page 858*

HES see hetastarch *on this page*

Hespan® [US] see hetastarch *on this page*

hetastarch (HET a starch)
Sound-Alike/Look-Alike Issues
Hespan® may be confused with heparin
Synonyms HES; hydroxyethyl starch
U.S./Canadian Brand Names Hespan® [US]; Hextend® [US/Can]; Voluven® [Can]
Therapeutic Category Plasma Volume Expander
Use Blood volume expander used in treatment of hypovolemia
Hespan®: Adjunct in leukapheresis to improve harvesting and increasing the yield of granulocytes by centrifugal means
Usual Dosage I.V. infusion (requires an infusion pump):
Plasma volume expansion: Adults: 500-1000 mL (up to 1500 mL/day) or 20 mL/kg/day (up to 1500 mL/day); larger volumes (15,000 mL/24 hours) have been used safely in small numbers of patients
Leukapheresis: 250-700 mL; **Note:** Citrate anticoagulant is added before use.
Dosage Forms
Infusion [premixed in lactated electrolyte injection]:
Hextend®: 6% (500 mL)
Infusion, solution [premixed in NaCl 0.9%]: 6% (500 mL)
Hespan®: 6% (500 mL)

Hexabrix™ [US] see ioxaglate meglumine and ioxaglate sodium *on page 469*

hexachlorocyclohexane see lindane *on page 509*

hexachlorophene (heks a KLOR oh feen)
Sound-Alike/Look-Alike Issues
pHisoHex® may be confused with Fostex®, pHisoDerm®
U.S./Canadian Brand Names pHisoHex® [US/Can]
Therapeutic Category Antibacterial, Topical
Use Surgical scrub and as a bacteriostatic skin cleanser; control an outbreak of gram-positive infection when other procedures have been unsuccessful
Usual Dosage Topical: Children and Adults: Apply 5 mL cleanser and water to area to be cleansed; lather and rinse thoroughly under running water
Dosage Forms
Liquid, topical:
pHisoHex®: 3% (150 mL, 500 mL, 3840 mL)

Hexalen® [US/Can] see altretamine *on page 36*

hexamethylenetetramine see methenamine *on page 551*

hexamethylmelamine see altretamine *on page 36*

Hexit™ [Can] see lindane *on page 509*

HEXM see altretamine *on page 36*

Hextend® [US/Can] see hetastarch *on this page*

hexylresorcinol (heks il re ZOR si nole)
U.S./Canadian Brand Names S.T. 37® [US-OTC]; Sucrets® Original [US-OTC]
Therapeutic Category Local Anesthetic
Use Minor antiseptic and local anesthetic for sore throat; topical antiseptic for minor cuts or abrasions
Usual Dosage Children ≥2 years and Adults:
Antiseptic: Topical: Solution: Apply to affected area 1-3 times/day
Sore throat: Oral:
Lozenge: May be used as needed, allow to dissolve slowly in mouth (maximum: 10 lozenges/day)
Solution: Gargle or swish in mouth up to 4 times/day
Dosage Forms
Lozenge:
Sucrets® Original [OTC]: 2.4 mg

Solution:
  S.T. 37® [OTC]: 0.1%

hFSH *see* urofollitropin *on page 878*

hGH *see* somatropin *on page 799*

Hib conjugate vaccine *see Haemophilus* B conjugate and hepatitis B vaccine *on page 411*

Hibiclens® [US-OTC] *see* chlorhexidine gluconate *on page 174*

Hibidil® 1:2000 [Can] *see* chlorhexidine gluconate *on page 174*

Hibistat® [US-OTC] *see* chlorhexidine gluconate *on page 174*

Hib polysaccharide conjugate *see Haemophilus* B conjugate vaccine *on page 411*

HibTITER® *(Discontinued)* *see Haemophilus* B conjugate vaccine *on page 411*

High Gamma Vitamin E Complete™ [US-OTC] *see* vitamin E *on page 894*

Hi-Kovite [US-OTC] *see* vitamins (multiple/oral) *on page 895*

Hiprex® [US/Can] *see* methenamine *on page 551*

hirulog *see* bivalirudin *on page 115*

Histacol™ BD [US] *see* brompheniramine, pseudoephedrine, and dextromethorphan *on page 122*

Histade™ *(Discontinued)* *see* chlorpheniramine and pseudoephedrine *on page 178*

Histalet® X *(Discontinued)* *see* guaifenesin and pseudoephedrine *on page 406*

Histatab® Plus *(Discontinued)* *see* chlorpheniramine and phenylephrine *on page 177*

Hista-Vent® DA [US] *see* chlorpheniramine, phenylephrine, and methscopolamine *on page 181*

Hista-Vent® PSE [US] *see* chlorpheniramine, pseudoephedrine, and methscopolamine *on page 184*

Histerone® Injection *(Discontinued)* *see* testosterone *on page 828*

Histex™ [US] *see* chlorpheniramine and pseudoephedrine *on page 178*

Histex™ I/E *(Discontinued)* *see* carbinoxamine *on page 151*

Histex™ HC [US] *see* hydrocodone, carbinoxamine, and pseudoephedrine *on page 430*

Histex™ SR *(Discontinued)* *see* brompheniramine and pseudoephedrine *on page 120*

Histinex® D Liquid *(Discontinued)* *see* hydrocodone and pseudoephedrine *on page 430*

Histinex® HC [US] *see* phenylephrine, hydrocodone, and chlorpheniramine *on page 678*

Histinex® PV [US] *see* pseudoephedrine, hydrocodone, and chlorpheniramine *on page 731*

Histor-D® Syrup *(Discontinued)* *see* chlorpheniramine and phenylephrine *on page 177*

Histor-D® Timecelles® *(Discontinued)* *see* chlorpheniramine, phenylephrine, and methscopolamine *on page 181*

Histrodrix® *(Discontinued)* *see* dexbrompheniramine and pseudoephedrine *on page 243*

Histussin D® *(Discontinued)* *see* hydrocodone and pseudoephedrine *on page 430*

Histussin® HC *(Discontinued)* *see* phenylephrine, hydrocodone, and chlorpheniramine *on page 678*

Hi-Vegi-Lip [US-OTC] *see* pancreatin *on page 648*

Hivid® *(Discontinued)*

hMG *see* menotropins *on page 541*

HMM *see* altretamine *on page 36*

HMR 3647 *see* telithromycin *on page 823*

HMS Liquifilm® *(Discontinued)* *see* medrysone *on page 537*

H5N1 influenza vaccine *see* influenza virus vaccine (H5N1) *on page 456*

HN₂ *see* mechlorethamine *on page 535*

Hold® DM [US-OTC] *see* dextromethorphan *on page 247*

homatropine (hoe MA troe peen)
  Synonyms homatropine hydrobromide
  U.S./Canadian Brand Names Isopto® Homatropine [US]
  Therapeutic Category Anticholinergic Agent
  Use Producing cycloplegia and mydriasis for refraction; treatment of acute inflammatory conditions of the uveal tract
  (Continued)

homatropine *(Continued)*

Usual Dosage Ophthalmic:
Children:
Mydriasis and cycloplegia for refraction: Instill 1 drop of 2% solution immediately before the procedure; repeat at 10-minute intervals as needed
Uveitis: Instill 1 drop of 2% solution 2-3 times/day
Adults:
Mydriasis and cycloplegia for refraction: Instill 1-2 drops of 2% solution or 1 drop of 5% solution before the procedure; repeat at 5- to 10-minute intervals as needed; maximum of 3 doses for refraction
Uveitis: Instill 1-2 drops of 2% or 5% 2-3 times/day up to every 3-4 hours as needed

Dosage Forms
Solution, ophthalmic:
Isopto® Homatropine: 2% (5 mL); 5% (5 mL, 15 mL)

homatropine and hydrocodone *see* hydrocodone and homatropine *on page 429*

homatropine hydrobromide *see* homatropine *on previous page*

horse antihuman thymocyte gamma globulin *see* antithymocyte globulin (equine) *on page 62*

H.P. Acthar® Gel [US] *see* corticotropin *on page 216*

Hp-PAC® [Can] *see* lansoprazole, amoxicillin, and clarithromycin *on page 493*

HPV Vaccine *see* papillomavirus (Types 6, 11, 16, 18) recombinant vaccine *on page 652*

HTF919 *see* tegaserod *on page 822*

hu1124 *see* efalizumab *on page 292*

Humalog® [US/Can] *see* insulin lispro *on page 459*

Humalog® Mix 25 [Can] *see* insulin lispro protamine and insulin lispro *on page 459*

Humalog® Mix 50/50™ [US] *see* insulin lispro protamine and insulin lispro *on page 459*

Humalog® Mix 50/50 Insulin *(Discontinued)*

Humalog® Mix 75/25™ [US] *see* insulin lispro protamine and insulin lispro *on page 459*

human antitumor necrosis factor alpha *see* adalimumab *on page 18*

human corticotrophin-releasing hormone, analogue *see* corticorelin *on page 216*

human diploid cell cultures rabies vaccine *see* rabies virus vaccine *on page 742*

human growth hormone *see* somatropin *on page 799*

humanized IgG1 anti-CD52 monoclonal antibody *see* alemtuzumab *on page 27*

human LFA-3/IgG(1) fusion protein *see* alefacept *on page 26*

human menopausal gonadotropin *see* menotropins *on page 541*

human papillomavirus vaccine *see* papillomavirus (Types 6, 11, 16, 18) recombinant vaccine *on page 652*

human thyroid stimulating hormone *see* thyrotropin alpha *on page 839*

Humate-P® [US/Can] *see* antihemophilic factor/von Willebrand factor complex (human) *on page 60*

Humatin® [US/Can] *see* paromomycin *on page 654*

Humatrope® [US/Can] *see* somatropin *on page 799*

Humegon® [Can] *see* chorionic gonadotropin (human) *on page 187*

Humegon® *(Discontinued)* *see* menotropins *on page 541*

Humibid® CS *(Discontinued)* *see* guaifenesin and dextromethorphan *on page 402*

Humibid® DM *(Discontinued)* *see* guaifenesin and dextromethorphan *on page 402*

Humibid® e *(Discontinued)* *see* guaifenesin *on page 401*

Humibid® LA *(Discontinued)* *see* guaifenesin *on page 401*

Humibid® LA *(reformulation)* [US] *see* guaifenesin and potassium guaiacolsulfonate *on page 405*

Humibid® Pediatric *(Discontinued)* *see* guaifenesin *on page 401*

Humibid® Sprinkle *(Discontinued)* *see* guaifenesin *on page 401*

Humira® [US/Can] *see* adalimumab *on page 18*

Humulin® 20/80 [Can] *see* insulin NPH and insulin regular *on page 460*

Humulin® 50/50 [US] *see* insulin NPH and insulin regular *on page 460*

Humulin® L *(Discontinued)*

Humulin® **70/30 [US/Can]** *see* insulin NPH and insulin regular *on page 460*

Humulin® **N [US/Can]** *see* insulin NPH *on page 459*

Humulin® **R [US/Can]** *see* insulin regular *on page 460*

Humulin® **R (Concentrated) U-500 [US]** *see* insulin regular *on page 460*

Humulin® **U** *(Discontinued)*

Hurricaine® **[US-OTC]** *see* benzocaine *on page 101*

HXM *see* altretamine *on page 36*

Hyalgan® **[US]** *see* hyaluronate and derivatives *on this page*

hyaluronan *see* hyaluronate and derivatives *on this page*

hyaluronate and derivatives (hye al yoor ON ate & dah RIV ah tives)

Sound-Alike/Look-Alike Issues
Healon® may be confused with Halcion®
Synvisc® may be confused with Synagis®

Synonyms hyaluronan; hyaluronic acid; hylan polymers; sodium hyaluronate

U.S./Canadian Brand Names Cystistat® [Can]; Durolane® [Can]; Euflexxa™ [US]; Eyestil [Can]; Healon GV® [US/Can]; Healon® [US/Can]; Healon®5 [US]; Hyalgan® [US]; Hylaform® Plus [US]; Hylaform® [US]; IPM Wound Gel™ [US-OTC]; Juvederm™ 24HV [US]; Juvederm™ 30 [US]; Juvederm™ 30HV [US]; Orthovisc® [US/Can]; Perlane® [US]; Provisc® [US]; Restylane® [US]; Supartz™ [US]; Suplasyn® [Can]; Synvisc® [US]; Vitrax® [US]

Therapeutic Category Antirheumatic Miscellaneous; Ophthalmic Agent, Viscoelastic; Skin and Mucous Membrane Agent

Use
Intra-articular injection: Treatment of pain in osteoarthritis in knee in patients who have failed nonpharmacologic treatment and simple analgesics
Intradermal: Correction of moderate-to-severe facial wrinkles or folds
Ophthalmic: Surgical aid in cataract extraction, intraocular implantation, corneal transplant, glaucoma filtration, and retinal attachment surgery
Topical: Management of skin ulcers and wounds

Usual Dosage Adults:
Osteoarthritis of the knee: Intra-articular:
Eulexxa™: Inject 20 mg (2 mL) once weekly for 3 weeks
Hyalgan®: Inject 20 mg (2 mL) once weekly for 5 weeks; some patients may benefit with a total of 3 injections
Orthovisc®: Inject 30 mg (2 mL) once weekly for 3-4 weeks
Supartz™: Inject 25 mg (2.5 mL) once weekly for 5 weeks
Synvisc®: Inject 16 mg (2 mL) once weekly for 3 weeks (total of 3 injections)
Facial wrinkles: Intradermal:
Note: Formulations differ in terms of recommended injection depth: Juvederm™, Hylaform®, and Restylane® are intended for mid to deep interdermal injection; Perlane® is intended for injection into the deep dermis to superficial subcutis
Hylaform®, Hylaform® Plus: Inject as required for cosmetic result; typical treatment regimen requires <2 mL; limit injection to ≤1.5 mL per injection site; maximum: 20 mL/60 kg/year
Juvederm™ (all formulations): Inject as required for cosmetic result; typical treatment regimen requires <2 mL; limit injection to 1.6 mL per injection site; maximum: 20 mL/60 kg/year
Perlane®: Inject as required into deep dermis/superficial subcutis for cosmetic result; typical treatment regimen requires 1.9-4.6 mL; maximum 6 mL per treatment
Restylane®: Inject as required for cosmetic result; typical treatment regimen requires <2 mL; limit injection to ≤1.5 mL per injection site
Ophthalmic (Biolon™, Healon®, Provisc®, Vitrax®): Depends upon procedure (slowly introduce a sufficient quantity into eye)
Topical (IPM Wound Gel™): Apply to clean dry ulcer or wound, and cover with nonstick dressing; repeat daily. Discontinue if wound size increase after 3-4 applications.

Dosage Forms
Hylan B:
Injection, gel:
Hylaform® [500 micron particle]: 5.5 mg/mL (0.75 mL)
Hylaform® Plus [700 micron particle]: 5.5 mg/mL (0.75 mL)
Hylan Polymers A and B (Hylan G-F 20):
Injection, solution, intra-articular:
Synvisc®: 8 mg/mL (2 mL)
Hyaluronate:
Gel, topical:
IPM Wound Gel™ [OTC]: 2.5% (10 g)
(Continued)

423

hyaluronate and derivatives *(Continued)*

Injection, gel, intradermal:
Juvederm™ 24HV, Juvederm™ 30, Juvederm™ 30HV: 24 mg/mL [prefilled syringe]
Perlane®: 20 mg/mL (1mL) [prefilled syringe]
Restylane®: 20 mg/mL
Injection, solution, intra-articular:
Euflexxa™, Hyalgan®: 10 mg/mL (2 mL)
Orthovisc®: 15 mg/mL (2 mL)
Supartz™: 10 mg/mL (2.5 mL)
Synvisc®: 8 mg/mL (2 mL)
Injection, solution, intraocular:
Healon®: 10 mg/mL (0.4 mL, 0.55 mL, 0.85 mL, 2 mL)
Healon®5: 23 mg/mL
Healon GV®: 14 mg/mL (0.55 mL, 0.85 mL)
Provisc®: 10 mg/mL (0.4 mL, 0.55 mL, 0.8 mL)
Vitrax®: 30 mg/mL (0.65 mL)

hyaluronic acid *see hyaluronate and derivatives on previous page*

hyaluronidase (hye al yoor ON i dase)

Sound-Alike/Look-Alike Issues
Wydase® may be confused with Lidex®, Wyamine®
U.S./Canadian Brand Names Amphadase™ [US]; Hydase™ [US]; Hylenex™ [US]; Vitrase® [US]
Therapeutic Category Enzyme
Use Increase the dispersion and absorption of other drugs; increase rate of absorption of parenteral fluids given by hypodermoclysis; adjunct in subcutaneous urography for improving resorption of radiopaque agents
Usual Dosage Note: A preliminary skin test for hypersensitivity can be performed. ACTH, antihistamines, corticosteroids, estrogens, and salicylates, when used in large doses, may cause tissues to be partly resistant to hyaluronidase. May require larger doses of hyaluronidase for the same effect.
Skin test: Intradermal: 0.02 mL (3 units) of a 150 units/mL solution. Positive reaction consists of a wheal with pseudopods appearing within 5 minutes and persisting for 20-30 minutes with localized itching.
Hypodermoclysis: SubQ: 15 units is added to each 100 mL of I.V. fluid to be administered; 150 units facilitates absorption of >1000 mL of solution
Premature Infants and Neonates: Volume of a single clysis should not exceed 25 mL/kg and the rate of administration should not exceed 2 mL/minute
Children <3 years: Volume of a single clysis should not exceed 200 mL
Children ≥3 years and Adults: Rate and volume of a single clysis should not exceed those used for infusion of I.V. fluids
Urography: Children and Adults: SubQ: 75 units over each scapula followed by injection of contrast medium at the same site; patient should be in the prone position.
Dosage Forms
Injection, powder for reconstitution:
Vitrase®: 6200 units
Injection, solution:
Amphadase™: 150 units/mL (1 mL)
Injection, solution [preservative free]:
Hydase™: 150 units/mL (1 mL)
Hylenex™: 150 units/mL (1 mL, 2 mL)
Vitrase®: 200 units/mL (2 mL)

hycamptamine *see topotecan on page 851*

Hycamtin® **[US/Can]** *see topotecan on page 851*

hycet™ **[US]** *see hydrocodone and acetaminophen on page 427*

HycoClear Tuss® *(Discontinued)* *see hydrocodone and guaifenesin on page 429*

Hycodan® **[US]** *see hydrocodone and homatropine on page 429*

Hycomine® **Compound [US]** *see hydrocodone, chlorpheniramine, phenylephrine, acetaminophen, and caffeine on page 431*

Hycomine® *(Discontinued)*

Hycomine® **Pediatric** *(Discontinued)*

Hycort™ **[Can]** *see hydrocortisone (topical) on page 434*

Hycotuss® **[US]** *see hydrocodone and guaifenesin on page 429*

Hydase™ **[US]** *see hyaluronidase on this page*

Hydeltra T.B.A.® **[Can]** *see* prednisolone (systemic) *on page 710*

Hydergine® **[Can]** *see* ergoloid mesylates *on page 306*

Hydergine® *(Discontinued)* *see* ergoloid mesylates *on page 306*

Hyderm [Can] *see* hydrocortisone (topical) *on page 434*

hydralazine (hye DRAL a zeen)

Sound-Alike/Look-Alike Issues
hydrALAZINE may be confused with hydrOXYzine

Synonyms hydralazine hydrochloride

Tall-Man hydr**ALAZINE**

U.S./Canadian Brand Names Apo-Hydralazine® [Can]; Apresoline® [Can]; Novo-Hylazin [Can]; Nu-Hydral [Can]

Therapeutic Category Vasodilator

Use Management of moderate to severe hypertension, congestive heart failure, hypertension secondary to preeclampsia/eclampsia; treatment of primary pulmonary hypertension

Usual Dosage

Children:

Oral: Initial: 0.75-1 mg/kg/day in 2-4 divided doses; increase over 3-4 weeks to maximum of 7.5 mg/kg/day in 2-4 divided doses; maximum daily dose: 200 mg/day

I.M., I.V.: 0.1-0.2 mg/kg/dose (not to exceed 20 mg) every 4-6 hours as needed, up to 1.7-3.5 mg/kg/day in 4-6 divided doses

Adults:

Oral:

Hypertension:

Initial dose: 10 mg 4 times/day for first 2-4 days; increase to 25 mg 4 times/day for the balance of the first week

Increase by 10-25 mg/dose gradually to 50 mg 4 times/day (maximum: 300 mg/day); usual dose range (JNC 7): 25-100 mg/day in 2 divided doses

Congestive heart failure:

Initial dose: 10-25 mg 3-4 times/day

Adjustment: Dosage must be adjusted based on individual response

Target dose: 225-300 mg/day in divided doses; use in combination with isosorbide dinitrate

I.M., I.V.:

Hypertension: Initial: 10-20 mg/dose every 4-6 hours as needed, may increase to 40 mg/dose; change to oral therapy as soon as possible.

Preeclampsia/eclampsia: 5 mg/dose then 5-10 mg every 20-30 minutes as needed.

Dosage Forms

Injection, solution: 20 mg/mL (1 mL)

Tablet: 10 mg, 25 mg, 50 mg, 100 mg

hydralazine and hydrochlorothiazide (hye DRAL a zeen & hye droe klor oh THYE a zide)

Synonyms hydrochlorothiazide and hydralazine

Therapeutic Category Antihypertensive Agent, Combination

Use Management of moderate to severe hypertension and treatment of congestive heart failure

Usual Dosage Oral: Adults: Hydralazine 25-100 mg/day and hydrochlorothiazide 25-50 mg/day in 2 divided doses (maximum: hydrochlorothiazide: 50 mg/day)

Dosage Forms

Capsule: 25/25: Hydralazine 25 mg and hydrochlorothiazide 25 mg; 50/50: Hydralazine 50 mg and hydrochlorothiazide 50 mg; 100/50: Hydralazine 100 mg and hydrochlorothiazide 50 mg

hydralazine and isosorbide dinitrate *see* isosorbide dinitrate and hydralazine *on page 476*

hydralazine hydrochloride *see* hydralazine *on this page*

Hydramine® **[US-OTC]** *see* diphenhydramine *on page 265*

hydrated chloral *see* chloral hydrate *on page 172*

Hydrate® *(Discontinued)* *see* dimenhydrinate *on page 262*

Hydrea® **[US/Can]** *see* hydroxyurea *on page 439*

Hydrisalic™ **[US-OTC]** *see* salicylic acid *on page 772*

Hydrocet® *(Discontinued)* *see* hydrocodone and acetaminophen *on page 427*

hydrochlorothiazide (hye droe klor oh THYE a zide)

Sound-Alike/Look-Alike Issues
hydrochlorothiazide may be confused with hydrocortisone, hydroflumethiazide
Esidrix may be confused with Lasix®
HCTZ is an error-prone abbreviation (mistaken as hydrocortisone)
Microzide™ may be confused with Micronase®

U.S./Canadian Brand Names Apo-Hydro® [Can]; Microzide™ [US]; Novo-Hydrazide [Can]; PMS-Hydrochlorothiazide [Can]

Therapeutic Category Diuretic, Thiazide

Use Management of mild to moderate hypertension; treatment of edema in congestive heart failure and nephrotic syndrome

Usual Dosage Oral (effect of drug may be decreased when used every day):
Children (in pediatric patients, chlorothiazide may be preferred over hydrochlorothiazide as there are more dosage formulations [eg, suspension] available): Edema, hypertension:
<6 months: 1-3 mg/kg/day in 2 divided doses
>6 months to 2 years: 1-3 mg/kg/day in 2 divided doses; maximum: 37.5 mg/day
>2-17 years: Initial: 1 mg/kg/day; maximum: 3 mg/kg/day (50 mg/day)
Adults:
Edema: 25-100 mg/day in 1-2 doses; maximum: 200 mg/day
Hypertension: 12.5-50 mg/day; minimal increase in response and more electrolyte disturbances are seen with doses >50 mg/day

Dosage Forms
Capsule: 12.5 mg
Microzide™: 12.5 mg
Tablet: 25 mg, 50 mg

hydrochlorothiazide and amiloride *see* amiloride and hydrochlorothiazide *on page 42*

hydrochlorothiazide and benazepril *see* benazepril and hydrochlorothiazide *on page 99*

hydrochlorothiazide and bisoprolol *see* bisoprolol and hydrochlorothiazide *on page 114*

hydrochlorothiazide and captopril *see* captopril and hydrochlorothiazide *on page 146*

hydrochlorothiazide and enalapril *see* enalapril and hydrochlorothiazide *on page 296*

hydrochlorothiazide and eprosartan *see* eprosartan and hydrochlorothiazide *on page 305*

hydrochlorothiazide and fosinopril *see* fosinopril and hydrochlorothiazide *on page 376*

hydrochlorothiazide and hydralazine *see* hydralazine and hydrochlorothiazide *on previous page*

hydrochlorothiazide and irbesartan *see* irbesartan and hydrochlorothiazide *on page 472*

hydrochlorothiazide and lisinopril *see* lisinopril and hydrochlorothiazide *on page 512*

hydrochlorothiazide and losartan *see* losartan and hydrochlorothiazide *on page 519*

hydrochlorothiazide and methyldopa *see* methyldopa and hydrochlorothiazide *on page 557*

hydrochlorothiazide and metoprolol *see* metoprolol and hydrochlorothiazide *on page 563*

hydrochlorothiazide and metoprolol tartrate *see* metoprolol and hydrochlorothiazide *on page 563*

hydrochlorothiazide and moexipril *see* moexipril and hydrochlorothiazide *on page 576*

hydrochlorothiazide and olmesartan medoxomil *see* olmesartan and hydrochlorothiazide *on page 627*

hydrochlorothiazide and propranolol *see* propranolol and hydrochlorothiazide *on page 724*

hydrochlorothiazide and quinapril *see* quinapril and hydrochlorothiazide *on page 739*

hydrochlorothiazide and ramipril *see* ramipril and hydrochlorothiazide *(Canada only) on page 743*

hydrochlorothiazide and spironolactone
(hye droe klor oh THYE a zide & speer on oh LAK tone)

Sound-Alike/Look-Alike Issues
Aldactazide® may be confused with Aldactone®

Synonyms spironolactone and hydrochlorothiazide

U.S./Canadian Brand Names Aldactazide 25® [Can]; Aldactazide 50® [Can]; Aldactazide® [US]; Novo-Spirozine [Can]

Therapeutic Category Antihypertensive Agent, Combination

Use Management of mild- to-moderate hypertension; treatment of edema in congestive heart failure and nephrotic syndrome, and cirrhosis of the liver accompanied by edema and/or ascites

Usual Dosage Oral:
Children: 1.5-3 mg/kg/day in 2-4 divided doses (maximum: 200 mg/day)

Adults: Hydrochlorothiazide 12.5-50 mg/day and spironolactone 12.5-50 mg/day; manufacturer labeling states hydrochlorothiazide maximum 200 mg/day, however, usual dose in JNC-7 is 12.5-50 mg/day

Dosage Forms

Tablet: Hydrochlorothiazide 25 mg and spironolactone 25 mg
Aldactazide®: 25/25: Hydrochlorothiazide 25 mg and spironolactone 25 mg; 50/50: Hydrochlorothiazide 50 mg and spironolactone 50 mg

hydrochlorothiazide and telmisartan *see* telmisartan and hydrochlorothiazide *on page 823*

hydrochlorothiazide and triamterene (hye droe klor oh THYE a zide & trye AM ter een)

Sound-Alike/Look-Alike Issues
Dyazide® may be confused with diazoxide, Dynacin®
Maxzide® may be confused with Maxidex®

Synonyms triamterene and hydrochlorothiazide

U.S./Canadian Brand Names Apo-Triazide® [Can]; Dyazide® [US]; Maxzide® [US]; Maxzide®-25 [US]; Novo-Triamzide [Can]; Nu-Triazide [Can]; Penta-Triamterene HCTZ [Can]; Riva-Zide [Can]

Therapeutic Category Antihypertensive Agent, Combination

Use Management of mild to moderate hypertension; treatment of edema in congestive heart failure and nephrotic syndrome

Usual Dosage Oral: Adults:
Hydrochlorothiazide 25 mg and triamterene 37.5 mg: 1-2 tablets/capsules once daily
Hydrochlorothiazide 50 mg and triamterene 75 mg: 1/2-1 tablet daily

Dosage Forms

Capsule: Hydrochlorothiazide 25 mg and triamterene 37.5 mg
Dyazide®: Hydrochlorothiazide 25 mg and triamterene 37.5 mg
Tablet: Hydrochlorothiazide 50 mg and triamterene 75 mg; hydrochlorothiazide 25 mg and triamterene 37.5 mg
Maxzide®: Hydrochlorothiazide 50 mg and triamterene 75 mg
Maxzide®-25: Hydrochlorothiazide 25 mg and triamterene 37.5 mg

hydrochlorothiazide and valsartan *see* valsartan and hydrochlorothiazide *on page 882*

Hydrocil® Instant [US-OTC] *see* psyllium *on page 732*

hydrocodone and acetaminophen (hye droe KOE done & a seet a MIN oh fen)

Sound-Alike/Look-Alike Issues
Lorcet® may be confused with Fioricet®
Lortab® may be confused with Cortef®, Lorabid®, Luride®
Vicodin® may be confused with Hycodan®, Hycomine®, Indocin®, Uridon®
Zydone® may be confused with Vytone®

Synonyms acetaminophen and hydrocodone

U.S./Canadian Brand Names Anexsia® [US]; Co-Gesic® [US]; hycet™ [US]; Lorcet® 10/650 [US]; Lorcet® Plus [US]; Lortab® [US]; Margesic® H [US]; Maxidone™ [US]; Norco® [US]; Stagesic® [US]; Vicodin® ES [US]; Vicodin® HP [US]; Vicodin® [US]; Xodol® 10/300 [US]; Xodol® 5/300 [US]; Xodol® 7.5/300 [US]; Zydone® [US]

Therapeutic Category Analgesic, Narcotic

Controlled Substance C-III

Use Relief of moderate to severe pain

Usual Dosage Oral (doses should be titrated to appropriate analgesic effect): Analgesic:
Children 2-13 years or <50 kg: Hydrocodone 0.135 mg/kg/dose every 4-6 hours; do not exceed 6 doses/day or the maximum recommended dose of acetaminophen
Children and Adults ≥50 kg: Average starting dose in opioid-naive patients: Hydrocodone 5-10 mg 4 times/day; the dosage of acetaminophen should be limited to ≤4 g/day (and possibly less in patients with hepatic impairment or ethanol use).
Dosage ranges (based on specific product labeling): Hydrocodone 2.5-10 mg every 4-6 hours; maximum: 60 mg hydrocodone/day (maximum dose of hydrocodone may be limited by the acetaminophen content of specific product)

Dosage Forms

Capsule: Hydrocodone 5 mg and acetaminophen 500 mg
Margesic® H, Stagesic®: Hydrocodone 5 mg and acetaminophen 500 mg
Elixir: Hydrocodone 7.5 mg and acetaminophen 500 mg per 15 mL
Lortab®: Hydrocodone 7.5 mg and acetaminophen 500 mg per 15 mL
Solution, oral: Hydrocodone 7.5 mg and acetaminophen 325 mg per 15 mL
hycet™: Hydrocodone 7.5 mg and acetaminophen 325 mg per 15 mL
Tablet:
Generics:
Hydrocodone 2.5 mg and acetaminophen 500 mg
(Continued)

427

hydrocodone and acetaminophen *(Continued)*

    Hydrocodone 5 mg and acetaminophen 325 mg
    Hydrocodone 5 mg and acetaminophen 500 mg
    Hydrocodone 7.5 mg and acetaminophen 325 mg
    Hydrocodone 7.5 mg and acetaminophen 500 mg
    Hydrocodone 7.5 mg and acetaminophen 650 mg
    Hydrocodone 7.5 mg and acetaminophen 750 mg
    Hydrocodone 10 mg and acetaminophen 325 mg
    Hydrocodone 10 mg and acetaminophen 500 mg
    Hydrocodone 10 mg and acetaminophen 650 mg
    Hydrocodone 10 mg and acetaminophen 660 mg
    Hydrocodone 10 mg and acetaminophen 750 mg
Brands:
Anexsia®:
    5/325: Hydrocodone 5 mg and acetaminophen 320 mg; 7.5/325: Hydrocodone 7.5 mg and acetaminophen 320 mg
Co-Gesic® 5/500: Hydrocodone 5 mg and acetaminophen 500 mg
Lorcet® 10/650: Hydrocodone 10 mg and acetaminophen 650 mg
Lorcet® Plus: Hydrocodone 7.5 mg and acetaminophen 650 mg
Lortab®: 5/500: Hydrocodone 5 mg and acetaminophen 500 mg; 7.5/500: Hydrocodone 7.5 mg and acetaminophen 500 mg; 10/500: Hydrocodone 10 mg and acetaminophen 500 mg
Maxidone™: Hydrocodone 10 mg and acetaminophen 750 mg
Norco®: Hydrocodone 5 mg and acetaminophen 325 mg; hydrocodone 7.5 mg and acetaminophen 325 mg; hydrocodone 10 mg and acetaminophen 325 mg
Vicodin®: Hydrocodone 5 mg and acetaminophen 500 mg
Vicodin® ES: Hydrocodone 7.5 mg and acetaminophen 750 mg
Vicodin® HP: Hydrocodone 10 mg and acetaminophen 660 mg
Xodol®: 10/300: Hydrocodone 10 mg and acetaminophen 300 mg; 5/300: Hydrocodone 5 mg and acetaminophen 300 mg; 7/300: Hydrocodone 7 mg and acetaminophen 300 mg
Zydone®: Hydrocodone 5 mg and acetaminophen 400 mg; hydrocodone 7.5 mg and acetaminophen 400 mg; hydrocodone 10 mg and acetaminophen 400 mg

hydrocodone and aspirin (hye droe KOE done & AS pir in)

Synonyms aspirin and hydrocodone
U.S./Canadian Brand Names Damason-P® [US]
Therapeutic Category Analgesic, Narcotic
Controlled Substance C-III
Use Relief of moderate to moderately severe pain
Usual Dosage Oral: Adults: 1-2 tablets every 4-6 hours as needed for pain
Dosage Forms
  Tablet:
    Damason-P®: Hydrocodone 5 mg and aspirin 500 mg

hydrocodone and chlorpheniramine (hye droe KOE done & klor fen IR a meen)

Synonyms chlorpheniramine maleate and hydrocodone bitartrate; hydrocodone tannate and chlorpheniramine tannate
U.S./Canadian Brand Names Tussionex® [US]
Therapeutic Category Antihistamine/Antitussive
Controlled Substance C-III
Use Symptomatic relief of cough and upper respiratory symptoms associated with cold and allergy
Usual Dosage Oral:
  Children 6-12 years:
    HyTan™: 5 mL every 12 hours; do not exceed 10 mL/24 hours
    Tussionex®: 2.5 mL every 12 hours; do not exceed 5 mL/24 hours
  Children >12 years and Adults:
    HyTan™: 10 mL every 12 hours; do not exceed 20 mL/24 hours
    Tussionex®: 5 mL every 12 hours; do not exceed 10 mL/24 hours
Dosage Forms
  Suspension, extended release:
    Tussionex®: Hydrocodone polistirex 10 mg and chlorpheniramine polistirex 8 mg per 5 mL

hydrocodone and guaifenesin (hye droe KOE done & gwye FEN e sin)

Synonyms guaifenesin and hydrocodone

U.S./Canadian Brand Names Atuss® HX [US]; Codiclear® DH [US]; EndaCof [US]; EndaCof-XP [US]; ExeClear [US]; ExeCof-XP [US]; Extendryl® HC [US]; Hycotuss® [US]; Kwelcof® [US]; Maxi-Tuss HCG [US]; Pancof-XP [US]; Phanatuss® HC [US]; Pneumotussin® [US]; Touro® HC [US]; Tusso-DF® [US]; Vitussin [US]; Xpect-HC™ [US]; Ztuss™ ZT [US]

Therapeutic Category Antitussive/Expectorant

Controlled Substance C-III

Use Symptomatic relief of nonproductive coughs associated with upper and lower respiratory tract congestion

Usual Dosage
Children:
6-12 years:
Atuss® Hx: One capsule every 8 hours
Codiclear® DH, ExeClear, Hycotuss®, Kwelcof®, Maxi-Tuss HCG: 2.5-5 mL every 4 hours, after meals and at bedtime
Hydro-Tussin™ HG: 2.5 mL after meals and at bedtime
Pneumotussin®: One tablet or 5 mL every 4-6 hours (maximum: 4 doses/24 hours)
>12 years:
Codiclear® DH, ExeClear, Hycotuss®, Kwelcof®, Maxi-Tuss HCG: 5-10 mL every 4 hours, after meals and at bedtime
Hydro-Tussin™ HG: 5 mL after meals and at bedtime; may increase to 10 mL/dose if needed (maximum: 30 mL/day)
Pneumotussin®: 1-2 tablets or 10 mL every 4-6 hours (maximum: 4 doses/24 hours)
Children ≥12 years and Adults (Atuss® HX): 1-2 capsules every 8 hours
Adults:
Codiclear® DH, Kwelcof®, ExeClear, Hycotuss®: 5-15 mL every 4 hours, after meals and at bedtime (maximum: 30 mL/24 hours)
Hydro-Tussin™ HG: 5 mL after meals and at bedtime; may increase to 15 mL/dose if needed (maximum: 30 mL/day)
Maxi-Tuss HCG: 5-10 mL every 4 hours, after meals and at bedtime
Pneumotussin®: 1-2 tablets or 10 mL every 4-6 hours (maximum: 4 doses/24 hours)

Dosage Forms
Caplet:
Ztuss™ ZT: Hydrocodone 5 mg and guaifenesin 300 mg
Capsule, variable release:
Atuss® HX: Hydrocodone 5 mg [immediate release] and guaifenesin 100 mg [sustained release]
Liquid: Hydrocodone 5 mg and guaifenesin 100 mg per 5 mL
ExeCof-XP, Pancof-XP: Hydrocodone 3 mg and guaifenesin 90 mg per 5 mL
Kwelcof®, Phanatuss® HC, Vitussin: Hydrocodone 5 mg and guaifenesin 100 mg per 5 mL
Tablet:
EndaCof: Hydrocodone 2.5 mg and guaifenesin 300 mg
Touro® HC: Hydrocodone 5 mg and guaifenesin 575 mg
Tablet, sustained release:
Extendryl® HC: Hydrocodone 10 mg and guaifenesin 1000 mg
Xpect-HC™: Hydrocodone 5 mg and guaifenesin 600 mg
Syrup: Hydrocodone 5 mg and guaifenesin 100 mg per 5 mL
Codiclear® DH: Hydrocodone 5 mg and guaifenesin 100 mg per 5 mL
EndaCof-XP, Pneumotussin®: Hydrocodone 2.5 mg and guaifenesin 200 mg per 5 mL
ExeClear: Hydrocodone 3.5 mg and guaifenesin 100 mg per 5 mL
Hycotuss®: Hydrocodone 5 mg and guaifenesin 100 mg per 5 mL
Maxi-Tuss HCG: Hydrocodone 6 mg and guaifenesin 200 mg per 5 mL
Tusso-DF®: Hydrocodone 2.5 mg and guaifenesin 100 mg per 5 mL

hydrocodone and homatropine (hye droe KOE done & hoe MA troe peen)

Sound-Alike/Look-Alike Issues
Hycodan® may be confused with Hycomine®, Vicodin®

Synonyms homatropine and hydrocodone

U.S./Canadian Brand Names Hycodan® [US]; Hydromet® [US]; Tussigon® [US]

Therapeutic Category Antitussive

Controlled Substance C-III

Use Symptomatic relief of cough

Usual Dosage Oral:
Children 6-12 years: ¹/₂ tablet or 2.5 mL every 4-6 hours as needed (maximum: 3 tablets or 15 mL/24 hours)
Children ≥12 years and Adults: 1 tablet or 5 mL every 4-6 hours as needed (maximum: 6 tablets/24 hours or 30 mL/24 hours)
(Continued)

hydrocodone and homatropine *(Continued)*

Dosage Forms
Syrup: Hydrocodone 5 mg and homatropine 1.5 mg per 5 mL
Hycodan®, Hydromet®: Hydrocodone 5 mg and homatropine 1.5 mg per 5 mL
Tablet:
Hycodan®, Tussigon®: Hydrocodone 5 mg and homatropine 1.5 mg

hydrocodone and ibuprofen (hye droe KOE done & eye byoo PROE fen)

Synonyms ibuprofen and hydrocodone
U.S./Canadian Brand Names Reprexain™ [US]; Vicoprofen® [US/Can]
Therapeutic Category Analgesic, Narcotic
Controlled Substance C-III
Use Short-term (generally <10 days) management of moderate to severe acute pain; is not indicated for treatment of such conditions as osteoarthritis or rheumatoid arthritis
Usual Dosage Oral: Adults: 1 tablet every 4-6 hours as needed for pain; maximum: 5 tablets/day
Dosage Forms
Tablet: Hydrocodone 5 mg and ibuprofen 200 mg; hydrocodone 7.5 mg and ibuprofen 200 mg
Reprexain®: Hydrocodone 5 mg and ibuprofen 200 mg; hydrocodone 7.5 mg and ibuprofen 200 mg
Vicoprofen®: Hydrocodone 7.5 mg and ibuprofen 200 mg

hydrocodone and pseudoephedrine (hye droe KOE done & soo doe e FED rin)

Synonyms pseudoephedrine and hydrocodone
U.S./Canadian Brand Names Coughcold HCM [US]; P-V Tussin Tablet [US]; Pancof-HC [US]
Therapeutic Category Cough and Cold Combination
Controlled Substance C-III
Use Symptomatic relief of cough due to colds, nasal congestion, and cough
Usual Dosage Oral: Adults: 5 mL 4 times/day
Dosage Forms
Syrup: Hydrocodone 5 mg and pseudoephedrine 60 mg per 5 mL
Coldcough HCM, Pancof-HC: Hydrocodone 3 mg and pseudoephedrine 15 mg per 5 mL
Tablet:
P-V Tussin: Hydrocodone 5 mg and pseudoephedrine 60 mg

hydrocodone bitartrate, carbinoxamine maleate, and pseudoephedrine hydrochloride *see* hydrocodone, carbinoxamine, and pseudoephedrine *on this page*

hydrocodone bitartrate, phenylephrine hydrochloride, and diphenhydramine hydrochloride *see* hydrocodone, phenylephrine, and diphenhydramine *on next page*

hydrocodone, carbinoxamine, and pseudoephedrine

(hye droe KOE done, kar bi NOKS a meen, & soo doe e FED rin)
Synonyms carbinoxamine, pseudoephedrine, and hydrocodone; hydrocodone bitartrate, carbinoxamine maleate, and pseudoephedrine hydrochloride; pseudoephedrine, hydrocodone, and carbinoxamine
U.S./Canadian Brand Names Histex™ HC [US]; Tri-Vent™ HC [US]
Therapeutic Category Antihistamine/Decongestant/Antitussive
Controlled Substance C-III
Use Symptomatic relief of cough, congestion, and rhinorrhea associated with the common cold, influenza, bronchitis, or sinusitis
Usual Dosage Oral: Relief of cough, congestion, and runny nose:
Children:
2-10 years: Dosing based on hydrocodone content: 0.6 mg/kg/day given in 4 divided doses. Alternately, the following dosing may be used based on age:
2-4 years: 1.25 mL every 4-6 hours; maximum dose: 7.5 mL/24 hours
4-10 years: 2.5 mL every 4-6 hours; maximum dose: 15 mL/24 hours
>10 years: Refer to Adults dosing
Adults: 5-10 mL every 4-6 hours; maximum dose: 30 mL/24 hours
Dosage Forms
Liquid:
Histex™ HC, Tri-Vent™ HC: Hydrocodone 5 mg, carbinoxamine 2 mg, and pseudoephedrine 30 mg per 5 mL

hydrocodone, chlorpheniramine, and pseudoephedrine *see* pseudoephedrine, hydrocodone, and chlorpheniramine *on page 731*

hydrocodone, chlorpheniramine, phenylephrine, acetaminophen, and caffeine

(hye droe KOE done, klor fen IR a meen, fen il EF rin, a seet a MIN oh fen, & KAF een)

Sound-Alike/Look-Alike Issues

Hycomine® may be confused with Byclomine®, Hycamtin®, Hycodan®, Vicodin®

Synonyms acetaminophen, caffeine, hydrocodone, chlorpheniramine, and phenylephrine; caffeine, hydroco-done, chlorpheniramine, phenylephrine, and acetaminophen; chlorpheniramine, hydrocodone, phenylephrine, acetaminophen, and caffeine; phenylephrine, hydrocodone, chlorpheniramine, acetaminophen, and caffeine

U.S./Canadian Brand Names Hycomine® Compound [US]

Therapeutic Category Antitussive

Controlled Substance C-III

Use Symptomatic relief of cough and symptoms of upper respiratory infection

Usual Dosage Oral: Adults: 1 tablet every 4 hours, up to 4 times/day

Dosage Forms

Tablet:

Hycomine® Compound: Hydrocodone 5 mg, chlorpheniramine 2 mg, phenylephrine 10 mg, acetaminophen 250 mg, and caffeine 30 mg

Hydrocodone PA® Syrup *(Discontinued)*

hydrocodone, phenylephrine, and chlorpheniramine *see* phenylephrine, hydrocodone, and chlor-pheniramine *on page 678*

hydrocodone, phenylephrine, and diphenhydramine

(hye droe KOE done, fen il EF rin, & dye fen HYE dra meen)

Sound-Alike/Look-Alike Issues

Endal® may be confused with Depen®, Intal®

Synonyms diphenhydramine, hydrocodone, and phenylephrine; hydrocodone bitartrate, phenylephrine hydro-chloride, and diphenhydramine hydrochloride; hydrocodone tannate, phenylephrine tannate, and diphenhy-dramine tannate; phenylephrine, diphenhydramine, and hydrocodone

U.S./Canadian Brand Names D-Tann HC [US]; Gentuss-HC [US]; Hydro DP [US]; Rindal HPD [US]; TussiNate™ [US]

Therapeutic Category Antihistamine/Decongestant/Antitussive; Antitussive; Decongestant

Controlled Substance C-III

Use Symptomatic relief of cough and congestion associated with the common cold, sinusitis, or acute upper respiratory tract infections

Usual Dosage Oral: Relief of cough, congestion:

D-Tann HC:

Children 6 to <12 years: 2.5-5 mL every 12 hours

Children ≥12 years and Adults: 5-10 mL every 12 hours

Rindal HPD, TussiNate™:

Children 6-12 years: 5 mL every 4 hours (maximum: 20 mL/24 hours)

Children >12 years and Adults: 10 mL every 4 hours (maximum: 40 mL/24 hours)

Dosage Forms

Suspension:

D-Tann HC: Hydrocodone 3.5 mg, phenylephrine 7.5 mg, and diphenhydramine 25 mg per 5 mL

Syrup:

Gestuss-HC: Hydrocodone 3 mg, phenylephrine 5 mg, and diphenhydramine 12.5 mg per 5 mL

Hydro DP, Rindal HPD: Hydrocodone 2 mg, phenylephrine 7.5 mg, and diphenhydramine 12.5 mg per 5 mL

TussiNate™: Hydrocodone 3.5 mg, phenylephrine 5 mg, and diphenhydramine 12.5 mg per 5 mL

hydrocodone, phenylephrine, and guaifenesin

(hye droe KOE done, fen il EF rin, & gwye FEN e sin)

Synonyms guaifenesin, hydrocodone bitartrate, and phenylephrine hydrochloride; phenylephrine, guaifenesin, and hydrocodone

U.S./Canadian Brand Names Crantex HC [US]; De-Chlor G [US]; Donatussin DC [US]; Duratuss® HD [US]; Gentex HC [US]; Giltuss HC® [US]; Guiaplex™ HC [US]; Hydro-GP [US]; HydroFed [US]; Levall 5.0 [US]; Mintuss G [US]; Tussafed® HC [US]; Tussafed® HCG [US]

Therapeutic Category Antitussive/Decongestant/Expectorant

Controlled Substance C-III

Use Temporary relief of cough, congestion, and other symptoms associated with colds or allergies

Usual Dosage Oral: Cough/congestion:

Children:

2-6 years (Crantex HC): 2.5 mL every 4-6 hours (maximum: 10 mL/24 hours)

3-6 years:

Giltuss HC®: 1.25 mL every 6 hours (maximum: 6 doses/24 hours)

(Continued)

hydrocodone, phenylephrine, and guaifenesin *(Continued)*

Tussafed® HC: 2.5 mL every 4-6 hours as needed (maximum: 6 doses/24 hours)
6-12 years:
Crantex HC: 5 mL every 4-6 hours (maximum: 4 doses/24 hours)
Giltuss HC®: 2.5 mL every 6 hours (maximum: 6 doses/24 hours)
Tussafed® HC: 5 mL every 4-6 hours as needed (maximum: 6 doses/24 hours)
Children ≥12 years and Adults:
Crantex HC: 5-10 mL every 4-6 hours (maximum: 40 mL/24 hours)
Giltuss HC®: 5 mL every 6 hours (maximum: 6 doses/24 hours)
Tussafed® HC: 10 mL every 4-6 hours as needed (maximum: 6 doses/24 hours)

Dosage Forms
Elixir:
Duratuss® HD: Hydrocodone 2.5 mg, phenylephrine 10 mg, and guaifenesin 225 mg per 5 mL
Liquid:
Crantex HC: Hydrocodone 5 mg, phenylephrine 7.5 mg, and guaifenesin 100 mg per 5 mL
De-Chlor G, Mintuss G: Hydrocodone 2 mg, phenylephrine 10 mg, and guaifenesin 100 mg per 5 mL
Gentex HC: Hydrocodone 2.5 mg, phenylephrine 7.5 mg, and guaifenesin 100 mg per 5 mL
Giltuss HC®: Hydrocodone 5 mg, phenylephrine 10 mg, and guaifenesin 300 mg per 5 mL
Guiaplex™ HC, Levall 5.0: Hydrocodone 5 mg, phenylephrine 15 mg, and guaifenesin 100 mg per 5 mL
Hydro-GP: Hydrocodone 2.5 mg, phenylephrine 7.5 mg, and guaifenesin 50 mg per 5 mL
Syrup:
Donatussin DC: Hydrocodone 2.5 mg, phenylephrine 6 mg, and guaifenesin 120 mg per 5 mL
HydroFed, Tussafed® HCG: Hydrocodone 2.5 mg, phenylephrine 6 mg, and guaifenesin 150 mg per 5 mL
Tussafed® HC: Hydrocodone 2.5 mg, phenylephrine 7.5 mg, and guaifenesin 50 mg per 5 mL

hydrocodone, pseudoephedrine, and guaifenesin

(hye droe KOE done, soo doe e FED rin & gwye FEN e sin)
Synonyms guaifenesin, hydrocodone, and pseudoephedrine; pseudoephedrine, hydrocodone, and guaifenesin
U.S./Canadian Brand Names Hydro-Tussin™ HD [US]; Hydro-Tussin™ XP [US]; Su-Tuss®-HD [US]; Ztuss™ Tablet [US]
Therapeutic Category Antitussive/Decongestant/Expectorant
Controlled Substance C-III
Use Symptomatic relief of irritating, nonproductive cough associated with upper respiratory conditions and allergies
Usual Dosage Oral: Cough/congestion:
Children:
2-6 years: Hydro-Tussin™ XP: 1.25-2.5 mL 4 times/day as needed
6-12 years:
Hydro-Tussin™ XP: 2.5-5 mL 4 times/day as needed
Tussend®, Hydro-Tussin™ HD: 5 mL every 4-6 hours as needed
Ztuss™: One-half to 1 tablet every 4-6 hours (maximum: 6 tablets/24 hours)
Children ≥12 years and Adults:
Hydro-Tussin™ XP: 5-10 mL 4 times/day as needed
Tussend®, Hydro-Tussin™ HD: 10 mL every 4-6 hours as needed
Ztuss™: 1-1¹/₂ tablets every 4-6 hours (maximum: 8 tablets/24 hours)
Dosage Forms
Elixir:
Su-Tuss®-HD: Hydrocodone 2.5 mg, pseudoephedrine 30 mg, and guaifenesin 100 mg per 5 mL
Liquid:
Entex® HC: Hydrocodone 3.75 mg, pseudoephedrine 22.5 mg, and guaifenesin 50 mg per 5 mL
Hydro-Tussin™ HD: Hydrocodone 2.5 mg, pseudoephedrine 30 mg, and guaifenesin 100 mg per 5 mL
Hydro-Tussin® XP: Hydrocodone 3 mg, pseudoephedrine 15 mg, and guaifenesin 100 mg per 5 mL
Tablet:
Ztuss™: Hydrocodone 5 mg, pseudoephedrine 30 mg, and guaifenesin 300 mg

hydrocodone tannate and chlorpheniramine tannate *see* hydrocodone and chlorpheniramine *on page 428*

hydrocodone tannate, phenylephrine tannate, and diphenhydramine tannate *see* hydrocodone, phenylephrine, and diphenhydramine *on previous page*

hydrocortisone acetate *see* hydrocortisone (rectal) *on next page*

hydrocortisone, acetic acid, and propylene glycol diacetate *see* acetic acid, propylene glycol diacetate, and hydrocortisone *on page 14*

hydrocortisone and benzoyl peroxide *see* benzoyl peroxide and hydrocortisone *on page 105*

hydrocortisone and ciprofloxacin *see* ciprofloxacin and hydrocortisone *on page 193*

hydrocortisone and iodoquinol *see* iodoquinol and hydrocortisone *on page 467*

hydrocortisone and lidocaine *see* lidocaine and hydrocortisone *on page 507*

hydrocortisone and pramoxine *see* pramoxine and hydrocortisone *on page 707*

hydrocortisone and urea *see* urea and hydrocortisone *on page 878*

hydrocortisone, bacitracin, neomycin, and polymyxin B *see* bacitracin, neomycin, polymyxin B, and hydrocortisone *on page 92*

hydrocortisone butyrate *see* hydrocortisone (topical) *on next page*

hydrocortisone, neomycin, and polymyxin B *see* neomycin, polymyxin B, and hydrocortisone *on page 597*

hydrocortisone, neomycin, colistin, and thonzonium *see* neomycin, colistin, hydrocortisone, and thonzonium *on page 597*

hydrocortisone probutate *see* hydrocortisone (topical) *on next page*

hydrocortisone (rectal) (hye droe KOR ti sone REK tal)

Sound-Alike/Look-Alike Issues
hydrocortisone may be confused with hydrocodone, hydroxychloroquine, hydrochlorothiazide
Anusol-HC® may be confused with Anusol®
Anusol® may be confused with Anusol-HC®, Aplisol®, Aquasol®
Proctocort® may be confused with ProctoCream®
ProctoCream® may be confused with Proctocort®

Synonyms hydrocortisone acetate

U.S./Canadian Brand Names Anucort-HC® [US]; Anusol-HC® [US]; Anusol® HC-1 [US-OTC]; Colocort® [US]; Cortenema® [Can]; Cortifoam® [US/Can]; Encort™ [US]; Hemril®-30 [US]; Nupercainal® Hydrocortisone Cream [US-OTC]; Preparation H® Hydrocortisone [US-OTC]; Procto-Kit™ [US]; Procto-Pak™ [US]; Proctocort® [US]; ProctoCream® HC [US]; Proctosert [US]; Proctosol-HC® [US]; Proctozone-HC™ [US]; Tucks® Anti-Itch [US-OTC]

Therapeutic Category Adrenal Corticosteroid

Use Adjunctive treatment of ulcerative colitis; rectal itching; hemorrhoids

Usual Dosage Rectal: Adults: Ulcerative colitis: 10-100 mg 1-2 times/day for 2-3 weeks

Dosage Forms
Aerosol, rectal:
Cortifoam®: 10% (15 g)
Cream, rectal: 1% (30 g)
Cortizone®-10 [OTC]: 1% (30 g)
Nupercainal® Hydrocortisone Cream [OTC]: 1% (27 g, 30 g)
Preparation H® Hydrocortisone [OTC]: 1% (27 g)
Suppository, rectal: 25 mg (12s, 24s, 100s)
Anucort-HC®, Tucks® Anti-Itch [OTC]: 25 mg (12s, 24s, 100s)
Anusol-HC®, Proctosol-HC®: 25 mg (12s, 24s)
Encort™, Proctocort®: 30 mg (12s)
Hemril®-30, Proctosert: 30 mg (12s, 24s)
Suspension, rectal: 100 mg/60 mL (7s)
Colocort®: 100 mg/60 mL (1s, 7s)

hydrocortisone sodium succinate *see* hydrocortisone (systemic) *on this page*

hydrocortisone (systemic) (hye droe KOR ti sone sis TEM ik)

Sound-Alike/Look-Alike Issues
hydrocortisone may be confused with hydrocodone, hydroxychloroquine, hydrochlorothiazide
Cortef® may be confused with Lortab®
HCT (occasional abbreviation for hydrocortisone) is an error-prone abbreviation (mistaken as hydrochlorothiazide)

Synonyms compound F; cortisol; hydrocortisone sodium succinate

U.S./Canadian Brand Names Cortef® [US/Can]; Solu-Cortef® [US/Can]

Therapeutic Category Adrenal Corticosteroid

Use Management of adrenocortical insufficiency

Usual Dosage Dose should be based on severity of disease and patient response
Acute adrenal insufficiency: I.M., I.V.:
Infants and young Children: Succinate: 1-2 mg/kg/dose bolus, then 25-150 mg/day in divided doses every 6-8 hours
Older Children: Succinate: 1-2 mg/kg bolus then 150-250 mg/day in divided doses every 6-8 hours
(Continued)

hydrocortisone (systemic) *(Continued)*

Adults: Succinate: 100 mg I.V. bolus, then 300 mg/day in divided doses every 8 hours or as a continuous infusion for 48 hours; once patient is stable change to oral, 50 mg every 8 hours for 6 doses, then taper to 30-50 mg/day in divided doses

Chronic adrenal corticoid insufficiency: Adults: Oral: 20-30 mg/day

Antiinflammatory or immunosuppressive:

Infants and Children:
Oral: 2.5-10 mg/kg/day **or** 75-300 mg/m^2/day every 6-8 hours
I.M., I.V.: Succinate: 1-5 mg/kg/day **or** 30-150 mg/m^2/day divided every 12-24 hours

Adolescents and Adults: Oral, I.M., I.V.: Succinate: 15-240 mg every 12 hours

Congenital adrenal hyperplasia: Oral: Initial: 10-20 mg/m^2/day in 3 divided doses; a variety of dosing schedules have been used. **Note:** Inconsistencies have occurred with liquid formulations; tablets may provide more reliable levels. Doses must be individualized by monitoring growth, bone age, and hormonal levels. Mineralocorticoid and sodium supplementation may be required based upon electrolyte regulation and plasma renin activity.

Physiologic replacement: Children:
Oral: 0.5-0.75 mg/kg/day **or** 20-25 mg/m^2/day every 8 hours
I.M.: Succinate: 0.25-0.35 mg/kg/day **or** 12-15 mg/m^2/day once daily

Shock: I.M., I.V.: Succinate:
Children: Initial: 50 mg/kg, then repeated in 4 hours and/or every 24 hours as needed
Adolescents and Adults: 500 mg to 2 g every 2-6 hours

Status asthmaticus: Children and Adults: I.V.: Succinate: 1-2 mg/kg/dose every 6 hours for 24 hours, then maintenance of 0.5-1 mg/kg every 6 hours

Adults:

Rheumatic diseases:

Intralesional, intra-articular, soft tissue injection: Acetate:
Large joints: 25 mg (up to 37.5 mg)
Small joints: 10-25 mg
Tendon sheaths: 5-12.5 mg
Soft tissue infiltration: 25-50 mg (up to 75 mg)
Bursae: 25-37.5 mg
Ganglia: 12.5-25 mg

Stress dosing (surgery) in patients known to be adrenally-suppressed or on chronic systemic steroids: I.V.:
Minor stress (ie, inguinal herniorrhaphy): 25 mg/day for 1 day
Moderate stress (ie, joint replacement, cholecystectomy): 50-75 mg/day (25 mg every 8-12 hours) for 1-2 days
Major stress (pancreatoduodenectomy, esophagogastrectomy, cardiac surgery): 100-150 mg/day (50 mg every 8-12 hours) for 2-3 days

Dosage Forms

Injection, powder for reconstitution:
Solu-Cortef®: 100 mg, 250 mg, 500 mg, 1 g
Tablet: 20 mg
Cortef®: 5 mg, 10 mg, 20 mg

hydrocortisone (topical) (hye droe KOR ti sone TOP i kal)

Sound-Alike/Look-Alike Issues

hydrocortisone may be confused with hydrocodone, hydroxychloroquine, hydrochlorothiazide

Cortizone® may be confused with cortisone

HCT (occasional abbreviation for hydrocortisone) is an error-prone abbreviation (mistaken as hydrochlorothiazide)

Hytone® may be confused with Vytone®

Synonyms hydrocortisone butyrate; hydrocortisone probutate; hydrocortisone valerate

U.S./Canadian Brand Names Aquacort® [Can]; Aquanil™ HC [US-OTC]; Beta-HC® [US]; Caldecort® [US-OTC]; Cetacort® [US]; Cortaid® Intensive Therapy [US-OTC]; Cortaid® Maximum Strength [US-OTC]; Cortaid® Sensitive Skin [US-OTC]; Cortamed® [Can]; Corticool® [US-OTC]; Cortizone®-10 Maximum Strength [US-OTC]; Cortizone®-10 Plus Maximum Strength [US-OTC]; Cortizone®-10 Quick Shot [US-OTC]; Dermarest Dricort® [US-OTC]; Dermtex® HC [US-OTC]; EarSol® HC [US]; Emo-Cort® [Can]; Hycort™ [Can]; Hyderm [Can]; HydroVal® [Can]; HydroZone Plus [US-OTC]; Hytone® [US]; IvySoothe® [US-OTC]; Locoid Lipocream® [US]; Locoid® [US/Can]; Nutracort® [US]; Pandel® [US]; Post Peel Healing Balm [US-OTC]; Prevex® HC [Can]; Sarna® HC [Can]; Sarnol®-HC [US-OTC]; Texacort® [US]; Westcort® [US/Can]

Therapeutic Category Corticosteroid, Topical

Use Relief of inflammation of corticosteroid-responsive dermatoses (low and medium potency topical corticosteroid)

Usual Dosage Topical: Children >2 years and Adults: Dermatosis: Apply to affected area 2-4 times/day (Buteprate: Apply once or twice daily). Therapy should be discontinued when control is achieved; if no improvement is seen, reassessment of diagnosis may be necessary.

Dosage Forms
  Cream, topical: 0.2% (15 g, 45 g, 60 g); 0.5% (9 g, 30 g, 60 g); 1% (1.5 g, 30 g, 114 g, 454 g); 2.5% (20 g, 30 g, 454 g)
    Anusol-HC®: 2.5% (30 g)
    Caldecort® [OTC], HydroZone Plus [OTC], IvySoothe® [OTC], Proctocort®, Procto-Pak™, Procto-Kit™: 1% (30 g)
    Cortaid® Intensive Therapy [OTC]: 1% (60 g)
    Cortaid® Maximum Strength [OTC]: 1% (15 g, 30 g, 40 g, 60 g)
    Cortaid® Sensitive Skin [OTC]: 0.5% (15 g)
    Cortizone®-10 Maximum Strength [OTC]: 1% (15 g, 30 g, 60 g)
    Cortizone®-10 Plus Maximum Strength [OTC]: 1% (30 g, 60 g)
    Dermarest® Dricort® [OTC]: 1% (15 g, 30 g)
    Hytone®: 2.5% (30 g, 60 g)
    Locoid®, Locoid Lipocream®: 0.1% (15 g, 45 g)
    Pandel®: 0.1% (15 g, 45 g, 80 g)
    Post Peel Healing Balm [OTC]: 1% (23 g)
    ProctoCream® HC, Proctosol-HC®, Proctozone-HC™: 2.5% (30 g)
    Westcort®: 0.2% (15 g, 45 g, 60 g)
  Gel, topical:
    Corticool®: 1% (45 g)
  Lotion, topical: 1% (120 mL); 2.5% (60 mL)
    Aquanil™ HC [OTC], HydroZone Plus: 1% (120 mL)
    Beta-HC®, Sarnol®-HC [OTC]: 1% (60 mL)
    Hytone®: 2.5% (60 mL)
    Nutracort®: 1% (60 mL, 120 mL); 2.5% (60 mL, 120 mL)
  Ointment, topical: 0.2% (15 g, 45 g, 60 g); 0.5% (30 g); 1% (30 g, 454 g); 2.5% (20 g, 30 g, 454 g)
    Anusol® HC-1 [OTC]: 1% (21 g)
    Cortaid® Maximum Strength [OTC]: 1% (15 g, 30 g)
    Cortizone®-10 Maximum Strength [OTC]: 1% (30 g, 60 g)
    Locoid®: 0.1% (15 g, 45 g)
    Westcort®: 0.2% (15 g, 45 g, 60 g)
  Solution, otic:
    EarSol® HC: 1% (30 mL)
  Solution, topical: 0.1% (20 mL, 60 mL); 2.5% (30 mL)
    Texacort®: 2.5% (30 mL)
    Locoid®: 0.1% (20 mL, 60 mL)
  Solution, topical spray:
    Cortaid® Intensive Therapy [OTC]: 1% (60 mL)
    Cortizone®-10 Quick Shot [OTC]: 1% (44 mL)
    Dermtex® HC [OTC]: 1% (52 mL)

hydrocortisone valerate *see* hydrocortisone (topical) *on previous page*

HydroDIURIL® *(Discontinued)* *see* hydrochlorothiazide *on page 426*

Hydro DP [US] *see* hydrocodone, phenylephrine, and diphenhydramine *on page 431*

HydroFed [US] *see* hydrocodone, phenylephrine, and guaifenesin *on page 431*

Hydrogesic® *(Discontinued)* *see* hydrocodone and acetaminophen *on page 427*

Hydro-GP [US] *see* hydrocodone, phenylephrine, and guaifenesin *on page 431*

Hydromet® [US] *see* hydrocodone and homatropine *on page 429*

Hydromorph Contin® [Can] *see* hydromorphone *on this page*

Hydromorph-IR® [Can] *see* hydromorphone *on this page*

hydromorphone (hye droe MOR fone)
Sound-Alike/Look-Alike Issues
hydromorphone may be confused with morphine; significant overdoses have occurred when hydromorphone products have been inadvertently administered instead of morphine sulfate. Commercially available prefilled syringes of both products looks similar and are often stored in close proximity to each other. **Note:** Hydromorphone 1 mg oral is approximately equal to morphine 4 mg oral; hydromorphone 1 mg I.V. is approximately equal to morphine 5 mg I.V.

Dilaudid® may be confused with Demerol®, Dilantin®

(Continued)

hydromorphone *(Continued)*

Dilaudid®, Dilaudid-HP®: Extreme caution should be taken to avoid confusing the highly-concentrated (Dilaudid-HP®) injection with the less-concentrated (Dilaudid®) injectable product.

Synonyms dihydromorphinone; hydromorphone hydrochloride

U.S./Canadian Brand Names Dilaudid-HP-Plus® [Can]; Dilaudid-HP® [US/Can]; Dilaudid-XP® [Can]; Dilaudid® Sterile Powder [Can]; Dilaudid® [US/Can]; Hydromorph Contin® [Can]; Hydromorph-IR® [Can]; Hydromorphone HP [Can]; Hydromorphone HP® 10 [Can]; Hydromorphone HP® 20 [Can]; Hydromorphone HP® 50 [Can]; Hydromorphone HP® Forte [Can]; Hydromorphone Hydrochloride Injection, USP [Can]; PMS-Hydromorphone [Can]

Therapeutic Category Analgesic, Narcotic

Controlled Substance C-II

Use Management of moderate-to-severe pain

Usual Dosage

Acute pain (moderate to severe): **Note:** These are guidelines and do not represent the maximum doses that may be required in all patients. Doses should be titrated to pain relief/prevention.

Children ≥6 months and <50 kg:

Oral: 0.03-0.08 mg/kg/dose every 3-4 hours as needed

I.V.: 0.015 mg/kg/dose every 3-6 hours as needed

Children >50 kg and Adults:

Oral: Initial: Opiate-naive: 2-4 mg every 3-6 hours as needed; elderly/debilitated patients may require lower doses; patients with prior opiate exposure may require higher initial doses; usual dosage range: 2-8 mg every 3-4 hours as needed

I.V.: Initial: Opiate-naive: 0.2-0.6 mg every 2-3 hours as needed; patients with prior opiate exposure may tolerate higher initial doses

Note: More frequent dosing may be needed.

Mechanically-ventilated patients (based on 70 kg patient): 0.7-2 mg every 1-2 hours as needed; infusion (based on 70 kg patient): 0.5-1 mg/hour

Patient-controlled analgesia (PCA): (Opiate-naive: Consider lower end of dosing range)

Usual concentration: 0.2 mg/mL

Demand dose: Usual: 0.1-0.2 mg; range: 0.05-0.5 mg

Lockout interval: 5-15 minutes

4-hour limit: 4-6 mg

Epidural:

Bolus dose: 1-1.5 mg

Infusion concentration: 0.05-0.075 mg/mL

Infusion rate: 0.04-0.4 mg/hour

Demand dose: 0.15 mg

Lockout interval: 30 minutes

I.M., SubQ: **Note:** I.M. use may result in variable absorption and a lag time to peak effect.

Initial: Opiate-naive: 0.8-1 mg every 4-6 hours as needed; patients with prior opiate exposure may require higher initial doses; usual dosage range: 1-2 mg every 3-6 hours as needed

Rectal: 3 mg every 4-8 hours as needed

Chronic pain: Adults: Oral: **Note:** Patients taking opioids chronically may become tolerant and require doses higher than the usual dosage range to maintain the desired effect. Tolerance can be managed by appropriate dose titration. There is no optimal or maximal dose for hydromorphone in chronic pain. The appropriate dose is one that relieves pain throughout its dosing interval without causing unmanageable side effects.

Controlled release formulation (Hydromorph Contin®, not available in U.S.): 3-30 mg every 12 hours. **Note:** A patient's hydromorphone requirement should be established using prompt release formulations; conversion to long acting products may be considered when chronic, continuous treatment is required. Higher dosages should be reserved for use only in opioid-tolerant patients.

Dosage Forms [CAN] = Canadian brand name

Capsule, controlled release:

Hydromorph Contin® [CAN]: 3 mg, 6 mg, 12 mg, 18 mg, 24 mg, 30 mg [not available in U.S.]

Injection, powder for reconstitution:

Dilaudid-HP®: 250 mg

Injection, solution: 1 mg/mL (1 mL); 2 mg/mL (1 mL, 20 mL); 4 mg/mL (1 mL); 10 mg/mL (1 mL, 5 mL, 10 mL)

Dilaudid®: 1 mg/mL (1 mL); 2 mg/mL (1 mL, 20 mL); 4 mg/mL (1 mL)

Dilaudid-HP®: 10 mg/mL (1 mL, 5 mL, 50 mL)

Liquid, oral:

Dilaudid®: 1 mg/mL

Suppository, rectal: 3 mg

Dilaudid®: 3 mg (6s)

Tablet: 2 mg, 4 mg, 8 mg

Dilaudid®: 2 mg, 4 mg, 8 mg

Hydromorphone HP [Can] *see* hydromorphone *on page 435*

Hydromorphone HP® 10 [Can] *see* hydromorphone *on page 435*

Hydromorphone HP® 20 [Can] *see* hydromorphone *on page 435*

Hydromorphone HP® 50 [Can] *see* hydromorphone *on page 435*

Hydromorphone HP® Forte [Can] *see* hydromorphone *on page 435*

hydromorphone hydrochloride *see* hydromorphone *on page 435*

Hydromorphone Hydrochloride Injection, USP [Can] *see* hydromorphone *on page 435*

Hydromox® *(Discontinued)*

Hydron CP [US] *see* phenylephrine, hydrocodone, and chlorpheniramine *on page 678*

Hydron PSC [US] *see* pseudoephedrine, hydrocodone, and chlorpheniramine *on page 731*

Hydro-Par® *(Discontinued)* *see* hydrochlorothiazide *on page 426*

Hydro-PC II [US] *see* phenylephrine, hydrocodone, and chlorpheniramine *on page 678*

Hydro PC II Plus [US] *see* phenylephrine, hydrocodone, and chlorpheniramine *on page 678*

hydroquinol *see* hydroquinone *on this page*

hydroquinone (HYE droe kwin one)
   Sound-Alike/Look-Alike Issues
      Eldopaque® may be confused with Eldoquin®
      Eldoquin® may be confused with Eldopaque®
      Eldopaque Forte® may be confused with Eldoquin Forte®
      Eldoquin Forte® may be confused with Eldopaque Forte®
   Synonyms hydroquinol; quinol
   U.S./Canadian Brand Names Alphaquin HP® [US]; Claripel™ [US]; Dermarest® Skin Correction Cream Plus [US-OTC]; Eldopaque Forte® [US]; Eldopaque® [US-OTC/Can]; Eldoquin Forte® [US]; Eldoquin® [US-OTC/Can]; EpiQuin™ Micro [US]; Esoterica® Regular [US-OTC]; Glyquin-XM™ [US/Can]; Glyquin® [US]; Lustra-AF™ [US]; Lustra® [US/Can]; Melanex® [US]; Melpaque HP® [US]; Melquin HP® [US]; Melquin-3® [US]; NeoStrata® AHA [US-OTC]; NeoStrata® HQ [Can]; Nuquin HP® [US]; Palmer's® Skin Success Eventone® Fade Cream [US-OTC]; Solaquin Forte® [US/Can]; Solaquin® [US-OTC/Can]; Ultraquin™ [Can]
   Therapeutic Category Topical Skin Product
   Use Gradual bleaching of hyperpigmented skin conditions
   Usual Dosage Topical: Children >12 years and Adults: Apply thin layer and rub in twice daily
   Dosage Forms
      Cream, topical: 4% (30 g)
       Alphaquin HP®: 4% (30 g, 60 g)
       Eldoquin® [OTC]: 2% (15 g, 30 g)
       Eldoquin Forte®, EpiQuin™ Micro, Lustra®: 4% (30 g)
       Esoterica® Regular [OTC]: 2% (85 g)
       Melquin HP®: 4% (15 g, 30 g)
      Cream, topical [with sunscreen]: 4% (30 g)
       Claripel™: 4% (30 g, 45 g)
       Dermarest® Skin Correcting Cream Plus [OTC]: 2% (85 g)
       Eldopaque® [OTC]: 2% (15 g, 30 g)
       Eldopaque Forte®, Glyquin®, Glyquin-XM™, Solaquin Forte®: 4% (30 g)
       Lustra-AF™: 4% (30 g, 60 g)
       Melpaque HP®: 4% (15 g, 30 g)
       Nuquin HP®: 4% (15 g, 30 g, 60 g)
       Palmer's® Skin Success Eventone® Fade Cream [OTC]: 2% (81 g, 132 g)
       Solaquin® [OTC]: 2% (30 g)
      Gel, topical:
       NeoStrata® AHA [OTC]: 2% (45 g)
      Gel, topical [with sunscreen]: 4% (30 g)
       Nuquin HP: 4% (15 g, 30 g)
       Solaquin Forte®: 4% (30 g)
      Solution, topical: 3% (30 mL)
       Melanex®, Melquin-3®: 3% (30 mL)

hydroquinone, fluocinolone acetonide, and tretinoin *see* fluocinolone, hydroquinone, and tretinoin *on page 360*

Hydrotropine® *(Discontinued)* *see* hydrocodone and homatropine *on page 429*

Hydro-Tussin™-CBX [US] *see* carbinoxamine and pseudoephedrine *on page 151*

Hydro-Tussin™ DHC [US] *see* pseudoephedrine, dihydrocodeine, and chlorpheniramine *on page 730*

Hydro-Tussin™ DM [US] *see* guaifenesin and dextromethorphan *on page 402*

Hydro-Tussin™ EXP [US] *see* dihydrocodeine, pseudoephedrine, and guaifenesin *on page 260*

Hydro-Tussin™ HC [US] *see* pseudoephedrine, hydrocodone, and chlorpheniramine *on page 731*

Hydro-Tussin™ HD [US] *see* hydrocodone, pseudoephedrine, and guaifenesin *on page 432*

Hydro-Tussin™ XP [US] *see* hydrocodone, pseudoephedrine, and guaifenesin *on page 432*

HydroVal® [Can] *see* hydrocortisone (topical) *on page 434*

hydroxyamphetamine and tropicamide (hye droks ee am FET a meen & troe PIK a mide)

Synonyms hydroxyamphetamine hydrobromide and tropicamide; tropicamide and hydroxyamphetamine

U.S./Canadian Brand Names Paremyd® [US]

Therapeutic Category Adrenergic Agonist Agent, Ophthalmic

Use Short-term pupil dilation for diagnostic procedures and exams

Usual Dosage Ophthalmic: Adults: Instill 1-2 drops into conjunctival sac(s)

Dosage Forms
Solution, ophthalmic:
Paremyd®: Hydroxyamphetamine 1% and tropicamide 0.25% (15 mL)

hydroxyamphetamine hydrobromide and tropicamide *see* hydroxyamphetamine and tropicamide *on this page*

4-hydroxybutyrate *see* sodium oxybate *on page 795*

hydroxycarbamide *see* hydroxyurea *on next page*

hydroxychloroquine (hye droks ee KLOR oh kwin)

Sound-Alike/Look-Alike Issues
hydroxychloroquine may be confused with hydrocortisone
Plaquenil® may be confused with Platinol®

Synonyms hydroxychloroquine sulfate

U.S./Canadian Brand Names Apo-Hydroxyquine® [Can]; Gen-Hydroxychloroquine [Can]; Plaquenil® [US/Can]

Therapeutic Category Aminoquinoline (Antimalarial)

Use Suppression and treatment of acute attacks of malaria; treatment of systemic lupus erythematosus and rheumatoid arthritis

Usual Dosage Note: Hydroxychloroquine sulfate 200 mg is equivalent to 155 mg hydroxychloroquine base and 250 mg chloroquine phosphate. Oral:
Children:
Chemoprophylaxis of malaria: 5 mg/kg (base) once weekly; should not exceed the recommended adult dose; begin 2 weeks before exposure; continue for 4-6 weeks after leaving endemic area; if suppressive therapy is not begun prior to the exposure, double the initial dose and give in 2 doses, 6 hours apart
Acute attack: 10 mg/kg (base) initial dose; followed by 5 mg/kg at 6, 24, and 48 hours
JRA or SLE: 3-5 mg/kg/day divided 1-2 times/day; avoid exceeding 7 mg/kg/day
Adults:
Chemoprophylaxis of malaria: 310 mg base weekly on same day each week; begin 2 weeks before exposure; continue for 4-6 weeks after leaving endemic area; if suppressive therapy is not begun prior to the exposure, double the initial dose and give in 2 doses, 6 hours apart
Acute attack: 620 mg first dose day 1; 310 mg in 6 hours day 1; 310 mg in 1 dose day 2; and 310 mg in 1 dose on day 3
Rheumatoid arthritis: 310-465 mg/day to start taken with food or milk; increase dose until optimum response level is reached; usually after 4-12 weeks dose should be reduced by $\frac{1}{2}$ and a maintenance dose of 155-310 mg/day given
Lupus erythematosus: 310 mg every day or twice daily for several weeks depending on response; 155-310 mg/day for prolonged maintenance therapy

Dosage Forms
Tablet: 200 mg
Plaquenil®: 200 mg

hydroxychloroquine sulfate *see* hydroxychloroquine *on this page*

hydroxydaunomycin hydrochloride *see* doxorubicin *on page 280*

1α-hydroxyergocalciferol *see* doxercalciferol *on page 280*

hydroxyethylcellulose *see* artificial tears *on page 75*

hydroxyethyl starch *see* hetastarch *on page 420*

hydroxyldaunorubicin hydrochloride *see* doxorubicin *on page 280*

hydroxypropyl cellulose (hye droks ee PROE pil SEL yoo lose)

U.S./Canadian Brand Names Lacrisert® [US/Can]

Therapeutic Category Ophthalmic Agent, Miscellaneous

Use Dry eyes (moderate to severe)

Usual Dosage Ophthalmic: Adults: Apply once daily into the inferior cul-de-sac beneath the base of tarsus, not in apposition to the cornea nor beneath the eyelid at the level of the tarsal plate

Dosage Forms

Insert, ophthalmic [preservative free]:

Lacrisert®: 5 mg

hydroxypropyl methylcellulose (hye droks ee PROE pil meth il SEL yoo lose)

Sound-Alike/Look-Alike Issues

Isopto® Tears may be confused with Isoptin®

Synonyms gonioscopic ophthalmic solution; hypromellose

U.S./Canadian Brand Names Cellugel® [US]; GenTeal® Mild [US-OTC]; GenTeal® [US-OTC/Can]; Gonak™ [US-OTC]; Goniosoft™ [US]; Isopto® Tears [US-OTC/Can]; Tearisol® [US-OTC]; Tears Again® MC [US-OTC]

Therapeutic Category Ophthalmic Agent, Miscellaneous

Use Relief of burning and minor irritation due to dry eyes; diagnostic agent in gonioscopic examination

Usual Dosage Ophthalmic: Adults: Dry eyes: Instill 1-2 drops in affected eye(s) as needed

Dosage Forms

Gel, ophthalmic:

GenTeal® [OTC]: 0.3% (10 mL)

Solution, ophthalmic: 0.4% (15 mL)

GenTeal® [OTC]: 0.3% (15 mL, 25 mL)

GenTeal® Mild [OTC]: 0.2% (15 mL, 25 mL)

Gonak™ [OTC], Goniosoft™: 2.5% (15 mL)

Isopto® Tears [OTC], Tearisol® [OTC]: 0.5% (15 mL)

Tears Again® MC [OTC]: 0.3% (15 mL)

Solution, ophthalmic [for injection]:

Cellugel®: 2% (1 mL)

9-hydroxy-risperidone *see* paliperidone *on page 646*

hydroxyurea (hye droks ee yoor EE a)

Sound-Alike/Look-Alike Issues

hydroxyurea may be confused with hydrOXYzine

Synonyms hydroxycarbamide

U.S./Canadian Brand Names Apo-Hydroxyurea® [Can]; Droxia® [US]; Gen-Hydroxyurea [Can]; Hydrea® [US/Can]; Mylocel™ [US]

Therapeutic Category Antineoplastic Agent

Use Treatment of melanoma, refractory chronic myelocytic leukemia (CML), relapsed and refractory metastatic ovarian cancer; radiosensitizing agent in the treatment of squamous cell head and neck cancer (excluding lip cancer); adjunct in the management of sickle cell patients who have had at least three painful crises in the previous 12 months (to reduce frequency of these crises and the need for blood transfusions)

Usual Dosage Oral (refer to individual protocols): All doses should be based on ideal or actual body weight, whichever is less:

Adults: Dose should always be titrated to patient response and WBC counts; usual oral doses range from 10-30 mg/kg/day or 500-3000 mg/day; if WBC count falls to <2500 cells/mm^3, or the platelet count to <100,000/mm^3, therapy should be stopped for at least 3 days and resumed when values rise toward normal

Solid tumors:

Intermittent therapy: 80 mg/kg as a single dose every third day

Continuous therapy: 20-30 mg/kg/day given as a single dose/day

Concomitant therapy with irradiation: 80 mg/kg as a single dose every third day starting at least 7 days before initiation of irradiation

Resistant chronic myelocytic leukemia: Continuous therapy: 20-30 mg/kg once daily

Sickle cell anemia (moderate/severe disease): Initial: 15 mg/kg/day, increased by 5 mg/kg every 12 weeks if blood counts are in an acceptable range until the maximum tolerated dose of 35 mg/kg/day is achieved or the dose that does not produce toxic effects

Acceptable range:

Neutrophils ≥2500 cells/mm^3

(Continued)

hydroxyurea *(Continued)*

Platelets ≥95,000/mm^3
Hemoglobin >5.3 g/dL, and
Reticulocytes ≥95,000/mm^3 if the hemoglobin concentration is <9 g/dL
Toxic range:
Neutrophils <2000 cells/mm^3
Platelets <80,000/mm^3
Hemoglobin <4.5 g/dL
Reticulocytes <80,000/mm^3 if the hemoglobin concentration is <9 g/dL
Monitor for toxicity every 2 weeks; if toxicity occurs, stop treatment until the bone marrow recovers; restart at 2.5 mg/kg/day less than the dose at which toxicity occurs; if no toxicity occurs over the next 12 weeks, then the subsequent dose should be increased by 2.5 mg/kg/day; reduced dosage of hydroxyurea alternating with erythropoietin may decrease myelotoxicity and increase levels of fetal hemoglobin in patients who have not been helped by hydroxyurea alone

Dosage Forms
Capsule: 500 mg
Droxia®: 200 mg, 300 mg, 400 mg
Hydrea®: 500 mg
Tablet:
Mylocel™: 1000 mg

hydroxyzine (hye DROKS i zeen)

Sound-Alike/Look-Alike Issues
hydrOXYzine may be confused with hydrALAZINE, hydroxyurea
Atarax® may be confused with amoxicillin, Ativan®
Vistaril® may be confused with Restoril®, Versed, Zestril®
Synonyms hydroxyzine hydrochloride; hydroxyzine pamoate
Tall-Man hydroOXYzine
U.S./Canadian Brand Names Apo-Hydroxyzine® [Can]; Atarax® [Can]; Hydroxyzine Hydrochloride Injection, USP [Can]; Novo-Hydroxyzin [Can]; PMS-Hydroxyzine [Can]; Vistaril® [US/Can]
Therapeutic Category Antiemetic; Antihistamine
Use Treatment of anxiety; preoperative sedative; antipruritic
Usual Dosage
Children:
Preoperative sedation:
Oral: 0.6 mg/kg/dose
I.M.: 0.5-1 mg/kg/dose
Pruritus, anxiety: Oral:
<6 years: 50 mg daily in divided doses
≥6 years: 50-100 mg daily in divided doses
Adults:
Anxiety: Oral, I.M.: 50-100 mg 4 times/day
Preoperative sedation:
Oral: 50-100 mg
I.M.: 25-100 mg
Pruritus: Oral, I.M.: 25 mg 3-4 times/day
Dosage Forms
Capsule: 25 mg, 50 mg, 100 mg
Vistaril®: 25 mg, 50 mg
Injection, solution: 25 mg/mL (1 mL); 50 mg/mL (1 mL, 2 mL, 10 mL)
Syrup: 10 mg/5 mL
Tablet: 10 mg, 25 mg, 50 mg

hydroxyzine hydrochloride *see* hydroxyzine *on this page*

Hydroxyzine Hydrochloride Injection, USP [Can] *see* hydroxyzine *on this page*

hydroxyzine pamoate *see* hydroxyzine *on this page*

HydroZone Plus [US-OTC] *see* hydrocortisone (topical) *on page 434*

Hyflex-DS® [US] *see* acetaminophen and phenyltoloxamine *on page 8*

Hygroton® *(Discontinued)* *see* chlorthalidone *on page 185*

Hylaform® [US] *see* hyaluronate and derivatives *on page 423*

Hylaform® Plus [US] *see* hyaluronate and derivatives *on page 423*

hylan polymers *see* hyaluronate and derivatives *on page 423*

Hylenex™ [US] *see* hyaluronidase *on page 424*

Hylutin Injection *(Discontinued)*

hyoscine butylbromide *see* scopolamine derivatives *on page 778*

hyoscine hydrobromide *see* scopolamine derivatives *on page 778*

hyoscyamine (hye oh SYE a meen)

Sound-Alike/Look-Alike Issues
Anaspaz® may be confused with Anaprox®, Antispas®
Levbid® may be confused with Lithobid®, Lopid®, Lorabid®
Levsinex® may be confused with Lanoxin®

Synonyms hyoscyamine sulfate; *l*-hyoscyamine sulfate

U.S./Canadian Brand Names Anaspaz® [US]; Cystospaz® [US/Can]; Hyosine [US]; Levbid® [US]; Levsin/SL® [US]; Levsinex® [US]; Levsin® [US/Can]; NuLev™ [US]; Symax SL [US]; Symax SR [US]

Therapeutic Category Anticholinergic Agent

Use
Oral: Adjunctive therapy for peptic ulcers, irritable bowel, neurogenic bladder/bowel; treatment of infant colic, GI tract disorders caused by spasm; to reduce rigidity, tremors, sialorrhea, and hyperhidrosis associated with parkinsonism; as a drying agent in acute rhinitis

Injection: Preoperative antimuscarinic to reduce secretions and block cardiac vagal inhibitory reflexes; to improve radiologic visibility of the kidneys; symptomatic relief of biliary and renal colic; reduce GI motility to facilitate diagnostic procedures (ie, endoscopy, hypotonic duodenography); reduce pain and hypersecretion in pancreatitis, certain cases of partial heart block associated with vagal activity; reversal of neuromuscular blockade

Usual Dosage
Oral: Children: Gastrointestinal disorders: Dose as listed, based on age and weight (kg) using 0.125 mg/mL drops; repeat dose every 4 hours as needed:

Children <2 years:
3.4 kg: 4 drops; maximum: 24 drops/24 hours
5 kg: 5 drops; maximum: 30 drops/24 hours
7 kg: 6 drops; maximum: 36 drops/24 hours
10 kg: 8 drops; maximum: 48 drops/24 hours

Oral, S.L.:
Children 2-12 years: Gastrointestinal disorders: Dose as listed, based on age and weight (kg); repeat dose every 4 hours as needed:
10 kg: 0.031-0.033 mg; maximum: 0.75 mg/24 hours
20 kg: 0.0625 mg; maximum: 0.75 mg/24 hours
40 kg: 0.0938 mg; maximum: 0.75 mg/24 hours
50 kg: 0.125 mg; maximum: 0.75 mg/24 hours
Children >12 years and Adults: Gastrointestinal disorders: 0.125-0.25 mg every 4 hours or as needed (before meals or food); maximum: 1.5 mg/24 hours
Cystospaz®: 0.15-0.3 mg up to 4 times/day

Oral (timed release): Children >12 years and Adults: Gastrointestinal disorders: 0.375-0.75 mg every 12 hours; maximum: 1.5 mg/24 hours

I.M., I.V., SubQ: Children >12 years and Adults: Gastrointestinal disorders: 0.25-0.5 mg; may repeat as needed up to 4 times/day, at 4-hour intervals

I.V.: Children >2 year and Adults: I.V.: Preanesthesia: 5 mcg/kg given 30-60 minutes prior to induction of anesthesia or at the time preoperative narcotics or sedatives are administered

I.V.: Adults: Diagnostic procedures: 0.25-0.5 mg given 5-10 minutes prior to procedure
To reduce drug-induced bradycardia during surgery: 0.125 mg; repeat as needed
To reverse neuromuscular blockade: 0.2 mg for every 1 mg neostigmine (or the physostigmine/pyridostigmine equivalent)

Dosage Forms
Capsule, timed release: 0.375 mg
Levsinex®: 0.375 mg
Elixir: 0.125 mg/5 mL
Hyosine, Levsin®: 0.125 mg/5 mL
Injection, solution: 0.5 mg/mL (1 mL)
Levsin®: 0.5 mg/mL (1 mL)
Liquid: 0.125 mg/5 mL
Solution, oral drops: 0.125 mg/mL
Hyosine, Levsin®: 0.125 mg/mL
Tablet: 0.125 mg, 0.15 mg
Anaspaz®, Levsin®: 0.125 mg
Cystospaz®: 0.15 mg
(Continued)

hyoscyamine *(Continued)*

Tablet, extended release: 0.375 mg
Levbid®, Symax SR: 0.375 mg
Tablet, orally disintegrating: 0.125 mg
NuLev™: 0.125 mg
Tablet, sublingual: 0.125 mg
Levsin/SL®, Symax SL: 0.125 mg

hyoscyamine, atropine, scopolamine, and phenobarbital

(hye oh SYE a meen, A troe peen, skoe POL a meen, & fee noe BAR bi tal)
Sound-Alike/Look-Alike Issues
Donnatal® may be confused with Donnagel®
Synonyms atropine, hyoscyamine, scopolamine, and phenobarbital; belladonna alkaloids with phenobarbital; phenobarbital, hyoscyamine, atropine, and scopolamine; scopolamine, hyoscyamine, atropine, and phenobarbital
U.S./Canadian Brand Names Donnatal Extentabs® [US]; Donnatal® [US]
Therapeutic Category Anticholinergic Agent
Use Adjunct in treatment of irritable bowel syndrome, acute enterocolitis, duodenal ulcer
Usual Dosage Oral:
Children: Donnatal® elixir: To be given every 4-6 hours; initial dose based on weight:
4.5 kg: 0.5 mL every 4 hours **or** 0.75 mL every 6 hours
10 kg: 1 mL every 4 hours **or** 1.5 mL every 6 hours
14 kg: 1.5 mL every 4 hours **or** 2 mL every 6 hours
23 kg: 2.5 mL every 4 hours **or** 3.8 mL every 6 hours
34 kg: 3.8 mL every 4 hours **or** 5 mL every 6 hours
≥45 kg: 5 mL every 4 hours **or** 7.5 mL every 6 hours
Adults:
Donnatal®: 1-2 tablets or 5-10 mL of elixir 3-4 times/day
Donnatal Extentabs®: 1 tablet every 12 hours; may increase to 1 tablet every 8 hours if needed
Dosage Forms
Elixir:
Donnatal®: Hyoscyamine 0.1037 mg, atropine 0.0194 mg, scopolamine 0.0065 mg, and phenobarbital 16.2 mg per 5 mL
Tablet: Hyoscyamine 0.1037 mg, atropine 0.0194 mg, scopolamine 0.0065 mg, and phenobarbital 16.2 mg
Donnatal®: Hyoscyamine 0.1037 mg, atropine 0.0194 mg, scopolamine 0.0065 mg, and phenobarbital 16.2 mg
Tablet, extended release:
Donnatal Extentabs®: Hyoscyamine 0.3111 mg, atropine 0.0582 mg, scopolamine 0.0195 mg, and phenobarbital 48.6 mg

hyoscyamine sulfate *see* hyoscyamine *on previous page*

Hyosine [US] *see* hyoscyamine *on previous page*

Hy-Pam® **Oral** *(Discontinued)* *see* hydroxyzine *on page 440*

Hypaque™-76 [US] *see* diatrizoate meglumine and diatrizoate sodium *on page 250*

Hypaque™ Meglumine [US] *see* diatrizoate meglumine *on page 249*

Hypaque™ Sodium [US] *see* diatrizoate sodium *on page 250*

Hyperab® *(Discontinued)* *see* rabies immune globulin (human) *on page 741*

hyperal *see* total parenteral nutrition *on page 853*

hyperalimentation *see* total parenteral nutrition *on page 853*

HyperHep B® **[Can]** *see* hepatitis B immune globulin *on page 417*

HyperHEP B™ S/D [US] *see* hepatitis B immune globulin *on page 417*

HyperRAB™ S/D [US/Can] *see* rabies immune globulin (human) *on page 741*

HyperRHO™ S/D Full Dose [US] *see* Rh₀(D) immune globulin *on page 753*

HyperRHO™ S/D Mini Dose [US] *see* Rh₀(D) immune globulin *on page 753*

Hyperstat® *(Discontinued)* *see* diazoxide *on page 252*

HyperTET™ S/D [US/Can] *see* tetanus immune globulin (human) *on page 829*

Hyphed [US] *see* pseudoephedrine, hydrocodone, and chlorpheniramine *on page 731*

Hy-Phen® *(Discontinued)* *see* hydrocodone and acetaminophen *on page 427*

HypoTears [US-OTC] *see* artificial tears *on page 75*

HypoTears PF [US-OTC] *see* artificial tears *on page 75*

HypRho®-D *(Discontinued)*

HypRho®-D Mini-Dose *(Discontinued)*

Hyprogest® 250 *(Discontinued)*

hypromellose *see* hydroxypropyl methylcellulose *on page 439*

Hytakerol® *(Discontinued)*

HyTan™ *(Discontinued)* *see* hydrocodone and chlorpheniramine *on page 428*

Hytone® [US] *see* hydrocortisone (topical) *on page 434*

Hytrin® [Can] *see* terazosin *on page 826*

Hytrin® *(Discontinued)* *see* terazosin *on page 826*

Hyzaar® [US/Can] *see* losartan and hydrochlorothiazide *on page 519*

Hyzaar® DS [Can] *see* losartan and hydrochlorothiazide *on page 519*

Hyzine® *(Discontinued)* *see* hydroxyzine *on page 440*

ibandronate (eye BAN droh nate)

Synonyms ibandronate sodium; ibandronic acid; NSC-722623
U.S./Canadian Brand Names Bondronat® [Can]; Boniva® [US]
Therapeutic Category Bisphosphonate Derivative
Use Treatment and prevention of osteoporosis in postmenopausal females
Usual Dosage
Oral:
Treatment of postmenopausal osteoporosis: 2.5 mg/day or 150 mg once a month
Prevention of postmenopausal osteoporosis: 2.5 mg/day; 150 mg once a month may be considered
I.V.: Treatment of postmenopausal osteoporosis: 3 mg every 3 months
Dosage Forms
Injection, solution:
Boniva®: 1 mg/mL (3 mL)
Tablet:
Boniva®: 2.5 mg [once-daily formulation]; 150 mg [once-monthly formulation]

ibandronate sodium *see* ibandronate *on this page*

ibandronic acid *see* ibandronate *on this page*

Iberet® [US-OTC] *see* vitamins (multiple/oral) *on page 895*

Iberet®-500 [US-OTC] *see* vitamins (multiple/oral) *on page 895*

ibidomide hydrochloride *see* labetalol *on page 486*

ibritumomab (ib ri TYOO mo mab)

Synonyms ibritumomab tiuxetan; IDEC-Y2B8; In-111 ibritumomab; In-111 zevalin; Y-90 ibritumomab; Y-90 zevalin
U.S./Canadian Brand Names Zevalin® [US/Can]
Therapeutic Category Antineoplastic Agent, Monoclonal Antibody; Radiopharmaceutical
Use Treatment of relapsed or refractory low-grade, follicular, or transformed B-cell non-Hodgkin lymphoma
Usual Dosage I.V.: Adults: Ibritumomab is administered **only** as part of the Zevalin™ therapeutic regimen (a combined treatment regimen with rituximab). The regimen consists of two steps:

Step 1:
Rituximab infusion: 250 mg/m^2 at an initial rate of 50 mg/hour. If hypersensitivity or infusion-related events do not occur, increase infusion in increments of 50 mg/hour every 30 minutes, to a maximum of 400 mg/hour. Infusions should be temporarily slowed or interrupted if hypersensitivity or infusion-related events occur. The infusion may be resumed at one-half the previous rate upon improvement of symptoms.
In-111 ibritumomab infusion: Within 4 hours of the completion of rituximab infusion, inject 5 mCi (1.6 mg total antibody dose) over 10 minutes.
Biodistribution of In-111 ibritumomab should be assessed by imaging at 48-72 hours postinjection. Optional additional imaging may be performed to resolve ambiguities. If biodistribution is not acceptable, the patient should not proceed to Step 2.

Step 2 (initiated 7-9 days following Step 1):
Rituximab infusion: 250 mg/m^2 at an initial rate of 100 mg/hour (50 mg/hour if infusion-related events occurred with the first infusion). If hypersensitivity or infusion-related events do not occur, increase infusion in increments of 100 mg/hour every 30 minutes, to a maximum of 400 mg/hour, as tolerated.
(Continued)

ibritumomab *(Continued)*

Y-90 ibritumomab infusion: Within 4 hours of the completion of rituximab infusion:

Platelet count >150,000 cells/mm^3: Inject 0.4 mCi/kg (14.8 MBq/kg actual body weight) over 10 minutes; maximum dose: 32 mCi (1184 MBq)

Platelet count between 100,000-149,000 cells/mm^3: Inject 0.3 mCi/kg (11.1 MBq/kg actual body weight) over 10 minutes; maximum dose: 32 mCi (1184 MBq)

Platelet count <100,000 cells/mm^3: Do **not** administer

Maximum dose: The prescribed, measured, and administered dose of Y-90 ibritumomab must not exceed 32 mCi (1184 MBq), regardless of the patient's body weight

Dosage Forms Each kit contains 4 vials for preparation of either In-111 or Y-90 conjugate (as indicated on container label)

Injection, solution:

Zevalin®: 1.6 mg/mL (2 mL)

ibritumomab tiuxetan *see ibritumomab on previous page*

Ibu-200 [US-OTC] *see ibuprofen on this page*

Ibuprin® *(Discontinued) see ibuprofen on this page*

ibuprofen (eye byoo PROE fen)

Sound-Alike/Look-Alike Issues

Haltran® may be confused with Halfprin®

Synonyms ibuprofen lysine; *p*-isobutylhydratropic acid

U.S./Canadian Brand Names Advil® Children's [US-OTC]; Advil® Infants' [US-OTC]; Advil® Junior [US-OTC]; Advil® Migraine [US-OTC]; Advil® [US-OTC/Can]; Apo-Ibuprofen® [Can]; ElixSure™ IB [US-OTC]; Genpril® [US-OTC]; I-Prin [US-OTC]; Ibu-200 [US-OTC]; Midol® Cramp and Body Aches [US-OTC]; Motrin® Children's [US-OTC/Can]; Motrin® IB [US-OTC/Can]; Motrin® Infants' [US-OTC]; Motrin® Junior Strength [US-OTC]; Motrin® [US]; NeoProfen® [US]; Novo-Profen [Can]; Nu-Ibuprofen [Can]; Proprinal [US-OTC]; Ultraprin [US-OTC]

Therapeutic Category Analgesic, Nonnarcotic; Antipyretic; Nonsteroidal Antiinflammatory Drug (NSAID)

Use

Oral: Inflammatory diseases and rheumatoid disorders including juvenile rheumatoid arthritis, mild-to-moderate pain, fever, dysmenorrhea

Injection: Ibuprofen lysine is for use in premature infants weighing between 500-1500 g and who are ≤32 weeks gestational age (GA) to induce closure of a clinically-significant patent ductus arteriosus (PDA) when usual treatments are ineffective

Usual Dosage

I.V.: Infants between 500-1500 g and ≤32 weeks GA: Patent ductus arteriosus: Initial dose: Ibuprofen 10 mg/kg, followed by two doses of 5 mg/kg at 24 and 48 hours. Dose should be based on birth weight.

Oral:

Children:

Antipyretic: 6 months to 12 years: Temperature <102.5°F (39°C): 5 mg/kg/dose; temperature >102.5°F: 10 mg/kg/dose given every 6-8 hours (maximum daily dose: 40 mg/kg/day)

Juvenile rheumatoid arthritis: 30-50 mg/kg/24 hours divided every 8 hours; start at lower end of dosing range and titrate upward (maximum: 2.4 g/day)

Analgesic: 4-10 mg/kg/dose every 6-8 hours

OTC labeling (analgesic, antipyretic):

Children 6 months to 11 years: See below; use of weight to select dose is preferred; doses may be repeated every 6-8 hours (maximum: 4 doses/day)

Children ≥12 years: 200 mg every 4-6 hours as needed (maximum: 1200 mg/24 hours)

Ibuprofen Dosing:

Weight 12-17 lbs (6-11 months of age): 50 mg

Weight 18-23 lbs (12-23 months of age): 75 mg

Weight 24-35 lbs (2-3 years of age): 100 mg

Weight 35-47 lbs (4-5 years of age): 150 mg

Weight 48-59 lbs (6-8 years of age): 200 mg

Weight 60-71 lbs (9-10 years of age): 250 mg

Weight 72-95 lbs (11 years of age): 300 mg

Adults:

Inflammatory disease: 400-800 mg/dose 3-4 times/day (maximum dose: 3.2 g/day)

Analgesia/pain/fever/dysmenorrhea: 200-400 mg/dose every 4-6 hours (maximum daily dose: 1.2 g, unless directed by physician)

OTC labeling (analgesic, antipyretic): 200 mg every 4-6 hours as needed (maximum: 1200 mg/24 hours)

Dosage Forms

Caplet: 200 mg [OTC]

Advil® [OTC], Ibu-200 [OTC], Motrin® IB [OTC]: 200 mg
Motrin® Junior Strength [OTC]: 100 mg
Capsule, liqui-gel:
Advil® [OTC], Advil® Migraine [OTC]: 200 mg
Gelcap:
Advil® [OTC]: 200 mg
Injection, solution, as lysine [preservative free]:
NeoProfen®: 17.1 mg/mL (2 mL) [equivalent to ibuprofen 10 mg/mL]
Suspension, oral: 100 mg/5 mL
Advil® Children's [OTC], ElixSure™ IB [OTC], Motrin® Children's [OTC]: 100 mg/5 mL
Suspension, oral drops: 40 mg/mL
Advil® Infants' [OTC], Motrin® Infants' [OTC]: 40 mg/mL
Tablet: 200 mg [OTC], 400 mg, 600 mg, 800 mg
Advil® [OTC], Genpril® [OTC], I-Prin [OTC], Midol® Cramp and Body Aches [OTC], Motrin® IB [OTC], Proprinal [OTC], Ultraprin [OTC]: 200 mg
Advil® Junior [OTC]: 100 mg
Motrin®: 600 mg, 800 mg
Tablet, chewable:
Advil® Children's [OTC], Motrin® Children's [OTC]: 50 mg
Advil® Junior [OTC], Motrin® Junior Strength [OTC]: 100 mg

ibuprofen and hydrocodone see hydrocodone and ibuprofen on page 430

ibuprofen and oxycodone see oxycodone and ibuprofen on page 642

ibuprofen and pseudoephedrine see pseudoephedrine and ibuprofen on page 729

ibuprofen lysine see ibuprofen on previous page

ibuprofen, pseudoephedrine, and chlorpheniramine
(eye byoo PROE fen, soo doe e FED rin, & klor fen IR a meen)
Synonyms chlorpheniramine maleate, ibuprofen, and pseudoephedrine; ibuprofen, pseudoephedrine, and chlorpheniramine maleate; pseudoephedrine, chlorpheniramine, and ibuprofen
U.S./Canadian Brand Names Advil® Allergy Sinus [US]; Advil® Cold and Sinus Plus [Can]; Advil® Multi-Symptom Cold [US]
Therapeutic Category Antihistamine/Decongestant/Analgesic
Use Temporary relief of symptoms associated with the common cold, hay fever, or other respiratory allergies
Usual Dosage Oral: Children ≥12 years and Adults: One caplet every 4-6 hours while symptoms persist (maximum: 6 caplets/24 hours)
Dosage Forms
Caplet:
Advil® Allergy Sinus, Advil® Multi-Symptom Cold: Ibuprofen 200 mg, pseudoephedrine 30 mg, and chlorpheniramine 2 mg

ibuprofen, pseudoephedrine, and chlorpheniramine maleate see ibuprofen, pseudoephedrine, and chlorpheniramine on this page

ibutilide (i BYOO ti lide)
Synonyms ibutilide fumarate
U.S./Canadian Brand Names Corvert® [US]
Therapeutic Category Antiarrhythmic Agent, Class III
Use Acute termination of atrial fibrillation or flutter of recent onset; the effectiveness of ibutilide has not been determined in patients with arrhythmias >90 days in duration
Usual Dosage I.V.: Initial: Adults:
<60 kg: 0.01 mg/kg over 10 minutes
≥60 kg: 1 mg over 10 minutes
If the arrhythmia does not terminate within 10 minutes after the end of the initial infusion, a second infusion of equal strength may be infused over a 10-minute period
Dosage Forms
Injection, solution:
Corvert®: 0.1 mg/mL (10 mL)

ibutilide fumarate see ibutilide on this page

Icar™ Prenatal [US] see vitamins (multiple/prenatal) on page 896

IC-Green™ [US] see indocyanine green on page 453

ICI-182,780 see fulvestrant on page 378

ICI-204,219 *see* zafirlukast *on page 902*

ICI-46474 *see* tamoxifen *on page 819*

ICI-118630 *see* goserelin *on page 399*

ICI-176334 *see* bicalutamide *on page 111*

ICI-D1033 *see* anastrozole *on page 56*

ICI-D1694 *see* raltitrexed *(Canada only) on page 743*

ICL670 *see* deferasirox *on page 234*

icodextrin (eye KOE dex trin)
U.S./Canadian Brand Names Adept® [US]; Extraneal® [US]
Therapeutic Category Adhesiolytic; Peritoneal Dialysate, Osmotic
Use
Adept®: Reduction of postsurgical adhesions in gynecologic laparoscopic procedures
Extraneal®: Daily exchange for the long dwell (8- to 16-hour) during continuous ambulatory peritoneal dialysis (CAPD) or automated peritoneal dialysis (APD) for the management of end-stage renal disease (ESRD); improvement of long-dwell ultrafiltration and clearance of creatinine and urea nitrogen (compared to 4.25% dextrose) in patients with high/average or greater transport characteristics as measured by peritoneal equilibration test (PET)
Usual Dosage Intraperitoneal: Adults:
CAPD or APD (Extraneal®): Given as a single daily exchange in CAPD or APD; dwell time of 8-16 hours is suggested
Laparoscopic gynecologic surgery (Adept®): Irrigate with at least 100 mL every 30 minutes during surgery; aspirate remaining fluid after surgery is completed, then instill 1 L into the cavity
Dosage Forms
  Solution, intraperitoneal:
  Adept®: 4% (1.5 L) [for laparoscopic surgery]
  Extraneal: 7.5% (1.5 L, 2 L, 2.5 L) [for peritoneal dialysis]

ICRF-187 *see* dexrazoxane *on page 245*

Idamycin® **[Can]** *see* idarubicin *on this page*

Idamycin® *(Discontinued)* *see* idarubicin *on this page*

Idamycin PFS® **[US]** *see* idarubicin *on this page*

Idarac® **[Can]** *see* floctafenine *(Canada only) on page 355*

idarubicin (eye da ROO bi sin)
Sound-Alike/Look-Alike Issues
idarubicin may be confused with DOXOrubicin, DAUNOrubicin, epirubicin
Idamycin PFS® may be confused with Adriamycin®
Synonyms 4-demethoxydaunorubicin; 4-DMDR; idarubicin hydrochloride; IDR; IMI 30; NSC-256439; SC 33428
U.S./Canadian Brand Names Idamycin PFS® [US]; Idamycin® [Can]
Therapeutic Category Antineoplastic Agent
Use Treatment of acute leukemias (AML, ANLL, ALL), accelerated phase or blast crisis of chronic myelogenous leukemia (CML), breast cancer
Usual Dosage I.V. (refer to individual protocols):
Children:
Leukemia: 10-12 mg/m^2/day for 3 days every 3 weeks
Solid tumors: 5 mg/m^2/day for 3 days every 3 weeks
Adults:
Leukemia induction: 12 mg/m^2/day for 3 days
Leukemia consolidation: 10-12 mg/m^2/day for 2 days
Dosage Forms
  Injection, solution [preservative free]: 1 mg/mL (5 mL, 10 mL, 20 mL)
  Idamycin PFS®: 1 mg/mL (5 mL, 10 mL, 20 mL)

idarubicin hydrochloride *see* idarubicin *on this page*

IDEC-C2B8 *see* rituximab *on page 762*

IDEC-Y2B8 *see* ibritumomab *on page 443*

IDR *see* idarubicin *on this page*

idursulfase (eye dur SUL fase)

Sound-Alike/Look-Alike Issues
Elaprase™ may be confused with Elspar®

U.S./Canadian Brand Names Elaprase™ [US]

Therapeutic Category Enzyme

Use Replacement therapy in mucopolysaccharidosis II (MPS II, Hunter syndrome) for improvement of walking capacity

Usual Dosage I.V.: MPS II: Children ≥5 years and Adults: 0.5 mg/kg once weekly; dose should be rounded up to the nearest whole vial

Dosage Forms
Injection, solution [preservative free]:
Elaprase™: 2 mg/mL (5 mL)

Ifex® [US/Can] *see* ifosfamide *on this page*

IFLrA *see* interferon alfa-2a *on page 462*

ifosfamide (eye FOSS fa mide)

Sound-Alike/Look-Alike Issues
ifosfamide may be confused with cyclophosphamide

Synonyms isophosphamide; NSC-109724; Z4942

U.S./Canadian Brand Names Ifex® [US/Can]

Therapeutic Category Antineoplastic Agent

Use Treatment of testicular cancer

Usual Dosage Refer to individual protocols. To prevent bladder toxicity, ifosfamide should be given with the urinary protector mesna and hydration of at least 2 L of oral or I.V. fluid per day.
I.V.: Adults: Testicular cancer: 1200 mg/m^2/day for 5 days every 3 weeks

Dosage Forms
Injection, powder for reconstitution: 1 g
Ifex®: 1 g, 3 g
Injection, solution:
50 mg/mL (20 mL, 60 mL)

IG *see* immune globulin (intramuscular) *on page 450*

IgG4-kappa monoclonal antibody *see* natalizumab *on page 593*

IGIM *see* immune globulin (intramuscular) *on page 450*

IL-1Ra *see* anakinra *on page 55*

IL-2 *see* aldesleukin *on page 26*

IL-11 *see* oprelvekin *on page 632*

Ilopan-Choline® Oral *(Discontinued)* *see* dexpanthenol *on page 244*

Ilopan® Injection *(Discontinued)* *see* dexpanthenol *on page 244*

iloprost (EYE loe prost)

Synonyms iloprost tromethamine; prostacyclin PGI$_2$

U.S./Canadian Brand Names Ventavis™ [US]

Therapeutic Category Prostaglandin

Use Treatment of idiopathic pulmonary arterial hypertension in patients with NYHA Class III or IV symptoms

Usual Dosage Inhalation: Adults: Initial: 2.5 mcg/dose; if tolerated, increase to 5 mcg/dose; administer 6-9 times daily (dosing at intervals ≥2 hours while awake); maintenance dose: 5 mcg/dose; maximum daily dose: 45 mcg

Dosage Forms
Solution for oral inhalation [preservative-free]:
Ventavis™: 10 mcg/mL (1 mL, 2 mL)

iloprost tromethamine *see* iloprost *on this page*

Ilozyme® *(Discontinued)* *see* pancrelipase *on page 648*

imatinib (eye MAT eh nib)

Synonyms CGP-57148B; glivec; imatinib mesylate; NSC-716051; STI571

U.S./Canadian Brand Names Gleevec® [US/Can]

Therapeutic Category Antineoplastic, Tyrosine Kinase Inhibitor

Use Treatment of:

Gastrointestinal stromal tumors (GIST) kit-positive (CD117) unresectable and/or (metastatic) malignant
Philadelphia chromosome-positive (Ph+) chronic myeloid leukemia (CML) in chronic phase (newly-diagnosed)
Ph+ CML in blast crisis, accelerated phase, or chronic phase after failure of interferon therapy
Ph+ acute lymphoblastic leukemia (ALL) (relapsed or refractory)
Ph+ ALL induction therapy (newly diagnosed) [**not** an approved indication in the U.S.]

Note: The following indications are **not** approved in Canada:
Aggressive systemic mastocytosis (ASM) without D816V c-Kit mutation (or c-Kit mutation status unknown)
Dermatofibrosarcoma protuberans (DFSP) (unresectable, recurrent and metastatic)
Hypereosinophilic syndrome (HES) and/or chronic eosinophilic leukemia (CEL)
Myelodysplastic/myeloproliferative disease (MDS/MPD) associated with platelet-derived growth factor receptor (PDGFR) gene rearrangements
Ph+ CML in chronic phase in pediatric patients recurring following stem cell transplant or who are resistant to interferon-alpha therapy

Usual Dosage Oral: **Note:** For concurrent use with a strong CYP3A4 enzyme-inducing agent (eg, rifampin, phenytoin), imatinib dosage should be increased by at least 50%.

Children ≥2 years: **Note:** May be administered once daily or in 2 divided doses.
  Ph+ CML (chronic phase, recurrent or resistant): 260 mg/m^2/day; maximum: 600 mg /day
  Ph+ CML (chronic phase, newly diagnosed): 340 mg/m^2/day; maximum: 600 mg /day

Adults:
  Ph+ CML:
   Chronic phase: 400 mg once daily; may be increased to 600 mg daily
   Accelerated phase or blast crisis: 600 mg once daily; may be increased to 800 mg daily (400 mg twice daily)
  Ph+ ALL: 600 mg once daily
  GIST: 400-600 mg/day
  ASM with eosinophilia: Initiate at 100 mg once daily; titrate up to a maximum of 400 mg once daily (if tolerated) for insufficient response to lower dose
  ASM without D816V c-Kit mutation or c-Kit mutation status unknown: 400 mg once daily
  DFSP: 400 mg twice daily
  HES/CEL: 400 mg once daily
  HES/CEL with FIP1L1-PDGFRα fusion kinase: Initiate at 100 mg once daily; titrate up to a maximum of 400 mg once daily (if tolerated) if insufficient response to lower dose
  MDS/MPD: 400 mg once daily

Dosage Forms
Tablet:
Gleevec®: 100 mg; 400 mg

imatinib mesylate *see imatinib on this page*

IMC-C225 *see cetuximab on page 170*

Imdur® [US/Can] *see isosorbide mononitrate on page 476*

IMI 30 *see idarubicin on page 446*

IMid-3 *see lenalidomide on page 495*

imidazole carboxamide *see dacarbazine on page 227*

imidazole carboxamide dimethyltriazene *see dacarbazine on page 227*

imiglucerase (i mi GLOO ser ace)

Sound-Alike/Look-Alike Issues
Cerezyme® may be confused with Cerebyx®, Ceredase®

U.S./Canadian Brand Names Cerezyme® [US/Can]

Therapeutic Category Enzyme

Use Long-term enzyme replacement therapy for patients with Type 1 Gaucher disease

Usual Dosage I.V.: Children ≥2 years and Adults: Initial: 30-60 units/kg every 2 weeks; dosing is individualized based on disease severity. Dosing range: 2.5 units/kg 3 times/week up to as much as 60 units/kg administered as frequently as once a week or as infrequently as every 4 weeks. Average dose: 60 units/kg administered every 2 weeks

Dosage Forms
Injection, powder for reconstitution:
Cerezyme®: 200 units, 400 units

imipemide *see* imipenem and cilastatin *on this page*

imipenem and cilastatin (i mi PEN em & sye la STAT in)

Sound-Alike/Look-Alike Issues
Primaxin® may be confused with Premarin®, Primacor®

Synonyms imipemide

U.S./Canadian Brand Names Primaxin® I.V. [Can]; Primaxin® [US/Can]

Therapeutic Category Carbapenem (Antibiotic)

Use Treatment of lower respiratory tract, urinary tract, intraabdominal, gynecologic, bone and joint, skin and skin structure, and polymicrobic infections as well as bacterial septicemia and endocarditis. Antibacterial activity includes resistant gram-negative bacilli (*Pseudomonas aeruginosa* and *Enterobacter* sp), gram-positive bacteria (methicillin-sensitive *Staphylococcus aureus* and *Streptococcus* sp) and anaerobes.

Usual Dosage
Usual dosage ranges: Note: Dosage based on **imipenem** content:
Neonates ≤3 months and weight ≥1500 g: Non-CNS infections: I.V.:
<1 week: 25 mg/kg every 12 hours
1-4 weeks: 25 mg/kg every 8 hours
4 weeks to 3 months: 25 mg/kg every 6 hours
Children >3 months: Non-CNS infections: I.V.: 15-25 mg/kg every 6 hours; maximum dosage: Susceptible infections: 2 g/day; moderately-susceptible organisms: 4 g/day
Adults:
I.M.: 500-750 mg every 12 hours; maximum: 1500 mg/day
I.V.: Weight ≥70 kg: 250-1000 mg every 6-8 hours; maximum: 4 g/day
Indication-specific dosing: Note: Doses based on imipenem content. I.M. administration is not intended for severe or life-threatening infections (eg, septicemia, endocarditis, shock), UTI, bone/joint or polymicrobic infections:
Children: I.V.: **Cystic fibrosis:** Doses up to 90 mg/kg/day have been used
Adults:
Intra-abdominal infections:
I.V.: Mild infection: 250-500 mg every 6 hours; severe: 500 mg every 6 hours
I.M.: Mild-to-moderate infection: 750 mg every 12 hours
Lower respiratory tract, skins/skin structure, gynecologic infections: I.M.: Mild/moderate: 500-750 mg every 12 hours
Mild infection: Note: Rarely a suitable option in mild infections; normally reserved for moderate-severe cases:
I.M.: 500 mg every 12 hours
I.V.:
Fully-susceptible organisms: 250 mg every 6 hours
Moderately-susceptible organisms: 500 mg every 6 hours
Moderate infection:
I.M.: 750 mg every 12 hours
I.V.:
Fully-susceptible organisms: 500 mg every 6-8 hours
Moderately-susceptible organisms: 500 mg every 6 hours or 1 g every 8 hours
***Pseudomonas* infections:** I.V.: 500 mg every 6 hours; **Note:** Higher doses may be required based on organism sensitivity.
Severe infection: I.V.:
Fully-susceptible organisms: 500 mg every 6 hours
Moderately-susceptible organisms: 1 g every 6-8 hours
Maximum daily dose should not exceed 50 mg/kg or 4 g/day, whichever is lower
Urinary tract infection: I.V.:
Uncomplicated: 250 mg every 6 hours
Complicated: 500 mg every 6 hours
Dosage Forms
Injection, powder for reconstitution [I.M.]:
Primaxin®: Imipenem 500 mg and cilastatin 500 mg
Injection, powder for reconstitution [I.V.]:
Primaxin®: Imipenem 250 mg and cilastatin 250 mg; imipenem 500 mg and cilastatin 500 mg

imipramine (im IP ra meen)

Sound-Alike/Look-Alike Issues
imipramine may be confused with amitriptyline, desipramine, Norpramin®

Synonyms imipramine hydrochloride; imipramine pamoate

U.S./Canadian Brand Names Apo-Imipramine® [Can]; Novo-Pramine [Can]; Tofranil-PM® [US]; Tofranil® [US/Can]

(Continued)

imipramine *(Continued)*
Therapeutic Category Antidepressant, Tricyclic (Tertiary Amine)
Use Treatment of depression; treatment of nocturnal enuresis in children
Usual Dosage Oral:
   Children: Enuresis: ≥6 years: Initial: 25 mg at bedtime, if inadequate response still seen after 1 week of therapy, increase by 25 mg/day; dose should not exceed 2.5 mg/kg/day or 50 mg at bedtime if 6-12 years of age or 75 mg at bedtime if ≥12 years of age
   Adolescents: Depression: Initial: 30-40 mg/day; increase gradually; maximum: 100 mg/day in single or divided doses
   Adults: Depression: Initial: 25 mg 3-4 times/day, increase dose gradually, total dose may be given at bedtime; maximum: 300 mg/day
Dosage Forms
   Capsule: 75 mg, 100 mg, 125 mg, 150 mg
      Tofranil-PM®: 75 mg, 100 mg, 125 mg, 150 mg
   Tablet: 10 mg, 25 mg, 50 mg
      Tofranil®: 10 mg, 25 mg, 50 mg

imipramine hydrochloride *see* imipramine *on previous page*

imipramine pamoate *see* imipramine *on previous page*

imiquimod (i mi KWI mod)
Sound-Alike/Look-Alike Issues
   Aldara™ may be confused with Alora®, Lialda™
U.S./Canadian Brand Names Aldara™ [US/Can]
Therapeutic Category Immune Response Modifier
Use Treatment of external genital and perianal warts/condyloma acuminata; nonhyperkeratotic, nonhypertrophic actinic keratosis on face or scalp; superficial basal cell carcinoma (sBCC) with a maximum tumor diameter of 2 cm located on the trunk, neck, or extremities (excluding hands or feet)
Usual Dosage Topical: **Note:** A rest period of several days may be taken if required by the patient's discomfort or severity of the local skin reaction. Treatment may resume once the reaction subsides.
   Children ≥12 years and Adults: Perianal warts/condyloma acuminata: Apply a thin layer 3 times/week prior to bedtime and leave on skin for 6-10 hours. Remove with mild soap and water. Examples of 3 times/week application schedules are: Monday, Wednesday, Friday; or Tuesday, Thursday, Saturday. Continue imiquimod treatment until there is total clearance of the genital/perianal warts for ≤16 weeks.
   Adults:
   Actinic keratosis: Apply twice weekly for 16 weeks to a treatment area on face or scalp (but not both concurrently); apply prior to bedtime and leave on skin for 8 hours. Remove with mild soap and water.
   Common oral warts (dental use): Apply once daily prior to bedtime
   Superficial basal cell carcinoma: Apply once daily prior to bedtime, 5 days/week for 6 weeks. Treatment area should include a 1 cm margin of skin around the tumor. Leave on skin for 8 hours. Remove with mild soap and water.
Dosage Forms
   Cream:
   Aldara™: 5% (12s)

Imitrex® [US/Can] *see* sumatriptan *on page 815*

Imitrex® DF [Can] *see* sumatriptan *on page 815*

Imitrex® Nasal Spray [Can] *see* sumatriptan *on page 815*

ImmuCyst® [Can] *see* BCG vaccine *on page 96*

immune globulin (intramuscular) (i MYUN GLOB yoo lin, IN tra MUS kyoo ler)
Synonyms gamma globulin; IG; IGIM; immune serum globulin; ISG
U.S./Canadian Brand Names BayGam® [Can]; GammaSTAN™ S/D [US]
Therapeutic Category Immune Globulin
Use To provide passive immunity in susceptible individuals under the following circumstances:
   Hepatitis A: Within 14 days of exposure and prior to manifestation of disease
   Measles: For use within 6 days of exposure in an unvaccinated person, who has not previously had measles
   Varicella: When Varicella Zoster Immune Globulin is not available
   Rubella: Post exposure prophylaxis (within 72 hours) to reduce the risk of infection in exposed pregnant women who will not consider therapeutic abortion
   Immunoglobulin deficiency: To help prevent serious infections

Usual Dosage I.M.: Children and Adults:
Hepatitis A:
Preexposure prophylaxis upon travel into endemic areas (hepatitis A vaccine preferred):
0.02 mL/kg for anticipated risk of exposure <3 months
0.06 mL/kg for anticipated risk of exposure ≥3 months
Repeat approximate dose every 5 months if exposure continues
Postexposure prophylaxis: 0.02 mL/kg given within 14 days of exposure. IG is not needed if at least 1 dose of hepatitis A vaccine was given at ≥1 month before exposure
Measles:
Prophylaxis, immunocompetent: 0.25 mL/kg/dose (maximum dose: 15 mL) given within 6 days of exposure followed by live attenuated measles vaccine in 5-6 months when indicated
Prophylaxis, immunocompromised: 0.5 mL/kg (maximum dose: 15 mL) immediately following exposure
Rubella: Prophylaxis during pregnancy: 0.55 mL/kg/dose within 72 hours of exposure
Varicella: Prophylaxis: 0.6-1.2 mL/kg (varicella zoster immune globulin preferred) within 72 hours of exposure
IgG deficiency: 0.66 mL/kg/dose every 3-4 weeks. A double dose may be given at onset of therapy; some patients may require more frequent injections.
Dosage Forms
Injection, solution [preservative free]:
GammaSTAN™ S/D: 15% to 18% (2 mL, 10 mL)

immune globulin (intravenous) (i MYUN GLOB yoo lin, IN tra VEE nus)
Sound-Alike/Look-Alike Issues
Gamimune® N may be confused with CytoGam®
Synonyms IVIG
U.S./Canadian Brand Names Carimune™ NF [US]; Flebogamma® [US]; Gamimune® N [Can]; Gammagard® Liquid [US/Can]; Gammagard® S/D [US/Can]; Gammar®-P I.V. [US]; Gamunex® [US/Can]; Iveegam EN [US]; Iveegam Immuno® [Can]; Octagam® [US]; Panglobulin® NF [US]; Polygam® S/D [US]
Therapeutic Category Immune Globulin
Use
Treatment of primary immunodeficiency syndromes (congenital agammaglobulinemia, severe combined immunodeficiency syndromes [SCIDS], common variable immunodeficiency, X-linked immunodeficiency, Wiskott-Aldrich syndrome); idiopathic thrombocytopenic purpura (ITP); Kawasaki disease (in combination with aspirin)
Prevention of bacterial infection in B-cell chronic lymphocytic leukemia (CLL); pediatric HIV infection; bone marrow transplant (BMT)
Usual Dosage Approved doses and regimens may vary between brands; check manufacturer guidelines. **Note:** Some clinicians dose IVIG on ideal body weight or an adjusted ideal body weight in morbidly obese patients.
Children: I.V.: Pediatric HIV: 400 mg/kg every 28 days
Children and Adults: I.V.:
Primary immunodeficiency disorders: 200-400 mg/kg every 4 weeks or as per monitored serum IgG concentrations
Flebogamma®, Gammagard® Liquid, Gamunex®, Octagam®: 300-600 mg/kg every 3-4 weeks; adjusted based on dosage and interval in conjunction with monitored serum IgG concentrations.
B-cell chronic lymphocytic leukemia (CLL): 400 mg/kg/dose every 3 weeks
Idiopathic thrombocytopenic purpura (ITP):
Acute: 400 mg/kg/day for 5 days or 1000 mg/kg/day for 1-2 days
Chronic: 400 mg/kg as needed to maintain platelet count >30,000/mm³; may increase dose to 800 mg/kg (1000 mg/kg if needed)
Kawasaki disease: Initiate therapy within 10 days of disease onset: 2 g/kg as a single dose administered over 10 hours, or 400 mg/kg/day for 4 days. **Note:** Must be used in combination with aspirin: 80-100 mg/kg/day in 4 divided doses for 14 days; when fever subsides, dose aspirin at 3-5 mg/kg once daily for ≥6-8 weeks
Bone marrow transplant: 500 mg/kg beginning on days 7 and 2 pretransplant, then 500 mg/kg/week for 90 days post-transplant
Dosage Forms
Injection, powder for reconstitution [preservative free]:
Gammar®-P I.V.: 5 g, 10 g
Iveegam EN: 5 g
Injection, powder for reconstitution [preservative free, nanofiltered]:
Carimune™ NF: 3 g, 6 g, 12 g
Panglobulin® NF: 6 g, 12 g
Injection, powder for reconstitution [preservative free, solvent detergent-treated]:
Gammagard® S/D: 2.5 g, 5 g, 10 g
Polygam® S/D: 5 g, 10 g
(Continued)

immune globulin (intravenous) *(Continued)*

Injection, solution [preservative free; solvent detergent-treated]:
Gammagard® Liquid: 10% (10 mL, 25 mL, 50 mL, 100 mL, 200 mL)
Octagam®: 5% (20 mL, 50 mL, 100 mL, 200 mL)
Injection, solution [preservative free]:
Flebogamma®: 5% (10 mL, 50 mL, 100 mL, 200 mL)
Gamunex®: 10% (10 mL, 25 mL, 50 mL, 100 mL, 200 mL)

immune globulin (subcutaneous) (i MYUN GLOB yoo lin sub kyoo TAY nee us)

Synonyms immune globulin subcutaneous (human); SCIG
U.S./Canadian Brand Names Vivaglobin® [US]
Therapeutic Category Immune Globulin
Use Treatment of primary immune deficiency (PID)
Usual Dosage Note: Consider premedicating with acetaminophen and diphenhydramine.
SubQ infusion: Children ≥2 years and Adults: 100-200 mg/kg weekly (maximum rate: 20 mL/hour; doses >15 mL should be divided between sites); adjust the dose over time to achieve desired clinical response or target IgG levels
Conversion from I.V. to SubQ: Multiply previous I.V. dose by 1.37, then divide into a weekly regimen by dividing by the previous I.V. dosing interval (eg, if the dosing interval was every 3 weeks, divide by 3); adjust the dose over time to achieve desired clinical response or target IgG levels. SubQ infusion administration should begin 1 week after the last I.V. dose.
Dosage Forms
Injection, solution [preservative free]:
Vivaglobin®: IgG 160 mg/mL (3 mL, 10 mL, 20 mL)

immune globulin subcutaneous (human) *see* immune globulin (subcutaneous) *on this page*

immune serum globulin *see* immune globulin (intramuscular) *on page 450*

Immunine® VH [Can] *see* factor IX *on page 340*

Imodium® [Can] *see* loperamide *on page 515*

Imodium® A-D [US-OTC] *see* loperamide *on page 515*

Imodium® Advanced [US] *see* loperamide and simethicone *on page 516*

Imogam® Rabies-HT [US] *see* rabies immune globulin (human) *on page 741*

Imogam® Rabies Pasteurized [Can] *see* rabies immune globulin (human) *on page 741*

Imovane® [Can] *see* zopiclone *(Canada only) on page 909*

Imovax® Rabies [US/Can] *see* rabies virus vaccine *on page 742*

Implanon™ [US] *see* etonogestrel *on page 336*

Imuran® [US/Can] *see* azathioprine *on page 87*

In-111 ibritumomab *see* ibritumomab *on page 443*

In-111 zevalin *see* ibritumomab *on page 443*

inamrinone (eye NAM ri none)

Sound-Alike/Look-Alike Issues
amrinone may be confused with amiloride, amiodarone
Synonyms amrinone lactate
Therapeutic Category Adrenergic Agonist Agent
Use Short-term therapy in patients with intractable heart failure
Usual Dosage Dosage is based on clinical response (**Note:** Dose should not exceed 10 mg/kg/24 hours).
Infants, Children, and Adults: 0.75 mg/kg I.V. bolus over 2-3 minutes followed by maintenance infusion of 5-10 mcg/kg/minute; I.V. bolus may need to be repeated in 30 minutes.
Dosage Forms
Injection, solution: 5 mg/mL (20 mL)

I-Naphline® Ophthalmic *(Discontinued)* *see* naphazoline *on page 590*

Inapsine® [US] *see* droperidol *on page 284*

Increlex™ [US] *see* mecasermin *on page 535*

indapamide (in DAP a mide)

Sound-Alike/Look-Alike Issues
indapamide may be confused with Iopidine®

U.S./Canadian Brand Names Apo-Indapamide® [Can]; Gen-Indapamide [Can]; Lozide® [Can]; Lozol® [Can]; Novo-Indapamide [Can]; Nu-Indapamide [Can]; PMS-Indapamide [Can]

Therapeutic Category Diuretic, Miscellaneous

Use Management of mild to moderate hypertension; treatment of edema in congestive heart failure and nephrotic syndrome

Usual Dosage Oral: Adults:
Edema: 2.5-5 mg/day. **Note:** There is little therapeutic benefit to increasing the dose >5 mg/day; there is, however, an increased risk of electrolyte disturbances
Hypertension: 1.25 mg in the morning, may increase to 5 mg/day by increments of 1.25-2.5 mg; consider adding another antihypertensive and decreasing the dose if response is not adequate

Dosage Forms
Tablet: 1.25 mg, 2.5 mg

indapamide and perindopril erbumine see perindopril erbumine and indapamide (Canada only) on page 669

Inderal® [US/Can] see propranolol on page 724

Inderal® LA [US/Can] see propranolol on page 724

Inderide® [US] see propranolol and hydrochlorothiazide on page 724

indinavir (in DIN a veer)

Sound-Alike/Look-Alike Issues
indinavir may be confused with Denavir®

Synonyms indinavir sulfate

U.S./Canadian Brand Names Crixivan® [US/Can]

Therapeutic Category Antiviral Agent

Use Treatment of HIV infection; should always be used as part of a multidrug regimen (at least three antiretroviral agents)

Usual Dosage Oral: Adults:
Unboosted regimen: 800 mg every 8 hours
Ritonavir-boosted regimens:
Ritonavir 100-200 mg twice daily plus indinavir 800 mg twice daily **or**
Ritonavir 400 mg twice daily plus indinavir 400 mg twice daily
Dosage adjustments for indinavir when administered in combination therapy:
Delavirdine, itraconazole, or ketoconazole: Reduce indinavir dose to 600 mg every 8 hours
Efavirenz: Increase indinavir dose to 1000 mg every 8 hours
Lopinavir and ritonavir (Kaletra™): Indinavir 600 mg twice daily
Nelfinavir: Increase indinavir dose to 1200 mg twice daily
Nevirapine: Increase indinavir dose to 1000 mg every 8 hours
Rifabutin: Reduce rifabutin to $1/2$ the standard dose plus increase indinavir to 1000 mg every 8 hours

Dosage Forms
Capsule:
Crixivan®: 100 mg, 200 mg, 333 mg, 400 mg

indinavir sulfate see indinavir on this page

Indocid® P.D.A. [Can] see indomethacin on next page

Indocin® [US/Can] see indomethacin on next page

Indocin® I.V. [US] see indomethacin on next page

indocyanine green (in doe SYE a neen green)

U.S./Canadian Brand Names IC-Green™ [US]

Therapeutic Category Diagnostic Agent

Use Determining hepatic function, cardiac output, and liver blood flow; ophthalmic angiography

Usual Dosage Adults:
Ophthalmic angiography: Use doses of up to 40 mg of dye in 2 mL of aqueous solvent, in some patients, half the volume (1 mL) has been found to produce angiograms of comparable resolution; immediately following the bolus dose of dye, a bolus of sodium chloride 0.9% 5 mL is given; this regimen will deliver a spatially limited dye bolus of optimal concentration to the choroidal vasculature following I.V. injection into the antecubital vein.
Cardiac output determination: Dye is injected as rapidly as possible through a cardiac catheter; the usual dose is 1.25 mg for infants, 2.5 mg for children, and 5 mg for adults; total dose should not exceed 2 mg/kg; the dye should be flushed from the catheter with sodium chloride 0.9% to prevent hemolysis
(Continued)

indocyanine green *(Continued)*

Dosage Forms
Injection, powder for reconstitution:
  IC-Green®: 25 mg

Indo-Lemmon [Can] *see* indomethacin *on this page*

indometacin *see* indomethacin *on this page*

indomethacin (in doe METH a sin)

Sound-Alike/Look-Alike Issues
  Indocin® may be confused with Imodium®, Lincocin®, Minocin®, Vicodin®
Synonyms indometacin; indomethacin sodium trihydrate
U.S./Canadian Brand Names Apo-Indomethacin® [Can]; Indo-Lemmon [Can]; Indocid® P.D.A. [Can]; Indocin® I.V. [US]; Indocin® [US/Can]; Indotec [Can]; Novo-Methacin [Can]; Nu-Indo [Can]; Rhodacine® [Can]
Therapeutic Category Analgesic, Nonnarcotic; Nonsteroidal Antiinflammatory Drug (NSAID)
Use Acute gouty arthritis, acute bursitis/tendonitis, moderate to severe osteoarthritis, rheumatoid arthritis, ankylosing spondylitis; I.V. form used as alternative to surgery for closure of patent ductus arteriosus in neonates
Usual Dosage
  Patent ductus arteriosus:
    Neonates: I.V.: Initial: 0.2 mg/kg, followed by 2 doses depending on postnatal age (PNA):
    PNA **at time of first dose** <48 hours: 0.1 mg/kg at 12- to 24-hour intervals
    PNA **at time of first dose** 2-7 days: 0.2 mg/kg at 12- to 24-hour intervals
    PNA **at time of first dose** >7 days: 0.25 mg/kg at 12- to 24-hour intervals
    In general, may use 12-hour dosing interval if urine output >1 mL/kg/hour after prior dose; use 24-hour dosing interval if urine output is <1 mL/kg/hour but >0.6 mL/kg/hour; doses should be withheld if patient has oliguria (urine output <0.6 mL/kg/hour) or anuria
  Inflammatory/rheumatoid disorders: Oral: Use lowest effective dose.
    Children ≥2 years: 1-2 mg/kg/day in 2-4 divided doses; maximum dose: 4 mg/kg/day; not to exceed 150-200 mg/day
    Adults: 25-50 mg/dose 2-3 times/day; maximum dose: 200 mg/day. In patients with arthritis and persistent night pain and/or morning stiffness may give the larger portion (up to 100 mg) of the total daily dose at bedtime.
  Bursitis/tendonitis: Oral: Adults: Initial dose: 75-150 mg/day in 3-4 divided doses; usual treatment is 7-14 days
  Acute gouty arthritis: Oral: Adults: 50 mg 3 times daily until pain is tolerable then reduce dose; usual treatment <3-5 days
Dosage Forms
  Capsule: 25 mg, 50 mg
  Injection, powder for reconstitution:
    Indocin® I.V.: 1 mg
  Suspension, oral: 25 mg/5 mL
    Indocin®: 25 mg/5 mL

indomethacin sodium trihydrate *see* indomethacin *on this page*

Indotec [Can] *see* indomethacin *on this page*

INF-alpha 2 *see* interferon alfa-2b *on page 462*

Infanrix® [US] *see* diphtheria, tetanus toxoids, and acellular pertussis vaccine *on page 269*

Infantaire [US-OTC] *see* acetaminophen *on page 5*

Infantaire Gas Drops [US-OTC] *see* simethicone *on page 786*

Infants' Tylenol® Cold Plus Cough Concentrated Drops *(Discontinued)* *see* acetaminophen, dextromethorphan, and pseudoephedrine *on page 12*

Infasurf® [US] *see* calfactant *on page 142*

INFeD® [US] *see* iron dextran complex *on page 473*

Infergen® [US] *see* interferon alfacon-1 *on page 464*

Inflamase® Mild [Can] *see* prednisolone (ophthalmic) *on page 709*

infliximab (in FLIKS e mab)

Sound-Alike/Look-Alike Issues
  infliximab may be confused with rituximab
  Remicade® may be confused with Renacidin®, Rituxan®

Synonyms infliximab, recombinant; NSC-728729

U.S./Canadian Brand Names Remicade® [US/Can]

Therapeutic Category Monoclonal Antibody

Use Treatment of rheumatoid arthritis (moderate-to-severe, with methotrexate); treatment of Crohn disease (moderate-to-severe with inadequate response to conventional therapy) for induction and maintenance of remission, and/or to reduce the number of draining enterocutaneous and rectovaginal fistulas, and to maintain fistula closure; treatment of psoriatic arthritis; treatment of plaque psoriasis (chronic severe); treatment of ankylosing spondylitis; treatment of and maintenance of healing of ulcerative colitis (moderately- to severely- active with inadequate response to conventional therapy)

Note: In Canada, infliximab is not approved for use in children.

Usual Dosage I.V.: **Note:** Premedication with antihistamines (anti-H_1 and/or anti-H_2), acetaminophen and/or corticosteroids may be considered to prevent and/or manage infusion-related reactions:

Children ≥6 years: Crohn disease: 5 mg/kg at 0, 2, and 6 weeks, followed by a maintenance dose of 5 mg/kg every 8 weeks

Adults:

Crohn disease: Induction regimen: 5 mg/kg at 0, 2, and 6 weeks, followed by 5 mg/kg every 8 weeks thereafter; dose may be increased to 10 mg/kg in patients who respond but then lose their response. If no response by week 14, consider discontinuing therapy.

Psoriatic arthritis (with or without methotrexate): 5 mg/kg at 0, 2, and 6 weeks, then every 8 weeks

Rheumatoid arthritis (in combination with methotrexate therapy): 3 mg/kg at 0, 2, and 6 weeks, then every 8 weeks thereafter; doses have ranged from 3-10 mg/kg intravenous infusion repeated at 4- to 8-week intervals

Ankylosing spondylitis: 5 mg/kg at 0, 2, and 6 weeks, followed by 5 mg/kg every 6 weeks thereafter

Plaque psoriasis: 5 mg/kg at 0, 2, and 6 weeks, then every 8 weeks thereafter

Ulcerative colitis: 5 mg/kg at 0, 2, and 6 weeks, followed by 5 mg/kg every 8 weeks thereafter

Dosage Forms

Injection, powder for reconstitution [preservative free]:

Remicade®: 100 mg

infliximab, recombinant *see* infliximab *on previous page*

influenza virus vaccine (in floo EN za VYE rus vak SEEN)

Sound-Alike/Look-Alike Issues

influenza virus vaccine (human strain) may be confused with the avian strain (H5N1) of influenza virus vaccine

Fluarix® may be confused with Flarex®

influenza virus vaccine may be confused with tetanus toxoid and tuberculin products. Medication errors have occurred when tuberculin skin tests (PPD) have been inadvertently administered instead of tetanus toxoid products and influenza virus vaccine. These products are refrigerated and often stored in close proximity to each other.

Synonyms influenza virus vaccine (purified surface antigen); influenza virus vaccine (split-virus); influenza virus vaccine (trivalent, live); live attenuated influenza vaccine (LAIV); trivalent inactivated influenza vaccine (TIV)

U.S./Canadian Brand Names Fluarix® [US]; FluLaval™ [US]; fluMist® [US]; Fluviral S/F® [Can]; Fluvirin® [US]; Fluzone® [US]; Vaxigrip® [Can]

Therapeutic Category Vaccine, Inactivated Virus

Use Provide active immunity to influenza virus strains contained in the vaccine

Groups at Increased Risk for Influenza-Related Complications: Recommendations for vaccination:

- Persons ≥65 years of age
- Residents of nursing homes and other chronic-care facilities that house persons of any age with chronic medical conditions
- Adults and children with chronic disorders of the pulmonary or cardiovascular systems, including children with asthma
- Adults and children who have required regular medical follow-up or hospitalization during the preceding year because of chronic metabolic diseases (including diabetes mellitus), renal dysfunction, hemoglobinopathies, or immunosuppression (including immunosuppression caused by medications or HIV)
- Adults and children with conditions which may compromise respiratory function, the handling of respiratory secretions, or that can increase the risk of aspiration (eg, cognitive dysfunction, spinal; cord injuries, seizure disorders, other neuromuscular disorders)
- Children and adolescents (6 months to 18 years of age) who are receiving long-term aspirin therapy and therefore, may be at risk for developing Reye syndrome after influenza
- Women who will be pregnant during the influenza season
- Children 6-23 months of age

(Continued)

influenza virus vaccine *(Continued)*

Vaccination is also recommended for persons 50-64 years of age, close contacts of children 0-23 months of age, healthy persons who may transmit influenza to those at risk, all healthcare workers, and persons who smoke.

Usual Dosage Optimal time to receive vaccine is October-November, prior to exposure to influenza; however, vaccination can continue into December and throughout the influenza season as long as vaccine is available.

Note: Children <9 years who are not previously vaccinated or who received only 1 dose of vaccine during the previous season should receive 2 doses, in order to achieve satisfactory antibody response.

I.M.:
Fluzone®:
  Children 6-35 months: 0.25 mL/dose (1 or 2 doses per season; see **Note**)
  Children 3-8 years: 0.5 mL/dose (1 or 2 doses per season; see **Note**)
  Children ≥9 years and Adults: 0.5 mL/dose (1 dose per season)
Fluvirin®:
  Children 4-8 years: 0.5 mL/dose (1 or 2 doses per season; see **Note**)
  Children ≥9 years and Adults: 0.5 mL/dose (1 dose per season)
Fluarix®, FluLaval™: Adults: 0.5 mL/dose (1 dose per season)
Intranasal (fluMist®):
  Children 5-8 years, previously **not vaccinated** with influenza vaccine: Initial season: Two 0.5 mL doses separated by 6-10 weeks
  Children 5-8 years, previously **vaccinated** with influenza vaccine: 0.5 mL/dose (1 or 2 doses separated by 6-10 weeks; see **Note**)
  Children ≥9 years and Adults ≤49 years: 0.5 mL/dose (1 dose per season)

Dosage Forms
Injection, solution, purified split-virus [preservative free]:
  Fluvirin®: 0.5 mL, 5 mL
Injection, suspension, purified split-virus:
  Afluria® [preservative free]: 0.5 mL
  Afluria® , FluLaval™, Fluzone®: 5 mL
  Fluzone® [preservative free]: 0.25 mL, 0.5 mL
  Fluarix® [preservative free]: 0.5 mL
Solution, intranasal [preservative free; trivalent; live virus; spray]:
  FluMist®: 0.2 mL

influenza virus vaccine (H5N1) (in floo EN za VYE rus vak SEEN H5N1)

Sound-Alike/Look-Alike Issues
influenza virus vaccine (H5N1) may be confused with the nonavian strain of influenza virus vaccine
Synonyms avian influenza virus vaccine; bird flu vaccine; H5N1 influenza vaccine; influenza virus vaccine (monovalent)
Therapeutic Category Vaccine
Use Active immunization of adults at increased risk of exposure to the H5N1 viral subtype of influenza
Usual Dosage I.M.: Adults 18-64 years: 1 mL, followed by second 1 mL dose given 28 days later (acceptable range: 21-35 days)
Dosage Forms Injection, suspension [monovalent]: Hemagglutinin (H5N1 strain) 90 mcg/1 mL (5 mL)

influenza virus vaccine (monovalent) *see* influenza virus vaccine (H5N1) *on this page*

influenza virus vaccine (purified surface antigen) *see* influenza virus vaccine *on previous page*

influenza virus vaccine (split-virus) *see* influenza virus vaccine *on previous page*

influenza virus vaccine (trivalent, live) *see* influenza virus vaccine *on previous page*

Infufer® [Can] *see* iron dextran complex *on page 473*

Infumorph® [US] *see* morphine sulfate *on page 578*

Infuvite® Adult [US] *see* vitamins (multiple/injectable) *on page 895*

Infuvite® Pediatric [US] *see* vitamins (multiple/injectable) *on page 895*

INH *see* isoniazid *on page 474*

inhaled insulin *see* insulin inhalation *on page 458*

Inhibace® [Can] *see* cilazapril *(Canada only) on page 189*

Innohep® [US/Can] *see* tinzaparin *on page 844*

InnoPran XL™ [US] *see* propranolol *on page 724*

Inocor® *(Discontinued)*

INOmax® **[US/Can]** *see* nitric oxide *on page 607*

insect sting kit *see* epinephrine and chlorpheniramine *on page 302*

insoluble prussian blue *see* ferric hexacyanoferrate *on page 349*

Inspra™ **[US]** *see* eplerenone *on page 303*

Insta-Glucose® **[US-OTC]** *see* glucose (instant) *on page 395*

Instat™ **[US]** *see* collagen hemostat *on page 213*

Instat™ **MCH [US]** *see* collagen hemostat *on page 213*

insulin aspart (IN soo lin AS part)

Sound-Alike/Look-Alike Issues
NovoLog® may be confused with Novolin®
NovoLog® Mix 70/30 may be confused with NovoLog®
Synonyms aspart insulin
U.S./Canadian Brand Names NovoLog® [US]; NovoRapid® [Can]
Therapeutic Category Antidiabetic Agent, Insulin
Use Treatment of type 1 diabetes mellitus (insulin-dependent, IDDM); type 2 diabetes mellitus (noninsulin-dependent, NIDDM) to control hyperglycemia
Usual Dosage Refer to insulin regular *on page 460*. Insulin aspart is a rapid-acting insulin analog which is normally administered as a premeal component of the insulin regimen. It is normally used along with a long-acting (basal) form of insulin.
SubQ: When used in a meal-related treatment regimen, 50% to 70% of total daily insulin requirement may be provided by insulin aspart and the remainder provided by an intermediate or long-acting insulin. Due to rapid onset and short duration, some patients may require more basal insulin to prevent premeal hypoglycemia when using insulin aspart as opposed to regular insulin.
SubQ infusion pump: ~50% of total dose given as meal related bolus and ~50% of total dose given as basal infusion; adjust dose as necessary
Dosage Forms
Injection, solution:
NovoLog®: 100 units/mL (3 mL) [FlexPen® prefilled syringe or PenFill® prefilled cartridge]; (10 mL)

insulin aspart and insulin aspart protamine *see* insulin aspart protamine and insulin aspart *on this page*

insulin aspart protamine and insulin aspart
(IN soo lin AS part PROE ta meen & IN soo lin AS part)
Sound-Alike/Look-Alike Issues
NovoLog® Mix 70/30 may be confused with Novolin® 70/30
Synonyms insulin aspart and insulin aspart protamine
U.S./Canadian Brand Names NovoLog® Mix 70/30 [US]; NovoMix® 30 [Can]
Therapeutic Category Antidiabetic Agent, Insulin
Use Treatment of type 1 diabetes mellitus (insulin-dependent, IDDM); type 2 diabetes mellitus (noninsulin-dependent, NIDDM) to control hyperglycemia
Usual Dosage Refer to insulin regular monograph *on page 460*. Fixed ratio insulins (such as insulin aspart protamine and insulin aspart combination) are normally administered in 2 daily doses.
Dosage Forms
Injection, suspension:
NovoLog® Mix 70/30: Insulin aspart protamine suspension 70% [intermediate acting] and insulin aspart solution 30% [rapid acting]: 100 units/mL (3 mL) [PenFill® prefilled cartridge or FlexPen® prefilled syringe]; (10 mL) [vial]

insulin detemir (IN soo lin DE te mir)
Synonyms detemir insulin
U.S./Canadian Brand Names Levemir® [US/Can]
Therapeutic Category Antidiabetic Agent, Insulin
Use Treatment of type 1 diabetes mellitus (insulin-dependent, IDDM); type 2 diabetes mellitus (noninsulin-dependent, NIDDM) to control hyperglycemia
Usual Dosage Also refer to insulin regular *on page 460*.

Note: Duration is dose-dependent. Dosage must be carefully titrated (adjustment of dose and timing. Adjustment of concomitant antidiabetic treatment (short-acting insulins or oral antidiabetic agents) may be required. In Canada, insulin detemir is not approved for use in children.
(Continued)

insulin detemir *(Continued)*

SubQ: Children ≥6 years and Adults:

Basal insulin or basal-bolus (Type 1 or type 2 diabetes): May be substituted on a unit-per-unit basis. Adjust dose to achieve glycemic targets.

Insulin-naive patients (type 2 diabetes only): 0.1-0.2 units/kg once daily in the evening or 10 units once or twice daily. Adjust dose to achieve glycemic targets. Note: Canadian labeling recommends 10 units once daily (twice daily dosing is not included).

Dosage Forms

Injection, solution:

Levemir®: 100 units/mL (3 mL) [FlexPen® prefilled syringe]; (10 mL) [vial]

insulin glargine (IN soo lin GLAR jeen)

Sound-Alike/Look-Alike Issues

Lantus® may be confused with Lente®

Synonyms glargine insulin

U.S./Canadian Brand Names Lantus® OptiSet® [Can]; Lantus® [US/Can]

Therapeutic Category Antidiabetic Agent, Insulin

Use Treatment of type 1 diabetes mellitus (insulin-dependent, IDDM); type 2 diabetes mellitus (noninsulin-dependent, NIDDM) requiring basal (long-acting) insulin to control hyperglycemia

Usual Dosage SubQ: Adults:

Type 1 diabetes: As a basal component of combination insulin regimen, normally 50% to 75% of daily insulin requirement is administered as a long-acting form. More rapid acting forms are usually used in association with meals. Refer to insulin regular *on page 460.*

Type 2 diabetes:

Patient not already on insulin: 10 units once daily, adjusted according to patient response (range in clinical study: 2-100 units/day)

Patient already receiving insulin: In clinical studies, when changing to insulin glargine from once-daily NPH or Ultralente® insulin, the initial dose was not changed; when changing from twice-daily NPH to once-daily insulin glargine, the total daily dose was reduced by 20% and adjusted according to patient response

Dosage Forms

Injection, solution:

Lantus®: 100 units/mL (3 mL) [cartridge or Solostar® prefilled disposable pen]; (10 mL) [vial]

insulin glulisine (IN soo lin gloo LIS een)

Synonyms glulisine insulin

U.S./Canadian Brand Names Apidra® [US/Can]

Therapeutic Category Antidiabetic Agent, Insulin

Use Treatment of type 1 diabetes mellitus (insulin-dependent, IDDM); type 2 diabetes mellitus (noninsulin-dependent, NIDDM) to control hyperglycemia

Usual Dosage Refer to insulin regular *on page 460.* Insulin glulisine is a rapid-acting insulin analog which is normally administered as a premeal component of the insulin regimen. It is normally used along with a long-acting (basal) form of insulin.

SubQ: When used in a meal-related treatment regimen, 50% to 70% of total daily insulin requirement may be provided by insulin glulisine (in divided doses) and the remainder provided by an intermediate- or long-acting insulin. Insulin glulisine may also be administered by external subcutaneous infusion pumps.

I.V.: Under close medical supervision, insulin glulisine may be administered by infusion.

Dosage Forms

Injection, solution:

Apidra®: 100 units/mL (3 mL [cartridge], 10 mL [vial])

insulin inhalation (IN soo lin in ha LAY shun)

Synonyms inhaled insulin

U.S./Canadian Brand Names Exubera® [US/Can]

Therapeutic Category Antidiabetic Agent, Insulin

Use Treatment of type 1 diabetes mellitus (insulin-dependent, IDDM); type 2 diabetes mellitus (noninsulin-dependent, NIDDM)

Usual Dosage Inhalation: Children ≥6 years and Adults:

Initial: 0.05 mg/kg (rounded down to nearest whole milligram) 3 times/daily administered within 10 minutes of a meal

Adjustment: Dosage may be increased or decreased based on serum glucose monitoring, meal size, nutrient composition, time of day, and exercise patterns.

Note: A 1 mg blister is approximately equivalent to 3 units of regular insulin, while a 3 mg blister is approximately equivalent to 8 units of regular insulin administered subcutaneously. Patients should combine

1 mg and 3 mg blisters so that the fewest blisters are required to achieve the prescribed dose. Consecutive inhalation of three 1 mg blisters results in significantly higher insulin levels as compared to inhalation of a single 3 mg blister (do not substitute). In a patient stabilized on a dosage which uses 3 mg blisters, if 3 mg blister is temporarily unavailable, inhalation of two 1 mg blisters may be substituted.

Dosage Forms
Combination package:
Exubera® Kit [packaged with inhaler, chamber and release unit]:
 Powder for oral inhalation: 1 mg/blister (180s) and 3 mg/blister (90s)
Exubera® Combination Pack 15 [packaged with 2 release units]:
 Powder for oral inhalation: 1 mg/blister (180s) and 3 mg/blister (90s)
Exubera® Combination Pack 12 [packaged with 2 release units:]
 Powder for oral inhalation 1 mg/blister (90s) and 3 mg/blister (90s)

insulin lispro (IN soo lin LYE sproe)

Sound-Alike/Look-Alike Issues
Humalog® may be confused with Humulin®, Humira®
Synonyms lispro insulin
U.S./Canadian Brand Names Humalog® [US/Can]
Therapeutic Category Antidiabetic Agent, Insulin
Use Treatment of type 1 diabetes mellitus (insulin-dependent, IDDM); type 2 diabetes mellitus (noninsulin-dependent, NIDDM) to control hyperglycemia
 Note: In type 1 diabetes mellitus (insulin dependent, IDDM), insulin lispro (Humalog®) should be used in combination with a long-acting insulin. However, in type 2 diabetes mellitus (noninsulin-dependent, NIDDM), insulin lispro (Humalog®) may be used without a long-acting insulin when used in combination with a sulfonylurea.
Usual Dosage Refer to insulin regular monograph *on page 460.* Insulin lispro is equipotent to insulin regular, but has a more rapid onset.
Dosage Forms
Injection, solution:
Humalog®: 100 units/mL (3 mL) [prefilled cartridge or prefilled disposable pen]; (10 mL) [vial]

insulin lispro and insulin lispro protamine *see* insulin lispro protamine and insulin lispro *on this page*

insulin lispro protamine and insulin lispro

(IN soo lin LYE sproe PROE ta meen & IN soo lin LYE sproe)
Sound-Alike/Look-Alike Issues
Humalog® Mix 75/25™ may be confused with Humulin® 70/30.
Synonyms insulin lispro and insulin lispro protamine
U.S./Canadian Brand Names Humalog® Mix 25 [Can]; Humalog® Mix 50/50™ [US]; Humalog® Mix 75/25™ [US]
Therapeutic Category Antidiabetic Agent, Insulin
Use Treatment of type 1 diabetes mellitus (insulin-dependent, IDDM); type 2 diabetes mellitus (noninsulin-dependent, NIDDM) to control hyperglycemia
Usual Dosage Refer to insulin regular monograph *on page 460.* Fixed ratio insulins (such as insulin lispro protamine and insulin lispro) are normally administered in 2 daily doses.
Dosage Forms
Injection, suspension:
Humalog® Mix 50/50™: Insulin lispro protamine suspension 50% [intermediate acting] and insulin lispro solution 50% [rapid acting]: 100 units/mL (3 mL) [disposable pen]
Humalog® Mix 75/25™: Insulin lispro protamine suspension 75% [intermediate acting] and insulin lispro solution 25% [rapid acting]: 100 units/mL (3 mL) [disposable pen]; (10 mL) [vial]

insulin NPH (IN soo lin N P H)

Sound-Alike/Look-Alike Issues
Humulin® may be confused with Humalog®, Humira®
Novolin® may be confused with NovoLog®
Synonyms isophane insulin; NPH insulin
U.S./Canadian Brand Names Humulin® N [US/Can]; Novolin® ge NPH [Can]; Novolin® N [US]
Therapeutic Category Insulin, Intermediate-Acting
Use Treatment of type 1 diabetes mellitus (insulin-dependent, IDDM); type 2 diabetes mellitus (noninsulin-dependent, NIDDM) to control hyperglycemia
Usual Dosage Refer to insulin regular monograph *on page 460.* Insulin NPH is usually administered 1-2 times daily.
(Continued)

459

insulin NPH *(Continued)*

Dosage Forms [CAN] = Canadian brand name
Injection, suspension:
Humulin® N, Novolin® N: 100 units/mL (3 mL, 10 mL)
Novolin® ge NPH [CAN]: 100 units/mL (3 mL, 10 mL) [not available in the U.S.]

insulin NPH and insulin regular (IN soo lin N P H & IN soo lin REG yoo ler)

Sound-Alike/Look-Alike Issues
Humulin® 70/30 may be confused with Humalog® Mix 75/25
Novolin® 70/30 may be confused with NovoLog® Mix 70/30

Synonyms insulin regular and insulin NPH; isophane insulin and regular insulin; NPH insulin and regular insulin

U.S./Canadian Brand Names Humulin® 20/80 [Can]; Humulin® 50/50 [US]; Humulin® 70/30 [US/Can]; Novolin® 70/30 [US]; Novolin® ge 10/90 [Can]; Novolin® ge 20/80 [Can]; Novolin® ge 30/70 [Can]; Novolin® ge 40/60 [Can]; Novolin® ge 50/50 [Can]

Therapeutic Category Antidiabetic Agent, Insulin

Use Treatment of type 1 diabetes mellitus (insulin-dependent, IDDM); type 2 diabetes mellitus (noninsulin-dependent, NIDDM) to control hyperglycemia

Usual Dosage Refer to insulin regular monograph *on page 460.* Fixed ratio insulins are normally administered in 1-2 daily doses.

Dosage Forms
Injection, suspension:
Humulin® 50/50: Insulin NPH suspension 50% [intermediate acting] and insulin regular solution 50% [short acting]: 100 units/mL (10 mL)
Humulin® 70/30: Insulin NPH suspension 70% [intermediate acting] and insulin regular solution 30% [short acting]: 100 units/mL (3 mL, 10 mL)
Novolin® 70/30: Insulin NPH suspension 70% [intermediate acting] and insulin regular solution 30% [short acting]: 100 units/mL (3 mL, 10 mL)
Additional formulations available in Canada [not available in the U.S.]:
Injection, suspension:
Humulin® 20/80: Insulin regular solution 20% [short acting] and insulin NPH suspension 80% [intermediate acting]: 100 units/mL (3 mL)
Novolin® ge 10/90: Insulin regular solution 10% [short acting] and insulin NPH suspension 90% [intermediate acting]: 100 units/mL (3 mL)
Novolin® ge 20/80: Insulin regular solution 20% [short acting] and insulin NPH suspension 80% [intermediate acting]: 100 units/mL (3 mL)
Novolin® ge 30/70: Insulin regular solution 30% [short acting] and insulin NPH suspension 70% [intermediate acting]: 100 units/mL (3 mL)
Novolin® ge 40/60: Insulin regular solution 40% [short acting] and insulin NPH suspension 60% [intermediate acting]: 100 units/mL (3 mL)
Novolin® ge 50/50: Insulin regular solution 50% [short acting] and insulin NPH suspension 50% [intermediate acting]: 100 units/mL (3 mL)

insulin regular (IN soo lin REG yoo ler)

Sound-Alike/Look-Alike Issues
Humulin® may be confused with Humalog®, Humira®
Novolin® may be confused with NovoLog®

Synonyms regular insulin

U.S./Canadian Brand Names Humulin® R (Concentrated) U-500 [US]; Humulin® R [US/Can]; Novolin® ge Toronto [Can]; Novolin® R [US]

Therapeutic Category Antidiabetic Agent, Insulin; Antidote

Use Treatment of type 1 diabetes mellitus (insulin-dependent, IDDM); type 2 diabetes mellitus (noninsulin-dependent, NIDDM) unresponsive to treatment with diet and/or oral hypoglycemics, to control hyperglycemia; adjunct to parenteral nutrition; diabetic ketoacidosis (DKA)

Usual Dosage SubQ (regular insulin may also be administered I.V.): The number and size of daily doses, time of administration, and diet and exercise require continuous medical supervision. In addition, specific formulations may require distinct administration procedures.

Type 1 Diabetes Mellitus: Children and Adults: **Note:** Multiple daily doses guided by blood glucose monitoring are the standard of diabetes care. Combinations of insulin are commonly used.

Initial dose: 0.2-0.6 units/kg/day in divided doses. Conservative initial doses of 0.2-0.4 units/kg/day are often recommended to avoid the potential for hypoglycemia.

Division of daily insulin requirement: Generally, 50% to 75% of the daily insulin dose is given as an intermediate- or long-acting form of insulin (in 1-2 daily injections). The remaining portion of the 24-hour insulin requirement is divided and administered as a rapid-acting or short-acting form of insulin. These may be given with meals (before or at the time of meals depending on the form of insulin) or at the same time as injections of intermediate forms (some premixed combinations are intended for this purpose).

Adjustment of dose: Dosage must be titrated to achieve glucose control and avoid hypoglycemia. Adjust dose to maintain premeal and bedtime glucose of 80-140 mg/dL (children <5 years: 100-200 mg/dL). Since combinations of agents are frequently used, dosage adjustment must address the individual component of the insulin regimen which most directly influences the blood glucose value in question, based on the known onset and duration of the insulin component.

Usual maintenance range: 0.5-1.2 units/kg/day in divided doses. An estimate of anticipated needs may be based on body weight and/or activity factors as follows:

Adolescents: May require ≤1.5 units/kg/day during growth spurts

Nonobese: 0.4-0.6 units/kg/day

Obese: 0.8-1.2 units/kg/day

Renal failure: Due to alterations in pharmacokinetics of insulin, may require <0.2 units/kg/day

Type 2 Diabetes Mellitus:

Augmentation therapy: Dosage must be carefully adjusted.

Insulins other than glargine: Initial dosage of 0.15-0.2 units/kg/day have been recommended

Insulin glargine: Initial dose: 10 units/day

Note: Administered when residual beta-cell function is present, as a supplemental agent when oral hypoglycemics have not achieved goal glucose control. Twice daily NPH, or an evening dose of NPH, lente, or glargine insulin may be added to oral therapy with metformin or a sulfonylurea. Augmentation to control postprandial glucose may be accomplished with regular, glulisine, aspart, or lispro insulin.

Monotherapy: Initial dose: Highly variable: See Augmentation therapy dosing.

Note: An empirically-defined scheme for dosage estimation based on fasting plasma glucose and degree of obesity has been published with recommended doses ranging from 6-77 units/day. In the setting of glucose toxicity (loss of beta-cell sensitivity to glucose concentrations), insulin therapy may be used for short-term management to restore sensitivity of beta-cells; in these cases, the dose may need to be rapidly reduced/ withdrawn when sensitivity is reestablished.

Diabetic ketoacidosis:

Children <20 years:

I.V.: Regular insulin infused at 0.1 units/kg/hour; continue until acidosis clears, then decrease to 0.05 units/ kg/hour until SubQ replacement dosing can be initiated

SubQ, I.M.: If no I.V. infusion access, regular insulin 0.1 units/kg I.M. bolus followed by 0.1 units/kg/hour SubQ or I.M.; continue until acidosis clears, then decrease to 0.05 units/kg/hour until SubQ replacement dosing can be initiated

Adults:

I.V.: Regular insulin 0.15 units/kg initially followed by an infusion of 0.1 units/kg/hour

SubQ, I.M.: Regular insulin 0.4 units/kg given half as I.V. bolus and half as SubQ or I.M., followed by 0.1 units/kg/hour SubQ or I.M.

If serum glucose does not fall by 50-70 mg/dL in the first hour, double insulin dose hourly until glucose falls at an hourly rate of 50-70 mg/dL. Decrease dose to 0.05-0.1 units/kg/hour once serum glucose reaches 250 mg/dL.

Note: Newly-diagnosed patients with IDDM presenting in DKA and patients with blood sugars <800 mg/dL may be relatively "sensitive" to insulin and should receive loading and initial maintenance doses ~50% of those indicated.

Infusion should continue until reversal of acid-base derangement/ketonemia. Serum glucose is not a direct indicator of these abnormalities, and may decrease more rapidly than correction of the range of metabolic abnormalities.

Dosage Forms

Injection, solution:

Humulin® R: 100 units/mL (10 mL) [vial]

Novolin® R: 100 units/mL (3 mL) [InnoLet® prefilled syringe or PenFill® prefilled cartridge]; (10 mL) [vial]

Injection, solution [concentrate]:

Humulin® R U-500: 500 units/mL (20 mL vial)

insulin regular and insulin NPH *see* insulin NPH and insulin regular *on previous page*

Intal® [US/Can] *see* cromolyn sodium *on page 218*

Integrilin® [US/Can] *see* eptifibatide *on page 305*

Intensol® Solution *(Discontinued)* *see* metoclopramide *on page 561*

α-2-interferon *see* interferon alfa-2b *on next page*

interferon alfa-2a (PEG conjugate) *see* peginterferon alfa-2a *on page 658*

interferon alfa-2b and ribavirin combination pack *see* interferon alfa-2b and ribavirin *on page 463*

interferon alfa-2b (PEG conjugate) *see* peginterferon alfa-2b *on page 658*

interferon alfa-2a (in ter FEER on AL fa too aye)

Sound-Alike/Look-Alike Issues
interferon alfa-2a may be confused with interferon alfa-2b, interferon alfa-n3, pegylated interferon alfa-2b
Roferon-A® may be confused with Rocephin®

Synonyms IFLrA; interferon alpha-2a; NSC-367982; rIFN-A

U.S./Canadian Brand Names Roferon-A® [US/Can]

Therapeutic Category Biological Response Modulator

Use
Patients >18 years of age: Treatment of hairy cell leukemia, chronic hepatitis C
Children and Adults: Treatment of Philadelphia chromosome-positive (Ph+) chronic myelogenous leukemia (CML) in chronic phase, within 1 year of diagnosis (limited experience in children)

Usual Dosage Refer to individual protocols
Children (limited data): Ph+ chronic myelogenous leukemia (CML): I.M.: 2.5-5 million units/m^2/day; **Note:** In juveniles, higher dosages (30 million units/m^2/day) have been associated with severe adverse events, including death
Adults:
Hairy cell leukemia: SubQ: 3 million units/day for 16-24 weeks, then 3 million units 3 times/week for up to 6-24 months
Ph+ chronic myelogenous leukemia (CML): SubQ: 9 million units/day, continue treatment until disease progression **or** 3 million units/day for 3 days, followed by 6 million units/day for 3 days, followed by 9 million units daily until disease progression
Chronic hepatitis C: SubQ: 3 million units 3 times/week for 12 months **or** 6 million units 3 times/week for 12 weeks followed by 3 million units 3 times/week for 36 weeks

Dosage Forms
Injection, solution
Roferon-A®: 3 million units/0.5 mL (0.5 mL); 6 million units/0.5 mL (0.5 mL); 9 million units/0.5 mL (0.5 mL)

interferon alfa-2b (in ter FEER on AL fa too bee)

Sound-Alike/Look-Alike Issues
interferon alfa-2b may be confused with interferon alfa-2a, interferon alfa-n3, pegylated interferon alfa-2b
Intron® A may be confused with PEG-Intron®

Synonyms α-2-interferon; INF-alpha 2; interferon alpha-2b; NSC-377523; rLFN-α2

U.S./Canadian Brand Names Intron® A [US/Can]

Therapeutic Category Biological Response Modulator

Use
Patients ≥1 year of age: Chronic hepatitis B
Patients ≥3 years of age: Chronic hepatitis C (in combination with ribavirin)
Patients ≥18 years of age: Condyloma acuminata, chronic hepatitis B, chronic hepatitis C, hairy cell leukemia, malignant melanoma, AIDS-related Kaposi sarcoma, follicular non-Hodgkin lymphoma

Usual Dosage Refer to individual protocols. **Note:** Withhold treatment for ANC <500/mm^3 or platelets <25,000/mm^3. Consider premedication with acetaminophen prior to administration to reduce the incidence of some adverse reactions. Not all dosage forms and strengths are appropriate for all indications; refer to product labeling for details.
Children 1-17 years: Chronic hepatitis B: SubQ: 3 million units/m^2 3 times/week for 1 week; then 6 million units/m^2 3 times/week; maximum: 10 million units 3 times/week; total duration of therapy 16-24 weeks
Children ≥3 years: Chronic hepatitis C: In combination with ribavirin (refer to interferon alfa-2b/ribavirin combination pack monograph)
Adults:
Hairy cell leukemia: I.M., SubQ: 2 million units/m^2 3 times/week for up to 6 months (may continue treatment with continued treatment response)
Lymphoma (follicular): SubQ: 5 million units 3 times/week for up to 18 months
Malignant melanoma: Induction: 20 million units/m^2 I.V. for 5 consecutive days per week for 4 weeks, followed by maintenance dosing of 10 million units/m^2 SubQ 3 times/week for 48 weeks
AIDS-related Kaposi sarcoma: I.M., SubQ: 30 million units/m^2 3 times/week
Chronic hepatitis B: I.M., SubQ: 5 million units/day or 10 million units 3 times/week for 16 weeks
Chronic hepatitis C: I.M., SubQ: 3 million units 3 times/week for 16 weeks. In patients with normalization of ALT at 16 weeks, continue treatment for 18-24 months; consider discontinuation if normalization does not occur at 16 weeks. **Note:** May be used in combination therapy with ribavirin in previously untreated patients or in patients who relapse following alpha interferon therapy.
Condyloma acuminata: Intralesionally: 1 million units/lesion (maximum: 5 lesions/treatment) 3 times/week (on alternate days) for 3 weeks; may administer a second course at 12-16 weeks

Dosage Forms
Injection, powder for reconstitution [preservative free]
Intron® A: 10 million units; 18 million units; 50 million units

Injection, solution [multidose prefilled pen]:
Intron® A:
Delivers 3 million units/0.2 mL (1.5 mL)
Delivers 5 million units/0.2 mL (1.5 mL)
Delivers 10 million units/0.2 mL (1.5 mL)
Injection, solution [multidose vial]:
Intron® A: 6 million units/mL (3 mL); 10 million units/mL (2.5 mL)
Injection, solution [single-dose vial]:
Intron® A: 10 million units/ mL (1 mL)

interferon alfa-2b and ribavirin (in ter FEER on AL fa too bee & rye ba VYE rin)

Synonyms interferon alfa-2b and ribavirin combination pack; ribavirin and interferon alfa-2b combination pack
U.S./Canadian Brand Names Rebetron® [US]
Therapeutic Category Antiviral Agent; Biological Response Modulator
Use Combination therapy for the treatment of chronic hepatitis C in patients with compensated liver disease previously untreated with alpha interferon or who have relapsed after alpha interferon therapy
Usual Dosage
Children ≥3 years: Chronic hepatitis C: **Note:** Treatment duration may vary. Consult current guidelines and literature. Combination therapy:
Intron® A: SubQ:
25-61 kg: 3 million int. units/m^2 3 times/week
>61 kg: Refer to Adults dosing
Rebetol®: Oral: **Note:** Oral solution should be used in children 3-5 years of age, children ≤25 kg, or those unable to swallow capsules.
Capsule/solution: 15 mg/kg/day in 2 divided doses (morning and evening)
Capsule dosing recommendations:
25-36 kg: 400 mg/day (200 mg morning and evening)
37-49 kg: 600 mg/day (200 mg in the morning and two 200 mg capsules in the evening)
50-61 kg: 800 mg/day (two 200 mg capsules morning and evening)
>61 kg: Refer to Adults dosing
Adults: Chronic hepatitis C: Recommended dosage of combination therapy:
Intron® A: SubQ: 3 million int. units 3 times/week **and**
Rebetol® capsule: Oral:
≤75 kg (165 lb): 1000 mg/day (two 200 mg capsules in the morning and three 200 mg capsules in the evening)
>75 kg: 1200 mg/day (three 200 mg capsules in the morning and three 200 mg capsules in the evening)
Note: Treatment duration may vary. Consult current guidelines and literature.
Dosage Forms
Combination package:
Rebetron®:
For patients ≤75 kg [contains single-dose vials]:
Injection, solution: Interferon alfa-2b (Intron® A): 3 million int. units/0.5 mL (0.5 mL)
Capsule: Ribavirin (Rebetol®): 200 mg (70s)
For patients ≤75 kg [contains multidose vials]:
Injection, solution: Interferon alfa-2b (Intron® A): 3 million int. units/0.5 mL (3.8 mL)
Capsule: Ribavirin (Rebetol®): 200 mg (70s)
For patients ≤75 kg [contains multidose pen]:
Injection, solution: Interferon alfa-2b (Intron® A): 3 million int. units/0.2 mL (1.5 mL)
Capsule: Ribavirin (Rebetol®): 200 mg (70s)
For patients >75 kg [contains single-dose vials]:
Injection, solution: Interferon alfa-2b (Intron® A): 3 million int. units/0.5 mL (0.5 mL)
Capsule: Ribavirin (Rebetol®): 200 mg (84s)
For patients >75 kg [contains multidose vials]:
Injection, solution: Interferon alfa-2b (Intron® A): 3 million int. units/0.5 mL (3.8 mL)
Capsule: Ribavirin (Rebetol®): 200 mg (84s)
For patients >75 kg [contains multidose pen]:
Injection, solution: Interferon alfa-2b (Intron® A): 3 million int. units/0.2 mL (1.5 mL)
Capsule: Ribavirin (Rebetol®): 200 mg (84s)
For Rebetol® dose reduction [contains single-dose vials]:
Injection, solution: Interferon alfa-2b (Intron® A): 3 million int. units/0.5 mL (0.5 mL)
Capsule: Ribavirin (Rebetol®): 200 mg (42s)
For Rebetol® dose reduction [contains multidose vials]:
Injection, solution: Interferon alfa-2b (Intron® A): 3 million int. units/0.5 mL (3.8 mL)
Capsule: Ribavirin (Rebetol®): 200 mg (42s)
For Rebetol® dose reduction [contains multidose pen]:
Injection, solution: Interferon alfa-2b (Intron® A): 3 million int. units/0.2 mL (1.5 mL)
Capsule: Ribavirin (Rebetol®): 200 mg (42s)

interferon alfacon-1 (in ter FEER on AL fa con one)
Sound-Alike/Look-Alike Issues
interferon alfacon-1 may be confused with interferon alfa-2a, interferon alfa-2b, interferon alfa-n3, peginterferon alfa-2b
U.S./Canadian Brand Names Infergen® [US]
Therapeutic Category Interferon
Use Treatment of chronic hepatitis C virus (HCV) infection in patients ≥18 years of age with compensated liver disease and anti-HCV serum antibodies or HCV RNA.
Usual Dosage SubQ: Adults ≥18 years:
Chronic HCV infection: 9 mcg 3 times/week for 24 weeks; allow 48 hours between doses
Patients who have previously tolerated interferon therapy but did not respond or relapsed: 15 mcg 3 times/week for up to 48 weeks
Dose reduction for toxicity: Dose should be held in patients who experience a severe adverse reaction, and treatment should be stopped or decreased if the reaction does not become tolerable.
Doses were reduced from 9 mcg to 7.5 mcg in the pivotal study.
For patients receiving 15 mcg/dose, doses were reduced in 3 mcg decrements. Efficacy is decreased with doses <7.5 mcg
Dosage Forms
Injection, solution [preservative free]:
Infergen®: 30 mcg/mL (0.3 mL, 0.5 mL)

interferon alfa-n3 (in ter FEER on AL fa en three)
Sound-Alike/Look-Alike Issues
Alferon® may be confused with Alkeran®
U.S./Canadian Brand Names Alferon® N [US/Can]
Therapeutic Category Biological Response Modulator
Use Patients ≥18 years of age: Intralesional treatment of refractory or recurring genital or venereal warts (condylomata acuminata)
Usual Dosage Adults: Inject 250,000 units (0.05 mL) in each wart twice weekly for a maximum of 8 weeks; therapy should not be repeated for at least 3 months after the initial 8-week course of therapy
Dosage Forms
Injection, solution:
Alferon® N: 5 million int. units (1 mL)

interferon alpha-2a see interferon alfa-2a on page 462

interferon alpha-2b see interferon alfa-2b on page 462

interferon beta-1a (in ter FEER on BAY ta won aye)
Sound-Alike/Look-Alike Issues
Avonex® may be confused with Avelox®
Synonyms rIFN beta-1a
U.S./Canadian Brand Names Avonex® [US/Can]; Rebif® [US/Can]
Therapeutic Category Biological Response Modulator
Use Treatment of relapsing forms of multiple sclerosis (MS)
Usual Dosage Adults: **Note:** Analgesics and/or antipyretics may help decrease flu-like symptoms on treatment days:
I.M. (Avonex®): 30 mcg once weekly
SubQ (Rebif®): Doses should be separated by at least 48 hours:
Target dose 44 mcg 3 times/week:
Initial: 8.8 mcg (20% of final dose) 3 times/week for 8 weeks
Titration: 22 mcg (50% of final dose) 3 times/week for 8 weeks
Final dose: 44 mcg 3 times/week
Target dose 22 mcg 3 times/week:
Initial: 4.4 mcg (20% of final dose) 3 times/week for 8 weeks
Titration: 11 mcg (50% of final dose) 3 times/week for 8 weeks
Final dose: 22 mcg 3 times/week
Dosage Forms
Combination package [preservative free]:
Rebif® Titration Pack:
Injection, solution: 8.8 mcg/0.2 mL (0.2 mL) [6 prefilled syringes]
Injection, solution: 22 mcg/0.5 mL (0.5 mL) [6 prefilled syringes]

Injection, powder for reconstitution:
Avonex®: 33 mcg [6.6 million units; provides 30 mcg/mL following reconstitution]
Injection, solution:
Avonex®: 30 mcg/0.5 mL (0.5 mL)
Injection, solution [preservative free]:
Rebif®: 22 mcg/0.5 mL (0.5 mL) [prefilled syringe]; 44 mcg/0.5 mL (0.5 mL) [prefilled syringe]

interferon beta-1b (in ter FEER on BAY ta won bee)
Synonyms rIFN beta-1b
U.S./Canadian Brand Names Betaseron® [US/Can]
Therapeutic Category Biological Response Modulator
Use Treatment of relapsing forms of multiple sclerosis (MS); treatment of first clinical episode with MRI features consistent with MS
Usual Dosage SubQ: **Note:** Gradual dose-titration, analgesics, and/or antipyretics may help decrease flu-like symptoms on treatment days:
Adults: Initial: 0.0625 mg (2 million units; 0.25 mL) every other day; gradually increase dose by 0.0625 every 2 weeks
Target dose: 0.25 mg (8 million units; 1 mL) every other day
Dosage Forms
Injection, powder for reconstitution [preservative free]:
Betaseron®: 0.3 mg [9.6 million units] [prefilled syringe]

interferon gamma-1b (in ter FEER on GAM ah won bee)
U.S./Canadian Brand Names Actimmune® [US/Can]
Therapeutic Category Biological Response Modulator
Use Reduce frequency and severity of serious infections associated with chronic granulomatous disease; delay time to disease progression in patients with severe, malignant osteopetrosis
Usual Dosage If severe reactions occur, reduce dose by 50% or therapy should be interrupted until adverse reaction abates.

Children: Severe, malignant osteopetrosis: SubQ:
BSA ≤0.5 m^2: 1.5 mcg/kg/dose 3 times/week
BSA >0.5 m^2: 50 mcg/m^2 (1 million int. units/m^2) 3 times/week
Children and Adults: Chronic granulomatous disease: SubQ:
BSA ≤0.5 m^2: 1.5 mcg/kg/dose 3 times/week
BSA >0.5 m^2: 50 mcg/m^2 (1 million int. units/m^2) 3 times/week

Note: Previously expressed as 1.5 million units/m^2; 50 mcg is equivalent to 1 million int. units/m^2.
Dosage Forms
Injection, solution [preservative free]:
Actimmune®: 100 mcg [2 million int. units] (0.5 mL)

interleukin-1 receptor antagonist *see* anakinra *on page 55*

interleukin-2 *see* aldesleukin *on page 26*

interleukin-11 *see* oprelvekin *on page 632*

Intralipid® [US/Can] *see* fat emulsion *on page 343*

intravenous fat emulsion *see* fat emulsion *on page 343*

intrifiban *see* eptifibatide *on page 305*

Intron® A [US/Can] *see* interferon alfa-2b *on page 462*

Intropaste [US] *see* barium *on page 94*

Intropin® *(Discontinued)* *see* dopamine *on page 276*

Invanz® [US/Can] *see* ertapenem *on page 308*

Invega™ [US] *see* paliperidone *on page 646*

Inversine® [US/Can] *see* mecamylamine *on page 534*

Invirase® [US/Can] *see* saquinavir *on page 776*

Iodex [US-OTC] *see* iodine *on this page*

Iodex-p® *(Discontinued)* *see* povidone-iodine *on page 704*

iodine (EYE oh dyne)
Sound-Alike/Look-Alike Issues
iodine may be confused with codeine, Iopidine®, Lodine®
(Continued)

iodine (Continued)

U.S./Canadian Brand Names Iodex [US-OTC]; Iodoflex™ [US]; Iodosorb® [US]

Therapeutic Category Topical Skin Product

Use Used topically as an antiseptic in the management of minor, superficial skin wounds and has been used to disinfect the skin preoperatively

Usual Dosage

Topical:

Cleaning wet ulcers and wounds (Iodosorb®, Iodoflex™): Apply to clean wound; maximum: 50 g/application and 150 g/week. Change dressing ~3 times/week; reduce applications as exudate decreases. Do not use for >3 months; discontinue when wound is free of exudate.

Antiseptic for minor cuts, scrapes, burns: Apply small amount to affected area 1- 3 times/day

Oral: RDA:

Children:

1-8 years: 90 mcg/day

9-13 years: 120 mcg/day

≥14 years: Refer to adult dosing

Adults: 150 mcg/day

Pregnancy: 220 mcg/day

Breast-feeding: 290 mcg/day

Dosage Forms

Dressing, topical [gel pad]:

Iodoflex™: 0.9% (5 g, 10 g)

Gel, topical:

Iodosorb®: 0.9% (40 g)

Ointment, topical:

Iodex [OTC]: 4.7% (30 g, 720 g)

Tincture, topical: 2% (30 mL, 480 mL); 7% (30 mL, 480 mL)

iodine *see* trace metals *on page 855*

iodine I 131 tositumomab and tositumomab *see* tositumomab and iodine I 131 tositumomab *on page 852*

iodipamide meglumine (eye oh DI pa mide MEG loo meen)

U.S./Canadian Brand Names Cholografin® Meglumine [US]

Therapeutic Category Iodinated Contrast Media; Radiological/Contrast Media, Ionic

Use Contrast medium for intravenous cholangiography and cholecystography

Dosage Forms

Injection, solution:

Cholografin® Meglumine: 52% (20 mL)

iodipamide meglumine and diatrizoate meglumine *see* diatrizoate meglumine and iodipamide meglumine *on page 250*

iodixanol (EYE oh dix an ole)

U.S./Canadian Brand Names Visipaque™ [US]

Therapeutic Category Iodinated Contrast Media; Radiological/Contrast Media, Nonionic

Use

Intra-arterial: Digital subtraction angiography, angiocardiography, peripheral arteriography, visceral arteriography, cerebral arteriography

Intravenous: Contrast enhanced computed tomography imaging, excretory urography, and peripheral venography

Usual Dosage

Children >1 year: **Note:** Maximum recommended total dose of iodine: Not been established

Intra-arterial (cerebral, cardiac chambers, and related major arteries and visceral studies): Iodixanol 320 mg iodine/mL: 1-2 mL/kg; maximum dose: 4 mL/kg

I.V. (contrast-enhanced computer tomography or excretory urography): Iodixanol 270 mg iodine /mL: 1-2 mL/kg; maximum dose: 2 mL/kg

Children >12 years and Adults: **Note:** Maximum recommended total dose of iodine: 80 g

Intra-arterial: Iodixanol 320 mg iodine/mL: Dose individualized based on injection site and study type; refer to product labeling

I.V.: Iodixanol 270 mg and 320 mg iodine/mL: concentration and dose vary based on study type; refer to product labeling.

Dosage Forms
Injection, solution [preservative free]:
Visipaque™ 270: 550 mg/mL (50 mL, 100 mL, 125 mL, 150 mL, 200 mL)
Visipaque™ 320: 652 mg/mL (50 mL, 100 mL, 125 mL, 150 mL, 200 mL)

iodochlorhydroxyquin and flumethasone *see* clioquinol and flumethasone *(Canada only) on*
page 201

Iodoflex™ [US] *see* iodine *on page 465*

Iodopen® [US] *see* trace metals *on page 855*

iodoquinol (eye oh doe KWIN ole)

Synonyms diiodohydroxyquin
U.S./Canadian Brand Names Diodoquin® [Can]; Yodoxin® [US]
Therapeutic Category Amebicide
Use Treatment of acute and chronic intestinal amebiasis; asymptomatic cyst passers; *Blastocystis hominis*
infections; ineffective for amebic hepatitis or hepatic abscess
Usual Dosage Oral:
Children: 30-40 mg/kg/day (maximum: 650 mg/dose) in 3 divided doses for 20 days; not to exceed 1.95 g/day
Adults: 650 mg 3 times/day after meals for 20 days; not to exceed 1.95 g/day
Dosage Forms
Tablet:
Yodoxin®: 210 mg, 650 mg

iodoquinol and hydrocortisone (eye oh doe KWIN ole & hye droe KOR ti sone)

Sound-Alike/Look-Alike Issues
Vytone® may be confused with Hytone®, Zydone®
Synonyms hydrocortisone and iodoquinol
U.S./Canadian Brand Names Dermazene® [US]; Vytone® [US]
Therapeutic Category Antifungal/Corticosteroid
Use Treatment of eczema; infectious dermatitis; chronic eczematoid otitis externa; mycotic dermatoses
Usual Dosage Apply 3-4 times/day
Dosage Forms
Cream: Iodoquinol 1% and hydrocortisone 1% (30 g)
Dermazene®: Iodoquinol 1% and hydrocortisone 1% (30 g, 45 g)
Vytone®: Iodoquinol 1% and hydrocortisone 1% (30 g)

Iodosorb® [US] *see* iodine *on page 465*

iohexol (eye oh HEX ole)

U.S./Canadian Brand Names Omnipaque™ [US]
Therapeutic Category Polypeptide Hormone; Radiological/Contrast Media, Nonionic
Use
Intrathecal: Myelography; contrast enhancement for computerized tomography
Intravascular: Angiocardiography, aortography, digital subtraction angiography, peripheral arteriography,
excretory urography; contrast enhancement for computed tomographic imaging
Oral/body cavity: Arthrography, GI tract examination, hysterosalpingography, pancreatography, cholangio-
pancreatography, herniography, cystourethrography; enhanced computed tomography of the abdomen
Dosage Forms
Solution, injection [preservative free]:
Omnipaque™:
140: 302 mg/mL (50 mL)
180: 388 mg/mL (10 mL, 20 mL)
240: 518 mg/mL (10 mL, 20 mL, 100 mL, 150 mL, 200 mL)
300: 647 mg/mL (10 mL, 30 mL, 50 mL, 75 mL, 100 mL, 125 mL, 150 mL, 200 mL)
350: 755 mg/mL (50 mL, 75 mL, 100 mL, 125 mL, 150 mL, 200 mL, 250 mL)

Ionamin® [US/Can] *see* phentermine *on page 674*

Ionil® [US-OTC] *see* salicylic acid *on page 772*

Ionil® Plus [US-OTC] *see* salicylic acid *on page 772*

Ionil T® [US-OTC] *see* coal tar *on page 208*

Ionil T® Plus [US-OTC] *see* coal tar *on page 208*

Ionsys™ [US] *see* fentanyl *on page 346*

iopamidol (eye oh PA mi dole)

U.S./Canadian Brand Names Isovue Multipack® [US]; Isovue-M® [US]; Isovue® [US]

Therapeutic Category Iodinated Contrast Media; Radiological/Contrast Media, Nonionic

Use

Intrathecal (Isovue-M®): Neuroradiology; contrast enhancement of computed tomographic cisternography and ventriculography; thoraco-lumbar myelography

Intravascular (Isovue®, Isovue Multipack®): Angiography, excretory urography; contrast enhancement of computed tomographic imaging; evaluation of certain malignancies; image enhancement of non-neoplastic lesions

Dosage Forms

Injection, solution:

Isovue®:

200: 41% (50 mL, 100 mL, 200 mL)

250: 51% (50 mL, 100 mL, 150 mL, 200 mL)

300: 61% (30 mL, 50 mL, 75 mL, 100 mL, 125 mL, 150 mL, 175 mL)

370: 76% (20 mL, 30 mL, 50 mL, 75 mL, 100 mL, 125 mL, 150 mL, 175 mL, 200 mL)

Isovue-M®:

200: 41% (10 mL, 20 mL)

300: 61% (15 mL)

Isovue Multipack® [pharmacy bulk package]:

250: 51% (200 mL)

300: 61% (200 mL, 500 mL)

370: 76% (200 mL, 500 mL)

Iopidine® [US/Can] see apraclonidine on page 70

iopromide (eye oh PROE mide)

U.S./Canadian Brand Names Ultravist® [US]

Therapeutic Category Radiological/Contrast Media, Nonionic

Use Enhance imaging in cerebral arteriography and peripheral arteriography; coronary arteriography and left ventriculography, visceral angiography and aortography; contrast-enhanced computed tomographic imaging of the head and body, excretory urography, intraarterial digital subtraction angiography, peripheral venography

Usual Dosage

Children >2 years: I.V.:

Cardiac chambers and related arteries: 370 mg iodine/mL (1-2 mL/kg); maximum dose for procedure: 4 mL/kg

Contrast-enhanced CT: 300 mg iodine/mL (1-2 mL/kg); maximum dose for procedure: 3 mL/kg

Adults: **Note:** Maximum recommended total dose of iodine is 86 g. Individualize dose based upon patient's age, body weight, size of the vessel and the rate of blood flow within the vessel.

Intravascular:

Aortography and visceral angiography: 370 mg iodine/mL; maximum dose for procedure: 225 mL

Cerebral arteriography: 300 mg iodine/mL; maximum dose for procedure: 150 mL

Carotid artery visualization: 4-12 mL

Vertebral artery visualization: 4-12 mL

Aortic arch injection: 20-50 mL

Coronary arteriography and left ventriculography: 370 mg iodine/mL; maximum dose for procedure: 225 mL

Left coronary: 3-14 mL

Right coronary: 3-14 mL

Left ventricle: 30-60 mL

Intraarterial digital subtraction angiography: 150 mg iodine/mL; maximum dose for procedure: 250 mL

Carotid arteries: 6-10 mL

Vertebral: 4-8 mL

Aorta: 20-50 mL

Major branches of the abdominal aorta: 2-20 mL

Peripheral arteriography: 300 mg iodine/mL; maximum dose for procedure: 250 mL. **Note:** The artery needs a pulse to be injected.

Subclavian or femoral artery: 5-40 mL

Aortic bifurcation for distal runoff 25-50 mL

I.V.:

Contrast-enhanced CT: 300 mg iodine/mL:

Head: 50-200 mL; maximum dose for procedure: 200 mL

Body: 50-200 mL (usual dose for infusion is 100-200 mL); **Note:** Can be given by bolus injection, by rapid infusion, or both; maximum dose for procedure: 200 mL

Excretory urography (normal renal function): 300 mg iodine/mL (300 mg iodine/kg); maximum dose for procedure: 100 mL

Peripheral venography: 240 mg iodine/mL (minimum amount to clearly visualize the structure under examination); maximum dose for procedure: 250 mL

Dosage Forms
Injection, solution:
Ultravist®:
Iodine 150 mg/mL (provides iopromide 311.7 mg/mL) (50 mL)
Iodine 240 mg/mL (provides iopromide 498.72 mg/mL) (50 mL, 100 mL, 200 mL)
Iodine 300 mg/mL (provides iopromide 623.4 mg/mL) (50 mL, 100 mL, 150 mL, 500 mL)
Iodine 370 mg/mL (provides iopromide 768.86 mg/mL) (50 mL, 100 mL, 150 mL, 200 mL, 500 mL)

Iosat™ [US-OTC] *see* potassium iodide *on page 702*

iothalamate meglumine (eye oh thal A mate MEG loo meen)

U.S./Canadian Brand Names Conray® 30 [US]; Conray® 43 [US]; Conray® [US]; Cysto-Conray® II [US]
Therapeutic Category Iodinated Contrast Media; Radiological/Contrast Media, Ionic
Use
Solution for injection: Arthrography, cerebral angiography, cranial computerized angiotomography, digital subtraction angiography, direct cholangiography, endoscopic retrograde cholangiopancreatography, excretory urography, peripheral arteriography, urography, venography; contrast enhancement of computed tomographic images
Solution for instillation: Retrograde cystography and cystourethrography
Dosage Forms
Injection, solution:
Conray®: 60% (30 mL, 50 mL, 100 mL, 150 mL)
Conray® 30: 30% (50 mL, 150 mL)
Conray® 43: 43% (50 mL, 100 mL, 200 mL, 250 mL)
Injection, solution for instillation:
Cysto-Conray® II: 17.2% (250 mL, 500 mL)

iothalamate sodium (eye oh thal A mate SOW dee um)

U.S./Canadian Brand Names Conray® 400 [US]
Therapeutic Category Iodinated Contrast Media; Radiological/Contrast Media, Ionic
Use Excretory urography, angiocardiography, aortography; contrast enhancement of computed tomographic brain images
Dosage Forms
Injection, solution:
Conray® 400: 66.8% (50 mL)

ioversol (EYE oh ver sole)

U.S./Canadian Brand Names Optiray® [US]
Therapeutic Category Iodinated Contrast Media; Radiological/Contrast Media, Nonionic
Use Arteriography, angiography, angiocardiography, ventriculography, excretory urography, and venography procedures; contrast enhanced tomographic imaging
Dosage Forms
Injection, solution [preservative free]:
Optiray®:
160: 34% (50 mL)
240: 51% (50 mL, 100 mL, 125 mL, 200 mL, 500 mL)
300: 64% (50 mL, 100 mL, 150 mL, 200 mL)
320: 68% (20 mL, 30 mL, 50 mL, 75 mL, 100 mL, 125 mL, 150 mL, 200 mL, 250 mL)
350: 74% (50 mL, 75 mL, 100 mL, 150 mL, 200 mL, 250 mL, 500 mL)

ioxaglate meglumine and ioxaglate sodium
(eye ox AG late MEG loo meen & eye ox AG late SOW dee um)
Synonyms ioxaglate sodium and ioxaglate meglumine
U.S./Canadian Brand Names Hexabrix™ [US]
Therapeutic Category Iodinated Contrast Media; Radiological/Contrast Media, Ionic
Use Angiocardiography, arteriography, aortography, arthrography, angiography, hysterosalpingography, venography, and urography procedures; contrast enhancement of computed tomographic imaging
(Continued)

ioxaglate meglumine and ioxaglate sodium *(Continued)*

Dosage Forms
Injection, solution:
Hexabrix™: Ioxaglate meglumine 39.3% and ioxaglate sodium 19.6% (20 mL, 50 mL, 100 mL, 150 mL, 200 mL)

ioxaglate sodium and ioxaglate meglumine *see* ioxaglate meglumine and ioxaglate sodium *on previous page*

ioxilan *(eye OKS ee lan)*

U.S./Canadian Brand Names Oxilan® 300 [Can]; Oxilan® 350 [Can]; Oxilan® [US]
Therapeutic Category Iodinated Contrast Media; Radiological/Contrast Media, Nonionic
Use
Intraarterial: Ioxilan 300 mgI/mL is indicated for cerebral arteriography. Ioxilan 350 mgI/mL is indicated for coronary arteriography and left ventriculography, visceral angiography, aortography, and peripheral arteriography

Intravenous: Both products are indicated for excretory urography and contrast-enhanced computed tomographic (CECT) imaging of the head and body
Usual Dosage Adults:
Intraarterial: Coronary arteriography and left ventriculography: For visualization of coronary arteries and left ventricle, ioxilan injection with a concentration of 350 mg iodine/mL is recommended
Usual injection volumes:
Left and right coronary: 2-10 mL (0.7-3.5 g iodine)
Left ventricle: 25-50 mL (8.75-17.5 g iodine)
Total doses should not exceed 250 mL; the injection rate of ioxilan should approximate the flow rate in the vessel injected
Cerebral arteriography: For evaluation of arterial lesions of the brain, a concentration of 300 mg iodine/mL is indicated
Recommended doses: 8-12 mL (2.4-3.6 g iodine)
Total dose should not exceed 150 mL
Dosage Forms
Injection, solution [preservative free]:
Oxilan®: 300: 62% (50 mL, 100 mL, 150 mL, 200 mL); 350: 73% (50 mL, 100 mL, 150 mL, 200 mL)

ipecac syrup *(IP e kak SIR up)*

Synonyms syrup of ipecac
Therapeutic Category Antidote
Use Treatment of acute oral drug overdosage and in certain poisonings
Usual Dosage Oral:
Children:
6-12 months: 5-10 mL followed by 10-20 mL/kg of water; repeat dose one time if vomiting does not occur within 20 minutes
1-12 years: 15 mL followed by 10-20 mL/kg of water; repeat dose one time if vomiting does not occur within 20 minutes
If emesis does not occur within 30 minutes after second dose, ipecac must be removed from stomach by gastric lavage
Adults: 15-30 mL followed by 200-300 mL of water; repeat dose one time if vomiting does not occur within 20 minutes
Dosage Forms
Syrup: 70 mg/mL (30 mL)

I-Pentolate® *(Discontinued)* *see* cyclopentolate *on page 221*

I-Phrine® Ophthalmic Solution *(Discontinued)* *see* phenylephrine *on page 675*

I-Picamide® *(Discontinued)* *see* tropicamide *on page 871*

Iplex™ [US] *see* mecasermin *on page 535*

IPM Wound Gel™ [US-OTC] *see* hyaluronate and derivatives *on page 423*

IPOL® [US/Can] *see* poliovirus vaccine (inactivated) *on page 693*

ipratropium *(i pra TROE pee um)*

Sound-Alike/Look-Alike Issues
Atrovent® may be confused with Alupent®

Synonyms ipratropium bromide

U.S./Canadian Brand Names Alti-Ipratropium [Can]; Apo-Ipravent® [Can]; Atrovent® HFA [US/Can]; Atrovent® [US/Can]; Gen-Ipratropium [Can]; Novo-Ipramide [Can]; Nu-Ipratropium [Can]; PMS-Ipratropium [Can]

Therapeutic Category Anticholinergic Agent

Use Anticholinergic bronchodilator used in bronchospasm associated with COPD, bronchitis, and emphysema; symptomatic relief of rhinorrhea associated with the common cold and allergic and nonallergic rhinitis

Usual Dosage
Nebulization:
Infants and Children ≤12 years: 125-250 mcg 3 times/day
Children >12 years and Adults: 500 mcg (one unit-dose vial) 3-4 times/day with doses 6-8 hours apart

Oral inhalation: MDI:
Children 3-12 years: 1-2 inhalations 3 times/day, up to 6 inhalations/24 hours
Children >12 years and Adults: 2 inhalations 4 times/day, up to 12 inhalations/24 hours

Intranasal: Nasal spray:
Symptomatic relief of rhinorrhea associated with the common cold (safety and efficacy of use beyond 4 days in patients with the common cold have not been established):
Children 5-11 years: 0.06%: 2 sprays in each nostril 3 times/day
Children ≥12 years and Adults: 0.06%: 2 sprays in each nostril 3-4 times/day
Symptomatic relief of rhinorrhea associated with allergic/nonallergic rhinitis: Children ≥6 years and Adults: 0.03%: 2 sprays in each nostril 2-3 times/day

Dosage Forms
Aerosol for oral inhalation:
Atrovent® HFA: 17 mcg/actuation (12.9 g)
Solution for nebulization: 0.02% (2.5 mL)
Solution, intranasal [spray]:
Atrovent®: 0.03% (30 mL); 0.06% (15 mL)

ipratropium and albuterol (i pra TROE pee um & al BYOO ter ole)

Sound-Alike/Look-Alike Issues
Combivent® may be confused with Combivir®

Synonyms albuterol and ipratropium; salbutamol and ipratropium

U.S./Canadian Brand Names CO Ipra-Sal [Can]; Combivent® [US/Can]; DuoNeb™ [US]; Gen-Combo Sterinebs [Can]

Therapeutic Category Bronchodilator

Use Treatment of COPD in those patients who are currently on a regular bronchodilator who continue to have bronchospasms and require a second bronchodilator

Usual Dosage Adults:
Inhalation: 2 inhalations 4 times/day (maximum: 12 inhalations/24 hours)
Inhalation via nebulization: Initial: 3 mL every 6 hours (maximum: 3 mL every 4 hours)

Dosage Forms
Aerosol for oral inhalation:
Combivent®: Ipratropium 18 mcg and albuterol 103 mcg per actuation [200 doses] (14.7 g)
Solution for nebulization: Ipratropium 0.5 mg [0.017%] and albuterol 2.5 mg [0.083%] per 3 mL (30s, 60s)
DuoNeb™: Ipratropium 0.5 mg [0.017%] and albuterol 2.5 mg [0.083%] per 3 mL (30s, 60s)

ipratropium bromide *see* ipratropium *on previous page*

I-Prin [US-OTC] *see* ibuprofen *on page 444*

iproveratril hydrochloride *see* verapamil *on page 887*

IPV *see* poliovirus vaccine (inactivated) *on page 693*

Iquix® [US] *see* levofloxacin *on page 501*

irbesartan (ir be SAR tan)

Sound-Alike/Look-Alike Issues
Avapro® may be confused with Anaprox®

U.S./Canadian Brand Names Avapro® [US/Can]

Therapeutic Category Angiotensin II Receptor Antagonist

Use Treatment of hypertension alone or in combination with other antihypertensives; treatment of diabetic nephropathy in patients with type 2 diabetes mellitus (noninsulin-dependent, NIDDM) and hypertension

Usual Dosage Oral:
Hypertension:
Children: ≥6-12 years: Initial: 75 mg once daily; may be titrated to a maximum of 150 mg once daily
Children ≥13 years and Adults: 150 mg once daily; patients may be titrated to 300 mg once daily
Note: Starting dose in volume-depleted patients should be 75 mg
(Continued)

irbesartan *(Continued)*

Nephropathy in patients with type 2 diabetes and hypertension: Adults: Target dose: 300 mg once daily

Dosage Forms
Tablet:
Avapro®: 75 mg, 150 mg, 300 mg

irbesartan and hydrochlorothiazide (ir be SAR tan & hye droe klor oh THYE a zide)

Sound-Alike/Look-Alike Issues
Avalide® may be confused with Avandia®
Synonyms Avapro® HCT; hydrochlorothiazide and irbesartan
U.S./Canadian Brand Names Avalide® [US/Can]
Therapeutic Category Antihypertensive Agent, Combination
Use Combination therapy for the management of hypertension

Note: In Canada, this combination product is approved for initial therapy in severe, essential hypertension (sitting diastolic blood pressure [DBP] ≥110 mmHg).

Usual Dosage Oral: Adults: Dose must be individualized. A patient who is not controlled with either agent alone may be switched to the combination product. Mean effect increases with the dose of each component. The lowest dosage available is irbesartan 150 mg/hydrochlorothiazide 12.5 mg. Dose increases should be made not more frequently than every 2-4 weeks.

Canadian dosing (not approved in U.S.): Severe hypertension: Initial: Combination product irbesartan 150 mg/hydrochlorothiazide 12.5 mg once daily. Titrate dose after 2-4 weeks, if needed, to a maximum dose of irbesartan 300 mg/hydrochlorothiazide 25 mg once daily.

Dosage Forms
Tablet:
Avalide®: Irbesartan 150 mg and hydrochlorothiazide 12.5 mg; irbesartan 300 mg and hydrochlorothiazide 12.5 mg; irbesartan 300 mg and hydrochlorothiazide 25 mg

Ircon® [US-OTC] *see* ferrous fumarate *on page 349*

IRESSA® [US] *see* gefitinib *on page 385*

irinotecan (eye rye no TEE kan)

Synonyms camptothecin-11; CPT-11; NSC-616348
U.S./Canadian Brand Names Camptosar® [US/Can]; Irinotecan Hydrochloride Trihydrate [Can]
Therapeutic Category Antineoplastic Agent
Use Treatment of metastatic carcinoma of the colon or rectum
Usual Dosage I.V. (Refer to individual protocols): **Note:** A reduction in the starting dose by one dose level should be considered for patients ≥65 years of age, prior pelvic/abdominal radiotherapy, performance status of 2, homozygosity for UGT1A1*28 allele, or increased bilirubin (dosing for patients with a bilirubin >2 mg/dL cannot be recommended based on lack of data per manufacturer).

Single-agent therapy:
125 mg/m^2 over 90 minutes on days 1, 8, 15, and 22, followed by a 2-week rest
Adjusted dose level -1: 100 mg/m^2
Adjusted dose level -2: 75 mg/m^2
Once-every-3-week regimen: 350 mg/m^2 over 90 minutes, once every 3 weeks
Adjusted dose level -1: 300 mg/m^2
Adjusted dose level -2: 250 mg/m^2
Depending on the patient's ability to tolerate therapy, doses should be adjusted in increments of 25-50 mg/m^2. Irinotecan doses may range from 50-150 mg/m^2 for the weekly regimen. Patients may be dosed as low as 200 mg/m^2 (in 50 mg/m^2 decrements) for the once-every-3-week regimen.

Combination therapy with fluorouracil and leucovorin: Six-week (42-day) cycle:
Regimen 1: 125 mg/m^2 over 90 minutes on days 1, 8, 15, and 22; to be given in combination with bolus leucovorin and fluorouracil (leucovorin administered immediately following irinotecan; fluorouracil immediately following leucovorin)
Adjusted dose level -1: 100 mg/m^2
Adjusted dose level -2: 75 mg/m^2
Regimen 2: 180 mg/m^2 over 90 minutes on days 1, 15, and 29; to be given in combination with infusional leucovorin and bolus/infusion fluorouracil (leucovorin administered immediately following irinotecan; fluorouracil immediately following leucovorin)
Adjusted dose level -1: 150 mg/m^2
Adjusted dose level -2: 120 mg/m^2

Note: For all regimens: It is recommended that new courses begin only after the granulocyte count recovers to ≥1500/mm^3, the platelet count recovers to ≥100,000/mm^3, and treatment-related diarrhea has fully resolved. Treatment should be delayed 1-2 weeks to allow for recovery from treatment-related toxicities. If the patient has not recovered after a 2-week delay, consideration should be given to discontinuing irinotecan.

Dosage Forms
Injection, solution:
Camptosar®: 20 mg/mL (2 mL, 5 mL)

Irinotecan Hydrochloride Trihydrate [Can] *see* irinotecan *on previous page*

iron dextran complex (EYE ern DEKS tran KOM pleks)

Sound-Alike/Look-Alike Issues
Dexferrum® may be confused with Desferal®

U.S./Canadian Brand Names Dexferrum® [US]; Dexiron™ [Can]; INFeD® [US]; Infufer® [Can]

Therapeutic Category Electrolyte Supplement, Oral

Use Treatment of microcytic hypochromic anemia resulting from iron deficiency in patients in whom oral administration is infeasible or ineffective

Usual Dosage I.M. (Z-track method should be used for I.M. injection), I.V.:
A 0.5 mL test dose (0.25 mL in infants) should be given prior to starting iron dextran therapy; total dose should be divided into a daily schedule for I.M., total dose may be given as a single continuous infusion
Iron-deficiency anemia:
Children 5-15 kg: Should not normally be given in the first 4 months of life:
Dose (mL) = 0.0442 (desired hemoglobin - observed hemoglobin) x W + (0.26 x W)
Desired hemoglobin: Usually 12 g/dL
W = Total body weight in kg
Children >15 kg and Adults:
Dose (mL) = 0.0442 (desired hemoglobin - observed hemoglobin) x LBW + (0.26 x LBW)
Desired hemoglobin: Usually 14.8 g/dL
LBW = Lean body weight in kg
Iron replacement therapy for blood loss: Replacement iron (mg) = blood loss (mL) x hematocrit

Maximum daily dosage:
Manufacturer's labeling: **Note:** Replacement of larger estimated iron deficits may be achieved by serial administration of smaller incremental dosages. Daily dosages should be limited to:
Children:
5-15 kg: 50 mg iron (1 mL)
15-50 kg: 100 mg iron (2 mL)
Adults >50 kg: 100 mg iron (2 mL)

Dosage Forms
Injection, solution:
Dexferrum®: 50 mg/mL (1 mL, 2 mL)
INFeD®: 50 mg/mL (2 mL)

iron fumarate *see* ferrous fumarate *on page 349*

iron gluconate *see* ferrous gluconate *on page 349*

iron-polysaccharide complex *see* polysaccharide-iron complex *on page 697*

iron sucrose (EYE ern SOO krose)

U.S./Canadian Brand Names Venofer® [US/Can]

Therapeutic Category Iron Salt

Use Treatment of iron-deficiency anemia in chronic renal failure, including nondialysis-dependent patients (with or without erythropoietin therapy) and dialysis-dependent patients receiving erythropoietin therapy

Usual Dosage Doses expressed in mg of **elemental** iron. **Note:** Test dose: Product labeling does not indicate need for a test dose in product-naive patients.
I.V.: Adults: Iron-deficiency anemia in chronic renal disease:
Hemodialysis-dependent patient: 100 mg (5 mL of iron sucrose injection) administered 1-3 times/week during dialysis; administer no more than 3 times/week to a cumulative total dose of 1000 mg (10 doses); may continue to administer at lowest dose necessary to maintain target hemoglobin, hematocrit, and iron storage parameters
Peritoneal dialysis-dependent patient: Slow intravenous infusion at the following schedule: Two infusions of 300 mg each over 1½ hours 14 days apart followed by a single 400 mg infusion over 2½ hours 14 days later (total cumulative dose of 1000 mg in 3 divided doses)
Nondialysis-dependent patient: 200 mg slow injection (over 2-5 minutes) on 5 different occasions within a 14-day period. Total cumulative dose: 1000 mg in 14-day period. **Note:** Dosage has also been administered as two infusions of 500 mg in a maximum of 250 mL 0.9% NaCl infused over 3.5-4 hours on day 1 and day 14 (limited experience)
(Continued)

iron sucrose *(Continued)*

Dosage Forms
  Injection, solution [preservative free]:
    Venofer®: 20 mg of elemental iron/mL (5 mL)

iron sulfate *see* ferrous sulfate *on page 350*

iron sulfate and vitamin C *see* ferrous sulfate and ascorbic acid *on page 350*

Isagel® [US-OTC] *see* alcohol (ethyl) *on page 25*

ISD *see* isosorbide dinitrate *on page 476*

ISDN *see* isosorbide dinitrate *on page 476*

ISG *see* immune globulin (intramuscular) *on page 450*

ISMN *see* isosorbide mononitrate *on page 476*

Ismo® [US] *see* isosorbide mononitrate *on page 476*

isoamyl nitrite *see* amyl nitrite *on page 55*

isobamate *see* carisoprodol *on page 154*

Isocal® [US-OTC] *see* nutritional formula, enteral/oral *on page 622*

isocarboxazid (eye soe kar BOKS a zid)

U.S./Canadian Brand Names Marplan® [US]
Therapeutic Category Antidepressant, Monoamine Oxidase Inhibitor
Use Treatment of depression
Usual Dosage Oral: Adults: 10 mg 2-3 times/day; reduce to 10-20 mg/day in divided doses when condition
  improves
Dosage Forms
  Tablet:
    Marplan®: 10 mg

Isochron™ [US] *see* isosorbide dinitrate *on page 476*

isoflurane (eye soe FLURE ane)

Sound-Alike/Look-Alike Issues
  isoflurane may be confused with enflurane, isoflurophate
U.S./Canadian Brand Names Forane® [US/Can]; Terrell™ [US]
Therapeutic Category General Anesthetic
Use Induction and maintenance of general anesthesia
Usual Dosage Inhalation: Adults:
  Anesthesia: Minimum alveolar concentration (MAC), the concentration at which 50% of patients do not
    respond to surgical incision, is 1.15% (44 years of age) for isoflurane.
  Induction: 1.5% to 3%
  Maintenance: In nitrous oxide: 1% to 2.5%; in oxygen: 1.5% to 3.5%
Dosage Forms
  Liquid, for inhalation: >99.9% (100 mL, 250 mL)
    Forane®, Terrell™: >99.9% (100 mL, 250 mL)

isometheptene, acetaminophen, and dichloralphenazone *see* acetaminophen, isometheptene,
and dichloralphenazone *on page 13*

isometheptene, dichloralphenazone, and acetaminophen *see* acetaminophen, isometheptene,
and dichloralphenazone *on page 13*

IsonaRif™ [US] *see* rifampin and isoniazid *on page 757*

isoniazid (eye soe NYE a zid)

Synonyms INH; isonicotinic acid hydrazide
U.S./Canadian Brand Names Isotamine® [Can]; PMS-Isoniazid [Can]
Therapeutic Category Antitubercular Agent
Use Treatment of susceptible tuberculosis infections; treatment of latent tuberculosis infection (LTBI)

Usual Dosage Recommendations often change due to resistant strains and newly-developed information; consult *MMWR* for current CDC recommendations:

Oral (injectable is available for patients who are unable to either take or absorb oral therapy):

Infants and Children:
Treatment of latent TB infection (LTBI): 10-20 mg/kg/day in 1-2 divided doses (maximum: 300 mg/day) or 20-40 mg/kg (maximum: 900 mg/dose) twice weekly for 9 months
Treatment of active TB infection:
Daily therapy: 10-15 mg/kg/day in 1-2 divided doses (maximum: 300 mg/day)
Twice weekly directly observed therapy (DOT): 20-30 mg/kg (maximum: 900 mg)

Adults:
Treatment of latent tuberculosis infection (LTBI): 300 mg/day or 900 mg twice weekly for 6-9 months in patients who do not have HIV infection (9 months is optimal, 6 months may be considered to reduce costs of therapy) and 9 months in patients who have HIV infection. Extend to 12 months of therapy if interruptions in treatment occur.
Treatment of active TB infection (drug susceptible):
Daily therapy: 5 mg/kg/day given daily (usual dose: 300 mg/day); 10 mg/kg/day in 1-2 divided doses in patients with disseminated disease
Twice weekly directly observed therapy (DOT): 15 mg/kg (maximum: 900 mg); 3 times/week therapy: 15 mg/kg (maximum: 900 mg)
Note: Treatment may be defined by the number of doses administered (eg, "six-month" therapy involves 192 doses of INH and rifampin, and 56 doses of pyrazinamide). Six months is the shortest interval of time over which these doses may be administered, assuming no interruption of therapy.
Note: Concomitant administration of 6-50 mg/day pyridoxine is recommended in malnourished patients or those prone to neuropathy (eg, alcoholics, diabetics)

Dosage Forms
Syrup: 50 mg/5 mL
Tablet: 100 mg, 300 mg

isoniazid and rifampin *see* rifampin and isoniazid *on page 757*

isoniazid, rifampin, and pyrazinamide *see* rifampin, isoniazid, and pyrazinamide *on page 758*

isonicotinic acid hydrazide *see* isoniazid *on previous page*

isonipecaine hydrochloride *see* meperidine *on page 542*

isophane insulin *see* insulin NPH *on page 459*

isophane insulin and regular insulin *see* insulin NPH and insulin regular *on page 460*

isophosphamide *see* ifosfamide *on page 447*

isoproterenol (eye soe proe TER e nole)

Sound-Alike/Look-Alike Issues
Isuprel® may be confused with Disophrol®, Ismelin®, Isordil®
Synonyms isoproterenol hydrochloride
U.S./Canadian Brand Names Isuprel® [US]
Therapeutic Category Adrenergic Agonist Agent
Use Ventricular arrhythmias due to AV nodal block; hemodynamically compromised bradyarrhythmias or atropine- and dopamine-resistant bradyarrhythmias (when transcutaneous/venous pacing is not available); temporary use in third-degree AV block until pacemaker insertion
Usual Dosage I.V.: Cardiac arrhythmias:
Children: Initial: 0.1 mcg/kg/minute (usual effective dose 0.2-2 mcg/kg/minute)
Adults: Initial: 2 mcg/minute; titrate to patient response (2-10 mcg/minute)
Dosage Forms
Injection, solution: 0.02 mg/mL (10 mL); 0.2 mg/mL (1:5000) (1 mL, 5 mL)
Isuprel®: 0.02 mg/mL (10 mL); 0.2 mg/mL (1:5000) (1 mL, 5 mL)

isoproterenol hydrochloride *see* isoproterenol *on this page*

Isoptin® *(Discontinued)* *see* verapamil *on page 887*

Isoptin® SR [US/Can] *see* verapamil *on page 887*

Isopto® Atropine [US/Can] *see* atropine *on page 83*

Isopto® Carbachol [US/Can] *see* carbachol *on page 146*

Isopto® Carpine [US/Can] *see* pilocarpine *on page 682*

Isopto® Cetapred® *(Discontinued)*

Isopto® Eserine [Can] *see* physostigmine *on page 681*

Isopto® Eserine *(Discontinued)* *see* physostigmine *on page 681*

Isopto® Frin Ophthalmic Solution *(Discontinued)* *see* phenylephrine *on page 675*

Isopto® **Homatropine [US]** *see* homatropine *on page 421*

Isopto® **Hyoscine [US]** *see* scopolamine derivatives *on page 778*

Isopto® **Plain Solution** *(Discontinued)* *see* artificial tears *on page 75*

Isopto® **Tears [US-OTC/Can]** *see* hydroxypropyl methylcellulose *on page 439*

Isordil® **[US]** *see* isosorbide dinitrate *on this page*

isosorbide dinitrate (eye soe SOR bide dye NYE trate)

Sound-Alike/Look-Alike Issues
Isordil® may be confused with Inderal®, Isuprel®
Synonyms ISD; ISDN
U.S./Canadian Brand Names Apo-ISDN® [Can]; Cedocard®-SR [Can]; Coronex® [Can]; Dilatrate®-SR [US]; Isochron™ [US]; Isordil® [US]; Novo-Sorbide [Can]; PMS-Isosorbide [Can]
Therapeutic Category Vasodilator
Use Prevention and treatment of angina pectoris; for congestive heart failure; to relieve pain, dysphagia, and spasm in esophageal spasm with GE reflux
Usual Dosage Oral: Adults:
Angina: 5-40 mg 4 times/day or 40 mg every 8-12 hours in sustained-release dosage form
Sublingual: 2.5-5 mg every 5-10 minutes for maximum of 3 doses in 15-30 minutes; may also use prophylactically 15 minutes prior to activities which may provoke an attack
Congestive heart failure:
Initial dose: 20 mg 3-4 times per day
Target dose: 120-160 mg/day in divided doses; use in combination with hydralazine
Tolerance to nitrate effects develops with chronic exposure: Dose escalation does not overcome this effect. Tolerance can only be overcome by short periods of nitrate absence from the body. Short periods (10-12 hours) of nitrate withdrawal help minimize tolerance. General recommendations are to take the last dose of short-acting agents no later than 7 PM; administer 2-3 times/day rather than 4 times/day. Sustained release preparations could be administered at times to allow a 15- to 17-hour interval between first and last daily dose. Example: Administer sustained release at 8 AM and 2 PM for a twice daily regimen.
Dosage Forms
Capsule, sustained release:
Dilatrate®-SR: 40 mg
Tablet: 5 mg, 10 mg, 20 mg, 30 mg
Isordil®: 5 mg, 40 mg
Tablet, extended release:
Isochron™: 40 mg
Tablet, sublingual: 2.5 mg, 5 mg

isosorbide dinitrate and hydralazine (eye soe SOR bide dye NYE trate & hye DRAL a zeen)

Synonyms hydralazine and isosorbide dinitrate
U.S./Canadian Brand Names BiDil® [US]
Therapeutic Category Vasodilator
Use Treatment of heart failure, adjunct to standard therapy, in self-identified African-Americans
Usual Dosage Oral: Adults: Initial: 1 tablet 3 times/day; titrate to a maximum dose of 2 tablets 3 times/day
Dosage Forms
Tablet:
BiDil®: Isosorbide 20 mg and hydralazine 37.5 mg

isosorbide mononitrate (eye soe SOR bide mon oh NYE trate)

Sound-Alike/Look-Alike Issues
Imdur® may be confused with Imuran®, Inderal LA®, K-Dur®
Monoket® may be confused with Monopril®
Synonyms ISMN
U.S./Canadian Brand Names Apo-ISMN [Can]; Imdur® [US/Can]; Ismo® [US]; Monoket® [US]
Therapeutic Category Vasodilator
Use Long-acting metabolite of the vasodilator isosorbide dinitrate used for the prophylactic treatment of angina pectoris
Usual Dosage Adults and Geriatrics (start with lowest recommended dose): Oral:
Regular tablet: 5-20 mg twice daily with the two doses given 7 hours apart (eg, 8 AM and 3 PM) to decrease tolerance development; then titrate to 10 mg twice daily in first 2-3 days.
Extended release tablet: Initial: 30-60 mg given in morning as a single dose; titrate upward as needed, giving at least 3 days between increases; maximum daily single dose: 240 mg
Tolerance to nitrate effects develops with chronic exposure. Dose escalation does not overcome this effect. Tolerance can only be overcome by short periods of nitrate absence from the body. Short periods (10-12

hours) of nitrate withdrawal help minimize tolerance. Recommended dosage regimens incorporate this interval. General recommendations are to take the last dose of short-acting agents no later than 7 PM; administer 2 times/day rather than 4 times/day. Administer sustained release tablet once daily in the morning.

Dosage Forms
Tablet: 10 mg, 20 mg
Ismo®: 20 mg
Monoket®: 10 mg, 20 mg
Tablet, extended release: 30 mg, 60 mg, 120 mg
Imdur®: 30 mg, 60 mg, 120 mg

Isotamine® [Can] *see* isoniazid *on page 474*

isotretinoin (eye soe TRET i noyn)
Sound-Alike/Look-Alike Issues
Accutane® may be confused with Accolate®, Accupril®
Synonyms 13-*cis*-retinoic acid
U.S./Canadian Brand Names Accutane® [US/Can]; Amnesteem™ [US]; Claravis™ [US]; Clarus™ [Can]; Isotrex® [Can]; Sotret® [US]
Therapeutic Category Retinoic Acid Derivative
Use Treatment of severe recalcitrant nodular acne unresponsive to conventional therapy
Usual Dosage Oral: Children 12-17 years and Adults: Severe recalcitrant nodular acne: 0.5-1 mg/kg/day in 2 divided doses (dosages as low as 0.05 mg/kg/day have been reported to be beneficial) for 15-20 weeks or until the total cyst count decreases by 70%, whichever is sooner. Adults with very severe disease/scarring or primarily involves the trunk may require dosage adjustment up to 2 mg/kg/day. A second course of therapy may be initiated after a period of ≥2 months off therapy.
Dosage Forms
Capsule:
Accutane®, Amnesteem™, Claravis™: 10 mg, 20 mg, 40 mg
Sotret®: 10 mg, 20 mg, 30 mg, 40 mg

Isotrex® [Can] *see* isotretinoin *on this page*

Isovue® [US] *see* iopamidol *on page 468*

Isovue-M® [US] *see* iopamidol *on page 468*

Isovue Multipack® [US] *see* iopamidol *on page 468*

isoxsuprine (eye SOKS syoo preen)
Sound-Alike/Look-Alike Issues
Vasodilan® may be confused with Vasocidin®
Synonyms isoxsuprine hydrochloride
Therapeutic Category Vasodilator
Use Treatment of peripheral vascular diseases, such as arteriosclerosis obliterans and Raynaud disease
Usual Dosage Oral: Adults: 10-20 mg 3-4 times/day
Dosage Forms
Tablet: 10 mg, 20 mg

isoxsuprine hydrochloride *see* isoxsuprine *on this page*

isradipine (iz RA di peen)
Sound-Alike/Look-Alike Issues
DynaCirc® may be confused with Dynabac®, Dynacin®
U.S./Canadian Brand Names DynaCirc® CR [US]; DynaCirc® [Can]
Therapeutic Category Calcium Channel Blocker
Use Treatment of hypertension
Usual Dosage Oral: Adults:
Capsule: 2.5 mg twice daily; antihypertensive response occurs in 2-3 hours; maximal response in 2-4 weeks; increase dose at 2- to 4-week intervals at 2.5-5 mg increments; usual dose range (JNC 7): 2.5-10 mg/day in 2 divided doses. **Note:** Most patients show no improvement with doses >10 mg/day except adverse reaction rate increases; therefore, maximal dose in older adults should be 10 mg/day.
Controlled release tablet: 5 mg once daily; antihypertensive response occurs in 2 hours. Adjust dose in increments of 5 mg at 2-4 week intervals. Maximum dose 20 mg/day; adverse events are increased at doses >10 mg/day.
(Continued)

isradipine *(Continued)*

Dosage Forms
Tablet, controlled release:
DynaCirc® CR: 5 mg, 10 mg

Istalol™ [US] *see* timolol *on page 843*

Isuprel® [US] *see* isoproterenol *on page 475*

Itch-X® [US-OTC] *see* pramoxine *on page 706*

itraconazole (i tra KOE na zole)

Sound-Alike/Look-Alike Issues
Sporanox® may be confused with Suprax®
U.S./Canadian Brand Names Sporanox® [US/Can]
Therapeutic Category Antifungal Agent
Use Treatment of susceptible fungal infections in immunocompromised and immunocompetent patients including blastomycosis and histoplasmosis; indicated for aspergillosis, and onychomycosis of the toenail; treatment of onychomycosis of the fingernail without concomitant toenail infection via a pulse-type dosing regimen; has activity against *Aspergillus, Candida, Coccidioides, Cryptococcus, Sporothrix,* tinea unguium

Oral: Useful in superficial mycoses including dermatophytoses (eg, tinea capitis), pityriasis versicolor, sebopsoriasis, vaginal and chronic mucocutaneous candidiases; systemic mycoses including candidiasis, meningeal and disseminated cryptococcal infections, paracoccidioidomycosis, coccidioidomycoses; miscellaneous mycoses such as sporotrichosis, chromomycosis, leishmaniasis, fungal keratitis, alternariosis, zygomycosis
Oral solution: Treatment of oral and esophageal candidiasis
Intravenous solution: Indicated in the treatment of blastomycosis, histoplasmosis (nonmeningeal), and aspergillosis (in patients intolerant or refractory to amphotericin B therapy); empiric therapy of febrile neutropenic fever

Usual Dosage
Usual dosage ranges:
Children: Efficacy and safety have not been established; a small number of patients 3-16 years of age have been treated with 100 mg/day for systemic fungal infections with no serious adverse effects reported. A dose of 5 mg/kg once daily was used in a pharmacokinetic study using the oral solution in patients 6 months to 12 years; duration of study was 2 weeks.
Adults: Oral, I.V.: 100-400 mg/day; doses >200 mg/day are given in 2 divided doses; length of therapy varies from 1 day to >6 months depending on the condition and mycological response
Indication-specific dosing:
Adults:
Aspergillosis:
Oral: 200-400 mg/day
I.V.: 200 mg twice daily for 4 doses, followed by 200 mg daily
Blastomycosis/histoplasmosis:
Oral: 200 mg once daily, if no obvious improvement or there is evidence of progressive fungal disease, increase the dose in 100 mg increments to a maximum of 400 mg/day; doses >200 mg/day are given in 2 divided doses; length of therapy varies from 1 day to >6 months depending on the condition and mycological response
I.V.: 200 mg twice daily for 4 doses, followed by 200 mg/day
Brain abscess: Cerebral phaeohyphomycosis (dematiaceous): Oral: 200 mg twice daily for at least 6 months with amphotericin
Candidiasis:
Oropharyngeal: Oral solution: 200 mg once daily for 1-2 weeks; in patients unresponsive or refractory to fluconazole: 100 mg twice daily (clinical response expected in 1-2 weeks)
Esophageal: Oral solution: 100-200 mg once daily for a minimum of 3 weeks; continue dosing for 2 weeks after resolution of symptoms
Coccidioides: Oral: 200 mg twice daily
Infections, life-threatening:
Oral: 200 mg 3 times/day (600 mg/day) should be given for the first 3 days of therapy
I.V.: 200 mg twice daily for 4 doses, followed by 200 mg/day
Meningitis: *Coccidioides:* Oral: 400-800 mg/day
Onychomycosis: Oral: 200 mg once daily for 12 consecutive weeks
Pneumonia: *Coccidioides:* Mild to moderate: Oral, I.V.: 200 mg twice daily
Protothecal infection: 200 mg once daily for 2 months
Sporotrichosis: Oral:
Lymphocutaneous: 100-200 mg/day for 3-6 months
Osteoarticular and pulmonary: 200 mg twice daily for 1-2 years (may use amphotericin B initially for stabilization)

Dosage Forms
Capsule:
Sporanox®: 100 mg
Injection, solution:
Sporanox®: 10 mg/mL (25 mL)
Solution, oral:
Sporanox®: 100 mg/10 mL

I-Tropine® *(Discontinued)* *see* atropine *on page 83*

Iveegam EN [US] *see* immune globulin (intravenous) *on page 451*

Iveegam Immuno® [Can] *see* immune globulin (intravenous) *on page 451*

ivermectin (eye ver MEK tin)
U.S./Canadian Brand Names Stromectol® [US]
Therapeutic Category Antibiotic, Miscellaneous
Use Treatment of the following infections: Strongyloidiasis of the intestinal tract due to the nematode parasite *Strongyloides stercoralis*. Onchocerciasis due to the nematode parasite *Onchocerca volvulus*. Ivermectin is only active against the immature form of *Onchocerca volvulus*, and the intestinal forms of *Strongyloides stercoralis*.
Usual Dosage Oral: Children ≥15 kg and Adults:
Strongyloidiasis: 200 mcg/kg as a single dose; follow-up stool examinations
Onchocerciasis: 150 mcg/kg as a single dose; retreatment may be required every 3-12 months until the adult worms die
Dosage Forms
Tablet [scored]:
Stromectol®: 3 mg

IVIG *see* immune globulin (intravenous) *on page 451*

IvyBlock® [US-OTC] *see* bentoquatam *on page 99*

Ivy-Rid® [US-OTC] *see* benzocaine *on page 101*

IvySoothe® [US-OTC] *see* hydrocortisone (topical) *on page 434*

Jamp® Travel Tablet [Can] *see* dimenhydrinate *on page 262*

Janimine® *(Discontinued)* *see* imipramine *on page 449*

Jantoven™ [US] *see* warfarin *on page 899*

Janumet™ [US] *see* sitagliptin and metformin *on page 789*

Januvia™ [US] *see* sitagliptin *on page 789*

Japanese encephalitis virus vaccine (inactivated)
(jap a NEESE en sef a LYE tis VYE rus vak SEEN, in ak ti VAY ted)
U.S./Canadian Brand Names JE-VAX® [US/Can]
Therapeutic Category Vaccine, Inactivated Virus
Use Active immunization against Japanese encephalitis
Usual Dosage U.S. recommended primary immunization schedule:
Children 1-3 years: SubQ: Three 0.5 mL doses given on days 0, 7, and 30
Children >3 years and Adults: SubQ: Three 1 mL doses given on days 0, 7, and 30
Booster dose: Give after 2 years, or according to current recommendation
Abbreviated dosing schedule: Three recommended doses, given on days 0, 7, and 14 with the last dose given at least 10 days before travel. Alternately, two doses given 1 week apart provide immunity in ~80% of patients. Abbreviated schedules should be used only when necessary due to time constraints.
Dosage Forms
Injection, powder for reconstitution:
JE-VAX®: Nakayama-NIH strain (1 mL)

Jenamicin® *(Discontinued)* *see* gentamicin *on page 390*

Jenest™-28 *(Discontinued)* *see* ethinyl estradiol and norethindrone *on page 328*

JE-VAX® [US/Can] *see* Japanese encephalitis virus vaccine (inactivated) *on this page*

Jolessa™ [US] *see* ethinyl estradiol and levonorgestrel *on page 325*

Jolivette™ [US] *see* norethindrone *on page 611*

Junel™ [US] *see* ethinyl estradiol and norethindrone *on page 328*

Junel™ Fe [US] *see* ethinyl estradiol and norethindrone *on page 328*

Just for Kids™ **[US-OTC]** *see* fluoride *on page 361*

Just Tears® **Solution** *(Discontinued) see* artificial tears *on page 75*

Juvederm™ **24HV [US]** *see* hyaluronate and derivatives *on page 423*

Juvederm™ **30 [US]** *see* hyaluronate and derivatives *on page 423*

Juvederm™ **30HV [US]** *see* hyaluronate and derivatives *on page 423*

K-10® **[Can]** *see* potassium chloride *on page 700*

Kabikinase® *(Discontinued) see* streptokinase *on page 806*

Kadian® **[US/Can]** *see* morphine sulfate *on page 578*

Kala® **[US-OTC]** *see* Lactobacillus *on page 488*

Kalcinate® *(Discontinued) see* calcium gluconate *on page 141*

Kaletra® **[US/Can]** *see* lopinavir and ritonavir *on page 516*

Kalmz [US-OTC] *see* fructose, dextrose, and phosphoric acid *on page 378*

kanamycin (kan a MYE sin)

Sound-Alike/Look-Alike Issues
kanamycin may be confused with Garamycin®, gentamicin

Synonyms kanamycin sulfate

U.S./Canadian Brand Names Kantrex® [US/Can]

Therapeutic Category Aminoglycoside (Antibiotic)

Use Treatment of serious infections caused by susceptible strains of *E. coli, Proteus* species, *Enterobacter aerogenes, Klebsiella pneumoniae, Serratia marcescens*, and *Acinetobacter* species; second-line treatment of *Mycobacterium tuberculosis*

Usual Dosage Note: Dosing should be based on ideal body weight
Children: Infections: I.M., I.V.: 15 mg/kg/day in divided doses every 8-12 hours
Adults:
Infections: I.M., I.V.: 5-7.5 mg/kg/dose in divided doses every 8-12 hours (<15 mg/kg/day)
Intraperitoneal: After contamination in surgery: 500 mg
Irrigating solution: 0.25%; maximum 1.5 g/day (via all administration routes)
Aerosol: 250 mg 2-4 times/day

Dosage Forms
Injection, solution:
Kantrex®: 1 g/3 mL (3 mL)

kanamycin sulfate *see* kanamycin *on this page*

Kanka® **Soft Brush**™ **[US-OTC]** *see* benzocaine *on page 101*

Kantrex® **[US/Can]** *see* kanamycin *on this page*

Kaochlor-Eff® *(Discontinued)*

Kaochlor® **SF** *(Discontinued) see* potassium chloride *on page 700*

Kaodene® *(Discontinued)*

Kaodene® **NN** *(Discontinued)*

Kaon-Cl-10® **[US]** *see* potassium chloride *on page 700*

Kaon-Cl® **20 [US]** *see* potassium chloride *on page 700*

Kao-Paverin® **[US-OTC]** *see* loperamide *on page 515*

Kaopectate® **[US-OTC]** *see* bismuth *on page 113*

Kaopectate® **II** *(Discontinued) see* loperamide *on page 515*

Kaopectate® **Advanced Formula** *(Discontinued)*

Kaopectate® **Extra Strength [US-OTC]** *see* bismuth *on page 113*

Kaopectate® **Maximum Strength Caplets** *(Discontinued)*

Kao-Spen® *(Discontinued)*

Kao-Tin [US-OTC] *see* bismuth *on page 113*

Kapectolin [US-OTC] *see* bismuth *on page 113*

Kapectolin® *(Discontinued)*

Karidium® *(Discontinued) see* fluoride *on page 361*

Karigel® *(Discontinued) see* fluoride *on page 361*

Karigel®-N *(Discontinued)* *see* fluoride *on page 361*

Kariva™ [US] *see* ethinyl estradiol and desogestrel *on page 322*

Kasof® *(Discontinued)* *see* docusate *on page 273*

Kaybovite-1000® *(Discontinued)* *see* cyanocobalamin *on page 220*

Kay Ciel® [US] *see* potassium chloride *on page 700*

Kayexalate® [US/Can] *see* sodium polystyrene sulfonate *on page 797*

K-Citra® [Can] *see* potassium citrate *on page 701*

KCl *see* potassium chloride *on page 700*

K-Dur® [Can] *see* potassium chloride *on page 700*

K-Dur® 10 [US] *see* potassium chloride *on page 700*

K-Dur® 20 [US] *see* potassium chloride *on page 700*

Keflex® [US] *see* cephalexin *on page 167*

Keftab® [Can] *see* cephalexin *on page 167*

Kefurox® Injection *(Discontinued)* *see* cefuroxime *on page 165*

Kefzol® *(Discontinued)* *see* cefazolin *on page 158*

K-Electrolyte® Effervescent *(Discontinued)* *see* potassium bicarbonate *on page 699*

Kelnor™ [US] *see* ethinyl estradiol and ethynodiol diacetate *on page 324*

Kemadrin® [US] *see* procyclidine *on page 717*

Kemsol® [Can] *see* dimethyl sulfoxide *on page 263*

Kenacort® Oral *(Discontinued)*

Kenaject® Injection *(Discontinued)*

Kenalog® [US/Can] *see* triamcinolone (topical) *on page 863*

Kenalog-10® [US] *see* triamcinolone (systemic) *on page 862*

Kenalog-40® [US] *see* triamcinolone (systemic) *on page 862*

Kenalog® in Orabase [Can] *see* triamcinolone (topical) *on page 863*

Kenonel® Topical *(Discontinued)*

keoxifene hydrochloride *see* raloxifene *on page 742*

Kepivance™ [US] *see* palifermin *on page 646*

Keppra® [US/Can] *see* levetiracetam *on page 498*

Keralac™ [US] *see* urea *on page 877*

Keralac™ Nailstik [US] *see* urea *on page 877*

Keralyt® [US-OTC] *see* salicylic acid *on page 772*

Kerlone® [US] *see* betaxolol *on page 109*

Kerr Insta-Char® [US-OTC] *see* charcoal *on page 171*

Ketalar® [US/Can] *see* ketamine *on this page*

ketamine (KEET a meen)

Sound-Alike/Look-Alike Issues
Ketalar® may be confused with Kenalog®

Synonyms ketamine hydrochloride

U.S./Canadian Brand Names Ketalar® [US/Can]; Ketamine Hydrochloride Injection, USP [Can]

Therapeutic Category General Anesthetic

Controlled Substance C-III

Use Induction and maintenance of general anesthesia, especially when cardiovascular depression must be avoided (ie, hypotension, hypovolemia, cardiomyopathy, constrictive pericarditis); sedation; analgesia

Usual Dosage Used in combination with anticholinergic agents to decrease hypersalivation

Children:

Oral: 6-10 mg/kg for 1 dose (mixed in 0.2-0.3 mL/kg of cola or other beverage) given 30 minutes before the procedure

I.M.: 3-7 mg/kg

I.V.: Range: 0.5-2 mg/kg, use smaller doses (0.5-1 mg/kg) for sedation for minor procedures; usual induction dosage: 1-2 mg/kg

Continuous I.V. infusion: Sedation: 5-20 mcg/kg/minute

(Continued)

ketamine *(Continued)*

Adults:
I.M.: 3-8 mg/kg
I.V.: Range: 1-4.5 mg/kg; usual induction dosage: 1-2 mg/kg
Children and Adults: Maintenance: Supplemental doses of $\frac{1}{3}$ to $\frac{1}{2}$ of initial dose

Dosage Forms
Injection, solution: 50 mg/mL (10 mL); 100 mg/mL (5 mL)
Ketalar®: 10 mg/mL (20 mL); 50 mg/mL (10 mL); 100 mg/mL (5 mL)

ketamine hydrochloride *see* ketamine *on previous page*

Ketamine Hydrochloride Injection, USP [Can] *see* ketamine *on previous page*

Ketek® [US/Can] *see* telithromycin *on page 823*

ketoconazole (kee toe KOE na zole)

Sound-Alike/Look-Alike Issues
Nizoral® may be confused with Nasarel®, Neoral®, Nitrol®
U.S./Canadian Brand Names Apo-Ketoconazole® [Can]; Extina® [US]; Ketoderm® [Can]; Kuric™ [US]; Nizoral® A-D [US-OTC]; Nizoral® [US]; Novo-Ketoconazole [Can]; Xolegel™ [US/Can]
Therapeutic Category Antifungal Agent
Use
Systemic: Treatment of susceptible fungal infections, including candidiasis, oral thrush, blastomycosis, histo-plasmosis, paracoccidioidomycosis, coccidioidomycosis, chromomycosis, candiduria, chronic mucocuta-neous candidiasis, as well as certain recalcitrant cutaneous dermatophytoses
Topical:
Cream: Treatment of tinea corporis, tinea cruris, tinea versicolor, cutaneous candidiasis, seborrheic derma-titis
Foam, gel: Treatment of seborrheic dermatitis
Shampoo: Treatment of dandruff, seborrheic dermatitis, tinea versicolor
Usual Dosage
Oral:
Fungal infections:
Children ≥2 years: 3.3-6.6 mg/kg/day as a single dose for 1-2 weeks for candidiasis, for at least 4 weeks in recalcitrant dermatophyte infections, and for up to 6 months for other systemic mycoses
Adults: 200-400 mg/day as a single daily dose for durations as stated above
Shampoo: Seborrheic dermatitis, tinea versicolor: Children ≥12 years and Adults: Apply twice weekly for 4 weeks with at least 3 days between each shampoo
Topical:
Tinea infections: Adults: Cream: Rub gently into the affected area once daily. Duration of treatment: Tinea corporis, cruris: 2 weeks; tinea pedis: 6 weeks
Seborrheic dermatitis: Children ≥12 years and Adults:
Cream: Rub gently into the affected area twice daily for 4 weeks or until clinical response is noted
Foam: Apply to affected area twice daily for 4 weeks
Gel: Rub gently into the affected area once daily for 2 weeks
Dosage Forms
Aerosol, topical [foam]:
Extina®: 2% (50 g, 100 g)
Cream, topical: 2% (15 g, 30 g, 60 g)
Kuric™: 2%: (75 g)
Gel, topical:
Xolegel™: 2% (15 g)
Shampoo, topical: 1% (120 mL), 2% (120 mL)
Nizoral®: 2% (120 mL)
Nizoral® A-D: 1% (120 mL, 210 mL)
Tablet: 200 mg
Nizoral®: 200 mg

Ketoderm® [Can] *see* ketoconazole *on this page*

3-keto-desogestrel *see* etonogestrel *on page 336*

ketoprofen (kee toe PROE fen)

Sound-Alike/Look-Alike Issues
Oruvail® may be confused with Clinoril®, Elavil®

U.S./Canadian Brand Names Apo-Keto SR® [Can]; Apo-Keto-E® [Can]; Apo-Keto® [Can]; Novo-Keto [Can]; Novo-Keto-EC [Can]; Nu-Ketoprofen [Can]; Nu-Ketoprofen-E [Can]; Oruvail® [Can]; Rhodis SR™ [Can]; Rhodis-EC™ [Can]; Rhodis™ [Can]

Therapeutic Category Analgesic, Nonnarcotic; Nonsteroidal Antiinflammatory Drug (NSAID)

Use Acute and long-term treatment of rheumatoid arthritis and osteoarthritis; primary dysmenorrhea; mild-to-moderate pain

Usual Dosage Oral: Children ≥16 years and Adults:

Rheumatoid arthritis or osteoarthritis:

Capsule: 50-75 mg 3-4 times/day up to a maximum of 300 mg/day

Capsule, extended release: 200 mg once daily

Mild to moderate pain: Capsule: 25-50 mg every 6-8 hours up to a maximum of 300 mg/day

OTC labeling: 12.5 mg every 4-6 hours, up to a maximum of 6 tablets/24 hours

Dosage Forms

Capsule, regular release: 50 mg, 75 mg

Capsule, extended release: 200 mg

ketorolac (KEE toe role ak)

Sound-Alike/Look-Alike Issues

Acular® may be confused with Acthar®, Ocular®

Toradol® may be confused with Foradil®, Inderal®, Tegretol®, Torecan®, tramadol

Synonyms ketorolac tromethamine

U.S./Canadian Brand Names Acular LS™ [US/Can]; Acular® PF [US]; Acular® [US/Can]; Apo-Ketorolac Injectable® [Can]; Apo-Ketorolac® [Can]; Ketorolac Tromethamine Injection, USP [Can]; Novo-Ketorolac [Can]; ratio-Ketorolac [Can]; Toradol® IM [Can]; Toradol® [US/Can]

Therapeutic Category Analgesic, Nonnarcotic; Nonsteroidal Antiinflammatory Drug (NSAID)

Use

Oral, injection: Short-term (≤5 days) management of moderate-to-severe acute pain requiring analgesia at the opioid level

Ophthalmic: Temporary relief of ocular itching due to seasonal allergic conjunctivitis; postoperative inflammation following cataract extraction; reduction of ocular pain and photophobia following incisional refractive surgery; reduction of ocular pain, burning, and stinging following corneal refractive surgery

Usual Dosage

Children 2-16 years: **Do not exceed adult doses**

Single-dose treatment:

I.M.: 1 mg/kg (maximum: 30 mg)

I.V.: 0.5 mg/kg (maximum: 15 mg)

Children ≥16 years and Adults (pain relief usually begins within 10 minutes with parenteral forms): **Note:** The maximum combined duration of treatment (for parenteral and oral) is 5 days; do not increase dose or frequency; supplement with low-dose opioids if needed for breakthrough pain.

I.M.: 60 mg as a single dose or 30 mg every 6 hours (maximum daily dose: 120 mg)

I.V.: 30 mg as a single dose or 30 mg every 6 hours (maximum daily dose: 120 mg)

Oral: 20 mg, followed by 10 mg every 4-6 hours; do not exceed 40 mg/day; oral dosing is intended to be a continuation of I.M. or I.V. therapy only

Ophthalmic: Children ≥3 years and Adults:

Allergic conjunctivitis (relief of ocular itching) (Acular®): Instill 1 drop (0.25 mg) 4 times/day for seasonal allergic conjunctivitis

Inflammation following cataract extraction (Acular®): Instill 1 drop (0.25 mg) to affected eye(s) 4 times/day beginning 24 hours after surgery; continue for 2 weeks

Pain and photophobia following incisional refractive surgery (Acular® PF): Instill 1 drop (0.25 mg) 4 times/day to affected eye for up to 3 days

Pain following corneal refractive surgery (Acular LS™): Instill 1 drop 4 times/day as needed to affected eye for up to 4 days

Dosage Forms

Injection, solution: 15 mg/mL (1 mL); 30 mg/mL (1 mL, 2 mL, 10 mL)

Solution, ophthalmic:

Acular®: 0.5% (3 mL, 5 mL, 10 mL)

Acular LS™: 0.4% (5 mL)

Acular® P.F. [preservative free]: 0.5% (0.4 mL)

Tablet: 10 mg

ketorolac tromethamine see ketorolac on this page

Ketorolac Tromethamine Injection, USP [Can] see ketorolac on this page

ketotifen (kee toe TYE fen)

Synonyms ketotifen fumarate

U.S./Canadian Brand Names Alaway™ [US-OTC]; Apo-Ketotifen® [Can]; Novo-Ketotifen [Can]; Zaditen® [Can]; Zaditor® [US-OTC/Can]

Therapeutic Category Antihistamine, H₁ Blocker, Ophthalmic

Use

Ophthalmic: Temporary prevention of eye itching due to allergic conjunctivitis

Oral (Canadian use - not approved in U.S.): Adjunctive therapy in the chronic treatment of pediatric patients ≥6 months of age with mild, atopic asthma

Usual Dosage Ophthalmic: Children ≥3 years and Adults: Instill 1 drop into the affected eye(s) twice daily, every 8-12 hours

Dosage Forms [CAN] = Canadian brand name

Solution, ophthalmic [drops]: 0.025% (5 mL)

Alaway™ [OTC]: 0.025% (10 mL)

Zaditor® [OTC]: 0.025% (5 mL)

Syrup: 1 mg/5 mL (250 mL) [not available in U.S.]

Novo-Ketotifen® [CAN]: 1 mg/5 mL (250 mL) [not available in U.S.]

Nu-Ketotifen® [CAN]: 1 mg/5 mL (250 mL) [not available in U.S.]

Zaditen® [CAN]: 1 mg/5 mL (250 mL) [not available in U.S.]

Tablet: 1 mg [not available in U.S.]

Novo-ketotifen® [CAN]: 1 mg [not available in U.S.]

Zaditen® [CAN]: 1 mg [not available in U.S.]

ketotifen fumarate see ketotifen on this page

Key-E® [US-OTC] see vitamin E on page 894

Key-E® Kaps [US-OTC] see vitamin E on page 894

Keygesic [US-OTC] see magnesium salicylate on page 528

Key-Pred® (Discontinued)

Key-Pred-SP® (Discontinued)

K-G® (Discontinued) see potassium gluconate on page 701

K-Gen® Effervescent (Discontinued) see potassium bicarbonate on page 699

KI see potassium iodide on page 702

K-Ide® (Discontinued)

Kidkare Cough and Cold [US-OTC] see chlorpheniramine, pseudoephedrine, and dextromethorphan on page 183

Kidkare Decongestant [US-OTC] see pseudoephedrine on page 727

Kidrolase® [Can] see asparaginase on page 77

Kinerase® (Discontinued) see hyaluronidase on page 424

Kineret® [US/Can] see anakinra on page 55

Kinesed® (Discontinued) see hyoscyamine, atropine, scopolamine, and phenobarbital on page 442

Kinevac® [US] see sincalide on page 787

Kionex™ [US] see sodium polystyrene sulfonate on page 797

Kivexa™ [Can] see abacavir and lamivudine on page 2

Klaron® [US] see sulfacetamide on page 810

Klean-Prep® [Can] see polyethylene glycol-electrolyte solution on page 695

K-Lease® (Discontinued) see potassium chloride on page 700

Klerist-D® Tablet (Discontinued) see chlorpheniramine and pseudoephedrine on page 178

Klonopin® [US/Can] see clonazepam on page 204

K-Lor® [US/Can] see potassium chloride on page 700

Klor-Con® [US] see potassium chloride on page 700

Klor-Con® 8 [US] see potassium chloride on page 700

Klor-Con® 10 [US] see potassium chloride on page 700

Klor-Con®/25 [US] see potassium chloride on page 700

Klor-Con® M [US] see potassium chloride on page 700

Klor-Con®/EF [US] see potassium bicarbonate and potassium citrate on page 699

Klorominr® Oral *(Discontinued)* *see* chlorpheniramine *on page 177*

Klorvess® *(Discontinued)* *see* potassium chloride *on page 700*

Klorvess® Effervescent *(Discontinued)*

K-Lyte® [US] *see* potassium bicarbonate and potassium citrate *on page 699*

K-Lyte/Cl® 50 *(Discontinued)* *see* potassium bicarbonate and potassium chloride *on page 699*

K-Lyte/Cl® [US] *see* potassium bicarbonate and potassium chloride *on page 699*

K-Lyte® DS [US] *see* potassium bicarbonate and potassium citrate *on page 699*

K-Lyte® Effervescent *(Discontinued)* *see* potassium bicarbonate *on page 699*

K-Norm® *(Discontinued)* *see* potassium chloride *on page 700*

Koāte®-DVI [US] *see* antihemophilic factor (human) *on page 58*

Koāte®-HP *(Discontinued)* *see* antihemophilic factor (human) *on page 58*

Kobee [US-OTC] *see* vitamin B complex combinations *on page 894*

Kodet SE [US-OTC] *see* pseudoephedrine *on page 727*

Koffex DM-D [Can] *see* pseudoephedrine and dextromethorphan *on page 728*

Koffex DM + Decongestant + Expectorant [Can] *see* guaifenesin, pseudoephedrine, and dextromethorphan *on page 408*

Koffex DM-Expectorant [Can] *see* guaifenesin and dextromethorphan *on page 402*

Koffex Expectorant [Can] *see* guaifenesin *on page 401*

Kogenate® [Can] *see* antihemophilic factor (recombinant) *on page 59*

Kogenate® *(Discontinued)* *see* antihemophilic factor (recombinant) *on page 59*

Kogenate® FS [US/Can] *see* antihemophilic factor (recombinant) *on page 59*

Kolephrin® [US-OTC] *see* acetaminophen, chlorpheniramine, and pseudoephedrine *on page 10*

Kolephrin® #1 [US] *see* guaifenesin and codeine *on page 402*

Kolephrin® GG/DM [US-OTC] *see* guaifenesin and dextromethorphan *on page 402*

Konakion [Can] *see* phytonadione *on page 681*

Konakion® Injection *(Discontinued)* *see* phytonadione *on page 681*

Kondon's Nasal® *(Discontinued)* *see* ephedrine *on page 299*

Konsyl® [US-OTC] *see* psyllium *on page 732*

Konsyl-D® [US-OTC] *see* psyllium *on page 732*

Konsyl® Easy Mix [US-OTC] *see* psyllium *on page 732*

Konsyl® Fiber Caplets [US-OTC] *see* polycarbophil *on page 694*

Konsyl® Orange [US-OTC] *see* psyllium *on page 732*

Kovia® [US] *see* papain and urea *on page 652*

K-Pek II [US-OTC] *see* loperamide *on page 515*

K-Pek® *(Discontinued)*

K-Phos® MF [US] *see* potassium phosphate and sodium phosphate *on page 703*

K-Phos® Neutral [US] *see* potassium phosphate and sodium phosphate *on page 703*

K-Phos® No. 2 [US] *see* potassium phosphate and sodium phosphate *on page 703*

K-Phos® Original [US] *see* potassium acid phosphate *on page 699*

KPN Prenatal [US] *see* vitamins (multiple/prenatal) *on page 896*

K+ Potassium [US] *see* potassium chloride *on page 700*

Kristalose® [US] *see* lactulose *on page 489*

Kronofed-A® [US] *see* chlorpheniramine and pseudoephedrine *on page 178*

Kronofed-A®-Jr [US] *see* chlorpheniramine and pseudoephedrine *on page 178*

K-Tab® [US] *see* potassium chloride *on page 700*

K-Tan [US] *see* phenylephrine and pyrilamine *on page 677*

K-Tan 4 [US] *see* phenylephrine and pyrilamine *on page 677*

kunecatechins *see* sinecatechins *on page 788*

Kuric™ [US] *see* ketoconazole *on page 482*

kutrase® **[US]** *see* pancreatin *on page 648*

ku-zyme® **[US]** *see* pancreatin *on page 648*

ku-zyme® **HP [US]** *see* pancrelipase *on page 648*

Kwelcof® **[US]** *see* hydrocodone and guaifenesin *on page 429*

Kwellada-P™ **[Can]** *see* permethrin *on page 670*

Kytril® **[US/Can]** *see* granisetron *on page 400*

L-749,345 *see* ertapenem *on page 308*

L-M-X™ **4 [US-OTC]** *see* lidocaine *on page 504*

L-M-X™ **5 [US-OTC]** *see* lidocaine *on page 504*

L 754030 *see* aprepitant *on page 71*

LA 20304a *see* gemifloxacin *on page 387*

labetalol (la BET a lole)

Sound-Alike/Look-Alike Issues
labetalol may be confused with betaxolol, Hexadrol®, lamotrigine
Trandate® may be confused with tramadol, Trendar®, Trental®, Tridrate®

Synonyms ibidomide hydrochloride; labetalol hydrochloride

U.S./Canadian Brand Names Apo-Labetalol® [Can]; Labetalol Hydrochloride Injection, USP [Can]; Normodyne® [Can]; Trandate® [US/Can]

Therapeutic Category Alpha-/Beta- Adrenergic Blocker

Use Treatment of mild to severe hypertension; I.V. for hypertensive emergencies

Usual Dosage
Children: Due to limited documentation of its use, labetalol should be initiated cautiously in pediatric patients with careful dosage adjustment and blood pressure monitoring.

I.V., intermittent bolus doses of 0.3-1 mg/kg/dose have been reported.

For treatment of pediatric hypertensive emergencies, initial continuous infusions of 0.4-1 mg/kg/hour with a maximum of 3 mg/kg/hour have been used. Administration requires the use of an infusion pump.

Adults:

Oral: Initial: 100 mg twice daily, may increase as needed every 2-3 days by 100 mg until desired response is obtained; usual dose: 200-400 mg twice daily; may require up to 2.4 g/day.

Usual dose range (JNC 7): 200-800 mg/day in 2 divided doses

I.V.: 20 mg (0.25 mg/kg for an 80 kg patient) IVP over 2 minutes; may administer 40-80 mg at 10-minute intervals, up to 300 mg total dose.

I.V. infusion (acute loading): Initial: 2 mg/minute; titrate to response up to 300 mg total dose, if needed. Administration requires the use of an infusion pump.

I.V. infusion (500 mg/250 mL D_5W) rates:

1 mg/minute: 30 mL/hour
2 mg/minute: 60 mL/hour
3 mg/minute: 90 mL/hour
4 mg/minute: 120 mL/hour
5 mg/minute: 150 mL/hour
6 mg/minute: 180 mL/hour

Note: Although loading infusions are well described in the product labeling, the labeling is silent in specific clinical situations, such as in the patient who has an initial response to labetalol infusions but cannot be converted to an oral route for subsequent dosing. There is limited documentation of prolonged continuous infusions. In rare clinical situations, higher dosages (up to 6 mg/minute) have been used in the critical care setting (eg, aortic dissection). At the other extreme, continuous infusions at relatively low doses (2-6 mg/hour - note difference in units) have been used in some settings (following loading infusion in patients who are unable to be converted to oral regimens or in some cases as a continuation of outpatient oral regimens). These prolonged infusions should not be confused with loading infusions. Because of wide variation in the use of infusions, an awareness of institutional policies and practices is extremely important. Careful clarification of orders and specific infusion rates/units is required to avoid confusion. Due to the prolonged duration of action, careful monitoring should be extended for the duration of the infusion and for several hours after the infusion. Excessive administration may result in prolonged hypotension and/or bradycardia.

Dosage Forms
Injection, solution: 5 mg/mL (4 mL, 20 mL, 40 mL)
Trandate®: 5 mg/mL (20 mL, 40 mL)
Tablet: 100 mg, 200 mg, 300 mg
Trandate®: 100 mg, 200 mg, 300 mg

labetalol hydrochloride *see* labetalol *on this page*

Labetalol Hydrochloride Injection, USP [Can] *see* labetalol *on this page*

Lac-Hydrin® **[US]** *see* lactic acid and ammonium hydroxide *on this page*

Lac-Hydrin® **Five [US-OTC]** *see* lactic acid and ammonium hydroxide *on this page*

LAClotion™ **[US]** *see* lactic acid and ammonium hydroxide *on this page*

Lacril® **Ophthalmic Solution** *(Discontinued) see* artificial tears *on page 75*

Lacrisert® **[US/Can]** *see* hydroxypropyl cellulose *on page 439*

Lactaid® **Extra Strength** *(Discontinued) see* lactase *on this page*

Lactaid® **Fast Act [US-OTC]** *see* lactase *on this page*

Lactaid® **Original [US-OTC]** *see* lactase *on this page*

Lactaid® **Ultra** *(Discontinued) see* lactase *on this page*

lactase (LAK tase)

U.S./Canadian Brand Names Dairyaid® [Can]; Lactaid® Fast Act [US-OTC]; Lactaid® Original [US-OTC]; Lactrase® [US-OTC]

Therapeutic Category Nutritional Supplement

Use Help digest lactose in milk for patients with lactose intolerance

Usual Dosage Oral:

Capsule: 1-2 capsules taken with milk or meal; pretreat milk with 1-2 capsules/quart of milk

Liquid: 5-15 drops/quart of milk

Tablet: 1-3 tablets with meals

Dosage Forms

Caplet:

Lactaid® Original [OTC]: 3000 FCC lactase units

Lactaid® Fast Act [OTC]: 9000 FCC lactase units

Capsule:

Lactrase® [OTC]: 250 mg standardized enzyme lactase

Tablet, chewable:

Lactaid® Fast Act [OTC]: 9000 FCC lactase units

lactic acid (LAK tik AS id)

Synonyms sodium-PCA and lactic acid

U.S./Canadian Brand Names LactiCare® [US-OTC]; Lactinol-E® [US]; Lactinol® [US]

Therapeutic Category Topical Skin Product

Use Lubricate and moisturize the skin counteracting dryness and itching

Usual Dosage Topical: Adults: Lubricant/moisturizer: Apply twice daily

Dosage Forms

Cream: 10% (120 g)

Lactinol-E®: 10% (120 g, 240 g)

Lotion: 10% (360 mL)

LactiCare® [OTC]: 5% (222 mL, 340 mL)

Lactinol®: 10% (360 mL, 480 mL)

lactic acid and ammonium hydroxide (LAK tik AS id & a MOE nee um hye DROKS ide)

Synonyms ammonium lactate

U.S./Canadian Brand Names AmLactin® [US-OTC]; Geri-Hydrolac™ [US-OTC]; Geri-Hydrolac™-12 [US-OTC]; Lac-Hydrin® Five [US-OTC]; Lac-Hydrin® [US]; LAClotion™ [US]

Therapeutic Category Topical Skin Product

Use Treatment of moderate to severe xerosis and ichthyosis vulgaris

Usual Dosage Topical: Children ≥2 years and Adults: Apply twice daily to affected area; rub in well

Dosage Forms

Cream, topical: Lactic acid 12% with ammonium hydroxide (140 g, 280 g, 385 g)

AmLactin® [OTC]: Lactic acid 12% with ammonium hydroxide (140 g)

Lac-Hydrin®: Lactic acid 12% with ammonium hydroxide (280 g, 385 g)

Lotion, topical: Lactic acid 12% with ammonium hydroxide (225 g, 400 g)

AmLactin® [OTC], Lac-Hydrin®, LAClotion™: Lactic acid 12% with ammonium hydroxide (225 g, 400 g)

Geri-Hydrolac™ [OTC], Lac-Hydrin® Five: Lactic acid 5% with ammonium hydroxide (120 mL, 240 mL)

Geri-Hydrolac™-12 [OTC]: Lactic acid 12% with ammonium hydroxide (120 mL, 240 mL)

LactiCare® **[US-OTC]** *see* lactic acid *on this page*

Lactinex™ **[US-OTC]** *see* Lactobacillus *on next page*

Lactinol® **[US]** *see* lactic acid *on this page*

Lactinol-E® **[US]** *see* lactic acid *on this page*

Lactobacillus (lak toe ba SIL us)

Synonyms *Lactobacillus acidophilus*; *Lactobacillus bifidus*; *Lactobacillus bulgaricus*; *Lactobacillus casei*; *Lactobacillus paracasei*; *Lactobacillus reuteri*; *Lactobacillus rhamnosus* GG

U.S./Canadian Brand Names Bacid® [US-OTC/Can]; Culturelle® [US-OTC]; Dofus [US-OTC]; Fermalac [Can]; Flora-Q™ [US-OTC]; Kala® [US-OTC]; Lactinex™ [US-OTC]; Lacto-Bifidus [US-OTC]; Lacto-Key [US-OTC]; Lacto-Pectin [US-OTC]; Lacto-TriBlend [US-OTC]; Megadophilus® [US-OTC]; MoreDophilus® [US-OTC]; Superdophilus® [US-OTC]

Therapeutic Category Gastrointestinal Agent, Miscellaneous

Use Promote normal bacterial flora of the intestinal tract

Usual Dosage Dietary supplement: Oral: Dosing varies by manufacturer; consult product labeling
Children (Culturelle®): 1 capsule daily
Adults:
Bacid®: 2 caplets/day
Culturelle®: 1 capsule daily; may increase to twice daily
Flora-Q™: 1 capsule/day
Lacto-Key 100 or 600: 1-2 capsules/day
Lactinex™: 1 packet or 4 tablets 3-4 times/day

Dosage Forms
Capsule:
Culturelle® [OTC]: *L. rhamnosus* GG 10 billion colony-forming units
Dofus [OTC]: *L. acidophilus* and *L. bifidus* 10:1 ratio
Flora-Q™ [OTC]: *L. acidophilus* and *L. paracasei* ≥8 billion colony-forming units
Lacto-Key [OTC]:
100: *L. acidophilus* 1 billion colony-forming units
600: *L. acidophilus* 6 billion colony-forming units
Lacto-Bifidus [OTC]:
100: *L. bifidus* 1 billion colony-forming units
600: *L. bifidus* 6 billion colony-forming units
Lacto-Pectin [OTC]: *L. acidophilus* and *L. casei* ≥5 billion colony-forming units
Lacto-TriBlend [OTC]:
100: *L. acidophilus*, *L. bifidus*, and *L. bulgaricus* 1 billion colony-forming units
600: *L. acidophilus*, *L. bifidus*, and *L. bulgaricus* 6 billion colony-forming units
Megadophilus® [OTC], Superdophilus® [OTC]: *L. acidophilus* 2 billion units
Capsule, softgel: *L. acidophilus* 100 active units
Caplet:
Bacid® [OTC]: *L. acidophilus 80%* and *L. bulgaricus* 10%
Granules:
Lactinex™ [OTC]: *L. acidophilus* and *L. bulgaricus* 100 million live cells per 1 g packet (12s)
Powder:
Lacto-TriBlend [OTC]: *L. acidophilus*, *L. bifidus*, and *L. bulgaricus* 10 billion colony-forming units per $\frac{1}{4}$ teaspoon
Megadophilus® [OTC], Superdophilus® [OTC]: *L. acidophilus* 2 billion units per half-teaspoon
MoreDophilus® [OTC]: *L. acidophilus* 12.4 billion units per teaspoon
Tablet:
Kala® [OTC]: *L. acidophilus* 200 million units
Lactinex™ [OTC]: *L. acidophilus* and *L. bulgaricus* 1 million live cells
Tablet, chewable: *L. reuteri* 100 million organisms
Wafer: *L. acidophilus* 90 mg and *L. bifidus* 25 mg (100s)

Lactobacillus acidophilus see Lactobacillus *on this page*

Lactobacillus bifidus see Lactobacillus *on this page*

Lactobacillus bulgaricus see Lactobacillus *on this page*

Lactobacillus casei see Lactobacillus *on this page*

Lactobacillus paracasei see Lactobacillus *on this page*

Lactobacillus reuteri see Lactobacillus *on this page*

Lactobacillus rhamnosus GG see Lactobacillus *on this page*

Lacto-Bifidus [US-OTC] see Lactobacillus *on this page*

lactoflavin see riboflavin *on page 756*

Lacto-Key [US-OTC] see Lactobacillus *on this page*

Lacto-Pectin [US-OTC] see Lactobacillus *on this page*

Lacto-TriBlend [US-OTC] see Lactobacillus *on this page*

Lactrase® **[US-OTC]** *see* lactase *on page 487*

lactulose (LAK tyoo lose)
Sound-Alike/Look-Alike Issues
lactulose may be confused with lactose
U.S./Canadian Brand Names Acilac [Can]; Apo-Lactulose® [Can]; Constulose [US]; Enulose [US]; Generlac [US]; Kristalose® [US]; Laxilose [Can]; PMS-Lactulose [Can]
Therapeutic Category Ammonium Detoxicant; Laxative
Use Adjunct in the prevention and treatment of portal-systemic encephalopathy; treatment of chronic constipation
Usual Dosage Diarrhea may indicate overdosage and responds to dose reduction
Prevention of portal systemic encephalopathy (PSE): Oral:
Infants: 2.5-10 mL/day divided 3-4 times/day; adjust dosage to produce 2-3 stools/day
Older Children: Daily dose of 40-90 mL divided 3-4 times/day; if initial dose causes diarrhea, then reduce it immediately; adjust dosage to produce 2-3 stools/day
Constipation: Oral:
Children: 5 g/day (7.5 mL) after breakfast
Adults: 15-30 mL/day increased to 60 mL/day in 1-2 divided doses if necessary
Acute PSE: Adults:
Oral: 20-30 g (30-45 mL) every 1-2 hours to induce rapid laxation; adjust dosage daily to produce 2-3 soft stools; doses of 30-45 mL may be given hourly to cause rapid laxation, then reduce to recommended dose; usual daily dose: 60-100 g (90-150 mL) daily
Rectal administration: 200 g (300 mL) diluted with 700 mL of H_2O or NS; administer rectally via rectal balloon catheter and retain 30-60 minutes every 4-6 hours
Dosage Forms
Crystals for solution, oral:
Kristalose®: 10 g/packet (30s), 20 g/packet (30s)
Syrup: 10 g/15 mL
Constulose, Enulose, Generlac: 10 g/15 mL

Lactulose PSE® *(Discontinued) see* lactulose *on this page*

ladakamycin *see* azacitidine *on page 87*

Lagesic™ **[US]** *see* acetaminophen and phenyltoloxamine *on page 8*

L-All 12 [US] *see* carbetapentane and phenylephrine *on page 149*

L-AmB *see* amphotericin B liposomal *on page 52*

Lamictal® **[US/Can]** *see* lamotrigine *on next page*

Lamisil® **Oral [US/Can]** *see* terbinafine (oral) *on page 826*

Lamisil® **Topical [US/Can]** *see* terbinafine (topical) *on page 826*

lamivudine (la MI vyoo deen)
Sound-Alike/Look-Alike Issues
lamivudine may be confused with lamotrigine
Epivir® may be confused with Combivir®
Synonyms 3TC
U.S./Canadian Brand Names 3TC® [Can]; Epivir-HBV® [US]; Epivir® [US]; Heptovir® [Can]
Therapeutic Category Antiviral Agent
Use
Epivir®: Treatment of HIV infection when antiretroviral therapy is warranted; should always be used as part of a multidrug regimen (at least three antiretroviral agents)
Epivir-HBV®: Treatment of chronic hepatitis B associated with evidence of hepatitis B viral replication and active liver inflammation
Usual Dosage Note: The formulation and dosage of Epivir-HBV® are not appropriate for patients infected with both HBV and HIV. Use with at least two other antiretroviral agents when treating HIV
Oral:
Children 3 months to 16 years: HIV: 4 mg/kg twice daily (maximum: 150 mg twice daily)
Children 2-17 years: Treatment of hepatitis B (Epivir-HBV®): 3 mg/kg once daily (maximum: 100 mg/day)
Adults:
HIV: 150 mg twice daily **or** 300 mg once daily
<50 kg: 4 mg/kg twice daily (maximum: 150 mg twice daily)
Treatment of hepatitis B (Epivir-HBV®): 100 mg/day
Dosage Forms
Solution, oral:
Epivir®: 10 mg/mL
(Continued)

lamivudine *(Continued)*
Epivir-HBV®: 5 mg/mL
Tablet:
Epivir®: 150 mg, 300 mg
Epivir-HBV®: 100 mg

lamivudine, abacavir, and zidovudine *see* abacavir, lamivudine, and zidovudine *on page 2*

lamivudine and abacavir *see* abacavir and lamivudine *on page 2*

lamivudine and zidovudine *see* zidovudine and lamivudine *on page 904*

lamotrigine *(la MOE tri jeen)*
Sound-Alike/Look-Alike Issues
lamotrigine may be confused with labetalol, Lamisil®, lamivudine, Lomotil®, ludiomil
Lamictal® may be confused with Lamisil®, Lomotil®, ludiomil
Synonyms BW-430C; LTG
U.S./Canadian Brand Names Apo-Lamotrigine® [Can]; Gen-Lamotrigine [Can]; Lamictal® [US/Can]; Novo-Lamotrigine [Can]; PMS-Lamotrigine [Can]; ratio-Lamotrigine [Can]
Therapeutic Category Anticonvulsant
Use Adjunctive therapy in the treatment of generalized seizures of Lennox-Gastaut syndrome, primary generalized tonic-clonic seizures, and partial seizures in adults and children ≥2 years of age; conversion to monotherapy in adults with partial seizures who are receiving treatment with valproic acid or a single enzyme-inducing antiepileptic drug (specifically carbamazepine, phenytoin, phenobarbital or primidone); maintenance treatment of bipolar I disorder
Usual Dosage Note: Only whole tablets should be used for dosing, round calculated dose down to the nearest whole tablet. Enzyme-inducing regimens specifically refer to those containing carbamazepine, phenytoin, phenobarbital, or primidone. Oral:

Children 2-12 years: Lennox-Gastaut (adjunctive), primary generalized tonic-clonic seizures (adjunctive), or partial seizures (adjunctive): **Note:** Children <30 kg will likely require maintenance doses to be increased as much as 50% based on clinical response regardless of regimen below:
Initial: 0.3 mg/kg/day in 1-2 divided doses for weeks 1 and 2, then increase to 0.6 mg/kg/day in 1-2 divided doses for weeks 3 and 4. Maintenance: Titrate dose to effect; after week 4, increase daily dose every 1-2 weeks by 0.6 mg/kg/day; usual maintenance: 4.5-7.5 mg/kg/day in 2 divided doses; maximum: 300 mg/day in 2 divided doses
Adjustment for AED regimens **containing** valproic acid (see "Note"): Initial: 0.15 mg/kg/day in 1-2 divided doses for weeks 1 and 2, then increase to 0.3 mg/kg/day in 1-2 divided doses for weeks 3 and 4. Maintenance: Titrate dose to effect; after week 4, increase daily dose every 1-2 weeks by 0.3 mg/kg/day; usual maintenance: 1-5 mg/kg/day in 2 divided doses; maximum: 200 mg/day in 1-2 divided doses
Note: For patients >6.7 kg and <14 kg, initial dosing should be 2 mg every other day for first 2 weeks, then increased to 2 mg daily for weeks 3-4. For patients taking lamotrigine with valproic acid alone, the usual maintenance dose is 1-3 mg/kg/day in 2 divided doses
Adjustment for **enzyme-inducing** AED regimens **without** valproic acid: Initial: 0.6 mg/kg/day in 2 divided doses for weeks 1 and 2, then increase to 1.2 mg/kg/day in 2 divided doses for weeks 3 and 4. Maintenance: Titrate dose to effect; after week 4, increase daily dose every 1-2 weeks by 1.2 mg/kg/day; usual maintenance: 5-15 mg/kg/day in 2 divided doses; maximum: 400 mg/day in 2 divided doses
Children >12 years: Lennox-Gastaut (adjunctive), primary generalized tonic-clonic seizures (adjunctive), or partial seizures (adjunctive): Refer to adult dosing.
Children ≥16 years: Conversion from adjunctive therapy with valproic acid or a single enzyme-inducing AED regimen to monotherapy with lamotrigine: Refer to adult dosing.

Adults:
Lennox-Gastaut (adjunctive), primary generalized tonic-clonic seizures (adjunctive) or partial seizures (adjunctive): Initial: 25 mg/day for weeks 1 and 2, then increase to 50 mg/day for weeks 3 and 4. Maintenance: Titrate dose to effect; after week 4 increase daily dose every 1-2 weeks by 50 mg/day; usual maintenance: 225-375 mg/day in 2 divided doses
Adjustment for AED regimens **containing** valproic acid (see "Note"): Initial: 25 mg every other day for weeks 1 and 2, then increase to 25 mg every day for weeks 3 and 4. Maintenance: Titrate dose to effect; after week 4 increase daily dose every 1-2 weeks by 25-50 mg/day; usual maintenance: 100-400 mg/day in 1 or 2 divided doses
Note: For patients taking lamotrigine with valproic acid alone, the usual maintenance dose is 100-200 mg/day
Adjustment for **enzyme-inducing** AED regimens **without** valproic acid: Initial: 50 mg/day for weeks 1 and 2, then increase to 100 mg/day in 2 divided doses for weeks 3 and 4. Maintenance: titrate dose to effect; after week 4 increase daily dose every 1-2 weeks by 100 mg/day; usual maintenance: 300-500 mg/day in 2 divided doses. Doses as high as 700 mg/day have been used, though additional benefit has not been established.

Conversion to monotherapy with lamotrigine:

Conversion from adjunctive therapy with valproic acid: Initiate and titrate as per recommendations to a lamotrigine dose of 200 mg/day. Then taper valproic acid dose in decrements of not >500 mg/day at intervals of 1 week (or longer) to a valproic acid dosage of 500 mg/day; this dosage should be maintained for 1 week. The lamotrigine dosage should then be increased to 300 mg/day while valproic acid is decreased to 250 mg/day; this dosage should be maintained for 1 week. Valproic acid may then be discontinued, while the lamotrigine dose is increased by 100 mg/day at weekly intervals to achieve a lamotrigine maintenance dose of 500 mg/day.

Conversion from adjunctive therapy with carbamazepine, phenytoin, phenobarbital, or primidone: Initiate and titrate as per recommendations to a lamotrigine dose of 500 mg/day. Concomitant enzyme-inducing AED should then be withdrawn by 20% decrements each week over a 4-week period. Patients should be monitored for rash.

Conversion from adjunctive therapy with AED other than carbamazepine, phenytoin, phenobarbital, primidone or valproic acid: No specific guidelines available

Bipolar disorder:

Initial: 25 mg/day for weeks 1 and 2, then increase to 50 mg/day for weeks 3 and 4, then increase to 100 mg/day for week 5; maintenance: increase dose to 200 mg/day beginning week 6

Adjustment for regimens **containing** valproic acid: Initial: 25 mg every other day for weeks 1 and 2, then increase to 25 mg every day for weeks 3 and 4, then increase to 50 mg/day for week 5; maintenance: 100 mg/day beginning week 6

Adjustment for **enzyme-inducing** regimens **without** valproic acid: Initial: 50 mg/day for weeks 1 and 2, then increase to 100 mg/day in divided doses for weeks 3 and 4, then increase to 200 mg/day in divided doses for week 5, then increase to 300 mg/day in divided dose for week 6; maintenance: 400 mg/day in divided doses beginning week 7

Adjustment following discontinuation of psychotropic medication:

Discontinuing valproic acid with current dose of lamotrigine 100 mg/day: 150 mg/day for week 1, then increase to 200 mg/day beginning week 2

Discontinuing carbamazepine, phenytoin, phenobarbital, primidone, or rifampin with current dose of lamotrigine 400 mg/day: 400 mg/day for week 1, then decrease to 300 mg/day for week 2, then decrease to 200 mg/day beginning week 3

Discontinuing therapy: Children and Adults: Decrease dose by ~50% per week, over at least 2 weeks unless safety concerns require a more rapid withdrawal. Discontinuing carbamazepine, phenytoin, phenobarbital, or primidone should prolong the half-life of lamotrigine; discontinuing valproic acid should shorten the half-life of lamotrigine

Restarting therapy after discontinuation: If lamotrigine has been withheld for >5 half-lives, consider restarting according to initial dosing recommendations.

Dosage Forms

Tablet:

Lamictal®: 25 mg, 100 mg, 150 mg, 200 mg

Tablet, combination package [each unit-dose starter kit contains]:

Lamictal® (blue kit; for patients taking valproic aid):

Tablet: Lamotrigine 25 mg (35s)

Lamictal® (green kit; for patients taking carbamazepine, phenytoin, phenobarbital, primidone, or rifampin and **not** taking valproic acid):

Tablet: Lamotrigine 25 mg (84s)

Tablet: Lamotrigine 100 mg (14s)

Lamictal® (orange kit; for patients **not** taking carbamazepine, phenytoin, phenobarbital, primidone, rifampin, or valproic acid):

Tablet: Lamotrigine 25 mg (42s)

Tablet: Lamotrigine 100 mg (7s)

Tablet, dispersible/chewable: 5 mg, 25 mg

Lamictal®: 2 mg, 5 mg, 25 mg

Lanacane® [US-OTC] see benzocaine on page 101

Lanacane® Maximum Strength [US-OTC] see benzocaine on page 101

Lanaphilic® [US-OTC] see urea on page 877

lanolin, cetyl alcohol, glycerin, petrolatum, and mineral oil

(LAN oh lin, SEE til AL koe hol, GLIS er in, pe troe LAY tum, & MIN er al oyl)

Synonyms mineral oil, petrolatum, lanolin, cetyl alcohol, and glycerin

U.S./Canadian Brand Names Lubriderm® Fragrance Free [US-OTC]; Lubriderm® [US-OTC]

Therapeutic Category Topical Skin Product

Use Treatment of dry skin

Usual Dosage Topical: Apply to skin as necessary

(Continued)

lanolin, cetyl alcohol, glycerin, petrolatum, and mineral oil *(Continued)*

Dosage Forms
Lotion, topical [bottle]: 180 mL, 300 mL, 480 mL
Lubriderm® Fragrance Free [OTC], Lubriderm® [OTC]: 180 mL, 300 mL, 480 mL
Lotion, topical [tube]: 100 mL
Lubriderm® Fragrance Free [OTC], Lubriderm® [OTC]: 100 mL

Lanorinal® *(Discontinued)*

Lanoxicaps® [US/Can] *see* digoxin *on page 257*

Lanoxin® [US/Can] *see* digoxin *on page 257*

lanreotide *(lan REE oh tide)*

Sound-Alike/Look-Alike Issues
Somatuline® may be confused with somatropin, sumatriptan
Synonyms lanreotide acetate
U.S./Canadian Brand Names Somatuline® Autogel® [Can]; Somatuline® Depot [US]
Therapeutic Category Somatostatin Analog
Use Long-term treatment of acromegaly in patients who are not candidates for or are unresponsive to surgery and/or radiotherapy

Note: Also approved in Canada for relief of symptoms of acromegaly
Usual Dosage SubQ: **Note: Differences in U.S. and Canadian labeled dosing:**
U.S. labeling: Adults: Acromegaly: 90 mg once every 4 weeks for 3 months; after initial 90 days of therapy, adjust dose based on clinical response of patient, growth hormone (GH) levels, and/or insulin-like growth factor 1 (IGF-1) levels as follows:
GH ≤1 ng/mL, IGF-1 normal, symptoms stable: 60 mg once every 4 weeks
GH >1-2.5 ng/mL, IGF-1 normal, symptoms stable: 90 mg once every 4 weeks
GH >2.5 ng/mL, IGF-1 elevated and/or uncontrolled symptoms: 120 mg once every 4 weeks

Canadian labeling: Children ≥16 years and Adults: Acromegaly: 90 mg once every 4 weeks for 3 months; after initial 90 days of therapy, adjust dose based on clinical response of patient, growth hormone (GH) levels, and/or insulin-like growth factor 1 (IGF-1) levels as follows:
GH = 1 ng/mL, IGF-1 normal, symptoms stable: 60 mg once every 4 weeks
GH >1-2.5 ng/mL, IGF-1 normal, symptoms stable: 90 mg once every 4 weeks
GH >2.5 ng/mL, IGF-1 elevated and/or uncontrolled symptoms: 120 mg once every 4 weeks
Dosage Forms Excipient information presented when available (limited, particularly for generics); consult specific product labeling. [CAN] = Canadian brand name
Injection, solution, as acetate [preservative free; prefilled syringe]:
Somatuline® Autogel® [CAN]: 60 mg/ 0.3 mL (0.3 mL); 90 mg/ 0.3 mL (0.3 mL); 120 mg/0.5 mL (0.5 mL)
Somatuline® Depot®: 60 mg/0.3 mL (0.3 mL); 90 mg/0.3 mL (0.3 mL); 120 mg/0.5 mL (0.5 mL)

lanreotide acetate *see* lanreotide *on this page*

lansoprazole *(lan SOE pra zole)*

Sound-Alike/Look-Alike Issues
Prevacid® may be confused with Pravachol®, Prevpac®, Prilosec®, Prinivil®
U.S./Canadian Brand Names Prevacid® SoluTab™ [US]; Prevacid® [US/Can]
Therapeutic Category Gastric Acid Secretion Inhibitor
Use
Oral: Short-term treatment of active duodenal ulcers; maintenance treatment of healed duodenal ulcers; as part of a multidrug regimen for *H. pylori* eradication to reduce the risk of duodenal ulcer recurrence; short-term treatment of active benign gastric ulcer; treatment of NSAID-associated gastric ulcer; to reduce the risk of NSAID-associated gastric ulcer in patients with a history of gastric ulcer who require an NSAID; short-term treatment of symptomatic GERD; short-term treatment for all grades of erosive esophagitis; to maintain healing of erosive esophagitis; long-term treatment of pathological hypersecretory conditions, including Zollinger-Ellison syndrome
I.V.: Short-term treatment (≤7 days) of erosive esophagitis in adults unable to take oral medications
Usual Dosage
Children 1-11 years: GERD, erosive esophagitis: Oral:
≤30 kg: 15 mg once daily
>30 kg: 30 mg once daily
Note: Doses were increased in some pediatric patients if still symptomatic after 2 or more weeks of treatment (maximum dose: 30 mg twice daily)
Children 12-17 years: Oral:
Nonerosive GERD: 15 mg once daily for up to 8 weeks

Erosive esophagitis: 30 mg once daily for up to 8 weeks

Adults:

Duodenal ulcer: Oral: Short-term treatment: 15 mg once daily for 4 weeks; maintenance therapy: 15 mg once daily

Gastric ulcer: Oral: Short-term treatment: 30 mg once daily for up to 8 weeks

NSAID-associated gastric ulcer (healing): Oral: 30 mg once daily for 8 weeks; controlled studies did not extend past 8 weeks of therapy

NSAID-associated gastric ulcer (to reduce risk): Oral: 15 mg once daily for up to 12 weeks; controlled studies did not extend past 12 weeks of therapy

Symptomatic GERD: Oral: Short-term treatment: 15 mg once daily for up to 8 weeks

Erosive esophagitis:

Oral: Short-term treatment: 30 mg once daily for up to 8 weeks; continued treatment for an additional 8 weeks may be considered for recurrence or for patients that do not heal after the first 8 weeks of therapy; maintenance therapy: 15 mg once daily

I.V.: 30 mg once daily for up to 7 days; patients should be switched to an oral formulation as soon as they can take oral medications

Hypersecretory conditions: Oral: Initial: 60 mg once daily; adjust dose based upon patient response and to reduce acid secretion to <10 mEq/hour (5 mEq/hour in patients with prior gastric surgery); doses of 90 mg twice daily have been used; administer doses >120 mg/day in divided doses

Helicobacter pylori eradication: Oral: Currently accepted recommendations (may differ from product labeling): Dose varies with regimen: 30 mg once daily or 60 mg/day in 2 divided doses; requires combination therapy with antibiotics

Dosage Forms

Capsule, delayed release:

Prevacid®: 15 mg, 30 mg

Granules, for oral suspension, delayed release:

Prevacid®: 15 mg/packet (30s), 30 mg/packet (30s)

Injection, powder for reconstitution:

Prevacid®: 30 mg

Tablet, orally disintegrating:

Prevacid® SoluTab™: 15 mg, 30 mg

lansoprazole, amoxicillin, and clarithromycin

(lan SOE pra zole, a moks i SIL in, & kla RITH roe mye sin)

Sound-Alike/Look-Alike Issues

Prevpac® may be confused with Prevacid®

Synonyms amoxicillin, lansoprazole, and clarithromycin; clarithromycin, lansoprazole, and amoxicillin

U.S./Canadian Brand Names Hp-PAC® [Can]; Prevpac® [US/Can]

Therapeutic Category Antibiotic, Macrolide Combination; Antibiotic, Penicillin; Gastrointestinal Agent, Miscellaneous

Use Eradication of *H. pylori* to reduce the risk of recurrent duodenal ulcer

Usual Dosage Oral: Adults: Lansoprazole 30 mg, amoxicillin 1 g, and clarithromycin 500 mg taken together twice daily for 10 or 14 days

Dosage Forms

Combination package [each administration card contains]:

Prevpac®:

Capsule: Amoxicillin 500 mg (4 capsules/day)

Capsule, delayed release (Prevacid®): Lansoprazole 30 mg (2 capsules/day)

Tablet (Biaxin®): Clarithromycin 500 mg (2 tablets/day)

lansoprazole and naproxen (lan SOE pra zole & na PROKS en)

Sound-Alike/Look-Alike Issues

Prevacid® may be confused with Pravachol®, Prevpac®, Prilosec®, Prinivil®

Synonyms NapraPAC™; naproxen and lansoprazole

U.S./Canadian Brand Names Prevacid® NapraPAC™ [US]

Therapeutic Category Gastric Acid Secretion Inhibitor; Nonsteroidal Antiinflammatory Drug (NSAID)

Use Reduction of the risk of NSAID-associated gastric ulcers in patients with history of gastric ulcer who require an NSAID for the treatment of rheumatoid arthritis, osteoarthritis, and ankylosing spondylitis

Usual Dosage Oral: Adults: Reduce NSAID-associated gastric ulcers during treatment for arthritis: Lansoprazole 15 mg once daily in the morning; naproxen 500 mg twice daily

Dosage Forms

Combination package:

Prevacid® NapraPAC™ 500 [each administration card contains]:

Capsule, delayed release (Prevacid®): Lansoprazole 15 mg (7 capsules per card)

Tablet (Naprosyn®): Naproxen 500 mg (14 tablets per card)

lanthanum (LAN tha num)
Synonyms lanthanum carbonate
U.S./Canadian Brand Names Fosrenol™ [US]
Therapeutic Category Phosphate Binder
Use Reduction of serum phosphate in patients with stage 5 chronic kidney disease (kidney failure: GFR <15 mL/minute/1.73 m² or dialysis)
Usual Dosage Oral: Adults: Initial: 750-1500 mg/day divided and taken with meals; typical increases of 750 mg/day every 2-3 weeks are suggested as needed to bring the serum phosphate level <6 mg/dL; usual dosage range: 1500-3000 mg; doses of up to 3750 mg have been used
Dosage Forms
Tablet, chewable:
Fosrenol™: 250 mg, 500 mg, 750 mg, 1000 mg

lanthanum carbonate *see* lanthanum *on this page*

Lantus® [US/Can] *see* insulin glargine *on page 458*

Lantus® OptiSet® [Can] *see* insulin glargine *on page 458*

Lanvis® [Can] *see* thioguanine *on page 837*

Lapase [US] *see* pancreatin *on page 648*

lapatinib (la PA ti nib)
Sound-Alike/Look-Alike Issues
lapatinib may be confused with dasatinib, erlotinib, imatinib
Synonyms GW572016; lapatinib ditosylate; NSC-727989
U.S./Canadian Brand Names Tykerb® [US]
Therapeutic Category Antineoplastic Agent, Tyrosine Kinase Inhibitor; Epidermal Growth Factor Receptor (EGFR) Inhibitor
Use Treatment (in combination with capecitabine) of HER2/neu overexpressing advanced or metastatic breast cancer, in patients who have received prior therapy (with an anthracycline, a taxane, and trastuzumab)
Usual Dosage Refer to individual protocols. **Note:** Dose reductions are likely to be needed when lapatinib is administered concomitantly with a strong CYP3A4 inhibitor (an alternate medication for CYP3A4 enzyme inhibitors should be investigated first).
Oral: Adults: 1250 mg once daily

lapatinib ditosylate *see* lapatinib *on this page*

Largactil® [Can] *see* chlorpromazine *on page 185*

Lariam® [US/Can] *see* mefloquine *on page 538*

laronidase (lair OH ni days)
Synonyms recombinant α-L-iduronidase (glycosaminoglycan α-L-iduronohydrolase)
U.S./Canadian Brand Names Aldurazyme® [US/Can]
Therapeutic Category Enzyme
Use Treatment of Hurler and Hurler-Scheie forms of mucopolysaccharidosis I (MPS I); treatment of Scheie form of MPS I in patients with moderate to severe symptoms
Usual Dosage Note: Premedicate with antipyretic and/or antihistamines 1 hour prior to start of infusion.
I.V.: Children ≥5 years and Adults: 0.58 mg/kg once weekly; dose should be rounded up to the nearest whole vial
Dosage Forms
Injection, solution [preservative free]:
Aldurazyme®: 2.9 mg/5 mL (5 mL)

Lasix® [US/Can] *see* furosemide *on page 379*

Lasix® Special [Can] *see* furosemide *on page 379*

L-asparaginase *see* asparaginase *on page 77*

lassar's zinc paste *see* zinc oxide *on page 906*

latanoprost (la TA noe prost)
Sound-Alike/Look-Alike Issues
Xalatan® may be confused with Travatan®, Zarontin®
U.S./Canadian Brand Names Xalatan® [US/Can]
Therapeutic Category Prostaglandin
Use Reduction of elevated intraocular pressure in patients with open-angle glaucoma or ocular hypertension

Usual Dosage Ophthalmic: Adults: 1 drop (1.5 mcg) in the affected eye(s) once daily in the evening; do not exceed the once daily dosage because it has been shown that more frequent administration may decrease the IOP lowering effect

Note: A medication delivery device (Xal-Ease™) is available for use with Xalatan®.

Dosage Forms
Solution, ophthalmic:
Xalatan®: 0.005% (2.5 mL)

Lavacol® [US-OTC] *see* alcohol (ethyl) *on page 25*

Laxilose [Can] *see* lactulose *on page 489*

***l*-bunolol hydrochloride** *see* levobunolol *on page 499*

L-carnitine *see* levocarnitine *on page 499*

LCD *see* coal tar *on page 208*

LCR *see* vincristine *on page 891*

L-deoxythymidine *see* telbivudine *on page 822*

L-deprenyl *see* selegiline *on page 780*

LDP-341 *see* bortezomib *on page 116*

Lectopam® [Can] *see* bromazepam *(Canada only) on page 119*

Leena™ [US] *see* ethinyl estradiol and norethindrone *on page 328*

leflunomide (le FLOO noh mide)

U.S./Canadian Brand Names Apo-Leflunomide® [Can]; Arava® [US/Can]; Novo-Leflunomide [Can]
Therapeutic Category Antiinflammatory Agent
Use Treatment of active rheumatoid arthritis; indicated to reduce signs and symptoms, and to retard structural damage and improve physical function
Orphan drug: Prevention of acute and chronic rejection in recipients of solid organ transplants
Usual Dosage Oral: Adults: Rheumatoid arthritis: Initial: 100 mg/day for 3 days, followed by 20 mg/day; dosage may be decreased to 10 mg/day in patients who have difficulty tolerating the 20 mg dose. Due to the long half-life of the active metabolite, plasma levels may require a prolonged period to decline after dosage reduction.
Dosage Forms
Tablet: 10 mg, 20 mg
Arava®: 10 mg, 20 mg

Legatrin PM® [US-OTC] *see* acetaminophen and diphenhydramine *on page 7*

lenalidomide (le na LID oh mide)

Synonyms CC-5013; IMid-3; NSC-703813
U.S./Canadian Brand Names Revlimid® [US]
Therapeutic Category Angiogenesis Inhibitor; Immunosuppressant Agent; Tumor Necrosis Factor (TNF) Blocking Agent
Use Treatment of myelodysplastic syndrome (MDS) in patients with deletion 5q (del 5q) cytogenetic abnormality; treatment of multiple myeloma
Usual Dosage Oral: Adults:
Myelodysplastic syndrome (MDS): 10 mg once daily
Multiple myeloma: 25 mg once daily for 21 days of a 28-day treatment cycle (in combination with dexamethasone)
Dosage Forms
Capsule:
Revlimid®: 5 mg, 10 mg, 15 mg, 25 mg

Lente® Iletin® II *(Discontinued)*

lepirudin (leh puh ROO din)

Synonyms lepirudin (rDNA); recombinant hirudin
U.S./Canadian Brand Names Refludan® [US/Can]
Therapeutic Category Anticoagulant (Other)
Use Indicated for anticoagulation in patients with heparin-induced thrombocytopenia (HIT) and associated thromboembolic disease in order to prevent further thromboembolic complications
Usual Dosage Adults: Maximum dose: Do not exceed 0.21 mg/kg/hour unless an evaluation of coagulation abnormalities limiting response has been completed. **Dosing is weight-based, however, patients weighing**
(Continued)

lepirudin (Continued)

>110 kg should not receive doses greater than the recommended dose for a patient weighing 110 kg (44 mg bolus and initial maximal infusion rate of 16.5 mg/hour).

Heparin-induced thrombocytopenia: Bolus dose: 0.4 mg/kg IVP (over 15-20 seconds), followed by continuous infusion at 0.15 mg/kg/hour; bolus and infusion must be reduced in renal insufficiency

Note: Due to potential renal insufficiency in critical care patients, some clinicians suggest that for isolated HIT (without thromboembolic complications), the initial infusion rate should be 0.1 mg/kg/hour (omit the initial bolus dose unless acute HITTS).

Concomitant use with thrombolytic therapy: Bolus dose: 0.2 mg/kg IVP (over 15-20 seconds), followed by continuous infusion at 0.1 mg/kg/hour

Dosing adjustments during infusions: Monitor first aPTT 4 hours after the start of the infusion. Subsequent determinations of aPTT should be obtained at least once daily during treatment. More frequent monitoring is recommended in renally- or hepatically-impaired patients. Any aPTT ratio measurement out of range (1.5-2.5) should be confirmed prior to adjusting dose, unless a clinical need for immediate reaction exists. If the aPTT is below target range, increase infusion by 20%. If the aPTT is in excess of the target range, stop infusion for 2 hours and when restarted the infusion rate should be decreased by 50%. A repeat aPTT should be obtained 4 hours after any dosing change.

Use in patients scheduled for switch to oral anticoagulants: Once platelets normalize, reduce lepirudin dose gradually to reach aPTT ratio just above 1.5 before starting warfarin therapy. Monitor PT/INR closely until results stabilize in therapeutic range. When lepirudin is discontinued, there may be a small reduction in INR.

Dosage Forms
Injection, powder for reconstitution:
Refludan®: 50 mg

lepirudin (rDNA) *see lepirudin on previous page*
Lescol® [US/Can] *see fluvastatin on page 370*
Lescol® XL [US/Can] *see fluvastatin on page 370*
Lessina™ [US] *see ethinyl estradiol and levonorgestrel on page 325*
Letairis™ [US] *see ambrisentan on page 39*

letrozole (LET roe zole)

Sound-Alike/Look-Alike Issues
Femara® may be confused with femhrt®
Synonyms CGS-20267; NSC-719345
U.S./Canadian Brand Names Femara® [US/Can]
Therapeutic Category Antineoplastic Agent, Hormone (Antiestrogen)
Use Adjuvant treatment of postmenopausal hormone receptor positive early breast cancer; treatment of postmenopausal hormone receptor positive or hormone receptor unknown, locally-advanced, or metastatic breast cancer
Usual Dosage Oral (refer to individual protocols): Adults: Female: Breast cancer: 2.5 mg once daily
Dosage Forms
Tablet:
Femara®: 2.5 mg

leucovorin (loo koe VOR in)

Sound-Alike/Look-Alike Issues
leucovorin may be confused with Leukeran®, Leukine®
folinic acid may be confused with folic acid
Synonyms calcium leucovorin; citrovorum factor; folinic acid; 5-formyl tetrahydrofolate; leucovorin calcium
Therapeutic Category Folic Acid Derivative
Use Antidote for folic acid antagonists (methotrexate, trimethoprim, pyrimethamine); treatment of megaloblastic anemias when folate is deficient as in infancy, sprue, pregnancy, and nutritional deficiency when oral folate therapy is not possible; in combination with fluorouracil in the treatment of colon cancer
Usual Dosage Children and Adults:
Treatment of folic acid antagonist overdosage: Oral: 2-15 mg/day for 3 days or until blood counts are normal, **or** 5 mg every 3 days; doses of 6 mg/day are needed for patients with platelet counts <100,000/mm^3
Folate-deficient megaloblastic anemia: I.M.: 1 mg/day
Megaloblastic anemia secondary to congenital deficiency of dihydrofolate reductase: I.M.: 3-6 mg/day
Rescue dose: Initial: I.V.: 10 mg/m^2, then:
Oral, I.M., I.V., SubQ: 10-15 mg/m^2 every 6 hours until methotrexate level <0.05 micromole/L; if methotrexate level remains >5 micromole/L at 48-72 hours after the end of the methotrexate infusion, increase to 20-100 mg/m^2 every 6 hours until methotrexate level <0.05 micromole/L

Dosage Forms
Injection, powder for reconstitution: 50 mg, 100 mg, 200 mg, 350 mg, 500 mg
Injection, solution: 10 mg/mL (50 mL)
Tablet: 5 mg, 10 mg, 15 mg, 25 mg

leucovorin calcium *see* leucovorin *on previous page*

Leukeran® [US/Can] *see* chlorambucil *on page 172*

Leukine® [US/Can] *see* sargramostim *on page 777*

leuprolide (loo PROE lide)

Sound-Alike/Look-Alike Issues
Lupron® may be confused with Nuprin®
Lupron Depot®-3 Month may be confused with Lupron Depot-Ped®
Synonyms abbott-43818; leuprolide acetate; leuprorelin acetate; NSC-377526; TAP-144
U.S./Canadian Brand Names Eligard® [US/Can]; Lupron Depot-Ped® [US]; Lupron Depot® [US/Can]; Lupron® [US/Can]; Viadur® [US/Can]
Therapeutic Category Antineoplastic Agent; Luteinizing Hormone-Releasing Hormone Analog
Use Palliative treatment of advanced prostate carcinoma; management of endometriosis; treatment of anemia caused by uterine leiomyomata (fibroids); central precocious puberty
Usual Dosage
Children: Precocious puberty (consider discontinuing by age 11 for females and by age 12 for males):
SubQ (Lupron®): Initial: 50 mcg/kg/day (per manufacturer, doses of 20-45 mcg/kg/day have also been reported); titrate dose upward by 10 mcg/kg/day if down-regulation is not achieved
I.M. (Lupron Depot-Ped®): 0.3 mg/kg/dose given every 28 days (minimum dose: 7.5 mg)
≤25 kg: 7.5 mg
>25-37.5 kg: 11.25 mg
>37.5 kg: 15 mg
Titrate dose upward in increments of 3.75 mg every 4 weeks if down-regulation is not achieved.
Adults:
Advanced prostatic carcinoma:
SubQ:
Eligard®: 7.5 mg monthly **or** 22.5 mg every 3 months **or** 30 mg every 4 months **or** 45 mg every 6 months
Lupron®: 1 mg/day
Viadur®: 65 mg implanted subcutaneously every 12 months
I.M.:
Lupron Depot®: 7.5 mg/dose given monthly (every 28-33 days) **or**
Lupron Depot®-3: 22.5 mg every 3 months **or**
Lupron Depot®-4: 30 mg every 4 months
Endometriosis: I.M.: Initial therapy may be with leuprolide alone or in combination with norethindrone; if retreatment for an additional 6 months is necessary, norethindrone should be used. Retreatment is not recommended for longer than one additional 6-month course.
Lupron Depot®: 3.75 mg/month for up to 6 months **or**
Lupron Depot®-3: 11.25 mg every 3 months for up to 2 doses (6 months total duration of treatment)
Uterine leiomyomata (fibroids): I.M. (in combination with iron):
Lupron Depot®: 3.75 mg/month for up to 3 months **or**
Lupron Depot®-3: 11.25 mg as a single injection
Dosage Forms
Implant, subcutaneous:
Viadur®: 65 mg [released over 12 months]
Injection, solution: 5 mg/mL (2.8 mL)
Lupron®: 5 mg/mL (2.8 mL)
Injection, powder for reconstitution [depot formulation]:
Eligard®:
7.5 mg [released over 1 month]
22.5 mg [released over 3 months]
30 mg [released over 4 months]
45 mg [released over 6 months]
Lupron Depot®: 3.75 mg, 7.5 mg [released over 1 month]
Lupron Depot®-3 Month: 11.25 mg, 22.5 mg [released over 3 months]
Lupron Depot®-4 Month: 30 mg [released over 4 months]
Lupron Depot-Ped®: 7.5 mg, 11.25 mg, 15 mg [released over 1 month]

leuprolide acetate *see* leuprolide *on this page*

leuprorelin acetate *see* leuprolide *on this page*

leurocristine sulfate *see* vincristine *on page 891*

Leustatin® **[US/Can]** *see* cladribine *on page 196*

levalbuterol (leve al BYOO ter ole)
Sound-Alike/Look-Alike Issues
Xopenex® may be confused with Xanax®
Synonyms levalbuterol hydrochloride; levalbuterol tartrate; R-albuterol
U.S./Canadian Brand Names Xopenex HFA™ [US]; Xopenex® [US/Can]
Therapeutic Category Adrenergic Agonist Agent; Beta$_2$-Adrenergic Agonist Agent; Bronchodilator
Use Treatment or prevention of bronchospasm in children and adults with reversible obstructive airway disease
Usual Dosage
Metered-dose inhalation: Aerosol: Children ≥4 years and Adults: 1-2 puffs every 4-6 hours
Nebulization:
Children 6-11 years: 0.31 mg 3 times/day (maximum dose: 0.63 mg 3 times/day)
Children >12 years and Adults: 0.63 mg 3 times/day at intervals of 6-8 hours; dosage may be increased to 1.25 mg 3 times/day with close monitoring for adverse effects. Most patients gain optimal benefit from regular use
Dosage Forms
Aerosol, oral:
Xopenex®, Xopenex HFA™: 45 mcg/actuation (15 g)
Solution for nebulization:
Xopenex®, Xopenex HFA™: 0.31 mg/3 mL (24s); 0.63 mg/3 mL (24s); 1.25 mg/3 mL (24s)
Solution for nebulization, concentrate:
Xopenex®, Xopenex HFA™: 1.25 mg/0.5 mL (30s)

levalbuterol hydrochloride *see* levalbuterol *on this page*

levalbuterol tartrate *see* levalbuterol *on this page*

Levall™ **[US]** *see* carbetapentane, guaifenesin, and phenylephrine *on page 149*

Levall 5.0 [US] *see* hydrocodone, phenylephrine, and guaifenesin *on page 431*

Levall G [US] *see* guaifenesin and pseudoephedrine *on page 406*

Levaquin® **[US/Can]** *see* levofloxacin *on page 501*

levarterenol bitartrate *see* norepinephrine *on page 611*

Levate® **[Can]** *see* amitriptyline *on page 44*

Levatol® **[US/Can]** *see* penbutolol *on page 660*

Levbid® **[US]** *see* hyoscyamine *on page 441*

Levemir® **[US/Can]** *see* insulin detemir *on page 457*

levetiracetam (lee va tye RA se tam)
Sound-Alike/Look-Alike Issues
Potential for dispensing errors between Keppra® and Kaletra™ (lopinavir/ritonavir)
U.S./Canadian Brand Names CO Levetiracetam [Can]; Keppra® [US/Can]
Therapeutic Category Anticonvulsant, Miscellaneous
Use Adjunctive therapy in the treatment of partial onset, myoclonic, and/or primary generalized tonic-clonic seizures
Usual Dosage
Oral:
Children 4-15 years: Partial onset seizures: 10 mg/kg/dose given twice daily; may increase every 2 weeks by 10 mg/kg/dose to a maximum of 30 mg/kg/dose twice daily
Children 6-15 years: Tonic-clonic seizures: Initial: 10 mg/kg dose given twice daily; may increase every 2 weeks by 10 mg/kg/dose to the recommended dose of 30 mg/kg twice daily. Efficacy of doses >60 mg/kg/day has not been established.
Children ≥12 years and Adults: Myoclonic seizures: Initial: 500 mg twice daily; may increase every 2 weeks by 500 mg/dose to the recommended dose of 1500 mg twice daily. Efficacy of doses >3000 mg/day has not been established.
Children ≥16 years and Adults:
Partial onset seizure: Initial: 500 mg twice daily; may increase every 2 weeks by 500 mg/dose to a maximum of 1500 mg twice daily. Doses >3000 mg/day have been used in trials; however, there is no evidence of increased benefit.
Tonic-clonic seizures: Initial: 500 mg twice daily; may increase every 2 weeks by 500 mg/dose to the recommended dose of 1500 mg twice daily. Efficacy of doses >3000 mg/day has not been established.

I.V.: Children ≥16 years and Adults: Partial onset seizure: Initial: 500 mg twice daily; may increase every 2 weeks by 500 mg/dose to a maximum of 1500 mg twice daily. Doses >3000 mg/day have been used in trials; however, there is no evidence of increased benefit.

Note: When switching from oral to I.V. formulations, the total daily dose should be the same.

Dosage Forms
Injection, solution:
Keppra®: 100 mg/mL (5 mL)
Solution, oral:
Keppra®: 100 mg/mL
Tablet:
Keppra®: 250 mg, 500 mg, 750 mg, 1000 mg

Levitra® [US/Can] *see* vardenafil *on page 884*

Levlen® [US] *see* ethinyl estradiol and levonorgestrel *on page 325*

Levlite™ [US] *see* ethinyl estradiol and levonorgestrel *on page 325*

levobunolol (lee voe BYOO noe lole)
Sound-Alike/Look-Alike Issues
levobunolol may be confused with levocabastine
Betagan® may be confused with Betadine®, Betoptic® S
Synonyms *l*-bunolol hydrochloride; levobunolol hydrochloride
U.S./Canadian Brand Names Apo-Levobunolol® [Can]; Betagan® [US/Can]; Novo-Levobunolol [Can]; Optho-Bunolol® [Can]; PMS-Levobunolol [Can]; Sandoz-Levobunolol [Can]
Therapeutic Category Beta-Adrenergic Blocker
Use To lower intraocular pressure in chronic open-angle glaucoma or ocular hypertension
Usual Dosage Ophthalmic: Adults: Instill 1 drop in the affected eye(s) 1-2 times/day
Dosage Forms
Solution, ophthalmic: 0.25% (5 mL, 10 mL); 0.5% (5 mL, 10 mL, 15 mL)
Betagan®: 0.25% (5 mL, 10 mL); 0.5% (2 mL, 5 mL, 10 mL, 15 mL)

levobunolol hydrochloride *see* levobunolol *on this page*

levocarnitine (lee voe KAR ni teen)
Sound-Alike/Look-Alike Issues
levocarnitine may be confused with levocabastine
Synonyms L-carnitine
U.S./Canadian Brand Names Carnitor® SF [US]; Carnitor® [US/Can]
Therapeutic Category Dietary Supplement
Use
Oral: Primary systemic carnitine deficiency; acute and chronic treatment of patients with an inborn error of metabolism which results in secondary carnitine deficiency
I.V.: Acute and chronic treatment of patients with an inborn error of metabolism which results in secondary carnitine deficiency; prevention and treatment of carnitine deficiency in patients with end-stage renal disease (ESRD) who are undergoing hemodialysis.
Usual Dosage
Carnitine deficiency:
Oral:
Infants/Children: Initial: 50 mg/kg/day; titrate to 50-100 mg/kg/day in divided doses with a maximum dose of 3 g/day
Adults: 990 mg (tablet) 2-3 times/day or 1-3 g/day (solution)
I.V.: Children and Adults: 50 mg/kg/day in divided doses; titrate based on patient response. Maximum reported dose: 300 mg/kg. An equivalent loading dose may be used in patients in severe metabolic crisis.
ESRD patients on hemodialysis: I.V.: Adults: 20 mg/kg dry body weight as a slow 2- to 3-minute bolus after each dialysis session
Note: Safety and efficacy of oral carnitine have not been established in ESRD. Chronic administration of high **oral** doses to patients with severely compromised renal function or ESRD patients on dialysis may result in accumulation of **potentially toxic** metabolites.
Dosage Forms
Capsule: 250 mg
Injection, solution: 200 mg/mL (5 mL, 12.5 mL)
Carnitor®: 200 mg/mL (5 mL)
Solution, oral: 100 mg/mL
Carnitor®: 100 mg/mL
Carnitor® SF: 100 mg/mL
(Continued)

levocarnitine *(Continued)*
Tablet: 330 mg, 500 mg
Carnitor®: 330 mg

levocetirizine (LEE vo se TI ra zeen)
Sound-Alike/Look-Alike Issues
levocetirizine may be confused with cetirizine
Synonyms levocetirizine dihydrochloride
U.S./Canadian Brand Names Xyzal® [US]
Therapeutic Category Antihistamine
Use Relief of symptoms of perennial and seasonal allergic rhinitis; treatment of skin manifestations (uncomplicated) of chronic idiopathic urticaria
Usual Dosage Oral: Allergic rhinitis, chronic urticaria:
Children 6-11 years: 2.5 mg once daily (in the evening); maximum: 2.5 mg/day
Children ≥12 years and Adults: 5 mg once daily (in the evening); some patients may experience relief of symptoms with 2.5 mg once daily
Dosage Forms
Tablet, as dihydrochloride [scored]:
Xyzal®: 5 mg

levocetirizine dihydrochloride *see* levocetirizine *on this page*

levodopa and benserazide *see* benserazide and levodopa *(Canada only)* on page 99

levodopa and carbidopa (lee voe DOE pa & kar bi DOE pa)
Synonyms carbidopa and levodopa
U.S./Canadian Brand Names Apo-Levocarb® CR [Can]; Apo-Levocarb® [Can]; Endo®-Levodopa/Carbidopa [Can]; Novo-Levocarbidopa [Can]; Nu-Levocarb [Can]; Parcopa™ [US]; Sinemet® CR [US/Can]; Sinemet® [US/Can]
Therapeutic Category Anti-Parkinson Agent (Dopamine Agonist)
Use Idiopathic Parkinson disease; postencephalitic parkinsonism; symptomatic parkinsonism
Usual Dosage Oral: Adults: Parkinson disease:
Immediate release tablet:
Initial: Carbidopa 25 mg/levodopa 100 mg 3 times/day
Dosage adjustment: Alternate tablet strengths may be substituted according to individual carbidopa/levodopa requirements. Increase by 1 tablet every other day as necessary, except when using the carbidopa 25 mg/levodopa 250 mg tablets where increases should be made using 1/2-1 tablet every 1-2 days. Use of more than 1 dosage strength or dosing 4 times/day may be required (maximum: 8 tablets of any strength/day or 200 mg of carbidopa and 2000 mg of levodopa)
Sustained release tablet:
Initial: Carbidopa 50 mg/levodopa 200 mg 2 times/day, at intervals not <6 hours
Dosage adjustment: May adjust every 3 days; intervals should be between 4-8 hours during the waking day (maximum: 8 tablets/day)
Dosage Forms
Tablet immediate release: 10/100: Carbidopa 10 mg and levodopa 100 mg; 25/100: Carbidopa 25 mg and levodopa 100 mg; 25/250: Carbidopa 25 mg and levodopa 250 mg
Sinemet®: 10/100: Carbidopa 10 mg and levodopa 100 mg; 25/100: Carbidopa 25 mg and levodopa 100 mg; 25/250: Carbidopa 25 mg and levodopa 250 mg
Tablet, immediate release, orally disintegrating:
Parcopa™: 10/100: Carbidopa 10 mg and levodopa 100 mg; 25/100: Carbidopa 25 mg and levodopa 100 mg; 25/250: Carbidopa 25 mg and levodopa 250 mg
Tablet, sustained release: Carbidopa 25 mg and levodopa 100 mg; carbidopa 50 mg and levodopa 200 mg
Sinemet® CR: Carbidopa 25 mg and levodopa 100 mg; carbidopa 50 mg and levodopa 200 mg

levodopa, carbidopa, and entacapone (lee voe DOE pa, kar bi DOE pa, & en TA ka pone)
Synonyms carbidopa, levodopa, and entacapone; entacapone, carbidopa, and levodopa
U.S./Canadian Brand Names Stalevo™ [US]
Therapeutic Category Anti-Parkinson Agent (Dopamine Agonist); Anti-Parkinson Agent, COMT Inhibitor
Use Treatment of idiopathic Parkinson disease
Usual Dosage Oral: Adults: Parkinson disease:
Note: All strengths of Stalevo™ contain a carbidopa/levodopa ratio of 1:4 plus entacapone 200 mg.
Dose should be individualized based on therapeutic response; doses may be adjusted by changing strength or adjusting interval. Fractionated doses are not recommended and only 1 tablet should be given at each dosing interval; maximum dose: 8 tablets/day (equivalent to entacapone 1600 mg/day)

Patients previously treated with carbidopa/levodopa immediate release tablets (ratio of 1:4):

With current entacapone therapy: May switch directly to corresponding strength of combination tablet. No data available on transferring patients from controlled release preparations or products with a 1:10 ratio of carbidopa/levodopa.

Without entacapone therapy:

If current levodopa dose is >600 mg/day: Levodopa dose reduction may be required when adding entacapone to therapy; therefore, titrate dose using individual products first (carbidopa/levodopa immediate release with a ratio of 1:4 plus entacapone 200 mg); then transfer to combination product once stabilized.

If current levodopa dose is <600 mg without dyskinesias: May transfer to corresponding dose of combination product; monitor, dose reduction of levodopa may be required.

Dosage Forms
Tablet:
Stalevo™: 50: Carbidopa 12.5 mg, levodopa 50 mg, and entacapone 200 mg; 100: Carbidopa 25 mg, levodopa 100 mg, and entacapone 200 mg; 150: Carbidopa 37.5 mg, levodopa 150 mg, and entacapone 200 mg

Levo-Dromoran® [US] *see* levorphanol *on next page*

levofloxacin (lee voe FLOKS a sin)
U.S./Canadian Brand Names Iquix® [US]; Levaquin® [US/Can]; Novo-Levofloxacin [Can]; Quixin™ [US]
Therapeutic Category Antibiotic, Ophthalmic; Antibiotic, Quinolone
Use
Systemic: Treatment of mild, moderate, or severe infections caused by susceptible organisms. Includes the treatment of community-acquired pneumonia, including multidrug resistant strains of *S. pneumoniae* (MDRSP); nosocomial pneumonia; chronic bronchitis (acute bacterial exacerbation); acute bacterial sinusitis; urinary tract infection (uncomplicated or complicated); acute pyelonephritis; skin or skin structure infections (uncomplicated or complicated); reduce incidence or disease progression of inhalational anthrax (postexposure)

Ophthalmic: Treatment of bacterial conjunctivitis caused by susceptible organisms (Quixin™ 0.5% ophthalmic solution); treatment of corneal ulcer caused by susceptible organisms (Iquix® 1.5% ophthalmic solution)

Usual Dosage Note: Sequential therapy (intravenous to oral) may be instituted based on prescriber's discretion.
Usual dosage range:
Children ≥1 year: Ophthalmic: 1-2 drops every 2-6 hours
Adults:
Ophthalmic: 1-2 drops every 2-6 hours
Oral, I.V.: 250-500 mg every 24 hours; severe or complicated infections: 750 mg every 24 hours
Indication-specific dosing:
Children ≥1 year and Adults: Ophthalmic:
Conjunctivitis (0.5% ophthalmic solution):
Treatment day 1 and day 2: Instill 1-2 drops into affected eye(s) every 2 hours while awake, up to 8 times/day
Treatment day 3 through day 7: Instill 1-2 drops into affected eye(s) every 4 hours while awake, up to 4 times/day
Children ≥6 years and Adults: Ophthalmic:
Corneal ulceration (1.5% ophthalmic solution): Treatment day 1 through day 3: Instill 1-2 drops into affected eye(s) every 30 minutes to 2 hours while awake and 4-6 hours after retiring.
Adults: Oral, I.V.:
Anthrax (inhalational): 500 mg every 24 hours for 60 days, beginning as soon as possible after exposure
Chronic bronchitis (acute bacterial exacerbation): 500 mg every 24 hours for at least 7 days
Pneumonia:
Community-acquired: 500 mg every 24 hours for 7-14 days or 750 mg every 24 hours for 5 days (efficacy of 5-day regimen for MDRSP not established)
Nosocomial: 750 mg every 24 hours for 7-14 days
Prostatitis (chronic bacterial): 500 mg every 24 hours for 28 days
Sinusitis (bacterial, acute): 500 mg every 24 hours for 10-14 days or 750 mg every 24 hours for 5 days
Skin and skin structure infections:
Uncomplicated: 500 mg every 24 hours for 7-10 days
Complicated: 750 mg every 24 hours for 7-14 days
Urinary tract infections:
Uncomplicated: 250 mg once daily for 3 days
Complicated, including pyelonephritis: 250 mg once daily for 10 days
Dosage Forms
Infusion [premixed in D₅W]:
Levaquin®: 250 mg (50 mL); 500 mg (100 mL); 750 mg (150 mL)
(Continued)

levofloxacin (Continued)

Injection, solution [preservative free]:
Levaquin®: 25 mg/mL (20 mL, 30 mL)
Solution, ophthalmic:
Iquix®: 1.5% (5 mL)
Quixin™: 0.5% (5 mL)
Solution, oral:
Levaquin®: 25 mg/mL
Tablet:
Levaquin®: 250 mg, 500 mg, 750 mg
Levaquin® Leva-Pak: 750 mg (5s)

levomepromazine see methotrimeprazine *(Canada only)* on page 554

levonordefrin and mepivacaine hydrochloride see mepivacaine and levonordefrin on page 544

levonorgestrel (LEE voe nor jes trel)

Synonyms LNg 20
U.S./Canadian Brand Names Mirena® [US/Can]; Norplant® Implant [Can]; Plan B® [US/Can]
Therapeutic Category Contraceptive, Implant (Progestin); Contraceptive, Progestin Only
Use Prevention of pregnancy
Usual Dosage Adults: Females:
  Long-term prevention of pregnancy: Intrauterine system: To be inserted into uterine cavity; should be inserted within 7 days of onset of menstruation or immediately after 1st trimester abortion; releases 20 mcg levonorgestrel/day over 5 years. May be removed and replaced with a new unit at anytime during menstrual cycle; do not leave any one system in place for >5 years
  Emergency contraception: Oral tablet: One 0.75 mg tablet as soon as possible within 72 hours of unprotected sexual intercourse; a second 0.75 mg tablet should be taken 12 hours after the first dose; may be used at any time during menstrual cycle
Dosage Forms
  Intrauterine device:
  Mirena®: 52 mg levonorgestrel/unit
  Tablet:
  Plan B®: 0.75 mg

levonorgestrel and estradiol see estradiol and levonorgestrel on page 315

levonorgestrel and ethinyl estradiol see ethinyl estradiol and levonorgestrel on page 325

Levophed® [US/Can] see norepinephrine on page 611

Levora® [US] see ethinyl estradiol and levonorgestrel on page 325

levorphanol (lee VOR fa nole)

Synonyms levorphanol tartrate; levorphan tartrate
U.S./Canadian Brand Names Levo-Dromoran® [US]
Therapeutic Category Analgesic, Narcotic
Controlled Substance C-II
Use Relief of moderate to severe pain; also used parenterally for preoperative sedation and an adjunct to nitrous oxide/oxygen anesthesia
Usual Dosage Adults: **Note:** These are guidelines and do not represent the maximum doses that may be required in all patients. Doses should be titrated to pain relief/prevention.
  Acute pain (moderate to severe):
  Oral: Initial: Opiate-naive: 2 mg every 6-8 hours as needed; patients with prior opiate exposure may require higher initial doses; usual dosage range: 2-4 mg every 6-8 hours as needed
  I.M., SubQ: Initial: Opiate-naive: 1 mg every 6-8 hours as needed; patients with prior opiate exposure may require higher initial doses; usual dosage range: 1-2 mg every 6-8 hours as needed
  Slow I.V.: Initial: Opiate-naive: Up to 1 mg/dose every 3-6 hours as needed; patients with prior opiate exposure may require higher initial doses
  Chronic pain: Patients taking opioids chronically may become tolerant and require doses higher than the usual dosage range to maintain the desired effect. Tolerance can be managed by appropriate dose titration. **There is no optimal or maximal dose for levorphanol in chronic pain. The appropriate dose is one that relieves pain throughout its dosing interval without causing unmanageable side effects.**
  Premedication: I.M., SubQ: 1-2 mg/dose 60-90 minutes prior to surgery; older or debilitated patients usually require less drug

Dosage Forms
Injection, solution:
Levo-Dromoran®: 2 mg/mL (1 mL, 10 mL)
Tablet: 2 mg
Levo-Dromoran®: 2 mg

levorphanol tartrate *see* levorphanol *on previous page*

levorphan tartrate *see* levorphanol *on previous page*

Levo-T™ *(Discontinued) see* levothyroxine *on this page*

Levothroid® [US] *see* levothyroxine *on this page*

levothyroxine (lee voe thye ROKS een)

Sound-Alike/Look-Alike Issues
levothyroxine may be confused with liothyronine
Levoxyl® may be confused with Lanoxin®, Luvox®
Synthroid® may be confused with Symmetrel®

Synonyms levothyroxine sodium; *L*-thyroxine sodium; T_4

U.S./Canadian Brand Names Eltroxin® [Can]; Gen-Levothyroxine [Can]; Levothroid® [US]; Levothyroxine Sodium [Can]; Levoxyl® [US]; Synthroid® [US/Can]; Unithroid® [US]

Therapeutic Category Thyroid Product

Use Replacement or supplemental therapy in hypothyroidism; pituitary TSH suppression

Usual Dosage Doses should be adjusted based on clinical response and laboratory parameters.

Oral:

Children: Hypothyroidism:

Newborns: Initial: 10-15 mcg/kg/day. Lower doses of 25 mcg/day should be considered in newborns at risk for cardiac failure. Newborns with T_4 levels <5 mcg/dL should be started at 50 mcg/day. Adjust dose at 4- to 6-week intervals.

Infants and Children: Dose based on body weight and age as listed below. Children with severe or chronic hypothyroidism should be started at 25 mcg/day; adjust dose by 25 mcg every 2-4 weeks. In older children, hyperactivity may be decreased by starting with $1/4$ of the recommended dose and increasing by $1/4$ dose each week until the full replacement dose is reached. Refer to adult dosing once growth and puberty are complete.

0-3 months: 10-15 mcg/kg/day
3-6 months: 8-10 mcg/kg/day
6-12 months: 6-8 mcg/kg/day
1-5 years: 5-6 mcg/kg/day
6-12 years: 4-5 mcg/kg/day
>12 years: 2-3 mcg/kg/day

Adults:

Hypothyroidism: 1.7 mcg/kg/day in otherwise healthy adults <50 years old, children in whom growth and puberty are complete, and older adults who have been recently treated for hyperthyroidism or who have been hypothyroid for only a few months. Titrate dose every 6 weeks. Average starting dose ~100 mcg; usual doses are ≤200 mcg/day; doses ≥300 mcg/day are rare (consider poor compliance, malabsorption, and/or drug interactions).

Severe hypothyroidism: Initial: 12.5-25 mcg/day; adjust dose by 25 mcg/day every 2-4 weeks as appropriate; **Note:** Oral agents are not recommended for myxedema (see I.V. dosing).

Subclinical hypothyroidism (if treated): 1 mcg/kg/day

TSH suppression:

Well-differentiated thyroid cancer: Highly individualized; Doses >2 mcg/kg/day may be needed to suppress TSH to <0.1 mU/L.

Benign nodules and nontoxic multinodular goiter: Goal TSH suppression: 0.1-0.3 mU/L

I.M., I.V.: Children, Adults: Hypothyroidism: 50% of the oral dose

I.V.: Adults: Myxedema coma or stupor: 200-500 mcg, then 100-300 mcg the next day if necessary; smaller doses should be considered in patients with cardiovascular disease

Dosage Forms
Capsule, soft gelatin:
Tirosint™: 13 mcg, 25 mcg, 50 mcg, 75 mcg, 100 mcg, 125 mcg, 150 mcg
Injection, powder for reconstitution: 0.2 mg, 0.5 mg
Tablet: 25 mcg, 50 mcg, 75 mcg, 88 mcg, 100 mcg, 112 mcg, 125 mcg, 150 mcg, 175 mcg, 200 mcg, 300 mcg
Levothroid®: 25 mcg, 50 mcg, 75 mcg, 88 mcg, 100 mcg, 112 mcg, 125 mcg, 150 mcg, 175 mcg, 200 mcg, 300 mcg
Levoxyl®: 25 mcg, 50 mcg, 75 mcg, 88 mcg, 100 mcg, 112 mcg, 125 mcg, 137 mcg, 150 mcg, 175 mcg, 200 mcg
(Continued)

levothyroxine *(Continued)*

Synthroid®: 25 mcg, 50 mcg, 75 mcg, 88 mcg, 100 mcg, 112 mcg, 125 mcg, 137 mcg, 150 mcg, 175 mcg, 200 mcg, 300 mcg

Unithroid®: 25 mcg, 50 mcg, 75 mcg, 88 mcg, 100 mcg, 112 mcg, 125 mcg, 150 mcg, 175 mcg, 200 mcg, 300 mcg

Levothyroxine Sodium [Can] *see* levothyroxine *on previous page*

levothyroxine sodium *see* levothyroxine *on previous page*

Levoxyl® [US] *see* levothyroxine *on previous page*

Levsin® [US/Can] *see* hyoscyamine *on page 441*

Levsinex® [US] *see* hyoscyamine *on page 441*

Levsin/SL® [US] *see* hyoscyamine *on page 441*

Levulan® [Can] *see* aminolevulinic acid *on page 42*

Levulan® Kerastick® [US] *see* aminolevulinic acid *on page 42*

levulose, dextrose and phosphoric acid *see* fructose, dextrose, and phosphoric acid *on page 378*

Lexapro® [US] *see* escitalopram *on page 311*

Lexiva® [US] *see* fosamprenavir *on page 374*

Lexxel® [US/Can] *see* enalapril and felodipine *on page 296*

LFA-3/IgG(1) fusion protein, human *see* alefacept *on page 26*

LHRH *see* gonadorelin *on page 399*

***l*-hyoscyamine sulfate** *see* hyoscyamine *on page 441*

Lialda™ [US] *see* mesalamine *on page 546*

Librax® [US/Can] *see* clidinium and chlordiazepoxide *on page 198*

Librax® *[reformulation] (Discontinued)*

Librium® [US] *see* chlordiazepoxide *on page 173*

Lice-Enz® Shampoo *(Discontinued)*

Licide® [US-OTC] *see* pyrethrins and piperonyl butoxide *on page 734*

LidaMantle® [US] *see* lidocaine *on this page*

Lida-Mantle® HC [US] *see* lidocaine and hydrocortisone *on page 507*

Lidemol® [Can] *see* fluocinonide *on page 360*

Lidex® [US/Can] *see* fluocinonide *on page 360*

Lidex-E® [US] *see* fluocinonide *on page 360*

lidocaine *(LYE doe kane)*

Synonyms lidocaine hydrochloride; lignocaine hydrochloride

U.S./Canadian Brand Names Anestacon® [US]; Band-Aid® Hurt-Free™ Antiseptic Wash [US-OTC]; Betacaine® [Can]; Burn Jel [US-OTC]; Burn-O-Jel [US-OTC]; Burnamycin [US-OTC]; L-M-X™ 4 [US-OTC]; L-M-X™ 5 [US-OTC]; LidaMantle® [US]; Lidodan™ [Can]; Lidoderm® [US/Can]; LTA® 360 [US]; Premjact® [US-OTC]; Solarcaine® Aloe Extra Burn Relief [US-OTC]; Topicaine® [US-OTC]; Xylocaine® MPF [US]; Xylocaine® Viscous [US]; Xylocaine® [US/Can]; Xylocard® [Can]; Zilactin-L® [US-OTC]; Zilactin® [Can]

Therapeutic Category Analgesic, Topical; Antiarrhythmic Agent, Class I-B; Local Anesthetic

Use Local anesthetic and acute treatment of ventricular arrhythmias from myocardial infarction, or cardiac manipulation

Rectal: Temporary relief of pain and itching due to anorectal disorders

Topical: Local anesthetic for use in laser, cosmetic, and outpatient surgeries; minor burns, cuts, and abrasions of the skin

Lidoderm® Patch: Relief of allodynia (painful hypersensitivity) and chronic pain in postherpetic neuralgia

Usual Dosage

Antiarrhythmic:

Children:

I.V., I.O.: **Note:** For use in pulseless VT or VF, give after defibrillation, CPR, and epinephrine:

Loading dose: 1 mg/kg (maximum 100 mg); follow with continuous infusion; may administer second bolus of 0.5-1 mg/kg if delay between bolus and start of infusion is >15 minutes

Continuous infusion: 20-50 mcg/kg/minute. Use 20 mcg/kg/minute in patients with shock, hepatic disease, cardiac arrest, mild CHF; moderate-to-severe CHF may require 1/2 loading dose and lower infusion rates to avoid toxicity.

E.T. (loading dose only): 2-10 times the I.V. bolus dose; dilute with NS to a volume of 3-5 mL and follow with several positive-pressure ventilations

Adults:

Ventricular fibrillation or pulseless ventricular tachycardia (after defibrillation, CPR, and vasopressor administration): I.V.: Initial: 1-1.5 mg/kg. Refractory ventricular tachycardia or ventricular fibrillation, a repeat 0.5-0.75 mg/kg bolus may be given every 5-10 minutes after initial dose for a maximum of 3 doses. Total dose should not exceed 3 mg/kg. Follow with continuous infusion (1-4 mg/minute) after return of perfusion. Reappearance of arrhythmia during constant infusion: 0.5 mg/kg bolus and reassessment of infusion.

E.T. (loading dose only): 2-2.5 times the recommended I.V. dose; dilute in 10 mL NS or distilled water.

Note: Absorption is greater with distilled water, but causes more adverse effects on PaO_2.

Hemodynamically stable VT: 0.5-0.75 mg/kg followed by synchronized cardioversion

Note: Decrease dose in patients with CHF, shock, or hepatic disease.

Anesthesia, topical:

Cream:

LidaMantle®: Skin irritation: Children and Adults: Apply to affected area 2-3 times/day as needed

L-M-X™ 4: Children ≥2 years and Adults: Apply 1/4 inch thick layer to intact skin. Leave on until adequate anesthetic effect is obtained. Remove cream and cleanse area before beginning procedure.

L-M-X™ 5: Relief of anorectal pain and itching: Children ≥12 years and Adults: Rectal: Apply topically to clean, dry area **or** using applicator, insert rectally, up to 6 times/day

Gel, ointment, solution: Adults: Apply to affected area ≤3 times/day as needed (maximum dose: 4.5 mg/kg, not to exceed 300 mg)

Jelly:

Children ≥10 years: Dose varies with age and weight (maximum dose: 4.5 mg/kg)

Adults (maximum dose: 30 mL [600 mg] in any 12-hour period):

Anesthesia of male urethra: 5-30 mL

Anesthesia of female urethra: 3-5 mL

Lubrication of endotracheal tube: Apply a moderate amount to external surface only

Liquid: Cold sores and fever blisters: Children ≥5 years and Adults: Apply to affected area every 6 hours as needed

Patch: Postherpetic neuralgia: Adults: Apply patch to most painful area. Up to 3 patches may be applied in a single application. Patch may remain in place for up to 12 hours in any 24-hour period.

Anesthetic, local injectable: Children and Adults: Varies with procedure, degree of anesthesia needed, vascularity of tissue, duration of anesthesia required, and physical condition of patient; maximum: 4.5 mg/kg/dose; do not repeat within 2 hours.

Dosage Forms

Cream, rectal: 5% (15 g, 30 g)

L-M-X™ 5 [OTC]: 5% (15 g,30 g)

Cream, topical: 3% (30 g); 4% (5 g, 15 g, 30 g)

LidaMantle®: 3% (30 g, 85 g)

L-M-X™ 4 [OTC]: 4% (5g, 15 g,30 g)

Gel, topical:

Burn Jel [OTC]: 2% (3.5 g, 120 g)

Burn-O-Jel [OTC]: 0.5% (90 g)

Solarcaine® Aloe Extra Burn Relief [OTC]: 0.5% (113 g, 226 g)

Topicaine® [OTC]: 4% (10 g, 30 g, 113 g)

Infusion [premixed in D_5W]: 0.4% [4 mg/mL] (250 mL, 500 mL); 0.8% [8 mg/mL] (250 mL, 500 mL)

Injection, solution: 0.5% [5 mg/mL] (50 mL); 1% [10 mg/mL] (2 mL, 10 mL, 20 mL, 30 mL, 50 mL); 2% [20 mg/mL] (2 mL, 5 mL, 20 mL, 50 mL)

Xylocaine®: 0.5% [5 mg/mL] (50 mL); 1% [10 mg/mL] (10 mL, 20 mL, 50 mL); 2% [20 mg/mL] (1.8 mL, 10 mL, 20 mL, 50 mL)

Injection, solution: [preservative free]: 0.5% [5 mg/mL] (50 mL); 1% [10 mg/mL] (2 mL, 5 mL, 30 mL); 1.5% [15 mg/mL] (20 mL); 2% [20 mg/mL] (2 mL, 5 mL, 10 mL); 4% [40 mg/mL] (5 mL)

Xylocaine®: 10% [100 mg/mL] (5 mL)

Xylocaine® MPF: 0.5% [5 mg/mL] (50 mL); 1% [10 mg/mL] (2 mL, 5 mL, 10 mL, 30 mL); 1.5% [15 mg/mL] (10 mL, 20 mL); 2% [20 mg/mL] (2 mL, 5 mL, 10 mL); 4% [40 mg/mL] (5 mL)

Injection, solution: [premixed in $D_{7.5}W$, preservative free]: 5% (2 mL)

Jelly, topical: 2% (5 mL, 30 mL)

Anestacon®: 2% (15 mL)

Xylocaine®: 2% (5 mL, 30 mL)

Liquid, topical:

Zilactin®-L [OTC]: 2.5% (7.5 mL)

Lotion, topical: 3% (177 mL)

LidaMantle®: 3% (177 mL)

Ointment, topical: 5% (37 g, 50 g)

(Continued)

lidocaine (Continued)

Solution, topical: 4% [40 mg/mL] (50 mL)
Band-Aid® Hurt-Free™ Antiseptic Wash [OTC]: 2% (180 mL)
LTA® 360: 4% [40 mg/mL] (4 mL)
Xylocaine®: 4% [40 mg/mL] (50 mL)
Solution, viscous: 2% [20 mg/mL] (20 mL, 100 mL)
Xylocaine® Viscous: 2% [20 mg/mL] (100 mL, 450 mL)
Spray, topical:
Burnamycin [OTC]: 0.5% (60 mL)
Premjact® [OTC]: 9.6% (13 mL)
Solarcaine® Aloe Extra Burn Relief [OTC]: 0.5% (127 g)
Transdermal system, topical:
Lidoderm®: 5% (30s)

lidocaine and bupivacaine (LYE doe kane & byoo PIV a kane)

Synonyms bupivacaine and lidocaine; lidocaine hydrochloride and bupivacaine hydrochloride
U.S./Canadian Brand Names Duocaine™ [US]
Therapeutic Category Local Anesthetic
Use Local or regional anesthesia in ophthalmologic surgery by peripheral nerve block techniques such as peribulbar, retrobulbar, and facial blocks; may be used with or without epinephrine
Usual Dosage Children ≥12 years and Adults: **Note:** Use lowest effective dose to limit toxic effects. Dosing based on lidocaine 1% and bupivacaine 0.375%
Retrobulbar injection: 2-5 mL; a portion of dose is injected retrobulbarly and remainder may be used to block the facial nerve
Peribulbar block: 6-12 mL
Maximum dose: 0.18 mL/kg or 12 mL; if used with epinephrine, the dose should not exceed 0.28 mL/kg or 20 mL
Dosage Forms
Injection, solution [preservative free]:
Duocaine™: Lidocaine 1% and bupivacaine 0.375% (10 mL)

lidocaine and epinephrine (LYE doe kane & ep i NEF rin)

Synonyms epinephrine and lidocaine
U.S./Canadian Brand Names LidoSite™ [US]; Xylocaine® MPF With Epinephrine [US]; Xylocaine® With Epinephrine [US/Can]
Therapeutic Category Local Anesthetic
Use Local infiltration anesthesia; AVS for nerve block; topical local analgesia for superficial dermatologic procedures
Usual Dosage Dosage varies with the anesthetic procedure, degree of anesthesia needed, vascularity of tissue, duration of anesthesia required, and physical condition of patient.
Dental anesthesia, infiltration, or conduction block:
Children <10 years: 20-30 mg (1-1.5 mL) of lidocaine hydrochloride as a 2% solution with epinephrine 1:100,000; maximum: 4-5 mg of lidocaine hydrochloride/kg of body weight or 100-150 mg as a single dose
Children >10 years and Adults: Do not exceed 6.6 mg/kg body weight or 300 mg of lidocaine hydrochloride and 3 mcg (0.003 mg) of epinephrine/kg of body weight or 0.2 mg epinephrine per dental appointment. The effective anesthetic dose varies with procedure, intensity of anesthesia needed, duration of anesthesia required, and physical condition of the patient. Always use the lowest effective dose along with careful aspiration.

For most routine dental procedures, lidocaine hydrochloride 2% with epinephrine 1:100,000 is preferred. When a more pronounced hemostasis is required, a 1:50,000 epinephrine concentration should be used.

Dermatologic procedure: Children ≥5 and Adults: Topical: Place 1 transdermal patch over area requiring analgesia; attach patch to iontophoretic controller and leave on for 10 minutes. Remove patch and perform procedure within 10-20 minutes of patch removal. Do not use another patch for 30 minutes.
Dosage Forms
Injection, solution:
Generics:
0.5% / 1:200,000: Lidocaine 0.5% and epinephrine 1:200,000 (50 mL)
1% / 1:100,000: Lidocaine 1% and epinephrine 1:100,000 (20 mL, 30 mL, 50 mL)
1% / 1:200,000: Lidocaine 1% and epinephrine 1:200,000 (30 mL)
1.5% / 1:200,000: Lidocaine 1.5% and epinephrine 1:200,000 (30 mL)
2% / 1:50,000: Lidocaine 2% and epinephrine 1:50,000 (1.8 mL)
2% / 1:100,000: Lidocaine 2% and epinephrine 1:100,000 (1.8 mL, 30 mL, 50 mL)
2% / 1:200,000: Lidocaine 2% and epinephrine 1:200,000 (20 mL)

Brands:
Xylocaine® with Epinephrine:
0.5% / 1:200,000: Lidocaine 0.5% and epinephrine 1:200,000 (50 mL)
1% / 1:100,000: Lidocaine 1% and epinephrine 1:100,000 (10 mL, 20 mL, 50 mL)
2% / 1:50,000: Lidocaine 2% and epinephrine 1:50,000 (1.8 mL)
2% / 1:100,000: Lidocaine 2% and epinephrine 1:100,000 (1.8 mL); (10 mL, 20 mL, 50 mL)
Xylocaine®-MPF with Epinephrine:
1% / 1:200,000: Lidocaine 1% and epinephrine 1:200,000 (5 mL, 10 mL, 30 mL)
1.5% / 1:200,000: Lidocaine 1.5% and epinephrine 1:200,000 (5 mL, 10 mL, 30 mL)
2% / 1:200,000: Lidocaine 2% and epinephrine 1:200,000 (5 mL, 10 mL, 20 mL)
Transdermal system:
LidoSite™: Lidocaine 10% and epinephrine 0.1% (25s)

lidocaine and hydrocortisone (LYE doe kane & hye droe KOR ti sone)
Synonyms hydrocortisone and lidocaine
U.S./Canadian Brand Names AnaMantle® HC [US]; Lida-Mantle® HC [US]
Therapeutic Category Anesthetic/Corticosteroid
Use Topical antiinflammatory and anesthetic for skin disorders; rectal for the treatment of hemorrhoids, anal fissures, pruritus ani, or similar conditions
Usual Dosage Adults:
Topical: Apply 2-3 times/day
Rectal: One applicatorful twice daily
Dosage Forms
Cream, rectal:
AnaMantle HC® Forte: Lidocaine 3% and hydrocortisone 1% (7 g)
AnaMantle® HC, Rectacreme HC: Lidocaine 3% and hydrocortisone 0.5% (7 g)
Peranex™ HC: Lidocaine 2% and hydrocortisone 2% (7 g)
Cream, topical: Lidocaine 3% and hydrocortisone 0.5% (30 g)
Lida-Mantle® HC: Lidocaine 3% and hydrocortisone 0.5% (30 g, 85 g)
Gel, rectal:
AnaMantle HC®: Lidocaine 3% and hydrocortisone 2.5% (7 g)
RectaGel™ HC: Lidocaine 2.8% and hydrocortisone 0.55% (20 g)
Lotion, topical: Lidocaine 3% and hydrocortisone 0.5% (177 mL)
Lida-Mantle® HC, Senatec HC: Lidocaine 3% and hydrocortisone 0.5% (177 mL)

lidocaine and prilocaine (LYE doe kane & PRIL oh kane)
Synonyms prilocaine and lidocaine
U.S./Canadian Brand Names EMLA® [US/Can]; Oraquix® [US]
Therapeutic Category Analgesic, Topical
Use Topical anesthetic for use on normal intact skin to provide local analgesia for minor procedures such as I.V. cannulation or venipuncture; has also been used for painful procedures such as lumbar puncture and skin graft harvesting; for superficial minor surgery of genital mucous membranes and as an adjunct for local infiltration anesthesia in genital mucous membranes.
Usual Dosage Although the incidence of systemic adverse effects with EMLA® is very low, caution should be exercised, particularly when applying over large areas and leaving on for >2 hours
Children (intact skin): EMLA® should **not** be used in neonates with a gestation age <37 weeks nor in infants <12 months of age who are receiving treatment with methemoglobin-inducing agents
Dosing is based on child's age and weight:
Age 0-3 months or <5 kg: Apply a maximum of 1 g over no more than 10 cm^2 of skin; leave on for no longer than 1 hour
Age 3 months to 12 months and >5 kg: Apply no more than a maximum 2 g total over no more than 20 cm^2 of skin; leave on for no longer than 4 hours
Age 1-6 years and >10 kg: Apply no more than a maximum of 10 g total over no more than 100 cm^2 of skin; leave on for no longer than 4 hours.
Age 7-12 years and >20 kg: Apply no more than a maximum 20 g total over no more than 200 cm^2 of skin; leave on for no longer than 4 hours.
Note: If a patient greater than 3 months old does not meet the minimum weight requirement, the maximum total dose should be restricted to the corresponding maximum based on patient weight.

Adults (intact skin):
EMLA® cream and EMLA® anesthetic disc: A thick layer of EMLA® cream is applied to intact skin and covered with an occlusive dressing, or alternatively, an EMLA® anesthetic disc is applied to intact skin
Minor dermal procedures (eg, I.V. cannulation or venipuncture): Apply 2.5 g of cream (1/2 of the 5 g tube) over 20-25 cm of skin surface area, or 1 anesthetic disc (1 g over 10 cm^2) for at least 1 hour. **Note:** In clinical trials, 2 sites were usually prepared in case there was a technical problem with cannulation or venipuncture at the first site.
(Continued)

lidocaine and prilocaine *(Continued)*

Major dermal procedures (eg, more painful dermatological procedures involving a larger skin area such as split thickness skin graft harvesting): Apply 2 g of cream per 10 cm² of skin and allow to remain in contact with the skin for at least 2 hours.

Adult male genital skin (eg, pretreatment prior to local anesthetic infiltration): Apply a thick layer of cream (1 g/10 cm²) to the skin surface for 15 minutes. Local anesthetic infiltration should be performed immediately after removal of EMLA® cream.

Note: Dermal analgesia can be expected to increase for up to 3 hours under occlusive dressing and persist for 1-2 hours after removal of the cream

Adult females: Genital mucous membranes: Minor procedures (eg, removal of condylomata acuminata, pretreatment for local anesthetic infiltration): Apply 5-10 g (thick layer) of cream for 5-10 minutes

Periodontal gel (Oraqix®): Adults: Apply on gingival margin around selected teeth using the blunt-tipped applicator included in package. Wait 30 seconds, then fill the periodontal pockets using the blunt-tipped applicator until gel becomes visible at the gingival margin. Wait another 30 seconds before starting treatment. Maximum recommended dose: One treatment session: 5 cartridges (8.5 g)

Dosage Forms

Cream, topical: Lidocaine 2.5% and prilocaine 2.5% (5 g, 30 g)
EMLA®: Lidocaine 2.5% and prilocaine 2.5% (5 g, 30 g)
Disc, topical:
EMLA®: Lidocaine 2.5% and prilocaine 2.5% per disc (2s, 10s)

lidocaine and tetracaine (LYE doe kane & TET ra kane)

Synonyms tetracaine and lidocaine
U.S./Canadian Brand Names Synera™ [US]
Therapeutic Category Analgesic, Topical; Local Anesthetic
Use Topical anesthetic for use on normal intact skin for minor procedures (eg, I.V. cannulation or venipuncture) and superficial dermatologic procedures
Usual Dosage Transdermal patch: Children ≥3 years and Adults:

Venipuncture or intravenous cannulation: Prior to procedure, apply to intact skin for 20-30 minutes
Superficial dermatological procedures: Prior to procedure, apply to intact skin for 30 minutes
Note: Adults can use another patch at a new location to facilitate venous access after a failed attempt; remove previous patch.

Dosage Forms

Transdermal system:
Synera™: Lidocaine 70 mg and tetracaine 70 mg (10s)

lidocaine hydrochloride *see* lidocaine *on page 504*

lidocaine hydrochloride and bupivacaine hydrochloride *see* lidocaine and bupivacaine *on page 506*

Lidodan™ [Can] *see* lidocaine *on page 504*

Lidoderm® [US/Can] *see* lidocaine *on page 504*

LidoPen® I.M. Injection Auto-Injector *(Discontinued) see* lidocaine *on page 504*

LidoSite™ [US] *see* lidocaine and epinephrine *on page 506*

LID-Pack® [Can] *see* bacitracin and polymyxin B *on page 91*

lignocaine hydrochloride *see* lidocaine *on page 504*

Limbitrol® [US/Can] *see* amitriptyline and chlordiazepoxide *on page 44*

Limbitrol® DS [US] *see* amitriptyline and chlordiazepoxide *on page 44*

Limbrel™ [US] *see* flavocoxid *on page 353*

Lin-Amox [Can] *see* amoxicillin *on page 48*

Lin-Buspirone [Can] *see* buspirone *on page 129*

Lincocin® [US/Can] *see* lincomycin *on this page*

lincomycin (lin koe MYE sin)

Sound-Alike/Look-Alike Issues
Lincocin® may be confused with Cleocin®, Indocin®, Minocin®
Synonyms lincomycin hydrochloride
U.S./Canadian Brand Names Lincocin® [US/Can]
Therapeutic Category Antibiotic, Lincosamide
Use Treatment of serious susceptible bacterial infections, mainly those caused by streptococci and staphylococci resistant to other agents

Usual Dosage Note: Frequency may be increased if needed due to severity of infection
Children >1 month:
I.M.: 10 mg/kg every 12-24 hours
I.V.: 10-20 mg/kg/day in divided doses every 8-12 hours
Adults:
I.M.: 600 mg every 12-24 hours
I.V.: 600 mg to 1 g every 8-12 hours; maximum dose: 8 g/day
Subconjuctival injection: 75 mg (ocular fluid levels with sufficient MICs last for at least 5 hours)
Dosage Forms
Injection, solution:
Lincocin®: 300 mg/mL (2 mL, 10 mL)

lincomycin hydrochloride *see* lincomycin *on previous page*

lindane (LIN dane)

Synonyms benzene hexachloride; gamma benzene hexachloride; hexachlorocyclohexane
U.S./Canadian Brand Names Hexit™ [Can]; PMS-Lindane [Can]
Therapeutic Category Scabicides/Pediculicides
Use Treatment of *Sarcoptes scabiei* (scabies), *Pediculus capitis* (head lice), and *Phthirus pubis* (crab lice); FDA recommends reserving lindane as a second-line agent or with inadequate response to other therapies
Usual Dosage Children and Adults: Topical:
Scabies: Apply a thin layer of lotion and massage it on skin from the neck to the toes; after 8-12 hours, bathe and remove the drug
Head lice, crab lice: Apply shampoo to dry hair and massage into hair for 4 minutes; add small quantities of water to hair until lather forms, then rinse hair thoroughly and comb with a fine tooth comb to remove nits. Amount of shampoo needed is based on length and density of hair; most patients will require 30 mL (maximum: 60 mL).
Dosage Forms
Lotion, topical: 1% (60 mL)
Shampoo, topical: 1% (60 mL)

Linessa® [Can] *see* ethinyl estradiol and desogestrel *on page 322*

linezolid (li NE zoh lid)

Sound-Alike/Look-Alike Issues
Zyvox® may be confused with Vioxx®, Ziox™, Zosyn®, Zovirax®
U.S./Canadian Brand Names Zyvoxam® [Can]; Zyvox® [US]
Therapeutic Category Antibiotic, Oxazolidinone
Use Treatment of vancomycin-resistant *Enterococcus faecium* (VRE) infections, nosocomial pneumonia caused by *Staphylococcus aureus* including MRSA or *Streptococcus pneumoniae* (including multidrug-resistant strains [MDRSP]), complicated and uncomplicated skin and skin structure infections (including diabetic foot infections without concomitant osteomyelitis), and community-acquired pneumonia caused by susceptible gram-positive organisms
Usual Dosage
VRE infections: Oral, I.V.:
Preterm neonates (<34 weeks gestational age): 10 mg/kg every 12 hours; neonates with a suboptimal clinical response can be advanced to 10 mg/kg every 8 hours. By day 7 of life, all neonates should receive 10 mg/kg every 8 hours.
Infants (excluding preterm neonates <1 week) and Children ≤11 years: 10 mg/kg every 8 hours for 14-28 days
Children ≥12 years and Adults: 600 mg every 12 hours for 14-28 days
Nosocomial pneumonia, complicated skin and skin structure infections, community-acquired pneumonia including concurrent bacteremia: Oral, I.V.:
Infants (excluding preterm neonates <1 week) and Children ≤11 years: 10 mg/kg every 8 hours for 10-14 days
Children ≥12 years and Adults: 600 mg every 12 hours for 10-14 days
Uncomplicated skin and skin structure infections: Oral:
Infants (excluding preterm neonates <1 week) and Children <5 years: 10 mg/kg every 8 hours for 10-14 days
Children 5-11 years: 10 mg/kg every 12 hours for 10-14 days
Children ≥12-18 years: 600 mg every 12 hours for 10-14 days
Adults: 400 mg every 12 hours for 10-14 days
Note: 400 mg dose is recommended in the product labeling; however, 600 mg dose is commonly employed clinically
(Continued)

linezolid *(Continued)*
Dosage Forms [CAN] = Canadian brand name
Infusion [premixed]:
Zyvox®: 200 mg (100 mL)
Zyvox® [CAN]: 600 mg (300 mL) [not available in the U.S.]
Powder for oral suspension:
Zyvox®: 20 mg/mL (150 mL)
Tablet:
Zyvox®: 600 mg

Lin-Sotalol [Can] *see* sotalol *on page 802*

Lioresal® [US/Can] *see* baclofen *on page 92*

Liotec [Can] *see* baclofen *on page 92*

liothyronine *(lye oh THYE roe neen)*
Sound-Alike/Look-Alike Issues
liothyronine may be confused with levothyroxine
T3 is an error-prone abbreviation (mistaken as acetaminophen and codeine [ie, Tylenol® #3])
Synonyms liothyronine sodium; sodium *L*-triiodothyronine
U.S./Canadian Brand Names Cytomel® [US/Can]; Triostat® [US]
Therapeutic Category Thyroid Product
Use
Oral: Replacement or supplemental therapy in hypothyroidism; management of nontoxic goiter; a diagnostic aid
I.V.: Treatment of myxedema coma/precoma
Usual Dosage Doses should be adjusted based on clinical response and laboratory parameters.
Children: Congenital hypothyroidism: Oral: 5 mcg/day increase by 5 mcg every 3-4 days until the desired response is achieved. Usual maintenance dose: 20 mcg/day for infants, 50 mcg/day for children 1-3 years of age, and adult dose for children >3 years.
Adults:
Hypothyroidism: Oral: 25 mcg/day increase by increments of 12.5-25 mcg/day every 1-2 weeks to a maximum of 100 mcg/day; usual maintenance dose: 25-75 mcg/day.
Patients with cardiovascular disease: Oral: 5 mcg/day; increase by 5 mcg/day every 2 weeks
T_3 suppression test: Oral: 75-100 mcg/day for 7 days
Myxedema: Oral: Initial: 5 mcg/day; increase in increments of 5-10 mcg/day every 1-2 weeks. When 25 mcg/day is reached, dosage may be increased at intervals of 5-25 mcg/day every 1-2 weeks. Usual maintenance dose: 50-100 mcg/day.
Myxedema coma: I.V.: 25-50 mcg
Patients with known or suspected cardiovascular disease: 10-20 mcg
Note: Normally, at least 4 hours should be allowed between doses to adequately assess therapeutic response and no more than 12 hours should elapse between doses to avoid fluctuations in hormone levels. Oral therapy should be resumed as soon as the clinical situation has been stabilized and the patient is able to take oral medication. If levothyroxine rather than liothyronine sodium is used in initiating oral therapy, the physician should bear in mind that there is a delay of several days in the onset of levothyroxine activity and that I.V. therapy should be discontinued gradually.
Simple (nontoxic) goiter: Oral: Initial: 5 mcg/day; increase by 5-10 mcg every 1-2 weeks; after 25 mcg/day is reached, may increase dose by 12.5-25 mcg. Usual maintenance dose: 75 mcg/day
Dosage Forms
Injection, solution:
Triostat®: 10 mcg/mL (1 mL)
Tablet:
Cytomel®: 5 mcg, 25 mcg, 50 mcg

liothyronine sodium *see* liothyronine *on this page*

liotrix *(LYE oh triks)*
Sound-Alike/Look-Alike Issues
liotrix may be confused with Klotrix®
Thyrolar® may be confused with Theolair™, Thyrogen®, Thytropar®
Synonyms T_3/T_4 liotrix
U.S./Canadian Brand Names Thyrolar® [US/Can]
Therapeutic Category Thyroid Product
Use Replacement or supplemental therapy in hypothyroidism (uniform mixture of $T_4:T_3$ in 4:1 ratio by weight); little advantage to this product exists and cost is not justified

Usual Dosage Oral:
  Congenital hypothyroidism:
   Children (dose of T_4 or levothyroxine/day):
    0-6 months: 8-10 mcg/kg or 25-50 mcg/day
    6-12 months: 6-8 mcg/kg or 50-75 mcg/day
    1-5 years: 5-6 mcg/kg or 75-100 mcg/day
    6-12 years: 4-5 mcg/kg or 100-150 mcg/day
    >12 years: 2-3 mcg/kg or >150 mcg/day
   Hypothyroidism (dose of thyroid equivalent): Adults: 30 mg/day (15 mg/day if cardiovascular impairment), increasing by increments of 15 mg/day at 2- to 3-week intervals to a maximum of 180 mg/day (usual maintenance dose: 60-120 mg/day)

Dosage Forms
  Tablet:
   Thyrolar®:
    1/4 [levothyroxine 12.5 mcg and liothyronine 3.1 mcg]
    1/2 [levothyroxine 25 mcg and liothyronine 6.25 mcg]
    1 [levothyroxine 50 mcg and liothyronine 12.5 mcg]
    2 [levothyroxine 100 mcg and liothyronine 25 mcg]
    3 [levothyroxine 150 mcg and liothyronine 37.5 mcg]

lipancreatin *see* pancrelipase *on page 648*

Lipidil EZ® **[Can]** *see* fenofibrate *on page 345*

Lipidil Micro® **[Can]** *see* fenofibrate *on page 345*

Lipidil Supra® **[Can]** *see* fenofibrate *on page 345*

Lipitor® **[US/Can]** *see* atorvastatin *on page 81*

Lipofen™ **[US]** *see* fenofibrate *on page 345*

liposomal DAUNOrubicin *see* daunorubicin citrate (liposomal) *on page 233*

liposomal DOXOrubicin *see* doxorubicin (liposomal) *on page 281*

Liposyn® **II [US/Can]** *see* fat emulsion *on page 343*

Liposyn® **III [US]** *see* fat emulsion *on page 343*

Lipram 4500 [US] *see* pancrelipase *on page 648*

Lipram-CR [US] *see* pancrelipase *on page 648*

Lipram-PN [US] *see* pancrelipase *on page 648*

Lipram-UL [US] *see* pancrelipase *on page 648*

Liqua-Cal [US-OTC] *see* calcium and vitamin D *on page 137*

Liquaemin® ***(Discontinued)*** *see* heparin *on page 415*

Liquibid-D [US] *see* guaifenesin and phenylephrine *on page 404*

Liquibid® **1200 *(Discontinued)*** *see* guaifenesin *on page 401*

Liquibid® ***(Discontinued)*** *see* guaifenesin *on page 401*

Liquibid-PD 1200 *(Discontinued)* *see* guaifenesin and phenylephrine *on page 404*

Liquibid-PD *(Discontinued)* *see* guaifenesin and phenylephrine *on page 404*

Liqui-Char® ***(Discontinued)*** *see* charcoal *on page 171*

Liqui-Coat HD® **[US]** *see* barium *on page 94*

liquid antidote *see* charcoal *on page 171*

Liquid Barosperse® **[US]** *see* barium *on page 94*

Liquid Pred® ***(Discontinued)*** *see* prednisone *on page 710*

Liquifilm® **Forte Solution *(Discontinued)*** *see* artificial tears *on page 75*

Liquifilm® **Tears [US-OTC]** *see* artificial tears *on page 75*

Liquifilm® **Tears Solution *(Discontinued)*** *see* artificial tears *on page 75*

lisdexamfetamine (lis dex am FET a meen)

Sound-Alike/Look-Alike Issues
  Vyvanse™ may be confused with Vytorin®, Glucovance®, Vivactil®

(Continued)

lisdexamfetamine *(Continued)*

Synonyms lisdexamfetamine dimesylate; NRP104
U.S./Canadian Brand Names Vyvanse™ [US]
Therapeutic Category Stimulant
Controlled Substance C-II
Use Treatment of attention-deficit/hyperactivity disorder (ADHD)
Usual Dosage Oral: Individualize dosage based on patient need and response to therapy. Administer at the lowest effective dose.
  Children: 6-12 years: Initial: 30 mg once daily; may increase in increments of 20 mg/day at weekly intervals until optimal response is obtained; maximum: 70 mg/day
Dosage Forms
  Capsule:
    Vyvanse™: 30 mg, 50 mg, 70 mg

lisdexamfetamine dimesylate *see* lisdexamfetamine *on previous page*

lisinopril *(lyse IN oh pril)*

Sound-Alike/Look-Alike Issues
  lisinopril may be confused with fosinopril, Lioresal®, Risperdal®
  Prinivil® may be confused with Plendil®, Pravachol®, Prevacid®, Prilosec®, Proventil®
  Zestril® may be confused with Desyrel®, Restoril®, Vistaril®, Zetia™, Zostrix®
U.S./Canadian Brand Names Apo-Lisinopril® [Can]; Prinivil® [US/Can]; Zestril® [US/Can]
Therapeutic Category Angiotensin-Converting Enzyme (ACE) Inhibitor
Use Treatment of hypertension, either alone or in combination with other antihypertensive agents; adjunctive therapy in treatment of CHF (afterload reduction); treatment of acute myocardial infarction within 24 hours in hemodynamically-stable patients to improve survival; treatment of left ventricular dysfunction after myocardial infarction
Usual Dosage Oral:
  Hypertension:
    Children ≥6 years: Initial: 0.07 mg/kg once daily (up to 5 mg); increase dose at 1- to 2-week intervals; doses >0.61 mg/kg or >40 mg have not been evaluated.
    Adults: Usual dosage range(JNC 7): 10-40 mg/day
    Not maintained on diuretic: Initial: 10 mg/day
    Maintained on diuretic: Initial: 5 mg/day
      Note: Antihypertensive effect may diminish toward the end of the dosing interval especially with doses of 10 mg/day. An increased dose may aid in extending the duration of antihypertensive effect. Doses up to 80 mg/day have been used, but do not appear to give greater effect (Zestril® Product Information, 12/04).
    Patients taking diuretics should have them discontinued 2-3 days prior to initiating lisinopril if possible. Restart diuretic after blood pressure is stable if needed. If diuretic cannot be discontinued prior to therapy, begin with 5 mg with close supervision until stable blood pressure. In patients with hyponatremia (<130 mEq/L), start dose at 2.5 mg/day
  Congestive heart failure: Adults: Initial: 2.5-5 mg once daily; then increase by no more than 10 mg increments at intervals no less than 2 weeks to a maximum daily dose of 40 mg. Usual maintenance: 5-40 mg/day as a single dose. Target dose: 20-40 mg once daily (ACC/AHA 2005 Heart Failure Guidelines)
    Note: If patient has hyponatremia (serum sodium <130 meq/L) or renal impairment (Cl_{cr} <30 mL/minute or creatinine >3 mg/dL), then initial dose should be 2.5 mg/day
  Acute myocardial infarction (within 24 hours in hemodynamically stable patients): Oral: 5 mg immediately, then 5 mg at 24 hours, 10 mg at 48 hours, and 10 mg every day thereafter for 6 weeks. Patients should continue to receive standard treatments such as thrombolytics, aspirin, and beta-blockers.
Dosage Forms
  Tablet: 2.5 mg, 5 mg, 10 mg, 20 mg, 30 mg, 40 mg
  Prinivil®: 5 mg, 10 mg, 20 mg, 30 mg
  Zestril®: 2.5 mg, 5 mg, 10 mg, 20 mg, 30 mg, 40 mg

lisinopril and hydrochlorothiazide *(lyse IN oh pril & hye droe klor oh THYE a zide)*

Synonyms hydrochlorothiazide and lisinopril
U.S./Canadian Brand Names Prinzide® [US/Can]; Zestoretic® [US/Can]
Therapeutic Category Antihypertensive Agent, Combination
Use Treatment of hypertension
Usual Dosage Oral: Adults: Dosage is individualized; see each component for appropriate dosing suggestions; doses >80 mg/day lisinopril or >50 mg/day hydrochlorothiazide are not recommended.
Dosage Forms
  Tablet: 10/12.5: Lisinopril 10 mg and hydrochlorothiazide 12.5 mg; 20/12.5: Lisinopril 20 mg and hydrochlorothiazide 12.5 mg; 20/25: Lisinopril 20 mg and hydrochlorothiazide 25 mg

Prinizide®:
10/12.5: Lisinopril 10 mg and hydrochlorothiazide 12.5 mg
20/25: Lisinopril 20 mg and hydrochlorothiazide 25 mg
Zestoretic®:
10/12.5: Lisinopril 10 mg and hydrochlorothiazide 12.5 mg
20/12.5: Lisinopril 20 mg and hydrochlorothiazide 12.5 mg
20/25: Lisinopril 20 mg and hydrochlorothiazide 25 mg

lispro insulin *see* insulin lispro *on page 459*

Listermint® With Fluoride *(Discontinued)* *see* fluoride *on page 361*

Lithane® [Can] *see* lithium *on this page*

Lithane® *(Discontinued)* *see* lithium *on this page*

lithium (LITH ee um)

Sound-Alike/Look-Alike Issues
Eskalith® may be confused with Estratest®
Lithobid® may be confused with Levbid®, Lithostat®

Synonyms lithium carbonate; lithium citrate

U.S./Canadian Brand Names Apo-Lithium® Carbonate SR [Can]; Apo-Lithium® Carbonate [Can]; Carbolith™ [Can]; Duralith® [Can]; Lithane® [Can]; Lithobid® [US]; PMS-Lithium Carbonate [Can]; PMS-Lithium Citrate [Can]

Therapeutic Category Antimanic Agent

Use Management of bipolar disorders; treatment of mania in individuals with bipolar disorder (maintenance treatment prevents or diminishes intensity of subsequent episodes)

Usual Dosage Oral: Monitor serum concentrations and clinical response (efficacy and toxicity) to determine proper dose

Children 6-12 years: Bipolar disorder: 15-60 mg/kg/day in 3-4 divided doses; dose not to exceed usual adult dosage

Adults: Bipolar disorder: 900-2400 mg/day in 3-4 divided doses or 900-1800 mg/day (sustained release) in 2 divided doses

Dosage Forms
Capsule, as carbonate: 150 mg, 300 mg, 600 mg
Solution: 300 mg/5 mL
Syrup: 300 mg/5 mL
Tablet: 300 mg
Tablet, controlled release: 450 mg
Tablet, slow release: 300 mg
Lithobid®: 300 mg

lithium carbonate *see* lithium *on this page*

lithium citrate *see* lithium *on this page*

Lithobid® [US] *see* lithium *on this page*

Lithonate® *(Discontinued)* *see* lithium *on this page*

Lithostat® [US/Can] *see* acetohydroxamic acid *on page 14*

Lithotabs® *(Discontinued)* *see* lithium *on this page*

Little Tummys® Gas Relief [US-OTC] *see* simethicone *on page 786*

Little Tummys® Laxative [US-OTC] *see* senna *on page 781*

live attenuated influenza vaccine (LAIV) *see* influenza virus vaccine *on page 455*

Livostin® *(Discontinued)*

l-lysine (el LYE seen)

Synonyms l-lysine hydrochloride

U.S./Canadian Brand Names Lysinyl [US-OTC]

Therapeutic Category Dietary Supplement

Use Improves utilization of vegetable proteins

Usual Dosage Oral: Adults: 334-1500 mg/day

Recurrent herpes simplex infection (dental use): 2000 mg every 4 hours until symptoms subside. Begin treatment during early stage of recurrence.

Dosage Forms
Capsule: 500 mg
Lysinyl [OTC]: 500 mg
Tablet: 500 mg, 1000 mg

l-lysine hydrochloride *see* l-lysine *on previous page*

LMD® **[US]** *see* dextran *on page 245*

LNg 20 *see* levonorgestrel *on page 502*

Locacorten® **Vioform®** **[Can]** *see* clioquinol and flumethasone *(Canada only) on page 201*

LoCHOLEST® *(Discontinued) see* cholestyramine resin *on page 186*

LoCHOLEST® **Light** *(Discontinued) see* cholestyramine resin *on page 186*

Locoid® **[US/Can]** *see* hydrocortisone (topical) *on page 434*

Locoid Lipocream® **[US]** *see* hydrocortisone (topical) *on page 434*

Lodine® **[Can]** *see* etodolac *on page 335*

Lodine® **XL** *(Discontinued) see* etodolac *on page 335*

Lodine® *(Discontinued) see* etodolac *on page 335*

Lodosyn® **[US]** *see* carbidopa *on page 151*

lodoxamide (loe DOKS a mide)
Synonyms lodoxamide tromethamine
U.S./Canadian Brand Names Alomide® [US/Can]
Therapeutic Category Mast Cell Stabilizer
Use Treatment of vernal keratoconjunctivitis, vernal conjunctivitis, and vernal keratitis
Usual Dosage Ophthalmic: Instill 1-2 drops in eye(s) 4 times/day for up to 3 months
Dosage Forms
  Solution, ophthalmic:
    Alomide®: 0.1% (10 mL)

Iodoxamide tromethamine *see* lodoxamide *on this page*

Lodrane® **[US]** *see* brompheniramine and pseudoephedrine *on page 120*

Lodrane® **12D [US]** *see* brompheniramine and pseudoephedrine *on page 120*

Lodrane® **12 Hour [US]** *see* brompheniramine *on page 120*

Lodrane® **24 [US]** *see* brompheniramine *on page 120*

Lodrane® **24D [US]** *see* brompheniramine and pseudoephedrine *on page 120*

Lodrane® **D [US]** *see* brompheniramine and pseudoephedrine *on page 120*

Lodrane® **XR [US]** *see* brompheniramine *on page 120*

Loestrin® **[US]** *see* ethinyl estradiol and norethindrone *on page 328*

Loestrin™ **1.5/30 [Can]** *see* ethinyl estradiol and norethindrone *on page 328*

Loestrin® **24 Fe [US]** *see* ethinyl estradiol and norethindrone *on page 328*

Loestrin® **Fe [US]** *see* ethinyl estradiol and norethindrone *on page 328*

Lofibra™ **[US]** *see* fenofibrate *on page 345*

Logen® *(Discontinued) see* diphenoxylate and atropine *on page 267*

LoHist-12 [US] *see* brompheniramine *on page 120*

LoHist 12D [US] *see* brompheniramine and pseudoephedrine *on page 120*

LoHist-D [US] *see* chlorpheniramine and pseudoephedrine *on page 178*

LoHist LQ [US] *see* brompheniramine and pseudoephedrine *on page 120*

LoHist PD [US] *see* brompheniramine and pseudoephedrine *on page 120*

L-OHP *see* oxaliplatin *on page 636*

LoKara™ **[US]** *see* desonide *on page 240*

Lomanate® *(Discontinued) see* diphenoxylate and atropine *on page 267*

Lomine [Can] *see* dicyclomine *on page 255*

Lomotil® **[US/Can]** *see* diphenoxylate and atropine *on page 267*

lomustine (loe MUS teen)

Sound-Alike/Look-Alike Issues
lomustine may be confused with carmustine

Synonyms CCNU; NSC-79037

U.S./Canadian Brand Names CeeNU® [US/Can]

Therapeutic Category Antineoplastic Agent

Use Treatment of brain tumors and Hodgkin disease

Usual Dosage Oral (refer to individual protocols):
Children: 75-150 mg/m^2 as a single dose once every 6 weeks; subsequent doses are readjusted after initial treatment according to platelet and leukocyte counts
Adults: 100-130 mg/m^2 as a single dose once every 6 weeks; readjust after initial treatment according to platelet and leukocyte counts
With compromised marrow function: Initial dose: 100 mg/m^2 as a single dose once every 6 weeks
Repeat courses should only be administered after adequate recovery: Leukocytes >4000/mm^3 and platelet counts >100,000/mm^3
Subsequent dosing adjustment based on nadir:
Leukocytes 2000-2999/mm^3, platelets 25,000-74,999/mm^3: Administer 70% of prior dose
Leukocytes <2000/mm^3, platelets <25,000/mm^3: Administer 50% of prior dose

Dosage Forms
Capsule:
CeeNU®: 10 mg, 40 mg, 100 mg
Capsule [dose pack]:
CeeNU®: 10 mg (2s); 40 mg (2s); 100 mg (2s)

Loniten® 2.5 mg Tablet (Discontinued) see minoxidil *on page 572*

Lonox® [US] see diphenoxylate and atropine *on page 267*

Lo/Ovral® [US] see ethinyl estradiol and norgestrel *on page 332*

Loperacap [Can] see loperamide *on this page*

loperamide (loe PER a mide)

Sound-Alike/Look-Alike Issues
Imodium® A-D may be confused with Indocin®, Ionamin®

Synonyms loperamide hydrochloride

U.S./Canadian Brand Names Apo-Loperamide® [Can]; Diamode [US-OTC]; Diarr-Eze [Can]; Imodium® A-D [US-OTC]; Imodium® [Can]; K-Pek II [US-OTC]; Kao-Paverin® [US-OTC]; Loperacap [Can]; Novo-Loperamide [Can]; PMS-Loperamide [Can]; Rho®-Loperamine [Can]; Riva-Loperamine [Can]

Therapeutic Category Antidiarrheal

Use Treatment of chronic diarrhea associated with inflammatory bowel disease; acute nonspecific diarrhea; increased volume of ileostomy discharge
OTC labeling: Control of symptoms of diarrhea, including traveler's diarrhea

Usual Dosage Oral:
Children:
Acute diarrhea: Initial doses (in first 24 hours):
2-5 years (13-20 kg): 1 mg 3 times/day
6-8 years (20-30 kg): 2 mg twice daily
8-12 years (>30 kg): 2 mg 3 times/day
Maintenance: After initial dosing, 0.1 mg/kg doses after each loose stool, but not exceeding initial dosage
Traveler's diarrhea:
6-8 years: 2 mg after first loose stool, followed by 1 mg after each subsequent stool (maximum dose: 4 mg/day)
9-11 years: 2 mg after first loose stool, followed by 1 mg after each subsequent stool (maximum dose: 6 mg/day)
≥12 years: See adult dosing.
Adults:
Acute diarrhea: Initial: 4 mg, followed by 2 mg after each loose stool, up to 16 mg/day
Chronic diarrhea: Initial: Follow acute diarrhea; maintenance dose should be slowly titrated downward to minimum required to control symptoms (typically, 4-8 mg/day in divided doses)
Traveler's diarrhea: Initial: 4 mg after first loose stool, followed by 2 mg after each subsequent stool (maximum dose: 8 mg/day)

Dosage Forms
Caplet: 2 mg
Diamode [OTC], Imodium® A-D [OTC], Kao-Paverin® [OTC]: 2 mg
Capsule: 2 mg
Liquid, oral: 1 mg/5 mL
(Continued)

loperamide *(Continued)*

Imodium® A-D [OTC]: 1 mg/5 mL
Imodium® A-D [OTC] [*new formulation*]: 1 mg/7.5 mL
Tablet: 2 mg
K-Pek II [OTC]: 2 mg

loperamide and simethicone (loe PER a mide & sye METH i kone)

Synonyms simethicone and loperamide hydrochloride
U.S./Canadian Brand Names Imodium® Advanced [US]
Therapeutic Category Antidiarrheal; Antiflatulent
Use Control of symptoms of diarrhea and gas (bloating, pressure, and cramps)
Usual Dosage Oral: Acute diarrhea (weight-based dosing is preferred):
Children:
6-8 years (48-59 lbs): 1 caplet or tablet after first loose stool, followed by ½ caplet/tablet with each subsequent loose stool (maximum: 2 caplets or tablets/24 hours)
9-11 years (60-95 lbs): 1 caplet or tablet after first loose stool, followed by ½ caplet or tablet with each subsequent loose stool (maximum: 3 caplets or tablets/24 hours)
Children >12 years and Adults: One caplet or tablet after first loose stool, followed by 1 caplet or tablet with each subsequent loose stool (maximum: 4 caplets or tablets/24 hours)
Dosage Forms
Caplet:
Imodium® Advanced: Loperamide 2 mg and simethicone 125 mg
Tablet, chewable:
Imodium® Advanced: Loperamide 2 mg and simethicone 125 mg

loperamide hydrochloride *see loperamide on previous page*

Lopid® [US/Can] *see gemfibrozil on page 387*

lopinavir and ritonavir (loe PIN a veer & rit ON uh veer)

Sound-Alike/Look-Alike Issues
Potential for dispensing errors between Kaletra™ and Keppra® (levetiracetam)
Synonyms ritonavir and lopinavir
U.S./Canadian Brand Names Kaletra® [US/Can]
Therapeutic Category Antiretroviral Agent, Nonnucleoside Reverse Transcriptase Inhibitor (NNRTI)
Use Treatment of HIV infection in combination with other antiretroviral agents
Usual Dosage Oral:
Children 6 months to 12 years: Dosage based on weight, presented based on mg of lopinavir (maximum dose: Lopinavir 400 mg/ritonavir 100 mg)
7-<15 kg: 12 mg/kg twice daily
15-40 kg: 10 mg/kg twice daily
>40 kg: Lopinavir 400 mg/ritonavir 100 mg twice daily
Note: For therapy-experienced patients with suspected reduced susceptibility to lopinavir, refer to adult dosing.
Children >12 years: Therapy-naive: Lopinavir 400 mg/ritonavir 100 mg twice daily (AIDS Info guidelines).
Note: For therapy-experienced patients with suspected reduced susceptibility to lopinavir, refer to adult dosing.
Adults:
Therapy-naive: Lopinavir 800 mg/ritonavir 200 mg once daily **or** lopinavir 400 mg/ritonavir 100 mg twice daily
Note: Once-daily dosing regimen should not be used with concurrent indinavir, saquinavir, phenytoin, carbamazepine, or phenobarbital therapy.
Therapy-experienced: Lopinavir 400 mg/ritonavir 100 mg twice daily (per manufacturer labeling)
Note: For therapy-experienced patients with suspected reduced susceptibility to lopinavir, clinicians may consider lopinavir 600 mg/ ritonavir 150 mg twice daily (AIDS Info guidelines)

Dosage adjustment for combination therapy:
When taken with amprenavir, efavirenz, fosamprenavir, nelfinavir, or nevirapine: **Note:** Once-daily dosing regimen should not be used
Children 6 months to 12 years: Solution:
7-<15 kg: 13 mg/kg twice daily
15-45 kg: 11 mg/kg twice daily
>45 kg: Refer to adult dosing
Note: In the USHHS AIDS Info guidelines, the cutoff for adult dosing is 50 kg. (Pediatric Guidelines - October 26, 2006, are available at http://www.aidsinfo.nih.gov)
Children >12 years and Adults:
Therapy-naive: Tablet: Lopinavir 400 mg/ritonavir 100 mg twice daily

Therapy-experienced:
   Solution: Lopinavir 533 mg/ritonavir 133 mg twice daily
   Tablet: Lopinavir 600 mg/ritonavir 150 mg twice daily
   When taken with saquinavir (Invirase®): Lopinavir 400 mg/ritonavir 100 mg twice daily
Dosage Forms
   Solution, oral:
   Kaletra®: Lopinavir 80 mg and ritonavir 20 mg per mL
   Tablet:
   Kaletra®: Lopinavir 200 mg and ritonavir 50 mg

Lopressor® [US/Can] *see* metoprolol *on page 562*

Lopressor HCT® [US] *see* metoprolol and hydrochlorothiazide *on page 563*

Loprox® [US/Can] *see* ciclopirox *on page 188*

Lorabid® [Can] *see* loracarbef *on this page*

Lorabid® *(Discontinued)* *see* loracarbef *on this page*

loracarbef (lor a KAR bef)

Sound-Alike/Look-Alike Issues
   Lorabid® may be confused with Levbid®, Lopid®, Lortab®, Slo-bid™
U.S./Canadian Brand Names Lorabid® [Can]
Therapeutic Category Antibiotic, Carbacephem
Use Treatment of infections caused by susceptible organisms involving the upper and lower respiratory tract, uncomplicated skin and skin structure, and urinary tract (including uncomplicated pyelonephritis)
Usual Dosage
   Usual dosage range:
   Children 6 months to 12 years: Oral: 7.5-15 mg/kg twice daily
   Adults: Oral: 200-400 mg every 12-24 hours
   Indication-specific dosing:
   Children 6 months to 12 years: Oral:
      Acute otitis media: 15 mg/kg twice daily for 10 days
      Pharyngitis and impetigo: 7.5-15 mg/kg twice daily for 10 days
   Adults: Oral:
      Bronchitis: 200-400 mg every 12 hours for 7 days
      Pharyngitis/tonsillitis: 200 mg every 12 hours for 10 days
      Pneumonia: 400 mg every 12 hours for 14 days
      Pyelonephritis (uncomplicated): 400 mg every 12 hours for 14 days
      Sinusitis: 400 mg every 12 hours for 10 days
      Skin and soft tissue: 200-400 mg every 12-24 hours
      Urinary tract infections (uncomplicated): 200 mg once daily for 7 days

loratadine (lor AT a deen)

Sound-Alike/Look-Alike Issues
   Dimetapp® may be confused with Dermatop®, Dimetabs®, Dimetane®
U.S./Canadian Brand Names Alavert® [US-OTC]; Apo-Loratadine® [Can]; Claritin® 24 Hour Allergy [US-OTC]; Claritin® Hives Relief [US-OTC]; Claritin® Kids [Can]; Claritin® [Can]; Tavist® ND [US-OTC]; Triaminic® Allerchews™ [US-OTC]
Therapeutic Category Antihistamine
Use Relief of nasal and nonnasal symptoms of seasonal allergic rhinitis; treatment of chronic idiopathic urticaria
Usual Dosage Oral: Seasonal allergic rhinitis, chronic idiopathic urticaria:
   Children 2-5 years: 5 mg once daily
   Children ≥6 years and Adults: 10 mg once daily
Dosage Forms
   Syrup: 5 mg/mL
   Claritin® [OTC]: 1 mg/mL
   Tablet: 10 mg
   Alavert® [OTC], Claritin® [OTC], Claritin® Hives Relief [OTC], Claritin® 24 Hour Allergy [OTC], Tavist® ND [OTC]: 10 mg
   Tablet, rapidly disintegrating: 10 mg
   Alavert® [OTC], Claritin® RediTabs® [OTC], Triaminic® Allerchews™ [OTC]: 10 mg

loratadine and pseudoephedrine (lor AT a deen & soo doe e FED rin)

Synonyms pseudoephedrine and loratadine

U.S./Canadian Brand Names Alavert™ Allergy and Sinus [US-OTC]; Chlor-Tripolon ND® [Can]; Claritin-D® 12-Hour [US-OTC]; Claritin-D® 24-Hour [US-OTC]; Claritin® Extra [Can]; Claritin® Liberator [Can]

Therapeutic Category Antihistamine/Decongestant Combination

Use Temporary relief of symptoms of seasonal allergic rhinitis, other upper respiratory allergies, or the common cold

Usual Dosage Oral: Children ≥12 years and Adults:

Claritin-D® 12-Hour: 1 tablet every 12 hours

Alavert™ Allergy and Sinus, Claritin-D® 24-Hour: 1 tablet daily

Dosage Forms

Tablet, extended release: Loratadine 10 mg and pseudoephedrine 240 mg

Alavert™ Allergy and Sinus [OTC], Claritin-D® 12-hour [OTC]: Loratadine 5 mg and pseudoephedrine 120 mg

Claritin-D® 24-hour [OTC]: Loratadine 10 mg and pseudoephedrine 240 mg

lorazepam (lor A ze pam)

Sound-Alike/Look-Alike Issues

lorazepam may be confused with alprazolam, clonazepam, clorazepate, diazepam, temazepam

Ativan® may be confused with Atarax®, Atgam®, Avitene®

U.S./Canadian Brand Names Apo-Lorazepam® [Can]; Ativan® [US/Can]; Lorazepam Injection, USP [Can]; Lorazepam Intensol® [US]; Novo-Lorazepam [Can]; Nu-Loraz [Can]; PMS-Lorazepam [Can]; Riva-Lorazepam [Can]

Therapeutic Category Benzodiazepine

Controlled Substance C-IV

Use

Oral: Management of anxiety disorders or short-term (≤4 months) relief of the symptoms of anxiety or anxiety associated with depressive symptoms

I.V.: Status epilepticus, preanesthesia for desired amnesia

Usual Dosage

Anxiety and sedation (unlabeled in children except for oral use in children >12 years):

Infants and Children: Oral, I.M., I.V.: Usual: 0.05 mg/kg/dose (range: 0.02-0.09 mg/kg) every 4-8 hours

I.V.: May use smaller doses (eg, 0.01-0.03 mg/kg) and repeat every 20 minutes, as needed to titrate to effect

Adults: Oral: 1-10 mg/day in 2-3 divided doses; usual dose: 2-6 mg/day in divided doses

Insomnia: Adults: Oral: 2-4 mg at bedtime

Preoperative: Adults:

I.M.: 0.05 mg/kg administered 2 hours before surgery (maximum: 4 mg/dose)

I.V.: 0.044 mg/kg 15-20 minutes before surgery (usual maximum: 2 mg/dose)

Preprocedural anxiety (dental use): Adults: Oral: 1-2 mg 1 hour before procedure

Operative amnesia: Adults: I.V.: Up to 0.05 mg/kg (maximum: 4 mg/dose)

Status epilepticus: I.V.:

Adolescents: 0.07 mg/kg slow I.V. over 2-5 minutes; maximum: 4 mg/dose; may repeat in 10-15 minutes

Adults: 4 mg/dose slow I.V. over 2-5 minutes; may repeat in 10-15 minutes; usual maximum dose: 8 mg

Rapid tranquilization of agitated patient (administer every 30-60 minutes): Adults:

Oral: 1-2 mg

I.M.: 0.5-1 mg

Average total dose for tranquilization: Oral, I.M.: 4-8 mg

Dosage Forms

Injection, solution: 2 mg/mL (1 mL, 10 mL); 4 mg/mL (1 mL, 10 mL)

Ativan®: 2 mg/mL (1 mL, 10 mL); 4 mg/mL (1 mL, 10 mL)

Solution, oral concentrate:

Lorazepam Intensol®: 2 mg/mL

Tablet: 0.5 mg, 1 mg, 2 mg

Ativan®: 0.5 mg, 1 mg, 2 mg

Lorazepam Injection, USP [Can] *see* lorazepam *on this page*

Lorazepam Intensol® [US] *see* lorazepam *on this page*

Lorcet® 10/650 [US] *see* hydrocodone and acetaminophen *on page 427*

Lorcet®-HD *(Discontinued) see* hydrocodone and acetaminophen *on page 427*

Lorcet® Plus [US] *see* hydrocodone and acetaminophen *on page 427*

Loroxide® [US-OTC] *see* benzoyl peroxide *on page 103*

Lorsin® *(Discontinued) see* acetaminophen, chlorpheniramine, and pseudoephedrine *on page 10*

Lortab® **[US]** *see* hydrocodone and acetaminophen *on page 427*

Lortab® **ASA** *(Discontinued) see* hydrocodone and aspirin *on page 428*

losartan (loe SAR tan)
Sound-Alike/Look-Alike Issues
losartan may be confused with valsartan
Cozaar® may be confused with Hyzaar®, Zocor®
Synonyms DuP 753; losartan potassium; MK594
U.S./Canadian Brand Names Cozaar® [US/Can]
Therapeutic Category Angiotensin II Receptor Antagonist
Use Treatment of hypertension (HTN); treatment of diabetic nephropathy in patients with type 2 diabetes mellitus (noninsulin-dependent, NIDDM) and a history of hypertension; stroke risk reduction in patients with HTN and left ventricular hypertrophy (LVH)
Usual Dosage Oral:
Hypertension:
Children 6-16 years: 0.7 mg/kg once daily (maximum: 50 mg/day); adjust dose based on response; doses >1.4 mg/kg (maximum: 100 mg) have not been studied
Adults: Usual starting dose: 50 mg once daily; can be administered once or twice daily with total daily doses ranging from 25-100 mg
Patients receiving diuretics or with intravascular volume depletion: Usual initial dose: 25 mg
Nephropathy in patients with type 2 diabetes and hypertension: Adults: Initial: 50 mg once daily; can be increased to 100 mg once daily based on blood pressure response
Stroke reduction (HTN with LVH): Adults: 50 mg once daily (maximum daily dose: 100 mg); may be used in combination with a thiazide diuretic
Dosage Forms
Tablet:
Cozaar®: 25 mg, 50 mg, 100 mg

losartan and hydrochlorothiazide (loe SAR tan & hye droe klor oh THYE a zide)
Sound-Alike/Look-Alike Issues
Hyzaar® may be confused with Cozaar®
Synonyms hydrochlorothiazide and losartan
U.S./Canadian Brand Names Hyzaar® DS [Can]; Hyzaar® [US/Can]
Therapeutic Category Antihypertensive Agent, Combination
Use Treatment of hypertension; stroke risk reduction in patients with HTN and left ventricular hypertrophy (LVH)
Usual Dosage Oral: Adults: Dose is individualized (combination substituted for individual components); dose may be titrated after 2-4 weeks of therapy
Hypertension/stroke reduction in hypertension (with LVH): Usual recommended starting dose of losartan: 50 mg once daily when used as monotherapy in patients who are not volume depleted
Dosage Forms
Tablet:
Hyzaar®: 50-12.5: Losartan 50 mg and hydrochlorothiazide 12.5 mg; 100-12.5: Losartan 100 mg and hydrochlorothiazide 12.5 mg; 100-25: Losartan 100 mg and hydrochlorothiazide 25 mg

losartan potassium *see* losartan *on this page*

Losec® **[Can]** *see* omeprazole *on page 629*

Losec MUPS® **[Can]** *see* omeprazole *on page 629*

Losopan® *(Discontinued) see* magaldrate and simethicone *on page 524*

Lotemax® **[US/Can]** *see* loteprednol *on this page*

Lotensin® **[US/Can]** *see* benazepril *on page 98*

Lotensin® **HCT [US]** *see* benazepril and hydrochlorothiazide *on page 99*

loteprednol (loe te PRED nol)
Synonyms loteprednol etabonate
U.S./Canadian Brand Names Alrex® [US/Can]; Lotemax® [US/Can]
Therapeutic Category Corticosteroid, Ophthalmic
Use
Suspension, 0.2% (Alrex®): Temporary relief of signs and symptoms of seasonal allergic conjunctivitis
Suspension, 0.5% (Lotemax®): Inflammatory conditions (treatment of steroid-responsive inflammatory conditions of the palpebral and bulbar conjunctiva, cornea, and anterior segment of the globe such as allergic conjunctivitis, acne rosacea, superficial punctate keratitis, herpes zoster keratitis, iritis, cyclitis, selected
(Continued)

519

loteprednol *(Continued)*

infective conjunctivitis, when the inherent hazard of steroid use is accepted to obtain an advisable diminution in edema and inflammation) and treatment of postoperative inflammation following ocular surgery

Usual Dosage Ophthalmic: Adults:

Suspension, 0.2% (Alrex®): Instill 1 drop into affected eye(s) 4 times/day

Suspension, 0.5% (Lotemax®):

Inflammatory conditions: Apply 1-2 drops into the conjunctival sac of the affected eye(s) 4 times/day. During the initial treatment within the first week, the dosing may be increased up to 1 drop every hour. Advise patients not to discontinue therapy prematurely. If signs and symptoms fail to improve after 2 days, re-evaluate the patient.

Postoperative inflammation: Apply 1-2 drops into the conjunctival sac of the operated eye(s) 4 times/day beginning 24 hours after surgery and continuing throughout the first 2 weeks of the postoperative period

Dosage Forms

Suspension, ophthalmic:

Alrex®: 0.2% (5 mL, 10 mL)

Lotemax®: 0.5% (2.5 mL, 5 mL, 10 mL, 15 mL)

loteprednol and tobramycin (loe te PRED nol & toe bra MYE sin)

Synonyms loteprednol etabonate and tobramycin; tobramycin and loteprednol etabonate

U.S./Canadian Brand Names Zylet™ [US]

Therapeutic Category Antibiotic/Corticosteroid, Ophthalmic

Use Treatment of steroid-responsive ocular inflammatory conditions where either a superficial bacterial ocular infection or the risk of a superficial bacterial ocular infection exists

Usual Dosage Ophthalmic: Adults: Instill 1-2 drops into the affected eye(s) every 4-6 hours; may increase frequency during the first 24-48 hours to every 1-2 hours. Interval should increase as signs and symptoms improve. Further evaluation should occur for use of greater than 20 mL.

Dosage Forms

Suspension, ophthalmic:

Zylet™: Loteprednol 0.5% and tobramycin 0.3% (2.5 mL, 5 mL, 10 mL)

loteprednol etabonate see loteprednol on previous page

loteprednol etabonate and tobramycin see loteprednol and tobramycin on this page

Lotrel® [US] see amlodipine and benazepril on page 46

Lotriderm® [Can] see betamethasone and clotrimazole on page 108

Lotrimin® AF Athlete's Foot Cream [US-OTC] see clotrimazole on page 206

Lotrimin® AF Athlete's Foot Solution [US-OTC] see clotrimazole on page 206

Lotrimin® AF Cream *(Discontinued)* see clotrimazole on page 206

Lotrimin® AF Jock Itch Cream [US-OTC] see clotrimazole on page 206

Lotrimin® AF Jock Itch Powder Spray [US-OTC] see miconazole on page 566

Lotrimin® AF Lotion *(Discontinued)* see clotrimazole on page 206

Lotrimin® AF Powder/Spray [US-OTC] see miconazole on page 566

Lotrimin® AF Solution *(Discontinued)* see clotrimazole on page 206

Lotrimin® Ultra™ [US-OTC] see butenafine on page 131

Lotrisone® [US] see betamethasone and clotrimazole on page 108

Lotronex® [US] see alosetron on page 31

lovastatin (LOE va sta tin)

Sound-Alike/Look-Alike Issues

lovastatin may be confused with Leustatin®, Livostin®, Lotensin®

Mevacor® may be confused with Mivacron®

Synonyms mevinolin; monacolin K

U.S./Canadian Brand Names Altoprev® [US]; Apo-Lovastatin® [Can]; CO Lovastatin [Can]; Gen-Lovastatin [Can]; Mevacor® [US/Can]; Novo-Lovastatin [Can]; Nu-Lovastatin [Can]; PMS-Lovastatin [Can]; RAN™-Lova-statin [Can]; ratio-Lovastatin [Can]; Riva-Lovastatin [Can]; Sandoz-Lovastatin [Can]

Therapeutic Category HMG-CoA Reductase Inhibitor

Use

Adjunct to dietary therapy to decrease elevated serum total and LDL-cholesterol concentrations in primary hypercholesterolemia

Primary prevention of coronary artery disease (patients without symptomatic disease with average to moderately elevated total and LDL-cholesterol and below average HDL-cholesterol); slow progression of coronary atherosclerosis in patients with coronary heart disease

Adjunct to dietary therapy in adolescent patients (10-17 years of age, females >1 year postmenarche) with heterozygous familial hypercholesterolemia having LDL >189 mg/dL, **or** LDL >160 mg/dL with positive family history of premature cardiovascular disease (CVD), **or** LDL >160 mg/dL with the presence of at least two other CVD risk factors

Usual Dosage Oral:

Adolescents 10-17 years: Immediate release tablet:

LDL reduction <20%: Initial: 10 mg/day with evening meal

LDL reduction ≥20%: Initial: 20 mg/day with evening meal

Usual range: 10-40 mg with evening meal, then adjust dose at 4-week intervals

Adults: Initial: 20 mg with evening meal, then adjust at 4-week intervals; maximum dose: 80 mg/day immediate release tablet **or** 60 mg/day extended release tablet

Dosage modification/limits based on concurrent therapy:

Cyclosporine and other immunosuppressant drugs: Initial dose: 10 mg/day with a maximum recommended dose of 20 mg/day

Concurrent therapy with fibrates, danazol, and/or lipid-lowering doses of niacin (>1 g/day): Maximum recommended dose: 20 mg/day. Concurrent use with fibrates should be avoided unless risk to benefit favors use.

Concurrent therapy with amiodarone or verapamil: Maximum recommended dose: 40 mg/day of regular release or 20 mg/day with extended release.

Dosage Forms

Tablet: 10 mg, 20 mg, 40 mg

Mevacor®: 20 mg, 40 mg

Tablet, extended release:

Altoprev®: 20 mg, 40 mg, 60 mg

lovastatin and niacin *see* niacin and lovastatin *on page 603*

Lovenox® [US/Can] *see* enoxaparin *on page 298*

Lovenox® HP [Can] *see* enoxaparin *on page 298*

Low-Ogestrel® [US] *see* ethinyl estradiol and norgestrel *on page 332*

Loxapac® IM [Can] *see* loxapine *on this page*

loxapine (LOKS a peen)

Sound-Alike/Look-Alike Issues

Loxitane® may be confused with Soriatane®

Synonyms loxapine succinate; oxilapine succinate

U.S./Canadian Brand Names Apo-Loxapine® [Can]; Loxapac® IM [Can]; Loxitane® [US]; Nu-Loxapine [Can]; PMS-Loxapine [Can]

Therapeutic Category Antipsychotic Agent, Dibenzoxazepine

Use Management of psychotic disorders

Usual Dosage Oral: Adults: 10 mg twice daily, increase dose until psychotic symptoms are controlled; usual dose range: 20-100 mg/day in divided doses 2-4 times/day; dosages >250 mg/day are not recommended

Dosage Forms

Capsule: 5 mg, 10 mg, 25 mg, 50 mg

Loxitane®: 5 mg, 10 mg, 25 mg, 50 mg

loxapine succinate *see* loxapine *on this page*

Loxitane® [US] *see* loxapine *on this page*

Loxitane® I.M. (Discontinued) *see* loxapine *on this page*

Lozide® [Can] *see* indapamide *on page 452*

Lozi-Flur™ [US] *see* fluoride *on page 361*

Lozi-Tab® (Discontinued) *see* fluoride *on page 361*

Lozol® [Can] *see* indapamide *on page 452*

Lozol® (Discontinued) *see* indapamide *on page 452*

L-PAM *see* melphalan *on page 539*

LRH *see* gonadorelin *on page 399*

L-sarcolysin *see* melphalan *on page 539*

LTA® 360 [US] *see* lidocaine *on page 504*

LTG *see* lamotrigine *on page 490*

L-thyroxine sodium *see* levothyroxine *on page 503*

Lu-26-054 *see* escitalopram *on page 311*

lubiprostone (loo bi PROS tone)
Synonyms RU 0211; SPI 0211
U.S./Canadian Brand Names Amitiza™ [US]
Therapeutic Category Gastrointestinal Agent, Miscellaneous
Use Treatment of chronic idiopathic constipation
Usual Dosage Oral: Adults: 24 mcg twice daily
Dosage Forms
Capsule:
Amitiza®: 24 mcg

Lubriderm® [US-OTC] *see* lanolin, cetyl alcohol, glycerin, petrolatum, and mineral oil *on page 491*

Lubriderm® Fragrance Free [US-OTC] *see* lanolin, cetyl alcohol, glycerin, petrolatum, and mineral oil *on page 491*

LubriTears® Solution *(Discontinued)* *see* artificial tears *on page 75*

Lucentis® [US] *see* ranibizumab *on page 744*

Ludiomil® *(Discontinued)* *see* maprotiline *on page 531*

Lufyllin® [US/Can] *see* dyphylline *on page 288*

Lufyllin®-GG [US] *see* dyphylline and guaifenesin *on page 288*

Lumigan® [US/Can] *see* bimatoprost *on page 112*

Luminal® Sodium [US] *see* phenobarbital *on page 672*

lumiracoxib *(Canada only)* (loo mye ra KOX ib)
U.S./Canadian Brand Names Prexige® [Can]
Therapeutic Category Nonsteroidal Antiinflammatory Drug (NSAID), COX-2 Selective
Use Acute and chronic treatment of signs and symptoms related to osteoarthritis of the knee
Usual Dosage Oral: Adults: 100 mg once daily; (maximum: 100 mg/day); no additional therapeutic benefit is derived with increased doses
Dosage Forms [CAN] = Canadian brand name
Tablet:
Prexige® [CAN]: 100mg [contains lactose; not available in the U.S.]

Lumitene™ [US] *see* beta-carotene *on page 107*

Lunesta™ [US] *see* eszopiclone *on page 320*

LupiCare™ II Psoriasis [US-OTC] *see* salicylic acid *on page 772*

LupiCare™ Dandruff [US-OTC] *see* salicylic acid *on page 772*

LupiCare™ Psoriasis [US-OTC] *see* salicylic acid *on page 772*

Lupron® [US/Can] *see* leuprolide *on page 497*

Lupron Depot® [US/Can] *see* leuprolide *on page 497*

Lupron Depot-Ped® [US] *see* leuprolide *on page 497*

Luride® [US] *see* fluoride *on page 361*

Luride® Lozi-Tab® [US] *see* fluoride *on page 361*

Luride®-SF *(Discontinued)* *see* fluoride *on page 361*

LuSonal™ [US] *see* phenylephrine *on page 675*

Lustra® [US/Can] *see* hydroquinone *on page 437*

Lustra-AF™ [US] *see* hydroquinone *on page 437*

luteinizing hormone releasing hormone *see* gonadorelin *on page 399*

Lutera™ [US] *see* ethinyl estradiol and levonorgestrel *on page 325*

Lutrepulse™ [Can] *see* gonadorelin *on page 399*

lutropin alfa (LOO troe pin AL fa)
Synonyms recombinant human luteinizing hormone; r-hLH
U.S./Canadian Brand Names Luveris® [US]
Therapeutic Category Gonadotropin; Ovulation Stimulator
Use Stimulation of follicular development in infertile hypogonadotropic hypogonadal (HH) women with profound luteinizing hormone (LH) deficiency; to be used in combination with follitropin alfa
Usual Dosage SubQ: Adults: Female: Infertility: 75 int. units daily until adequate follicular development is noted; maximum duration of treatment: 14 days; to be used concomitantly with follitropin alfa
Dosage Forms
Injection, powder for reconstitution:
Luveris®: 75 int. units

Luveris® [US] *see* lutropin alfa *on this page*

Luvox® [Can] *see* fluvoxamine *on page 370*

Luvox® (Discontinued) *see* fluvoxamine *on page 370*

Luxiq® [US] *see* betamethasone (topical) *on page 109*

LY139603 *see* atomoxetine *on page 81*

LY146032 *see* daptomycin *on page 231*

LY170053 *see* olanzapine *on page 626*

LY231514 *see* pemetrexed *on page 660*

LY248686 *see* duloxetine *on page 286*

LY303366 *see* anidulafungin *on page 57*

LY2148568 *see* exenatide *on page 338*

Lybrel™ [US] *see* ethinyl estradiol and levonorgestrel *on page 325*

Lycolan® Elixir (Discontinued) *see* l-lysine *on page 513*

Lyderm® [Can] *see* fluocinonide *on page 360*

LYMErix™ (Discontinued)

lymphocyte immune globulin *see* antithymocyte globulin (equine) *on page 62*

lymphocyte mitogenic factor *see* aldesleukin *on page 26*

Lyphocin® Injection (Discontinued) *see* vancomycin *on page 883*

Lyrica® [US/Can] *see* pregabalin *on page 712*

Lysinyl [US-OTC] *see* l-lysine *on page 513*

Lysodren® [US/Can] *see* mitotane *on page 573*

Maalox® [US-OTC] *see* aluminum hydroxide, magnesium hydroxide, and simethicone *on page 37*

Maalox® Anti-Gas (Discontinued) *see* aluminum hydroxide, magnesium hydroxide, and simethicone *on page 37*

Maalox® Anti-Gas Extra Strength (Discontinued) *see* aluminum hydroxide, magnesium hydroxide, and simethicone *on page 37*

Maalox® Extra Strength (Discontinued) *see* aluminum hydroxide and magnesium hydroxide *on page 37*

Maalox® Max [US-OTC] *see* aluminum hydroxide, magnesium hydroxide, and simethicone *on page 37*

Maalox® Plus (Discontinued) *see* aluminum hydroxide, magnesium hydroxide, and simethicone *on page 37*

Maalox® Regular Chewable [US-OTC] *see* calcium carbonate *on page 138*

Maalox® TC (Therapeutic Concentrate) (Discontinued) *see* aluminum hydroxide and magnesium hydroxide *on page 37*

Maalox® Total Stomach Relief® [US-OTC] *see* bismuth *on page 113*

MabCampath® [Can] *see* alemtuzumab *on page 27*

Macrobid® [US/Can] *see* nitrofurantoin *on page 607*

Macrodantin® [US/Can] *see* nitrofurantoin *on page 607*

Macrodex® (Discontinued) *see* dextran *on page 245*

Macugen® [US/Can] *see* pegaptanib *on page 657*

mafenide (MA fe nide)

Synonyms mafenide acetate

U.S./Canadian Brand Names Sulfamylon® [US]

Therapeutic Category Antibacterial, Topical

Use Cream: Adjunctive antibacterial agent in the treatment of second- and third-degree burns

Solution: Adjunctive antibacterial agent for use under moist dressings over meshed autografts on excised burn wounds

Usual Dosage Topical: Children and Adults:

Cream: Apply once or twice daily with a sterile-gloved hand; apply to a thickness of approximately ¹/₁₆ inch; the burned area should be covered with cream at all times

Solution: Cover graft area with 1 layer of fine mesh gauze. Wet an 8-ply burn dressing with mafenide solution and cover graft area. Keep dressing wet using syringe or irrigation tubing every 4 hours (or as necessary), or by moistening dressing every 6-8 hours (or as necessary). Irrigation dressing should be secured with bolster dressing and wrapped as appropriate. May leave dressings in place for up to 5 days.

Dosage Forms

Cream, topical:

Sulfamylon®: 85 mg/g (60 g, 120 g, 454 g)

Powder, for topical solution, as acetate:

Sulfamylon®: 50 g/packet (5s)

mafenide acetate *see* mafenide *on this page*

Mag 64™ [US-OTC] *see* magnesium chloride *on this page*

magaldrate and simethicone (MAG al drate & sye METH i kone)

Sound-Alike/Look-Alike Issues

Riopan Plus® may be confused with Repan®

Synonyms simethicone and magaldrate

Therapeutic Category Antacid; Antiflatulent

Use Relief of hyperacidity associated with peptic ulcer, gastritis, peptic esophagitis and hiatal hernia which are accompanied by symptoms of gas

Usual Dosage Oral: Adults: 540-1080 mg magaldrate between meals and at bedtime

Dosage Forms

Suspension, oral: Magaldrate 540 mg and simethicone 20 mg per 5 mL

Magalox Plus® *(Discontinued)* *see* aluminum hydroxide, magnesium hydroxide, and simethicone *on page 37*

Magan® *(Discontinued)* *see* magnesium salicylate *on page 528*

Mag-Caps [US-OTC] *see* magnesium oxide *on page 528*

Mag Delay® [US-OTC] *see* magnesium chloride *on this page*

Mag G® [US-OTC] *see* magnesium gluconate *on page 526*

MagGel™ [US-OTC] *see* magnesium oxide *on page 528*

Maginex™ [US-OTC] *see* magnesium L-aspartate hydrochloride *on page 527*

Maginex™ DS [US-OTC] *see* magnesium L-aspartate hydrochloride *on page 527*

Magnacal® [US-OTC] *see* nutritional formula, enteral/oral *on page 622*

Magnacet™ [US] *see* oxycodone and acetaminophen *on page 641*

Magnelium® [Can] *see* magnesium glucoheptonate *on next page*

magnesia magma *see* magnesium hydroxide *on page 526*

magnesium carbonate and aluminum hydroxide *see* aluminum hydroxide and magnesium carbonate *on page 36*

magnesium chloride (mag NEE zhum KLOR ide)

U.S./Canadian Brand Names Chloromag® [US]; Mag 64™ [US-OTC]; Mag Delay® [US-OTC]; Slow-Mag® [US-OTC]

Therapeutic Category Electrolyte Supplement, Oral

Use Correction or prevention of hypomagnesemia; dietary supplement

Usual Dosage Note: Serum magnesium is poor reflection of repletional status as the majority of magnesium is intracellular; serum levels may be transiently normal for a few hours after a dose is given, therefore, aim for consistently high normal serum levels in patients with normal renal function for most efficient repletion.

Dietary supplement: Adults: Oral (Mag 64™, Mag Delay®, Slow-Mag®): 2 tablets once daily

Parenteral nutrition supplementation: I.V. (elemental magnesium):
Children:
<50 kg: 0.3-0.5 mEq/kg/day
>50 kg: 10-30 mEq/day
Adults: 8-20 mEq/day

RDA (elemental magnesium):
Children:
1-3 years: 80 mg/day
4-8 years: 130 mg/day
9-13 years: 240 mg/day
14-18 years:
Female: 360 mg/day
Pregnant female: 400 mg/day
Male: 410 mg/day
Adults:
19-30 years:
Female: 310 mg/day
Pregnant female: 350 mg/day
Male: 400 mg/day
≥31 years:
Female: 320 mg/day
Pregnant female: 360 mg/day
Male: 420 mg/day

Dosage Forms
Injection, solution: 200 mg/mL [1.97 mEq/mL] (50 mL)
Chloromag®: 200 mg/mL [1.97 mEq/mL] (50 mL)
Tablet [enteric coated]:
Slow-Mag® [OTC]: Elemental magnesium 64 mg
Tablet, extended release:
Mag 64™ [OTC], Mag Delay® [OTC]: Magnesium chloride 535 mg

magnesium citrate (mag NEE zhum SIT rate)

Synonyms citrate of magnesia
U.S./Canadian Brand Names Citro-Mag® [Can]; Citroma® [US-OTC]
Therapeutic Category Laxative
Use Evacuation of bowel prior to certain surgical and diagnostic procedures or overdose situations
Usual Dosage Cathartic: Oral:
Children:
<6 years: 0.5 mL/kg up to a maximum of 200 mL repeated every 4-6 hours until stools are clear
6-12 years: 100-150 mL
Children ≥12 years and Adults: $^1/_2$ to 1 full bottle (120-300 mL)
Dosage Forms
Solution, oral: 290 mg/5 mL
Citroma®: 290 mg/5 mL (300 mL)
Tablet: 100 mg [as elemental magnesium]

magnesium gluceptate *see* magnesium glucoheptonate *on this page*

magnesium glucoheptonate (mag NEE zhum gloo koh HEP toh nate)

Synonyms magnesium gluceptate
U.S./Canadian Brand Names Magnelium® [Can]; Magnolex® [Can]; Magnorol® Sirop [Can]; ratio-Magnesium [Can]
Therapeutic Category Electrolyte Supplement, Parenteral; Magnesium Salt
Use Treatment and prevention of hypomagnesemia
Usual Dosage The recommended dietary allowance (RDA) of magnesium is 4.5 mg/kg which is a total daily allowance of 350-400 mg for adult men and 280-300 mg for adult women. During pregnancy the RDA is 300 mg and during lactation the RDA is 355 mg. Average daily intakes of dietary magnesium have declined in recent years due to processing of food. The latest estimate of the average American dietary intake was 349 mg/day. Dose represented as magnesium sulfate unless stated otherwise.

Note: Serum magnesium is poor reflection of repletional status as the majority of magnesium is intracellular; serum levels may be transiently normal for a few hours after a dose is given, therefore, aim for consistently high normal serum levels in patients with normal renal function for most efficient repletion
Hypomagnesemia: Adults: Oral: 100-600 mg (5-30 mg elemental magnesium) 1-2 times/day with food.
(Continued)

magnesium glucoheptonate *(Continued)*

Maintenance electrolyte requirements:
Daily requirements: 0.2-0.5 mEq/kg/24 hours or 3-10 mEq/1000 kcal/24 hours
Maximum: 8-16 mEq/24 hours

Dosage Forms [CAN] = Canadian brand name
Capsule: 20 mg, 300 mg [not available in the U.S.]
Magnelium® [CAN], Magnorol® [CAN]: 20 mg [not available in the U.S.]
Magnolex® [CAN]: 300 mg [not available in the U.S.]
Solution, oral: 100 mg/mL [not available in the U.S.]
ratio-Magnesium [CAN]: 100 mg/mL [not available in the U.S.]
Syrup: 90 mg/mL [not available in the U.S.]
Magnorol® Sirop [CAN]: 90 mg/mL [not available in the U.S.]

magnesium gluconate *(mag NEE zhum GLOO koe nate)*

U.S./Canadian Brand Names Almora® [US-OTC]; Mag G® [US-OTC]; Magonate® [US-OTC]; Magtrate® [US-OTC]

Therapeutic Category Electrolyte Supplement, Oral

Use Dietary supplement

Usual Dosage RDA (elemental magnesium):
Children:
1-3 years: 80 mg/day
4-8 years: 130 mg/day
9-13 years: 240 mg/day
14-18 years:
Female: 360 mg/day
Pregnant female: 400 mg/day
Male: 410 mg/day
Adults:
19-30 years:
Female: 310 mg/day
Pregnant female: 350 mg/day
Male: 400 mg/day
≥31 years:
Female: 320 mg/day
Pregnant female: 360 mg/day
Male: 420 mg/day

Dosage Forms
Solution:
Magonate® [OTC], Magonate® Sport [OTC]: 1000 mg/5 mL
Tablet: 500 mg
Almora® [OTC], Mag G® [OTC], Magonate® [OTC], Magtrate® [OTC]: 500 mg

magnesium hydroxide *(mag NEE zhum hye DROKS ide)*

Synonyms magnesia magma; milk of magnesia; MOM

U.S./Canadian Brand Names Phillips'® Chews [US-OTC]; Phillips'® Milk of Magnesia [US-OTC]

Therapeutic Category Antacid; Electrolyte Supplement, Oral; Laxative

Use Short-term treatment of occasional constipation and symptoms of hyperacidity, laxative; dietary supplement

Usual Dosage Oral:
Laxative:
Liquid:
Children: Magnesium hydroxide 400 mg/5 mL: 1-3 mL/kg/day; adjust dose to induce daily bowel movement
OTC labeling:
2-5 years: Magnesium hydroxide 400 mg/5 mL: 5-15 mL/day once daily at bedtime or in divided doses
6-11 years:
Magnesium hydroxide 400 mg/5 mL: 15-30 mL/day once daily at bedtime or in divided doses
Magnesium hydroxide 800 mg/5 mL: 7.5-15 mL/day once daily at bedtime or in divided doses
Children ≥12 years and Adults:
Magnesium hydroxide 400 mg/5 mL: 30-60 mL/day once daily at bedtime or in divided doses
Magnesium hydroxide 800 mg/5 mL: 15-30 mL/day once daily at bedtime or in divided doses
Tablet: OTC labeling:
Children:
3-5 years: Magnesium hydroxide 311 mg/tablet: 2 tablets/day once daily at bedtime or in divided doses
6-11 years: Magnesium hydroxide 311 mg/tablet: 4 tablets/day once daily at bedtime or in divided doses

Children ≥12 years and Adults: Magnesium hydroxide 311 mg/tablet: 8 tablets/day once daily at bedtime or in divided doses
Antacid: OTC labeling:
Liquid: Children ≥12 years and Adults: Magnesium hydroxide 400 mg/5 mL: 5-15 mL as needed up to 4 times/day
Tablet: Children ≥12 years and Adults: Magnesium hydroxide 311 mg/tablet: 2-4 tablets every 4 hours up to 4 times/day
Dietary supplement: OTC labeling (Phillips'® Chews): Children ≥12 years and Adults: Magnesium 500 mg: 2-4 tablets/day once daily at bedtime or in divided doses
Dosage Forms
Liquid, oral: 400 mg/5 mL
Phillips'® Milk of Magnesia [OTC]: 400 mg/5 mL
Liquid, oral concentrate: 800 mg/5 mL
Phillips'® Milk of Magnesia [OTC] [concentrate]: 800 mg/5 mL
Tablet, chewable:
Phillips'® Chews [OTC]: Magnesium 500 mg
Phillips'® Milk of Magnesia [OTC]: 311 mg

magnesium hydroxide, aluminum hydroxide, and simethicone *see* aluminum hydroxide, magnesium hydroxide, and simethicone *on page 37*

magnesium hydroxide and aluminum hydroxide *see* aluminum hydroxide and magnesium hydroxide *on page 37*

magnesium hydroxide and calcium carbonate *see* calcium carbonate and magnesium hydroxide *on page 139*

magnesium hydroxide and mineral oil (mag NEE zhum hye DROKS ide & MIN er al oyl)
Synonyms Haley's M-O; MOM/mineral oil emulsion
U.S./Canadian Brand Names Phillips'® M-O [US-OTC]
Therapeutic Category Laxative
Use Short-term treatment of occasional constipation
Usual Dosage Oral: Laxative: OTC labeling:
Children 6-11 years: 20-30 mL at bedtime
Children ≥12 years and Adults: 45-60 mL at bedtime
Dosage Forms
Suspension, oral:
Phillips'® M-O [OTC]: Magnesium hydroxide 300 mg and mineral oil 1.25 mL per 5 mL

magnesium hydroxide, famotidine, and calcium carbonate *see* famotidine, calcium carbonate, and magnesium hydroxide *on page 342*

magnesium L-aspartate hydrochloride (mag NEE zhum el as PAR tate hye droe KLOR ide)
Synonyms MAH
U.S./Canadian Brand Names Maginex™ DS [US-OTC]; Maginex™ [US-OTC]
Therapeutic Category Electrolyte Supplement, Oral
Use Dietary supplement
Usual Dosage
RDA (elemental magnesium):
Children:
1-3 years: 80 mg/day
4-8 years: 130 mg/day
9-13 years: 240 mg/day
14-18 years:
Female: 360 mg/day
Pregnant female: 400 mg/day
Male: 410 mg/day
Adults:
19-30 years:
Female: 310 mg/day
Pregnant female: 350 mg/day
Male: 400 mg/day
≥31 years:
Female: 320 mg/day
Pregnant female: 360 mg/day
Male: 420 mg/day
Dietary supplement: Adults: Oral: Magnesium-L-aspartate 1230 mg (magnesium 122 mg) up to 3 times/day
(Continued)

magnesium L-aspartate hydrochloride *(Continued)*

Dosage Forms
Granules:
Maginex™ DS [OTC]: 1230 mg
Tablet:
Maginex™ [OTC]: 615 mg

magnesium oxide (mag NEE zhum OKS ide)

U.S./Canadian Brand Names Mag-Caps [US-OTC]; Mag-Ox® 400 [US-OTC]; MagGel™ [US-OTC]; Uro-Mag® [US-OTC]

Therapeutic Category Antacid; Electrolyte Supplement, Oral; Laxative

Use Electrolyte replacement

Usual Dosage
RDA (elemental magnesium):
Children:
1-3 years: 80 mg/day
4-8 years: 130 mg/day
9-13 years: 240 mg/day
14-18 years:
Female: 360 mg/day
Pregnant female: 400 mg/day
Male: 410 mg/day
Adults:
19-30 years:
Female: 310 mg/day
Pregnant female: 350 mg/day
Male: 400 mg/day
≥31 years:
Female: 320 mg/day
Pregnant female: 360 mg/day
Male: 420 mg/day

Dietary supplement: Adults: Oral:
Mag-Ox 400®: 2 tablets daily with food
Mag-Caps, Uro-Mag®: 4-5 capsules daily with food
Dosage Forms
Capsule:
Mag-Caps: Elemental magnesium 85 mg
Uro-Mag® [OTC]: 140 mg
Capsule, softgel:
MagGel™: 600 mg
Tablet: 400 mg
Mag-Ox® 400 [OTC]: 400 mg

magnesium salicylate (mag NEE zhum sa LIS i late)

U.S./Canadian Brand Names Doan's® Extra Strength [US-OTC]; Keygesic [US-OTC]; Momentum® [US-OTC]; Novasal™ [US]

Therapeutic Category Nonsteroidal Antiinflammatory Drug (NSAID)

Use Mild-to-moderate pain, fever, various inflammatory conditions; relief of pain and inflammation of rheumatoid arthritis and osteoarthritis

Usual Dosage Oral:
Children ≥12 years and Adults: Relief of mild-to-moderate pain:
Doan's® Extra Strength, Momentum®: Two caplets every 6 hours as needed (maximum: 8 caplets/24 hours)
Keygesic: One tablet every 4 hours as needed (maximum 4 tablets/24 hours)
Adults: Treatment of arthritis (Novasal™): Initial: 1 tablet 3-4 times/day. Maximum: 8 tablets/day
Dosage Forms
Caplet: 467 mg
Doan's® Extra Strength [OTC]: 467 mg
Momentum® [OTC]: 467 mg
Tablet, chelated:
Keygesic [OTC]: 650 mg
Tablet, as tetrahydrate [scored]:
Novasal™: 600 mg

magnesium sulfate (mag NEE zhum SUL fate)

Sound-Alike/Look-Alike Issues
magnesium sulfate may be confused with manganese sulfate, morphine sulfate
$MgSO_4$ is an error-prone abbreviation (mistaken as morphine sulfate)

Synonyms epsom salts

Therapeutic Category Anticonvulsant; Electrolyte Supplement, Oral; Laxative

Use Treatment and prevention of hypomagnesemia; prevention and treatment of seizures in severe pre-eclampsia or eclampsia, pediatric acute nephritis; torsade de pointes; treatment of cardiac arrhythmias (VT/VF) caused by hypomagnesemia; short-term treatment of constipation; soaking aid

Usual Dosage Dose represented as magnesium sulfate unless stated otherwise. **Note:** Serum magnesium is poor reflection of repletional status as the majority of magnesium is intracellular; serum levels may be transiently normal for a few hours after a dose is given, therefore, aim for consistently high normal serum levels in patients with normal renal function for most efficient repletion.

Hypomagnesemia: Note: Treatment depends on severity and clinical status:
Children: I.V., I.O.: 25-50 mg/kg/dose (0.2-0.4 mEq/kg/dose) over 10-20 minutes (faster in torsade); maximum single dose: 2000 mg (16 mEq)
Adults:
Mild deficiency: I.M.: 1 g every 6 hours for 4 doses, or as indicated by serum magnesium levels
Severe deficiency:
I.M.: Up to 250 mg/kg within a 4-hour period
I.V.: 5 g over 3 hours
Severe or symptomatic deficiency: I.V.: 1-2 g over 5-60 minutes
Hypomagnesemia with seizures: I.V.: 2 g over 10 minutes; calcium administration may also be appropriate
Eclampsia, preeclampsia: Adults: I.V.: 4-6 g over 15-20 minutes followed by 2 g/hour continuous infusion
Torsade de pointes: Adults: I.V.:
Pulseless: 1-2 g over 5-20 minutes
With pulse: 1-2 g over 5-60 minutes. **Note:** Slower administration preferable for stable patients.
Cathartic: Oral:
Children:
2-5 years: 2.5-5 g/kg/day in divided doses
6-11 years: 5-10 g/day in divided doses
Children ≥12 years and Adults: 10-30 g/day in divided doses
Parenteral nutrition supplementation (elemental magnesium): I.V.:
Children:
<50 kg: 0.3-0.5 mEq/kg/day
>50 kg: 10-30 mEq/day
Adults: 8-20 mEq/day
Soaking aid: Topical: Adults: Dissolve 2 cupfuls of powder per gallon of warm water

RDA (elemental magnesium):
Children:
1-3 years: 80 mg/day
4-8 years: 130 mg/day
9-13 years: 240 mg/day
14-18 years:
Female: 360 mg/day
Pregnant female: 400 mg/day
Male: 410 mg/day
Adults:
19-30 years:
Female: 310 mg/day
Pregnant female: 350 mg/day
Male: 400 mg/day
≥31 years:
Female: 320 mg/day
Pregnant female: 360 mg/day
Male: 420 mg/day

Dosage Forms
Infusion [premixed in D_5W]: 10 mg/mL (100 mL); 20 mg/mL (500 mL, 1000 mL)
Infusion [premixed in water for injection]: 40 mg/mL (100 mL, 500 mL, 1000 mL); 80 mg/mL (50 mL)
Injection, solution: 125 mg/mL (8 mL); 500 mg/mL (2 mL, 5 mL, 10 mL, 20 mL, 50 mL)
Powder, oral/topical: Magnesium sulfate USP (227 g, 454 g, 480 g, 1810 g, 1920 g, 2720 g)

magnesium trisilicate and aluminum hydroxide *see* aluminum hydroxide and magnesium trisilicate *on page 37*

Magnevist® [US/Can] *see* gadopentetate dimeglumine *on page 382*

Magnolex® **[Can]** *see* magnesium glucoheptonate *on page 525*

Magnorol® **Sirop [Can]** *see* magnesium glucoheptonate *on page 525*

Magonate® **[US-OTC]** *see* magnesium gluconate *on page 526*

Magonate® **Sport** *(Discontinued) see* magnesium gluconate *on page 526*

Mag-Ox® **400 [US-OTC]** *see* magnesium oxide *on page 528*

Magsal® *(Discontinued) see* magnesium salicylate *on page 528*

Magtrate® **[US-OTC]** *see* magnesium gluconate *on page 526*

MAH *see* magnesium L-aspartate hydrochloride *on page 527*

Majeptil® **[Can]** *see* thioproperazine *(Canada only) on page 837*

Malarone® **[US/Can]** *see* atovaquone and proguanil *on page 82*

Malarone® **Pediatric [Can]** *see* atovaquone and proguanil *on page 82*

malathion (mal a THYE on)

U.S./Canadian Brand Names Ovide® [US]

Therapeutic Category Scabicides/Pediculicides

Use Treatment of head lice and their ova

Usual Dosage Sprinkle Ovide® lotion on dry hair and rub gently until the scalp is thoroughly moistened; pay special attention to the back of the head and neck. Allow to dry naturally - use no heat and leave uncovered. After 8-12 hours, the hair should be washed with a nonmedicated shampoo; rinse and use a fine-toothed comb to remove dead lice and eggs. If required, repeat with second application in 7-9 days. Further treatment is generally not necessary. Other family members should be evaluated to determine if infested and if so, receive treatment.

Dosage Forms
  Lotion:
  Ovide®: 0.5% (59 mL)

Maldemar™ **[US]** *see* scopolamine derivatives *on page 778*

Mallisol® *(Discontinued) see* povidone-iodine *on page 704*

maltodextrin (mal toe DEK strin)

U.S./Canadian Brand Names Multidex® [US-OTC]; OraRinse™ [US-OTC]

Therapeutic Category Skin and Mucous Membrane Agent

Use Topical: Treatment of infected or noninfected wounds

Usual Dosage Adults:

  Oral: Management of pain due to oral lesions: OraRinse™: 1 tablespoonful, swish or gargle for ~1 minute, 4 times/day or more if needed

  Topical: Wound dressing: Multidex®: After debridement and irrigation of wound, apply and cover with a nonadherent, nonocclusive dressing. May be applied to moist or dry, infected or noninfected wounds.

Dosage Forms
  Gel, topical dressing:
  Multidex® [OTC]: (4 mL, 7 mL, 14 mL, 85 mL)
  Powder, for oral suspension:
  OraRinse™ [OTC]: (19 g)
  Powder, topical dressing:
  Multidex®: (6 g, 12 g, 25 g, 45 g)

Mandelamine® **[US/Can]** *see* methenamine *on page 551*

mandrake *see* podophyllum resin *on page 693*

Manerix® **[Can]** *see* moclobemide *(Canada only) on page 575*

manganese *see* trace metals *on page 855*

mannitol (MAN i tole)

Sound-Alike/Look-Alike Issues

  Osmitrol® may be confused with esmolol

Synonyms *D*-mannitol

U.S./Canadian Brand Names Osmitrol® [US/Can]; Resectisol® [US]

Therapeutic Category Diuretic, Osmotic

Use Reduction of increased intracranial pressure associated with cerebral edema; promotion of diuresis in the prevention and/or treatment of oliguria or anuria due to acute renal failure; reduction of increased intraocular pressure; promoting urinary excretion of toxic substances; genitourinary irrigant in transurethral prostatic resection or other transurethral surgical procedures

Usual Dosage

Children: I.V.:

Test dose (to assess adequate renal function): 200 mg/kg over 3-5 minutes to produce a urine flow of at least 1 mL/kg for 1-3 hours

Initial: 0.25-1 g/kg

Maintenance: 0.25-0.5 g/kg given every 4-6 hours

Adults:

I.V.:

Test dose (to assess adequate renal function): 12.5 g (200 mg/kg) over 3-5 minutes to produce a urine flow of at least 30-50 mL of urine per hour. If urine flow does not increase, a second test dose may be given. If test dose does not produce an acceptable urine output, then need to reassess management.

Initial: 0.5-1 g/kg

Maintenance: 0.25-0.5 g/kg every 4-6 hours; usual daily dose: 20-200 g/24 hours

Intracranial pressure: Cerebral edema: 0.25-1.5 g/kg/dose I.V. as a 15% to 20% solution over ≥30 minutes; maintain serum osmolality 310 to <320 mOsm/kg

Prevention of acute renal failure (oliguria): 50-100 g dose

Treatment of oliguria: 100 g dose

Preoperative for neurosurgery: 1.5-2 g/kg administered 1-1.5 hours prior to surgery

Reduction of intraocular pressure: 1.5-2 g/kg as a 15% to 20% solution; administer over 30 minutes

Topical: Transurethral irrigation: Use urogenital solution as required for irrigation

Dosage Forms

Injection, solution: 5% [50 mg/mL] (1000 mL); 10% [100 mg/mL] (500 mL, 1000 mL); 15% [150 mg/mL] (500 mL); 20% [200 mg/mL] (150 mL, 250 mL, 500 mL); 25% [250 mg/mL] (50 mL)

Osmitrol®: 5% [50 mg/mL] (1000 mL); 10% [100 mg/mL] (500 mL, 1000 mL); 15% [150 mg/mL] (500 mL); 20% [200 mg/mL] (250 mL, 500 mL)

Solution, urogenital: 5% [50 mg/mL] (2000 mL, 4000 mL)

Resectisol®: 5% [50 mg/mL] (2000 mL, 4000 mL)

mantoux *see* tuberculin tests *on page 872*

Maox® *(Discontinued)* *see* magnesium oxide *on page 528*

Mapap [US-OTC] *see* acetaminophen *on page 5*

Mapap Children's [US-OTC] *see* acetaminophen *on page 5*

Mapap Extra Strength [US-OTC] *see* acetaminophen *on page 5*

Mapap Infants [US-OTC] *see* acetaminophen *on page 5*

Mapap Sinus Maximum Strength [US-OTC] *see* acetaminophen and pseudoephedrine *on page 8*

Mapezine® [Can] *see* carbamazepine *on page 147*

maprotiline (ma PROE ti leen)

Sound-Alike/Look-Alike Issues

Ludiomil® may be confused with Lamictal®, lamotrigine, Lomotil®

Synonyms maprotiline hydrochloride

U.S./Canadian Brand Names Novo-Maprotiline [Can]

Therapeutic Category Antidepressant, Tetracyclic

Use Treatment of depression and anxiety associated with depression

Usual Dosage Oral: Adults: Depression/anxiety: 75 mg/day to start, increase by 25 mg every 2 weeks up to 150-225 mg/day; given in 3 divided doses or in a single daily dose

Dosage Forms

Tablet: 25 mg, 50 mg, 75 mg

maprotiline hydrochloride *see* maprotiline *on this page*

maraviroc (mah RAV er rock)

Synonyms UK-427,857

U.S./Canadian Brand Names Selzentry™ [US]

Therapeutic Category Antiretroviral Agent, CCR5 Antagonist

Use Treatment of CCR5-tropic HIV-1 infection, in combination with other antiretroviral agents in treatment-experienced patients with evidence of viral replication and HIV-1 strains resistant to multiple antiretroviral therapy

Usual Dosage Oral: Adolescents ≥16 years and Adults: 300 mg twice daily

(Continued)

maraviroc *(Continued)*
Dosage Forms Tablet:
Selzentry™: 150 mg, 300 mg

Marcaine® **[US/Can]** *see* bupivacaine *on page 125*

Marcaine® **Spinal [US]** *see* bupivacaine *on page 125*

Marcaine® **with Epinephrine [US]** *see* bupivacaine and epinephrine *on page 126*

Margesic® **H [US]** *see* hydrocodone and acetaminophen *on page 427*

Marinol® **[US/Can]** *see* dronabinol *on page 284*

Marmine® **Injection** *(Discontinued) see* dimenhydrinate *on page 262*

Marmine® **Oral** *(Discontinued) see* dimenhydrinate *on page 262*

Marplan® **[US]** *see* isocarboxazid *on page 474*

Marthritic® *(Discontinued) see* salsalate *on page 775*

Marvelon® **[Can]** *see* ethinyl estradiol and desogestrel *on page 322*

Matulane® **[US/Can]** *see* procarbazine *on page 716*

3M™ Avagard® *(Discontinued) see* chlorhexidine gluconate *on page 174*

Mavik® **[US/Can]** *see* trandolapril *on page 857*

Maxair™ **Autohaler**™ **[US]** *see* pirbuterol *on page 686*

Maxalt® **[US/Can]** *see* rizatriptan *on page 763*

Maxalt-MLT® **[US]** *see* rizatriptan *on page 763*

Maxalt RPD™ **[Can]** *see* rizatriptan *on page 763*

Maxaquin® *(Discontinued)*

Maxidex® **[US/Can]** *see* dexamethasone (ophthalmic) *on page 241*

Maxidone™ **[US]** *see* hydrocodone and acetaminophen *on page 427*

Maxifed® **[US]** *see* guaifenesin and pseudoephedrine *on page 406*

Maxifed DM [US] *see* guaifenesin, pseudoephedrine, and dextromethorphan *on page 408*

Maxifed DMX [US] *see* guaifenesin, pseudoephedrine, and dextromethorphan *on page 408*

Maxifed-G® **[US]** *see* guaifenesin and pseudoephedrine *on page 406*

Maxiflor® *(Discontinued) see* diflorasone *on page 257*

Maximum Strength Desenex® **Antifungal Cream** *(Discontinued) see* miconazole *on page 566*

Maximum Strength Dex-A-Diet® *(Discontinued)*

Maximum Strength Dexatrim® *(Discontinued)*

Maxiphen DM [US] *see* guaifenesin, dextromethorphan, and phenylephrine *on page 407*

Maxipime® **[US/Can]** *see* cefepime *on page 160*

Maxitrol® **[US/Can]** *see* neomycin, polymyxin B, and dexamethasone *on page 597*

Maxi-Tuss HC® **[US]** *see* phenylephrine, hydrocodone, and chlorpheniramine *on page 678*

Maxi-Tuss HCG [US] *see* hydrocodone and guaifenesin *on page 429*

Maxi-Tuss HCX [US] *see* phenylephrine, hydrocodone, and chlorpheniramine *on page 678*

Maxivate® **[US]** *see* betamethasone (topical) *on page 109*

Maxolon® *(Discontinued) see* metoclopramide *on page 561*

Maxzide® **[US]** *see* hydrochlorothiazide and triamterene *on page 427*

Maxzide®**-25 [US]** *see* hydrochlorothiazide and triamterene *on page 427*

may apple *see* podophyllum resin *on page 693*

3M™ Cavilon™ **Skin Cleanser** *(Discontinued) see* benzalkonium chloride *on page 100*

MCH *see* collagen hemostat *on page 213*

m-cresyl acetate *(em-KREE sil AS e tate)*
U.S./Canadian Brand Names Cresylate® [US]
Therapeutic Category Otic Agent, Antiinfective
Use Provides an acid medium; for external otitis infections caused by susceptible bacteria or fungus
Usual Dosage Otic: Instill 2-4 drops as required

Dosage Forms
Solution, otic:
Cresylate®: 25% (15 mL)

MCT *see* medium chain triglycerides *on page 536*

MCT Oil® [US-OTC/Can] *see* medium chain triglycerides *on page 536*

MCV4 *see* meningococcal polysaccharide (Groups A / C / Y and W-135) diphtheria toxoid conjugate vaccine *on page 540*

MD-76®R [US] *see* diatrizoate meglumine and diatrizoate sodium *on page 250*

MD-Gastroview® [US] *see* diatrizoate meglumine and diatrizoate sodium *on page 250*

MDL 73,147EF *see* dolasetron *on page 274*

measles, mumps, and rubella vaccines, combined

(MEE zels, mumpz & roo BEL a vak SEENS, kom BINED)

Synonyms MMR; mumps, measles, and rubella vaccines, combined; rubella, measles, and mumps vaccines, combined

U.S./Canadian Brand Names M-M-R® II [US/Can]; Priorix™ [Can]

Therapeutic Category Vaccine, Live Virus

Use Measles, mumps, and rubella prophylaxis

Usual Dosage SubQ:

Infants <12 months: If there is risk of exposure to measles, single-antigen measles vaccine should be administered at 6-11 months of age with a second dose (of MMR) at >12 months of age.

Children ≥12 months:

Primary immunization: 0.5 mL at 12-15 months

Revaccination: 0.5 mL at 4-6 years of age; revaccination is recommended prior to elementary school. If the second dose was not received, the schedule should be completed by the 11- to 12-year old visit. During a mumps outbreak, children ages 1-4 should consider a second dose of a live mumps virus vaccine. (Minimum interval between doses is 28 days.)

Adults:

Birth year ≥1957 without evidence of immunity: 1 or 2 doses (0.5 mL/dose); minimum interval between doses is 28 days

Routine vaccination of healthcare workers:

Birth year ≥1957 without evidence of immunity: 2 doses of a live mumps virus vaccine; minimum interval between doses is 28 days

Birth year <1957 without evidence of immunity: 1 dose of a live mumps virus vaccine.

Mumps outbreak:

Healthcare workers born <1957 without other evidence of immunity: Consider 2 doses of a live mumps virus vaccine; minimum interval between doses is 28 days

Low-risk adults: A second dose of a live mumps virus vaccine should be considered in adults who previously received 1 dose; minimum interval between doses is 28 days

Dosage Forms

Injection, powder for reconstitution [preservative free]:

M-M-R® II: Measles virus 1000 TCID50, mumps virus 20,000 $TCID_{50}$, and rubella virus 1000 $TCID_{50}$

measles, mumps, rubella, and varicella virus vaccine

(MEE zels, mumpz, roo BEL a, & var i SEL a VYE rus vak SEEN)

Synonyms MMRV; mumps, rubella, varicella, and measles vaccine; rubella, varicella, measles, and mumps vaccine; varicella, measles, mumps, and rubella vaccine

U.S./Canadian Brand Names ProQuad® [US]

Therapeutic Category Vaccine, Live Virus

Use To provide simultaneous active immunization against measles, mumps, rubella, and varicella

Usual Dosage SubQ: Children 12 months to 12 years: One dose (0.5 mL)

Administer on or after the first birthday, as soon as child becomes eligible for vaccination. Use of the combined MMRV vaccine is preferred in order to decrease the number of injections. It may be used whenever all components of the vaccine are needed in children within this age group. (Refer to current CDC Recommended Immunization Schedule)

Allow at least 1 month between administering a dose of a measles containing vaccine (eg, M-M-R® II) and ProQuad®.

Allow at least 3 months between administering a varicella containing vaccine (eg, Varivax®) and ProQuad®.

Dosage Forms

Injection, powder for reconstitution [preservative free]:

ProQuad®: Measles virus ≥3.00 $\log_{10}$ TCID50, mumps virus ≥4.3 $\log_{10}$ TCID50, rubella virus ≥3.0 $\log_{10}$ TCID50, and varicella virus ≥3.99 $\log_{10}$ plaque-forming units

measles virus vaccine (live) (MEE zels VYE rus vak SEEN, live)

Sound-Alike/Look-Alike Issues
Attenuvax® may be confused with Meruvax®

Synonyms more attenuated enders strain; rubeola vaccine

U.S./Canadian Brand Names Attenuvax® [US]

Therapeutic Category Vaccine, Live Virus

Use Active immunization against measles (rubeola)

Note: Trivalent measles - mumps - rubella (MMR) is the vaccine of choice if recipients are likely to be susceptible to rubella and/or mumps as well as to measles.

Usual Dosage Note: Trivalent measles - mumps - rubella (MMR) vaccine should be used unless contraindicated in adults and children ≥12 months of age.

Children ≥6 months and Adults: SubQ: 0.5 mL in outer aspect of the upper arm

Primary vaccination recommended at 12-15 months of age and repeated at 4-6 years of age. Children requiring vaccination with measles virus vaccine prior to 12 months of age (eg, during local outbreak, international travel to endemic area) should receive another dose between 12-15 months and again prior to elementary school.

Adults born in or after 1957 without documentation of live vaccine on or after first birthday, without physician-diagnosed measles, or without laboratory evidence of immunity should be vaccinated, ideally with 2 doses of vaccine separated by no less than 1 month. For those previously vaccinated with 1 dose of measles vaccine, revaccination is recommended for students entering colleges and other institutions of higher education, for healthcare workers at the time of employment, and for international travelers who visit endemic areas. Persons vaccinated between 1963 and 1967 with a killed measles vaccine, followed by live vaccine within 3 months, or with a vaccine of unknown type should be revaccinated with live measles virus vaccine.

Dosage Forms
Injection, powder for reconstitution [preservative free]:
Attenuvax®: ≥1000 $TCID_{50}$

Measurin® *(Discontinued)* see aspirin *on page 78*

Mebaral® [US/Can] see mephobarbital *on page 543*

mebendazole (me BEN da zole)

U.S./Canadian Brand Names Vermox® [Can]

Therapeutic Category Anthelmintic

Use Treatment of pinworms (*Enterobius vermicularis*), whipworms (*Trichuris trichiura*), roundworms (*Ascaris lumbricoides*), and hookworms (*Ancylostoma duodenale*)

Usual Dosage Oral: Children ≥2 years and Adults:
Pinworms: 100 mg as a single dose; may need to repeat after 2 weeks; treatment should include family members in close contact with patient
Whipworms, roundworms, hookworms: One tablet twice daily, morning and evening on 3 consecutive days; if patient is not cured within 3-4 weeks, a second course of treatment may be administered
Capillariasis: 200 mg twice daily for 20 days

Dosage Forms
Tablet, chewable: 100 mg

mecamylamine (mek a MIL a meen)

Sound-Alike/Look-Alike Issues
mecamylamine may be confused with mesalamine

Synonyms mecamylamine hydrochloride

U.S./Canadian Brand Names Inversine® [US/Can]

Therapeutic Category Ganglionic Blocking Agent

Use Treatment of moderately severe to severe hypertension and in uncomplicated malignant hypertension

Usual Dosage Oral: Adults: 2.5 mg twice daily after meals for 2 days; increased by increments of 2.5 mg at intervals ≥2 days until desired blood pressure response is achieved; average daily dose: 25 mg (usually in 3 divided doses)

Note: Reduce dosage of other antihypertensives when combined with mecamylamine with exception of thiazide diuretics which may be maintained at usual dose while decreasing mecamylamine by 50%

Dosage Forms
Tablet:
Inversine®: 2.5 mg

mecamylamine hydrochloride see mecamylamine *on this page*

mecasermin (mek a SER min)

Synonyms mecasermin (rDNA origin); mecasermin rinfabate; recombinant human insulin-like growth factor-1; rhIGF-1; rhIGF-1/rhIGFBP-3

U.S./Canadian Brand Names Increlex™ [US]; Iplex™ [US]

Therapeutic Category Growth Hormone

Use Treatment of growth failure in children with severe primary insulin-like growth factor-1 deficiency (IGF-1 deficiency; primary IGFD), or with growth hormone (GH) gene deletions who have developed neutralizing antibodies to GH

Usual Dosage Primary IGFD: SubQ:

Increlex™: Children ≥2 years: Initial: 0.04-0.08 mg/kg twice daily; if tolerated for 7 days, may increase by 0.04 mg/kg/dose (maximum dose: 0.12 mg/kg given twice daily). Must be administered within 20 minutes of a meal or snack; omit dose if patient is unable to eat. Reduce dose if hypoglycemia occurs despite adequate food intake.

Iplex™: Children ≥3 years: Initial: 0.5 mg/kg once daily; dose may be increased to 1-2 mg/kg/day, given once daily. Withhold dose if hypoglycemia is present.

Dosage Forms

Injection, solution:

Increlex™: 10 mg/mL (4 mL)

Injection, solution [preservative free]:

Iplex™: 36 mg/0.6 mL (0.6 mL)

mecasermin (rDNA origin) *see* mecasermin *on this page*

mecasermin rinfabate *see* mecasermin *on this page*

mechlorethamine (me klor ETH a meen)

Synonyms chlorethazine; chlorethazine mustard; HN$_2$; mechlorethamine hydrochloride; mustine; nitrogen mustard; NSC-762

U.S./Canadian Brand Names Mustargen® [US/Can]

Therapeutic Category Antineoplastic Agent

Use Combination therapy of Hodgkin disease and malignant lymphomas; non-Hodgkin lymphoma; may be used by intracavitary injection for treatment of metastatic tumors; pleural and other malignant effusions; topical treatment of mycosis fungoides

Usual Dosage Refer to individual protocols.

Children and Adults: I.V.: 6 mg/m^2 on days 1 and 8 of a 28-day cycle (MOPP regimen)

Adults:

I.V.: 0.4 mg/kg **or** 12-16 mg/m^2 for one dose **or** divided into 0.1 mg/kg/day for 4 days, repeated at 4- to 6-week intervals

Intracavitary: 0.2-0.4 mg/kg (10-20 mg) as a single dose; may be repeated if fluid continues to accumulate.

Intrapericardially: 0.2-0.4 mg/kg as a single dose; may be repeated if fluid continues to accumulate.

Topical: 0.01% to 0.02% solution, lotion, or ointment

Dosage Forms

Injection, powder for reconstitution:

Mustargen®: 10 mg

mechlorethamine hydrochloride *see* mechlorethamine *on this page*

meclizine (MEK li zeen)

Sound-Alike/Look-Alike Issues

Antivert® may be confused with Axert™

Synonyms meclizine hydrochloride; meclozine hydrochloride

U.S./Canadian Brand Names Antivert® [US]; Bonamine™ [Can]; Bonine® [US-OTC/Can]; Dramamine® Less Drowsy Formula [US-OTC]

Therapeutic Category Antihistamine

Use Prevention and treatment of symptoms of motion sickness; management of vertigo with diseases affecting the vestibular system

Usual Dosage Oral: Children >12 years and Adults:

Motion sickness: 12.5-25 mg 1 hour before travel, repeat dose every 12-24 hours if needed; doses up to 50 mg may be needed

Vertigo: 25-100 mg/day in divided doses

Dosage Forms

Tablet: 12.5 mg, 25 mg

Antivert®: 12.5 mg, 25 mg, 50 mg

Dramamine® Less Drowsy Formula [OTC]: 25 mg

Tablet, chewable: 25 mg

Bonine® [OTC]: 25 mg

meclizine hydrochloride *see* meclizine *on previous page*

meclofenamate (me kloe fen AM ate)
Synonyms meclofenamate sodium
U.S./Canadian Brand Names Meclomen® [Can]
Therapeutic Category Analgesic, Nonnarcotic; Nonsteroidal Antiinflammatory Drug (NSAID)
Use Treatment of inflammatory disorders, arthritis, mild to moderate pain, dysmenorrhea
Usual Dosage Oral: Children >14 years and Adults:
  Mild to moderate pain: 50 mg every 4-6 hours; increases to 100 mg may be required; maximum dose: 400 mg
  Rheumatoid arthritis and osteoarthritis: 50 mg every 4-6 hours; increase, over weeks, to 200-400 mg/day in 3-4 divided doses; do not exceed 400 mg/day; maximal benefit for any dose may not be seen for 2-3 weeks
Dosage Forms
  Capsule: 50 mg, 100 mg

meclofenamate sodium *see* meclofenamate *on this page*

Meclomen® [Can] *see* meclofenamate *on this page*

meclozine hydrochloride *see* meclizine *on previous page*

Med-Diltiazem [Can] *see* diltiazem *on page 261*

Medebar® Plus [US] *see* barium *on page 94*

Medent-DM [US] *see* guaifenesin, pseudoephedrine, and dextromethorphan *on page 408*

medicinal carbon *see* charcoal *on page 171*

medicinal charcoal *see* charcoal *on page 171*

Medicone® Suppositories [US-OTC] *see* phenylephrine *on page 675*

Medidin® Liquid *(Discontinued)* *see* hydrocodone and guaifenesin *on page 429*

Medigesic® [US] *see* butalbital, acetaminophen, and caffeine *on page 130*

Medihaler-Iso® *(Discontinued)* *see* isoproterenol *on page 475*

Medipain 5® *(Discontinued)* *see* hydrocodone and acetaminophen *on page 427*

Medi-Phenyl [US-OTC] *see* phenylephrine *on page 675*

Mediplast® [US-OTC] *see* salicylic acid *on page 772*

Medipren® *(Discontinued)* *see* ibuprofen *on page 444*

Medi-Quick® Topical Ointment *(Discontinued)* *see* bacitracin, neomycin, and polymyxin B *on page 91*

Medispaz® *(Discontinued)* *see* hyoscyamine *on page 441*

Medi-Synal [US-OTC] *see* acetaminophen and pseudoephedrine *on page 8*

Medi-Tuss® *(Discontinued)* *see* guaifenesin *on page 401*

medium chain triglycerides (mee DEE um chane trye GLIS er ides)
Synonyms MCT; triglycerides, medium chain
U.S./Canadian Brand Names MCT Oil® [US-OTC/Can]
Therapeutic Category Nutritional Supplement
Use Dietary supplement for those who cannot digest long chain fats; malabsorption associated with disorders such as pancreatic insufficiency, bile salt deficiency, short bowel syndrome, and bacterial overgrowth of the small bowel; induce ketosis as a prevention for seizures
Usual Dosage Oral:
  Infants: Nutritional supplement: Initial: 0.5 mL every other feeding, then advance to every feeding, then increase in increments of 0.25-0.5 mL/feeding at intervals of 2-3 days as tolerated
  Children: Seizures: About 40 mL with each meal or 50% to 70% (800-1120 kcal) of total calories (1600 kcal) as the oil will induce ketosis necessary for seizure control
  Children and Adults: Cystic fibrosis: 3 tablespoons/day in divided doses
  Adults: Malabsorption syndromes: 15 mL 3-4 times/day
Dosage Forms
  Oil:
  MCT Oil® [OTC]: 14 g/15 mL

Medralone® Injection *(Discontinued)* *see* methylprednisolone *on page 559*

Medrol® **[US/Can]** *see* methylprednisolone *on page 559*

medroxyprogesterone (me DROKS ee proe JES te rone)

Sound-Alike/Look-Alike Issues

medroxyPROGESTERone may be confused with hydroxyprogesterone, methylPREDNISolone, methylTES-TOSTERone

Provera® may be confused with Covera®, Parlodel®, Premarin®

Synonyms acetoxymethylprogesterone; medroxyprogesterone acetate; methylacetoxyprogesterone

Tall-Man medroxy**PROGESTER**one

U.S./Canadian Brand Names Alti-MPA [Can]; Apo-Medroxy® [Can]; Depo-Prevera® [Can]; Depo-Provera® Contraceptive [US]; Depo-Provera® [US/Can]; depo-subQ provera 104™ [US]; Gen-Medroxy [Can]; Novo-Medrone [Can]; Provera-Pak [Can]; Provera® [US/Can]

Therapeutic Category Contraceptive, Progestin Only; Progestin

Use Endometrial carcinoma or renal carcinoma; secondary amenorrhea or abnormal uterine bleeding due to hormonal imbalance; reduction of endometrial hyperplasia in nonhysterectomized postmenopausal women receiving conjugated estrogens; prevention of pregnancy; management of endometriosis-associated pain

Usual Dosage

Adolescents and Adults:

Amenorrhea: Oral: 5-10 mg/day for 5-10 days

Abnormal uterine bleeding: Oral: 5-10 mg for 5-10 days starting on day 16 or 21 of cycle

Contraception:

Depo-Provera® Contraceptive: I.M.: 150 mg every 3 months

depo-subQ provera 104™: SubQ: 104 mg every 3 months (every 12-14 weeks)

Endometriosis: depo-subQ provera 104™: SubQ: 104 mg every 3 months (every 12-14 weeks)

Adults:

Endometrial or renal carcinoma (Depo-Provera®): I.M.: 400-1000 mg/week

Accompanying cyclic estrogen therapy, postmenopausal: Oral: 5-10 mg for 12-14 consecutive days each month, starting on day 1 or day 16 of the cycle; lower doses may be used if given with estrogen continuously throughout the cycle

Dosage Forms

Injection, suspension: 150 mg/mL (1 mL)

Depo-Provera®: 400 mg/mL (2.5 mL)

Depo-Provera® Contraceptive: 150 mg/mL (1 mL)

depo-subQ provera 104™: 104 mg/0.65 mL (0.65 mL)

Tablet: 2.5 mg, 5 mg, 10 mg

Provera®: 2.5 mg, 5 mg, 10 mg

medroxyprogesterone acetate *see* medroxyprogesterone *on this page*

medroxyprogesterone and estrogens (conjugated) *see* estrogens (conjugated/equine) and medroxyprogesterone *on page 318*

medrysone (ME dri sone)

Therapeutic Category Adrenal Corticosteroid

Use Treatment of allergic conjunctivitis, vernal conjunctivitis, episcleritis, ophthalmic epinephrine sensitivity reaction

Usual Dosage Ophthalmic: Children ≥3 years and Adults: Instill 1 drop in conjunctival sac 2-4 times/day up to every 4 hours; may use every 1-2 hours during first 1-2 days

Mefenamic-250 [Can] *see* mefenamic acid *on this page*

mefenamic acid (me fe NAM ik AS id)

Sound-Alike/Look-Alike Issues

Ponstel® may be confused with Pronestyl®

U.S./Canadian Brand Names Apo-Mefenamic® [Can]; Dom-Mefenamic Acid [Can]; Mefenamic-250 [Can]; Nu-Mefenamic [Can]; PMS-Mefenamic Acid [Can]; Ponstan® [Can]; Ponstel® [US]

Therapeutic Category Analgesic, Nonnarcotic; Nonsteroidal Antiinflammatory Drug (NSAID)

Use Short-term relief of mild to moderate pain including primary dysmenorrhea

Usual Dosage Oral: Children >14 years and Adults: 500 mg to start then 250 mg every 4 hours as needed; maximum therapy: 1 week

Dosage Forms

Capsule: 250 mg

Ponstel®: 250 mg

mefloquine (ME floe kwin)

Synonyms mefloquine hydrochloride
U.S./Canadian Brand Names Apo-Mefloquine® [Can]; Lariam® [US/Can]
Therapeutic Category Antimalarial Agent
Use Treatment of acute malarial infections and prevention of malaria
Usual Dosage Oral (dose expressed as mg of mefloquine hydrochloride):
Children ≥6 months and >5 kg:
Malaria treatment: 20-25 mg/kg in 2 divided doses, taken 6-8 hours apart (maximum: 1250 mg) Take with food and an ample amount of water. If clinical improvement is not seen within 48-72 hours, an alternative therapy should be used for retreatment.
Malaria prophylaxis: 5 mg/kg/once weekly (maximum dose: 250 mg) starting 1 week before, arrival in endemic area, continuing weekly during travel and for 4 weeks after leaving endemic area. Take with food and an ample amount of water.
Adults:
Malaria treatment (mild to moderate infection): 5 tablets (1250 mg) as a single dose. Take with food and at least 8 oz of water. If clinical improvement is not seen within 48-72 hours, an alternative therapy should be used for retreatment.
Malaria prophylaxis: 1 tablet (250 mg) weekly starting 1 week before, arrival in endemic area, continuing weekly during travel and for 4 weeks after leaving endemic area. Take with food and at least 8 oz of water.
Dosage Forms
Tablet: 250 mg
Lariam®: 250 mg

mefloquine hydrochloride *see* mefloquine *on this page*

Mefoxin® [US] *see* cefoxitin *on page 161*

Megace® [US/Can] *see* megestrol *on this page*

Megace® ES [US] *see* megestrol *on this page*

Megace® OS [Can] *see* megestrol *on this page*

Megadophilus® [US-OTC] *see* Lactobacillus *on page 488*

megestrol (me JES trole)

Sound-Alike/Look-Alike Issues
Megace® may be confused with Reglan®
Synonyms 5071-1DL(6); megestrol acetate; NSC-71423
U.S./Canadian Brand Names Apo-Megestrol® [Can]; Megace® ES [US]; Megace® OS [Can]; Megace® [US/Can]; Nu-Megestrol [Can]
Therapeutic Category Antineoplastic Agent; Progestin
Use Palliative treatment of breast and endometrial carcinoma; treatment of anorexia, cachexia, or unexplained significant weight loss in patients with AIDS
Usual Dosage Oral: Adults: **Note:** Megace® ES suspension is not equivalent to other formulations on a mg-per-mg basis:
Tablet: Female (refer to individual protocols):
Breast carcinoma: 40 mg 4 times/day
Endometrial carcinoma: 40-320 mg/day in divided doses; use for 2 months to determine efficacy; maximum doses used have been up to 800 mg/day
Suspension: Male/Female: HIV-related cachexia:
Megace®: Initial dose: 800 mg/day; daily doses of 400 and 800 mg/day were found to be clinically effective
Megace® ES: 625 mg/day
Dosage Forms
Suspension, oral: 40 mg/mL
Megace®: 40 mg/mL
Megace® ES: 125 mg/mL
Tablet: 20 mg, 40 mg

megestrol acetate *see* megestrol *on this page*

Melanex® [US] *see* hydroquinone *on page 437*

Melfiat® (Discontinued) *see* phendimetrazine *on page 671*

Mellaril® [Can] *see* thioridazine *on page 838*

Mellaril® (all products) (Discontinued) *see* thioridazine *on page 838*

Mellaril-S® (Discontinued) *see* thioridazine *on page 838*

meloxicam (mel OKS i kam)

U.S./Canadian Brand Names Apo-Meloxicam® [Can]; CO Meloxicam [Can]; Gen-Meloxicam [Can]; Mobicox® [Can]; Mobic® [US/Can]; Novo-Meloxicam [Can]; PMS-Meloxicam [Can]

Therapeutic Category Nonsteroidal Antiinflammatory Drug (NSAID)

Use Relief of signs and symptoms of osteoarthritis, rheumatoid arthritis, and juvenile rheumatoid arthritis (JRA)

Usual Dosage Oral:

Children ≥2 years: JRA: 0.125 mg/kg/day; maximum dose: 7.5 mg/day

Adults: Osteoarthritis, rheumatoid arthritis: Initial: 7.5 mg once daily; some patients may receive additional benefit from an increased dose of 15 mg once daily; maximum dose: 15 mg/day

Dosage Forms

Suspension: 7.5 mg/5 mL (100 mL)

Mobic®: 7.5 mg/5 mL

Tablet: 7.5 mg, 15 mg

Mobic®: 7.5 mg, 15 mg

Melpaque HP® [US] *see* hydroquinone *on page 437*

melphalan (MEL fa lan)

Sound-Alike/Look-Alike Issues

melphalan may be confused with Mephyton®, Myleran®

Alkeran® may be confused with Alferon®, Leukeran®

Synonyms L-PAM; L-sarcolysin; NSC-8806; phenylalanine mustard

U.S./Canadian Brand Names Alkeran® [US/Can]

Therapeutic Category Antineoplastic Agent

Use Palliative treatment of multiple myeloma and nonresectable epithelial ovarian carcinoma

Usual Dosage Adults: Refer to individual protocols.

Oral: Dose should always be adjusted to patient response and weekly blood counts:

Multiple myeloma (multiple regimens have been employed): **Note:** Response is gradual; may require repeated courses to realize benefit:

6 mg daily for 2-3 weeks initially, followed by up to 4 weeks rest, then a maintenance dose of 2 mg daily as hematologic recovery begins **or**

10 mg daily for 7-10 days; institute 2 mg daily maintenance dose after WBC >4000 cells/mcL and platelets >100,000 cells/mcL (~4-8 weeks); titrate maintenance dose to hematologic response **or**

0.15 mg/kg/day for 7 days, with a 2-6 week rest, followed by a maintenance dose of ≤0.05 mg/kg/day as hematologic recovery begins **or**

0.25 mg/kg/day for 4 days (or 0.2 mg/kg/day for 5 days); repeat at 4- to 6-week intervals as ANC and platelet counts return to normal

Ovarian carcinoma: 0.2 mg/kg/day for 5 days, repeat every 4-5 weeks.

I.V.: Multiple myeloma: 16 mg/m^2 administered at 2-week intervals for 4 doses, then administer at 4-week intervals after adequate hematologic recovery.

Dosage Forms

Injection, powder for reconstitution:

Alkeran®: 50 mg

Tablet:

Alkeran®: 2 mg

Melquin-3® [US] *see* hydroquinone *on page 437*

Melquin HP® [US] *see* hydroquinone *on page 437*

memantine (me MAN teen)

Synonyms memantine hydrochloride

U.S./Canadian Brand Names Ebixa® [Can]; Namenda™ [US]

Therapeutic Category N-Methyl-D-Aspartate Receptor Antagonist

Use Treatment of moderate-to-severe dementia of the Alzheimer type

Usual Dosage Oral: Adults:

Alzheimer disease: Initial: 5 mg/day; increase dose by 5 mg/day to a target dose of 20 mg/day; wait at least 1 week between dosage changes. Doses >5 mg/day should be given in 2 divided doses.

Suggested titration: 5 mg/day for ≥1 week; 5 mg twice daily for ≥1 week; 15 mg/day given in 5 mg and 10 mg separated doses for ≥1 week; then 10 mg twice daily

Dosage Forms

Solution, oral:

Namenda™: 2 mg/mL

(Continued)

memantine *(Continued)*

Tablet:
Namenda™: 5 mg, 10 mg
Combination package [titration pack contains two separate tablet formulations]:
Namenda™: Memantine 5 mg (28s), 10 mg (21s)

memantine hydrochloride *see* memantine *on previous page*

Menactra® [US] *see* meningococcal polysaccharide (Groups A / C / Y and W-135) diphtheria toxoid conjugate vaccine *on this page*

Menadol® *(Discontinued)* *see* ibuprofen *on page 444*

Menest® [US/Can] *see* estrogens (esterified) *on page 319*

Meni-D® *(Discontinued)* *see* meclizine *on page 535*

meningococcal polysaccharide (Groups A / C / Y and W-135) diphtheria toxoid conjugate vaccine

(me NIN joe kok al pol i SAK a ride groops aye, see, why & dubl yoo won thur tee fyve dif THEER ee a TOKS oyds KON joo gate vak SEEN)

Synonyms MCV4; quadrivalent meningococcal conjugate vaccine
U.S./Canadian Brand Names Menactra® [US]
Therapeutic Category Vaccine
Use Provide active immunization of adolescents and adults (11-55 years of age) against invasive meningococcal disease caused by *N. meningitidis* serogroups A, C, Y and W-135

The ACIP recommends routine vaccination of all persons 11-18 years of age at the earliest opportunity. Adolescents should be vaccinated at the 11-12 year visit. For adolescents not previously vaccinated, vaccine should be administered prior to high school entry (~15 years of age).

The ACIP also recommends routine vaccination for persons at increased risk for meningococcal disease. (MCV4 is preferred for persons aged 11-55 years; MPSV4 may be used if MCV4 is not available). Persons at increased risk include:
College freshmen living in dormitories
Microbiologists routinely exposed to isolates of *N. meningitides*
Military recruits
Persons traveling to or who reside in countries where *N. meningitides* is hyperendemic or epidemic, particularly if contact with local population will be prolonged
Persons with terminal complement component deficiencies
Persons with anatomic or functional asplenia
Use is also recommended during meningococcal outbreaks caused by vaccine preventable serogroups.

Usual Dosage I.M.: Adolescents 11-18 years and Adults ≤55 years: 0.5 mL
Note: Revaccination: May be indicated in patients previously vaccinated with MPSV4 who remain at increased risk for infection. The ACIP recommends the use of MCV4 for revaccination in patients 11-55 years, however use of MPSV4 is also acceptable. Consider revaccination after 3-5 years. The need for revaccination in patients previously vaccinated with MCV4 is currently under study.

Dosage Forms
Injection, solution:
Menactra®: 4 mcg each of polysaccharide antigen groups A, C, Y, and W-135 per 0.5 mL

meningococcal polysaccharide vaccine (groups A / C / Y and W-135)

(me NIN joe kok al pol i SAK a ride vak SEEN groops aye, see, why & dubl yoo won thur tee fyve)
Synonyms MPSV4
U.S./Canadian Brand Names Menomune®-A/C/Y/W-135 [US]
Therapeutic Category Vaccine, Live Bacteria
Use Provide active immunity to meningococcal serogroups contained in the vaccine

The ACIP recommends routine vaccination for persons at increased risk for meningococcal disease. (Use of MPSV4 is recommended in children 2-10 years and adults >55 years. MCV4 is preferred for persons aged 11-55 years; MPSV4 may be used if MCV4 is not available). Persons at increased risk include:
College freshmen living in dormitories
Microbiologists routinely exposed to isolates of *N. meningitides*
Military recruits
Persons traveling to or who reside in countries where *N. meningitides* is hyperendemic or epidemic, particularly if contact with local population will be prolonged
Persons with terminal complement component deficiencies
Persons with anatomic or functional asplenia
Use is also recommended during meningococcal outbreaks caused by vaccine preventable serogroups.

Usual Dosage SubQ:

Children <2 years: Not usually recommended. Two doses (0.5 mL/dose), 3 months apart, may be considered in children 3-18 months to elicit short-term protection against serogroup A disease. A single dose may be considered in children 19-23 months.

Children ≥2 years and Adults: 0.5 mL

Note: Revaccination: May be indicated in patients previously vaccinated with MPSV4 who remain at increased risk for infection. The ACIP recommends the use of MCV4 for revaccination in patients 11-55 years, however use of MPSV4 is also acceptable.

Children first vaccinated at <4 years: Revaccinate after 2-3 years.

Adults: Not determined, consider revaccination after 3-5 years.

Dosage Forms

Injection, powder for reconstitution:

Menomune®-A/C/Y/W-135: 50 mcg each of polysaccharide antigen groups A, C, Y, and W-135

Menomune®-A/C/Y/W-135 [US] *see* meningococcal polysaccharide vaccine (groups A / C / Y and W-135) *on previous page*

Menopur® [US] *see* menotropins *on this page*

Menostar™ [US/Can] *see* estradiol *on page 313*

menotropins (men oh TROE pins)

Sound-Alike/Look-Alike Issues

Repronex® may be confused with Regranex®

Synonyms hMG; human menopausal gonadotropin

U.S./Canadian Brand Names Menopur® [US]; Repronex® [US/Can]

Therapeutic Category Gonadotropin

Use Female:

In conjunction with hCG to induce ovulation and pregnancy in infertile females experiencing oligoanovulation or anovulation when the cause of anovulation is functional and not caused by primary ovarian failure (Repronex®)

Stimulation of multiple follicle development in ovulatory patients as part of an assisted reproductive technology (ART) (Menopur®, Repronex®)

Usual Dosage Adults:

Repronex®: I.M., SubQ:

Induction of ovulation in patients with oligoanovulation (Female): Initial: 150 int. units daily for the first 5 days of treatment. Adjustments should not be made more frequently than once every 2 days and should not exceed 75-150 int. units per adjustment. Maximum daily dose should not exceed 450 int. units and dosing beyond 12 days is not recommended. If patient's response is appropriate, hCG 5000-10,000 units should be given one day following the last dose of Repronex®. Hold dose if serum estradiol is >2000 pg/mL, if the ovaries are abnormally enlarged, or if abdominal pain occurs; the patient should also be advised to refrain from intercourse. May repeat process if follicular development is inadequate or if pregnancy does not occur.

Assisted reproductive technologies (Female): Initial (in patients who have received GnRH agonist or antagonist pituitary suppression): 225 int. units; adjustments in dose should not be made more frequently than once every 2 days and should not exceed more than 75-150 int. units per adjustment. The maximum daily doses of Repronex® given should not exceed 450 int. units and dosing beyond 12 days is not recommended. Once adequate follicular development is evident, hCG (5000-10,000 units) should be administered to induce final follicular maturation in preparation for oocyte retrieval. Withhold treatment when ovaries are abnormally enlarged on last day of therapy (to reduce chance of developing OHSS).

Menopur®: SubQ: *Assisted reproductive technologies (ART):* Initial (in patients who have received GnRH agonist for pituitary suppression): 225 int. units; adjustments in dose should not be made more frequently than once every 2 days and should not exceed more than 150 int. units per adjustment. The maximum daily dose given should not exceed 450 int. units and dosing beyond 20 days is not recommended. Once adequate follicular development is evident, hCG should be administered to induce final follicular maturation in preparation for oocyte retrieval. Withhold treatment when ovaries are abnormally enlarged on last day of therapy (to reduce chance of developing OHSS).

Dosage Forms

Injection, powder for reconstitution:

Menopur®, Repronex®: Follicle stimulating hormone activity 75 int. units and luteinizing hormone activity 75 int. units

Mentax® [US] *see* butenafine *on page 131*

292 MEP® [Can] *see* meprobamate and aspirin *on page 544*

mepenzolate (me PEN zoe late)
Sound-Alike/Look-Alike Issues
Cantil® may be confused with Bentyl®
Synonyms mepenzolate bromide
U.S./Canadian Brand Names Cantil® [Can]
Therapeutic Category Anticholinergic Agent
Use Adjunctive treatment of peptic ulcer disease
Usual Dosage Oral: Adults: 25-50 mg 4 times/day with meals and at bedtime

mepenzolate bromide *see* mepenzolate *on this page*

mepergan *see* meperidine and promethazine *on this page*

meperidine (me PER i deen)
Sound-Alike/Look-Alike Issues
meperidine may be confused with meprobamate
Demerol® may be confused with Demulen®, Desyrel®, dicumarol, Dilaudid®, Dymelor®, Pamelor®
Synonyms isonipecaine hydrochloride; meperidine hydrochloride; pethidine hydrochloride
U.S./Canadian Brand Names Demerol® [US/Can]; Meperitab® [US]
Therapeutic Category Analgesic, Narcotic
Controlled Substance C-II
Use Management of moderate-to-severe pain; adjunct to anesthesia and preoperative sedation
Usual Dosage Note: Doses should be titrated to necessary analgesic effect. When changing route of administration, note that oral doses are about half as effective as parenteral dose. Not recommended for chronic pain. These are guidelines and do not represent the maximum doses that may be required in all patients. In patients with normal renal function, doses of ≤600 mg/24 hours and use for ≤48 hours are recommended.

Children: Pain: Oral, I.M., I.V., SubQ: 1-1.5 mg/kg/dose every 3-4 hours as needed; 1-2 mg/kg as a single dose preoperative medication may be used; maximum 100 mg/dose (**Note:** Oral route is not recommended for acute pain.)
Adults: Pain:
Oral: Initial: Opiate-naive: 50 mg every 3-4 hours as needed; usual dosage range: 50-150 mg every 2-4 hours as needed (manufacturers recommendation; oral route is not recommended for acute pain)
I.M., SubQ: Initial: Opiate-naive: 50-75 mg every 3-4 hours as needed; patients with prior opiate exposure may require higher initial doses
Preoperatively: 50-100 mg given 30-90 minutes before the beginning of anesthesia
Slow I.V.: Initial: 5-10 mg every 5 minutes as needed
Patient-controlled analgesia (PCA): Usual concentration: 10 mg/mL
Initial dose: 10 mg
Demand dose: 1-5 mg (manufacturer recommendations); range 5-25 mg
Lockout interval: 5-10 minutes
Dosage Forms
Injection, solution [ampul]: 25 mg/0.5 mL (0.5 mL); 25 mg/mL (1 mL); 50 mg/mL (1 mL, 1.5 mL, 2 mL); 75 mg/mL (1 mL); 100 mg/mL (1 mL)
Injection, solution [prefilled syringe]: 25 mg/mL (1 mL); 50 mg/mL (1 mL); 75 mg/mL (1 mL); 100 mg/mL (1 mL)
Injection, solution [for PCA pump]: 10 mg/mL (30 mL, 50 mL, 60 mL)
Injection, solution [vial]: 25 mg/mL (1 mL); 50 mg/mL (1 mL, 30 mL); 75 mg/mL (1 mL); 100 mg/mL (1 mL, 20 mL)
Solution, oral: 50 mg/5 mL (500 mL)
Syrup: 50 mg/5 mL
Demerol®: 50 mg/5 mL
Tablet: 50 mg, 100 mg
Demerol®, Meperitab®: 50 mg, 100 mg

meperidine and promethazine (me PER i deen & proe METH a zeen)
Sound-Alike/Look-Alike Issues
mepergan may be confused with meprobamate
Synonyms mepergan; promethazine and meperidine
Therapeutic Category Analgesic, Narcotic
Controlled Substance C-II
Use Management of moderate pain
Usual Dosage Oral: Adults: One (1) capsule every 4-6 hours as needed
Dosage Forms
Capsule: Meperidine 50 mg and promethazine 25 mg

meperidine hydrochloride *see* meperidine *on previous page*

Meperitab® **[US]** *see* meperidine *on previous page*

mephobarbital (me foe BAR bi tal)
Sound-Alike/Look-Alike Issues
mephobarbital may be confused with methocarbamol
Mebaral® may be confused with Medrol®, Mellaril®, Tegretol®
Synonyms methylphenobarbital
U.S./Canadian Brand Names Mebaral® [US/Can]
Therapeutic Category Barbiturate
Controlled Substance C-IV
Use Sedative; treatment of grand mal and petit mal epilepsy
Usual Dosage Oral:
Epilepsy:
Children: 6-12 mg/kg/day in 2-4 divided doses
Adults: 200-600 mg/day in 2-4 divided doses
Sedation:
Children:
<5 years: 16-32 mg 3-4 times/day
>5 years: 32-64 mg 3-4 times/day
Adults: 32-100 mg 3-4 times/day
Dosage Forms
Tablet:
Mebaral®: 32 mg, 50 mg, 100 mg

Mephyton® **[US/Can]** *see* phytonadione *on page 681*

mepivacaine (me PIV a kane)
Sound-Alike/Look-Alike Issues
mepivacaine may be confused with bupivacaine
Polocaine® may be confused with prilocaine
Synonyms mepivacaine hydrochloride
U.S./Canadian Brand Names Carbocaine® [US/Can]; Polocaine® Dental [US]; Polocaine® MPF [US]; Polocaine® [US/Can]
Therapeutic Category Local Anesthetic
Use Local or regional analgesia; anesthesia by local infiltration, peripheral and central neural techniques including epidural and caudal blocks; **not** for use in spinal anesthesia
Usual Dosage
Injectable local anesthetic: Dose varies with procedure, degree of anesthesia needed, vascularity of tissue, duration of anesthesia required, and physical condition of patient. The smallest dose and concentration required to produce the desired effect should be used.
Children: Maximum dose: 5-6 mg/kg; only concentrations <2% should be used in children <3 years or <14 kg (30 lbs)
Adults: Maximum dose: 400 mg; do not exceed 1000 mg/24 hours
Cervical, brachial, intercostal, pudendal nerve block: 5-40 mL of a 1% solution (maximum: 400 mg) **or** 5-20 mL of a 2% solution (maximum: 400 mg). For pudendal block, inject ¹/₂ the total dose each side.
Transvaginal block (paracervical plus pudendal): Up to 30 mL (both sides) of a 1% solution (maximum: 300 mg). Inject ¹/₂ the total dose each side.
Paracervical block: Up to 20 mL (both sides) of a 1% solution (maximum: 200 mg). Inject ¹/₂ the total dose to each side. This is the maximum recommended dose per 90-minute procedure; inject slowly with 5 minutes between sides.
Caudal and epidural block (preservative free solutions only): 15-30 mL of a 1% solution (maximum: 300 mg) **or** 10-25 mL of a 1.5% solution (maximum: 375 mg) **or** 10-20 mL of a 2% solution (maximum: 400 mg)
Infiltration: Up to 40 mL of a 1% solution (maximum: 400 mg)
Therapeutic block (pain management): 1-5 mL of a 1% solution (maximum: 50 mg) **or** 1-5 mL of a 2% solution (maximum: 100 mg)
Dental anesthesia: Adults:
Single site in upper or lower jaw: 54 mg (1.8 mL) as a 3% solution
Infiltration and nerve block of entire oral cavity: 270 mg (9 mL) as a 3% solution. Manufacturer's maximum recommended dose is not more than 400 mg to normal healthy adults.
Dosage Forms
Injection, solution:
Carbocaine®: 1% (50 mL); 2% (50 mL)
Polocaine®: 1% (50 mL); 2% (50 mL)
(Continued)

mepivacaine *(Continued)*

Injection, solution [preservative free]:
Carbocaine®: 1% (30 mL); 1.5% (30 mL); 2% (20 mL); 3% (1.8 mL)
Polocaine® Dental: 3% (1.8 mL)
Polocaine® MPF: 1% (30 mL); 1.5% (30 mL); 2% (20 mL)

mepivacaine and levonordefrin (me PIV a kane & lee voe nor DEF rin)

Synonyms levonordefrin and mepivacaine hydrochloride
U.S./Canadian Brand Names Carbocaine® 2% with Neo-Cobefrin® [US]; Polocaine® 2% and Levonordefrin 1:20,000 [Can]
Therapeutic Category Local Anesthetic
Usual Dosage
Children <10 years: Maximum pediatric dosage must be carefully calculated on the basis of patient's weight but should not exceed 6.6 mg/kg of body weight or 180 mg of mepivacaine hydrochloride as a 2% solution with levonordefrin 1:20,000

Children >10 years and Adults:
Dental infiltration and nerve block, single site: 36 mg (1.8 mL) of mepivacaine hydrochloride as a 2% solution with levonordefrin 1:20,000
Entire oral cavity: 180 mg (9 mL) of mepivacaine hydrochloride as a 2% solution with levonordefrin 1:20,000; up to a maximum of 6.6 mg/kg of body weight but not to exceed 400 mg of mepivacaine hydrochloride per appointment. The effective anesthetic dose varies with procedure, intensity of anesthesia needed, duration of anesthesia required, and physical condition of the patient. Always use the lowest effective dose along with careful aspiration.
Dosage Forms
Injection, solution:
Carbocaine® 2% with Neo-Cobefrin®: Mepivacaine 2% and levonordefrin 1:20,000 (1.8 mL)

mepivacaine hydrochloride *see mepivacaine on previous page*

meprobamate (me proe BA mate)

Sound-Alike/Look-Alike Issues
meprobamate may be confused with Mepergan, meperidine
U.S./Canadian Brand Names Novo-Mepro [Can]
Therapeutic Category Antianxiety Agent, Miscellaneous
Controlled Substance C-IV
Use Management of anxiety disorders
Usual Dosage Oral:
Children 6-12 years: Anxiety: 100-200 mg 2-3 times/day
Adults: Anxiety: 400 mg 3-4 times/day, up to 2400 mg/day
Dosage Forms
Tablet: 200 mg, 400 mg

meprobamate and aspirin (me proe BA mate & AS pir in)

Synonyms aspirin and meprobamate
U.S./Canadian Brand Names 292 MEP® [Can]; Equagesic® [US]
Therapeutic Category Skeletal Muscle Relaxant
Controlled Substance C-IV
Use Adjunct to the short-term treatment of pain in patients with skeletal-muscular disease exhibiting tension and/or anxiety
Usual Dosage Oral: Children ≥12 years and Adults: 1-2 tablets 3-4 times/day for up to 10 days
Dosage Forms
Tablet:
Equagesic®: Meprobamate 200 mg and aspirin 325 mg

Mepron® [US/Can] *see atovaquone on page 82*

mequinol and tretinoin (ME kwi nole & TRET i noyn)

Synonyms tretinoin and mequinol
U.S./Canadian Brand Names Solagé™ [US/Can]
Therapeutic Category Retinoic Acid Derivative; Vitamin A Derivative; Vitamin, Topical
Use Treatment of solar lentigines; the efficacy of using Solagé™ daily for >24 weeks has not been established. The local cutaneous safety of Solagé™ in non-Caucasians has not been adequately established.

Usual Dosage Solar lentigines: Topical: Apply twice daily to solar lentigines using the applicator tip while avoiding application to the surrounding skin. Separate application by at least 8 hours or as directed by physician.

Dosage Forms

Liquid, topical:

Solagé™: Mequinol 2% and tretinoin 0.01% (30 mL)

mercaptopurine (mer kap toe PYOOR een)

Sound-Alike/Look-Alike Issues

Purinethol® may be confused with propylthiouracil

Synonyms 6-mercaptopurine; 6-MP; NSC-755

U.S./Canadian Brand Names Purinethol® [US/Can]

Therapeutic Category Antineoplastic Agent

Use Treatment (maintenance and induction) of acute lymphoblastic leukemia (ALL)

Usual Dosage Oral (refer to individual protocols):

Children: ALL:

Induction: 2.5-5 mg/kg/day **or** 70-100 mg/m^2/day given once daily

Maintenance: 1.5-2.5 mg/kg/day **or** 50-75 mg/m^2/day given once daily

Adults:

ALL:

Induction: 2.5-5 mg/kg/day (100-200 mg)

Maintenance: 1.5-2.5 mg/kg/day **or** 80-100 mg/m^2/day given once daily

Dosage adjustment with concurrent allopurinol: Reduce mercaptopurine dosage to $1/4$ to $1/3$ the usual dose.

Dosage adjustment in TPMT-deficiency: Not established; substantial reductions are generally required only in homozygous deficiency.

Dosage Forms

Tablet [scored]: 50 mg

Purinethol®: 50 mg

6-mercaptopurine see mercaptopurine on this page

mercapturic acid see acetylcysteine on page 15

Meridia® [US/Can] see sibutramine on page 784

meropenem (mer oh PEN em)

U.S./Canadian Brand Names Merrem® I.V. [US]; Merrem® [Can]

Therapeutic Category Carbapenem (Antibiotic)

Use Treatment of intraabdominal infections (complicated appendicitis and peritonitis); treatment of bacterial meningitis in pediatric patients ≥3 months of age caused by *S. pneumoniae*, *H. influenzae*, and *N. meningitidis*; treatment of complicated skin and skin structure infections caused by susceptible organisms

Usual Dosage

Usual dosage ranges:

Neonates: I.V.:

Postnatal age 0-7 days: 20 mg/kg/dose every 12 hours

Postnatal age >7 days:

Weight 1200-2000 g: 20 mg/kg/dose every 12 hours

Weight >2000 g: 20 mg/kg/dose every 8 hours

Children ≥3 months: I.V.: 60 mg/kg/day divided every 8 hours (maximum dose: 6 g/day)

Adults: I.V.: 1.5-6 g/day divided every 8 hours

Indication-specific dosing:

Children ≥3 months (<50 kg): I.V.:

Intraabdominal infections: 20 mg/kg every 8 hours (maximum dose: 1 g every 8 hours)

Meningitis: 40 mg/kg every 8 hours (maximum dose: 2 g every 8 hours)

Skin and skin structure infections (complicated): 10 mg/kg every 8 hours (maximum dose: 500 mg every 8 hours)

Children >50 kg and Adults: I.V.:

Cholangitis, intraabdominal infections, febrile neutropenia: 1 g every 8 hours

Skin and skin structure infections (complicated): 500 mg every 8 hours; diabetic foot: 1 g every 8 hours

Dosage Forms

Injection, powder for reconstitution:

Merrem® I.V.: 500 mg, 1 g

Merrem® [Can] see meropenem on this page

Merrem® I.V. [US] see meropenem on this page

Mersyndol® With Codeine [Can] *see* acetaminophen, codeine, and doxylamine *(Canada only) on page 11*

Meruvax® II [US] *see* rubella virus vaccine (live) *on page 770*

mesalamine (me SAL a meen)
Sound-Alike/Look-Alike Issues
mesalamine may be confused with mecamylamine
Asacol® may be confused with Ansaid®, Os-Cal®
Lialda™ may be confused with Aldara™
Synonyms 5-aminosalicylic acid; 5-ASA; fisalamine; mesalazine
U.S./Canadian Brand Names Asacol® 800 [Can]; Asacol® [US/Can]; Canasa™ [US]; Lialda™ [US]; Mesasal® [Can]; Novo-5 ASA [Can]; Pendo-5 ASA [Can]; Pentasa® [US/Can]; Quintasa® [Can]; Rowasa® [US/Can]; Salofalk® [Can]
Therapeutic Category 5-Aminosalicylic Acid Derivative
Use
Oral: Treatment and maintenance of remission of mildly to moderately active ulcerative colitis
Rectal: Treatment of active mild to moderate distal ulcerative colitis, proctosigmoiditis, or proctitis
Usual Dosage Adults (usual course of therapy is 3-8 weeks):
Oral:
Treatment of ulcerative colitis:
Capsule: 1 g 4 times/day
Tablet: Initial:
Asacol®: 800 mg 3 times/day for 6 weeks
Lialda™ (once-daily formulation): 2.4"4.8 g/day for up to 8 weeks (treatment only)
Maintenance of remission of ulcerative colitis:
Capsule: 1 g 4 times/day
Tablet (Asacol®): 1.6 g/day in divided doses
Rectal:
Retention enema: 60 mL (4 g) at bedtime, retained overnight, approximately 8 hours
Rectal suppository (Canasa™):
500 mg: Insert 1 suppository in rectum twice daily; may increase to 3 times/day if inadequate response is seen after 2 weeks
1000 mg: Insert 1 suppository in rectum daily at bedtime
Note: Suppositories should be retained for at least 1-3 hours to achieve maximum benefit.
Note: Some patients may require rectal and oral therapy concurrently.
Dosage Forms
Capsule, controlled release:
Pentasa®: 250 mg, 500 mg
Suppository, rectal:
Canasa®: 1000 mg
Suspension, rectal: 4 g/60 mL (7s, 28s)
Rowasa®: 4 g/60 mL (7s, 28s)
Tablet, delayed release [enteric coated]:
Asacol®: 400 mg
Lialda™: 1.2 g

mesalazine *see* mesalamine *on this page*

Mesasal® [Can] *see* mesalamine *on this page*

M-Eslon® [Can] *see* morphine sulfate *on page 578*

mesna (MES na)
Synonyms sodium 2-mercaptoethane sulfonate
U.S./Canadian Brand Names Mesnex® [US/Can]; Uromitexan [Can]
Therapeutic Category Antidote
Use Orphan drug: Prevention of hemorrhagic cystitis induced by ifosfamide
Usual Dosage Children and Adults (refer to individual protocols):
I.V.: Recommended dose is 60% of the ifosfamide dose given in 3 divided doses (0, 4, and 8 hours after the start of ifosfamide)
Alternative I.V. regimens include 80% of the ifosfamide dose given in 4 divided doses (0, 3, 6, and 9 hours after the start of ifosfamide) and continuous infusions
I.V./Oral: Recommended dose is 100% of the ifosfamide dose, given as 20% of the ifosfamide dose I.V. at hour 0, followed by 40% of the ifosfamide dose given orally 2 and 6 hours after start of ifosfamide
Dosage Forms
Injection, solution: 100 mg/mL (10 mL)

Mesnex®: 100 mg/mL (10 mL)
Tablet: 400 mg
Mesnex®: 400 mg

Mesnex® [US/Can] *see* mesna *on previous page*

Mestinon® [US/Can] *see* pyridostigmine *on page 735*

Mestinon® Injection *(Discontinued)* *see* pyridostigmine *on page 735*

Mestinon®-SR [Can] *see* pyridostigmine *on page 735*

Mestinon® Timespan® [US] *see* pyridostigmine *on page 735*

mestranol and norethindrone (MES tra nole & nor eth IN drone)

Sound-Alike/Look-Alike Issues
Norinyl® may be confused with Nardil®
Synonyms norethindrone and mestranol
U.S./Canadian Brand Names Necon® 1/50 [US]; Norinyl® 1+50 [US]; Ortho-Novum® 1/50 [US/Can]
Therapeutic Category Contraceptive, Oral
Use Prevention of pregnancy
Usual Dosage Oral: Adults: Female: Contraception:
Schedule 1 (Sunday starter): Dose begins on first Sunday after onset of menstruation; if the menstrual period starts on Sunday, take first tablet that very same day. **With a Sunday start, an additional method of contraception should be used until after the first 7 days of consecutive administration.**
For 21-tablet package: Dosage is 1 tablet daily for 21 consecutive days, followed by 7 days off of the medication; a new course begins on the 8th day after the last tablet is taken.
For 28-tablet package: Dosage is 1 tablet daily without interruption.
Schedule 2 (Day 1 starter): Dose starts on first day of menstrual cycle taking 1 tablet daily.
For 21-tablet package: Dosage is 1 tablet daily for 21 consecutive days, followed by 7 days off of the medication; a new course begins on the 8th day after the last tablet is taken.
For 28-tablet package: Dosage is 1 tablet daily without interruption.
If all doses have been taken on schedule and one menstrual period is missed, continue dosing cycle. If two consecutive menstrual periods are missed, pregnancy test is required before new dosing cycle is started.
Missed doses **monophasic formulations** (refer to package insert for complete information):
One dose missed: Take as soon as remembered or take 2 tablets next day
Two consecutive doses missed in the first 2 weeks: Take 2 tablets as soon as remembered or 2 tablets next 2 days. **An additional method of contraception should be used for 7 days after missed dose.**
Two consecutive doses missed in week 3 or three consecutive doses missed at any time: **An additional method of contraception must be used for 7 days after a missed dose:**
Schedule 1 (Sunday starter): Continue dose of 1 tablet daily until Sunday, then discard the rest of the pack, and a new pack should be started that same day.
Schedule 2 (Day 1 starter): Current pack should be discarded, and a new pack should be started that same day.
Dosage Forms
Tablet, monophasic formulations:
Necon® 1/50: Norethindrone 1 mg and mestranol 0.05 mg [21 light blue tablets and 7 white inactive tablets] (28s)
Norinyl® 1+50: Norethindrone 1 mg and mestranol 0.05 mg [21 white tablets and 7 orange inactive tablets] (28s)
Ortho-Novum® 1/50: Norethindrone 1 mg and mestranol 0.05 mg [21 yellow tablets and 7 green inactive tablets] (28s)

metacortandralone *see* prednisolone (systemic) *on page 710*

Metadate® CD [US] *see* methylphenidate *on page 558*

Metadate® ER [US] *see* methylphenidate *on page 558*

Metadol™ [Can] *see* methadone *on page 550*

Metaglip™ [US] *see* glipizide and metformin *on page 394*

Metamucil® [US-OTC/Can] *see* psyllium *on page 732*

Metamucil® Plus Calcium [US-OTC] *see* psyllium *on page 732*

Metamucil® Smooth Texture [US-OTC] *see* psyllium *on page 732*

Metanx™ [US] *see* vitamin B complex combinations *on page 894*

metaproterenol (met a proe TER e nol)

Sound-Alike/Look-Alike Issues
metaproterenol may be confused with metipranolol, metoprolol
Alupent® may be confused with Atrovent®

Synonyms metaproterenol sulfate; orciprenaline sulfate

U.S./Canadian Brand Names Alupent® [US]; Apo-Orciprenaline® [Can]; Ratio-Orciprenaline® [Can]; Tanta-Orciprenaline® [Can]

Therapeutic Category Adrenergic Agonist Agent

Use Bronchodilator in reversible airway obstruction due to asthma or COPD; because of its delayed onset of action (1 hour) and prolonged effect (4 or more hours), this may not be the drug of choice for assessing response to a bronchodilator

Usual Dosage
Oral:
Children:
<2 years: 0.4 mg/kg/dose given 3-4 times/day; in infants, the dose can be given every 8-12 hours
2-6 years: 1-2.6 mg/kg/day divided every 6 hours
6-9 years: 10 mg/dose 3-4 times/day
Children >9 years and Adults: 20 mg 3-4 times/day
Inhalation: Children >12 years and Adults: 2-3 inhalations every 3-4 hours, up to 12 inhalations in 24 hours
Nebulizer:
Infants and Children: 0.01-0.02 mL/kg of 5% solution; minimum dose: 0.1 mL; maximum dose: 0.3 mL diluted in 2-3 mL normal saline every 4-6 hours (may be given more frequently according to need)
Adolescents and Adults: 5-20 breaths of full strength 5% metaproterenol **or** 0.2 to 0.3 mL 5% metaproterenol in 2.5-3 mL normal saline until nebulized every 4-6 hours (can be given more frequently according to need)

Dosage Forms
Aerosol for oral inhalation:
Alupent®: 0.65 mg/inhalation (14 g)
Solution for nebulization [preservative free]: 0.4% [4 mg/mL] (2.5 mL); 0.6% [6 mg/mL] (2.5 mL)
Syrup: 10 mg/5 mL
Tablet: 10 mg, 20 mg

metaproterenol sulfate see metaproterenol on this page

Metasep® *(Discontinued)*

Metastron® [US/Can] see strontium-89 on page 807

metaxalone (me TAKS a lone)

Sound-Alike/Look-Alike Issues
metaxalone may be confused with metolazone

U.S./Canadian Brand Names Skelaxin® [US/Can]

Therapeutic Category Skeletal Muscle Relaxant

Use Relief of discomfort associated with acute, painful musculoskeletal conditions

Usual Dosage Oral: Children >12 years and Adults: 800 mg 3-4 times/day

Dosage Forms
Tablet:
Skelaxin®: 800 mg

metformin (met FOR min)

Sound-Alike/Look-Alike Issues
metformin may be confused with metronidazole
Glucophage® may be confused with Glucotrol®, Glutofac®

Synonyms metformin hydrochloride

U.S./Canadian Brand Names Alti-Metformin [Can]; Apo-Metformin® [Can]; BCI-Metformin [Can]; Fortamet® [US]; Gen-Metformin [Can]; Glucophage® XR [US]; Glucophage® [US/Can]; Glumetza™ [US/Can]; Glycon [Can]; Novo-Metformin [Can]; Nu-Metformin [Can]; PMS-Metformin [Can]; RAN™-Metformin [Can]; ratio-Metformin [Can]; Rho®-Metformin [Can]; Riomet™ [US]; Sandoz-Metformin FC [Can]

Therapeutic Category Antidiabetic Agent, Oral

Use Management of type 2 diabetes mellitus (noninsulin-dependent, NIDDM) as monotherapy when hyperglycemia cannot be managed on diet alone. May be used concomitantly with a sulfonylurea or insulin to improve glycemic control.

Usual Dosage Type 2 diabetes management: **Note:** Allow 1-2 weeks between dose titrations: Generally, clinically significant responses are not seen at doses <1500 mg daily; however, a lower recommended starting dose and gradual increased dosage is recommended to minimize gastrointestinal symptoms.

Immediate release tablet or solution: Oral:

Children 10-16 years: Initial: 500 mg twice daily (given with the morning and evening meals); increases in daily dosage should be made in increments of 500 mg at weekly intervals, given in divided doses, up to a maximum of 2000 mg/day

Adults ≥17 years: Initial: 500 mg twice daily (give with the morning and evening meals) **or** 850 mg once daily; increase dosage incrementally.

Incremental dosing recommendations based on dosage form:

500 mg tablet: One tablet/day at weekly intervals

850 mg tablet: One tablet/day every other week

Oral solution: 500 mg twice daily every other week

Doses of up to 2000 mg/day may be given twice daily. If a dose >2000 mg/day is required, it may be better tolerated in three divided doses. Maximum recommended dose 2550 mg/day.

Extended release tablet: Oral: **Note:** If glycemic control is not achieved at maximum dose, may divide dose and administer twice daily.

Children ≥17 years and Adults:

Fortamet®: Initial: 1000 mg once daily; dosage may be increased by 500 mg weekly; maximum dose: 2500 mg once daily

Glucophage® XR: Initial: 500 mg once daily (with the evening meal); dosage may be increased by 500 mg weekly; maximum dose: 2000 mg once daily

Adults: Glumetza™: Initial: 1000 mg once daily; dosage may be increased by 500 mg weekly; maximum dose: 2000 mg once daily

Transfer from other antidiabetic agents: No transition period is generally necessary except when transferring from chlorpropamide. When transferring from chlorpropamide, care should be exercised during the first 2 weeks because of the prolonged retention of chlorpropamide in the body, leading to overlapping drug effects and possible hypoglycemia.

Concomitant metformin and oral sulfonylurea therapy: If patients have not responded to 4 weeks of the maximum dose of metformin monotherapy, consider a gradual addition of an oral sulfonylurea, even if prior primary or secondary failure to a sulfonylurea has occurred. Continue metformin at the maximum dose.

Failed sulfonylurea therapy: Patients with prior failure on glyburide may be treated by gradual addition of metformin. Initiate with glyburide 20 mg and metformin 500 mg daily. Metformin dosage may be increased by 500 mg/day at weekly intervals, up to a maximum metformin dose (dosage of glyburide maintained at 20 mg/day).

Concomitant metformin and insulin therapy: Initial: 500 mg metformin once daily, continue current insulin dose; increase by 500 mg metformin weekly until adequate glycemic control is achieved

Maximum daily dose: Immediate release and solution: 2550 mg metformin; Extended release: 2000-2500 mg (varies by product)

Decrease insulin dose 10% to 25% when FPG <120 mg/dL; monitor and make further adjustments as needed

Dosage Forms

Solution, oral:

Riomet™: 100 mg/mL

Tablet: 500 mg, 850 mg, 1000 mg

Glucophage®: 500 mg, 850 mg, 1000 mg

Tablet, extended release: 500 mg, 750 mg

Fortamet®: 500 mg, 1000 mg

Glucophage® XR: 500 mg, 750 mg

Glumetza™: 500 mg

metformin and glipizide *see* glipizide and metformin *on page 394*

metformin and glyburide *see* glyburide and metformin *on page 396*

metformin and rosiglitazone *see* rosiglitazone and metformin *on page 767*

metformin and sitagliptin *see* sitagliptin and metformin *on page 789*

metformin hydrochloride *see* metformin *on previous page*

metformin hydrochloride and pioglitazone hydrochloride *see* pioglitazone and metformin *on page 685*

metformin hydrochloride and rosiglitazone maleate *see* rosiglitazone and metformin *on page 767*

methacholine (meth a KOLE leen)

Synonyms methacholine chloride

U.S./Canadian Brand Names Methacholine Omega [Can]; Provocholine® [US/Can]

Therapeutic Category Diagnostic Agent

Use Diagnosis of bronchial airway hyperactivity

(Continued)

methacholine (Continued)

Usual Dosage Before inhalation challenge, perform baseline pulmonary function tests; the patient must have an FEV_1 of at least 70% of the predicted value. The following is a suggested schedule for administration of methacholine challenge. Calculate cumulative units by multiplying number of breaths by concentration given. Total cumulative units is the sum of cumulative units for each concentration given. See table.

Methacholine

Vial	Serial Concentration (mg/mL)	No. of Breaths	Cumulative Units per Concentration	Total Cumulative Units
E	0.025	5	0.125	0.125
D	0.25	5	1.25	1.375
C	2.5	5	12.5	13.88
B	10	5	50	63.88
A	25	5	125	188.88

Dosage Forms
Powder for oral inhalation:
Provocholine®: 100 mg

methacholine chloride see methacholine on previous page

Methacholine Omega [Can] see methacholine on previous page

methadone (METH a done)

Sound-Alike/Look-Alike Issues
methadone may be confused with Mephyton®, methylphenidate, Metadate®, and Metadate® ER
Synonyms methadone hydrochloride
U.S./Canadian Brand Names Dolophine® [US]; Metadol™ [Can]; Methadone Diskets® [US]; Methadone Intensol™ [US]; Methadose® [US]
Therapeutic Category Analgesic, Narcotic
Controlled Substance C-II
Use Management of moderate-to-severe pain; detoxification and maintenance treatment of opioid addiction (if used for detoxification and maintenance treatment of narcotic addiction, it must be part of an FDA-approved program)
Usual Dosage Note: These are guidelines and do not represent the maximum doses that may be required in all patients. Methadone accumulates with repeated doses and dosage may need reduction after 3-5 days to prevent CNS depressant effects. Some patients may benefit from every 8-12 hour dosing interval for chronic pain management. Doses should be titrated to appropriate effects.
Adults:
Acute pain (moderate-to-severe):
Oral: Opioid-naive: Initial: 2.5-10 mg every 8-12 hours; more frequent administration may be required during initiation to maintain adequate analgesia. Dosage interval may range from 4-12 hours, since duration of analgesia is relatively short during the first days of therapy, but increases substantially with continued administration.
Chronic pain (opioid-tolerant): **Conversion from oral morphine to oral methadone:**
Daily oral morphine dose <100 mg: Estimated daily oral methadone dose: 20% to 30% of total daily morphine dose
Daily oral morphine dose 100-300 mg: Estimated daily oral methadone dose: 10% to 20% of total daily morphine dose
Daily oral morphine dose 300-600 mg: Estimated daily oral methadone dose: 8% to 12% of total daily morphine dose
Daily oral morphine dose 600-1000 mg: Estimated daily oral methadone dose: 5% to 10% of total daily morphine dose.
Daily oral morphine dose >1000 mg: Estimated daily oral methadone dose: <5% of total daily morphine dose.
Note: The total daily methadone dose should then be divided to reflect the intended dosing schedule.
I.V.: Manufacturers labeling: Initial: 2.5-10 mg every 8-12 hours in opioid-naive patients; titrate slowly to effect; may also be administered by SubQ or I.M. injection
Conversion from oral methadone to parenteral methadone dose: Initial dose: Parenteral:Oral ratio: 1:2 (eg, 5 mg parenteral methadone equals 10 mg oral methadone)
Detoxification: Oral:
Initial: A single dose of 20-30 mg is generally sufficient to suppress symptoms. Should not exceed 30 mg; lower doses should be considered in patients with low tolerance at initiation (eg, absence of opioids ≥5 days); an additional 5-10 mg of methadone may be provided if withdrawal symptoms have not been suppressed or if symptoms reappear after 2-4 hours; total daily dose on the first day should not exceed 40 mg,

unless the program physician documents in the patient's record that 40 mg did not control opiate abstinence symptoms.

Maintenance: Titrate to a dosage which attenuates craving, blocks euphoric effects of other opiates, and tolerance to sedative effect of methadone. Usual range: 80-120 mg/day (titration should occur cautiously)

Withdrawal: Dose reductions should be <10% of the maintenance dose, every 10-14 days

Detoxification (short-term): Oral:

Initial: Titrate to ~40 mg/day in divided doses to achieve stabilization, may continue 40 mg dose for 2-3 days

Maintenance: Titrate to a dosage which prevents/attenuates euphoric effects of self-administered opioids, reduces drug craving, and withdrawal symptoms are prevented for 24 hours.

Withdrawal: Requires individualization. Decrease daily or every other day, keeping withdrawal symptoms tolerable; hospitalized patients may tolerate a 20% reduction/day; ambulatory patients may require a slower reduction

Dosage Forms
Injection, solution: 10 mg/mL (20 mL)
Solution, oral: 5 mg/5 mL, 10 mg/5 mL
Solution, oral, as hydrochloride [concentrate]: 10 mg/mL
Methadone Intensol™, Methadose®: 10 mg/mL
Tablet: 5 mg, 10 mg
Dolophine®: 5 mg, 10 mg
Methadose®: 5 mg, 10 mg [DSC]
Tablet, dispersible: 40 mg
Methadose®, Methadone Diskets®: 40 mg

Methadone Diskets® [US] *see* methadone *on previous page*

methadone hydrochloride *see* methadone *on previous page*

Methadone Intensol™ [US] *see* methadone *on previous page*

Methadose® [US] *see* methadone *on previous page*

methaminodiazepoxide hydrochloride *see* chlordiazepoxide *on page 173*

methamphetamine (meth am FET a meen)
Sound-Alike/Look-Alike Issues
Desoxyn® may be confused with digoxin
Synonyms desoxyephedrine hydrochloride; methamphetamine hydrochloride
U.S./Canadian Brand Names Desoxyn® [US/Can]
Therapeutic Category Amphetamine
Controlled Substance C-II
Use Treatment of attention-deficit/hyperactivity disorder (ADHD); exogenous obesity (short-term adjunct)
Usual Dosage Oral:
Children ≥6 years and Adults: ADHD: 5 mg 1-2 times/day; may increase by 5 mg increments at weekly intervals until optimum response is achieved, usually 20-25 mg/day
Children ≥12 years and Adults: Exogenous obesity: 5 mg 30 minutes before each meal; treatment duration should not exceed a few weeks
Dosage Forms
Tablet: 5 mg
Desoxyn®: 5 mg

methamphetamine hydrochloride *see* methamphetamine *on this page*

methazolamide (meth a ZOE la mide)
Sound-Alike/Look-Alike Issues
methazolamide may be confused with methenamine, metolazone
Neptazane® may be confused with Nesacaine®
U.S./Canadian Brand Names Apo-Methazolamide® [Can]
Therapeutic Category Carbonic Anhydrase Inhibitor
Use Adjunctive treatment of open-angle or secondary glaucoma; short-term therapy of narrow-angle glaucoma when delay of surgery is desired
Usual Dosage Oral: Adults: 50-100 mg 2-3 times/day
Dosage Forms
Tablet: 25 mg, 50 mg

methenamine (meth EN a meen)
Sound-Alike/Look-Alike Issues
methenamine may be confused with methazolamide, methionine
(Continued)

methenamine *(Continued)*

Urex® may be confused with Eurax®, Serax®

Synonyms hexamethylenetetramine; methenamine hippurate; methenamine mandelate

U.S./Canadian Brand Names Dehydral® [Can]; Hiprex® [US/Can]; Mandelamine® [US/Can]; Urasal® [Can]; Urex® [US/Can]

Therapeutic Category Antibiotic, Miscellaneous

Use Prophylaxis or suppression of recurrent urinary tract infections; urinary tract discomfort secondary to hypermotility

Usual Dosage Oral:

Children:

>2-6 years: *Mandelate:* 50-75 mg/kg/day in 3-4 doses or 0.25 g/30 lb 4 times/day

6-12 years:

Hippurate: 0.5-1 g twice daily

Mandelate: 50-75 mg/kg/day in 3-4 doses or 0.5 g 4 times/day

Children >12 years and Adults:

Hippurate: 0.5-1 g twice daily

Mandelate: 1 g 4 times/day after meals and at bedtime

Dosage Forms

Tablet: 1 g

Hiprex®, Urex®: 1 g

Tablet, enteric coated: 500 mg, 1 g

Mandelamine®: 500 mg, 1 g

methenamine hippurate *see* methenamine *on previous page*

methenamine mandelate *see* methenamine *on previous page*

Methergine® [US/Can] *see* methylergonovine *on page 558*

methimazole *(meth IM a zole)*

Sound-Alike/Look-Alike Issues

methimazole may be confused with metolazone

Synonyms thiamazole

U.S./Canadian Brand Names Dom-Methimazole [Can]; PHL-Methimazole [Can]; Tapazole® [US/Can]

Therapeutic Category Antithyroid Agent

Use Palliative treatment of hyperthyroidism, return the hyperthyroid patient to a normal metabolic state prior to thyroidectomy, and to control thyrotoxic crisis that may accompany thyroidectomy

Usual Dosage Oral: Administer in 3 equally divided doses at approximately 8-hour intervals

Children: Initial: 0.4 mg/kg/day in 3 divided doses; maintenance: 0.2 mg/kg/day in 3 divided doses up to 30 mg/24 hours maximum

Alternatively: Initial: 0.5-0.7 mg/kg/day **or** 15-20 mg/m^2/day in 3 divided doses

Maintenance: $1/3$ to $2/3$ of the initial dose beginning when the patient is euthyroid

Maximum: 30 mg/24 hours

Adults: Initial: 15 mg/day for mild hyperthyroidism; 30-40 mg/day in moderately severe hyperthyroidism; 60 mg/day in severe hyperthyroidism; maintenance: 5-15 mg/day

Adjust dosage as required to achieve and maintain serum T_3, T_4, and TSH levels in the normal range. An elevated T_3 may be the sole indicator of inadequate treatment. An elevated TSH indicates excessive antithyroid treatment.

Dosage Forms

Tablet: 5 mg, 10 mg, 20 mg

Tapazole® 5 mg, 10 mg

Methitest™ [US] *see* methyltestosterone *on page 560*

methocarbamol *(meth oh KAR ba mole)*

Sound-Alike/Look-Alike Issues

methocarbamol may be confused with mephobarbital

Robaxin® may be confused with Rubex®

U.S./Canadian Brand Names Robaxin® [US/Can]

Therapeutic Category Skeletal Muscle Relaxant

Use Treatment of muscle spasm associated with acute painful musculoskeletal conditions; supportive therapy in tetanus

Usual Dosage

Tetanus: I.V.:

Children: Recommended **only** for use in tetanus: 15 mg/kg/dose or 500 mg/m^2/dose, may repeat every 6 hours if needed; maximum dose: 1.8 g/m^2/day for 3 days only

Adults: Initial dose: 1-3 g; may repeat dose every 6 hours until oral dosing is possible; injection should not be used for more than 3 consecutive days

Muscle spasm: Children ≥16 years and Adults:

Oral: 1.5 g 4 times/day for 2-3 days (up to 8 g/day may be given in severe conditions), then decrease to 4-4.5 g/day in 3-6 divided doses

I.M., I.V.: 1 g every 8 hours if oral not possible; injection should not be used for more than 3 consecutive days. If condition persists, may repeat course of therapy after a drug-free interval of 48 hours.

Dosage Forms
Injection, solution:
Robaxin®: 100 mg/mL (10 mL)
Tablet: 500 mg, 750 mg
Robaxin®: 500 mg, 750 mg

methohexital (meth oh HEKS i tal)
Sound-Alike/Look-Alike Issues
Brevital® may be confused with Brevibloc®
Synonyms methohexital sodium
U.S./Canadian Brand Names Brevital® Sodium [US]; Brevital® [Can]
Therapeutic Category Barbiturate
Controlled Substance C-IV
Use Induction and maintenance of general anesthesia for short procedures
Can be used in pediatric patients ≥1 month of age as follows: For rectal or intramuscular induction of anesthesia prior to the use of other general anesthetic agents, as an adjunct to subpotent inhalational anesthetic agents for short surgical procedures, or for short surgical, diagnostic, or therapeutic procedures associated with minimal painful stimuli
Usual Dosage Doses must be titrated to effect
Manufacturer's recommendations:
Infants ≥1 month and Children:
I.M.: Induction: 6.6-10 mg/kg of a 5% solution
Rectal: Induction: Usual: 25 mg/kg of a 1% solution
Alternative pediatric dosing:
Children 3-12 years:
I.M.: Preoperative: 5-10 mg/kg/dose
I.V.: Induction: 1-2 mg/kg/dose
Rectal: Preoperative/induction: 20-35 mg/kg/dose; usual: 25 mg/kg/dose; maximum dose: 500 mg/dose; give as 10% aqueous solution
Adults: I.V.: Induction: 50-120 mg to start; 20-40 mg every 4-7 minutes
Dosage Forms
Injection, powder for reconstitution:
Brevital® Sodium: 500 mg, 2.5 g, 5 g

methohexital sodium see methohexital on this page

methotrexate (meth oh TREKS ate)
Sound-Alike/Look-Alike Issues
methotrexate may be confused with metolazone, mitoxantrone
MTX is an error-prone abbreviation (mistaken as mitoxantrone)
Synonyms amethopterin; methotrexate sodium; NSC-740
U.S./Canadian Brand Names Apo-Methotrexate® [Can]; ratio-Methotrexate [Can]; Rheumatrex® Dose Pack® [US]; Trexall™ [US]
Therapeutic Category Antineoplastic Agent
Use Treatment of trophoblastic neoplasms; leukemias; psoriasis; rheumatoid arthritis (RA), including polyartic-ular-course juvenile rheumatoid arthritis (JRA); breast, head and neck, and lung carcinomas; osteosarcoma; soft-tissue sarcomas; carcinoma of gastrointestinal tract, esophagus, testes; lymphomas
Usual Dosage Refer to individual protocols.
Note: Doses between 100-500 mg/m^2 **may require** leucovorin rescue. Doses >500 mg/m^2 **require** leucovorin rescue: Oral, I.M., I.V.: Leucovorin 10-15 mg/m^2 every 6 hours for 8 or 10 doses, starting 24 hours after the start of methotrexate infusion. Continue until the methotrexate level is ≤0.1 micromolar (10^{-7}M). Some clinicians continue leucovorin until the methotrexate level is <0.05 micromolar (5×10^{-8}M) or 0.01 micromolar (10^{-8}M).
If the 48-hour methotrexate level is >1 micromolar (10^{-7}M) or the 72-hour methotrexate level is >0.2 micro-molar (2×10^{-7}M): I.V., I.M, Oral: Leucovorin 100 mg/m^2 every 6 hours until the methotrexate level is ≤0.1 micromolar (10^{-7}M). Some clinicians continue leucovorin until the methotrexate level is <0.05 micromolar (5×10^{-8}M) or 0.01 micromolar (10^{-8}M).
(Continued)

methotrexate *(Continued)*

Children:
Dermatomyositis: Oral: 15-20 mg/m^2/week as a single dose once weekly **or** 0.3-1 mg/kg/dose once weekly
Juvenile rheumatoid arthritis: Oral, I.M.: 10 mg/m^2 once weekly, then 5-15 mg/m^2/week as a single dose **or** as 3 divided doses given 12 hours apart
Antineoplastic dosage range:
Oral, I.M.: 7.5-30 mg/m^2/week **or** every 2 weeks
I.V.: 10-18,000 mg/m^2 bolus dosing **or** continuous infusion over 6-42 hours
Pediatric solid tumors (high-dose): I.V.:
<12 years: 12-25 g/m^2
≥12 years: 8 g/m^2
Acute lymphocytic leukemia (intermediate-dose): I.V.: Loading: 100 mg/m^2 bolus dose, followed by 900 mg/m^2/day infusion over 23-41 hours.
Meningeal leukemia: I.T.: 10-15 mg/m^2 (maximum dose: 15 mg) **or** an age-based dosing regimen; one possible system is:
≤3 months: 3 mg/dose
4-11 months: 6 mg/dose
1 year: 8 mg/dose
2 years: 10 mg/dose
≥3 years: 12 mg/dose

Adults: I.V.: Range is wide from 30-40 mg/m^2/week to 100-12,000 mg/m^2 with leucovorin rescue
Trophoblastic neoplasms:
Oral, I.M.: 15-30 mg/day for 5 days; repeat in 7 days for 3-5 courses
I.V.: 11 mg/m^2 days 1 through 5 every 3 weeks
Head and neck cancer: Oral, I.M., I.V.: 25-50 mg/m^2 once weekly
Mycosis fungoides (cutaneous T-cell lymphoma): Oral, I.M.: Initial (early stages):
5-50 mg once weekly **or**
15-37.5 mg twice weekly
Bladder cancer: I.V.:
30 mg/m^2 day 1 and 8 every 3 weeks **or**
30 mg/m^2 day 1, 15, and 22 every 4 weeks
Breast cancer: I.V.: 30-60 mg/m^2 days 1 and 8 every 3-4 weeks
Gastric cancer: I.V.: 1500 mg/m^2 every 4 weeks
Lymphoma, non-Hodgkin's: I.V.:
30 mg/m^2 days 3 and 10 every 3 weeks **or**
120 mg/m^2 day 8 and 15 every 3-4 weeks **or**
200 mg/m^2 day 8 and 15 every 3 weeks **or**
400 mg/m^2 every 4 weeks for 3 cycles **or**
1 g/m^2 every 3 weeks **or**
1.5 g/m^2 every 4 weeks
Sarcoma: I.V.: 8-12 g/m^2 weekly for 2-4 weeks
Rheumatoid arthritis: Oral: 7.5 mg once weekly **or** 2.5 mg every 12 hours for 3 doses/week, not to exceed 20 mg/week
Psoriasis:
Oral: 2.5-5 mg/dose every 12 hours for 3 doses given weekly **or**
Oral, I.M.: 10-25 mg/dose given once weekly

Dosage Forms
Injection, powder for reconstitution [preservative free]: 20 mg, 1 g
Injection, solution: 25 mg/mL (2 mL, 10 mL)
Injection, solution [preservative free]: 25 mg/mL (2 mL, 4 mL, 8 mL, 10 mL, 40 mL)
Tablet: 2.5 mg
Trexall™: 5 mg, 7.5 mg, 10 mg, 15 mg
Tablet [dose pack]: 2.5 mg (4 cards with 2, 3, 4, 5, or 6 tablets each)
Rheumatrex® Dose Pack: 2.5 mg (4 cards with 2, 3, 4, 5, or 6 tablets each)

methotrexate sodium *see* methotrexate *on previous page*

methotrexate *(Canada only)* (meth oh trye MEP ra zeen)

Synonyms levomepromazine; methotrimeprazine hydrochloride
U.S./Canadian Brand Names Apo-Methoprazine® [Can]; Novo Meprazine [Can]; Nozinan® [Can]; PMS-Methotrimeprazine [Can]
Therapeutic Category Neuroleptic Agent
Use Treatment of schizophrenia or psychosis; management of pain, including pain caused by neuralgia or cancer; adjunct to general anesthesia; management of nausea and vomiting; sedation

Usual Dosage
Children >2 years:
Oral: 0.25 mg/kg/day in 2-3 divided doses; may increase gradually based on response.
Maximum dose: 40 mg/day in children <12 years
I.M.: 0.06-0.125 mg/kg/day in 1-3 divided doses
Adults:
Oral:
Anxiety, mild-moderate pain: 6-25 mg/day in 3 divided doses
Psychoses, severe pain: 50-75 mg/day in 2-3 divided doses; titrate to effect (doses up to 1000 mg/day or greater have been used in treatment of some patients with psychoses). If higher dosages are used to initiate therapy (100-200 mg/day), patients should be restricted to bed for the first few days of therapy.
Sedative: 10-25 mg at bedtime
I.M.:
Psychoses, severe pain: 75-100 mg (administered in 3-4 deep I.M. injections)
Analgesia (postoperative): 10-25 mg every 8 hours (2.5-7.5 mg every 4-6 hours is suggested postoperatively if residual effects of anesthetic may be present)
Premedication: 10-25 mg every 8 hours (final preoperative dose may be 25-50 mg administered ~1 hour prior to surgery)
I.V.: During surgical procedures/labor: 20-50 mcg/minute (some patients may require up to 100 mcg/minute)
SubQ (continuous infusion): Palliative care: 25-200 mcg/day (via syringe driver)
Dosage Forms [CAN] = Canadian brand name
Injection, solution:
Nozinan® [CAN]: 25 mg/mL (1 mL) [not available in the U.S.]
Solution, oral:
Nozinan® [CAN]: 5 mg/mL [not available in the U.S.]
Solution, oral drops:
Nozinan® [CAN]: 40 mg/mL [not available in the U.S.]
Tablet:
Apo-Methoprazine® [CAN]: 2 mg, 5 mg, 25 mg, 50 mg [not available in the U.S.]
Nozinan® [CAN]: 5 mg, 25 mg, 50 mg [not available in the U.S.]

methotrimeprazine hydrochloride *see* methotrimeprazine *(Canada only)* on previous page

methotrimeprazine (meth OKS a len)

Synonyms methoxypsoralen; 8-methoxypsoralen
U.S./Canadian Brand Names 8-MOP® [US/Can]; Oxsoralen-Ultra® [US/Can]; Oxsoralen® [US/Can]; Ultramop™ [Can]; Uvadex® [US/Can]
Therapeutic Category Psoralen
Use
Oral: Symptomatic control of severe, recalcitrant disabling psoriasis; repigmentation of idiopathic vitiligo; palliative treatment of skin manifestations of cutaneous T-cell lymphoma (CTCL)
Topical: Repigmentation of idiopathic vitiligo
Extracorporeal: Palliative treatment of skin manifestations of CTCL
Usual Dosage Note: Refer to treatment protocols for UVA exposure guidelines.
Children >12 years and Adults: Vitiligo: Topical: Apply lotion 1-2 hours before exposure to UVA light, no more than once weekly
Adults:
Psoriasis: Oral: 10-70 mg 11/2-2 hours before exposure to UVA light; dose may be repeated 2-3 times per week, based on UVA exposure; doses must be given at least 48 hours apart; dosage is based upon patient's body weight and skin type:
<30 kg: 10 mg
30-50 kg: 20 mg
51-65 kg: 30 mg
66-80 kg: 40 mg
81-90 kg: 50 mg
91-115 kg: 60 mg
>115 kg: 70 mg
Vitiligo: (8-MOP®): Oral: 20 mg 2-4 hours before exposure to UVA light; dose may be repeated based on erythema and tenderness of skin; do not give on 2 consecutive days
CTCL: Extracorporeal (Uvadex®): 200 mcg injected into the photoactivation bag during the collection cycle using the UVAR® photopheresis system (consult user's guide). Treatment schedule: Two consecutive days every 4 weeks for a minimum of 7 treatment cycles
Dosage Forms
Capsule:
8-MOP®, Oxsoralen-Ultra®: 10 mg
(Continued)

methoxsalen *(Continued)*

Lotion:
Oxsoralen®: 1% (30 mL)
Solution, for extracorporeal administration:
Uvadex®: 20 mcg/mL (10 mL) **[not for injection]**

methoxypsoralen *see* methoxsalen *on previous page*

8-methoxypsoralen *see* methoxsalen *on previous page*

methscopolamine (meth skoe POL a meen)

Synonyms methscopolamine bromide
U.S./Canadian Brand Names Pamine® Forte [US]; Pamine® [US/Can]
Therapeutic Category Anticholinergic Agent
Use Adjunctive therapy in the treatment of peptic ulcer
Usual Dosage Oral: Adults: 2.5 mg 30 minutes before meals or food and 2.5-5 mg at bedtime; may increase dose to 5 mg twice daily
Dosage Forms
Tablet: 2.5 mg, 5 mg
Pamine®: 2.5 mg
Pamine® Forte: 5 mg

methscopolamine and pseudoephedrine *see* pseudoephedrine and methscopolamine *on page 730*

methscopolamine bromide *see* methscopolamine *on this page*

methscopolamine, chlorpheniramine, and pseudoephedrine *see* chlorpheniramine, pseudoephedrine, and methscopolamine *on page 184*

methscopolamine nitrate, chlorpheniramine maleate, and phenylephrine hydrochloride *see* chlorpheniramine, phenylephrine, and methscopolamine *on page 181*

methscopolamine, pseudoephedrine, and chlorpheniramine *see* chlorpheniramine, pseudoephedrine, and methscopolamine *on page 184*

methsuximide (meth SUKS i mide)

Sound-Alike/Look-Alike Issues
methsuximide may be confused with ethosuximide
U.S./Canadian Brand Names Celontin® [US/Can]
Therapeutic Category Anticonvulsant
Use Control of absence (petit mal) seizures that are refractory to other drugs
Usual Dosage Oral: Anticonvulsant:
Children: Initial: 10-15 mg/kg/day in 3-4 divided doses; increase weekly up to maximum of 30 mg/kg/day
Adults: 300 mg/day for the first week; may increase by 300 mg/day at weekly intervals up to 1.2 g/day in 2-4 divided doses/day
Dosage Forms
Capsule:
Celontin®: 150 mg, 300 mg

methyclothiazide (meth i kloe THYE a zide)

Sound-Alike/Look-Alike Issues
Enduron® may be confused with Empirin®, Imuran®, Inderal®
U.S./Canadian Brand Names Aquatensen® [Can]; Enduron® [Can]
Therapeutic Category Diuretic, Thiazide
Use Management of mild to moderate hypertension; treatment of edema in congestive heart failure and nephrotic syndrome
Usual Dosage Oral: Adults:
Edema: 2.5-10 mg/day
Hypertension: 2.5-5 mg/day; may add another antihypertensive if 5 mg is not adequate after a trial of 8-12 weeks of therapy
Dosage Forms
Tablet: 5 mg

methylacetoxyprogesterone *see* medroxyprogesterone *on page 537*

methylcellulose (meth il SEL yoo lose)
Sound-Alike/Look-Alike Issues
Citrucel® may be confused with Citracal®
U.S./Canadian Brand Names Citrucel® Fiber Shake [US-OTC]; Citrucel® Fiber Smoothie [US-OTC]; Citrucel® [US-OTC]
Therapeutic Category Laxative
Use Adjunct in treatment of constipation
Usual Dosage Oral:
Children 6-12 years:
Citrucel® caplet: 1 caplet up to 6 times/day; follow each dose with 8 oz of water
Citrucel® powder: Half the adult dose in 4 oz of cold water, 1-3 times/day
Children ≥12 years and Adults:
Citrucel® caplet: 2-4 caplets 1-3 times/day; follow each dose with 8 oz of water
Citrucel® powder: 1 heaping tablespoon (19 g) in 8 oz of cold water, 1-3 times/day
FiberEase™: 2 tablespoonsful mixed in 7 oz of water, 1-3 times/day
Dosage Forms
Caplet:
Citrucel® [OTC]: 500 mg
Powder: 2 g/level scoop
Citrucel® Fiber Smoothie: 2 g/level scoop (275 g, 539 g)
Citrucel®: 2 g/level scoop (448 g, 840 g, 1418g, 1843 g)
Citrucel® [sugar free formulation]: 2 g/level scoop (473 g, 907g, 1190 g)
Citrucel® Fiber Shake: 2 g/level scoop (204 g, 413 g)

methylcellulose, gelatin, and pectin *see* gelatin, pectin, and methylcellulose *on page 386*

methyldopa (meth il DOE pa)
Sound-Alike/Look-Alike Issues
methyldopa may be confused with L-dopa, levodopa
Synonyms methyldopate hydrochloride
U.S./Canadian Brand Names Apo-Methyldopa® [Can]; Nu-Medopa [Can]
Therapeutic Category Alpha-Adrenergic Blocking Agent
Use Management of moderate to severe hypertension
Usual Dosage
Children:
Oral: Initial: 10 mg/kg/day in 2-4 divided doses; increase every 2 days as needed to maximum dose of 65 mg/kg/day; do not exceed 3 g/day.
I.V.: 5-10 mg/kg/dose every 6-8 hours up to a total dose of 65 mg/kg/24 hours or 3 g/24 hours
Adults:
Oral: Initial: 250 mg 2-3 times/day; increase every 2 days as needed (maximum dose: 3 g/day): usual dose range (JNC 7): 250-1000 mg/day in 2 divided doses
I.V.: 250-500 mg every 6-8 hours; maximum dose: 1 g every 6 hours
Dosage Forms
Injection, solution: 50 mg/mL (5 mL)
Tablet: 250 mg, 500 mg

methyldopa and hydrochlorothiazide (meth il DOE pa & hye droe klor oh THYE a zide)
Sound-Alike/Look-Alike Issues
Aldoril® may be confused with Aldoclor®, Aldomet®, Elavil®
Synonyms hydrochlorothiazide and methyldopa
U.S./Canadian Brand Names Aldoril® [US]; Apo-Methazide® [Can]
Therapeutic Category Antihypertensive Agent, Combination
Use Management of moderate to severe hypertension
Usual Dosage Oral: Dosage titrated on individual components, then switch to combination product; no more than methyldopa 3 g/day and/or hydrochlorothiazide 50 mg/day; maintain initial dose for first 48 hours, then decrease or increase at intervals of not less than 2 days until an adequate response is achieved
Methyldopa 250 mg and hydrochlorothiazide 15 mg: 2-3 times/day
Methyldopa 250 mg and hydrochlorothiazide 25 mg: Twice daily
Dosage Forms
Tablet: Methyldopa 250 mg and hydrochlorothiazide 15 mg; methyldopa 250 mg and hydrochlorothiazide 25 mg
Aldoril® 25: Methyldopa 250 mg and hydrochlorothiazide 25 mg

methyldopate hydrochloride *see* methyldopa *on this page*

methylene blue (METH i leen bloo)

U.S./Canadian Brand Names Urolene Blue® [US]

Therapeutic Category Antidote

Use Antidote for cyanide poisoning and drug-induced methemoglobinemia, indicator dye

Usual Dosage

Children: NADPH-methemoglobin reductase deficiency: Oral: 1-1.5 mg/kg/day (maximum: 300 mg/day) given with 5-8 mg/kg/day of ascorbic acid

Children and Adults: Methemoglobinemia: I.V.: 1-2 mg/kg or 25-50 mg/m^2 over several minutes; may be repeated in 1 hour if necessary

Adults: Genitourinary antiseptic: Oral: 65-130 mg 3 times/day with a full glass of water (maximum: 390 mg/day)

Dosage Forms

Injection, solution: 10 mg/mL (1 mL, 10 mL)

Tablet: 65 mg

Urolene Blue®: 65 mg

methylergometrine maleate *see* methylergonovine *on this page*

methylergonovine (meth il er goe NOE veen)

Sound-Alike/Look-Alike Issues

methylergonovine and terbutaline parenteral dosage forms look similar. Due to their contrasting indications, use care when administering these agents.

Synonyms methylergometrine maleate; methylergonovine maleate

U.S./Canadian Brand Names Methergine® [US/Can]

Therapeutic Category Ergot Alkaloid and Derivative

Use Prevention and treatment of postpartum and postabortion hemorrhage caused by uterine atony or subinvolution

Usual Dosage Adults:

Oral: 0.2 mg 3-4 times/day in the puerperium for 2-7 days

I.M., I.V.: 0.2 mg after delivery of anterior shoulder, after delivery of placenta, or during puerperium; may be repeated as required at intervals of 2-4 hours

Dosage Forms

Injection, solution:

Methergine®: 0.2 mg/mL (1 mL)

Tablet:

Methergine®: 0.2 mg

methylergonovine maleate *see* methylergonovine *on this page*

Methylin® [US] *see* methylphenidate *on this page*

Methylin® ER [US] *see* methylphenidate *on this page*

methylmorphine *see* codeine *on page 210*

methylphenidate (meth il FEN i date)

Sound-Alike/Look-Alike Issues

methylphenidate may be confused with methadone

Ritalin® may be confused with Ismelin®, Rifadin®

Synonyms methylphenidate hydrochloride

U.S./Canadian Brand Names Apo-Methylphenidate® SR [Can]; Apo-Methylphenidate® [Can]; Biphentin® [Can]; Concerta® [US/Can]; Daytrana™ [US]; Metadate® CD [US]; Metadate® ER [US]; Methylin® ER [US]; Methylin® [US]; PMS-Methylphenidate [Can]; Riphenidate [Can]; Ritalin-SR® [US/Can]; Ritalin® LA [US]; Ritalin® [US/Can]

Therapeutic Category Central Nervous System Stimulant, Nonamphetamine

Controlled Substance C-II

Use Treatment of attention-deficit/hyperactivity disorder (ADHD); symptomatic management of narcolepsy

Usual Dosage

ADHD:

Oral:

Immediate release products Children ≥6 years and Adults: Initial: 5 mg/dose (~0.3 mg/kg/dose) given twice daily before breakfast and lunch; increase by 5-10 mg/day (0.2 mg/kg/day) at weekly intervals; maximum dose: 60 mg/day (2 mg/kg/day). **Note:** Discontinue periodically to re-evaluate or if no improvement occurs within 1 month.

Extended release products:
Children ≥6 years and Adults:
Metadate® ER, Methylin® ER, Ritalin® SR: May be given in place of immediate release products, once the daily dose is titrated and the titrated 8-hour dosage corresponds to sustained or extended release tablet size; maximum: 60 mg/day
Metadate® CD, Ritalin® LA: Initial: 20 mg once daily; may be adjusted in 10-20 mg increments at weekly intervals; maximum: 60 mg/day
Children 6-12 years and Adolescents 13-17 years: *Concerta®:*
Patients not currently taking methylphenidate: Initial dose: 18 mg once daily in the morning
Patients currently taking methylphenidate: **Note:** Initial dose: Dosing based on current regimen and clinical judgment; suggested dosing listed below:
— Patients taking methylphenidate 5 mg 2-3 times/day **or** 20 mg/day sustained release formulation: 18 mg once every morning
— Patients taking methylphenidate 10 mg 2-3 times/day **or** 40 mg/day sustained release formulation: 36 mg once every morning
— Patients taking methylphenidate 15 mg 2-3 times/day **or** 60 mg/day sustained release formulation: 54 mg once every morning
Dose adjustment: May increase dose in increments of 18 mg; dose may be adjusted at weekly intervals. A dosage strength of 27 mg is available for situations in which a dosage between 18-36 mg is desired. Maximum dose should not exceed 2 mg/kg/day **or** 54 mg/day in children 6-12 years or 72 mg/day in children 13-17 years.
Transdermal (Daytrana™): Children 6-12 years: Initial: 10 mg patch once daily; remove up to 9 hours after application. Titrate based on response and tolerability; may increase to next transdermal dose no more frequently than every week. **Note:** Application should occur 2 hours prior to desired effect. Drug absorption may continue for a period of time after patch removal.

Narcolepsy: Oral: Adults: 10 mg 2-3 times/day, up to 60 mg/day

Dosage Forms
Capsule, extended release:
Metadate® CD: 10 mg, 20 mg, 30 mg, 40 mg, 50 mg, 60 mg
Ritalin® LA: 10 mg, 20 mg, 30 mg, 40 mg
Solution, oral:
Methylin®: 5 mg/5 mL, 10 mg/5 mL
Tablet: 5 mg, 10 mg, 20 mg
Methylin®, Ritalin®: 5 mg, 10 mg, 20 mg
Tablet, chewable:
Methylin®: 2.5 mg, 5 mg, 10 mg
Tablet, extended release: 20 mg
Concerta®: 18 mg, 27 mg, 36 mg, 54 mg
Metadate® ER, Methylin® ER: 10 mg, 20 mg
Tablet, sustained release: 20 mg
Ritalin-SR®: 20 mg
Transdermal system [once-daily patch]:
Daytrana™: 10 mg/9 hours (10s, 30s); 15 mg/9 hours (10s, 30s); 20 mg/9 hours (10s, 30s); 30 mg/9 hours (10s, 30s)

methylphenidate hydrochloride *see* methylphenidate *on previous page*

methylphenobarbital *see* mephobarbital *on page 543*

methylphenoxy-benzene propanamine *see* atomoxetine *on page 81*

methylphenyl isoxazolyl penicillin *see* oxacillin *on page 636*

methylphytyl napthoquinone *see* phytonadione *on page 681*

methylprednisolone (meth il pred NIS oh lone)
Sound-Alike/Look-Alike Issues
methylPREDNISolone may be confused with medroxyPROGESTERone, predniSONE
Depo-Medrol® may be confused with Solu-Medrol®
Medrol® may be confused with Mebaral®
Solu-Medrol® may be confused with Depo-Medrol®
Synonyms 6-α-methylprednisolone; A-methapred; methylprednisolone acetate; methylprednisolone sodium succinate
Tall-Man methyl**PREDNIS**olone
U.S./Canadian Brand Names Depo-Medrol® [US/Can]; Medrol® [US/Can]; Methylprednisolone Acetate [Can]; Solu-Medrol® [US/Can]
(Continued)

methylprednisolone *(Continued)*

Therapeutic Category Adrenal Corticosteroid

Use Primarily as an antiinflammatory or immunosuppressant agent in the treatment of a variety of diseases including those of hematologic, allergic, inflammatory, neoplastic, and autoimmune origin. Prevention and treatment of graft-versus-host disease following allogeneic bone marrow transplantation.

Usual Dosage Dosing should be based on the lesser of ideal body weight or actual body weight

Only sodium succinate may be given I.V.; methylprednisolone sodium succinate is highly soluble and has a rapid effect by I.M. and I.V. routes. Methylprednisolone acetate has a low solubility and has a sustained I.M. effect.

Children:

Antiinflammatory or immunosuppressive: Oral, I.M., I.V. (sodium succinate): 0.5-1.7 mg/kg/day **or** 5-25 mg/m²/day in divided doses every 6-12 hours; "Pulse" therapy: 15-30 mg/kg/dose over ≥30 minutes given once daily for 3 days

Status asthmaticus: I.V. (sodium succinate): Loading dose: 2 mg/kg/dose, then 0.5-1 mg/kg/dose every 6 hours for up to 5 days

Acute spinal cord injury: I.V. (sodium succinate): 30 mg/kg over 15 minutes, followed in 45 minutes by a continuous infusion of 5.4 mg/kg/hour for 23 hours

Lupus nephritis: I.V. (sodium succinate): 30 mg/kg over ≥30 minutes every other day for 6 doses

Adults: **Only sodium succinate may be given I.V.;** methylprednisolone sodium succinate is highly soluble and has a rapid effect by I.M. and I.V. routes. Methylprednisolone acetate has a low solubility and has a sustained I.M. effect.

Acute spinal cord injury: I.V. (sodium succinate): 30 mg/kg over 15 minutes, followed in 45 minutes by a continuous infusion of 5.4 mg/kg/hour for 23 hours

Antiinflammatory or immunosuppressive:

Oral: 2-60 mg/day in 1-4 divided doses to start, followed by gradual reduction in dosage to the lowest possible level consistent with maintaining an adequate clinical response.

I.M. (sodium succinate): 10-80 mg/day once daily

I.M. (acetate): 10-80 mg every 1-2 weeks

I.V. (sodium succinate): 10-40 mg over a period of several minutes and repeated I.V. or I.M. at intervals depending on clinical response; when high dosages are needed, give 30 mg/kg over a period ≥30 minutes and may be repeated every 4-6 hours for 48 hours.

Status asthmaticus: I.V. (sodium succinate): Loading dose: 2 mg/kg/dose, then 0.5-1 mg/kg/dose every 6 hours for up to 5 days

Lupus nephritis: High-dose "pulse" therapy: I.V. (sodium succinate): 1 g/day for 3 days

Aplastic anemia: I.V. (sodium succinate): 1 mg/kg/day or 40 mg/day (whichever dose is higher), for 4 days. After 4 days, change to oral and continue until day 10 or until symptoms of serum sickness resolve, then rapidly reduce over approximately 2 weeks.

Pneumocystis pneumonia in AIDs patients: I.V.: 40-60 mg every 6 hours for 7-10 days

Intraarticular (acetate): Administer every 1-5 weeks.

Large joints: 20-80 mg

Small joints: 4-10 mg

Intralesional (acetate): 20-60 mg every 1-5 weeks

Dosage Forms

Injection, powder for reconstitution: 40 mg, 125 mg, 500 mg, 1 g

Solu-Medrol®: 40 mg, 125 mg, 500 mg, 1 g, 2 g

Solu-Medrol®: 500 mg, 1 g

Injection, suspension: 40 mg/mL (5 mL, 10 mL); 80 mg/mL (5 mL)

Depo-Medrol®: 20 mg/mL (5 mL); 40 mg/mL (5 mL); 80 mg/mL (5 mL)

Injection, suspension [single-dose vial]: 40 mg/mL (1 mL); 80 mg/mL (1 mL)

Depo-Medrol®: 40 mg/mL (1 mL, 10 mL); 80 mg/mL (1 mL)

Tablet: 4 mg

Medrol®: 2 mg, 4 mg, 8 mg, 16 mg, 32 mg

Tablet, dose-pack: 4 mg (21s)

Medrol® Dosepak™: 4 mg (21s)

6-α-methylprednisolone *see* methylprednisolone *on previous page*

Methylprednisolone Acetate [Can] *see* methylprednisolone *on previous page*

methylprednisolone acetate *see* methylprednisolone *on previous page*

methylprednisolone sodium succinate *see* methylprednisolone *on previous page*

4-methylpyrazole *see* fomepizole *on page 373*

methyltestosterone *(meth il tes TOS te rone)*

Sound-Alike/Look-Alike Issues

methylTESTOSTERone may be confused with medroxyPROGESTERone

Virilon® may be confused with Verelan®

Tall-Man methyl**TESTOSTER**one

U.S./Canadian Brand Names Android® [US]; Methitest™ [US]; Testred® [US]; Virilon® [US]

Therapeutic Category Androgen

Controlled Substance C-III

Use
Male: Hypogonadism; delayed puberty; impotence and climacteric symptoms
Female: Palliative treatment of metastatic breast cancer

Usual Dosage Adults (buccal absorption produces twice the androgenic activity of oral tablets):
Male:
Hypogonadism, male climacteric and impotence: Oral: 10-40 mg/day
Androgen deficiency:
Oral: 10-50 mg/day
Buccal: 5-25 mg/day
Postpubertal cryptorchidism: Oral: 30 mg/day
Female:
Breast pain/engorgement:
Oral: 80 mg/day for 3-5 days
Buccal: 40 mg/day for 3-5 days
Breast cancer:
Oral: 50-200 mg/day
Buccal: 25-100 mg/day

Dosage Forms
Capsule:
Android®, Testred®, Virilon®: 10 mg
Tablet:
Methitest™: 10 mg

Meticorten® *(Discontinued)* see prednisone *on page 710*

Metimyd Ophthalmic Ointment *(Discontinued)*

metipranolol (met i PRAN oh lol)
Sound-Alike/Look-Alike Issues
metipranolol may be confused with metaproterenol
Synonyms metipranolol hydrochloride
U.S./Canadian Brand Names OptiPranolol® [US/Can]
Therapeutic Category Beta-Adrenergic Blocker
Use Agent for lowering intraocular pressure in patients with chronic open-angle glaucoma
Usual Dosage Ophthalmic: Adults: Instill 1 drop in the affected eye(s) twice daily
Dosage Forms
Solution, ophthalmic: 0.3% (5 mL, 10 mL)
OptiPranolol®: 0.3% (5 mL, 10 mL)

metipranolol hydrochloride see metipranolol *on this page*

metoclopramide (met oh KLOE pra mide)
Sound-Alike/Look-Alike Issues
metoclopramide may be confused with metolazone
Reglan® may be confused with Megace®, Regonol®, Renagel®
U.S./Canadian Brand Names Apo-Metoclop® [Can]; Metoclopramide Hydrochloride Injection [Can]; Nu-Metoclopramide [Can]; Reglan® [US]
Therapeutic Category Gastrointestinal Agent, Prokinetic
Use
Oral: Symptomatic treatment of diabetic gastric stasis; gastroesophageal reflux
I.V., I.M.: Symptomatic treatment of diabetic gastric stasis; postpyloric placement of enteral feeding tubes; prevention and/or treatment of nausea and vomiting associated with chemotherapy, or postsurgery; to stimulate gastric emptying and intestinal transit of barium during radiological examination
Usual Dosage
Children:
Postpyloric feeding tube placement: I.V.:
<6 years: 0.1 mg/kg
6-14 years: 2.5-5 mg
>14 years: Refer to Adults dosing.
(Continued)

metoclopramide (Continued)

Adults:

Gastroesophageal reflux: Oral: 10-15 mg/dose up to 4 times/day 30 minutes before meals or food and at bedtime; single doses of 20 mg are occasionally needed for provoking situations. Treatment >12 weeks has not been evaluated.

Diabetic gastric stasis:

Oral: 10 mg 30 minutes before each meal and at bedtime

I.M., I.V. (for severe symptoms): 10 mg over 1-2 minutes; 10 days of I.V. therapy may be necessary for best response

Chemotherapy-induced emesis:

I.V.: 1-2 mg/kg 30 minutes before chemotherapy and repeated every 2 hours for 2 doses, then every 3 hours for 3 doses (manufacturer labeling)

Alternate dosing (with or without diphenhydramine):

Moderate emetic risk chemotherapy: 0.5 mg/kg every 6 hours on days 2-4

Low and minimal risk chemotherapy: 1-2 mg/kg every 3-4 hours

Breakthrough treatment: 1-2 mg/kg every 3-4 hours

Postoperative nausea and vomiting: I.M., I.V.: 10-20 mg near end of surgery

Postpyloric feeding tube placement, radiological exam: I.V.: 10 mg

Dosage Forms

Injection, solution: 5 mg/mL (2 mL, 10 mL, 30 mL)

Reglan®: 5 mg/mL (2 mL, 10 mL, 30 mL)

Syrup: 5 mg/5 mL

Tablet: 5 mg, 10 mg

Reglan®: 5 mg, 10 mg

Metoclopramide Hydrochloride Injection [Can] *see* metoclopramide *on previous page*

metolazone (me TOLE a zone)

Sound-Alike/Look-Alike Issues

metolazone may be confused with metaxalone, methazolamide, methimazole, methotrexate, metoclopramide, metoprolol, minoxidil

Zaroxolyn® may be confused with Zarontin®

U.S./Canadian Brand Names Zaroxolyn® [US/Can]

Therapeutic Category Diuretic, Miscellaneous

Use Management of mild to moderate hypertension; treatment of edema in congestive heart failure and nephrotic syndrome, impaired renal function

Usual Dosage Oral: Adults:

Edema: 2.5-20 mg/dose every 24 hours (ACC/AHA 2005 Heart Failure Guidelines)

Hypertension: 2.5-5 mg/dose every 24 hours

Dosage Forms

Tablet: 2.5 mg, 5 mg, 10 mg

Zaroxolyn®: 2.5 mg, 5 mg, 10 mg

Metopirone® [US] *see* metyrapone *on page 565*

metoprolol (me toe PROE lole)

Sound-Alike/Look-Alike Issues

metoprolol may be confused with metaproterenol, metolazone, misoprostol

Toprol-XL® may be confused with Tegretol®, Tegretol®-XR, Topamax®

Synonyms metoprolol succinate; metoprolol tartrate

U.S./Canadian Brand Names Apo-Metoprolol® [Can]; Betaloc® Durules® [Can]; Betaloc® [Can]; Lopressor® [US/Can]; Metoprolol Tartrate Injection, USP [Can]; Novo-Metoprolol [Can]; Nu-Metop [Can]; PMS-Metoprolol [Can]; Sandoz-Metoprolol [Can]; Toprol-XL® [US/Can]

Therapeutic Category Beta-Adrenergic Blocker

Use Treatment of hypertension and angina pectoris; prevention of myocardial infarction, atrial fibrillation, flutter, symptomatic treatment of hypertrophic subaortic stenosis

Extended release: To reduce mortality/hospitalization in patients with congestive heart failure (stable NYHA Class II or III) in patients already receiving ACE inhibitors, diuretics, and/or digoxin

Usual Dosage

Children: Hypertension: Oral:

1-17 years: Nonextended release tablet: Initial: 1-2 mg/kg/day; maximum 6 mg/kg/day (≤200 mg/day); administer in 2 divided doses

≥6 years: Extended release tablet: Initial: 1 mg/kg/ once daily (maximum 50 mg/day). Adjust dose based on patient response (maximum 2 mg/kg or 200 mg/day)

Adults:
Hypertension: Oral: 100-450 mg/day in 2-3 divided doses, begin with 50 mg twice daily and increase doses at weekly intervals to desired effect; usual dosage range (JNC 7): 50-100 mg/day
Extended release: Initial: 25-100 mg/day (maximum: 400 mg/day)
Angina, SVT, MI prophylaxis: Oral: 100-450 mg/day in 2-3 divided doses, begin with 50 mg twice daily and increase doses at weekly intervals to desired effect
Extended release: Initial: 100 mg/day (maximum: 400 mg/day)
Hypertension/ventricular rate control: I.V. (in patients having nonfunctioning GI tract): Initial: 1.25-5 mg every 6-12 hours; titrate initial dose to response. Initially, low doses may be appropriate to establish response; however, up to 15 mg every 3-6 hours has been employed.
Congestive heart failure: Oral (extended release): Initial: 25 mg once daily (reduce to 12.5 mg once daily in NYHA class higher than class II); may double dosage every 2 weeks as tolerated, up to 200 mg/day
Myocardial infarction (acute): I.V.: 5 mg every 2 minutes for 3 doses in early treatment of myocardial infarction; thereafter give 50 mg orally every 6 hours 15 minutes after last I.V. dose and continue for 48 hours; then administer a maintenance dose of 100 mg twice daily.
Note: When switching from immediate release metoprolol to extended release, the same total daily dose of metoprolol should be used.
Dosage Forms
Injection, solution: 1 mg/mL (5 mL)
Lopressor®: 1 mg/mL (5 mL)
Tablet: 25 mg, 50 mg, 100 mg
Lopressor®: 50 mg, 100 mg
Tablet, extended release: 25 mg, 50 mg, 100 mg, 200 mg
Toprol-XL®: 25 mg, 50 mg, 100 mg, 200 mg

metoprolol and hydrochlorothiazide (me toe PROE lole & hye droe klor oh THYE a zide)
Synonyms hydrochlorothiazide and metoprolol; hydrochlorothiazide and metoprolol tartrate; metoprolol tartrate and hydrochlorothiazide
U.S./Canadian Brand Names Lopressor HCT® [US]
Therapeutic Category Beta Blocker, Beta₁ Selective; Diuretic, Thiazide
Use Treatment of hypertension
Usual Dosage Oral: Adults: Hypertension: Dosage should be determined by titration of the individual agents and the combination product substituted based upon the daily requirements.
Usual dose: Metoprolol 50-100 mg and hydrochlorothiazide 25-50 mg administered daily as single or divided doses (twice daily)
Note: Hydrochlorothiazide >50 mg/day is not recommended.
Concomitant therapy: It is recommended that if an additional antihypertensive agent is required, gradual titration should occur using ½ the usual starting dose of the other agent to avoid hypotension.
Dosage Forms
Tablet: 50/25: Metoprolol 50 mg and hydrochlorothiazide 25 mg; 100/25: Metoprolol 100 mg and hydrochlorothiazide 25 mg; 100/50: Metoprolol 100 mg and hydrochlorothiazide 50 mg
Lopressor HCT®: 50/25: Metoprolol 50 mg and hydrochlorothiazide 25 mg; 100/25: Metoprolol 100 mg and hydrochlorothiazide 25 mg; 100/50: Metoprolol 100 mg and hydrochlorothiazide 50 mg

metoprolol succinate see metoprolol on previous page

metoprolol tartrate see metoprolol on previous page

metoprolol tartrate and hydrochlorothiazide see metoprolol and hydrochlorothiazide on this page

Metoprolol Tartrate Injection, USP [Can] see metoprolol on previous page

Metreton® (Discontinued)

MetroCream® [US/Can] see metronidazole on this page

MetroGel® [US/Can] see metronidazole on this page

MetroGel-Vaginal® [US] see metronidazole on this page

Metro I.V.® Injection (Discontinued) see metronidazole on this page

MetroLotion® [US] see metronidazole on this page

metronidazole (met roe NYE da zole)
Sound-Alike/Look-Alike Issues
metronidazole may be confused with metformin.
Synonyms metronidazole hydrochloride
U.S./Canadian Brand Names Apo-Metronidazole® [Can]; Flagyl ER® [US]; Flagyl® [US/Can]; Florazole® ER [Can]; MetroCream® [US/Can]; MetroGel-Vaginal® [US]; MetroGel® [US/Can]; MetroLotion® [US]; Nidagel™ [Can]; Noritate® [US/Can]; Trikacide [Can]; Vandazole™ [US]
(Continued)

metronidazole *(Continued)*

Therapeutic Category Amebicide; Antibiotic, Miscellaneous; Antibiotic, Topical; Antiprotozoal

Use Treatment of susceptible anaerobic bacterial and protozoal infections in the following conditions: Amebiasis, symptomatic and asymptomatic trichomoniasis; skin and skin structure infections; CNS infections; intra-abdominal infections (as part of combination regimen); systemic anaerobic infections; treatment of antibiotic-associated pseudomembranous colitis (AAPC), bacterial vaginosis; as part of a multidrug regimen for *H. pylori* eradication to reduce the risk of duodenal ulcer recurrence

Topical: Treatment of inflammatory lesions and erythema of rosacea

Usual Dosage

Infants and Children:

Amebiasis: Oral: 35-50 mg/kg/day in divided doses every 8 hours for 10 days

Trichomoniasis: Oral: 15-30 mg/kg/day in divided doses every 8 hours for 7 days

Anaerobic infections:

Oral: 15-35 mg/kg/day in divided doses every 8 hours

I.V.: 30 mg/kg/day in divided doses every 6 hours

Clostridium difficile (antibiotic-associated colitis): Oral: 20 mg/kg/day divided every 6 hours

Maximum dose: 2 g/day

Adults:

Anaerobic infections (diverticulitis, intraabdominal, peritonitis, cholangitis, or abscess): Oral, I.V.: 500 mg every 6-8 hours, not to exceed 4 g/day

Acne rosacea: Topical:

0.75%: Apply and rub a thin film twice daily, morning and evening, to entire affected areas after washing. Significant therapeutic results should be noticed within 3 weeks. Clinical studies have demonstrated continuing improvement through 9 weeks of therapy.

1%: Apply thin film to affected area once daily

Amebiasis: Oral: 500-750 mg every 8 hours for 5-10 days

Antibiotic-associated pseudomembranous colitis: Oral: 250-500 mg 3-4 times/day for 10-14 days

Note: Due to the emergence of a new strain of *C. difficile*, some clinicians recommend converting to oral vancomycin therapy if the patient does not show a clear clinical response after 2 days of metronidazole therapy.

Giardiasis: 500 mg twice daily for 5-7 days

Helicobacter pylori eradication: Oral: 250-500 mg with meals and at bedtime for 14 days; requires combination therapy with at least one other antibiotic and an acid-suppressing agent (proton pump inhibitor or H_2 blocker)

Bacterial vaginosis or vaginitis due to *Gardnerella, Mobiluncus*:

Oral: 500 mg twice daily (regular release) or 750 mg once daily (extended release tablet) for 7 days

Vaginal: 1 applicatorful (~37.5 mg metronidazole) intravaginally once or twice daily for 5 days; apply once in morning and evening if using twice daily, if daily, use at bedtime

Trichomoniasis: Oral: 250 mg every 8 hours for 7 days **or** 375 mg twice daily for 7 days **or** 2 g as a single dose

Dosage Forms

Capsule: 375 mg

Flagyl®: 375 mg

Cream, topical: 0.75% (45 g)

MetroCream®: 0.75% (45 g)

Noritate®: 1% (60 g)

Gel, topical: 1% (45 g)

MetroGel®: 1% (46 g, 60 g)

Gel, vaginal: 0.75% (70 g)

MetroGel-Vaginal®, Vandazole™: 0.75% (70 g)

Infusion [premixed iso-osmotic sodium chloride solution]: 500 mg (100 mL)

Lotion, topical: 0.75% (60 mL)

MetroLotion®: 0.75% (60 mL)

Tablet: 250 mg, 500 mg

Flagyl®: 250 mg, 500 mg

Tablet, extended release:

Flagyl® ER: 750 mg

metronidazole and nystatin *(Canada only)* (met roe NYE da zole & nye STAT in)

U.S./Canadian Brand Names Flagystatin® [Can]

Therapeutic Category Antifungal Agent, Vaginal; Antiprotozoal, Nitroimidazole

Use Treatment of mixed vaginal infection due to *T. vaginalis* and *C. albicans*

Usual Dosage Intravaginal: Adults:

Vaginal tablet (ovule): Insert 1 tablet/day at bedtime for 10 consecutive days. May repeat for an additional 10 days if cure is not achieved.

Vaginal cream: Insert 1 applicatorful daily at bedtime for 10 consecutive days. May repeat for an additional 10 days if cure is not achieved.

Note: If *Trichomonas vaginalis* is not completely eliminated, oral (systemic) metronidazole (250 mg twice daily for 10 days) should be administered.

Dosage Forms [CAN] = Canadian brand name
Cream, vaginal:
Flagystatin® [CAN]: Metronidazole 500 mg and nystatin 100,000 units per applicatorful (55 g) [not available in the U.S.]
Tablet, vaginal:
Flagystatin® Ovule [CAN]: Metronidazole 500 mg and nystatin 100,000 units (10s) [not available in the U.S.]

metronidazole, bismuth subcitrate potassium, and tetracycline *see* bismuth, metronidazole, and tetracycline *on page 113*

metronidazole, bismuth subsalicylate, and tetracycline *see* bismuth, metronidazole, and tetracycline *on page 113*

metronidazole hydrochloride *see* metronidazole *on page 563*

metyrapone (me TEER a pone)
Sound-Alike/Look-Alike Issues
metyrapone may be confused with metyrosine
U.S./Canadian Brand Names Metopirone® [US]
Therapeutic Category Diagnostic Agent
Use Diagnostic test for hypothalamic-pituitary ACTH function
Usual Dosage Oral:
Children: 15 mg/kg every 4 hours for 6 doses; minimum dose: 250 mg
Adults: 750 mg every 4 hours for 6 doses
Dosage Forms
Capsule:
Metopirone®: 250 mg

metyrosine (me TYE roe seen)
Sound-Alike/Look-Alike Issues
metyrosine may be confused with metyrapone
Synonyms AMPT; OGMT
U.S./Canadian Brand Names Demser® [US/Can]
Therapeutic Category Tyrosine Hydroxylase Inhibitor
Use Short-term management of pheochromocytoma before surgery, long-term management when surgery is contraindicated or when chronic malignant pheochromocytoma exists
Usual Dosage Oral: Children >12 years and Adults: Initial: 250 mg 4 times/day, increased by 250-500 mg/day up to 4 g/day; maintenance: 2-3 g/day in 4 divided doses; for preoperative preparation, administer optimum effective dosage for 5-7 days
Dosage Forms
Capsule:
Demser®: 250 mg

Mevacor® [US/Can] *see* lovastatin *on page 520*

mevinolin *see* lovastatin *on page 520*

Mexar™ Wash [US] *see* sulfacetamide *on page 810*

mexiletine (meks IL e teen)
U.S./Canadian Brand Names Novo-Mexiletine [Can]
Therapeutic Category Antiarrhythmic Agent, Class I-B
Use Management of serious ventricular arrhythmias; suppression of PVCs
Usual Dosage Oral: Adults: Initial: 200 mg every 8 hours (may load with 400 mg if necessary); adjust dose every 2-3 days; usual dose: 200-300 mg every 8 hours; maximum dose: 1.2 g/day (some patients respond to every 12-hour dosing). When switching from another antiarrhythmic, initiate a 200 mg dose 6-12 hours after stopping former agents, 3-6 hours after stopping procainamide.
Dosage Forms
Capsule: 150 mg, 200 mg, 250 mg

Mexitil® *(Discontinued)* *see* mexiletine *on this page*

MG 217® [US-OTC] *see* coal tar *on page 208*

MG 217® Medicated Tar [US-OTC] *see* coal tar *on page 208*

MG217 Sal-Acid® **[US-OTC]** *see* salicylic acid *on page 772*

Miacalcin® **[US]** *see* calcitonin *on page 135*

Miacalcin® **NS [Can]** *see* calcitonin *on page 135*

Mi-Acid [US-OTC] *see* aluminum hydroxide, magnesium hydroxide, and simethicone *on page 37*

Mi-Acid™ **Double Strength [US-OTC]** *see* calcium carbonate and magnesium hydroxide *on page 139*

Mi-Acid Maximum Strength [US-OTC] *see* aluminum hydroxide, magnesium hydroxide, and simethicone *on page 37*

Micaderm® **[US-OTC]** *see* miconazole *on this page*

micafungin (mi ka FUN gin)

Synonyms micafungin sodium

U.S./Canadian Brand Names Mycamine® [US]

Therapeutic Category Antifungal Agent, Parental; Drug-induced Neuritis, Treatment Agent

Use Esophageal candidiasis; *Candida* prophylaxis in patients undergoing hematopoietic stem cell transplant

Usual Dosage I.V.: Adults:

Esophageal candidiasis: 150 mg daily; median duration of therapy (from clinical trials) was 14 days

Prophylaxis of *Candida* infection in hematopoietic stem cell transplantation: 50 mg daily; median duration of therapy (from clinical trials) was 18 days

Dosage Forms

Injection, powder for reconstitution [preservative-free]:

Mycamine®: 50 mg, 100 mg [contains lactose]

micafungin sodium *see* micafungin *on this page*

Micanol® **[Can]** *see* anthralin *on page 57*

Micardis® **[US/Can]** *see* telmisartan *on page 823*

Micardis® **HCT [US]** *see* telmisartan and hydrochlorothiazide *on page 823*

Micardis® **Plus [Can]** *see* telmisartan and hydrochlorothiazide *on page 823*

Micatin® **[Can]** *see* miconazole *on this page*

Micatin® **Athlete's Foot [US-OTC]** *see* miconazole *on this page*

Micatin® **Jock Itch [US-OTC]** *see* miconazole *on this page*

miconazole (mi KON a zole)

Sound-Alike/Look-Alike Issues

miconazole may be confused with Micronase®, Micronor®

Lotrimin® may be confused with Lotrisone®, Otrivin®

Micatin® may be confused with Miacalcin®

Synonyms miconazole nitrate

U.S./Canadian Brand Names Aloe Vesta® 2-n-1 Antifungal [US-OTC]; Baza® Antifungal [US-OTC]; Carrington Antifungal [US-OTC]; DermaFungal [US-OTC]; Dermagran® AF [US-OTC]; Dermazole [Can]; DiabetAid™ Antifungal Foot Bath [US-OTC]; Fungoid® Tincture [US-OTC]; Lotrimin® AF Jock Itch Powder Spray [US-OTC]; Lotrimin® AF Powder/Spray [US-OTC]; Micaderm® [US-OTC]; Micatin® Athlete's Foot [US-OTC]; Micatin® Jock Itch [US-OTC]; Micatin® [Can]; Micozole [Can]; Micro-Guard® [US-OTC]; Mitrazol™ [US-OTC]; Monistat® 1 Combination Pack [US-OTC]; Monistat® 3 Combination Pack [US-OTC]; Monistat® 3 [US-OTC/Can]; Monistat® 7 [US-OTC]; Monistat® [Can]; Neosporin® AF [US-OTC]; Podactin Cream [US-OTC]; Secura® Antifungal [US-OTC]; Zeasorb®-AF [US-OTC]

Therapeutic Category Antifungal Agent

Use Treatment of vulvovaginal candidiasis and a variety of skin and mucous membrane fungal infections

Usual Dosage

Topical: Children and Adults: **Note:** Not for OTC use in children <2 years:

Tinea corporis: Apply twice daily for 4 weeks

Tinea pedis: Apply twice daily for 4 weeks

Effervescent tablet: Dissolve 1 tablet in ~1 gallon of water; soak feet for 15-30 minutes; pat dry

Tinea cruris: Apply twice daily for 2 weeks

Vaginal: Children ≥12 years and Adults: Vulvovaginal candidiasis:

Cream, 2%: Insert 1 applicatorful at bedtime for 7 days

Cream, 4%: Insert 1 applicatorful at bedtime for 3 days

Suppository, 100 mg: Insert 1 suppository at bedtime for 7 days

Suppository, 200 mg: Insert 1 suppository at bedtime for 3 days

Suppository, 1200 mg: Insert 1 suppository (a one-time dose); may be used at bedtime or during the day

Note: Many products are available as a combination pack, with a suppository for vaginal instillation and cream to relieve external symptoms. External cream may be used twice daily, as needed, for up to 7 days.

Dosage Forms

Combination products: Miconazole vaginal suppository 200 mg (3s) and miconazole external cream 2%
Monistat® 1 Combination Pack: Miconazole vaginal insert 1200 mg (1) and miconazole external cream 2% (5 g) [**Note:** Do not confuse with 1-Day™ (formerly Monistat® 1) which contains tioconazole]
Monistat® 3 Combination Pack:
 Miconazole vaginal insert 200 mg (3s) and miconazole external cream 2%
 Miconazole vaginal cream 4% and miconazole external cream 2%
Monistat® 7 Combination Pack:
 Miconazole vaginal suppository 100 mg (7s) and miconazole external cream 2%
 Miconazole vaginal cream 2% (7 prefilled applicators) and miconazole external cream 2%
Cream, topical: 2% (15 g, 30 g, 45 g)
 Baza® Antifungal: 2% (4 g, 57 g, 142 g)
 Carrington Antifungal: 2% (150 g)
 Micaderm®, Neosporin® AF, Podactin: 2% (30 g)
 Micatin® Athlete's Foot, Micatin® Jock Itch: 2% (15 g)
 Micro-Guard®, Mitrazol™: 2% (60 g)
 Secura® Antifungal: 2% (60 g, 98 g)
Cream, vaginal [prefilled or refillable applicator]: 2% (45 g)
 Monistat® 3: 4% (15 g, 25 g)
 Monistat® 7: 2% (45 g)
Liquid, spray, topical:
 Micatin® Athlete's Foot: 2% (90 mL)
 Neosporin AF®: 2% (105 mL)
Lotion, powder:
 Zeasorb®-AF: 2% (56 g)
Ointment, topical:
 Aloe Vesta® 2-n-1 Antifungal: 2% (60 g, 150 g)
 DermaFungal: 2% (113 g)
 Dermagran® AF: (113 g)
Powder, topical:
 Lotrimin® AF: 2% (160 g)
 Micro-Guard®: 2% (90 g)
 Mitrazol™: 2% (30 g)
 Zeasorb®-AF: 2% (70 g)
Powder spray, topical:
 Lotrimin® AF, Lotrimin® AF Jock Itch: 2% (140 g)
 Micatin® Athlete's Foot, Micatin® Jock Itch: 2% (90 g)
 Neosporin® AF: 2% (85 g)
Suppository, vaginal: 100 mg (7s); 200 mg (3s)
 Monistat® 3: 200 mg (3s)
 Monistat® 7: 100 mg (7s)
Tablet, for solution, topical [effervescent]:
 DiabetAid™ Antifungal Foot Bath: 2% (10s)
Tincture, topical:
 Fungoid®: 2% (30 mL, 473 mL)

miconazole and zinc oxide (mi KON a zole & zink OKS ide)
Synonyms zinc oxide and miconazole nitrate
U.S./Canadian Brand Names Vusion™ [US]
Therapeutic Category Antifungal Agent, Topical
Use Adjunctive treatment of diaper dermatitis complicated by *Candida albicans* infection
Usual Dosage Topical: Children ≥4 weeks: Diaper dermatitis: Apply to affected area with each diaper change for 7 days. Treatment should continue for 7 days, even with initial improvement. Do not use for >7 days.
Dosage Forms
 Ointment, topical:
  Vusion®: Miconazole 0.25% and zinc oxide 15% (60 g)

miconazole nitrate *see* miconazole *on previous page*

Micozole [Can] *see* miconazole *on previous page*

MICRhoGAM® [US] *see* Rh₀(D) immune globulin *on page 753*

microfibrillar collagen hemostat *see* collagen hemostat *on page 213*

Microgestin™ [US] *see* ethinyl estradiol and norethindrone *on page 328*

Microgestin™ Fe [US] *see* ethinyl estradiol and norethindrone *on page 328*

Micro-Guard® [US-OTC] *see* miconazole *on page 566*

microK® [US] *see* potassium chloride *on page 700*

microK® 10 [US] *see* potassium chloride *on page 700*

Micro-K Extencaps® [Can] *see* potassium chloride *on page 700*

Micro-K® LS *(Discontinued) see* potassium chloride *on page 700*

Microlipid™ [US-OTC] *see* nutritional formula, enteral/oral *on page 622*

Micronase® [US] *see* glyburide *on page 396*

microNefrin® *(Discontinued) see* epinephrine *on page 300*

Micronor® [Can] *see* norethindrone *on page 611*

Microzide™ [US] *see* hydrochlorothiazide *on page 426*

Midamor® *(Discontinued) see* amiloride *on page 41*

midazolam (MID aye zoe lam)

Sound-Alike/Look-Alike Issues
Versed® may be confused with VePesid®, Vistaril®

Synonyms midazolam hydrochloride

U.S./Canadian Brand Names Apo-Midazolam® [Can]; Midazolam Injection [Can]

Therapeutic Category Benzodiazepine

Controlled Substance C-IV

Use Preoperative sedation and provides conscious sedation prior to diagnostic or radiographic procedures; ICU sedation (continuous infusion); intravenous anesthesia (induction); intravenous anesthesia (maintenance)

Usual Dosage The dose of midazolam needs to be individualized based on the patient's age, underlying diseases, and concurrent medications. Decrease dose (by ~30%) if narcotics or other CNS depressants are administered concomitantly. **Personnel and equipment needed for standard respiratory resuscitation should be immediately available during midazolam administration.**

Children <6 years may require higher doses and closer monitoring than older children; calculate dose on ideal body weight

Conscious sedation for procedures or preoperative sedation:

Oral: 0.25-0.5 mg/kg as a single dose preprocedure, up to a maximum of 20 mg; administer 30-45 minutes prior to procedure. Children <6 years or less cooperative patients may require as much as 1 mg/kg as a single dose; 0.25 mg/kg may suffice for children 6-16 years of age.

I.M.: 0.1-0.15 mg/kg 30-60 minutes before surgery or procedure; range 0.05-0.15 mg/kg; doses up to 0.5 mg/kg have been used in more anxious patients; maximum total dose: 10 mg

I.V.:

Infants <6 months: Limited information is available in nonintubated infants; dosing recommendations not clear; infants <6 months are at higher risk for airway obstruction and hypoventilation; titrate dose in small increments to desired effect; monitor carefully

Infants 6 months to Children 5 years: Initial: 0.05-0.1 mg/kg; titrate dose carefully; total dose of 0.6 mg/kg may be required; usual maximum total dose: 6 mg

Children 6-12 years: Initial: 0.025-0.05 mg/kg; titrate dose carefully; total doses of 0.4 mg/kg may be required; usual maximum total dose: 10 mg

Children 12-16 years: Dose as adults; usual maximum total dose: 10 mg

Conscious sedation during mechanical ventilation: Children: Loading dose: 0.05-0.2 mg/kg, followed by initial continuous infusion: 0.06-0.12 mg/kg/hour (1-2 mcg/kg/minute); titrate to the desired effect; usual range: 0.4-6 mcg/kg/minute

Adults:

Preoperative sedation:

I.M.: 0.07-0.08 mg/kg 30-60 minutes prior to surgery/procedure; usual dose: 5 mg; **Note:** Reduce dose in patients with COPD, high-risk patients, patients ≥60 years of age, and patients receiving other narcotics or CNS depressants

I.V.: 0.02-0.04 mg/kg; repeat every 5 minutes as needed to desired effect or up to 0.1-0.2 mg/kg

Conscious sedation: I.V.: Initial: 0.5-2 mg slow I.V. over at least 2 minutes; slowly titrate to effect by repeating doses every 2-3 minutes if needed; usual total dose: 2.5-5 mg

Healthy Adults <60 years: Some patients respond to doses as low as 1 mg; no more than 2.5 mg should be administered over a period of 2 minutes. Additional doses of midazolam may be administered after a 2-minute waiting period and evaluation of sedation after each dose increment. A total dose >5 mg is generally not needed. If narcotics or other CNS depressants are administered concomitantly, the midazolam dose should be reduced by 30%.

Anesthesia: I.V.:
Induction:
 Unpremedicated patients: 0.3-0.35 mg/kg (up to 0.6 mg/kg in resistant cases)
 Premedicated patients: 0.15-0.35 mg/kg
 Maintenance: 0.05-0.3 mg/kg as needed, or continuous infusion 0.25-1.5 mcg/kg/minute
 Sedation in mechanically-ventilated patients: I.V. continuous infusion: 100 mg in 250 mL D_5W or NS (if patient is fluid-restricted, may concentrate up to a maximum of 0.5 mg/mL); initial dose: 0.02-0.08 mg/kg ($\sim$1 mg to 5 mg in 70 kg adult) initially and either repeated at 5-15 minute intervals until adequate sedation is achieved or continuous infusion rates of 0.04-0.2 mg/kg/hour and titrate to reach desired level of sedation

Dosage Forms
 Injection, solution: 1 mg/mL (2 mL, 5 mL, 10 mL); 5 mg/mL (1 mL, 2 mL, 5 mL, 10 mL)
 Injection, solution [preservative free]: 1 mg/mL (2 mL, 5 mL); 5 mg/mL (1 mL, 2 mL)
 Syrup: 2 mg/mL

midazolam hydrochloride *see* midazolam *on previous page*

Midazolam Injection [Can] *see* midazolam *on previous page*

midodrine (MI doe dreen)
 Sound-Alike/Look-Alike Issues
  ProAmatine® may be confused with protamine
 Synonyms midodrine hydrochloride
 U.S./Canadian Brand Names Amatine® [Can]; Apo-Midodrine® [Can]; Orvaten™ [US]; ProAmatine® [US]
 Therapeutic Category Alpha-Adrenergic Agonist
 Use Orphan drug: Treatment of symptomatic orthostatic hypotension
 Usual Dosage Oral: Adults: 10 mg 3 times/day during daytime hours (every 3-4 hours) when patient is upright (maximum: 40 mg/day)
 Dosage Forms
  Tablet: 2.5 mg, 5 mg, 10 mg
  Orvaten™, ProAmatine®: 2.5 mg, 5 mg, 10 mg

midodrine hydrochloride *see* midodrine *on this page*

Midol® Cramp and Body Aches [US-OTC] *see* ibuprofen *on page 444*

Midol® Extended Relief [US] *see* naproxen *on page 591*

Midrin® [US] *see* acetaminophen, isometheptene, and dichloralphenazone *on page 13*

Mifeprex® [US] *see* mifepristone *on this page*

mifepristone (mi FE pris tone)
 Sound-Alike/Look-Alike Issues
  Mifeprex® may be confused with Mirapex®
 Synonyms RU-486; RU-38486
 U.S./Canadian Brand Names Mifeprex® [US]
 Therapeutic Category Abortifacient; Antineoplastic Agent, Hormone Antagonist; Antiprogestin
 Use Medical termination of intrauterine pregnancy, through day 49 of pregnancy. Patients may need treatment with misoprostol and possibly surgery to complete therapy
 Usual Dosage Oral: Adults:
  Termination of pregnancy: Treatment consists of three office visits by the patient; the patient must read medication guide and sign patient agreement prior to treatment:
  Day 1: 600 mg (three 200 mg tablets) taken as a single dose under physician supervision
  Day 3: Patient must return to the healthcare provider 2 days following administration of mifepristone; unless abortion has occurred (confirmed using ultrasound or clinical examination): 400 mcg (two 200 mcg tablets) of misoprostol; patient may need treatment for cramps or gastrointestinal symptoms at this time
  Day 14: Patient must return to the healthcare provider $\sim$14 days after administration of mifepristone; confirm complete termination of pregnancy by ultrasound or clinical exam. Surgical termination is recommended to manage treatment failures.
 Dosage Forms
  Tablet:
  Mifeprex®: 200 mg

Migergot [US] *see* ergotamine and caffeine *on page 307*

miglitol (MIG li tol)
U.S./Canadian Brand Names Glyset® [US/Can]
Therapeutic Category Antidiabetic Agent, Oral
Use Type 2 diabetes mellitus (noninsulin-dependent, NIDDM):
Monotherapy adjunct to diet to improve glycemic control in patients with type 2 diabetes mellitus (noninsulin-dependent, NIDDM) whose hyperglycemia cannot be managed with diet alone
Combination therapy with a sulfonylurea when diet plus either miglitol or a sulfonylurea alone do not result in adequate glycemic control. The effect of miglitol to enhance glycemic control is additive to that of sulfonylureas when used in combination.
Usual Dosage Oral: Adults: 25 mg 3 times/day with the first bite of food at each meal; the dose may be increased to 50 mg 3 times/day after 4-8 weeks; maximum recommended dose: 100 mg 3 times/day
Dosage Forms
Tablet:
Glyset®: 25 mg, 50 mg, 100 mg

miglustat (MIG loo stat)
Synonyms OGT-918
U.S./Canadian Brand Names Zavesca® [US/Can]
Therapeutic Category Enzyme Inhibitor
Use Treatment of mild-to-moderate type 1 Gaucher disease when enzyme replacement therapy is not a therapeutic option
Usual Dosage Oral: Adults: Type 1 Gaucher disease: 100 mg 3 times/day; dose may be reduced to 100 mg 1-2 times/day in patients with adverse effects (ie, tremor, GI distress)
Dosage Forms
Capsule:
Zavesca®: 100 mg

Migquin *(Discontinued)* see acetaminophen, isometheptene, and dichloralphenazone on page 13

Migranal® **[US/Can]** see dihydroergotamine on page 260

Migrapap® *(Discontinued)* see acetaminophen, isometheptene, and dichloralphenazone on page 13

Migratine [US] see acetaminophen, isometheptene, and dichloralphenazone on page 13

Migrazone® *(Discontinued)* see acetaminophen, isometheptene, and dichloralphenazone on page 13

Migrin-A *(Discontinued)* see acetaminophen, isometheptene, and dichloralphenazone on page 13

Mild-C® **[US-OTC]** see ascorbic acid on page 76

milk of magnesia see magnesium hydroxide on page 526

Milontin® *(Discontinued)*

Milophene® **[Can]** see clomiphene on page 203

Milophene® *(Discontinued)* see clomiphene on page 203

milrinone (MIL ri none)
Sound-Alike/Look-Alike Issues
Primacor® may be confused with Primaxin®
Synonyms milrinone lactate
U.S./Canadian Brand Names Milrinone Lactate Injection [Can]; Primacor® [US/Can]
Therapeutic Category Cardiovascular Agent, Other
Use Short-term I.V. therapy of acutely-decompensated heart failure
Usual Dosage I.V.: Adults: Loading dose: 50 mcg/kg administered over 10 minutes followed by a maintenance dose titrated according to the hemodynamic and clinical response
Dosage Forms
Infusion [premixed in D_5W]: 200 mcg/mL (100 mL, 200 mL)
Primacor®: 200 mcg/mL (200 mL)
Injection, solution: 1 mg/mL (10 mL, 20 mL, 50 mL)
Primacor®: 1 mg/mL (10 mL, 20 mL)

milrinone lactate see milrinone on this page

Milrinone Lactate Injection [Can] see milrinone on this page

Miltown® *(Discontinued)* see meprobamate on page 544

Mindal DM *(Discontinued)* see guaifenesin and dextromethorphan on page 402

mineral oil, petrolatum, lanolin, cetyl alcohol, and glycerin *see* lanolin, cetyl alcohol, glycerin, petrolatum, and mineral oil *on page 491*

Minestrin™ 1/20 [Can] *see* ethinyl estradiol and norethindrone *on page 328*

Minidyne® [US-OTC] *see* povidone-iodine *on page 704*

Mini-Gamulin® Rh *(Discontinued)*

Mini-Prenatal [US] *see* vitamins (multiple/prenatal) *on page 896*

Minipress® [US/Can] *see* prazosin *on page 708*

Minirin® [Can] *see* desmopressin acetate *on page 239*

Minitran™ [US/Can] *see* nitroglycerin *on page 608*

Minocin® [Can] *see* minocycline *on this page*

Minocin® PAC [US] *see* minocycline *on this page*

minocycline (mi noe SYE kleen)

Sound-Alike/Look-Alike Issues
Dynacin® may be confused with Dyazide®, Dynabac®, DynaCirc®, Dynapen®
Minocin® may be confused with Indocin®, Lincocin®, Minizide®, Mithracin®, niacin

Synonyms minocycline hydrochloride

U.S./Canadian Brand Names Alti-Minocycline [Can]; Apo-Minocycline® [Can]; Dynacin® [US]; Gen-Minocycline [Can]; Minocin® PAC [US]; Minocin® [Can]; myrac™ [US]; Novo-Minocycline [Can]; PMS-Minocycline [Can]; Rhoxal-minocycline [Can]; Sandoz-Minocycline [Can]; Solodyn™ [US]

Therapeutic Category Tetracycline Derivative

Use Treatment of susceptible bacterial infections of both gram-negative and gram-positive organisms; treatment of anthrax (inhalational, cutaneous, and gastrointestinal); acne; meningococcal (asymptomatic) carrier state; Rickettsial diseases (including Rocky Mountain spotted fever, Q fever); nongonococcal urethritis, gonorrhea; acute intestinal amebiasis

Usual Dosage

Usual dosage range:
Children >8 years: Oral: Initial: 4 mg/kg, followed by 2 mg/kg/dose every 12 hours
Adults: Oral: Initial: 200 mg, followed by 100 mg every 12 hours (maximum: 400 mg/day)

Indication-specific dosing:
Children ≥12 years: **Acne** *(inflammatory, nonnodular, moderate-to-severe)* (Solodyn™): Oral:
45-59 kg: 45 mg once daily
60-90 kg: 90 mg once daily
91-136 kg: 135 mg once daily
Note: Therapy should be continued for 12 weeks. Higher doses do not confer greater efficacy, and safety of use beyond 12 weeks has not been established.

Adults: Oral:
Acne: Capsule or immediate-release tablet: 50-100 mg daily
Inflammatory, nonnodular, moderate-to-severe (Solodyn™):
45-59 kg: 45 mg once daily
60-90 kg: 90 mg once daily
91-136 kg: 135 mg once daily
Note: Therapy should be continued for 12 weeks. Higher doses do not confer greater efficacy, and safety of use beyond 12 weeks has not been established.

Chlamydial or *Ureaplasma urealyticum* infection, uncomplicated: Urethral, endocervical, or rectal: 100 mg every 12 hours for at least 7 days

Gonococcal infection, uncomplicated (males):
Without urethritis or anorectal infection: Initial: 200 mg, followed by 100 mg every 12 hours for at least 4 days (cultures 2-3 days post-therapy)
Urethritis: 100 mg every 12 hours for 5 days

Meningococcal carrier state: 100 mg every 12 hours for 5 days

***Mycobacterium marinum*:** 100 mg every 12 hours for 6-8 weeks

Nocardiosis, cutaneous (non-CNS): 100 mg every 12 hours

Syphilis: Initial: 200 mg, followed by 100 mg every 12 hours for 10-15 days

Dosage Forms
Capsule: 50 mg, 75 mg, 100 mg
Dynacin®: 75 mg, 100 mg
Capsule, pellet filled: 50 mg, 100 mg
Minocin® PAC: 50 mg, 100 mg
Tablet: 50 mg, 75 mg, 100 mg
Dynacin®, myrac™: 50 mg, 75 mg, 100 mg
(Continued)

minocycline *(Continued)*

Tablet, extended release:
Solodyn™: 45 mg, 90 mg, 135 mg

minocycline hydrochloride *see* minocycline *on previous page*

Min-Ovral® [Can] *see* ethinyl estradiol and levonorgestrel *on page 325*

Minox [Can] *see* minoxidil *on this page*

minoxidil *(mi NOKS i dil)*

Sound-Alike/Look-Alike Issues
minoxidil may be confused with metolazone, Monopril®, Noxafil®

U.S./Canadian Brand Names Apo-Gain® [Can]; Minox [Can]; Rogaine® Extra Strength for Men [US-OTC]; Rogaine® for Men [US-OTC]; Rogaine® for Women [US-OTC]; Rogaine® [Can]

Therapeutic Category Topical Skin Product; Vasodilator

Use Management of severe hypertension (usually in combination with a diuretic and beta-blocker); treatment (topical formulation) of alopecia androgenetica in males and females

Usual Dosage
Children <12 years: Hypertension: Oral: Initial: 0.1-0.2 mg/kg once daily; maximum: 5 mg/day; increase gradually every 3 days; usual dosage: 0.25-1 mg/kg/day in 1-2 divided doses; maximum: 50 mg/day
Children >12 years and Adults: Hypertension: Oral: Initial: 5 mg once daily, increase gradually every 3 days (maximum: 100 mg/day); usual dose range (JNC 7): 2.5-80 mg/day in 1-2 divided doses
Adults: Alopecia: Topical: Apply twice daily; 4 months of therapy may be necessary for hair growth.

Dosage Forms
Aerosol, topical [foam]:
Men's Rogaine®: 5% (60 g)
Solution, topical: 2% (60 mL); 5% (60 mL)
Rogaine® for Men [OTC], Rogaine® for Women [OTC]: 2% (60 mL)
Rogaine® Extra Strength for Men [OTC]: 5% (60 mL)
Tablet: 2.5 mg, 10 mg

Mintab DM [US] *see* guaifenesin and dextromethorphan *on page 402*

Mintezol® [US] *see* thiabendazole *on page 836*

Mintox Extra Strength [US-OTC] *see* aluminum hydroxide, magnesium hydroxide, and simethicone *on page 37*

Mintox Plus [US-OTC] *see* aluminum hydroxide, magnesium hydroxide, and simethicone *on page 37*

Mintuss G [US] *see* hydrocodone, phenylephrine, and guaifenesin *on page 431*

Mintuss HC [US] *see* phenylephrine, hydrocodone, and chlorpheniramine *on page 678*

Mintuss MS [US] *see* phenylephrine, hydrocodone, and chlorpheniramine *on page 678*

Minute-Gel® *(Discontinued)* *see* fluoride *on page 361*

Miochol-E® [US/Can] *see* acetylcholine *on page 14*

Miostat® [US/Can] *see* carbachol *on page 146*

MiraLax® [US-OTC] *see* polyethylene glycol 3350 *on page 694*

Mirapex® [US/Can] *see* pramipexole *on page 706*

Mircette® [US] *see* ethinyl estradiol and desogestrel *on page 322*

Mirena® [US/Can] *see* levonorgestrel *on page 502*

mirtazapine *(mir TAZ a peen)*

Sound-Alike/Look-Alike Issues
Remeron® may be confused with Premarin®, Zemuron®

U.S./Canadian Brand Names CO Mirtazapine [Can]; Gen-Mirtazapine [Can]; Novo-Mirtazapine [Can]; PMS-Mirtazapine [Can]; ratio-Mirtazapine [Can]; Remeron SolTab® [US]; Remeron® RD [Can]; Remeron® [US/Can]; Rhoxal-mirtazapine FC [Can]; Rhoxal-mirtazapine [Can]; Riva-Mirtazapine [Can]; Sandoz-Mirtazapine FC [Can]; Sandoz-Mirtazapine [Can]

Therapeutic Category Antidepressant, Alpha-2 Antagonist

Use Treatment of depression

Usual Dosage Oral: Adults: Treatment of depression: Initial: 15 mg nightly, titrate up to 15-45 mg/day with dose increases made no more frequently than every 1-2 weeks; there is an inverse relationship between dose and sedation

Dosage Forms
Tablet: 15 mg, 30 mg, 45 mg
Remeron®: 15 mg, 30 mg, 45 mg
Tablet, orally disintegrating: 15 mg, 30 mg
Remeron SolTab®: 15 mg, 30 mg, 45 mg

misoprostol (mye soe PROST ole)
Sound-Alike/Look-Alike Issues
misoprostol may be confused with metoprolol
Cytotec® may be confused with Cytoxan®, Sytobex®
U.S./Canadian Brand Names Apo-Misoprostol® [Can]; Cytotec® [US]; Novo-Misoprostol [Can]
Therapeutic Category Prostaglandin
Use Prevention of NSAID-induced gastric ulcers; medical termination of pregnancy of ≤49 days (in conjunction with mifepristone)
Usual Dosage Oral: Adults:
Prevention of NSAID-induced gastric ulcers: 200 mcg 4 times/day with food; if not tolerated, may decrease dose to 100 mcg 4 times/day with food or 200 mcg twice daily with food; last dose of the day should be taken at bedtime
Medical termination of pregnancy: Refer to mifepristone monograph.
Dosage Forms
Tablet: 100 mcg, 200 mcg
Cytotec®: 100 mcg, 200 mcg

misoprostol and diclofenac *see diclofenac and misoprostol on page 254*

Mito-Carn® *(Discontinued)* *see levocarnitine on page 499*

mitomycin (mye toe MYE sin)
Sound-Alike/Look-Alike Issues
mitomycin may be confused with mithramycin, mitotane, mitoxantrone
Synonyms mitomycin-C; mitomycin-X; MTC; NSC-26980
U.S./Canadian Brand Names Mutamycin® [US/Can]
Therapeutic Category Antineoplastic Agent
Use Treatment of adenocarcinoma of stomach or pancreas, bladder cancer, breast cancer, or colorectal cancer
Usual Dosage Refer to individual protocols. Adults:
Single agent therapy: I.V.: 20 mg/m^2 every 6-8 weeks
Combination therapy: I.V.: 10 mg/m^2 every 6-8 weeks
Bladder carcinoma: Intravesicular instillation (unapproved route): 20-40 mg instilled into the bladder and retained for 3 hours up to 3 times/week for up to 20 procedures per course
Dosage Forms
Injection, powder for reconstitution: 5 mg, 20 mg, 40 mg
Mutamycin®: 5 mg, 20 mg, 40 mg

mitomycin-X *see mitomycin on this page*

mitomycin-C *see mitomycin on this page*

mitotane (MYE toe tane)
Sound-Alike/Look-Alike Issues
mitotane may be confused with mitomycin
Synonyms NSC-38721; o,p'-DDD
U.S./Canadian Brand Names Lysodren® [US/Can]
Therapeutic Category Antineoplastic Agent
Use Treatment of adrenocortical carcinoma
Usual Dosage Oral: Adults: Adrenocortical carcinoma: Start at 2-6 g/day in 3-4 divided doses, then increase incrementally to 9-10 g/day in 3-4 divided doses (maximum daily dose: 18 g)
Dosage Forms
Tablet [scored]:
Lysodren®: 500 mg

mitoxantrone (mye toe ZAN trone)
Sound-Alike/Look-Alike Issues
mitoxantrone may be confused with methotrexate, mitomycin
Synonyms DAD; DHAD; DHAQ; dihydroxyanthracenedione dihydrochloride; mitoxantrone hydrochloride CL-232315; mitozantrone; NSC-301739
(Continued)

mitoxantrone *(Continued)*

U.S./Canadian Brand Names Mitoxantrone Injection® [Can]; Novantrone® [US/Can]

Therapeutic Category Antineoplastic Agent

Use Treatment of acute leukemias, lymphoma, breast cancer, pediatric sarcoma, secondary progressive or relapsing-remitting multiple sclerosis, prostate cancer

Usual Dosage Refer to individual protocols. I.V. (dilute in D_5W or NS): Adults:

Acute leukemias:

Induction: 12 mg/m^2 once daily for 3 days; for incomplete response, may repeat at 12 mg/m^2 once daily for 2 days

Consolidation: 12 mg/m^2 once daily for 2 days, repeat in 4 weeks

Solid tumors: 12-14 mg/m^2 every 3-4 weeks **or** 2-4 mg/m^2/day for 5 days every 4 weeks

Hormone-refractory prostate cancer: 12-14 mg/m^2 every 3 weeks

Multiple sclerosis: 12 mg/m^2 every 3 months (maximum lifetime cumulative dose: 140 mg/m^2

Dosage Forms

Injection, solution: 2 mg/mL (10 mL, 12.5 mL, 15 mL)

Novantrone®: 2 mg/mL (10 mL, 15 mL)

mitoxantrone hydrochloride CL-232315 *see* mitoxantrone *on previous page*

Mitoxantrone Injection® [Can] *see* mitoxantrone *on previous page*

mitozantrone *see* mitoxantrone *on previous page*

Mitran® Oral *(Discontinued)* *see* chlordiazepoxide *on page 173*

Mitrazol™ [US-OTC] *see* miconazole *on page 566*

Mivacron® [Can] *see* mivacurium *on this page*

Mivacron® *(Discontinued)* *see* mivacurium *on this page*

mivacurium *(mye va KYOO ree um)*

Sound-Alike/Look-Alike Issues

Mivacron® may be confused with Mevacor®

Synonyms mivacurium chloride

U.S./Canadian Brand Names Mivacron® [Can]

Therapeutic Category Skeletal Muscle Relaxant

Use Adjunct to general anesthesia to facilitate endotracheal intubation and to relax skeletal muscles during surgery; to facilitate mechanical ventilation in ICU patients; does not relieve pain or produce sedation

Usual Dosage Continuous infusion requires an infusion pump; dose to effect; doses will vary due to interpatient variability; use ideal body weight for obese patients

Children 2-12 years (duration of action is shorter and dosage requirements are higher): 0.2 mg/kg I.V. followed by average infusion rate of 14 mcg/kg/minute (range: 5-31 mcg/kg/minute) upon evidence of spontaneous recovery from initial dose

Adults: Initial: I.V.: 0.15-0.25 mg/kg bolus followed by maintenance doses of 0.1 mg/kg at approximately 15-minute intervals; for prolonged neuromuscular block, initial infusion of 9-10 mcg/kg/minute is used upon evidence of spontaneous recovery from initial dose, usual infusion rate of 6-7 mcg/kg/minute (1-15 mcg/kg/minute) under balanced anesthesia; initial dose after succinylcholine for intubation (balanced anesthesia): Adults: 0.1 mg/kg

Pretreatment/priming: 10% of intubating dose given 3-5 minutes before initial dose

mivacurium chloride *see* mivacurium *on this page*

MK-191 *see* pivampicillin *(Canada only) on page 687*

MK383 *see* tirofiban *on page 846*

MK-0431 *see* sitagliptin *on page 789*

MK462 *see* rizatriptan *on page 763*

MK594 *see* losartan *on page 519*

MK0826 *see* ertapenem *on page 308*

MK 869 *see* aprepitant *on page 71*

MLN341 *see* bortezomib *on page 116*

MMF *see* mycophenolate *on page 584*

MMR *see* measles, mumps, and rubella vaccines, combined *on page 533*

M-M-R® II [US/Can] *see* measles, mumps, and rubella vaccines, combined *on page 533*

MMRV *see* measles, mumps, rubella, and varicella virus vaccine *on page 533*

Moban® **[US/Can]** *see* molindone *on next page*

Mobic® **[US/Can]** *see* meloxicam *on page 539*

Mobicox® **[Can]** *see* meloxicam *on page 539*

Mobidin® *(Discontinued)* *see* magnesium salicylate *on page 528*

Mobisyl® **[US-OTC]** *see* trolamine *on page 870*

moclobemide *(Canada only)* (moe KLOE be mide)
U.S./Canadian Brand Names Alti-Moclobemide [Can]; Apo-Moclobemide® [Can]; Dom-Moclobemide [Can]; Manerix® [Can]; Novo-Moclobemide [Can]; Nu-Moclobemide [Can]; PMS-Moclobemide [Can]
Therapeutic Category Antidepressant, Monoamine Oxidase Inhibitor
Use Symptomatic relief of depressive illness
Usual Dosage Oral: Adults: Initial: 300 mg/day in 2 divided doses; increase gradually to maximum of 600 mg/day; **Note:** Individual patient response may allow a reduction in daily dose in long-term therapy.
Dosage Forms [CAN] = Canadian brand name
  Tablet: 150 mg, 300 mg [not available in the U.S.]
  Alti-Moclobemide [CAN], Apo-Moclobemide® [CAN], Dom-Moclobemide® [CAN], Manerix®e [CAN], Novo-Moclobemidee [CAN], Nu-Moclobemidee [CAN], PMS-Moclobemide [CAN]: 150 mg, 300 mg [not available in the U.S.]

modafinil (moe DAF i nil)
U.S./Canadian Brand Names Alertec® [Can]; Provigil® [US/Can]
Therapeutic Category Central Nervous System Stimulant, Nonamphetamine
Controlled Substance C-IV
Use Improve wakefulness in patients with excessive daytime sleepiness associated with narcolepsy and shift work sleep disorder (SWSD); adjunctive therapy for obstructive sleep apnea/hypopnea syndrome (OSAHS)
Usual Dosage Oral: Adults:
  Narcolepsy, OSAHS: Initial: 200 mg as a single daily dose in the morning
  SWSD: Initial: 200 mg as a single dose taken ~1 hour prior to start of work shift
  Note: Doses of 400 mg/day, given as a single dose, have been well tolerated, but there is no consistent evidence that this dose confers additional benefit
Dosage Forms
  Tablet:
  Provigil®: 100 mg, 200 mg

Modane® **Bulk [US-OTC]** *see* psyllium *on page 732*

Modane® **Soft** *(Discontinued)* *see* docusate *on page 273*

Modecate® **[Can]** *see* fluphenazine *on page 365*

Modecate® **Concentrate [Can]** *see* fluphenazine *on page 365*

Modicon® **[US]** *see* ethinyl estradiol and norethindrone *on page 328*

modified Dakin's solution *see* sodium hypochlorite solution *on page 794*

Modical® **[US-OTC]** *see* glucose polymers *on page 395*

Modulon® **[Can]** *see* trimebutine *(Canada only)* *on page 866*

Moduret [Can] *see* amiloride and hydrochlorothiazide *on page 42*

Moduretic® *(Discontinued)* *see* amiloride and hydrochlorothiazide *on page 42*

moexipril (mo EKS i pril)
Sound-Alike/Look-Alike Issues
  moexipril may be confused with Monopril®
Synonyms moexipril hydrochloride
U.S./Canadian Brand Names Univasc® [US]
Therapeutic Category Angiotensin-Converting Enzyme (ACE) Inhibitor
Use Treatment of hypertension, alone or in combination with thiazide diuretics; treatment of left ventricular dysfunction after myocardial infarction
Usual Dosage Oral: Adults: Initial: 7.5 mg once daily (in patients **not** receiving diuretics), 1 hour prior to a meal **or** 3.75 mg once daily (when combined with thiazide diuretics); maintenance dose: 7.5-30 mg/day in 1 or 2 divided doses 1 hour before meals
Dosage Forms
  Tablet [scored]: 7.5 mg, 15 mg
  Univasc®: 7.5 mg, 15 mg

moexipril and hydrochlorothiazide (mo EKS i pril & hye droe klor oh THYE a zide)

Synonyms hydrochlorothiazide and moexipril

U.S./Canadian Brand Names Uniretic® [US/Can]

Therapeutic Category Angiotensin-Converting Enzyme (ACE) Inhibitor; Diuretic, Thiazide

Use Combination therapy for hypertension, however, not indicated for initial treatment of hypertension; replacement therapy in patients receiving separate dosage forms (for patient convenience); when monotherapy with one component fails to achieve desired antihypertensive effect, or when dose-limiting adverse effects limit upward titration of monotherapy

Usual Dosage Oral: Adults: 7.5-30 mg of moexipril, taken either in a single or divided dose one hour before meals; hydrochlorothiazide dose should be ≤50 mg/day

Dosage Forms

Tablet [scored]:

7.5/12.5: Moexipril 7.5 mg and hydrochlorothiazide 12.5

15/12.5: Moexipril 15 mg and hydrochlorothiazide 12.5

15/25: Moexipril 15 mg and hydrochlorothiazide 25

Uniretic®: 7.5/12.5: Moexipril 7.5 mg and hydrochlorothiazide 12.5 mg; 15/12.5: Moexipril 15 mg and hydrochlorothiazide 12.5 mg; 15/25: Moexipril 15 mg and hydrochlorothiazide 25 mg

moexipril hydrochloride see moexipril on previous page

Mogadon [Can] see nitrazepam (Canada only) on page 607

Moi-Stir® [US-OTC] see saliva substitute on page 774

Moisture® Eyes [US-OTC] see artificial tears on page 75

Moisture® Eyes PM [US-OTC] see artificial tears on page 75

molindone (moe LIN done)

Sound-Alike/Look-Alike Issues

molindone may be confused with Mobidin®

Moban® may be confused with Mobidin®, Modane®

Synonyms molindone hydrochloride

U.S./Canadian Brand Names Moban® [US/Can]

Therapeutic Category Antipsychotic Agent, Dihydroindoline

Use Management of schizophrenia

Usual Dosage Oral: Adults: Schizophrenia/psychoses: 50-75 mg/day increase at 3- to 4-day intervals up to 225 mg/day

Dosage Forms

Tablet:

Moban®: 5 mg, 10 mg, 25 mg, 50 mg

molindone hydrochloride see molindone on this page

molybdenum see trace metals on page 855

Molypen® [US] see trace metals on page 855

MOM see magnesium hydroxide on page 526

Momentum® [US-OTC] see magnesium salicylate on page 528

mometasone (moe MET a sone)

Sound-Alike/Look-Alike Issues

Elocon® lotion may be confused with ophthalmic solutions. Manufacturer's labeling emphasizes the product is **NOT** for use in the eyes.

Synonyms mometasone furoate

U.S./Canadian Brand Names Asmanex® Twisthaler® [US]; Elocom® [Can]; Elocon® [US]; Nasonex® [US/Can]; PMS-Mometasone [Can]; ratio-Mometasone [Can]; Taro-Mometasone [Can]

Therapeutic Category Corticosteroid, Intranasal; Corticosteroid, Topical

Use Relief of the inflammatory and pruritic manifestations of corticosteroid-responsive dermatoses (medium potency topical corticosteroid); treatment of nasal symptoms of seasonal and perennial allergic rhinitis; prevention of nasal symptoms associated with seasonal allergic rhinitis; treatment of nasal polyps in adults; maintenance treatment of asthma as prophylactic therapy or as a supplement in asthma patients requiring oral corticosteroids for the purpose of decreasing or eliminating the oral corticosteroid requirement

Usual Dosage

Oral inhalation: Children ≥12 years and Adults: Previous therapy:

Bronchodilators or inhaled corticosteroids: Initial: 1 inhalation (220 mcg) daily (maximum 2 inhalations or 440 mcg/day); may be given in the evening or in divided doses twice daily

Oral corticosteroids: Initial: 440 mcg twice daily (maximum 880 mcg/day); prednisone should be reduced no faster than 2.5 mg/day on a weekly basis, beginning after at least 1 week of mometasone furoate use

Note: Maximum effects may not be evident for 1-2 weeks or longer; dose should be titrated to effect, using the lowest possible dose

Nasal spray:

Allergic rhinitis:

Children 2-11 years: 1 spray (50 mcg) in each nostril daily

Children ≥12 years and Adults: 2 sprays (100 mcg) in each nostril daily; when used for the prevention of allergic rhinitis, treatment should begin 2-4 weeks prior to pollen season

Nasal polyps: Adults: 2 sprays (100 mcg) in each nostril twice daily; 2 sprays (100 mcg) once daily may be effective in some patients

Topical: Apply sparingly, do not use occlusive dressings. Therapy should be discontinued when control is achieved; if no improvement is seen in 2 weeks, reassessment of diagnosis may be necessary.

Cream, ointment: Children ≥2 years and Adults: Apply a thin film to affected area once daily; do not use in pediatric patients for longer than 3 weeks

Lotion: Children ≥12 years and Adults: Apply a few drops to affected area once daily

Dosage Forms

Cream, topical: 0.1% (15 g, 45 g)

Elocon®: 0.1% (15 g, 45 g)

Lotion, topical: 0.1% (30 mL, 60 mL)

Elocon®: 0.1% (30 mL, 60 mL)

Ointment, topical: 0.1% (15 g, 45 g)

Elocon®: 0.1% (15 g, 45 g)

Powder for oral inhalation:

Asmanex® Twisthaler®: 220 mcg (14 units, 30 units, 60 units, 120 units)

Suspension, intranasal [spray]:

Nasonex®: 50 mcg/spray (17 g)

mometasone furoate *see* mometasone *on previous page*

MOM/mineral oil emulsion *see* magnesium hydroxide and mineral oil *on page 527*

monacolin K *see* lovastatin *on page 520*

Monafed® *(Discontinued) see* guaifenesin *on page 401*

Monafed® DM *(Discontinued) see* guaifenesin and dextromethorphan *on page 402*

Monarc-M™ [US] *see* antihemophilic factor (human) *on page 58*

Monilia skin test *see* Candida albicans (Monilia) *on page 144*

Monistat® [Can] *see* miconazole *on page 566*

Monistat® 1 Combination Pack [US-OTC] *see* miconazole *on page 566*

Monistat® 3 [US-OTC/Can] *see* miconazole *on page 566*

Monistat® 3 Combination Pack [US-OTC] *see* miconazole *on page 566*

Monistat® 7 [US-OTC] *see* miconazole *on page 566*

Monistat-Derm® *(Discontinued) see* miconazole *on page 566*

Monistat i.v.™ Injection *(Discontinued) see* miconazole *on page 566*

Monitan® [Can] *see* acebutolol *on page 4*

monobenzone (mon oh BEN zone)

U.S./Canadian Brand Names Benoquin® [US]

Therapeutic Category Topical Skin Product

Use Final depigmentation in extensive vitiligo

Usual Dosage Topical: Children ≥12 years and Adults: Apply 2-3 times daily; once desired degree of pigmentation is obtained, may apply as needed (usually 2 times/week)

Dosage Forms

Cream, topical:

Benoquin®: 20% (35 g)

Monocaps [US-OTC] *see* vitamins (multiple/oral) *on page 895*

Monoclate-P® [US] *see* antihemophilic factor (human) *on page 58*

monoclonal antibody *see* muromonab-CD3 *on page 583*

Monocor® [Can] *see* bisoprolol *on page 114*

Monodox® [US] *see* doxycycline *on page 281*

monoethanolamine *see* ethanolamine oleate *on page 322*

Monoket® [US] *see* isosorbide mononitrate *on page 476*

MonoNessa™ [US] *see* ethinyl estradiol and norgestimate *on page 331*

Mononine® [US/Can] *see* factor IX *on page 340*

Monopril® [US/Can] *see* fosinopril *on page 376*

Monopril-HCT® [US/Can] *see* fosinopril and hydrochlorothiazide *on page 376*

montelukast (mon te LOO kast)

Sound-Alike/Look-Alike Issues
Singulair® may be confused with Sinequan®
Synonyms montelukast sodium
U.S./Canadian Brand Names Singulair® [US/Can]
Therapeutic Category Leukotriene Receptor Antagonist
Use Prophylaxis and chronic treatment of asthma; relief of symptoms of seasonal allergic rhinitis and perennial allergic rhinitis; prevention of exercise-induced bronchospasm
Usual Dosage Oral:
Children:
6-23 months: Perennial allergic rhinitis: 4 mg (oral granules) once daily
12-23 months: Asthma: 4 mg (oral granules) once daily, taken in the evening
2-5 years: Asthma, seasonal or perennial allergic rhinitis: 4 mg (chewable tablet or oral granules) once daily, taken in the evening
6-14 years: Asthma, seasonal or perennial allergic rhinitis: 5 mg (chewable tablet) once daily, taken in the evening
Children ≥15 years and Adults:
Asthma, seasonal or perennial allergic rhinitis: 10 mg/day, taken in the evening
Bronchoconstriction, exercise-induced (prevention): 10 mg at least 2 hours prior to exercise; additional doses should not be administered within 24 hours. Daily administration to prevent exercise-induced bronchoconstriction has not been evaluated.
Dosage Forms
Granules:
Singulair®: 4 mg/packet
Tablet:
Singulair®: 10 mg
Tablet, chewable:
Singulair®: 4 mg, 5 mg

montelukast sodium *see* montelukast *on this page*

Monurol™ [US/Can] *see* fosfomycin *on page 375*

8-MOP® [US/Can] *see* methoxsalen *on page 555*

more attenuated enders strain *see* measles virus vaccine (live) *on page 534*

MoreDophilus® [US-OTC] *see* Lactobacillus *on page 488*

moricizine (mor I siz een)

Sound-Alike/Look-Alike Issues
Ethmozine® may be confused with Erythrocin®, erythromycin
Synonyms moricizine hydrochloride
U.S./Canadian Brand Names Ethmozine® [US/Can]
Therapeutic Category Antiarrhythmic Agent, Class I
Use Treatment of ventricular tachycardia and life-threatening ventricular arrhythmias
Usual Dosage Oral: Adults: 200-300 mg every 8 hours, adjust dosage at 150 mg/day at 3-day intervals.

moricizine hydrochloride *see* moricizine *on this page*

morning after pill *see* ethinyl estradiol and norgestrel *on page 332*

Morphine HP® [Can] *see* morphine sulfate *on this page*

Morphine LP® Epidural [Can] *see* morphine sulfate *on this page*

morphine sulfate (MOR feen SUL fate)

Sound-Alike/Look-Alike Issues
morphine may be confused with hydromorphone
morphine sulfate may be confused with magnesium sulfate
MSO$_4$ is an error-prone abbreviation (mistaken as magnesium sulfate)

Avinza® may be confused with Evista®, Invanz®

Roxanol™ may be confused with OxyFast®, Roxicet™

U.S./Canadian Brand Names Astramorph/PF™ [US]; Avinza® [US]; DepoDur™ [US]; Duramorph® [US]; Infumorph® [US]; Kadian® [US/Can]; M-Eslon® [Can]; M.O.S.-SR® [Can]; M.O.S.-Sulfate® [Can]; M.O.S.® 10 [Can]; M.O.S.® 20 [Can]; M.O.S.® 30 [Can]; Morphine HP® [Can]; Morphine LP® Epidural [Can]; MS Contin® [US/Can]; MS-IR® [Can]; Oramorph SR® [US]; PMS-Morphine Sulfate SR [Can]; ratio-Morphine SR [Can]; Roxanol™ [US]; Statex® [Can]; Zomorph® [Can]

Therapeutic Category Analgesic, Narcotic

Controlled Substance C-II

Use Relief of moderate to severe acute and chronic pain; relief of pain of myocardial infarction; relief of dyspnea of acute left ventricular failure and pulmonary edema; preanesthetic medication

DepoDur™: Epidural (lumbar) single-dose management of surgical pain

Infumorph®: Used in microinfusion devices for intraspinal administration in treatment of intractable chronic pain

Usual Dosage Note: These are guidelines and do not represent the doses that may be required in all patients. Doses should be titrated to pain relief/prevention.

Children >6 months and <50 kg: Acute pain (moderate-to-severe):

Oral (prompt release): 0.15-0.3 mg/kg every 3-4 hours as needed

I.M.: 0.1 mg/kg every 3-4 hours as needed

I.V.: 0.05-0.1 mg/kg every 3-4 hours as needed

I.V. infusion: Range: 10-30 mcg/kg/hour

Adolescents >12 years: Sedation/analgesia for procedures: I.V.: 3-4 mg and repeat in 5 minutes if necessary

Adults:

Acute pain (moderate-to-severe):

Oral: Prompt release formulations: Opiate-naive: Initial: 10 mg every 3-4 hours as needed; patients with prior opiate exposure may require higher initial doses: usual dosage range: 10-30 mg every 3-4 hours as needed

I.M., SubQ: **Note:** Repeated SubQ administration causes local tissue irritation, pain, and induration.

Initial: Opiate-naive: 5-10 mg every 3-4 hours as needed; patients with prior opiate exposure may require higher initial doses; usual dosage range: 5-20 mg every 3-4 hours as needed

Rectal: 10-20 mg every 3-4 hours

I.V.: Initial: Opiate-naive: 2.5-5 mg every 3-4 hours; patients with prior opiate exposure may require higher initial doses. **Note:** Repeated doses (up to every 5 minutes if needed) in small increments (eg, 1-4 mg) may be preferred to larger and less frequent doses.

I.V., SubQ continuous infusion: 0.8-10 mg/hour; usual range: Up to 80 mg/hour

Mechanically-ventilated patients (based on 70 kg patient): 0.7-10 mg every 1-2 hours as needed; infusion: 5-35 mg/hour

Patient-controlled analgesia (PCA): (Opiate-naive: Consider lower end of dosing range):

Usual concentration: 1 mg/mL

Demand dose: Usual: 1 mg; range: 0.5-2.5 mg

Lockout interval: 5-10 minutes

Intrathecal (I.T.): **Note:** Administer with extreme caution and in reduced dosage to geriatric or debilitated patients.

Opioid-naive: 0.2-0.25 mg/dose (may provide adequate relief for 24 hours); repeat doses are **not** recommended.

Epidural: **Note:** Administer with extreme caution and in reduced dosage to geriatric or debilitated patients. Vigilant monitoring is particularly important in these patients.

Pain management:

Single-dose (Duramorph®): Initial: 3-5 mg

Infusion:

Bolus dose: 1-6 mg

Infusion rate: 0.1-0.2 mg/hour

Maximum dose: 10 mg/24 hours

Surgical anesthesia: Epidural: Single-dose (extended-release, Depo-Dur™): Lumbar epidural only; not recommended in patients <18 years of age:

Cesarean section: 10 mg

Lower abdominal/pelvic surgery: 10-15 mg

Major orthopedic surgery of lower extremity: 15 mg

For Depo-Dur™: To minimize the pharmacokinetic interaction resulting in higher peak serum concentrations of morphine, administer the test dose of the local anesthetic at least 15 minutes prior to Depo-Dur™ administration. Use of Depo-Dur™ with epidural local anesthetics has not been studied. Other medications should not be administered into the epidural space for at least 48 hours after administration of DepoDur™.

Note: Some patients may benefit from a 20 mg dose, however, the incidence of adverse effects may be increased.

Chronic pain: Note: Patients taking opioids chronically may become tolerant and require doses higher than the usual dosage range to maintain the desired effect. Tolerance can be managed by appropriate dose (Continued)

579

morphine sulfate (Continued)

titration. There is no optimal or maximal dose for morphine in chronic pain. The appropriate dose is one that relieves pain throughout its dosing interval without causing unmanageable side effects.

Oral: Controlled-, extended-, or sustained-release formulations: A patient's morphine requirement should be established using prompt-release formulations. Conversion to long-acting products may be considered when chronic, continuous treatment is required. Higher dosages should be reserved for use only in opioid-tolerant patients.

Capsules, extended-release (Avinza™): Daily dose administered once daily (for best results, administer at same time each day)

Capsules, sustained-release (Kadian®): Daily dose administered once daily or in 2 divided doses daily (every 12 hours)

Tablets, controlled-release (MS Contin®), sustained-release (Oramorph SR®), or extended-release: Daily dose divided and administered every 8 or every 12 hours

Dosage Forms
Capsule, extended release:
Avinza®: 30 mg, 60 mg, 90 mg, 120 mg
Capsule, sustained release:
Kadian®: 20 mg, 30 mg, 50 mg, 60 mg, 80 mg, 100 mg, 200 mg
Infusion [premixed in D_5W]: 1 mg/mL (100 mL, 250 mL)
Injection, extended release liposomal suspension [lumbar epidural injection, preservative free]:
DepoDur™: 10 mg/mL (1 mL, 1.5 mL, 2 mL)
Injection, solution: 2 mg/mL (1 mL); 4 mg/mL (1 mL); 5 mg/mL (1 mL); 8 mg/mL (1 mL); 10 mg/0.7 mL (0.7 mL); 10 mg/mL (1 mL, 10 mL); 15 mg/mL (1 mL, 20 mL); 25 mg/mL (4 mL, 10 mL, 20 mL, 40 mL, 50 mL, 100 mL, 250 mL); 50 mg/mL (20 mL, 40 mL)
Injection, solution [epidural, intrathecal, or I.V. infusion; preservative free]:
Astramorph/PF™: 0.5 mg/mL (2 mL, 10 mL); 1 mg/mL (2 mL, 10 mL)
Duramorph®: 0.5 mg/mL (10 mL); 1 mg/mL (10 mL)
Injection, solution [epidural or intrathecal infusion via microinfusion device; preservative free]: 10 mg/mL (20 mL); 25 mg/mL (20 mL)
Infumorph®: 10 mg/mL (20 mL); 25 mg/mL (20 mL)
Injection, solution [I.V. infusion via PCA pump]: 0.5 mg/mL (30 mL); 1 mg/mL (30 mL, 50 mL); 2 mg/mL (30 mL); 5 mg/mL (30 mL, 50 mL)
Injection, solution [preservative free]: 0.5 mg/mL (10 mL); 1 mg/mL (10 mL); 25 mg/mL (4 mL, 10 mL, 20 mL)
Solution, oral: 10 mg/5 mL, 20 mg/5 mL, 20 mg/mL
Roxanol™: 20 mg/mL
Solution, oral [concentrate]: 5 mg/0.25 mL (0.25 mL); 10 mg/0.5 mL (0.5 mL); 20 mg/mL (1 mL)
Suppository, rectal: 5 mg (12s), 10 mg (12s), 20 mg (12s), 30 mg (12s)
Tablet: 10 mg, 15 mg, 30 mg
Tablet, controlled release:
MS Contin®: 15 mg, 30 mg, 60 mg, 100 mg, 200 mg
Tablet, extended release: 15 mg, 30 mg, 60 mg, 100 mg, 200 mg
Tablet, sustained release:
Oramorph SR®: 15 mg, 30 mg, 60 mg, 100 mg

morrhuate sodium (MOR yoo ate SOW dee um)
U.S./Canadian Brand Names Scleromate® [US]
Therapeutic Category Sclerosing Agent
Use Treatment of small, uncomplicated varicose veins of the lower extremities
Usual Dosage I.V.: Adults: 50-250 mg, repeated at 5- to 7-day intervals (50-100 mg for small veins, 150-250 mg for large veins)
Dosage Forms
Injection, solution: 50 mg/mL (30 mL)
Scleromate®: 50 mg/mL (30 mL)

M.O.S.® 10 [Can] see morphine sulfate on page 578

M.O.S.® 20 [Can] see morphine sulfate on page 578

M.O.S.® 30 [Can] see morphine sulfate on page 578

Mosco® Corn and Callus Remover [US-OTC] see salicylic acid on page 772

M.O.S.-SR® [Can] see morphine sulfate on page 578

M.O.S.-Sulfate® [Can] see morphine sulfate on page 578

Motilium® [Can] see domperidone (Canada only) on page 276

Motofen® [US] see difenoxin and atropine on page 256

Motrin® **[US]** *see* ibuprofen *on page 444*

Motrin® **Children's [US-OTC/Can]** *see* ibuprofen *on page 444*

Motrin® **Cold and Sinus [US-OTC]** *see* pseudoephedrine and ibuprofen *on page 729*

Motrin® **Cold, Children's [US-OTC]** *see* pseudoephedrine and ibuprofen *on page 729*

Motrin® **IB [US-OTC/Can]** *see* ibuprofen *on page 444*

Motrin® **IB Sinus** *(Discontinued)* *see* pseudoephedrine and ibuprofen *on page 729*

Motrin® **Infants' [US-OTC]** *see* ibuprofen *on page 444*

Motrin® **Junior Strength [US-OTC]** *see* ibuprofen *on page 444*

Mouthkote® **[US-OTC]** *see* saliva substitute *on page 774*

MoviPrep® **[US]** *see* polyethylene glycol-electrolyte solution *on page 695*

moxifloxacin (moxs i FLOKS a sin)

Sound-Alike/Look-Alike Issues
Avelox® may be confused with Avonex®

Synonyms moxifloxacin hydrochloride

U.S./Canadian Brand Names Avelox® I.V. [US/Can]; Avelox® [US/Can]; Vigamox™ [US/Can]

Therapeutic Category Antibiotic, Quinolone

Use Treatment of mild-to-moderate community-acquired pneumonia, including multidrug-resistant *Streptococcus pneumoniae* (MDRSP); acute bacterial exacerbation of chronic bronchitis; acute bacterial sinusitis; complicated and uncomplicated skin and skin structure infections; complicated intraabdominal infections; bacterial conjunctivitis (ophthalmic formulation)

Usual Dosage
Usual dosage range:
Children ≥1 year and Adults: Ophthalmic: Instill 1 drop into affected eye(s) 3 times/day for 7 days
Adults: Oral, I.V.: 400 mg every 24 hours

Indication-specific dosing:
Children ≥1 year and Adults: Ophthalmic:
Bacterial conjunctivitis: Instill 1 drop into affected eye(s) 3 times/day for 7 days
Adults: Oral, I.V.:
Acute bacterial sinusitis: 400 mg every 24 hours for 10 days
Chronic bronchitis, acute bacterial exacerbation: 400 mg every 24 hours for 5 days
Intraabdominal infections (complicated): 400 mg every 24 hours for 5-14 days (initiate with I.V.)
Pneumonia, community-acquired (including MDRSP): 400 mg every 24 hours for 7-14 days
Skin and skin structure infections:
Complicated: 400 mg every 24 hours for 7-21 days
Uncomplicated: 400 mg every 24 hours for 7 days

Dosage Forms
Infusion [premixed in sodium chloride 0.8%]:
Avelox® I.V.: 400 mg (250 mL)
Solution, ophthalmic:
Vigamox™: 0.5% (3 mL)
Tablet:
Avelox®: 400 mg
Avelox® ABC Pack [unit-dose pack]: 400 mg (5s)

moxifloxacin hydrochloride *see* moxifloxacin *on this page*

4-MP *see* fomepizole *on page 373*

6-MP *see* mercaptopurine *on page 545*

MPA *see* mycophenolate *on page 584*

MPA and estrogens (conjugated) *see* estrogens (conjugated/equine) and medroxyprogesterone *on page 318*

M-Prednisol® **Injection** *(Discontinued)* *see* methylprednisolone *on page 559*

MPSV4 *see* meningococcal polysaccharide vaccine (groups A / C / Y and W-135) *on page 540*

MS Contin® **[US/Can]** *see* morphine sulfate *on page 578*

MS-IR® **[Can]** *see* morphine sulfate *on page 578*

MTA *see* pemetrexed *on page 660*

MTC *see* mitomycin *on page 573*

M.T.E.-4® **[US]** *see* trace metals *on page 855*

MUMPS VIRUS VACCINE, LIVE, ATTENUATED

M.T.E.-5® **[US]** *see* trace metals *on page 855*

M.T.E.-6® **[US]** *see* trace metals *on page 855*

M.T.E.-7® **[US]** *see* trace metals *on page 855*

Mucinex® **[US-OTC]** *see* guaifenesin *on page 401*

Mucinex®-D [US-OTC] *see* guaifenesin and pseudoephedrine *on page 406*

Mucinex® D Maximum Strength [US-OTC] *see* guaifenesin and pseudoephedrine *on page 406*

Mucinex®, Children's [US-OTC] *see* guaifenesin *on page 401*

Mucinex® Children's Cough [US-OTC] *see* guaifenesin and dextromethorphan *on page 402*

Mucinex®, Children's Mini-Melts™ [US-OTC] *see* guaifenesin *on page 401*

Mucinex® DM [US-OTC] *see* guaifenesin and dextromethorphan *on page 402*

Mucinex® DM Maximum Strength [US-OTC] *see* guaifenesin and dextromethorphan *on page 402*

Mucinex®, Junior Mini-Melts™ [US-OTC] *see* guaifenesin *on page 401*

Mucinex® Maximum Strength [US-OTC] *see* guaifenesin *on page 401*

Mucomyst® [Can] *see* acetylcysteine *on page 15*

Mucosil™ *(Discontinued) see* acetylcysteine *on page 15*

Multidex® [US-OTC] *see* maltodextrin *on page 530*

Multihance® [US] *see* gadobenate dimeglumine *on page 380*

Multihance® Multipak™ [US] *see* gadobenate dimeglumine *on page 380*

multiple vitamins *see* vitamins (multiple/oral) *on page 895*

multitargeted antifolate *see* pemetrexed *on page 660*

Multitest CMI® *(Discontinued)*

Multitrace™-4 [US] *see* trace metals *on page 855*

Multitrace™-4 Neonatal [US] *see* trace metals *on page 855*

Multitrace™-4 Pediatric [US] *see* trace metals *on page 855*

Multitrace™-5 [US] *see* trace metals *on page 855*

multivitamins/fluoride *see* vitamins (multiple/pediatric) *on page 896*

mumps, measles, and rubella vaccines, combined *see* measles, mumps, and rubella vaccines, combined *on page 533*

mumps, rubella, varicella, and measles vaccine *see* measles, mumps, rubella, and varicella virus vaccine *on page 533*

Mumpsvax® [US] *see* mumps virus vaccine, live, attenuated *on this page*

mumps virus vaccine, live, attenuated (mumpz VYE rus vak SEEN, live, a ten YOO ate ed)

U.S./Canadian Brand Names Mumpsvax® [US]

Therapeutic Category Vaccine, Live Virus

Use Mumps prophylaxis by promoting active immunity

Note: Trivalent measles-mumps-rubella (MMR) vaccine is the preferred agent for most children and many adults; persons born prior to 1957 are generally considered immune and need not be vaccinated

Usual Dosage SubQ: Children ≥12-15 months and Adults: 0.5 mL as a single dose

Dosage Forms

Injection, powder for reconstitution [preservative free]:
Mumpsvax®: $TCID_{50}$ 20,000

mupirocin (myoo PEER oh sin)

Sound-Alike/Look-Alike Issues

Bactroban® may be confused with bacitracin, baclofen

Synonyms mupirocin calcium; pseudomonic acid A

U.S./Canadian Brand Names Bactroban® Nasal [US]; Bactroban® [US/Can]; Centany™ [US]

Therapeutic Category Antibiotic, Topical

Use

Intranasal: Eradication of nasal colonization with MRSA in adult patients and healthcare workers

Topical: Treatment of impetigo or secondary infected traumatic skin lesions due to *S. aureus* and *S. pyogenes*

Usual Dosage
Intranasal: Children ≥12 years and Adults: Eradication of nasal MRSA: Approximately one-half of the ointment from the single-use tube should be applied into one nostril and the other half into the other nostril twice daily for 5 days

Topical:
Children ≥2 months and Adults: Impetigo: Ointment: Apply to affected area 3 times/day; re-evaluate after 3-5 days if no clinical response

Children ≥3 months and Adults: Secondary skin infections: Cream: Apply to affected area 3 times/day for 10 days; re-evaluate after 3-5 days if no clinical response

Dosage Forms
Cream, topical:
Bactroban®: 2% (15 g, 30 g)
Ointment, intranasal, topical:
Bactroban® Nasal: 2% (1 g)
Ointment, topical: 2% (0.9 g, 22 g)
Bactroban®: 2% (22 g)
Centany™: 2% (15 g, 30 g)

mupirocin calcium see mupirocin on previous page

Murine® Ear Wax Removal System [US-OTC] see carbamide peroxide on page 148

Murine® Tears [US-OTC] see artificial tears on page 75

Murine® Tears Plus [US-OTC] see tetrahydrozoline on page 832

Muro 128® [US-OTC] see sodium chloride on page 792

Murocel® [US-OTC] see artificial tears on page 75

Murocoll-2® [US] see phenylephrine and scopolamine on page 677

muromonab-CD3 (myoo roe MOE nab see dee three)
Synonyms monoclonal antibody; OKT3
U.S./Canadian Brand Names Orthoclone OKT® 3 [US/Can]
Therapeutic Category Immunosuppressant Agent
Use Treatment of acute allograft rejection in renal transplant patients; treatment of acute hepatic, kidney, and pancreas rejection episodes resistant to conventional treatment. Acute graft-versus-host disease following bone marrow transplantation resistant to conventional treatment.
Usual Dosage I.V. (refer to individual protocols):
Children <30 kg: 2.5 mg/day once daily for 7-14 days
Children >30 kg: 5 mg/day once daily for 7-14 days
OR
Children <12 years: 0.1 mg/kg/day once daily for 10-14 days
Children ≥12 years and Adults: 5 mg/day once daily for 10-14 days
Dosage Forms
Injection, solution:
Orthoclone OKT® 3: 1 mg/mL (5 mL)

Muroptic-5® *(Discontinued)* see sodium chloride on page 792

Muse® [US] see alprostadil on page 33

Muse® Pellet [Can] see alprostadil on page 33

Mustargen® [US/Can] see mechlorethamine on page 535

mustine see mechlorethamine on page 535

Mutamycin® [US/Can] see mitomycin on page 573

M.V.I.®-12 *(Discontinued)* see vitamins (multiple/injectable) on page 895

M.V.I. Adult™ [US] see vitamins (multiple/injectable) on page 895

M.V.I® Pediatric [US] see vitamins (multiple/injectable) on page 895

Myadec® [US-OTC] see vitamins (multiple/oral) on page 895

Myambutol® [US] see ethambutol on page 321

Mycamine® [US] see micafungin on page 566

Mycelex® [US] see clotrimazole on page 206

Mycelex®-7 [US-OTC] see clotrimazole on page 206

Mycelex®-G *(Discontinued)* see clotrimazole on page 206

Mycelex® Twin Pack [US-OTC] *see* clotrimazole *on page 206*

Mycifradin® Sulfate *(Discontinued)* *see* neomycin *on page 596*

Mycinaire™ [US-OTC] *see* sodium chloride *on page 792*

Mycinettes® [US-OTC] *see* benzocaine *on page 101*

Mycobutin® [US/Can] *see* rifabutin *on page 757*

Mycocide® NS [US-OTC] *see* tolnaftate *on page 849*

Mycolog®-II *(Discontinued)* *see* nystatin and triamcinolone *on page 623*

Myco-Nail [US-OTC] *see* triacetin *on page 861*

Myconel® Topical *(Discontinued)* *see* nystatin and triamcinolone *on page 623*

mycophenolate (mye koe FEN oh late)

Synonyms MMF; MPA; mycophenolate mofetil; mycophenolate sodium; mycophenolic acid

U.S./Canadian Brand Names CellCept® [US/Can]; Myfortic® [US/Can]

Therapeutic Category Immunosuppressant Agent

Use Prophylaxis of organ rejection concomitantly with cyclosporine and corticosteroids in patients receiving allogenic renal (CellCept®, Myfortic®), cardiac (CellCept®), or hepatic (CellCept®) transplants

Usual Dosage

Children: Renal transplant: Oral:
CellCept® suspension: 600 mg/m²/dose twice daily; maximum dose: 1 g twice daily
Alternatively, may use solid dosage forms according to BSA as follows:
BSA 1.25-1.5 m²: 750 mg capsule twice daily
BSA >1.5 m²: 1 g capsule or tablet twice daily
Myfortic®: 400 mg/m²/dose twice daily; maximum dose: 720 mg twice daily
BSA <1.19 m²: Use of this formulation is not recommended
BSA 1.19-1.58 m²: 540 mg twice daily (maximum: 1080 mg/day)
BSA >1.58 m²: 720 mg twice daily (maximum: 1440 mg/day)

Adults:
Renal transplant:
CellCept®:
Oral: 1 g twice daily. Doses >2 g/day are not recommended.
I.V.: 1 g twice daily
Myfortic®: Oral: 720 mg twice daily (1440 mg/day)
Cardiac transplantation:
Oral (CellCept®): 1.5 g twice daily
I.V. (CellCept®): 1.5 g twice daily
Hepatic transplantation:
Oral (CellCept®): 1.5 g twice daily
I.V. (CellCept®): 1 g twice daily

Dosage Forms

Capsule:
CellCept®: 250 mg

Injection, powder for reconstitution:
CellCept®: 500 mg

Powder for oral suspension:
CellCept®: 200 mg/mL

Tablet:
CellCept®: 500 mg

Tablet, delayed release:
Myfortic®: 180 mg, 360 mg

mycophenolate mofetil *see* mycophenolate *on this page*

mycophenolate sodium *see* mycophenolate *on this page*

mycophenolic acid *see* mycophenolate *on this page*

Mycostatin® [US] *see* nystatin *on page 623*

Mydfrin® [US/Can] *see* phenylephrine *on page 675*

Mydral™ [US] *see* tropicamide *on page 871*

Mydriacyl® [US/Can] *see* tropicamide *on page 871*

My First Flintstones® [US-OTC] *see* vitamins (multiple/pediatric) *on page 896*

Myfortic® [US/Can] *see* mycophenolate *on this page*

MyKidz Iron FL™ [US-OTC] *see* vitamins (multiple/pediatric) *on page 896*

Mykrox® *(Discontinued)* *see* metolazone *on page 562*

Mylanta™ [Can] *see* aluminum hydroxide and magnesium hydroxide *on page 37*

Mylanta®-II *(Discontinued)* *see* aluminum hydroxide, magnesium hydroxide, and simethicone *on page 37*

Mylanta AR® *(Discontinued)* *see* famotidine *on page 341*

Mylanta® Children's [US-OTC] *see* calcium carbonate *on page 138*

Mylanta® Double Strength [Can] *see* aluminum hydroxide, magnesium hydroxide, and simethicone *on page 37*

Mylanta® Extra Strength [Can] *see* aluminum hydroxide, magnesium hydroxide, and simethicone *on page 37*

Mylanta® Gas [US-OTC] *see* simethicone *on page 786*

Mylanta® Gas Maximum Strength [US-OTC] *see* simethicone *on page 786*

Mylanta® Gelcaps® [US-OTC] *see* calcium carbonate and magnesium hydroxide *on page 139*

Mylanta® Liquid [US-OTC] *see* aluminum hydroxide, magnesium hydroxide, and simethicone *on page 37*

Mylanta® Maximum Strength Liquid [US-OTC] *see* aluminum hydroxide, magnesium hydroxide, and simethicone *on page 37*

Mylanta® Regular Strength [Can] *see* aluminum hydroxide, magnesium hydroxide, and simethicone *on page 37*

Mylanta® Supreme [US-OTC] *see* calcium carbonate and magnesium hydroxide *on page 139*

Mylanta® Ultra [US-OTC] *see* calcium carbonate and magnesium hydroxide *on page 139*

Myleran® [US/Can] *see* busulfan *on page 129*

Mylicon® Infants [US-OTC] *see* simethicone *on page 786*

Mylocel™ [US] *see* hydroxyurea *on page 439*

Mylotarg® [US/Can] *see* gemtuzumab ozogamicin *on page 388*

Myminic® Expectorant *(Discontinued)*

Myobloc® [US] *see* botulinum toxin type B *on page 117*

Myochrysine® [US/Can] *see* gold sodium thiomalate *on page 398*

Myoflex® [US-OTC/Can] *see* trolamine *on page 870*

Myotonachol® [Can] *see* bethanechol *on page 110*

Myotonachol® *(Discontinued)* *see* bethanechol *on page 110*

Myozyme® [US] *see* alglucosidase alfa *on page 29*

Myphetane DX [US] *see* brompheniramine, pseudoephedrine, and dextromethorphan *on page 122*

myrac™ [US] *see* minocycline *on page 571*

Mysoline® [US] *see* primidone *on page 714*

Mytelase® [US/Can] *see* ambenonium *on page 39*

Mytrex *(Discontinued)* *see* nystatin and triamcinolone *on page 623*

Mytussin® AC [US] *see* guaifenesin and codeine *on page 402*

Mytussin® DAC [US] *see* guaifenesin, pseudoephedrine, and codeine *on page 408*

N-9 *see* nonoxynol 9 *on page 610*

N-0923 *see* rotigotine *on page 769*

Na2EDTA *see* edetate disodium *on page 291*

Nabi-HB® [US] *see* hepatitis B immune globulin *on page 417*

NAB-paclitaxel *see* paclitaxel (protein bound) *on page 646*

nabumetone (na BYOO me tone)

U.S./Canadian Brand Names Apo-Nabumetone® [Can]; Gen-Nabumetone [Can]; Novo-Nabumetone [Can]; Relafen® [Can]; Rhoxal-nabumetone [Can]; Sandoz-Nabumetone [Can]

Therapeutic Category Analgesic, Nonnarcotic; Nonsteroidal Antiinflammatory Drug (NSAID)

Use Management of osteoarthritis and rheumatoid arthritis

Usual Dosage Oral: Adults: 1000 mg/day; an additional 500-1000 mg may be needed in some patients to obtain more symptomatic relief; may be administered once or twice daily (maximum dose: 2000 mg/day)

Note: Patients <50 kg are less likely to require doses >1000 mg/day.

Dosage Forms Tablet: 500 mg, 750 mg

NAC *see* acetylcysteine *on page 15*

n-acetyl-L-cysteine *see* acetylcysteine *on page 15*

n-acetylcysteine *see* acetylcysteine *on page 15*

n-acetyl-p-aminophenol *see* acetaminophen *on page 5*

NaCl *see* sodium chloride *on page 792*

nadolol (NAY doe lol)
Sound-Alike/Look-Alike Issues
nadolol may be confused with Mandol®
Corgard® may be confused with Cognex®
U.S./Canadian Brand Names Alti-Nadolol [Can]; Apo-Nadol® [Can]; Corgard® [US/Can]; Novo-Nadolol [Can]
Therapeutic Category Beta-Adrenergic Blocker
Use Treatment of hypertension and angina pectoris; prophylaxis of migraine headaches
Usual Dosage Oral: Adults: Initial: 40 mg/day, increase dosage gradually by 40-80 mg increments at 3- to 7-day intervals until optimum clinical response is obtained with profound slowing of heart rate; doses up to 160-240 mg/day in angina and 240-320 mg/day in hypertension may be necessary.
Hypertension: Usual dosage range (JNC 7): 40-120 mg once daily
Dosage Forms
Tablet: 20 mg, 40 mg, 80 mg, 120 mg, 160 mg
Corgard®: 20 mg, 40 mg, 80 mg

nadolol and bendroflumethiazide (NAY doe lol & ben droe floo meth EYE a zide)
Synonyms bendroflumethiazide and nadolol
U.S./Canadian Brand Names Corzide® [US]
Therapeutic Category Antihypertensive Agent, Combination; Beta-Adrenergic Blocker, Nonselective; Diuretic, Thiazide
Use Treatment of hypertension; combination product should not be used for initial therapy
Usual Dosage Oral: Adults: Treatment of hypertension: Initial: Nadolol 40 mg and bendroflumethiazide 5 mg once daily. May increase dose to nadolol 80 mg and bendroflumethiazide 5 mg once daily if needed.
Dosage Forms
Tablet [scored]:
Corzide®: 40/5: Nadolol 40 mg and bendroflumethiazide 5 mg; 80/5: Nadolol 80 mg and bendroflumethiazide 5 mg

nadroparin calcium *see* nadroparin *(Canada only)* *on this page*

nadroparin *(Canada only)* (nad roe PA rin)
Synonyms nadroparin calcium
U.S./Canadian Brand Names Fraxiparine™ Forte [Can]; Fraxiparine™ [Can]
Therapeutic Category Low Molecular Weight Heparin
Use Prophylaxis of thromboembolic disorders (particularly deep venous thrombosis and pulmonary embolism) in general and orthopedic surgery; treatment of deep venous thrombosis; prevention of clotting during hemodialysis
Usual Dosage SubQ: Adults:
Prophylaxis of thromboembolic disorders in general surgery: 2850 anti-Xa int. units once daily; begin 2-4 hours before surgery and continue for 7 days
Prophylaxis of thromboembolic disorders in hip replacement: 38 anti-Xa int. units/kg 12 hours before and 12 hours after surgery, **followed by** 38 anti-Xa int. units/kg/day up to and including day 3, **then** 57 anti-Xa int. units/kg/day for up to 10 days total therapy
Treatment of thromboembolic disorders: 171 anti-Xa int. units/kg/day to a maximum of 17,100 int. units; plasma anti-Xa levels should be 1.2-1.8 anti-Xa int. units/mL 3-4 hours postinjection
Patients at increased risk of bleeding: 86 anti-Xa int. units/kg twice daily; plasma anti-Xa levels should be 0.5-1.1 anti-Xa int. units/mL 3-4 hours postinjection
Prevention of clotting during hemodialysis: Single dose of 65 anti-Xa int. units/kg into arterial line at start of each dialysis session; may give additional dose if session lasts longer than 4 hours
Patients at risk of hemorrhage: Administer 50% of dose
Dosage Forms [CAN] = Canadian brand name
Injection, solution:
Fraxiparine™ [CAN]: 9500 anti-Xa int. units/mL (0.2 mL, 0.3 mL, 0.4 mL, 0.6 mL, 0.8 mL, 1 mL) [not available in the U.S.]
Fraxiparine™ Forte [CAN]: 19,000 anti-Xa int. units/mL (0.6 mL, 0.8 mL, 1 mL) [not available in the U.S.]

nafarelin (naf a REL in)

Sound-Alike/Look-Alike Issues
nafarelin may be confused with Anafranil®, enalapril
Synonyms nafarelin acetate
U.S./Canadian Brand Names Synarel® [US/Can]
Therapeutic Category Hormone, Posterior Pituitary
Use Treatment of endometriosis, including pain and reduction of lesions; treatment of central precocious puberty (CPP; gonadotropin-dependent precocious puberty) in children of both sexes
Usual Dosage Intranasal:

Endometriosis: Adults: Female: 1 spray (200 mcg) in 1 nostril each morning and the other nostril each evening starting on days 2-4 of menstrual cycle (total: 2 sprays/day). Dose may be increased to 2 sprays (400 mcg; 1 spray in each nostril) in the morning and evening if amenorrhea is not achieved (total: 8 sprays [1600 mcg]/day). Total duration of therapy should not exceed 6 months due to decreases in bone mineral density; retreatment is not recommended by the manufacturer.

Central precocious puberty: Children: Male/Female: 2 sprays (400 mcg) into each nostril in the morning and 2 sprays (400 mcg) into each nostril in the evening (total: 8 sprays [1600 mcg]/day). If inadequate suppression, may increase dose to 3 sprays (600 mcg) into alternating nostrils 3 times/day (total: 9 sprays [1800 mcg]/day).

Dosage Forms
Solution, intranasal [spray]:
Synarel®: 2 mg/mL (8 mL)

nafarelin acetate *see* nafarelin *on this page*

Nafazair® Ophthalmic *(Discontinued)* *see* naphazoline *on page 590*

nafcillin (naf SIL in)

Synonyms ethoxynaphthamido penicillin sodium; nafcillin sodium; sodium nafcillin
U.S./Canadian Brand Names Nallpen® [Can]; Unipen® [Can]
Therapeutic Category Penicillin
Use Treatment of infections such as osteomyelitis, septicemia, endocarditis, and CNS infections caused by susceptible strains of staphylococci species
Usual Dosage
Usual dosage range:
Neonates: I.M., I.V.:
1200-2000 g, <7 days: 50 mg/kg/day divided every 12 hours
>2000 g, <7 days: 75 mg/kg/day divided every 8 hours
1200-2000 g, ≥7 days: 75 mg/kg/day divided every 8 hours
>2000 g, ≥7 days: 100-140 mg/kg/day divided every 6 hours
Children:
I.M.: 25 mg/kg twice daily
I.V.: 50-200 mg/kg/day in divided doses every 4-6 hours (maximum: 12 g/day)
Adults:
I.M.: 500 mg every 4-6 hours
I.V.: 500-2000 mg every 4-6 hours
Indication-specific dosing:
Children:
Mild-to-moderate infections: I.M., I.V.: 50-100 mg/kg/day in divided doses every 6 hours
Severe infections: I.M., I.V.: 100-200 mg/kg/day in divided doses every 4-6 hours (maximum dose: 12 g/day
Staphylococcal endocarditis: I.V.:
Native valve: 200 mg/kg/day in divided doses every 4-6 hours for 6 weeks
Prosthetic valve: 200 mg/kg/day in divided doses every 4-6 hours for ≥6 weeks (use with rifampin and gentamicin)
Adults: I.V.:
Endocarditis: MSSA:
Native valve: 12 g/24 hours in 4-6 divided doses for 6 weeks
Prosthetic valve: 12 g/24 hours in 4-6 divided doses for ≥6 weeks (use with rifampin and gentamicin)
Joint:
Bursitis, septic: 2 g every 4 hours
Prosthetic: 2 g every 4-6 hours with rifampin for 6 weeks
***Staphylococcus aureus,* methicillin-susceptible infections, including brain abscess, empyema, erysipelas, mastitis, myositis, osteomyelitis, pneumonia, toxic shock, urinary tract (perinephric abscess):** 2 g every 4 hours
(Continued)

nafcillin *(Continued)*

Dosage Forms
Infusion [premixed iso-osmotic dextrose solution]: 1 g (50 mL); 2 g (100 mL)
Injection, powder for reconstitution: 1 g, 2 g, 10 g

nafcillin sodium *see* nafcillin *on previous page*

naftifine *(NAF ti feen)*

Synonyms naftifine hydrochloride
U.S./Canadian Brand Names Naftin® [US]
Therapeutic Category Antifungal Agent
Use Topical treatment of tinea cruris (jock itch), tinea corporis (ringworm), and tinea pedis (athlete's foot)
Usual Dosage Topical: Adults: Apply cream once daily and gel twice daily (morning and evening) for up to 4 weeks
Dosage Forms
Cream:
Naftin®: 1% (15 g, 30 g, 60 g, 90 g)
Gel:
Naftin®: 1% (20 g, 40 g, 60 g, 90 g)

naftifine hydrochloride *see* naftifine *on this page*

Naftin® [US] *see* naftifine *on this page*

Naglazyme™ [US] *see* galsulfase *on page 383*

NaHCO₃ *see* sodium bicarbonate *on page 791*

nalbuphine *(NAL byoo feen)*

Sound-Alike/Look-Alike Issues
Nubain® may be confused with Navane®, Nebcin®
Synonyms nalbuphine hydrochloride
U.S./Canadian Brand Names Nubain® [US]
Therapeutic Category Analgesic, Narcotic
Use Relief of moderate to severe pain; preoperative analgesia, postoperative and surgical anesthesia, and obstetrical analgesia during labor and delivery
Usual Dosage Adults:
Pain management: I.M., I.V., SubQ: 10 mg/70 kg every 3-6 hours; maximum single dose in nonopioid-tolerant patients: 20 mg; maximum daily dose: 160 mg
Surgical anesthesia supplement: I.V.: Induction: 0.3-3 mg/kg over 10-15 minutes; maintenance doses of 0.25-0.5 mg/kg may be given as required
Dosage Forms
Injection, solution: 10 mg/mL (10 mL); 20 mg/mL (10 mL)
Nubain®: 20 mg/mL (10 mL)
Injection, solution [preservative free]: 10 mg/mL (1 mL); 20 mg/mL (1 mL)
Nubain®: 10 mg/mL (1 mL); 20 mg/mL (1 mL)

nalbuphine hydrochloride *see* nalbuphine *on this page*

Nalcrom® [Can] *see* cromolyn sodium *on page 218*

Naldecon® DX Adult Liquid *(Discontinued)*

Naldecon-EX® Children's Syrup *(Discontinued)*

Naldecon Senior EX® *(Discontinued)* *see* guaifenesin *on page 401*

Nalex®-A [US] *see* chlorpheniramine, phenylephrine, and phenyltoloxamine *on page 182*

Nalfon® [US/Can] *see* fenoprofen *on page 345*

Nallpen® [Can] *see* nafcillin *on previous page*

Nallpen® *(Discontinued)* *see* nafcillin *on previous page*

N-allylnoroxymorphine hydrochloride *see* naloxone *on next page*

nalmefene *(NAL me feen)*

Sound-Alike/Look-Alike Issues
Revex® may be confused with Nimbex®, ReVia®, Rubex®

Synonyms nalmefene hydrochloride
U.S./Canadian Brand Names Revex® [US]
Therapeutic Category Antidote
Use Complete or partial reversal of opioid drug effects, including respiratory depression induced by natural or synthetic opioids; reversal of postoperative opioid depression; management of known or suspected opioid overdose
Usual Dosage I.M., I.V., SubQ:
Reversal of postoperative opioid depression: Blue-labeled product (100 mcg/mL): Titrate to reverse the undesired effects of opioids; initial dose for nonopioid dependent patients: 0.25 mcg/kg followed by 0.25 mcg/kg incremental doses at 2- to 5-minute intervals; after a total dose >1 mcg/kg, further therapeutic response is unlikely
Note: In patients with increased cardiovascular risks, dilute 1:1 in NS or SWFI, and initiate/titrate with 0.1 mcg/kg doses.
Management of known/suspected opioid overdose: Green-labeled product (1 mg/mL): Initial dose: 0.5 mg/70 kg; may repeat with 1 mg/70 kg in 2-5 minutes; further increase beyond a total dose of 1.5 mg/70 kg will not likely result in improved response and may result in cardiovascular stress and precipitated withdrawal syndrome. (If opioid dependency is suspected, administer a challenge dose of 0.1 mg/70 kg; if no withdrawal symptoms are observed in 2 minutes, the recommended doses can be administered.)
Note: If recurrence of respiratory depression is noted, dose may again be titrated to clinical effect using incremental doses.
Note: If I.V. access is lost or not readily obtainable, a single SubQ or I.M. dose of 1 mg may be effective in 5-15 minutes.
Dosage Forms
Injection, solution:
Revex®: 100 mcg/mL (1 mL) [blue label]; 1 mg/mL (2 mL) [green label]

nalmefene hydrochloride *see* nalmefene *on previous page*

naloxone (nal OKS one)
Sound-Alike/Look-Alike Issues
naloxone may be confused with naltrexone
Narcan® may be confused with Marcaine®, Norcuron®
Synonyms *N*-allylnoroxymorphine hydrochloride; naloxone hydrochloride
U.S./Canadian Brand Names Naloxone Hydrochloride Injection® [Can]
Therapeutic Category Antidote
Use
Complete or partial reversal of opioid depression, including respiratory depression, induced by natural and synthetic opioids, including propoxyphene, methadone, and certain mixed agonist-antagonist analgesics: nalbuphine, pentazocine, and butorphanol
Diagnosis of suspected opioid tolerance or acute opioid overdose
Adjunctive agent to increase blood pressure in the management of septic shock
Usual Dosage I.M., I.V. (preferred), intratracheal, SubQ:
Postanesthesia narcotic reversal: Infants and Children: 0.01 mg/kg; may repeat every 2-3 minutes, as needed based on response
Opiate intoxication:
Children:
Birth (including premature infants) to 5 years or <20 kg: 0.1 mg/kg; repeat every 2-3 minutes if needed; may need to repeat doses every 20-60 minutes
>5 years or ≥20 kg: 2 mg/dose; if no response, repeat every 2-3 minutes; may need to repeat doses every 20-60 minutes
Children and Adults: Continuous infusion: I.V.: If continuous infusion is required, calculate dosage/hour based on effective intermittent dose used and duration of adequate response seen, titrate dose 0.04-0.16 mg/kg/hour for 2-5 days in children, adult dose typically 0.25-6.25 mg/hour (short-term infusions as high as 2.4 mg/kg/hour have been tolerated in adults during treatment for septic shock); alternatively, continuous infusion utilizes $2/3$ of the initial naloxone bolus on an hourly basis; add 10 times this dose to each liter of D_5W and infuse at a rate of 100 mL/hour; $1/2$ of the initial bolus dose should be readministered 15 minutes after initiation of the continuous infusion to prevent a drop in naloxone levels; increase infusion rate as needed to assure adequate ventilation
Narcotic overdose: Adults: I.V.: 0.4-2 mg every 2-3 minutes as needed; may need to repeat doses every 20-60 minutes, if no response is observed after 10 mg, question the diagnosis. **Note:** Use 0.1-0.2 mg increments in patients who are opioid dependent and in postoperative patients to avoid large cardiovascular changes.
Dosage Forms
Injection, solution: 0.4 mg/mL (1 mL, 10 mL); 1 mg/mL (2 mL)

naloxone and buprenorphine *see* buprenorphine and naloxone *on page 127*

naloxone hydrochloride *see* naloxone *on previous page*

naloxone hydrochloride and pentazocine hydrochloride *see* pentazocine *on page 665*

naloxone hydrochloride dihydrate and buprenorphine hydrochloride *see* buprenorphine and naloxone *on page 127*

Naloxone Hydrochloride Injection® **[Can]** *see* naloxone *on previous page*

naltrexone (nal TREKS one)

Sound-Alike/Look-Alike Issues
naltrexone may be confused with naloxone
ReVia® may be confused with Revex®

Synonyms naltrexone hydrochloride

U.S./Canadian Brand Names Depade® [US]; ReVia® [US/Can]; Vivitrol™ [US]

Therapeutic Category Antidote

Use Treatment of ethanol dependence; blockade of the effects of exogenously administered opioids

Usual Dosage Adults: Do not give until patient is opioid-free for 7-10 days as determined by urinalysis
Oral: Alcohol dependence, opioid antidote: 25 mg; if no withdrawal signs within 1 hour give another 25 mg; maintenance regimen is flexible, variable and individualized (50 mg/day to 100-150 mg 3 times/week for 12 weeks); up to 800 mg/day has been tolerated in a small number of healthy adults without an adverse effect
I.M.: Alcohol dependence: 380 mg once every 4 weeks

Dosage Forms
Injection, powder for suspension [extended-release microspheres]:
Vivitrol™: 380 mg
Tablet: 50 mg
Depade®: 25 mg, 50 mg, 100 mg
ReVia®: 50 mg

naltrexone hydrochloride *see* naltrexone *on this page*

Namenda™ **[US]** *see* memantine *on page 539*

nandrolone (NAN droe lone)

Synonyms nandrolone decanoate; nandrolone phenpropionate

U.S./Canadian Brand Names Deca-Durabolin® [Can]; Durabolin® [Can]

Therapeutic Category Androgen

Controlled Substance C-III

Use Control of metastatic breast cancer; management of anemia of renal insufficiency

Usual Dosage Deep I.M. (into gluteal muscle):
Children 2-13 years (decanoate): 25-50 mg every 3-4 weeks
Adults:
Male:
Breast cancer (phenpropionate): 50-100 mg/week
Anemia of renal insufficiency (decanoate): 100-200 mg/week
Female: 50-100 mg/week
Breast cancer (phenpropionate): 50-100 mg/week
Anemia of renal insufficiency (decanoate): 50-100 mg/week

nandrolone decanoate *see* nandrolone *on this page*

nandrolone phenpropionate *see* nandrolone *on this page*

NAPA and NABZ *see* sodium phenylacetate and sodium benzoate *on page 795*

naphazoline (naf AZ oh leen)

Synonyms naphazoline hydrochloride

U.S./Canadian Brand Names AK-Con™ [US]; Albalon® [US]; Clear eyes® for Dry Eyes and ACR Relief [US-OTC]; Clear eyes® for Dry Eyes and Redness Relief [US-OTC]; Clear eyes® Redness Relief [US-OTC]; Clear eyes® Seasonal Relief [US-OTC]; Naphcon Forte® [Can]; Naphcon® [US-OTC]; Privine® [US-OTC]; Vasocon® [Can]

Therapeutic Category Adrenergic Agonist Agent

Use Topical ocular vasoconstrictor; temporary relief of nasal congestion associated with the common cold, upper respiratory allergies or sinusitis; relief of redness of the eye due to minor irritation

Usual Dosage
Nasal: Children ≥12 years and Adults: 0.05% instill 1-2 drops or sprays every 6 hours if needed; therapy should not exceed 3 days
Ophthalmic: Adults:
0.1% (prescription): 1-2 drops into conjuctival sac every 3-4 hours as needed

0.012% or 0.025% (OTC): 1-2 drops into affected eye(s) up to 4 times a day; therapy should not exceed 3 days

Dosage Forms
   Solution, intranasal drops:
   Privine® [OTC]: 0.05% (25 mL)
   Solution, intranasal spray:
   Privine® [OTC]: 0.05% (20 mL)
   Solution, ophthalmic:
   AK-Con™, Albalon®: 0.1% (15 mL)
   Clear eyes® for Dry Eyes and ACR Relief [OTC]: 0.025% (15 mL)
   Clear eyes® for Dry Eyes and Redness Relief [OTC], Naphcon® [OTC]: 0.012% (15 mL)
   Clear eyes® Redness Relief [OTC]: 0.012% (6 mL, 15 mL, 30 mL)
   Clear eyes® Seasonal Relief [OTC]: 0.012% (15 mL, 30 mL)

naphazoline and pheniramine (naf AZ oh leen & fen NIR a meen)

Sound-Alike/Look-Alike Issues
   Visine® may be confused with Visken®
Synonyms pheniramine and naphazoline
U.S./Canadian Brand Names Naphcon-A® [US-OTC/Can]; Opcon-A® [US-OTC]; Visine-A® [US-OTC]; Visine® Advanced Allergy [Can]
Therapeutic Category Antihistamine/Decongestant Combination
Use Treatment of ocular congestion, irritation, and itching
Usual Dosage Ophthalmic: Children ≥6 years and Adults: 1-2 drops up to 4 times/day
Dosage Forms
   Solution, ophthalmic:
   Naphcon-A®: Naphazoline 0.025% and pheniramine 0.3%
   Opcon-A®: Naphazoline 0.027% and pheniramine 0.3%
   Visine-A®: Naphazoline 0.025% and pheniramine 0.3%

naphazoline hydrochloride *see* naphazoline *on previous page*

Naphcon® [US-OTC] *see* naphazoline *on previous page*

Naphcon-A® [US-OTC/Can] *see* naphazoline and pheniramine *on this page*

Naphcon Forte® [Can] *see* naphazoline *on previous page*

Naphcon Forte® Ophthalmic *(Discontinued)* *see* naphazoline *on previous page*

NapraPAC™ *see* lansoprazole and naproxen *on page 493*

Naprelan® [US] *see* naproxen *on this page*

Naprosyn® [US/Can] *see* naproxen *on this page*

naproxen (na PROKS en)

Sound-Alike/Look-Alike Issues
   naproxen may be confused with Natacyn®, Nebcin®
   Aleve® may be confused with Alesse®
   Anaprox® may be confused with Anaspaz®, Avapro®
   Naprelan® may be confused with Naprosyn®
   Naprosyn® may be confused with Naprelan®, Natacyn®, Nebcin®
Synonyms naproxen sodium
U.S./Canadian Brand Names Aleve® [US-OTC]; Anaprox® DS [US/Can]; Anaprox® [US/Can]; Apo-Napro-Na DS® [Can]; Apo-Napro-Na® [Can]; Apo-Naproxen EC® [Can]; Apo-Naproxen SR® [Can]; Apo-Naproxen® [Can]; EC-Naprosyn® [US]; Gen-Naproxen EC [Can]; Midol® Extended Relief [US]; Naprelan® [US]; Naprosyn® [US/Can]; Naxen® EC [Can]; Naxen® [Can]; Novo-Naproc EC [Can]; Novo-Naprox Sodium DS [Can]; Novo-Naprox Sodium [Can]; Novo-Naprox SR [Can]; Novo-Naprox [Can]; Nu-Naprox [Can]; Pamprin® Maximum Strength All Day Relief [US-OTC]; Riva-Naproxen [Can]
Therapeutic Category Analgesic, Nonnarcotic; Antipyretic; Nonsteroidal Antiinflammatory Drug (NSAID)
Use Management of ankylosing spondylitis, osteoarthritis, and rheumatoid disorders (including juvenile rheumatoid arthritis); acute gout; mild-to-moderate pain; tendonitis, bursitis; dysmenorrhea; fever
Usual Dosage Note: Dosage expressed as naproxen base; 200 mg naproxen base is equivalent to 220 mg naproxen sodium.

Oral:
Children >2 years: Juvenile arthritis: 10 mg/kg/day in 2 divided doses
Adults:
   Gout, acute: Initial: 750 mg, followed by 250 mg every 8 hours until attack subsides. **Note:** EC-Naprosyn® is not recommended.
(Continued)

591

naproxen (Continued)

Pain (mild-to-moderate), dysmenorrhea, acute tendonitis, bursitis: Initial: 500 mg, then 250 mg every 6-8 hours; maximum: 1250 mg/day naproxen base

Rheumatoid arthritis, osteoarthritis, and ankylosing spondylitis: 500-1000 mg/day in 2 divided doses; may increase to 1.5 g/day of naproxen base for limited time period

OTC labeling: Pain/fever:

Children ≥12 years and Adults ≤65 years: 200 mg naproxen base every 8-12 hours; if needed, may take 400 mg naproxen base for the initial dose; maximum: 600 mg naproxen base/24 hours

Adults >65 years: 200 mg naproxen base every 12 hours

Dosage Forms

Caplet: 220 mg

Aleve® [OTC], Midol® Extended Relief, Pamprin® Maximum Strength All Day Relief [OTC]: 220 mg

Capsule, liquid gel: 220 mg

Aleve®: 220 mg

Gelcap: 220 mg

Aleve® [OTC]: 220 mg

Suspension, oral: 125 mg/5 mL

Naprosyn®: 125 mg/5 mL

Tablet: 220 mg, 250 mg, 275 mg, 375 mg, 500 mg, 550 mg

Aleve® [OTC]: 220 mg

Anaprox®: 275 mg

Anaprox® DS: 550 mg

Naprosyn®: 250 mg, 375 mg, 500 mg

Tablet, controlled release: 550 mg

Naprelan®: 421.5 mg, 550 mg

Tablet, delayed release: 375 mg, 500 mg

EC-Naprosyn®: 375 mg, 500 mg

naproxen and lansoprazole *see* lansoprazole and naproxen *on page 493*

naproxen and pseudoephedrine (na PROKS en & soo doe e FED rin)

Synonyms naproxen sodium and pseudoephedrine; pseudoephedrine and naproxen

U.S./Canadian Brand Names Aleve® Cold & Sinus [US-OTC]; Aleve® Sinus & Headache [US-OTC]

Therapeutic Category Decongestant/Analgesic

Use Temporary relief of cold, sinus, and flu symptoms (including nasal congestion, sinus congestion/pressure, headache, minor body aches and pains, and fever)

Usual Dosage Oral: Children ≥12 years and Adults: Aleve® Cold & Sinus, Aleve® Sinus & Headache: One caplet every 12 hours (maximum dose: 2 caplets/24 hours)

Dosage Forms

Caplet, extended release:

Aleve® Cold & Sinus, Aleve ® Sinus & Headache: Naproxen sodium 220 mg [equivalent to naproxen 200 mg and sodium 20 mg] and pseudoephedrine hydrochloride 120 mg

naproxen sodium *see* naproxen *on previous page*

naproxen sodium and pseudoephedrine *see* naproxen and pseudoephedrine *on this page*

naratriptan (NAR a trip tan)

Sound-Alike/Look-Alike Issues

Amerge® may be confused with Altace®, Amaryl®

Synonyms naratriptan hydrochloride

U.S./Canadian Brand Names Amerge® [US/Can]

Therapeutic Category Antimigraine Agent; Serotonin Agonist

Use Treatment of acute migraine headache with or without aura

Usual Dosage Oral: Adults: 1-2.5 mg at the onset of headache; it is recommended to use the lowest possible dose to minimize adverse effects. If headache returns or does not fully resolve, the dose may be repeated after 4 hours; do not exceed 5 mg in 24 hours.

Dosage Forms

Tablet:

Amerge®: 1 mg, 2.5 mg

naratriptan hydrochloride *see* naratriptan *on this page*

Narcan® (Discontinued) *see* naloxone *on page 589*

Nardil® [US/Can] *see* phenelzine *on page 672*

Naropin® **[US/Can]** *see* ropivacaine *on page 766*

Nasacort® **AQ [US/Can]** *see* triamcinolone (inhalation, nasal) *on page 861*

Nasacort® **HFA [US]** *see* triamcinolone (inhalation, nasal) *on page 861*

Nasahist B® *(Discontinued)* *see* brompheniramine *on page 120*

NaSal™ **[US-OTC]** *see* sodium chloride *on page 792*

NasalCrom® **[US-OTC]** *see* cromolyn sodium *on page 218*

Nasalide® **[Can]** *see* flunisolide *on page 359*

Nasal Moist® **[US-OTC]** *see* sodium chloride *on page 792*

Nasarel® **[US]** *see* flunisolide *on page 359*

Nasatab® **LA [US]** *see* guaifenesin and pseudoephedrine *on page 406*

Nascobal® **[US]** *see* cyanocobalamin *on page 220*

Nasex-G **[US]** *see* guaifenesin and phenylephrine *on page 404*

Nasonex® **[US/Can]** *see* mometasone *on page 576*

Nāsop™ **[US]** *see* phenylephrine *on page 675*

Natabec® *(Discontinued)*

Natabec® **FA** *(Discontinued)*

Natabec® **Rx** *(Discontinued)*

NataCaps™ **[US]** *see* vitamins (multiple/prenatal) *on page 896*

NataChew™ **[US]** *see* vitamins (multiple/prenatal) *on page 896*

Natacyn® **[US/Can]** *see* natamycin *on this page*

NataFort® **[US]** *see* vitamins (multiple/prenatal) *on page 896*

NatalCare® **CFe 60** *(Discontinued)* *see* vitamins (multiple/prenatal) *on page 896*

NatalCare® **GlossTabs™ [US]** *see* vitamins (multiple/prenatal) *on page 896*

NatalCare® **PIC [US]** *see* vitamins (multiple/prenatal) *on page 896*

NatalCare® **PIC Forte [US]** *see* vitamins (multiple/prenatal) *on page 896*

NatalCare® **Plus [US]** *see* vitamins (multiple/prenatal) *on page 896*

NatalCare® **Rx [US]** *see* vitamins (multiple/prenatal) *on page 896*

NatalCare® **Three [US]** *see* vitamins (multiple/prenatal) *on page 896*

Natalins® **Rx** *(Discontinued)*

natalizumab (na ta LIZ u mab)
Synonyms AN100226; anti-4 alpha integrin; IgG4-kappa monoclonal antibody
U.S./Canadian Brand Names Tysabri® [US]
Therapeutic Category Monoclonal Antibody, Selective Adhesion-Molecule Inhibitor
Use Treatment of relapsing forms of multiple sclerosis
Usual Dosage I.V.: Adults: Multiple sclerosis: 300 mg infused over 1 hour every 4 weeks
Dosage Forms
Injection, solution [preservative free]:
Tysabri®: 300 mg/15 mL (15 mL)

natamycin (na ta MYE sin)
Sound-Alike/Look-Alike Issues
Natacyn® may be confused with Naprosyn®
Synonyms pimaricin
U.S./Canadian Brand Names Natacyn® [US/Can]
Therapeutic Category Antifungal Agent
Use Treatment of blepharitis, conjunctivitis, and keratitis caused by susceptible fungi (*Aspergillus*, *Candida*), *Cephalosporium*, *Curvularia*, *Fusarium*, *Penicillium*, *Microsporum*, *Epidermophyton*, *Blastomyces dermatitidis*, *Coccidioides immitis*, *Cryptococcus neoformans*, *Histoplasma capsulatum*, *Sporothrix schenckii*, and *Trichomonas vaginalis*
Usual Dosage Ophthalmic: Adults: Instill 1 drop in conjunctival sac every 1-2 hours, after 3-4 days reduce to one drop 6-8 times/day; usual course of therapy is 2-3 weeks.
Dosage Forms
Suspension, ophthalmic:
Natacyn®: 5% (15 mL)

NataTab™ **CFe [US]** *see* vitamins (multiple/prenatal) *on page 896*

NataTab™ **FA [US]** *see* vitamins (multiple/prenatal) *on page 896*

NataTab™ **Rx [US]** *see* vitamins (multiple/prenatal) *on page 896*

nateglinide (na te GLYE nide)
U.S./Canadian Brand Names Starlix® [US/Can]
Therapeutic Category Antidiabetic Agent
Use Management of type 2 diabetes mellitus (noninsulin-dependent, NIDDM) as monotherapy when hyperglycemia cannot be managed by diet and exercise alone; in combination with metformin or a thiazolidinedione to lower blood glucose in patients whose hyperglycemia cannot be controlled by exercise, diet, or a single agent alone
Usual Dosage Oral: Adults: Management of type 2 diabetes mellitus: Initial and maintenance dose: 120 mg 3 times/day, 1-30 minutes before meals; may be given alone or in combination with metformin or a thiazolidinedione; patients close to Hb A_{1c} goal may be started at 60 mg 3 times/day
Dosage Forms
Tablet:
Starlix®: 60 mg, 120 mg

Natrecor® **[US]** *see* nesiritide *on page 600*

natriuretic peptide *see* nesiritide *on page 600*

Natulan® **[Can]** *see* procarbazine *on page 716*

Natural Fiber Therapy [US-OTC] *see* psyllium *on page 732*

natural lung surfactant *see* beractant *on page 106*

Nature's Tears® **[US-OTC]** *see* artificial tears *on page 75*

Nature-Throid® **NT [US]** *see* thyroid *on page 839*

Naus-A-Way® **(Discontinued)**

Nausea Relief [US-OTC] *see* fructose, dextrose, and phosphoric acid *on page 378*

Nauseatol [Can] *see* dimenhydrinate *on page 262*

Nausetrol® **[US-OTC]** *see* fructose, dextrose, and phosphoric acid *on page 378*

Navane® **[US/Can]** *see* thiothixene *on page 838*

Navelbine® **[US/Can]** *see* vinorelbine *on page 891*

Naxen® **[Can]** *see* naproxen *on page 591*

Naxen® **EC [Can]** *see* naproxen *on page 591*

Na-Zone® **[US-OTC]** *see* sodium chloride *on page 792*

NC-722665 *see* bicalutamide *on page 111*

***n*-docosanol** *see* docosanol *on page 273*

Nebcin® **(Discontinued)** *see* tobramycin *on page 846*

NebuPent® **[US]** *see* pentamidine *on page 665*

Necon® **0.5/35 [US]** *see* ethinyl estradiol and norethindrone *on page 328*

Necon® **1/35 [US]** *see* ethinyl estradiol and norethindrone *on page 328*

Necon® **1/50 [US]** *see* mestranol and norethindrone *on page 547*

Necon® **7/7/7 [US]** *see* ethinyl estradiol and norethindrone *on page 328*

Necon® **10/11 [US]** *see* ethinyl estradiol and norethindrone *on page 328*

nedocromil (inhalation) (ne doe KROE mil in hil LA shun)
U.S./Canadian Brand Names Tilade® [US/Can]
Therapeutic Category Mast Cell Stabilizer
Use Maintenance therapy in patients with mild to moderate bronchial asthma
Usual Dosage Children >6 years and Adults: 2 inhalations 4 times/day; may reduce dosage to 2-3 times/day once desired clinical response to initial dose is observed
Dosage Forms
Aerosol for oral inhalation:
Tilade®: 1.75 mg/activation (16.2 g)

nedocromil (ophthalmic) (ne doe KROE mil op THAL mik)
U.S./Canadian Brand Names Alocril® [US/Can]
Therapeutic Category Mast Cell Stabilizer
Use Treatment of itching associated with allergic conjunctivitis
Usual Dosage Ophthalmic: Adults: 1-2 drops in eye(s) twice daily
Dosage Forms
Solution, ophthalmic:
Alocril®: 2% (5 mL)

nefazodone (nef AY zoe done)
Sound-Alike/Look-Alike Issues
Serzone® may be confused with selegiline, Serentil®, Seroquel®, sertraline
Synonyms nefazodone hydrochloride
Therapeutic Category Antidepressant, Miscellaneous
Use Treatment of depression
Usual Dosage Oral: Adults: Depression: 200 mg/day, administered in 2 divided doses initially, with a range of 300-600 mg/day in 2 divided doses thereafter
Dosage Forms
Tablet: 50 mg, 100 mg, 150 mg, 200 mg, 250 mg

nefazodone hydrochloride see nefazodone on this page

NegGram® (Discontinued)

nelarabine (nel AY re been)
Synonyms 2-amino-6-methoxypurine arabinoside; GW506U78; 506U78
U.S./Canadian Brand Names Arranon® [US]
Therapeutic Category Antineoplastic Agent, Antimetabolite
Use Treatment of relapsed or refractory T-cell acute lymphoblastic leukemia (ALL) and T-cell lymphoblastic lymphoma
Usual Dosage I.V.: T-cell ALL, T-cell lymphoblastic lymphoma:
Children: 650 mg/m^2/day on days 1 through 5; repeat every 21 days
Adults: 1500 mg/m^2/day on days 1, 3, and 5; repeat every 21 days
Dosage Forms
Injection, solution:
Arranon®: 5 mg/mL (50 mL)

nelfinavir (nel FIN a veer)
Sound-Alike/Look-Alike Issues
nelfinavir may be confused with nevirapine
Viracept® may be confused with Viramune®
Synonyms NFV
U.S./Canadian Brand Names Viracept® [US/Can]
Therapeutic Category Antiviral Agent
Use In combination with other antiretroviral therapy in the treatment of HIV infection
Usual Dosage Oral:
Children 2-13 years: 45-55 mg/kg twice daily **or** 25-35 mg/kg 3 times/day (maximum: 2500 mg/day). If tablets are unable to be taken, use oral powder in small amount of water, milk, formula, or dietary supplements; do not use acidic food/juice or store for >6 hours.
Adults: 750 mg 3 times/day or 1250 mg twice daily with meals in combination with other antiretroviral therapies
Dosage Forms
Powder, oral:
Viracept®: 50 mg/g
Tablet:
Viracept®: 250 mg, 625 mg

Nelova™ 0.5/35E (Discontinued) see ethinyl estradiol and norethindrone on page 328

Nelova™ 1/35E (Discontinued) see ethinyl estradiol and norethindrone on page 328

Nelova™ 1/50M (Discontinued) see mestranol and norethindrone on page 547

Nelova™ 10/11 (Discontinued) see ethinyl estradiol and norethindrone on page 328

Nembutal® [US] see pentobarbital on page 666

Nembutal® Sodium [Can] see pentobarbital on page 666

Neo-Calglucon® *(Discontinued)* see calcium glubionate *on page 140*

NeoCeuticals™ Acne Spot Treatment [US-OTC] see salicylic acid *on page 772*

Neo-Dexameth® Ophthalmic *(Discontinued)*

Neo DM [US] see chlorpheniramine, phenylephrine, and dextromethorphan *on page 180*

Neo-Durabolic® *(Discontinued)* see nandrolone *on page 590*

Neofed® *(Discontinued)* see pseudoephedrine *on page 727*

Neo-Fradin™ [US] see neomycin *on this page*

Neofrin™ [US] see phenylephrine *on page 675*

Neomixin® Topical *(Discontinued)* see bacitracin, neomycin, and polymyxin B *on page 91*

neomycin (nee oh MYE sin)

Sound-Alike/Look-Alike Issues
myciguent may be confused with Mycitracin®

Synonyms neomycin sulfate

U.S./Canadian Brand Names Neo-Fradin™ [US]; Neo-Rx [US]

Therapeutic Category Aminoglycoside (Antibiotic); Antibiotic, Topical

Use Orally to prepare GI tract for surgery; topically to treat minor skin infections; treatment of diarrhea caused by *E. coli*; adjunct in the treatment of hepatic encephalopathy; bladder irrigation; ocular infections

Usual Dosage
Children: Oral:
Preoperative intestinal antisepsis: 90 mg/kg/day divided every 4 hours for 2 days; or 25 mg/kg at 1 PM, 2 PM, and 11 PM on the day preceding surgery as an adjunct to mechanical cleansing of the intestine and in combination with erythromycin base
Hepatic encephalopathy: 50-100 mg/kg/day in divided doses every 6-8 hours or 2.5-7 g/m^2/day divided every 4-6 hours for 5-6 days not to exceed 12 g/day
Children and Adults: Topical: Topical solutions containing 0.1% to 1% neomycin have been used for irrigation
Adults: Oral:
Preoperative intestinal antisepsis: 1 g each hour for 4 doses then 1 g every 4 hours for 5 doses; or 1 g at 1 PM, 2 PM, and 11 PM on day preceding surgery as an adjunct to mechanical cleansing of the bowel and oral erythromycin; or 6 g/day divided every 4 hours for 2-3 days
Hepatic encephalopathy: 500-2000 mg every 6-8 hours or 4-12 g/day divided every 4-6 hours for 5-6 days
Chronic hepatic insufficiency: 4 g/day for an indefinite period

Dosage Forms
Powder, micronized [for prescription compounding]: (10 g, 100 g)
Neo-Rx: (10 g, 100 g)
Solution, oral: 125 mg/5 mL
Neo-Fradin™: 125 mg/5 mL
Tablet: 500 mg

neomycin and polymyxin B (nee oh MYE sin & pol i MIKS in bee)

Synonyms polymyxin B and neomycin

U.S./Canadian Brand Names Neosporin® G.U. Irrigant [US]; Neosporin® Irrigating Solution [Can]

Therapeutic Category Antibiotic, Topical; Genitourinary Irrigant

Use Short-term as a continuous irrigant or rinse in the urinary bladder to prevent bacteriuria and gram-negative rod septicemia associated with the use of indwelling catheters; to help prevent infection in minor cuts, scrapes, and burns

Usual Dosage Children and Adults: Bladder irrigation: **Not for injection**; add 1 mL irrigant to 1 liter isotonic saline solution and connect container to the inflow of lumen of 3-way catheter. Continuous irrigant or rinse in the urinary bladder for up to a maximum of 10 days with administration rate adjusted to patient's urine output; usually no more than 1 L of irrigant is used per day.

Dosage Forms
Solution, irrigant: Neomycin 40 mg and polymyxin B 200,000 units per mL (1 mL)
Neosporin® G.U. Irrigant: Neomycin 40 mg and polymyxin B 200,000 units per mL (1 mL, 20 mL)

neomycin, bacitracin, and polymyxin B see bacitracin, neomycin, and polymyxin B *on page 91*

neomycin, bacitracin, polymyxin B, and hydrocortisone see bacitracin, neomycin, polymyxin B, and hydrocortisone *on page 92*

neomycin, bacitracin, polymyxin B, and pramoxine see bacitracin, neomycin, polymyxin B, and pramoxine *on page 92*

neomycin, colistin, hydrocortisone, and thonzonium
(nee oh MYE sin, koe LIS tin, hye droe KOR ti sone, & thon ZOE nee um)

Synonyms colistin, neomycin, hydrocortisone, and thonzonium; hydrocortisone, neomycin, colistin, and thonzonium; thonzonium, neomycin, colistin, and hydrocortisone

U.S./Canadian Brand Names Coly-Mycin® S [US]; Cortisporin®-TC [US]

Therapeutic Category Antibiotic/Corticosteroid, Otic

Use Treatment of superficial and susceptible bacterial infections of the external auditory canal; for treatment of susceptible bacterial infections of mastoidectomy and fenestration cavities

Usual Dosage Otic:
Calibrated dropper:
Children: 4 drops in affected ear 3-4 times/day
Adults: 5 drops in affected ear 3-4 times/day
Dropper bottle:
Children: 3 drops in affected ear 3-4 times/day
Adults: 4 drops in affected ear 3-4 times/day
Note: Alternatively, a cotton wick may be inserted in the ear canal and saturated with suspension every 4 hours; wick should be replaced at least every 24 hours

Dosage Forms
Suspension, otic [drops]:
Coly-Mycin® S: Neomycin 0.33%, colistin 0.3%, hydrocortisone 1%, and thonzonium 0.05% (5 mL)
Cortisporin®-TC: Neomycin 0.33%, colistin 0.3%, hydrocortisone 1%, and thonzonium 0.05% (10 mL)

neomycin, polymyxin B, and dexamethasone
(nee oh MYE sin, pol i MIKS in bee, & deks a METH a sone)

Sound-Alike/Look-Alike Issues
AK-Trol® may be confused with AKTob®

Synonyms dexamethasone, neomycin, and polymyxin B; polymyxin B, neomycin, and dexamethasone

U.S./Canadian Brand Names Dioptrol® [Can]; Maxitrol® [US/Can]; Poly-Dex™ [US]

Therapeutic Category Antibiotic/Corticosteroid, Ophthalmic

Use Steroid-responsive inflammatory ocular conditions in which a corticosteroid is indicated and where bacterial infection or a risk of bacterial infection exists

Usual Dosage Ophthalmic: Children and Adults:
Ointment: Place a small amount (~½") in the affected eye 3-4 times/day or apply at bedtime as an adjunct with drops
Suspension: Instill 1-2 drops into affected eye(s) every 3-4 hours; in severe disease, drops may be used hourly and tapered to discontinuation

Dosage Forms
Ointment, ophthalmic: Neomycin 3.5 mg, polymyxin B 10,000 units, and dexamethasone 0.1% per g (3.5 g)
Maxitrol®, Poly-Dex™: Neomycin 3.5 mg, polymyxin B 10,000 units, and dexamethasone 0.1% per g (3.5 g)
Suspension, ophthalmic: Neomycin 3.5 mg, polymyxin B 10,000 units, and dexamethasone 0.1% per mL (5 mL)
Maxitrol®, Poly-Dex™: Neomycin 3.5 mg, polymyxin B10,000 units, and dexamethasone 0.1% per mL (5 mL)

neomycin, polymyxin B, and gramicidin
(nee oh MYE sin, pol i MIKS in bee, & gram i SYE din)

Synonyms gramicidin, neomycin, and polymyxin B; polymyxin B, neomycin, and gramicidin

U.S./Canadian Brand Names Neosporin® Ophthalmic Solution [US]; Neosporin® [Can]; Optimyxin Plus® [Can]

Therapeutic Category Antibiotic, Ophthalmic

Use Treatment of superficial ocular infection

Usual Dosage Ophthalmic: Children and Adults: Instill 1-2 drops 4-6 times/day or more frequently as required for severe infections

Dosage Forms
Solution, ophthalmic: Neomycin 1.75 mg, polymyxin B 10,000 units, and gramicidin 0.025 mg per mL (10 mL)
Neosporin® Ophthalmic Solution: Neomycin 1.75 mg, polymyxin B 10,000 units, and gramicidin 0.025 mg per mL (10 mL)

neomycin, polymyxin B, and hydrocortisone
(nee oh MYE sin, pol i MIKS in bee, & hye droe KOR ti sone)

Synonyms hydrocortisone, neomycin, and polymyxin B; polymyxin B, neomycin, and hydrocortisone

U.S./Canadian Brand Names Cortimyxin® [Can]; Cortisporin® Cream [US]; Cortisporin® Ophthalmic [US]; Cortisporin® Otic [US/Can]; PediOtic® [US]
(Continued)

neomycin, polymyxin B, and hydrocortisone *(Continued)*

Therapeutic Category Antibiotic/Corticosteroid, Ophthalmic; Antibiotic/Corticosteroid, Otic; Antibiotic/Corticosteroid, Topical

Use Steroid-responsive inflammatory condition for which a corticosteroid is indicated and where bacterial infection or a risk of bacterial infection exists

Usual Dosage Duration of use should be limited to 10 days unless otherwise directed by the physician
Otic solution is used **only** for swimmer's ear (infections of external auditory canal)
Otic:
Children: Instill 3 drops into affected ear 3-4 times/day
Adults: Instill 4 drops 3-4 times/day; otic suspension is the preferred otic preparation
Children and Adults:
Ophthalmic: Drops: Instill 1-2 drops 2-4 times/day, or more frequently as required for severe infections; in acute infections, instill 1-2 drops every 15-30 minutes gradually reducing the frequency of administration as the infection is controlled
Topical: Apply a thin layer 1-4 times/day. Therapy should be discontinued when control is achieved; if no improvement is seen, reassessment of diagnosis may be necessary.

Dosage Forms
Cream, topical: Neomycin 3.5 mg, polymyxin B 10,000 units, and hydrocortisone 5 mg per g (7.5 g)
Cortisporin®: Neomycin 3.5 mg, polymyxin B 10,000 units, and hydrocortisone 5 mg per g (7.5 g)
Solution, otic: Neomycin 3.5 mg, polymyxin B 10,000 units, and hydrocortisone 10 mg per mL (10 mL)
Cortisporin®: Neomycin 3.5 mg, polymyxin B 10,000 units, and hydrocortisone 10 mg per mL (10 mL)
Suspension, ophthalmic: Neomycin 3.5 mg, polymyxin B 10,000 units, and hydrocortisone 10 mg per mL (7.5 mL)
Cortisporin®: Neomycin 3.5 mg, polymyxin B 10,000 units, and hydrocortisone 10 mg per mL (7.5 mL)
Suspension, otic: Neomycin 3.5 mg, polymyxin B 10,000 units, and hydrocortisone 10 mg per mL (10 mL)
Cortisporin®: Neomycin 3.5 mg, polymyxin B 10,000 units, and hydrocortisone 10 mg per mL (10 mL)
PediOtic®: Neomycin 3.5 mg, polymyxin B 10,000 units, and hydrocortisone 10 mg per mL (7.5 mL)

neomycin, polymyxin B, and prednisolone

(nee oh MYE sin, pol i MIKS in bee, & pred NIS oh lone)

Synonyms polymyxin B, neomycin, and prednisolone; prednisolone, neomycin, and polymyxin B

U.S./Canadian Brand Names Poly-Pred® [US]

Therapeutic Category Antibiotic/Corticosteroid, Ophthalmic

Use Steroid-responsive inflammatory ocular condition in which bacterial infection or a risk of bacterial ocular infection exists

Usual Dosage Ophthalmic: Children and Adults: Instill 1-2 drops every 3-4 hours; acute infections may require every 30-minute instillation initially with frequency of administration reduced as the infection is brought under control. To treat the lids: Instill 1-2 drops every 3-4 hours, close the eye and rub the excess on the lids and lid margins.

Dosage Forms
Suspension, ophthalmic:
Poly-Pred®: Neomycin 0.35%, polymyxin B 10,000 units per mL, and prednisolone 0.5% (5 mL)

neomycin sulfate *see neomycin on page 596*

neonatal trace metals *see trace metals on page 855*

NeoProfen® [US] *see ibuprofen on page 444*

Neoral® [US/Can] *see cyclosporine on page 223*

Neo-Rx [US] *see neomycin on page 596*

Neosporin® [Can] *see neomycin, polymyxin B, and gramicidin on previous page*

Neosporin® AF [US-OTC] *see miconazole on page 566*

Neosporin® G.U. Irrigant [US] *see neomycin and polymyxin B on page 596*

Neosporin® Irrigating Solution [Can] *see neomycin and polymyxin B on page 596*

Neosporin® Neo To Go® [US-OTC] *see bacitracin, neomycin, and polymyxin B on page 91*

Neosporin® Ophthalmic Ointment [Can] *see bacitracin, neomycin, and polymyxin B on page 91*

Neosporin® Ophthalmic Ointment *(Discontinued)* *see bacitracin, neomycin, and polymyxin B on page 91*

Neosporin® Ophthalmic Solution [US] *see neomycin, polymyxin B, and gramicidin on previous page*

Neosporin® + Pain Relief Ointment [US-OTC] *see bacitracin, neomycin, polymyxin B, and pramoxine on page 92*

Neosporin® Topical [US-OTC] *see bacitracin, neomycin, and polymyxin B on page 91*

neostigmine (nee oh STIG meen)

Sound-Alike/Look-Alike Issues
Prostigmin® may be confused with physostigmine
Synonyms neostigmine bromide; neostigmine methylsulfate
U.S./Canadian Brand Names Prostigmin® [US/Can]
Therapeutic Category Cholinergic Agent
Use Diagnosis and treatment of myasthenia gravis; prevention and treatment of postoperative bladder distention and urinary retention; reversal of the effects of nondepolarizing neuromuscular-blocking agents after surgery
Usual Dosage
Myasthenia gravis: Diagnosis: I.M.:
Children: 0.04 mg/kg as a single dose
Adults: 0.02 mg/kg as a single dose
Myasthenia gravis: Treatment:
Children:
Oral: 2 mg/kg/day divided every 3-4 hours
I.M., I.V., SubQ: 0.01-0.04 mg/kg every 2-4 hours
Adults:
Oral: 15 mg/dose every 3-4 hours up to 375 mg/day maximum; interval between doses must be individualized to maximal response
I.M., I.V., SubQ: 0.5-2.5 mg every 1-3 hours up to 10 mg/24 hours maximum
Reversal of nondepolarizing neuromuscular blockade after surgery in conjunction with atropine (must administer atropine several minutes prior to neostigmine): I.V.:
Infants: 0.025-0.1 mg/kg/dose
Children: 0.025-0.08 mg/kg/dose
Adults: 0.5-2.5 mg; total dose not to exceed 5 mg
Bladder atony: Adults: I.M., SubQ:
Prevention: 0.25 mg every 4-6 hours for 2-3 days
Treatment: 0.5-1 mg every 3 hours for 5 doses after bladder has emptied
Dosage Forms
Injection, solution: 0.5 mg/mL (1 mL, 10 mL); 1 mg/mL (10 mL)
Prostigmin®: 0.5 mg/mL (1 mL, 10 mL); 1 mg/mL (10 mL)
Tablet:
Prostigmin®: 15 mg

neostigmine bromide *see* neostigmine *on this page*

neostigmine methylsulfate *see* neostigmine *on this page*

NeoStrata® AHA [US-OTC] *see* hydroquinone *on page 437*

NeoStrata® HQ [Can] *see* hydroquinone *on page 437*

Neo-Synephrine® [Can] *see* phenylephrine *on page 675*

Neo-Synephrine® 12 Hour [US-OTC] *see* oxymetazoline *on page 643*

Neo-Synephrine® 12 Hour Extra Moisturizing [US-OTC] *see* oxymetazoline *on page 643*

Neo-Synephrine® Extra Strength [US-OTC] *see* phenylephrine *on page 675*

Neo-Synephrine® Injection [US] *see* phenylephrine *on page 675*

Neo-Synephrine® Mild [US-OTC] *see* phenylephrine *on page 675*

Neo-Synephrine® Ophthalmic (Discontinued) *see* phenylephrine *on page 675*

Neo-Synephrine® Regular Strength [US-OTC] *see* phenylephrine *on page 675*

Neo-Tabs® (Discontinued) *see* neomycin *on page 596*

Neotrace-4® [US] *see* trace metals *on page 855*

NeoVadrin® (Discontinued)

nepafenac (ne pa FEN ak)

U.S./Canadian Brand Names Nevanac™ [US]
Therapeutic Category Nonsteroidal Antiinflammatory Drug (NSAID), Ophthalmic
Use Treatment of pain and inflammation associated with cataract surgery
Usual Dosage Ophthalmic: Children ≥10 years and Adults: Instill 1 drop into affected eye(s) 3 times/day, beginning 1 day prior to surgery, the day of surgery, and through the first 2 weeks of the postoperative period
Dosage Forms
Suspension, ophthalmic:
Nevanac™: 0.1% (3 mL)

NephPlex® Rx [US] *see* vitamin B complex combinations *on page 894*

Nephro-Calci® [US-OTC] *see* calcium carbonate *on page 138*

Nephrocaps® [US] *see* vitamin B complex combinations *on page 894*

Nephro-Fer® [US-OTC] *see* ferrous fumarate *on page 349*

Nephronex® [US] *see* vitamin B complex combinations *on page 894*

Nephron FA® [US] *see* vitamin B complex combinations *on page 894*

Nephro-Vite® [US-OTC] *see* vitamin B complex combinations *on page 894*

Nephro-Vite® Rx [US] *see* vitamin B complex combinations *on page 894*

Nephrox Suspension *(Discontinued)* *see* aluminum hydroxide *on page 36*

Neptazane® *(Discontinued)* *see* methazolamide *on page 551*

Nervocaine® Injection *(Discontinued)* *see* lidocaine *on page 504*

Nesacaine® [US] *see* chloroprocaine *on page 175*

Nesacaine®-CE [Can] *see* chloroprocaine *on page 175*

Nesacaine®-MPF [US] *see* chloroprocaine *on page 175*

nesiritide (ni SIR i tide)
    Synonyms B-type natriuretic peptide (human); hBNP; natriuretic peptide
    U.S./Canadian Brand Names Natrecor® [US]
    Therapeutic Category Natriuretic Peptide, B-type, Human; Vasodilator
    Use Treatment of acutely decompensated congestive heart failure (CHF) in patients with dyspnea at rest or with minimal activity
    Usual Dosage I.V.: Adults: Initial: 2 mcg/kg (bolus); followed by continuous infusion at 0.01 mcg/kg/minute. **Note:** Should not be initiated at a dosage higher than initial recommended dose. There is limited experience with larger doses; in one trial, a limited number of patients received higher doses that were increased no faster than every 3 hours by 0.005 mcg/kg/minute (preceded by a bolus of 1 mcg/kg), up to a maximum of 0.03 mcg/kg/minute. Increases beyond the initial infusion rate should be limited to selected patients and accompanied by close hemodynamic and renal function monitoring.
    Patients experiencing hypotension during the infusion: Infusion should be interrupted. May attempt to restart at a lower dose (reduce initial infusion dose by 30% and omit bolus).
    Dosage Forms
    Injection, powder for reconstitution:
      Natrecor®: 1.5 mg

Nestrex® *(Discontinued)* *see* pyridoxine *on page 735*

Netromycin® *(Discontinued)*

Neucalm-50® Injection *(Discontinued)* *see* hydroxyzine *on page 440*

Neulasta® [US/Can] *see* pegfilgrastim *on page 657*

Neuleptil® [Can] *see* pericyazine *(Canada only) on page 669*

Neumega® [US] *see* oprelvekin *on page 632*

Neupogen® [US/Can] *see* filgrastim *on page 352*

Neupro® [US] *see* rotigotine *on page 769*

Neuramate® *(Discontinued)* *see* meprobamate *on page 544*

Neurontin® [US/Can] *see* gabapentin *on page 380*

Neut® [US] *see* sodium bicarbonate *on page 791*

NeutraCare® [US] *see* fluoride *on page 361*

NeutraGard® [US-OTC] *see* fluoride *on page 361*

NeutraGard® Advanced [US] *see* fluoride *on page 361*

NeutraGard® Plus [US] *see* fluoride *on page 361*

Neutra-Phos® [US-OTC] *see* potassium phosphate and sodium phosphate *on page 703*

Neutra-Phos®-K [US-OTC] *see* potassium phosphate *on page 703*

Neutrogena® Acne Mask [US-OTC] *see* benzoyl peroxide *on page 103*

Neutrogena® Acne Wash [US-OTC] *see* salicylic acid *on page 772*

Neutrogena® Body Clear™ [US-OTC] *see* salicylic acid *on page 772*

Neutrogena® Clear Pore [US-OTC] *see* salicylic acid *on page 772*

Neutrogena® Clear Pore Shine Control [US-OTC] *see* salicylic acid *on page 772*

Neutrogena® Healthy Scalp [US-OTC] *see* salicylic acid *on page 772*

Neutrogena® Maximum Strength T/Sal® [US-OTC] *see* salicylic acid *on page 772*

Neutrogena® On The Spot® Acne Patch [US-OTC] *see* salicylic acid *on page 772*

Neutrogena® On The Spot® Acne Treatment [US-OTC] *see* benzoyl peroxide *on page 103*

Neutrogena® T/Gel [US-OTC] *see* coal tar *on page 208*

Neutrogena® T/Gel Extra Strength [US-OTC] *see* coal tar *on page 208*

Neutrogena® T/Gel Stubborn Itch Control [US-OTC] *see* coal tar *on page 208*

Nevanac™ [US] *see* nepafenac *on page 599*

nevirapine (ne VYE ra peen)
Sound-Alike/Look-Alike Issues
nevirapine may be confused with nelfinavir
Viramune® may be confused with Viracept®
Synonyms NVP
U.S./Canadian Brand Names Viramune® [US/Can]
Therapeutic Category Antiviral Agent
Use In combination therapy with other antiretroviral agents for the treatment of HIV-1
Usual Dosage Oral:
HIV infection:
Children 2 months to <8 years: Initial: 4 mg/kg/dose once daily for first 14 days; increase dose to 7 mg/kg/dose every 12 hours if no rash or other adverse effects occur; maximum dose: 200 mg/dose every 12 hours
Children ≥8 years: Initial: 4 mg/kg/dose once daily for first 14 days; increase dose to 4 mg/kg/dose every 12 hours if no rash or other adverse effects occur; maximum dose: 200 mg/dose every 12 hours
Note: *Alternative pediatric dosing (AIDSinfo guidelines):* 120-200 mg/m² every 12 hours; this dosing has been proposed due to the fact that dosing based on mg/kg may result in an abrupt decrease in dose at the 8th birthday, which may be inappropriate.
Adults: Initial: 200 mg once daily for first 14 days; maintenance: 200 mg twice daily (in combination with an additional antiretroviral agent)
Note: If patient experiences a rash during the 14-day lead-in period, dose should not be increased until the rash has resolved. Discontinue if severe rash, or rash with constitutional symptoms, is noted. If therapy is interrupted for >7 days, restart with initial dose for 14 days. Use of prednisone to prevent nevirapine-associated rash is not recommended. Permanently discontinue if symptomatic hepatic events occur.

Prevention of maternal-fetal HIV transmission in women with no prior antiretroviral therapy (AIDS information guidelines):
Mother: 200 mg as a single dose at onset of labor. May be used in combination with zidovudine.
Infant: 2 mg/kg as a single dose at age 48-72 hours. If a maternal dose was given <1 hour prior to delivery, administer a 2 mg/kg dose as soon as possible after birth and repeat at 48-72 hours. May be used in combination with zidovudine.
Dosage Forms
Suspension, oral:
Viramune®: 50 mg/5 mL
Tablet:
Viramune®: 200 mg

Nexavar® [US] *see* sorafenib *on page 802*

Nexium® [US/Can] *see* esomeprazole *on page 312*

Nexphen PD [US] *see* guaifenesin and phenylephrine *on page 404*

NFV *see* nelfinavir *on page 595*

N.G.A.® Topical (Discontinued) *see* nystatin and triamcinolone *on page 623*

niacin (NYE a sin)
Sound-Alike/Look-Alike Issues
niacin may be confused with Minocin®, Niaspan®, Nispan®
Niaspan® may be confused with niacin
Nicobid® may be confused with Nitro-Bid®
(Continued)

niacin (Continued)

Synonyms nicotinic acid; vitamin B$_3$

U.S./Canadian Brand Names Niacin-Time® [US]; Niacor® [US]; Niaspan® [US/Can]; Slo-Niacin® [US-OTC]

Therapeutic Category Vitamin, Water Soluble

Use Adjunctive treatment of dyslipidemias (types IIa and IIb or primary hypercholesterolemia) to lower the risk of recurrent MI and/or slow progression of coronary artery disease, including combination therapy with other antidyslipidemic agents when additional triglyceride-lowering or HDL-increasing effects are desired; treatment of hypertriglyceridemia in patients at risk of pancreatitis; treatment of peripheral vascular disease and circulatory disorders; treatment of pellagra; dietary supplement

Usual Dosage Note: Formulations of niacin (regular release versus extended release) are not interchangeable.

Children: Oral:

Pellagra: 50-100 mg/dose 3 times/day

Recommended daily allowances:

0-0.5 years: 5 mg/day

0.5-1 year: 6 mg/day

1-3 years: 9 mg/day

4-6 years: 12 mg/day

7-10 years: 13 mg/day

Children and Adolescents: Recommended daily allowances:

Male:

11-14 years: 17 mg/day

15-18 years: 20 mg/day

19-24 years: 19 mg/day

Female: 11-24 years: 15 mg/day

Adults: Oral:

Recommended daily allowances:

Male: 25-50 years: 19 mg/day; >51 years: 15 mg/day

Female: 25-50 years: 15 mg/day; >51 years: 13 mg/day

Hyperlipidemia: Usual target dose: 1.5-6 g/day in 3 divided doses with or after meals using a dosage titration schedule; extended release: 375 mg to 2 g once daily at bedtime

Regular release formulation (Niacor®): Initial: 250 mg once daily (with evening meal); increase frequency and/or dose every 4-7 days to desired response or first-level therapeutic dose (1.5-2 g/day in 2-3 divided doses); after 2 months, may increase at 2- to 4-week intervals to 3 g/day in 3 divided doses

Extended release formulation (Niaspan®): 500 mg at bedtime for 4 weeks, then 1 g at bedtime for 4 weeks; adjust dose to response and tolerance; can increase to a maximum of 2 g/day, but only at 500 mg/day at 4-week intervals

With lovastatin: Maximum lovastatin dose: 40 mg/day

Pellagra: 50-100 mg 3-4 times/day, maximum: 500 mg/day

Niacin deficiency: 10-20 mg/day, maximum: 100 mg/day

Dosage Forms

Capsule, extended release: 125 mg, 250 mg, 400 mg, 500 mg

Capsule, timed release: 250 mg, 500 mg

Tablet: 50 mg, 100 mg, 250 mg, 500 mg

Niacor®: 500 mg

Tablet, controlled release: 250 mg, 500 mg, 750 mg

Slo-Niacin® [OTC]: 250 mg, 500 mg, 750 mg

Tablet, extended release: 500 mg, 750 mg, 1000 mg

Niaspan®: 500 mg, 750 mg, 1000 mg

Tablet, timed release: 250 mg, 500 mg, 750 mg, 1000 mg

Niacin-Time®: 500 mg

niacinamide (nye a SIN a mide)

Sound-Alike/Look-Alike Issues

niacinamide may be confused with niCARdipine

Synonyms nicotinamide; nicotinic acid amide; vitamin B$_3$

U.S./Canadian Brand Names Nicomide-T™ [US]

Therapeutic Category Vitamin, Water Soluble

Use

Oral: Prophylaxis and treatment of pellagra

Topical: Improve the appearance of acne and decrease visible inflammation and irritation caused by acne medications

Usual Dosage

Pellagra: Oral:

Children: 100-300 mg/day in divided doses

Adults: 300-500 mg/day
Acne: Topical: Adults: Apply to affected area on face twice daily
Dosage Forms
Cream:
Nicomide-T™: 4% (30 g)
Gel:
Nicomide-T™: 4% (30 g)
Tablet: 100 mg, 250 mg, 500 mg

niacin and lovastatin (NYE a sin & LOE va sta tin)
Sound-Alike/Look-Alike Issues
Advicor® may be confused with Advair, Altocor™
Synonyms lovastatin and niacin
U.S./Canadian Brand Names Advicor® [US/Can]
Therapeutic Category HMG-CoA Reductase Inhibitor; Vitamin, Water Soluble
Use For use when treatment with both extended-release niacin and lovastatin is appropriate in combination with a standard cholesterol-lowering diet:
Extended-release niacin: Adjunctive treatment of dyslipidemias (types IIa and IIb or primary hypercholesterolemia) to lower the risk of recurrent MI and/or slow progression of coronary artery disease, including combination therapy with other antidyslipidemic agents when additional triglyceride-lowering or HDL-increasing effects are desired; treatment of hypertriglyceridemia in patients at risk of pancreatitis
Lovastatin: Treatment of primary hypercholesterolemia (Frederickson types IIa and IIb); primary and secondary prevention of cardiovascular disease
Usual Dosage Dosage forms are a fixed combination of niacin and lovastatin.
Oral: Adults: Lowest dose: Niacin 500 mg/lovastatin 20 mg; may increase by not more than 500 mg (niacin) at 4-week intervals (maximum dose: Niacin 2000 mg/lovastatin 40 mg daily); should be taken at bedtime with a low-fat snack
Not for use as initial therapy of dyslipidemias. May be substituted for equivalent dose of Niaspan®, however, manufacturer does not recommend direct substitution with other niacin products.
Dosage Forms
Tablet, variable release:
Advicor®: 500/20: Niacin 500 mg [extended release] and lovastatin 20 mg [immediate release]; 750/20: Niacin 750 mg [extended release] and lovastatin 20 mg [immediate release]; 1000/20: Niacin 1000 mg [extended release] and lovastatin 20 mg [immediate release]; 1000/40: Niacin 1000 mg [extended release] and lovastatin 40 mg [immediate release]

Niacin-Time® [US] *see* niacin *on page 601*

Niacor® [US] *see* niacin *on page 601*

Niaspan® [US/Can] *see* niacin *on page 601*

Niastase® [Can] *see* factor VIIa (recombinant) *on page 339*

nicardipine (nye KAR de peen)
Sound-Alike/Look-Alike Issues
niCARdipine may be confused with niacinamide, NIFEdipine, nimodipine
Cardene® may be confused with Cardizem®, Cardura®, codeine
Synonyms nicardipine hydrochloride
Tall-Man niCARdipine
U.S./Canadian Brand Names Cardene® I.V. [US]; Cardene® SR [US]; Cardene® [US]
Therapeutic Category Calcium Channel Blocker
Use Chronic stable angina (immediate-release product only); management of essential hypertension (immediate and sustained release; parenteral only for short time that oral treatment is not feasible)
Usual Dosage Adults:
Oral:
Immediate release: Initial: 20 mg 3 times/day; usual: 20-40 mg 3 times/day (allow 3 days between dose increases)
Sustained release: Initial: 30 mg twice daily, titrate up to 60 mg twice daily
Note: The total daily dose of immediate-release product may not automatically be equivalent to the daily sustained-release dose; use caution in converting.
I.V. (dilute to 0.1 mg/mL):
Acute hypertension: Initial: 5 mg/hour increased by 2.5 mg/hour every 15 minutes to a maximum of 15 mg/hour; consider reduction to 3 mg/hour after response is achieved. Monitor and titrate to lowest dose necessary to maintain stable blood pressure.
Substitution for oral therapy (approximate equivalents):
20 mg every 8 hours oral, equivalent to 0.5 mg/hour I.V. infusion
(Continued)

nicardipine *(Continued)*

30 mg every 8 hours oral, equivalent to 1.2 mg/hour I.V. infusion
40 mg every 8 hours oral, equivalent to 2.2 mg/hour I.V. infusion

Dosage Forms

Capsule: 20 mg, 30 mg
Cardene®: 20 mg, 30 mg

Capsule, sustained release:
Cardene® SR: 30 mg, 45 mg, 60 mg

Injection, solution:
Cardene® IV: 2.5 mg/mL (10 mL)

nicardipine hydrochloride *see* nicardipine *on previous page*

N'ice® *(Discontinued) see* ascorbic acid *on page 76*

Nicobid® *(Discontinued) see* niacin *on page 601*

Nicoderm® [Can] *see* nicotine *on this page*

NicoDerm® CQ® [US-OTC] *see* nicotine *on this page*

Nicolar® *(Discontinued) see* niacin *on page 601*

Nicomide-T™ [US] *see* niacinamide *on page 602*

Nicorette® [US-OTC/Can] *see* nicotine *on this page*

Nicorette® Plus [Can] *see* nicotine *on this page*

nicotinamide *see* niacinamide *on page 602*

nicotine (nik oh TEEN)

Sound-Alike/Look-Alike Issues
NicoDerm® may be confused with Nitroderm®
Nicorette® may be confused with Nordette®

U.S./Canadian Brand Names Commit® [US-OTC]; Habitrol® [Can]; NicoDerm® CQ® [US-OTC]; Nicoderm® [Can]; Nicorette® Plus [Can]; Nicorette® [US-OTC/Can]; Nicotrol® Inhaler [US]; Nicotrol® NS [US]; Nicotrol® [Can]

Therapeutic Category Smoking Deterrent

Use Treatment to aid smoking cessation for the relief of nicotine withdrawal symptoms (including nicotine craving)

Usual Dosage

Smoking deterrent: Patients should be advised to completely stop smoking upon initiation of therapy.

Oral:

Gum: Chew 1 piece of gum when urge to smoke, up to 24 pieces/day. Patients who smoke <25 cigarettes/day should start with 2-mg strength; patients smoking ≥25 cigarettes/day should start with the 4-mg strength. Use according to the following 12-week dosing schedule:

Weeks 1-6: Chew 1 piece of gum every 1-2 hours; to increase chances of quitting, chew at least 9 pieces/day during the first 6 weeks

Weeks 7-9: Chew 1 piece of gum every 2-4 hours

Weeks 10-12: Chew 1 piece of gum every 4-8 hours

Inhaler: Usually 6 to 16 cartridges per day; best effect was achieved by frequent continuous puffing (20 minutes); recommended duration of treatment is 3 months, after which patients may be weaned from the inhaler by gradual reduction of the daily dose over 6-12 weeks

Lozenge: Patients who smoke their first cigarette within 30 minutes of waking should use the 4 mg strength; otherwise the 2 mg strength is recommended. Use according to the following 12-week dosing schedule:

Weeks 1-6: One lozenge every 1-2 hours

Weeks 7-9: One lozenge every 2-4 hours

Weeks 10-12: One lozenge every 4-8 hours

Note: Use at least 9 lozenges/day during first 6 weeks to improve chances of quitting; do not use more than one lozenge at a time (maximum: 5 lozenges every 6 hours, 20 lozenges/day)

Topical:

Transdermal patch: Apply new patch every 24 hours to nonhairy, clean, dry skin on the upper body or upper outer arm; each patch should be applied to a different site. **Note:** Adjustment may be required during initial treatment (move to higher dose if experiencing withdrawal symptoms; lower dose if side effects are experienced).

NicoDerm CQ®:

Patients smoking ≥10 cigarettes/day: Begin with **step 1** (21 mg/day) for 4-6 weeks, followed by **step 2** (14 mg/day) for 2 weeks; finish with **step 3** (7 mg/day) for 2 weeks

Patients smoking <10 cigarettes/day: Begin with **step 2** (14 mg/day) for 6 weeks, followed by **step 3** (7 mg/day) for 2 weeks

Note: Initial starting dose for patients <100 pounds, history of cardiovascular disease: 14 mg/day for 4-6 weeks, followed by 7 mg/day for 2-4 weeks

Note: Patients receiving >600 mg/day of cimetidine: Decrease to the next lower patch size

Note: Benefits of use of nicotine transdermal patches beyond 3 months have not been demonstrated.

Nasal: Spray: 1-2 sprays/hour; do not exceed more than 5 doses (10 sprays) per hour [maximum: 40 doses/day (80 sprays); each dose (2 sprays) contains 1 mg of nicotine

Dosage Forms

Gum, chewing: 2 mg (20s, 50s, 110s); 4 mg (20s, 50s, 110s)

Nicorette®: 2 mg (40s, 48s, 50s, 100s, 108s, 110s, 168s, 170s, 192s, 200s, 216s); 4 mg (40s, 48s, 50s, 100s, 108s, 110s, 168s, 170s, 192s, 200s, 216s)

Lozenge:

Commit®: 2 mg (48s, 72s, 84s, 108s, 168s); 4 mg (48s, 72s, 84s, 108s, 168s, 192s)

Oral inhalation system:

Nicotrol® Inhaler: 10 mg cartridge [cartridge delivers 4 mg nicotine] (168s)

Patch, transdermal: 7 mg/24 (30s); 14 mg/24 hours (30s); 21 mg/24 hours (30s)

NicoDerm® CQ® [OTC]: 7 mg/24 hours (14s); 14 mg/24 hours (14s); 21 mg/24 hours (14s)

Solution, intranasal spray:

Nicotrol® NS: 10 mg/mL (10 mL)

nicotinic acid *see* niacin *on page 601*

nicotinic acid amide *see* niacinamide *on page 602*

Nicotrol® [Can] *see* nicotine *on previous page*

Nicotrol® Inhaler [US] *see* nicotine *on previous page*

Nicotrol® NS [US] *see* nicotine *on previous page*

Nico-Vert® *(Discontinued)* *see* meclizine *on page 535*

Nidagel™ [Can] *see* metronidazole *on page 563*

Nifediac™ CC [US] *see* nifedipine *on this page*

Nifedical™ XL [US] *see* nifedipine *on this page*

nifedipine (nye FED i peen)

Sound-Alike/Look-Alike Issues

NIFEdipine may be confused with niCARdipine, nimodipine, nisoldipine

Procardia XL® may be confused with Cartia® XT

Tall-Man NIFEdipine

U.S./Canadian Brand Names Adalat® CC [US]; Adalat® XL® [Can]; Afeditab™ CR [US]; Apo-Nifed PA® [Can]; Apo-Nifed® [Can]; Nifediac™ CC [US]; Nifedical™ XL [US]; Novo-Nifedin [Can]; Nu-Nifed [Can]; Procardia XL® [US]; Procardia® [US/Can]

Therapeutic Category Calcium Channel Blocker

Use Angina and hypertension (sustained release only), pulmonary hypertension

Usual Dosage Oral:

Children:

Hypertrophic cardiomyopathy: 0.6-0.9 mg/kg/24 hours in 3-4 divided doses

Hypertension: Children 1-17 years: Extended release tablet: Initial: 0.25-0.5 mg/kg/day once daily or in 2 divided doses; maximum: 3 mg/kg/day up to 120 mg/day

Adults: (**Note:** When switching from immediate release to sustained release formulations, total daily dose will start the same)

Initial: 30 mg once daily as sustained release formulation, or if indicated, 10 mg 3 times/day as capsules

Usual dose: 10-30 mg 3 times/day as capsules or 30-60 mg once daily as sustained release

Maximum dose: 120-180 mg/day

Increase sustained release at 7- to 14-day intervals

Dosage Forms

Capsule, softgel: 10 mg, 20 mg

Procardia®: 10 mg

Tablet, extended release: 30 mg, 60 mg, 90 mg

Adalat® CC, Nifediac™ CC, Procardia XL®: 30 mg, 60 mg, 90 mg

Afeditab™ CR, Nifedical™ XL: 30 mg, 60 mg

Niferex® [US-OTC] *see* polysaccharide-iron complex *on page 697*

niftolid *see* flutamide *on page 367*

Nilandron® [US] *see* nilutamide *on next page*

Nilstat [Can] *see* nystatin *on page 623*

Nilstat® *(Discontinued) see* nystatin *on page 623*

nilutamide (ni LOO ta mide)
Synonyms NSC-684588; RU-23908
U.S./Canadian Brand Names Anandron® [Can]; Nilandron® [US]
Therapeutic Category Antineoplastic Agent
Use Treatment of metastatic prostate cancer
Usual Dosage Oral (refer to individual protocols): Adults: 300 mg daily for 30 days starting the same day or day after surgical castration, then 150 mg/day
Dosage Forms
 Tablet:
 Nilandron®: 150 mg

Nimbex® [US/Can] *see* cisatracurium *on page 193*

nimodipine (nye MOE di peen)
Sound-Alike/Look-Alike Issues
 nimodipine may be confused with niCARdipine, NIFEdipine
U.S./Canadian Brand Names Nimotop® [US/Can]
Therapeutic Category Calcium Channel Blocker
Use Spasm following subarachnoid hemorrhage from ruptured intracranial aneurysms regardless of the patients neurological condition postictus (Hunt and Hess grades I-V)
Usual Dosage Note: Capsules and contents are for oral administration **ONLY.** Oral: Adults: 60 mg every 4 hours for 21 days, start therapy within 96 hours after subarachnoid hemorrhage.
Dosage Forms
 Capsule, liquid filled: 30 mg
 Nimotop®: 30 mg

Nimotop® [US/Can] *see* nimodipine *on this page*

Nipent® [US/Can] *see* pentostatin *on page 667*

Niravam™ [US] *see* alprazolam *on page 32*

nisoldipine (nye SOL di peen)
Sound-Alike/Look-Alike Issues
 nisoldipine may be confused with NIFEdipine
U.S./Canadian Brand Names Sular® [US]
Therapeutic Category Calcium Channel Blocker
Use Management of hypertension, alone or in combination with other antihypertensive agents
Usual Dosage Oral: Adults: Initial: 20 mg once daily, then increase by 10 mg/week (or longer intervals) to attain adequate control of blood pressure; usual dose range (JNC 7): 10-40 mg once daily; doses >60 mg once daily are not recommended.
Dosage Forms
 Tablet, extended release:
 Sular®: 10 mg, 20 mg, 30 mg, 40 mg

nitalapram *see* citalopram *on page 194*

nitazoxanide (nye ta ZOX a nide)
Synonyms NTZ
U.S./Canadian Brand Names Alinia® [US]
Therapeutic Category Antiprotozoal
Use Treatment of diarrhea caused by *Cryptosporidium parvum* or *Giardia lamblia*
Usual Dosage Diarrhea caused by *Cryptosporidium parvum* or *Giardia lamblia*:
 Children 1-3 years: 100 mg every 12 hours for 3 days
 Children 4-11 years: 200 mg every 12 hours for 3 days
 Children ≥12 years and Adults: 500 mg every 12 hours for 3 days
Dosage Forms
 Powder for oral suspension:
 Alinia®: 100 mg/5 mL
 Tablet:
 Alinia®: 500 mg
 Alinia® 3-Day Therapy Packs™ [unit-dose pack]: 500 mg (6s)

nitisinone (ni TIS i known)
  U.S./Canadian Brand Names Orfadin® [US]
  Therapeutic Category 4-Hydroxyphenylpyruvate Dioxygenase Inhibitor
  Use Treatment of hereditary tyrosinemia type 1 (HT-1); to be used with dietary restriction of tyrosine and phenylalanine
  Usual Dosage Oral: **Note:** Must be used in conjunction with a low protein diet restricted in tyrosine and phenylalanine.
    Infants: See dosing for Children and Adults; infants may require maximal dose once liver function has improved
    Children and Adults: Initial: 1 mg/kg/day in divided doses, given in the morning and evening, 1 hour before meals; doses do not need to be divided evenly
  Dosage Forms
    Capsule:
      Orfadin®: 2 mg, 5 mg, 10 mg

Nitoman™ **[Can]** *see* tetrabenazine *(Canada only)* on page 830

Nitrazadon [Can] *see* nitrazepam *(Canada only)* on this page

nitrazepam *(Canada only)* (nye TRA ze pam)
  Synonyms nitrozepamum
  U.S./Canadian Brand Names Apo-Nitrazepam® [Can]; Mogadon [Can]; Nitrazadon [Can]; Nitrazepam (Pro-Doc) [Can]; Sandoz-Nitrazepam [Can]
  Therapeutic Category Benzodiazepine
  Controlled Substance CDSA IV
  Use Short-term management of insomnia; treatment of myoclonic seizures
  Usual Dosage Oral:
    Children ≤30 kg: Myoclonic seizures: 0.3-1 mg/kg/day in 3 divided doses
    Adults: Insomnia: 5-10 mg at bedtime; treatment should not exceed 7-10 consecutive days; use for more than 2-3 consecutive weeks requires complete reevaluation of patient
  Dosage Forms [CAN] = Canadian brand name
    Tablet:
      Apo-Nitrazepam® [CAN], Mogadon [CAN], Nitrazadon [CAN], Nitrazepam [CAN], Sandoz-Nitrazepam [CAN]: 5 mg, 10 mg [not available in the U.S.]

Nitrazepam (Pro-Doc) [Can] *see* nitrazepam *(Canada only)* on this page

Nitrek® *(Discontinued)* *see* nitroglycerin on next page

nitric oxide (NYE trik OKS ide)
  U.S./Canadian Brand Names INOmax® [US/Can]
  Therapeutic Category Vasodilator, Pulmonary
  Use Treatment of term and near-term (>34 weeks) neonates with hypoxic respiratory failure associated with pulmonary hypertension; used concurrently with ventilatory support and other agents
  Usual Dosage Inhalation: Neonates (up to 14 days old): 20 ppm. Treatment should be maintained up to 14 days or until the underlying oxygen desaturation has resolved and the neonate is ready to be weaned from therapy. In the CINRGI trial, patients whose oxygenation improved had their dose reduced to 5 ppm at the end of 4 hours of treatment. Doses above 20 ppm should not be used because of the risk of methemoglobinemia and elevated NO_2.
  Dosage Forms
    Gas, for inhalation:
      INOmax®: 100 ppm [nitric oxide 0.01% and nitrogen 99.99%] (353 L, 1963 L); 800 ppm [nitric oxide 0.08% and nitrogen 99.92%] (353 L, 1963 L)

4′-nitro-3′-trifluoromethylisobutyrantide *see* flutamide on page 367

Nitro-Bid® **[US]** *see* nitroglycerin on next page

Nitrodisc® **Patch** *(Discontinued)* *see* nitroglycerin on next page

Nitro-Dur® **[US/Can]** *see* nitroglycerin on next page

nitrofurantoin (nye troe fyoor AN toyn)
  U.S./Canadian Brand Names Apo-Nitrofurantoin® [Can]; Furadantin® [US]; Macrobid® [US/Can]; Macrodantin® [US/Can]; Novo-Furantoin [Can]
  Therapeutic Category Antibiotic, Miscellaneous
  Use Prevention and treatment of urinary tract infections caused by susceptible strains of *E. coli, S. aureus, Enterococcus, Klebsiella,* and *Enterobacter*
  (Continued)

nitrofurantoin *(Continued)*

Usual Dosage Oral:

Children >1 month:

UTI treatment (Furadantin®, Macrodantin®): 5-7 mg/kg/day in divided doses every 6 hours; maximum: 400 mg/day. Administer for 7 days or at least 3 days after obtaining sterile urine

UTI prophylaxis (Furadantin®, Macrodantin®): 1-2 mg/kg/day in divided doses every 12-24 hours; maximum: 100 mg/day

Children >12 years: UTI treatment (Macrobid®): 100 mg twice daily for 7 days

Adults:

UTI treatment:

Furadantin®, Macrodantin®: 50-100 mg/dose every 6 hours; administer for 7 days or at least 3 days after obtaining sterile urine

Macrobid®: 100 mg twice daily for 7 days

UTI prophylaxis (Furadantin®, Macrodantin®): 50-100 mg/dose at bedtime

Dosage Forms

Capsule, macrocrystal: 50 mg, 100 mg

Macrodantin®: 25 mg, 50 mg, 100 mg

Capsule, macrocrystal/monohydrate: 100 mg

Macrobid®: 100 mg

Suspension, oral:

Furadantin®: 25 mg/5 mL

nitrogen mustard *see* mechlorethamine *on page 535*

nitroglycerin (nye troe GLI ser in)

Sound-Alike/Look-Alike Issues

nitroglycerin may be confused with nitroprusside

Nitro-Bid® may be confused with Nicobid®

Nitroderm may be confused with NicoDerm®

Nitrol® may be confused with Nizoral®

Nitrostat® may be confused with Hyperstat®, Nilstat®, nystatin

Synonyms glyceryl trinitrate; nitroglycerol; NTG

U.S./Canadian Brand Names Gen-Nitro [Can]; Minitran™ [US/Can]; Nitro-Bid® [US]; Nitro-Dur® [US/Can]; Nitroglycerin Injection, USP [Can]; Nitrolingual® [US]; Nitrol® [Can]; NitroMist™ [US]; NitroQuick® [US]; Nitrostat® [US/Can]; NitroTime® [US]; Rho®-Nitro [Can]; Transderm-Nitro® [Can]; Trinipatch® 0.2 [Can]; Trinipatch® 0.4 [Can]; Trinipatch® 0.6 [Can]

Therapeutic Category Vasodilator

Use Treatment of angina pectoris; I.V. for congestive heart failure (especially when associated with acute myocardial infarction); pulmonary hypertension; hypertensive emergencies occurring perioperatively (especially during cardiovascular surgery)

Usual Dosage Note: Hemodynamic and antianginal tolerance often develop within 24-48 hours of continuous nitrate administration. Nitrate-free interval (10-12 hours/day) is recommended to avoid tolerance development; gradually decrease dose in patients receiving NTG for prolonged period to avoid withdrawal reaction.

Children: Pulmonary hypertension: Continuous infusion: Start 0.25-0.5 mcg/kg/minute and titrate by 1 mcg/kg/minute at 20- to 60-minute intervals to desired effect; usual dose: 1-3 mcg/kg/minute; maximum: 5 mcg/kg/minute

Adults:

Oral: 2.5-9 mg 2-4 times/day (up to 26 mg 4 times/day)

I.V.: 5 mcg/minute, increase by 5 mcg/minute every 3-5 minutes to 20 mcg/minute; if no response at 20 mcg/minute increase by 10 mcg/minute every 3-5 minutes, up to 200 mcg/minute

Ointment: 1/2" upon rising and 1/2" 6 hours later; the dose may be doubled and even doubled again as needed

Patch, transdermal: Initial: 0.2-0.4 mg/hour, titrate to doses of 0.4-0.8 mg/hour; tolerance is minimized by using a patch-on period of 12-14 hours and patch-off period of 10-12 hours

Sublingual: 0.2-0.6 mg every 5 minutes for maximum of 3 doses in 15 minutes; may also use prophylactically 5-10 minutes prior to activities which may provoke an attack

Translingual: 1-2 sprays into mouth under tongue every 5 minutes for maximum of 3 doses in 15 minutes, may also be used 5-10 minutes prior to activities which may provoke an attack prophylactically

Dosage Forms

Capsule, extended release: 2.5 mg, 6.5 mg, 9 mg

Nitro-Time®: 2.5 mg, 6.5 mg, 9 mg

Infusion [premixed in D_5W]: 25 mg (250 mL) [0.1 mg/mL]; 50 mg (250 mL) [0.2 mg/mL]; 50 mg (500 mL) [0.1 mg/mL]; 100 mg (250 mL) [0.4 mg/mL]; 200 mg (500 mL) [0.4 mg/mL]

Injection, solution: 5 mg/mL (5 mL, 10 mL)

Ointment, topical:

Nitro-Bid®: 2% [20 mg/g] (1 g, 30 g, 60 g)

Solution, translingual [spray]:
Nitrolingual®: 0.4 mg/metered spray (4.9 g, 12 g)
NitroMist™:0.4 mg/metered spray (8.5 g)
Tablet, sublingual: 0.3 mg, 0.4 mg, 0.6 mg
NitroQuick®, Nitrostat®, Nitro-Tab®: 0.3 mg, 0.4 mg, 0.6 mg
Transdermal system [once-daily patch]: 0.1 mg/hour (30s); 0.2 mg/hour (30s); 0.4 mg/hour (30s); 0.6 mg/hour (30s)
Minitran™: 0.1 mg/hour (30s); 0.2 mg/hour (30s); 0.4 mg/hour (30s); 0.6 mg/hour (30s)
Nitro-Dur®: 0.1 mg/hour (30s); 0.2 mg/hour (30s); 0.3 mg/hour (30s); 0.4 mg/hour (30s); 0.6 mg/hour (30s); 0.8 mg/hour (30s)

Nitroglycerin Injection, USP [Can] *see* nitroglycerin *on previous page*

nitroglycerol *see* nitroglycerin *on previous page*

Nitrol® [Can] *see* nitroglycerin *on previous page*

Nitrol® (Discontinued) *see* nitroglycerin *on previous page*

Nitrolingual® [US] *see* nitroglycerin *on previous page*

NitroMist™ [US] *see* nitroglycerin *on previous page*

Nitrong® Oral Tablet (Discontinued) *see* nitroglycerin *on previous page*

Nitropress® [US] *see* nitroprusside *on this page*

nitroprusside (nye troe PRUS ide)
Sound-Alike/Look-Alike Issues
nitroprusside may be confused with nitroglycerin
Synonyms nitroprusside sodium; sodium nitroferricyanide; sodium nitroprusside
U.S./Canadian Brand Names Nitropress® [US]
Therapeutic Category Vasodilator
Use Management of hypertensive crises; congestive heart failure; used for controlled hypotension to reduce bleeding during surgery
Usual Dosage Administration requires the use of an infusion pump. Average dose: 5 mcg/kg/minute.

Children: Pulmonary hypertension: I.V.: Initial: 1 mcg/kg/minute by continuous I.V. infusion; increase in increments of 1 mcg/kg/minute at intervals of 20-60 minutes; titrating to the desired response; usual dose: 3 mcg/kg/minute, rarely need >4 mcg/kg/minute; maximum: 5 mcg/kg/minute.
Adults: I.V. Initial: 0.3-0.5 mcg/kg/minute; increase in increments of 0.5 mcg/kg/minute, titrating to the desired hemodynamic effect or the appearance of headache or nausea; usual dose: 3 mcg/kg/minute; rarely need >4 mcg/kg/minute; maximum: 10 mcg/kg/minute. When administered by prolonged infusion faster than 2 mcg/kg/minute, cyanide is generated faster than an unaided patient can handle.
Dosage Forms
Injection, solution: 25 mg/mL (2 mL)
Nitropress®: 25 mg/mL (2 mL)

nitroprusside sodium *see* nitroprusside *on this page*

NitroQuick® [US] *see* nitroglycerin *on previous page*

Nitrostat® [US/Can] *see* nitroglycerin *on previous page*

NitroTime® [US] *see* nitroglycerin *on previous page*

nitrous oxide (NYE trus OKS ide)
Therapeutic Category Anesthetic, Gas
Use Produces sedation and analgesia; principal adjunct to inhalation and intravenous general anesthesia
Usual Dosage Children and Adults:
Surgical: For sedation and analgesia: Concentrations of 25% to 50% nitrous oxide with oxygen. For general anesthesia, concentrations of 40% to 70% via mask or endotracheal tube. Minimal alveolar concentration (MAC), which can be considered the ED_{50} of inhalational anesthetics, is 105%; therefore delivery in a hyperbaric chamber is necessary to use as a complete anesthetic. When administered at 70%, reduces the MAC of other anesthetics by half.
Dental: For sedation and analgesia: Concentrations of 25% to 50% nitrous oxide with oxygen
Dosage Forms
Supplied in blue cylinders

nitrozepamum *see* nitrazepam *(Canada only) on page 607*

Nix® [US-OTC/Can] *see* permethrin *on page 670*

nizatidine (ni ZA ti deen)

Sound-Alike/Look-Alike Issues
Axid® may be confused with Ansaid®

U.S./Canadian Brand Names Apo-Nizatidine® [Can]; Axid® AR [US-OTC]; Axid® [US/Can]; Gen-Nizatidine [Can]; Novo-Nizatidine [Can]; Nu-Nizatidine [Can]; PMS-Nizatidine [Can]

Therapeutic Category Histamine H_2 Antagonist

Use Treatment and maintenance of duodenal ulcer; treatment of benign gastric ulcer; treatment of gastroesophageal reflux disease (GERD); OTC tablet used for the prevention of meal-induced heartburn, acid indigestion, and sour stomach

Usual Dosage Oral:
Children ≥12 years:
GERD: Refer to Adults dosing
Meal-induced heartburn, acid indigestion and sour stomach: Refer to Adults dosing
Adults:
Duodenal ulcer:
Treatment of active ulcer: 300 mg at bedtime or 150 mg twice daily
Maintenance of healed ulcer: 150 mg/day at bedtime
Gastric ulcer: 150 mg twice daily or 300 mg at bedtime
GERD: 150 mg twice daily
Meal-induced heartburn, acid indigestion, and sour stomach: 75 mg tablet [OTC] twice daily, 30 to 60 minutes prior to consuming food or beverages

Dosage Forms
Capsule: 150 mg, 300 mg
Axid®: 150 mg, 300 mg
Solution, oral:
Axid®: 15 mg/mL
Tablet:
Axid® AR [OTC]: 75 mg

Nizoral® [US] *see* ketoconazole *on page 482*

Nizoral® A-D [US-OTC] *see* ketoconazole *on page 482*

N-methylhydrazine *see* procarbazine *on page 716*

No Doz® Maximum Strength [US-OTC] *see* caffeine *on page 133*

NoHist [US] *see* chlorpheniramine and phenylephrine *on page 177*

Nolahist® (Discontinued)

Nolex® LA (Discontinued)

Nolvadex® [Can] *see* tamoxifen *on page 819*

Nolvadex®-D [Can] *see* tamoxifen *on page 819*

Nolvadex® (Discontinued) *see* tamoxifen *on page 819*

nonoxynol 9 (non OKS i nole nine)

Sound-Alike/Look-Alike Issues
Delfen® may be confused with Delsym®

Synonyms N-9

U.S./Canadian Brand Names Advantage-S™ [US-OTC]; Conceptrol® [US-OTC]; Delfen® [US-OTC]; Encare® [US-OTC]; Gynol II® [US-OTC]; Today® Sponge [US-OTC]; VCF™ [US-OTC]

Therapeutic Category Spermicide

Use Prevention of pregnancy

Usual Dosage Note: Prior to use, refer to specific product labeling for complete instructions.
Prevention of pregnancy: Vaginal:
Advantage-S®, Conceptrol®: Insert 1 applicatorful vaginally up to 1 hour prior to intercourse
Encare®: Unwrap and insert 1 suppository vaginally at least 10 minutes prior to intercourse; effective for 1 hour
Today® Sponge: Insert 1 sponge vaginally prior to intercourse; allow to remain in place for 6 hours after intercourse before removing; effective for use up to 24 continuous hours. Do not leave in place for >30 hours.
VCF®:
Film: Insert 1 film vaginally at least 15 minutes, but no more than 3 hours, prior to intercourse. Insert new film for each act of intercourse or if more than 3 hours have elapsed.
Foam: Insert 1 applicatorful at least 15 minutes prior to intercourse; effective for up to 1 hour

Dosage Forms
  Film, vaginal:
   VCF™ [OTC]: 28% (3s, 6s,12s)
  Foam, vaginal:
   Delfen® [OTC]: 12.5% (18 g)
   VCF™ [OTC]: 12.5% (40 g)
  Gel, vaginal:
   Advantage-S™ [OTC]: 3.5% (1.5 g, 30 g)
   Conceptrol® [OTC]: 4% (2.7 g)
   Gynol II® [OTC]: 2% (85 g, 114 g)
  Sponge, vaginal:
   Today® [OTC]: 1 g (3s, 6s, 12s)
  Suppository, vaginal:
   Encare® [OTC]: 100 mg (12s, 18s)

No Pain-HP® *(Discontinued)* see capsaicin *on page 145*

Nora-BE™ [US] see norethindrone *on this page*

noradrenaline see norepinephrine *on this page*

noradrenaline acid tartrate see norepinephrine *on this page*

Norcet® *(Discontinued)* see hydrocodone and acetaminophen *on page 427*

Norco® [US] see hydrocodone and acetaminophen *on page 427*

Norcuron® [Can] see vecuronium *on page 886*

Norcuron® *(Discontinued)* see vecuronium *on page 886*

nordeoxyguanosine see ganciclovir *on page 383*

Nordette® [US] see ethinyl estradiol and levonorgestrel *on page 325*

Norditropin® [US] see somatropin *on page 799*

Norditropin® NordiFlex® [US] see somatropin *on page 799*

Nordryl® Injection *(Discontinued)* see diphenhydramine *on page 265*

Nordryl® Oral *(Discontinued)* see diphenhydramine *on page 265*

norel® EX [US] see guaifenesin and phenylephrine *on page 404*

norelgestromin and ethinyl estradiol see ethinyl estradiol and norelgestromin *on page 328*

norepinephrine (nor ep i NEF rin)
  Synonyms levarterenol bitartrate; noradrenaline; noradrenaline acid tartrate; norepinephrine bitartrate
  U.S./Canadian Brand Names Levophed® [US/Can]
  Therapeutic Category Adrenergic Agonist Agent
  Use Treatment of shock which persists after adequate fluid volume replacement
  Usual Dosage Administration requires the use of an infusion pump!
    Note: Norepinephrine dosage is stated in terms of norepinephrine base and intravenous formulation is norepinephrine bitartrate
    Norepinephrine bitartrate 2 mg = Norepinephrine base 1 mg
    Continuous I.V. infusion:
     Children: Initial: 0.05-0.1 mcg/kg/minute; titrate to desired effect; maximum dose: 1-2 mcg/kg/minute
     Adults: Initial: 0.5-1 mcg/minute and titrate to desired response; 8-30 mcg/minute is usual range; range used in clinical trials: 0.01-3 mcg/kg/minute; ACLS dosage range: 0.5-30 mcg/minute
  Dosage Forms
    Injection, solution: 1 mg/mL (4 mL)
     Levophed®: 1 mg/mL (4 mL)

norepinephrine bitartrate see norepinephrine *on this page*

Norethin™ 1/35E *(Discontinued)* see ethinyl estradiol and norethindrone *on page 328*

norethindrone (nor ETH in drone)
  Sound-Alike/Look-Alike Issues
    Micronor® may be confused with miconazole, Micronase®
  Synonyms norethindrone acetate; norethisterone
  U.S./Canadian Brand Names Aygestin® [US]; Camila™ [US]; Errin™ [US]; Jolivette™ [US]; Micronor® [Can]; Nor-QD® [US]; Nora-BE™ [US]; Norlutate® [Can]; Ortho Micronor® [US]
  Therapeutic Category Contraceptive, Progestin Only; Progestin
  Use Treatment of amenorrhea; abnormal uterine bleeding; endometriosis; prevention of pregnancy
  (Continued)

norethindrone (Continued)

Usual Dosage Oral: Adolescents and Adults: Female:

Contraception: Progesterone only: Norethindrone 0.35 mg every day (no missed days)

Initial dose: Start on first day of menstrual period or the day after a miscarriage or abortion. If switching from a combined oral contraceptive, begin the day after finishing the last active combined tablet.

Missed dose: Take as soon as remembered. A back up method of contraception should be used for 48 hours if dose is taken ≥3 hours late.

Amenorrhea and abnormal uterine bleeding: Norethindrone acetate: 2.5-10 mg/day for 5-10 days during the second half of the menstrual cycle

Endometriosis: Norethindrone acetate: 5 mg/day for 14 days; increase at increments of 2.5 mg/day every 2 weeks to reach 15 mg/day; continue for 6-9 months or until breakthrough bleeding demands temporary termination

Dosage Forms

Tablet: 0.35 mg, 5 mg

Aygestin®: 5 mg

Camila™, Errin™, Jolivette™, Micronor®, Nora-BE™, Nor-QD®: 0.35 mg

norethindrone acetate *see* norethindrone *on previous page*

norethindrone acetate and ethinyl estradiol *see* ethinyl estradiol and norethindrone *on page 328*

norethindrone and estradiol *see* estradiol and norethindrone *on page 316*

norethindrone and mestranol *see* mestranol and norethindrone *on page 547*

norethisterone *see* norethindrone *on previous page*

Norflex™ [US/Can] *see* orphenadrine *on page 634*

norfloxacin (nor FLOKS a sin)

Sound-Alike/Look-Alike Issues

norfloxacin may be confused with Norflex™, Noroxin®

Noroxin® may be confused with Neurontin®, Norflex™, norfloxacin

U.S./Canadian Brand Names Apo-Norflox® [Can]; CO Norfloxacin [Can]; Norfloxacine® [Can]; Noroxin® [US/Can]; Novo-Norfloxacin [Can]; PMS-Norfloxacin [Can]; Riva-Norfloxacin [Can]

Therapeutic Category Quinolone

Use Uncomplicated and complicated urinary tract infections caused by susceptible gram-negative and gram-positive bacteria; sexually-transmitted disease (eg, uncomplicated urethral and cervical gonorrhea) caused by *N. gonorrhoeae*; prostatitis due to *E. coli*

Note: As of April 2007, the CDC no longer recommends the use of fluoroquinolones for the treatment of gonococcal disease.

Usual Dosage

Usual dosage range:

Adults: Oral: 400 mg every 12 hours (maximum: 800 mg/day)

Indication-specific dosing:

Adults: Oral:

Prostatitis: 400 mg every 12 hours for 4-6 weeks

Uncomplicated gonorrhea: 800 mg as a single dose. **Note:** As of April 2007, the CDC no longer recommends the use of fluoroquinolones for the treatment of uncomplicated gonococcal disease.

Urinary tract infections:

Uncomplicated: 400 mg twice daily for 3-14 days

Uncomplicated due to *E. coli, K. pneumoniae, P. mirabilis*: 400 mg twice daily for 7-10 days

Complicated: 400 mg twice daily for 10-21 days

Dosage Forms

Tablet:

Noroxin®: 400 mg

Norfloxacine® [Can] *see* norfloxacin *on this page*

Norgesic™ [Can] *see* orphenadrine, aspirin, and caffeine *on page 634*

Norgesic™ (Discontinued) *see* orphenadrine, aspirin, and caffeine *on page 634*

Norgesic™ Forte [Can] *see* orphenadrine, aspirin, and caffeine *on page 634*

Norgesic™ Forte (Discontinued) *see* orphenadrine, aspirin, and caffeine *on page 634*

norgestimate and estradiol *see* estradiol and norgestimate *on page 316*

norgestimate and ethinyl estradiol *see* ethinyl estradiol and norgestimate *on page 331*

norgestrel and ethinyl estradiol *see* ethinyl estradiol and norgestrel *on page 332*

Norinyl® 1+35 [US] *see* ethinyl estradiol and norethindrone *on page 328*

Norinyl® 1+50 [US] *see* mestranol and norethindrone *on page 547*

Noritate® [US/Can] *see* metronidazole *on page 563*

Norlutate® [Can] *see* norethindrone *on page 611*

normal human serum albumin *see* albumin *on page 22*

normal saline *see* sodium chloride *on page 792*

normal serum albumin (human) *see* albumin *on page 22*

Normiflo® *(Discontinued)*

Normodyne® [Can] *see* labetalol *on page 486*

Noroxin® [US/Can] *see* norfloxacin *on previous page*

Norpace® [US/Can] *see* disopyramide *on page 271*

Norpace® CR [US] *see* disopyramide *on page 271*

Norplant® Implant [Can] *see* levonorgestrel *on page 502*

Norplant® Implant *(Discontinued)* *see* levonorgestrel *on page 502*

Norpramin® [US/Can] *see* desipramine *on page 238*

Nor-QD® [US] *see* norethindrone *on page 611*

Nortemp Children's [US-OTC] *see* acetaminophen *on page 5*

North American coral snake antivenin *see* antivenin *(Micrurus fulvius) on page 64*

North and South American antisnake-bite serum *see* antivenin *(Crotalidae)* polyvalent *on page 63*

Nortrel™ [US] *see* ethinyl estradiol and norethindrone *on page 328*

Nortrel™ 7/7/7 [US] *see* ethinyl estradiol and norethindrone *on page 328*

nortriptyline (nor TRIP ti leen)

Sound-Alike/Look-Alike Issues
  nortriptyline may be confused with amitriptyline, desipramine, Norpramin®
  Aventyl® HCl may be confused with Bentyl®
  Pamelor® may be confused with Demerol®, Dymelor®
Synonyms nortriptyline hydrochloride
U.S./Canadian Brand Names Alti-Nortriptyline [Can]; Apo-Nortriptyline® [Can]; Aventyl® [Can]; Gen-Nortrip-tyline [Can]; Norventyl [Can]; Novo-Nortriptyline [Can]; Nu-Nortriptyline [Can]; Pamelor® [US]; PMS-Nortripty-line [Can]
Therapeutic Category Antidepressant, Tricyclic (Secondary Amine)
Use Treatment of symptoms of depression
Usual Dosage Oral:
  Depression: Adults: 25 mg 3-4 times/day up to 150 mg/day
  Myofascial pain, neuralgia, burning mouth syndrome (dental use): Initial: 10-25 mg at bedtime; dosage may be increased by 25 mg/day weekly, if tolerated; usual maintenance dose: 75 mg as a single bedtime dose or 2 divided doses
Dosage Forms
  Capsule: 10 mg, 25 mg, 50 mg, 75 mg
  Pamelor®: 10 mg, 25 mg, 50 mg, 75 mg
  Solution:
  Pamelor®: 10 mg/5 mL

nortriptyline hydrochloride *see* nortriptyline *on this page*

Norvasc® [US/Can] *see* amlodipine *on page 45*

Norventyl [Can] *see* nortriptyline *on this page*

Norvir® [US/Can] *see* ritonavir *on page 761*

Norvir® SEC [Can] *see* ritonavir *on page 761*

Nöstrilla® [US-OTC] *see* oxymetazoline *on page 643*

Novacet® *(Discontinued)* *see* sulfur and sulfacetamide *on page 815*

Novafed® A *(Discontinued)* *see* chlorpheniramine and pseudoephedrine *on page 178*

Novahistex® DM Decongestant [Can] *see* pseudoephedrine and dextromethorphan *on page 728*

Novahistex® DM Decongestant Expectorant [Can] *see* guaifenesin, pseudoephedrine, and dextro-methorphan *on page 408*

Novahistex® Expectorant with Decongestant [Can] *see* guaifenesin and pseudoephedrine *on page 406*

Novahistine® DM Decongestant [Can] *see* pseudoephedrine and dextromethorphan *on page 728*

Novahistine® DM Decongestant Expectorant [Can] *see* guaifenesin, pseudoephedrine, and dextromethorphan *on page 408*

Novamilor [Can] *see* amiloride and hydrochlorothiazide *on page 42*

Novamoxin® [Can] *see* amoxicillin *on page 48*

Novantrone® [US/Can] *see* mitoxantrone *on page 573*

Novarel® [US] *see* chorionic gonadotropin (human) *on page 187*

Novasal™ [US] *see* magnesium salicylate *on page 528*

Novasen [Can] *see* aspirin *on page 78*

Nove-Desmopressin® [Can] *see* desmopressin acetate *on page 239*

Novo-5 ASA [Can] *see* mesalamine *on page 546*

Novo-Acebutolol [Can] *see* acebutolol *on page 4*

Novo-Alendronate [Can] *see* alendronate *on page 27*

Novo-Alprazol [Can] *see* alprazolam *on page 32*

Novo-Amiodarone [Can] *see* amiodarone *on page 43*

Novo-Ampicillin [Can] *see* ampicillin *on page 53*

Novo-Atenol [Can] *see* atenolol *on page 80*

Novo-Azathioprine [Can] *see* azathioprine *on page 87*

Novo-Azithromycin [Can] *see* azithromycin *on page 88*

Novo-Benzydamine [Can] *see* benzydamine *(Canada only) on page 105*

Novo-Bicalutamide [Can] *see* bicalutamide *on page 111*

Novo-Bisoprolol [Can] *see* bisoprolol *on page 114*

Novo-Bromazepam [Can] *see* bromazepam *(Canada only) on page 119*

Novo-Bupropion SR [Can] *see* bupropion *on page 127*

Novo-Buspirone [Can] *see* buspirone *on page 129*

Novocain® [US] *see* procaine *on page 716*

Novo-Captopril [Can] *see* captopril *on page 145*

Novo-Carbamaz [Can] *see* carbamazepine *on page 147*

Novo-Carvedilol [Can] *see* carvedilol *on page 155*

Novo-Cefaclor [Can] *see* cefaclor *on page 157*

Novo-Cefadroxil [Can] *see* cefadroxil *on page 158*

Novo-Chloroquine [Can] *see* chloroquine *on page 176*

Novo-Chlorpromazine [Can] *see* chlorpromazine *on page 185*

Novo-Cholamine [Can] *see* cholestyramine resin *on page 186*

Novo-Cholamine Light [Can] *see* cholestyramine resin *on page 186*

Novo-Cilazapril [Can] *see* cilazapril *(Canada only) on page 189*

Novo-Cimetidine [Can] *see* cimetidine *on page 189*

Novo-Ciprofloxacin [Can] *see* ciprofloxacin *on page 190*

Novo-Citalopram [Can] *see* citalopram *on page 194*

Novo-Clavamoxin [Can] *see* amoxicillin and clavulanate potassium *on page 49*

Novo-Clindamycin [Can] *see* clindamycin *on page 198*

Novo-Clobazam [Can] *see* clobazam *(Canada only) on page 201*

Novo-Clobetasol [Can] *see* clobetasol *on page 201*

Novo-Clonazepam [Can] *see* clonazepam *on page 204*

Novo-Clonidine [Can] *see* clonidine *on page 204*

Novo-Clopate [Can] *see* clorazepate *on page 206*

Novo-Cloxin [Can] *see* cloxacillin *on page 207*

Novo-Cycloprine [Can] *see* cyclobenzaprine *on page 221*

Novo-Cyproterone [Can] *see* cyproterone *(Canada only)* *on page 225*

Novo-Difenac [Can] *see* diclofenac *on page 253*

Novo-Difenac K [Can] *see* diclofenac *on page 253*

Novo-Difenac-SR [Can] *see* diclofenac *on page 253*

Novo-Diflunisal [Can] *see* diflunisal *on page 257*

Novo-Digoxin [Can] *see* digoxin *on page 257*

Novo-Diltazem [Can] *see* diltiazem *on page 261*

Novo-Diltazem-CD [Can] *see* diltiazem *on page 261*

Novo-Diltiazem HCl ER [Can] *see* diltiazem *on page 261*

Novo-Dimenate [Can] *see* dimenhydrinate *on page 262*

Novo-Dipam [Can] *see* diazepam *on page 251*

Novo-Divalproex [Can] *see* valproic acid and derivatives *on page 881*

Novo-Docusate Calcium [Can] *see* docusate *on page 273*

Novo-Docusate Sodium [Can] *see* docusate *on page 273*

Novo-Domperidone [Can] *see* domperidone *(Canada only)* *on page 276*

Novo-Doxazosin [Can] *see* doxazosin *on page 278*

Novo-Doxepin [Can] *see* doxepin *on page 279*

Novo-Doxylin [Can] *see* doxycycline *on page 281*

Novo-Famotidine [Can] *see* famotidine *on page 341*

Novo-Fenofibrate [Can] *see* fenofibrate *on page 345*

Novo-Fenofibrate-S [Can] *see* fenofibrate *on page 345*

Novo-Ferrogluc [Can] *see* ferrous gluconate *on page 349*

Novo-Fluconazole [Can] *see* fluconazole *on page 356*

Novo-Flunarizine [Can] *see* flunarizine *(Canada only)* *on page 359*

Novo-Fluoxetine [Can] *see* fluoxetine *on page 364*

Novo-Flurprofen [Can] *see* flurbiprofen *on page 366*

Novo-Flutamide [Can] *see* flutamide *on page 367*

Novo-Fluvoxamine [Can] *see* fluvoxamine *on page 370*

Novo-Fosinopril [Can] *see* fosinopril *on page 376*

Novo-Furantoin [Can] *see* nitrofurantoin *on page 607*

Novo-Gabapentin [Can] *see* gabapentin *on page 380*

Novo-Gemfibrozil [Can] *see* gemfibrozil *on page 387*

Novo-Gesic [Can] *see* acetaminophen *on page 5*

Novo-Gliclazide [Can] *see* gliclazide *(Canada only)* *on page 393*

Novo-Glimepiride [Can] *see* glimepiride *on page 393*

Novo-Glyburide [Can] *see* glyburide *on page 396*

Novo-Hydrazide [Can] *see* hydrochlorothiazide *on page 426*

Novo-Hydroxyzin [Can] *see* hydroxyzine *on page 440*

Novo-Hylazin [Can] *see* hydralazine *on page 425*

Novo-Indapamide [Can] *see* indapamide *on page 452*

Novo-Ipramide [Can] *see* ipratropium *on page 470*

Novo-Keto [Can] *see* ketoprofen *on page 482*

Novo-Ketoconazole [Can] *see* ketoconazole *on page 482*

Novo-Keto-EC [Can] *see* ketoprofen *on page 482*

Novo-Ketorolac [Can] *see* ketorolac *on page 483*

Novo-Ketotifen [Can] *see* ketotifen *on page 484*

Novo-Lamotrigine [Can] *see* lamotrigine *on page 490*

Novo-Leflunomide [Can] *see* leflunomide *on page 495*

Novo-Levobunolol [Can] *see* levobunolol *on page 499*

Novo-Levocarbidopa [Can] *see* levodopa and carbidopa *on page 500*

Novo-Levofloxacin [Can] *see* levofloxacin *on page 501*

Novo-Lexin [Can] *see* cephalexin *on page 167*

Novolin® L Insulin *(Discontinued)*

Novolin® 70/30 [US] *see* insulin NPH and insulin regular *on page 460*

Novolin® ge 10/90 [Can] *see* insulin NPH and insulin regular *on page 460*

Novolin® ge 20/80 [Can] *see* insulin NPH and insulin regular *on page 460*

Novolin® ge 30/70 [Can] *see* insulin NPH and insulin regular *on page 460*

Novolin® ge 40/60 [Can] *see* insulin NPH and insulin regular *on page 460*

Novolin® ge 50/50 [Can] *see* insulin NPH and insulin regular *on page 460*

Novolin® ge NPH [Can] *see* insulin NPH *on page 459*

Novolin® ge Toronto [Can] *see* insulin regular *on page 460*

Novolin® N [US] *see* insulin NPH *on page 459*

Novolin® R [US] *see* insulin regular *on page 460*

NovoLog® [US] *see* insulin aspart *on page 457*

NovoLog® Mix 70/30 [US] *see* insulin aspart protamine and insulin aspart *on page 457*

Novo-Loperamide [Can] *see* loperamide *on page 515*

Novo-Lorazepam [Can] *see* lorazepam *on page 518*

Novo-Lovastatin [Can] *see* lovastatin *on page 520*

Novo-Maprotiline [Can] *see* maprotiline *on page 531*

Novo-Medrone [Can] *see* medroxyprogesterone *on page 537*

Novo-Meloxicam [Can] *see* meloxicam *on page 539*

Novo Meprazine [Can] *see* methotrimeprazine *(Canada only) on page 554*

Novo-Mepro [Can] *see* meprobamate *on page 544*

Novo-Metformin [Can] *see* metformin *on page 548*

Novo-Methacin [Can] *see* indomethacin *on page 454*

Novo-Metoprolol [Can] *see* metoprolol *on page 562*

Novo-Mexiletine [Can] *see* mexiletine *on page 565*

Novo-Minocycline [Can] *see* minocycline *on page 571*

Novo-Mirtazapine [Can] *see* mirtazapine *on page 572*

Novo-Misoprostol [Can] *see* misoprostol *on page 573*

NovoMix® 30 [Can] *see* insulin aspart protamine and insulin aspart *on page 457*

Novo-Moclobemide [Can] *see* moclobemide *(Canada only) on page 575*

Novo-Nabumetone [Can] *see* nabumetone *on page 585*

Novo-Nadolol [Can] *see* nadolol *on page 586*

Novo-Naproc EC [Can] *see* naproxen *on page 591*

Novo-Naprox [Can] *see* naproxen *on page 591*

Novo-Naprox Sodium [Can] *see* naproxen *on page 591*

Novo-Naprox Sodium DS [Can] *see* naproxen *on page 591*

Novo-Naprox SR [Can] *see* naproxen *on page 591*

Novo-Nifedin [Can] *see* nifedipine *on page 605*

Novo-Nizatidine [Can] *see* nizatidine *on page 610*

Novo Nordisk® (all products) *(Discontinued)*

Novo-Norfloxacin [Can] *see* norfloxacin *on page 612*

Novo-Nortriptyline [Can] *see* nortriptyline *on page 613*

Novo-Ofloxacin [Can] *see* ofloxacin *on page 625*

Novo-Oxybutynin [Can] *see* oxybutynin *on page 639*

Novo-Paroxetine [Can] *see* paroxetine *on page 654*

Novo-Pen-VK [Can] *see* penicillin V potassium *on page 664*

Novo-Peridol [Can] *see* haloperidol *on page 413*
Novo-Pheniram [Can] *see* chlorpheniramine *on page 177*
Novo-Pindol [Can] *see* pindolol *on page 683*
Novo-Pirocam [Can] *see* piroxicam *on page 687*
Novo-Pramine [Can] *see* imipramine *on page 449*
Novo-Pramipexole [Can] *see* pramipexole *on page 706*
Novo-Pranol [Can] *see* propranolol *on page 724*
Novo-Pravastatin [Can] *see* pravastatin *on page 707*
Novo-Prazin [Can] *see* prazosin *on page 708*
Novo-Prednisolone [Can] *see* prednisolone (systemic) *on page 710*
Novo-Prednisone [Can] *see* prednisone *on page 710*
Novo-Profen [Can] *see* ibuprofen *on page 444*
Novo-Propamide [Can] *see* chlorpropamide *on page 185*
Novo-Purol [Can] *see* allopurinol *on page 30*
Novo-Quinidin [Can] *see* quinidine *on page 740*
Novo-Quinine [Can] *see* quinine *on page 740*
Novo-Ranidine [Can] *see* ranitidine *on page 744*
NovoRapid® [Can] *see* insulin aspart *on page 457*
Novo-Rythro Estolate [Can] *see* erythromycin *on page 309*
Novo-Rythro Ethylsuccinate [Can] *see* erythromycin *on page 309*
Novo-Selegiline [Can] *see* selegiline *on page 780*
Novo-Semide [Can] *see* furosemide *on page 379*
Novo-Sertraline [Can] *see* sertraline *on page 783*
NovoSeven® [US] *see* factor VIIa (recombinant) *on page 339*
Novo-Simvastatin [Can] *see* simvastatin *on page 787*
Novo-Sorbide [Can] *see* isosorbide dinitrate *on page 476*
Novo-Sotalol [Can] *see* sotalol *on page 802*
Novo-Soxazole [Can] *see* sulfisoxazole *on page 814*
Novo-Spiroton [Can] *see* spironolactone *on page 804*
Novo-Spirozine [Can] *see* hydrochlorothiazide and spironolactone *on page 426*
Novo-Sucralate [Can] *see* sucralfate *on page 808*
Novo-Sumatriptan [Can] *see* sumatriptan *on page 815*
Novo-Sundac [Can] *see* sulindac *on page 815*
Novo-Tamoxifen [Can] *see* tamoxifen *on page 819*
Novo-Temazepam [Can] *see* temazepam *on page 823*
Novo-Terazosin [Can] *see* terazosin *on page 826*
Novo-Theophyl SR [Can] *see* theophylline *on page 834*
Novo-Tiaprofenic [Can] *see* tiaprofenic acid *(Canada only) on page 840*
Novo-Ticlopidine [Can] *see* ticlopidine *on page 842*
Novo-Topiramate [Can] *see* topiramate *on page 851*
Novo-Trazodone [Can] *see* trazodone *on page 859*
Novo-Triamzide [Can] *see* hydrochlorothiazide and triamterene *on page 427*
Novo-Trifluzine [Can] *see* trifluoperazine *on page 865*
Novo-Trimel [Can] *see* sulfamethoxazole and trimethoprim *on page 813*
Novo-Trimel D.S. [Can] *see* sulfamethoxazole and trimethoprim *on page 813*
Novo-Triptyn [Can] *see* amitriptyline *on page 44*
Novo-Venlafaxine XR [Can] *see* venlafaxine *on page 887*
Novo-Veramil SR [Can] *see* verapamil *on page 887*
Novo-Warfarin [Can] *see* warfarin *on page 899*

Novoxapram® **[Can]** *see* oxazepam *on page 637*

Novo-Zopiclone [Can] *see* zopiclone *(Canada only) on page 909*

Noxafil® **[US]** *see* posaconazole *on page 698*

Nozinan® **[Can]** *see* methotrimeprazine *(Canada only) on page 554*

NP-27® *(Discontinued) see* tolnaftate *on page 849*

NPH Iletin® **II** *(Discontinued)*

NPH Iletin® **Insulin** *(Discontinued)*

NPH insulin *see* insulin NPH *on page 459*

NPH insulin and regular insulin *see* insulin NPH and insulin regular *on page 460*

NRP104 *see* lisdexamfetamine *on page 511*

NRS® **[US-OTC]** *see* oxymetazoline *on page 643*

NSC-740 *see* methotrexate *on page 553*

NSC-750 *see* busulfan *on page 129*

NSC-752 *see* thioguanine *on page 837*

NSC-755 *see* mercaptopurine *on page 545*

NSC-762 *see* mechlorethamine *on page 535*

NSC-3053 *see* dactinomycin *on page 228*

NSC-3088 *see* chlorambucil *on page 172*

NSC-8806 *see* melphalan *on page 539*

NSC-13875 *see* altretamine *on page 36*

NSC-26271 *see* cyclophosphamide *on page 222*

NSC-26980 *see* mitomycin *on page 573*

NSC-27640 *see* floxuridine *on page 356*

NSC-38721 *see* mitotane *on page 573*

NSC-49842 *see* vinblastine *on page 890*

NSC-63878 *see* cytarabine *on page 226*

NSC-66847 *see* thalidomide *on page 833*

NSC-67574 *see* vincristine *on page 891*

NSC-71423 *see* megestrol *on page 538*

NSC-77213 *see* procarbazine *on page 716*

NSC-79037 *see* lomustine *on page 515*

NSC-82151 *see* daunorubicin hydrochloride *on page 233*

NSC-85998 *see* streptozocin *on page 807*

NSC-89199 *see* estramustine *on page 317*

NSC-102816 *see* azacitidine *on page 87*

NSC-105014 *see* cladribine *on page 196*

NSC-106977 (Erwinia) *see* asparaginase *on page 77*

NSC-109229 (E. coli) *see* asparaginase *on page 77*

NSC-109724 *see* ifosfamide *on page 447*

NSC-122758 *see* tretinoin (oral) *on page 860*

NSC-123127 *see* doxorubicin *on page 280*

NSC-125066 *see* bleomycin *on page 115*

NSC-125973 *see* paclitaxel *on page 645*

NSC-127716 *see* decitabine *on page 234*

NSC-147834 *see* flutamide *on page 367*

NSC-169780 *see* dexrazoxane *on page 245*

NSC-180973 *see* tamoxifen *on page 819*

NSC-218321 *see* pentostatin *on page 667*

NSC-241240 *see* carboplatin *on page 153*

NSC-721631 *see* rasburicase *on page 746*

NSC-722623 *see* ibandronate *on page 443*

NSC-722848 *see* oprelvekin *on page 632*

NSC-724223 *see* epoetin alfa *on page 303*

NSC-724772 *see* sorafenib *on page 802*

NSC-725961 *see* pegfilgrastim *on page 657*

NSC-727989 *see* lapatinib *on page 494*

NSC-728729 *see* infliximab *on page 454*

NSC-729969 *see* darbepoetin alfa *on page 232*

NSC-732517 *see* dasatinib *on page 233*

NSC-736511 *see* sunitinib *on page 816*

NSC-736631 *see* paclitaxel (protein bound) *on page 646*

NSC-742319 *see* panitumumab *on page 650*

NTG *see* nitroglycerin *on page 608*

NTZ *see* nitazoxanide *on page 606*

NTZ® Long Acting Nasal Solution *(Discontinued)* *see* oxymetazoline *on page 643*

Nu-Acebutolol [Can] *see* acebutolol *on page 4*

Nu-Acyclovir [Can] *see* acyclovir *on page 17*

Nu-Alprax [Can] *see* alprazolam *on page 32*

Nu-Amilzide [Can] *see* amiloride and hydrochlorothiazide *on page 42*

Nu-Amoxi [Can] *see* amoxicillin *on page 48*

Nu-Ampi [Can] *see* ampicillin *on page 53*

Nu-Atenol [Can] *see* atenolol *on page 80*

Nu-Baclo [Can] *see* baclofen *on page 92*

Nubain® [US] *see* nalbuphine *on page 588*

Nu-Beclomethasone [Can] *see* beclomethasone *on page 97*

Nu-Bromazepam [Can] *see* bromazepam *(Canada only) on page 119*

Nu-Buspirone [Can] *see* buspirone *on page 129*

Nu-Capto [Can] *see* captopril *on page 145*

Nu-Carbamazepine [Can] *see* carbamazepine *on page 147*

Nu-Cefaclor [Can] *see* cefaclor *on page 157*

Nu-Cephalex [Can] *see* cephalexin *on page 167*

Nu-Cimet [Can] *see* cimetidine *on page 189*

Nu-Clonazepam [Can] *see* clonazepam *on page 204*

Nu-Clonidine [Can] *see* clonidine *on page 204*

Nu-Cloxi [Can] *see* cloxacillin *on page 207*

Nucofed® Expectorant *(Discontinued)* *see* guaifenesin, pseudoephedrine, and codeine *on page 408*

Nucofed® Pediatric Expectorant *(Discontinued)* *see* guaifenesin, pseudoephedrine, and codeine *on page 408*

Nu-Cotrimox [Can] *see* sulfamethoxazole and trimethoprim *on page 813*

Nu-Cromolyn [Can] *see* cromolyn sodium *on page 218*

Nu-Cyclobenzaprine [Can] *see* cyclobenzaprine *on page 221*

Nu-Desipramine [Can] *see* desipramine *on page 238*

Nu-Diclo [Can] *see* diclofenac *on page 253*

Nu-Diclo-SR [Can] *see* diclofenac *on page 253*

Nu-Diflunisal [Can] *see* diflunisal *on page 257*

Nu-Diltiaz [Can] *see* diltiazem *on page 261*

Nu-Diltiaz-CD [Can] *see* diltiazem *on page 261*

Nu-Divalproex [Can] *see* valproic acid and derivatives *on page 881*

Nu-Domperidone [Can] *see* domperidone *(Canada only) on page 276*

Nu-Doxycycline [Can] *see* doxycycline *on page 281*

Nu-Erythromycin-S [Can] *see* erythromycin *on page 309*

Nu-Famotidine [Can] *see* famotidine *on page 341*

Nu-Fenofibrate [Can] *see* fenofibrate *on page 345*

Nu-Fluoxetine [Can] *see* fluoxetine *on page 364*

Nu-Flurprofen [Can] *see* flurbiprofen *on page 366*

Nu-Fluvoxamine [Can] *see* fluvoxamine *on page 370*

Nu-Gabapentin [Can] *see* gabapentin *on page 380*

Nu-Gemfibrozil [Can] *see* gemfibrozil *on page 387*

Nu-Glyburide [Can] *see* glyburide *on page 396*

Nu-Hydral [Can] *see* hydralazine *on page 425*

Nu-Ibuprofen [Can] *see* ibuprofen *on page 444*

Nu-Indapamide [Can] *see* indapamide *on page 452*

Nu-Indo [Can] *see* indomethacin *on page 454*

Nu-Ipratropium [Can] *see* ipratropium *on page 470*

Nu-Iron® 150 [US-OTC] *see* polysaccharide-iron complex *on page 697*

Nu-Ketoprofen [Can] *see* ketoprofen *on page 482*

Nu-Ketoprofen-E [Can] *see* ketoprofen *on page 482*

NuLev™ [US] *see* hyoscyamine *on page 441*

Nu-Levocarb [Can] *see* levodopa and carbidopa *on page 500*

Nullo® [US-OTC] *see* chlorophyll *on page 175*

Nu-Loraz [Can] *see* lorazepam *on page 518*

Nu-Lovastatin [Can] *see* lovastatin *on page 520*

Nu-Loxapine [Can] *see* loxapine *on page 521*

NuLYTELY® [US] *see* polyethylene glycol-electrolyte solution *on page 695*

Nu-Medopa [Can] *see* methyldopa *on page 557*

Nu-Mefenamic [Can] *see* mefenamic acid *on page 537*

Nu-Megestrol [Can] *see* megestrol *on page 538*

Nu-Metformin [Can] *see* metformin *on page 548*

Nu-Metoclopramide [Can] *see* metoclopramide *on page 561*

Nu-Metop [Can] *see* metoprolol *on page 562*

Nu-Moclobemide [Can] *see* moclobemide *(Canada only) on page 575*

Numoisyn™ [US] *see* saliva substitute *on page 774*

Numorphan® *(Discontinued)* *see* oxymorphone *on page 643*

Numzident® *(Discontinued)* *see* benzocaine *on page 101*

Nu-Naprox [Can] *see* naproxen *on page 591*

Nu-Nifed [Can] *see* nifedipine *on page 605*

Nu-Nizatidine [Can] *see* nizatidine *on page 610*

Nu-Nortriptyline [Can] *see* nortriptyline *on page 613*

Nu-Oxybutyn [Can] *see* oxybutynin *on page 639*

Nu-Pentoxifylline SR [Can] *see* pentoxifylline *on page 667*

Nu-Pen-VK [Can] *see* penicillin V potassium *on page 664*

Nupercainal® [US-OTC] *see* dibucaine *on page 252*

Nupercainal® Hydrocortisone Cream [US-OTC] *see* hydrocortisone (rectal) *on page 433*

Nu-Pindol [Can] *see* pindolol *on page 683*

Nu-Pirox [Can] *see* piroxicam *on page 687*

Nu-Prazo [Can] *see* prazosin *on page 708*

Nuprin® *(Discontinued)* *see* ibuprofen *on page 444*

Nu-Prochlor [Can] *see* prochlorperazine *on page 716*

Nu-Propranolol [Can] *see* propranolol *on page 724*

Nuquin HP® **[US]** *see* hydroquinone *on page 437*

Nu-Ranit [Can] *see* ranitidine *on page 744*

Nuromax® **[US]** *see* doxacurium *on page 278*

Nu-Selegiline [Can] *see* selegiline *on page 780*

Nu-Sertraline [Can] *see* sertraline *on page 783*

Nu-Sotalol [Can] *see* sotalol *on page 802*

Nu-Sucralate [Can] *see* sucralfate *on page 808*

Nu-Sulfinpyrazone [Can] *see* sulfinpyrazone *on page 814*

Nu-Sundac [Can] *see* sulindac *on page 815*

Nu-Tears® **[US-OTC]** *see* artificial tears *on page 75*

Nu-Tears® **II [US-OTC]** *see* artificial tears *on page 75*

Nu-Temazepam [Can] *see* temazepam *on page 823*

Nu-Terazosin [Can] *see* terazosin *on page 826*

Nu-Tetra [Can] *see* tetracycline *on page 831*

Nu-Tiaprofenic [Can] *see* tiaprofenic acid *(Canada only) on page 840*

Nu-Ticlopidine [Can] *see* ticlopidine *on page 842*

Nu-Timolol [Can] *see* timolol *on page 843*

Nutracort® **[US]** *see* hydrocortisone (topical) *on page 434*

Nutralox® **[US-OTC]** *see* calcium carbonate *on page 138*

Nutraplus® **[US-OTC]** *see* urea *on page 877*

Nu-Trazodone [Can] *see* trazodone *on page 859*

Nu-Triazide [Can] *see* hydrochlorothiazide and triamterene *on page 427*

Nu-Trimipramine [Can] *see* trimipramine *on page 868*

NutriNate® **[US]** *see* vitamins (multiple/prenatal) *on page 896*

NutriSpire™ **[US]** *see* vitamins (multiple/prenatal) *on page 896*

nutritional formula, enteral/oral (noo TRISH un al FOR myoo la, EN ter al/OR al)

Synonyms dietary supplements

U.S./Canadian Brand Names Carnation Instant Breakfast® [US-OTC]; Citrotein® [US-OTC]; Criticare HN® [US-OTC]; Ensure Plus® [US-OTC]; Ensure® [US-OTC]; Isocal® [US-OTC]; Magnacal® [US-OTC]; Microlipid™ [US-OTC]; Osmolite® HN [US-OTC]; Pedialyte® [US-OTC]; Portagen® [US-OTC]; Pregestimil® [US-OTC]; Propac™ [US-OTC]; Soyalac® [US-OTC]; Vital HN® [US-OTC]; Vitaneed™ [US-OTC]; Vivonex® T.E.N. [US-OTC]; Vivonex® [US-OTC]

Therapeutic Category Nutritional Supplement

Dosage Forms

Liquid: Calcium and sodium caseinate, maltodextrin, sucrose, partially hydrogenated soy oil, soy lecithin

Powder: Amino acids, predigested carbohydrates, safflower oil

Nutropin® **[US]** *see* somatropin *on page 799*

Nutropin AQ® **[US/Can]** *see* somatropin *on page 799*

Nutropine® **[Can]** *see* somatropin *on page 799*

NuvaRing® **[US/Can]** *see* ethinyl estradiol and etonogestrel *on page 325*

Nu-Verap [Can] *see* verapamil *on page 887*

Nu-Zopiclone [Can] *see* zopiclone *(Canada only) on page 909*

NVB *see* vinorelbine *on page 891*

NVP *see* nevirapine *on page 601*

Nyaderm [Can] *see* nystatin *on next page*

Nyamyc™ **[US]** *see* nystatin *on next page*

Nydrazid® *(Discontinued) see* isoniazid *on page 474*

nystatin (nye STAT in)

Sound-Alike/Look-Alike Issues
nystatin may be confused with Nilstat®, Nitrostat®
Nilstat® may be confused with Nitrostat®, nystatin

U.S./Canadian Brand Names Bio-Statin® [US]; Candistatin® [Can]; Mycostatin® [US]; Nilstat [Can]; Nyaderm [Can]; Nyamyc™ [US]; Nystat-Rx® [US]; Nystop® [US]; Pedi-Dri® [US]; PMS-Nystatin [Can]

Therapeutic Category Antifungal Agent

Use Treatment of susceptible cutaneous, mucocutaneous, and oral cavity fungal infections normally caused by the *Candida* species

Usual Dosage
Oral candidiasis:
Suspension (swish and swallow orally):
Premature infants: 100,000 units 4 times/day
Infants: 200,000 units 4 times/day or 100,000 units to each side of mouth 4 times/day
Children and Adults: 400,000-600,000 units 4 times/day
Powder for compounding: Children and Adults: $1/8$ teaspoon (500,000 units) to equal approximately $1/2$ cup of water; give 4 times/day
Mucocutaneous infections: Children and Adults: Topical: Apply 2-3 times/day to affected areas; very moist topical lesions are treated best with powder
Intestinal infections: Adults: Oral: 500,000-1,000,000 units every 8 hours
Vaginal infections: Adults: Vaginal tablets: Insert 1 tablet/day at bedtime for 2 weeks

Dosage Forms
Capsule:
Bio-Statin®: 500,000 units, 1 million units
Cream: 100,000 units/g (15 g, 30 g)
Mycostatin®: 100,000 units/g (30 g)
Ointment, topical: 100,000 units/g (15 g, 30 g)
Powder, for prescription compounding: 50 million units (10 g); 150 million units (30 g); 500 million units (100 g); 2 billion units (400 g)
Nystat-Rx®: 50 million units (10 g); 150 million units (30 g); 500 million units (100 g); 1 billion units (190 g); 2 billion units (350 g)
Powder, topical: 100,000 units/g (15 g, 30 g, 60 g)
Mycostatin®: 100,000 units/g (15 g)
Nyamyc™: 100,000 units/g (15 g, 30 g)
Nystop®: 100,000 units/g (15 g, 30 g, 60 g)
Pedi-Dri®: 100,000 units/g (56.7 g)
Suspension, oral: 100,000 units/mL
Tablet: 500,000 units
Tablet, vaginal: 100,000 units (15s)

nystatin and triamcinolone (nye STAT in & trye am SIN oh lone)

Sound-Alike/Look-Alike Issues
Mycolog®-II may be confused with Halog®

Synonyms triamcinolone and nystatin

Therapeutic Category Antifungal/Corticosteroid

Use Treatment of cutaneous candidiasis

Usual Dosage Topical: Children and Adults: Apply sparingly 2-4 times/day. Therapy should be discontinued when control is achieved; if no improvement is seen, reassessment of diagnosis may be necessary.

Dosage Forms
Cream: Nystatin 100,000 units and triamcinolone 0.1% (15 g, 30 g, 60 g)
Ointment: Nystatin 100,000 units and triamcinolone 0.1% (15 g, 30 g, 60 g)

Nystat-Rx® [US] *see* nystatin *on this page*

Nystex® (Discontinued) *see* nystatin *on this page*

Nystop® [US] *see* nystatin *on this page*

Nytol® [Can] *see* diphenhydramine *on page 265*

Nytol® Extra Strength [Can] *see* diphenhydramine *on page 265*

Nytol® Quick Caps [US-OTC] *see* diphenhydramine *on page 265*

Nytol® Quick Gels [US-OTC] *see* diphenhydramine *on page 265*

Obezine® (Discontinued) *see* phendimetrazine *on page 671*

OCBZ *see* oxcarbazepine *on page 638*

Occlusal®-HP [US-OTC/Can] *see* salicylic acid *on page 772*

Ocean® [US-OTC] *see* sodium chloride *on page 792*

Ocean® for Kids [US-OTC] *see* sodium chloride *on page 792*

OCL® (Discontinued) *see* polyethylene glycol-electrolyte solution *on page 695*

Octagam® [US] *see* immune globulin (intravenous) *on page 451*

Octamide® (Discontinued) *see* metoclopramide *on page 561*

Octicair® Otic (Discontinued) *see* neomycin, polymyxin B, and hydrocortisone *on page 597*

Octocaine® (Discontinued) *see* lidocaine and epinephrine *on page 506*

Octostim® [Can] *see* desmopressin acetate *on page 239*

octreotide (ok TREE oh tide)

Sound-Alike/Look-Alike Issues
Sandostatin® may be confused with Sandimmune®

Synonyms NSC-671663; octreotide acetate

U.S./Canadian Brand Names Octreotide Acetate Injection [Can]; Octreotide Acetate Omega [Can]; Sandostatin LAR® [US/Can]; Sandostatin® [US/Can]

Therapeutic Category Somatostatin Analog

Use Control of symptoms in patients with metastatic carcinoid and vasoactive intestinal peptide-secreting tumors (VIPomas); acromegaly

Usual Dosage Adults: SubQ, I.V.: Initial: 50 mcg 2-3 times/day and titrate dose based on patient tolerance, response, and indication

Carcinoid: Initial 2 weeks: 100-600 mcg/day in 2-4 divided doses; usual range 50-1500 mcg/day

VIPomas: Initial 2 weeks: 200-300 mcg/day in 2-4 divided doses; usual range 150-750 mcg/day

Acromegaly: Initial: SubQ: 50 mcg 3 times/day; titrate to achieve growth hormone levels <5 ng/mL or IGF-I (somatomedin C) levels <1.9 U/mL in males and <2.2 U/mL in females; usual effective dose 100 mcg 3 times/day; range 300-1500 mcg/day

Note: Should be withdrawn yearly for a 4-week interval (8 weeks for depot injection) in patients who have received irradiation. Resume if levels increase and signs/symptoms recur.

Acromegaly, carcinoid tumors, and VIPomas (depot injection): Patients must be stabilized on subcutaneous octreotide for at least 2 weeks before switching to the long-acting depot: Upon switch: 20 mg I.M. intragluteally every 4 weeks for 2-3 months, then the dose may be modified based upon response. Patients receiving depot injection for carcinoid tumor or VIPoma should continue to receive their SubQ injections for the first 2 weeks at the same dose in order to maintain therapeutic levels.

Dosage adjustment for acromegaly: After 3 months of depot injections the dosage may be continued or modified as follows:

GH ≤2.5 ng/mL, IGF-1 is normal, symptoms controlled: Maintain octreotide LAR® at 20 mg I.M. every 4 weeks

GH >2.5 ng/mL, IGF-1 is elevated, and/or symptoms uncontrolled: Increase octreotide LAR® to 30 mg I.M. every 4 weeks

GH ≤1 ng/mL, IGF-1 is normal, symptoms controlled: Reduce octreotide LAR® to 10 mg I.M. every 4 weeks

Note: Patients not adequately controlled may increase dose to 40 mg every 4 weeks. Dosages >40 mg are not recommended

Dosage adjustment for carcinoid tumors and VIPomas: After 2 months of depot injections the dosage may be continued or modified as follows:

Increase to 30 mg I.M. every 4 weeks if symptoms are inadequately controlled

Decrease to 10 mg I.M. every 4 weeks, for a trial period, if initially responsive to 20 mg dose

Dosage >30 mg is not recommended

Dosage Forms

Injection, microspheres for suspension [depot formulation]:
Sandostatin LAR®: 10 mg, 20 mg, 30 mg

Injection, solution: 0.2 mg/mL (5 mL); 1 mg/mL (5 mL)
Sandostatin®: 0.2 mg/mL (5 mL); 1 mg/mL (5 mL)

Injection, solution [preservative free]: 0.05 mg/mL (1 mL); 0.1 mg/mL (1 mL); 0.5 mg/mL (1 mL)
Sandostatin®: 0.05 mg/mL (1 mL); 0.1 mg/mL (1 mL); 0.5 mg/mL (1 mL)

octreotide acetate *see* octreotide *on this page*

Octreotide Acetate Injection [Can] *see* octreotide *on this page*

Octreotide Acetate Omega [Can] *see* octreotide *on this page*

OcuClear® (Discontinued) *see* oxymetazoline *on page 643*

OcuCoat® [US-OTC] *see* artificial tears *on page 75*

OcuCoat® PF [US-OTC] *see* artificial tears *on page 75*

Ocufen® [US/Can] *see* flurbiprofen *on page 366*

Ocuflox® **[US/Can]** *see* ofloxacin *on this page*

OcuNefrin™ **[US-OTC]** *see* phenylephrine *on page 675*

Ocupress® *(Discontinued)* *see* carteolol *on page 155*

Ocupress® **Ophthalmic [Can]** *see* carteolol *on page 155*

Ocusert Pilo-20® *(Discontinued)* *see* pilocarpine *on page 682*

Ocusert Pilo-40® *(Discontinued)* *see* pilocarpine *on page 682*

Ocu-Sul® *(Discontinued)* *see* sulfacetamide *on page 810*

Ocutricin® **Topical Ointment** *(Discontinued)* *see* bacitracin, neomycin, and polymyxin B *on page 91*

Ocuvite® **[US-OTC]** *see* vitamins (multiple/oral) *on page 895*

Ocuvite® **Adult [US-OTC]** *see* vitamins (multiple/oral) *on page 895*

Ocuvite® **Adult 50+ [US-OTC]** *see* vitamins (multiple/oral) *on page 895*

Ocuvite® **Extra**® **[US-OTC]** *see* vitamins (multiple/oral) *on page 895*

Ocuvite® **Lutein [US-OTC]** *see* vitamins (multiple/oral) *on page 895*

Oesclim® **[Can]** *see* estradiol *on page 313*

ofloxacin (oh FLOKS a sin)

Sound-Alike/Look-Alike Issues
Floxin® may be confused with Flexeril®
Ocuflox® may be confused with Ocufen®

U.S./Canadian Brand Names Apo-Ofloxacin® [Can]; Apo-Oflox® [Can]; Floxin® [US/Can]; Novo-Ofloxacin [Can]; Ocuflox® [US/Can]; PMS-Ofloxacin [Can]

Therapeutic Category Antibiotic, Ophthalmic; Antibiotic, Otic; Quinolone

Use Quinolone antibiotic for the treatment of acute exacerbations of chronic bronchitis, community-acquired pneumonia, skin and skin structure infections (uncomplicated), urethral and cervical gonorrhea (acute, uncomplicated), urethritis and cervicitis (nongonococcal), mixed infections of the urethra and cervix, pelvic inflammatory disease (acute), cystitis (uncomplicated), urinary tract infections (complicated), prostatitis

Note: As of April 2007, the CDC no longer recommends the use of fluoroquinolones for the treatment of gonococcal disease.

Ophthalmic: Treatment of superficial ocular infections involving the conjunctiva or cornea due to strains of susceptible organisms

Otic: Otitis externa, chronic suppurative otitis media, acute otitis media

Usual Dosage

Usual dosage range:
Children ≥6 months: Otic: 5 drops daily
Children >1 year: Ophthalmic: 1-2 drops every 30 minutes to 4 hours initially, decreasing to every 4-6 hours
Children >12 years: Otic: 10 drops once or twice daily
Adults:
 Ophthalmic: 1-2 drops every 30 minutes to 4 hours initially, decreasing to every 4-6 hours
 Oral: 200-400 mg every 12 hours
 Otic: 10 drops once or twice daily

Indication-specific dosing:
Children 6 months to 13 years: Otic:
 Otitis externa: Instill 5 drops (or the contents of 1 single-dose container) into affected ear(s) once daily for 7 days
Children 1-12 years: Otic:
 Acute otitis media with tympanostomy tubes: Instill 5 drops (or the contents of 1 single-dose container) into affected ear(s) twice daily for 10 days
Children >1 year and Adults: Ophthalmic:
 Conjunctivitis: Instill 1-2 drops in affected eye(s) every 2-4 hours for the first 2 days, then use 4 times/day for an additional 5 days
 Corneal ulcer: Instill 1-2 drops every 30 minutes while awake and every 4-6 hours after retiring for the first 2 days; beginning on day 3, instill 1-2 drops every hour while awake for 4-6 additional days; thereafter, 1-2 drops 4 times/day until clinical cure.
Children >12 years and Adults: Otic:
 Otitis media, chronic suppurative with perforated tympanic membranes: Instill 10 drops (or the contents of 2 single-dose containers) into affected ear twice daily for 14 days
Children ≥13 years and Adults: Otic:
 Otitis externa: Instill 10 drops (or the contents of 2 single-dose containers) into affected ear(s) once daily for 7 days
(Continued)

ofloxacin *(Continued)*

Adults: Oral:

Cervicitis/urethritis:

Nongonococcal: 300 mg every 12 hours for 7 days

Gonococcal (acute, uncomplicated): 400 mg as a single dose; **Note:** As of April 2007, the CDC no longer recommends the use of fluoroquinolones for the treatment of uncomplicated gonococcal disease.

Chronic bronchitis (acute exacerbation), community-acquired pneumonia, skin and skin structure infections (uncomplicated): 400 mg every 12 hours for 10 days

Pelvic inflammatory disease (acute): 400 mg every 12 hours for 10-14 days with or without metronidazole; **Note:** The CDC recommends use only if standard cephalosporin therapy is not feasible and community prevalence of quinolone-resistant gonococcal organisms is low. Culture sensitivity must be confirmed.

Prostatitis:

Acute: 400 mg for 1 dose, then 300 mg twice daily for 10 days

Chronic: 200 mg every 12 hours for 6 weeks

UTI:

Uncomplicated: 200 mg every 12 hours for 3-7 days

Complicated: 200 mg every 12 hours for 10 days

Dosage Forms

Solution, ophthalmic: 0.3% (5 mL)

Ocuflox®: 0.3% (5 mL)

Solution, otic:

Floxin®: 0.3% (5 mL, 10 mL)

Floxin® Otic Singles™: 0.3% (0.25 mL)

Tablet: 200 mg, 300 mg, 400 mg

Floxin®: 200 mg, 300 mg, 400 mg

Ogen® [US/Can] *see* estropipate *on page 320*

Ogestrel® [US] *see* ethinyl estradiol and norgestrel *on page 332*

OGMT *see* metyrosine *on page 565*

OGT-918 *see* miglustat *on page 570*

9-OH-risperidone *see* paliperidone *on page 646*

OKT3 *see* muromonab-CD3 *on page 583*

olanzapine *(oh LAN za peen)*

Sound-Alike/Look-Alike Issues

olanzapine may be confused with olsalazine

Zyprexa® may be confused with Celexa®, Zyrtec®

Synonyms LY170053

U.S./Canadian Brand Names Zyprexa® Zydis® [US/Can]; Zyprexa® [US/Can]

Therapeutic Category Antipsychotic Agent

Use Treatment of the manifestations of schizophrenia; treatment of acute or mixed mania episodes associated with Bipolar I Disorder (as monotherapy or in combination with lithium or valproate); maintenance treatment of bipolar disorder; acute agitation (patients with schizophrenia or bipolar mania)

Usual Dosage Adults:

Schizophrenia: Oral: Initial: 5-10 mg once daily (increase to 10 mg once daily within 5-7 days); thereafter, adjust by 5 mg/day at 1-week intervals, up to a recommended maximum of 20 mg/day. Maintenance: 10-20 mg once daily. **Note:** Doses of 30-50 mg/day have been used; however, doses >10 mg/day have not demonstrated better efficacy, and safety and efficacy of doses >20 mg/day have not been evaluated.

Bipolar I acute mixed or manic episodes: Oral:

Monotherapy: Initial: 10-15 mg once daily; increase by 5 mg/day at intervals of not less than 24 hours. Maintenance: 5-20 mg/day; recommended maximum dose: 20 mg/day.

Combination therapy (with lithium or valproate): Initial: 10 mg once daily; dosing range: 5-20 mg/day

Agitation (acute, associated with bipolar I mania or schizophrenia): I.M.: Initial dose: 5-10 mg (a lower dose of 2.5 mg may be considered when clinical factors warrant); additional doses (2.5-10 mg) may be considered; however, 2-4 hours should be allowed between doses to evaluate response (maximum total daily dose: 30 mg, per manufacturer's recommendation)

Dosage Forms

Injection, powder for reconstitution:

Zyprexa® IntraMuscular: 10 mg

Tablet:

Zyprexa®: 2.5 mg, 5 mg, 7.5 mg, 10 mg, 15 mg, 20 mg

Tablet, orally disintegrating:

Zyprexa® Zydis®: 5 mg, 10 mg, 15 mg, 20 mg

olanzapine and fluoxetine (oh LAN za peen & floo OKS e teen)

Synonyms fluoxetine and olanzapine; olanzapine and fluoxetine hydrochloride

U.S./Canadian Brand Names Symbyax® [US]

Therapeutic Category Antidepressant, Selective Serotonin Reuptake Inhibitor; Antipsychotic Agent, Thienobenzodiaepine

Use Treatment of depressive episodes associated with bipolar disorder

Usual Dosage Oral: Adults: Depression associated with bipolar disorder: Initial: Olanzapine 3-6 mg/fluoxetine 25 mg once daily in the evening. Dosing range: Olanzapine 6-12 mg/fluoxetine 25-50 mg. Lower doses (olanzapine 3 mg/fluoxetine 25 mg) should be used in patients predisposed to hypotension, in hepatic impairment, with combined factors for reduced metabolism (females, the elderly, nonsmokers), or enhanced sensitivity to olanzapine; use caution in dose adjustments in these patients. Safety of daily doses of olanzapine >18 mg/fluoxetine >75 mg have not been evaluated.

Dosage Forms
Capsule:
Symbyax®:
3/25: Olanzapine 3 mg and fluoxetine 25 mg
6/25: Olanzapine 6 mg and fluoxetine 25 mg
6/50: Olanzapine 6 mg and fluoxetine 50 mg
12/25: Olanzapine 12 mg and fluoxetine 25 mg
12/50: Olanzapine 12 mg and fluoxetine 50 mg

olanzapine and fluoxetine hydrochloride *see* olanzapine and fluoxetine *on this page*

Olay® Vitamins Complete Women's [US-OTC] *see* vitamins (multiple/oral) *on page 895*

Olay® Vitamins Complete Women's 50+ [US-OTC] *see* vitamins (multiple/oral) *on page 895*

oleovitamin A *see* vitamin A *on page 892*

oleum ricini *see* castor oil *on page 157*

olmesartan (ole me SAR tan)

Synonyms olmesartan medoxomil

U.S./Canadian Brand Names Benicar® [US]

Therapeutic Category Angiotensin II Receptor Antagonist

Use Treatment of hypertension with or without concurrent use of other antihypertensive agents

Usual Dosage Oral: Adults: Initial: Usual starting dose is 20 mg once daily; if initial response is inadequate, may be increased to 40 mg once daily after 2 weeks. May administer with other antihypertensive agents if blood pressure inadequately controlled with olmesartan. Consider lower starting dose in patients with possible depletion of intravascular volume (eg, patients receiving diuretics).

Dosage Forms
Tablet:
Benicar®: 5 mg, 20 mg, 40 mg

olmesartan and hydrochlorothiazide (ole me SAR tan & hye droe klor oh THYE a zide)

Synonyms hydrochlorothiazide and olmesartan medoxomil; olmesartan medoxomil and hydrochlorothiazide

U.S./Canadian Brand Names Benicar HCT® [US]

Therapeutic Category Angiotensin II Receptor Antagonist; Diuretic, Thiazide

Use Treatment of hypertension (not recommended for initial treatment)

Usual Dosage Oral: Adults: One tablet daily; dosage must be individualized (see below). May be titrated at 2- to 4-week intervals.
Replacement therapy: May be substituted for previously titrated dosages of the individual components.
Patients not controlled with single-agent therapy: Initiate by adding the lowest available dose of the alternative component (hydrochlorothiazide 12.5 mg or olmesartan 20 mg). Titrate to effect (maximum daily hydrochlorothiazide dose: 25 mg; maximum daily olmesartan dose: 40 mg).

Dosage Forms
Tablet:
Benicar HCT®: 20/12.5: Olmesartan 20 mg and hydrochlorothiazide 12.5 mg; 40/12.5: Olmesartan 40 mg and hydrochlorothiazide 12.5 mg; 40/25: Olmesartan 40 mg and hydrochlorothiazide 25 mg

olmesartan medoxomil *see* olmesartan *on this page*

olmesartan medoxomil and hydrochlorothiazide *see* olmesartan and hydrochlorothiazide *on this page*

olopatadine (oh la PAT a deen)

Sound-Alike/Look-Alike Issues
Patanol® may be confused with Platinol®
(Continued)

olopatadine *(Continued)*
Synonyms olopatadine hydrochloride
U.S./Canadian Brand Names Pataday™ [US]; Patanol® [US/Can]
Therapeutic Category Antihistamine
Use Treatment of the signs and symptoms of allergic conjunctivitis
Usual Dosage Ophthalmic: Children ≥3 years and Adults:
  Patanol®: Instill 1 drop into affected eye(s) twice daily (allowing 6-8 hours between doses); results from an environmental study demonstrated that olopatadine was effective when dosed twice daily for up to 6 weeks
  Pataday™: Instill 1 drop into affected eye(s) once daily
Dosage Forms
  Solution, ophthalmic:
  Patanol®: 0.1% (5 mL)
  Pataday™: 0.2% (2.5 mL)

olopatadine hydrochloride *see* olopatadine *on previous page*

olsalazine *(ole SAL a zeen)*
Sound-Alike/Look-Alike Issues
  olsalazine may be confused with olanzapine
  Dipentum® may be confused with Dilantin®
Synonyms olsalazine sodium
U.S./Canadian Brand Names Dipentum® [US/Can]
Therapeutic Category 5-Aminosalicylic Acid Derivative
Use Maintenance of remission of ulcerative colitis in patients intolerant to sulfasalazine
Usual Dosage Oral: Adults: 1 g/day in 2 divided doses
Dosage Forms
  Capsule:
  Dipentum®: 250 mg

olsalazine sodium *see* olsalazine *on this page*

Olux® [US] *see* clobetasol *on page 201*

Olux-E™ [US] *see* clobetasol *on page 201*

Omacor® [US] *see* omega-3-acid ethyl esters *on next page*

omalizumab *(oh mah lye ZOO mab)*
Synonyms rhuMAb-E25
U.S./Canadian Brand Names Xolair® [US/Can]
Therapeutic Category Monoclonal Antibody
Use Treatment of moderate-to-severe, persistent allergic asthma not adequately controlled with inhaled corticosteroids
Usual Dosage SubQ: Children ≥12 years and Adults: Asthma: Dose is based on pretreatment IgE serum levels and body weight. Dosing should not be adjusted based on IgE levels taken during treatment or <1 year following discontinuation of therapy; doses should be adjusted during treatment for significant changes in body weight
IgE ≥30-100 int. units/mL:
  30-90 kg: 150 mg every 4 weeks
  >90-150 kg: 300 mg every 4 weeks
IgE >100-200 int. units/mL:
  30-90 kg: 300 mg every 4 weeks
  >90-150 kg: 225 mg every 2 weeks
IgE >200-300 int. units/mL:
  30-60 kg: 300 mg every 4 weeks
  >60-90 kg: 225 mg every 2 weeks
  >90-150 kg: 300 mg every 2 weeks
IgE >300-400 int. units/mL:
  30-70 kg: 225 mg every 2 weeks
  >70-90 kg: 300 mg every 2 weeks
  >90 kg: Do not administer dose
IgE >400-500 int. units/mL:
  30-70 kg: 300 mg every 2 weeks
  >70-90 kg: 375 mg every 2 weeks
  >90 kg: Do not administer dose

IgE >500-600 int. units/mL:
30-60 kg: 300 mg every 2 weeks
>60-70 kg: 375 mg every 2 weeks
>70 kg: Do not administer dose
IgE >600-700 int. units/mL:
30-60 kg: 375 mg every 2 weeks
>60 kg: Do not administer dose

Dosage Forms
Injection, powder for reconstitution [preservative free]:
Xolair®: 150 mg

omega-3-acid ethyl esters (oh MEG a three AS id ETH il ES ters)

Sound-Alike/Look-Alike Issues
Omacor® may be confused with Amicar®

Synonyms ethyl esters of omega-3 fatty acids; fish oil

U.S./Canadian Brand Names Omacor® [US]

Therapeutic Category Antilipemic Agent, Miscellaneous

Use Omacor®: Treatment of hypertriglyceridemia (≥500 mg/dL)
Note: A number of OTC formulations containing omega-3 fatty acids are marketed as nutritional supplements; these do not have FDA-approved indications.

Usual Dosage Oral: Adults: Hypertriglyceridemia: 4 g/day as a single daily dose or in 2 divided doses

Dosage Forms
Capsule:
Lovaza™: 1 g

omeprazole (oh MEP ra zole)

Sound-Alike/Look-Alike Issues
Prilosec® may be confused with Plendil®, Prevacid®, predniSONE, prilocaine, Prinivil®, Proventil®, Prozac®

U.S./Canadian Brand Names Apo-Omeprazole® [Can]; Losec MUPS® [Can]; Losec® [Can]; Prilosec OTC™ [US-OTC]; Prilosec® [US]

Therapeutic Category Gastric Acid Secretion Inhibitor

Use Short-term (4-8 weeks) treatment of active duodenal ulcer disease or active benign gastric ulcer; treatment of heartburn and other symptoms associated with gastroesophageal reflux disease (GERD); short-term (4-8 weeks) treatment of endoscopically-diagnosed erosive esophagitis; maintenance healing of erosive esophagitis; long-term treatment of pathological hypersecretory conditions; as part of a multidrug regimen for *H. pylori* eradication to reduce the risk of duodenal ulcer recurrence

OTC labeling: Short-term treatment of frequent, uncomplicated heartburn occurring ≥2 days/week

Usual Dosage Oral:
Children ≥2 years: GERD or other acid-related disorders:
<20 kg: 10 mg once daily
≥20 kg: 20 mg once daily
Adults:
Active duodenal ulcer: 20 mg/day for 4-8 weeks
Gastric ulcers: 40 mg/day for 4-8 weeks
Symptomatic GERD: 20 mg/day for up to 4 weeks
Erosive esophagitis: 20 mg/day for 4-8 weeks; maintenance of healing: 20 mg/day for up to 12 months total therapy (including treatment period of 4-8 weeks)
Helicobacter pylori eradication: Dose varies with regimen: 20 mg once daily **or** 40 mg/day as single dose or in 2 divided doses; requires combination therapy with antibiotics
Pathological hypersecretory conditions: Initial: 60 mg once daily; doses up to 120 mg 3 times/day have been administered; administer daily doses >80 mg in divided doses
Frequent heartburn (OTC labeling): 20 mg/day for 14 days; treatment may be repeated after 4 months if needed

Dosage Forms
Capsule, delayed release: 10 mg, 20 mg
Prilosec®: 10 mg, 20 mg, 40 mg
Tablet, delayed release:
Prilosec OTC™ [OTC]: 20 mg

omeprazole and sodium bicarbonate (oh MEP ra zole & SOW dee um bye KAR bun ate)

U.S./Canadian Brand Names Zegerid® [US]

Therapeutic Category Proton Pump Inhibitor; Substituted Benzimidazole

Use Short-term (4-8 weeks) treatment of active duodenal ulcer disease or active benign gastric ulcer; treatment of heartburn and other symptoms associated with gastroesophageal reflux disease (GERD); short-term (4-8 (Continued)

omeprazole and sodium bicarbonate *(Continued)*

weeks) treatment of endoscopically-diagnosed erosive esophagitis; maintenance healing of erosive esophagitis; reduction of risk of upper gastrointestinal bleeding in critically-ill patients

Usual Dosage Oral: Adults:

Active duodenal ulcer: 20 mg/day for 4-8 weeks

Gastric ulcers: 40 mg/day for 4-8 weeks

Symptomatic GERD: 20 mg/day for up to 4 weeks

Erosive esophagitis: 20 mg/day for 4-8 weeks; maintenance of healing: 20 mg/day for up to 12 months total therapy (including treatment period of 4-8 weeks)

Risk reduction of upper GI bleeding in critically-ill patients (Zegerid® powder for oral suspension):

Loading dose: Day 1: 40 mg every 6-8 hours for two doses

Maintenance dose: 40 mg/day for up to 14 days; therapy >14 days has not been evaluated

Dosage Forms

Capsule, immediate release:

Zegerid®: 20 mg, 40 mg

Powder for oral suspension:

Zegerid®: 20 mg, 40 mg

Omnaris™ **[US]** *see* ciclesonide *on page 188*

Omnicef® **[US/Can]** *see* cefdinir *on page 159*

OMNIhist® **II L.A. [US]** *see* chlorpheniramine, phenylephrine, and methscopolamine *on page 181*

Omnii Gel™ **[US-OTC]** *see* fluoride *on page 361*

Omnipaque™ **[US]** *see* iohexol *on page 467*

Omnipen® *(Discontinued) see* ampicillin *on page 53*

Omnipen®**-N** *(Discontinued) see* ampicillin *on page 53*

Omniscan™ **[US]** *see* gadodiamide *on page 381*

Omnitrope™ **[US]** *see* somatropin *on page 799*

Oncaspar® **[US]** *see* pegaspargase *on page 657*

Oncet® *(Discontinued) see* hydrocodone and homatropine *on page 429*

Oncotice™ **[Can]** *see* BCG vaccine *on page 96*

Oncovin® *(Discontinued) see* vincristine *on page 891*

ondansetron (on DAN se tron)

Sound-Alike/Look-Alike Issues

ondansetron may be confused with dolasetron, granisetron, palonosetron

Zofran® may be confused with Zantac®, Zosyn®

Synonyms GR38032R; ondansetron hydrochloride

U.S./Canadian Brand Names Apo-Ondansetron® [Can]; Zofran® ODT [US/Can]; Zofran® [US/Can]

Therapeutic Category Selective 5-HT$_3$ Receptor Antagonist

Use Prevention of nausea and vomiting associated with moderately- to highly-emetogenic cancer chemotherapy; radiotherapy in patients receiving total body irradiation or fractions to the abdomen; prevention of postoperative nausea and vomiting (PONV); treatment of PONV if no prophylactic dose received

Usual Dosage Note: Studies in adults have shown a single daily dose of 8-12 mg I.V. or 8-24 mg orally to be as effective as mg/kg dosing, and should be considered for **all** patients whose mg/kg dose exceeds 8-12 mg I.V.; oral solution and ODT formulations are bioequivalent to corresponding doses of tablet formulation

Children:

I.V.:

Prevention of chemotherapy-induced emesis: 6 months to 18 years: 0.15 mg/kg/dose administered 30 minutes prior to chemotherapy, 4 and 8 hours after the first dose **or** 0.45 mg/kg/day as a single dose

Prevention of postoperative nausea and vomiting: 1 month to 12 years:

≤40 kg: 0.1 mg/kg as a single dose

>40 kg: 4 mg as a single dose

Oral: Prevention of chemotherapy-induced emesis:

4-11 years: 4 mg 30 minutes before chemotherapy; repeat 4 and 8 hours after initial dose, then 4 mg every 8 hours for 1-2 days after chemotherapy completed

≥12 years: Refer to adult dosing.

Adults:

I.V.:

Prevention of chemotherapy-induced emesis:

0.15 mg/kg 3 times/day beginning 30 minutes prior to chemotherapy **or**

0.45 mg/kg once daily **or**
8-10 mg 1-2 times/day **or**
24 mg or 32 mg once daily
I.M., I.V.: Postoperative nausea and vomiting: 4 mg as a single dose approximately 30 minutes before the end of anesthesia, or as treatment if vomiting occurs after surgery
Note: Repeat doses given in response to inadequate control of nausea/vomiting from preoperative doses are generally ineffective.
Oral:
Chemotherapy-induced emesis:
Highly-emetogenic agents/single-day therapy: 24 mg given 30 minutes prior to the start of therapy
Moderately-emetogenic agents: 8 mg every 12 hours beginning 30 minutes before chemotherapy, continuously for 1-2 days after chemotherapy completed
Total body irradiation: 8 mg 1-2 hours before daily each fraction of radiotherapy
Single high-dose fraction radiotherapy to abdomen: 8 mg 1-2 hours before irradiation, then 8 mg every 8 hours after first dose for 1-2 days after completion of radiotherapy
Daily fractionated radiotherapy to abdomen: 8 mg 1-2 hours before irradiation, then 8 mg 8 hours after first dose for each day of radiotherapy
Postoperative nausea and vomiting: 16 mg given 1 hour prior to induction of anesthesia
Dosage Forms
Infusion [premixed in D_5W, preservative free]: 32 mg (50 mL)
Zofran®: 32 mg (50 mL)
Injection, solution: 2 mg/mL (2 mL, 20 mL)
Zofran®: 2 mg/mL (2 mL, 20 mL)
Solution, oral: 4 mg/5 mL (50 mL)
Zofran®: 4 mg/5 mL
Tablet: 4 mg; 8 mg
Zofran®: 4 mg, 8 mg
Tablet, orally disintegrating: 4 mg; 8 mg
Zofran® ODT: 4 mg, 8 mg

ondansetron hydrochloride *see* ondansetron *on previous page*

One-A-Day® **50 Plus Formula [US-OTC]** *see* vitamins (multiple/oral) *on page 895*

One-A-Day® **Active Formula [US-OTC]** *see* vitamins (multiple/oral) *on page 895*

One-A-Day® **All Day Energy [US-OTC]** *see* vitamins (multiple/oral) *on page 895*

One-A-Day® **Cholesterol Plus**™ **[US-OTC]** *see* vitamins (multiple/oral) *on page 895*

One-A-Day® **Essential Formula [US-OTC]** *see* vitamins (multiple/oral) *on page 895*

One-A-Day® **Kids Bugs Bunny and Friends Complete [US-OTC]** *see* vitamins (multiple/pediatric) *on page 896*

One-A-Day® **Kids Scooby-Doo! Complete [US-OTC]** *see* vitamins (multiple/pediatric) *on page 896*

One-A-Day® **Kids Scooby-Doo! Plus Calcium [US-OTC]** *see* vitamins (multiple/pediatric) *on page 896*

One-A-Day® **Maximum Formula [US-OTC]** *see* vitamins (multiple/oral) *on page 895*

One-A-Day® **Men's Health Formula [US-OTC]** *see* vitamins (multiple/oral) *on page 895*

One-A-Day® **Scooby-Doo! Gummies [US-OTC]** *see* vitamins (multiple/pediatric) *on page 896*

One-A-Day® **Weight Smart [US-OTC]** *see* vitamins (multiple/oral) *on page 895*

One-A-Day® **Women's Formula [US-OTC]** *see* vitamins (multiple/oral) *on page 895*

One Gram C [US-OTC] *see* ascorbic acid *on page 76*

ONTAK® **[US]** *see* denileukin diftitox *on page 236*

Onxol™ **[US]** *see* paclitaxel *on page 645*

Ony-Clear *(Discontinued) see* benzalkonium chloride *on page 100*

Opana® **[US]** *see* oxymorphone *on page 643*

Opana® **ER [US]** *see* oxymorphone *on page 643*

OPC-13013 *see* cilostazol *on page 189*

OPC-14597 *see* aripiprazole *on page 73*

OP-CCK *see* sincalide *on page 787*

Opcon-A® **[US-OTC]** *see* naphazoline and pheniramine *on page 591*

Opcon® **Ophthalmic** *(Discontinued) see* naphazoline *on page 590*

o,p′-DDD *see* mitotane *on page 573*

Operand® **[US-OTC]** *see* povidone-iodine *on page 704*

Operand® **Chlorhexidine Gluconate [US-OTC]** *see* chlorhexidine gluconate *on page 174*

Ophthalgan® **Ophthalmic** *(Discontinued)* *see* glycerin *on page 397*

Ophthetic® **[US]** *see* proparacaine *on page 721*

Ophthifluor® *(Discontinued)* *see* fluorescein *on page 361*

Ophthochlor® **Ophthalmic** *(Discontinued)* *see* chloramphenicol *on page 173*

Ophtho-Dipivefrin™ **[Can]** *see* dipivefrin *on page 270*

Ophtho-Tate® **[Can]** *see* prednisolone (ophthalmic) *on page 709*

opium and belladonna *see* belladonna and opium *on page 97*

opium tincture (OH pee um TING chur)

Sound-Alike/Look-Alike Issues
opium tincture may be confused with camphorated tincture of opium (paregoric)
DTO is an error-prone abbreviation (mistaken as Diluted Tincture of Opium; dose equivalency of paregoric)
Synonyms opium tincture, deodorized
Therapeutic Category Analgesic, Narcotic
Controlled Substance C-II
Use Treatment of diarrhea or relief of pain
Usual Dosage Oral: **Note:** Opium tincture 10% contains morphine 10 mg/mL. use caution in ordering, dispensing, and/or administering.
Children:
Diarrhea: 0.005-0.01 mL/kg/dose every 3-4 hours for a maximum of 6 doses/24 hours
Analgesia: 0.01-0.02 mL/kg/dose every 3-4 hours
Adults:
Diarrhea: 0.3-1 mL/dose every 2-6 hours to maximum of 6 mL/24 hours
Analgesia: 0.6-1.5 mL/dose every 3-4 hours
Dosage Forms
Liquid: 10%

opium tincture, deodorized *see* opium tincture *on this page*

oprelvekin (oh PREL ve kin)

Sound-Alike/Look-Alike Issues
oprelvekin may be confused with aldesleukin, Proleukin®
Neumega® may be confused with Neulasta®, Neupogen®
Synonyms IL-11; interleukin-11; NSC-722848; recombinant human interleukin-11; recombinant interleukin-11; rhIL-11; rIL-11
U.S./Canadian Brand Names Neumega® [US]
Therapeutic Category Platelet Growth Factor
Use Prevention of severe thrombocytopenia; reduce the need for platelet transfusions following myelosuppressive chemotherapy
Usual Dosage SubQ: Administer first dose ~6-24 hours after the end of chemotherapy. Discontinue at least 48 hours before beginning the next cycle of chemotherapy.
Adults: 50 mcg/kg once daily for ~10-21 days (until postnadir platelet count ≥50,000 cells/µL)
Dosage Forms
Injection, powder for reconstitution:
Neumega®: 5 mg

Optase™ **[US]** *see* trypsin, balsam peru, and castor oil *on page 872*

Optho-Bunolol® **[Can]** *see* levobunolol *on page 499*

Opticrom® **[US/Can]** *see* cromolyn sodium *on page 218*

Optigene® **3 [US-OTC]** *see* tetrahydrozoline *on page 832*

OptiMARK® **[US]** *see* gadoversetamide *on page 382*

Optimine® **[Can]** *see* azatadine *(Canada only)* *on page 87*

Optimine® *(Discontinued)*

Optimoist® **Solution** *(Discontinued)* *see* saliva substitute *on page 774*

Optimyxin® **[Can]** *see* bacitracin and polymyxin B *on page 91*

Optimyxin Plus® **[Can]** *see* neomycin, polymyxin B, and gramicidin *on page 597*

OptiPranolol® **[US/Can]** *see* metipranolol *on page 561*

Optiray® **[US]** *see* ioversol *on page 469*

Optivar® **[US]** *see* azelastine *on page 88*

Optivite® **P.M.T. [US-OTC]** *see* vitamins (multiple/oral) *on page 895*

Orabase® **with Benzocaine [US-OTC]** *see* benzocaine *on page 101*

Oracea™ **[US]** *see* doxycycline *on page 281*

Oracort [Can] *see* triamcinolone (systemic) *on page 862*

Oradex-C® *(Discontinued)* *see* dyclonine *on page 287*

Orajel® **Baby Teething [US-OTC]** *see* benzocaine *on page 101*

Orajel® **Baby Teething Daytime and Nighttime [US-OTC]** *see* benzocaine *on page 101*

Orajel® **Baby Teething Nighttime [US-OTC]** *see* benzocaine *on page 101*

Orajel® **Brace-Aid Oral Anesthetic** *(Discontinued)* *see* benzocaine *on page 101*

Orajel® **Denture Plus [US-OTC]** *see* benzocaine *on page 101*

Orajel® **Maximum Strength [US-OTC]** *see* benzocaine *on page 101*

Orajel® **Medicated Toothache [US-OTC]** *see* benzocaine *on page 101*

Orajel® **Mouth Sore [US-OTC]** *see* benzocaine *on page 101*

Orajel® **Multi-Action Cold Sore [US-OTC]** *see* benzocaine *on page 101*

Orajel® **Perioseptic**® **Spot Treatment [US-OTC]** *see* carbamide peroxide *on page 148*

Orajel PM® **[US-OTC]** *see* benzocaine *on page 101*

Orajel® **Ultra Mouth Sore [US-OTC]** *see* benzocaine *on page 101*

Oramorph SR® **[US]** *see* morphine sulfate *on page 578*

Oranyl [US-OTC] *see* pseudoephedrine *on page 727*

Oranyl Plus [US-OTC] *see* acetaminophen and pseudoephedrine *on page 8*

Orap® **[US/Can]** *see* pimozide *on page 683*

Orapred® **[US]** *see* prednisolone (systemic) *on page 710*

Oraquix® **[US]** *see* lidocaine and prilocaine *on page 507*

OraRinse™ **[US-OTC]** *see* maltodextrin *on page 530*

Orasone® *(Discontinued)* *see* prednisone *on page 710*

Orazinc® **[US-OTC]** *see* zinc sulfate *on page 906*

orciprenaline sulfate *see* metaproterenol *on page 548*

Orencia® **[US]** *see* abatacept *on page 3*

Oreton® **Methyl** *(Discontinued)* *see* methyltestosterone *on page 560*

Orfadin® **[US]** *see* nitisinone *on page 607*

ORG 946 *see* rocuronium *on page 764*

Orgalutran® **[Can]** *see* ganirelix *on page 384*

Organidin® **NR [US]** *see* guaifenesin *on page 401*

Orgaran® **[Can]** *see* danaparoid *(Canada only)* *on page 230*

Orgaran® *(Discontinued)* *see* danaparoid *(Canada only)* *on page 230*

ORG NC 45 *see* vecuronium *on page 886*

Orinase Diagnostic® *(Discontinued)* *see* tolbutamide *on page 849*

Orinase® **Oral** *(Discontinued)* *see* tolbutamide *on page 849*

ORLAAM® *(Discontinued)*

orlistat (OR li stat)
  Sound-Alike/Look-Alike Issues
    Xenical® may be confused with Xeloda®
  U.S./Canadian Brand Names Alli™ [US-OTC]; Xenical® [US/Can]
  Therapeutic Category Lipase Inhibitor
  Use Management of obesity, including weight loss and weight management, when used in conjunction with a reduced-calorie and low-fat diet; reduce the risk of weight regain after prior weight loss; indicated for obese patients with an initial body mass index (BMI) ≥30 kg/m^2 or ≥27 kg/m^2 in the presence of other risk factors
(Continued)

orlistat *(Continued)*

Usual Dosage Oral:

Children ≥12 years and Adults (Xenical®): 120 mg 3 times/day with each main meal containing fat (during or up to 1 hour after the meal); omit dose if meal is occasionally missed or contains no fat.

Adults (Alli™): OTC labeling: 60 mg 3 times/day with each main meal containing fat

Dosage Forms

Capsule:

Alli™ [OTC]: 60 mg

Xenical®: 120 mg

Ormazine® *(Discontinued)* *see* chlorpromazine *on page 185*

Ornex® [US-OTC] *see* acetaminophen and pseudoephedrine *on page 8*

Ornex® Maximum Strength [US-OTC] *see* acetaminophen and pseudoephedrine *on page 8*

Ornidyl® Injection *(Discontinued)* *see* eflornithine *on page 293*

ORO-Clense [Can] *see* chlorhexidine gluconate *on page 174*

Orphenace® [Can] *see* orphenadrine *on this page*

orphenadrine *(or FEN a dreen)*

Sound-Alike/Look-Alike Issues

Norflex™ may be confused with norfloxacin, Noroxin®

Synonyms orphenadrine citrate

U.S./Canadian Brand Names Norflex™ [US/Can]; Orphenace® [Can]; Rhoxal-orphendrine [Can]

Therapeutic Category Skeletal Muscle Relaxant

Use Treatment of muscle spasm associated with acute painful musculoskeletal conditions

Usual Dosage Adults:

Oral: 100 mg twice daily

I.M., I.V.: 60 mg every 12 hours

Dosage Forms

Injection, solution: 30 mg/mL (2 mL)

Norflex™: 30 mg/mL (2 mL)

Tablet, extended release: 100 mg

Norflex™: 100 mg

orphenadrine, aspirin, and caffeine *(or FEN a dreen, AS pir in, & KAF een)*

Sound-Alike/Look-Alike Issues

Norgesic™ Forte may be confused with Norgesic 40®

Synonyms aspirin, orphenadrine, and caffeine; caffeine, orphenadrine, and aspirin

U.S./Canadian Brand Names Norgesic™ Forte [Can]; Norgesic™ [Can]

Therapeutic Category Analgesic, Nonnarcotic; Skeletal Muscle Relaxant

Use Relief of discomfort associated with skeletal muscular conditions

Usual Dosage Oral: 1-2 tablets 3-4 times/day

Dosage Forms

Tablet: Orphenadrine 25 mg, aspirin 385 mg, and caffeine 30 mg; orphenadrine 50 mg, aspirin 770 mg, and caffeine 60 mg

orphenadrine citrate *see* orphenadrine *on this page*

Orphengesic *(Discontinued)* *see* orphenadrine, aspirin, and caffeine *on this page*

Orphengesic Forte *(Discontinued)* *see* orphenadrine, aspirin, and caffeine *on this page*

Ortho® 0.5/35 [Can] *see* ethinyl estradiol and norethindrone *on page 328*

Ortho® 1/35 [Can] *see* ethinyl estradiol and norethindrone *on page 328*

Ortho® 7/7/7 [Can] *see* ethinyl estradiol and norethindrone *on page 328*

Ortho-Cept® [US/Can] *see* ethinyl estradiol and desogestrel *on page 322*

Orthoclone OKT® 3 [US/Can] *see* muromonab-CD3 *on page 583*

Ortho-Cyclen® [US] *see* ethinyl estradiol and norgestimate *on page 331*

Ortho-Est® [US] *see* estropipate *on page 320*

Ortho Evra® [US] *see* ethinyl estradiol and norelgestromin *on page 328*

Ortho Micronor® [US] *see* norethindrone *on page 611*

Ortho-Novum® [US] *see* ethinyl estradiol and norethindrone *on page 328*

Ortho-Novum® **1/50 [US/Can]** *see* mestranol and norethindrone *on page 547*

ortho prefest *see* estradiol and norgestimate *on page 316*

Ortho Tri-Cyclen® **[US]** *see* ethinyl estradiol and norgestimate *on page 331*

Ortho Tri-Cyclen® **Lo [US]** *see* ethinyl estradiol and norgestimate *on page 331*

Orthovisc® **[US/Can]** *see* hyaluronate and derivatives *on page 423*

Or-Tyl® **Injection** *(Discontinued) see* dicyclomine *on page 255*

Orudis® **KT** *(Discontinued) see* ketoprofen *on page 482*

Oruvail® **[Can]** *see* ketoprofen *on page 482*

Orvaten™ **[US]** *see* midodrine *on page 569*

Os-Cal® **[Can]** *see* calcium carbonate *on page 138*

Os-Cal® **500+D [US-OTC]** *see* calcium and vitamin D *on page 137*

Os-Cal® **500** *(Discontinued) see* calcium carbonate *on page 138*

oseltamivir (oh sel TAM i vir)

Sound-Alike/Look-Alike Issues
Tamiflu® may be confused with Thera-Flu®

U.S./Canadian Brand Names Tamiflu® [US/Can]

Therapeutic Category Antiviral Agent, Oral

Use Treatment of uncomplicated acute illness due to influenza (A or B) infection in children ≥1 year of age and adults who have been symptomatic for no more than 2 days; prophylaxis against influenza (A or B) infection in children ≥1 year of age and adults

Usual Dosage Oral:

Treatment: Initiate treatment within 2 days of onset of symptoms; duration of treatment: 5 days:

Children: 1-12 years:

≤15 kg: 30 mg twice daily

>15 kg to ≤23 kg: 45 mg twice daily

>23 kg to ≤40 kg: 60 mg twice daily

>40 kg: 75 mg twice daily

Adolescents ≥13 years and Adults: 75 mg twice daily

Prophylaxis: Initiate treatment within 2 days of contact with an infected individual; duration of treatment: 10 days

Children: 1-12 years:

≤15 kg: 30 mg once daily

>15 kg to ≤23 kg: 45 mg once daily

>23 kg to ≤40 kg: 60 mg once daily

>40 kg: 75 mg once daily

Adolescents ≥13 years and Adults: 75 mg once daily. During community outbreaks, dosing is 75 mg once daily. May be used for up to 6 weeks; duration of protection lasts for length of dosing period

Dosage Forms

Capsule:
Tamiflu®: 75 mg

Powder for oral suspension:
Tamiflu®: 12 mg/mL

OSI-774 *see* erlotinib *on page 307*

Osmitrol® **[US/Can]** *see* mannitol *on page 530*

Osmoglyn® *(Discontinued) see* glycerin *on page 397*

Osmolite® **HN [US-OTC]** *see* nutritional formula, enteral/oral *on page 622*

OsmoPrep™ **[US]** *see* sodium phosphates *on page 796*

Ostac® **[Can]** *see* clodronate *(Canada only) on page 202*

Osteocalcin® *(Discontinued) see* calcitonin *on page 135*

Osteocit® **[Can]** *see* calcium citrate *on page 140*

Ostoforte® **[Can]** *see* ergocalciferol *on page 305*

OTFC (oral transmucosal fentanyl citrate) *see* fentanyl *on page 346*

Oticaine [US] *see* benzocaine *on page 101*

Otic-Care® **Otic** *(Discontinued) see* neomycin, polymyxin B, and hydrocortisone *on page 597*

Otobiotic Otic Solution *(Discontinued)*

Otocaine™ [US] *see* benzocaine *on page 101*

Otocort® Otic *(Discontinued) see* neomycin, polymyxin B, and hydrocortisone *on page 597*

Otosporin® Otic *(Discontinued) see* neomycin, polymyxin B, and hydrocortisone *on page 597*

Otrivin® *(Discontinued)*

Otrivin® Pediatric *(Discontinued)*

Outgro® [US-OTC] *see* benzocaine *on page 101*

Ovace® [US] *see* sulfacetamide *on page 810*

Ovace® Wash [US] *see* sulfacetamide *on page 810*

Ovcon® [US] *see* ethinyl estradiol and norethindrone *on page 328*

Ovide® [US] *see* malathion *on page 530*

Ovidrel® [US/Can] *see* chorionic gonadotropin (recombinant) *on page 187*

ovine corticotrophin-releasing hormone *see* corticorelin *on page 216*

Ovol® [Can] *see* simethicone *on page 786*

Ovral® [Can] *see* ethinyl estradiol and norgestrel *on page 332*

Ovral® *(Discontinued) see* ethinyl estradiol and norgestrel *on page 332*

Ovrette® *(Discontinued)*

O-V Staticin® *(Discontinued) see* nystatin *on page 623*

oxacillin (oks a SIL in)
Synonyms methylphenyl isoxazolyl penicillin; oxacillin sodium
Therapeutic Category Penicillin
Use Treatment of infections such as osteomyelitis, septicemia, endocarditis, and CNS infections caused by susceptible strains of *Staphylococcus*
Usual Dosage
Usual dosage range:
Infants and Children: I.M., I.V.: 100-200 mg/kg/day in divided doses every 6 hours (maximum: 12 g/day)
Adults: I.M., I.V.: 250-2000 mg every 4-6 hours
Indication-specific dosing:
Children:
Arthritis (septic): I.V.: 37 mg/kg every 6 hours
Epiglottitis: I.V.: 150-200 mg/kg/day divided every 6 hours
Mild-to-moderate infections: I.M., I.V.: 100-150 mg/kg/day in divided doses every 6 hours (maximum: 4 g/day)
Severe infections: I.M., I.V.: 150-200 mg/kg/day in divided doses every 6 hours (maximum: 12 g/day)
Staphylococcal scalded-skin syndrome: I.V.: 150 mg/kg/day divided every 6 hours for 5-7 days
Adults:
Endocarditis: I.V.: 2 g every 4 hours with gentamicin
Mild-to-moderate infections: I.M., I.V.: 250-500 mg every 4-6 hours
Prosthetic joint infection: I.V.: 2 g every 4 hours with rifampin
Severe infections: I.M., I.V.: 1-2 g every 4-6 hours
***Staphylococcus aureus,* methicillin-susceptible infections, including brain abscess, bursitis, erysipelas, mastitis, mastoiditis, osteomyelitis, perinephric abscess, pneumonia, pyomyositis, scalded skin syndrome, toxic shock syndrome:** I.V.: 2 g every 4 hours
Dosage Forms
Infusion [premixed iso-osmotic dextrose solution]: 1 g (50 mL); 2 g (50 mL)
Injection, powder for reconstitution: 1 g, 2 g, 10 g

oxacillin sodium *see* oxacillin *on this page*

oxaliplatin (ox AL i pla tin)
Sound-Alike/Look-Alike Issues
oxaliplatin may be confused with Aloxi®, carboplatin
Synonyms diaminocyclohexane oxalatoplatinum; L-OHP; NSC-266046
U.S./Canadian Brand Names Eloxatin® [US]
Therapeutic Category Antineoplastic Agent, Alkylating Agent
Use Treatment of stage III colon cancer and advanced colorectal cancer
Usual Dosage I.V. (refer to individual protocols): Adults: Stage III colon cancer and colorectal cancer: 85 mg/m^2 every 2 weeks

Dosage Forms
Injection, solution [preservative free]:
Eloxatin™: 5 mg/mL (10 mL, 20 mL, 40 mL)

Oxandrin® [US] *see* oxandrolone *on this page*

oxandrolone (oks AN droe lone)
U.S./Canadian Brand Names Oxandrin® [US]
Therapeutic Category Androgen
Controlled Substance C-III
Use Adjunctive therapy to promote weight gain after weight loss following extensive surgery, chronic infections, or severe trauma, and in some patients who, without definite pathophysiologic reasons, fail to gain or to maintain normal weight; to offset protein catabolism with prolonged corticosteroid administration; relief of bone pain associated with osteoporosis
Usual Dosage
Children: Total daily dose: ≤0.1 mg/kg **or** ≤0.045 mg/lb
Adults: 2.5-20 mg in divided doses 2-4 times/day based on individual response; a course of therapy of 2-4 weeks is usually adequate. This may be repeated intermittently as needed.
Dosage Forms
Tablet: 2.5 mg, 10 mg
Oxandrin®: 2.5 mg, 10 mg

oxaprozin (oks a PROE zin)
Sound-Alike/Look-Alike Issues
oxaprozin may be confused with oxazepam
Daypro® may be confused with Diupres®
U.S./Canadian Brand Names Apo-Oxaprozin® [Can]; Daypro® [US/Can]
Therapeutic Category Analgesic, Nonnarcotic; Nonsteroidal Antiinflammatory Drug (NSAID)
Use Acute and long-term use in the management of signs and symptoms of osteoarthritis and rheumatoid arthritis; juvenile rheumatoid arthritis
Usual Dosage Oral (individualize dosage to lowest effective dose to minimize adverse effects):
Children 6-16 years: Juvenile rheumatoid arthritis:
22-31 kg: 600 mg once daily
32-54 kg: 900 mg once daily
≥55 kg: 1200 mg once daily
Adults:
Osteoarthritis: 600-1200 mg once daily; patients should be titrated to lowest dose possible; patients with low body weight should start with 600 mg daily
Rheumatoid arthritis: 1200 mg once daily; a one-time loading dose of up to 1800 mg/day or 26 mg/kg (whichever is lower) may be given
Maximum doses:
Patient <50 kg: Maximum: 1200 mg/day
Patient >50 kg with normal renal/hepatic function and low risk of peptic ulcer: Maximum: 1800 mg or 26 mg/kg (whichever is lower) in divided doses
Dosage Forms
Tablet: 600 mg
Daypro®: 600 mg

oxazepam (oks A ze pam)
Sound-Alike/Look-Alike Issues
oxazepam may be confused with oxaprozin, quazepam
Serax® may be confused with Eurax®, Urex®, Zyrtec®
U.S./Canadian Brand Names Apo-Oxazepam® [Can]; Novoxapram® [Can]; Oxpam® [Can]; Oxpram® [Can]; PMS-Oxazepam [Can]; Riva-Oxazepam [Can]; Serax® [US]
Therapeutic Category Anticonvulsant; Benzodiazepine
Controlled Substance C-IV
Use Treatment of anxiety; management of ethanol withdrawal
Usual Dosage Oral: Adults:
Anxiety: 10-30 mg 3-4 times/day
Ethanol withdrawal: 15-30 mg 3-4 times/day
Hypnotic: 15-30 mg
Dosage Forms
Capsule: 10 mg, 15 mg, 30 mg
Serax®: 10 mg, 15 mg, 30 mg
(Continued)

oxazepam *(Continued)*

Tablet:
Serax®: 15 mg

oxcarbazepine (ox car BAZ e peen)

Synonyms GP 47680; OCBZ

U.S./Canadian Brand Names Trileptal® [US/Can]

Therapeutic Category Anticonvulsant, Miscellaneous

Use Monotherapy or adjunctive therapy in the treatment of partial seizures in adults and children ≥4 years of age with epilepsy; adjunctive therapy in the treatment of partial seizures in children ≥2 years of age with epilepsy

Usual Dosage Oral:

Children 2-3 years:

Adjunctive therapy: 8-10 mg/kg/day, not to exceed 600 mg/day, given in 2 divided daily doses. Maintenance dose should be achieved over 2 weeks, and is dependent upon patient weight.

<20 kg: Consider initiating dose at 16-20 mg/kg/day; maximum maintenance dose should be achieved over 2-4 weeks and should not exceed 60 mg/kg/day

Children 4-16 years:

Adjunctive therapy: 8-10 mg/kg/day, not to exceed 600 mg/day, given in 2 divided daily doses. Maintenance dose should be achieved over 2 weeks, and is dependent upon patient weight, according to the following:

20-29 kg: 900 mg/day in 2 divided doses

29.1-39 kg: 1200 mg/day in 2 divided doses

>39 kg: 1800 mg/day in 2 divided doses

Children 4-16 years:

Conversion to monotherapy: Oxcarbazepine 8-10 mg/kg/day in twice daily divided doses, while simultaneously initiating the reduction of the dose of the concomitant antiepileptic drug; the concomitant drug should be withdrawn over 3-6 weeks. Oxcarbazepine dose may be increased by a maximum of 10 mg/kg/day at weekly intervals. See below for recommended total daily dose by weight.

Initiation of monotherapy: Oxcarbazepine should be initiated at 8-10 mg/kg/day in twice daily divided doses; doses may be titrated by 5 mg/kg/day every third day. See below for recommended total daily dose by weight.

Range of maintenance doses by weight during monotherapy:

20 kg: 600-900 mg/day

25-30 kg: 900-1200 mg/day

35-40 kg: 900-1500 mg/day

45 kg: 1200-1500 mg/day

50-55 kg: 1200-1800 mg/day

60-65 kg: 1200-2100 mg/day

70 kg: 1500-2100 mg/day

Adults:

Adjunctive therapy: Initial: 300 mg twice daily; dose may be increased by as much as 600 mg/day at weekly intervals; recommended daily dose: 1200 mg/day in 2 divided doses. Although daily doses >1200 mg/day demonstrated greater efficacy, most patients were unable to tolerate 2400 mg/day (due to CNS effects).

Conversion to monotherapy: Oxcarbazepine 600 mg/day in twice daily divided doses while simultaneously initiating the reduction of the dose of the concomitant antiepileptic drug. The concomitant dosage should be withdrawn over 3-6 weeks, while the maximum dose of oxcarbazepine should be reached in about 2-4 weeks. Recommended daily dose: 2400 mg/day.

Initiation of monotherapy: Oxcarbazepine should be initiated at a dose of 600 mg/day in twice daily divided doses; doses may be titrated upward by 300 mg/day every third day to a final dose of 1200 mg/day given in 2 daily divided doses

Dosage Forms

Suspension, oral:

Trileptal®: 300 mg/5 mL

Tablet:

Trileptal®: 150 mg, 300 mg, 600 mg

Oxeze® Turbuhaler® [Can] *see* formoterol *on page 374*

oxiconazole (oks i KON a zole)

Synonyms oxiconazole nitrate

U.S./Canadian Brand Names Oxistat® [US/Can]

Therapeutic Category Antifungal Agent

Use Treatment of tinea pedis (athlete's foot), tinea cruris (jock itch), tinea corporis (ringworm), and tinea (pityriasis) versicolor

Usual Dosage Topical:
Children and Adults:
Tinea corporis/tinea cruris: Cream, lotion: Apply to affected areas 1-2 times daily for 2 weeks
Tinea pedis: Cream, lotion: Apply to affected areas 1-2 times daily for 1 month
Adults: Tinea versicolor: Cream: Apply to affected areas once daily for 2 weeks
Dosage Forms
Cream:
Oxistat®: 1% (15 g, 30 g, 60 g)
Lotion:
Oxistat®: 1% (30 mL)

oxiconazole nitrate *see* oxiconazole *on previous page*

oxidized regenerated cellulose *see* cellulose, oxidized regenerated *on page 167*

Oxilan® [US] *see* ioxilan *on page 470*

Oxilan® 300 [Can] *see* ioxilan *on page 470*

Oxilan® 350 [Can] *see* ioxilan *on page 470*

oxilapine succinate *see* loxapine *on page 521*

Oxipor® VHC [US-OTC] *see* coal tar *on page 208*

Oxistat® [US/Can] *see* oxiconazole *on previous page*

Oxpam® [Can] *see* oxazepam *on page 637*

oxpentifylline *see* pentoxifylline *on page 667*

Oxpram® [Can] *see* oxazepam *on page 637*

oxprenolol *(Canada only)* (ox PREN oh lole)
Synonyms oxprenolol hydrochloride
U.S./Canadian Brand Names Slow-Trasicor® [Can]; Trasicor® [Can]
Therapeutic Category Beta-Adrenergic Blocker
Use Treatment of mild or moderate hypertension
Usual Dosage Oral: Adults:
Initial: 20 mg 3 times/day (regular-release formulation); increase by 60 mg/day (in 3 divided doses) at 1-2 week intervals until adequate control is obtained
Maintenance: 120-320 mg/day; do not exceed 480 mg; may switch to slow-release formulation once-daily dosing at this time
Dosage Forms [CAN] = Canadian brand name
Tablet:
Trasicor® [CAN]: 40 mg, 80 mg [not available in the U.S.]

oxprenolol hydrochloride *see* oxprenolol *(Canada only)* *on this page*

Oxsoralen® [US/Can] *see* methoxsalen *on page 555*

Oxsoralen-Ultra® [US/Can] *see* methoxsalen *on page 555*

Oxy-5® *(Discontinued)* *see* benzoyl peroxide *on page 103*

Oxy 10® Balanced Medicated Face Wash [US-OTC] *see* benzoyl peroxide *on page 103*

Oxy 10® Balance Spot Treatment [US-OTC] *see* benzoyl peroxide *on page 103*

Oxy Balance® [US-OTC] *see* salicylic acid *on page 772*

Oxy Balance® Deep Pore [US-OTC] *see* salicylic acid *on page 772*

oxybutynin (oks i BYOO ti nin)
Sound-Alike/Look-Alike Issues
oxybutynin may be confused with OxyContin®
Ditropan® may be confused with Detrol®, diazepam, Diprivan®, dithranol
Synonyms oxybutynin chloride
U.S./Canadian Brand Names Apo-Oxybutynin® [Can]; Ditropan® XL [US/Can]; Ditropan® [US/Can]; Gen-Oxybutynin [Can]; Novo-Oxybutynin [Can]; Nu-Oxybutyn [Can]; Oxytrol® [US/Can]; PMS-Oxybutynin [Can]; Uromax® [Can]
Therapeutic Category Antispasmodic Agent, Urinary
Use Antispasmodic for neurogenic bladder (urgency, frequency, urge incontinence) and uninhibited bladder
(Continued)

oxybutynin *(Continued)*

Usual Dosage
Oral:
Children:
>5 years: 5 mg twice daily, up to 5 mg 3 times/day maximum
>6 years: Extended release: 5 mg once daily; maximum dose: 20 mg/day
Adults: 5 mg 2-3 times/day up to 5 mg 4 times/day maximum
Extended release: Initial: 5-10 mg once daily, may increase in 5-10 mg increments; maximum: 30 mg daily
Transdermal: Adults: Apply one 3.9 mg/day patch twice weekly (every 3-4 days)

Note: Should be discontinued periodically to determine whether the patient can manage without the drug and to minimize resistance to the drug

Dosage Forms
Syrup: 5 mg/5 mL
Ditropan®: 5 mg/5 mL
Tablet: 5 mg
Ditropan®: 5 mg
Tablet, extended release: 5 mg, 10 mg, 15 mg
Ditropan® XL: 5 mg, 10 mg, 15 mg
Transdermal system:
Oxytrol®: 3.9 mg/day (8s)

oxybutynin chloride *see* oxybutynin *on previous page*

oxychlorosene (oks i KLOR oh seen)

Synonyms oxychlorosene sodium
U.S./Canadian Brand Names Clorpactin® WCS-90 [US-OTC]
Therapeutic Category Antibiotic, Topical
Use Treatment of localized infections
Usual Dosage Topical (0.1% to 0.5% solutions): Apply by irrigation, instillation, spray, soaks, or wet compresses
Dosage Forms
Powder for solution:
Clorpactin® WCS-90 [OTC]: 2 g

oxychlorosene sodium *see* oxychlorosene *on this page*

Oxycocet® [Can] *see* oxycodone and acetaminophen *on next page*

Oxycodan® [Can] *see* oxycodone and aspirin *on page 642*

oxycodone (oks i KOE done)

Sound-Alike/Look-Alike Issues
oxycodone may be confused with OxyContin®, oxymorphone
OxyContin® may be confused with oxybutynin
OxyFast® may be confused with Roxanol™
Synonyms dihydrohydroxycodeinone; oxycodone hydrochloride
U.S./Canadian Brand Names ETH-Oxydose™ [Can]; Oxy.IR® [Can]; OxyContin® [US/Can]; OxyFast® [US]; OxyIR® [US]; Roxicodone® [US]; Supeudol® [Can]
Therapeutic Category Analgesic, Narcotic
Controlled Substance C-II
Use Management of moderate-to-severe pain, normally used in combination with nonopioid analgesics

OxyContin® is indicated for around-the-clock management of moderate-to-severe pain when an analgesic is needed for an extended period of time.

Usual Dosage Oral:
Children: Immediate release:
6-12 years: 1.25 mg every 6 hours as needed
>12 years: 2.5 mg every 6 hours as needed
Adults:
Immediate release: 5 mg every 6 hours as needed
Controlled release:
Opioid naive: 10 mg every 12 hours
Concurrent CNS depressants: Reduce usual dose by $^1/_3$ to $^1/_2$
Conversion from transdermal fentanyl: For each 25 mcg/hour transdermal dose, substitute 10 mg controlled release oxycodone every 12 hours; should be initiated 18 hours after the removal of the transdermal fentanyl patch

Currently on opioids: Use standard conversion chart to convert daily dose to oxycodone equivalent. Divide daily dose in 2 (for twice-daily dosing, usually every 12 hours) and round down to nearest dosage form.

Note: 60 mg, 80 mg, or 160 mg tablets are for use **only** in opioid-tolerant patients. Special safety considerations must be addressed when converting to OxyContin® doses ≥160 mg every 12 hours. Dietary caution must be taken when patients are initially titrated to 160 mg tablets. Using different strengths to obtain the same daily dose is equivalent (eg, four 40 mg tablets, two 80 mg tablets, one 160 mg tablet); all produce similar blood levels.

Multiplication factors for converting the daily dose of current oral opioid to the daily dose of oral oxycodone:

Current opioid mg/day dose x factor = Oxycodone mg/day dose

Codeine mg/day oral dose **x** 0.15 = Oxycodone mg/day dose
Hydrocodone mg/day oral dose **x** 0.9 = Oxycodone mg/day dose
Hydromorphone mg/day oral dose **x** 4 = Oxycodone mg/day dose
Levorphanol mg/day oral dose **x** 7.5 = Oxycodone mg/day dose
Meperidine mg/day oral dose **x** 0.1 = Oxycodone mg/day dose
Methadone mg/day oral dose **x** 1.5 = Oxycodone mg/day dose
Morphine mg/day oral dose **x** 0.5 = Oxycodone mg/day dose

Note: Divide the oxycodone mg/day dose into the appropriate dosing interval for the specific form being used.

Dosage Forms

Capsule: 5 mg
OxyIR®: 5 mg
Solution, oral: 5 mg/5 mL
Roxicodone®: 5 mg/5 mL
Solution, oral [concentrate]: 20 mg/mL
ETH-Oxydose™,Oxydose®, OxyFast®, Roxicodone®: 20 mg/mL
Tablet: 5 mg, 15 mg, 30 mg
Roxicodone®: 5 mg, 15 mg, 30 mg
Tablet, controlled release: 10 mg, 20 mg, 40 mg, 80 mg, 160 mg
OxyContin®: 10 mg, 20 mg, 40 mg, 60 mg, 80 mg, 160 mg
Tablet, extended release: 10 mg, 20 mg, 40 mg, 80 mg

oxycodone and acetaminophen (oks i KOE done & a seet a MIN oh fen)

Sound-Alike/Look-Alike Issues

Percocet® may be confused with Percodan®
Roxicet™ may be confused with Roxanol™
Tylox® may be confused with Trimox®, Tylenol®, Wymox®, Xanax®

Synonyms acetaminophen and oxycodone

U.S./Canadian Brand Names Endocet® [US/Can]; Magnacet™ [US]; Oxycocet® [Can]; Percocet® [US/Can]; Percocet®-Demi [Can]; PMS-Oxycodone-Acetaminophen [Can]; Roxicet™ 5/500 [US]; Roxicet™ [US]; Tylox® [US]

Therapeutic Category Analgesic, Narcotic

Controlled Substance C-II

Use Management of moderate-to-severe pain

Usual Dosage Oral: Doses should be given every 4-6 hours as needed and titrated to appropriate analgesic effects. **Note:** Initial dose is based on the **oxycodone** content; however, the maximum daily dose is based on the **acetaminophen** content.

Children: Maximum acetaminophen dose: Children <45 kg: 90 mg/kg/day; children >45 kg: 4 g/day
Mild-to-moderate pain: Initial dose, **based on oxycodone content:** 0.05-0.1 mg/kg/dose
Severe pain: Initial dose, **based on oxycodone content:** 0.3 mg/kg/dose
Adults:
Mild-to-moderate pain: Initial dose, **based on oxycodone content:** 2.5-5 mg
Severe pain: Initial dose, **based on oxycodone content:** 10-30 mg. Do not exceed acetaminophen 4 g/day.

Dosage Forms

Caplet: Oxycodone 5 mg and acetaminophen 500 mg
Roxicet™ 5/500: Oxycodone 5 mg and acetaminophen 500 mg
Capsule: Oxycodone 5 mg and acetaminophen 500 mg
Tylox®: Oxycodone 5 mg and acetaminophen 500 mg
Solution, oral: Oxycodone 5 mg and acetaminophen 325 mg per 5 mL
Roxicet™: Oxycodone 5 mg and acetaminophen 325 mg per 5 mL
Tablet:
Generics:
Oxycodone 5 mg and acetaminophen 325 mg
Oxycodone 7.5 mg and acetaminophen 325 mg
Oxycodone 7.5 mg and acetaminophen 500 mg
(Continued)

641

oxycodone and acetaminophen (Continued)

Oxycodone 10 mg and acetaminophen 325 mg
Oxycodone 10 mg and acetaminophen 650 mg
Brands:
Endocet®:
5/325 [scored]: Oxycodone 5 mg and acetaminophen 325 mg
7.5/325: Oxycodone 7.5 mg and acetaminophen 325 mg
7.5/500: Oxycodone 7.5 mg and acetaminophen 500 mg
10/325: Oxycodone 10 mg and acetaminophen 325 mg
10/650: Oxycodone 10 mg and acetaminophen 650 mg
Magnacet™
2.5/400: Oxycodone 2.5 mg and acetaminophen 400 mg
5/400: Oxycodone 5 mg and acetaminophen 400 mg
7.5/400: Oxycodone 7.5 mg and acetaminophen 400 mg
10/400: Oxycodone 10 mg and acetaminophen 400 mg
Percocet®:
2.5/325: Oxycodone 2.5 mg and acetaminophen 325 mg
5/325 [scored]: Oxycodone 5 mg and acetaminophen 325 mg
7.5/325: Oxycodone 7.5 mg and acetaminophen 325 mg
7.5/500: Oxycodone 7.5 mg and acetaminophen 500 mg
10/325: Oxycodone 10 mg and acetaminophen 325 mg
10/650: Oxycodone 10 mg and acetaminophen 650 mg
Roxicet™ [scored]: Oxycodone 5 mg and acetaminophen 325 mg

oxycodone and aspirin (oks i KOE done & AS pir in)

Sound-Alike/Look-Alike Issues
Percodan® may be confused with Decadron®, Percocet®, Percogesic®, Periactin®
Synonyms aspirin and oxycodone
U.S./Canadian Brand Names Endodan® [US/Can]; Oxycodan® [Can]; Percodan® [US/Can]
Therapeutic Category Analgesic, Narcotic
Controlled Substance C-II
Use Management of moderate-to-severe pain
Usual Dosage Oral (based on oxycodone combined salts):
Children: Maximum oxycodone: 5 mg/dose; maximum aspirin dose should not exceed 4 g/day. Doses should be given every 6 hours as needed.
Mild-to-moderate pain: Initial dose, **based on oxycodone content:** 0.05-0.1 mg/kg/dose
Severe pain: Initial dose, **based on oxycodone content:** 0.3 mg/kg/dose
Adults: Percodan®: 1 tablet every 6 hours as needed for pain; maximum aspirin dose should not exceed 4 g/day.
Dosage Forms
Tablet: Oxycodone hydrochloride 4.5 mg, oxycodone terephthalate 0.38 mg, and aspirin 325 mg
Endodan®, Percodan®: Oxycodone hydrochloride 4.8355 mg and aspirin 325 mg

oxycodone and ibuprofen (oks i KOE done & eye byoo PROE fen)

Synonyms ibuprofen and oxycodone
U.S./Canadian Brand Names Combunox™ [US]
Therapeutic Category Analgesic, Opioid; Nonsteroidal Antiinflammatory Drug (NSAID), Oral
Controlled Substance C-II
Use Short-term (≤7 days) management of acute, moderate-to-severe pain
Usual Dosage Oral: Adults: Pain: Take 1 tablet every 6 hours as needed (maximum: 4 tablets/24 hours); do not take for longer than 7 days
Dosage Forms
Tablet:
Combunox™: 5/400: Oxycodone 5 mg and ibuprofen 400 mg

oxycodone hydrochloride *see* oxycodone *on page 640*

OxyContin® [US/Can] *see* oxycodone *on page 640*

Oxyderm™ [Can] *see* benzoyl peroxide *on page 103*

OxyFast® [US] *see* oxycodone *on page 640*

Oxy.IR® [Can] *see* oxycodone *on page 640*

oxymetazoline (oks i met AZ oh leen)

Sound-Alike/Look-Alike Issues
oxymetazoline may be confused with oxymetholone
Afrin® may be confused with aspirin
Visine® may be confused with Visken®

Synonyms oxymetazoline hydrochloride

U.S./Canadian Brand Names 4-Way® 12 Hour [US-OTC]; Afrin® Extra Moisturizing [US-OTC]; Afrin® Original [US-OTC]; Afrin® Severe Congestion [US-OTC]; Afrin® Sinus [US-OTC]; Claritin® Allergic Decongestant [Can]; Dristan® Long Lasting Nasal [Can]; Dristan™ 12-Hour [US-OTC]; Drixoral® Nasal [Can]; Duramist® Plus [US-OTC]; Duration® [US-OTC]; Genasal [US-OTC]; Neo-Synephrine® 12 Hour Extra Moisturizing [US-OTC]; Neo-Synephrine® 12 Hour [US-OTC]; NRS® [US-OTC]; Nōstrilla® [US-OTC]; Vicks® Sinex® 12 Hour Ultrafine Mist [US-OTC]; Vicks® Sinex® 12 Hour [US-OTC]; Visine® L.R. [US-OTC]

Therapeutic Category Adrenergic Agonist Agent

Use Adjunctive therapy of middle ear infections, associated with acute or chronic rhinitis, the common cold, sinusitis, hay fever, or other allergies
Ophthalmic: Relief of redness of eye due to minor eye irritations

Usual Dosage
Intranasal (therapy should not exceed 3 days): Children ≥6 years and Adults: 0.05% solution: Instill 2-3 sprays into each nostril twice daily
Ophthalmic: Children ≥6 years and Adults: 0.025% solution: Instill 1-2 drops in affected eye(s) every 6 hours as needed or as directed by healthcare provider

Dosage Forms
Solution, intranasal [spray]: 0.05% (15 mL, 30 mL)
Afrin® Extra Moisturizing [OTC], Afrin® Severe Congestion [OTC], Afrin® Sinus [OTC], Dristan™ 12-Hour, Duramist® Plus [OTC], Neo-Synephrine® 12 Hour [OTC], Neo-Synephrine® 12 Hour Extra Moisturizing [OTC], Nōstrilla® [OTC], Vicks Sinex® 12 Hour Ultrafine Mist [OTC], Vicks Sinex® 12 Hour [OTC], 4-Way® 12 Hour [OTC]: 0.05% (15 mL)
Afrin® Original [OTC], Genasal [OTC], NRS® [OTC]: 0.05% (15 mL, 30 mL)
Duration® [OTC]: 0.05% (30 mL)
Solution, ophthalmic:
Visine® L.R. [OTC]: 0.025% (15 mL, 30 mL)

oxymetazoline hydrochloride *see oxymetazoline on this page*

oxymetholone (oks i METH oh lone)

Sound-Alike/Look-Alike Issues
oxymetholone may be confused with oxymetazoline, oxymorphone

U.S./Canadian Brand Names Anadrol® [US]

Therapeutic Category Anabolic Steroid

Controlled Substance C-III

Use Treatment of anemias caused by deficient red cell production

Usual Dosage Oral: Children and Adults: Erythropoietic effects: 1-5 mg/kg/day in one daily dose; usual effective dose: 1-2 mg/kg/day; give for a minimum trial of 3-6 months because response may be delayed

Dosage Forms
Tablet:
Anadrol®-50: 50 mg

oxymorphone (oks i MOR fone)

Sound-Alike/Look-Alike Issues
oxymorphone may be confused with oxymetholone

Synonyms oxymorphone hydrochloride

U.S./Canadian Brand Names Opana® ER [US]; Opana® [US]

Therapeutic Category Analgesic, Narcotic

Controlled Substance C-II

Use
Parenteral: Management of moderate-to-severe pain and preoperatively as a sedative and/or supplement to anesthesia
Oral, regular release: Management of moderate-to-severe pain
Oral, extended release: Management of moderate-to-severe pain in patients requiring around-the-clock opioid treatment for an extended period of time

Usual Dosage Adults: **Note:** Dosage must be individualized.
I.M., SubQ: Initial: 1-1.5 mg; may repeat every 4-6 hours as needed
Labor analgesia: I.M.: 0.5-1 mg
I.V.: Initial: 0.5 mg
(Continued)

oxymorphone *(Continued)*

Oral:

Immediate release:

Opioid-naive: 10-20 mg every 4-6 hours as needed. Initial dosages as low as 5 mg may be considered in selected patients and/or patients with renal impairment. Dosage adjustment should be based on level of analgesia, side effects, and pain intensity. Initiation of therapy with initial dose >20 mg is **not** recommended.

Currently on stable dose of parenteral oxymorphone: ~10 times the daily parenteral requirement. The calculated amount should be divided and given in 4-6 equal doses.

Currently on other opioids: Use standard conversion chart to convert daily dose to oxymorphone equivalent. Generally start with 1/2 the calculated daily oxymorphone dosage and administered in divided doses every 4-6 hours.

Extended release (Opana® ER):

Opioid-naive: Initial: 5 mg every 12 hours. Supplemental doses of immediate-release oxymorphone may be used as "rescue" medication as dosage is titrated.

Note: Continued requirement for supplemental dosing may be used to titrate the dose of extended-release continuous therapy. Adjust therapy incrementally, by 5-10 mg every 12 hours at intervals of every 3-7 days. Ideally, basal dosage may be titrated to generally mild pain or no pain with the regular use of fewer than 2 supplemental doses per 24 hours.

Currently on stable dose of parenteral oxymorphone: Approximately 10 times the daily parenteral requirement. The calculated amount should be given in 2 divided doses (every 12 hours).

Currently on opioids: Use conversion chart (see Note below) to convert daily dose to oxymorphone equivalent. Generally start with 1/2 the calculated daily oxymorphone dosage. Divide daily dose in 2 (for every 12-hour dosing) and round down to nearest dosage form. **Note:** Per manufacturer, the following approximate oral dosages are equivalent to oxymorphone 10 mg:

Hydrocodone 20 mg
Oxycodone 20 mg
Methadone 20 mg
Morphine 30 mg

Conversion of stable dose of immediate-release oxymorphone to extended-release oxymorphone: Administer 1/2 of the daily dose of immediate-release oxymorphone (Opana®) as the extended-release formulation (Opana® ER) every 12 hours

Dosage Forms

Injection, solution:
Opana®: 1 mg/mL (1 mL)

Tablet:
Opana®: 5 mg, 10 mg

Tablet, extended release:
Opana® ER: 5 mg, 10 mg, 20 mg, 40 mg

oxymorphone hydrochloride *see oxymorphone on previous page*

oxytetracycline (oks i tet ra SYE kleen)

Sound-Alike/Look-Alike Issues
Terramycin® may be confused with Garamycin®

Synonyms oxytetracycline hydrochloride

U.S./Canadian Brand Names Terramycin® [Can]

Therapeutic Category Tetracycline Derivative

Use Treatment of susceptible bacterial infections; both gram-positive and gram-negative, as well as, *Rickettsia* and *Mycoplasma* organisms

Usual Dosage I.M.:
Children >8 years: 15-25 mg/kg/day (maximum: 250 mg/dose) in divided doses every 8-12 hours
Adults: 250 mg every 24 hours or 300 mg/day divided every 8-12 hours

oxytetracycline hydrochloride *see oxytetracycline on this page*

oxytocin (oks i TOE sin)

Sound-Alike/Look-Alike Issues
Pitocin® may be confused with Pitressin®

Synonyms pit

U.S./Canadian Brand Names Pitocin® [US/Can]; Syntocinon® [Can]

Therapeutic Category Oxytocic Agent

Use Induction of labor at term; control of postpartum bleeding; adjunctive therapy in management of abortion

Usual Dosage I.V. administration requires the use of an infusion pump. Adults:

Induction of labor: I.V.: 0.5-1 milliunits/minute; gradually increase dose in increments of 1-2 milliunits/minute until desired contraction pattern is established; dose may be decreased after desired frequency of contractions is reached and labor has progressed to 5-6 cm dilation. Infusion rates of 6 milliunits/minute provide oxytocin levels similar to those at spontaneous labor; rates >9-10 milliunits/minute are rarely required.

Postpartum bleeding:

I.M.: Total dose of 10 units after delivery

I.V.: 10-40 units by I.V. infusion in 1000 mL of intravenous fluid at a rate sufficient to control uterine atony

Adjunctive treatment of abortion: I.V.: 10-20 milliunits/minute; maximum total dose: 30 units/12 hours

Dosage Forms

Injection, solution: 10 units/mL (1 mL, 10 mL)

Pitocin®: 10 units/mL (1 mL)

Oxytrol® [US/Can] *see* oxybutynin *on page 639*

Oysco D [US-OTC] *see* calcium and vitamin D *on page 137*

Oysco 500 [US-OTC] *see* calcium carbonate *on page 138*

Oysco 500+D [US-OTC] *see* calcium and vitamin D *on page 137*

Oyst-Cal-D [US-OTC] *see* calcium and vitamin D *on page 137*

Oyst-Cal 500 [US-OTC] *see* calcium carbonate *on page 138*

Oyst-Cal-D 500 [US-OTC] *see* calcium and vitamin D *on page 137*

P2E1 *(Discontinued)*

P-V-Tussin® Syrup [US] *see* pseudoephedrine, hydrocodone, and chlorpheniramine *on page 731*

P-V Tussin Tablet [US] *see* hydrocodone and pseudoephedrine *on page 430*

P-071 *see* cetirizine *on page 169*

Pacerone® [US] *see* amiodarone *on page 43*

Pacis™ [Can] *see* BCG vaccine *on page 96*

paclitaxel (pac li TAKS el)

Sound-Alike/Look-Alike Issues

paclitaxel may be confused with paroxetine, Paxil®

paclitaxel (conventional) may be confused with paclitaxel (protein-bound)

Taxol® may be confused with Abraxane®, Paxil®, Taxotere®

Synonyms NSC-125973; NSC-673089

U.S./Canadian Brand Names Apo-Paclitaxel® [Can]; Onxol™ [US]; Taxol® [US/Can]

Therapeutic Category Antineoplastic Agent

Use Treatment of breast, lung (nonsmall cell), and ovarian cancers; treatment of AIDS-related Kaposi sarcoma (KS)

Usual Dosage Premedication with dexamethasone (20 mg orally or I.V. at 12 and 6 hours **or** 14 and 7 hours before the dose; reduce dexamethasone dose to 10 mg orally with advanced HIV disease), diphenhydramine (50 mg I.V. 30-60 minutes prior to the dose), and cimetidine, famotidine or ranitidine (I.V. 30-60 minutes prior to the dose) is recommended.

Adults: I.V.: Refer to individual protocols

Ovarian carcinoma: 135-175 mg/m^2 over 3 hours every 3 weeks **or**

135 mg/m^2 over 24 hours every 3 weeks **or**

50-80 mg/m^2 over 1-3 hours weekly **or**

1.4-4 mg/m^2/day continuous infusion for 14 days every 4 weeks

Metastatic breast cancer: 175-250 mg/m^2 over 3 hours every 3 weeks **or**

50-80 mg/m^2 weekly **or**

1.4-4 mg/m^2/day continuous infusion for 14 days every 4 weeks

Nonsmall cell lung carcinoma: 135 mg/m^2 over 24 hours every 3 weeks

AIDS-related Kaposi sarcoma: 135 mg/m^2 over 3 hours every 3 weeks **or**

100 mg/m^2 over 3 hours every 2 weeks

Dosage modification for toxicity (solid tumors, including ovary, breast, and lung carcinoma): Courses of paclitaxel should not be repeated until the neutrophil count is ≥1500 cells/mm^3 and the platelet count is ≥100,000 cells/mm^3; reduce dosage by 20% for patients experiencing severe peripheral neuropathy or severe neutropenia (neutrophil <500 cells/mm^3 for a week or longer)

Dosage modification for immunosuppression in advanced HIV disease: Paclitaxel should not be given to patients with HIV if the baseline or subsequent neutrophil count is <1000 cells/mm^3. Additional modifications include: Reduce dosage of dexamethasone in premedication to 10 mg orally; reduce dosage by 20% in patients experiencing severe peripheral neuropathy or severe neutropenia (neutrophil <500 cells/mm^3 for a week or longer); initiate concurrent hematopoietic growth factor (G-CSF) as clinically indicated

(Continued)

paclitaxel *(Continued)*

Dosage Forms
Injection, solution: 6 mg/mL (5 mL, 16.7 mL, 25 mL, 50 mL)
Onxol™: 6 mg/mL (5 mL, 25 mL, 50 mL)
Taxol®: 6 mg/mL (5 mL, 16.7 mL, 50 mL)

paclitaxel (protein bound) (pac li TAKS el PROE teen bownd)

Sound-Alike/Look-Alike Issues
paclitaxel (protein bound) may be confused with paclitaxel (conventional)
Abraxane® may be confused with Paxil®, Taxol®, Taxotere®
Synonyms ABI-007; albumin-bound paclitaxel; NAB-paclitaxel; NSC-736631; protein-bound paclitaxel
U.S./Canadian Brand Names Abraxane® [US]
Therapeutic Category Antineoplastic Agent, Antimicrotubular; Antineoplastic Agent, Natural Source (Plant) Derivative
Use Treatment of relapsed or refractory breast cancer
Usual Dosage I.V.: Adults: Breast cancer: 260 mg/m^2 every 3 weeks
Dosage Forms
Injection, powder for reconstitution:
Abraxane®: 100 mg

Pain-A-Lay® **[US-OTC]** *see* phenol *on page 673*

Pain Eze [US-OTC] *see* acetaminophen *on page 5*

Pain-Off [US-OTC] *see* acetaminophen, aspirin, and caffeine *on page 9*

Palafer® **[Can]** *see* ferrous fumarate *on page 349*

Palcaps [US] *see* pancrelipase *on page 648*

Palgic® **[US]** *see* carbinoxamine *on page 151*

Palgic®**-D** *(Discontinued) see* carbinoxamine and pseudoephedrine *on page 151*

Palgic®**-DS** *(Discontinued) see* carbinoxamine and pseudoephedrine *on page 151*

palifermin (pal ee FER min)

Synonyms AMJ 9701; rHu-KGF
U.S./Canadian Brand Names Kepivance™ [US]
Therapeutic Category Keratinocyte Growth Factor
Use Decrease the incidence and severity of severe oral mucositis associated with hematologic malignancies in patients receiving myelotoxic therapy requiring hematopoietic stem cell support
Usual Dosage I.V.: Adults: 60 mcg/kg/day for 3 consecutive days before and after myelotoxic therapy; total of 6 doses
Note: Administer first 3 doses prior to myelotoxic therapy, with the 3rd dose given 24-48 hours before therapy begins. The last 3 doses should be administered after myelotoxic therapy, with the first of these doses after but on the same day of hematopoietic stem cell infusion and at least 4 days after the most recent dose of palifermin.
Dosage Forms
Injection, powder for reconstitution [preservative free]:
Kepivance™: 6.25 mg

paliperidone (pal ee PER i done)

Synonyms 9-hydroxy-risperidone; 9-OH-risperidone
U.S./Canadian Brand Names Invega™ [US]
Therapeutic Category Antipsychotic Agent, Atypical
Use Treatment of schizophrenia
Usual Dosage Oral: Adults: Schizophrenia: Initial: 6 mg once daily in the morning; titration not required, though some may benefit from higher or lower doses. If exceeding 6 mg/day, increases of 3 mg/day are recommended no more frequently than every 5 days, up to a maximum of 12 mg/day.
Dosage Forms
Tablet, extended-release:
Invega™: 3 mg, 6 mg, 9 mg

palivizumab (pah li VIZ u mab)

Sound-Alike/Look-Alike Issues
Synagis® may be confused with Synalgos®-DC, Synvisc®

U.S./Canadian Brand Names Synagis® [US/Can]

Therapeutic Category Monoclonal Antibody

Use Prevention of serious lower respiratory tract disease caused by respiratory syncytial virus (RSV) in infants and children at high risk of RSV disease

Usual Dosage I.M.: Infants and Children <2 years: 15 mg/kg of body weight, monthly throughout RSV season (First dose administered prior to commencement of RSV season)

Dosage Forms
Injection, solution [preservative free]:
Synagis®: 50 mg/0.5 mL (0.5 mL); 100 mg/mL (1 mL)

Palladone™ *(Discontinued)* see hydromorphone *on page 435*

Palmer's® Skin Success Acne [US-OTC] *see* benzoyl peroxide *on page 103*

Palmer's® Skin Success Acne Cleanser [US-OTC] *see* salicylic acid *on page 772*

Palmer's® Skin Success Eventone® Fade Cream [US-OTC] *see* hydroquinone *on page 437*

Palmitate-A® [US-OTC] *see* vitamin A *on page 892*

palonosetron (pal oh NOE se tron)

Sound-Alike/Look-Alike Issues
palonosetron may be confused with dolasetron, granisetron, ondansetron
Aloxi® may be confused with oxaliplatin

Synonyms palonosetron hydrochloride; RS-25259; RS-25259-197

U.S./Canadian Brand Names Aloxi® [US]

Therapeutic Category Antiemetic; Selective 5-HT$_3$ Receptor Antagonist

Use Prevention of chemotherapy-associated nausea and vomiting; indicated for prevention of acute (highly-emetogenic therapy) as well as acute and delayed (moderately-emetogenic therapy) nausea and vomiting

Usual Dosage I.V.: Adults:
Chemotherapy-induced nausea and vomiting: 0.25 mg 30 minutes prior to chemotherapy administration, day 1 of each cycle (doses should not be given more than once weekly)
Breakthrough: Palonosetron has not been shown to be effective in terminating nausea or vomiting once it occurs and should not be used for this purpose.

Dosage Forms
Injection, solution:
Aloxi®: 0.05 mg/mL (5 mL)

palonosetron hydrochloride see palonosetron *on this page*

2-PAM see pralidoxime *on page 705*

Pamelor® [US] see nortriptyline *on page 613*

pamidronate (pa mi DROE nate)

Sound-Alike/Look-Alike Issues
Aredia® may be confused with Adriamycin®, Meridia®

Synonyms pamidronate disodium

U.S./Canadian Brand Names Aredia® [US/Can]; Pamidronate Disodium® [Can]; Rhoxal-pamidronate [Can]

Therapeutic Category Bisphosphonate Derivative

Use Treatment of hypercalcemia associated with malignancy; treatment of osteolytic bone lesions associated with multiple myeloma or metastatic breast cancer; moderate to severe Paget disease of bone

Usual Dosage Drug must be diluted properly before administration and infused intravenously slowly. Due to risk of nephrotoxicity, doses should not exceed 90 mg. I.V.: Adults:
Hypercalcemia of malignancy:
Moderate cancer-related hypercalcemia (corrected serum calcium: 12-13.5 mg/dL): 60-90 mg, as a single dose
Severe cancer-related hypercalcemia (corrected serum calcium: >13.5 mg/dL): 90 mg, as a single dose
A period of 7 days should elapse before the use of second course; repeat infusions every 2-3 weeks have been suggested, however, could be administered every 2-3 months according to the degree and of severity of hypercalcemia and/or the type of malignancy.
Osteolytic bone lesions with multiple myeloma: 90 mg monthly
Osteolytic bone lesions with metastatic breast cancer: 90 mg repeated every 3-4 weeks
Paget disease: 30 mg daily for 3 consecutive days

Dosage Forms
Injection, powder for reconstitution: 30 mg, 90 mg
Aredia®: 30 mg, 90 mg
Injection, solution: 3 mg/mL (10 mL); 6 mg/mL (10 mL); 9 mg/mL (10 mL)

Pamidronate Disodium® **[Can]** *see* pamidronate *on previous page*

pamidronate disodium *see* pamidronate *on previous page*

Pamine® **[US/Can]** *see* methscopolamine *on page 556*

Pamine® **Forte [US]** *see* methscopolamine *on page 556*

p-aminoclonidine *see* apraclonidine *on page 70*

Pamprin IB® *(Discontinued) see* ibuprofen *on page 444*

Pamprin® **Maximum Strength All Day Relief [US-OTC]** *see* naproxen *on page 591*

Pan-2400™ **[US-OTC]** *see* pancreatin *on this page*

Panadol® *(Discontinued) see* acetaminophen *on page 5*

Panafil® **[US]** *see* chlorophyllin, papain, and urea *on page 175*

Panafil® **SE [US]** *see* chlorophyllin, papain, and urea *on page 175*

Panasal® **5/500** *(Discontinued) see* hydrocodone and aspirin *on page 428*

pan-B antibody *see* rituximab *on page 762*

Pancof® *(Discontinued) see* pseudoephedrine, dihydrocodeine, and chlorpheniramine *on page 730*

Pancof®**-EXP [US]** *see* dihydrocodeine, pseudoephedrine, and guaifenesin *on page 260*

Pancof-HC [US] *see* hydrocodone and pseudoephedrine *on page 430*

Pancof®**-PD [US]** *see* dihydrocodeine, chlorpheniramine, and phenylephrine *on page 259*

Pancof-XP [US] *see* hydrocodone and guaifenesin *on page 429*

Pancrease® **[Can]** *see* pancrelipase *on this page*

Pancrease® **MT [US/Can]** *see* pancrelipase *on this page*

pancreatin (PAN kree a tin)

Sound-Alike/Look-Alike Issues
pancreatin may be confused with Panretin®

U.S./Canadian Brand Names Dygase [US]; Hi-Vegi-Lip [US-OTC]; ku-zyme® [US]; kutrase® [US]; Lapase [US]; Pan-2400™ [US-OTC]; Pancreatin 4X [US-OTC]; Pancreatin 8X [US-OTC]; Veg-Pancreatin 4X [US-OTC]

Therapeutic Category Enzyme

Use Relief of functional indigestion due to enzyme deficiency or imbalance

Usual Dosage Oral: Adults: Actual dose varies with condition of patient and is usually given with each meal or snack.
ku-zyme®: 1-2 capsules with each meal or snack
kutrase®: 1 capsule with each meal or snack

Dosage Forms
Capsule: Lipase 8500 units, protease 50,000 units, amylase 50,000 units
Dygase, kutrase®: Lipase 2400 units, protease 30,000 units, amylase 30,000 units
ku-zyme®: Lipase 1200 units, protease 15,000 units, amylase 15,000 units
Lapase: Lipase 1200 units, protease 15,000 units, and amylase 15,000 units [contains tartrazine]
Pan-2400™ [OTC]: Lipase 9816 units, protease 60,214 units, amylase 75,900 units
Tablet: Lipase 565 units, protease 8200 units, amylase 8200 units [pancreatin 325 mg]; lipase 2400 units, protease 30,000 units, amylase 30,000 units
Hi-Vegi-Lip [OTC], Pancreatin 4X [OTC]: Lipase 4800 units, protease 60,000 units, amylase 60,000 units
Pancreatin 8X [OTC]: Lipase 14,400 units, protease 180,000 units, amylase 180,000 units
Veg-Pancreatin 4X [OTC]: Lipase 5500 units, protease 690,000 units, amylase 690,000 units

Pancreatin 4X [US-OTC] *see* pancreatin *on this page*

Pancreatin 8X [US-OTC] *see* pancreatin *on this page*

Pancrecarb MS® **[US]** *see* pancrelipase *on this page*

pancrelipase (pan kre LYE pase)

Synonyms lipancreatin

U.S./Canadian Brand Names Cotazym® [Can]; Creon® [US/Can]; ku-zyme® HP [US]; Lipram 4500 [US]; Lipram-CR [US]; Lipram-PN [US]; Lipram-UL [US]; Palcaps [US]; Pancrease® MT [US/Can]; Pancrease® [Can]; Pancrecarb MS® [US]; Pangestyme™ CN [US]; Pangestyme™ EC [US]; Pangestyme™ MT [US]; Pangestyme™ UL [US]; Panocaps MT [US]; Panocaps [US]; Panokase® 16 [US]; Panokase® [US]; Plaretase® 8000 [US]; Ultracaps MT [US]; Ultrase® MT [US/Can]; Ultrase® [US/Can]; Viokase® [US/Can]

Therapeutic Category Enzyme

Use Replacement therapy in symptomatic treatment of malabsorption syndrome caused by pancreatic insufficiency

Usual Dosage Oral:

Powder: Actual dose depends on the condition being treated and the digestive requirements of the patient

Children <1 year: Start with $\frac{1}{8}$ teaspoonful with feedings

Adults: 0.7 g ($\frac{1}{4}$ teaspoonful) with meals

Capsules/tablets: The following dosage recommendations are only an approximation for initial dosages. The actual dosage will depend on the condition being treated and the digestive requirements of the individual patient. Adjust dose based on body weight and stool fat content. Total daily dose reflects ~3 meals/day and 2-3 snacks/day, with half the mealtime dose given with a snack. Older patients may need less units/kg due to increased weight, but decreased ingestion of fat/kg. Maximum dose: 2500 units of lipase/kg/meal (10,000 units of lipase/kg/day)

Children:

<1 year: 2000 units of lipase with meals

1-6 years: 4000-8000 units of lipase with meals and 4000 units with snacks

7-12 years: 4000-12,000 units of lipase with meals and snacks

Adults: 4000-48,000 units of lipase with meals and with snacks

Occluded feeding tubes: One tablet of Viokase® crushed with one 325 mg tablet of sodium bicarbonate (to activate the Viokase®) in 5 mL of water can be instilled into the nasogastric tube and clamped for 5 minutes; then, flushed with 50 mL of tap water

Dosage Forms

Capsule:

ku-zyme® HP: Lipase 8000 units, protease 30,000 units, and amylase 30,000 units

Capsule, delayed release, enteric coated granules:

Pangestyme™ CN-10: Lipase 10,000 units, protease 37,500 units, amylase 33,200 units

Pangestyme™ CN-20: Lipase 20,000 units, protease 75,000 units, amylase 66,400 units

Pangestyme™ EC: Lipase 4500 units, protease 25,000 units, and amylase 20,000 units

Pangestyme™ MT16: Lipase 16,000 units, protease 48,000 units, and amylase 48,000 units

Pangestyme™ UL 12: Lipase 12,000 units, protease 39,000 units, and amylase 39,000 units

Pangestyme™ UL 18: Lipase 18,000 units, protease 58,500 units, and amylase 58,500 units

Pangestyme™ UL 20: Lipase 20,000 units, protease 65,000 units, and amylase 65,000 units

Capsule, delayed release, enteric coated microspheres: Lipase 4500 units, protease 25,000 units, and amylase 20,000 units

Creon® 5: Lipase 5000 units, protease 18,750 units, and amylase 16,600 units

Creon® 10, Lipram-CR10, Palcaps 10: Lipase 10,000 units, protease 37,500 units, and amylase 33,200 units

Creon® 20, Lipram-CR20, Palcaps 20: Lipase 20,000 units, protease 75,000 units, and amylase 66,400 units

Lipram 4500, Panocaps: Lipase 4500 units, protease 25,000 units, and amylase 20,000 units

Lipram-PN10: Lipase 10,000 units, protease 30,000 units, and amylase 30,000 units

Lipram-PN16, Panocap MT 16: Lipase 16,000 units, protease 48,000 units, and amylase 48,000 units

Lipram-PN20, Panocap MT 20: Lipase 20,000 units, protease 44,000 units, and amylase 56,000 units

Lipram-UL20, Ultracaps MT 20: Lipase 20,000 units, protease 65,000 units, and amylase 65,000 units

Pancrecarb MS-4®: Lipase 4000 units, protease 25,000 units, and amylase 25,000 units [buffered]

Pancrecarb MS-8®: Lipase 8000 units, protease 45,000 units, and amylase 40,000 units [buffered]

Pancrecarb MS-16®: Lipase 16,000 units, protease 52,000 units, and amylase 52,000 units [buffered]

Capsule, enteric coated microspheres: Lipase 4500 units, protease 25,000 units, and amylase 20,000 units

Ultrase®: Lipase 4500 units, protease 25,000 units, and amylase 20,000 units

Capsule, enteric coated microtablets:

Pancrease® MT 4: Lipase 4000 units, protease 12,000 units, and amylase 12,000 units

Pancrease® MT 10: Lipase 10,000 units, protease 30,000 units, and amylase 30,000 units

Pancrease® MT 16: Lipase 16,000 units, protease 48,000 units, and amylase 48,000 units

Pancrease® MT 20: Lipase 20,000 units, protease 44,000 units, and amylase 56,000 units

Capsule, enteric coated minitablets:

Ultrase® MT12: Lipase 12,000 units, protease 39,000 units, and amylase 39,000 units

Ultrase® MT18: Lipase 18,000 units, protease 58,500 units, and amylase 58,500 units

Ultrase® MT20: Lipase 20,000 units, protease 65,000 units, and amylase 65,000 units

Powder:

Viokase®: Lipase 16,800 units, protease 70,000 units, and amylase 70,000 units per 0.7 g (227 g)

Tablet: Lipase 8000 units, protease 30,000 units, and amylase 30,000 units

Panokase®, Plaretase™ 8000, Viokase® 8: Lipase 8000 units, protease 30,000 units, and amylase 30,000 units

Panokase® 16, Viokase® 16: Lipase 16,000 units, protease 60,000 units, and amylase 60,000 units

pancuronium (pan kyoo ROE nee um)

Sound-Alike/Look-Alike Issues
pancuronium may be confused with pipecuronium

Synonyms pancuronium bromide

U.S./Canadian Brand Names Pancuronium Bromide® [Can]

Therapeutic Category Skeletal Muscle Relaxant

Use Adjunct to general anesthesia to facilitate endotracheal intubation and to relax skeletal muscles during surgery; to facilitate mechanical ventilation in ICU patients; does not relieve pain or produce sedation

Drug of choice for neuromuscular blockade except in patients with renal failure, hepatic failure, or cardiovascular instability or in situations not suited for pancuronium's long duration of action

Usual Dosage Administer I.V.; dose to effect; doses will vary due to interpatient variability; use ideal body weight for obese patients
Surgery:
Neonates <1 month:
Test dose: 0.02 mg/kg to measure responsiveness
Initial: 0.03 mg/kg/dose repeated twice at 5- to 10-minute intervals as needed; maintenance: 0.03-0.09 mg/kg/dose every 30 minutes to 4 hours as needed
Infants >1 month, Children, and Adults: Initial: 0.06-0.1 mg/kg or 0.05 mg/kg after initial dose of succinylcholine for intubation; maintenance dose: 0.01 mg/kg 60-100 minutes after initial dose and then 0.01 mg/kg every 25-60 minutes
Pretreatment/priming: 10% of intubating dose given 3-5 minutes before initial dose
ICU: 0.05-0.1 mg/kg bolus followed by 0.8-1.7 mcg/kg/minute once initial recovery from bolus observed or 0.1-0.2 mg/kg every 1-3 hours

Dosage Forms
Injection, solution: 1 mg/mL (10 mL); 2 mg/mL (2 mL, 5 mL)

Pancuronium Bromide® [Can] *see* pancuronium *on this page*

pancuronium bromide *see* pancuronium *on this page*

Pandel® [US] *see* hydrocortisone (topical) *on page 434*

Panectyl® [Can] *see* trimeprazine *(Canada only) on page 867*

Pangestyme™ CN [US] *see* pancrelipase *on page 648*

Pangestyme™ EC [US] *see* pancrelipase *on page 648*

Pangestyme™ MT [US] *see* pancrelipase *on page 648*

Pangestyme™ UL [US] *see* pancrelipase *on page 648*

Panglobulin® NF [US] *see* immune globulin (intravenous) *on page 451*

Panhematin® [US] *see* hemin *on page 414*

panitumumab (pan i TOOM yoo mab)

Synonyms ABX-EGF; NSC-742319; rHuMAb-EGFr

U.S./Canadian Brand Names Vectibix™ [US]

Therapeutic Category Antineoplastic Agent, Monoclonal Antibody; Epidermal Growth Factor Receptor (EGFR) Inhibitor

Use Treatment of refractory (EGFR positive) metastatic colorectal cancer

Usual Dosage I.V.: Adults: Colorectal cancer: 6 mg/kg every 2 weeks
Dosing adjustment for toxicity:
Infusion reactions, mild-to-moderate (grade 1 or 2): Reduce the infusion rate by 50% for the duration of infusion
Infusion reactions, severe (grade 3 or 4): Immediately and permanently discontinue treatment
Skin toxicity (grade 3 or 4): Withhold treatment; if skin toxicity does not improve to ≤ grade 2 within 1 month, permanently discontinue. If skin toxicity improves to ≤ grade 2 within 1 month (with patient missing ≤2 doses), resume treatment at 50% of the original dose. Dose may be increased in increments of 25% of the original dose (up to 6 mg/kg) if skin toxicities do not recur. For recurrent skin toxicity, permanently discontinue.

Dosage Forms
Injection, solution [preservative free]:
Vectibix™: 20 mg/mL (5 mL, 10 mL, 20 mL)

Panixine DisperDose™ *(Discontinued)* *see* cephalexin *on page 167*

Panlor® DC [US] *see* acetaminophen, caffeine, and dihydrocodeine *on page 10*

Panlor® SS [US] *see* acetaminophen, caffeine, and dihydrocodeine *on page 10*

Panocaps [US] *see* pancrelipase *on page 648*

Panocaps MT [US] *see* pancrelipase *on page 648*

Panokase® [US] *see* pancrelipase *on page 648*

Panokase® 16 [US] *see* pancrelipase *on page 648*

PanOxyl® [US/Can] *see* benzoyl peroxide *on page 103*

PanOxyl®-AQ [US] *see* benzoyl peroxide *on page 103*

PanOxyl® Aqua Gel [US] *see* benzoyl peroxide *on page 103*

PanOxyl® Bar [US-OTC] *see* benzoyl peroxide *on page 103*

Panretin® [US/Can] *see* alitretinoin *on page 29*

Panscol® Lotion *(Discontinued)* *see* salicylic acid *on page 772*

Panscol® Ointment *(Discontinued)* *see* salicylic acid *on page 772*

Panthoderm® [US-OTC] *see* dexpanthenol *on page 244*

Panto™ IV [Can] *see* pantoprazole *on this page*

Panto-250 [US] *see* pantothenic acid *on this page*

Pantoloc® [Can] *see* pantoprazole *on this page*

Pantoloc® M [Can] *see* pantoprazole *on this page*

Pantopon® *(Discontinued)*

pantoprazole (pan TOE pra zole)

Sound-Alike/Look-Alike Issues
Protonix® may be confused with Lotronex®, Lovenox®, protamine

U.S./Canadian Brand Names Pantoloc® M [Can]; Pantoloc® [Can]; Panto™ IV [Can]; PMS-Pantoprazole [Can]; Protonix® [US/Can]

Therapeutic Category Proton Pump Inhibitor

Use

Oral: Treatment and maintenance of healing of erosive esophagitis associated with GERD; reduction in relapse rates of daytime and nighttime heartburn symptoms in GERD; hypersecretory disorders associated with Zollinger-Ellison syndrome or other neoplastic disorders

I.V.: Short-term treatment (7-10 days) of patients with gastroesophageal reflux disease (GERD) and a history of erosive esophagitis; hypersecretory disorders associated with Zollinger-Ellison syndrome or other neoplastic disorders

Usual Dosage Adults:

Oral:

Erosive esophagitis associated with GERD:

Treatment: 40 mg once daily for up to 8 weeks; an additional 8 weeks may be used in patients who have not healed after an 8-week course

Maintenance of healing: 40 mg once daily

Note: Lower doses (20 mg once daily) have been used successfully in mild GERD treatment and maintenance of healing

Hypersecretory disorders (including Zollinger-Ellison): Initial: 40 mg twice daily; adjust dose based on patient needs; doses up to 240 mg/day have been administered

I.V.:

Erosive esophagitis associated with GERD: 40 mg once daily for 7-10 days

Hypersecretory disorders: 80 mg twice daily; adjust dose based on acid output measurements; 160-240 mg/day in divided doses has been used for a limited period (up to 7 days)

Dosage Forms

Injection, powder for reconstitution:

Protonix®: 40 mg

Tablet, delayed release:

Protonix®: 20 mg, 40 mg

Tablet, enteric coated, as magnesium:

Pantoloc® M [CAN]: 40 mg [not available in the U.S.]

pantothenic acid (pan toe THEN ik AS id)

Synonyms calcium pantothenate; vitamin B_5

U.S./Canadian Brand Names Panto-250 [US]

Therapeutic Category Vitamin, Water Soluble

Use Pantothenic acid deficiency

Usual Dosage Oral: Adults: Recommended daily dose 4-7 mg/day

(Continued)

pantothenic acid *(Continued)*

Dosage Forms
Capsule:
Panto-250: 250 mg [contains calcium 23 mg]
Liquid: 200 mg/5 mL (240 mL)
Tablet: 100 mg, 200 mg, 250 mg, 500 mg
Tablet, sustained release: 500 mg

pantothenyl alcohol *see* dexpanthenol *on page 244*

papain and urea (pa PAY in & yoor EE a)

U.S./Canadian Brand Names Accuzyme® [US]; Allanzyme 650 [US]; Allanzyme [US]; Ethezyme™ 830 [US]; Ethezyme™ [US]; Gladase® [US]; Kovia® [US]
Therapeutic Category Enzyme, Topical Debridement; Topical Skin Product
Use Debridement of necrotic tissue and liquefaction of slough in acute and chronic lesions such as pressure ulcers, varicose and diabetic ulcers, burns, postoperative wounds, pilonidal cyst wounds, carbuncles, and miscellaneous traumatic or infected wounds
Usual Dosage Topical: Adults: Apply with each dressing change. Daily or twice daily dressing changes are preferred, but may be every 2-3 days. Cover with dressing following application.
Ointment: Apply $^1/_8$-inch thickness over the wound with clean applicator.
Spray: Completely cover the wound site so that the wound is not visible.
Dosage Forms
Emulsion, topical [spray]:
Accuzyme® SE: Papain 8.3 x 10^5 units/g and urea 10% (34 mL)
Ointment, topical:
Accuzyme®: Papain 8.3 x 10^5 units/g and urea 10% (6 g, 30 g)
AllanEnzyme 650: Papain 8.3 x 10^5 units/g and urea 10% (30 g)
Ethezyme™: Papain 1.1 x 10^6 units and urea 10% (30 g)
Ethezyme™ 650: Papain 6.5 x 10^5 units/g and urea 10% (30 g)
Ethezyme™ 830: Papain 8.3 x 10^5 units/g and urea 10% (30 g)
Kovia®: Papain 8.3 x 10^5 units/g and urea 10% (3.5 g) [single-dose packet]; 30 g
Solution, topical [spray]:
AllanEnzyme: Papain 8.3 x 10^5 units/g and urea 10% (33 mL)

papain, urea, and chlorophyllin *see* chlorophyllin, papain, and urea *on page 175*

papaverine (pa PAV er een)

Synonyms papaverine hydrochloride
U.S./Canadian Brand Names Para-Time S.R.® [US]
Therapeutic Category Vasodilator
Use Oral: Relief of peripheral and cerebral ischemia associated with arterial spasm and myocardial ischemia complicated by arrhythmias
Usual Dosage
I.M., I.V.:
Children: 6 mg/kg/day in 4 divided doses
Adults: 30-65 mg (rarely up to 120 mg); may repeat every 3 hours
Oral, sustained release: Adults: 150-300 mg every 12 hours; in difficult cases: 150 mg every 8 hours
Dosage Forms
Capsule, sustained release: 150 mg
Para-Time SR®: 150 mg
Injection, solution: 30 mg/mL (2 mL, 10 mL)

papaverine hydrochloride *see* papaverine *on this page*

papillomavirus (Types 6, 11, 16, 18) recombinant vaccine

(pap ih LO ma VYE rus typs six e LEV en SIX teen aye teen ree KOM be nant vak SEEN)
Synonyms HPV Vaccine; human papillomavirus vaccine; papillomavirus vaccine, recombinant; quadrivalent human papillomavirus vaccine
U.S./Canadian Brand Names Gardasil® [US]
Therapeutic Category Vaccine
Use Females: Prevention of cervical cancer, genital warts, cervical adenocarcinoma *in situ*, and vulvar, vaginal, or cervical intraepithelial neoplasia caused by human papillomavirus (HPV) types 6, 11, 16, 18
Usual Dosage I.M.: Females: Children ≥9 years and Adults ≤26 years: 0.5 mL followed by 0.5 mL at 2 and 6 months after initial dose

CDC recommended immunization schedule: Administer first dose to females at age 11-12 years; begin series in females aged 13-26 years if not previously vaccinated. Minimum interval between first and second doses is 4 weeks; the minimum interval between second and third doses is 12 weeks.

Dosage Forms

Injection, suspension [preservative free]:

Gardasil®: HPV 6 L1 protein 20 mcg, HPV 11 L1 protein 40 mcg, HPV 16 L1 protein 40 mcg, and HPV 18 L1 protein 20 mcg per 0.5 mL (0.5 mL)

papillomavirus vaccine, recombinant *see* papillomavirus (Types 6, 11, 16, 18) recombinant vaccine *on previous page*

para-aminosalicylate sodium *see* aminosalicylic acid *on page 43*

paracetamol *see* acetaminophen *on page 5*

Paraflex® *(Discontinued) see* chlorzoxazone *on page 186*

Parafon Forte® **[Can]** *see* chlorzoxazone *on page 186*

Parafon Forte® *(Discontinued) see* chlorzoxazone *on page 186*

Parafon Forte® **DSC [US]** *see* chlorzoxazone *on page 186*

Paraplatin-AQ [Can] *see* carboplatin *on page 153*

Paraplatin® *(Discontinued) see* carboplatin *on page 153*

parathyroid hormone (1-34) *see* teriparatide *on page 827*

Para-Time S.R.® **[US]** *see* papaverine *on previous page*

Parcopa™ [US] *see* levodopa and carbidopa *on page 500*

Paredrine® *(Discontinued)*

paregoric (par e GOR ik)

Sound-Alike/Look-Alike Issues

paregoric may be confused with Percogesic®

camphorated tincture of opium is an error-prone synonym (mistaken as opium tincture)

Therapeutic Category Analgesic, Narcotic

Controlled Substance C-III

Use Treatment of diarrhea or relief of pain; neonatal opiate withdrawal

Usual Dosage Oral:

Neonatal opiate withdrawal: 3-6 drops every 3-6 hours as needed, or initially 0.2 mL every 3 hours; increase dosage by approximately 0.05 mL every 3 hours until withdrawal symptoms are controlled; it is rare to exceed 0.7 mL/dose. Stabilize withdrawal symptoms for 3-5 days, then gradually decrease dosage over a 2- to 4-week period.

Children: 0.25-0.5 mL/kg 1-4 times/day

Adults: 5-10 mL 1-4 times/day

Dosage Forms

Liquid, oral: Morphine equivalent 2 mg/5 mL

Paremyd® **[US]** *see* hydroxyamphetamine and tropicamide *on page 438*

parenteral nutrition *see* total parenteral nutrition *on page 853*

Parepectolin® *(Discontinued)*

paricalcitol (pah ri KAL si tole)

U.S./Canadian Brand Names Zemplar® [US/Can]

Therapeutic Category Vitamin D Analog

Use

I.V.: Prevention and treatment of secondary hyperparathyroidism associated with stage 5 chronic kidney disease (CKD)

Oral: Prevention and treatment of secondary hyperparathyroidism associated with stage 3 and 4 CKD

Usual Dosage Note: If hypercalcemia or Ca x P >75 is observed, reduce or interrupt dosing until parameters are normalized.

Secondary hyperparathyroidism associated with chronic renal failure (stage 5 CKD): Children ≥5 years and Adults: I.V.: 0.04-0.1 mcg/kg (2.8-7 mcg) given as a bolus dose no more frequently than every other day at any time during dialysis; dose may be increased by 2-4 mcg every 2-4 weeks; doses as high as 0.24 mcg/kg (16.8 mcg) have been administered safely; the dose of paricalcitol should be adjusted based on serum intact PTH (iPTH) levels, as follows:

Same or increasing iPTH level: Increase paricalcitol dose

iPTH level decreased by <30%: Increase paricalcitol dose

iPTH level decreased by >30% and <60%: Maintain paricalcitol dose

(Continued)

paricalcitol *(Continued)*

iPTH level decrease by >60%: Decrease paricalcitol dose
iPTH level 1.5-3 times upper limit of normal: Maintain paricalcitol dose

Secondary hyperparathyroidism associated with stage 3 and 4 CKD: Adults: Oral: Initial dose based on baseline iPTH:
iPTH ≤500 pg/mL: 1 mcg/day or 2 mcg 3 times/week
iPTH >500 pg/mL: 2 mcg/day or 4 mcg 3 times/week

Dosage adjustment based on iPTH level relative to baseline, adjust dose at 2-4 week intervals:
iPTH same or increased: Increase paricalcitol dose by 1 mcg/day or 2 mcg 3 times/week
iPTH decreased by <30%: Increase paricalcitol dose by 1 mcg/day or 2 mcg 3 times//week
iPTH decreased by ≥30% or ≤60%: Maintain paricalcitol dose
iPTH decreased by >60%: Decrease paricalcitol dose by 1 mcg/day* or 2 mcg 3 times/week
iPTH <60 pg/mL: Decrease paricalcitol dose by 1 mcg/day* or 2 mcg 3 times/week
*If patient is taking the lowest dose on a once-daily regimen, but further dose reduction is needed, decrease dose to 1 mcg 3 times/week. If further dose reduction is required, withhold drug as needed and restart at a lower dose. If applicable, calcium-phosphate binder dosing may also be adjusted or withheld, or switch to noncalcium-based binder

Dosage Forms
Capsule, gelatin:
Zemplar®: 1 mcg, 2 mcg, 4 mcg
Injection, solution:
Zemplar®: 2 mcg/mL (1 mL); 5 mcg/mL (1 mL, 2 mL)

Pariet® [Can] *see* rabeprazole *on page 741*

pariprazole *see* rabeprazole *on page 741*

Parlodel® [US/Can] *see* bromocriptine *on page 119*

Parnate® [US/Can] *see* tranylcypromine *on page 858*

paromomycin *(par oh moe MYE sin)*

Synonyms paromomycin sulfate
U.S./Canadian Brand Names Humatin® [US/Can]
Therapeutic Category Amebicide
Use Treatment of acute and chronic intestinal amebiasis; hepatic coma
Usual Dosage Oral:
Intestinal amebiasis: Children and Adults: 25-35 mg/kg/day in 3 divided doses for 5-10 days
Dientamoeba fragilis: Children and Adults: 25-30 mg/kg/day in 3 divided doses for 7 days
Tapeworm (fish, dog, bovine, porcine):
Children: 11 mg/kg every 15 minutes for 4 doses
Adults: 1 g every 15 minutes for 4 doses
Hepatic coma: Adults: 4 g/day in 2-4 divided doses for 5-6 days
Dwarf tapeworm: Children and Adults: 45 mg/kg/dose every day for 5-7 days
Dosage Forms
Capsule: 250 mg
Humatin®: 250 mg

paromomycin sulfate *see* paromomycin *on this page*

paroxetine *(pa ROKS e teen)*

Sound-Alike/Look-Alike Issues
paroxetine may be confused with paclitaxel, pyridoxine
Paxil® may be confused with Doxil®, paclitaxel, Plavix®, Taxol®
Synonyms paroxetine hydrochloride; paroxetine mesylate
U.S./Canadian Brand Names Apo-Paroxetine® [Can]; CO Paroxetine [Can]; Gen-Paroxetine [Can]; Novo-Paroxetine [Can]; Paxil CR® [US/Can]; Paxil® [US/Can]; Pexeva® [US]; PMS-Paroxetine [Can]; ratio-Paroxetine [Can]; Rhoxal-paroxetine [Can]; Sandoz-Paroxetine [Can]
Therapeutic Category Antidepressant, Selective Serotonin Reuptake Inhibitor
Use Treatment of major depressive disorder (MDD); treatment of panic disorder with or without agoraphobia; obsessive-compulsive disorder (OCD); social anxiety disorder (social phobia); generalized anxiety disorder (GAD); post-traumatic stress disorder (PTSD); premenstrual dysphoric disorder (PMDD)
Usual Dosage Oral: Adults:
MDD:
Paxil®, Pexeva®: Initial: 20 mg once daily, preferably in the morning; increase if needed by 10 mg/day increments at intervals of at least 1 week; maximum dose: 50 mg/day

Paxil CR®: Initial: 25 mg once daily; increase if needed by 12.5 mg/day increments at intervals of at least 1 week; maximum dose: 62.5 mg/day

GAD (Paxil®, Pexeva®): Initial: 20 mg once daily, preferably in the morning (if dose is increased, adjust in increments of 10 mg/day at 1-week intervals); doses of 20-50 mg/day were used in clinical trials, however, no greater benefit was seen with doses >20 mg.

OCD (Paxil®, Pexeva™): Initial: 20 mg once daily, preferably in the morning; increase if needed by 10 mg/day increments at intervals of at least 1 week; recommended dose: 40 mg/day; range: 20-60 mg/day; maximum dose: 60 mg/day

Panic disorder:

Paxil®, Pexeva®: Initial: 10 mg once daily, preferably in the morning; increase if needed by 10 mg/day increments at intervals of at least 1 week; recommended dose: 40 mg/day; range: 10-60 mg/day; maximum dose: 60 mg/day

Paxil CR®: Initial: 12.5 mg once daily; increase if needed by 12.5 mg/day at intervals of at least 1 week; maximum dose: 75 mg/day

PMDD (Paxil CR®): Initial: 12.5 mg once daily in the morning; may be increased to 25 mg/day; dosing changes should occur at intervals of at least 1 week. May be given daily throughout the menstrual cycle or limited to the luteal phase.

PTSD (Paxil®): Initial: 20 mg once daily, preferably in the morning; increase if needed by 10 mg/day increments at intervals of at least 1 week; range: 20-50 mg. Limited data suggest doses of 40 mg/day were not more efficacious than 20 mg/day.

Social anxiety disorder:

Paxil®: Initial: 20 mg once daily, preferably in the morning; recommended dose: 20 mg/day; range: 20-60 mg/day; doses >20 mg may not have additional benefit

Paxil CR®: Initial: 12.5 mg once daily, preferably in the morning; may be increased by 12.5 mg/day at intervals of at least 1 week; maximum dose: 37.5 mg/day

Note: Upon discontinuation of paroxetine therapy, gradually taper dose:

Paxil®, Pexeva®: 10 mg/day at weekly intervals; when 20 mg/day dose is reached, continue for 1 week before treatment is discontinued. Some patients may need to be titrated to 10 mg/day for 1 week before discontinuation.

Paxil CR®: Patients receiving 37.5 mg/day in clinical trials had their dose decreased by 12.5 mg/day to a dose of 25 mg/day and remained at a dose of 25 mg/day for 1 week before treatment was discontinued.

Dosage Forms Note: Strength expressed as base:

Suspension, oral:

Paxil®: 10 mg/5 mL (250 mL)

Tablet: 10 mg, 20 mg, 30 mg, 40 mg

Paxil®, Pexeva®: 10 mg, 20 mg, 30 mg, 40 mg

Tablet, controlled release:

Paxil CR®: 12.5 mg, 25 mg, 37.5 mg

paroxetine hydrochloride *see* paroxetine *on previous page*

paroxetine mesylate *see* paroxetine *on previous page*

Partuss® LA *(Discontinued)*

Parvolex® [Can] *see* acetylcysteine *on page 15*

PAS *see* aminosalicylic acid *on page 43*

Paser® [US] *see* aminosalicylic acid *on page 43*

Pataday™ [US] *see* olopatadine *on page 627*

Patanol® [US/Can] *see* olopatadine *on page 627*

Pathilon® *(Discontinued)*

Pathocil® [Can] *see* dicloxacillin *on page 254*

Pathocil® *(Discontinued)* *see* dicloxacillin *on page 254*

Pavabid® *(Discontinued)* *see* papaverine *on page 652*

Pavatine® *(Discontinued)*

Pavulon® *(Discontinued)* *see* pancuronium *on page 650*

Paxene® *(Discontinued)* *see* paclitaxel *on page 645*

Paxil® [US/Can] *see* paroxetine *on previous page*

Paxil CR® [US/Can] *see* paroxetine *on previous page*

PCE® [US/Can] *see* erythromycin *on page 309*

PCEC *see* rabies virus vaccine *on page 742*

P Chlor GG [US] *see* chlorpheniramine, phenylephrine, and guaifenesin *on page 181*

PCM [US] *see* chlorpheniramine, phenylephrine, and methscopolamine *on page 181*

PCM Allergy [US] *see* chlorpheniramine, phenylephrine, and methscopolamine *on page 181*

PCV7 *see* pneumococcal conjugate vaccine (7-valent) *on page 691*

PD-Cof [US] *see* chlorpheniramine, phenylephrine, and dextromethorphan *on page 180*

PD-Hist-D [US] *see* chlorpheniramine and phenylephrine *on page 177*

pectin, gelatin, and methylcellulose *see* gelatin, pectin, and methylcellulose *on page 386*

Pedameth® *(Discontinued)*

Pediacare® Children's Long Acting Cough Plus Cold *(Discontinued)* *see* pseudoephedrine and dextromethorphan *on page 728*

PediaCare® Children's Medicated Freezer Pops Long Acting Cough *(Discontinued)* *see* dextromethorphan *on page 247*

PediaCare® Cold and Allergy *(Discontinued)* *see* chlorpheniramine and pseudoephedrine *on page 178*

PediaCare® Decongestant Infants [US-OTC] *see* pseudoephedrine *on page 727*

Pediacare® Infants' Decongestant & Cough [US-OTC] *see* pseudoephedrine and dextromethorphan *on page 728*

PediaCare® Infants' Long-Acting Cough [US-OTC] *see* dextromethorphan *on page 247*

PediaCare® Multi-Symptom Cold *(Discontinued)* *see* chlorpheniramine, pseudoephedrine, and dextromethorphan *on page 183*

PediaCare® NightRest Cough and Cold *(Discontinued)* *see* chlorpheniramine, pseudoephedrine, and dextromethorphan *on page 183*

Pediacof® *(Discontinued)* *see* chlorpheniramine, phenylephrine, codeine, and potassium iodide *on page 183*

Pediaflor® *(Discontinued)* *see* fluoride *on page 361*

PediaHist DM [US] *see* brompheniramine, pseudoephedrine, and dextromethorphan *on page 122*

Pedialyte® [US-OTC] *see* nutritional formula, enteral/oral *on page 622*

PediaPatch Transdermal Patch *(Discontinued)* *see* salicylic acid *on page 772*

Pediapred® [US/Can] *see* prednisolone (systemic) *on page 710*

Pedia-Profen™ *(Discontinued)* *see* ibuprofen *on page 444*

Pedia Relief Cough and Cold [US-OTC] *see* pseudoephedrine and dextromethorphan *on page 728*

Pedia Relief Infants [US-OTC] *see* pseudoephedrine and dextromethorphan *on page 728*

Pediarix® [US/Can] *see* diphtheria, tetanus toxoids, acellular pertussis, hepatitis B (recombinant), and poliovirus (inactivated) vaccine *on page 268*

PediaTan™ [US] *see* chlorpheniramine *on page 177*

PediaTan™D [US] *see* chlorpheniramine and phenylephrine *on page 177*

Pediatex™ 12 *(Discontinued)* *see* carbinoxamine *on page 151*

Pediatex™-D *(Discontinued)* *see* carbinoxamine and pseudoephedrine *on page 151*

Pediatex™ *(Discontinued)* *see* carbinoxamine *on page 151*

Pediatex™ DM *(Discontinued)* *see* carbinoxamine, pseudoephedrine, and dextromethorphan *on page 152*

Pediatex™ HC [US] *see* pseudoephedrine, hydrocodone, and chlorpheniramine *on page 731*

Pediatric Digoxin CSD [Can] *see* digoxin *on page 257*

Pediatric Triban® *(Discontinued)*

Pediatrix [Can] *see* acetaminophen *on page 5*

Pediazole® [Can] *see* erythromycin and sulfisoxazole *on page 310*

Pediazole® *(Discontinued)* *see* erythromycin and sulfisoxazole *on page 310*

Pedi-Boro® [US-OTC] *see* aluminum sulfate and calcium acetate *on page 38*

Pedi-Dri® [US] *see* nystatin *on page 623*

PediOtic® [US] *see* neomycin, polymyxin B, and hydrocortisone *on page 597*

Pedi-Pro® [US] *see* benzalkonium chloride *on page 100*

Pedisilk® [US-OTC] *see* salicylic acid *on page 772*

Pedtrace-4® **[US]** *see* trace metals *on page 855*

PedvaxHIB® **[US/Can]** *see Haemophilus* B conjugate vaccine *on page 411*

PEG *see* polyethylene glycol 3350 *on page 694*

PEG-L-asparaginase *see* pegaspargase *on this page*

pegademase (bovine) (peg A de mase BOE vine)
U.S./Canadian Brand Names Adagen® [US/Can]
Therapeutic Category Enzyme
Use Orphan drug: Enzyme replacement therapy for adenosine deaminase (ADA) deficiency in patients with severe combined immunodeficiency disease (SCID) who can not benefit from bone marrow transplant; not a cure for SCID, unlike bone marrow transplants, injections must be used the rest of the child's life, therefore is not really an alternative
Usual Dosage I.M.: Children: Dose given every 7 days, 10 units/kg the first dose, 15 units/kg the second dose, and 20 units/kg the third dose; maintenance dose: 20 units/kg/week is recommended depending on patient's ADA level; maximum single dose: 30 units/kg
Dosage Forms
Injection, solution [preservative free]:
Adagen®: 250 units/mL (1.5 mL)

Peganone® **[US/Can]** *see* ethotoin *on page 333*

pegaptanib (peg AP ta nib)
Synonyms EYE001; pegaptanib sodium
U.S./Canadian Brand Names Macugen® [US/Can]
Therapeutic Category Ophthalmic Agent; Vaccine, Recombinant
Use Treatment of neovascular (wet) age-related macular degeneration (AMD)
Usual Dosage Intravitreous injection: Adults: AMD: 0.3 mg into affected eye every 6 weeks
Dosage Forms
Injection, solution [preservative free; prefilled syringe]:
Macugen®: 0.3 mg/90 µL (90 µL)

pegaptanib sodium *see* pegaptanib *on this page*

pegaspargase (peg AS par jase)
Sound-Alike/Look-Alike Issues
pegaspargase may be confused with asparaginase
Synonyms NSC-644954; PEG-L-asparaginase
U.S./Canadian Brand Names Oncaspar® [US]
Therapeutic Category Antineoplastic Agent
Use Treatment of acute lymphocytic leukemia (ALL); treatment of ALL with previous hypersensitivity to native L-asparaginase
Usual Dosage Usually administered as part of a combination chemotherapy regimen.
I.M. administration is **preferred** over I.V. administration due to lower incidence of hepatotoxicity, coagulopathy, gastrointestinal, and renal disorders with I.M. administration.
Children: I.M., I.V.:
Body surface area <0.6 m^2: 82.5 int. units/kg every 14 days
Body surface area ≥0.6 m^2: 2500 int. units/m^2 every 14 days
Adults: I.M., I.V.: 2500 int. units/m^2 every 14 days
Hemodialysis: Significant drug removal is unlikely based on physiochemical characteristics
Peritoneal dialysis: Significant drug removal is unlikely based on physiochemical characteristics
Dosage Forms
Injection, solution [preservative free]:
Oncaspar®: 750 units/mL (5 mL)

Pegasys® **[US/Can]** *see* peginterferon alfa-2a *on next page*

Pegasys [Can] *see* peginterferon alfa-2b and ribavirin *(Canada only) on page 659*

Pegasys® **RBV [Can]** *see* peginterferon alfa-2b and ribavirin *(Canada only) on page 659*

Pegetron™ **[Can]** *see* peginterferon alfa-2b and ribavirin *(Canada only) on page 659*

pegfilgrastim (peg fil GRA stim)
Sound-Alike/Look-Alike Issues
Neulasta® may be confused with Neumega® and Lunesta™
(Continued)

pegfilgrastim (Continued)

Synonyms G-CSF (PEG conjugate); granulocyte colony stimulating factor (PEG conjugate); NSC-725961; SD/01

U.S./Canadian Brand Names Neulasta® [US/Can]

Therapeutic Category Colony-Stimulating Factor

Use To decrease the incidence of infection, by stimulation of granulocyte production, in patients with nonmyeloid malignancies receiving myelosuppressive therapy associated with a significant risk of febrile neutropenia

Usual Dosage SubQ: Adolescents >45 kg and Adults: 6 mg once per chemotherapy cycle; do not administer in the period between 14 days before and 24 hours after administration of cytotoxic chemotherapy; do not use in infants, children, and smaller adolescents weighing <45 kg

Dosage Forms

Injection, solution [preservative free]:

Neulasta®: 10 mg/mL (0.6 mL)

peginterferon alfa-2a (peg in ter FEER on AL fa too aye)

Synonyms interferon alfa-2a (PEG conjugate); pegylated interferon alfa-2a

U.S./Canadian Brand Names Pegasys® [US/Can]

Therapeutic Category Interferon

Use Treatment of chronic hepatitis C (CHC), alone or in combination with ribavirin, in patients with compensated liver disease and histological evidence of cirrhosis (Child-Pugh class A) and patients with clinically-stable HIV disease; treatment of patients with HBeAg positive and HBeAg negative chronic hepatitis B with compensated liver disease and evidence of viral replication and liver inflammation

Usual Dosage SubQ: Adults:

Chronic hepatitis C (monoinfection or coinfection with HIV):

Monotherapy: 180 mcg once weekly for 48 weeks

Combination therapy with ribavirin: Recommended dosage: 180 mcg once/week with ribavirin (Copegus®)

Duration of therapy: Monoinfection (based on genotype):

Genotype 1,4: 48 weeks

Genotype 2,3: 24 weeks

Duration of therapy: Coinfection with HIV: 48 weeks

Chronic hepatitis B: 180 mcg once weekly for 48 weeks

Dose modifications for adverse reactions/toxicity:

For moderate-to-severe adverse reactions: Initial: 135 mcg/week; may need decreased to 90 mcg/week in some cases

Based on hematologic parameters:

ANC <750/mm^3: 135 mcg/week

ANC <500/mm^3: Suspend therapy until >1000/mm^3, then restart at 90 mcg/week and monitor

Platelet count <50,000/mm^3: 90 mcg/week

Platelet count <25,000/mm^3: Discontinue therapy

Depression (severity based on DSM-IV criteria):

Mild depression: No dosage adjustment required; evaluate once weekly by visit/phone call. If depression remains stable, continue weekly visits. If depression improves, resume normal visit schedule

Moderate depression: Decrease interferon dose to 90-135 mcg once/week; evaluate once weekly with an office visit at least every other week. If depression remains stable, consider psychiatric evaluation and continue with reduced dosing. If symptoms improve and remain stable for 4 weeks, resume normal visit schedule; continue reduced dosing or return to normal dose.

Severe depression: Discontinue interferon permanently. Obtain immediate psychiatric consultation. Discontinue ribavirin if using concurrently.

Dosage Forms

Injection, solution:

Pegasys®

180 mcg/0.5 mL (0.5 mL) [prefilled syringe; contains benzyl alcohol and polysorbate 80; packaged with needles and alcohol swabs]

180 mcg/mL (1 mL) [vial; contains benzyl alcohol and polysorbate 80]

peginterferon alfa-2b (peg in ter FEER on AL fa too bee)

Synonyms interferon alfa-2b (PEG conjugate); pegylated interferon alfa-2b

U.S./Canadian Brand Names PEG-Intron® [US/Can]

Therapeutic Category Interferon

Use Treatment of chronic hepatitis C (as monotherapy or in combination with ribavirin) in adult patients who have never received interferon alpha and have compensated liver disease

Usual Dosage SubQ: Adults: Chronic hepatitis C: Administer dose once weekly; **Note:** Treatment duration may vary. Consult current guidelines and literature.

Monotherapy: Initial:
  ≤45 kg: 40 mcg
  46-56 kg: 50 mcg
  57-72 kg: 64 mcg
  73-88 kg: 80 mcg
  89-106 kg: 96 mcg
  107-136 kg: 120 mcg
  137-160 kg: 150 mcg
  Combination therapy with ribavirin (400 mg twice daily): Initial: 1.5 mcg/kg/week
  <40 kg: 50 mcg
  40-50 kg: 64 mcg
  51-60 kg: 80 mcg
  61-75 kg: 96 mcg
  76-85 kg: 120 mcg
  >85 kg: 150 mcg
Dosage Forms
  Injection, powder for reconstitution:
  PegIntron™: 50 mcg, 80 mcg, 120 mcg, 150 mcg
  PegIntron™ Redipen®: 50 mcg, 80 mcg, 120 mcg, 150 mcg

peginterferon alfa-2b and ribavirin *(Canada only)*
  (peg in ter FEER on AL fa too bee & rye ba VYE rin)
Synonyms ribavirin and peginterferon alfa-2b
U.S./Canadian Brand Names Pegasys [Can]; Pegasys® RBV [Can]; Pegetron™ [Can]
Therapeutic Category Antiviral Agent; Interferon
Use Combination therapy for the treatment of chronic hepatitis C in patients with compensated liver disease
Usual Dosage Chronic hepatitis C:
  Recommended dosage of combination therapy:
  Intron® A: SubQ: 1.5 mcg/kg/week
  and
  Rebetol®: Oral:
    ≤64 kg: 800 mg/day (two 200 mg capsules in the morning and two 200 mg capsules in the evening)
    64-84 kg: 1000 mg/day (two 200 mg capsules in the morning and three 200 mg capsules in the evening)
    ≥85 kg: 1200 mg/day (three 200 mg capsules in the morning and three 200 mg capsules in the evening)
  Note: Treatment duration may vary. Consult current guidelines and literature.
Dosage Forms Combination package:
  Pegasys® RBV [CAN], Pegetron™ [CAN] [not available in the U.S.]:
  Injection, powder for reconstitution (Peginterferon alfa-2b): 50 mcg/0.5 mL
  Capsules: Ribavirin (Rebetol®): 200 mg (56s)

  Injection, powder for reconstitution (Peginterferon alfa-2b): 80 mcg/0.5 mL
  Capsules: Ribavirin (Rebetol®): 200 mg (56s)

  Injection, powder for reconstitution (Peginterferon alfa-2b): 100 mcg/0.5 mL
  Capsules: Ribavirin (Rebetol®): 200 mg (70s)

  Injection, powder for reconstitution (Peginterferon alfa-2b): 120 mcg/0.5 mL
  Capsules: Ribavirin (Rebetol®): 200 mg (70s)

  Injection, powder for reconstitution (Peginterferon alfa-2b): 150 mcg/0.5 mL
  Capsules: Ribavirin (Rebetol®): 200 mg (84s)

PEG-Intron® [US/Can] *see* peginterferon alfa-2b *on previous page*

PegLyte® [Can] *see* polyethylene glycol-electrolyte solution *on page 695*

pegvisomant (peg VI soe mant)
Synonyms B2036-PEG
U.S./Canadian Brand Names Somavert® [US]
Therapeutic Category Growth Hormone Receptor Antagonist
Use Treatment of acromegaly in patients resistant to or unable to tolerate other therapies
Usual Dosage SubQ: Adults: Initial loading dose: 40 mg; maintenance dose: 10 mg once daily; doses may be adjusted by 5 mg in 4- to 6-week intervals based on IGF-I concentrations (maximum dose: 30 mg/day)
Dosage Forms
  Injection, powder for reconstitution [preservative free]:
  Somavert®: 10 mg, 15 mg, 20 mg

pegylated interferon alfa-2a *see* peginterferon alfa-2a *on page 658*

pegylated interferon alfa-2b *see* peginterferon alfa-2b *on page 658*

pegylated liposomal DOXOrubicin *see* doxorubicin (liposomal) *on page 281*

pemetrexed (pem e TREKS ed)
Synonyms LY231514; MTA; multitargeted antifolate; NSC-698037; pemetrexed disodium
U.S./Canadian Brand Names Alimta® [US/Can]
Therapeutic Category Antineoplastic Agent, Antimetabolite; Antineoplastic Agent, Antimetabolite (Antifolate)
Use Treatment of malignant pleural mesothelioma; treatment of nonsmall cell lung cancer
Usual Dosage I.V.: Adults: Refer to individual protocols:
Nonsmall cell lung cancer: 500 mg/m^2 on day 1 of each 21-day cycle
Malignant pleural mesothelioma: 500 mg/m^2 on day 1 of each 21-day cycle (in combination with cisplatin)
Note: Start vitamin supplements 1 week before initial dose of pemetrexed. Folic acid 350-1000 mcg/day orally (continuing for 21 days after last dose of pemetrexed) and vitamin B$_{12}$ 1000 mcg I.M. every 9 weeks. Dexamethasone 4 mg twice daily can be started the day before therapy, and continued the day of and the day after to minimize cutaneous reactions.
Dosage Forms
  Injection, powder for reconstitution:
  Alimta®: 500 mg

pemetrexed disodium *see* pemetrexed *on this page*

pemirolast (pe MIR oh last)
U.S./Canadian Brand Names Alamast® [US/Can]
Therapeutic Category Mast Cell Stabilizer; Ophthalmic Agent, Miscellaneous
Use Prevention of itching of the eye due to allergic conjunctivitis
Usual Dosage Children >3 years and Adults: 1-2 drops instilled in affected eye(s) 4 times/day
Dosage Forms
  Solution, ophthalmic:
  Alamast®: 0.1% (10 mL)

pemoline *(Discontinued)*

penbutolol (pen BYOO toe lole)
Sound-Alike/Look-Alike Issues
  Levatol® may be confused with Lipitor®
Synonyms penbutolol sulfate
U.S./Canadian Brand Names Levatol® [US/Can]
Therapeutic Category Beta-Adrenergic Blocker
Use Treatment of mild to moderate arterial hypertension
Usual Dosage Oral: Adults: Initial: 20 mg once daily, full effect of a 20 or 40 mg dose is seen by the end of a 2-week period, doses of 40-80 mg have been tolerated but have shown little additional antihypertensive effects; usual dose range (JNC 7): 10-40 mg once daily
Dosage Forms
  Tablet:
  Levatol®: 20 mg

penbutolol sulfate *see* penbutolol *on this page*

penciclovir (pen SYE kloe veer)
Sound-Alike/Look-Alike Issues
  Denavir® may be confused with indinavir
U.S./Canadian Brand Names Denavir® [US]
Therapeutic Category Antiviral Agent
Use Topical treatment of herpes simplex labialis (cold sores)
Usual Dosage Topical: Children ≥12 years and Adults: Apply cream at the first sign or symptom of cold sore (eg, tingling, swelling); apply every 2 hours during waking hours for 4 days
Dosage Forms
  Cream:
  Denavir®: 1% (1.5 g)

Pendex [US] *see* guaifenesin and phenylephrine *on page 404*

Pendo-5 ASA [Can] *see* mesalamine *on page 546*

Penetrex® *(Discontinued)*

penicillamine (pen i SIL a meen)
Sound-Alike/Look-Alike Issues
penicillamine may be confused with penicillin
Depen® may be confused with Endal®
Synonyms β,β-dimethylcysteine; D-3-mercaptovaline; D-penicillamine
U.S./Canadian Brand Names Cuprimine® [US/Can]; Depen® [US/Can]
Therapeutic Category Chelating Agent
Use Treatment of Wilson disease, cystinuria; adjunctive treatment of rheumatoid arthritis
Usual Dosage Oral:
Rheumatoid arthritis:
Adults: 125-250 mg/day, may increase dose at 1- to 3-month intervals up to 1-1.5 g/day; maximum in older adults: 750 mg/day
Wilson disease (doses titrated to maintain urinary copper excretion >2 mg/day); decrease dose for surgery and during last trimester of pregnancy
Children <12 years: 20 mg/kg/day in 2-3 divided doses, round off to the nearest 250 mg dose; maximum 1 g/day
Adults: 250 mg 4 times/day (maximum in older adults: 750 mg/day)
Cystinuria: **Note:** Adjust dose to limit cystine excretion to 100-200 mg/day (<100 mg/day with history of stone formation)
Children: 30 mg/kg/day in 4 divided doses
Adults: 1-4 g/day in divided doses every 6 hours; usual dose: 2 g/day
Dosage Forms
Capsule:
Cuprimine®: 250 mg
Tablet:
Depen®: 250 mg

penicillin G benzathine (pen i SIL in jee BENZ a theen)
Sound-Alike/Look-Alike Issues
penicillin may be confused with penicillamine
Bicillin® may be confused with Wycillin®
Bicillin® C-R (penicillin G benzathine and penicillin G procaine) may be confused with Bicillin® L-A (penicillin G benzathine). Penicillin G benzathine is the only product currently approved for the treatment of syphilis. Administration of penicillin G benzathine and penicillin G procaine combination instead of Bicillin® L-A may result in inadequate treatment response.
Synonyms benzathine benzylpenicillin; benzathine penicillin G; benzylpenicillin benzathine
U.S./Canadian Brand Names Bicillin® L-A [US/Can]
Therapeutic Category Penicillin
Use Active against some gram-positive organisms, few gram-negative organisms such as *Neisseria gonorrhoeae*, and some anaerobes and spirochetes; used in the treatment of syphilis; used only for the treatment of mild to moderately severe infections caused by organisms susceptible to low concentrations of penicillin G or for prophylaxis of infections caused by these organisms
Usual Dosage Note: Administer undiluted injection; higher doses result in more sustained rather than higher levels. Use a penicillin G benzathine-penicillin G procaine combination to achieve early peak levels in acute infections.
Usual dosage range:
Children: I.M.: 25,000-50,000 units/kg as a single dose (maximum: 2.4 million units)
Adults: I.M.: 1.2-2.4 million units as a single dose
Indication-specific dosing:
Neonates >1200 g: I.M.:
Congenital syphilis (asymptomatic): 50,000 units/kg as a single dose
Infants and Children: I.M.:
Group A streptococcal upper respiratory infection: 25,000-50,000 units/kg as a single dose (maximum: 1.2 million units)
Prophylaxis of recurrent rheumatic fever: 25,000-50,000 units/kg every 3-4 weeks (maximum: 1.2 million units/dose)
Syphilis:
Early: 50,000 units/kg as a single injection (maximum: 2.4 million units)
More than 1-year duration: 50,000 units/kg every week for 3 doses (maximum: 2.4 million units/dose)
Adults: I.M.:
Group A streptococcal upper respiratory infection: 1.2 million units as a single dose
Prophylaxis of recurrent rheumatic fever: 1.2 million units every 3-4 weeks or 600,000 units twice monthly
(Continued)

penicillin G benzathine *(Continued)*

Syphilis:
Early: 2.4 million units as a single dose in 2 injection sites
More than 1-year duration: 2.4 million units in 2 injection sites once weekly for 3 doses
Neurosyphilis: Not indicated as single-drug therapy, but may be given once weekly for 3 weeks following
I.V. treatment; refer to penicillin G parenteral/aqueous monograph for dosing

Dosage Forms
Injection, suspension [prefilled syringe]:
Bicillin® L-A: 600,000 units/mL (1 mL, 2 mL, 4 mL)

penicillin G benzathine and penicillin G procaine

(pen i SIL in jee BENZ a theen & pen i SIL in jee PROE kane)

Sound-Alike/Look-Alike Issues
penicillin may be confused with penicillamine
Bicillin® may be confused with Wycillin®
Bicillin® C-R (penicillin G benzathine and penicillin G procaine) may be confused with Bicillin® L-A (penicillin G benzathine). Penicillin G benzathine is the only product currently approved for the treatment of syphilis. Administration of penicillin G benzathine and penicillin G procaine combination instead of Bicillin® L-A may result in inadequate treatment response.

Synonyms penicillin G procaine and benzathine combined
U.S./Canadian Brand Names Bicillin® C-R 900/300 [US]; Bicillin® C-R [US]
Therapeutic Category Penicillin
Use May be used in specific situations in the treatment of streptococcal infections
Usual Dosage
Usual dosage range and indication-specific dosing:
Streptococcal infections:
Children: I.M.:
<14 kg: 600,000 units in a single dose
14-27 kg: 900,000 units to 1.2 million units in a single dose
Children >27 kg and Adults: 2.4 million units in a single dose

Dosage Forms
Injection, suspension [prefilled syringe]:
Bicillin® C-R:
600,000 units: Penicillin G benzathine 300,000 units and penicillin G procaine 300,000 units per 1 mL (1 mL)
1,200,000 units: Penicillin G benzathine 600,000 units and penicillin G procaine 600,000 units per 2 mL (2 mL)
2,400,000 units: Penicillin G benzathine 1,200,000 units and penicillin G procaine 1,200,000 units per 4 mL (4 mL)
Bicillin® C-R 900/300: 1,200,000 units: Penicillin G benzathine 900,000 units and penicillin G procaine 300,000 units per 2 mL (2 mL)

penicillin G (parenteral/aqueous) (pen i SIL in jee, pa REN ter al, AYE kwee us)

Sound-Alike/Look-Alike Issues
penicillin may be confused with penicillamine
Synonyms benzylpenicillin potassium; benzylpenicillin sodium; crystalline penicillin; penicillin G potassium; penicillin G sodium
U.S./Canadian Brand Names Pfizerpen® [US/Can]
Therapeutic Category Penicillin
Use Active against some gram-positive organisms, generally not *Staphylococcus aureus*; some gram-negative organisms such as *Neisseria gonorrhoeae*, and some anaerobes and spirochetes
Usual Dosage
Usual dosage range:
Neonates: I.M., I.V.:
<7 days, <2000 g: 25,000-50,000 units/kg every 12 hours
<7 days, >2000 g: 25,000-50,000 units/kg every 8 hours
>7 days, <2000 g: 25,000-50,000 units/kg every 8 hours
>7 days, >2000 g: 25,000-50,000 units/kg every 6 hours
Infants and Children: I.M., I.V.: 25,000-400,000 units/kg/day in divided doses every 4-6 hours (maximum dose: 24 million units/day)
Adults: I.M., I.V.: 2-24 million units/day in divided doses every 4 hours depending on sensitivity of the organism and severity of the infection

Indication-specific dosing:
Infants and Children:
Gonococcal:
Disseminated or ophthalmia: I.V.: 100,000 units/kg/day in 2 divided doses (>1 week of age: 4 divided doses)
Meningitis: I.V.: 150,000 units/kg in 2 divided doses (>1 week of age: 4 divided doses)
Mild infections: I.M., I.V.: 25,000-50,000 units/kg/day in 4 divided doses
Moderate infections: I.M., I.V.: 100,000-200,000 units/kg/day in 4 divided doses
Severe infections: I.M., I.V.: 250,000-400,000 units/kg/day in divided doses every 4-6 hours (maximum dose: 24 million units/day)
Syphilis (congenital):
Neonates:
≤7 days: 50,000 units/kg I.V. every 12 hours for a total of 10 days
>7 days: 50,000 units/kg I.V. every 8 hours for a total of 10 days
Infants: I.V.: 50,000 units/kg every 4-6 hours for 10 days
Adults:
***Actinomyces* species:** I.V.: 10-20 million units/day divided every 4-6 hours for 4-6 weeks
Anthrax (cutaneous): I.V.: 2 million units every 3 hours for 5-7 days
Clostridium perfringens: I.V.: 24 million units/day divided every 4-6 hours with clindamycin
Corynebacterium diphtheriae: I.V.: 25,000-50,000 units/kg to maximum 1.2 million units every 12 hours, until oral therapy tolerated
Erysipelas: I.V.: 1-2 million units every 4-6 hours
Erysipelothrix: I.V.: 2-4 million units every 4 hours
Fascial space infections: I.V.: 2-4 million units every 4-6 hours with metronidazole
Leptospirosis: I.V.: 1.5 million units every 6 hours for 7 days
Listeria: I.V.: 300,000 units/kg/day every 4 hours
Lyme disease (meningitis): I.V.: 20 million units/day in divided doses
Neurosyphilis: I.M., I.V.: 18-24 million units/day in divided doses every 4 hours (or by continuous infusion) for 10-14 days
Streptococcus:
Brain abscess: I.V.: 20-24 million units/day in divided doses with metronidazole
Endocarditis or osteomyelitis: I.V.: 3-4 million units every 4 hours for at least 4 weeks
Meningitis: I.V.: 3-4 million units every 4 hours for 2-3 weeks
Pregnancy (prophylaxis GBS): I.V.: 5-6 million units x 1 dose, then 2.5-3 million units every 4 hours until delivery
Skin and soft tissue: I.V.: 3-4 million units every 4 hours for 10 days
Toxic shock: I.V.: 24 million units/day in divided doses with clindamycin
Streptococcal pneumonia:
Meningitis: I.V.: 2-4 million units every 2-4 hours
Nonmeningitis: I.V.: 2-3 million units every 4 hours
Whipple disease: I.V.: 2 million units every 4 hours (with streptomycin) for 10-14 days, followed by oral trimethoprim/sulfamethoxazole or doxycycline for 1 year
Dosage Forms
Infusion, as potassium [premixed iso-osmotic dextrose solution, frozen]: 1 million units (50 mL), 2 million units (50 mL), 3 million units (50 mL)
Injection, powder for reconstitution: 5 million units, 20 million units
Pfizerpen®: 5 million units, 20 million units

penicillin G potassium *see* penicillin G (parenteral/aqueous) *on previous page*

penicillin G procaine (pen i SIL in jee PROE kane)
Sound-Alike/Look-Alike Issues
penicillin G procaine may be confused with penicillin V potassium
Wycillin® may be confused with Bicillin®
Synonyms APPG; aqueous procaine penicillin G; procaine benzylpenicillin; procaine penicillin G
U.S./Canadian Brand Names Pfizerpen-AS® [Can]; Wycillin® [Can]
Therapeutic Category Penicillin
Use Moderately severe infections due to *Treponema pallidum* and other penicillin G-sensitive microorganisms that are susceptible to low, but prolonged serum penicillin concentrations; anthrax due to *Bacillus anthracis* (postexposure) to reduce the incidence or progression of disease following exposure to aerolized *Bacillus anthracis*
Usual Dosage
Usual dosage range:
Infants and Children: I.M.: 25,000-50,000 units/kg/day in divided doses 1-2 times/day; (maximum: 4.8 million units/day)
Adults: I.M.: 0.6-4.8 million units/day in divided doses every 12-24 hours
(Continued)

penicillin G procaine *(Continued)*

Indication-specific dosing:

Children: I.M.:

Anthrax, inhalational (postexposure prophylaxis): 25,000 units/kg every 12 hours (maximum: 1,200,000 units every 12 hours); see "Note" in Adults dosing

Syphilis (congenital): 50,000 units/kg/day for 10 days; if more than 1 day of therapy is missed, the entire course should be restarted

Adults: I.M.:

Anthrax:

Inhalational (postexposure prophylaxis): 1,200,000 units every 12 hours

Note: Overall treatment duration should be 60 days. Available safety data suggest continued administration of penicillin G procaine for longer than 2 weeks may incur additional risk for adverse reactions. Clinicians may consider switching to effective alternative treatment for completion of therapy beyond 2 weeks.

Cutaneous (treatment): 600,000-1,200,000 units/day; alternative therapy is recommended in severe cutaneous or other forms of anthrax infection

Endocarditis caused by susceptible viridans *Streptococcus* (when used in conjunction with an aminoglycoside): 1.2 million units every 6 hours for 2-4 weeks

Gonorrhea (uncomplicated): 4.8 million units as a single dose divided in 2 sites given 30 minutes after probenecid 1 g orally

Neurosyphilis: 2.4 million units/day with 500 mg probenecid by mouth 4 times/day for 10-14 days; **Note: Penicillin G aqueous I.V. is the preferred agent**

Whipple disease: 1.2 million units/day (with streptomycin) for 10-14 days, followed by oral trimethoprim/sulfamethoxazole or doxycycline for 1 year

Dosage Forms

Injection, suspension: 600,000 units/mL (1 mL, 2 mL)

penicillin G procaine and benzathine combined *see* penicillin G benzathine and penicillin G procaine *on page 662*

penicillin G sodium *see* penicillin G (parenteral/aqueous) *on page 662*

penicillin V potassium (pen i SIL in vee poe TASS ee um)

Sound-Alike/Look-Alike Issues

penicillin V procaine may be confused with penicillin G potassium

Synonyms pen VK; phenoxymethyl penicillin

U.S./Canadian Brand Names Apo-Pen VK® [Can]; Novo-Pen-VK [Can]; Nu-Pen-VK [Can]

Therapeutic Category Penicillin

Use Treatment of infections caused by susceptible organisms involving the respiratory tract, otitis media, sinusitis, skin, and urinary tract; prophylaxis in rheumatic fever

Usual Dosage

Usual dosage range:

Children <12 years: Oral: 25-50 mg/kg/day in divided doses every 6-8 hours (maximum dose: 3 g/day)

Children ≥12 years and Adults: Oral: 125-500 mg every 6-8 hours

Indication-specific dosing:

Children: Oral:

Pharyngitis (streptococcal): 250 mg 2-3 times/day for 10 days

Prophylaxis of pneumococcal infections:

Children <5 years: 125 mg twice daily

Children ≥5 years: 250 mg twice daily

Prophylaxis of recurrent rheumatic fever:

Children <5 years: 125 mg twice daily

Children ≥5 years: 250 mg twice daily

Adults: Oral:

Acintomycosis:

Mild: 2-4 g/day in 4 divided doses for 8 weeks

Surgical: 2-4 g/day in 4 divided doses for 6-12 months (after I.V. penicillin G therapy of 4-6 weeks)

Erysipelas: 500 mg 4 times/day

Periodontal infections: 250-500 mg every 6 hours for 5-7 days

Note: Efficacy of antimicrobial therapy in periapical abscess is questionable; the American Academy of Periodontology recommends use of antibiotic therapy only when systemic symptoms (eg, fever, lymphadenopathy) are present or in immunocompromised patients.

Pharyngitis (streptococcal): 500 mg 3-4 times/day for 10 days

Prophylaxis of pneumococcal or recurrent rheumatic fever infections: 250 mg twice daily

Dosage Forms 250 mg = 400,000 units

Powder for oral solution: 125 mg/5 mL; 250 mg/5 mL

Tablet: 250 mg, 500 mg

penicilloyl-polylysine *see* benzylpenicilloyl-polylysine *on page 106*

Penlac® **[US/Can]** *see* ciclopirox *on page 188*

Pennsaid® **[Can]** *see* diclofenac *on page 253*

Pentacarinat® **Injection** *(Discontinued)* *see* pentamidine *on this page*

pentahydrate *see* sodium thiosulfate *on page 798*

Pentam-300® **[US]** *see* pentamidine *on this page*

pentamidine (pen TAM i deen)
  Synonyms pentamidine isethionate
  U.S./Canadian Brand Names NebuPent® [US]; Pentam-300® [US]
  Therapeutic Category Antiprotozoal
  Use Treatment and prevention of pneumonia caused by *Pneumocystis carinii* (PCP)
  Usual Dosage
    Children:
      Treatment of PCP pneumonia: I.M., I.V. (I.V. preferred): 4 mg/kg/day once daily for 10-14 days
      Prevention of PCP pneumonia:
        I.M., I.V.: 4 mg/kg monthly or every 2 weeks
        Inhalation (aerosolized pentamidine in children ≥5 years): 300 mg/dose given every 3-4 weeks via Respir-gard® II inhaler (8 mg/kg dose has also been used in children <5 years)
    Adults:
      Treatment: I.M., I.V. (I.V. preferred): 4 mg/kg/day once daily for 14-21 days
      Prevention: Inhalation: 300 mg every 4 weeks via Respirgard® II nebulizer
  Dosage Forms
    Injection, powder for reconstitution: [preservative free]:
    Pentam-300®: 300 mg
    Powder for nebulization: [preservative free]:
    NebuPent®: 300 mg

pentamidine isethionate *see* pentamidine *on this page*

Pentamycetin® **[Can]** *see* chloramphenicol *on page 173*

Pentasa® **[US/Can]** *see* mesalamine *on page 546*

pentasodium colistin methanesulfonate *see* colistimethate *on page 212*

Pentaspan® **[US/Can]** *see* pentastarch *on this page*

pentastarch (PEN ta starch)
  U.S./Canadian Brand Names Pentaspan® [US/Can]
  Therapeutic Category Blood Modifiers
  Use Orphan drug: Adjunct in leukapheresis to improve harvesting and increase yield of leukocytes by centrifugal means
  Usual Dosage 250-700 mL to which citrate anticoagulant has been added is administered by adding to the input line of the centrifugation apparatus at a ratio of 1:8-1:13 to venous whole blood
  Dosage Forms
    Infusion [premixed in NS]:
    Pentaspan®: 10% (500 mL)

Penta-Triamterene HCTZ [Can] *see* hydrochlorothiazide and triamterene *on page 427*

pentavalent human-bovine reassortant rotavirus vaccine *see* rotavirus vaccine *on page 769*

pentazocine (pen TAZ oh seen)
  Synonyms naloxone hydrochloride and pentazocine hydrochloride; pentazocine hydrochloride; pentazocine hydrochloride and naloxone hydrochloride; pentazocine lactate
  U.S./Canadian Brand Names Talwin® NX [US]; Talwin® [US/Can]
  Therapeutic Category Analgesic, Narcotic
  Controlled Substance C-IV
  Use Relief of moderate to severe pain; has also been used as a sedative prior to surgery and as a supplement to surgical anesthesia
  Usual Dosage
    Preoperative/preanesthetic: Children 1-16 years: I.M.: 0.5 mg/kg
    (Continued)

pentazocine *(Continued)*

Analgesia:
Children: I.M.:
5-8 years: 15 mg
8-14 years: 30 mg
Children >12 years and Adults: Oral: 50 mg every 3-4 hours; may increase to 100 mg/dose if needed, but should not exceed 600 mg/day
Adults:
I.M., SubQ: 30-60 mg every 3-4 hours; do not exceed 60 mg/dose (maximum: 360 mg/day)
I.V.: 30 mg every 3-4 hours; do not exceed 30 mg/dose (maximum: 360 mg/day)

Dosage Forms
Injection, solution:
Talwin®: 30 mg/mL (1 mL, 10 mL)
Tablet: Pentazocine 50 mg and naloxone 0.5 mg
Talwin® NX: Pentazocine 50 mg and naloxone 0.5 mg

pentazocine and acetaminophen (pen TAZ oh seen & a seet a MIN oh fen)

Sound-Alike/Look-Alike Issues
Talacen® may be confused with Tegison®, Timoptic®, Tinactin®
Synonyms acetaminophen and pentazocine; pentazocine hydrochloride and acetaminophen
U.S./Canadian Brand Names Talacen® [US]
Therapeutic Category Analgesic Combination (Opioid)
Controlled Substance C-IV
Use Relief of mild to moderate pain
Usual Dosage Oral: Adults: Analgesic: 1 caplet every 4 hours, up to a maximum of 6 caplets
Dosage Forms
Caplet: Pentazocine 25 mg and acetaminophen 650 mg
Talacen®: Pentazocine 25 mg and acetaminophen 650 mg
Tablet: Pentazocine 25 mg and acetaminophen 650 mg

pentazocine hydrochloride *see* pentazocine *on previous page*

pentazocine hydrochloride and acetaminophen *see* pentazocine and acetaminophen *on this page*

pentazocine hydrochloride and naloxone hydrochloride *see* pentazocine *on previous page*

pentazocine lactate *see* pentazocine *on previous page*

pentetate calcium trisodium *see* diethylene triamine penta-acetic acid *on page 256*

pentetate zinc trisodium *see* diethylene triamine penta-acetic acid *on page 256*

Penthrane® *(Discontinued)*

pentobarbital (pen toe BAR bi tal)

Sound-Alike/Look-Alike Issues
pentobarbital may be confused with phenobarbital
Nembutal® may be confused with Myambutol®
Synonyms pentobarbital sodium
U.S./Canadian Brand Names Nembutal® Sodium [Can]; Nembutal® [US]
Therapeutic Category Barbiturate
Controlled Substance C-II
Use Sedative/hypnotic; preanesthetic; high-dose barbiturate coma for treatment of increased intracranial pressure or status epilepticus unresponsive to other therapy
Usual Dosage
Children:
Hypnotic: I.M.: 2-6 mg/kg; maximum: 100 mg/dose
Preoperative/preprocedure sedation: ≥6 months:
Note: Limited information is available for infants <6 months of age.
I.M.: 2-6 mg/kg; maximum: 100 mg/dose
I.V.: 1-3 mg/kg to a maximum of 100 mg until asleep
Conscious sedation prior to a procedure: Children 5-12 years: I.V.: 2 mg/kg 5-10 minutes before procedures, may repeat one time
Adolescents: Conscious sedation: I.V.: 100 mg prior to a procedure
Children and Adults: Barbiturate coma in head injury patients: I.V.: Loading dose: 5-10 mg/kg given slowly over 1-2 hours; monitor blood pressure and respiratory rate; Maintenance infusion: Initial: 1 mg/kg/hour; may increase to 2-3 mg/kg/hour; maintain burst suppression on EEG

Status epilepticus: I.V.: **Note**: Intubation required; monitor hemodynamics
　Children: Loading dose: 5-15 mg/kg given slowly over 1-2 hours; maintenance infusion: 0.5-5 mg/kg/hour
　Adults: Loading dose: 2-15 mg/kg given slowly over 1-2 hours; maintenance infusion: 0.5-3 mg/kg/hour
　Adults:
　Hypnotic:
　I.M.: 150-200 mg
　I.V.: Initial: 100 mg, may repeat every 1-3 minutes up to 200-500 mg total dose
　Preoperative sedation: I.M.: 150-200 mg
Dosage Forms
Injection, solution:
Nembutal®: 50 mg/mL (20 mL, 50 mL)

pentobarbital sodium *see* pentobarbital *on previous page*

pentosan polysulfate sodium (PEN toe san pol i SUL fate SOW dee um)
Sound-Alike/Look-Alike Issues
pentosan may be confused with pentostatin
Elmiron® may be confused with Imuran®
Synonyms PPS
U.S./Canadian Brand Names Elmiron® [US/Can]
Therapeutic Category Analgesic, Urinary
Use Orphan drug: Relief of bladder pain or discomfort due to interstitial cystitis
Usual Dosage Adults: Oral: 100 mg 3 times/day taken with water 1 hour before or 2 hours after meals
Patients should be evaluated at 3 months and may be continued an additional 3 months if there has been no improvement and if there are no therapy-limiting side effects. **The risks and benefits of continued use beyond 6 months in patients who have not responded is not yet known.**
Dosage Forms
Capsule:
Elmiron®: 100 mg

pentostatin (pen toe STAT in)
Sound-Alike/Look-Alike Issues
pentostatin may be confused with pentosan
Synonyms CL-825; co-vidarabine; dCF; deoxycoformycin; NSC-218321; 2'-deoxycoformycin
U.S./Canadian Brand Names Nipent® [US/Can]
Therapeutic Category Antineoplastic Agent
Use Treatment of hairy cell leukemia; non-Hodgkin lymphoma, cutaneous T-cell lymphoma
Usual Dosage Refractory hairy cell leukemia: Adults (refer to individual protocols):
4 mg/m^2 every other week **or**
4 mg/m^2 weekly for 3 weeks, then every 2 weeks **or**
5 mg/m^2 daily for 3 days every 3 weeks
Dosage Forms
Injection, powder for reconstitution [preservative free]:
Nipent®: 10 mg

Pentothal® [US/Can] *see* thiopental *on page 837*

Pentothal® Sodium Rectal Suspension *(Discontinued)* *see* thiopental *on page 837*

pentoxifylline (pen toks IF i lin)
Sound-Alike/Look-Alike Issues
pentoxifylline may be confused with tamoxifen
Trental® may be confused with Bentyl®, Tegretol®, Trandate®
Synonyms oxpentifylline
U.S./Canadian Brand Names Albert® Pentoxifylline [Can]; Apo-Pentoxifylline SR® [Can]; Nu-Pentoxifylline SR [Can]; Pentoxil® [US]; ratio-Pentoxifylline [Can]; Trental® [US/Can]
Therapeutic Category Blood Viscosity Reducer Agent
Use Treatment of intermittent claudication on the basis of chronic occlusive arterial disease of the limbs; may improve function and symptoms, but not intended to replace more definitive therapy
Usual Dosage Oral: Adults: 400 mg 3 times/day with meals; maximal therapeutic benefit may take 2-4 weeks to develop; recommended to maintain therapy for at least 8 weeks. May reduce to 400 mg twice daily if GI or CNS side effects occur.
Dosage Forms
Tablet, controlled release:
Trental®: 400 mg
(Continued)

pentoxifylline *(Continued)*

Tablet, extended release: 400 mg
Pentoxil®: 400 mg

Pentoxil® [US] *see* pentoxifylline *on previous page*

Pen.Vee® K *(Discontinued)* *see* penicillin V potassium *on page 664*

pen VK *see* penicillin V potassium *on page 664*

Pepcid® [US/Can] *see* famotidine *on page 341*

Pepcid® AC [US-OTC/Can] *see* famotidine *on page 341*

Pepcid® Complete [US-OTC/Can] *see* famotidine, calcium carbonate, and magnesium hydroxide *on page 342*

Pepcid® I.V. [Can] *see* famotidine *on page 341*

Pepcid RPD® *(Discontinued)* *see* famotidine *on page 341*

Peptic Relief [US-OTC] *see* bismuth *on page 113*

Pepto-Bismol® [US-OTC] *see* bismuth *on page 113*

Pepto-Bismol® Maximum Strength [US-OTC] *see* bismuth *on page 113*

Pepto® Diarrhea Control *(Discontinued)* *see* loperamide *on page 515*

Pepto Relief [US-OTC] *see* bismuth *on page 113*

Perchloracap® *(Discontinued)*

Percocet® [US/Can] *see* oxycodone and acetaminophen *on page 641*

Percocet®-Demi [Can] *see* oxycodone and acetaminophen *on page 641*

Percodan® [US/Can] *see* oxycodone and aspirin *on page 642*

Percodan®-Demi *(Discontinued)* *see* oxycodone and aspirin *on page 642*

Percogesic® [US-OTC] *see* acetaminophen and phenyltoloxamine *on page 8*

Percogesic® Extra Strength [US-OTC] *see* acetaminophen and diphenhydramine *on page 7*

Percolone® *(Discontinued)* *see* oxycodone *on page 640*

Perdiem® Overnight Relief [US-OTC] *see* senna *on page 781*

Perfectoderm® Gel *(Discontinued)* *see* benzoyl peroxide *on page 103*

perflutren lipid microspheres (per FLOO tren LIP id MIKE roe sfeers)

U.S./Canadian Brand Names Definity® [US/Can]

Therapeutic Category Diagnostic Agent

Use Opacification of left ventricular chamber and improvement of delineation of the left ventricular endocardial border in patients with suboptimal echocardiograms

Usual Dosage Adults: Dose should be given following baseline noncontrast echocardiography. Imaging should begin immediately following dose and compared to noncontrast image. Mechanical index for the ultrasound device should be set at ≤0.8.

I.V. bolus: 10 µL/kg of activated product, followed by 10 mL saline flush. May repeat in 30 minutes if needed (maximum dose: 2 bolus infusions).

I.V. infusion: Initial: 4 mL/minute of prepared infusion; titrate to achieve optimal image; maximum rate: 10 mL/minute (maximum dose: 1 intravenous infusion).

Dosage Forms

Injection, solution [preservative free]:
Definity®: OFP 6.52 mg/mL and lipid blend 0.75 mg/mL (2 mL)

pergolide *(Canada only)* (PER go lide)

Sound-Alike/Look-Alike Issues

Permax® may be confused with Bumex®, Pentrax®, Pernox®

Synonyms pergolide mesylate

U.S./Canadian Brand Names Permax® [Can]

Therapeutic Category Anti-Parkinson Agent (Dopamine Agonist); Ergot Alkaloid and Derivative

Use Adjunctive treatment to levodopa/carbidopa in the management of Parkinson disease

Usual Dosage When adding pergolide to levodopa/carbidopa, the dose of the latter can usually and should be decreased. Patients no longer responsive to bromocriptine may benefit by being switched to pergolide.

Oral: Adults: Parkinson disease: Start with 0.05 mg/day for 2 days, then increase dosage by 0.1 or 0.15 mg/day every 3 days over next 12 days, increase dose by 0.25 mg/day every 3 days until optimal therapeutic dose is achieved, up to 5 mg/day maximum; usual dosage range: 2-3 mg/day in 3 divided doses

pergolide mesylate *see* pergolide *(Canada only)* *on previous page*

Pergonal® *(Discontinued)* *see* menotropins *on page 541*

Periactin® *(Discontinued)* *see* cyproheptadine *on page 224*

Peri-Colace® **[US-OTC]** *see* docusate and senna *on page 274*

pericyazine *(Canada only)* (per ee CYE ah zeen)

U.S./Canadian Brand Names Neuleptil® [Can]

Therapeutic Category Phenothiazine Derivative

Use As adjunctive medication in some psychotic patients, for the control of residual prevailing hostility, impulsiveness and aggressiveness

Usual Dosage Oral:

Children >5 years: 2.5-10 mg in the morning and 5-30 mg in the evening. In general, lower dosage should be used on initiation and gradually increased based on effect and tolerance.

Adults: 5-20 mg in the morning followed by 10-40 mg in the evening. In dividing doses, it is suggested that the larger dose should be administered in the evening. In general, lower dosage should be used on initiation and gradually increased based on effect and tolerance.

Dosage Forms [CAN] = Canadian brand name

Capsule:

Neuleptil® [CAN]: 5 mg, 10 mg, 20 mg [not available in the U.S.]

Solution, oral drops:

Neuleptil® [CAN]: 10 mg/mL [not available in the U.S.]

Peridex® **[US]** *see* chlorhexidine gluconate *on page 174*

Peridol [Can] *see* haloperidol *on page 413*

perindopril and indapamide *see* perindopril erbumine and indapamide *(Canada only)* *on this page*

perindopril erbumine (per IN doe pril er BYOO meen)

U.S./Canadian Brand Names Aceon® [US]; Apo-Perindopril® [Can]; Coversyl® [Can]

Therapeutic Category Miscellaneous Product

Use Treatment of essential hypertension; reduction of cardiovascular mortality or nonfatal myocardial infarction in patients with stable coronary artery disease

Usual Dosage Oral: Adults:

Essential hypertension: Initial: 4 mg/day but may be titrated to response; usual range: 4-8 mg/day (may be given in 2 divided doses); increase at 1- to 2-week intervals (maximum: 16 mg/day)

Concomitant therapy with diuretics: To reduce the risk of hypotension, discontinue diuretic, if possible, 2-3 days prior to initiating perindopril. If unable to stop diuretic, initiate perindopril at 2-4 mg/day and monitor blood pressure closely for the first 2 weeks of therapy, and after any dose adjustment of perindopril or diuretic.

Stable coronary artery disease: Initial: 4 mg once daily for 2 weeks; increase as tolerated to 8 mg once daily.

Dosage Forms

Tablet:

Aceon®: 2 mg, 4 mg, 8 mg

perindopril erbumine and indapamide *(Canada only)*

(per IN doe pril er BYOO meen & in DAP a mide)

Synonyms indapamide and perindopril erbumine; perindopril and indapamide

U.S./Canadian Brand Names Coversyl® Plus [Can]

Therapeutic Category Angiotensin-Converting Enzyme (ACE) Inhibitor; Antihypertensive Agent, Combination; Diuretic, Thiazide-Related

Use Maintenance treatment of mild-moderate essential hypertension

Usual Dosage Note: Not for initial therapy. Titration of individual components to an appropriate clinical response is required prior to converting to an equivalent dose of the combination product.

Oral: Adults: Hypertension: Usual maintenance dose: Perindopril 4 mg/indapamide 1.25 mg once daily

Dosage Forms [CAN] = Canadian brand name

Tablet:

Coversyl® Plus [CAN]: Perindopril erbumine 4 mg and indapamide 1.25 mg [not available in the U.S.]

PerioChip® **[US]** *see* chlorhexidine gluconate *on page 174*

PerioGard® **[US]** *see* chlorhexidine gluconate *on page 174*

PerioMed™ **[US]** *see* fluoride *on page 361*

Periostat® **[US/Can]** *see* doxycycline *on page 281*

Perlane® **[US]** *see* hyaluronate and derivatives *on page 423*

Permax® **[Can]** *see* pergolide *(Canada only) on page 668*

Permax® *(Discontinued)* *see* pergolide *(Canada only) on page 668*

permethrin (per METH rin)

U.S./Canadian Brand Names A200® Lice [US-OTC]; Acticin® [US]; Elimite® [US]; Kwellada-P™ [Can]; Nix® [US-OTC/Can]; Rid® Spray [US-OTC]

Therapeutic Category Scabicides/Pediculicides

Use Single-application treatment of infestation with *Pediculus humanus capitis* (head louse) and its nits or *Sarcoptes scabiei* (scabies); indicated for prophylactic use during epidemics of lice

Usual Dosage Topical:

Head lice: Children >2 months and Adults: After hair has been washed with shampoo, rinsed with water, and towel dried, apply a sufficient volume of topical liquid (lotion or cream rinse) to saturate the hair and scalp. Leave on hair for 10 minutes before rinsing off with water; remove remaining nits; may repeat in 1 week if lice or nits still present.

Scabies: Apply cream from head to toe; leave on for 8-14 hours before washing off with water; for infants, also apply on the hairline, neck, scalp, temple, and forehead; may reapply in 1 week if live mites appear

Permethrin 5% cream was shown to be safe and effective when applied to an infant <1 month of age with neonatal scabies; time of application was limited to 6 hours before rinsing with soap and water

Dosage Forms

Cream, topical: 5% (60 g)

Acticin®, Elimite®: 5% (60 g)

Lotion, topical: 1% (59 mL)

Liquid, topical [creme rinse formulation]: 1% (60 mL)

Nix® [OTC]: 1% (60 mL)

Solution, spray [for bedding and furniture]:

A200® Lice [OTC]: 0.5% (180 mL)

Nix® [OTC]: 0.25% (148 mL)

Rid® [OTC]: 0.5% (150 mL)

Permitil® **Oral** *(Discontinued)* *see* fluphenazine *on page 365*

Peroxin A5® *(Discontinued)* *see* benzoyl peroxide *on page 103*

Peroxin A10® *(Discontinued)* *see* benzoyl peroxide *on page 103*

perphenazine (per FEN a zeen)

Sound-Alike/Look-Alike Issues

Trilafon® may be confused with Tri-Levlen®

U.S./Canadian Brand Names Apo-Perphenazine® [Can]

Therapeutic Category Phenothiazine Derivative

Use Treatment of schizophrenia; nausea and vomiting

Usual Dosage Oral: Adults:

Schizophrenia/psychoses: 4-16 mg 2-4 times/day not to exceed 64 mg/day

Nausea/vomiting: 8-16 mg/day in divided doses up to 24 mg/day

Dosage Forms

Tablet: 2 mg, 4 mg, 8 mg, 16 mg

perphenazine and amitriptyline hydrochloride *see* amitriptyline and perphenazine *on page 45*

Persa-Gel® *(Discontinued)* *see* benzoyl peroxide *on page 103*

Persantine® **[US/Can]** *see* dipyridamole *on page 270*

Pertussin® **CS** *(Discontinued)* *see* dextromethorphan *on page 247*

Pertussin® **ES** *(Discontinued)* *see* dextromethorphan *on page 247*

pethidine hydrochloride *see* meperidine *on page 542*

Pexeva® **[US]** *see* paroxetine *on page 654*

Pexicam® **[Can]** *see* piroxicam *on page 687*

PFA *see* foscarnet *on page 375*

Pfizerpen® **[US/Can]** *see* penicillin G (parenteral/aqueous) *on page 662*

Pfizerpen-AS® **[Can]** *see* penicillin G procaine *on page 663*

PGE$_1$ *see* alprostadil *on page 33*

PGE$_2$ *see* dinoprostone *on page 264*

PGI$_2$ *see* epoprostenol *on page 304*

PGX *see* epoprostenol *on page 304*

Phanasin® **[US-OTC]** *see* guaifenesin *on page 401*

Phanasin® **Diabetic Choice [US-OTC]** *see* guaifenesin *on page 401*

Phanatuss® **DM [US-OTC]** *see* guaifenesin and dextromethorphan *on page 402*

Phanatuss® **HC [US]** *see* hydrocodone and guaifenesin *on page 429*

Pharmaflur® **[US]** *see* fluoride *on page 361*

Pharmaflur® **1.1 [US]** *see* fluoride *on page 361*

Pharmorubicin® **[Can]** *see* epirubicin *on page 302*

Phazyme® **[Can]** *see* simethicone *on page 786*

Phazyme® *(Discontinued)* *see* simethicone *on page 786*

Phazyme® **Quick Dissolve [US-OTC]** *see* simethicone *on page 786*

Phazyme® **Ultra Strength [US-OTC]** *see* simethicone *on page 786*

Phenabid® **[US]** *see* chlorpheniramine and phenylephrine *on page 177*

Phenabid DM® **[US]** *see* chlorpheniramine, phenylephrine, and dextromethorphan *on page 180*

Phenadex® **Senior** *(Discontinued)* *see* guaifenesin and dextromethorphan *on page 402*

Phenadoz™ **[US]** *see* promethazine *on page 719*

Phenagesic [US-OTC] *see* acetaminophen and phenyltoloxamine *on page 8*

Phenameth® **DM** *(Discontinued)* *see* promethazine and dextromethorphan *on page 719*

Phenaphen® *(Discontinued)* *see* acetaminophen *on page 5*

Phenaseptic [US-OTC] *see* phenol *on page 673*

PhenaVent™ **[US]** *see* guaifenesin and phenylephrine *on page 404*

PhenaVent™ **D [US]** *see* guaifenesin and phenylephrine *on page 404*

PhenaVent™ **LA [US]** *see* guaifenesin and phenylephrine *on page 404*

PhenaVent™ **Ped [US]** *see* guaifenesin and phenylephrine *on page 404*

Phenazine® **Injection** *(Discontinued)* *see* promethazine *on page 719*

Phenazo™ **[Can]** *see* phenazopyridine *on this page*

phenazopyridine (fen az oh PEER i deen)

Sound-Alike/Look-Alike Issues
Pyridium® may be confused with Dyrenium®, Perdiem®, pyridoxine, pyrithione
Synonyms phenazopyridine hydrochloride; phenylazo diamino pyridine hydrochloride
U.S./Canadian Brand Names AZO-Gesic® [US-OTC]; AZO-Standard® Maximum Strength [US-OTC]; AZO-Standard® [US-OTC]; Baridium® [US-OTC]; Phenazo™ [Can]; Prodium® [US-OTC]; Pyridium® [US]; ReAzo [US-OTC]; Uristat® [US-OTC]; UTI Relief® [US-OTC]
Therapeutic Category Analgesic, Urinary
Use Symptomatic relief of urinary burning, itching, frequency and urgency in association with urinary tract infection or following urologic procedures
Usual Dosage Oral:
Children: 12 mg/kg/day in 3 divided doses administered after meals for 2 days
Adults: 100-200 mg 3 times/day after meals for 2 days when used concomitantly with an antibacterial agent
Dosage Forms
Tablet: 100 mg, 200 mg
AZO-Gesic® [OTC], AZO-Standard® [OTC], Prodium® [OTC], ReAzo [OTC], Uristat® [OTC]: 95 mg
AZO Standard® Maximum Strength [OTC]: 97.5 mg
Baridium® [OTC], UTI Relief® [OTC]: 97.2 mg
Pyridium®: 100 mg, 200 mg

phenazopyridine hydrochloride *see* phenazopyridine *on this page*

Phencarb GG [US] *see* carbetapentane, guaifenesin, and phenylephrine *on page 149*

phendimetrazine (fen dye ME tra zeen)

Sound-Alike/Look-Alike Issues
Bontril PDM® may be confused with Bentyl®
Synonyms phendimetrazine tartrate
U.S./Canadian Brand Names Bontril PDM® [US]; Bontril® Slow-Release [US]; Bontril® [Can]; Plegine® [Can]; Statobex® [Can]
(Continued)

phendimetrazine *(Continued)*

Therapeutic Category Anorexiant
Controlled Substance C-III
Use Short-term (few weeks) adjunct in exogenous obesity
Usual Dosage Oral: Adults:
  Capsule: 105 mg once daily in the morning before breakfast
  Tablet: 17.5-35 mg 2 or 3 times daily, 1 hour before meals (maximum: 70 mg 3 times/day)
Dosage Forms
  Capsule, slow release: 105 mg
   Bontril® Slow Release: 105 mg
  Tablet: 35 mg
   Bontril PDM®: 35 mg

phendimetrazine tartrate *see* phendimetrazine *on previous page*

Phendry® Oral *(Discontinued)* *see* diphenhydramine *on page 265*

phenelzine (FEN el zeen)

Sound-Alike/Look-Alike Issues
  phenelzine may be confused with phenytoin
  Nardil® may be confused with Norinyl®
Synonyms phenelzine sulfate
U.S./Canadian Brand Names Nardil® [US/Can]
Therapeutic Category Antidepressant, Monoamine Oxidase Inhibitor
Use Symptomatic treatment of atypical, nonendogenous, or neurotic depression
Usual Dosage Oral: Adults: Depression: 15 mg 3 times/day; may increase to 60-90 mg/day during early phase of treatment, then reduce dose for maintenance therapy slowly after maximum benefit is obtained; takes 2-4 weeks for a significant response to occur
Dosage Forms
  Tablet:
   Nardil®: 15 mg

phenelzine sulfate *see* phenelzine *on this page*

Phenerbel-S® *(Discontinued)*

Phenergan® [US/Can] *see* promethazine *on page 719*

Phenergan® VC With Codeine *(Discontinued)* *see* promethazine, phenylephrine, and codeine *on page 720*

Phenergan® With Dextromethorphan *(Discontinued)* *see* promethazine and dextromethorphan *on page 719*

pheniramine and naphazoline *see* naphazoline and pheniramine *on page 591*

phenobarbital (fee noe BAR bi tal)

Sound-Alike/Look-Alike Issues
  phenobarbital may be confused with pentobarbital
  Luminal® may be confused with Tuinal®
Synonyms phenobarbital sodium; phenobarbitone; phenylethylmalonylurea
U.S./Canadian Brand Names Luminal® Sodium [US]; PMS-Phenobarbital [Can]
Therapeutic Category Anticonvulsant; Barbiturate
Controlled Substance C-IV
Use Management of generalized tonic-clonic (grand mal) and partial seizures; sedative
Usual Dosage
  Children:
   Sedation: Oral: 2 mg/kg 3 times/day
   Hypnotic: I.M., I.V., SubQ: 3-5 mg/kg at bedtime
   Preoperative sedation: Oral, I.M., I.V.: 1-3 mg/kg 1-1.5 hours before procedure
  Adults:
   Sedation: Oral, I.M.: 30-120 mg/day in 2-3 divided doses
   Hypnotic: Oral, I.M., I.V., SubQ: 100-320 mg at bedtime
   Preoperative sedation: I.M.: 100-200 mg 1-1.5 hours before procedure

  Anticonvulsant: Status epilepticus: **Loading dose:** I.V.:
   Infants and Children: 10-20 mg/kg in a single or divided dose; in select patients may administer additional 5 mg/kg/dose every 15-30 minutes until seizure is controlled or a total dose of 40 mg/kg is reached

Adults: 300-800 mg initially followed by 120-240 mg/dose at 20-minute intervals until seizures are controlled or a total dose of 1-2 g

Anticonvulsant maintenance dose: Oral, I.V.:

Infants: 5-8 mg/kg/day in 1-2 divided doses

Children:

1-5 years: 6-8 mg/kg/day in 1-2 divided doses

5-12 years: 4-6 mg/kg/day in 1-2 divided doses

Children >12 years and Adults: 1-3 mg/kg/day in divided doses or 50-100 mg 2-3 times/day

Dosage Forms

Elixir: 20 mg/5 mL

Injection, solution: 65 mg/mL (1 mL); 130 mg/mL (1 mL)

Luminal® Sodium: 60 mg/mL (1 mL); 130 mg/mL (1 mL)

Tablet: 15 mg, 30 mg, 60 mg, 100 mg

phenobarbital, belladonna, and ergotamine tartrate *see* belladonna, phenobarbital, and ergotamine *on page 98*

phenobarbital, hyoscyamine, atropine, and scopolamine *see* hyoscyamine, atropine, scopolamine, and phenobarbital *on page 442*

phenobarbital sodium *see* phenobarbital *on previous page*

phenobarbitone *see* phenobarbital *on previous page*

phenol (FEE nol)

Sound-Alike/Look-Alike Issues

Cēpastat® may be confused with Capastat®

Synonyms carbolic acid

U.S./Canadian Brand Names Castellani Paint Modified [US-OTC]; Cheracol® [US-OTC]; Chloraseptic® Gargle [US-OTC]; Chloraseptic® Mouth Pain [US-OTC]; Chloraseptic® Pocket Pump [US-OTC]; Chloraseptic® Spray for Kids [US-OTC]; Chloraseptic® Spray [US-OTC]; Cēpastat® Extra Strength [US-OTC]; Cēpastat® [US-OTC]; P & S™ Liquid Phenol [Can]; Pain-A-Lay® [US-OTC]; Phenaseptic [US-OTC]; Phenol EZ® [US-OTC]; Ulcerease® [US-OTC]; Vicks® Formula 44® Sore Throat [US-OTC]

Therapeutic Category Pharmaceutical Aid

Use Relief of sore throat pain, mouth, gum, and throat irritations; antiseptic; topical anesthetic

Usual Dosage

Oral: Sore throat:

Children 2-12 years:

Chloraseptic®: Three sprays onto throat or affected area; may repeat every 2 hours

Chloraseptic® for Kids: Five sprays onto throat or affected area; may repeat every 2 hours

Children >3 year (Ulcerease®): Refer to adult dosing.

Children 6-12 years:

Cēpastat®: Up to 1 lozenge every 2 hours as needed (maximum: 18 lozenges/24 hours)

Cēpastat® Extra Strength: Up to 1 lozenge every 2 hours as needed (maximum: 10 lozenges/24 hours)

Pain-A-Lay® Gargle: Using gauze pad, apply 10 mL to affected area, or gargle or swish for 15 seconds, then expectorate

Children ≥12 years and Adults:

Cēpastat® Extra Strength, Cēpastat®: Up to 2 lozenges every 2 hours as needed

Cheracol®, Pain-A-Lay® Spray: Spray directly in throat; rinse for 15 seconds then expectorate; may repeat every 2 hours

Chloraseptic®: Five sprays onto throat or affected area; may repeat every 2 hours

Chloraseptic® Gargle, Chloraseptic® Mouth Pain, Pain-A-Lay® Gargle, Ulcerease®: Gargle or swish for 15 seconds, then expectorate; may repeat every 2 hours

Topical: Antiseptic: Adults: Castellani Paint Modified: Apply small amount to affected area 1-3 times/day

Dosage Forms

Lozenge, oral:

Cēpastat® [OTC]: 14.5 mg (18s)

Cēpastat® Extra Strength [OTC]: 29 mg (18s)

Solution, oral [gargle]:

Chloraseptic® [OTC]: 1.4% (296 mL)

Pain-A-Lay® [OTC]: 1.4% (240 mL, 540 mL)

Ulcerease® [OTC]: 0.6% (180 mL)

Solution, oral: [spray]

Cheracol® [OTC], Chloraseptic® [OTC], Pain-A-Lay® [OTC], Phenaseptic [OTC], Vicks® Formula 44® Sore Throat [OTC]: 1.4% (180 mL)

Chloraseptic® for Kids [OTC]: 0.5% (177 mL)

Chloraseptic® Mouth Pain [OTC]: 1.4% (30 mL)

(Continued)

phenol *(Continued)*

Chloraseptic® Pocket Pump [OTC]: 1.4% (20 mL)
Solution, topical:
Castellani Paint Modified [OTC]: Phenol 1.5% (30 mL)
Castellani Paint Modified [OTC] [colorless]: Phenol 1.5% (30 mL)
Swabs, topical:
Phenol EZ® [OTC]: 89% (30s) [~0.2 mL]

phenol and camphor *see* camphor and phenol *on page 143*

Phenol EZ® [US-OTC] *see* phenol *on previous page*

Phenoxine® *(Discontinued)*

phenoxybenzamine (fen oks ee BEN za meen)

Synonyms phenoxybenzamine hydrochloride
U.S./Canadian Brand Names Dibenzyline® [US/Can]
Therapeutic Category Alpha-Adrenergic Blocking Agent
Use Symptomatic management of pheochromocytoma; treatment of hypertensive crisis caused by sympatho-mimetic amines
Usual Dosage Oral:
Children: Initial: 0.2 mg/kg (maximum: 10 mg) once daily, increase by 0.2 mg/kg increments; usual mainte-nance dose: 0.4-1.2 mg/kg/day every 6-8 hours, higher doses may be necessary
Adults: Initial: 10 mg twice daily, increase by 10 mg every other day until optimum dose is achieved; usual range: 20-40 mg 2-3 times/day
Dosage Forms
Capsule:
Dibenzyline®: 10 mg

phenoxybenzamine hydrochloride *see* phenoxybenzamine *on this page*

phenoxymethyl penicillin *see* penicillin V potassium *on page 664*

phentermine (FEN ter meen)

Sound-Alike/Look-Alike Issues
phentermine may be confused with phentolamine, phenytoin
Ionamin® may be confused with Imodium®
Synonyms phentermine hydrochloride
U.S./Canadian Brand Names Adipex-P® [US]; Ionamin® [US/Can]
Therapeutic Category Anorexiant
Controlled Substance C-IV
Use Short-term (few weeks) adjunct in exogenous obesity
Usual Dosage Oral: Children >16 years and Adults: Obesity:
Phentermine hydrochloride: 18.75-37.5 mg/day
Phentermine resin: 15-30 mg/day
Dosage Forms
Capsule: 30 mg
Adipex-P®: 37.5 mg
Capsule, resin complex:
Ionamin®: 15 mg
Tablet: 37.5 mg
Adipex-P®: 37.5 mg

phentermine hydrochloride *see* phentermine *on this page*

phentolamine (fen TOLE a meen)

Sound-Alike/Look-Alike Issues
phentolamine may be confused with phentermine, Ventolin®
Synonyms phentolamine mesylate
U.S./Canadian Brand Names Regitine® [Can]; Rogitine® [Can]
Therapeutic Category Alpha-Adrenergic Blocking Agent; Diagnostic Agent
Use Diagnosis of pheochromocytoma and treatment of hypertension associated with pheochromocytoma or other forms of hypertension caused by excess sympathomimetic amines; as treatment of dermal necrosis after extravasation of drugs with alpha-adrenergic effects (norepinephrine, dopamine, epinephrine)

Usual Dosage

Treatment of alpha-adrenergic drug extravasation: SubQ:

Children: 0.1-0.2 mg/kg diluted in 10 mL 0.9% sodium chloride infiltrated into area of extravasation within 12 hours

Adults: Infiltrate area with small amount of solution made by diluting 5-10 mg in 10 mL 0.9% sodium chloride within 12 hours of extravasation; do not exceed 0.1-0.2 mg/kg or 5 mg total

If dose is effective, normal skin color should return to the blanched area within 1 hour

Diagnosis of pheochromocytoma: I.M., I.V.:

Children: 0.05-0.1 mg/kg/dose, maximum single dose: 5 mg

Adults: 5 mg

Surgery for pheochromocytoma: Hypertension: I.M., I.V.:

Children: 0.05-0.1 mg/kg/dose given 1-2 hours before procedure; repeat as needed every 2-4 hours until hypertension is controlled; maximum single dose: 5 mg

Adults: 5 mg given 1-2 hours before procedure and repeated as needed every 2-4 hours

Hypertensive crisis: Adults: 5-20 mg

Dosage Forms

Injection, powder for reconstitution: 5 mg

phentolamine mesylate *see* phentolamine *on previous page*

phenylalanine mustard *see* melphalan *on page 539*

phenylazo diamino pyridine hydrochloride *see* phenazopyridine *on page 671*

Phenyldrine® *(Discontinued)*

phenylephrine (fen il EF rin)

Sound-Alike/Look-Alike Issues

Mydfrin® may be confused with Midrin®

Synonyms phenylephrine hydrochloride; phenylephrine tannate

U.S./Canadian Brand Names 4 Way® Fast Acting [US-OTC]; 4 Way® Menthol [US-OTC]; 4 Way® No Drip [US-OTC]; Ah-Chew D® [US]; AK-Dilate® [US]; Altafrin [US]; Anu-Med [US-OTC]; Dimetapp® Toddler's [US-OTC]; Dionephrine® [Can]; Formulation R™ [US-OTC]; LuSonal™ [US]; Medi-Phenyl [US-OTC]; Medicone® Suppositories [US-OTC]; Mydfrin® [US/Can]; Neo-Synephrine® Extra Strength [US-OTC]; Neo-Synephrine® Injection [US]; Neo-Synephrine® Mild [US-OTC]; Neo-Synephrine® Regular Strength [US-OTC]; Neo-Synephrine® [Can]; Neofrin™ [US]; Nāsop™ [US]; OcuNefrin™ [US-OTC]; Preparation H® [US-OTC]; Rectacaine [US-OTC]; Relief® [US-OTC]; Rhinall [US-OTC]; Sudafed PE™ [US-OTC]; Triaminic® Infant Thin Strips® Decongestant [US-OTC]; Triaminic® Thin Strips® Cold [US-OTC]; Tronolane® Suppository [US-OTC]; Tur-bi-kal® [US-OTC]; Vicks® Sinex® Nasal Spray [US-OTC]; Vicks® Sinex® UltraFine Mist [US-OTC]

Therapeutic Category Adrenergic Agonist Agent

Use Treatment of hypotension, vascular failure in shock; as a vasoconstrictor in regional analgesia; as a mydriatic in ophthalmic procedures and treatment of wide-angle glaucoma; supraventricular tachycardia

For OTC use as symptomatic relief of nasal and nasopharyngeal mucosal congestion, treatment of hemorrhoids, relief of redness of the eye due to irritation

Usual Dosage

Hemorrhoids: Children ≥12 years and Adults: Rectal:

Cream/ointment: Apply to clean dry area, up to 4 times/day; may be used externally or inserted rectally using applicator.

Suppository: Insert 1 suppository rectally, up to 4 times/day

Hypotension/shock:

Children:

I.V. bolus: 5-20 mcg/kg/dose every 10-15 minutes as needed

I.V. infusion: 0.1-0.5 mcg/kg/minute

Adults:

I.V. bolus: 0.1-0.5 mg/dose every 10-15 minutes as needed (initial dose should not exceed 0.5 mg)

I.V. infusion: Initial dose: 100-180 mcg/minute; when blood pressure is stabilized, maintenance rate: 40-60 mcg/minute; rates up to 360 mcg/minute have been reported; dosing range: 0.4-9.1 mcg/kg/minute

Nasal decongestant:

Children:

2-6 years:

Intranasal: Instill 1 drop every 2-4 hours of 0.125% solution as needed. (**Note:** Therapy should not exceed 3 continuous days.)

Oral: Tannate salt (NāSop™ suspension): 1.87-3.75 mg every 12 hours

6-12 years:

Intranasal: Instill 1-2 sprays or instill 1-2 drops every 4 hours of 0.25% solution as needed. (**Note:** Therapy should not exceed 3 continuous days.)

(Continued)

phenylephrine *(Continued)*

Oral:
  Hydrochloride salt: 10 mg every 4 hours
  Tannate salt (NāSop™ suspension): 3.75-7.5 mg every 12 hours
Children >12 years and Adults:
  Intranasal: Instill 1-2 sprays or instill 1-2 drops every 4 hours of 0.25% to 0.5% solution as needed; 1% solution may be used in adult in cases of extreme nasal congestion; do not use nasal solutions more than 3 days
  Oral:
    Hydrochloride salt: 10-20 mg every 4 hours
    Tannate salt (NāSop™ suspension): 7.5-15 mg every 12 hours
  Ocular procedures:
    Infants <1 year: Instill 1 drop of 2.5% 15-30 minutes before procedures
    Children and Adults: Instill 1 drop of 2.5% or 10% solution, may repeat in 10-60 minutes as needed
  Ophthalmic irritation (OTC formulation for relief of eye redness): Adults: Instill 1-2 drops 0.12% solution into affected eye, up to 4 times/day; do not use for >72 hours
  Paroxysmal supraventricular tachycardia: I.V.:
    Children: 5-10 mcg/kg/dose over 20-30 seconds
    Adults: 0.25-0.5 mg/dose over 20-30 seconds

Dosage Forms

Cream, rectal:
  Formulation R™ [OTC]: 0.25% (54 g)
Filmstrip, orally disintegrating:
  Sudafed PE™ [OTC]: 10 mg (5s, 10s)
  Triaminic® Thin Strips® Cold [OTC]: 2.5 mg
Injection, solution: 1% [10 mg/mL] (1 mL, 5 mL, 10 mL)
  Neo-Synephrine®: 1% (1 mL)
Liquid, oral:
  LuSonal™: 7.5 mg/5 mL
Liquid, oral [drops]:
  Dimetapp® Toddler's [OTC]: 1.25 mg/0.8 mL
Ointment, rectal:
  Formulation R™ [OTC], Preparation H® [OTC]: 0.25% (30 g, 60 g)
  Rectacaine [OTC]: 0.25% (30 g)
Solution, intranasal [drops]:
  Little Noses® Decongestant [OTC]: 0.125% (15 mL)
  Neo-Synephrine® Extra Strength [OTC]: 1% (15 mL)
  Neo-Synephrine® Regular Strength [OTC]: 0.5% (15 mL)
  Rhinall [OTC]: 0.25% (30 mL)
  Tur-bi-kal® [OTC]: 0.17% (30 mL)
Solution, intranasal [spray]:
  4 Way® Fast Acting [OTC]: 1% (15 mL, 30 mL) [contains benzalkonium chloride]
  4 Way® Menthol [OTC], 4 Way® No Drip [OTC], Neo-Synephrine® Extra Strength [OTC]: 1% (15 mL)
  Neo-Synephrine® Mild [OTC]: 0.25% (15 mL)
  Neo-Synephrine® Regular Strength [OTC], Vicks® Sinex® [OTC], Vicks® Sinex® UltraFine Mist [OTC]: 0.5% (15 mL)
  Rhinall [OTC]: 0.25% (40 mL)
Solution, ophthalmic: 2.5% (2 mL, 3 mL, 5 mL, 15 mL)
  AK-Dilate®: 2.5% (2 mL, 15 mL); 10% (5 mL)
  Altrafin: 0.12% (15 mL) [OTC]; 2.5% (15 mL); 10% (5 mL)
  Mydfrin® [OTC]: 2.5% (3 mL, 5 mL)
  Neofrin™: 2.5% (15 mL); 10% (15 mL)
  OcuNefrin™ [OTC], Relief® [OTC]: 0.12% (15 mL)
Suppository, rectal: 0.25% (12s)
  Anu-Med [OTC]: 0.25% (12s)
  Formulation R™ [OTC], Preparation H® [OTC]: 0.25% (12s, 24s, 48s)
  Medicone® [OTC], Tronolane® [OTC]: 0.25% (12s, 24s)
  Rectacaine [OTC]: 0.25% (12s)
Suspension, oral:
  Ah-Chew D®: Phenylephrine tannate [equivalent to phenylephrine hydrochloride 10 mg/5 mL]
  NāSop™: 7.5 mg/5 mL
Tablet: 10 mg
  Medi-Phenyl [OTC]: 5 mg
  Sudafed PE™ [OTC]: 10 mg
Tablet, orally dissolving:
  NāSop™: 10 mg

Phenylephrine CM [US] *see* chlorpheniramine, phenylephrine, and methscopolamine *on page 181*

phenylephrine, acetaminophen, and dextromethorphan *see* acetaminophen, dextromethorphan, and phenylephrine *on page 11*

phenylephrine and chlorpheniramine *see* chlorpheniramine and phenylephrine *on page 177*

phenylephrine and cyclopentolate *see* cyclopentolate and phenylephrine *on page 221*

phenylephrine and promethazine *see* promethazine and phenylephrine *on page 720*

phenylephrine and pyrilamine (fen il EF rin & peer IL a meen)
Synonyms pyrilamine tannate and phenylephrine tannate
U.S./Canadian Brand Names Aldex® D [US]; AllanVan-S [US]; Deconsal® CT [US]; K-Tan 4 [US]; K-Tan [US]; Pyrilafen Tannate-12™ [US]; Ry-T 12 [US]; Ryna-12 S™ [US]; Ryna-12™ [US]; Rynesa 12S™ [US]; V-Tann [US]; Viravan® [US]
Therapeutic Category Antihistamine; Antihistamine/Decongestant Combination; Sympathomimetic
Use Symptomatic relief of nasal congestion and discharge associated with the common cold, sinusitis, allergic rhinitis, and other respiratory tract conditions
Usual Dosage Oral: Relief of cough, congestion (Viravan®):
Children 2-6 years: 2.5 mL of the suspension or 1/2 tablet every 12 hours
Children 6-12 years: 5 mL of the suspension or 1/2 to 1 tablet every 12 hours
Children >12 years and Adults: 5-10 mL of the suspension or 1-2 tablets every 12 hours
Dosage Forms
  Suspension:
  Aldex® D: Phenylephrine 5 mg and pyrilamine 16 mg
  AllanVan-S, V-Tann™, Viravan®: Phenylephrine 12.5 mg and pyrilamine 30 mg per 5 mL
  K-Tan 4, Pyrilafen Tannate-12™, Ryna-12 S™, Rynesa 12S™, Ry-T 12: Phenylephrine 5 mg and pyrilamine 30 mg per 5 mL
  Tablet:
  K-Tan, Ryna-12™: Phenylephrine 25 mg and pyrilamine 60 mg
  Tablet, chewable:
  Deconsal® CT: Phenylephrine 10 mg and pyrilamine 16 mg
  Viravan®: Phenylephrine 25 mg and pyrilamine 30 mg

phenylephrine and scopolamine (fen il EF rin & skoe POL a meen)
Sound-Alike/Look-Alike Issues
  Murocoll-2® may be confused with Murocel®
Synonyms scopolamine and phenylephrine
U.S./Canadian Brand Names Murocoll-2® [US]
Therapeutic Category Anticholinergic/Adrenergic Agonist
Use Mydriasis, cycloplegia, and to break posterior synechiae in iritis
Usual Dosage Ophthalmic: Instill 1-2 drops into eye(s); repeat in 5 minutes
Dosage Forms
  Solution, ophthalmic:
  Murocoll-2®: Phenylephrine 10% and scopolamine 0.3% (5 mL)

phenylephrine and zinc sulfate *(Canada only)* (fen il EF rin & zingk SUL fate)
Synonyms zinc sulfate and phenylephrine
U.S./Canadian Brand Names Zincfrin® [Can]
Therapeutic Category Adrenergic Agonist Agent
Use Soothe, moisturize, and remove redness due to minor eye irritation
Usual Dosage Ophthalmic: Instill 1-2 drops in eye(s) 2-4 times/day as needed
Dosage Forms
  Solution, ophthalmic:
  Zincfrin® [OTC; CAN]: Phenylephrine 0.12% and zinc sulfate 0.25% (15 mL)

phenylephrine, chlorpheniramine, and carbetapentane *see* carbetapentane, phenylephrine, and chlorpheniramine *on page 150*

phenylephrine, chlorpheniramine, and dextromethorphan *see* chlorpheniramine, phenylephrine, and dextromethorphan *on page 180*

phenylephrine, chlorpheniramine, and dihydrocodeine *see* dihydrocodeine, chlorpheniramine, and phenylephrine *on page 259*

phenylephrine, chlorpheniramine, and guaifenesin *see* chlorpheniramine, phenylephrine, and guaifenesin *on page 181*

phenylephrine, chlorpheniramine, and phenyltoloxamine *see* chlorpheniramine, phenylephrine, and phenyltoloxamine *on page 182*

phenylephrine, chlorpheniramine, codeine, and potassium iodide *see* chlorpheniramine, phenylephrine, codeine, and potassium iodide *on page 183*

phenylephrine, dextromethorphan, and acetaminophen *see* acetaminophen, dextromethorphan, and phenylephrine *on page 11*

phenylephrine, diphenhydramine, and hydrocodone *see* hydrocodone, phenylephrine, and diphenhydramine *on page 431*

phenylephrine, ephedrine, chlorpheniramine, and carbetapentane *see* chlorpheniramine, ephedrine, phenylephrine, and carbetapentane *on page 179*

phenylephrine, guaifenesin, and hydrocodone *see* hydrocodone, phenylephrine, and guaifenesin *on page 431*

phenylephrine hydrochloride *see* phenylephrine *on page 675*

phenylephrine hydrochloride and guaifenesin *see* guaifenesin and phenylephrine *on page 404*

phenylephrine hydrochloride, carbetapentane citrate, and guaifenesin *see* carbetapentane, guaifenesin, and phenylephrine *on page 149*

phenylephrine hydrochloride, chlorpheniramine maleate, dextromethorphan hydrobromide, and guaifenesin *see* dextromethorphan, chlorpheniramine, phenylephrine, and guaifenesin *on page 248*

phenylephrine hydrochloride, guaifenesin, and dextromethorphan hydrobromide *see* guaifenesin, dextromethorphan, and phenylephrine *on page 407*

phenylephrine hydrochloride, hydrocodone bitartrate, and chlorpheniramine maleate *see* phenylephrine, hydrocodone, and chlorpheniramine *on this page*

phenylephrine, hydrocodone, and chlorpheniramine

(fen il EF rin, hye droe KOE done, & klor fen IR a meen)

Synonyms chlorpheniramine, phenylephrine, and hydrocodone; dihydrocodeine bitartrate, phenylephrine hydrochloride, and chlorpheniramine maleate; hydrocodone, phenylephrine, and chlorpheniramine; phenylephrine hydrochloride, hydrocodone bitartrate, and chlorpheniramine maleate

U.S./Canadian Brand Names B-Tuss™ [US]; Coughtuss [US]; Cytuss HC [US]; De-Chlor HC [US]; De-Chlor HD [US]; DroTuss-CP [US]; ED-TLC [US]; ED-Tuss HC [US]; Histinex® HC [US]; Hydro PC II Plus [US]; Hydro-PC II [US]; Hydron CP [US]; Maxi-Tuss HCX [US]; Maxi-Tuss HC® [US]; Mintuss HC [US]; Mintuss MS [US]; Relacon-HC NR [US]; Relacon-HC [US]; Rindal HD Plus [US]; Triant-HC™ [US]; Tusana-D [US]; Z-Cof HC [US]

Therapeutic Category Antihistamine; Antihistamine/Decongestant/Antitussive; Antitussive; Decongestant

Controlled Substance C-III

Use Symptomatic relief of cough and congestion associated with the common cold, sinusitis, or acute upper respiratory tract infections

Usual Dosage Oral:

Children 2-6 years: Z-Cof HC: 1.25-2.5 mL every 4-6 hours (maximum: 10 mL/24 hours)

Children 6-12 years:

Histinex® HC, Cytuss HC: 5 mL every 4 hours (maximum: 20 mL/24 hours)

Maxi-Tuss HC®, Maxi-Tuss HCX: 2.5 mL every 4 hours (maximum: 15 mL/24 hours)

Z-Cof HC: 2.5-5 mL every 4-6 hours as needed (maximum: 20 mL/24 hours)

Adults:

Histinex® HC, Cytuss HC: 10 mL every 4 hours (maximum: 40 mL/24 hours)

Maxi-Tuss HC®, Maxi-Tuss HCX: 5 mL every 4 hours (maximum: 30 mL/24 hours)

Z-Cof HC: 5-10 mL every 4-6 hours (maximum: 40 mL/24 hours)

Dosage Forms

Liquid:

B-Tuss™: Phenylephrine 5 mg, hydrocodone 5 mg, and chlorpheniramine 2 mg per 5 mL

Coughtuss, DroTuss-CP: Phenylephrine 5 mg, hydrocodone 5 mg, and chlorpheniramine 2 mg per 5 mL

De-Chlor HC: Phenylephrine 10 mg, hydrocodone 2.5 mg, and chlorpheniramine 2 mg per 5 mL

De-Chlor HD: Phenylephrine 10 mg, hydrocodone 2.5 mg, and chlorpheniramine 4 mg per 5 mL

ED-Tuss HC: Phenylephrine 10 mg, hydrocodone 3.5 mg, and chlorpheniramine 4 mg per 5 mL

ED-TLC: Phenylephrine 5 mg, hydrocodone 1.67 mg, and chlorpheniramine 2 mg per 5 mL

Hydro PC II Plus: Phenylephrine 7.5 mg, hydrocodone 3.5 mg, and chlorpheniramine 2 mg per 5 mL

Hydron CP: Phenylephrine 10 mg, hydrocodone 5 mg, and chlorpheniramine 2 mg per 5 mL

Maxi-Tuss HCX, Tusana-D: Phenylephrine 12 mg, hydrocodone 6 mg and chlorpheniramine 2 mg per 5 mL

Relacon-HC: Phenylephrine 10 mg, hydrocodone 3.5 mg, and chlorpheniramine 2.5 mg per 5 mL

Relacon-HC NR: Phenylephrine 8 mg, hydrocodone 3.5 mg, and chlorpheniramine 2 mg per 5 mL

Triant-HC™: Phenylephrine 5 mg, hydrocodone 1.67 mg, and chlorpheniramine 2 mg per 5 mL

Syrup:

Cytuss HC, H-C Tussive, Histinex® HC: Phenylephrine 5 mg, hydrocodone 2.5 mg, and chlorpheniramine 2 mg per 5 mL

Hydro-PC II: Phenylephrine 7.5 mg, hydrocodone 2 mg, and chlorpheniramine 2 mg per 5 mL

Maxi-Tuss HC®, Mintuss HD: Phenylephrine 10 mg, hydrocodone 2.5 mg, and chlorpheniramine 4 mg per 5 mL

Mintuss HC: Phenylephrine 10 mg, hydrocodone 2.5 mg, and chlorpheniramine 2 mg per 5 mL

Mintuss MS: Phenylephrine 10 mg, hydrocodone 5 mg, and chlorpheniramine 2 mg per 5 mL

PolyTussin HD: Phenylephrine 5 mg, hydrocodone 6 mg, and chlorpheniramine 2 mg per 5 mL

Rindal HD Plus: Phenylephrine 7.5 mg, hydrocodone 3.5 mg, and chlorpheniramine 2 mg per 5 mL

Z-Cof HC: Phenylephrine 8 mg, hydrocodone 3.25 mg, and chlorpheniramine 2.5 mg per 5 mL

phenylephrine, hydrocodone, chlorpheniramine, acetaminophen, and caffeine *see* hydrocodone, chlorpheniramine, phenylephrine, acetaminophen, and caffeine *on page 431*

phenylephrine, promethazine, and codeine *see* promethazine, phenylephrine, and codeine *on page 720*

phenylephrine, pyrilamine, and dextromethorphan

(fen il EF rin, peer IL a meen, & deks troe meth OR fan)

Synonyms dextromethorphan tannate, pyrilamine tannate, and phenylephrine tannate; pyrilamine maleate, dextromethorphan hydrobromide, and phenylephrine hydrochloride

U.S./Canadian Brand Names Aldex® DM [US]; AllanVan-DM [US]; Codal-DM [US-OTC]; codimal® DM [US-OTC]; Codituss DM [US-OTC]; Poly-Hist DM [US]; Tannate-V-DM [US]; Viravan®-DM [US]

Therapeutic Category Antihistamine; Antihistamine/Decongestant/Antitussive; Antitussive; Sympathomimetic

Use Symptomatic relief of cough, nasal congestion, and discharge associated with the common cold, sinusitis, allergic rhinitis, and other respiratory tract conditions

Usual Dosage Oral: Relief of cough, congestion:

Children 2-6 years (Viravan®-DM): 2.5 mL of the suspension or ¹/₂ tablet every 12 hours

Children 6-12 years:

codimal® DM: 5 mL every 4 hours; maximum: 30 mL/24 hours

Viravan®-DM: 5 mL of the suspension or ¹/₂ to 1 tablet every 12 hours

Children >12 years and Adults:

codimal® DM: 10 mL every 4 hours; maximum: 60 mL/24 hours

Viravan®-DM: 5-10 mL of the suspension or 1-2 tablets every 12 hours

Dosage Forms

Suspension:

AllanVan-DM, Tannate-V-DM, Viravan®-DM: Phenylephrine 12.5 mg, pyrilamine 30 mg, and dextromethorphan 25 mg per 5 mL

Aldex® DM: Phenylephrine 5 mg, pyrilamine 16 mg, and dextromethorphan 15 mg per 5 mL

Syrup:

Codal-DM [OTC], Codimal® DM [OTC], Codituss DM [OTC]: Phenylephrine 5 mg, pyrilamine 8.33 mg, and dextromethorphan 10 mg

Poly Hist DM: Phenylephrine 7.5 mg, pyrilamine 8.33 mg, and dextromethorphan 10 mg

Tablet, chewable [scored]:

Deconsal® DM: Phenylephrine 10 mg, pyrilamine 16 mg, and dextromethorphan 15 mg

Viravan®-DM: Phenylephrine 25 mg, pyrilamine 30 mg, and dextromethorphan 25 mg

phenylephrine tannate *see* phenylephrine *on page 675*

phenylephrine tannate and carbetapentane tannate *see* carbetapentane and phenylephrine *on page 149*

phenylephrine tannate, carbetapentane tannate, and pyrilamine tannate *see* carbetapentane, phenylephrine, and pyrilamine *on page 150*

phenylephrine tannate, chlorpheniramine tannate, and methscopolamine nitrate *see* chlorpheniramine, phenylephrine, and methscopolamine *on page 181*

phenylethylmalonylurea *see* phenobarbital *on page 672*

Phenylfenesin® L.A. *(Discontinued)*

Phenylgesic [US-OTC] *see* acetaminophen and phenyltoloxamine *on page 8*

phenyltoloxamine, chlorpheniramine, and phenylephrine *see* chlorpheniramine, phenylephrine, and phenyltoloxamine *on page 182*

phenyltoloxamine citrate and acetaminophen *see* acetaminophen and phenyltoloxamine *on page 8*

Phenytek® [US] *see* phenytoin *on this page*

phenytoin (FEN i toyn)

Sound-Alike/Look-Alike Issues
phenytoin may be confused with phenelzine, phentermine
Dilantin® may be confused with Dilaudid®, diltiazem, Dipentum®

Synonyms diphenylhydantoin; DPH; phenytoin sodium; phenytoin sodium, extended; phenytoin sodium, prompt

U.S./Canadian Brand Names Dilantin® [US/Can]; Phenytek® [US]

Therapeutic Category Antiarrhythmic Agent, Class I-B; Hydantoin

Use Management of generalized tonic-clonic (grand mal), complex partial seizures; prevention of seizures following head trauma/neurosurgery

Usual Dosage
Status epilepticus: I.V.:
Infants and Children: Loading dose: 15-20 mg/kg in a single or divided dose; maintenance dose: Initial: 5 mg/kg/day in 2 divided doses; usual doses:
6 months to 3 years: 8-10 mg/kg/day
4-6 years: 7.5-9 mg/kg/day
7-9 years: 7-8 mg/kg/day
10-16 years: 6-7 mg/kg/day, some patients may require every 8 hours dosing
Adults: Loading dose: Manufacturer recommends 10-15 mg/kg, however, 15-25 mg/kg has been used clinically; maintenance dose: 300 mg/day or 5-6 mg/kg/day in 3 divided doses or 1-2 divided doses using extended release
Anticonvulsant: Children and Adults: Oral:
Loading dose: 15-20 mg/kg; based on phenytoin serum concentrations and recent dosing history; administer oral loading dose in 3 divided doses given every 2-4 hours to decrease GI adverse effects and to ensure complete oral absorption; maintenance dose: same as I.V.
Neurosurgery (prophylactic): 100-200 mg at approximately 4-hour intervals during surgery and during the immediate postoperative period

Dosage Forms
Capsule, extended release: 100 mg
Dilantin®: 30 mg, 100 mg
Phenytek®: 200 mg, 300 mg
Capsule, prompt release: 100 mg
Injection, solution: 50 mg/mL (2 mL, 5 mL)
Suspension, oral: 100 mg/4 mL, 125 mg/5 mL
Dilantin®: 125 mg/5 mL
Tablet, chewable:
Dilantin®: 50 mg

phenytoin sodium *see* phenytoin *on this page*

phenytoin sodium, extended *see* phenytoin *on this page*

phenytoin sodium, prompt *see* phenytoin *on this page*

Pherazine® VC With Codeine *(Discontinued)* *see* promethazine, phenylephrine, and codeine *on page 720*

Pherazine® With Codeine *(Discontinued)* *see* promethazine and codeine *on page 719*

Pherazine® With DM *(Discontinued)* *see* promethazine and dextromethorphan *on page 719*

Phillips'® M-O [US-OTC] *see* magnesium hydroxide and mineral oil *on page 527*

Phillips'® Chews [US-OTC] *see* magnesium hydroxide *on page 526*

Phillips'® Milk of Magnesia [US-OTC] *see* magnesium hydroxide *on page 526*

Phillips'® Stool Softener Laxative [US-OTC] *see* docusate *on page 273*

pHisoHex® [US/Can] *see* hexachlorophene *on page 420*

PHL-Amoxicillin [Can] *see* amoxicillin *on page 48*

PHL-Azithromycin [Can] *see* azithromycin *on page 88*

PHL-Citalopram [Can] *see* citalopram *on page 194*

PHL-Domperidone [Can] *see* domperidone *(Canada only) on page 276*

Phlemex [US] *see* guaifenesin and dextromethorphan *on page 402*

PHL-Fenofibrate Supra [Can] *see* fenofibrate *on page 345*

PHL-Methimazole [Can] *see* methimazole *on page 552*

PHL-Sumatriptan [Can] *see* sumatriptan *on page 815*

PHL-Topiramate [Can] *see* topiramate *on page 851*

Phos-Flur® [US] *see* fluoride *on page 361*

Phos-Flur® Rinse [US-OTC] *see* fluoride *on page 361*

PhosLo® [US] *see* calcium acetate *on page 137*

Phos-NaK [US] *see* potassium phosphate and sodium phosphate *on page 703*

Phospha 250™ Neutral [US] *see* potassium phosphate and sodium phosphate *on page 703*

phosphate, potassium *see* potassium phosphate *on page 703*

Phospholine Iodide® [US] *see* echothiophate iodide *on page 289*

phosphonoformate *see* foscarnet *on page 375*

phosphonoformic acid *see* foscarnet *on page 375*

phosphorated carbohydrate solution *see* fructose, dextrose, and phosphoric acid *on page 378*

phosphoric acid, levulose and dextrose *see* fructose, dextrose, and phosphoric acid *on page 378*

Photofrin® [US/Can] *see* porfimer *on page 698*

Phoxal-timolol [Can] *see* timolol *on page 843*

Phrenilin® [US] *see* butalbital and acetaminophen *on page 131*

Phrenilin® Forte [US] *see* butalbital and acetaminophen *on page 131*

Phrenilin® with Caffeine and Codeine [US] *see* butalbital, acetaminophen, caffeine, and codeine *on page 130*

p-hydroxyampicillin *see* amoxicillin *on page 48*

Phyllocontin® [Can] *see* aminophylline *on page 43*

Phyllocontin®-350 [Can] *see* aminophylline *on page 43*

phylloquinone *see* phytonadione *on this page*

physostigmine (fye zoe STIG meen)

Sound-Alike/Look-Alike Issues
physostigmine may be confused with Prostigmin®, pyridostigmine

Synonyms eserine salicylate; physostigmine salicylate; physostigmine sulfate

U.S./Canadian Brand Names Eserine® [Can]; Isopto® Eserine [Can]

Therapeutic Category Cholinesterase Inhibitor

Use Reverse toxic CNS effects caused by anticholinergic drugs

Usual Dosage
Children: Anticholinergic drug overdose: Reserve for life-threatening situations only: I.V.: 0.01-0.03 mg/kg/dose (maximum: 0.5 mg/minute); may repeat after 5-10 minutes to a maximum total dose of 2 mg or until response occurs or adverse cholinergic effects occur

Adults: Anticholinergic drug overdose:
I.M., I.V., SubQ: 0.5-2 mg to start, repeat every 20 minutes until response occurs or adverse effect occurs
Repeat 1-4 mg every 30-60 minutes as life-threatening signs (arrhythmias, seizures, deep coma) recur; maximum I.V. rate: 1 mg/minute

Dosage Forms
Injection, solution: 1 mg/mL (2 mL)

physostigmine salicylate *see* physostigmine *on this page*

physostigmine sulfate *see* physostigmine *on this page*

phytomenadione *see* phytonadione *on this page*

phytonadione (fye toe na DYE one)

Sound-Alike/Look-Alike Issues
Mephyton® may be confused with melphalan, methadone

Synonyms methylphytyl napthoquinone; phylloquinone; phytomenadione; vitamin K_1

U.S./Canadian Brand Names AquaMEPHYTON® [Can]; Konakion [Can]; Mephyton® [US/Can]

Therapeutic Category Vitamin, Fat Soluble

Use Prevention and treatment of hypoprothrombinemia caused by coumarin derivative-induced or other drug-induced vitamin K deficiency, hypoprothrombinemia caused by malabsorption or inability to synthesize vitamin K; hemorrhagic disease of the newborn

Usual Dosage SubQ is the preferred (per manufacturer) parenteral route; I.V. route should be restricted for emergency use only
(Continued)

phytonadione *(Continued)*

Minimum daily requirement: Not well established
Infants: 1-5 mcg/kg/day
Adults: 0.03 mcg/kg/day
Hemorrhagic disease of the newborn:
Prophylaxis: I.M.: 0.5-1 mg within 1 hour of birth
Treatment: I.M., SubQ: 1-2 mg/dose/day
Oral anticoagulant overdose:
Infants and Children:
No bleeding, rapid reversal needed, patient **will require** further oral anticoagulant therapy: SubQ, I.V.: 0.5-2 mg
No bleeding, rapid reversal needed, patient **will not require** further oral anticoagulant therapy: SubQ, I.V.: 2-5 mg
Significant bleeding, not life-threatening: SubQ, I.V.: 0.5-2 mg
Significant bleeding, life-threatening: I.V.: 5 mg over 10-20 minutes
Adults: Oral, I.V., SubQ: 1-10 mg/dose depending on degree of INR elevation
Serious bleeding or major overdose: 10 mg I.V. (slow infusion); may repeat every 12 hours (have required doses up to 25 mg)
Vitamin K deficiency: Due to drugs, malabsorption, or decreased synthesis of vitamin K
Infants and Children:
Oral: 2.5-5 mg/24 hours
I.M., I.V., SubQ: 1-2 mg/dose as a single dose
Adults:
Oral: 5-25 mg/24 hours
I.M., I.V., SubQ: 10 mg
Dosage Forms
Injection, aqueous colloidal: 2 mg/mL (0.5 mL); 10 mg/mL (1 mL)
Tablet: 100 mcg [OTC]
Mephyton®: 5 mg

α₁-PI *see* alpha₁-proteinase inhibitor *on page 32*

pidorubicin *see* epirubicin *on page 302*

pidorubicin hydrochloride *see* epirubicin *on page 302*

Pilagan® Ophthalmic *(Discontinued)* *see* pilocarpine *on this page*

pilocarpine (pye loe KAR peen)

Sound-Alike/Look-Alike Issues
Isopto® Carpine may be confused with Isopto® Carbachol
Salagen® may be confused with Salacid®, selegiline
Synonyms pilocarpine hydrochloride
U.S./Canadian Brand Names Diocarpine [Can]; Isopto® Carpine [US/Can]; Pilopine HS® [US/Can]; Salagen® [US/Can]
Therapeutic Category Cholinergic Agent
Use
Ophthalmic: Management of chronic simple glaucoma, chronic and acute angle-closure glaucoma
Oral: Symptomatic treatment of xerostomia caused by salivary gland hypofunction resulting from radiotherapy for cancer of the head and neck or Sjögren syndrome
Usual Dosage Adults:
Ophthalmic: Glaucoma:
Solution: Instill 1-2 drops up to 6 times/day; adjust the concentration and frequency as required to control elevated intraocular pressure
Gel: Instill 0.5" ribbon into lower conjunctival sac once daily at bedtime
Oral: Xerostomia:
Following head and neck cancer: 5 mg 3 times/day, titration up to 10 mg 3 times/day may be considered for patients who have not responded adequately; do not exceed 2 tablets/dose
Sjögren's syndrome: 5 mg 4 times/day
Dosage Forms
Gel, ophthalmic:
Pilopine HS®: 4% (4 g)
Solution, ophthalmic: 0.5% (15 mL); 1% (2 mL, 15 mL); 2% (2 mL, 15 mL); 3% (15 mL); 4% (2 mL, 15 mL); 6% (15 mL)
Isopto® Carpine: 1% (15 mL); 2% (15 mL); 4% (15 mL)
Tablet: 5 mg, 7.5 mg
Salagen®: 5 mg, 7.5 mg

pilocarpine hydrochloride *see* pilocarpine *on previous page*

Pilopine HS® **[US/Can]** *see* pilocarpine *on previous page*

Pilostat® **Ophthalmic** *(Discontinued)* *see* pilocarpine *on previous page*

Pima® **[US]** *see* potassium iodide *on page 702*

pimaricin *see* natamycin *on page 593*

pimecrolimus (pim e KROE li mus)
U.S./Canadian Brand Names Elidel® [US/Can]
Therapeutic Category Immunosuppressant Agent; Topical Skin Product
Use Short-term and intermittent long-term treatment of mild to moderate atopic dermatitis in patients not responsive to conventional therapy or when conventional therapy is not appropriate
Usual Dosage Topical: Children ≥2 years and Adults: Apply thin layer to affected area twice daily; rub in gently and completely. **Note:** Limit application to involved areas. Continue as long as signs and symptoms persist; discontinue if resolution occurs; reevaluate if symptoms persist >6 weeks.
Dosage Forms
Cream, topical:
Elidel®: 1% (30 g, 60 g, 100 g)

pimozide (PI moe zide)
U.S./Canadian Brand Names Apo-Pimozide® [Can]; Orap® [US/Can]
Therapeutic Category Neuroleptic Agent
Use Suppression of severe motor and phonic tics in patients with Tourette disorder who have failed to respond satisfactorily to standard treatment
Usual Dosage Oral: **Note:** An ECG should be performed baseline and periodically thereafter, especially during dosage adjustment:
Children ≤12 years: Tourette disorder: Initial: 0.05 mg/kg preferably once at bedtime; may be increased every third day; usual range: 2-4 mg/day; do not exceed 10 mg/day (0.2 mg/kg/day)
Children >12 years and Adults: Tourette disorder: Initial: 1-2 mg/day in divided doses, then increase dosage as needed every other day; range is usually 7-16 mg/day, maximum dose: 10 mg/day or 0.2 mg/kg/day are not generally recommended
Note: Sudden unexpected deaths have occurred in patients taking doses >10 mg. Therefore, dosages exceeding 10 mg/day are generally not recommended.
Dosage Forms
Tablet:
Orap®: 1 mg, 2 mg

Pin-X® **[US-OTC]** *see* pyrantel pamoate *on page 733*

pinaverium bromide *see* pinaverium *(Canada only) on this page*

pinaverium *(Canada only)* (pin ah VEER ee um)
Synonyms pinaverium bromide
U.S./Canadian Brand Names Dicetel® [Can]
Therapeutic Category Calcium Antagonist; Gastrointestinal Agent, Miscellaneous
Use Treatment and relief of symptoms associated with irritable bowel syndrome (IBS); treatment of symptoms related to functional disorders of the biliary tract
Usual Dosage Oral: Adults: 50 mg 3 times/day; in exceptional cases, the dosage may be increased up to 100 mg 3 times/day (maximum dose: 300 mg/day). Tablets should be taken with a full glass of water during a meal/snack.
Dosage Forms [CAN] = Canadian brand name
Tablet:
Dicetel® [CAN]: 50 mg, 100 mg [not available in the U.S.]

pindolol (PIN doe lole)
Sound-Alike/Look-Alike Issues
pindolol may be confused with Parlodel®, Plendil®
Visken® may be confused with Visine®
U.S./Canadian Brand Names Apo-Pindol® [Can]; Gen-Pindolol [Can]; Novo-Pindol [Can]; Nu-Pindol [Can]; PMS-Pindolol [Can]; Visken® [Can]
Therapeutic Category Beta-Adrenergic Blocker
Use Management of hypertension
(Continued)

pindolol (Continued)

Usual Dosage Oral: Adults:

Hypertension: Initial: 5 mg twice daily, increase as necessary by 10 mg/day every 3-4 weeks (maximum daily dose: 60 mg); usual dose range (JNC 7): 10-40 mg twice daily

Antidepressant augmentation: 2.5 mg 3 times/day

Dosage Forms

Tablet: 5 mg, 10 mg

pink bismuth see bismuth on page 113

Pin-Rid® *(Discontinued)* see pyrantel pamoate on page 733

pioglitazone (pye oh GLI ta zone)

Sound-Alike/Look-Alike Issues

Actos® may be confused with Actidose®, Actonel®

U.S./Canadian Brand Names Actos® [US/Can]

Therapeutic Category Antidiabetic Agent; Thiazolidinedione Derivative

Use

Type 2 diabetes mellitus (noninsulin dependent, NIDDM), monotherapy: Adjunct to diet and exercise, to improve glycemic control

Type 2 diabetes mellitus (noninsulin dependent, NIDDM), combination therapy with sulfonylurea, metformin, or insulin: When diet, exercise, and a single agent alone does not result in adequate glycemic control

Usual Dosage Oral: Adults:

Monotherapy: Initial: 15-30 mg once daily; if response is inadequate, the dosage may be increased in increments up to 45 mg once daily; maximum recommended dose: 45 mg once daily

Combination therapy: Maximum recommended dose: 45 mg/day

With sulfonylureas: Initial: 15-30 mg once daily; dose of sulfonylurea should be reduced if the patient reports hypoglycemia

With metformin: Initial: 15-30 mg once daily; it is unlikely that the dose of metformin will need to be reduced due to hypoglycemia

With insulin: Initial: 15-30 mg once daily; dose of insulin should be reduced by 10% to 25% if the patient reports hypoglycemia or if the plasma glucose falls to <100 mg/dL.

Dosage adjustment in patients with CHF (NYHA Class II) in mono- or combination therapy: Initial: 15 mg once daily; may be increased after several months of treatment, with close attention to heart failure symptoms

Dosage Forms

Tablet:

Actos®: 15 mg, 30 mg, 45 mg

pioglitazone and glimepiride (pye oh GLI ta zone & GLYE me pye ride)

Synonyms glimepiride and pioglitazone; glimepiride and pioglitazone hydrochloride

U.S./Canadian Brand Names Duetact™ [US]

Therapeutic Category Antidiabetic Agent, Sulfonylurea; Antidiabetic Agent, Thiazolidinedione; Hypoglycemic Agent, Oral

Use Management of type 2 diabetes mellitus (noninsulin dependent, NIDDM) as an adjunct to diet and exercise

Usual Dosage Oral: Type 2 diabetes mellitus:

Adults: Initial dose should be based on current dose of pioglitazone and/or sulfonylurea.

Patients inadequately controlled on **glimepiride** alone: Initial dose: 30 mg/2 mg or 30 mg/4 mg once daily

Patients inadequately controlled on **pioglitazone** alone: Initial dose: 30 mg/2 mg once daily

Patients with systolic dysfunction (eg, NYHA Class I and II): Initiate only after patient has been safely titrated to 30 mg of pioglitazone. Initial dose: 30 mg/2 mg or 30 mg/4 mg once daily.

Note: No exact dosing relationship exists between glimepiride and other sulfonlyureas. Dosing should be limited to less than or equal to the maximum initial dose of glimepiride (2 mg). When converting patients from other sulfonylureas with longer half lives (eg, chlorpropamide) to glimepiride, observe patient carefully for 1-2 weeks due to overlapping hypoglycemic effects.

Dosing adjustment: Dosage may be increased up to max dose and formulation strengths available; tablet should not be given more than once daily; see individual agents for frequency of adjustments. Dosage adjustments in patients with systolic dysfunction should be done carefully and patient monitored for symptoms of worsening heart failure.

Maximum dose: Pioglitazone 45 mg/glimepiride 8 mg daily

Dosage Forms

Tablet:

Duetact™: 30 mg/2 mg: Pioglitazone 30 mg and glimepiride 2 mg; 30 mg/4 mg: Pioglitazone 30 mg and glimepiride 4 mg

pioglitazone and metformin (pye oh GLI ta zone & met FOR min)

Synonyms metformin hydrochloride and pioglitazone hydrochloride

U.S./Canadian Brand Names Actoplus Met™ [US]

Therapeutic Category Antidiabetic Agent, Biguanide; Antidiabetic Agent, Thiazolidinedione

Use Management of type 2 diabetes mellitus (noninsulin-dependent, NIDDM)

Usual Dosage Oral: Type 2 diabetes mellitus:

Adults: Initial dose should be based on current dose of pioglitazone and/or metformin; daily dose should be divided and given with meals

Patients inadequately controlled on **metformin alone**: Initial dose: Pioglitazone 15-30 mg/day plus current dose of metformin

Patients inadequately controlled on **pioglitazone alone**: Initial dose: Metformin 1000-1700 mg/day plus current dose of pioglitazone

Note: When switching from combination pioglitazone and metformin as separate tablets: Use current dose.

Dosing adjustment: Doses may be increased as increments of pioglitazone 15 mg and/or metformin 500-850 mg, up to the maximum dose; doses should be titrated gradually. Guidelines for frequency of adjustment (adapted from rosiglitazone/metformin combination labeling):

After a change in the **metformin** dosage, titration can be done after 1-2 weeks

After a change in the **pioglitazone** dosage, titration can be done after 8-12 weeks

Maximum dose: Pioglitazone 45 mg/metformin 2550 mg daily

Dosage Forms

Tablet:

Actoplus Met™: 15/500: Pioglitazone 15 mg and metformin 500 mg; 15/850: Pioglitazone 15 mg and metformin 850 mg

piperacillin (pi PER a sil in)

Synonyms piperacillin sodium

U.S./Canadian Brand Names Piperacillin for Injection, USP [Can]

Therapeutic Category Penicillin

Use Treatment of susceptible infections such as septicemia, acute and chronic respiratory tract infections, skin and soft tissue infections, and urinary tract infections due to susceptible strains of *Pseudomonas*, *Proteus*, and *Escherichia coli* and *Enterobacter*; active against some streptococci and some anaerobic bacteria; febrile neutropenia (as part of combination regimen)

Usual Dosage

Usual dosage range:

Neonates: I.M., I.V.: 100 mg/kg every 12 hours

Infants and Children: I.M., I.V.: 200-300 mg/kg/day in divided doses every 4-6 hours

Adults: I.M., I.V.: 2-4 g/dose every 4-6 hours (maximum: 24 g/day)

Indication-specific dosing:

Children: I.M., I.V.:

Cystic fibrosis: 350-500 mg/kg/day in divided doses every 4-6 hours

Adults:

Burn wound sepsis: I.V.: 4 g every 4 hours with vancomycin and amikacin

Cholangitis, acute: I.V.: 4 g every 6 hours

Keratitis *(Pseudomonas):* Ophthalmic: 6-12 mg/mL every 15-60 minutes around the clock for 24-72 hours, then slow reduction

Malignant otitis externa: I.V.: 4-6 g every 4-6 hours with tobramycin

Moderate infections: I.M., I.V.: 2-3 g/dose every 6-12 hours (maximum: 2 g I.M./site)

Prosthetic joint *(Pseudomonas):* I.V.: 3 g every 6 hours with aminoglycoside

***Pseudomonas* infections:** I.V.: 4 g every 4 hours

Severe infections: I.M., I.V.: 3-4 g/dose every 4-6 hours (maximum: 24 g/24 hours)

Urinary tract infections: I.V.: 2-3 g/dose every 6-12 hours

Uncomplicated gonorrhea: I.M.: 2 g in a single dose accompanied by 1 g probenecid 30 minutes prior to injection

Dosage Forms

Injection, powder for reconstitution: 2 g, 3 g, 4 g, 40 g

piperacillin and tazobactam sodium (pi PER a sil in & ta zoe BAK tam SOW dee um)

Sound-Alike/Look-Alike Issues

Zosyn® may be confused with Zofran®, Zyvox™

(Continued)

piperacillin and tazobactam sodium *(Continued)*

Synonyms piperacillin sodium and tazobactam sodium; tazobactam and piperacillin

U.S./Canadian Brand Names Tazocin® [Can]; Zosyn® [US]

Therapeutic Category Penicillin

Use Treatment of moderate-to-severe infections caused by susceptible organisms, including infections of the lower respiratory tract (community-acquired pneumonia, nosocomial pneumonia); urinary tract; uncomplicated and complicated skin and skin structures; gynecologic (endometritis, pelvic inflammatory disease); bone and joint infections; intra-abdominal infections (appendicitis with rupture/abscess, peritonitis); and septicemia. Tazobactam expands activity of piperacillin to include beta-lactamase producing strains of *S. aureus*, *H. influenzae*, *Bacteroides*, and other gram-negative bacteria.

Usual Dosage

Usual dosage range:

Children: I.V.:

2-8 months: 80 mg of piperacillin component/kg every 8 hours

≥9 months and ≤40 kg: 100 mg of piperacillin component/kg every 8 hours

Adults: I.V.: 3.375 g every 6 hours **or** 4.5 g every 6-8 hours; maximum: Piperacillin 18 g/day

Indication-specific dosing: I.V.:

Children: **Note:** Dosing based on piperacillin component:

Appendicitis, peritonitis:

2-8 months: 80 mg/kg every 8 hours

≥9 months and ≤40 kg: 100 mg/kg every 8 hours

>40 kg: refer to Adult dosing

Adults:

Diverticulitis, intra-abdominal abscess, peritonitis: I.V.: 3.375 g every 6 hours; **Note:** Some clinicians use 4.5 g every 8 hours for empiric coverage since the %time>MIC is similar between the regimens for most pathogens; however, this regimen is NOT recommended for nosocomial pneumonia or *Pseudomonas* coverage.

Pneumonia (nosocomial): I.V.: 4.5 g every 6 hours for 7-14 days (when used empirically, combination with an aminoglycoside is recommended; consider discontinuation of aminoglycoside if *P. aeruginosa* is not isolated)

Severe infections: I.V.: 3.375 g every 6 hours for 7-10 days; **Note:** Some clinicians use 4.5 g every 8 hours for empiric coverage since the %time>MIC is similar between the regimens for most pathogens; however, this regimen is NOT recommended for nosocomial pneumonia or *Pseudomonas* coverage.

Dosage Forms 8:1 ratio of piperacillin sodium/tazobactam sodium

Infusion [premixed iso-osmotic solution, frozen]:

Zosyn®

2.25 g: Piperacillin 2 g and tazobactam 0.25 g (50 mL)

3.375 g: Piperacillin 3 g and tazobactam 0.375 g (50 mL)

4.5 g: Piperacillin 4 g and tazobactam 0.5 g (50 mL)

Injection, powder for reconstitution:

Zosyn®

2.25 g: Piperacillin 2 g and tazobactam 0.25 g

3.375 g: Piperacillin 3 g and tazobactam 0.375 g

4.5 g: Piperacillin 4 g and tazobactam 0.5 g

40.5 g: Piperacillin 36 g and tazobactam 4.5 g

Piperacillin for Injection, USP [Can] *see* piperacillin *on previous page*

piperacillin sodium *see* piperacillin *on previous page*

piperacillin sodium and tazobactam sodium *see* piperacillin and tazobactam sodium *on previous page*

piperazine estrone sulfate *see* estropipate *on page 320*

piperonyl butoxide and pyrethrins *see* pyrethrins and piperonyl butoxide *on page 734*

Pipracil® *(Discontinued)* *see* piperacillin *on previous page*

pirbuterol (peer BYOO ter ole)

Synonyms pirbuterol acetate

U.S./Canadian Brand Names Maxair™ Autohaler™ [US]

Therapeutic Category Adrenergic Agonist Agent

Use Prevention and treatment of reversible bronchospasm including asthma

Usual Dosage Children ≥12 years and Adults: 2 inhalations every 4-6 hours for prevention; two inhalations at an interval of at least 1-3 minutes, followed by a third inhalation in treatment of bronchospasm, not to exceed 12 inhalations/day

Dosage Forms
Aerosol for oral inhalation:
Maxair™ Autohaler™: 200 mcg/actuation (14 g)

pirbuterol acetate *see* pirbuterol *on previous page*

piroxicam (peer OKS i kam)

U.S./Canadian Brand Names Apo-Piroxicam® [Can]; Feldene® [US]; Gen-Piroxicam [Can]; Novo-Pirocam [Can]; Nu-Pirox [Can]; Pexicam® [Can]

Therapeutic Category Analgesic, Nonnarcotic; Nonsteroidal Antiinflammatory Drug (NSAID)

Use Symptomatic treatment of acute and chronic rheumatoid arthritis and osteoarthritis

Usual Dosage Oral: Adults: 10-20 mg/day once daily; although associated with increase in GI adverse effects, doses >20 mg/day have been used (ie, 30-40 mg/day)

Dosage Forms
Capsule: 10 mg, 20 mg
Feldene®: 10 mg, 20 mg

p-**isobutylhydratropic acid** *see* ibuprofen *on page 444*

pit *see* oxytocin *on page 644*

Pitocin® **[US/Can]** *see* oxytocin *on page 644*

Pitressin® **[US]** *see* vasopressin *on page 886*

Pitrex [Can] *see* tolnaftate *on page 849*

pit viper antivenin *see* antivenin *(Crotalidae)* polyvalent *on page 63*

pivampicilin *see* pivampicillin *(Canada only) on this page*

pivampicillin *(Canada only)* (piv am pi SIL in)

Synonyms MK-191; pivampicilin

U.S./Canadian Brand Names Pondocillin® [Can]

Therapeutic Category Penicillin

Use Treatment of susceptible bacterial infections (nonbeta-lactamase-producing organisms); susceptible bacterial infections caused by streptococci, pneumococci, nonpenicillinase-producing staphylococci, *H. influenzae*, *N. gonorrhoeae*, *E. coli*, *P. mirabilis*, *Listeria*, *Salmonella*, *Shigella*, *Enterobacter*, and *Klebsiella*

Usual Dosage Oral:
Infants and Children: Bacterial infections: Oral suspension:
Infants <3 months: Use of pivampicillin in this age group should be avoided
Infants 3-12 months: Dosage range: 40-60 mg/kg/day in 2 divided doses
Children ≤10 years: Dosage range: 25-35 mg/kg/day, not to exceed recommended daily adult dose of 500 mg twice daily
Alternatively: Children:
1-3 years: 175 mg twice daily
4-6 years: 262.5 mg twice daily
7-10 years: 350 mg twice daily
Children >10 years and Adults: Usual dose: 500 mg (tablet) or 525 mg (suspension) twice daily; dosage may be doubled in severe infections
Gonococcal urethritis: 1.5 g as a single dose with 1 g probenecid concurrently

Dosage Forms [CAN] = Canadian brand name
Powder for oral suspension:
Pondocillin® [CAN]: 175 mg/5 mL (100 mL, 150 mL, 200 mL) [not available in the U.S.]
Tablet:
Pondocillin® [CAN]: 500 mg [equivalent to 377 mg ampicillin; not available in the U.S.]

pix carbonis *see* coal tar *on page 208*

pizotifen *(Canada only)* (pi ZOE ti fen)

Synonyms pizotifen malate

U.S./Canadian Brand Names Sandomigran DS® [Can]; Sandomigran® [Can]

Therapeutic Category Antimigraine Agent

Use Migraine prophylaxis

Usual Dosage Oral: Children ≥12 years and Adults: Migraine prophylaxis: Initial: 0.5 mg at bedtime; increase gradually to 0.5 mg 3 times/day; usual dosage range: 1-6 mg/day

Note: Therapeutic response may require several weeks of therapy. Do not discontinue abruptly (reduce gradually over 2-week period).

Dosage Forms [CAN] = Canadian brand name

Tablet:

Sandomigran® [CAN]: 0.5 mg [not available in the U.S.]

Tablet, double strength:

Sandomigran® DS [CAN]: 1 mg [not available in the U.S.]

pizotifen malate *see* pizotifen *(Canada only) on this page*

Plan B® [US/Can] *see* levonorgestrel *on page 502*

plantago seed *see* psyllium *on page 732*

plantain seed *see* psyllium *on page 732*

Plaquase® *(Discontinued)* *see* collagenase *on page 213*

Plaquenil® [US/Can] *see* hydroxychloroquine *on page 438*

Plaretase® 8000 [US] *see* pancrelipase *on page 648*

Plasbumin® [US] *see* albumin *on page 22*

Plasbumin®-5 [Can] *see* albumin *on page 22*

Plasbumin®-25 [Can] *see* albumin *on page 22*

Plasmanate® [US] *see* plasma protein fraction *on this page*

Plasma-Plex® *(Discontinued)* *see* plasma protein fraction *on this page*

plasma protein fraction (PLAS mah PROE teen FRAK shun)

U.S./Canadian Brand Names Plasmanate® [US]

Therapeutic Category Blood Product Derivative

Use Plasma volume expansion and maintenance of cardiac output in the treatment of certain types of shock or impending shock

Usual Dosage I.V.: Adults: Usual minimum dose: 250-500 mL; adjust dose based on response

Dosage Forms

Injection, solution [human, preservative free]:

Plasmanate®: 5% (50 mL, 250 mL)

Plasmatein® *(Discontinued)* *see* plasma protein fraction *on this page*

Platinol®-AQ *(Discontinued)* *see* cisplatin *on page 194*

Plavix® [US/Can] *see* clopidogrel *on page 205*

Plegine® [Can] *see* phendimetrazine *on page 671*

Plegine® *(Discontinued)* see phendimetrazine *on page 671*

Plenaxis™ *(Discontinued)* see abarelix *on page 2*

Plendil® [US/Can] *see* felodipine *on page 344*

Pletal® [US/Can] *see* cilostazol *on page 189*

Plexion® [US] *see* sulfur and sulfacetamide *on page 815*

Plexion SCT® [US] *see* sulfur and sulfacetamide *on page 815*

Plexion TS® [US] *see* sulfur and sulfacetamide *on page 815*

PMPA *see* tenofovir *on page 825*

PMS-Alendronate [Can] *see* alendronate *on page 27*

PMS-Amantadine [Can] *see* amantadine *on page 38*

PMS-Amiodarone [Can] *see* amiodarone *on page 43*

PMS-Amitriptyline [Can] *see* amitriptyline *on page 44*

PMS-Amoxicillin [Can] *see* amoxicillin *on page 48*

PMS-Anagrelide [Can] *see* anagrelide *on page 55*

PMS-Atenolol [Can] *see* atenolol *on page 80*

PMS-Azithromycin [Can] *see* azithromycin *on page 88*

PMS-Baclofen [Can] *see* baclofen *on page 92*

PMS-Benzydamine [Can] *see* benzydamine *(Canada only) on page 105*

PMS-Bethanechol [Can] *see* bethanechol *on page 110*

PMS-Bezafibrate [Can] *see* bezafibrate *(Canada only) on page 111*

PMS-Bicalutamide [Can] *see* bicalutamide *on page 111*

PMS-Brimonidine Tartrate [Can] *see* brimonidine *on page 118*

PMS-Bromocriptine [Can] *see* bromocriptine *on page 119*

PMS-Buspirone [Can] *see* buspirone *on page 129*

PMS-Butorphanol [Can] *see* butorphanol *on page 132*

PMS-Captopril [Can] *see* captopril *on page 145*

PMS-Carbamazepine [Can] *see* carbamazepine *on page 147*

PMS-Carvedilol [Can] *see* carvedilol *on page 155*

PMS-Cefaclor [Can] *see* cefaclor *on page 157*

PMS-Chloral Hydrate [Can] *see* chloral hydrate *on page 172*

PMS-Cholestyramine [Can] *see* cholestyramine resin *on page 186*

PMS-Cimetidine [Can] *see* cimetidine *on page 189*

PMS-Ciprofloxacin [Can] *see* ciprofloxacin *on page 190*

PMS-Citalopram [Can] *see* citalopram *on page 194*

PMS-Clobazam [Can] *see* clobazam *(Canada only) on page 201*

PMS-Clonazepam [Can] *see* clonazepam *on page 204*

PMS-Deferoxamine [Can] *see* deferoxamine *on page 235*

PMS-Desipramine [Can] *see* desipramine *on page 238*

PMS-Desonide [Can] *see* desonide *on page 240*

PMS-Dexamethasone [Can] *see* dexamethasone (systemic) *on page 241*

PMS-Diclofenac [Can] *see* diclofenac *on page 253*

PMS-Diclofenac SR [Can] *see* diclofenac *on page 253*

PMS-Diphenhydramine [Can] *see* diphenhydramine *on page 265*

PMS-Dipivefrin [Can] *see* dipivefrin *on page 270*

PMS-Docusate Calcium [Can] *see* docusate *on page 273*

PMS-Docusate Sodium [Can] *see* docusate *on page 273*

PMS-Domperidone [Can] *see* domperidone *(Canada only) on page 276*

PMS-Erythromycin [Can] *see* erythromycin *on page 309*

PMS-Famciclovir [Can] *see* famciclovir *on page 341*

PMS-Fenofibrate Micro [Can] *see* fenofibrate *on page 345*

PMS-Fenofibrate Supra [Can] *see* fenofibrate *on page 345*

PMS-Flunisolide [Can] *see* flunisolide *on page 359*

PMS-Fluorometholone [Can] *see* fluorometholone *on page 363*

PMS-Fluoxetine [Can] *see* fluoxetine *on page 364*

PMS-Fluphenazine Decanoate [Can] *see* fluphenazine *on page 365*

PMS-Fluvoxamine [Can] *see* fluvoxamine *on page 370*

PMS-Gabapentin [Can] *see* gabapentin *on page 380*

PMS-Gemfibrozil [Can] *see* gemfibrozil *on page 387*

PMS-Glyburide [Can] *see* glyburide *on page 396*

PMS-Haloperidol LA [Can] *see* haloperidol *on page 413*

PMS-Hydrochlorothiazide [Can] *see* hydrochlorothiazide *on page 426*

PMS-Hydromorphone [Can] *see* hydromorphone *on page 435*

PMS-Hydroxyzine [Can] *see* hydroxyzine *on page 440*

PMS-Indapamide [Can] *see* indapamide *on page 452*

PMS-Ipratropium [Can] *see* ipratropium *on page 470*

PMS-Isoniazid [Can] *see* isoniazid *on page 474*

PMS-Isosorbide [Can] *see* isosorbide dinitrate *on page 476*

PMS-Lactulose [Can] *see* lactulose *on page 489*

PMS-Lamotrigine [Can] *see* lamotrigine *on page 490*

PMS-Levobunolol [Can] *see* levobunolol *on page 499*

PMS-Lindane [Can] *see* lindane *on page 509*

PMS-Lithium Carbonate [Can] *see* lithium *on page 513*

PMS-Lithium Citrate [Can] *see* lithium *on page 513*

PMS-Loperamine [Can] *see* loperamide *on page 515*

PMS-Lorazepam [Can] *see* lorazepam *on page 518*

PMS-Lovastatin [Can] *see* lovastatin *on page 520*

PMS-Loxapine [Can] *see* loxapine *on page 521*

PMS-Mefenamic Acid [Can] *see* mefenamic acid *on page 537*

PMS-Meloxicam [Can] *see* meloxicam *on page 539*

PMS-Metformin [Can] *see* metformin *on page 548*

PMS-Methotrimeprazine [Can] *see* methotrimeprazine *(Canada only) on page 554*

PMS-Methylphenidate [Can] *see* methylphenidate *on page 558*

PMS-Metoprolol [Can] *see* metoprolol *on page 562*

PMS-Minocycline [Can] *see* minocycline *on page 571*

PMS-Mirtazapine [Can] *see* mirtazapine *on page 572*

PMS-Moclobemide [Can] *see* moclobemide *(Canada only) on page 575*

PMS-Mometasone [Can] *see* mometasone *on page 576*

PMS-Morphine Sulfate SR [Can] *see* morphine sulfate *on page 578*

PMS-Nizatidine [Can] *see* nizatidine *on page 610*

PMS-Norfloxacin [Can] *see* norfloxacin *on page 612*

PMS-Nortriptyline [Can] *see* nortriptyline *on page 613*

PMS-Nystatin [Can] *see* nystatin *on page 623*

PMS-Ofloxacin [Can] *see* ofloxacin *on page 625*

PMS-Oxazepam [Can] *see* oxazepam *on page 637*

PMS-Oxybutynin [Can] *see* oxybutynin *on page 639*

PMS-Oxycodone-Acetaminophen [Can] *see* oxycodone and acetaminophen *on page 641*

PMS-Pantoprazole [Can] *see* pantoprazole *on page 651*

PMS-Paroxetine [Can] *see* paroxetine *on page 654*

PMS-Phenobarbital [Can] *see* phenobarbital *on page 672*

PMS-Pindolol [Can] *see* pindolol *on page 683*

PMS-Polytrimethoprim [Can] *see* trimethoprim and polymyxin B *on page 868*

PMS-Pramipexole [Can] *see* pramipexole *on page 706*

PMS-Pravastatin [Can] *see* pravastatin *on page 707*

PMS-Procyclidine [Can] *see* procyclidine *on page 717*

PMS-Pseudoephedrine [Can] *see* pseudoephedrine *on page 727*

PMS-Ranitidine [Can] *see* ranitidine *on page 744*

PMS-Risperidone ODT [Can] *see* risperidone *on page 760*

PMS-Salbutamol [Can] *see* albuterol *on page 23*

PMS-Sertraline [Can] *see* sertraline *on page 783*

PMS-Simvastatin [Can] *see* simvastatin *on page 787*

PMS-Sodium Polystyrene Sulfonate [Can] *see* sodium polystyrene sulfonate *on page 797*

PMS-Sotalol [Can] *see* sotalol *on page 802*

PMS-Sucralate [Can] *see* sucralfate *on page 808*

PMS-Sumatriptan [Can] *see* sumatriptan *on page 815*

PMS-Temazepam [Can] *see* temazepam *on page 823*

PMS-Terazosin [Can] *see* terazosin *on page 826*

PMS-Theophylline [Can] *see* theophylline *on page 834*

PMS-Tiaprofenic [Can] *see* tiaprofenic acid *(Canada only) on page 840*

PMS-Timolol [Can] *see* timolol *on page 843*

PMS-Tobramycin [Can] *see* tobramycin *on page 846*

PMS-Topiramate [Can] *see* topiramate *on page 851*

PMS-Trazodone [Can] *see* trazodone *on page 859*

PMS-Trifluoperazine [Can] *see* trifluoperazine *on page 865*

PMS-Valproic Acid [Can] *see* valproic acid and derivatives *on page 881*

PMS-Valproic Acid E.C. [Can] *see* valproic acid and derivatives *on page 881*

PMS-Yohimbine [Can] *see* yohimbine *on page 901*

PMS-Zopiclone [Can] *see* zopiclone *(Canada only) on page 909*

PN *see* total parenteral nutrition *on page 853*

Pneumo 23™ [Can] *see* pneumococcal polysaccharide vaccine (polyvalent) *on next page*

pneumococcal 7-valent conjugate vaccine *see* pneumococcal conjugate vaccine (7-valent) *on this page*

pneumococcal conjugate vaccine (7-valent)
(noo moe KOK al KON ju gate vak SEEN, seven vay lent)
Sound-Alike/Look-Alike Issues
Prevnar® may be confused with PREVEN®
Synonyms diphtheria CRM_{197} protein; PCV7; pneumococcal 7-valent conjugate vaccine
U.S./Canadian Brand Names Prevnar® [US/Can]
Therapeutic Category Vaccine
Use Immunization of infants and toddlers against *Streptococcus pneumoniae* infection caused by serotypes included in the vaccine

Advisory Committee on Immunization Practices (ACIP) guidelines also recommend PCV7 for use in:
All children 2-23 months
Children ≥2-59 months with cochlear implants
Children ages 24-59 months with: Sickle cell disease (including other sickle cell hemoglobinopathies, asplenia, splenic dysfunction), HIV infection, immunocompromising conditions (congenital immunodeficiencies, renal failure, nephrotic syndrome, diseases associated with immunosuppressive or radiation therapy, solid organ transplant), chronic illnesses (cardiac disease, cerebrospinal fluid leaks, diabetes mellitus, pulmonary disease excluding asthma unless on high dose corticosteroids)
Consider use in all children 24-59 months with priority given to:
Children 24-35 months
Children 24-59 months who are of Alaska native, American Indian, or African-American descent
(Continued)

pneumococcal conjugate vaccine (7-valent) *(Continued)*

Children 24-59 months who attend group day care centers

Usual Dosage I.M.:

Infants: 2-6 months: 0.5 mL at approximately 2-month intervals for 3 consecutive doses, followed by a fourth dose of 0.5 mL at 12-15 months of age; first dose may be given as young as 6 weeks of age, but is typically given at 2 months of age. In case of a moderate shortage of vaccine, defer the fourth dose until shortage is resolved; in case of a severe shortage of vaccine, defer third and fourth doses until shortage is resolved.

Previously Unvaccinated Older Infants and Children:

7-11 months: 0.5 mL for a total of 3 doses; 2 doses at least 4 weeks apart, followed by a third dose after the 1-year birthday (12-15 months), separated from the second dose by at least 2 months. In case of a severe shortage of vaccine, defer the third dose until shortage is resolved.

12-23 months: 0.5 mL for a total of 2 doses, separated by at least 2 months. In case of a severe shortage of vaccine, defer the second dose until shortage is resolved.

24-59 months:

Healthy Children: 0.5 mL as a single dose. In case of a severe shortage of vaccine, defer dosing until shortage is resolved.

Children with sickle cell disease, asplenia, HIV infection, chronic illness or immunocompromising conditions (not including bone marrow transplants - results pending; use PPV23 [pneumococcal polysaccharide vaccine, polyvalent] at 12- and 24-months until studies are complete): 0.5 mL for a total of 2 doses, separated by 2 months

Previously Vaccinated Children with a lapse in vaccine administration:

7-11 months: Previously received 1 or 2 doses PCV7: 0.5 mL dose at 7-11 months of age, followed by a second dose ≥2 months later at 12-15 months of age

12-23 months:

Previously received 1 dose before 12 months of age: 0.5 mL dose, followed by a second dose ≥2 months later

Previously received 2 doses before age 12 months: 0.5 mL dose ≥2 months after the most recent dose

24-59 months: Any incomplete schedule: 0.5 mL as a single dose; **Note:** Patients with chronic diseases or immunosuppressing conditions should receive 2 doses ≥2 months apart

Dosage Forms

Injection, suspension:

Prevnar®: 2 mcg of each saccharide for serotypes 4, 9V, 14, 18C, 19F, and 23F, and 4 mcg of serotype 6B per 0.5 mL (0.5 mL)

pneumococcal polysaccharide vaccine (polyvalent)

(noo moe KOK al pol i SAK a ride vak SEEN, pol i VAY lent)

Synonyms PPV23; 23PS; 23-valent pneumococcal polysaccharide vaccine

U.S./Canadian Brand Names Pneumo 23™ [Can]; Pneumovax® 23 [US/Can]

Therapeutic Category Vaccine, Inactivated Bacteria

Use Children ≥2 years of age and adults who are at increased risk of pneumococcal disease and its complications because of underlying health conditions (including patients with cochlear implants); routine use in older adults >50 years of age, including all those ≥65 years

Current Advisory Committee on Immunization Practices (ACIP) guidelines recommend **pneumococcal 7-valent conjugate vaccine (PCV7)** be used for children 2-23 months of age and, in certain situations, children up to 59 months of age

Usual Dosage I.M., SubQ:

Children >2 years and Adults: 0.5 mL

Previously vaccinated with PCV7 vaccine: Children ≥2 years and Adults:

With sickle cell disease, asplenia, immunocompromised or HIV infection: 0.5 mL at ≥2 years of age and ≥2 months after last dose of PCV7; revaccination with PPV23 should be given ≥5 years for children >10 years of age and every 3-5 years for children ≤10 years of age; revaccination should not be administered <3 years after the previous PPV23 dose

With chronic illness: 0.5 mL at ≥2 years of age and ≥2 months after last dose of PCV7; revaccination with PPV23 is not recommended

Following bone marrow transplant (use of PCV7 under study): Administer one dose PPV23 at 12- and 24-months following BMT

Revaccination should be considered:

1. If ≥6 years since initial vaccination has elapsed, or
2. In patients who received 14-valent pneumococcal vaccine and are at highest risk (asplenic) for fatal infection or
3. At ≥6 years in patients with nephrotic syndrome, renal failure, or transplant recipients, or
4. 3-5 years in children with nephrotic syndrome, asplenia, or sickle cell disease

Pneumomist® *(Discontinued)* see guaifenesin on page 401

Pneumotussin® **[US]** *see* hydrocodone and guaifenesin *on page 429*

Pneumovax® **23 [US/Can]** *see* pneumococcal polysaccharide vaccine (polyvalent) *on previous page*

PNU-140690E *see* tipranavir *on page 845*

Pnu-Imune® **23** *(Discontinued)*

Pnu-Imune 23 Injection *(Discontinued) see* pneumococcal polysaccharide vaccine (polyvalent) *on previous page*

Podactin Cream [US-OTC] *see* miconazole *on page 566*

Podactin Powder [US-OTC] *see* tolnaftate *on page 849*

Pod-Ben-25® *(Discontinued) see* podophyllum resin *on this page*

Podocon-25® **[US]** *see* podophyllum resin *on this page*

Podofilm® **[Can]** *see* podophyllum resin *on this page*

podofilox (poe DOF il oks)
U.S./Canadian Brand Names Condyline™ [Can]; Condylox® [US]; Wartec® [Can]
Therapeutic Category Keratolytic Agent
Use Treatment of external genital warts
Usual Dosage Topical: Adults: Apply twice daily (morning and evening) for 3 consecutive days, then withhold use for 4 consecutive days; this cycle may be repeated up to 4 times until there is no visible wart tissue
Dosage Forms
Gel:
Condylox®: 0.5% (3.5 g)
Solution, topical: 0.5% (3.5 mL)
Condylox®: 0.5% (3.5 mL)

Podofin® *(Discontinued) see* podophyllum resin *on this page*

podophyllin *see* podophyllum resin *on this page*

podophyllum resin (po DOF fil um REZ in)
Synonyms mandrake; may apple; podophyllin
U.S./Canadian Brand Names Podocon-25® [US]; Podofilm® [Can]
Therapeutic Category Keratolytic Agent
Use Topical treatment of benign growths including external genital and perianal warts, papillomas, fibroids; compound benzoin tincture generally is used as the medium for topical application
Usual Dosage Topical:
Children and Adults: 10% to 25% solution in compound benzoin tincture; apply drug to dry surface, use 1 drop at a time allowing drying between drops until area is covered; total volume should be limited to <0.5 mL per treatment session
Condylomata acuminatum: 25% solution is applied daily; use a 10% solution when applied to or near mucous membranes
Verrucae: 25% solution is applied 3-5 times/day directly to the wart
Dosage Forms
Liquid, topical:
Podocon-25®: 25% (15 mL)

Point-Two® *(Discontinued) see* fluoride *on page 361*

Poladex® *(Discontinued) see* dexchlorpheniramine *on page 243*

Polaramine® *(Discontinued) see* dexchlorpheniramine *on page 243*

poliovirus vaccine (inactivated) (POE lee oh VYE rus vak SEEN, in ak ti VAY ted)
Synonyms enhanced-potency inactivated poliovirus vaccine; IPV; salk vaccine
U.S./Canadian Brand Names IPOL® [US/Can]
Therapeutic Category Vaccine, Live Virus and Inactivated Virus
Use Active immunization against poliomyelitis caused by poliovirus types 1, 2 and 3. Routine immunization of adults in the United States is generally not recommended. Adults with previous wild poliovirus disease, who have never been immunized, or those who are incompletely immunized may receive inactivated poliovirus vaccine if they fall into one of the following categories:
- Travelers to regions or countries where poliomyelitis is endemic or epidemic
- Healthcare workers in close contact with patients who may be excreting poliovirus
- Laboratory workers handling specimens that may contain poliovirus
- Members of communities or specific population groups with diseases caused by wild poliovirus

(Continued)

poliovirus vaccine (inactivated) *(Continued)*

- Incompletely vaccinated or unvaccinated adults in a household or with other close contact with children receiving oral poliovirus (may be at increased risk of vaccine associated paralytic poliomyelitis)

Usual Dosage I.M., SubQ:

Children:

Primary immunization: Administer three 0.5 mL doses, preferably 8 or more weeks apart, at 2,4, and 6-18 months of age. First dose may be given as early as 6 weeks of age. Do not administer more frequently than 4 weeks apart.

Booster dose: 0.5 mL at 4-6 years of age

Adults:

Previously unvaccinated: Two 0.5 mL doses administered at 1- to 2-month intervals, followed by a third dose 6-12 months later. If <3 months, but at least 2 months are available before protection is needed, 3 doses may be administered at least 1 month apart. If administration must be completed within 1-2 months, give 2 doses at least 1 month apart. If <1 month is available, give 1 dose.

Incompletely vaccinated: Adults with at least 1 previous dose of OPV, <3 doses of IPV, or a combination of OPV and IPV equaling <3 doses, administer at least one 0.5 mL dose of IPV. Additional doses to complete the series may be given if time permits.

Completely vaccinated: One 0.5 mL dose

Dosage Forms

Injection, suspension:

IPOL®: Type 1 poliovirus 40 D antigen units, type 2 poliovirus 8 D antigen units, and type 3 poliovirus 32 D antigen units per 0.5 mL (0.5 mL, 5 mL)

Polocaine® [US/Can] *see* mepivacaine *on page 543*

Polocaine® 2% and Levonordefrin 1:20,000 [Can] *see* mepivacaine and levonordefrin *on page 544*

Polocaine® Dental [US] *see* mepivacaine *on page 543*

Polocaine® MPF [US] *see* mepivacaine *on page 543*

polycarbophil *(pol i KAR boe fil)*

U.S./Canadian Brand Names Equalactin® [US-OTC]; Fiber-Lax® [US-OTC]; Fiber-Tabs™ [US-OTC]; FiberCon® [US-OTC]; Konsyl® Fiber Caplets [US-OTC]

Therapeutic Category Gastrointestinal Agent, Miscellaneous; Laxative

Use Treatment of constipation or diarrhea

Usual Dosage Oral: General dosing guidelines (OTC labeling):

Children 6-12 years: 625 mg calcium polycarbophil 1-4 times/day

Children ≥12 years and Adults: 1250 mg calcium polycarbophil 1-4 times/day

Dosage Forms

Caplet: Calcium polycarbophil 625 mg [equivalent to polycarbophil 500 mg]

FiberCon® [OTC], Konsyl® Fiber [OTC]: Calcium polycarbophil 625 mg

Captab:

Fiber-Lax® [OTC]: Calcium polycarbophil 625 mg

Tablet: Calcium polycarbophil 625 mg

Fiber-Tabs™: Calcium polycarbophil 625 mg

Tablet, chewable:

Equalactin® [OTC]: Calcium polycarbophil 625 mg

Polycitra® [US] *see* citric acid, sodium citrate, and potassium citrate *on page 195*

Polycitra®-K [US] *see* potassium citrate and citric acid *on page 701*

Polycitra®-LC [US] *see* citric acid, sodium citrate, and potassium citrate *on page 195*

Polycose® [US-OTC] *see* glucose polymers *on page 395*

Poly-Dex™ [US] *see* neomycin, polymyxin B, and dexamethasone *on page 597*

polyethylene glycol 3350 *(pol i ETH i leen GLY kol 3350)*

Sound-Alike/Look-Alike Issues

MiraLax® may be confused with Mirapex®

Synonyms PEG

U.S./Canadian Brand Names GlycoLax® [US]; MiraLax® [US-OTC]

Therapeutic Category Laxative, Osmotic

Use Treatment of occasional constipation in adults

Usual Dosage Oral: Adults: Occasional constipation: 17 g of powder (~1 heaping tablespoon) dissolved in 8 oz of water, once daily; do not use for >2 weeks.

Dosage Forms
Powder, for oral solution: PEG 3350 17 g/packet (12s); PEG 3350 255 g (14 oz); PEG 3350 527 g (26 oz)
GlycoLax™: PEG 3350 17 g/packet (14s); PEG 3350 255 g (16 oz); PEG 3350 527 g (24 oz)
MiraLax® [OTC]: PEG 3350 255 g (14 oz)

polyethylene glycol-electrolyte solution
(pol i ETH i leen GLY kol ee LEK troe lite soe LOO shun)

Sound-Alike/Look-Alike Issues
GoLYTELY® may be confused with NuLYTELY®
NuLYTELY® may be confused with GoLYTELY®

Synonyms electrolyte lavage solution

U.S./Canadian Brand Names Colyte® [US/Can]; GoLYTELY® [US]; Klean-Prep® [Can]; MoviPrep® [US]; NuLYTELY® [US]; PegLyte® [Can]; TriLyte™ [US]

Therapeutic Category Laxative

Use Bowel cleansing prior to GI examination or following toxic ingestion

Usual Dosage
Oral:
Children ≥6 months: Bowel cleansing prior to GI exam (CoLyte®, GoLYTELY®, NuLYTELY®, TriLyte®): 25-40 mL/kg/hour for 4-10 hours (until rectal effluent is clear). Ideally, patients should fast for ~3-4 hours prior to administration; absolutely no solid food for at least 2 hours before the solution is given. The solution may be given via nasogastric tube to patients who are unwilling or unable to drink the solution. Patients <2 years should be monitored closely.

Adults: Bowel cleansing prior to GI exam:
CoLyte®, GoLYTELY®, NuLYTELY®, TriLyte®: 240 mL (8 oz) every 10 minutes, until 4 L are consumed or the rectal effluent is clear; rapid drinking of each portion is preferred to drinking small amounts continuously. Ideally, patients should fast for ~3-4 hours prior to administration; absolutely no solid food for at least 2 hours before the solution is given. The solution may be given via nasogastric tube to patients who are unwilling or unable to drink the solution.

MoviPrep®: Administer 2 L total with an additional L of clear fluid prior to colonoscopy.
Split dose: Evening before and morning of the colonoscopy: 240 mL (8 oz) every 15 minutes until 1L is consumed. Then drink 16 oz of clear liquid. On the morning of the colonoscopy, repeat process at least 1 hour before the procedure.
Full dose: Evening before colonoscopy (6 PM): 240 mL (8 oz every 15 minutes) until 1 L is consumed; 90 minutes later (~7:30 PM), repeat dose. Then drink 32 oz of clear liquid.
Note: Patient should not eat solid food from start of solution administration until after colonoscopy. Clear liquid/plain yogurt for dinner; finishing 1 hour before start of colon prep.

Nasogastric tube (CoLyte®, GoLYTELY®, NuLYTELY®, TriLyte®):
Children ≥6 months: Bowel cleansing prior to GI exam: 25 mL/kg/hour until rectal effluent is clear. Ideally, patients should fast for ~3-4 hours prior to administration; absolutely no solid food for at least 2 hours before the solution is given.
Adults: Bowel cleansing prior to GI exam: 20-30 mL/minute (1.2-1.8 L/hour); the first bowel movement should occur ~1 hour after the start of administration. Ideally, patients should fast for ~3-4 hours prior to administration; absolutely no solid food for at least 2 hours before the solution is given.

Dosage Forms
Powder, for oral solution: PEG 3350 240 g, sodium sulfate 22.72 g, sodium bicarbonate 6.72 g, sodium chloride 5.84 g, and potassium2.98 g
Colyte®: PEG 3350 240 g, sodium sulfate 22.72 g, sodium bicarbonate 6.72 g, sodium chloride 5.84 g, and potassium 2.98 g
GoLYTELY®:
Disposable jug: PEG 3350 236 g, sodium sulfate 22.74 g, sodium bicarbonate 6.74 g, sodium chloride 5.86 g, and potassium2.97 g
Packets: PEG 3350 227.1 g, sodium sulfate 21.5 g, sodium bicarbonate 6.36 g, sodium chloride 5.53 g, and potassium 2.82 g
MoviPrep® [disposable jug]: Pouch A: PEG 3350 100g, sodium sulfate 7.5 g, sodium chloride 2.69 g, potassium chloride 1.015 g; Pouch B: Ascorbic acid 4.7 g, sodium ascorbate 5.9 g
NuLYTELY®: PEG 3350 420 g, sodium bicarbonate 5.72 g, sodium chloride 11.2 g, and potassium 1.48
TriLyte™: PEG 3350 420 g, sodium bicarbonate 5.72 g, sodium chloride 11.2 g, and potassium 1.48

polyethylene glycol-electrolyte solution and bisacodyl
(pol i ETH i leen GLY kol ee LEK troe lite soe LOO shun & bis a KOE dil)

U.S./Canadian Brand Names HalfLytely® and Bisacodyl [US]

Therapeutic Category Laxative, Bowel Evacuant; Laxative, Stimulant

Use Bowel cleansing prior to GI examination
(Continued)

polyethylene glycol-electrolyte solution and bisacodyl *(Continued)*

Usual Dosage Oral: Adults: Bowel cleansing:

Bisacodyl: 4 tablets as a single dose. After bowel movement or 6 hours (whichever occurs first), initiate polyethylene glycol-electrolyte solution

Polyethylene glycol-electrolyte solution: 8 ounces every 10 minutes until 2 L are consumed

Dosage Forms

Kit:

HalfLytely® and Bisacodyl [each kit contains]:

Powder for oral solution (HalfLytely®): PEG 3350 210 g, sodium bicarbonate 2.86 g, sodium chloride 5.6 g, potassium 0.74 g

Tablet, delayed release (Bisacodyl): 5 mg (4s)

Polygam® S/D [US] *see* immune globulin (intravenous) *on page 451*

Poly-Hist DM [US] *see* phenylephrine, pyrilamine, and dextromethorphan *on page 679*

Poly-Histine-D® Capsule *(Discontinued)*

polymyxin B (pol i MIKS in bee)

Synonyms polymyxin B sulfate

U.S./Canadian Brand Names Poly-Rx [US]

Therapeutic Category Antibiotic, Irrigation; Antibiotic, Miscellaneous

Use Treatment of acute infections caused by susceptible strains of *Pseudomonas aeruginosa*; used occasionally for gut decontamination; parenteral use of polymyxin B has mainly been replaced by less toxic antibiotics, reserved for life-threatening infections caused by organisms resistant to the preferred drugs (eg, pseudomonal meningitis - intrathecal administration)

Usual Dosage

Otic (in combination with other drugs): 1-2 drops, 3-4 times/day; should be used sparingly to avoid accumulation of excess debris

Infants <2 years:

I.M.: Up to 40,000 units/kg/day divided every 6 hours (not routinely recommended due to pain at injection sites)

I.V.: Up to 40,000 units/kg/day divided every 12 hours

Intrathecal: 20,000 units/day for 3-4 days, then 25,000 units every other day for at least 2 weeks after CSF cultures are negative and CSF (glucose) has returned to within normal limits

Children ≥2 years and Adults:

I.M.: 25,000-30,000 units/kg/day divided every 4-6 hours (not routinely recommended due to pain at injection sites)

I.V.: 15,000-25,000 units/kg/day divided every 12 hours

Intrathecal: 50,000 units/day for 3-4 days, then every other day for at least 2 weeks after CSF cultures are negative and CSF (glucose) has returned to within normal limits

Total daily dose should not exceed 2,000,000 units/day

Bladder irrigation: Continuous irrigant or rinse in the urinary bladder for up to 10 days using 20 mg (equal to 200,000 units) added to 1 L of normal saline; usually no more than 1 L of irrigant is used per day unless urine flow rate is high; administration rate is adjusted to patient's urine output

Topical irrigation or topical solution: 500,000 units/L of normal saline; topical irrigation should not exceed 2 million units/day in adults

Gut sterilization: Oral: 15,000-25,000 units/kg/day in divided doses every 6 hours

Clostridium difficile enteritis: Oral: 25,000 units every 6 hours for 10 days

Ophthalmic: A concentration of 0.1% to 0.25% is administered as 1-3 drops every hour, then increasing the interval as response indicates to 1-2 drops 4-6 times/day

Dosage Forms

Injection, powder for reconstitution: 500,000 units

Powder [for prescription compounding]:

Poly-Rx: 100 million units (13 g)

polymyxin B and bacitracin *see* bacitracin and polymyxin B *on page 91*

polymyxin B and neomycin *see* neomycin and polymyxin B *on page 596*

polymyxin B and trimethoprim *see* trimethoprim and polymyxin B *on page 868*

polymyxin B, bacitracin, and neomycin *see* bacitracin, neomycin, and polymyxin B *on page 91*

polymyxin B, bacitracin, neomycin, and hydrocortisone *see* bacitracin, neomycin, polymyxin B, and hydrocortisone *on page 92*

polymyxin B, neomycin, and dexamethasone *see* neomycin, polymyxin B, and dexamethasone *on page 597*

polymyxin B, neomycin, and gramicidin *see* neomycin, polymyxin B, and gramicidin *on page 597*

polymyxin B, neomycin, and hydrocortisone *see* neomycin, polymyxin B, and hydrocortisone *on page 597*

polymyxin B, neomycin, and prednisolone *see* neomycin, polymyxin B, and prednisolone *on page 598*

polymyxin B, neomycin, bacitracin, and pramoxine *see* bacitracin, neomycin, polymyxin B, and pramoxine *on page 92*

polymyxin B sulfate *see* polymyxin B *on previous page*

polyphenols *see* sinecatechins *on page 788*

polyphenon E *see* sinecatechins *on page 788*

Poly-Pred® [US] *see* neomycin, polymyxin B, and prednisolone *on page 598*

Poly-Rx [US] *see* polymyxin B *on previous page*

polysaccharide-iron complex (pol i SAK a ride-EYE ern KOM pleks)
Sound-Alike/Look-Alike Issues
Niferex® may be confused with Nephrox®
Synonyms iron-polysaccharide complex
U.S./Canadian Brand Names Ferrex 150 [US-OTC]; Niferex® [US-OTC]; Nu-Iron® 150 [US-OTC]
Therapeutic Category Electrolyte Supplement, Oral
Use Prevention and treatment of iron-deficiency anemias
Usual Dosage
Children ≥6 years: Tablets/elixir: 50-100 mg/day; may be given in divided doses
Adults:
Elixir: 50-100 mg twice daily
Capsules: 150-300 mg/day
Dosage Forms
Capsule: Elemental iron 150 mg
Ferrex 150 [OTC], Nu-Iron® 150 [OTC]: Elemental iron 150 mg
Niferex®: Elemental iron 60 mg
Elixir:
Niferex® [OTC]: Elemental iron 100 mg/5 mL

Polysporin® [US-OTC] *see* bacitracin and polymyxin B *on page 91*

Polytar® [US-OTC] *see* coal tar *on page 208*

Polytrim® [US/Can] *see* trimethoprim and polymyxin B *on page 868*

Poly-Vi-Flor® *(Discontinued)* *see* vitamins (multiple/pediatric) *on page 896*

Poly-Vi-Flor® With Iron [US] *see* vitamins (multiple/pediatric) *on page 896*

polyvinyl alcohol *see* artificial tears *on page 75*

polyvinylpyrrolidone with iodine *see* povidone-iodine *on page 704*

Poly-Vi-Sol® [US-OTC] *see* vitamins (multiple/pediatric) *on page 896*

Poly-Vi-Sol® with Iron [US-OTC] *see* vitamins (multiple/pediatric) *on page 896*

Pondocillin® [Can] *see* pivampicillin *(Canada only) on page 687*

Ponstan® [Can] *see* mefenamic acid *on page 537*

Ponstel® [US] *see* mefenamic acid *on page 537*

Pontocaine® [US/Can] *see* tetracaine *on page 831*

Pontocaine® Niphanoid® [US] *see* tetracaine *on page 831*

poractant alfa (por AKT ant AL fa)
U.S./Canadian Brand Names Curosurf® [US/Can]
Therapeutic Category Lung Surfactant
Use Orphan drug: Treatment and prevention of respiratory distress syndrome (RDS) in premature infants
Usual Dosage Intratracheal use **only**: Premature infant with RDS: Initial dose is 2.5 mL/kg of birth weight. Up to 2 subsequent doses of 1.25 mL/kg birth weight can be administered at 12-hour intervals if needed in infants who continue to require mechanical ventilation and supplemental oxygen.
Dosage Forms
Suspension, intratracheal [preservative free; porcine derived]:
Curosurf®: 80 mg/mL

Porcelana® Sunscreen *(Discontinued)* *see* hydroquinone *on page 437*

porfimer (POR fi mer)

Synonyms CL-184116; dihematoporphyrin ether; porfimer sodium

U.S./Canadian Brand Names Photofrin® [US/Can]

Therapeutic Category Antineoplastic Agent

Use Adjunct to laser light therapy for obstructing esophageal cancer, obstructing endobronchial nonsmall cell lung cancer (NSCLC), ablation of high-grade dysplasia in Barrett esophagus

Usual Dosage I.V. (refer to individual protocols):
Children: Safety and efficacy have not been established
Adults: 2 mg/kg, followed by exposure to the appropriate laser light; repeat courses must be separated by at least 30 days (esophageal or endobronchial cancer) or 90 days (Barrett esophagus) for a maximum of 3 courses

Dosage Forms
Injection, powder for reconstitution:
Photofrin®: 75 mg

porfimer sodium *see* porfimer *on this page*

Portagen® [US-OTC] *see* nutritional formula, enteral/oral *on page 622*

Portia™ [US] *see* ethinyl estradiol and levonorgestrel *on page 325*

posaconazole (poe sa KON a zole)

Sound-Alike/Look-Alike Issues
Noxafil® may be confused with minoxidil

Synonyms SCH 56592

U.S./Canadian Brand Names Noxafil® [US]

Therapeutic Category Antifungal Agent, Oral

Use Prophylaxis of invasive *Aspergillus* and *Candida* infections in severely-immunocompromised patients [eg, hematopoietic stem cell transplant (HSCT) recipients with graft-versus-host disease (GVHD) or those with prolonged neutropenia secondary to chemotherapy for hematologic malignancies]; treatment of oropharyngeal candidiasis (including patients refractory to itraconazole and/or fluconazole)

Usual Dosage Oral: Children ≥13 years and Adults:
Prophylaxis of invasive *Aspergillus* and *Candida* species: 200 mg 3 times/day
Treatment of oropharyngeal candidiasis: Initial: 100 mg twice daily for 1 day; maintenance: 100 mg once daily for 13 days
Treatment of refractory oropharyngeal candidiasis: 400 mg twice daily

Dosage Forms
Suspension, oral:
Noxafil®: 40 mg/mL

Post Peel Healing Balm [US-OTC] *see* hydrocortisone (topical) *on page 434*

Posture® [US-OTC] *see* calcium phosphate (tribasic) *on page 142*

Potasalan® *(Discontinued)* *see* potassium chloride *on page 700*

potassium acetate (poe TASS ee um AS e tate)

Therapeutic Category Electrolyte Supplement, Oral

Use Potassium deficiency; to avoid chloride when high concentration of potassium is needed, source of bicarbonate

Usual Dosage I.V. doses should be incorporated into the patient's maintenance I.V. fluids, intermittent I.V. potassium administration should be reserved for severe depletion situations and requires ECG monitoring; doses listed as mEq of potassium

Children:
Treatment of hypokalemia: I.V.: 2-5 mEq/kg/day
I.V. intermittent infusion (must be diluted prior to administration): 0.5-1 mEq/kg/dose (maximum: 30 mEq/dose) to infuse at 0.3-0.5 mEq/kg/hour (maximum: 1 mEq/kg/hour)
Note: Use caution in premature neonates; potassium acetate for injection contains aluminum.
Adults:
Treatment of hypokalemia: I.V.: 40-100 mEq/day
I.V. intermittent infusion (must be diluted prior to administration): 5-10 mEq/dose (maximum: 40 mEq/dose) to infuse over 2-3 hours (maximum: 40 mEq over 1 hour)
Note: Continuous cardiac monitor recommended for rates >0.5 mEq/hour
Potassium dosage/rate of infusion guidelines:
Serum potassium >2.5 mEq/L: Maximum infusion rate: 10 mEq/hour; maximum concentration: 40 mEq/L; maximum 24-hour dose: 200 mEq

Serum potassium <2.5 mEq/L: Maximum infusion rate: 40 mEq/hour; maximum concentration: 80 mEq/L; maximum 24-hour dose: 400 mEq

Dosage Forms

Injection, solution: 2 mEq/mL (20 mL, 50 mL, 100 mL) [contains aluminum]

Injection, solution [concentrate]: 4 mEq/mL (50 mL) [contains aluminum]

potassium acid phosphate (poe TASS ee um AS id FOS fate)

U.S./Canadian Brand Names K-Phos® Original [US]

Therapeutic Category Urinary Acidifying Agent

Use Acidifies urine and lowers urinary calcium concentration; reduces odor and rash caused by ammoniacal urine; increases the antibacterial activity of methenamine

Usual Dosage Oral: Adults: 1000 mg dissolved in 6-8 oz of water 4 times/day with meals and at bedtime; for best results, soak tablets in water for 2-5 minutes, then stir and swallow

Dosage Forms

Tablet [scored]:

K-Phos® Original: 500 mg

potassium bicarbonate (poe TASS ee um bye KAR bun ate)

Therapeutic Category Electrolyte Supplement, Oral

Use Potassium deficiency, hypokalemia

Usual Dosage Oral:

Children: 1-4 mEq/kg/day

Adults: 25 mEq 2-4 times/day

Dosage Forms

Tablet for oral solution, effervescent: Potassium 25 mEq

potassium bicarbonate and potassium chloride

(poe TASS ee um bye KAR bun ate & poe TASS ee um KLOR ide)

Synonyms potassium bicarbonate and potassium chloride (effervescent)

U.S./Canadian Brand Names K-Lyte/Cl® [US]

Therapeutic Category Electrolyte Supplement, Oral

Use Treatment or prevention of hypokalemia

Usual Dosage Oral:

Children: 1-4 mEq/kg/24 hours in divided doses as required to maintain normal serum potassium

Adults:

Prevention: 16-24 mEq/day in 2-4 divided doses

Treatment: 40-100 mEq/day in 2-4 divided doses

Dosage Forms

Tablet for solution, oral [effervescent]: Potassium chloride 25 mEq

K-Lyte/Cl®: Potassium chloride 25 mEq

potassium bicarbonate and potassium chloride (effervescent) *see* potassium bicarbonate and potassium chloride *on this page*

potassium bicarbonate and potassium citrate

(poe TASS ee um bye KAR bun ate & poe TASS ee um SIT rate)

Sound-Alike/Look-Alike Issues

Klor-Con® may be confused with Klaron®, K-Lor®

Synonyms potassium bicarbonate and potassium citrate (effervescent)

U.S./Canadian Brand Names Effer-K™ [US]; K-Lyte® DS [US]; K-Lyte® [US]; Klor-Con®/EF [US]

Therapeutic Category Electrolyte Supplement, Oral

Use Treatment or prevention of hypokalemia

Usual Dosage Oral:

Children: 1-4 mEq/kg/24 hours in divided doses as required to maintain normal serum potassium

Adults:

Prevention: 16-24 mEq/day in 2-4 divided doses

Treatment: 40-100 mEq/day in 2-4 divided doses

Dosage Forms

Tablet, effervescent:

Effer-K™, Klor-Con®/EF, K-Lyte®: Potassium 25 mEq

K-Lyte® DS: Potassium 50 mEq

potassium bicarbonate and potassium citrate (effervescent) *see* potassium bicarbonate and potassium citrate *on this page*

potassium chloride (poe TASS ee um KLOR ide)

Sound-Alike/Look-Alike Issues
Kaon-Cl-10® may be confused with kaolin

KCl may be confused with HCl

K-Dur® may be confused with Cardura®, Imdur®

K-Lor® may be confused with Kaochlor®, Klor-Con®

Klor-Con® may be confused with Klaron®, K-Lor®

Klotrix® may be confused with liotrix

microK® may be confused with Micronase®

Synonyms KCl

U.S./Canadian Brand Names Apo-K® [Can]; K+ Potassium [US]; K-10® [Can]; K-Dur® 10 [US]; K-Dur® 20 [US]; K-Dur® [Can]; K-Lor® [US/Can]; K-Tab® [US]; Kaon-Cl-10® [US]; Kaon-Cl® 20 [US]; Kay Ciel® [US]; Klor-Con® 10 [US]; Klor-Con® 8 [US]; Klor-Con® M [US]; Klor-Con® [US]; Klor-Con®/25 [US]; Micro-K Extencaps® [Can]; microK® 10 [US]; microK® [US]; Roychlor® [Can]; Rum-K® [US]; Slo-Pot [Can]; Slow-K® [Can]

Therapeutic Category Electrolyte Supplement, Oral

Use Treatment or prevention of hypokalemia

Usual Dosage I.V. doses should be incorporated into the patient's maintenance I.V. fluids; intermittent I.V. potassium administration should be reserved for severe depletion situations in patients undergoing ECG monitoring.

Normal daily requirements: Oral, I.V.:
 Premature infants: 2-6 mEq/kg/24 hours
 Term infants 0-24 hours: 0-2 mEq/kg/24 hours
 Infants >24 hours: 1-2 mEq/kg/24 hours
 Children: 2-3 mEq/kg/day
 Adults: 40-80 mEq/day

Prevention during diuretic therapy: Oral:
 Children: 1-2 mEq/kg/day in 1-2 divided doses
 Adults: 20-40 mEq/day in 1-2 divided doses

Treatment of hypokalemia: Children:
 Oral: 1-2 mEq/kg initially, then as needed based on frequently obtained lab values. If deficits are severe or ongoing losses are great, I.V. route should be considered.
 I.V.: 1 mEq/kg over 1-2 hours initially, then repeated as needed based on frequently obtained lab values; severe depletion or ongoing losses may require >200% of normal limit needs
 I.V. intermittent infusion: Dose should not exceed 1 mEq/kg/hour, or 40 mEq/hour; if it exceeds 0.5 mEq/kg/hour, physician should be at bedside and patient should have continuous ECG monitoring; usual pediatric maximum: 3 mEq/kg/day or 40 mEq/m^2/day

Treatment of hypokalemia: Adults:
 I.V. intermittent infusion: 5-10 mEq/hour (continuous cardiac monitor recommended for rates >5 mEq/hour), not to exceed 40 mEq/hour; usual adult maximum per 24 hours: 400 mEq/day.
 Potassium dosage/rate of infusion guidelines:
  Serum potassium >2.5 mEq/L: Maximum infusion rate: 10 mEq/hour; maximum concentration: 40 mEq/L; maximum 24-hour dose: 200 mEq
  Serum potassium <2.5 mEq/L: Maximum infusion rate: 40 mEq/hour; maximum concentration: 80 mEq/L; maximum 24-hour dose: 400 mEq
 Potassium >2.5 mEq/L:
 Oral: 60-80 mEq/day plus additional amounts if needed
 I.V.: 10 mEq over 1 hour with additional doses if needed
 Potassium <2.5 mEq/L:
 Oral: Up to 40-60 mEq initial dose, followed by further doses based on lab values
 I.V.: Up to 40 mEq over 1 hour, with doses based on frequent lab monitoring; deficits at a plasma level of 2 mEq/L may be as high as 400-800 mEq of potassium

Dosage Forms
Capsule, extended release, microencapsulated: 10 mEq [750 mg]
 microK®: 8 mEq [600 mg]
 microK® 10: 10 mEq [750 mg]

Infusion [premixed in D$_5$W]: 20 mEq (1000 mL); 30 mEq (1000 mL); 40 mEq (1000 mL)

Infusion [premixed in D$_5$W and LR]: 20 mEq (1000 mL); 30 mEq (1000 mL); 40 mEq (1000 mL)

Infusion [premixed in D$_5$W and sodium chloride 0.2%]: 5 mEq (250 mL); 10 mEq (500 mL, 1000 mL); 20 mEq (1000 mL); 30 mEq (1000 mL); 40 mEq (1000 mL)

Infusion [premixed in D$_5$W and sodium chloride 0.225%]: 10 mEq (500 mL, 1000 mL); 20 mEq (1000 mL); 30 mEq (1000 mL); 40 mEq (1000 mL)

Infusion [premixed in D$_5$W and sodium chloride 0.3%]: 10 mEq (500 mL); 20 mEq (1000 mL)

Infusion [premixed in D$_5$W and sodium chloride 0.33%]: 10 mEq (500 mL); 20 mEq (1000 mL)

Infusion [premixed in D$_5$W and sodium chloride 0.45%]: 10 mEq (500 mL, 1000 mL); 20 mEq (1000 mL); 30 mEq (1000 mL); 40 mEq (1000 mL)

Infusion [premixed in D_5W and NS]: 20 mEq (1000 mL); 40 mEq (1000 mL)
Infusion [premixed in $D_{10}W$ and sodium chloride 0.2%]: 5 mEq (250 mL)
Infusion [premixed in sodium chloride 0.45%]: 20 mEq (1000 mL); 40 mEq (1000 mL)
Infusion [premixed in NS]: 20 mEq (1000 mL); 40 mEq (1000 mL)
Infusion [premixed in SWFI; highly concentrated]: 10 mEq (50 mL, 100 mL); 20 mEq (50 mL, 100 mL); 30 mEq (100 mL); 40 mEq (100 mL)
Injection, solution [concentrate]: 2 mEq/mL (5 mL, 10 mL, 15 mL, 20 mL, 30 mL, 250 mL, 500 mL)
Powder, for oral solution: 20 mEq/packet
K-Lor™, Kay Ciel® 10%, Klor-Con®: 20 mEq/packet
Klor-Con®/25: 25 mEq/packet
Solution, oral: 20 mEq/15 mL, 40 mEq/15 mL
Tablet, extended release: 8 mEq [600 mg]; 10 mEq [750 mg]; 20 mEq [1500 mg]
K-Tab®, Kaon-Cl®: 10 mEq
Tablet, extended release, microencapsulated: 10 mEq, 20 mEq
Klor-Con® M10: 10 mEq
Klor-Con® M15: 15 mEq
Klor-Con® M20: 20 mEq
Tablet, extended release, wax matrix: 8 mEq, 10 mEq
Klor-Con® 8: 8 mEq [600 mg]
Klor-Con® 10: 10 mEq)750 mg]

potassium citrate (poe TASS ee um SIT rate)

Sound-Alike/Look-Alike Issues
Urocit®-K may be confused with Urised®
U.S./Canadian Brand Names K-Citra® [Can]; Urocit®-K [US]
Therapeutic Category Alkalinizing Agent
Use Prevention of uric acid nephrolithiasis; prevention of calcium renal stones in patients with hypocitraturia; urinary alkalinizer when sodium citrate is contraindicated
Usual Dosage Oral: Adults: 10-20 mEq 3 times/day with meals up to 100 mEq/day
Dosage Forms
Tablet: 540 mg [5 mEq]; 1080 mg [10 mEq]
Urocit®-K: 540 mg [5 mEq]; 1080 mg [10 mEq]
Tablet, extended release: 540 mg [5 mEq]; 1080 mg [10 mEq]

potassium citrate and citric acid (poe TASS ee um SIT rate & SI trik AS id)

Synonyms citric acid and potassium citrate
U.S./Canadian Brand Names Cytra-K [US]; Polycitra®-K [US]
Therapeutic Category Alkalinizing Agent
Use Treatment of metabolic acidosis; alkalinizing agent in conditions where long-term maintenance of an alkaline urine is desirable
Usual Dosage Urine alkalizing agent:
Children: Solution: 5-15 mL after meals and at bedtime; adjust dose based on urinary pH
Adults:
Powder: One packet dissolved in water after meals and at bedtime; adjust dose to urinary pH
Solution: 15-30 mL after meals and at bedtime; adjust dose based on urinary pH
Dosage Forms Equivalent to potassium 2 mEq/mL and bicarbonate 2 mEq/mL
Powder for solution, oral:
Cytra-K: Potassium citrate 3300 mg and citric acid 1002 mg per packet (100s)
Polycitra®-K: Potassium citrate 3300 mg and citric acid 1002 mg per packet (100s)
Solution:
Cytra-K: Potassium citrate 1100 mg and citric acid 334 mg per 5 mL
Polycitra®-K: Potassium citrate 1100 mg and citric acid 334 mg per 5 mL

potassium citrate, citric acid, and sodium citrate *see* citric acid, sodium citrate, and potassium citrate *on page 195*

potassium gluconate (poe TASS ee um GLOO coe nate)

Therapeutic Category Electrolyte Supplement, Oral
Use Treatment or prevention of hypokalemia
Usual Dosage Oral (doses listed as mEq of potassium):
Normal daily requirement:
Children: 2-3 mEq/kg/day
Adults: 40-80 mEq/day
Prevention of hypokalemia during diuretic therapy:
Children: 1-2 mEq/kg/day in 1-2 divided doses
(Continued)

potassium gluconate *(Continued)*

Adults: 16-24 mEq/day in 1-2 divided doses
Treatment of hypokalemia:
Children: 2-5 mEq/kg/day in 2-4 divided doses
Adults: 40-100 mEq/day in 2-4 divided doses

Dosage Forms
Caplet: 595 mg
Capsule: 99 mg
Tablet: 99 mg, 550 mg, 595 mg
Tablet, timed release: 95 mg

potassium guaiacolsulfonate and guaifenesin *see* guaifenesin and potassium guaiacolsulfonate *on page 405*

potassium iodide (poe TASS ee um EYE oh dide)

Sound-Alike/Look-Alike Issues
Potassium iodide products, including saturated solution of potassium iodide (SSKI®) may be confused with potassium iodide and iodine (Strong Iodide Solution or Lugol's solution)

Synonyms KI

U.S./Canadian Brand Names Iosat™ [US-OTC]; Pima® [US]; SSKI® [US]; ThyroSafe™ [US-OTC]; ThyroShield™ [US-OTC]

Therapeutic Category Antithyroid Agent; Expectorant

Use Expectorant for the symptomatic treatment of chronic pulmonary diseases complicated by mucous; reduce thyroid vascularity prior to thyroidectomy and management of thyrotoxic crisis; block thyroidal uptake of radioactive isotopes of iodine in a radiation emergency or other exposure to radioactive iodine

Usual Dosage Oral:
Adults: RDA: 150 mcg (iodine)
Expectorant:
Children (Pima®):
<3 years: 162 mg 3 times/day
>3 years: 325 mg 3 times/day
Adults:
Pima®: 325-650 mg 3 times/day
SSKI®: 300-600 mg 3-4 times/day
Preoperative thyroidectomy: Children and Adults: 50-250 mg (1-5 drops SSKI®) 3 times/day; administer for 10 days before surgery
Radiation protectant to radioactive isotopes of iodine (Pima®):
Children:
Infants up to 1 year: 65 mg once daily for 10 days; start 24 hours prior to exposure
>1 year: 130 mg once daily for 10 days; start 24 hours prior to exposure
Adults: 195 mg once daily for 10 days; start 24 hours prior to exposure 7
To reduce risk of thyroid cancer following nuclear accident (Iosat™, ThyroSafe™, ThyroShield™): Dosing should continue until risk of exposure has passed or other measures are implemented:
Children (see adult dose for children >68 kg):
Infants <1 month: 16.25 mg once daily
1 month to 3 years: 32.5 mg once daily
3-18 years: 65 mg once daily
Children >68 kg and Adults (including pregnant/lactating women): 130 mg once daily
Thyrotoxic crisis:
Infants <1 year: 150-250 mg (3-5 drops SSKI®) 3 times/day
Children and Adults: 300-500 mg (6-10 drops SSKI®) 3 times/day

Dosage Forms
Solution, oral:
SSKI®: 1 g/mL
ThyroShield™ [OTC]: 65 mg/mL
Syrup:
Pima®: 325 mg/5 mL
Tablet:
Iosat™ [OTC]: 130 mg
ThyroSafe™ [OTC]: 65 mg

potassium iodide, chlorpheniramine, phenylephrine, and codeine *see* chlorpheniramine, phenylephrine, codeine, and potassium iodide *on page 183*

potassium phosphate (poe TASS ee um FOS fate)

Sound-Alike/Look-Alike Issues
Neutra-Phos®-K may be confused with K-Phos® Neutral
Synonyms phosphate, potassium
U.S./Canadian Brand Names Neutra-Phos®-K [US-OTC]
Therapeutic Category Electrolyte Supplement, Oral
Use Treatment and prevention of hypophosphatemia or hypokalemia
Usual Dosage
Oral:
Normal Requirements Elemental Phosphorus:
0-6 months: 240 mg
6-12 months: 360 mg
1-10 years: 800 mg
>10 years: 1200 mg
Pregnancy lactation: Additional 400 mg/day
Adults: 800 mg
Oral Maintenance:
Children <4 years: 1 capsule (250 mg phosphorus/8 mmol) 4 times/day; dilute as instructed
Children >4 years and Adults: 1-2 capsules (250-500 mg phosphorus/8-16 mmol) 4 times/day; dilute as instructed

I.V.: Doses listed as mmol of phosphate. **Caution: With orders for I.V. phosphate, there is considerable confusion associated with the use of millimoles (mmol) versus milliequivalents (mEq) to express the phosphate requirement.** The most reliable method of ordering I.V. phosphate is by millimoles, then specifying the potassium or sodium salt.

Acute treatment of hypophosphatemia: It is recommended that repletion of severe hypophosphatemia be done I.V. because large doses of oral phosphate may cause diarrhea and intestinal absorption may be unreliable. Intermittent I.V. infusion should be reserved for severe depletion situations; requires continuous cardiac monitoring. Guidelines differ based on degree of illness, need/use of TPN, and severity of hypophosphatemia. If potassium >4.0 mEq/L consider phosphate replacement strategy without potassium (eg, sodium phosphates). Obese patients and/or severe renal impairment were excluded from phosphate supplement trials.

Children and Adults: **Note:** There are no prospective studies of parenteral phosphate replacement in children. The following weight-based guidelines for adult dosing may be cautiously employed in pediatric patients.

General replacement guidelines:
Low dose: 0.08 mmol/kg over 6 hours; use if losses are recent and uncomplicated
Intermediate dose: 0.16-0.24 mmol/kg over 4-6 hours; use if serum phosphorus level 0.5-1 mg/dL (0.16-0.32 mmoles/L)
Note: The initial dose may be increased by 25% to 50% if the patient is symptomatic secondary to hypophosphatemia and lowered by 25% to 50% if the patient is hypercalcemic.
Patients receiving TPN; supplemental dose:
Low dose: 0.16 mmol/kg over 4-6 hours; use if serum phosphorus level 2.3-3 mg/dL (0.73-0.96 mmoles/L)
Intermediate dose: 0.32 mmol/kg over 4-6 hours; use if serum phosphorus level 1.6-2.2 mg/dL (0.51-0.72 mmoles/L)
High dose: 0.64 mmol/kg over 8-12 hours; use if serum phosphorus <1.5 mg/dL (<0.5 mmoles/L)
Critically-ill adult trauma patients receiving TPN:
Low dose: 0.32 mmol/kg over 4-6 hours; use if serum phosphorus level 2.3-3 mg/dL (0.73-0.96 mmoles/L)
Intermediate dose: 0.64 mmol/kg over 4-6 hours; use if serum phosphorus level 1.6-2.2 mg/dL (0.51-0.72 mmoles/L)
High dose: 1 mmol/kg over 8-12 hours; use if serum phosphorus <1.5 mg/dL (<0.5 mmoles/L)

Maintenance: I.V. solutions: Doses may be incorporated into the patient's maintenance I.V. fluids.
Children: 0.5-1.5 mmol/kg/24 hours I.V. or 2-3 mmol/kg/24 hours orally in divided doses
Adults: 15-30 mmol/24 hours I.V. or 50-150 mmol/24 hours orally in divided doses
Dosage Forms
Injection, solution: Potassium 4.4 mEq and phosphorus 3 mmol per mL (5 mL, 15 mL, 50 mL)
Powder for oral solution:
Neutra-Phos®-K [OTC]: Monobasic potassium phosphate and dibasic potassium phosphate per packet (100s)

potassium phosphate and sodium phosphate
(poe TASS ee um FOS fate & SOW dee um FOS fate)
Sound-Alike/Look-Alike Issues
K-Phos® Neutral may be confused with Neutra-Phos®-K

(Continued)

potassium phosphate and sodium phosphate *(Continued)*

Synonyms sodium phosphate and potassium phosphate

U.S./Canadian Brand Names K-Phos® MF [US]; K-Phos® Neutral [US]; K-Phos® No. 2 [US]; Neutra-Phos® [US-OTC]; Phos-NaK [US]; Phospha 250™ Neutral [US]; Uro-KP-Neutral® [US]

Therapeutic Category Electrolyte Supplement, Oral

Use Treatment of conditions associated with excessive renal phosphate loss or inadequate GI absorption of phosphate; to acidify the urine to lower calcium concentrations; to increase the antibacterial activity of methenamine; reduce odor and rash caused by ammonia in urine

Usual Dosage All dosage forms to be mixed in 6-8 oz of water prior to administration

Children ≥4 years: Elemental phosphorus 250 mg 4 times/day after meals and at bedtime

Adults: Elemental phosphorus 250-500 mg 4 times/day after meals and at bedtime

Dosage Forms

Caplet:

Uro-KP-Neutral®: Dipotassium phosphate, disodium phosphate, and monobasic sodium phosphate

Powder, for oral solution:

Neutra-Phos® [OTC], Phos-NaK: Dibasic potassium phosphate, monobasic potassium phosphate, dibasic sodium phosphate, and monosodium phosphate per packet (100s)

Tablet:

K-Phos® MF: Potassium phosphate 155 mg and sodium phosphate 350 mg

K-Phos® Neutral: Monobasic potassium phosphate 155 mg, dibasic sodium phosphate 852 mg, and monobasic sodium phosphate 130 mg

K-Phos® No. 2: Potassium phosphate 305 mg and sodium phosphate 700 mg

Phospha 250™ Neutral: Monobasic potassium phosphate 155 mg, dibasic sodium phosphate 852 mg, and monobasic sodium phosphate 130 mg

Povidine™ [US-OTC] *see* povidone-iodine *on this page*

povidone-iodine (POE vi done EYE oh dyne)

Sound-Alike/Look-Alike Issues

Betadine® may be confused with Betagan®, betaine

Synonyms polyvinylpyrrolidone with iodine; PVP-I

U.S./Canadian Brand Names Betadine® Ophthalmic [US]; Betadine® [US-OTC/Can]; Minidyne® [US-OTC]; Operand® [US-OTC]; Povidine™ [US-OTC]; Proviodine [Can]; Summer's Eve® Medicated Douche [US-OTC]; Vagi-Gard® [US-OTC]

Therapeutic Category Antibacterial, Topical

Use External antiseptic with broad microbicidal spectrum for the prevention or treatment of topical infections associated with surgery, burns, minor cuts/scrapes; relief of minor vaginal irritation

Usual Dosage

Antiseptic: Apply topically to affected area as needed. Ophthalmic solution may be used to irrigate the eye or applied to area around the eye such as skin, eyelashes, or lid margins.

Surgical scrub: Topical: Apply solution to wet skin or hands, scrub for ~5 minutes, rinse; refer to product labeling for specific procedure-related instructions.

Vaginal irritation: Douche: Insert 0.3% solution vaginally once daily for 5-7 days

Dosage Forms

Gel, topical: 10% (120 g)

Operand® [OTC]: 10% (120 g)

Liquid, topical [prep-swab ampule]: 10% (0.65 mL)

Ointment, topical: 10% (1 g, 30 g)

Povidine™ [OTC]: 10% (30 g)

Pad [prep pads]: 10% (200s)

Betadine® SwabAids [OTC]: 10% (100s)

Solution, ophthalmic: 5% (30 mL)

Betadine® [OTC]: 5% (30 mL)

Solution, perineal [concentrate]:

Operand® [OTC]: 10% (240 mL)

Solution, topical: 10% (22 mL, 60 mL, 90 mL, 240 mL, 480 mL, 3840 mL)

Betadine® [OTC]: 10% (15 mL, 120 mL, 240 mL, 480 mL, 960 mL, 3840 mL)

Operand® [OTC]: 10% (60 mL, 120 mL, 240 mL, 480 mL, 960 mL, 3840 mL)

Povidine™ [OTC}: 10% (240 mL)

Solution, topical [cleanser]:

Betadine® Skin Cleanser [OTC]: 7.5% (120 mL)

Solution, topical [paint sponge]: 10% (50s)

Solution, topical [paint]: 10% (60 mL, 90 mL, 120 mL)

Solution, topical [surgical scrub]: 7.5% (60 mL, 120 mL)

Betadine® Surgical Scrub [OTC]: 7.5% (120 mL, 480 mL, 960 mL, 3840 mL)

Operand® [OTC]: 7.5% (60 mL, 120 mL, 240 mL, 480 mL, 960 mL, 3840 mL)
Solution, topical [spray]: 10% (60 mL)
Betadine® [OTC]: 5% (90 mL)
Operand® [OTC]: 10% (59 mL)
Solution, topical [surgical scrub sponge]: 10% (50s)
Solution, vaginal [concentrate, douche]:
Operand® [OTC]: 10% (240 mL)
Vagi-Gard® [OTC]: 10% (180 mL, 240 mL)
Solution, vaginal [douche]:
Summer's Eve® Medicated Douche [OTC]: 0.3% (135 mL) [contains sodium benzoate]
Solution [concentrate, whirlpool]:
Operand® [OTC]: 10% (3840 mL)
Swabsticks: 10% (25s, 50s, 1000s)
Betadine® [OTC]: 10% (50s, 200s)
Swabsticks [gel saturated]: 10% (50s)
Swabsticks, topical [surgical scrub]: 7.5% (25s, 50s, 1000s)

PPD *see* tuberculin tests *on page 872*

PPI-149 *see* abarelix *on page 2*

PPL *see* benzylpenicilloyl-polylysine *on page 106*

PPS *see* pentosan polysulfate sodium *on page 667*

PPV23 *see* pneumococcal polysaccharide vaccine (polyvalent) *on page 692*

pralidoxime (pra li DOKS eem)
Sound-Alike/Look-Alike Issues
pralidoxime may be confused with pramoxine, pyridoxine
Protopam® may be confused with Proloprim®, protamine, Protropin®
Synonyms 2-PAM; pralidoxime chloride; 2-pyridine aldoxime methochloride
U.S./Canadian Brand Names Protopam® [US/Can]
Therapeutic Category Antidote
Use Reverse muscle paralysis caused by toxic exposure to organophosphate anticholinesterase pesticides and chemicals; control of overdose of anticholinesterase medications used to treat myasthenia gravis (ambenonium, neostigmine, pyridostigmine)
Usual Dosage
Organic phosphorus poisoning (use in conjunction with atropine; atropine effects should be established before pralidoxime is administered): I.V. (may be given I.M. or SubQ if I.V. is not feasible):
Children: 20-50 mg/kg/dose; repeat in 1-2 hours if muscle weakness has not been relieved, then at 8- to 12-hour intervals if cholinergic signs recur
Adults: 1-2 g; repeat in 1 hour if muscle weakness has not been relieved, then at 8- to 12-hour intervals if cholinergic signs recur. When the poison has been ingested, continued absorption from the lower bowel may require additional doses; patients should be titrated as long as signs of poisoning recur; dosing may need repeated every 3-8 hours.
Treatment of acetylcholinesterase inhibitor toxicity: Adults: I.V.: Initial: 1-2 g followed by increments of 250 mg every 5 minutes until response is observed
Infants and Children:
Prehospital ("in the field"): Mild-to-moderate symptoms: I.M.: 15 mg/kg; severe symptoms: 25 mg/kg
Hospital/emergency department: Mild-to-severe symptoms: I.V.: 15 mg/kg (up to 1 g)
Adults:
Prehospital ("in the field"): Mild-to-moderate symptoms: I.M.: 600 mg; severe symptoms: 1800 mg
Hospital/emergency department: Mild-to-severe symptoms: I.V.: 15 mg/kg (up to 1 g)
Frail patients:
Prehospital ("in the field"): Mild-to-moderate symptoms: I.M.: 10 mg/kg; severe symptoms: 25 mg/kg
Hospital/emergency department: Mild-to-severe symptoms: I.V.: 5-10 mg/kg
Dosage Forms
Injection, powder for reconstitution:
Protopam®: 1 g
Injection, solution: 300 mg/mL (2 mL)

pralidoxime and atropine *see* atropine and pralidoxime *on page 84*

pralidoxime chloride *see* pralidoxime *on this page*

Pramet® FA *(Discontinued)*

Pramilet® FA *(Discontinued)*

pramipexole (pra mi PEKS ole)

Sound-Alike/Look-Alike Issues
Mirapex® may be confused with Mifeprex®, MiraLax®

U.S./Canadian Brand Names Apo-Pramipexole [Can]; Mirapex® [US/Can]; Novo-Pramipexole [Can]; PMS-Pramipexole [Can]

Therapeutic Category Anti-Parkinson Agent (Dopamine Agonist)

Use Treatment of the signs and symptoms of idiopathic Parkinson disease; treatment of moderate-to-severe primary Restless Legs Syndrome (RLS)

Usual Dosage Oral: Adults:
Parkinson disease: Initial: 0.375 mg/day given in 3 divided doses, increase gradually by 0.125 mg/dose every 5-7 days; range: 1.5-4.5 mg/day
Restless legs syndrome: Initial: 0.125 mg once daily 2-3 hours before bedtime. Dose may be doubled every 4-7 days up to 0.5 mg/day. Maximum dose: 0.5 mg/day (manufacturer's recommendation).
Note: Most patients require <0.5 mg/day, but higher doses have been used (2 mg/day). If augmentation occurs, dose earlier in the day.

Dosage Forms
Tablet:
Mirapex®: 0.125 mg, 0.25 mg, 0.5 mg, 1 mg, 1.5 mg

pramlintide (PRAM lin tide)

Synonyms pramlintide acetate

U.S./Canadian Brand Names Symlin® [US]

Therapeutic Category Antidiabetic Agent

Use
Adjunctive treatment with mealtime insulin in type 1 diabetes mellitus (insulin-dependent, IDDM) patients who have failed to achieve desired glucose control despite optimal insulin therapy
Adjunctive treatment with mealtime insulin in type 2 diabetes mellitus (noninsulin-dependent, NIDDM) patients who have failed to achieve desired glucose control despite optimal insulin therapy, with or without concurrent sulfonylurea and/or metformin

Usual Dosage SubQ: Adults: **Note:** When initiating pramlintide, reduce current insulin dose (including rapidly- and mixed-acting preparations) by 50% to avoid hypoglycemia.
Type 1 diabetes mellitus (insulin-dependent, IDDM): Initial: 15 mcg immediately prior to meals; titrate in 15 mcg increments every 3 days (if no significant nausea occurs) to target dose of 30-60 mcg (consider discontinuation if intolerant of 30 mcg dose)
Type 2 diabetes mellitus (noninsulin-dependent, NIDDM): Initial: 60 mcg immediately prior to meals; after 3-7 days, increase to 120 mcg prior to meals if no significant nausea occurs (if nausea occurs at 120 mcg dose, reduce to 60 mcg)
If pramlintide is discontinued for any reason, restart therapy with same initial titration protocol.

Dosage Forms
Injection, solution:
Symlin®: Pramlintide 0.6 mg/mL (5 mL)

pramlintide acetate see pramlintide on this page

Pramosone® [US] see pramoxine and hydrocortisone on next page

Pramox® HC [Can] see pramoxine and hydrocortisone on next page

pramoxine (pra MOKS een)

Sound-Alike/Look-Alike Issues
pramoxine may be confused with pralidoxime
Anusol® may be confused with Anusol-HC®, Aplisol®, Aquasol®

Synonyms pramoxine hydrochloride

U.S./Canadian Brand Names Anusol® Ointment [US-OTC]; Caladryl® Clear [US-OTC]; CalaMycin® Cool and Clear [US-OTC]; Callergy Clear [US-OTC]; Curasore [US-OTC]; Itch-X® [US-OTC]; Prax® [US-OTC]; ProctoFoam® NS [US-OTC]; Sarna® Sensitive [US-OTC]; Soothing Care™ Itch Relief [US-OTC]; Summer's Eve® Anti-Itch Maximum Strength [US-OTC]; Tronolane® [US-OTC]; Tucks® Hemorrhoidal [US-OTC]

Therapeutic Category Local Anesthetic

Use Temporary relief of pain and itching associated with anogenital pruritus or irritation; dermatosis, minor burns, or hemorrhoids

Usual Dosage Adults: Topical: Apply as directed, usually every 3-4 hours to affected area (maximum adult dose: 200 mg)

Dosage Forms
Aerosol, topical [foam]:
ProctoFoam® NS [OTC]: 1% (15 g)

Cloth:
Summer's Eve® Anti-Itch Maximum Strength [OTC]: 1% (12s)
Cream, topical:
Tronolane® [OTC]: 1% (30 g, 60 g)
Gel, topical:
Itch-X® [OTC]: 1% (35.4 g)
Summer's Eve® Anti-Itch Maximum Strength [OTC]: 1% (30 mL)
Liquid, topical:
Curasore® [OTC]: 1% (15 mL)
Lotion, topical:
Caladryl® Clear [OTC]: 1% (177 mL)
Callergy Clear [OTC]: 1% (180 mL)
Prax® [OTC]: 1% (15 mL, 120 mL, 240 mL)
Sarna® Sensitive: 1% (222 mL)
Ointment, rectal:
Anusol® [OTC], Tucks® Hemorrhoidal [OTC]: 1% (30 g)
Solution, topical [spray]:
CalaMycin® Cool and Clear [OTC], Itch-X® [OTC]: 1% (60 mL)
Soothing Care™ Itch Relief: 1% (74 mL)

pramoxine and hydrocortisone (pra MOKS een & hye droe KOR ti sone)
Sound-Alike/Look-Alike Issues
Pramosone® may be confused with predniSONE
Zone-A Forte® may be confused with Zonalon®
Synonyms hydrocortisone and pramoxine; pramoxine hydrochloride and hydrocortisone acetate
U.S./Canadian Brand Names Analpram-HC® [US]; Epifoam® [US]; Pramosone® [US]; Pramox® HC [Can];
ProctoFoam®-HC [US/Can]
Therapeutic Category Anesthetic/Corticosteroid
Use Relief of inflammatory and pruritic manifestations of corticosteroid-responsive dermatoses
Usual Dosage Topical/rectal: Apply to affected areas 3-4 times/day
Dosage Forms
Cream, topical:
Analpram-HC®: Pramoxine 1% and hydrocortisone 1% (4 g, 30 g); pramoxine 1% and hydrocortisone 2.5%
(4 g, 30 g)
Pramosone®: Pramoxine 1% and hydrocortisone 1% (30 g, 60 g); pramoxine 1% and hydrocortisone 2.5%
(30 g, 60 g)
Foam, rectal;
ProctoFoam®-HC: Pramoxine 1% and hydrocortisone 1% (10 g)
Foam, topical:
Epifoam®: Pramoxine 1% and hydrocortisone 1% (10 g)
Lotion, topical:
Analpram-HC®: Pramoxine 1% and hydrocortisone 2.5% (60 mL)
Pramosone®: Pramoxine 1% and hydrocortisone 1% (60 mL, 120 mL, 240 mL); pramoxine 1% and hydrocortisone 2.5% (60 mL, 120 mL)
Ointment, topical:
Pramosone®: Pramoxine 1% and hydrocortisone 1% (30 g); pramoxine 1% and hydrocortisone 2.5% (30 g)

pramoxine hydrochloride *see* pramoxine *on previous page*

pramoxine hydrochloride and hydrocortisone acetate *see* pramoxine and hydrocortisone *on this page*

pramoxine, neomycin, bacitracin, and polymyxin B *see* bacitracin, neomycin, polymyxin B, and pramoxine *on page 92*

Prandase® [Can] *see* acarbose *on page 4*

Prandin® [US/Can] *see* repaglinide *on page 750*

Pravachol® [US/Can] *see* pravastatin *on this page*

pravastatin (prav a STAT in)
Sound-Alike/Look-Alike Issues
Pravachol® may be confused with Prevacid®, Prinivil®, propranolol
Synonyms pravastatin sodium
U.S./Canadian Brand Names Apo-Pravastatin® [Can]; CO Pravastatin [Can]; Novo-Pravastatin [Can]; PMS-Pravastatin [Can]; Pravachol® [US/Can]; ratio-Pravastatin [Can]; Riva-Pravastatin [Can]; Sandoz-Pravastatin [Can]
(Continued)

pravastatin *(Continued)*

Therapeutic Category HMG-CoA Reductase Inhibitor

Use Use with dietary therapy for the following:

Primary prevention of coronary events: In hypercholesterolemic patients without established coronary heart disease to reduce cardiovascular morbidity (myocardial infarction, coronary revascularization procedures) and mortality.

Secondary prevention of cardiovascular events in patients with established coronary heart disease: To slow the progression of coronary atherosclerosis; to reduce cardiovascular morbidity (myocardial infarction, coronary vascular procedures) and to reduce mortality; to reduce the risk of stroke and transient ischemic attacks

Hyperlipidemias: Reduce elevations in total cholesterol, LDL-C, apolipoprotein B, and triglycerides (elevations of 1 or more components are present in Fredrickson type IIa, IIb, III, and IV hyperlipidemias)

Heterozygous familial hypercholesterolemia (HeFH): In pediatric patients, 8-18 years of age, with HeFH having LDL-C ≥190 mg/dL **or** LDL ≥160 mg/dL with positive family history of premature cardiovascular disease (CVD) or 2 or more CVD risk factors in the pediatric patient

Usual Dosage Oral: **Note:** Doses should be individualized according to the baseline LDL-cholesterol levels, the recommended goal of therapy, and patient response; adjustments should be made at intervals of 4 weeks or more; doses may need adjusted based on concomitant medications

Children: HeFH:

8-13 years: 20 mg/day

14-18 years: 40 mg/day

Dosage adjustment for pravastatin based on concomitant cyclosporine: Refer to adult dosing section

Adults: Hyperlipidemias, primary prevention of coronary events, secondary prevention of cardiovascular events: Initial: 40 mg once daily; titrate dosage to response; usual range: 10-80 mg; (maximum dose: 80 mg once daily)

Dosage adjustment for pravastatin based on concomitant cyclosporine: Initial: 10 mg/day, titrate with caution (maximum dose: 20 mg/day)

Dosage Forms

Tablet: 10 mg, 20 mg, 40 mg, 80 mg

Pravachol®: 10 mg, 20 mg, 40 mg, 80 mg

pravastatin sodium *see pravastatin on previous page*

Pravigard™ PAC *(Discontinued)*

Prax® [US-OTC] *see pramoxine on page 706*

praziquantel *(pray zi KWON tel)*

U.S./Canadian Brand Names Biltricide® [US/Can]

Therapeutic Category Anthelmintic

Use All stages of schistosomiasis caused by all *Schistosoma* species pathogenic to humans; clonorchiasis and opisthorchiasis

Usual Dosage Oral: Children >4 years and Adults:

Schistosomiasis: 20 mg/kg/dose 2-3 times/day for 1 day at 4- to 6-hour intervals

Clonorchiasis/opisthorchiasis: 3 doses of 25 mg/kg as a 1-day treatment

Dosage Forms

Tablet [tri-scored]:

Biltricide®: 600 mg

prazosin *(PRAZ oh sin)*

Sound-Alike/Look-Alike Issues

prazosin may be confused with predniSONE

Synonyms furazosin; prazosin hydrochloride

U.S./Canadian Brand Names Apo-Prazo® [Can]; Minipress® [US/Can]; Novo-Prazin [Can]; Nu-Prazo [Can]

Therapeutic Category Alpha-Adrenergic Blocking Agent

Use Treatment of hypertension

Usual Dosage Oral: Adults:

Hypertension: Initial: 1 mg/dose 2-3 times/day; usual maintenance dose: 3-15 mg/day in divided doses 2-4 times/day; maximum daily dose: 20 mg

Hypertensive urgency: 10-20 mg once, may repeat in 30 minutes

Dosage Forms

Capsule: 1 mg, 2 mg, 5 mg

Minipress®: 1 mg, 2 mg, 5 mg

prazosin hydrochloride *see prazosin on this page*

PreCare® [US] *see vitamins (multiple/prenatal) on page 896*

PreCare® Conceive™ [US] *see* vitamins (multiple/prenatal) *on page 896*

PreCare Premier™ [US] *see* vitamins (multiple/prenatal) *on page 896*

PreCare® Prenatal [US] *see* vitamins (multiple/prenatal) *on page 896*

Precedex™ [US/Can] *see* dexmedetomidine *on page 243*

Precose® [US] *see* acarbose *on page 4*

Pred Forte® [US/Can] *see* prednisolone (ophthalmic) *on this page*

Pred-G® [US] *see* prednisolone and gentamicin *on this page*

Pred Mild® [US/Can] *see* prednisolone (ophthalmic) *on this page*

prednicarbate (pred ni KAR bate)
Sound-Alike/Look-Alike Issues
Dermatop® may be confused with Dimetapp®
U.S./Canadian Brand Names Dermatop® [US/Can]
Therapeutic Category Corticosteroid, Topical
Use Relief of the inflammatory and pruritic manifestations of corticosteroid-responsive dermatoses (medium potency topical corticosteroid)
Usual Dosage Topical: Adults: Apply a thin film to affected area twice daily. Therapy should be discontinued when control is achieved; if no improvement is seen, reassessment of diagnosis may be necessary.
Dosage Forms
Cream: 0.1% (15 g, 60 g)
Dermatop®: 0.1% (15 g, 60 g)
Ointment:
Dermatop®: 0.1% (15 g, 60 g)

Prednicen-M® *(Discontinued)* *see* prednisone *on next page*

prednisolone acetate *see* prednisolone (systemic) *on next page*

prednisolone acetate, ophthalmic *see* prednisolone (ophthalmic) *on this page*

prednisolone and gentamicin (pred NIS oh lone & jen ta MYE sin)
Synonyms gentamicin and prednisolone
U.S./Canadian Brand Names Pred-G® [US]
Therapeutic Category Antibiotic/Corticosteroid, Ophthalmic
Use Treatment of steroid responsive inflammatory conditions and superficial ocular infections due to microorganisms susceptible to gentamicin
Usual Dosage Ophthalmic: Children and Adults:
Ointment: Apply ½ inch ribbon in the conjunctival sac 1-3 times/day
Suspension: 1 drop 2-4 times/day; during the initial 24-48 hours, the dosing frequency may be increased if necessary up to 1 drop every hour
Dosage Forms
Ointment, ophthalmic:
Pred-G®: Prednisolone 0.6% and gentamicin 0.3% (3.5 g)
Suspension, ophthalmic:
Pred-G®: Prednisolone 1% and gentamicin 0.3% (5 mL, 10 mL)

prednisolone and sulfacetamide *see* sulfacetamide and prednisolone *on page 811*

prednisolone, neomycin, and polymyxin B *see* neomycin, polymyxin B, and prednisolone *on page 598*

prednisolone (ophthalmic) (pred NISS oh lone op THAL mik)
Sound-Alike/Look-Alike Issues
prednisoLONE may be confused with predniSONE
Synonyms prednisolone acetate, ophthalmic; prednisolone sodium phosphate, ophthalmic
Tall-Man prednisoLONE (ophthalmic)
U.S./Canadian Brand Names AK-Pred® [US]; Econopred® Plus [US]; Inflamase® Mild [Can]; Ophtho-Tate® [Can]; Pred Forte® [US/Can]; Pred Mild® [US/Can]
Therapeutic Category Adrenal Corticosteroid
Use Treatment of palpebral and bulbar conjunctivitis; corneal injury from chemical, radiation, thermal burns, or foreign body penetration
Usual Dosage Ophthalmic suspension/solution: Children and Adults: Conjunctivitis, corneal injury: Instill 1-2 drops into conjunctival sac every hour during day, every 2 hours at night until favorable response is obtained, then use 1 drop every 4 hours.
(Continued)

prednisolone (ophthalmic) *(Continued)*

Dosage Forms
Solution, ophthalmic: 1% (5 mL, 10 mL, 15 mL)
Suspension, ophthalmic: 1% (5 mL, 10 mL, 15 mL)
Econopred® Plus: 1% (5 mL, 10 mL)
Pred Forte®: 1% (1 mL, 5 mL, 10 mL, 15 mL)
Pred Mild®: 0.12% (5 mL, 10 mL)

prednisolone sodium phosphate *see* prednisolone (systemic) *on this page*

prednisolone sodium phosphate, ophthalmic *see* prednisolone (ophthalmic) *on previous page*

prednisolone (systemic) (pred NISS oh lone sis TEM ik)

Sound-Alike/Look-Alike Issues
prednisoLONE may be confused with predniSONE
Pediapred® may be confused with Pediazole®

Synonyms deltahydrocortisone; metacortandralone; prednisolone acetate; prednisolone sodium phosphate

Tall-Man prednisoLONE (systemic)

U.S./Canadian Brand Names Bubbli-Pred™ [US]; Diopred® [Can]; Hydeltra T.B.A.® [Can]; Novo-Predniso-lone [Can]; Orapred® [US]; Pediapred® [US/Can]; Prelone® [US]; Sab-Prenase [Can]

Therapeutic Category Adrenal Corticosteroid

Use Treatment of endocrine disorders, rheumatic disorders, collagen diseases, dermatologic diseases, allergic states, ophthalmic diseases, respiratory diseases, hematologic disorders, neoplastic diseases, edematous states, and gastrointestinal diseases; resolution of acute exacerbations of multiple sclerosis

Usual Dosage Dose depends upon condition being treated and response of patient; dosage for infants and children should be based on severity of the disease and response of the patient rather than on strict adherence to dosage indicated by age, weight, or body surface area. Consider alternate day therapy for long-term therapy. Discontinuation of long-term therapy requires gradual withdrawal by tapering the dose. Patients undergoing unusual stress while receiving corticosteroids, should receive increased doses prior to, during, and after the stressful situation.

Children: Oral:
Acute asthma: 1-2 mg/kg/day in divided doses 1-2 times/day for 3-5 days
Antiinflammatory or immunosuppressive dose: 0.1-2 mg/kg/day in divided doses 1-4 times/day
Nephrotic syndrome:
Initial (first 3 episodes): 2 mg/kg/day **or** 60 mg/m^2/day (maximum: 80 mg/day) in divided doses 3-4 times/day until urine is protein free for 3 consecutive days (maximum: 28 days); followed by 1-1.5 mg/kg/dose **or** 40 mg/m^2/dose given every other day for 4 weeks
Maintenance (long-term maintenance dose for frequent relapses): 0.5-1 mg/kg/dose given every other day for 3-6 months
Adults: Oral:
Usual range: 5-60 mg/day
Multiple sclerosis: 200 mg/day for 1 week followed by 80 mg every other day for 1 month
Rheumatoid arthritis: Initial: 5-7.5 mg/day; adjust dose as necessary

Dosage Forms
Solution, oral: Prednisolone 15 mg/5 mL
Solution, oral: Prednisolone 5 mg/5 mL
Orapred®: 20 mg/5 mL
Pediapred®: 6.7 mg/5 mL
Syrup: 5 mg/5 m, 15 mg/5 mL
Prelone®: 15 mg/5 mL
Tablet: 5 mg
Tablet, orally disintegrating:
Orapred ODT™: 10 mg, 15 mg, 30 mg [grape flavor]

prednisone (PRED ni sone)

Sound-Alike/Look-Alike Issues
predniSONE may be confused with methylPREDNISolone, Pramosone®, prazosin, prednisoLONE, Prilosec®, primidone, promethazine

Synonyms deltacortisone; deltadehydrocortisone

Tall-Man predniSONE

U.S./Canadian Brand Names Apo-Prednisone® [Can]; Novo-Prednisone [Can]; Prednisone Intensol™ [US]; Sterapred® DS [US]; Sterapred® [US]; Winpred™ [Can]

Therapeutic Category Adrenal Corticosteroid

Use Treatment of a variety of diseases including adrenocortical insufficiency, hypercalcemia, rheumatic, and collagen disorders; dermatologic, ocular, respiratory, gastrointestinal, and neoplastic diseases; organ transplantation and a variety of diseases including those of hematologic, allergic, inflammatory, and autoimmune in origin; not available in injectable form, prednisolone must be used

Usual Dosage Oral: Dose depends upon condition being treated and response of patient; dosage for infants and children should be based on severity of the disease and response of the patient rather than on strict adherence to dosage indicated by age, weight, or body surface area. Consider alternate day therapy for long-term therapy. Discontinuation of long-term therapy requires gradual withdrawal by tapering the dose.

Children:
Antiinflammatory or immunosuppressive dose: 0.05-2 mg/kg/day divided 1-4 times/day
Acute asthma: 1-2 mg/kg/day in divided doses 1-2 times/day for 3-5 days
Alternatively (for 3- to 5-day "burst"):
<1 year: 10 mg every 12 hours
1-4 years: 20 mg every 12 hours
5-13 years: 30 mg every 12 hours
>13 years: 40 mg every 12 hours
Asthma long-term therapy (alternative dosing by age):
<1 year: 10 mg every other day
1-4 years: 20 mg every other day
5-13 years: 30 mg every other day
>13 years: 40 mg every other day
Nephrotic syndrome:
Initial (first 3 episodes): 2 mg/kg/day **or** 60 mg/m^2/day (maximum: 80 mg/day) in divided doses 3-4 times/day until urine is protein free for 3 consecutive days (maximum: 28 days); followed by 1-1.5 mg/kg/dose **or** 40 mg/m^2/dose given every other day for 4 weeks
Maintenance dose (long-term maintenance dose for frequent relapses): 0.5-1 mg/kg/dose given every other day for 3-6 months
Children and Adults: Physiologic replacement: 4-5 mg/m^2/day
Children ≥5 years and Adults: Asthma:
Moderate persistent: Inhaled corticosteroid (medium dose) or inhaled corticosteroid (low-medium dose) with a long-acting bronchodilator
Severe persistent: Inhaled corticosteroid (high dose) and corticosteroid tablets or syrup long term: 2 mg/kg/day, generally not to exceed 60 mg/day
Adults:
Immunosuppression/chemotherapy adjunct: Range: 5-60 mg/day in divided doses 1-4 times/day
Allergic reaction (contact dermatitis):
Day 1: 30 mg divided as 10 mg before breakfast, 5 mg at lunch, 5 mg at dinner, 10 mg at bedtime
Day 2: 5 mg at breakfast, 5 mg at lunch, 5 mg at dinner, 10 mg at bedtime
Day 3: 5 mg 4 times/day (with meals and at bedtime)
Day 4: 5 mg 3 times/day (breakfast, lunch, bedtime)
Day 5: 5 mg 2 times/day (breakfast, bedtime)
Day 6: 5 mg before breakfast
Pneumocystis carinii pneumonia (PCP):
40 mg twice daily for 5 days **followed by**
40 mg once daily for 5 days **followed by**
20 mg once daily for 11 days or until antimicrobial regimen is completed
Thyrotoxicosis: Oral: 60 mg/day
Chemotherapy (refer to individual protocols): Oral: Range: 20 mg/day to 100 mg/m^2/day
Rheumatoid arthritis: Oral: Use lowest possible daily dose (often ≤7.5 mg/day)
Idiopathic thrombocytopenia purpura (ITP): Oral: 60 mg daily for 4-6 weeks, gradually tapered over several weeks
Systemic lupus erythematosus (SLE): Oral:
Acute: 1-2 mg/kg/day in 2-3 divided doses
Maintenance: Reduce to lowest possible dose, usually <1 mg/kg/day as single dose (morning)

Dosage Forms
Solution, oral: 1 mg/mL
Solution, oral [concentrate]:
PredniSONE Intensol™: 5 mg/mL
Tablet: 1 mg, 2.5 mg, 5 mg, 10 mg, 20 mg, 50 mg
Sterapred®: 5 mg
Sterapred® DS: 10 mg

Prednisone Intensol™ [US] *see* prednisone *on previous page*

Prefest™ [US] *see* estradiol and norgestimate *on page 316*

Prefrin™ *(Discontinued)* *see* phenylephrine *on page 675*

pregabalin (pre GAB a lin)

Synonyms CI-1008; S-(+)-3-isobutylgaba
U.S./Canadian Brand Names Lyrica® [US/Can]
Therapeutic Category Analgesic, Miscellaneous; Anticonvulsant, Miscellaneous
Controlled Substance C-V
Use Management of pain associated with diabetic peripheral neuropathy; management of postherpetic neuralgia; adjunctive therapy for partial-onset seizure disorder in adults; management of fibromyalgia
Usual Dosage Oral: Adults:

Fibromyalgia: Initial: 150 mg/day in divided doses (75 mg 2 times/day); may be increased to 300 mg/day (150 mg 2 times/day) within 1 week based on tolerability and effect; may be further increased to 450 mg/day (225 mg 2 times/day). Maximum dose: 450 mg/day (dosages up to 600 mg/day were evaluated with no significant additional benefit and an increase in adverse effects)

Neuropathic pain (diabetes-associated): Initial: 150 mg/day in divided doses (50 mg 3 times/day); may be increased within 1 week based on tolerability and effect; maximum dose: 300 mg/day (dosages up to 600 mg/day were evaluated with no significant additional benefit and an increase in adverse effects)

Postherpetic neuralgia: Initial: 150 mg/day in divided doses (75 mg 2 times/day or 50 mg 3 times/day); may be increased to 300 mg/day within 1 week based on tolerability and effect; further titration (to 600 mg/day) after 2-4 weeks may be considered in patients who do not experience sufficient relief of pain provided they are able to tolerate pregabalin. Maximum dose: 600 mg/day

Partial-onset seizures (adjunctive therapy): Initial: 150 mg per day in divided doses (75 mg 2 times/day or 50 mg 3 times/day); may be increased based on tolerability and effect (optimal titration schedule has not been defined). Maximum dose: 600 mg/day

Discontinuing therapy: Pregabalin should not be abruptly discontinued; taper dosage over at least 1 week
Dosage Forms
Capsule:
Lyrica®: 25 mg, 50 mg, 75 mg, 100 mg, 150 mg, 200 mg, 225 mg, 300 mg

Pregestimil® [US-OTC] *see* nutritional formula, enteral/oral *on page 622*

pregnenedione *see* progesterone *on page 718*

Pregnyl® [US/Can] *see* chorionic gonadotropin (human) *on page 187*

Prelone® [US] *see* prednisolone (systemic) *on page 710*

Prelu-2® *(Discontinued)* *see* phendimetrazine *on page 671*

Premarin® [US/Can] *see* estrogens (conjugated/equine) *on page 318*

Premarin® With Methyltestosterone *(Discontinued)*

Premjact® [US-OTC] *see* lidocaine *on page 504*

Premphase® [US/Can] *see* estrogens (conjugated/equine) and medroxyprogesterone *on page 318*

Premplus® [Can] *see* estrogens (conjugated/equine) and medroxyprogesterone *on page 318*

Prempro™ [US/Can] *see* estrogens (conjugated/equine) and medroxyprogesterone *on page 318*

Prenatal AD [US] *see* vitamins (multiple/prenatal) *on page 896*

Prenatal H [US] *see* vitamins (multiple/prenatal) *on page 896*

Prenatal MR 90 Fe™ [US] *see* vitamins (multiple/prenatal) *on page 896*

Prenatal MTR with Selenium [US] *see* vitamins (multiple/prenatal) *on page 896*

Prenatal Plus [US] *see* vitamins (multiple/prenatal) *on page 896*

Prenatal Rx 1 [US] *see* vitamins (multiple/prenatal) *on page 896*

Prenatal U [US] *see* vitamins (multiple/prenatal) *on page 896*

prenatal vitamins *see* vitamins (multiple/prenatal) *on page 896*

Prenatal Z [US] *see* vitamins (multiple/prenatal) *on page 896*

Prenate DHA™ [US] *see* vitamins (multiple/prenatal) *on page 896*

Prenate Elite™ [US] *see* vitamins (multiple/prenatal) *on page 896*

Preparation H® [US-OTC] *see* phenylephrine *on page 675*

Preparation H® Cleansing Pads [Can] *see* witch hazel *on page 900*

Preparation H® Hydrocortisone [US-OTC] *see* hydrocortisone (rectal) *on page 433*

Preparation H® Medicated Wipes [US-OTC] *see* witch hazel *on page 900*

Prepcat [US] *see* barium *on page 94*

Pre-Pen® *(Discontinued)* *see* benzylpenicilloyl-polylysine *on page 106*

Prepidil® **[US/Can]** *see* dinoprostone *on page 264*

Prescription Strength Desenex® *(Discontinued)* *see* miconazole *on page 566*

Preservative-Free Cosopt® **[Can]** *see* dorzolamide and timolol *on page 277*

PreserVision® **AREDS [US-OTC]** *see* vitamins (multiple/oral) *on page 895*

PreserVision® **Lutein [US-OTC]** *see* vitamins (multiple/oral) *on page 895*

Pressyn® **[Can]** *see* vasopressin *on page 886*

Pressyn® **AR [Can]** *see* vasopressin *on page 886*

Pretz® **[US-OTC]** *see* sodium chloride *on page 792*

Pretz-D® **[US-OTC]** *see* ephedrine *on page 299*

Prevacare® **[US-OTC]** *see* alcohol (ethyl) *on page 25*

Prevacid® **[US/Can]** *see* lansoprazole *on page 492*

Prevacid® **NapraPAC**™ **[US]** *see* lansoprazole and naproxen *on page 493*

Prevacid® **SoluTab**™ **[US]** *see* lansoprazole *on page 492*

Prevalite® **[US]** *see* cholestyramine resin *on page 186*

Prevex® **B [Can]** *see* betamethasone (topical) *on page 109*

Prevex® **HC [Can]** *see* hydrocortisone (topical) *on page 434*

PreviDent® **[US]** *see* fluoride *on page 361*

PreviDent® **5000 Plus**™ **[US]** *see* fluoride *on page 361*

Previfem™ **[US]** *see* ethinyl estradiol and norgestimate *on page 331*

Prevnar® **[US/Can]** *see* pneumococcal conjugate vaccine (7-valent) *on page 691*

Prevpac® **[US/Can]** *see* lansoprazole, amoxicillin, and clarithromycin *on page 493*

Prexige® **[Can]** *see* lumiracoxib *(Canada only) on page 522*

Prezista™ **[US]** *see* darunavir *on page 232*

Prialt® **[US]** *see* ziconotide *on page 903*

Priftin® **[US/Can]** *see* rifapentine *on page 758*

prilocaine (PRIL oh kane)

Sound-Alike/Look-Alike Issues
prilocaine may be confused with Polocaine®, Prilosec®

U.S./Canadian Brand Names Citanest® Plain [US/Can]

Therapeutic Category Local Anesthetic

Usual Dosage
Children <10 years: Doses >40 mg (1 mL) as a 4% solution per procedure rarely needed

Children >10 years and Adults: Dental anesthesia, infiltration, or conduction block: Initial: 40-80 mg (1-2 mL) as a 4% solution; up to a maximum of 400 mg (10 mL) as a 4% solution within a 2-hour period. Manufacturer's maximum recommended dose is not more than 600 mg to normal healthy adults. The effective anesthetic dose varies with procedure, intensity of anesthesia needed, duration of anesthesia required and physical condition of the patient. Always use the lowest effective dose along with careful aspiration.

Note: Adult and children doses of prilocaine hydrochloride cited from USP Dispensing Information (USP DI), 17th ed, The United States Pharmacopeial Convention, Inc, Rockville, MD, 1997, 139.

Dosage Forms
Injection, solution:
Citanest® Plain Dental: Prilocaine 4% (1.8 mL)

prilocaine and lidocaine *see* lidocaine and prilocaine *on page 507*

Prilosec® **[US]** *see* omeprazole *on page 629*

Prilosec OTC™ **[US-OTC]** *see* omeprazole *on page 629*

PrimaCare® **[US]** *see* vitamins (multiple/prenatal) *on page 896*

PrimaCare® **One [US]** *see* vitamins (multiple/prenatal) *on page 896*

primaclone *see* primidone *on next page*

Primacor® **[US/Can]** *see* milrinone *on page 570*

primaquine (PRIM a kween)

Synonyms primaquine phosphate; prymaccone

Therapeutic Category Aminoquinoline (Antimalarial)

Use Treatment of malaria

Usual Dosage Oral: Dosage expressed as mg of base (15 mg base = 26.3 mg primaquine phosphate):

Treatment of malaria (decrease risk of delayed primary attacks and prevent relapse):

Children: 0.3 mg base/kg/day once daily for 14 days (not to exceed 15 mg/day) or 0.9 mg base/kg once weekly for 8 weeks not to exceed 45 mg base/week

Adults: 15 mg/day (base) once daily for 14 days or 45 mg base once weekly for 8 weeks

CDC treatment recommendations: Begin therapy during last 2 weeks of, or following a course of, suppression with chloroquine or a comparable drug

Note: A second course (30 mg/day) for 14 days may be required in patients with relapse. Higher initial doses (30 mg/day) have also been used following exposure in S.E. Asia or Somalia.

Dosage Forms

Tablet: 26.3 mg

primaquine phosphate *see* primaquine *on this page*

Primatene® Mist [US-OTC] *see* epinephrine *on page 300*

Primaxin® [US/Can] *see* imipenem and cilastatin *on page 449*

Primaxin® I.V. [Can] *see* imipenem and cilastatin *on page 449*

primidone (PRI mi done)

Sound-Alike/Look-Alike Issues

primidone may be confused with predniSONE

Synonyms desoxyphenobarbital; primaclone

U.S./Canadian Brand Names Apo-Primidone® [Can]; Mysoline® [US]

Therapeutic Category Anticonvulsant; Barbiturate

Use Management of grand mal, psychomotor, and focal seizures

Usual Dosage Oral:

Children <8 years: Initial: 50-125 mg/day given at bedtime; increase by 50-125 mg/day increments every 3-7 days; usual dose: 10-25 mg/kg/day in divided doses 3-4 times/day

Children ≥8 years and Adults: Initial: 125-250 mg/day at bedtime; increase by 125-250 mg/day every 3-7 days; usual dose: 750-1500 mg/day in divided doses 3-4 times/day with maximum dosage of 2 g/day

Dosage Forms [CAN] = Canadian brand name

Tablet: 50 mg [U.S. only], 125 [CAN only], 250 mg

Mysoline®: 50 mg, 250 mg

Primsol® [US] *see* trimethoprim *on page 867*

Prinivil® [US/Can] *see* lisinopril *on page 512*

Prinzide® [US/Can] *see* lisinopril and hydrochlorothiazide *on page 512*

Priorix™ [Can] *see* measles, mumps, and rubella vaccines, combined *on page 533*

Priscoline® *(Discontinued)*

pristinamycin *see* quinupristin and dalfopristin *on page 741*

Privine® [US-OTC] *see* naphazoline *on page 590*

ProAir™ HFA [US] *see* albuterol *on page 23*

ProAmatine® [US] *see* midodrine *on page 569*

Pro-Banthine® *(Discontinued) see* propantheline *on page 721*

probenecid (proe BEN e sid)

Sound-Alike/Look-Alike Issues

probenecid may be confused with Procanbid®

U.S./Canadian Brand Names Benuryl™ [Can]

Therapeutic Category Uricosuric Agent

Use Prevention of hyperuricemia associated with gout or gouty arthritis; prolongation and elevation of beta-lactam plasma levels

Usual Dosage Oral:

Children:

<2 years: Contraindicated

2-14 years: Prolong penicillin serum levels: Initial: 25 mg/kg, then 40 mg/kg/day given 4 times/day (maximum: 500 mg/dose)

Gonorrhea: >45 kg: Refer to adult guidelines

Adults:

Hyperuricemia with gout: 250 mg twice daily for one week; increase to 250-500 mg/day; may increase by 500 mg/month, if needed, to maximum of 2-3 g/day (dosages may be increased by 500 mg every 6 months if serum urate concentrations are controlled)

Prolong penicillin serum levels: 500 mg 4 times/day

Gonorrhea: CDC guidelines (alternative regimen): Probenecid 1 g orally with cefoxitin 2 g I.M.

Pelvic inflammatory disease: CDC guidelines: Cefoxitin 2 g I.M. plus probenecid 1 g orally as a single dose

Neurosyphilis: CDC guidelines (alternative regimen): Procaine penicillin 2.4 million units/day I.M. plus probenecid 500 mg 4 times/day; both administered for 10-14 days

Dosage Forms

Tablet: 500 mg

probenecid and colchicine *see* colchicine and probenecid *on page 211*

Pro-Bionate® *(Discontinued)*

procainamide (pro KANE a mide)

Sound-Alike/Look-Alike Issues

Procanbid® may be confused with probenecid

Pronestyl® may be confused with Ponstel®

PCA is an error-prone abbreviation (mistaken as patient controlled analgesia)

Synonyms procainamide hydrochloride; procaine amide hydrochloride

U.S./Canadian Brand Names Apo-Procainamide® [Can]; Procainamide Hydrochloride Injection, USP [Can]; Procanbid® [US]; Procan® SR [Can]; Pronestyl®-SR [Can]

Therapeutic Category Antiarrhythmic Agent, Class I-A

Use Treatment of ventricular tachycardia (VT), premature ventricular contractions, paroxysmal atrial tachycardia (PSVT), and atrial fibrillation (AF); prevent recurrence of ventricular tachycardia, paroxysmal supraventricular tachycardia, atrial fibrillation or flutter

Usual Dosage Must be titrated to patient's response

Children:

Oral: 15-50 mg/kg/24 hours divided every 3-6 hours

I.M.: 50 mg/kg/24 hours divided into doses of $1/8$ to $1/4$ every 3-6 hours in divided doses until oral therapy is possible

I.V. (infusion requires use of an infusion pump):

Load: 3-6 mg/kg/dose over 5 minutes not to exceed 100 mg/dose; may repeat every 5-10 minutes to maximum of 15 mg/kg/load

Maintenance as continuous I.V. infusion: 20-80 mcg/kg/minute; maximum: 2 g/24 hours

Possible VT (pulses and poor perfusion) [PALS 2005 Guidelines]: I.V.; I.O.: 15 mg/kg over 30-60 minutes

Adults:

Oral: Usual dose: 50 mg/kg/24 hours: maximum: 5 g/24 hours (**Note:** Twice-daily dosing approved for Procanbid®.)

Immediate release formulation: 250-500 mg/dose every 3-6 hours

Extended release formulation: 500 mg to 1 g every 6 hours; Procanbid®: 1000-2500 mg every 12 hours

I.M.: 0.5-1 g every 4-8 hours until oral therapy is possible

I.V. (infusion requires use of an infusion pump):

Loading dose: 15-18 mg/kg administered as slow infusion over 25-30 minutes **or** 100-200 mg/dose repeated every 5 minutes as needed to a total dose of 1 g. Reduce loading dose to 12 mg/kg in severe renal or cardiac impairment.

Maintenance dose: 1-4 mg/minute by continuous infusion. Maintenance infusions should be reduced by one-third in patients with moderate renal or cardiac impairment and by two-thirds in patients with severe renal or cardiac impairment.

ACLS guidelines: Infuse 20 mg/minute until arrhythmia is controlled, hypotension occurs, QRS complex widens by 50% of its original width, or total of 17 mg/kg is given.

Dosage Forms

Capsule: 250 mg, 500 mg

Injection, solution: 100 mg/mL (10 mL); 500 mg/mL (2 mL)

Tablet, extended release: 500 mg, 750 mg, 1000 mg

Procanbid®: 500 mg, 1000 mg

procainamide hydrochloride *see* procainamide *on this page*

Procainamide Hydrochloride Injection, USP [Can] *see* procainamide *on this page*

procaine (PROE kane)
Synonyms procaine hydrochloride
U.S./Canadian Brand Names Novocain® [US]
Therapeutic Category Local Anesthetic
Use Produces spinal anesthesia
Usual Dosage Dose varies with procedure, desired depth, and duration of anesthesia, desired muscle relaxation, vascularity of tissues, physical condition, and age of patient
Adults: Spinal analgesia: Extent of anesthesia:
Perineum: Total dose: 50 mg; Procaine 10%: 0.5 mL with 0.5 mL diluent
Perineum and lower extremities: Total dose: 100 mg; Procaine 10%: 1 mL with 1 mL diluent
Up to costal margin: Total dose: 200 mg; Procaine 10%: 2 mL with 1 mL diluent
Dosage Forms
Injection, solution:
Novocain®: 10% (2 mL)

procaine amide hydrochloride see procainamide on previous page

procaine benzylpenicillin see penicillin G procaine on page 663

procaine hydrochloride see procaine on this page

procaine penicillin G see penicillin G procaine on page 663

Pro-Cal-Sof® *(Discontinued)* see docusate on page 273

Procanbid® [US] see procainamide on previous page

Procan® SR [Can] see procainamide on previous page

procarbazine (proe KAR ba zeen)
Sound-Alike/Look-Alike Issues
procarbazine may be confused with dacarbazine
Matulane® may be confused with Modane®
Synonyms benzmethyzin; N-methylhydrazine; NSC-77213; procarbazine hydrochloride
U.S./Canadian Brand Names Matulane® [US/Can]; Natulan® [Can]
Therapeutic Category Antineoplastic Agent
Use Treatment of Hodgkin disease
Usual Dosage Refer to individual protocols. Manufacturer states that the dose is based on patient's ideal weight if the patient is obese or has abnormal fluid retention. Other studies suggest that ideal body weight may not be necessary. Oral (may be given as a single daily dose or in 2-3 divided doses):
Children:
BMT aplastic anemia conditioning regimen: 12.5 mg/kg/day every other day for 4 doses
Hodgkin's disease: MOPP/IC-MOPP regimens: 100 mg/m^2/day for 14 days and repeated every 4 weeks
Neuroblastoma and medulloblastoma: Doses as high as 100-200 mg/m^2/day once daily have been used
Adults: Initial: 2-4 mg/kg/day in single or divided doses for 7 days then increase dose to 4-6 mg/kg/day until response is obtained or leukocyte count decreased <4000/mm^3 or the platelet count decreased <100,000/mm^3; maintenance: 1-2 mg/kg/day
Dosage Forms
Capsule:
Matulane®: 50 mg

procarbazine hydrochloride see procarbazine on this page

Procardia® [US/Can] see nifedipine on page 605

Procardia XL® [US] see nifedipine on page 605

procetofene see fenofibrate on page 345

Prochieve® [US] see progesterone on page 718

prochlorperazine (proe klor PER a zeen)
Sound-Alike/Look-Alike Issues
prochlorperazine may be confused with chlorproMAZINE
Compazine® may be confused with Copaxone®, Coumadin®
CPZ (occasional abbreviation for Compazine®) is an error-prone abbreviation (mistaken as chlorpromazine)
Synonyms chlormeprazine; prochlorperazine edisylate; prochlorperazine maleate
U.S./Canadian Brand Names Apo-Prochlorperazine® [Can]; Compazine® [Can]; Compro™ [US]; Nu-Prochlor [Can]; Stemetil® [Can]
Therapeutic Category Phenothiazine Derivative
Use Management of nausea and vomiting; psychotic disorders including schizophrenia; anxiety

Usual Dosage
Antiemetic: Children (therapy >1 day usually not required): **Note:** Not recommended for use in children <9 kg or <2 years:
Oral, rectal: >9 kg: 0.4 mg/kg/24 hours in 3-4 divided doses; **or**
9-13 kg: 2.5 mg every 12-24 hours as needed; maximum: 7.5 mg/day
13.1-17 kg: 2.5 mg every 8-12 hours as needed; maximum: 10 mg/day
17.1-37 kg: 2.5 mg every 8 hours or 5 mg every 12 hours as needed; maximum: 15 mg/day
I.M.: 0.13 mg/kg/dose; change to oral as soon as possible
Antiemetic: Adults:
Oral (tablet): 5-10 mg 3-4 times/day; usual maximum: 40 mg/day; larger doses may rarely be required
I.M. (deep): 5-10 mg every 3-4 hours; usual maximum: 40 mg/day
I.V.: 2.5-10 mg; maximum 10 mg/dose or 40 mg/day; may repeat dose every 3-4 hours as needed
Rectal: 25 mg twice daily
Surgical nausea/vomiting: Adults: **Note:** Should not exceed 40 mg/day
I.M.: 5-10 mg 1-2 hours before induction or to control symptoms during or after surgery; may repeat once if necessary
I.V. (administer slow IVP <5 mg/minute): 5-10 mg 15-30 minutes before induction or to control symptoms during or after surgery; may repeat once if necessary
Antipsychotic:
Children 2-12 years (not recommended in children <9 kg or <2 years):
Oral, rectal: 2.5 mg 2-3 times/day; do not give more than 10 mg the first day; increase dosage as needed to maximum daily dose of 20 mg for 2-5 years and 25 mg for 6-12 years
I.M.: 0.13 mg/kg/dose; change to oral as soon as possible
Adults:
Oral: 5-10 mg 3-4 times/day; titrate dose slowly every 2-3 days; doses up to 150 mg/day may be required in some patients for treatment of severe disturbances
I.M.: Initial: 10-20 mg; if necessary repeat initial dose every 1-4 hours to gain control; more than 3-4 doses are rarely needed. If parenteral administration is still required; give 10-20 mg every 4-6 hours; change to oral as soon as possible.
Nonpsychotic anxiety: Oral (tablet): Adults: Usual dose: 15-20 mg/day in divided doses; do not give doses >20 mg/day or for longer than 12 weeks
Dosage Forms
Injection, solution: 5 mg/mL (2 mL, 10 mL)
Suppository, rectal: 2.5 mg (12s), 5 mg (12s), 25 mg (12s)
Compro™: 25 mg (12s)
Tablet: 5 mg, 10 mg

prochlorperazine edisylate see prochlorperazine on previous page

prochlorperazine maleate see prochlorperazine on previous page

Procrit® [US] see epoetin alfa on page 303

Proctocort® [US] see hydrocortisone (rectal) on page 433

ProctoCream® HC [US] see hydrocortisone (rectal) on page 433

proctofene see fenofibrate on page 345

ProctoFoam®-HC [US/Can] see pramoxine and hydrocortisone on page 707

ProctoFoam® NS [US-OTC] see pramoxine on page 706

Procto-Kit™ [US] see hydrocortisone (rectal) on page 433

Procto-Pak™ [US] see hydrocortisone (rectal) on page 433

Proctosert [US] see hydrocortisone (rectal) on page 433

Proctosol-HC® [US] see hydrocortisone (rectal) on page 433

Proctozone-HC™ [US] see hydrocortisone (rectal) on page 433

procyclidine (proe SYE kli deen)
Sound-Alike/Look-Alike Issues
Kemadrin® may be confused with Coumadin®
Synonyms procyclidine hydrochloride
U.S./Canadian Brand Names Kemadrin® [US]; PMS-Procyclidine [Can]
Therapeutic Category Anti-Parkinson Agent; Anticholinergic Agent
Use Relieves symptoms of parkinsonian syndrome and drug-induced extrapyramidal symptoms
Usual Dosage Oral: Adults: 2.5 mg 3 times/day after meals; if tolerated, gradually increase dose, maximum of 20 mg/day if necessary
(Continued)

procyclidine *(Continued)*

Dosage Forms
Tablet [scored]:
Kemadrin®: 5 mg

procyclidine hydrochloride *see* procyclidine *on previous page*

Procytox® [Can] *see* cyclophosphamide *on page 222*

Prodium® [US-OTC] *see* phenazopyridine *on page 671*

Pro Doc Limitee [Can] *see* bromazepam *(Canada only) on page 119*

Profasi® HP [Can] *see* chorionic gonadotropin (human) *on page 187*

Profen II DM® [US] *see* guaifenesin, pseudoephedrine, and dextromethorphan *on page 408*

Profen Forte™ DM [US] *see* guaifenesin, pseudoephedrine, and dextromethorphan *on page 408*

Profen LA® *(Discontinued)*

Profilnine® SD [US] *see* factor IX complex (human) *on page 341*

Proflavanol C™ [Can] *see* ascorbic acid *on page 76*

progesterone *(proe JES ter one)*

Synonyms pregnenedione; progestin
U.S./Canadian Brand Names Crinone® [US/Can]; Endometrin® [US]; Prochieve® [US]; Prometrium® [US/Can]
Therapeutic Category Progestin
Use
Oral: Prevention of endometrial hyperplasia in nonhysterectomized, postmenopausal women who are receiving conjugated estrogen tablets; secondary amenorrhea
I.M.: Amenorrhea; abnormal uterine bleeding due to hormonal imbalance
Intravaginal gel: Part of assisted reproductive technology (ART) for infertile women with progesterone deficiency; secondary amenorrhea
Vaginal tablet: Part of ART for infertile women with progesterone deficiency
Usual Dosage Adults:
I.M.: Female:
Amenorrhea: 5-10 mg/day for 6-8 consecutive days
Functional uterine bleeding: 5-10 mg/day for 6 doses
Oral: Female:
Prevention of endometrial hyperplasia (in postmenopausal women with a uterus who are receiving daily conjugated estrogen tablets): 200 mg as a single daily dose every evening for 12 days sequentially per 28-day cycle
Amenorrhea: 400 mg every evening for 10 days
Intravaginal gel: Female:
ART in women who require progesterone supplementation: 90 mg (8% gel) once daily; if pregnancy occurs, may continue treatment for up to 10-12 weeks
ART in women with partial or complete ovarian failure: 90 mg (8% gel) intravaginally twice daily; if pregnancy occurs, may continue up to 10-12 weeks
Secondary amenorrhea: 45 mg (4% gel) intravaginally every other day for up to 6 doses; women who fail to respond may be increased to 90 mg (8% gel) every other day for up to 6 doses
Intravaginal tablet: Female: ART: 100 mg 2-3 times daily starting at oocyte retrieval and continuing for up to 10 weeks.
Dosage Forms
Capsule:
Prometrium®: 100 mg, 200 mg
Gel, vaginal:
Crinone®, Prochieve®: 4% (45 mg); 8% (90 mg)
Injection, oil: 50 mg/mL (10 mL)
Tablet, vaginal:
Endometrin®: 100 mg (21s)

progestin *see* progesterone *on this page*

Proglycem® [US/Can] *see* diazoxide *on page 252*

Prograf® [US/Can] *see* tacrolimus *on page 818*

proguanil and atovaquone *see* atovaquone and proguanil *on page 82*

ProHance® [US] *see* gadoteridol *on page 382*

ProHIBiT® *(Discontinued)*

Prolastin® **[US/Can]** *see* alpha₁-proteinase inhibitor *on page 32*

Proleukin® **[US/Can]** *see* aldesleukin *on page 26*

Prolex®**-D [US]** *see* guaifenesin and phenylephrine *on page 404*

Prolex®**-PD [US]** *see* guaifenesin and phenylephrine *on page 404*

Prolixin Decanoate® **[US]** *see* fluphenazine *on page 365*

Prolixin® *(Discontinued) see* fluphenazine *on page 365*

Prolixin Enanthate® *(Discontinued) see* fluphenazine *on page 365*

Prolopa® **[Can]** *see* benserazide and levodopa *(Canada only) on page 99*

Proloprim® **[US]** *see* trimethoprim *on page 867*

Promacet [US] *see* butalbital and acetaminophen *on page 131*

Prometa® *(Discontinued)*

promethazine (proe METH a zeen)

Sound-Alike/Look-Alike Issues
promethazine may be confused with chlorproMAZINE, predniSONE, promazine
Phenergan® may be confused with Phenaphen®, Phrenilin®, Theragran®
Synonyms promethazine hydrochloride
U.S./Canadian Brand Names Phenadoz™ [US]; Phenergan® [US/Can]; Promethegan™ [US]
Therapeutic Category Antiemetic; Phenothiazine Derivative
Use Symptomatic treatment of various allergic conditions; antiemetic; motion sickness; sedative; postoperative pain (adjunctive therapy); anesthetic (adjunctive therapy); anaphylactic reactions (adjunctive therapy)
Usual Dosage
Children ≥2 years:
Allergic conditions: Oral, rectal: 0.1 mg/kg/dose (maximum: 12.5 mg) every 6 hours during the day and 0.5 mg/kg/dose (maximum: 25 mg) at bedtime as needed
Antiemetic: Oral, I.M., I.V., rectal: 0.25-1 mg/kg 4-6 times/day as needed (maximum: 25 mg/dose)
Motion sickness: Oral, rectal: 0.5 mg/kg/dose 30 minutes to 1 hour before departure, then every 12 hours as needed (maximum dose: 25 mg twice daily)
Sedation: Oral, I.M., I.V., rectal: 0.5-1 mg/kg/dose every 6 hours as needed (maximum: 50 mg/dose)
Adults:
Allergic conditions (including allergic reactions to blood or plasma):
Oral, rectal: 25 mg at bedtime **or** 12.5 mg before meals and at bedtime (range: 6.25-12.5 mg 3 times/day)
I.M., I.V.: 25 mg, may repeat in 2 hours when necessary; switch to oral route as soon as feasible
Antiemetic: Oral, I.M., I.V., rectal: 12.5-25 mg every 4-6 hours as needed
Motion sickness: Oral, rectal: 25 mg 30-60 minutes before departure, then every 12 hours as needed
Sedation: Oral, I.M., I.V., rectal: 12.5-50 mg/dose
Dosage Forms
Injection, solution: 25 mg/mL (1 mL); 50 mg/mL (1 mL)
Phenergan®: 25 mg/mL (1 mL); 50 mg/mL (1 mL)
Suppository, rectal: 12.5 mg, 25 mg, 50 mg
Phenadoz™: 12.5 mg, 25 mg
Promethegan™: 12.5 mg, 25 mg, 50 mg
Syrup: 6.25 mg/5 mL
Tablet: 12.5 mg, 25 mg, 50 mg

promethazine and codeine (proe METH a zeen & KOE deen)

Synonyms codeine and promethazine
Therapeutic Category Antihistamine/Antitussive
Controlled Substance C-V
Use Temporary relief of coughs and upper respiratory symptoms associated with allergy or the common cold
Usual Dosage Oral: Children ≥16 years and Adults: 5 mL every 4-6 hours (maximum: 30 mL/24 hours)
Dosage Forms
Syrup: Promethazine 6.25 mg and codeine 10 mg per 5 mL

promethazine and dextromethorphan (proe METH a zeen & deks troe meth OR fan)

Synonyms dextromethorphan and promethazine
Therapeutic Category Antihistamine/Antitussive
Use Temporary relief of coughs and upper respiratory symptoms associated with allergy or the common cold
(Continued)

promethazine and dextromethorphan *(Continued)*
Usual Dosage Oral:
Children:
2-6 years: 1.25-2.5 mL every 4-6 hours up to 10 mL in 24 hours
6-12 years: 2.5-5 mL every 4-6 hours up to 20 mL in 24 hours
Adults: 5 mL every 4-6 hours up to 30 mL in 24 hours
Dosage Forms
Syrup: Promethazine 6.25 mg and dextromethorphan 15 mg per 5 mL

promethazine and meperidine *see* meperidine and promethazine *on page 542*

promethazine and phenylephrine (proe METH a zeen & fen il EF rin)
Synonyms phenylephrine and promethazine
Therapeutic Category Antihistamine/Decongestant Combination
Use Temporary relief of upper respiratory symptoms associated with allergy or the common cold
Usual Dosage Oral:
Children:
2-6 years: 1.25-2.5 mL every 4-6 hours, not to exceed 7.5 mL in 24 hours
6-12 years: 2.5-5 mL every 4-6 hours, not to exceed 30 mL in 24 hours
Children >12 years and Adults: 5 mL every 4-6 hours, not to exceed 30 mL in 24 hours
Dosage Forms
Syrup: Promethazine 6.25 mg and phenylephrine 5 mg per 5 mL

promethazine hydrochloride *see* promethazine *on previous page*

promethazine, phenylephrine, and codeine (proe METH a zeen, fen il EF rin, & KOE deen)
Synonyms codeine, promethazine, and phenylephrine; phenylephrine, promethazine, and codeine
Therapeutic Category Antihistamine/Decongestant/Antitussive
Controlled Substance C-V
Use Temporary relief of coughs and upper respiratory symptoms including nasal congestion associated with allergy or the common cold
Usual Dosage Oral: Children ≥16 years and Adults: 5 mL every 4-6 hours, not to exceed 30 mL/24 hours
Dosage Forms
Syrup: Promethazine 6.25 mg, phenylephrine 5 mg, and codeine 10 mg per 5 mL

Promethegan™ [US] *see* promethazine *on previous page*

Promethist® With Codeine *(Discontinued)* *see* promethazine, phenylephrine, and codeine *on this page*

Prometh® VC Plain Liquid *(Discontinued)* *see* promethazine and phenylephrine *on this page*

Prometh® VC With Codeine *(Discontinued)* *see* promethazine, phenylephrine, and codeine *on this page*

Prometrium® [US/Can] *see* progesterone *on page 718*

Promit® *(Discontinued)* *see* dextran 1 *on page 245*

Pronap-100® [US] *see* propoxyphene and acetaminophen *on page 723*

Pronestyl® *(Discontinued)* *see* procainamide *on page 715*

Pronestyl®-SR [Can] *see* procainamide *on page 715*

Pronto® Complete Lice Removal System [US-OTC] *see* pyrethrins and piperonyl butoxide *on page 734*

Pronto® Lice Control [Can] *see* pyrethrins and piperonyl butoxide *on page 734*

Pronto® Plus Hair and Scalp Masque *(Discontinued)* *see* pyrethrins and piperonyl butoxide *on page 734*

Pronto® Plus Lice Egg Remover Kit [US-OTC] *see* benzalkonium chloride *on page 100*

Pronto® Plus Lice Killing Mousse Plus Vitamin E [US-OTC] *see* pyrethrins and piperonyl butoxide *on page 734*

Pronto® Plus Lice Killing Mousse Shampoo Plus Natural Extracts and Oils [US-OTC] *see* pyrethrins and piperonyl butoxide *on page 734*

Pronto® Plus Warm Oil Treatment and Conditioner [US-OTC] *see* pyrethrins and piperonyl butoxide *on page 734*

Propac™ [US-OTC] *see* nutritional formula, enteral/oral *on page 622*

Propacet® *(Discontinued)* *see* propoxyphene and acetaminophen *on page 723*

Propaderm® **[Can]** *see* beclomethasone *on page 97*

propafenone (pro PAF en one)

Synonyms propafenone hydrochloride

U.S./Canadian Brand Names Apo-Propafenone® [Can]; Rythmol® Gen-Propafenone [Can]; Rythmol® SR [US]; Rythmol® [US]

Therapeutic Category Antiarrhythmic Agent, Class I-C

Use Treatment of life-threatening ventricular arrhythmias

Rythmol® SR: Maintenance of normal sinus rhythm in patients with symptomatic atrial fibrillation

Usual Dosage Oral: Adults: **Note:** Patients who exhibit significant widening of QRS complex or second- or third-degree AV block may need dose reduction.

Ventricular arrhythmias:

Immediate release tablet: Initial: 150 mg every 8 hours, increase at 3- to 4-day intervals up to 300 mg every 8 hours.

Extended release capsule: Initial: 225 mg every 12 hours; dosage increase may be made at a minimum of 5-day intervals; may increase to 325 mg every 12 hours; if further increase is necessary, may increase to 425 mg every 12 hours

Dosage Forms

Capsule, extended release:

Rythmol® SR: 225 mg, 325 mg, 425 mg

Tablet: 150 mg, 225 mg, 300 mg

Rythmol®: 150 mg, 225 mg, 300 mg

propafenone hydrochloride *see* propafenone *on this page*

Propagest® *(Discontinued)*

propantheline (proe PAN the leen)

Synonyms propantheline bromide

Therapeutic Category Anticholinergic Agent

Use Adjunctive treatment of peptic ulcer, irritable bowel syndrome, pancreatitis, ureteral and urinary bladder spasm; reduce duodenal motility during diagnostic radiologic procedures

Usual Dosage Oral:

Antisecretory:

Children: 1-2 mg/kg/day in 3-4 divided doses

Adults: 15 mg 3 times/day before meals or food and 30 mg at bedtime

Antispasmodic:

Children: 2-3 mg/kg/day in divided doses every 4-6 hours and at bedtime

Adults: 15 mg 3 times/day before meals or food and 30 mg at bedtime

Dosage Forms

Tablet: 15 mg

propantheline bromide *see* propantheline *on this page*

Propa pH [US-OTC] *see* salicylic acid *on page 772*

proparacaine (proe PAR a kane)

Sound-Alike/Look-Alike Issues

proparacaine may be confused with propoxyphene

Synonyms proparacaine hydrochloride; proxymetacaine

U.S./Canadian Brand Names Alcaine® [US/Can]; Diocaine® [Can]; Ophthetic® [US]

Therapeutic Category Local Anesthetic

Use Anesthesia for tonometry, gonioscopy; suture removal from cornea; removal of corneal foreign body; cataract extraction, glaucoma surgery; short operative procedure involving the cornea and conjunctiva

Usual Dosage Children and Adults:

Ophthalmic surgery: Instill 1 drop of 0.5% solution in eye every 5-10 minutes for 5-7 doses

Tonometry, gonioscopy, suture removal: Instill 1-2 drops of 0.5% solution in eye just prior to procedure

Dosage Forms

Solution, ophthalmic: 0.5% (15 mL)

Alcaine®, Ophthetic®: 0.5% (15 mL)

proparacaine and fluorescein (proe PAR a kane & FLURE e seen)

Synonyms fluorescein and proparacaine

U.S./Canadian Brand Names Flucaine® [US]; Fluoracaine® [US]

Therapeutic Category Diagnostic Agent; Local Anesthetic

Use Anesthesia for tonometry, gonioscopy; suture removal from cornea; removal of corneal foreign body; cataract extraction, glaucoma surgery

Usual Dosage

Ophthalmic surgery: Children and Adults: Instill 1 drop in each eye every 5-10 minutes for 5-7 doses

Tonometry, gonioscopy, suture removal: Adults: Instill 1-2 drops in each eye just prior to procedure

Dosage Forms

Solution, ophthalmic: Proparacaine 0.5% and fluorescein 0.25% (5 mL)

Flucaine®: Proparacaine 0.5% and fluorescein 0.25% (5 mL)

proparacaine hydrochloride *see* proparacaine *on previous page*

Propecia® [US/Can] *see* finasteride *on page 353*

Propine® [US/Can] *see* dipivefrin *on page 270*

Proplex® T (Discontinued) *see* factor IX complex (human) *on page 341*

propofol (PROE po fole)

Sound-Alike/Look-Alike Issues

Diprivan® may be confused with Diflucan®, Ditropan®

U.S./Canadian Brand Names Diprivan® [US/Can]

Therapeutic Category General Anesthetic

Use Induction of anesthesia for inpatient or outpatient surgery in patients ≥3 years of age; maintenance of anesthesia for inpatient or outpatient surgery in patients >2 months of age; in adults, for the induction and maintenance of monitored anesthesia care sedation during diagnostic procedures; treatment of agitation in intubated, mechanically-ventilated ICU patients

Usual Dosage Dosage must be individualized based on total body weight and titrated to the desired clinical effect; wait at least 3-5 minutes between dosage adjustments to clinically assess drug effects; smaller doses are required when used with narcotics; the following are general dosing guidelines:

General anesthesia:

Induction: I.V.:

Children (healthy) 3-16 years, ASA-PS 1 or 2: 2.5-3.5 mg/kg over 20-30 seconds; use a lower dose for children ASA-PS 3 or 4

Adults (healthy), ASA-PS 1 or 2, <55 years: 2-2.5 mg/kg (~40 mg every 10 seconds until onset of induction)

Cardiac anesthesia: 0.5-1.5 mg/kg (~20 mg every 10 seconds until onset of induction)

Neurosurgical patients: 1-2 mg/kg (~20 mg every 10 seconds until onset of induction)

Maintenance: I.V. infusion:

Children (healthy) 2 months to 16 years, ASA-PS 1 or 2: Initial: 125-300 mcg/kg/minute; decrease dose after 30 minutes if clinical signs of light anesthesia are absent; usual infusion rate: 125-150 mcg/kg/minute (range: 125-300 mcg/kg/minute; 7.5-18 mg/kg/hour); children ≤5 years may require larger infusion rates compared to older children

Adults (healthy), ASA-PS 1 or 2, <55 years: Initial: 150-200 mcg/kg/minute for 10-15 minutes; decrease by 30% to 50% during first 30 minutes of maintenance; usual infusion rate: 50-100 mcg/kg/minute (3-6 mg/kg/hour) to optimize recovery time

Cardiac anesthesia:

Low-dose propofol with primary opioid: 50-100 mcg/kg/minute (see manufacturer's labeling)

Primary propofol with secondary opioid: 100-150 mcg/kg/minute

Neurosurgical patients: 100-200 mcg/kg/minute (6-12 mg/kg/hour)

Maintenance: I.V. intermittent bolus: Adults (healthy), ASA-PS 1 or 2, <55 years: 20-50 mg increments as needed

Monitored anesthesia care sedation:

Initiation: Adults (healthy), ASA-PS 1 or 2, <55 years: Slow I.V. infusion: 100-150 mcg/kg/minute for 3-5 minutes **or** slow injection: 0.5 mg/kg over 3-5 minutes

Maintenance: Adults (healthy), ASA-PS 1 or 2, <55 years: I.V. infusion using variable rates (preferred over intermittent boluses): 25-75 mcg/kg/minute **or** incremental bolus doses: 10 mg or 20 mg

ICU sedation in intubated mechanically-ventilated patients: Avoid rapid bolus injection; individualize dose and titrate to response. Continuous infusion: Initial: 0.3 mg/kg/hour (5 mcg/kg/minute); increase by 0.3-0.6 mg/kg/hour (5-10 mcg/kg/minute) every 5-10 minutes until desired sedation level is achieved; usual maintenance: 0.3-3 mg/kg/hour (5-50 mcg/kg/minute) or higher; use 80% of healthy adult dose in elderly, debilitated, and ASA-PS 3 or 4 patients; reduce dose after adequate sedation established and adjust to response (eg, evaluate frequently to use minimum dose for sedation). Some clinicians recommend daily interruption of infusion to perform clinical evaluation.

Dosage Forms
  Injection, emulsion: 10 mg/mL (20 mL, 50 mL, 100 mL)
  Diprivan®: 10 mg/mL (20 mL, 50 mL, 100 mL)

Propoxacet-N® *(Discontinued)* *see* propoxyphene and acetaminophen *on this page*

propoxyphene (proe POKS i feen)
Sound-Alike/Look-Alike Issues
  propoxyphene may be confused with proparacaine
  Darvon® may be confused with Devrom®, Diovan®
  Darvon-N® may be confused with Darvocet-N®
Synonyms dextropropoxyphene; propoxyphene hydrochloride; propoxyphene napsylate
U.S./Canadian Brand Names 642® Tablet [Can]; Darvon-N® [US/Can]; Darvon® [US]
Therapeutic Category Analgesic, Narcotic
Controlled Substance C-IV
Use Management of mild to moderate pain
Usual Dosage Oral:
  Children: Doses for children are not well established; doses of the hydrochloride of 2-3 mg/kg/day divided every 6 hours have been used
  Adults:
    Hydrochloride: 65 mg every 3-4 hours as needed for pain; maximum: 390 mg/day
    Napsylate: 100 mg every 4 hours as needed for pain; maximum: 600 mg/day
Dosage Forms
  Capsule: 65 mg
  Darvon®: 65 mg
  Tablet:
  Darvon-N®: 100 mg

propoxyphene and acetaminophen (proe POKS i feen & a seet a MIN oh fen)
Sound-Alike/Look-Alike Issues
  Darvocet-N® may be confused with Darvon-N®
Synonyms acetaminophen and propoxyphene; propoxyphene hydrochloride and acetaminophen; propoxyphene napsylate and acetaminophen
U.S./Canadian Brand Names Balacet 325™ [US]; Darvocet A500™ [US]; Darvocet-N® 100 [US/Can]; Darvocet-N® 50 [US/Can]; Pronap-100® [US]
Therapeutic Category Analgesic, Narcotic
Controlled Substance C-IV
Use Management of mild to moderate pain
Usual Dosage Oral: Adults:
  Darvocet A500™, Darvocet-N® 100: 1 tablet every 4 hours as needed; maximum: 600 mg propoxyphene napsylate/day
  Darvocet-N® 50: 1-2 tablets every 4 hours as needed; maximum: 600 mg propoxyphene napsylate/day
  Propoxyphene hydrochloride 65 mg and acetaminophen 650 mg: 1 tablet every 4 hours as needed; maximum: 390 mg/day propoxyphene hydrochloride, 4 g/day acetaminophen)
  Note: Dosage of acetaminophen should not exceed 4 g/day (6 tablets of Darvocet-N® 100); possibly less in patients with ethanol
Dosage Forms
  Tablet: 65/650: Propoxyphene 65 mg and acetaminophen 650 mg; 100/500: Propoxyphene 100 mg and acetaminophen 500 mg; 100/650: Propoxyphene 100 mg and acetaminophen 650 mg
  Balacet 325™: Propoxyphene 100 mg and acetaminophen 325 mg
  Darvocet A500®: Propoxyphene 100 mg and acetaminophen 500 mg
  Darvocet-N® 50: Propoxyphene 50 mg and acetaminophen 325 mg
  Darvocet-N® 100: Propoxyphene 100 mg and acetaminophen 650 mg

propoxyphene, aspirin, and caffeine (proe POKS i feen, AS pir in, & KAF een)
Sound-Alike/Look-Alike Issues
  Darvon® may be confused with Devrom®, Diovan®
Synonyms aspirin, caffeine, and propoxyphene; caffeine, propoxyphene, and aspirin; propoxyphene hydrochloride, aspirin, and caffeine
Therapeutic Category Analgesic Combination (Narcotic)
Controlled Substance C-IV
Use Treatment of mild-to-moderate pain
  (Continued)

propoxyphene, aspirin, and caffeine *(Continued)*

Usual Dosage Oral: Adults: Pain: One capsule (providing propoxyphene 65 mg) every 4 hours as needed; maximum propoxyphene 390 mg/day. This will also provide aspirin 389 mg and caffeine 32.4 mg per capsule.

propoxyphene hydrochloride *see* propoxyphene *on previous page*

propoxyphene hydrochloride and acetaminophen *see* propoxyphene and acetaminophen *on previous page*

propoxyphene hydrochloride, aspirin, and caffeine *see* propoxyphene, aspirin, and caffeine *on previous page*

propoxyphene napsylate *see* propoxyphene *on previous page*

propoxyphene napsylate and acetaminophen *see* propoxyphene and acetaminophen *on previous page*

propranolol (proe PRAN oh lole)

Sound-Alike/Look-Alike Issues

propranolol may be confused with Pravachol®, Propulsid®

Inderal® may be confused with Adderall®, Enduron®, Enduronyl®, Imdur®, Imuran®, Inderide®, Isordil®, Toradol®

Inderal® 40 may be confused with Enduronyl® Forte

Synonyms propranolol hydrochloride

U.S./Canadian Brand Names Apo-Propranolol® [Can]; Inderal® LA [US/Can]; Inderal® [US/Can]; InnoPran XL™ [US]; Novo-Pranol [Can]; Nu-Propranolol [Can]; Propranolol Hydrochloride Injection, USP [Can]

Therapeutic Category Antiarrhythmic Agent, Class II; Beta-Adrenergic Blocker

Use Management of hypertension; angina pectoris; pheochromocytoma; essential tremor; supraventricular arrhythmias (such as atrial fibrillation and flutter, AV nodal reentrant tachycardias), ventricular tachycardias (catecholamine-induced arrhythmias, digoxin toxicity); prevention of myocardial infarction; migraine headache prophylaxis; symptomatic treatment of hypertrophic subaortic stenosis

Usual Dosage Adults:

Essential tremor: Oral: 20-40 mg twice daily initially; maintenance doses: usually 120-320 mg/day

Hypertension:

Oral:

Initial: 40 mg twice daily; increase dosage every 3-7 days; usual dose: ≤320 mg divided in 2-3 doses/day; maximum daily dose: 640 mg; usual dosage range (JNC 7): 40-160 mg/day in 2 divided doses

Long-acting formulation: Initial: 80 mg once daily; usual maintenance: 120-160 mg once daily; maximum daily dose: 640 mg; usual dosage range (JNC 7): 60-180 mg/day once daily

Hypertrophic subaortic stenosis: Oral: 20-40 mg 3-4 times/day

Long-acting formulation: 80-160 mg once daily

Migraine headache prophylaxis: Oral:

Initial: 80 mg/day divided every 6-8 hours; increase by 20-40 mg/dose every 3-4 weeks to a maximum of 160-240 mg/day given in divided doses every 6-8 hours; if satisfactory response not achieved within 6 weeks of starting therapy, drug should be withdrawn gradually over several weeks

Long-acting formulation: Initial: 80 mg once daily; effective dose range: 160-240 mg once daily

Post-MI mortality reduction: Oral: 180-240 mg/day in 3-4 divided doses

Pheochromocytoma: Oral: 30-60 mg/day in divided doses

Stable angina: Oral: 80-320 mg/day in doses divided 2-4 times/day

Long-acting formulation: Initial: 80 mg once daily; maximum dose: 320 mg once daily

Tachyarrhythmias:

Oral: 10-30 mg/dose every 6-8 hours

I.V.: Patients having nonfunctional GI tract: 1 mg/dose slow IVP; repeat every 5 minutes up to a total of 5 mg; titrate initial dose to desired response

Dosage Forms

Capsule, extended release: 60 mg, 80 mg, 120 mg, 160 mg

InnoPran XL™: 80 mg, 120 mg

Capsule, sustained release:

Inderal® LA: 60 mg, 80 mg, 120 mg, 160 mg

Injection, solution: 1 mg/mL (1 mL)

Inderal®: 1 mg/mL (1 mL)

Solution, oral: 4 mg/mL, 8 mg/mL

Tablet: 10 mg, 20 mg, 40 mg, 80 mg

Inderal®: 40 mg, 60 mg, 80 mg

propranolol and hydrochlorothiazide (proe PRAN oh lole & hye droe klor oh THYE a zide)

Sound-Alike/Look-Alike Issues

Inderide® may be confused with Inderal®

Synonyms hydrochlorothiazide and propranolol

U.S./Canadian Brand Names Inderide® [US]

Therapeutic Category Antihypertensive Agent, Combination

Use Management of hypertension

Usual Dosage Oral: Adults: Hypertension: Dose is individualized; typical dosages of **hydrochlorothiazide**: 12.5-50 mg/day; initial dose of **propranolol**: 80 mg/day

Daily dose of tablet form should be divided into 2 daily doses; may be used to maximum dosage of up to 160 mg of propranolol; higher dosages would result in higher than optimal thiazide dosages.

Dosage Forms

Tablet: Propranolol 40 mg and hydrochlorothiazide 25 mg; propranolol 80 mg and hydrochlorothiazide 25 mg

Inderide®: 40/25: Propranolol 40 mg and hydrochlorothiazide 25 mg

propranolol hydrochloride *see* propranolol *on previous page*

Propranolol Hydrochloride Injection, USP [Can] *see* propranolol *on previous page*

Proprinal [US-OTC] *see* ibuprofen *on page 444*

Proprinal® Cold and Sinus [US-OTC] *see* pseudoephedrine and ibuprofen *on page 729*

Propulsid® [US] *see* cisapride *on page 193*

propylene glycol diacetate, acetic acid, and hydrocortisone *see* acetic acid, propylene glycol diacetate, and hydrocortisone *on page 14*

propylhexedrine (proe pil HEKS e dreen)

U.S./Canadian Brand Names Benzedrex® [US-OTC]

Therapeutic Category Adrenergic Agonist Agent

Use Topical nasal decongestant

Usual Dosage Nasal: Children 6-12 years and Adults: Two inhalations in each nostril, not more frequently than every 2 hours

Dosage Forms

Inhaler, nasal:

Benzedrex® [OTC]: 0.4-0.5 mg/inhalation (1s)

2-propylpentanoic acid *see* valproic acid and derivatives *on page 881*

propylthiouracil (proe pil thye oh YOOR a sil)

Sound-Alike/Look-Alike Issues

propylthiouracil may be confused with Purinethol®

PTU is an error-prone abbreviation (mistaken as mercaptopurine [Purinethol®; 6-MP])

U.S./Canadian Brand Names Propyl-Thyracil® [Can]

Therapeutic Category Antithyroid Agent

Use Palliative treatment of hyperthyroidism as an adjunct to ameliorate hyperthyroidism in preparation for surgical treatment or radioactive iodine therapy; management of thyrotoxic crisis

Usual Dosage Oral: Administer in 3 equally divided doses at approximately 8-hour intervals. Adjust dosage to maintain T_3, T_4, and TSH levels in normal range; elevated T_3 may be sole indicator of inadequate treatment. Elevated TSH indicates excessive antithyroid treatment.

Children: Initial: 5-7 mg/kg/day **or** 150-200 mg/m^2/day in divided doses every 8 hours

or

6-10 years: 50-150 mg/day

>10 years: 150-300 mg/day

Maintenance: Determined by patient response **or** $1/3$ to $2/3$ of the initial dose in divided doses every 8-12 hours. This usually begins after 2 months on an effective initial dose.

Adults: Initial: 300 mg/day in divided doses every 8 hours. In patients with severe hyperthyroidism, very large goiters, or both, the initial dosage is usually 450 mg/day; an occasional patient will require 600-900 mg/day; maintenance: 100-150 mg/day in divided doses every 8-12 hours

Withdrawal of therapy: Therapy should be withdrawn gradually with evaluation of the patient every 4-6 weeks for the first 3 months then every 3 months for the first year after discontinuation of therapy to detect any reoccurrence of a hyperthyroid state.

Dosage Forms

Tablet: 50 mg

Propyl-Thyracil® [Can] *see* propylthiouracil *on this page*

2-propylvaleric acid *see* valproic acid and derivatives *on page 881*

ProQuad® [US] *see* measles, mumps, rubella, and varicella virus vaccine *on page 533*

Proquin® XR [US] *see* ciprofloxacin *on page 190*

Proscar® **[US/Can]** *see* finasteride *on page 353*

ProSom® *(Discontinued)* *see* estazolam *on page 313*

prostacyclin *see* epoprostenol *on page 304*

prostacyclin PGI₂ *see* iloprost *on page 447*

prostaglandin E₁ *see* alprostadil *on page 33*

prostaglandin E₂ *see* dinoprostone *on page 264*

prostaglandin F₂ *see* carboprost tromethamine *on page 153*

ProStep® **Patch** *(Discontinued)* *see* nicotine *on page 604*

Prostigmin® **[US/Can]** *see* neostigmine *on page 599*

Prostin E₂® **[US/Can]** *see* dinoprostone *on page 264*

Prostin F₂ Alpha® *(Discontinued)*

Prostin® **VR [Can]** *see* alprostadil *on page 33*

Prostin VR Pediatric® **[US]** *see* alprostadil *on page 33*

protamine sulfate (PROE ta meen SUL fate)

Sound-Alike/Look-Alike Issues
  protamine may be confused with ProAmatine®, protamine, Protopam®, Protropin®
Therapeutic Category Antidote
Use Treatment of heparin overdosage; neutralize heparin during surgery or dialysis procedures
Usual Dosage
  Heparin neutralization: I.V.: Protamine dosage is determined by the dosage of heparin; 1 mg of protamine neutralizes 90 USP units of heparin (lung) and 115 USP units of heparin (intestinal); maximum dose: 50 mg
  Heparin overdosage, following intravenous administration: I.V.: Since blood heparin concentrations decrease rapidly **after** administration, adjust the protamine dosage depending upon the duration of time since heparin administration.
  Note: Excessive protamine doses may worsen bleeding potential.
Dosage Forms
  Injection, solution [preservative free]: 10 mg/mL (5 mL, 25 mL)

Protection Plus® **[US-OTC]** *see* alcohol (ethyl) *on page 25*

protein C *see* protein C concentrate (human) *on this page*

protein C (activated), human, recombinant *see* drotrecogin alfa *on page 285*

protein-bound paclitaxel *see* paclitaxel (protein bound) *on page 646*

protein C concentrate (human) (PROE teen cee KON suhn trate HYU man)

Sound-Alike/Look-Alike Issues
  protein C concentrate (human) may be confused with activated protein C (human, recombinant) which refers to drotrecogin alfa
  Ceprotin may be confused with aprotinin, Cipro®
Synonyms protein C
U.S./Canadian Brand Names Ceprotin [US]
Therapeutic Category Anticoagulant
Use Replacement therapy for severe congenital protein C deficiency for the prevention and/or treatment of venous thromboembolism and purpura fulminans
Usual Dosage Patient variables (including age, clinical condition, and plasma levels of protein C) will influence dosing and duration of therapy. Individualize dosing based on protein C activity and patient pharmacokinetic profile. Dosing is dependent on the severity of protein C deficiency, age of patient, clinical condition, and patient's level of protein C. The frequency, duration, and dose should be individualized.

  I.V.: Children and Adults: Severe congenital protein C deficiency:
    Acute episode/short-term prophylaxis: Initial dose: 100-120 int. units/kg (for determination of recovery and half-life)
      Subsequent 3 doses: 60-80 int. units/kg every 6 hours (adjust to maintain peak protein C activity of 100%)
      Maintenance dose: 45-60 int. units/kg every 6 or 12 hours (adjust to maintain recommended maintenance trough protein C activity levels >25%)
    Long-term prophylaxis: Maintenance dose: 45-60 int. units/kg every 12 hours (recommended maintenance trough protein C activity levels >25%)

  Note: Maintain target peak protein C activity of 100% during acute episodes and short-term prophylaxis. Maintain trough levels of protein C activity >25%. Higher peak levels of protein C may be necessary in prophylactic therapy of patients at increased risk for thrombosis (eg, infection, trauma, surgical intervention).

Dosage Forms
Injection, powder for reconstitution:
Ceprotin: ~500 int. units, ~1000 int. units

Protenate® *(Discontinued)* *see* plasma protein fraction *on page 688*

Prothazine-DC® *(Discontinued)* *see* promethazine and codeine *on page 719*

prothrombin complex concentrate *see* factor IX complex (human) *on page 341*

Protilase® *(Discontinued)* *see* pancrelipase *on page 648*

Protonix® **[US/Can]** *see* pantoprazole *on page 651*

Protopam® **[US/Can]** *see* pralidoxime *on page 705*

Protopic® **[US/Can]** *see* tacrolimus *on page 818*

Protostat® **Oral** *(Discontinued)* *see* metronidazole *on page 563*

protriptyline (proe TRIP ti leen)
Sound-Alike/Look-Alike Issues
Vivactil® may be confused with Vyvanse™
Synonyms protriptyline hydrochloride
U.S./Canadian Brand Names Vivactil® [US]
Therapeutic Category Antidepressant, Tricyclic (Secondary Amine)
Use Treatment of depression
Usual Dosage Oral:
Adolescents: 15-20 mg/day
Adults: 15-60 mg in 3-4 divided doses
Dosage Forms
Tablet:
Vivactil®: 5 mg, 10 mg

protriptyline hydrochloride *see* protriptyline *on this page*

Protuss®**-DM** *(Discontinued)* *see* guaifenesin, pseudoephedrine, and dextromethorphan *on page 408*

Proventil® **[US]** *see* albuterol *on page 23*

Proventil® **HFA [US]** *see* albuterol *on page 23*

Proventil® **Inhaler** *(Discontinued)* *see* albuterol *on page 23*

Proventil® **Solution** *(Discontinued)* *see* albuterol *on page 23*

Proventil® **Tablet** *(Discontinued)* *see* albuterol *on page 23*

Provera® **[US/Can]** *see* medroxyprogesterone *on page 537*

Provera-Pak [Can] *see* medroxyprogesterone *on page 537*

Provigil® **[US/Can]** *see* modafinil *on page 575*

Proviodine [Can] *see* povidone-iodine *on page 704*

Provisc® **[US]** *see* hyaluronate and derivatives *on page 423*

Provocholine® **[US/Can]** *see* methacholine *on page 549*

proxymetacaine *see* proparacaine *on page 721*

Prozac® **[US/Can]** *see* fluoxetine *on page 364*

Prozac® **Weekly**™ **[US]** *see* fluoxetine *on page 364*

PRP-OMP *see* Haemophilus B conjugate vaccine *on page 411*

PRP-T *see* Haemophilus B conjugate vaccine *on page 411*

Prudoxin™ **[US]** *see* doxepin *on page 279*

prussian blue *see* ferric hexacyanoferrate *on page 349*

prymaccone *see* primaquine *on page 714*

23PS *see* pneumococcal polysaccharide vaccine (polyvalent) *on page 692*

PS-341 *see* bortezomib *on page 116*

pseudoephedrine (soo doe e FED rin)
Sound-Alike/Look-Alike Issues
Dimetapp® may be confused with Dermatop®, Dimetabs®, Dimetane®
Sudafed® may be confused with Sufenta®
(Continued)

pseudoephedrine *(Continued)*

Synonyms *d*-isoephedrine hydrochloride; pseudoephedrine hydrochloride; pseudoephedrine sulfate

U.S./Canadian Brand Names Balminil Decongestant [Can]; Benylin® D for Infants [Can]; Contac® Cold 12 Hour Relief Non Drowsy [Can]; Drixoral® ND [Can]; Eltor® [Can]; Genaphed® [US-OTC]; Kidkare Decongestant [US-OTC]; Kodet SE [US-OTC]; Oranyl [US-OTC]; PediaCare® Decongestant Infants [US-OTC]; PMS-Pseudoephedrine [Can]; Pseudofrin [Can]; Robidrine® [Can]; Silfedrine Children's [US-OTC]; Sudafed® 12 Hour [US-OTC]; Sudafed® 24 Hour [US-OTC]; Sudafed® Children's [US-OTC]; Sudafed® Decongestant [Can]; Sudafed® Maximum Strength Nasal Decongestant [US-OTC]; Sudo-Tab® [US-OTC]; Sudodrin [US-OTC]; SudoGest [US-OTC]

Therapeutic Category Adrenergic Agonist Agent

Use Temporary symptomatic relief of nasal congestion due to common cold, upper respiratory allergies, and sinusitis; also promotes nasal or sinus drainage

Usual Dosage Oral: General dosing guidelines:

Children:

<2 years: 4 mg/kg/day in divided doses every 6 hours

2-5 years: 15 mg every 4-6 hours; maximum: 60 mg/24 hours

6-12 years: 30 mg every 4-6 hours; maximum: 120 mg/24 hours

Adults: 30-60 mg every 4-6 hours, sustained release: 120 mg every 12 hours; maximum: 240 mg/24 hours

Dosage Forms

Caplet, extended release:

Sudafed® 12 Hour [OTC]: 120 mg

Liquid: 30 mg/5 mL

Silfedrine Children's [OTC], Sudafed® Children's [OTC]: 15 mg/5 mL

Unifed [OTC]: 30 mg/5 mL

Liquid, oral [drops]:

Kidkare Decongestant [OTC]: 7.5 mg/0.8 mL

Syrup: 30 mg/5 mL

Tablet: 30 mg, 60 mg

Genaphed® [OTC], Oranyl [OTC], Sudafed® [OTC], Sudo-Tab® [OTC]: 30 mg

SudoGest [OTC]: 30 mg, 60 mg

Tablet, chewable:

Sudafed® Children's [OTC]: 15 mg

Tablet, extended release:

Sudafed® 24 Hour [OTC]: 240 mg

pseudoephedrine, acetaminophen, and chlorpheniramine *see* acetaminophen, chlorpheniramine, and pseudoephedrine *on page 10*

pseudoephedrine, acetaminophen, and dextromethorphan *see* acetaminophen, dextromethorphan, and pseudoephedrine *on page 12*

pseudoephedrine and acetaminophen *see* acetaminophen and pseudoephedrine *on page 8*

pseudoephedrine and brompheniramine *see* brompheniramine and pseudoephedrine *on page 120*

pseudoephedrine and carbetapentane *see* carbetapentane and pseudoephedrine *on page 149*

pseudoephedrine and carbinoxamine *see* carbinoxamine and pseudoephedrine *on page 151*

pseudoephedrine and chlorpheniramine *see* chlorpheniramine and pseudoephedrine *on page 178*

pseudoephedrine and desloratadine *see* desloratadine and pseudoephedrine *on page 239*

pseudoephedrine and dexbrompheniramine *see* dexbrompheniramine and pseudoephedrine *on page 243*

pseudoephedrine and dextromethorphan (soo doe e FED rin & deks troe meth OR fan)

Synonyms dextromethorphan and pseudoephedrine

U.S./Canadian Brand Names Balminil DM D [Can]; Benylin® DM-D [Can]; Koffex DM-D [Can]; Novahistex® DM Decongestant [Can]; Novahistine® DM Decongestant [Can]; Pedia Relief Cough and Cold [US-OTC]; Pedia Relief Infants [US-OTC]; Pediacare® Infants' Decongestant & Cough [US-OTC]; Robitussin® Childrens Cough & Cold [Can]; Sudafed® Children's Cold & Cough [US-OTC]; SudoGest Children's [US-OTC]

Therapeutic Category Antitussive/Decongestant

Use Temporary symptomatic relief of nasal congestion and cough due to common cold, hay fever, upper respiratory allergies

Usual Dosage Relief of nasal congestion and cough: Oral:

General dosing guidelines base on pseudoephedrine component:

Children 2-6 years: 15 mg every 4-6 hours (maximum: 60 mg/24 hours)

Children 6-12 years: 30 mg every 4-6 hours (maximum: 120 mg/24 hours)

Children ≥12 years and Adults: 60 mg every 4-6 hours (maximum: 240 mg/24 hours)

Product-specific dosing:

Children 2-3 years (PediaCare® Infants Decongestant & Cough): 1.6 mL every 4-6 hours (maximum: 6.4 mL/ 24 hours)

Children 2-6 years:

Pediacare® Children's Long Acting Cough Plus Cold: One chewable tablet or 5 mL every 6-8 hours (maximum: 4 doses/24 hours)

Robitussin® Pediatric Cough & Cold, Triaminic® Cough and Nasal Congestion: 5 mL every 6 hours (maximum: 20 mL/24 hours)

Sudafed® Children's Cold & Cough: 5 mL every 4 hours (maximum: 20 mL/24 hours)

Triaminic® Cough: 5 mL every 4-6 hours (maximum: 20 mL/24 hours)

Children 6-12 years:

Pediacare® Children's Long Acting Cough Plus Cold: Two chewable tablets or 10 mL every 6-8 hours (maximum: 4 doses/24 hours)

Robitussin® Pediatric Cough & Cold, Triaminic® Cough and Nasal Congestion: 10 mL every 6 hours (maximum: 40 mL/24 hours)

Sudafed® Children's Cold & Cough: 10 mL every 4 hours (maximum: 40 mL/24 hours)

Triaminic Cough: 10 mL every 4-6 hours (maximum: 40 mL/24 hours)

Vicks® 44D Cough & Head Congestion: 7.5 mL every 6 hours (maximum: 30 mL/24 hours)

Children ≥12 years and Adults:

Robitussin® Maximum Strength Cough & Cold: 10 mL every 6 hours as needed (maximum: 40 mL/24 hours)

Sudafed® Children's Cold & Cough: 20 mL every 4 hours (maximum: 80 mL/24 hours)

Vicks® 44D Cough & Head Congestion: 15 mL every 6 hours (maximum: 60 mL/24 hours)

Dosage Forms

Liquid:

Sudafed® Children's Cold & Cough [OTC]: Pseudoephedrine 15 mg and dextromethorphan 5 mg per 5 mL

Liquid, oral [drops]:

Pedia Relief Infants [OTC]: Pseudoephedrine 7.5 mg and dextromethorphan 2.5 mg per 0.8 mL

Syrup:

Pedia Relief Cough and Cold [OTC]: Pseudoephedrine 15 mg and dextromethorphan 7.5 mg per 5 mL

SudoGest Children's [OTC]: Pseudoephedrine 15 mg and dextromethorphan 5 mg per 5 mL

pseudoephedrine and diphenhydramine see diphenhydramine and pseudoephedrine *on page 266*

pseudoephedrine and fexofenadine see fexofenadine and pseudoephedrine *on page 351*

pseudoephedrine and guaifenesin see guaifenesin and pseudoephedrine *on page 406*

pseudoephedrine and hydrocodone see hydrocodone and pseudoephedrine *on page 430*

pseudoephedrine and ibuprofen (soo doe e FED rin & eye byoo PROE fen)

Synonyms ibuprofen and pseudoephedrine

U.S./Canadian Brand Names Advil® Cold & Sinus [US-OTC/Can]; Advil® Cold, Children's [US-OTC]; Children's Advil® Cold [Can]; Motrin® Cold and Sinus [US-OTC]; Motrin® Cold, Children's [US-OTC]; Proprinal® Cold and Sinus [US-OTC]; Sudafed® Sinus Advance [Can]

Therapeutic Category Decongestant/Analgesic

Use For temporary relief of cold, sinus, and flu symptoms (including nasal congestion, headache, sore throat, minor body aches and pains, and fever)

Usual Dosage OTC labeling: Oral:

Children: Ibuprofen 100 mg and pseudoephedrine 15 mg per 5 mL: May repeat dose every 6 hours (maximum: 4 doses/24 hours); dose should be based on weight when possible. Contact healthcare provider if symptoms have not improved within 3 days (2 days if treating sore throat accompanied by fever).

2-5 years or 11 to <22 kg (24-47 pounds): 5 mL

6-11 years or 22-43 kg (48-95 pounds): 10 mL

Children ≥12 years and Adults: Ibuprofen 200 mg and pseudoephedrine 30 mg per dose: One dose every 4-6 hours as needed; may increase to 2 doses if necessary (maximum: 6 doses/24 hours). Contact healthcare provider if symptoms have not improved within 7 days when treating cold symptoms or within 3 days when treating fever.

Dosage Forms

Caplet:

Advil® Cold and Sinus [OTC], Proprinal® Cold and Sinus [OTC]: Pseudoephedrine 30 mg and ibuprofen 200 mg

Capsule, liquid filled:

Advil® Cold and Sinus [OTC]: Pseudoephedrine 30 mg and ibuprofen 200 mg

Suspension:

Advil® Cold, Children's [OTC]: Pseudoephedrine 15 mg and ibuprofen 100 mg per 5 mL

pseudoephedrine and loratadine *see* loratadine and pseudoephedrine *on page 518*

pseudoephedrine and methscopolamine (soo doe e FED rin & meth skoe POL a meen)

Synonyms methscopolamine and pseudoephedrine; pseudoephedrine hydrochloride and methscopolamine nitrate

U.S./Canadian Brand Names AlleRx™-D [US]; Amdry-D [US]; Extendryl PSE [US]

Therapeutic Category Decongestant/Anticholingeric Combination

Use Relief of symptoms of allergic rhinitis, vasomotor rhinitis, sinusitis, and the common cold

Usual Dosage Oral: Children ≥12 years and Adults (Allerx™-D, Amdry-D): One tablet every 12 hours (maximum: 2 tablets/24 hours)

Dosage Forms

Tablet: Pseudoephedrine hydrochloride 120 mg and methscopolamine nitrate 2.5 mg

Allerx™-D, Amdry-D: Pseudoephedrine 120 mg and methscopolamine 2.5 mg

Tablet, extended release:

Extendryl PSE: Pseudoephedrine 120 mg and methscopolamine 2.5 mg

pseudoephedrine and naproxen *see* naproxen and pseudoephedrine *on page 592*

pseudoephedrine and triprolidine *see* triprolidine and pseudoephedrine *on page 869*

pseudoephedrine, carbinoxamine, and dextromethorphan *see* carbinoxamine, pseudoephedrine, and dextromethorphan *on page 152*

pseudoephedrine, chlorpheniramine, and acetaminophen *see* acetaminophen, chlorpheniramine, and pseudoephedrine *on page 10*

pseudoephedrine, chlorpheniramine, and codeine *see* chlorpheniramine, pseudoephedrine, and codeine *on page 183*

pseudoephedrine, chlorpheniramine, and dextromethorphan *see* chlorpheniramine, pseudoephedrine, and dextromethorphan *on page 183*

pseudoephedrine, chlorpheniramine, and dihydrocodeine *see* pseudoephedrine, dihydrocodeine, and chlorpheniramine *on this page*

pseudoephedrine, chlorpheniramine, and ibuprofen *see* ibuprofen, pseudoephedrine, and chlorpheniramine *on page 445*

pseudoephedrine, codeine, and triprolidine *see* triprolidine, pseudoephedrine, and codeine *(Canada only) on page 869*

pseudoephedrine, dextromethorphan, and acetaminophen *see* acetaminophen, dextromethorphan, and pseudoephedrine *on page 12*

pseudoephedrine, dextromethorphan, and carbinoxamine *see* carbinoxamine, pseudoephedrine, and dextromethorphan *on page 152*

pseudoephedrine, dextromethorphan, and guaifenesin *see* guaifenesin, pseudoephedrine, and dextromethorphan *on page 408*

pseudoephedrine, dihydrocodeine, and chlorpheniramine

(soo doe e FED rin, dye hye droe KOE deen, & klor fen IR a meen)

Synonyms chlorpheniramine, pseudoephedrine, and dihydrocodeine; dihydrocodeine bitartrate, pseudoephedrine hydrochloride, and chlorpheniramine maleate; pseudoephedrine, chlorpheniramine, and dihydrocodeine

U.S./Canadian Brand Names Coldcough [US]; DiHydro-CP [US]; Hydro-Tussin™ DHC [US]

Therapeutic Category Antihistamine/Decongestant/Antitussive

Controlled Substance C-III

Use Temporary relief of cough, congestion, and sneezing due to colds, respiratory infections, or hay fever

Usual Dosage Oral:

Children:

2-6 years: 1.25-2.5 mL every 4-6 hours; do not exceed 4 doses in 24 hours

6-12 years: 2.5-5 mL every 4-6 hours; do not exceed 4 doses in 24 hours

Children >12 years and Adults: 5-10 mL every 4-6 hours; do not exceed 4 doses in 24 hours

Dosage Forms

Syrup:

Coldcough, DiHydro-CP, Hydro-Tussin™ DHC: Pseudoephedrine 15 mg, dihydrocodeine 7.5 mg, and chlorpheniramine 2 mg per 5 mL

pseudoephedrine, guaifenesin, and codeine *see* guaifenesin, pseudoephedrine, and codeine *on page 408*

pseudoephedrine hydrochloride *see* pseudoephedrine *on page 727*

pseudoephedrine hydrochloride and acrivastine *see* acrivastine and pseudoephedrine *on page 16*

pseudoephedrine hydrochloride and cetirizine hydrochloride *see* cetirizine and pseudoephedrine *on page 169*

pseudoephedrine hydrochloride and methscopolamine nitrate *see* pseudoephedrine and methscopolamine *on previous page*

pseudoephedrine hydrochloride, guaifenesin, and dihydrocodeine bitartrate *see* dihydrocodeine, pseudoephedrine, and guaifenesin *on page 260*

pseudoephedrine hydrochloride, hydrocodone bitartrate, and chlorpheniramine maleate *see* pseudoephedrine, hydrocodone, and chlorpheniramine *on this page*

pseudoephedrine hydrochloride, methscopolamine nitrate, and chlorpheniramine maleate *see* chlorpheniramine, pseudoephedrine, and methscopolamine *on page 184*

pseudoephedrine, hydrocodone, and carbinoxamine *see* hydrocodone, carbinoxamine, and pseudoephedrine *on page 430*

pseudoephedrine, hydrocodone, and chlorpheniramine
(soo doe e FED rin, hye droe KOE done, & klor fen IR a meen)

Synonyms chlorpheniramine, pseudoephedrine, and hydrocodone; hydrocodone, chlorpheniramine, and pseudoephedrine; pseudoephedrine hydrochloride, hydrocodone bitartrate, and chlorpheniramine maleate

U.S./Canadian Brand Names Atuss® HD [US]; Coldcough HC [US]; Cordron-HC NR [US]; Detuss [US]; Histinex® PV [US]; Hydro-Tussin™ HC [US]; Hydron PSC [US]; Hyphed [US]; P-V-Tussin® Syrup [US]; Pediatex™ HC [US]; Vasophrinic DH [Can]

Therapeutic Category Antihistamine; Antihistamine/Decongestant/Antitussive; Antitussive; Decongestant

Controlled Substance C-III

Use Temporary relief of cough, congestion, and sneezing due to colds, respiratory infections, or hay fever

Usual Dosage Oral:

Children:

2-6 years:

Hydro-Tussin™ HC: 1.25-2.5 mL every 4-6 hours; do not exceed 4 doses in 24 hours

Histinex® PV, P-V-Tussin®: 2.5 mL every 4-6 hours; do not exceed 4 doses in 24 hours

6-12 years:

Histinex® PV, P-V-Tussin®: 5 mL or 1/2 tablet every 4-6 hours; do not exceed 4 doses in 24 hours

Hydro-Tussin™ HC: 2.5-5 mL or 1/2 tablet every 4-6 hours; do not exceed 4 doses in 24 hours

Children >12 years and Adults:

Histinex® PV, P-V-Tussin®: 10 mL or 1 tablet every 4-6 hours; do not exceed 4 doses in 24 hours

Hydro-Tussin™ HC: 5-10 mL or 1 tablet every 4-6 hours; do not exceed 4 doses in 24 hours

Dosage Forms

Capsule, variable release:

Atuss® HD: Pseudoephedrine 30 mg [sustained release], hydrocodone 5 mg [immediate release], and chlorpheniramine 2 mg [sustained release]

Liquid:

Cordron-HC: Pseudoephedrine 20 mg, hydrocodone 1.67 mg, and chlorpheniramine 2.5 mg per 5 mL

Detuss, Hydron PSC: Pseudoephedrine 30 mg, hydrocodone 5 mg, and chlorpheniramine 2 mg per 5 mL

Pediatex™ HC: Pseudoephedrine 17.5 mg, hydrocodone 1.67 mg, and chlorpheniramine 2.5 mg per 5 mL

Syrup:

Coldcough HC, Hydro-Tussin™ HC: Pseudoephedrine 15 mg, hydrocodone 3 mg, and chlorpheniramine 2 mg per 5 mL

Cordron-HC NR: Pseudoephedrine 17.5 mg, hydrocodone 1.67 mg, and chlorpheniramine 2.5 mg per 5 mL

Histinex® PV, Hyphed, P-V-Tussin®: Pseudoephedrine 30 mg, hydrocodone 2.5 mg, and chlorpheniramine 2 mg per 5 mL

pseudoephedrine, hydrocodone, and guaifenesin *see* hydrocodone, pseudoephedrine, and guaifenesin *on page 432*

pseudoephedrine, methscopolamine, and chlorpheniramine *see* chlorpheniramine, pseudoephedrine, and methscopolamine *on page 184*

pseudoephedrine sulfate *see* pseudoephedrine *on page 727*

pseudoephedrine tannate and dexchlorpheniramine tannate *see* dexchlorpheniramine and pseudoephedrine *on page 243*

pseudoephedrine tannate, dextromethorphan tannate, and brompheniramine tannate *see* brompheniramine, pseudoephedrine, and dextromethorphan *on page 122*

pseudoephedrine, triprolidine, and codeine *see* triprolidine, pseudoephedrine, and codeine *(Canada only) on page 869*

Pseudofrin [Can] *see* pseudoephedrine *on page 727*

Pseudo-Gest Plus® Tablet *(Discontinued)* *see* chlorpheniramine and pseudoephedrine *on page 178*

Pseudo GG TR [US] *see* guaifenesin and pseudoephedrine *on page 406*

Pseudo Max [US] *see* guaifenesin and pseudoephedrine *on page 406*

Pseudo Max DMX [US] *see* guaifenesin, pseudoephedrine, and dextromethorphan *on page 408*

pseudomonic acid A *see* mupirocin *on page 582*

Pseudovent™ [US] *see* guaifenesin and pseudoephedrine *on page 406*

Pseudovent™ 400 [US] *see* guaifenesin and pseudoephedrine *on page 406*

Pseudovent™ DM [US] *see* guaifenesin, pseudoephedrine, and dextromethorphan *on page 408*

Pseudovent™-Ped [US] *see* guaifenesin and pseudoephedrine *on page 406*

P & S™ Liquid Phenol [Can] *see* phenol *on page 673*

Psorcon® [Can] *see* diflorasone *on page 257*

Psorcon® *(Discontinued)* *see* diflorasone *on page 257*

Psorcon® e™ *(Discontinued)* *see* diflorasone *on page 257*

Psoriatec™ [US] *see* anthralin *on page 57*

PsoriGel® *(Discontinued)* *see* coal tar *on page 208*

Psorion® Topical *(Discontinued)*

psyllium (SIL i yum)
  Sound-Alike/Look-Alike Issues
    Fiberall® may be confused with Feverall®
    Hydrocil® may be confused with Hydrocet®
    Modane® may be confused with Matulane®, Moban®
  Synonyms plantago seed; plantain seed; psyllium hydrophilic mucilloid
  U.S./Canadian Brand Names Fiberall® [US]; Fibro-Lax [US-OTC]; Fibro-XL [US-OTC]; Genfiber® [US-OTC]; Hydrocil® Instant [US-OTC]; Konsyl-D® [US-OTC]; Konsyl® Easy Mix [US-OTC]; Konsyl® Orange [US-OTC]; Konsyl® [US-OTC]; Metamucil® Plus Calcium [US-OTC]; Metamucil® Smooth Texture [US-OTC]; Metamucil® [US-OTC/Can]; Modane® Bulk [US-OTC]; Natural Fiber Therapy [US-OTC]; Reguloid® [US-OTC]; Serutan® [US-OTC]
  Therapeutic Category Laxative
  Use Treatment of chronic atonic or spastic constipation and in constipation associated with rectal disorders; management of irritable bowel syndrome; labeled for OTC use as fiber supplement, treatment of constipation
  Usual Dosage Oral (administer at least 2 hours before or after other drugs):
    Children 6-11 years: Approximately ¹/₂ adult dosage
    Children ≥12 years and Adults: Take 1 dose up to 3 times/day; all doses should be followed with 8 oz of water or liquid
    Capsule: 4 capsules/dose (range: 2-6); swallow capsules one at a time
    Powder: 1 rounded tablespoonful/dose (1 teaspoonful/dose for many sugar free or select concentrated products) mixed in 8 oz liquid
    Tablet: 1 tablet/dose
    Wafer: 2 wafers/dose
  Dosage Forms
    Capsule:
      Fibro XL [OTC]: 675 mg
      Metamucil® [OTC]: 0.52 g
      Metamucil® Plus Calcium [OTC]: 0.42 g
    Granules:
      Serutan® [OTC]: 2.5 g/teaspoon
    Powder: 3.4 g/dose
      Bulk-K [OTC], Fibro-Lax [OTC]: 4.725 g/dose
      Fiberall®: 3.5 g/dose
      Genfiber® [OTC], Konsyl-D® [OTC], Konsyl® Orange [OTC], Konsyl® Orange [OTC], Metamucil® [OTC], Metamucil® Smooth Texture [OTC], Modane® Bulk [OTC], Natural Fiber Therapy [OTC], Reguloid® [OTC]: 3.4 g/dose
      Genfiber® [OTC], Hydrocil® Instant: [OTC]: 3.5 g/dose
      Konsyl® [OTC], Konsyl® Easy Mix [OTC]: 6 g/dose

Wafers:
Metamucil® [OTC]: 3.4 g/dose (24s)

psyllium hydrophilic mucilloid *see* psyllium *on previous page*

P.T.E.-4® [US] *see* trace metals *on page 855*

P.T.E.-5® [US] *see* trace metals *on page 855*

pteroylglutamic acid *see* folic acid *on page 371*

Pulmicort® [Can] *see* budesonide *on page 123*

Pulmicort Flexhaler® [US] *see* budesonide *on page 123*

Pulmicort Respules® [US] *see* budesonide *on page 123*

Pulmicort Turbuhaler® [US] *see* budesonide *on page 123*

Pulmophylline [Can] *see* theophylline *on page 834*

Pulmozyme® [US/Can] *see* dornase alfa *on page 277*

Puralube® Tears [US-OTC] *see* artificial tears *on page 75*

Puregon® [Can] *see* follitropin beta *on page 372*

Purell® [US-OTC] *see* alcohol (ethyl) *on page 25*

Purell® 2 in 1 [US-OTC] *see* alcohol (ethyl) *on page 25*

Purell® with Aloe [US-OTC] *see* alcohol (ethyl) *on page 25*

purified chick embryo cell *see* rabies virus vaccine *on page 742*

Purinethol® [US/Can] *see* mercaptopurine *on page 545*

PVP-I *see* povidone-iodine *on page 704*

Pylera™ [US] *see* bismuth, metronidazole, and tetracycline *on page 113*

pyrantel pamoate (pi RAN tel PAM oh ate)

U.S./Canadian Brand Names Combantrin™ [Can]; Pin-X® [US-OTC]; Reese's® Pinworm Medicine [US-OTC]
Therapeutic Category Anthelmintic
Use Treatment of pinworms (*Enterobius vermicularis*) and roundworms (*Ascaris lumbricoides*)
Usual Dosage Children and Adults (purgation is not required prior to use): Oral: **Note:** Dose is expressed as pyrantel base: Roundworm, pinworm, or trichostrongyliasis: 11 mg/kg administered as a single dose; maximum dose: 1 g. **(Note:** For pinworm infection, dosage should be repeated in 2 weeks and all family members should be treated).
Dosage Forms
Caplet:
Reese's® Pinworm Medicine [OTC]: 180 mg
Suspension, oral:
Pin-X® [OTC], Reese's® Pinworm Medicine [OTC]: 144 mg/mL
Tablet:
Pin-X® [OTC]: 720.5 mg

pyrazinamide (peer a ZIN a mide)

Synonyms pyrazinoic acid amide
U.S./Canadian Brand Names Tebrazid™ [Can]
Therapeutic Category Antitubercular Agent
Use Adjunctive treatment of tuberculosis in combination with other antituberculosis agents
Usual Dosage Oral: Treatment of tuberculosis:
Note: Used as part of a multidrug regimen. Treatment regimens consist of an initial 2-month phase, followed by a continuation phase of 4 or 7 additional months; frequency of dosing may differ depending on phase of therapy.
Children:
Daily therapy: 15-30 mg/kg/day (maximum: 2 g/day)
Twice weekly directly observed therapy (DOT): 50 mg/kg/dose (maximum: 4 g/dose)
Adults (dosing is based on lean body weight):
Daily therapy: 15-30 mg/kg/day
40-55 kg: 1000 mg
56-75 kg: 1500 mg
76-90 kg: 2000 mg (maximum dose regardless of weight)
Twice weekly directly observed therapy (DOT): 50 mg/kg
40-55 kg: 2000 mg
56-75 kg: 3000 mg
(Continued)

pyrazinamide *(Continued)*

76-90 kg: 4000 mg (maximum dose regardless of weight)
Three times/week DOT: 25-30 mg/kg (maximum: 2.5 g)
40-55 kg: 1500 mg
56-75 kg: 2500 mg
76-90 kg: 3000 mg (maximum dose regardless of weight)

Dosage Forms
Tablet: 500 mg

pyrazinamide, rifampin, and isoniazid *see* rifampin, isoniazid, and pyrazinamide *on page 758*

pyrazinoic acid amide *see* pyrazinamide *on previous page*

pyrethrins and piperonyl butoxide (pye RE thrins & pi PER oh nil byo TOKS ide)

Synonyms piperonyl butoxide and pyrethrins

U.S./Canadian Brand Names A-200® Lice Treatment Kit [US-OTC]; A-200® Maximum Strength [US-OTC]; Licide® [US-OTC]; Pronto® Complete Lice Removal System [US-OTC]; Pronto® Lice Control [Can]; Pronto® Plus Lice Killing Mousse Plus Vitamin E [US-OTC]; Pronto® Plus Lice Killing Mousse Shampoo Plus Natural Extracts and Oils [US-OTC]; Pronto® Plus Warm Oil Treatment and Conditioner [US-OTC]; R & C™ II [Can]; R & C™ Shampoo/Conditioner [Can]; RID® Maximum Strength [US-OTC]; RID® Mousse [Can]; Tisit® Blue Gel [US-OTC]; Tisit® [US-OTC]

Therapeutic Category Scabicides/Pediculicides

Use Treatment of *Pediculus humanus* infestations (head lice, body lice, pubic lice and their eggs)

Usual Dosage Application of pyrethrins:

Topical products:
Apply enough solution to completely wet infested area, including hair
Allow to remain on area for 10 minutes
Wash and rinse with large amounts of warm water.
Use fine-toothed comb to remove lice and eggs from hair
Shampoo hair to restore body and luster
Treatment may be repeated if necessary once in a 24-hour period
Repeat treatment in 7-10 days to kill newly hatched lice
Note: Keep out of eyes when rinsing hair; protect eyes with a washcloth or towel
Solution for furniture, bedding: Spray on entire area to be treated; allow to dry before use. Intended for use on items which cannot be laundered or dry cleaned. **Not for use on humans or animals.**

Dosage Forms
Gel, topical:
Tisit® Blue Gel [OTC]: Pyrethrins 0.33% and piperonyl butoxide 3% (30 g)
Kit:
A-200® Lice Treatment Kit [OTC]:
Shampoo: Pyrethrins 0.33% and piperonyl butoxide 4% (120 mL)
Solution: Permethrin 0.5% (180 mL)
Pronto® Complete Lice Removal System [OTC]:
Shampoo: Pyrethrins 0.33% and piperonyl butoxide 4% (60 mL)
Solution, topical: Benzalkonium chloride 0.1% (60 mL)
Liquid, topical:
Tisit® [OTC]: Pyrethrins 0.33% and piperonyl butoxide 2% (60 mL, 120 mL)
Oil, topical:
Pronto® Plus Warm Oil Treatment and Conditioner [OTC]: Pyrethrins 0.33% and piperonyl butoxide 4% (36 mL)
Shampoo: Pyrethrins 0.33% and piperonyl butoxide 4% (60 mL, 120 mL)
A-200® Maximum Strength [OTC], Tisit® [OTC]: Pyrethrins 0.33% and piperonyl butoxide 4% (60 mL, 120 mL)
Licide® [OTC], Pronto® Plus Lice Killing Mousse Shampoo Plus Vitamin E: Pyrethrins 0.33% and piperonyl butoxide 4% (120 mL)
Pronto® Plus Lice Killing Mousse Shampoo Plus Natural Extracts and Oils: Pyrethrins 0.33% and piperonyl butoxide 4% (60 mL)
Pronto® Plus Lice Killing Mousse Shampoo Plus Vitamin E: Pyrethrins 0.33% and piperonyl butoxide 4% (120 mL)
RID® Maximum Strength [OTC]: Pyrethrins 0.33% and piperonyl butoxide 4% (60 mL, 120 mL, 180 mL, 240 mL)
Solution:
Tisit® [OTC]: Pyrethrins 0.4% and piperonyl butoxide 2% (150 mL)

Pyri-500 [US-OTC] *see* pyridoxine *on next page*

2-pyridine aldoxime methochloride *see* pralidoxime *on page 705*

Pyridium® **[US]** *see* phenazopyridine *on page 671*

pyridostigmine (peer id oh STIG meen)

Sound-Alike/Look-Alike Issues
pyridostigmine may be confused with physostigmine
Mestinon® may be confused with Metatensin®
Regonol® may be confused with Reglan®, Renagel®

Synonyms pyridostigmine bromide

U.S./Canadian Brand Names Mestinon® Timespan® [US]; Mestinon® [US/Can]; Mestinon®-SR [Can]; Regonol® [US]

Therapeutic Category Cholinergic Agent

Use Symptomatic treatment of myasthenia gravis; antidote for nondepolarizing neuromuscular blockers
Military use: Pretreatment for soman nerve gas exposure

Usual Dosage
Myasthenia gravis:
Oral:
Children: 7 mg/kg/24 hours divided into 5-6 doses
Adults: Highly individualized dosing ranges: 60-1500 mg/day, usually 600 mg/day divided into 5-6 doses, spaced to provide maximum relief
Sustained release formulation: Highly individualized dosing ranges: 180-540 mg once or twice daily (doses separated by at least 6 hours); **Note:** Most clinicians reserve sustained release dosage form for bedtime dose only.
I.M., slow I.V. push:
Children: 0.05-0.15 mg/kg/dose
Adults: To supplement oral dosage pre- and postoperatively during labor and postpartum, during myasthenic crisis, or when oral therapy is impractical: ~1/30th of oral dose; observe patient closely for cholinergic reactions
or
I.V. infusion: Initial: 2 mg/hour with gradual titration in increments of 0.5-1 mg/hour, up to a maximum rate of 4 mg/hour
Pretreatment for soman nerve gas exposure (military use): Oral: Adults: 30 mg every 8 hours beginning several hours prior to exposure; discontinue at first sign of nerve agent exposure, then begin atropine and pralidoxime
Reversal of nondepolarizing muscle relaxants: **Note:** Atropine sulfate (0.6-1.2 mg) I.V. immediately prior to pyridostigmine to minimize side effects: I.V.:
Children: Dosing range: 0.1-0.25 mg/kg/dose*
Adults: 0.1-0.25 mg/kg/dose; 10-20 mg is usually sufficient*
*Full recovery usually occurs ≤15 minutes, but ≥30 minutes may be required

Dosage Forms
Injection, solution:
Regonol®: 5 mg/mL (2 mL)
Syrup:
Mestinon®: 60 mg/5 mL
Tablet: 60 mg
Mestinon®: 60 mg
Tablet, sustained release:
Mestinon® Timespan®: 180 mg

pyridostigmine bromide *see* pyridostigmine *on this page*

pyridoxine (peer i DOKS een)

Sound-Alike/Look-Alike Issues
pyridoxine may be confused with paroxetine, pralidoxime, Pyridium®

Synonyms pyridoxine hydrochloride; vitamin B$_6$

U.S./Canadian Brand Names Aminoxin [US-OTC]; Pyri-500 [US-OTC]

Therapeutic Category Vitamin, Water Soluble

Use Prevention and treatment of vitamin B$_6$ deficiency, pyridoxine-dependent seizures in infants; adjunct to treatment of acute toxicity from isoniazid, cycloserine, or hydrazine overdose

Usual Dosage
Recommended daily allowance (RDA):
Children:
1-3 years: 0.9 mg
4-6 years: 1.3 mg
7-10 years: 1.6 mg
(Continued)

pyridoxine *(Continued)*

Adults:
Male: 1.7-2.0 mg
Female: 1.4-1.6 mg
Pyridoxine-dependent Infants:
Oral: 2-100 mg/day
I.M., I.V., SubQ: 10-100 mg
Dietary deficiency: Oral:
Children: 5-25 mg/24 hours for 3 weeks, then 1.5-2.5 mg/day in multiple vitamin product
Adults: 10-20 mg/day for 3 weeks
Drug-induced neuritis (eg, isoniazid, hydralazine, penicillamine, cycloserine): Oral:
Children:
Treatment: 10-50 mg/24 hours
Prophylaxis: 1-2 mg/kg/24 hours
Adults:
Treatment: 100-200 mg/24 hours
Prophylaxis: 25-100 mg/24 hours
Treatment of seizures and/or coma from acute isoniazid toxicity, a dose of pyridoxine hydrochloride equal to the amount of INH ingested can be given I.M./I.V. in divided doses together with other anticonvulsants; if the amount INH ingested is not known, administer 5 g I.V. pyridoxine
Treatment of acute hydrazine toxicity, a pyridoxine dose of 25 mg/kg in divided doses I.M./I.V. has been used

Dosage Forms
Capsule: 50 mg, 250 mg
Aminoxin [OTC]: 20 mg
Injection, solution: 100 mg/mL (1 mL)
Liquid, oral: 200 mg/5 mL (120 mL)
Tablet: 25 mg, 50 mg, 100 mg, 250 mg, 500 mg
Tablet, sustained release:
Pyri-500 [OTC]: 500 mg

pyridoxine and doxylamine *see* doxylamine and pyridoxine *(Canada only) on page 283*

pyridoxine, folic acid, and cyanocobalamin *see* folic acid, cyanocobalamin, and pyridoxine *on page 371*

pyridoxine hydrochloride *see* pyridoxine *on previous page*

Pyrilafen Tannate-12™ [US] *see* phenylephrine and pyrilamine *on page 677*

pyrilamine maleate, dextromethorphan hydrobromide, and phenylephrine hydrochloride *see* phenylephrine, pyrilamine, and dextromethorphan *on page 679*

pyrilamine, phenylephrine, and carbetapentane *see* carbetapentane, phenylephrine, and pyrilamine *on page 150*

pyrilamine tannate and phenylephrine tannate *see* phenylephrine and pyrilamine *on page 677*

pyrimethamine *(peer i METH a meen)*

Sound-Alike/Look-Alike Issues
Daraprim® may be confused with Dantrium®, Daranide®
U.S./Canadian Brand Names Daraprim® [US/Can]
Therapeutic Category Folic Acid Antagonist (Antimalarial)
Use Prophylaxis of malaria due to susceptible strains of plasmodia; used in conjunction with quinine and sulfadiazine for the treatment of uncomplicated attacks of chloroquine-resistant *P. falciparum* malaria; used in conjunction with fast-acting schizonticide to initiate transmission control and suppression cure; synergistic combination with sulfonamide in treatment of toxoplasmosis
Usual Dosage
Malaria chemoprophylaxis (for areas where chloroquine-resistant *P. falciparum* exists): Begin prophylaxis 2 weeks before entering endemic area:
Children: 0.5 mg/kg once weekly; not to exceed 25 mg/dose
or
Children:
<4 years: 6.25 mg once weekly
4-10 years: 12.5 mg once weekly
Children >10 years and Adults: 25 mg once weekly
Dosage should be continued for all age groups for at least 6-10 weeks after leaving endemic areas
Chloroquine-resistant *P. falciparum* malaria (when used in conjunction with quinine and sulfadiazine):
Children:
<10 kg: 6.25 mg/day once daily for 3 days

10-20 kg: 12.5 mg/day once daily for 3 days
20-40 kg: 25 mg/day once daily for 3 days
Adults: 25 mg twice daily for 3 days
Toxoplasmosis:
Infants (congenital toxoplasmosis): Oral: 1 mg/kg once daily for 6 months with sulfadiazine then every other month with sulfa, alternating with spiramycin.
Children: Loading dose: 2 mg/kg/day divided into 2 equal daily doses for 1-3 days (maximum: 100 mg/day) followed by 1 mg/kg/day divided into 2 doses for 4 weeks; maximum: 25 mg/day
With sulfadiazine or trisulfapyrimidines: 2 mg/kg/day divided every 12 hours for 3 days, followed by 1 mg/kg/day once daily or divided twice daily for 4 weeks given with trisulfapyrimidines or sulfadiazine
Adults: 50-75 mg/day together with 1-4 g of a sulfonamide for 1-3 weeks depending on patient's tolerance and response, then reduce dose by 50% and continue for 4-5 weeks **or** 25-50 mg/day for 3-4 weeks
Prophylaxis for first episode of *Toxoplasma gondii*:
Children ≥1 month of age: 1 mg/kg/day once daily with dapsone, plus oral folinic acid 5 mg every 3 days
Adolescents and Adults: 50 mg once weekly with dapsone, plus oral folinic acid 25 mg once weekly
Prophylaxis to prevent recurrence of *Toxoplasma gondii*:
Children ≥1 month of age: 1 mg/kg/day once daily given with sulfadiazine or clindamycin, plus oral folinic acid 5 mg every 3 days
Adolescents and Adults: 25-50 mg once daily in combination with sulfadiazine or clindamycin, plus oral folinic acid 10-25 mg daily; atovaquone plus oral folinic acid has also been used in combination with pyrimethamine.

Dosage Forms
Tablet:
Daraprim®: 25 mg

pyrimethamine and sulfadoxine *see* sulfadoxine and pyrimethamine *on page 812*

pyrithione zinc (peer i THYE one zingk)

Sound-Alike/Look-Alike Issues
pyrithione may be confused with Pyridium®
U.S./Canadian Brand Names BetaMed [US-OTC]; DermaZinc™ [US-OTC]; DHS™ Zinc [US-OTC]; Head & Shoulders® Citrus Breeze [US-OTC]; Head & Shoulders® Classic Clean 2-In-1 [US-OTC]; Head & Shoulders® Classic Clean [US-OTC]; Head & Shoulders® Dry Scalp Care [US-OTC]; Head & Shoulders® Extra Volume [US-OTC]; Head & Shoulders® Leave-in Treatment [US-OTC]; Head & Shoulders® Refresh [US-OTC]; Head & Shoulders® Sensitive Care [US-OTC]; Head & Shoulders® Smooth & Silky 2-In-1 [US-OTC]; Skin Care™ [US-OTC]; Zincon® [US-OTC]; ZNP® Bar [US-OTC]
Therapeutic Category Antiseborrheic Agent, Topical
Use Relieves the itching, irritation and scalp flaking associated with dandruff and/or seborrheal dermatitis
Usual Dosage Adults: Products should be used at least twice weekly for best results, but may be used with each washing.
Bar: May be used on body and or scalp; wet area, massage in, and rinse.
Shampoo: Should be applied to wet hair and massaged into scalp; rinse. May be followed with conditioner
Dosage Forms
Conditioner, topical:
DermaZinc™ [OTC]: 0.25% (120 g)
Head & Shoulders® Dry Scalp Care [OTC]: 0.5% (400 mL)
Head & Shoulders® Extra Volume [OTC]: 0.5% (200 mL, 400 mL)
Lotion, topical:
Head & Shoulders® Leave-in Treatment [OTC]: 0.1% (200 mL)
Skin Care™ [OTC]: 0.25% (120 mL)
Shampoo, topical:
BetaMed [OTC]: 2% (480 mL)
DermaZinc™ [OTC]: 2% (240 mL)
DHS™ Zinc [OTC]: 2% (240 mL, 360 mL)
Head & Shoulders® Citrus Breeze [OTC], Head & Shoulders® Extra Volume [OTC]: 1% (400 mL, 700 mL)
Head & Shoulders® Classic Clean [OTC]: 1% (50 mL, 200 mL, 400 mL, 700 mL, 1000 mL, 1200 mL)
Head & Shoulders® Dry Scalp Care [OTC], Head & Shoulders® Refresh [OTC], Head & Shoulders® Sensitive Care [OTC]: 1% (400 mL, 700 mL, 1200 mL)
Zincon® [OTC]: 1% (120 mL, 240 mL)
Shampoo, topical [with conditioner]:
Head & Shoulders® Classic Clean 2-in-1 [OTC]: 1% (200 mL, 400 mL, 700 mL)
Head & Shoulders® Dry Scalp Care [OTC]: 0.5% (400 mL, 700 mL)
Head & Shoulders® Smooth and Silky 2-in-1 [OTC]: 1% (400 mL)
Soap, topical:
ZNP® [OTC]) 2% (119 g) [bar]
(Continued)

pyrithione zinc *(Continued)*
Solution, topical:
DermaZinc™ [OTC]: 0.25% (120 mL)

QDALL® [US] *see* chlorpheniramine and pseudoephedrine *on page 178*

QDALL® AR [US] *see* chlorpheniramine *on page 177*

Q-Naftate [US-OTC] *see* tolnaftate *on page 849*

quadrivalent human papillomavirus vaccine *see* papillomavirus (Types 6, 11, 16, 18) recombinant vaccine *on page 652*

quadrivalent meningococcal conjugate vaccine *see* meningococcal polysaccharide (Groups A / C / Y and W-135) diphtheria toxoid conjugate vaccine *on page 540*

Qualaquin™ [US] *see* quinine *on page 740*

Quasense™ [US] *see* ethinyl estradiol and levonorgestrel *on page 325*

quaternium-18 bentonite *see* bentoquatam *on page 99*

quazepam *(KWAZ e pam)*
Sound-Alike/Look-Alike Issues
quazepam may be confused with oxazepam
U.S./Canadian Brand Names Doral® [US/Can]
Therapeutic Category Benzodiazepine
Controlled Substance C-IV
Use Treatment of insomnia
Usual Dosage Oral: Adults: Initial: 15 mg at bedtime, in some patients the dose may be reduced to 7.5 mg after a few nights
Dosage Forms
Tablet:
Doral®: 7.5 mg, 15 mg

Quelicin® [US/Can] *see* succinylcholine *on page 808*

Queltuss® *(Discontinued)* *see* guaifenesin and dextromethorphan *on page 402*

Questran® [US/Can] *see* cholestyramine resin *on page 186*

Questran® Light [US] *see* cholestyramine resin *on page 186*

Questran® Light Sugar Free [Can] *see* cholestyramine resin *on page 186*

quetiapine *(kwe TYE a peen)*
Sound-Alike/Look-Alike Issues
Seroquel® may be confused with Serentil®, Serzone®, Sinequan®
Synonyms quetiapine fumarate
U.S./Canadian Brand Names Seroquel® XR [US]; Seroquel® [US/Can]
Therapeutic Category Antipsychotic Agent
Use Treatment of schizophrenia; treatment of acute manic episodes associated with bipolar disorder (as monotherapy or in combination with lithium or valproate); treatment of depressive episodes associated with bipolar disorder
Usual Dosage Oral: Adults:
Bipolar depression: Immediate release tablet: Initial: 50 mg/day the first day; increase to 100 mg/day on day 2, further increasing by 100 mg/day each day to a target of 300 mg/day by day 4. Further increases up to 600 mg/day by day 8 have been evaluated in clinical trials, but no additional antidepressant efficacy was noted.
Bipolar mania: Immediate release tablet: Initial: 50 mg twice daily on day 1, increase dose in increments of 100 mg/day to 200 mg twice daily on day 4; may increase to a target dose of 800 mg/day by day 6 at increments ≤200 mg/day. Usual dosage range: 400-800 mg/day.
Schizophrenia/psychoses:
Immediate release tablet: Initial: 25 mg twice daily; increase in increments of 25-50 mg 2-3 times/day on the second and third day, if tolerated, to a target dose of 300-400 mg in 2-3 divided doses by day 4. Make further adjustments as needed at intervals of at least 2 days in adjustments of 25-50 mg twice daily. Usual maintenance range: 300-800 mg/day.
Extended release tablet: Initial: 300 mg once daily; increase in increments of up to 300 mg/day (in intervals of ≥1 day). For dosage requirements <200 mg during initial titration, the immediate release formulation should be used. Usual maintenance range: 400-800 mg/day.
Note: Dose reductions should be attempted periodically to establish lowest effective dose in patients with psychosis. Patients being restarted after 1 week of no drug need to be titrated as above.

Dosage Forms
  Tablet:
    Seroquel®: 25 mg, 50 mg, 100 mg, 200 mg, 300 mg, 400 mg
  Tablet, extended release:
    Seroquel® XR: 200 mg, 300 mg, 400 mg

quetiapine fumarate *see* quetiapine *on previous page*

Quibron® *(Discontinued)* *see* theophylline and guaifenesin *on page 835*

Quibron®-T *(Discontinued)* *see* theophylline *on page 834*

Quibron®-T/SR *(Discontinued)* *see* theophylline *on page 834*

Quiess® Injection *(Discontinued)* *see* hydroxyzine *on page 440*

Quinaglute® Dura-Tabs® *(Discontinued)* *see* quinidine *on next page*

quinagolide *(Discontinued)*

Quinalan® *(Discontinued)* *see* quinidine *on next page*

quinalbarbitone sodium *see* secobarbital *on page 779*

quinapril (KWIN a pril)
  Sound-Alike/Look-Alike Issues
    Accupril® may be confused with Accolate®, Accutane®, AcipHex®, Monopril®
  Synonyms quinapril hydrochloride
  U.S./Canadian Brand Names Accupril® [US/Can]; GD-Quinapril [Can]
  Therapeutic Category Angiotensin-Converting Enzyme (ACE) Inhibitor
  Use Management of hypertension; treatment of congestive heart failure
  Usual Dosage Oral: Adults:
    Hypertension: Initial: 10-20 mg once daily, adjust according to blood pressure response at peak and trough blood levels; initial dose may be reduced to 5 mg in patients receiving diuretic therapy if the diuretic is continued; usual dose range (JNC 7): 10-40 mg once daily
    Congestive heart failure or post-MI: Initial: 5 mg once or twice daily, titrated at weekly intervals to 20-40 mg daily in 2 divided doses; target dose (heart failure): 20 mg twice daily (ACC/AHA 2005 Heart Failure Guidelines)
  Dosage Forms
    Tablet: 5 mg, 10 mg, 20 mg, 40 mg
    Accupril®: 5 mg, 10 mg, 20 mg, 40 mg

quinapril and hydrochlorothiazide (KWIN a pril & hye droe klor oh THYE a zide)
  Synonyms hydrochlorothiazide and quinapril
  U.S./Canadian Brand Names Accuretic® [US/Can]; Quinaretic [US]
  Therapeutic Category Antihypertensive Agent, Combination
  Use Treatment of hypertension (not for initial therapy)
  Usual Dosage Oral:
    Children: Safety and efficacy have not been established.
    Adults: Initial:
    Patients who have failed quinapril monotherapy:
    Quinapril 10 mg/hydrochlorothiazide 12.5 mg **or**
    Quinapril 20 mg/hydrochlorothiazide 12.5 mg once daily
    Patients with adequate blood pressure control on hydrochlorothiazide 25 mg/day, but significant potassium loss:
    Quinapril 10 mg/hydrochlorothiazide 12.5 mg **or**
    Quinapril 20 mg/hydrochlorothiazide 12.5 mg once daily
    Note: Clinical trials of quinapril/hydrochlorothiazide combinations used quinapril doses of 2.5-40 mg/day and hydrochlorothiazide doses of 6.25-25 mg/day.
  Dosage Forms
    Tablet: 10/12.5: Quinapril 10 mg and hydrochlorothiazide 12.5 mg; 20/12.5: Quinapril 20 mg and hydrochlorothiazide 12.5 mg; 20/25: Quinapril 20 mg and hydrochlorothiazide 25 mg
    Accuretic®, Quinaretic: 10/12.5: Quinapril 10 mg and hydrochlorothiazide 12.5 mg; 20/12.5: Quinapril 20 mg and hydrochlorothiazide 12.5 mg; 20/25: Quinapril 20 mg and hydrochlorothiazide 25 mg

quinapril hydrochloride *see* quinapril *on this page*

Quinaretic [US] *see* quinapril and hydrochlorothiazide *on this page*

Quinate® [Can] *see* quinidine *on next page*

Quin B Strong [US-OTC] *see* vitamin B complex combinations *on page 894*

Quin B Strong with C and Zinc [US-OTC] *see* vitamin B complex combinations *on page 894*

quinidine (KWIN i deen)
Sound-Alike/Look-Alike Issues
  quinidine may be confused with clonidine, quinine, Quinora®
Synonyms quinidine gluconate; quinidine polygalacturonate; quinidine sulfate
U.S./Canadian Brand Names Apo-Quinidine® [Can]; BioQuin® Durules™ [Can]; Novo-Quinidin [Can]; Quinate® [Can]
Therapeutic Category Antiarrhythmic Agent, Class I-A
Use Prophylaxis after cardioversion of atrial fibrillation and/or flutter to maintain normal sinus rhythm; prevent recurrence of paroxysmal supraventricular tachycardia, paroxysmal AV junctional rhythm, paroxysmal ventricular tachycardia, paroxysmal atrial fibrillation, and atrial or ventricular premature contractions; has activity against *Plasmodium falciparum* malaria
Usual Dosage Dosage expressed in terms of the salt: 267 mg of quinidine gluconate = 200 mg of quinidine sulfate.

  Children: Test dose for idiosyncratic reaction (sulfate, oral or gluconate, I.M.): 2 mg/kg or 60 mg/m²
    Oral (quinidine sulfate): 15-60 mg/kg/day in 4-5 divided doses or 6 mg/kg every 4-6 hours; usual 30 mg/kg/day or 900 mg/m²/day given in 5 daily doses
    I.V. **not** recommended (quinidine gluconate): 2-10 mg/kg/dose given at a rate ≤10 mg/minute every 3-6 hours as needed
  Adults: Test dose: Oral, I.M.: 200 mg administered several hours before full dosage (to determine possibility of idiosyncratic reaction)
    Oral (for malaria):
    Sulfate: 100-600 mg/dose every 4-6 hours; begin at 200 mg/dose and titrate to desired effect (maximum daily dose: 3-4 g)
    Gluconate: 324-972 mg every 8-12 hours
    I.M.: 400 mg/dose every 2-6 hours; initial dose: 600 mg (gluconate)
    I.V.: 200-400 mg/dose diluted and given at a rate ≤10 mg/minute; may require as much as 500-750 mg
Dosage Forms
  Injection, solution: 80 mg/mL (10 mL)
  Tablet: 200 mg, 300 mg
  Tablet, extended release: 300 mg, 324 mg

quinidine gluconate *see* quinidine *on this page*

quinidine polygalacturonate *see* quinidine *on this page*

quinidine sulfate *see* quinidine *on this page*

quinine (KWYE nine)
Sound-Alike/Look-Alike Issues
  quinine may be confused with quinidine
Synonyms quinine sulfate
U.S./Canadian Brand Names Apo-Quinine® [Can]; Novo-Quinine [Can]; Qualaquin™ [US]; Quinine-Odan™ [Can]
Therapeutic Category Antimalarial Agent
Use In conjunction with other antimalarial agents, treatment of uncomplicated chloroquine-resistant *P. falciparum* malaria
Usual Dosage Note: Actual duration of treatment for malaria may be dependent upon the geographic region or pathogen. Oral:
  Children: Treatment of chloroquine-resistant malaria (CDC guidelines): 30 mg/kg/day in divided doses every 8 hours for 3-7 days with tetracycline, doxycycline, or clindamycin (consider risk versus benefit of using tetracycline or doxycycline in children <8 years of age)
  Adults: Treatment of chloroquine-resistant malaria: 648 mg every 8 hours for 7 days with tetracycline, doxycycline, or clindamycin
Dosage Forms
  Capsule:
  Qualaquin™: 324 mg

Quinine-Odan™ [Can] *see* quinine *on this page*

quinine sulfate *see* quinine *on this page*

quinol *see* hydroquinone *on page 437*

Quinora® *(Discontinued)* *see* quinidine *on this page*

Quintabs [US-OTC] *see* vitamins (multiple/oral) *on page 895*

Quintabs-M [US-OTC] *see* vitamins (multiple/oral) *on page 895*

Quintasa® **[Can]** *see* mesalamine *on page 546*

quinupristin and dalfopristin (kwi NYOO pris tin & dal FOE pris tin)

Synonyms pristinamycin; RP-59500

U.S./Canadian Brand Names Synercid® [US/Can]

Therapeutic Category Antibiotic, Streptogramin

Use Treatment of serious or life-threatening infections associated with vancomycin-resistant *Enterococcus faecium* bacteremia; treatment of complicated skin and skin structure infections caused by methcillin-suscep-tible *Staphylococcus aureus* or *Streptococcus pyogenes*

Has been studied in the treatment of a variety of infections caused by *Enterococcus faecium* (not *E. fecalis*) including vancomycin-resistant strains. May also be effective in the treatment of serious infections caused by *Staphylococcus* species including those resistant to methicillin.

Usual Dosage I.V.:

Children (limited information): Dosages similar to adult dosing have been used in the treatment of complicated skin/soft tissue infections and infections caused by vancomycin-resistant *Enterococcus faecium*

CNS shunt infection due to vancomycin-resistant *Enterococcus faecium*: 7.5 mg/kg/dose every 8 hours; concurrent intrathecal doses of 1-2 mg/day have been administered for up to 68 days

Adults:

Vancomycin-resistant *Enterococcus faecium*: 7.5 mg/kg every 8 hours

Complicated skin and skin structure infection: 7.5 mg/kg every 12 hours

Dosage Forms

Injection, powder for reconstitution:

Synercid®: 500 mg: Quinupristin 150 mg and dalfopristin 350 mg; 600 mg: Quinupristin 180 mg and dalfopristin 420 mg

Quixin™ **[US]** *see* levofloxacin *on page 501*

QVAR® **[US/Can]** *see* beclomethasone *on page 97*

R 14-15 *see* erlotinib *on page 307*

R & C™ **II [Can]** *see* pyrethrins and piperonyl butoxide *on page 734*

R & C® **Lice** *(Discontinued)* *see* permethrin *on page 670*

R & C™ **Shampoo/Conditioner [Can]** *see* pyrethrins and piperonyl butoxide *on page 734*

R-3827 *see* abarelix *on page 2*

RabAvert® **[US/Can]** *see* rabies virus vaccine *on next page*

rabeprazole (ra BEP ra zole)

Sound-Alike/Look-Alike Issues

rabeprazole may be confused with aripiprazole

AcipHex® may be confused with Acephen®, Accupril®, Aricept®

Synonyms pariprazole

U.S./Canadian Brand Names AcipHex® [US/Can]; Pariet® [Can]

Therapeutic Category Gastric Acid Secretion Inhibitor

Use Short-term (4-8 weeks) treatment and maintenance of erosive or ulcerative gastroesophageal reflux disease (GERD); symptomatic GERD; short-term (up to 4 weeks) treatment of duodenal ulcers; long-term treatment of pathological hypersecretory conditions, including Zollinger-Ellison syndrome; *H. pylori* eradica-tion (in combination with amoxicillin and clarithromycin)

Usual Dosage Oral: Adults >18 years:

GERD: 20 mg once daily for 4-8 weeks; maintenance: 20 mg once daily

Duodenal ulcer: 20 mg/day before breakfast for 4 weeks

H. pylori eradication: 20 mg twice daily for 7 days; to be administered with amoxicillin 1000 mg and clarithromycin 500 mg, also given twice daily for 7 days.

Hypersecretory conditions: 60 mg once daily; dose may need to be adjusted as necessary. Doses as high as 100 mg once daily and 60 mg twice daily have been used.

Dosage Forms

Tablet, delayed release, enteric coated:

AcipHex®: 20 mg

rabies immune globulin (human) (RAY beez i MYUN GLOB yoo lin, HYU man)

Synonyms RIG

U.S./Canadian Brand Names HyperRAB™ S/D [US/Can]; Imogam® Rabies Pasteurized [Can]; Imogam® Rabies-HT [US]

(Continued)

rabies immune globulin (human) *(Continued)*

Therapeutic Category Immune Globulin

Use Part of postexposure prophylaxis of persons with rabies exposure who lack a history of pre-exposure or postexposure prophylaxis with rabies vaccine or a recently documented neutralizing antibody response to previous rabies vaccination; although it is preferable to administer RIG with the first dose of vaccine, it can be given up to 8 days after vaccination

Usual Dosage Children and Adults: Postexposure prophylaxis: Local wound infiltration: 20 units/kg in a single dose, RIG should always be administered as part of rabies vaccine (HDCV) regimen as soon as possible (after the first dose of vaccine, up to 8 days). If anatomically feasible, the full rabies immune globulin dose should be infiltrated around and into the wound(s); remaining volume should be administered I.M. at a site distant from the vaccine administration site. If rabies vaccine was initiated without rabies immune globulin, rabies immune globulin may be administered through the seventh day after the first vaccine dose.

Note: Persons known to have an adequate titer or who have been completely immunized with rabies vaccine should not receive RIG, only booster doses of HDCV

Dosage Forms

Injection, solution [preservative free]:

HyperRAB™ S/D, Imogam® Rabies-HT: 150 int. units/mL (2 mL, 10 mL)

rabies virus vaccine (RAY beez VYE rus vak SEEN)

Synonyms HDCV; human diploid cell cultures rabies vaccine; PCEC; purified chick embryo cell

U.S./Canadian Brand Names Imovax® Rabies [US/Can]; RabAvert® [US/Can]

Therapeutic Category Vaccine, Inactivated Virus

Use Preexposure immunization: Vaccinate persons with greater than usual risk due to occupation or avocation including veterinarians, rangers, animal handlers, certain laboratory workers, and persons living in or visiting countries for longer than 1 month where rabies is a constant threat.

Postexposure prophylaxis: If a bite from a carrier animal is unprovoked, if it is not captured and rabies is present in that species and area, administer rabies immune globulin (RIG) and the vaccine as indicated

Usual Dosage

Preexposure prophylaxis: 1 mL I.M. on days 0, 7, and 21 to 28. **Note:** Prolonging the interval between doses does not interfere with immunity achieved after the concluding dose of the basic series.

Postexposure prophylaxis: All postexposure treatment should begin with immediate cleansing of the wound with soap and water

Persons not previously immunized as above: I.M.: 5 doses (1 mL each) on days 0, 3, 7, 14, 28. In addition, patients should receive rabies immune globulin 20 units/kg body weight, half infiltrated at bite site if possible, remainder I.M.)

Persons who have previously received postexposure prophylaxis with rabies vaccine, received a recommended I.M. pre-exposure series of rabies vaccine or have a previously documented rabies antibody titer considered adequate: 1 mL of either vaccine I.M. only on days 0 and 3; do not administer RIG

Booster (for occupational or other continuing risk): 1 mL I.M. every 2-5 years or based on antibody titers

Dosage Forms

Injection, powder for reconstitution:

Imovax® Rabies: 2.5 int. units [HDCV]

RabAvert®: 2.5 int. units [PCEC]

racepinephrine *see* epinephrine *on page 300*

Radiogardase™ [US] *see* ferric hexacyanoferrate *on page 349*

rAHF *see* antihemophilic factor (recombinant) *on page 59*

R-albuterol *see* levalbuterol *on page 498*

Ralix [US] *see* chlorpheniramine, phenylephrine, and methscopolamine *on page 181*

raloxifene (ral OKS i feen)

Sound-Alike/Look-Alike Issues

Evista® may be confused with Avinza™

Synonyms keoxifene hydrochloride; NSC-706725; raloxifene hydrochloride

U.S./Canadian Brand Names Evista® [US/Can]

Therapeutic Category Selective Estrogen Receptor Modulator (SERM)

Use Prevention and treatment of osteoporosis in postmenopausal women; risk reduction for invasive breast cancer in postmenopausal women with osteoporosis and in postmenopausal women with high risk for invasive breast cancer

Usual Dosage Oral: Adults: Female: Osteoporosis: 60 mg/day

Dosage Forms
Tablet:
Evista®: 60 mg

raloxifene hydrochloride *see* raloxifene *on previous page*

raltitrexed *(Canada only)* (ral ti TREX ed)
Synonyms ICI-D1694; NSC-639186; raltitrexed disodium; ZD1694
U.S./Canadian Brand Names Tomudex® [Can]
Therapeutic Category Antineoplastic Agent
Use Treatment of advanced colorectal neoplasms
Usual Dosage I.V. (refer to individual protocols): 3 mg/m² every 3 weeks
Dosage Forms
Injection, powder for reconstitution:
2 mg [not available in the U.S.; investigational]

raltitrexed disodium *see* raltitrexed *(Canada only)* on this page

ramelteon (ra MEL tee on)
Sound-Alike/Look-Alike Issues
Rozerem™ may be confused with Razadyne™
Synonyms TAK-375
U.S./Canadian Brand Names Rozerem™ [US]
Therapeutic Category Hypnotic, Nonbenzodiazepine
Use Treatment of insomnia characterized by difficulty with sleep onset
Usual Dosage Oral: Adults: One 8 mg tablet within 30 minutes of bedtime
Dosage Forms
Tablet:
Rozerem™: 8 mg

ramipril (RA mi pril)
Sound-Alike/Look-Alike Issues
ramipril may be confused with enalapril, Monopril®
Altace® may be confused with alteplase, Amaryl®, Amerge®, Artane®
U.S./Canadian Brand Names Altace® [US/Can]; Apo-Ramipril® [Can]
Therapeutic Category Angiotensin-Converting Enzyme (ACE) Inhibitor
Use Treatment of hypertension, alone or in combination with thiazide diuretics; treatment of left ventricular dysfunction after myocardial infarction; to reduce risk of heart attack, stroke, and death in patients at increased risk for these problems
Usual Dosage Oral: Adults:
Hypertension: 2.5-5 mg once daily, maximum: 20 mg/day
Reduction in risk of MI, stroke, and death from cardiovascular causes: Initial: 2.5 mg once daily for 1 week, then 5 mg once daily for the next 3 weeks, then increase as tolerated to 10 mg once daily (may be given as divided dose)
Heart failure postmyocardial infarction: Initial: 2.5 mg twice daily titrated upward, if possible, to 5 mg twice daily.
Note: The dose of any concomitant diuretic should be reduced. If the diuretic cannot be discontinued, initiate therapy with 1.25 mg. After the initial dose, the patient should be monitored carefully until blood pressure has stabilized.
Dosage Forms
Capsule:
Altace®: 1.25 mg, 2.5 mg, 5 mg, 10 mg

ramipril and hydrochlorothiazide *(Canada only)*
(RA mi pril & hye droe klor oh THYE a zide)
Sound-Alike/Look-Alike Issues
Altace® HCT may be confused with alteplase, Artane®, Altace®
Synonyms hydrochlorothiazide and ramipril
U.S./Canadian Brand Names Altace® HCT [Can]
Therapeutic Category Angiotensin-Converting Enzyme (ACE) Inhibitor; Antihypertensive Agent, Combination; Diuretic, Thiazide
Use Treatment of essential hypertension (not for initial therapy)
Usual Dosage Oral: Adults: **Note:** Not for initial therapy; titration of individual agents to an appropriate clinical response is required before patient is converted over to an equivalent dose of the combination product.
(Continued)

743

ramipril and hydrochlorothiazide *(Canada only)* *(Continued)*

Usual dosage: Ramipril 2.5 mg/hydrochlorothiazide 12.5 mg once daily; titrate to maximum ramipril 10 mg/hydrochlorothiazide 50 mg once daily

Dosage Forms

Tablet:

Altace® HCT 2.5/12.5 [CAN]: Ramipril 2.5 mg and hydrochlorothiazide 12.5 mg [not available in the U.S.]

Altace® HCT 5/12.5 [CAN]: Ramipril 5 mg and hydrochlorothiazide 12.5 mg [not available in the U.S.]

Altace® HCT 5/25 [CAN]: Ramipril 5 mg and hydrochlorothiazide 25 mg [not available in the U.S.]

Altace® HCT 10/12.5 [CAN]: Ramipril 10 mg and hydrochlorothiazide 12.5 mg [not available in the U.S.]

Altace® HCT 10/25 [CAN]: Ramipril 10 mg and hydrochlorothiazide 25 mg [not available in the U.S.]

RAN™-Atenolol [Can] *see* atenolol *on page 80*

RAN™-Carvedilol [Can] *see* carvedilol *on page 155*

RAN™-Ciprofloxacin [Can] *see* ciprofloxacin *on page 190*

RAN™-Citalopram [Can] *see* citalopram *on page 194*

RAN™-Domperidone [Can] *see* domperidone *(Canada only) on page 276*

Ranexa® [US] *see* ranolazine *on next page*

ranibizumab (ra ni BIZ oo mab)

Synonyms rhuFabV2

U.S./Canadian Brand Names Lucentis® [US]

Therapeutic Category Monoclonal Antibody; Ophthalmic Agent; Vascular Endothelial Growth Factor (VEGF) Inhibitor

Use Treatment of neovascular (wet) age-related macular degeneration (AMD)

Usual Dosage Ophthalmic: Adults: AMD: Intravitreal injection: 0.5 mg once a month. Although not as effective, frequency may be reduced after the first 4 injections to once every 3 months if monthly injections are not feasible. Dosing every 3 months will lead to an ~5 letter (1 line) loss of visual acuity over 9 months, as compared to monthly dosing.

Dosage Forms

Injection, solution [preservative free]:

Lucentis®: 10 mg/mL (0.05 mL)

Raniclor™ [US] *see* cefaclor *on page 157*

ranitidine (ra NI ti deen)

Sound-Alike/Look-Alike Issues

ranitidine may be confused with amantadine, rimantadine

Zantac® may be confused with Xanax®, Zarontin®, Zofran®, Zyrtec®

Synonyms ranitidine hydrochloride

U.S./Canadian Brand Names Alti-Ranitidine [Can]; Apo-Ranitidine® [Can]; BCI-Ranitidine [Can]; CO Ranitidine [Can]; Gen-Ranidine [Can]; Novo-Ranidine [Can]; Nu-Ranit [Can]; PMS-Ranitidine [Can]; Ranitidine Injection, USP [Can]; Rhoxal-ranitidine [Can]; Sandoz-Ranitidine [Can]; Zantac 150™ [US-OTC]; Zantac 75® [US-OTC/Can]; Zantac® EFFERdose® [US]; Zantac® [US/Can]

Therapeutic Category Histamine H_2 Antagonist

Use

Zantac®: Short-term and maintenance therapy of duodenal ulcer, gastric ulcer, gastroesophageal reflux, active benign ulcer, erosive esophagitis, and pathological hypersecretory conditions; as part of a multidrug regimen for *H. pylori* eradication to reduce the risk of duodenal ulcer recurrence

Zantac® 75 [OTC]: Relief of heartburn, acid indigestion, and sour stomach

Usual Dosage

Children 1 month to 16 years:

Duodenal and gastric ulcer:

Oral:

Treatment: 2-4 mg/kg/day divided twice daily; maximum treatment dose: 300 mg/day

Maintenance: 2-4 mg/kg once daily; maximum maintenance dose: 150 mg/day

I.V.: 2-4 mg/kg/day divided every 6-8 hours; maximum: 200 mg/day

GERD and erosive esophagitis: Oral: 5-10 mg/kg/day divided twice daily; maximum: GERD: 300 mg/day, erosive esophagitis: 600 mg/day

Children ≥12 years: Prevention of heartburn: Oral: Zantac® 75 [OTC]: 75 mg 30-60 minutes before eating food or drinking beverages which cause heartburn; maximum: 150 mg/24 hours; do not use for more than 14 days

Adults:

Duodenal ulcer: Oral: Treatment: 150 mg twice daily, or 300 mg once daily after the evening meal or at bedtime; maintenance: 150 mg once daily at bedtime

Helicobacter pylori eradication: 150 mg twice daily; requires combination therapy

Pathological hypersecretory conditions:

Oral: 150 mg twice daily; adjust dose or frequency as clinically indicated; doses of up to 6 g/day have been used

I.V.: Continuous infusion for Zollinger-Ellison: 1 mg/kg/hour; measure gastric acid output at 4 hours, if >10 mEq or if patient is symptomatic, increase dose in increments of 0.5 mg/kg/hour; doses of up to 2.5 mg/kg/hour have been used

Gastric ulcer, benign: Oral: 150 mg twice daily; maintenance: 150 mg once daily at bedtime

Erosive esophagitis: Oral: Treatment: 150 mg 4 times/day; maintenance: 150 mg twice daily

Prevention of heartburn: Oral: Zantac® 75 [OTC]: 75 mg 30-60 minutes before eating food or drinking beverages which cause heartburn; maximum: 150 mg in 24 hours; do not use for more than 14 days

Patients not able to take oral medication:

I.M.: 50 mg every 6-8 hours

I.V.: Intermittent bolus or infusion: 50 mg every 6-8 hours

Continuous I.V. infusion: 6.25 mg/hour

Dosage Forms

Capsule: 150 mg, 300 mg

Infusion [premixed in NaCl 0.45%; preservative free]: 50 mg (50 mL)

Zantac®: 50 mg (50 mL)

Injection, solution: 25 mg/mL (2 mL, 6 mL)

Zantac®: 25 mg/mL (2 mL, 6 mL, 40 mL)

Syrup: 15 mg/mL

Zantac®: 15 mg/mL

Tablet: 75 mg [OTC], 150 mg, 300 mg

Zantac®: 150 mg, 300 mg

Zantac 75® [OTC]: 75 mg

Zantac 150™ [OTC]: 150 mg

Tablet, effervescent:

Zantac® EFFERdose®: 25 mg

ranitidine hydrochloride *see* ranitidine *on previous page*

Ranitidine Injection, USP [Can] *see* ranitidine *on previous page*

RAN™-Lovastatin [Can] *see* lovastatin *on page 520*

RAN™-Metformin [Can] *see* metformin *on page 548*

ranolazine (ra NOE la zeen)

Sound-Alike/Look-Alike Issues

Ranexa® may be confused with Celexa®

U.S./Canadian Brand Names Ranexa® [US]

Therapeutic Category Cardiovascular Agent, Miscellaneous

Use Treatment of chronic angina in combination with amlodipine, beta-blockers, or nitrates

Usual Dosage Oral: Adults: Chronic angina: Initial: 500 mg twice daily; maximum recommended dose: 1000 mg twice daily

Dosage Forms

Tablet, extended release:

Ranexa®: 500 mg, 1000 mg

RAN™-Zopiclone [Can] *see* zopiclone *(Canada only) on page 909*

Rapamune® [US/Can] *see* sirolimus *on page 788*

Raphon [US-OTC] *see* epinephrine *on page 300*

Raplon® *(Discontinued)*

Raptiva® [US] *see* efalizumab *on page 292*

rasagiline (ra SA ji leen)

Sound-Alike/Look-Alike Issues

Azilect® may be confused with Aricept®

Synonyms AGN 1135; rasagiline mesylate; TVP-1012

U.S./Canadian Brand Names Azilect® [US]

Therapeutic Category Anti-Parkinson Agent, MAO Type B Inhibitor

Use Initial monotherapy or as adjunct to levodopa in the treatment of idiopathic Parkinson disease

Usual Dosage Oral: Adults: Parkinson disease:

Monotherapy: 1 mg once daily

(Continued)

rasagiline *(Continued)*

Adjunctive therapy with levodopa: Initial: 0.5 mg once daily; may increase to 1 mg once daily based on response and tolerability

Note: When added to existing levodopa therapy, a dose reduction of levodopa may be required to avoid exacerbation of dyskinesias; typical dose reductions of ~9% to 13% were employed in clinical trials

Dosage Forms

Tablet, as mesylate:

Azilect®: 0.5 mg, 1 mg

rasagiline mesylate *see* rasagiline *on previous page*

rasburicase *(ras BYOOR i kayse)*

Synonyms NSC-721631; recombinant urate oxidase

U.S./Canadian Brand Names Elitek™ [US]; Fasturtec® [Can]

Therapeutic Category Enzyme

Use Initial management of uric acid levels in pediatric patients with leukemia, lymphoma, and solid tumor malignancies receiving anticancer therapy expected to result in tumor lysis and elevation of plasma uric acid

Usual Dosage I.V.:

Children: Management of uric acid levels: 0.15 mg/kg or 0.2 mg/kg once daily for 5 days (manufacturer-recommended duration); begin chemotherapy 4-24 hours after the first dose

Limited data suggest that a single prechemotherapy dose (versus multiple-day administration) may be sufficiently efficacious. Monitoring electrolytes, hydration status, and uric acid concentrations are necessary to identify the need for additional doses. Other clinical manifestations of tumor lysis syndrome (eg, hyperphosphatemia, hypocalcemia, and hyperkalemia) may occur.

Adults: Refer to pediatric dosing; insufficient data collected in adult/geriatric patients to determine response to treatment

Dosage Forms

Injection, powder for reconstitution:

Elitek™: 1.5 mg, 7.5 mg

ratio-Aclavulanate [Can] *see* amoxicillin and clavulanate potassium *on page 49*

ratio-Acyclovir [Can] *see* acyclovir *on page 17*

ratio-Alendronate [Can] *see* alendronate *on page 27*

ratio-Amcinonide [Can] *see* amcinonide *on page 39*

ratio-Azithromycin [Can] *see* azithromycin *on page 88*

ratio-Benzydamine [Can] *see* benzydamine *(Canada only) on page 105*

ratio-Bicalutamide [Can] *see* bicalutamide *on page 111*

ratio-Brimonidine [Can] *see* brimonidine *on page 118*

ratio-Carvedilol [Can] *see* carvedilol *on page 155*

ratio-Cefuroxime [Can] *see* cefuroxime *on page 165*

ratio-Ciprofloxacin [Can] *see* ciprofloxacin *on page 190*

ratio-Citalopram [Can] *see* citalopram *on page 194*

ratio-Clarithromycin [Can] *see* clarithromycin *on page 196*

ratio-Clobazam [Can] *see* clobazam *(Canada only) on page 201*

ratio-Cotridin [Can] *see* triprolidine, pseudoephedrine, and codeine *(Canada only) on page 869*

ratio-Diltiazem CD [Can] *see* diltiazem *on page 261*

ratio-Domperidone [Can] *see* domperidone *(Canada only) on page 276*

ratio-Emtec [Can] *see* acetaminophen and codeine *on page 6*

ratio-Famotidine [Can] *see* famotidine *on page 341*

ratio-Fenofibrate MC [Can] *see* fenofibrate *on page 345*

ratio-Fosinopril [Can] *see* fosinopril *on page 376*

ratio-Glimepiride [Can] *see* glimepiride *on page 393*

ratio-Glyburide [Can] *see* glyburide *on page 396*

ratio-Inspra-Sal [Can] *see* albuterol *on page 23*

ratio-Ketorolac [Can] *see* ketorolac *on page 483*

ratio-Lamotrigine [Can] *see* lamotrigine *on page 490*

ratio-Lenoltec [Can] *see* acetaminophen and codeine *on page 6*

ratio-Lovastatin [Can] *see* lovastatin *on page 520*

ratio-Magnesium [Can] *see* magnesium glucoheptonate *on page 525*

ratio-Metformin [Can] *see* metformin *on page 548*

ratio-Methotrexate [Can] *see* methotrexate *on page 553*

ratio-Mirtazapine [Can] *see* mirtazapine *on page 572*

ratio-Mometasone [Can] *see* mometasone *on page 576*

ratio-Morphine SR [Can] *see* morphine sulfate *on page 578*

Ratio-Orciprenaline® [Can] *see* metaproterenol *on page 548*

ratio-Paroxetine [Can] *see* paroxetine *on page 654*

ratio-Pentoxifylline [Can] *see* pentoxifylline *on page 667*

ratio-Pravastatin [Can] *see* pravastatin *on page 707*

ratio-Salbutamol [Can] *see* albuterol *on page 23*

ratio-Sertraline [Can] *see* sertraline *on page 783*

ratio-Simvastatin [Can] *see* simvastatin *on page 787*

ratio-Sumatriptan [Can] *see* sumatriptan *on page 815*

ratio-Temazepam [Can] *see* temazepam *on page 823*

ratio-Theo-Bronc [Can] *see* theophylline *on page 834*

ratio-Topiramate [Can] *see* topiramate *on page 851*

ratio-Trazodone [Can] *see* trazodone *on page 859*

Ratio-Zopiclone [Can] *see* zopiclone *(Canada only) on page 909*

Raudixin® *(Discontinued)*

Rauverid® *(Discontinued)*

Razadyne™ [US] *see* galantamine *on page 382*

Razadyne™ ER [US] *see* galantamine *on page 382*

Reactine™ [Can] *see* cetirizine *on page 169*

Reactine® Allergy and Sinus [Can] *see* cetirizine and pseudoephedrine *on page 169*

Readi-Cat® [US] *see* barium *on page 94*

Readi-Cat® 2 [US] *see* barium *on page 94*

Rea-Lo® [US-OTC] *see* urea *on page 877*

ReAzo [US-OTC] *see* phenazopyridine *on page 671*

Rebetol® [US] *see* ribavirin *on page 755*

Rebetron® [US] *see* interferon alfa-2b and ribavirin *on page 463*

Rebif® [US/Can] *see* interferon beta-1a *on page 464*

Reclast® [US] *see* zoledronic acid *on page 907*

Reclipsen™ [US] *see* ethinyl estradiol and desogestrel *on page 322*

recombinant α-L-iduronidase (glycosaminoglycan α-L-iduronohydrolase) *see* laronidase *on page 494*

recombinant hirudin *see* lepirudin *on page 495*

recombinant human deoxyribonuclease *see* dornase alfa *on page 277*

recombinant human insulin-like growth factor-1 *see* mecasermin *on page 535*

recombinant human interleukin-11 *see* oprelvekin *on page 632*

recombinant human luteinizing hormone *see* lutropin alfa *on page 523*

recombinant human parathyroid hormone (1-34) *see* teriparatide *on page 827*

recombinant human platelet-derived growth factor B *see* becaplermin *on page 96*

recombinant interleukin-11 *see* oprelvekin *on page 632*

recombinant N-acetylgalactosamine 4-sulfatase *see* galsulfase *on page 383*

recombinant plasminogen activator *see* reteplase *on page 751*

recombinant urate oxidase *see* rasburicase *on previous page*

Recombinate [US/Can] *see* antihemophilic factor (recombinant) *on page 59*

Recombivax HB® [US/Can] *see* hepatitis B vaccine *on page 418*

Rectacaine [US-OTC] *see* phenylephrine *on page 675*

Red Cross™ Canker Sore [US-OTC] *see* benzocaine *on page 101*

Redisol® *(Discontinued) see* cyanocobalamin *on page 220*

Reese's® Pinworm Medicine [US-OTC] *see* pyrantel pamoate *on page 733*

ReFacto® [US/Can] *see* antihemophilic factor (recombinant) *on page 59*

Refenesen Plus [US-OTC] *see* guaifenesin and pseudoephedrine *on page 406*

Refludan® [US/Can] *see* lepirudin *on page 495*

Refresh® [US-OTC] *see* artificial tears *on page 75*

Refresh Liquigel™ [US-OTC] *see* carboxymethylcellulose *on page 153*

Refresh Plus® [US-OTC] *see* artificial tears *on page 75*

Refresh Plus® [US-OTC/Can] *see* carboxymethylcellulose *on page 153*

Refresh Tears® [US-OTC] *see* artificial tears *on page 75*

Refresh Tears® [US-OTC/Can] *see* carboxymethylcellulose *on page 153*

Regitine® [Can] *see* phentolamine *on page 674*

Regitine® *(Discontinued) see* phentolamine *on page 674*

Reglan® [US] *see* metoclopramide *on page 561*

Reglan® Syrup *(Discontinued) see* metoclopramide *on page 561*

Regonol® [US] *see* pyridostigmine *on page 735*

Regranex® [US/Can] *see* becaplermin *on page 96*

Regular Iletin® II *(Discontinued)*

regular insulin *see* insulin regular *on page 460*

Regulax SS® *(Discontinued) see* docusate *on page 273*

Regulex® [Can] *see* docusate *on page 273*

Reguloid® [US-OTC] *see* psyllium *on page 732*

Rejuva-A® [Can] *see* tretinoin (topical) *on page 861*

Relacon-DM NR [US] *see* guaifenesin, pseudoephedrine, and dextromethorphan *on page 408*

Relacon-HC [US] *see* phenylephrine, hydrocodone, and chlorpheniramine *on page 678*

Relacon-HC NR [US] *see* phenylephrine, hydrocodone, and chlorpheniramine *on page 678*

Relafen® [Can] *see* nabumetone *on page 585*

Relafen® *(Discontinued) see* nabumetone *on page 585*

Relenza® [US/Can] *see* zanamivir *on page 902*

Relera [US] *see* chlorpheniramine and phenylephrine *on page 177*

Relief® [US-OTC] *see* phenylephrine *on page 675*

Relief® Ophthalmic Solution *(Discontinued) see* phenylephrine *on page 675*

Relpax® [US/Can] *see* eletriptan *on page 294*

Remeron® [US/Can] *see* mirtazapine *on page 572*

Remeron® RD [Can] *see* mirtazapine *on page 572*

Remeron SolTab® [US] *see* mirtazapine *on page 572*

Reme-T™ [US-OTC] *see* coal tar *on page 208*

Remicade® [US/Can] *see* infliximab *on page 454*

remifentanil (rem i FEN ta nil)

Sound-Alike/Look-Alike Issues
remifentanil may be confused with alfentanil
Synonyms GI87084B
U.S./Canadian Brand Names Ultiva® [US/Can]
Therapeutic Category Analgesic, Narcotic
Controlled Substance C-II

Use Analgesic for use during the induction and maintenance of general anesthesia; for continued analgesia into the immediate postoperative period; analgesic component of monitored anesthesia

Usual Dosage I.V. continuous infusion: Dose should be based on ideal body weight (IBW) in obese patients (>30% over IBW).

Children birth to 2 months: Maintenance of anesthesia with nitrous oxide (70%): 0.4 mcg/kg/minute (range: 0.4-1 mcg/kg/minute); supplemental bolus dose of 1 mcg/kg may be administered, smaller bolus dose may be required with potent inhalation agents, potent neuraxial anesthesia, significant comorbidities, significant fluid shifts, or without atropine pretreatment. Clearance in neonates is highly variable; dose should be carefully titrated.

Children 1-12 years: Maintenance of anesthesia with halothane, sevoflurane or isoflurane: 0.25 mcg/kg/minute (range 0.05-1.3 mcg/kg/minute); supplemental bolus dose of 1 mcg/kg may be administered every 2-5 minutes. Consider increasing concomitant anesthetics with infusion rate >1 mcg/kg/minute. Infusion rate can be titrated upward in increments up to 50% or titrated downward in decrements of 25% to 50%. May titrate every 2-5 minutes.

Adults:

Induction of anesthesia: 0.5-1 mcg/kg/minute; if endotracheal intubation is to occur in <8 minutes, an initial dose of 1 mcg/kg may be given over 30-60 seconds

Coronary bypass surgery: 1 mcg/kg/minute

Maintenance of anesthesia: **Note:** Supplemental bolus dose of 1 mcg/kg may be administered every 2-5 minutes. Consider increasing concomitant anesthetics with infusion rate >1 mcg/kg/minute. Infusion rate can be titrated upward in increments of 25% to 100% or downward in decrements of 25% to 50%. May titrate every 2-5 minutes.

With nitrous oxide (66%): 0.4 mcg/kg/minute (range: 0.1-2 mcg/kg/minute)

With isoflurane: 0.25 mcg/kg/minute (range: 0.05-2 mcg/kg/minute)

With propofol: 0.25 mcg/kg/minute (range: 0.05-2 mcg/kg/minute)

Coronary bypass surgery: 1 mcg/kg/minute (range: 0.125-4 mcg/kg/minute); supplemental dose: 0.5-1 mcg/kg

Continuation as an analgesic in immediate postoperative period: 0.1 mcg/kg/minute (range: 0.025-0.2 mcg/kg/minute). Infusion rate may be adjusted every 5 minutes in increments of 0.025 mcg/kg/minute. Bolus doses are not recommended. Infusion rates >0.2 mcg/kg/minute are associated with respiratory depression.

Coronary bypass surgery, continuation as an analgesic into the ICU: 1 mcg/kg/minute (range: 0.05-1 mcg/kg/minute)

Analgesic component of monitored anesthesia care: **Note:** Supplemental oxygen is recommended:

Single I.V. dose given 90 seconds prior to local anesthetic:

Remifentanil alone: 1 mcg/kg over 30-60 seconds

With midazolam: 0.5 mcg/kg over 30-60 seconds

Continuous infusion beginning 5 minutes prior to local anesthetic:

Remifentanil alone: 0.1 mcg/kg minute

With midazolam: 0.05 mcg/kg/minute

Continuous infusion given after local anesthetic:

Remifentanil alone: 0.05 mcg/kg/minute (range: 0.025-0.2 mcg/kg/minute)

With midazolam: 0.025 mcg/kg/minute (range: 0.025-0.2 mcg/kg/minute)

Note: Following local or anesthetic block, infusion rate should be decreased to 0.05 mcg/kg/minute; rate adjustments of 0.025 mcg/kg/minute may be done at 5-minute intervals

Dosage Forms
Injection, powder for reconstitution:
Ultiva®: 1 mg, 2 mg, 5 mg

Reminyl® [Can] *see* galantamine *on page 382*

Reminyl® (Discontinued) *see* galantamine *on page 382*

Reminyl® ER [Can] *see* galantamine *on page 382*

Remodulin® [US/Can] *see* treprostinil *on page 860*

Renacidin® [US] *see* citric acid, magnesium carbonate, and glucono-delta-lactone *on page 195*

Renagel® [US/Can] *see* sevelamer *on page 783*

Renal Caps [US] *see* vitamin B complex combinations *on page 894*

Rena-Vite [US-OTC] *see* vitamin B complex combinations *on page 894*

Rena-Vite RX [US] *see* vitamin B complex combinations *on page 894*

Renedil® [Can] *see* felodipine *on page 344*

Reno-30® [US] *see* diatrizoate meglumine *on page 249*

Reno-60® [US] *see* diatrizoate meglumine *on page 249*

RenoCal-76® [US] *see* diatrizoate meglumine and diatrizoate sodium *on page 250*

Reno-Dip® [US] *see* diatrizoate meglumine *on page 249*

Renografin®-60 [US] *see* diatrizoate meglumine and diatrizoate sodium *on page 250*

Renoquid® *(Discontinued)*

Renova® [US] *see* tretinoin (topical) *on page 861*

ReoPro® [US/Can] *see* abciximab *on page 3*

repaglinide (re PAG li nide)

Sound-Alike/Look-Alike Issues
Prandin® may be confused with Avandia®

U.S./Canadian Brand Names GlucoNorm® [Can]; Prandin® [US/Can]

Therapeutic Category Hypoglycemic Agent, Oral

Use Management of type 2 diabetes mellitus (noninsulin-dependent, NIDDM); may be used in combination with metformin or thiazolidinediones

Usual Dosage Oral: Adults: Should be taken within 15 minutes of the meal, but time may vary from immediately preceding the meal to as long as 30 minutes before the meal

Initial: For patients not previously treated or whose Hb A_{1c} is <8%, the starting dose is 0.5 mg. For patients previously treated with blood glucose-lowering agents whose Hb A_{1c} is ≥8%, the initial dose is 1 or 2 mg before each meal.

Dose adjustment: Determine dosing adjustments by blood glucose response, usually fasting blood glucose. Double the preprandial dose up to 4 mg until satisfactory blood glucose response is achieved. At least 1 week should elapse to assess response after each dose adjustment.

Dose range: 0.5-4 mg taken with meals. Repaglinide may be dosed preprandial 2, 3 or 4 times/day in response to changes in the patient's meal pattern. Maximum recommended daily dose: 16 mg.

Patients receiving other oral hypoglycemic agents: When repaglinide is used to replace therapy with other oral hypoglycemic agents, it may be started the day after the final dose is given. Observe patients carefully for hypoglycemia because of potential overlapping of drug effects. When transferred from longer half-life sulfonylureas (eg, chlorpropamide), close monitoring may be indicated for up to ≥1 week.

Combination therapy: If repaglinide monotherapy does not result in adequate glycemic control, metformin or a thiazolidinedione may be added. Or, if metformin or thiazolidinedione therapy does not provide adequate control, repaglinide may be added. The starting dose and dose adjustments for combination therapy are the same as repaglinide monotherapy. Carefully adjust the dose of each drug to determine the minimal dose required to achieve the desired pharmacologic effect. Failure to do so could result in an increase in the incidence of hypoglycemic episodes. Use appropriate monitoring of FPG and Hb A_{1c} measurements to ensure that the patient is not subjected to excessive drug exposure or increased probability of secondary drug failure. If glucose is not achieved after a suitable trial of combination therapy, consider discontinuing these drugs and using insulin.

Dosage Forms
Tablet:
Prandin®: 0.5 mg, 1 mg, 2 mg

Repan® [US] *see* butalbital, acetaminophen, and caffeine *on page 130*

Replace [US-OTC] *see* vitamins (multiple/oral) *on page 895*

Replace with Iron [US-OTC] *see* vitamins (multiple/oral) *on page 895*

Replagal™ [Can] *see* agalsidase alfa *(Canada only) on page 21*

Repliva 21/7™ [US] *see* vitamins (multiple/oral) *on page 895*

Reposans-10® Oral *(Discontinued) see* chlordiazepoxide *on page 173*

Reprexain™ [US] *see* hydrocodone and ibuprofen *on page 430*

Repronex® [US/Can] *see* menotropins *on page 541*

Requip® [US/Can] *see* ropinirole *on page 765*

Resa® *(Discontinued) see* reserpine *on next page*

Rescon® [US] *see* chlorpheniramine, phenylephrine, and methscopolamine *on page 181*

Rescon® MX [US] *see* chlorpheniramine, phenylephrine, and methscopolamine *on page 181*

Rescon DM [US-OTC] *see* chlorpheniramine, pseudoephedrine, and dextromethorphan *on page 183*

Rescon GG [US] *see* guaifenesin and phenylephrine *on page 404*

Rescon-Jr [US] *see* chlorpheniramine and phenylephrine *on page 177*

Rescriptor® [US/Can] *see* delavirdine *on page 235*

Rescula® *(Discontinued)*

Resectisol® [US] *see* mannitol *on page 530*

reserpine (re SER peen)

Sound-Alike/Look-Alike Issues
reserpine may be confused with Risperdal®, risperidone

Therapeutic Category Rauwolfia Alkaloid

Use Management of mild-to-moderate hypertension; treatment of agitated psychotic states (schizophrenia)

Usual Dosage Note: When used for management of hypertension, full antihypertensive effects may take as long as 3 weeks.

Oral:
Children: Hypertension: 0.01-0.02 mg/kg/24 hours divided every 12 hours; maximum dose: 0.25 mg/day (not recommended in children)

Adults:
Hypertension:
Manufacturer's labeling: Initial: 0.5 mg/day for 1-2 weeks; maintenance: 0.1-0.25 mg/day
Note: Clinically, the need for a "loading" period (as recommended by the manufacturer) is not well supported, and alternative dosing is preferred.
Usual dose range (JNC 7): 0.05-0.25 mg once daily; 0.1 mg every other day may be given to achieve 0.05 mg once daily
Schizophrenia: Dosing recommendations vary; initial dose recommendations generally range from 0.05-0.25 mg (although manufacturer recommends 0.5 mg once daily initially in schizophrenia). May be increased in increments of 0.1-0.25 mg.

Dosage Forms
Tablet: 0.1 mg, 0.25 mg

Respa®-1st [US] see guaifenesin and pseudoephedrine on page 406

Respa-DM® [US] see guaifenesin and dextromethorphan on page 402

Respa-GF® (Discontinued) see guaifenesin on page 401

Respahist® [US] see brompheniramine and pseudoephedrine on page 120

Respaire®-60 SR [US] see guaifenesin and pseudoephedrine on page 406

Respaire®-120 SR [US] see guaifenesin and pseudoephedrine on page 406

Respa® PE [US] see guaifenesin and phenylephrine on page 404

Respbid® (Discontinued) see theophylline on page 834

Respi-Tann™ [US] see carbetapentane and pseudoephedrine on page 149

Resporal® (Discontinued) see dexbrompheniramine and pseudoephedrine on page 243

Restall® (Discontinued) see hydroxyzine on page 440

Restasis® [US] see cyclosporine on page 223

Restoril® [US/Can] see temazepam on page 823

Restylane® [US] see hyaluronate and derivatives on page 423

retapamulin (re te PAM ue lin)

U.S./Canadian Brand Names Altabax™ [US]

Therapeutic Category Antibiotic, Pleuromutilin; Antibiotic, Topical

Use Treatment of impetigo caused by susceptible strains of S. pyogenes or methicillin-susceptible S. aureus

Usual Dosage Topical: Impetigo:
Children ≥9 months: Apply to affected area twice daily for 5 days. Total treatment area should not exceed 2% of total body surface area.
Adults: Apply to affected area twice daily for 5 days. Total treatment area should not exceed 100 cm² total body surface area.

Dosage Forms
Ointment, topical:
Altabax™: 1% (5 g, 10 g, 15 g)

Retavase® [US/Can] see reteplase on this page

reteplase (RE ta plase)

Synonyms recombinant plasminogen activator; r-PA

U.S./Canadian Brand Names Retavase® [US/Can]

Therapeutic Category Fibrinolytic Agent

Use Management of acute myocardial infarction (AMI); improvement of ventricular function; reduction of the incidence of CHF and the reduction of mortality following AMI

(Continued)

reteplase *(Continued)*

Usual Dosage Adults: 10 units I.V. over 2 minutes, followed by a second dose 30 minutes later of 10 units I.V. over 2 minutes

Withhold second dose if serious bleeding or anaphylaxis occurs

Dosage Forms

Injection, powder for reconstitution [preservative free]:
Retavase®: 10.4 units

Retin-A® [US/Can] *see* tretinoin (topical) *on page 861*

Retin-A® Micro [US/Can] *see* tretinoin (topical) *on page 861*

retinoic acid *see* tretinoin (topical) *on page 861*

Retinova® [Can] *see* tretinoin (topical) *on page 861*

Retisert™ [US] *see* fluocinolone *on page 359*

Retrovir® [US/Can] *see* zidovudine *on page 904*

Revatio™ [US] *see* sildenafil *on page 785*

Reversol® [US] *see* edrophonium *on page 291*

Revex® [US] *see* nalmefene *on page 588*

Rēv-Eyes™ [US] *see* dapiprazole *on page 231*

ReVia® [US/Can] *see* naltrexone *on page 590*

Revitalose C-1000® [Can] *see* ascorbic acid *on page 76*

Revlimid® [US] *see* lenalidomide *on page 495*

Rexigen Forte® *(Discontinued) see* phendimetrazine *on page 671*

Reyataz® [US/Can] *see* atazanavir *on page 80*

Rezulin® *(Discontinued)*

rFSH-alpha *see* follitropin alfa *on page 372*

rFSH-beta *see* follitropin beta *on page 372*

rFVIIa *see* factor VIIa (recombinant) *on page 339*

R-Gel® *(Discontinued) see* capsaicin *on page 145*

R-Gene® [US] *see* arginine *on page 73*

rGM-CSF *see* sargramostim *on page 777*

rhASB *see* galsulfase *on page 383*

r-hCG *see* chorionic gonadotropin (recombinant) *on page 187*

rhDNase *see* dornase alfa *on page 277*

Rheaban® *(Discontinued)*

Rheomacrodex® *(Discontinued) see* dextran *on page 245*

Rheumatrex® Dose Pack® [US] *see* methotrexate *on page 553*

rhFSH-alpha *see* follitropin alfa *on page 372*

rhFSH-beta *see* follitropin beta *on page 372*

rhGAA *see* alglucosidase alfa *on page 29*

r-h α-GAL *see* agalsidase beta *on page 21*

RhIG *see* Rh$_o$(D) immune globulin *on next page*

rhIGF-1 *see* mecasermin *on page 535*

rhIGF-1/rhIGFBP-3 *see* mecasermin *on page 535*

rhIL-11 *see* oprelvekin *on page 632*

Rhinalar® [Can] *see* flunisolide *on page 359*

Rhinall [US-OTC] *see* phenylephrine *on page 675*

Rhinocort® Aqua® [US] *see* budesonide *on page 123*

Rhinocort® Nasal Inhaler *(Discontinued) see* budesonide *on page 123*

Rhinocort® Turbuhaler® [Can] *see* budesonide *on page 123*

RhinoFlex™ [US] *see* acetaminophen and phenyltoloxamine *on page 8*

RhinoFlex 650 [US] *see* acetaminophen and phenyltoloxamine *on page 8*

r-hLH *see* lutropin alfa *on page 523*

Rho(D) immune globulin (human) *see* Rh$_o$(D) immune globulin *on this page*

Rho®-Clonazepam [Can] *see* clonazepam *on page 204*

Rhodacine® [Can] *see* indomethacin *on page 454*

Rh$_o$(D) immune globulin (ar aych oh (dee) i MYUN GLOB yoo lin)

Synonyms RhIG; Rho(D) immune globulin (human); RhoIGIV; RhoIVIM

U.S./Canadian Brand Names HyperRHO™ S/D Full Dose [US]; HyperRHO™ S/D Mini Dose [US]; MICRhoGAM® [US]; RhoGAM® [US]; Rhophylac® [US]; WinRho® SDF [US/Can]

Therapeutic Category Immune Globulin

Use

Suppression of Rh isoimmunization: Use in the following situations when an Rh$_o$(D)-negative individual is exposed to Rh$_o$(D)-positive blood: During delivery of an Rh$_o$(D)-positive infant; abortion; amniocentesis; chorionic villus sampling; ruptured tubal pregnancy; abdominal trauma; hydatidiform mole; transplacental hemorrhage. Used when the mother is Rh$_o$(D) negative, the father of the child is either Rh$_o$(D) positive or Rh$_o$(D) unknown, the baby is either Rh$_o$(D) positive or Rh$_o$(D) unknown.

Transfusion: Suppression of Rh isoimmunization in Rh$_o$(D)-negative individuals transfused with Rh$_o$(D) antigen-positive RBCs or blood components containing Rh$_o$(D) antigen-positive RBCs

Treatment of idiopathic thrombocytopenic purpura (ITP): Used in the following nonsplenectomized Rh$_o$(D) positive individuals: Children with acute or chronic ITP, adults with chronic ITP, children and adults with ITP secondary to HIV infection

Usual Dosage

ITP: Children and Adults:

Rhophylac®: I.V.: 50 mcg/kg

WinRho® SDF: I.V.:

Initial: 50 mcg/kg as a single injection, or can be given as a divided dose on separate days. If hemoglobin is <10 g/dL: Dose should be reduced to 25-40 mcg/kg.

Subsequent dosing: 25-60 mcg/kg can be used if required to elevate platelet count

Maintenance dosing if patient **did respond** to initial dosing: 25-60 mcg/kg based on platelet and hemoglobin levels

Maintenance dosing if patient **did not respond** to initial dosing:

Hemoglobin 8-10 g/dL: Redose between 25-40 mcg/kg

Hemoglobin >10 g/dL: Redose between 50-60 mcg/kg

Hemoglobin <8 g/dL: Use with caution

Rh$_o$(D) suppression: Adults: **Note:** One "full dose" (300 mcg) provides enough antibody to prevent Rh sensitization if the volume of RBC entering the circulation is ≤15 mL. When >15 mL is suspected, a fetal red cell count should be performed to determine the appropriate dose.

Pregnancy:

Antepartum prophylaxis: In general, dose is given at 28 weeks. If given early in pregnancy, administer every 12 weeks to ensure adequate levels of passively acquired anti-Rh

HyperRHO™ S/D Full Dose, RhoGAM®: I.M.: 300 mcg

Rhophylac®, WinRho® SDF: I.M., I.V.: 300 mcg

Postpartum prophylaxis: In general, dose is administered as soon as possible after delivery, preferably within 72 hours. Can be given up to 28 days following delivery

HyperRHO™ S/D Full Dose, RhoGAM®: I.M.: 300 mcg

Rhophylac®: I.M., I.V.: 300 mcg

WinRho® SDF: I.M., I.V.: 120 mcg

Threatened abortion, any time during pregnancy (with continuation of pregnancy):

HyperRHO™ S/D Full Dose, RhoGAM®: I.M.: 300 mcg; administer as soon as possible

Rhophylac®, WinRho® SDF: I.M., I.V.: 300 mcg; administer as soon as possible

Abortion, miscarriage, termination of ectopic pregnancy:

RhoGAM®: I.M.: ≥13 weeks gestation: 300 mcg.

HyperRHO™ S/D Mini Dose, MICRhoGAM®: <13 weeks gestation: I.M.: 50 mcg

Rhophylac®: I.M., I.V.: 300 mcg

WinRho® SDF: I.M., I.V.: After 34 weeks gestation: 120 mcg; administer immediately or within 72 hours

Amniocentesis, chorionic villus sampling:

HyperRHO™ S/D Full Dose, RhoGAM®: I.M.: At 15-18 weeks gestation or during the 3rd trimester: 300 mcg. If dose is given between 13-18 weeks, repeat at 26-28 weeks and within 72 hours of delivery.

Rhophylac®: I.M., I.V.: 300 mcg

WinRho® SDF: I.M., I.V.: Before 34 weeks gestation: 300 mcg; administer immediately, repeat dose every 12 weeks during pregnancy; After 34 weeks gestation: 120 mcg, administered immediately or within 72 hours

(Continued)

Rh_o(D) immune globulin *(Continued)*

Excessive fetomaternal hemorrhage (>15 mL): Rhophylac®: I.M., I.V.: 300 mcg within 72 hours plus 20 mcg/ mL fetal RBCs in excess of 15 mL if excess transplacental bleeding is quantified **or** 300 mcg/dose if bleeding cannot be quantified

Abdominal trauma, manipulation:

HyperRHO™ S/D Full Dose, RhoGAM®: I.M.: 2nd or 3rd trimester: 300 mcg. If dose is given between 13-18 weeks, repeat at 26-28 weeks and within 72 hours of delivery

Rhophylac®: I.M., I.V.: 300 mcg within 72 hours

WinRho® SDF: I.M./I.V.: After 34 weeks gestation: 120 mcg; administer immediately or within 72 hours

Transfusion:

Children and Adults: WinRho® SDF: Administer within 72 hours after exposure of incompatible blood transfusions or massive fetal hemorrhage.

I.V.: Calculate dose as follows; administer 600 mcg every 8 hours until the total dose is administered:

Exposure to Rh_o(D) positive whole blood: 9 mcg/mL blood

Exposure to Rh_o(D) positive red blood cells: 18 mcg/mL cells

I.M.: Calculate dose as follows; administer 1200 mcg every 12 hours until the total dose is administered:

Exposure to Rh_o(D) positive whole blood: 12 mcg/mL blood

Exposure to Rh_o(D) positive red blood cells: 24 mcg/mL cells

Adults:

HyperRHO™ S/D Full Dose, RhoGAM®: I.M.: Multiply the volume of Rh positive whole blood administered by the hematocrit of the donor unit to equal the volume of RBCs transfused. The volume of RBCs is then divided by 15 mL, providing the number of 300 mcg doses (vials/syringes) to administer. If the dose calculated results in a fraction, round up to the next higher whole 300 mcg dose (vial/syringe).

Rhophylac®: I.M., I.V.: 20 mcg/2 mL transfused blood or 20 mcg/mL erythrocyte concentrate

Dosage Forms

Injection, solution [preservative free]:

HyperRHO™ S/D Full Dose, RhoGAM®: 300 mcg [I.M. use only]

HyperRHO™ S/D Mini Dose, MICRhoGAM®: 50 mcg [I.M. use only]

WinRho® SDF:

120 mcg/~0.5 mL (~0.5 mL)

300 mcg/~1.3 mL (~1.3 mL)

500 mcg/~2.2 mL (~2.2 mL)

1000 mcg/~4.4 mL (~4.4 mL)

3000 mcg/~13 mL (~13 mL)

Rhodis™ [Can] *see* ketoprofen *on page 482*

Rhodis-EC™ [Can] *see* ketoprofen *on page 482*

Rhodis SR™ [Can] *see* ketoprofen *on page 482*

RhoGAM® [US] *see* Rh_o(D) immune globulin *on previous page*

RhoIGIV *see* Rh_o(D) immune globulin *on previous page*

RhoIVIM *see* Rh_o(D) immune globulin *on previous page*

Rho®-Loperamine [Can] *see* loperamide *on page 515*

Rho®-Metformin [Can] *see* metformin *on page 548*

Rho®-Nitro [Can] *see* nitroglycerin *on page 608*

Rhophylac® [US] *see* Rh_o(D) immune globulin *on previous page*

Rho®-Sotalol [Can] *see* sotalol *on page 802*

Rhotral [Can] *see* acebutolol *on page 4*

Rhotrimine® [Can] *see* trimipramine *on page 868*

Rhovane® [Can] *see* zopiclone *(Canada only) on page 909*

Rhoxal-acebutolol [Can] *see* acebutolol *on page 4*

Rhoxal-amiodarone [Can] *see* amiodarone *on page 43*

Rhoxal-anagrelide [Can] *see* anagrelide *on page 55*

Rhoxal-atenolol [Can] *see* atenolol *on page 80*

Rhoxal-ciprofloxacin [Can] *see* ciprofloxacin *on page 190*

Rhoxal-citalopram [Can] *see* citalopram *on page 194*

Rhoxal-cyclosporine [Can] *see* cyclosporine *on page 223*

Rhoxal-diltiazem CD [Can] *see* diltiazem *on page 261*

Rhoxal-diltiazem SR [Can] *see* diltiazem *on page 261*

Rhoxal-diltiazem T [Can] *see* diltiazem *on page 261*

Rhoxal-fluoxetine [Can] *see* fluoxetine *on page 364*

Rhoxal-fluvoxamine [Can] *see* fluvoxamine *on page 370*

Rhoxal-glimepiride [Can] *see* glimepiride *on page 393*

Rhoxal-minocycline [Can] *see* minocycline *on page 571*

Rhoxal-mirtazapine [Can] *see* mirtazapine *on page 572*

Rhoxal-mirtazapine FC [Can] *see* mirtazapine *on page 572*

Rhoxal-nabumetone [Can] *see* nabumetone *on page 585*

Rhoxal-orphendrine [Can] *see* orphenadrine *on page 634*

Rhoxal-pamidronate [Can] *see* pamidronate *on page 647*

Rhoxal-paroxetine [Can] *see* paroxetine *on page 654*

Rhoxal-ranitidine [Can] *see* ranitidine *on page 744*

Rhoxal-salbutamol [Can] *see* albuterol *on page 23*

Rhoxal-Sertraline [Can] *see* sertraline *on page 783*

Rhoxal-sumatriptan [Can] *see* sumatriptan *on page 815*

Rhoxal-ticlopidine [Can] *see* ticlopidine *on page 842*

Rhoxal-topiramate [Can] *see* topiramate *on page 851*

Rhoxal-valproic [Can] *see* valproic acid and derivatives *on page 881*

Rhoxal-zopiclone [Can] *see* zopiclone *(Canada only) on page 909*

rhPTH(1-34) *see* teriparatide *on page 827*

*r*HuEPO-α *see* epoetin alfa *on page 303*

rhuFabV2 *see* ranibizumab *on page 744*

rHu-KGF *see* palifermin *on page 646*

Rhulicaine® *(Discontinued) see* benzocaine *on page 101*

rhuMAb-E25 *see* omalizumab *on page 628*

rHuMAb-EGFr *see* panitumumab *on page 650*

rhuMAb-VEGF *see* bevacizumab *on page 110*

RibaPak™ [US] *see* ribavirin *on this page*

Ribasphere™ [US] *see* ribavirin *on this page*

ribavirin (rye ba VYE rin)

Sound-Alike/Look-Alike Issues
ribavirin may be confused with riboflavin

Synonyms RTCA; tribavirin

U.S./Canadian Brand Names Copegus® [US]; Rebetol® [US]; RibaPak™ [US]; Ribasphere™ [US]; Virazole® [US/Can]

Therapeutic Category Antiviral Agent

Use

Inhalation: Treatment of patients with respiratory syncytial virus (RSV) infections; specially indicated for treatment of severe lower respiratory tract RSV infections in patients with an underlying compromising condition (prematurity, bronchopulmonary dysplasia and other chronic lung conditions, congenital heart disease, immunodeficiency, immunosuppression), and recent transplant recipients

Oral capsule:

In combination with interferon alfa-2b (Intron® A) injection for the treatment of chronic hepatitis C in patients with compensated liver disease who have relapsed after alpha interferon therapy or were previously untreated with alpha interferons

In combination with peginterferon alfa-2b (PEG-Intron®) injection for the treatment of chronic hepatitis C in patients with compensated liver disease who were previously untreated with alpha interferons

Oral solution: In combination with interferon alfa 2b (Intron® A) injection for the treatment of chronic hepatitis C in patients ≥3 years of age with compensated liver disease who were previously untreated with alpha interferons or patients ≥18 years of age who have relapsed after alpha interferon therapy

Oral tablet: In combination with peginterferon alfa-2a (Pegasys®) injection for the treatment of chronic hepatitis C in patients with compensated liver disease who were previously untreated with alpha interferons (includes patients with histological evidence of cirrhosis [Child-Pugh class A] and patients with clinically-stable HIV disease)

(Continued)

ribavirin *(Continued)*

Usual Dosage
Aerosol inhalation: Infants and children: Use with Viratek® small particle aerosol generator (SPAG-2) at a concentration of 20 mg/mL (6 g reconstituted with 300 mL of sterile water without preservatives). Continuous aerosol administration: 12-18 hours/day for 3 days, up to 7 days in length

Oral capsule or solution: Children ≥3 years: Chronic hepatitis C (in combination with interferon alfa-2b): Rebetol®: Oral: **Note:** Oral solution should be used in children 3-5 years of age, children ≤25 kg, or those unable to swallow capsules.

Capsule/solution: 15 mg/kg/day in 2 divided doses (morning and evening)

Capsule dosing recommendations:
26-36 kg: 400 mg/day (200 mg morning and evening)
37-49 kg: 600 mg/day (200 mg in the morning and two 200 mg capsules in the evening)
50-61 kg: 800 mg/day (two 200 mg capsules morning and evening)
>61 kg: Refer to adult dosing
Note: Treatment duration may vary. Consult current guidelines and literature.

Oral capsule (Rebetol®, Ribasphere™): Adults:
Chronic hepatitis C (in combination with interferon alfa-2b):
≤75 kg: 400 mg in the morning, then 600 mg in the evening
>75 kg: 600 mg in the morning, then 600 mg in the evening
Chronic hepatitis C (in combination with peginterferon alfa-2b): 400 mg twice daily
Note: Treatment duration may vary. Consult current guidelines and literature.

Oral tablet (Copegus®, in combination with peginterferon alfa-2b): Adults: Chronic hepatitis C:
Monoinfection, genotype 1,4:
<75kg: 1000 mg/day in 2 divided doses
≥75kg: 1200 mg/day in 2 divided doses
Monoinfection, genotype 2,3: 800 mg/day in 2 divided doses
Coinfection with HIV: 800 mg/day in 2 divided doses
Note: Treatment duration may vary. Consult current guidelines and literature.

Dosage Forms
Capsule: 200 mg
Rebetol®, Ribasphere™: 200 mg
Powder for solution, inhalation [for aerosol administration]:
Virazole®: 6 g
Solution, oral:
Rebetol®: 40 mg/mL
Tablet: 200 mg
Copegus®: 200 mg
Tablet [dose pack]:
RibaPak™: 400 mg (14s), 600 mg (14s)

ribavirin and interferon alfa-2b combination pack *see* interferon alfa-2b and ribavirin *on* *page 463*

ribavirin and peginterferon alfa-2b *see* peginterferon alfa-2b and ribavirin *(Canada only) on* *page 659*

Ribo-100 [US] *see* riboflavin *on this page*

riboflavin *(RYE boe flay vin)*
Sound-Alike/Look-Alike Issues
riboflavin may be confused with ribavirin
Synonyms lactoflavin; vitamin B$_2$; vitamin G
U.S./Canadian Brand Names Ribo-100 [US]
Therapeutic Category Vitamin, Water Soluble
Use Prevention of riboflavin deficiency and treatment of ariboflavinosis
Usual Dosage Oral:
Riboflavin deficiency:
Children: 2.5-10 mg/day in divided doses
Adults: 5-30 mg/day in divided doses
Recommended daily allowance:
Children: 0.4-1.8 mg
Adults: 1.2-1.7 mg
Dosage Forms
Tablet: 25 mg, 50 mg, 100 mg
Ribo-100: 100 mg

Rid-A-Pain Dental Drops [US-OTC] *see* benzocaine *on page 101*

Ridaura® **[US/Can]** *see* auranofin *on page 85*

RID® *(Discontinued) see* pyrethrins and piperonyl butoxide *on page 734*

RID® **Maximum Strength [US-OTC]** *see* pyrethrins and piperonyl butoxide *on page 734*

RID® **Mousse [Can]** *see* pyrethrins and piperonyl butoxide *on page 734*

Rid® **Spray [US-OTC]** *see* permethrin *on page 670*

rifabutin (rif a BYOO tin)
Sound-Alike/Look-Alike Issues
rifabutin may be confused with rifampin
Synonyms ansamycin
U.S./Canadian Brand Names Mycobutin® [US/Can]
Therapeutic Category Antibiotic, Miscellaneous
Use Prevention of disseminated *Mycobacterium avium* complex (MAC) in patients with advanced HIV infection
Usual Dosage Oral:
Children >1 year: Prophylaxis: 5 mg/kg daily; higher dosages have been used in limited trials
Adults: Prophylaxis: 300 mg once daily (alone or in combination with azithromycin)
Dosage Forms
Capsule:
Mycobutin®: 150 mg

Rifadin® **[US/Can]** *see* rifampin *on this page*

Rifamate® **[US/Can]** *see* rifampin and isoniazid *on this page*

rifampicin *see* rifampin *on this page*

rifampin (rif AM pin)
Sound-Alike/Look-Alike Issues
rifampin may be confused with rifabutin, Rifamate®, rifapentine, rifaximin
Rifadin® may be confused with Ritalin®
Synonyms rifampicin
U.S./Canadian Brand Names Rifadin® [US/Can]; Rofact™ [Can]
Therapeutic Category Antibiotic, Miscellaneous
Use Management of active tuberculosis in combination with other agents; elimination of meningococci from the nasopharynx in asymptomatic carriers
Usual Dosage Oral (I.V. infusion dose is the same as for the oral route):
Tuberculosis therapy (drug susceptible): Note: A four-drug regimen (isoniazid, rifampin, pyrazinamide, and ethambutol) is preferred for the initial, empiric treatment of TB. When the drug susceptibility results are available, the regimen should be altered as appropriate.
Infants and Children <12 years:
Daily therapy: 10-20 mg/kg/day usually as a single dose (maximum: 600 mg/day)
Twice weekly directly observed therapy (DOT): 10-20 mg/kg (maximum: 600 mg)
Adults:
Daily therapy: 10 mg/kg/day (maximum: 600 mg/day)
Twice weekly directly observed therapy (DOT): 10 mg/kg (maximum: 600 mg); 3 times/week: 10 mg/kg (maximum: 600 mg)
Latent tuberculosis infection (LTBI): As an alternative to isoniazid:
Children: 10-20 mg/kg/day (maximum: 600 mg/day) for 6 months
Adults: 10 mg/kg/day (maximum: 600 mg/day) for 4 months. **Note:** Combination with pyrazinamide should not generally be offered
Meningococcal meningitis prophylaxis:
Infants <1 month: 10 mg/kg/day in divided doses every 12 hours for 2 days
Infants ≥1 month and Children: 20 mg/kg/day in divided doses every 12 hours for 2 days (maximum: 600 mg/dose)
Meningitis *(Pneumococcus* or *Staphylococcus):* I.V.: Adults: 600 mg once daily
Adults: 600 mg every 12 hours for 2 days
Dosage Forms
Capsule: 150 mg, 300 mg
Rifadin®: 150 mg, 300 mg
Injection, powder for reconstitution: 600 mg
Rifadin®: 600 mg

rifampin and isoniazid (rif AM pin & eye soe NYE a zid)
Sound-Alike/Look-Alike Issues
Rifamate® may be confused with rifampin
(Continued)

rifampin and isoniazid (Continued)

Synonyms isoniazid and rifampin
U.S./Canadian Brand Names IsonaRif™ [US]; Rifamate® [US/Can]
Therapeutic Category Antibiotic, Miscellaneous
Use Management of active tuberculosis; see individual agents for additional information
Usual Dosage Oral: 2 capsules/day
Dosage Forms
Capsule:
IsonaRif™, Rifamate®: 300/150: Rifampin 300 mg and isoniazid 150 mg

rifampin, isoniazid, and pyrazinamide (rif AM pin, eye soe NYE a zid, & peer a ZIN a mide)

Synonyms isoniazid, rifampin, and pyrazinamide; pyrazinamide, rifampin, and isoniazid
U.S./Canadian Brand Names Rifater® [US/Can]
Therapeutic Category Antibiotic, Miscellaneous
Use Initial phase, short-course treatment of pulmonary tuberculosis; see individual agents for additional information
Usual Dosage Oral: Adults: Patients weighing:
≤44 kg: 4 tablets
45-54 kg: 5 tablets
≥55 kg: 6 tablets
Doses should be administered in a single daily dose
Dosage Forms
Tablet:
Rifater®: Rifampin 120 mg, isoniazid 50 mg, and pyrazinamide 300 mg

rifapentine (rif a PEN teen)

Sound-Alike/Look-Alike Issues
rifapentine may be confused with rifampin
U.S./Canadian Brand Names Priftin® [US/Can]
Therapeutic Category Antitubercular Agent
Use Treatment of pulmonary tuberculosis; rifapentine must always be used in conjunction with at least one other antituberculosis drug to which the isolate is susceptible; it may also be necessary to add a third agent (either streptomycin or ethambutol) until susceptibility is known.
Usual Dosage
Children: No dosing information available
Adults: **Rifapentine should not be used alone**; initial phase should include a 3- to 4-drug regimen
Intensive phase (initial 2 months) of short-term therapy: 600 mg (four 150 mg tablets) given twice weekly (with an interval of not less than 72 hours between doses); following the intensive phase, treatment should continue with rifapentine 600 mg once weekly for 4 months in combination with INH or appropriate agent for susceptible organisms
Dosage Forms
Tablet:
Priftin®: 150 mg

Rifater® **[US/Can]** see rifampin, isoniazid, and pyrazinamide on this page

rifaximin (rif AX i min)

Sound-Alike/Look-Alike Issues
rifaximin may be confused with rifampin
U.S./Canadian Brand Names Xifaxan™ [US]
Therapeutic Category Antibiotic, Miscellaneous
Use Treatment of traveler's diarrhea caused by noninvasive strains of E. coli
Usual Dosage Oral: Children ≥12 years and Adults: Traveler's diarrhea: 200 mg 3 times/day for 3 days
Dosage Forms
Tablet:
Xifaxan™: 200 mg

rIFN-A see interferon alfa-2a on page 462

rIFN beta-1a see interferon beta-1a on page 464

rIFN beta-1b see interferon beta-1b on page 465

RIG see rabies immune globulin (human) on page 741

rIL-11 see oprelvekin on page 632

Rilutek® **[US/Can]** *see* riluzole *on this page*

riluzole (RIL yoo zole)
Synonyms 2-amino-6-trifluoromethoxy-benzothiazole; RP-54274
U.S./Canadian Brand Names Rilutek® [US/Can]
Therapeutic Category Miscellaneous Product
Use Treatment of amyotrophic lateral sclerosis (ALS); riluzole can extend survival or time to tracheostomy
Usual Dosage Oral: Adults: 50 mg every 12 hours; no increased benefit can be expected from higher daily doses, but adverse events are increased
  Dosage adjustment in smoking: Cigarette smoking is known to induce CYP1A2; patients who smoke cigarettes would be expected to eliminate riluzole faster. There is no information, however, on the effect of, or need for, dosage adjustment in these patients.
  Dosage adjustment in special populations: Females and Japanese patients may possess a lower metabolic capacity to eliminate riluzole compared with male and Caucasian subjects, respectively
Dosage Forms
  Tablet:
    Rilutek®: 50 mg

rimantadine (ri MAN ta deen)
Sound-Alike/Look-Alike Issues
    rimantadine may be confused with amantadine, ranitidine, Rimactane®
    Flumadine® may be confused with fludarabine, flunisolide, flutamide
Synonyms rimantadine hydrochloride
U.S./Canadian Brand Names Flumadine® [US/Can]
Therapeutic Category Antiviral Agent
Use Prophylaxis (adults and children >1 year of age) and treatment (adults) of influenza A viral infection (per manufacturer labeling; also refer to current CDC guidelines for recommendations during current flu season)
Usual Dosage Oral:
  Prophylaxis:
    Children 1-10 years: 5 mg/kg/day; maximum: 150 mg/day
    Children >10 years and Adults: 100 mg twice daily
  Treatment: Adults: 100 mg twice daily
Dosage Forms
  Syrup:
    Flumadine®: 50 mg/5 mL
  Tablet: 100 mg
    Flumadine®: 100 mg

rimantadine hydrochloride *see* rimantadine *on this page*

rimexolone (ri MEKS oh lone)
Sound-Alike/Look-Alike Issues
    Vexol® may be confused with VoSol®
U.S./Canadian Brand Names Vexol® [US/Can]
Therapeutic Category Adrenal Corticosteroid
Use Treatment of inflammation after ocular surgery and the treatment of anterior uveitis
Usual Dosage Ophthalmic: Adults: Instill 1 drop in conjunctival sac 2-4 times/day up to every 4 hours; may use every 1-2 hours during first 1-2 days
Dosage Forms
  Suspension, ophthalmic:
    Vexol®: 1% (5 mL, 10 mL)

Rimso®**-50 [US/Can]** *see* dimethyl sulfoxide *on page 263*

Rindal HD Plus [US] *see* phenylephrine, hydrocodone, and chlorpheniramine *on page 678*

Rindal HPD [US] *see* hydrocodone, phenylephrine, and diphenhydramine *on page 431*

Riobin® *(Discontinued)* *see* riboflavin *on page 756*

Riomet™ **[US]** *see* metformin *on page 548*

Riopan® **Plus** *(Discontinued)* *see* magaldrate and simethicone *on page 524*

Riopan® **Plus Double Strength** *(Discontinued)* *see* magaldrate and simethicone *on page 524*

Riphenidate [Can] *see* methylphenidate *on page 558*

risedronate (ris ED roe nate)

Synonyms risedronate sodium

U.S./Canadian Brand Names Actonel® [US/Can]

Therapeutic Category Bisphosphonate Derivative

Use Paget disease of the bone; treatment and prevention of glucocorticoid-induced osteoporosis; treatment and prevention of osteoporosis in postmenopausal women; treatment of osteoporosis in men

Usual Dosage Oral: Adults:

Paget disease of bone: 30 mg once daily for 2 months

Retreatment may be considered (following post-treatment observation of at least 2 months) if relapse occurs, or if treatment fails to normalize serum alkaline phosphatase. For retreatment, the dose and duration of therapy are the same as for initial treatment. No data are available on more than one course of retreatment.

Osteoporosis (postmenopausal) prevention and treatment: 5 mg once daily **or** 35 mg once weekly **or** one 75 mg tablet taken on 2 consecutive days once a month (total of 2 tablets/month)

Osteoporosis (male) treatment: 35 mg once weekly

Osteoporosis (glucocorticoid-induced) prevention and treatment: 5 mg once daily

Dosage Forms

Tablet:

Actonel®: 5 mg, 30 mg, 35 mg, 75 mg

risedronate and calcium (ris ED roe nate & KAL see um)

Synonyms calcium and risedronate; risedronate sodium and calcium carbonate

U.S./Canadian Brand Names Actonel® and Calcium [US]

Therapeutic Category Bisphosphonate Derivative; Calcium Salt

Use Treatment and prevention of osteoporosis in postmenopausal women

Usual Dosage Oral: Adults: Osteoporosis in postmenopausal females:

Risedronate: 35 mg once weekly on day 1 of 7-day treatment cycle

Calcium carbonate: 1250 mg (elemental calcium 500 mg) once daily on days 2 through 7 of 7-day treatment cycle

Dosage Forms

Combination package [each package contains]:

Actonel® and Calcium:

Tablet (Actonel®): Risedronate 35 mg (4s)

Tablet: Calcium 1250 mg (24s)

risedronate sodium see risedronate on this page

risedronate sodium and calcium carbonate see risedronate and calcium on this page

Risperdal® [US/Can] see risperidone on this page

Risperdal® M-Tab® [US/Can] see risperidone on this page

Risperdal® Consta® [US/Can] see risperidone on this page

risperidone (ris PER i done)

Sound-Alike/Look-Alike Issues

risperidone may be confused with reserpine

Risperdal® may be confused with lisinopril, reserpine

U.S./Canadian Brand Names Apo-Risperidone® [Can]; PMS-Risperidone ODT [Can]; Risperdal® Consta® [US/Can]; Risperdal® M-Tab® [US/Can]; Risperdal® [US/Can]; Sandoz Risperidone [Can]

Therapeutic Category Antipsychotic Agent, Benzisoxazole

Use Treatment of schizophrenia; treatment of acute mania or mixed episodes associated with bipolar I disorder (as monotherapy in children or adults, or in combination with lithium or valproate in adults); treatment of irritability/aggression associated with autistic disorder

Usual Dosage

Oral:

Children ≥5 years and Adolescents: Autism:

<15 kg: Use with caution; specific dosing recommendations not available

<20 kg: Initial: 0.25 mg/day; may increase dose to 0.5 mg/day after ≥4 days, maintain dose for ≥14 days. In patients not achieving sufficient clinical response, may increase dose by 0.25 mg/day in ≥2-week intervals. Therapeutic effect reached plateau at 1 mg/day in clinical trials. Following clinical response, consider gradually lowering dose. May be administered once daily or in divided doses twice daily.

≥20 kg: Initial: 0.5 mg/day; may increase dose to 1 mg/day after ≥4 days, maintain dose for ≥14 days. In patients not achieving sufficient clinical response, may increase dose by 0.5 mg/day in ≥2-week intervals. Therapeutic effect reached plateau at 2.5 mg/day (3 mg/day in children >45 kg) in clinical trials. Following clinical response, consider gradually lowering dose. May be administered once daily or in divided doses twice daily.

Adults:

Schizophrenia:

Initial: 1 mg twice daily; may be increased by 2 mg/day to a target dose of 6 mg/day; usual range: 4-8 mg/day; may be given as a single daily dose once maintenance dose is achieved; daily dosages >6 mg do not appear to confer any additional benefit, and the incidence of extrapyramidal symptoms is higher than with lower doses. Further dose adjustments should be made in increments/decrements of 1-2 mg/day on a weekly basis. Dose range studied in clinical trials: 4-16 mg/day.

Maintenance: Target dose: 4 mg once daily (range 2-8 mg/day)

Bipolar mania:

Initial: 2-3 mg once daily; if needed, adjust dose by 1 mg/day in intervals ≥24 hours; dosing range: 1-6 mg/day

Maintenance: No dosing recommendation available for treatment >3 weeks duration.

I.M.: Adults: Schizophrenia (Risperdal® Consta®): 25 mg every 2 weeks; some patients may benefit from larger doses; maximum dose not to exceed 50 mg every 2 weeks. Dosage adjustments should not be made more frequently than every 4 weeks. A lower initial dose of 12.5 mg may be appropriate in some patients.

Note: Oral risperidone (or other antipsychotic) should be administered with the initial injection of Risperdal® Consta® and continued for 3 weeks (then discontinued) to maintain adequate therapeutic plasma concentrations prior to main release phase of risperidone from injection site. When switching from depot administration to a short-acting formulation, administer short-acting agent in place of the next regularly-scheduled depot injection.

Dosage Forms

Injection, microspheres for reconstitution, extended release:

Risperdal® Consta®: 12.5 mg, 25 mg, 37.5 mg, 50 mg

Solution, oral:

Risperdal®: 1 mg/mL

Tablet:

Risperdal®: 0.25 mg, 0.5 mg, 1 mg, 2 mg, 3 mg, 4 mg

Tablet, orally disintegrating:

Risperdal® M-Tabs®: 0.5 mg, 1 mg, 2 mg, 3 mg, 4 mg

Ritalin® [US/Can] *see* methylphenidate *on page 558*

Ritalin® LA [US] *see* methylphenidate *on page 558*

Ritalin-SR® [US/Can] *see* methylphenidate *on page 558*

ritonavir (ri TOE na veer)

Sound-Alike/Look-Alike Issues

ritonavir may be confused with Retrovir®

Norvir® may be confused with Norvasc®

U.S./Canadian Brand Names Norvir® SEC [Can]; Norvir® [US/Can]

Therapeutic Category Antiviral Agent

Use Treatment of HIV infection; should always be used as part of a multidrug regimen (at least three antiretroviral agents); may be used as a pharmacokinetic "booster" for other protease inhibitors

Usual Dosage Treatment of HIV infection: Oral:

Children >1 month: 350-400 mg/m² twice daily (maximum dose: 600 mg twice daily). Initiate dose at 250 mg/m² twice daily; titrate dose upward every 2-3 days by 50 mg/m² twice daily.

Adults: 600 mg twice daily; dose escalation tends to avoid nausea that many patients experience upon initiation of full dosing. Escalate the dose as follows: 300 mg twice daily for 1 day, 400 mg twice daily for 2 days, 500 mg twice daily for 1 day, then 600 mg twice daily. Ritonavir may be better tolerated when used in combination with other antiretrovirals by initiating the drug alone and subsequently adding the second agent within 2 weeks.

Pharmacokinetic "booster" in combination with other protease inhibitors: 100-400 mg/day

Refer to individual monographs; specific dosage recommendations often require adjustment of both agents.

Note: Dosage adjustments for ritonavir when administered in combination therapy:

Amprenavir: Adjustments necessary for each agent:

Amprenavir 1200 mg with ritonavir 200 mg once daily **or**

Amprenavir 600 mg with ritonavir 100 mg twice daily

Amprenavir plus efavirenz (3-drug regimen): Amprenavir 1200 mg twice daily plus ritonavir 200 mg twice daily plus efavirenz at standard dose

Indinavir: Adjustments necessary for both agents:

Indinavir 800 mg twice daily plus ritonavir 100-200 mg twice daily **or**

Indinavir 400 mg twice daily plus ritonavir 400 mg twice daily

Nelfinavir or saquinavir: Ritonavir 400 mg twice daily

Rifabutin: Decrease rifabutin dose to 150 mg every other day

Saquinavir: Ritonavir 400 mg twice daily

(Continued)

ritonavir (Continued)

Dosage Forms
Capsule:
Norvir®: 100 mg
Oral Solution:
Norvir®: 80 mg/mL

ritonavir and lopinavir see lopinavir and ritonavir on page 516

Rituxan® [US/Can] see rituximab on this page

rituximab (ri TUK si mab)

Sound-Alike/Look-Alike Issues
rituximab may be confused with infliximab
Rituxan® may be confused with Remicade®

Synonyms anti-CD20 monoclonal antibody; C2B8; C2B8 monoclonal antibody; IDEC-C2B8; NSC-687451; pan-B antibody

U.S./Canadian Brand Names Rituxan® [US/Can]

Therapeutic Category Antineoplastic Agent

Use Treatment of low-grade or follicular CD20-positive, B-cell non-Hodgkin lymphoma (NHL); treatment of diffuse large B-cell CD20-positive NHL; treatment of rheumatoid arthritis (RA) in combination with methotrexate

Usual Dosage Note: Pretreatment with acetaminophen and diphenhydramine is recommended.
Adults: I.V. infusion (refer to individual protocols):
NHL (relapsed/refractory, low-grade or follicular CD20-positive, B-cell): 375 mg/m^2 once weekly for 4 or 8 doses
Retreatment following disease progression: 375 mg/m^2 once weekly for 4 doses
NHL (diffuse large B-cell): 375 mg/m^2 given on day 1 of each chemotherapy cycle for up to 8 doses
NHL (follicular, CD20-positive, B-cell, previously untreated): 375 mg/m^2 given on day 1 of each chemotherapy cycle for up to 8 doses
NHL (low-grade, CD20-positive, B-cell, previously untreated): 375 mg/m^2 once weekly for 4 doses every 6 months for up to 4 cycles (initiate after 6-8 cycles of chemotherapy are completed)
Rheumatoid arthritis: 1000 mg on days 1 and 15 in combination with methotrexate
Note: Premedication with a corticosteroid (eg, methylprednisolone 100 mg I.V.) prior to each rituximab dose is recommended. In clinical trials, patients received oral corticosteroids on a tapering schedule from baseline through day 16.
Combination therapy with ibritumomab: 250 mg/m^2 I.V. day 1; repeat in 7-9 days with ibritumomab (also see ibritumomab monograph):

Dosage Forms
Injection, solution [preservative free]:
Rituxan®: 10 mg/mL (10 mL, 50 mL)

Riva-Alendronate [Can] see alendronate on page 27

Riva-Atenolol [Can] see atenolol on page 80

Riva-Clindamycin [Can] see clindamycin on page 198

Riva-Cloxacillin [Can] see cloxacillin on page 207

Riva-Diclofenac [Can] see diclofenac on page 253

Riva-Diclofenac-K [Can] see diclofenac on page 253

Riva-Dicyclomine [Can] see dicyclomine on page 255

Riva-Famotidine [Can] see famotidine on page 341

Riva-Fluconazole [Can] see fluconazole on page 356

Riva-Fosinopril [Can] see fosinopril on page 376

Riva-Loperamine [Can] see loperamide on page 515

Riva-Lorazepam [Can] see lorazepam on page 518

Riva-Lovastatin [Can] see lovastatin on page 520

Riva-Mirtazapine [Can] see mirtazapine on page 572

Riva-Naproxen [Can] see naproxen on page 591

Rivanase AQ [Can] see beclomethasone on page 97

Riva-Norfloxacin [Can] see norfloxacin on page 612

Riva-Oxazepam [Can] see oxazepam on page 637

Riva-Pravastatin [Can] *see* pravastatin *on page 707*

Riva-Simvastatin [Can] *see* simvastatin *on page 787*

Rivasol [Can] *see* zinc sulfate *on page 906*

Riva-Sotalol [Can] *see* sotalol *on page 802*

rivastigmine (ri va STIG meen)

Synonyms ENA 713; rivastigmine tartrate; SDZ ENA 713

U.S./Canadian Brand Names Exelon® [US/Can]

Therapeutic Category Acetylcholinesterase Inhibitor; Cholinergic Agent

Use Treatment of mild-to-moderate dementia associated with Alzheimer disease or Parkinson disease

Usual Dosage Adults:

Oral: **Note:** Exelon® oral solution and capsules are bioequivalent.

Mild-to-moderate Alzheimer dementia: Initial: 1.5 mg twice daily; may increase by 3 mg/day (1.5 mg/dose) every 2 weeks based on tolerability (maximum recommended dose: 6 mg twice daily)

Note: If GI adverse events occur, discontinue treatment for several doses then restart at the same or next lower dosage level; antiemetics have been used to control GI symptoms. If treatment is interrupted for longer than several days, restart the treatment at the lowest dose and titrate as previously described.

Mild-to-moderate Parkinson-related dementia: Initial: 1.5 mg twice daily; may increase by 3 mg/day (1.5 mg/dose) every 4 weeks based on tolerability (maximum recommended dose: 6 mg twice daily)

Transdermal patch: Mild-to-moderate Alzheimer- or Parkinson-related dementia:

Initial: 4.6 mg/24 hours; if well tolerated, may be increased (after at least 4 weeks) to 9.5 mg/24 hours (recommended effective dose)

Maintenance: 9.5 mg/24 hours (maximum dose: 9.5 mg/24 hours)

Note: If intolerance is noted (nausea, vomiting), patch should be removed and treatment interrupted for several days then restarted at the same or lower dosage. If interrupted for more than several days, reinitiate at lowest dosage and increase to maintenance dose after 4 weeks.

Conversion from oral therapy: If oral daily dose <6 mg, switch to 4.6 mg/24 hours patch; if oral daily dose 6-12 mg, switch to 9.5 mg/24 hours patch. Apply patch on the next day following last oral dose.

Dosage Forms

Capsule:

Exelon®: 1.5 mg, 3 mg, 4.5 mg, 6 mg

Solution, oral:

Exelon®: 2 mg/mL

Transdermal system [once-daily patch]:

Exelon®: 4.6 mg/24hours (30s); 9.5 mg/24hours (30s)

rivastigmine tartrate *see* rivastigmine *on this page*

Riva-Sumatriptan [Can] *see* sumatriptan *on page 815*

Riva-Verapamil SR [Can] *see* verapamil *on page 887*

Riva-Zide [Can] *see* hydrochlorothiazide and triamterene *on page 427*

Riva-Zopiclone [Can] *see* zopiclone *(Canada only) on page 909*

Rivotril® [Can] *see* clonazepam *on page 204*

rizatriptan (rye za TRIP tan)

Synonyms MK462

U.S./Canadian Brand Names Maxalt RPD™ [Can]; Maxalt-MLT® [US]; Maxalt® [US/Can]

Therapeutic Category Antimigraine Agent; Serotonin Agonist

Use Acute treatment of migraine with or without aura

Usual Dosage Note: In patients with risk factors for coronary artery disease, following adequate evaluation to establish the absence of coronary artery disease, the initial dose should be administered in a setting where response may be evaluated (physician's office or similarly staffed setting). ECG monitoring may be considered.

Oral: 5-10 mg, repeat after 2 hours if significant relief is not attained; maximum: 30 mg in a 24-hour period (use 5 mg dose in patients receiving propranolol with a maximum of 15 mg in 24 hours)

Note: For orally-disintegrating tablets (Maxalt-MLT®): Patient should be instructed to place tablet on tongue and allow to dissolve. Dissolved tablet will be swallowed with saliva.

Dosage Forms

Tablet:

Maxalt®: 5 mg, 10 mg

Tablet, orally disintegrating:

Maxalt-MLT®: 5 mg, 10 mg

rLFN-α2 *see* interferon alfa-2b *on page 462*

RMS® *(Discontinued) see* morphine sulfate *on page 578*

Ro 5488 *see* tretinoin (oral) *on page 860*

Robafen® **AC [US]** *see* guaifenesin and codeine *on page 402*

Robafen® **CF** *(Discontinued)*

Robafen DM [US-OTC] *see* guaifenesin and dextromethorphan *on page 402*

Robafen DM Clear [US-OTC] *see* guaifenesin and dextromethorphan *on page 402*

Robaxin® **[US/Can]** *see* methocarbamol *on page 552*

Robidrine® **[Can]** *see* pseudoephedrine *on page 727*

Robinul® **[US]** *see* glycopyrrolate *on page 397*

Robinul® **Forte [US]** *see* glycopyrrolate *on page 397*

Robitussin® **[US-OTC/Can]** *see* guaifenesin *on page 401*

Robitussin® **A-C** *(Discontinued) see* guaifenesin and codeine *on page 402*

Robitussin® **Childrens Cough & Cold [Can]** *see* pseudoephedrine and dextromethorphan *on page 728*

Robitussin® **Cough and Cold**® **[US-OTC/Can]** *see* guaifenesin, pseudoephedrine, and dextromethorphan *on page 408*

Robitussin® **Cough and Cold CF [US-OTC]** *see* guaifenesin, pseudoephedrine, and dextromethorphan *on page 408*

Robitussin® **Cough and Cold Infant CF [US-OTC]** *see* guaifenesin, pseudoephedrine, and dextromethorphan *on page 408*

Robitussin® **Cough and Congestion [US-OTC]** *see* guaifenesin and dextromethorphan *on page 402*

Robitussin® **CoughGels**™ **[US-OTC]** *see* dextromethorphan *on page 247*

Robitussin®**-DAC** *(Discontinued) see* guaifenesin, pseudoephedrine, and codeine *on page 408*

Robitussin® **DM [US-OTC/Can]** *see* guaifenesin and dextromethorphan *on page 402*

Robitussin® **DM Infant [US-OTC]** *see* guaifenesin and dextromethorphan *on page 402*

Robitussin® **Maximum Strength Cough [US-OTC]** *see* dextromethorphan *on page 247*

Robitussin® **Maximum Strength Cough & Cold** *(Discontinued) see* pseudoephedrine and dextromethorphan *on page 728*

Robitussin® **Pediatric Cough [US-OTC]** *see* dextromethorphan *on page 247*

Robitussin® **Pediatric Cough & Cold** *(Discontinued) see* pseudoephedrine and dextromethorphan *on page 728*

Robitussin® **Pediatric Night Relief** *(Discontinued) see* chlorpheniramine, pseudoephedrine, and dextromethorphan *on page 183*

Robitussin-PE® *(Discontinued) see* guaifenesin and pseudoephedrine *on page 406*

Robitussin® **Severe Congestion** *(Discontinued) see* guaifenesin and pseudoephedrine *on page 406*

Robitussin® **Sugar Free Cough [US-OTC]** *see* guaifenesin and dextromethorphan *on page 402*

Rocaltrol® **[US/Can]** *see* calcitriol *on page 135*

Rocephin® **[US/Can]** *see* ceftriaxone *on page 164*

rocuronium (roe kyoor OH nee um)

  Sound-Alike/Look-Alike Issues

    Zemuron® may be confused with Remeron®

  Synonyms ORG 946; rocuronium bromide

  U.S./Canadian Brand Names Zemuron® [US/Can]

  Therapeutic Category Skeletal Muscle Relaxant

  Use Adjunct to general anesthesia to facilitate both rapid sequence and routine endotracheal intubation and to relax skeletal muscles during surgery; to facilitate mechanical ventilation in ICU patients; does not relieve pain or produce sedation

  Usual Dosage Administer I.V.; dose to effect; doses will vary due to interpatient variability; use ideal body weight for obese patients

Children:

Initial: 0.6 mg/kg under halothane anesthesia produce excellent to good intubating conditions within 1 minute and will provide a median time of 41 minutes of clinical relaxation in children 3 months to 1 year of age, and 27 minutes in children 1-12 years

Maintenance: 0.075-0.125 mg/kg administered upon return of T_1 to 25% of control provides clinical relaxation for 7-10 minutes

Adults:

Tracheal intubation: I.V.:

Initial: 0.6 mg/kg is expected to provide approximately 31 minutes of clinical relaxation under opioid/nitrous oxide/oxygen anesthesia with neuromuscular block sufficient for intubation attained in 1-2 minutes; lower doses (0.45 mg/kg) may be used to provide 22 minutes of clinical relaxation with median time to neuromuscular block of 1-3 minutes; maximum blockade is achieved in <4 minutes

Maximum: 0.9-1.2 mg/kg may be given during surgery under opioid/nitrous oxide/oxygen anesthesia without adverse cardiovascular effects and is expected to provide 58-67 minutes of clinical relaxation; neuromuscular blockade sufficient for intubation is achieved in <2 minutes with maximum blockade in <3 minutes

Maintenance: 0.1, 0.15, and 0.2 mg/kg administered at 25% recovery of control T_1 (defined as 3 twitches of train-of-four) provides a median of 12, 17, and 24 minutes of clinical duration under anesthesia

Rapid sequence intubation: 0.6-1.2 mg/kg in appropriately premedicated and anesthetized patients with excellent or good intubating conditions within 2 minutes

Continuous infusion: Initial: 0.01-0.012 mg/kg/minute only after early evidence of spontaneous recovery of neuromuscular function is evident; infusion rates have ranged from 4-16 mcg/kg/minute

ICU: 10 mcg/kg/minute; adjust dose to maintain appropriate degree of neuromuscular blockade (eg, 1 or 2 twitches on train-of-four)

Dosage Forms

Injection, solution:

Zemuron®: 10 mg/mL (5 mL, 10 mL)

rocuronium bromide *see rocuronium on previous page*

Rofact™ [Can] *see rifampin on page 757*

Roferon-A® [US/Can] *see interferon alfa-2a on page 462*

Rogaine® [Can] *see minoxidil on page 572*

Rogaine® Extra Strength for Men [US-OTC] *see minoxidil on page 572*

Rogaine® for Men [US-OTC] *see minoxidil on page 572*

Rogaine® for Women [US-OTC] *see minoxidil on page 572*

Rogitine® [Can] *see phentolamine on page 674*

Rolaids® [US-OTC] *see calcium carbonate and magnesium hydroxide on page 139*

Rolaids® Extra Strength [US-OTC] *see calcium carbonate and magnesium hydroxide on page 139*

Rolaids® Softchews [US-OTC] *see calcium carbonate on page 138*

Rolatuss® Plain Liquid *(Discontinued)* *see chlorpheniramine and phenylephrine on page 177*

Romazicon® [US/Can] *see flumazenil on page 358*

Romilar® AC [US] *see guaifenesin and codeine on page 402*

Romycin® [US] *see erythromycin on page 309*

Rondec® [US] *see chlorpheniramine and phenylephrine on page 177*

Rondec®-DM [US] *see chlorpheniramine, phenylephrine, and dextromethorphan on page 180*

Rondec®-DM Drops *(Discontinued)* *see carbinoxamine, pseudoephedrine, and dextromethorphan on page 152*

Rondec®-DM Syrup *(Discontinued)* *see brompheniramine, pseudoephedrine, and dextromethorphan on page 122*

Rondec® Drops *(Discontinued)* *see carbinoxamine and pseudoephedrine on page 151*

Rondec® Syrup *(Discontinued)* *see brompheniramine and pseudoephedrine on page 120*

Rondomycin® Capsule *(Discontinued)*

ropinirole (roe PIN i role)

Sound-Alike/Look-Alike Issues

ropinirole may be confused with ropivacaine

(Continued)

ropinirole *(Continued)*

Synonyms ropinirole hydrochloride

U.S./Canadian Brand Names Requip® [US/Can]

Therapeutic Category Anti-Parkinson Agent (Dopamine Agonist)

Use Treatment of idiopathic Parkinson disease; in patients with early Parkinson disease who were not receiving concomitant levodopa therapy as well as in patients with advanced disease on concomitant levodopa; treatment of moderate-to-severe primary restless legs syndrome (RLS)

Usual Dosage Oral: Adults:

Parkinson disease: The dosage should be increased to achieve a maximum therapeutic effect, balanced against the principal side effects of nausea, dizziness, somnolence and dyskinesia. Recommended starting dose is 0.25 mg 3 times/day; based on individual patient response, the dosage should be titrated with weekly increments as described below:

- Week 1: 0.25 mg 3 times/day; total daily dose: 0.75 mg
- Week 2: 0.5 mg 3 times/day; total daily dose: 1.5 mg
- Week 3: 0.75 mg 3 times/day; total daily dose: 2.25 mg
- Week 4: 1 mg 3 times/day; total daily dose: 3 mg

Note: After week 4, if necessary, daily dosage may be increased by 1.5 mg per day on a weekly basis up to a dose of 9 mg/day, and then by up to 3 mg/day weekly to a total of 24 mg/day

Parkinson disease discontinuation taper: Ropinirole should be gradually tapered over 7 days as follows: reduce frequency of administration from 3 times daily to twice daily for 4 days, then reduce to once daily for remaining 3 days.

Restless Legs Syndrome: Initial: 0.25 mg once daily 1-3 hours before bedtime. Dose may be increased after 2 days to 0.5 mg daily, and after 7 days to 1 mg daily. Dose may be further titrated upward in 0.5 mg increments every week until reaching a daily dose of 3 mg during week 6. If symptoms persist or reappear, the daily dose may be increased to a maximum of 4 mg beginning week 7.

Note: Doses up to 4 mg per day may be discontinued without tapering.

Dosage Forms

Tablet:

Requip®: 0.25 mg, 0.5 mg, 1 mg, 2 mg, 3 mg, 4 mg, 5 mg

ropinirole hydrochloride *see* ropinirole *on previous page*

ropivacaine *(roe PIV a kane)*

Sound-Alike/Look-Alike Issues

ropivacaine may be confused with bupivacaine, ropinirole

Synonyms ropivacaine hydrochloride

U.S./Canadian Brand Names Naropin® [US/Can]

Therapeutic Category Local Anesthetic

Use Local anesthetic for use in surgery, postoperative pain management, and obstetrical procedures when local or regional anesthesia is needed

Usual Dosage Dose varies with procedure, onset and depth of anesthesia desired, vascularity of tissues, duration of anesthesia, and condition of patient: Adults:

Surgical anesthesia:

Lumbar epidural: 15-30 mL of 0.5% to 1% solution

Lumbar epidural block for cesarean section:

  20-30 mL dose of 0.5% solution

  15-20 mL dose of 0.75% solution

Thoracic epidural block: 5-15 mL dose of 0.5% to 0.75% solution

Major nerve block:

  35-50 mL dose of 0.5% solution (175-250 mg)

  10-40 mL dose of 0.75% solution (75-300 mg)

Field block: 1-40 mL dose of 0.5% solution (5-200 mg)

Labor pain management: Lumbar epidural: Initial: 10-20 mL 0.2% solution; continuous infusion dose: 6-14 mL/hour of 0.2% solution with incremental injections of 10-15 mL/hour of 0.2% solution

Postoperative pain management:

Lumbar or thoracic epidural: Continuous infusion dose: 6-14 mL/hour of 0.2% solution

Infiltration/minor nerve block:

  1-100 mL dose of 0.2% solution

  1-40 mL dose of 0.5% solution

Dosage Forms

Infusion:

Naropin®: 2 mg/mL (100 mL, 200 mL)

Injection, solution [preservative free]:

Naropin®: 2 mg/mL (10 mL, 20 mL); 5 mg/mL (20 mL, 30 mL); 7.5 mg/mL (20 mL); 10 mg/mL (10 mL, 20 mL)

ropivacaine hydrochloride *see* ropivacaine *on previous page*

Rosac® **[US]** *see* sulfur and sulfacetamide *on page 815*

Rosanil® **[US]** *see* sulfur and sulfacetamide *on page 815*

rosiglitazone (roh si GLI ta zone)

Sound-Alike/Look-Alike Issues
Avandia® may be confused with Avalide®, Coumadin®, Prandin®

U.S./Canadian Brand Names Avandia® [US/Can]

Therapeutic Category Hypoglycemic Agent, Oral; Thiazolidinedione Derivative

Use Type 2 diabetes mellitus (noninsulin dependent, NIDDM):
Monotherapy: Improve glycemic control as an adjunct to diet and exercise
Combination therapy: In combination with a sulfonylurea, metformin, or insulin, or sulfonylurea plus metformin when diet, exercise, and a single agent do not result in adequate glycemic control

Usual Dosage Oral: Adults: **Note:** All patients should be initiated at the lowest recommended dose.
Monotherapy: Initial: 4 mg daily as a single daily dose or in divided doses twice daily. If response is inadequate after 8-12 weeks of treatment, the dosage may be increased to 8 mg daily as a single daily dose or in divided doses twice daily. In clinical trials, the 4 mg twice-daily regimen resulted in the greatest reduction in fasting plasma glucose and Hb A_{1c}.
Combination therapy: When adding rosiglitazone to existing therapy, continue current dose(s) of previous agents:
With sulfonylureas or metformin (or sulfonylurea plus metformin): Initial: 4 mg daily as a single daily dose or in divided doses twice daily. If response is inadequate after 8-12 weeks of treatment, the dosage may be increased to 8 mg daily as a single daily dose or in divided doses twice daily. Reduce dose of sulfonylurea if hypoglycemia occurs. It is unlikely that the dose of metformin will need to be reduced to hypoglycemia.
With insulin: Initial: 4 mg daily as a single daily dose or in divided doses twice daily. Dose of insulin should be reduced by 10% to 25% if the patient reports hypoglycemia or if the plasma glucose falls to <100 mg/dL. Doses of rosiglitazone >4 mg/day are not indicated in combination with insulin.

Dosage Forms
Tablet:
Avandia®: 2 mg, 4 mg, 8 mg

rosiglitazone and glimepiride (roh si GLI ta zone & GLYE me pye ride)

Synonyms glimepiride and rosiglitazone maleate

U.S./Canadian Brand Names Avandaryl™ [US]

Therapeutic Category Antidiabetic Agent, Sulfonylurea; Antidiabetic Agent, Thiazolidinedione

Use Management of type 2 diabetes mellitus (noninsulin-dependent, NIDDM) as an adjunct to diet and exercise

Usual Dosage Oral: Adults: Type 2 diabetes mellitus:
Initial: Rosiglitazone 4 mg and glimepiride 1 mg once daily **or** rosiglitazone 4 mg and glimepiride 2 mg once daily (for patients previously treated with sulfonylurea or thiazolidinedione monotherapy)
Patients switching from combination rosiglitazone and glimepiride as separate tablets: Use current dose.
Maximum: Rosiglitazone 8 mg and glimepiride 4 mg once daily
Titration:
Dose adjustment in patients previously on sulfonylurea monotherapy: May take 2 weeks to observe decreased blood glucose and 2-3 months to see full effects of rosiglitazone component. If not adequately controlled after 8-12 weeks, increase daily dose of rosiglitazone component. Maximum: Rosiglitazone 8 mg and glimepiride 4 mg once daily
Dose adjustment in patients previously on thiazolidinedione monotherapy: If not adequately controlled after 1-2 weeks, increase daily dose of glimepiride component in ≤2 mg increments in 1-2 week intervals.
Maximum: Rosiglitazone 8 mg and glimepiride 4 mg once daily

Dosage Forms
Tablet:
Avandaryl™: 4 mg/1 mg: Rosiglitazone 4 mg and glimepiride 1 mg; 4 mg/2 mg: Rosiglitazone 4 mg and glimepiride 2 mg; 4 mg/4 mg: Rosiglitazone 4 mg and glimepiride 4 mg; 8 mg/2 mg: Rosiglitazone 8 mg and glimepiride 2 mg; 8 mg/4 mg: Rosiglitazone 8 mg and glimepiride 4 mg

rosiglitazone and metformin (roh si GLI ta zone & met FOR min)

Synonyms metformin and rosiglitazone; metformin hydrochloride and rosiglitazone maleate; rosiglitazone maleate and metformin hydrochloride

U.S./Canadian Brand Names Avandamet® [US/Can]

Therapeutic Category Antidiabetic Agent (Biguanide); Antidiabetic Agent (Thiazolidinedione)

Use Management of type 2 diabetes mellitus (noninsulin-dependent, NIDDM) as an adjunct to diet and exercise in patients where dual rosiglitazone and metformin therapy is appropriate
(Continued)

rosiglitazone and metformin *(Continued)*

Usual Dosage Oral:

Adults: Type 2 diabetes mellitus: Daily dose should be divided and given with meals:

First-line therapy (drug-naive patients): Initial: Rosiglitazone 2 mg and metformin 500 mg once or twice daily; may increase by 2 mg/500 mg per day after 4 weeks to a maximum of 8 mg/2000 mg per day.

Second-line therapy:

Patients inadequately controlled on **metformin alone**: Initial dose: Rosiglitazone 4 mg/day plus current dose of metformin

Patients inadequately controlled on **rosiglitazone alone**: Initial dose: Metformin 1000 mg/day plus current dose of rosiglitazone

Note: When switching from combination rosiglitazone and metformin as separate tablets: Use current dose

Dose adjustment: Doses may be increased as increments of rosiglitazone 4 mg and/or metformin 500 mg, up to the maximum dose; doses should be titrated gradually.

After a change in the metformin dosage, titration can be done after 1-2 weeks

After a change in the rosiglitazone dosage, titration can be done after 8-12 weeks

Maximum dose: Rosiglitazone 8 mg/metformin 2000 mg daily

Dosage Forms

Tablet:

Avandamet®: 2/500: Rosiglitazone 2 mg and metformin 500 mg

Avandamet®: 4/500: Rosiglitazone 4 mg and metformin 500 mg

Avandamet®: 2/1000: Rosiglitazone 2 mg and metformin 1000 mg

Avandamet®: 4/1000: Rosiglitazone 4 mg and metformin 1000 mg

rosiglitazone maleate and metformin hydrochloride *see* rosiglitazone and metformin *on previous page*

Rosula® [US] *see* sulfur and sulfacetamide *on page 815*

Rosula® NS [US] *see* sulfacetamide *on page 810*

rosuvastatin (roe soo va STAT in)

Synonyms rosuvastatin calcium

U.S./Canadian Brand Names Crestor® [US/Can]

Therapeutic Category Antilipemic Agent, HMG-CoA Reductase Inhibitor

Use Used with dietary therapy for hyperlipidemias to reduce elevations in total cholesterol (TC), LDL-C, apolipoprotein B, and triglycerides (TG) in patients with primary hypercholesterolemia (elevations of 1 or more components are present in Fredrickson type IIa, IIb, and IV hyperlipidemias); treatment of homozygous familial hypercholesterolemia (FH)

Usual Dosage Oral: Adults:

Heterozygous familial and nonfamilial hypercholesterolemia; mixed dyslipidemia:

Initial dose:

General dosing: 10 mg once daily (20 mg in patients with severe hypercholesterolemia)

Conservative dosing: Patients requiring less aggressive treatment or predisposed to myopathy (including patients of Asian descent): 5 mg once daily

Titration: After 2 weeks, may be increased by 5-10 mg once daily; dosing range: 5-40 mg/day (maximum dose: 40 mg once daily)

Note: The 40 mg dose should be reserved for patients who have not achieved goal cholesterol levels on a dose of 20 mg/day, including patients switched from another HMG-CoA reductase inhibitor.

Homozygous FH: Initial: 20 mg once daily (maximum dose: 40 mg/day)

Dosage adjustment with concomitant medications:

Cyclosporine: Rosuvastatin dose should not exceed 5 mg/day

Gemfibrozil: Rosuvastatin dose should not exceed 10 mg/day

Dosage adjustment for persistent, unexplained proteinuria while on 40 mg/day: Reduce dose and evaluate causes

Dosage Forms

Tablet:

Crestor®: 5 mg, 10 mg, 20 mg, 40 mg

rosuvastatin calcium *see* rosuvastatin *on this page*

RotaShield® *(Discontinued)*

RotaTeq® [US] *see* rotavirus vaccine *on next page*

rotavirus vaccine (ROE ta vye rus vak SEEN)

Synonyms pentavalent human-bovine reassortant rotavirus vaccine; rotavirus vaccine, pentavalent

U.S./Canadian Brand Names RotaTeq® [US]

Therapeutic Category Vaccine

Use Prevention of rotavirus gastroenteritis in infants and children

Usual Dosage Oral: Children 6-32 weeks: Three 2 mL doses at 2-, 4-, and 6 months of age, the first given at 6-12 weeks of age, followed by subsequent doses at 4- to 10-week intervals. Routine administration of the first dose at >12 weeks of age is not recommended (insufficient data). Administer all doses by 32 weeks of age. Infants who have had rotavirus gastroenteritis before getting the full course of vaccine should still initiate or complete the 3-dose schedule; initial infection provides only partial immunity.

Dosage Forms

Suspension, oral [preservative free]:

RotaTeq®: G1 $\geq$2.2 10^6 infectious units, G2 $\geq$2.8 10^6 infectious units, G3 $\geq$2.2 10^6 infectious units, G4 $\geq$2.0 10^6 infectious units, and P1 [8] $\geq$2.3 10^6 infectious units (2 mL)

rotavirus vaccine, pentavalent *see* rotavirus vaccine *on this page*

rotigotine (roe TIG oh teen)

Sound-Alike/Look-Alike Issues

Neupro® may be confused with Neupogen®

Synonyms N-0923

U.S./Canadian Brand Names Neupro® [US]

Therapeutic Category Anti-Parkinson Agent (Dopamine Agonist)

Use Treatment of the signs and symptoms of early-stage idiopathic Parkinson disease

Usual Dosage Topical: Transdermal: Adults: Initial: Apply 2 mg/24 hours patch once daily; may increase by 2 mg/24 hours weekly, based on clinical response and tolerability (maximum: 6 mg/24 hours)

Dosage reductions or discontinuation: Decrease by 2 mg/24 hours every other day

Note: In clinical trials, the lowest effective dose was 4 mg/24 hours and doses >6 mg/24 hours did not provide any additional therapeutic benefit and increased incidence of adverse effects

Dosage Forms

Transdermal system [once-daily patch]:

Neupro®: 2 mg/24 hours (7s, 30s); 4 mg/24 hours (7s, 30s); 6 mg/24 hours (7s, 30s)

Rowasa® [US/Can] *see* mesalamine *on page 546*

Roxanol™ [US] *see* morphine sulfate *on page 578*

Roxanol SR™ Oral *(Discontinued)* *see* morphine sulfate *on page 578*

Roxanol™-T *(Discontinued)* *see* morphine sulfate *on page 578*

Roxicet™ [US] *see* oxycodone and acetaminophen *on page 641*

Roxicet™ 5/500 [US] *see* oxycodone and acetaminophen *on page 641*

Roxicodone® [US] *see* oxycodone *on page 640*

Roxiprin® *(Discontinued)* *see* oxycodone and aspirin *on page 642*

Roychlor® [Can] *see* potassium chloride *on page 700*

Rozerem™ [US] *see* ramelteon *on page 743*

RP-6976 *see* docetaxel *on page 272*

RP-54274 *see* riluzole *on page 759*

RP-59500 *see* quinupristin and dalfopristin *on page 741*

r-PA *see* reteplase *on page 751*

rPDGF-BB *see* becaplermin *on page 96*

(R,R)-formoterol L-tartrate *see* arformoterol *on page 72*

RS-25259 *see* palonosetron *on page 647*

RS-25259-197 *see* palonosetron *on page 647*

R-Tanna [US] *see* chlorpheniramine and phenylephrine *on page 177*

RTCA *see* ribavirin *on page 755*

RU 0211 *see* lubiprostone *on page 522*

RU-486 *see* mifepristone *on page 569*

RU-23908 *see* nilutamide *on page 606*

RU-38486 *see* mifepristone *on page 569*

rubella, measles, and mumps vaccines, combined *see* measles, mumps, and rubella vaccines, combined *on page 533*

rubella, varicella, measles, and mumps vaccine *see* measles, mumps, rubella, and varicella virus vaccine *on page 533*

rubella virus vaccine (live) (rue BEL a VYE rus vak SEEN, live)

Sound-Alike/Look-Alike Issues
Meruvax® II may be confused with Attenuvax®

Synonyms German measles vaccine

U.S./Canadian Brand Names Meruvax® II [US]

Therapeutic Category Vaccine, Live Virus

Use Selective active immunization against rubella
Note: Trivalent measles - mumps - rubella (MMR) vaccine is the preferred immunizing agent for most children and many adults.

Usual Dosage SubQ: Children ≥12 months and Adults: 0.5 mL
Primary immunization is recommended at 12-15 months; revaccination with MMR-II at 4-6 years of age is recommended prior to elementary school. Previously unvaccinated children of susceptible pregnant women should be vaccinated.

Adults without documentation of immunity: Vaccination is recommended for students entering colleges and other institutions of higher education, for military personal, for healthcare workers, for international travelers who visit endemic areas, and to women of childbearing potential. Do not administer to women who may become pregnant within 4 weeks of receiving vaccine; administer following completion or termination of pregnancy

Dosage Forms
Injection, powder for reconstitution [preservative free]:
Meruvax® II: ≥1000 $TCID_{50}$ (Wistar RA 27/3 Strain)

rubeola vaccine *see* measles virus vaccine (live) *on page 534*

Rubex® *(Discontinued)* *see* doxorubicin *on page 280*

rubidomycin hydrochloride *see* daunorubicin hydrochloride *on page 233*

Rubramin-PC® *(Discontinued)* *see* cyanocobalamin *on page 220*

Rulox [US-OTC] *see* aluminum hydroxide and magnesium hydroxide *on page 37*

Rulox No. 1 *(Discontinued)* *see* aluminum hydroxide and magnesium hydroxide *on page 37*

Rum-K® [US] *see* potassium chloride *on page 700*

Ru-Tuss DM [US] *see* guaifenesin, pseudoephedrine, and dextromethorphan *on page 408*

Ru-Tuss® Liquid *(Discontinued)* *see* chlorpheniramine and phenylephrine *on page 177*

Ru-Vert-M® *(Discontinued)* *see* meclizine *on page 535*

Rylosol [Can] *see* sotalol *on page 802*

Rymed® *(Discontinued)* *see* guaifenesin and pseudoephedrine *on page 406*

Rymed-TR® *(Discontinued)*

Ryna-12™ [US] *see* phenylephrine and pyrilamine *on page 677*

Ryna-12 S™ [US] *see* phenylephrine and pyrilamine *on page 677*

Ryna-C® *(Discontinued)* *see* chlorpheniramine, pseudoephedrine, and codeine *on page 183*

Ryna® *(Discontinued)* *see* chlorpheniramine, pseudoephedrine, and codeine *on page 183*

Rynatan® [US] *see* chlorpheniramine and phenylephrine *on page 177*

Rynatan® Pediatric Suspension [US] *see* chlorpheniramine and phenylephrine *on page 177*

Rynatuss® [US] *see* chlorpheniramine, ephedrine, phenylephrine, and carbetapentane *on page 179*

Rynatuss® Pediatric *(Discontinued)* *see* chlorpheniramine, ephedrine, phenylephrine, and carbetapentane *on page 179*

Rynesa 12S™ [US] *see* phenylephrine and pyrilamine *on page 677*

Ry-T 12 [US] *see* phenylephrine and pyrilamine *on page 677*

Rythmodan® [Can] *see* disopyramide *on page 271*

Rythmodan®-LA [Can] *see* disopyramide *on page 271*

Rythmol® [US] *see* propafenone *on page 721*

Rythmol® Gen-Propafenone [Can] *see* propafenone *on page 721*

Rythmol® SR [US] *see* propafenone *on page 721*

S2® **[US-OTC]** *see* epinephrine *on page 300*

S-(+)-3-isobutylgaba *see* pregabalin *on page 712*

SAB-Dimenhydrinate [Can] *see* dimenhydrinate *on page 262*

SAB-Gentamicin [Can] *see* gentamicin *on page 390*

Sab-Prenase [Can] *see* prednisolone (systemic) *on page 710*

Sabril® **[Can]** *see* vigabatrin *(Canada only)* *on page 890*

SAB-Trifluridine [Can] *see* trifluridine *on page 866*

Saccharomyces boulardii (sak roe MYE sees boo LAR dee)

Synonyms *Saccharomyces boulardii lyo*; *S. boulardii*
U.S./Canadian Brand Names Florastor® Kids [US-OTC]; Florastor® [US-OTC]
Therapeutic Category Dietary Supplement; Probiotic
Use Promote maintenance of normal microflora in the gastrointestinal tract; used in management of bloating, gas, and diarrhea, particularly to decrease the incidence of diarrhea associated with antibiotic use
Usual Dosage Oral: Dietary supplement: Dosing varies by manufacturer; consult product labeling.
Children (Florastor® Kids): 250 mg twice daily
Adults (Florastor®): 250 mg twice daily
Dosage Forms
Capsule:
Florastor®: *S. boulardii lyo* 250 mg
Powder:
Florastor® Kids: *S. boulardii lyo* 250 mg

Saccharomyces boulardii lyo *see Saccharomyces boulardii on this page*

sacrosidase (sak ROE si dase)

U.S./Canadian Brand Names Sucraid® [US/Can]
Therapeutic Category Enzyme
Use Orphan drug: Oral replacement therapy in sucrase deficiency, as seen in congenital sucrase-isomaltase deficiency (CSID)
Usual Dosage Oral:
Infants ≥5 months and Children <15 kg: 8500 int. units (1 mL) per meal or snack
Children >15 kg and Adults: 17,000 int. units (2 mL) per meal or snack
Doses should be diluted with 2-4 oz of water, milk, or formula with each meal or snack. Approximately one-half of the dose may be taken before, and the remainder of a dose taken at the completion of each meal or snack.
Dosage Forms
Solution, oral:
Sucraid®: 8500 int. units per mL

Safe Tussin® **[US-OTC]** *see* guaifenesin and dextromethorphan *on page 402*

SAHA *see* vorinostat *on page 898*

Saizen® **[US/Can]** *see* somatropin *on page 799*

SalAc® **[US-OTC]** *see* salicylic acid *on next page*

Sal-Acid® **[US-OTC]** *see* salicylic acid *on next page*

Salacid® **Ointment *(Discontinued)*** *see* salicylic acid *on next page*

Salactic® **[US-OTC]** *see* salicylic acid *on next page*

Salagen® **[US/Can]** *see* pilocarpine *on page 682*

Salazopyrin® **[Can]** *see* sulfasalazine *on page 814*

Salazopyrin En-Tabs® **[Can]** *see* sulfasalazine *on page 814*

Salbu-2 [Can] *see* albuterol *on page 23*

Salbu-4 [Can] *see* albuterol *on page 23*

salbutamol *see* albuterol *on page 23*

salbutamol and ipratropium *see* ipratropium and albuterol *on page 471*

salbutamol sulphate *see* albuterol *on page 23*

Saleto-200® ***(Discontinued)*** *see* ibuprofen *on page 444*

Saleto-400® ***(Discontinued)*** *see* ibuprofen *on page 444*

Salflex® **[Can]** *see* salsalate *on page 775*

Salgesic® *(Discontinued)* *see* salsalate *on page 775*

salicylazosulfapyridine *see* sulfasalazine *on page 814*

salicylic acid (sal i SIL ik AS id)

U.S./Canadian Brand Names Compound W® One Step Wart Remover [US-OTC]; Compound W® [US-OTC]; DHS™ Sal [US-OTC]; Dr. Scholl's® Callus Remover [US-OTC]; Dr. Scholl's® Clear Away [US-OTC]; DuoFilm® [US-OTC/Can]; Duoforte® 27 [Can]; Freezone® [US-OTC]; Fung-O® [US-OTC]; Gordofilm® [US-OTC]; Hydrisalic™ [US-OTC]; Ionil® Plus [US-OTC]; Ionil® [US-OTC]; Keralyt® [US-OTC]; LupiCare™ Dandruff [US-OTC]; LupiCare™ II Psoriasis [US-OTC]; LupiCare™ Psoriasis [US-OTC]; Mediplast® [US-OTC]; MG217 Sal-Acid® [US-OTC]; Mosco® Corn and Callus Remover [US-OTC]; NeoCeuticals™ Acne Spot Treatment [US-OTC]; Neutrogena® Acne Wash [US-OTC]; Neutrogena® Body Clear™ [US-OTC]; Neutrogena® Clear Pore Shine Control [US-OTC]; Neutrogena® Clear Pore [US-OTC]; Neutrogena® Healthy Scalp [US-OTC]; Neutrogena® Maximum Strength T/Sal® [US-OTC]; Neutrogena® On The Spot® Acne Patch [US-OTC]; Occlusal®-HP [US-OTC/Can]; Oxy Balance® Deep Pore [US-OTC]; Oxy Balance® [US-OTC]; Palmer's® Skin Success Acne Cleanser [US-OTC]; Pedisilk® [US-OTC]; Propa pH [US-OTC]; Sal-Acid® [US-OTC]; Sal-Plant® [US-OTC]; Salactic® [US-OTC]; SalAc® [US-OTC]; Sebcur® [Can]; Soluver® Plus [Can]; Soluver® [Can]; Stri-dex® Body Focus [US-OTC]; Stri-dex® Facewipes To Go™ [US-OTC]; Stri-dex® Maximum Strength [US-OTC]; Stri-dex® [US-OTC]; Tinamed® [US-OTC]; Tiseb® [US-OTC]; Trans-Plantar® [Can]; Trans-Ver-Sal® [US-OTC/Can]; Wart-Off® Maximum Strength [US-OTC]; Zapzyt® Acne Wash [US-OTC]; Zapzyt® Pore Treatment [US-OTC]

Therapeutic Category Keratolytic Agent

Use Topically for its keratolytic effect in controlling seborrheic dermatitis or psoriasis of body and scalp, dandruff, and other scaling dermatoses; also used to remove warts, corns, and calluses; acne

Usual Dosage Children and Adults (consult specific product labeling for use in children <12 years):

Acne:

Cream, cloth, foam, or liquid cleansers (2%): Use to cleanse skin once or twice daily. Massage gently into skin, work into lather and rinse thoroughly. Cloths should be wet with water prior to using and disposed of (not flushed) after use.

Gel (0.5% or 2%): Apply small amount to face in the morning or evening; if peeling occurs, may be used every other day. Some products may be labeled for OTC use up to 3 or 4 times per day. Apply to clean, dry skin

Pads (0.5% or 2%): Use pad to cover affected area with thin layer of salicylic acid one to three times a day. Apply to clean, dry skin. Do not leave pad on skin.

Patch (2%): At bedtime, after washing face, allow skin to dry at least 5 minutes. Apply patch directly over pimple being treated. Remove in the morning.

Shower/bath gels or soap (2%): Use once daily in shower or bath to massage over skin prone to acne. Rinse well.

Callus, corns, or warts:

Gel or liquid (17%): Apply to each wart and allow to dry. May repeat once or twice daily, up to 12 weeks. Apply to clean dry area.

Gel (6%): Apply to affected area once daily, generally used at night and rinsed off in the morning.

Plaster or transdermal patch (40%): Apply directly over affected area, leave in place for 48 hours. Some products may be cut to fit area or secured with adhesive strips. May repeat procedure for up to 12 weeks. Apply to clean, dry skin

Transdermal patch (15%): Apply directly over affected area at bedtime, leave in place overnight and remove in the morning. Patch should be trimmed to cover affected area. May repeat daily for up to 12 weeks.

Dandruff, psoriasis, or seborrheic dermatitis:

Cream (2.5%): Apply to affected area 3-4 times daily. Apply to clean, dry skin. Some products may be left in place overnight.

Ointment (3%): Apply to scales or plaques on skin up to 4 times per day (not for scalp or face)

Shampoo (1.8% to 3%): Massage into wet hair or affected area; leave in place for several minutes; rinse thoroughly. Labeled for OTC use 2-3 times a week, or as directed by healthcare provider. Some products may be left in place overnight.

Dosage Forms

Cloths:

Neutrogena® Acne Wash [OTC]: 2% (30s)

Cream:

Akurza: 6% (340 g)

LupiCare™ Dandruff [OTC], LupiCare™ Psoriasis [OTC]: 2.5% (120 g, 240 g)

LupiCare™ II Psoriasis [OTC]: 2.5% (60 g, 240 g)

Neutrogena® Acne Wash [OTC]: 2% (200 mL)

Salex™: 6% (400 g)

Foam:

Neutrogena® Acne Wash [OTC]: 2% (150 mL)

SalAc® [OTC]: 2% (100 g)
Gel: 17% (15 g)
Compound W® [OTC]: 17% (7 g)
Hydrisalic™ [OTC]: 6% (28 g)
Keralyt® [OTC]: 6% (30 g)
NeoCeuticals™ Acne Spot Treatment [OTC]: 2% (15 g)
Neutrogena® Clear Pore [OTC]: 2% (60 g)
Neutrogena® Clear Pore Shine Control [OTC]: 0.5% (10 g)
Oxy Balance® [OTC]: 2% (240 mL)
Sal-Plant® [OTC]: 17% (14 g)
Stri-dex® Body Focus™ [OTC]: 2% (300 mL)
Zapzyt® Acne Wash [OTC]: 2% (190 mL)
Zapzyt® Pore Treatment [OTC]: 2% (23 g)
Liquid, topical:
Compound W® [OTC]: 17% (9 mL)
DuoFilm® [OTC], Pedisilk® [OTC], Fung-O® [OTC], Salactic® [OTC], Tinamed® [OTC]: 17% (15 mL)
Freezone® [OTC]: 17.6% (9.3 mL)
Gordofilm® [OTC]: 16.7% (15 mL)
Mosco® Corn and Callus Remover [OTC]: 17.6% (10 mL)
NeoCeuticals™ Acne Spot Treatment [OTC]: 2% (60 mL)
Neutrogena® Acne Wash [OTC], SalAc® [OTC]: 2% (180 mL)
Neutrogena® Body Clear™ [OTC] [body scrub with microbeads], Neutrogena® Body Clear™ [OTC] [body wash]: 2% (250 mL)
Occlusal®-HP [OTC]: 17% (10 mL)
Palmer's® Skin Success Acne Cleanser [OTC]: 0.5% (240 mL)
Propa pH [OTC]: 2% (80 mL)
Wart-Off® [OTC]: 17% (13 mL)
Lotion, topical:
Akurza: 6% (355 mL)
Salex™: 6% (414 mL)
Ointment:
MG217 Sal-Acid® [OTC]: 3% (56 g) [contains vitamin E]
Pads:
Oxy Balance® [OTC], Oxy Balance® Deep Pore [OTC]: 0.5% (55s, 90s)
Stri-dex® [OTC]: 0.5% (55s)
Stri-dex® Facewipes To Go™ [OTC]: 0.5% (32s)
Stri-dex® Maximum Strength [OTC]: 2% (32s, 55s, 90s)
Patch, transdermal:
Compound W® One Step Wart Remover [OTC]: 40% (12s, 14s)
Dr. Scholl's® Callus Remover [OTC]: 40% (4s)
Dr. Scholl's® Clear Away [OTC]: 40% (14s, 16s, 18s, 24s)
DuoFilm® [OTC]: 40% (18s)
Neutrogena® On The Spot® Acne Patch [OTC]: 2% (27s)
Trans-Ver-Sal® [OTC]: 15% [6 mm PediaPatch, 12 mm AdultPatch, 20 mm PlantarPatch] (10s, 12s, 15s, 25s, 40s)
Plaster:
Mediplast® [OTC]: 40% (25s)
Sal-Acid® [OTC]: 40% (14s)
Tinamed® [OTC]: 40% (24s)
Shampoo:
DHS™ Sal [OTC]: 3% (120 mL)
Ionil® [OTC]: 2% (240 mL, 480 mL, 960 mL)
Ionil® Plus [OTC]: 2% (240 mL)
LupiCare™ Dandruff [OTC], LupiCare™ Psoriasis [OTC]: 2% (120 mL, 240 mL)
Neutrogena® Healthy Scalp [OTC]: 1.8% (90 mL, 180 mL)
Neutrogena® Maximum Strength T/Sal® [OTC]: 3% (135 mL)
Salex™: 6% (177 mL)
Tiseb® [OTC]: 2% (240 mL)
Soap: 2% (114 g)

salicylic acid and coal tar *see* coal tar and salicylic acid *on page 209*

salicylsalicylic acid *see* salsalate *on page 775*

SalineX® [US-OTC] *see* sodium chloride *on page 792*

Salivart® [US-OTC] *see* saliva substitute *on next page*

saliva substitute (sa LYE va SUB stee tute)

U.S./Canadian Brand Names Aquoral™ [US]; Caphasol [US]; Entertainer's Secret® [US-OTC]; Moi-Stir® [US-OTC]; Mouthkote® [US-OTC]; Numoisyn™ [US]; Saliva Substitute™ [US-OTC]; Salivart® [US-OTC]; SalivaSure™ [US-OTC]

Therapeutic Category Gastrointestinal Agent, Miscellaneous

Use Relief of dry mouth and throat in xerostomia

Usual Dosage Use as needed

Dosage Forms

Liquid:

Numoisyn™: Water, sorbitol, linseed extract, *Chondrus crispus*, methylparaben, sodium benzoate, potassium sorbate, dipotassium phosphate, propylparaben

Lozenge:

Numoisyn™: Sorbitol 0.3 g/lozenge, polyethylene glycol, malic acid, sodium citrate, calcium phosphate dibasic, hydrogenated cottonseed oil, citric acid, magnesium stearate, silicon dioxide

SalivaSure™: Xylitol, citric acid, apple acid, sodium citrate dihydrate, sodium carboxymethylcellulose, dibasic calcium phosphate, silica colloidal, magnesium stearate, stearic acid

Solution, oral:

Caphosol: Dibasic sodium phosphate 0.032%, monobasic sodium phosphate 0.009%, calcium chloride 0.052%, sodium chloride 0.569%, purified water

Entertainer's Secret®: Sodium carboxymethylcellulose, aloe vera gel, glycerin (60 mL) [honey-apple flavor]

Saliva Substitute®: Sorbitol, sodium carboxymethylcellulose, methylparaben (120 mL)

Solution, oral [spray]:

Aquoral™: Oxidized glycerol triesters and silicon dioxide

Moi-Stir [OTC]: Water, sorbitol, sodium carboxymethylcellulose, methylparaben, propylparaben, potassium chloride, dibasic sodium phosphate, calcium chloride, magnesium chloride, sodium chloride

Mouthkote® [OTC]: Water, xylitol, sorbitol, yerba santa, citric acid, ascorbic acid, sodium saccharin, sodium benzoate

Salivart® [OTC]: Water, sodium carboxymethylcellulose, sorbitol, sodium chloride, potassium chloride, calcium chloride, magnesium chloride, potassium phosphate

Saliva Substitute™ [US-OTC] *see* saliva substitute *on this page*

SalivaSure™ [US-OTC] *see* saliva substitute *on this page*

salk vaccine *see* poliovirus vaccine (inactivated) *on page 693*

salmeterol (sal ME te role)

Sound-Alike/Look-Alike Issues

salmeterol may be confused with salbutamol

Serevent® may be confused with Serentil®

Synonyms salmeterol xinafoate

U.S./Canadian Brand Names Serevent® Diskus® [US]; Serevent® [Can]

Therapeutic Category Adrenergic Agonist Agent

Use Maintenance treatment of asthma and in prevention of bronchospasm with reversible obstructive airway disease, including patients with symptoms of nocturnal asthma; prevention of exercise-induced bronchospasm; maintenance treatment of bronchospasm associated with COPD

Usual Dosage Inhalation, powder (Serevent® Diskus®):

Asthma, maintenance and prevention: Children ≥4 years and Adults: One inhalation (50 mcg) twice daily (~12 hours apart); maximum: 1 inhalation twice daily

Exercise-induced asthma, prevention: Children ≥4 years and Adults: One inhalation (50 mcg) at least 30 minutes prior to exercise; additional doses should not be used for 12 hours; should not be used in individuals already receiving salmeterol twice daily

COPD (maintenance treatment of associated bronchospasm): Adults: One inhalation (50 mcg) twice daily (~12 hours apart); maximum: 1 inhalation twice daily

Dosage Forms

Powder for oral inhalation:

Serevent® Diskus®: 50 mcg (28s, 60s)

salmeterol and fluticasone *see* fluticasone and salmeterol *on page 367*

salmeterol xinafoate *see* salmeterol *on this page*

Salmonella typhi Vi capsular polysaccharide vaccine *(Canada only)*

(sal mo NEL la TI fi vi CAP su lar po le SAK ar ide VAK seen)

U.S./Canadian Brand Names Typherix™ [Can]

Therapeutic Category Vaccine

Use For active immunization against typhoid fever in persons 2 years of age and older.

Usual Dosage One dose administered I.M. ensures protection for at least 3 years. The vaccine must be given at least 2 weeks prior to travel to endemic areas.

Dosage Forms Injection: Vi polysaccharide vaccine of *S. typhi* 25 mcg (0.5 mL)

Salmonine® *(Discontinued)* see calcitonin *on page 135*

Salofalk® **[Can]** see mesalamine *on page 546*

Sal-Plant® **[US-OTC]** see salicylic acid *on page 772*

salsalate (SAL sa late)

Sound-Alike/Look-Alike Issues
salsalate may be confused with sucralfate, sulfasalazine

Synonyms disalicylic acid; salicylsalicylic acid

U.S./Canadian Brand Names Amigesic® [US/Can]; Salflex® [Can]

Therapeutic Category Analgesic, Nonnarcotic; Antipyretic; Nonsteroidal Antiinflammatory Drug (NSAID)

Use Treatment of minor pain or fever; arthritis

Usual Dosage Oral: Adults: 3 g/day in 2-3 divided doses

Dosage Forms
Tablet: 500 mg, 750 mg
Amigesic®: 500 mg, 750 mg

Salsitab® *(Discontinued)* see salsalate *on this page*

salt see sodium chloride *on page 792*

salt-poor albumin see albumin *on page 22*

Sal-Tropine™ **[US]** see atropine *on page 83*

Sanctura® **[US]** see trospium *on page 872*

Sandimmune® **[US]** see cyclosporine *on page 223*

Sandimmune® **I.V. [Can]** see cyclosporine *on page 223*

Sandomigran® **[Can]** see pizotifen *(Canada only) on page 688*

Sandomigran DS® **[Can]** see pizotifen *(Canada only) on page 688*

Sandostatin® **[US/Can]** see octreotide *on page 624*

Sandostatin LAR® **[US/Can]** see octreotide *on page 624*

Sandoz-Acebutolol [Can] see acebutolol *on page 4*

Sandoz Alendronate [Can] see alendronate *on page 27*

Sandoz-Amiodarone [Can] see amiodarone *on page 43*

Sandoz-Anagrelide [Can] see anagrelide *on page 55*

Sandoz-Atenolol [Can] see atenolol *on page 80*

Sandoz-Azithromycin [Can] see azithromycin *on page 88*

Sandoz-Betaxolol [Can] see betaxolol *on page 109*

Sandoz-Bicalutamide [Can] see bicalutamide *on page 111*

Sandoz-Bisoprolol [Can] see bisoprolol *on page 114*

Sandoz-Ciprofloxacin [Can] see ciprofloxacin *on page 190*

Sandoz-Citalopram [Can] see citalopram *on page 194*

Sandoz-Clonazepam [Can] see clonazepam *on page 204*

Sandoz-Cyclosporine [Can] see cyclosporine *on page 223*

Sandoz-Diltiazem CD [Can] see diltiazem *on page 261*

Sandoz-Diltiazem T [Can] see diltiazem *on page 261*

Sandoz-Estradiol Derm 50 [Can] see estradiol *on page 313*

Sandoz-Estradiol Derm 75 [Can] see estradiol *on page 313*

Sandoz-Estradiol Derm 100 [Can] see estradiol *on page 313*

Sandoz Fenofibrate S [Can] see fenofibrate *on page 345*

Sandoz-Fluoxetine [Can] see fluoxetine *on page 364*

Sandoz-Fluvoxamine [Can] see fluvoxamine *on page 370*

Sandoz-Gliclazide [Can] see gliclazide *(Canada only) on page 393*

Sandoz-Glimepiride [Can] *see* glimepiride *on page 393*

Sandoz-Glyburide [Can] *see* glyburide *on page 396*

Sandoz-Levobunolol [Can] *see* levobunolol *on page 499*

Sandoz-Lovastatin [Can] *see* lovastatin *on page 520*

Sandoz-Metformin FC [Can] *see* metformin *on page 548*

Sandoz-Metoprolol [Can] *see* metoprolol *on page 562*

Sandoz-Minocycline [Can] *see* minocycline *on page 571*

Sandoz-Mirtazapine [Can] *see* mirtazapine *on page 572*

Sandoz-Mirtazapine FC [Can] *see* mirtazapine *on page 572*

Sandoz-Nabumetone [Can] *see* nabumetone *on page 585*

Sandoz-Nitrazepam [Can] *see* nitrazepam *(Canada only) on page 607*

Sandoz-Paroxetine [Can] *see* paroxetine *on page 654*

Sandoz-Pravastatin [Can] *see* pravastatin *on page 707*

Sandoz-Ranitidine [Can] *see* ranitidine *on page 744*

Sandoz Risperidone [Can] *see* risperidone *on page 760*

Sandoz-Sertraline [Can] *see* sertraline *on page 783*

Sandoz-Simvastatin [Can] *see* simvastatin *on page 787*

Sandoz-Sumatriptan [Can] *see* sumatriptan *on page 815*

Sandoz-Ticlopidine [Can] *see* ticlopidine *on page 842*

Sandoz-Timolol [Can] *see* timolol *on page 843*

Sandoz-Tobramycin [Can] *see* tobramycin *on page 846*

Sandoz-Topiramate [Can] *see* topiramate *on page 851*

Sandoz-Trifluridine [Can] *see* trifluridine *on page 866*

Sandoz-Valporic [Can] *see* valproic acid and derivatives *on page 881*

Sandoz-Zopiclone [Can] *see* zopiclone *(Canada only) on page 909*

SangCya™ *(Discontinued)* *see* cyclosporine *on page 223*

Sani-Supp® [US-OTC] *see* glycerin *on page 397*

Sans Acne® [Can] *see* erythromycin *on page 309*

Santyl® [US] *see* collagenase *on page 213*

saquinavir (sa KWIN a veer)

Sound-Alike/Look-Alike Issues
saquinavir may be confused with Sinequan®

Synonyms saquinavir mesylate

U.S./Canadian Brand Names Invirase® [US/Can]

Therapeutic Category Antiviral Agent

Use Treatment of HIV infection; used in combination with at least two other antiretroviral agents

Usual Dosage Oral:

Children >16 years and Adults (Invirase®): 1000 mg (five 200 mg capsules or two 500 mg tablets) twice daily given in combination with ritonavir 100 mg twice daily. This combination should be given together and within 2 hours after a full meal in combination with a nucleoside analog. **Note:** Saquinavir hard-gel capsules (Invirase®) should not be used in "unboosted regimens."

Dosage adjustments when administered in combination therapy: Lopinavir and ritonavir (Kaletra™): Invirase® 1000 mg twice daily

Dosage Forms Strength expressed as base

Capsule:
Invirase®: 200 mg

Tablet:
Invirase®: 500 mg

saquinavir mesylate *see* saquinavir *on this page*

Sarafem® [US] *see* fluoxetine *on page 364*

sargramostim (sar GRAM oh stim)

Sound-Alike/Look-Alike Issues
Leukine® may be confused with Leukeran®, leucovorin
Synonyms GM-CSF; granulocyte-macrophage colony stimulating factor; NSC-613795; rGM-CSF
U.S./Canadian Brand Names Leukine® [US/Can]
Therapeutic Category Colony-Stimulating Factor

Use

Myeloid reconstitution after autologous bone marrow transplantation: Non-Hodgkin lymphoma (NHL), acute lymphoblastic leukemia (ALL), Hodgkin lymphoma, metastatic breast cancer

Myeloid reconstitution after allogeneic bone marrow transplantation

Peripheral stem cell transplantation: Metastatic breast cancer, non-Hodgkin lymphoma, Hodgkin lymphoma, multiple myeloma

Orphan drug:

Acute myelogenous leukemia (AML) following induction chemotherapy in older adults to shorten time to neutrophil recovery and to reduce the incidence of severe and life-threatening infections and infections resulting in death

Bone marrow transplant (allogeneic or autologous) failure or engraftment delay

Safety and efficacy of GM-CSF given simultaneously with cytotoxic chemotherapy have not been established. Concurrent treatment may increase myelosuppression.

Usual Dosage

Adults: I.V. infusion over ≥2 hours or SubQ: **Rounding the dose to the nearest vial size enhances patient convenience and reduces costs without clinical detriment**

Myeloid reconstitution after peripheral stem cell, allogeneic or autologous bone marrow transplant: I.V.: 250 mcg/m^2/day (over 2 hours), begin 2-4 hours after the marrow infusion and ≥24 hours after chemotherapy or radiotherapy, when the post marrow infusion ANC is <500 cells/mm^3, and continue until ANC >1500 cells/mm^3 for 3 consecutive days

If a severe adverse reaction occurs, reduce or temporarily discontinue the dose until the reaction abates

If blast cells appear or progression of the underlying disease occurs, disrupt treatment

Interrupt or reduce the dose by half if ANC is >20,000 cells/mm^3

Neutrophil recovery following chemotherapy in AML: I.V.: 250 mcg/m^2/day (over 4 hours) starting approximately day 11 or 4 days following the completion of induction chemotherapy, if day 10 bone marrow is hypoblastic with <5% blasts

If a second cycle of chemotherapy is necessary, administer ~4 days after the completion of chemotherapy if the bone marrow is hypoblastic with <5% blasts

Continue sargramostim until ANC is >1500 cells/mm^3 for 3 consecutive days or a maximum of 42 days

Discontinue sargramostim immediately if leukemic regrowth occurs

If a severe adverse reaction occurs, reduce the dose by 50% or temporarily discontinue the dose until the reaction abates

Mobilization of peripheral blood progenitor cells: I.V., SubQ: 250 mcg/m^2/day I.V. over 24 hours or SubQ once daily

Continue the same dose through the period of PBPC collection

The optimal schedule for PBPC collection has not been established (usually begun by day 5 and performed daily until protocol specified targets are achieved)

If WBC >50,000 cells/mm^3, reduce the dose by 50%

If adequate numbers of progenitor cells are not collected, consider other mobilization therapy

Postperipheral blood progenitor cell transplantation: I.V., SubQ: 250 mcg/m^2/day I.V. over 24 hours or SubQ once daily beginning immediately following infusion of progenitor cells and continuing until ANC is >1500 cells/mm^3 for 3 consecutive days is attained

BMT failure or engraftment delay: I.V.: 250 mcg/m^2/day over 2 hours for 14 days

May be repeated after 7 days off therapy if engraftment has not occurred

If engraftment still has not occurred, a third course of 500 mcg/m^2/day for 14 days may be tried after another 7 days off therapy; if there is still no improvement, it is unlikely that further dose escalation will be beneficial

If a severe adverse reaction occurs, reduce or temporarily discontinue the dose until the reaction abates

If blast cells appear or disease progression occurs, discontinue treatment

Dosage Forms

Injection, powder for reconstitution:
Leukine®: 250 mcg
Injection, solution:
Leukine®: 500 mcg/mL (1 mL)

Sarna® HC [Can] *see* hydrocortisone (topical) *on page 434*

Sarna® Sensitive [US-OTC] *see* pramoxine *on page 706*

Sarnol®-HC [US-OTC] *see* hydrocortisone (topical) *on page 434*

Sativex® [Can] *see* tetrahydrocannabinol and cannabidiol *(Canada only) on page 832*

SB-265805 *see* gemifloxacin *on page 387*

S. boulardii *see Saccharomyces boulardii on page 771*

SC 33428 *see* idarubicin *on page 446*

SCH 13521 *see* flutamide *on page 367*

SCH 56592 *see* posaconazole *on page 698*

SCIG *see* immune globulin (subcutaneous) *on page 452*

S-citalopram *see* escitalopram *on page 311*

Scleromate® **[US]** *see* morrhuate sodium *on page 580*

Scopace™ **[US]** *see* scopolamine derivatives *on this page*

scopolamine and phenylephrine *see* phenylephrine and scopolamine *on page 677*

scopolamine base *see* scopolamine derivatives *on this page*

scopolamine butylbromide *see* scopolamine derivatives *on this page*

scopolamine derivatives (skoe POL a meen dah RIV ah tives)

Synonyms hyoscine butylbromide; hyoscine hydrobromide; scopolamine base; scopolamine butylbromide; scopolamine hydrobromide

U.S./Canadian Brand Names Buscopan® [Can]; Isopto® Hyoscine [US]; Maldemar™ [US]; Scopace™ [US]; Transderm Scōp® [US]; Transderm-V® [Can]

Therapeutic Category Anticholinergic Agent

Use

Scopolamine base:

Transdermal: Prevention of nausea/vomiting associated with motion sickness and recovery from anesthesia and surgery

Scopolamine hydrobromide:

Injection: Preoperative medication to produce amnesia, sedation, tranquilization, antiemetic effects, and decrease salivary and respiratory secretions

Ophthalmic: Produce cycloplegia and mydriasis; treatment of iridocyclitis

Oral: Symptomatic treatment of postencephalitic parkinsonism and paralysis agitans; in spastic states; inhibits excessive motility and hypertonus of the gastrointestinal tract in such conditions as the irritable colon syndrome, mild dysentery, diverticulitis, pylorospasm, and cardiospasm

Scopolamine butylbromide [not available in the U.S.]:

Oral/injection: Treatment of smooth muscle spasm of the genitourinary or gastrointestinal tract; injection may also be used to prior to radiological/diagnostic procedures to prevent spasm

Usual Dosage Note: Scopolamine (hyoscine) hydrobromide should not be interchanged with scopolamine butylbromide formulations. Dosages are not equivalent.

Scopolamine base: Transdermal patch: Adults:

Preoperative: Apply 1 patch to hairless area behind ear the night before surgery or 1 hour prior to cesarean section (apply no sooner than 1 hour before surgery to minimize newborn exposure); remove 24 hours after surgery

Motion sickness: Apply 1 patch behind the ear at least 4 hours prior to exposure and every 3 days as needed; effective if applied as soon as 2-3 hours before anticipated need, best if 12 hours before

Scopolamine hydrobromide:

Antiemetic: SubQ:

Children: 0.006 mg/kg

Adults: 0.6-1 mg

Preoperative: I.M., I.V., SubQ:

Children 6 months to 3 years: 0.1-0.15 mg

Children 3-6 years: 0.2-0.3 mg

Adults: 0.3-0.65 mg

Sedation, tranquilization: I.M., I.V., SubQ: Adults: 0.6 mg 3-4 times/day

Refraction: Ophthalmic:

Children: Instill 1 drop of 0.25% to eye(s) twice daily for 2 days before procedure

Adults: Instill 1-2 drops of 0.25% to eye(s) 1 hour before procedure

Iridocyclitis: Ophthalmic:

Children: Instill 1 drop of 0.25% to eye(s) up to 3 times/day

Adults: Instill 1-2 drops of 0.25% to eye(s) up to 4 times/day

Parkinsonism, spasticity, motion sickness: Adults: Oral: 0.4-0.8 mg. May repeat every 8-12 hours as needed; the dosage may be cautiously increased in parkinsonism and spastic states. For motion sickness, administration at least 1 hour before exposure is recommended.

Scopolamine butylbromide:
Gastrointestinal/genitourinary spasm (Buscopan® [CAN]; not available in the U.S.): Adults:
Oral: 10-20 mg daily (1-2 tablets); maximum: 6 tablets/day
I.M., I.V., SubQ: 10-20 mg; maximum: 100 mg/day. Intramuscular injections should be administered 10-15 minutes prior to radiological/diagnostic procedures
Dosage Forms [CAN] = Canadian brand name
Injection, solution: 0.4 mg/mL (1 mL)
Buscopan® [CAN]: 20 mg/mL [not available in the U.S.]
Solution, ophthalmic:
Isopto® Hyoscine: 0.25% (5 mL, 15 mL)
Tablet:
Buscopan® [CAN]: 10 mg [not available in the U.S.]
Tablet, soluble:
Maldemar™, Scopace™: 0.4 mg
Transdermal system:
Transderm Scōp®: 1.5 mg (4s, 10s, 24s)

scopolamine hydrobromide *see* scopolamine derivatives *on previous page*

scopolamine, hyoscyamine, atropine, and phenobarbital *see* hyoscyamine, atropine, scopolamine, and phenobarbital *on page 442*

Scot-Tussin DM® Cough Chasers [US-OTC] *see* dextromethorphan *on page 247*

Scot-Tussin® Expectorant [US-OTC] *see* guaifenesin *on page 401*

Scot-Tussin® Senior [US-OTC] *see* guaifenesin and dextromethorphan *on page 402*

SD/01 *see* pegfilgrastim *on page 657*

SDZ ENA 713 *see* rivastigmine *on page 763*

Seasonale® [US] *see* ethinyl estradiol and levonorgestrel *on page 325*

Seasonique™ [US] *see* ethinyl estradiol and levonorgestrel *on page 325*

Seba-Gel™ [US] *see* benzoyl peroxide *on page 103*

Sebcur® [Can] *see* salicylic acid *on page 772*

Sebcur/T® [Can] *see* coal tar and salicylic acid *on page 209*

Sebivo™ [Can] *see* telbivudine *on page 822*

Sebizon® *(Discontinued)* *see* sulfacetamide *on page 810*

secobarbital (see koe BAR bi tal)
Sound-Alike/Look-Alike Issues
Seconal® may be confused with Sectral®
Synonyms quinalbarbitone sodium; secobarbital sodium
U.S./Canadian Brand Names Seconal® [US]
Therapeutic Category Barbiturate
Controlled Substance C-II
Use Preanesthetic agent; short-term treatment of insomnia
Usual Dosage Oral:
Children:
Preoperative sedation: 2-6 mg/kg (maximum dose: 100 mg/dose) 1-2 hours before procedure
Sedation: 6 mg/kg/day divided every 8 hours
Adults:
Hypnotic: Usual: 100 mg/dose at bedtime; range 100-200 mg/dose
Preoperative sedation: 100-300 mg 1-2 hours before procedure
Dosage Forms
Capsule:
Seconal®: 100 mg

secobarbital sodium *see* secobarbital *on this page*

Seconal® [US] *see* secobarbital *on this page*

Secran® *(Discontinued)*

SecreFlo™ [US] *see* secretin *on next page*

secretin (SEE kr tin)

Synonyms secretin, human; secretin, porcine

U.S./Canadian Brand Names ChiRhoStim® [US]; SecreFlo™ [US]

Therapeutic Category Diagnostic Agent

Use Secretin-stimulation testing to aid in diagnosis of pancreatic exocrine dysfunction; diagnosis of gastrinoma (Zollinger-Ellison syndrome); facilitation of endoscopic retrograde cholangiopancreatography (ERCP) visualization

Usual Dosage I.V.: Adults: **Note:** A test dose of 0.1 mL (0.2-0.4 mcg) is injected to test for possible allergy. Dosing may be completed if no reaction occurs after 1 minute.
Diagnosis of pancreatic dysfunction, facilitation of ERCP: 0.2 mcg/kg over 1 minute
Diagnosis of gastrinoma: 0.4 mcg/kg over 1 minute

Dosage Forms

Injection, powder for reconstitution [human]:
ChiRhoStim®: 16 mcg, 40 mcg

Injection, powder for reconstitution [porcine]:
SecreFlo™: 16 mcg

secretin, human *see* secretin *on this page*

secretin, porcine *see* secretin *on this page*

Sectral® [US/Can] *see* acebutolol *on page 4*

Secura® Antifungal [US-OTC] *see* miconazole *on page 566*

Sedapap® [US] *see* butalbital and acetaminophen *on page 131*

Selax® [Can] *see* docusate *on page 273*

Select™ 1/35 [Can] *see* ethinyl estradiol and norethindrone *on page 328*

selegiline (se LE ji leen)

Sound-Alike/Look-Alike Issues

selegiline may be confused with Salagen®, Serentil®, sertraline, Serzone®, Stelazine®
Eldepryl® may be confused with Elavil®, enalapril
Zelapar™ may be confused with zaleplon, Zemplar®

Synonyms deprenyl; L-deprenyl; selegiline hydrochloride

U.S./Canadian Brand Names Apo-Selegiline® [Can]; Eldepryl® [US]; Emsam® [US]; Gen-Selegiline [Can]; Novo-Selegiline [Can]; Nu-Selegiline [Can]; Zelapar™ [US]

Therapeutic Category Anti-Parkinson Agent; Dopaminergic Agent (Anti-Parkinson)

Use Adjunct in the management of parkinsonian patients in which levodopa/carbidopa therapy is deteriorating (oral products); treatment of major depressive disorder (transdermal product)

Usual Dosage Adults:

Capsule/tablet: Parkinson disease: 5 mg twice daily with breakfast and lunch or 10 mg in the morning
Orally disintegrating tablet (Zelapar™): Parkinson disease: Initial 1.25 mg daily for at least 6 weeks; may increase to 2.5 mg daily based on clinical response (maximum: 2.5 mg daily)
Transdermal (Emsam®): Depression: Initial: 6 mg/24 hours once daily; may titrate based on clinical response in increments of 3 mg/day every 2 weeks up to a maximum of 12 mg/24 hours

Dosage Forms

Capsule: 5 mg
Eldepryl®: 5 mg

Tablet: 5 mg

Tablet, orally-disintegrating:
Zelapar™: 1.25 mg

Transdermal system [once-daily patch]:
Emsam®: 6 mg/24 hours (30s); 9 mg/24 hours (30s); 12 mg/24 hours (30s)

selegiline hydrochloride *see* selegiline *on this page*

selenium *see* trace metals *on page 855*

selenium sulfide (se LEE nee um SUL fide)

U.S./Canadian Brand Names Head & Shoulders® Intensive Treatment [US-OTC]; Selsun Blue® 2-in-1 Treatment [US-OTC]; Selsun Blue® Balanced Treatment [US-OTC]; Selsun Blue® Medicated Treatment [US-OTC]; Selsun Blue® Moisturizing Treatment [US-OTC]; Selsun® [US]; Versel® [Can]

Therapeutic Category Antiseborrheic Agent, Topical

Use Treatment of itching and flaking of the scalp associated with dandruff, to control scalp seborrheic dermatitis; treatment of tinea versicolor

Usual Dosage Topical:
Dandruff, seborrhea: Massage 5-10 mL into wet scalp, leave on scalp 2-3 minutes, rinse thoroughly
Tinea versicolor: Apply the 2.5% lotion to affected area and lather with small amounts of water; leave on skin for 10 minutes, then rinse thoroughly; apply every day for 7 days

Dosage Forms
Lotion, topical: 2.5% (120 mL)
Shampoo, topical: 1% (210 mL)
Head & Shoulders® Intensive Treatment [OTC]: 1% (400 mL)
Selsun®: 2.5% (120 mL)
Selsun Blue® Balanced Treatment [OTC], Selsun Blue® Medicated Treatment [OTC], Selsun Blue® Moisturizing Treatment [OTC], Selsun Blue® 2-in-1 Treatment [OTC]: 1% (120 mL, 210 mL, 330 mL)

Selepen® [US] see trace metals on page 855

Selpak® (Discontinued) see selegiline on previous page

Selsun® [US] see selenium sulfide on previous page

Selsun Blue® 2-in-1 Treatment [US-OTC] see selenium sulfide on previous page

Selsun Blue® Balanced Treatment [US-OTC] see selenium sulfide on previous page

Selsun Blue® Medicated Treatment [US-OTC] see selenium sulfide on previous page

Selsun Blue® Moisturizing Treatment [US-OTC] see selenium sulfide on previous page

Selsun Gold® for Women (Discontinued) see selenium sulfide on previous page

Selzentry™ [US] see maraviroc on page 531

Semprex®-D [US] see acrivastine and pseudoephedrine on page 16

Senexon [US-OTC] see senna on this page

Senilezol [US] see vitamin B complex combinations on page 894

senna (SEN na)
Sound-Alike/Look-Alike Issues
Perdiem® may be confused with Pyridium®
Senexon may be confused with Cenestin®
Senokot® may be confused with Depakote®
U.S./Canadian Brand Names Black-Draught Tablets [US-OTC]; Evac-U-Gen [US-OTC]; ex-lax® Maximum Strength [US-OTC]; ex-lax® [US-OTC]; Fletcher's® [US-OTC]; Little Tummys® Laxative [US-OTC]; Perdiem® Overnight Relief [US-OTC]; Senexon [US-OTC]; Senna-Gen® [US-OTC]; Sennatural™ [US-OTC]; SenokotXTRA® [US-OTC]; Senokot® [US-OTC]; Uni-Senna [US-OTC]
Therapeutic Category Laxative
Use Short-term treatment of constipation; evacuate the colon for bowel or rectal examinations
Usual Dosage Oral:
Bowel evacuation: OTC labeling: Children ≥12 years and Adults: Usual dose: Sennosides 130 mg (X-Prep® 75 mL) between 2-4 PM the afternoon of the day prior to procedure
Constipation: OTC ranges:
Children :
2-6 years:
Sennosides: Initial: 3.75 mg once daily (maximum: 15 mg/day, divided twice daily)
Senna concentrate: 33.3 mg/mL: 5-10 mL up to twice daily
6-12 years:
Sennosides: Initial: 8.6 mg once daily (maximum: 50 mg/day, divided twice daily)
Senna concentrate: 33.3 mg/mL: 10-30 mL up to twice daily
Children ≥12 years and Adults: Sennosides 15 mg once daily (maximum: 70-100 mg/day, divided twice daily)
Dosage Forms
Liquid:
Senexon [OTC]: Sennosides 8.8 mg/5 mL
Liquid [concentrate]:
Fletcher's® [OTC]: Senna concentrate 33.3 mg/mL
Liquid [concentrate; drops]:
Little Tummys® Laxative [OTC]: Sennosides 8.8 mg/1 mL
Syrup: Sennosides 8.8 mg/5 mL
Tablet: Sennosides 8.6 mg
ex-lax® [OTC], Perdiem® Overnight Relief [OTC]: Sennosides USP 15 mg
ex-lax® Maximum Strength [OTC]: Sennosides USP 25 mg
Sennatural™ [OTC], Senokot® [OTC], Senexon® [OTC], Senna-Gen® [OTC], Uni-Senna [OTC]: Sennosides 8.6 mg
SenokotXTRA® [OTC]: Sennosides 17 mg
(Continued)

senna *(Continued)*

Tablet, chewable:
Black-Draught™ [OTC]: Sennosides 10 mg
ex-lax® [OTC]: Sennosides USP 15 mg
Evac-U-Gen [OTC]: Sennosides 10 mg

senna and docusate *see* docusate and senna *on page 274*

Senna-Gen® [US-OTC] *see* senna *on previous page*

senna-S *see* docusate and senna *on page 274*

Sennatural™ [US-OTC] *see* senna *on previous page*

Senokot® [US-OTC] *see* senna *on previous page*

Senokot-S® [US-OTC] *see* docusate and senna *on page 274*

SenokotXTRA® [US-OTC] *see* senna *on previous page*

SenoSol™-SS [US-OTC] *see* docusate and senna *on page 274*

Sensipar™ [US] *see* cinacalcet *on page 190*

Sensorcaine® [US/Can] *see* bupivacaine *on page 125*

Sensorcaine®-MPF [US] *see* bupivacaine *on page 125*

Sensorcaine®-MPF Spinal [US] *see* bupivacaine *on page 125*

Sensorcaine®-MPF with Epinephrine [US] *see* bupivacaine and epinephrine *on page 126*

Sensorcaine® with Epinephrine [US/Can] *see* bupivacaine and epinephrine *on page 126*

Septanest® N [Can] *see* articaine and epinephrine *on page 75*

Septanest® SP [Can] *see* articaine and epinephrine *on page 75*

Septa® Topical Ointment *(Discontinued)* *see* bacitracin, neomycin, and polymyxin B *on page 91*

Septisol® *(Discontinued)* *see* hexachlorophene *on page 420*

Septocaine® with epinephrine 1:100,000 [US] *see* articaine and epinephrine *on page 75*

Septocaine® with epinephrine 1:200,000 [US] *see* articaine and epinephrine *on page 75*

Septra® [US] *see* sulfamethoxazole and trimethoprim *on page 813*

Septra® DS [US] *see* sulfamethoxazole and trimethoprim *on page 813*

Septra® Injection [Can] *see* sulfamethoxazole and trimethoprim *on page 813*

Serax® [US] *see* oxazepam *on page 637*

Serc® [Can] *see* betahistine *(Canada only) on page 107*

Serevent® [Can] *see* salmeterol *on page 774*

Serevent® *(Discontinued)* *see* salmeterol *on page 774*

Serevent® Diskus® [US] *see* salmeterol *on page 774*

sermorelin acetate (ser moe REL in AS e tate)

U.S./Canadian Brand Names Geref® Diagnostic [US]

Therapeutic Category Diagnostic Agent

Use Geref® Diagnostic: For evaluation of the ability of the pituitary gland to secrete growth hormone (GH)

Usual Dosage I.V.: Children and Adults: Diagnostic: 1 mcg/kg as a single dose in the morning following an overnight fast

Note: Response to diagnostic test may be decreased in patients >40 years

Dosage Forms

Injection, powder for reconstitution:
Geref® Diagnostic: 50 mcg

Seromycin® [US] *see* cycloserine *on page 222*

Serophene® [US/Can] *see* clomiphene *on page 203*

Seroquel® [US/Can] *see* quetiapine *on page 738*

Seroquel® XR [US] *see* quetiapine *on page 738*

Serostim® [US/Can] *see* somatropin *on page 799*

Serpalan® *(Discontinued)* *see* reserpine *on page 751*

Serpatabs® *(Discontinued)* *see* reserpine *on page 751*

sertaconazole (ser ta KOE na zole)
Synonyms sertaconazole nitrate
U.S./Canadian Brand Names Ertaczo™ [US]
Therapeutic Category Antifungal Agent, Topical
Use Topical treatment of tinea pedis (athlete's foot)
Usual Dosage Topical: Children ≥12 years and Adults: Apply between toes and to surrounding healthy skin twice daily for 4 weeks
Dosage Forms
  Cream, topical:
    Ertaczo®: 2% (30 g, 60 g)

sertaconazole nitrate *see sertaconazole on this page*

sertraline (SER tra leen)
Sound-Alike/Look-Alike Issues
  sertraline may be confused with selegiline, Serentil®
  Zoloft® may be confused with Zocor®
Synonyms sertraline hydrochloride
U.S./Canadian Brand Names Apo-Sertraline® [Can]; Gen-Sertraline [Can]; GMD-Sertraline [Can]; Novo-Sertraline [Can]; Nu-Sertraline [Can]; PMS-Sertraline [Can]; ratio-Sertraline [Can]; Rhoxal-Sertraline [Can]; Sandoz-Sertraline [Can]; Zoloft® [US/Can]
Therapeutic Category Antidepressant, Selective Serotonin Reuptake Inhibitor
Use Treatment of major depression; obsessive-compulsive disorder (OCD); panic disorder; posttraumatic stress disorder (PTSD); premenstrual dysphoric disorder (PMDD); social anxiety disorder
Usual Dosage Oral:
  Children and Adolescents: OCD:
    6-12 years: Initial: 25 mg once daily
    13-17 years: Initial: 50 mg once daily
    Note: May increase daily dose, at intervals of not less than 1 week, to a maximum of 200 mg/day. If somnolence is noted, give at bedtime.
  Adults:
    Depression/OCD: Oral: Initial: 50 mg/day (see "Note" above)
    Panic disorder, PTSD, social anxiety disorder: Initial: 25 mg once daily; increase to 50 mg once daily after 1 week (see "Note" above)
    PMDD: 50 mg/day either daily throughout menstrual cycle **or** limited to the luteal phase of menstrual cycle, depending on physician assessment. Patients not responding to 50 mg/day may benefit from dose increases (50 mg increments per menstrual cycle) up to 150 mg/day when dosing throughout menstrual cycle **or** up to 100 mg day when dosing during luteal phase only. If a 100 mg/day dose has been established with luteal phase dosing, a 50 mg/day titration step for 3 days should be utilized at the beginning of each luteal phase dosing period.
Dosage Forms
  Solution, oral [concentrate]: 20 mg/mL (60 mL)
    Zoloft®: 20 mg/mL
  Tablet: 25 mg, 50 mg, 100 mg
    Zoloft®: 25 mg, 50 mg, 100 mg

sertraline hydrochloride *see sertraline on this page*

Serutan® [US-OTC] *see psyllium on page 732*

Serzone® (Discontinued) *see nefazodone on page 595*

sevelamer (se VEL a mer)
Sound-Alike/Look-Alike Issues
  Renagel® may be confused with Reglan®, Regonol®
Synonyms sevelamer hydrochloride
U.S./Canadian Brand Names Renagel® [US/Can]
Therapeutic Category Phosphate Binder
Use Reduction of serum phosphorous in patients with chronic kidney disease on hemodialysis
Usual Dosage
  Adults: Oral: Patients not taking a phosphate binder: 800-1600 mg 3 times/day with meals; the initial dose may be based on serum phosphorous levels:
    >5.5 mg/dL to <7.5 mg/dL: 800 mg 3 times/day
    ≥7.5 mg/dL to <9.0 mg/dL: 1200-1600 mg 3 times/day
    ≥9.0 mg/dL: 1600 mg 3 times/day
  (Continued)

sevelamer *(Continued)*

Maintenance dose adjustment based on serum phosphorous concentration (goal of lowering to <5.5 mg/dL; maximum daily dose studied was equivalent to 13 g/day):
>5.5 mg/dL: Increase by 1 tablet per meal every 2 weeks
3.5-5.5 mg/dL: Maintain current dose
<3.5 mg/dL: Decrease by 1 tablet per meal
Dosage adjustment when switching between phosphate binder products: 667 mg of calcium acetate is equivalent to 800 mg sevelamer

Dosage Forms
Tablet:
Renagel®: 400 mg, 800 mg

sevelamer hydrochloride *see* sevelamer *on previous page*

sevoflurane (see voe FLOO rane)

Sound-Alike/Look-Alike Issues
Ultane® may be confused with Ultram®
U.S./Canadian Brand Names Sevorane™ [Can]; Ultane® [US]
Therapeutic Category General Anesthetic
Use Induction and maintenance of general anesthesia
Usual Dosage Minimum alveolar concentration (MAC), the concentration that abolishes movement in response to a noxious stimulus (surgical incision) in 50% of patients, is 2.6% (25 years of age) for sevoflurane. Surgical levels of anesthesia are generally achieved with concentrations from 0.5% to 3%; the concentration at which amnesia and loss of awareness occur is 0.6%.
Minimum alveolar concentrations (MAC) values for surgical levels of anesthesia:
0 to 1 month old full-term neonates: Sevoflurane in oxygen: 3.3%
1 to <6 months: Sevoflurane in oxygen: 3%
6 months to <3 years:
 Sevoflurane in oxygen: 2.8%
 Sevoflurane in 60% N_2O/40% oxygen: 2%
3-12 years: Sevoflurane in oxygen: 2.5%
25 years:
 Sevoflurane in oxygen: 2.6%
 Sevoflurane in 65% N_2O/35% oxygen: 1.4%
40 years:
 Sevoflurane in oxygen: 2.1%
 Sevoflurane in 65% N_2O/35% oxygen: 1.1%
60 years:
 Sevoflurane in oxygen: 1.7%
 Sevoflurane in 65% N_2O/35% oxygen: 0.9%
80 years:
 Sevoflurane in oxygen: 1.4%
 Sevoflurane in 65% N_2O/35% oxygen: 0.7%

Dosage Forms
Liquid for inhalation: 100% (250 mL)
Sojourn™, Ultane®: 100% (250 mL)

Sevorane™ [Can] *see* sevoflurane *on this page*

shingles vaccine *see* zoster vaccine *on page 909*

Shur-Seal® *(Discontinued)* *see* nonoxynol 9 *on page 610*

Sibelium® [Can] *see* flunarizine *(Canada only) on page 359*

sibutramine (si BYOO tra meen)

Sound-Alike/Look-Alike Issues
Meridia® may be confused with Aredia®
Synonyms sibutramine hydrochloride monohydrate
U.S./Canadian Brand Names Meridia® [US/Can]
Therapeutic Category Anorexiant
Controlled Substance C-IV
Use Management of obesity
Usual Dosage Children ≥16 years and Adults:
Initial: 10 mg once daily; after 4 weeks may titrate up to 15 mg once daily as needed and tolerated (may be used for up to 2 years, per manufacturer labeling)
Maintenance: 5-15 mg once daily

Dosage Forms
  Capsule:
  Meridia®: 5 mg, 10 mg, 15 mg

sibutramine hydrochloride monohydrate *see* sibutramine *on previous page*

Silace [US-OTC] *see* docusate *on page 273*

Siladryl® **Allergy [US-OTC]** *see* diphenhydramine *on page 265*

Silafed® **[US-OTC]** *see* triprolidine and pseudoephedrine *on page 869*

Silain® *(Discontinued) see* simethicone *on next page*

Silaminic® **Expectorant** *(Discontinued)*

Silapap® **Children's [US-OTC]** *see* acetaminophen *on page 5*

Silapap® **Infants [US-OTC]** *see* acetaminophen *on page 5*

Sildec *(Discontinued) see* carbinoxamine and pseudoephedrine *on page 151*

Sildec-DM *(Discontinued) see* carbinoxamine, pseudoephedrine, and dextromethorphan *on page 152*

Sildec PE [US] *see* chlorpheniramine and phenylephrine *on page 177*

Sildec PE-DM [US] *see* chlorpheniramine, phenylephrine, and dextromethorphan *on page 180*

Sildec Syrup [US] *see* brompheniramine and pseudoephedrine *on page 120*

sildenafil (sil DEN a fil)
  Sound-Alike/Look-Alike Issues
    Viagra® may be confused with Allegra®, Vaniqa™
  Synonyms UK92480
  U.S./Canadian Brand Names GD-Sildenafil [US]; Revatio™ [US]; Viagra® [US/Can]
  Therapeutic Category Phosphodiesterase (Type 5) Enzyme Inhibitor
  Use Treatment of erectile dysfunction; treatment of pulmonary arterial hypertension
  Usual Dosage Oral: Adults:
    Erectile dysfunction (Viagra®): For most patients, the recommended dose is 25-50 mg taken as needed, approximately 1 hour before sexual activity. However, sildenafil may be taken anywhere from 30 minutes to 4 hours before sexual activity. Based on effectiveness and tolerance, the dose may be increased to a maximum recommended dose of 100 mg or decreased to 25 mg. The maximum recommended dosing frequency is once daily.
    Pulmonary arterial hypertension (Revatio™): 20 mg 3 times/day, taken 4-6 hours apart
  Dosage Forms
    Tablet:
    Revatio™: 20 mg
    Viagra®: 25 mg, 50 mg, 100 mg

Sildicon-E® *(Discontinued)*

Silexin® **[US-OTC]** *see* guaifenesin and dextromethorphan *on page 402*

Silfedrine Children's [US-OTC] *see* pseudoephedrine *on page 727*

Silphen® **[US-OTC]** *see* diphenhydramine *on page 265*

Silphen DM® **[US-OTC]** *see* dextromethorphan *on page 247*

Sil-Tex [US] *see* guaifenesin and phenylephrine *on page 404*

Siltussin-CF® *(Discontinued)*

Siltussin DAS [US-OTC] *see* guaifenesin *on page 401*

Siltussin DM [US-OTC] *see* guaifenesin and dextromethorphan *on page 402*

Siltussin DM DAS [US-OTC] *see* guaifenesin and dextromethorphan *on page 402*

Siltussin SA [US-OTC] *see* guaifenesin *on page 401*

Silvadene® **[US]** *see* silver sulfadiazine *on next page*

silver nitrate (SIL ver NYE trate)
  Synonyms AgNO$_3$
  Therapeutic Category Topical Skin Product
  Use Cauterization of wounds and sluggish ulcers, removal of granulation tissue and warts; aseptic prophylaxis of burns
  (Continued)

silver nitrate *(Continued)*

Usual Dosage Children and Adults:

Sticks: Apply to mucous membranes and other moist skin surfaces only on area to be treated 2-3 times/week for 2-3 weeks

Topical solution: Apply a cotton applicator dipped in solution on the affected area 2-3 times/week for 2-3 weeks

Dosage Forms

Applicator sticks, topical: Silver nitrate 75% and potassium 25% (6", 12", 18")

Solution, topical: 10% (30 mL); 25% (30 mL); 50% (30 mL)

silver sulfadiazine (SIL ver sul fa DYE a zeen)

U.S./Canadian Brand Names Flamazine® [Can]; Silvadene® [US]; SSD® AF [US]; SSD® [US]; Thermazene® [US]

Therapeutic Category Antibacterial, Topical

Use Prevention and treatment of infection in second and third degree burns

Usual Dosage Topical: Children and Adults: Apply once or twice daily with a sterile-gloved hand; apply to a thickness of $1/_{16}$"; burned area should be covered with cream at all times

Dosage Forms

Cream, topical: 1% (25 g, 50 g, 85 g, 400 g)

Silvadene®, Thermazene®: 1% (20 g, 50 g, 85 g, 400 g, 1000 g)

SSD®: 1% (25 g, 50 g, 85 g, 400 g)

SSD® AF: 1% (50 g, 400 g)

simethicone (sye METH i kone)

Sound-Alike/Look-Alike Issues

simethicone may be confused with cimetidine

Mylanta® may be confused with Mynatal®

Mylicon® may be confused with Modicon®, Myleran®

Phazyme® may be confused with Pherazine®

Synonyms activated dimethicone; activated methylpolysiloxane

U.S./Canadian Brand Names Equalizer Gas Relief [US-OTC]; Gas-X® Extra Strength [US-OTC]; Gas-X® Maximum Strength [US-OTC]; Gas-X® [US-OTC]; GasAid [US-OTC]; Genasyme® [US-OTC]; Infantaire Gas Drops [US-OTC]; Little Tummys® Gas Relief [US-OTC]; Mylanta® Gas Maximum Strength [US-OTC]; Mylanta® Gas [US-OTC]; Mylicon® Infants [US-OTC]; Ovol® [Can]; Phazyme® Quick Dissolve [US-OTC]; Phazyme® Ultra Strength [US-OTC]; Phazyme® [Can]

Therapeutic Category Antiflatulent

Use Relieves flatulence and functional gastric bloating, and postoperative gas pains

Usual Dosage Oral:

Infants: 20 mg 4 times/day

Children <12 years: 40 mg 4 times/day

Children >12 years and Adults: 40-120 mg after meals and at bedtime as needed, not to exceed 500 mg/day

Dosage Forms

Softgels: 125 mg

GasAid [OTC], Gas-X® Extra Strength [OTC], Mylanta® Gas Maximum Strength [OTC]: 125 mg

Gas-X® Maximum Strength [OTC]: 166 mg

Phazyme® Ultra Strength [OTC]: 180 mg

Suspension, oral [drops]: 40 mg/0.6 mL

Equalizer Gas Relief [OTC], Genasyme® [OTC], Infantaire Gas [OTC], Little Tummys® Gas Relief [OTC], Mylicon® Infants [OTC]: 40 mg/0.6 mL

Tablet, chewable: 80 mg, 125 mg

Gas-X® [OTC], Genasyme® [OTC], Mylanta® Gas [OTC]: 80 mg

Mylanta® Gas Maximum Strength [OTC], Phazyme® Quick Dissolve [OTC], Gas-X® Extra Strength [OTC]: 125 mg

simethicone, aluminum hydroxide, and magnesium hydroxide *see* aluminum hydroxide, magnesium hydroxide, and simethicone *on page 37*

simethicone and calcium carbonate *see* calcium carbonate and simethicone *on page 139*

simethicone and loperamide hydrochloride *see* loperamide and simethicone *on page 516*

simethicone and magaldrate *see* magaldrate and simethicone *on page 524*

Simply Cough® *(Discontinued)* *see* dextromethorphan *on page 247*

Simply Saline® [US-OTC] *see* sodium chloride *on page 792*

Simply Saline® Baby [US-OTC] *see* sodium chloride *on page 792*

Simply Saline® **Nasal Moist**® **[US-OTC]** *see* sodium chloride *on page 792*

Simply Sleep® **[US-OTC/Can]** *see* diphenhydramine *on page 265*

Simply Stuffy™ *(Discontinued) see* pseudoephedrine *on page 727*

Simuc [US] *see* guaifenesin and phenylephrine *on page 404*

Simuc-DM [US] *see* guaifenesin and dextromethorphan *on page 402*

Simulect® **[US/Can]** *see* basiliximab *on page 95*

simvastatin (sim va STAT in)

Sound-Alike/Look-Alike Issues
Zocor® may be confused with Cozaar®, Yocon®, Zoloft®

U.S./Canadian Brand Names Apo-Simvastatin® [Can]; BCI-Simvastatin [Can]; CO Simvastatin [Can]; Gen-Simvastatin [Can]; Novo-Simvastatin [Can]; PMS-Simvastatin [Can]; ratio-Simvastatin [Can]; Riva-Simvastatin [Can]; Sandoz-Simvastatin [Can]; Taro-Simvastatin [Can]; Zocor® [US/Can]

Therapeutic Category HMG-CoA Reductase Inhibitor

Use Used with dietary therapy for the following:
Secondary prevention of cardiovascular events in hypercholesterolemic patients with established coronary heart disease (CHD) or at high risk for CHD: To reduce cardiovascular morbidity (myocardial infarction, coronary revascularization procedures) and mortality; to reduce the risk of stroke and transient ischemic attacks

Hyperlipidemias: To reduce elevations in total cholesterol, LDL-C, apolipoprotein B, and triglycerides in patients with primary hypercholesterolemia (elevations of 1 or more components are present in Fredrickson type IIa, IIb, III, and IV hyperlipidemias); treatment of homozygous familial hypercholesterolemia

Heterozygous familial hypercholesterolemia (HeFH): In adolescent patients (10-17 years of age, females >1 year postmenarche) with HeFH having LDL-C ≥190 mg/dL **or** LDL ≥160 mg/dL with positive family history of premature cardiovascular disease (CVD), or 2 or more CVD risk factors in the adolescent patient

Usual Dosage Oral: **Note:** Doses should be individualized according to the baseline LDL-cholesterol levels, the recommended goal of therapy, and the patient's response; adjustments should be made at intervals of 4 weeks or more; doses may need adjusted based on concomitant medications
Children 10-17 years (females >1 year postmenarche): HeFH: 10 mg once daily in the evening; range: 10-40 mg/day (maximum: 40 mg/day)

Dosage adjustment for simvastatin with concomitant cyclosporine, danazol, fibrates, niacin, amiodarone, or verapamil: Refer to drug-specific dosing in adult dosing section
Adults:
Homozygous familial hypercholesterolemia: 40 mg once daily in the evening **or** 80 mg/day (given as 20 mg, 20 mg, and 40 mg evening dose)

Prevention of cardiovascular events, hyperlipidemias: 20-40 mg once daily in the evening; range: 5-80 mg/day
Patients requiring only moderate reduction of LDL-cholesterol may be started at 10 mg once daily
Patients requiring reduction of >45% in low-density lipoprotein (LDL) cholesterol may be started at 40 mg once daily in the evening
Patients with CHD or at high risk for CHD: Dosing should be started at 40 mg once daily in the evening; simvastatin may be started simultaneously with diet

Dosage adjustment with concomitant medications:
Cyclosporine or danazol (patient must first demonstrate tolerance to simvastatin ≥5 mg once daily): Initial: 5 mg simvastatin, should **not** exceed 10 mg/day
Fibrates or niacin: Simvastatin dose should **not** exceed 10 mg/day
Amiodarone or verapamil: Simvastatin dose should **not** exceed 20 mg/day

Dosage Forms
Tablet: 5 mg, 10 mg, 20 mg, 40 mg, 80 mg
Zocor®: 5 mg, 10 mg, 20 mg, 40 mg, 80 mg

Sina-12X [US] *see* guaifenesin and phenylephrine *on page 404*

sincalide (SIN ka lide)

Synonyms C8-CCK; OP-CCK

U.S./Canadian Brand Names Kinevac® [US]

Therapeutic Category Diagnostic Agent

Use Postevacuation cholecystography; gallbladder bile sampling; stimulate pancreatic secretion for analysis; accelerate the transit of barium through the small bowel

Usual Dosage Adults:
Contraction of gallbladder:
I.V.: 0.02 mcg/kg over 30-60 seconds; may repeat in 15 minutes with a 0.04 mcg/kg dose
Infusion: 0.12 mcg/kg in 100 mL of NS; administer over 50 minutes
(Continued)

sincalide *(Continued)*

I.M.: 0.1 mcg/kg
Pancreatic function: I.V.: 0.02 mcg/kg over 30 minutes
Accelerate barium transit through small bowel:
I.V.: 0.04 mcg/kg over 30-60 seconds; if movement of barium has not occurred in 30 minutes, may repeat dose
Infusion: 0.12 mcg/kg in 30 mL of NS; administer over 30 minutes

Dosage Forms
Injection, powder for reconstitution:
Kinevac®: 5 mcg

Sine-Aid® IB *(Discontinued)* *see* pseudoephedrine and ibuprofen *on page 729*

sinecatechins *(sin e KAT e kins)*

Synonyms catechins; green tea extract; kunecatechins; polyphenols; polyphenon E
U.S./Canadian Brand Names Veregen™ [US]
Therapeutic Category Immunomodulator, Topical; Topical Skin Product
Use Treatment of external genital and perianal warts secondary to *Condylomata acuminata*
Usual Dosage Topical: Adults: Apply a thin layer (~0.5 cm strand) 3 times/day to all external genital and perianal warts until all warts have been cleared (maximum duration: 16 weeks)
Dosage Forms
Ointment, topical:
Veregen ™: 15% (15 g)

Sinemet® [US/Can] *see* levodopa and carbidopa *on page 500*

Sinemet® CR [US/Can] *see* levodopa and carbidopa *on page 500*

Sinequan® [Can] *see* doxepin *on page 279*

Sinequan® *(Discontinued)* *see* doxepin *on page 279*

Singulair® [US/Can] *see* montelukast *on page 578*

Sinografin® [US] *see* diatrizoate meglumine and iodipamide meglumine *on page 250*

Sinubid® *(Discontinued)*

Sinufed® Timecelles® *(Discontinued)* *see* guaifenesin and pseudoephedrine *on page 406*

Sinumed® *(Discontinued)* *see* acetaminophen, chlorpheniramine, and pseudoephedrine *on page 10*

Sinumist®-SR Capsulets® *(Discontinued)* *see* guaifenesin *on page 401*

Sinus-Relief *(Discontinued)* *see* acetaminophen and pseudoephedrine *on page 8*

Sinutab® Non Drowsy [Can] *see* acetaminophen and pseudoephedrine *on page 8*

Sinutab® Non-Drying [US-OTC] *see* guaifenesin and pseudoephedrine *on page 406*

Sinutab® Sinus & Allergy [Can] *see* acetaminophen, chlorpheniramine, and pseudoephedrine *on page 10*

Sinutab® Sinus Allergy Maximum Strength [US-OTC] *see* acetaminophen, chlorpheniramine, and pseudoephedrine *on page 10*

SINUtuss® DM [US] *see* guaifenesin, dextromethorphan, and phenylephrine *on page 407*

SINUvent® PE [US] *see* guaifenesin and phenylephrine *on page 404*

Sirdalud® *(Discontinued)* *see* tizanidine *on page 846*

sirolimus *(sir OH li mus)*

Sound-Alike/Look-Alike Issues
sirolimus may be confused with tacrolimus, temsirolimus
U.S./Canadian Brand Names Rapamune® [US/Can]
Therapeutic Category Immunosuppressant Agent
Use Prophylaxis of organ rejection in patients receiving renal transplants, in combination with corticosteroids and cyclosporine (cyclosporine may be withdrawn in low-to-moderate immunological risk patients after 2-4 months, in conjunction with an increase in sirolimus dosage)
Usual Dosage Oral:
Combination therapy with cyclosporine: Doses should be taken 4 hours after cyclosporine, and should be taken consistently either with or without food.

Low- to moderate-risk renal transplant patients: Children ≥13 years and Adults: Dosing by body weight:
<40 kg: Loading dose: 3 mg/m^2 on day 1, followed by maintenance dosing of 1 mg/m^2 once daily

≥40 kg: Loading dose: 6 mg on day 1; maintenance: 2 mg once daily

High-risk renal transplant patients: Adults: Loading dose: Up to 15 mg on day 1; maintenance: 5 mg/day; obtain trough concentration between days 5-7. Continue concurrent cyclosporine/sirolimus therapy for 1 year following transplantation. Further adjustment of the regimen must be based on clinical status.

Dosage adjustment: Sirolimus dosages should be adjusted to maintain trough concentrations within desired range based on risk and concomitant therapy. Maximum daily dose: 40 mg. Dosage should be adjusted at intervals of 7-14 days to account for the long half-life of sirolimus. In general, dose proportionality may be assumed. New sirolimus dose **equals** current dose **multiplied by** (target concentration/current concentration). **Note:** If large dose increase is required, consider loading dose calculated as:

Loading dose **equals** (new maintenance dose **minus** current maintenance dose) **multiplied by** 3

Doses >40 mg (with inclusion of loading dose) may be administered over 2 days. Serum concentrations should not be used as the sole basis for dosage adjustment (monitor clinical signs/symptoms, tissue biopsy, and laboratory parameters).

Maintenance therapy after withdrawal of cyclosporine: Cyclosporine withdrawal is not recommended in high immunological risk patients. Following 2-4 months of combined therapy, withdrawal of cyclosporine may be considered in low-to-moderate risk patients. Cyclosporine should be discontinued over 4-8 weeks, and a necessary increase in the dosage of sirolimus (up to fourfold) should be anticipated due to removal of metabolic inhibition by cyclosporine and to maintain adequate immunosuppressive effects. Dose-adjusted trough target concentrations are typically 16-24 ng/mL for the first year post-transplant and 12-20 ng/mL thereafter (measured by chromatographic methodology).

Dosage Forms
Solution, oral:
Rapamune®: 1 mg/mL
Tablet:
Rapamune®: 1 mg, 2 mg

sitagliptin (sit a GLIP tin)

Sound-Alike/Look-Alike Issues
Januvia™ may be confused with Jantoven™

Synonyms MK-0431; sitagliptin phosphate

U.S./Canadian Brand Names Januvia™ [US]

Therapeutic Category Antidiabetic Agent, Dipeptidyl Peptidase IV (DPP-IV) Inhibitor

Use Management of type 2 diabetes mellitus (noninsulin dependent, NIDDM) as an adjunct to diet and exercise as monotherapy or in combination therapy with metformin or a peroxisome proliferator-actived receptor (PPAR) gamma agonist (eg, a thiazolidinedione)

Usual Dosage Oral: Adults: Type 2 diabetes: 100 mg once daily

Dosage Forms
Tablet:
Januvia™: 25 mg, 50 mg, 100 mg

sitagliptin and metformin (sit a GLIP tin & met FOR min)

Synonyms metformin and sitagliptin; sitagliptin phosphate and metformin hydrochloride

U.S./Canadian Brand Names Janumet™ [US]

Therapeutic Category Antidiabetic Agent, Biguanide; Antidiabetic Agent, Dipeptidyl Peptidase IV (DPP-IV) Inhibitor; Hypoglycemic Agent, Oral

Use Management of type 2 diabetes mellitus (noninsulin-dependent, NIDDM) as an adjunct to diet and exercise

Usual Dosage Oral: Type 2 diabetes mellitus:
Adults: Initial doses should be based on current dose of sitagliptin and metformin; daily doses should be divided and given twice daily with meals. Maximum: Sitagliptin 100 mg/metformin 2000 mg daily

Patients inadequately controlled on metformin alone: Initial dose: Sitagliptin 100 mg/day plus current dose of metformin. **Note:** Per manufacturer labeling, patients currently receiving metformin 850 mg twice daily should receive an initial dose of sitagliptin 50 mg and metformin 1000 mg twice daily

Patients inadequately controlled on sitagliptin alone: Initial dose: Metformin 1000 mg/day plus sitagliptin 100 mg/day. **Note:** Patients currently receiving a renally adjusted dose of sitagliptin should not be switched to combination product.

Dosing adjustment: Metformin component may be gradually increased up to the maximum dose. Maximum dose: Sitagliptin 100 mg/metformin 2000 mg daily

Dosage Forms
Tablet:
Janumet™:
50/500: Sitagliptin 50 mg and metformin 500 mg
50/1000: Sitagliptin 50 mg and metformin 1000 mg

sitagliptin phosphate *see* sitagliptin *on this page*

sitagliptin phosphate and metformin hydrochloride *see* sitagliptin and metformin *on previous page*

sitaxsentan *(Canada only)* (sye TACKS en tan)
Sound-Alike/Look-Alike Issues
Thelin™ may be confused with Theolair™
Synonyms sitaxsentan sodium
U.S./Canadian Brand Names Thelin™ [Can]
Therapeutic Category Endothelin Antagonist
Use Treatment of primary pulmonary arterial hypertension (PAH) or pulmonary hypertension secondary to connective tissue disease, in World Health Organization (WHO) class III patients unresponsive to conventional therapy; treatment of PAH in WHO class II patients who are unresponsive to conventional therapy and have no alternative treatment options
Usual Dosage Oral: Adults: 100 mg once daily. (**Note:** Doses above 100 mg/day are not recommended; higher doses have not been shown to provide additional benefit and may increase risk of hepatic toxicity).
Dosage Forms CAN = Canadian brand name
Tablet:
Thelin™ [CAN]: 100 mg [not available in U.S.]

sitaxsentan sodium *see* sitaxsentan *(Canada only) on this page*

SK *see* streptokinase *on page 806*

SK and F 104864 *see* topotecan *on page 851*

Skeeter Stik [US-OTC] *see* benzocaine *on page 101*

Skelaxin® [US/Can] *see* metaxalone *on page 548*

Skelid® [US] *see* tiludronate *on page 843*

SKF 104864 *see* topotecan *on page 851*

SKF 104864-A *see* topotecan *on page 851*

Skin Care™ [US-OTC] *see* pyrithione zinc *on page 737*

Sleep-ettes D [US-OTC] *see* diphenhydramine *on page 265*

Sleep-eze 3® Oral *(Discontinued)* *see* diphenhydramine *on page 265*

Sleepinal® [US-OTC] *see* diphenhydramine *on page 265*

Sleepwell 2-nite® *(Discontinued)* *see* diphenhydramine *on page 265*

Slim-Mint® *(Discontinued)* *see* benzocaine *on page 101*

Slo-bid™ *(Discontinued)* *see* theophylline *on page 834*

Slo-Niacin® [US-OTC] *see* niacin *on page 601*

Slo-Phyllin® (all products) *(Discontinued)* *see* theophylline *on page 834*

Slo-Phyllin® GG *(Discontinued)* *see* theophylline and guaifenesin *on page 835*

Slo-Pot [Can] *see* potassium chloride *on page 700*

Slow FE® [US-OTC] *see* ferrous sulfate *on page 350*

Slow-K® [Can] *see* potassium chloride *on page 700*

Slow-K® *(Discontinued)* *see* potassium chloride *on page 700*

Slow-Mag® [US-OTC] *see* magnesium chloride *on page 524*

Slow-Trasicor® [Can] *see* oxprenolol *(Canada only) on page 639*

smallpox vaccine (SMAL poks vak SEEN)
Synonyms dried smallpox vaccine; vaccinia vaccine
U.S./Canadian Brand Names Dryvax® [US]
Therapeutic Category Vaccine
Use Active immunization against vaccinia virus, the causative agent of smallpox in persons determined to be at risk for smallpox infection. The ACIP recommends vaccination of laboratory workers at risk of exposure from cultures or contaminated animals which may be a source of vaccinia or related Orthopoxviruses capable of causing infections in humans (monkeypox, cowpox, or variola). The ACIP also recommends that consideration be given for vaccination in healthcare workers having contact with clinical specimens, contaminated material, or patients receiving vaccinia or recombinant vaccinia viruses. ACIP recommends revaccination every 10 years. The Armed Forces recommend vaccination of certain personnel categories. Recommendations for use in response to bioterrorism are regularly updated by the CDC, and may be found at www.cdc.gov.

Usual Dosage Not for I.M., I.V., or SubQ injection: Vaccination by scarification (multiple-puncture technique) only: **Note:** A trace of blood should appear at vaccination site after 15-20 seconds; if no trace of blood is visible, an additional 3 insertions should be made using the same needle, without reinserting the needle into the vaccine bottle.

Adults (children ≥12 months in emergency conditions only):

Primary vaccination: Use a single drop of vaccine suspension and 2 or 3 needle punctures (using the same needle) into the superficial skin

Revaccination: Use a single drop of vaccine suspension and 15 needle punctures (using the same needle) into the superficial skin

Dosage Forms

Injection, powder for reconstitution [calf liver source]:

Dryvax®: ~1 x 10^8 vaccinia virions per mL

Injection, powder for reconstitution [purified monkey cell source]:

ACAM2000™: 1-5 x 10^8 plaque-forming units per mL

smelling salts *see* ammonia spirit (aromatic) *on page 47*

SMZ-TMP *see* sulfamethoxazole and trimethoprim *on page 813*

snake (pit vipers) antivenin *see* antivenin *(Crotalidae)* polyvalent *on page 63*

Snaplets-EX® *(Discontinued)*

(+)-(*S*)-*N*-methyl-γ-(1-naphthyloxy)-2-thiophenepropylamine hydrochloride *see* duloxetine *on page 286*

sodium 2-mercaptoethane sulfonate *see* mesna *on page 546*

sodium 4-hydroxybutyrate *see* sodium oxybate *on page 795*

sodium *L*-triiodothyronine *see* liothyronine *on page 510*

sodium acetate (SOW dee um AS e tate)

Therapeutic Category Alkalinizing Agent; Electrolyte Supplement, Oral

Use Sodium source in large volume I.V. fluids to prevent or correct hyponatremia in patients with restricted intake; used to counter acidosis through conversion to bicarbonate

Usual Dosage Sodium acetate is metabolized to bicarbonate on an equimolar basis outside the liver; administer in large volume I.V. fluids as a sodium source. Refer to sodium bicarbonate monograph.

Maintenance electrolyte requirements of sodium in parenteral nutrition solutions:

Daily requirements: 3-4 mEq/kg/24 hours or 25-40 mEq/1000 kcal/24 hours

Maximum: 100-150 mEq/24 hours

Dosage Forms

Injection, solution: 2 mEq/mL (20 mL, 50 mL, 100 mL); 4 mEq/mL (50 mL, 100 mL)

sodium acid carbonate *see* sodium bicarbonate *on this page*

sodium aurothiomalate *see* gold sodium thiomalate *on page 398*

sodium benzoate and caffeine *see* caffeine *on page 133*

sodium benzoate and sodium phenylacetate *see* sodium phenylacetate and sodium benzoate *on page 795*

sodium bicarbonate (SOW dee um bye KAR bun ate)

Synonyms baking soda; NaHCO₃; sodium acid carbonate; sodium hydrogen carbonate

U.S./Canadian Brand Names Brioschi® [US-OTC]; Neut® [US]

Therapeutic Category Alkalinizing Agent; Antacid; Electrolyte Supplement, Oral

Use Management of metabolic acidosis; gastric hyperacidity; as an alkalinization agent for the urine; treatment of hyperkalemia; management of overdose of certain drugs, including tricyclic antidepressants and aspirin

Usual Dosage

Cardiac arrest: **Routine use of NaHCO₃ is not recommended and should be given only after adequate alveolar ventilation has been established and effective cardiac compressions are provided**

Infants and Children: I.V.: 0.5-1 mEq/kg/dose repeated every 10 minutes or as indicated by arterial blood gases; rate of infusion should not exceed 10 mEq/minute; neonates and children <2 years of age should receive 4.2% (0.5 mEq/mL) solution

Adults: I.V.: Initial: 1 mEq/kg/dose one time; maintenance: 0.5 mEq/kg/dose every 10 minutes or as indicated by arterial blood gases

Metabolic acidosis: Infants, Children, and Adults: Dosage should be based on the following formula if blood gases and pH measurements are available:

HCO_3^- (mEq) = 0.3 x weight (kg) x base deficit (mEq/L)

Administer ½ dose initially, then remaining ½ dose over the next 24 hours; monitor pH, serum HCO_3^-, and clinical status

(Continued)

sodium bicarbonate *(Continued)*

Note: If acid-base status is not available: Dose for older Children and Adults: 2-5 mEq/kg I.V. infusion over 4-8 hours; subsequent doses should be based on patient's acid-base status

Chronic renal failure: Oral: Initiate when plasma HCO_3^- <15 mEq/L

Children: 1-3 mEq/kg/day

Adults: Start with 20-36 mEq/day in divided doses, titrate to bicarbonate level of 18-20 mEq/L

Hyperkalemia: Adults: I.V.: 1 mEq/kg over 5 minutes

Renal tubular acidosis: Oral:

Distal:

Children: 2-3 mEq/kg/day

Adults: 0.5-2 mEq/kg/day in 4-5 divided doses

Proximal: Children and Adults: Initial: 5-10 mEq/kg/day; maintenance: Increase as required to maintain serum bicarbonate in the normal range

Urine alkalinization: Oral:

Children: 1-10 mEq (84-840 mg)/kg/day in divided doses every 4-6 hours; dose should be titrated to desired urinary pH

Adults: Initial: 48 mEq (4 g), then 12-24 mEq (1-2 g) every 4 hours; dose should be titrated to desired urinary pH; doses up to 16 g/day (200 mEq) in patients <60 years and 8 g (100 mEq) in patients >60 years

Antacid: Adults: Oral: 325 mg to 2 g 1-4 times/day

Dosage Forms

Granules, effervescent:

Brioschi® [OTC]: 2.69 g/packet, 2.69 g/capful

Infusion [premixed in sterile water]: 5% (500 mL)

Injection, solution:

Generics:

4.2% [42 mg/mL = 5 mEq/10 mL] (10 mL)

7.5% [75 mg/mL = 8.92 mEq/10 mL] (50 mL)

8.4% [84 mg/mL = 10 mEq/10 mL] (10 mL, 50 mL)

Brands:

Neut®: 4% [40 mg/mL = 2.4 mEq/5 mL] (5 mL)

Powder: Sodium bicarbonate USP (120 g, 480 g)

Tablet: 325 mg [3.8 mEq]; 650 mg [7.6 mEq]

sodium chloride *(SOW dee um KLOR ide)*

Synonyms NaCl; normal saline; salt

U.S./Canadian Brand Names 4-Way® Saline Moisturizing Mist [US-OTC]; Altachlore [US-OTC]; Altamist [US-OTC]; Ayr® Baby Saline [US-OTC]; Ayr® Saline No-Drip [US-OTC]; Ayr® Saline [US-OTC]; Breathe Right® Saline [US-OTC]; Deep Sea [US-OTC]; Entsol® [US-OTC]; Muro 128® [US-OTC]; Mycinaire™ [US-OTC]; Na-Zone® [US-OTC]; Nasal Moist® [US-OTC]; NaSal™ [US-OTC]; Ocean® for Kids [US-OTC]; Ocean® [US-OTC]; Pretz® [US-OTC]; SalineX® [US-OTC]; Simply Saline® Baby [US-OTC]; Simply Saline® Nasal Moist® [US-OTC]; Simply Saline® [US-OTC]; Syrex [US]; Wound Wash Saline™ [US-OTC]

Therapeutic Category Electrolyte Supplement, Oral; Lubricant, Ocular

Use

Parenteral: Restores sodium ion in patients with restricted oral intake (especially hyponatremia states or low salt syndrome). In general, parenteral saline uses:

Bacteriostatic sodium chloride: Dilution or dissolving drugs for I.M., I.V., or SubQ injections

Concentrated sodium chloride: Additive for parenteral fluid therapy

Hypertonic sodium chloride: For severe hyponatremia and hypochloremia

Hypotonic sodium chloride: Hydrating solution

Normal saline: Restores water/sodium losses

Pharmaceutical aid/diluent for infusion of compatible drug additives

Ophthalmic: Reduces corneal edema

Inhalation: Restores moisture to pulmonary system; loosens and thins congestion caused by colds or allergies; diluent for bronchodilator solutions that require dilution before inhalation

Intranasal: Restores moisture to nasal membranes

Irrigation: Wound cleansing, irrigation, and flushing

Usual Dosage

Children: I.V.: Hypertonic solutions (>0.9%) should only be used for the initial treatment of acute serious symptomatic hyponatremia; maintenance: 3-4 mEq/kg/day; maximum: 100-150 mEq/day; dosage varies widely depending on clinical condition

Replacement: Determined by laboratory determinations mEq

Sodium deficiency (mEq/kg) = [% dehydration (L/kg)/100 x 70 (mEq/L)] + [0.6 (L/kg) x (140 - serum sodium) (mEq/L)]

Children ≥2 years and Adults:

Intranasal: 2-3 sprays in each nostril as needed

Irrigation: Spray affected area

Children and Adults: Inhalation: Bronchodilator diluent: 1-3 sprays (1-3 mL) to dilute bronchodilator solution in nebulizer prior to administration

Adults:

GU irrigant: 1-3 L/day by intermittent irrigation

Replacement I.V.: Determined by laboratory determinations mEq

Sodium deficiency (mEq/kg) = [% dehydration (L/kg)/100 x 70 (mEq/L)] + [0.6 (L/kg) x (140 - serum sodium) (mEq/L)]

To correct acute, serious hyponatremia: mEq sodium = [desired sodium (mEq/L) - actual sodium (mEq/L)] x [0.6 x wt (kg)]; for acute correction use 125 mEq/L as the desired serum sodium; acutely correct serum sodium in 5 mEq/L/dose increments; more gradual correction in increments of 10 mEq/L/day is indicated in the asymptomatic patient

Chloride maintenance electrolyte requirement in parenteral nutrition: 2-4 mEq/kg/24 hours or 25-40 mEq/ 1000 kcals/24 hours; maximum: 100-150 mEq/24 hours

Sodium maintenance electrolyte requirement in parenteral nutrition: 3-4 mEq/kg/24 hours or 25-40 mEq/ 1000 kcals/24 hours; maximum: 100-150 mEq/24 hours.

Ophthalmic:

Ointment: Apply once daily or more often

Solution: Instill 1-2 drops into affected eye(s) every 3-4 hours

Dosage Forms

Gel, intranasal:

Ayr® Saline No-Drip [OTC]: 0.5% (22 mL)

Ayr® Saline [OTC]: 0.5% (14 g)

Entsol® [OTC]: 3% (20 g)

Simply Saline® Nasal Moist® [OTC]: 0.65% (30 g)

Injection, solution [preservative free]: 0.9% (2 mL, 5 mL, 10 mL, 20 mL, 100 mL)

Injection, solution [preservative free, prefilled I.V. flush syringe]: 0.9% (2 mL, 2.5 mL, 3 mL, 5 mL, 10 mL)

Injection, solution: 0.45% (25 mL, 50 mL, 100 mL, 250 mL, 500 mL, 1000 mL); 0.9% (3 mL, 5 mL, 10 mL, 20 mL, 25 mL, 30 mL, 50 mL, 100 mL, 150 mL, 250 mL, 500 mL, 1000 mL); 3% (500 mL); 5% (500 mL)

Syrex: 0.9% (2.5 mL, 5 mL, 10 mL)

Injection, solution [bacteriostatic]: 0.9% (10 mL, 20 mL, 30 mL)

Injection, solution [concentrate]: 14.6% (2.5 mEq/mL) (20 mL, 40 mL); 23.4% (4 mEq/mL) (30 mL, 100 mL, 200 mL, 250 mL)

Ointment, ophthalmic: 5% (3.5 g)

Altachlore [OTC], Muro 128® [OTC]: 5% (3.5 g)

Powder for nasal solution:

Entsol® [OTC]: 3% (10.5 g)

Solution for inhalation: 0.45% (3 mL, 5 mL); 0.9% (3 mL, 5 mL, 15 mL); 3% (15 mL); 10% (15 mL)

Solution, intranasal: 0.65% (45 mL)

Altamist [OTC], Na-Zone® [OTC]: 0.65% (60 mL)

Ayr® Baby Saline [OTC], Mycinaire™ [OTC]: 0.65% (30 mL)

Ayr® Saline [OTC]: 0.65% (50 mL)

Breathe Right® Saline [OTC]: 0.65% (44 mL)

Deep Sea [OTC], Nasal Moist® [OTC]: 0.65% (45 mL)

Entsol® Mist [OTC]: 3% (30 mL)

Entsol® [OTC] [preservative free]: 3% (100 mL, 240 mL)

Little Noses® Saline: 0.65% (30 mL)

Little Noses® Stuffy Nose Kit: 0.65% (15 mL)

NaSal™ [OTC]: 0.65% (15 mL, 30 mL)

Ocean® [OTC]: 0.65% (45 mL, 473 mL)

Ocean® for Kids [OTC]: 0.65% (37.5 mL)

Pretz® [OTC]: 0.75% (50 mL, 240 mL, 960 mL)

SalineX® [OTC]: 0.4% (15 mL, 50 mL)

Simply Saline® [OTC]: 0.9% (44 mL, 90 mL)

Simply Saline® Baby [OTC]: 0.9% (45 mL)

4-Way® Saline Moisturizing Mist [OTC]: 0.74% (30 mL)

Solution for irrigation: 0.45% (1500 mL, 2000 mL); 0.9% (250 mL, 500 mL, 1000 mL, 1500 mL, 2000 mL, 3000 mL, 4000 mL, 5000 mL)

Wound Wash Saline™ [OTC]: 0.9% (90 mL, 210 mL)

Solution, ophthalmic: 5% (15 mL)

Altachlore [OTC]: 5% (15 mL, 30 mL)

Muro 128® [OTC]: 2% (15 mL); 5% (15 mL, 30 mL)

sodium chondroitin sulfate and sodium hyaluronate
(SOW de um kon DROY tin SUL fate & SOW de um hye al yoor ON ate)

Synonyms chondroitin sulfate and sodium hyaluronate; sodium hyaluronate and chondroitin sulfate

U.S./Canadian Brand Names DisCoVisc™ [US]; Viscoat® [US]

Therapeutic Category Ophthalmic Agent, Viscoelastic

Use Ophthalmic surgical aid in the anterior segment during cataract extraction and intraocular lens implantation

Usual Dosage Ophthalmic: Adults: Carefully introduce (using a 27-gauge cannula) into anterior chamber during surgery

Dosage Forms
  Injection, solution, intraocular:
  DisCoVisc™: Sodium chondroitin sulfate ≤4% and sodium hyaluronate ≤1.7% (0.5 mL, 1 mL)
  Viscoat®: Sodium chondroitin sulfate ≤4% and sodium hyaluronate ≤3% (0.5 mL, 0.75 mL)

sodium citrate, citric acid, and potassium citrate *see* citric acid, sodium citrate, and potassium citrate *on page 195*

sodium edetate *see* edetate disodium *on page 291*

sodium etidronate *see* etidronate disodium *on page 335*

sodium ferric gluconate *see* ferric gluconate *on page 348*

sodium fluorescein *see* fluorescein *on page 361*

sodium fluoride *see* fluoride *on page 361*

sodium fusidate *see* fusidic acid *(Canada only) on page 379*

sodium hyaluronate *see* hyaluronate and derivatives *on page 423*

sodium hyaluronate and chondroitin sulfate *see* sodium chondroitin sulfate and sodium hyaluronate *on this page*

sodium hydrogen carbonate *see* sodium bicarbonate *on page 791*

sodium hypochlorite solution (SOW dee um hye poe KLOR ite soe LOO shun)

Synonyms modified Dakin's solution

U.S./Canadian Brand Names Dakin's Solution [US]; Di-Dak-Sol [US]

Therapeutic Category Disinfectant

Use Treatment of athlete's foot (0.5%); wound irrigation (0.5%); disinfection of utensils and equipment (5%)

Usual Dosage Topical irrigation

Dosage Forms
  Solution, topical:
  Dakin's: 0.25% (480 mL); 0.5% (480 mL, 3840 mL)
  Di-Dak-Sol: 0.0125% (480 mL)

sodium hyposulfate *see* sodium thiosulfate *on page 798*

sodium lactate (SOW dee um LAK tate)

Therapeutic Category Alkalinizing Agent

Use Source of bicarbonate for prevention and treatment of mild to moderate metabolic acidosis

Usual Dosage Dosage depends on degree of acidosis

Dosage Forms
  Injection, solution: 560 mg/mL (10 mL)

sodium nafcillin *see* nafcillin *on page 587*

sodium nitrite, sodium thiosulfate, and amyl nitrite
(SOW dee um NYE trite, SOW dee um thye oh SUL fate, & AM il NYE trite)

Synonyms amyl nitrite, sodium thiosulfate, and sodium nitrite; cyanide antidote kit; sodium thiosulfate, sodium nitrite, and amyl nitrite

U.S./Canadian Brand Names Cyanide Antidote Package [US]

Therapeutic Category Antidote

Use Treatment of cyanide poisoning

Usual Dosage Cyanide poisoning:
  Children: 0.3 mL ampul of amyl nitrite is crushed every minute and vapor is inhaled for 15-30 seconds until an I.V. sodium nitrite infusion is available. Following administration of sodium nitrite I.V. 6-8 mL/m^2 (~0.2 mL/kg, maximum: 10 mL), inject sodium thiosulfate I.V. 7 g/m^2 (maximum 12.5 g) over ~10 minutes, if needed; injection of both may be repeated at $^1/_2$ the original dose.

Adults: 0.3 mL ampul of amyl nitrite is crushed every minute and vapor is inhaled for 15-30 seconds until an I.V. sodium nitrite infusion is available. Following administration of 300 mg I.V. sodium nitrite, inject 12.5 g sodium thiosulfate I.V. (over ~10 minutes), if needed; injection of both may be repeated at $^1/_2$ the original dose.

Dosage Forms Kit [each kit contains]:

Cyanide Antidote Package:

Injection, solution:

Sodium nitrite 300 mg/10 mL (2)

Sodium thiosulfate 12.5 g/50 mL (2)

Inhalant: Amyl nitrite 0.3 mL (12)

sodium nitroferricyanide *see* nitroprusside *on page 609*

sodium nitroprusside *see* nitroprusside *on page 609*

sodium oxybate (SOW dee um ox i BATE)

Synonyms gamma hydroxybutyric acid; GHB; 4-hydroxybutyrate; sodium 4-hydroxybutyrate

U.S./Canadian Brand Names Xyrem® [US/Can]

Therapeutic Category Central Nervous System Depressant

Controlled Substance C-I (illicit use); C-III (medical use)

Use Treatment of cataplexy and daytime sleepiness in patients with narcolepsy

Usual Dosage Oral: Children ≥16 years and Adults: Narcolepsy: Initial: 4.5 g/day, in 2 equal doses; first dose to be given at bedtime after the patient is in bed, and second dose to be given 2.5-4 hours later. Dose may be increased or adjusted in 2-week intervals; average dose: 6-9 g/day (maximum: 9 g/day)

Dosage Forms

Solution, oral:

Xyrem®: 500 mg/mL

sodium PAS *see* aminosalicylic acid *on page 43*

sodium-PCA and lactic acid *see* lactic acid *on page 487*

sodium phenylacetate and sodium benzoate
(SOW dee um fen il AS e tate & SOW dee um BENZ oh ate)

Synonyms NAPA and NABZ; sodium benzoate and sodium phenylacetate

U.S./Canadian Brand Names Ammonul® [US]

Therapeutic Category Ammonium Detoxicant

Use Adjunct to treatment of acute hyperammonemia and encephalopathy in patients with urea cycle disorders involving partial or complete deficiencies of carbamyl-phosphate synthetase (CPS), ornithine transcarbamoylase (OTC), argininosuccinate lysase (ASL), or argininosuccinate synthetase (ASS); for use with hemodialysis in acute neonatal hyperammonemic coma, moderate-to-severe hyperammonemic encephalopathy and hyperammonemia which fails to respond to initial therapy

Usual Dosage Administer as a loading dose over 90-120 minutes, followed by an equivalent maintenance infusion given over 24 hours. Dosage based on weight and specific enzyme deficiency; therapy should continue until ammonia levels are in normal range.

≤20 kg:

CPS and OTC deficiency: Ammonul® 2.5 mL/kg and arginine 10% 2 mL/kg (provides sodium phenylacetate 250 mg/kg, sodium benzoate 250 mg/kg, and arginine hydrochloride 200 mg/kg).

ASS and ASL deficiency: Ammonul® 2.5 mL/kg and arginine 10% 6 mL/kg (provides sodium phenylacetate 250 mg/kg, sodium benzoate 250 mg/kg, and arginine hydrochloride 600 mg/kg)

Note: Pending a specific diagnosis in infants, the bolus and maintenance dose of arginine should be 6 mL/kg. If ASS or ASL are excluded as diagnostic possibilities, reduce dose of arginine to 2 mL/kg/day.

>20 kg:

CPS and OTC deficiency: Ammonul® 55 mL/m^2 and arginine 10% 2 mL/kg (provides sodium phenylacetate 5.5 g/m^2, sodium benzoate 5.5 g/m^2, and arginine hydrochloride 200 mg/kg)

ASS and ASL deficiency: Ammonul® 55 mL/m^2 and arginine 10% 6 mL/kg (provides sodium phenylacetate 5.5 g/m^2, sodium benzoate 5.5 g/m^2, and arginine hydrochloride 600 mg/kg)

Dosage Forms

Injection, solution:

Ammonul®: Sodium phenylacetate 100 mg and sodium benzoate 100 mg per mL (50 mL)

sodium phenylbutyrate (SOW dee um fen il BYOO ti rate)

Synonyms ammonapse

U.S./Canadian Brand Names Buphenyl® [US]

Therapeutic Category Miscellaneous Product

Use Orphan drug: Adjunctive therapy in the chronic management of patients with urea cycle disorder involving deficiencies of carbamoylphosphate synthetase, ornithine transcarbamylase, or argininosuccinic acid synthetase

Usual Dosage Oral:

Powder: Patients weighing <20 kg: 450-600 mg/kg/day or 9.9-13 g/m^2/day, administered in equally divided amounts with each meal or feeding, four to six times daily; safety and efficacy of doses >20 g/day has not been established

Tablet: Children >20 kg and Adults: 450-600 mg/kg/day or 9.9-13 g/m^2/day, administered in equally divided amounts with each meal; safety and efficacy of doses >20 g/day have not been established

Dosage Forms

Powder, for oral solution:

Buphenyl®: 3 g/level teaspoon

Tablet:

Buphenyl®: 500 mg

sodium phosphate and potassium phosphate *see* potassium phosphate and sodium phosphate *on page 703*

sodium phosphates (SOW dee um FOS fates)

Sound-Alike/Look-Alike Issues

Visicol® may be confused with VESIcare®

U.S./Canadian Brand Names Fleet Enema® [Can]; Fleet® Accu-Prep® [US-OTC]; Fleet® Enema [US-OTC]; Fleet® Phospho-Soda® Oral Laxative [Can]; Fleet® Phospho-Soda® [US-OTC]; OsmoPrep™ [US]; Visicol® [US]

Therapeutic Category Electrolyte Supplement, Oral; Laxative

Use

Oral, rectal: Short-term treatment of constipation and to evacuate the colon for rectal and bowel exams

I.V.: Source of phosphate in large volume I.V. fluids and parenteral nutrition; treatment and prevention of hypophosphatemia

Usual Dosage

Normal requirements elemental phosphorus: Oral:

0-6 months: Adequate intake: 100 mg/day

6-12 months: Adequate intake: 275 mg/day

1-3 years: RDA: 460 mg

4-8 years: RDA: 500 mg

9-18 years: RDA: 1250 mg

≥19 years: RDA: 700 mg

Hypophosphatemia: It is difficult to provide concrete guidelines for the treatment of severe hypophosphatemia because the extent of total body deficits and response to therapy are difficult to predict. Aggressive doses of phosphate may result in a transient serum elevation followed by redistribution into intracellular compartments or bone tissue. Intermittent I.V. infusion should be reserved for severe depletion situations (<1 mg/dL in adults); large doses of oral phosphate may cause diarrhea and intestinal absorption may be unreliable. I.V. solutions should be infused slowly. Use caution when mixing with calcium and magnesium, precipitate may form. The following dosages are empiric guidelines. **Note:** 1 mmol phosphate = 31 mg phosphorus; 1 mg phosphorus = 0.032 mmol phosphate

Hypophosphatemia treatment: Doses listed as mmol of phosphate:

Intermittent I.V. infusion: Acute repletion or replacement:

Children:

Low dose: 0.08 mmol/kg over 6 hours; use if losses are recent and uncomplicated

Intermediate dose: 0.16-0.24 mmol/kg over 4-6 hours; use if serum phosphorus level 0.5-1 mg/dL

High dose: 0.36 mmol/kg over 6 hours; use if serum phosphorus <0.5 mg/dL

Adults: Varying dosages: 0.15-0.3 mmol/kg/dose over 12 hours; may repeat as needed to achieve desired serum level **or**

15 mmol/dose over 2 hours; use if serum phosphorus <2 mg/dL **or**

Low dose: 0.16 mmol/kg over 4-6 hours; use if serum phosphorus level 2.3-3 mg/dL

Intermediate dose: 0.32 mmol/kg over 4-6 hours; use if serum phosphorus level 1.6-2.2 mg/dL

High dose: 0.64 mmol/kg over 8-12 hours; use if serum phosphorus <1.5 mg/dL

Oral: Adults: 0.5-1 g elemental phosphorus 2-3 times/day may be used when serum phosphorus level is 1-2.5 mg/dL

Maintenance: Doses listed as mmol of phosphate:
Children:
 Oral: 2-3 mmol/kg/day in divided doses
 I.V.: 0.5-1.5 mmol/kg/day
Adults:
 Oral: 50-150 mmol/day in divided doses
 I.V.: 50-70 mmol/day

Laxative (Fleet®): Rectal:
Children 2-<5 years: One-half contents of one 2.25 oz pediatric enema
Children 5-12 years: Contents of one 2.25 oz pediatric enema, may repeat
Children ≥12 years and Adults: Contents of one 4.5 oz enema as a single dose, may repeat

Laxative (Fleet® Phospho-Soda®): Oral: Take on an empty stomach; dilute dose with 8 ounces cool water, then follow dose with 8 ounces water; **do not repeat dose within 24 hours**
Children 5-9 years: 7.5 mL as a single dose; maximum daily dose: 7.5 mL
Children 10-12 years: 15 mL as a single dose; maximum daily dose: 15 mL
Children ≥12 years and Adults: 15 mL as a single dose; maximum daily dose: 45 mL

Bowel cleansing prior to colonoscopy: Adults: **Note:** Each dose should be taken with a minimum of 8 ounces of clear liquids. Do not repeat treatment within 7 days. Do not use additional agents, especially sodium phosphate products.
Fleet® Phospho-Soda®: Oral: Prior to procedure (timing of doses determined by prescriber): One dose is equal to 45 mL (2 doses are recommended): Each dose is diluted as follows:
Mix 45 mL with 120 mL clear liquid; drink, then follow with at least 240 mL of clear liquid; **or**
Mix 15 mL with 240 mL clear liquid; drink, then follow with 240 mL clear liquid; repeat every 10 minutes for a total of 45 mL
Visicol™: Oral: Adults: A total of 40 tablets divided as follows:
Evening before colonoscopy: 3 tablets every 15 minutes for 6 doses, then 2 additional tablets in 15 minutes (total of 20 tablets)
3-5 hours prior to colonoscopy: 3 tablets every 15 minutes for 6 doses, then 2 additional tablets in 15 minutes (total of 20 tablets)
OsmoPrep™: A total of 32 tablets divided as follows:
Evening before colonoscopy: 4 tablets every 15 minutes for 5 doses (total of 20 tablets)
3-5 hours prior to colonoscopy: 4 tablets every 15 minutes for 3 doses (total of 12 tablets)
Dosage Forms
Kit:
Fleet® Accu-Prep® [OTC]:
Solution, oral (Fleet® Phosph-Soda® [OTC]): Monobasic sodium phosphate 2.4 g and dibasic sodium phosphate 0.9 g per 5 mL (15 mL)
Pads, anorectal (Fleet® Relief™ [OTC]): Pramoxine 1% and glycerin 12% (4s)
Injection, solution [preservative free]: Phosphorus 3 mmol and sodium 4 mEq per mL (5 mL, 15 mL, 50 mL)
Solution, oral:
Fleet® Phospho-Soda® [OTC]: Monobasic sodium phosphate 2.4 g and dibasic sodium phosphate 0.9 g per 5 mL
Solution, rectal [enema]: Monobasic sodium phosphate 19 g and dibasic sodium phosphate 7 g per 118 mL delivered dose (135 mL)
Fleet® Enema [OTC]: Monobasic sodium phosphate 19 g and dibasic sodium phosphate 7 g per 118 mL delivered dose (135 mL)
Fleet® Enema for Children [OTC]: Monobasic sodium phosphate 9.5 g and dibasic sodium phosphate 3.5 g per 59 mL delivered dose (68 mL)
Tablet, oral:
OsmoPrep™: Sodium phosphate monobasic monohydrate 1.102 g and sodium phosphate dibasic anhydrous 0.398 g
Visicol®: Monobasic sodium phosphate 1.102 g and dibasic sodium phosphate 0.398 g

sodium polystyrene sulfonate (SOW dee um pol ee STYE reen SUL fon ate)
Sound-Alike/Look-Alike Issues
Kayexalate® may be confused with Kaopectate®
U.S./Canadian Brand Names Kayexalate® [US/Can]; Kionex™ [US]; PMS-Sodium Polystyrene Sulfonate [Can]; SPS® [US]
Therapeutic Category Antidote
Use Treatment of hyperkalemia
Usual Dosage
Children:
Oral: 1 g/kg/dose every 6 hours
Rectal: 1 g/kg/dose every 2-6 hours (In small children and infants, employ lower doses by using the practical exchange ratio of 1 mEq K+/g of resin as the basis for calculation)
(Continued)

sodium polystyrene sulfonate *(Continued)*
Adults: Hyperkalemia:
Oral: 15 g (60 mL) 1-4 times/day
Rectal: 30-50 g every 6 hours
Dosage Forms
Powder for suspension, oral/rectal: 15 g/4 level teaspoons
Kayexalate®, Kionex™: 15 g/4 level teaspoons
Suspension, oral/rectal: 15 g/60 mL
SPS®: 15 g/60 mL

sodium sulfacetamide *see* sulfacetamide *on page 810*

sodium sulfacetamide and sulfur *see* sulfur and sulfacetamide *on page 815*

sodium tetradecyl (SOW dee um tetra DEK il)
Synonyms sodium tetradecyl sulfate
U.S./Canadian Brand Names Sotradecol® [US]; Trombovar® [Can]
Therapeutic Category Sclerosing Agent
Use Treatment of small, uncomplicated varicose veins of the lower extremities
Usual Dosage I.V.: Test dose: 0.5 mL given several hours prior to administration of larger dose; 0.5-2 mL (preferred maximum: 1 mL) in each vein, maximum: 10 mL per treatment session; 3% solution reserved for large varices
Dosage Forms
Injection:
Sotradecol®: 1% [10 mg/mL] (2 mL); 3% [30 mg/mL] (2 mL)

sodium tetradecyl sulfate *see* sodium tetradecyl *on this page*

sodium thiosulfate (SOW dee um thye oh SUL fate)
Synonyms disodium thiosulfate pentahydrate; pentahydrate; sodium hyposulfate; sodium thiosulphate; thiosulfuric acid disodium salt
U.S./Canadian Brand Names Versiclear™ [US]
Therapeutic Category Antidote; Antifungal Agent
Use
Parenteral: Used alone or with sodium nitrite or amyl nitrite in cyanide poisoning; reduce the risk of nephrotoxicity associated with cisplatin therapy
Topical: Treatment of tinea versicolor
Usual Dosage
Cyanide and nitroprusside antidote: I.V.:
Children <25 kg: 50 mg/kg after receiving 4.5-10 mg/kg sodium nitrite; a half dose of each may be repeated if necessary
Children >25 kg and Adults: 12.5 g after 300 mg of sodium nitrite; a half dose of each may be repeated if necessary
Cyanide poisoning: I.V.: Dose should be based on determination as with nitrite, at rate of 2.5-5 mL/minute to maximum of 50 mL.
Cisplatin rescue should be given before or during cisplatin administration: I.V. infusion (in sterile water): 12 g/m^2 over 6 hours or 9 g/m^2 I.V. push followed by 1.2 g/m^2 continuous infusion for 6 hours
Tinea versicolor: Children and Adults: Topical: 20% to 25% solution: Apply a thin layer to affected areas twice daily
Dosage Forms
Injection, solution [preservative free]: 100 mg/mL (10 mL); 250 mg/mL (50 mL)
Versiclear™: 100 mg/mL (10 mL); 250 mg/mL (50 mL)
Lotion:
Versiclear™: Sodium thiosulfate 25% and salicylic acid 1% (120 mL)

sodium thiosulfate, sodium nitrite, and amyl nitrite *see* sodium nitrite, sodium thiosulfate, and amyl nitrite *on page 794*

sodium thiosulphate *see* sodium thiosulfate *on this page*

Soflax™ [Can] *see* docusate *on page 273*

Sofra-Tulle® [Can] *see* framycetin *(Canada only) on page 377*

Solagé™ [US/Can] *see* mequinol and tretinoin *on page 544*

Solaquin® [US-OTC/Can] *see* hydroquinone *on page 437*

Solaquin Forte® [US/Can] *see* hydroquinone *on page 437*

Solaraze® **[US]** *see* diclofenac *on page 253*

Solarcaine® **Aloe Extra Burn Relief [US-OTC]** *see* lidocaine *on page 504*

Solfoton® ***(Discontinued)*** *see* phenobarbital *on page 672*

Solia™ **[US]** *see* ethinyl estradiol and desogestrel *on page 322*

solifenacin (sol i FEN a sin)
Sound-Alike/Look-Alike Issues
　VESIcare® may be confused with Visicol®
Synonyms solifenacin succinate
U.S./Canadian Brand Names VESIcare® [US]
Therapeutic Category Anticholinergic Agent
Use Treatment of overactive bladder with symptoms of urinary frequency, urgency, or urge incontinence
Usual Dosage Oral:
　Children: Use is not recommended.
　Adults: 5 mg/day; if tolerated, may increase to 10 mg/day
Dosage Forms
　Tablet:
　　VESIcare®: 5 mg, 10 mg

solifenacin succinate *see* solifenacin *on this page*

Soliris™ **[US]** *see* eculizumab *on page 290*

Solodyn™ **[US]** *see* minocycline *on page 571*

Soltamox™ **[US]** *see* tamoxifen *on page 819*

soluble fluorescein *see* fluorescein *on page 361*

Solu-Cortef® **[US/Can]** *see* hydrocortisone (systemic) *on page 433*

Solugel® **[Can]** *see* benzoyl peroxide *on page 103*

Solu-Medrol® **[US/Can]** *see* methylprednisolone *on page 559*

Soluver® **[Can]** *see* salicylic acid *on page 772*

Soluver® **Plus [Can]** *see* salicylic acid *on page 772*

Soma® **[US/Can]** *see* carisoprodol *on page 154*

Soma® **Compound [US]** *see* carisoprodol and aspirin *on page 154*

Soma® **Compound w/Codeine [US]** *see* carisoprodol, aspirin, and codeine *on page 154*

somatostatin *(Canada only)* (soe mat oh STA tin)
U.S./Canadian Brand Names Stilamin® [Can]
Therapeutic Category Variceal Bleeding (Acute) Agent
Use For the symptomatic treatment of acute bleeding from esophageal varices. Other treatment options for long-term management of the condition may be considered if necessary, once initial control has been established.
Usual Dosage Slow 250 mcg I.V. bolus injection over 3 to 5 minutes, followed by a continuous infusion at a rate of 250 mcg/hour until bleeding from the varices has stopped (usually within 12 to 24 hours). Once bleeding has been controlled, it is recommended that the infusion be continued for at least another 48 to 72 hours, or out to a maximum of 120 hours to prevent recurrent bleeding.
Dosage Forms
　Injection: 250 mcg, 3 mg

somatrem *see* somatropin *on this page*

somatropin (soe ma TROE pin)
Sound-Alike/Look-Alike Issues
　somatropin may be confused with somatrem, sumatriptan
　somatrem may be confused with somatropin
Synonyms hGH; human growth hormone; somatrem
U.S./Canadian Brand Names Genotropin Miniquick® [US]; Genotropin® [US]; Humatrope® [US/Can]; Nordi-tropin® NordiFlex® [US]; Norditropin® [US]; Nutropin AQ® [US/Can]; Nutropine® [Can]; Nutropin® [US]; Omni-trope™ [US]; Saizen® [US/Can]; Serostim® [US/Can]; Tev-Tropin® [US]; Zorbtive® [US]
(Continued)

somatropin *(Continued)*

Therapeutic Category Growth Hormone

Use

Children:

Treatment of growth failure due to inadequate endogenous growth hormone secretion (Genotropin®, Humatrope®, Norditropin®, Nutropin®, Nutropin AQ®, Omnitrope™, Saizen®, Tev-Tropin®)

Treatment of short stature associated with Turner syndrome (Genotropin®, Humatrope®, Nutropin®, Nutropin AQ®)

Treatment of Prader-Willi syndrome (Genotropin®)

Treatment of growth failure associated with chronic renal insufficiency (CRI) up until the time of renal transplantation (Nutropin®, Nutropin AQ®)

Treatment of growth failure in children born small for gestational age who fail to manifest catch-up growth by 2 years of age (Genotropin®)

Treatment of idiopathic short stature (nongrowth hormone-deficient short stature) defined by height standard deviation score (SDS) less than or equal to -2.25 and growth rate not likely to attain normal adult height (Humatrope®, Nutropin®, Nutropin AQ®)

Treatment of short stature or growth failure associated with short stature homeobox gene (SHOX) deficiency (Humatrope®)

Treatment of short stature associated with Noonan syndrome (Norditropin®)

Adults:

HIV patients with wasting or cachexia with concomitant antiviral therapy (Serostim®)

Replacement of endogenous growth hormone in patients with adult growth hormone deficiency who meet both of the following criteria (Genotropin®, Humatrope®, Norditropin®, Nutropin®, Nutropin AQ®, Omnitrope™, Saizen®):

Biochemical diagnosis of adult growth hormone deficiency by means of a subnormal response to a standard growth hormone stimulation test (peak growth hormone ≤5 mcg/L). Confirmatory testing may not be required in patients with congenital/genetic growth hormone deficiency or multiple pituitary hormone deficiencies due to organic diseases.

and

Adult-onset: Patients who have adult growth hormone deficiency whether alone or with multiple hormone deficiencies (hypopituitarism) as a result of pituitary disease, hypothalamic disease, surgery, radiation therapy, or trauma

or

Childhood-onset: Patients who were growth hormone deficient during childhood, confirmed as an adult before replacement therapy is initiated

Treatment of short-bowel syndrome (Zorbtive®)

Usual Dosage

Children (individualize dose):

Chronic renal insufficiency (CRI): Nutropin®, Nutropin® AQ: SubQ: Weekly dosage: 0.35 mg/kg divided into daily injections; continue until the time of renal transplantation

Dosage recommendations in patients treated for CRI who require dialysis:

Hemodialysis: Administer dose at night prior to bedtime or at least 3-4 hours after hemodialysis to prevent hematoma formation from heparin

CCPD: Administer dose in the morning following dialysis

CAPD: Administer dose in the evening at the time of overnight exchange

Growth hormone deficiency:

Genotropin®, Omnitrope™: SubQ: Weekly dosage: 0.16-0.24 mg/kg divided into 6-7 doses

Humatrope®: I.M., SubQ: Weekly dosage: 0.18 mg/kg; maximum replacement dose: 0.3 mg/kg/week; dosing should be divided into equal doses given 3 times/week on alternating days, 6 times/week, or daily

Norditropin®: SubQ: 0.024-0.034 mg/kg/day, 6-7 times/week

Nutropin®, Nutropin® AQ: SubQ: Weekly dosage: 0.3 mg/kg divided into daily doses; pubertal patients: ≤0.7 mg/kg/week divided daily

Tev-Tropin®: SubQ: Up to 0.1 mg/kg administered 3 times/week

Saizen®: I.M., SubQ: 0.06 mg/kg/dose administered 3 times/week

Note: Therapy should be discontinued when patient has reached satisfactory adult height, when epiphyses have fused, or when the patient ceases to respond. Growth of 5 cm/year or more is expected, if growth rate does not exceed 2.5 cm in a 6-month period, double the dose for the next 6 months; if there is still no satisfactory response, discontinue therapy

Idiopathic short stature:

Humatrope®: SubQ: Weekly dosage: 0.37 mg/kg divided into equal doses 6-7 times per week

Nutropin®, Nutropin AQ®: SubQ: Weekly dosage: Up to 0.3 mg/kg divided into daily doses

Noonan syndrome: Nortidropin®: SubQ: Up to 0.066 mg/kg/day

Prader-Willi syndrome: Genotropin®: SubQ: Weekly dosage: 0.24 mg/kg divided into 6-7 doses

SHOX deficiency: Humatrope®: SubQ: 0.35 mg/kg/week divided into equal daily doses

Small for gestational age: Genotropin®: SubQ: Weekly dosage: 0.48 mg/kg divided into 6-7 doses

Turner syndrome:
Genotropin®: SubQ: Weekly dosage: 0.33 mg/kg divided into 6-7 doses
Humatrope®, Nutropin®, Nutropin® AQ: SubQ: Weekly dosage: ≤0.375 mg/kg divided into equal doses 3-7 times per week

Adults:
Growth hormone deficiency: Adjust dose based on individual requirements: To minimize adverse events in older or overweight patients, reduced dosages may be necessary. During therapy, dosage should be decreased if required by the occurrence of side effects or excessive IGF-I levels.
Norditropin®: SubQ: Initial dose ≤0.004 mg/kg/day; after 6 weeks of therapy, may increase dose up to 0.016 mg/kg/day
Nutropin®, Nutropin® AQ: SubQ: ≤0.006 mg/kg/day; dose may be increased up to a maximum of 0.025 mg/kg/day in patients <35 years of age, or up to a maximum of 0.0125 mg/kg/day in patients ≥35 years of age
Humatrope®: SubQ: ≤0.006 mg/kg/day; dose may be increased up to a maximum of 0.0125 mg/kg/day
Genotropin®, Omnitrope™: SubQ: Weekly dosage: ≤0.04 mg/kg divided into 6-7 doses; dose may be increased at 4- to 8-week intervals to a maximum of 0.08 mg/kg/week
Saizen®: SubQ: ≤0.005 mg/kg/day; dose may be increased to not more than 0.01 mg/kg/day after 4 weeks
Alternate dosing (growth hormone deficiency): SubQ: Initial: 0.2 mg/day (range: 0.15-0.3 mg/day); may increase every 1-2 months by 0.1-0.2 mg/day
Dosage adjustment with estrogen supplementation (growth hormone deficiency): Larger doses of somatropin may be needed for women taking oral estrogen replacement products; dosing not affected by topical products
HIV patients with wasting or cachexia: Serostim®: SubQ: 0.1 mg/kg once daily at bedtime (maximum 6 mg/day). Alternately, patients at risk for side effects may be started at 0.1 mg/kg every other day. Patients who continue to lose weight after 12 weeks should be re-evaluated for opportunistic infections or other clinical events; rotate injection sites to avoid lipodystrophy Adjust dose if needed to manage side effects.
Daily dose based on body weight:
<35 kg: 0.1 mg/kg
35-45 kg: 4 mg
45-55 kg: 5 mg
>55 kg: 6 mg
Short-bowel syndrome (Zorbtive®): SubQ: 0.1 mg/kg once daily for 4 weeks (maximum: 8 mg/day)
Fluid retention (moderate) or arthralgias: Treat symptomatically or reduce dose by 50%
Severe toxicity: Discontinue therapy for up to 5 days; when symptoms resolve, restart at 50% of dose. If severe toxicity recurs or does not disappear within 5 days after discontinuation, permanently discontinue treatment.

Dosage Forms

Injection, powder for reconstitution [rDNA origin]:
Genotropin®: 5.8 mg [~15 int. units/mL]; 13.8 mg [~36 int. units/mL]
Genotropin Miniquick® [preservative free]: 0.2 mg, 0.4 mg, 0.6 mg, 0.8 mg, 1 mg, 1.2 mg, 1.4 mg, 1.6 mg, 1.8 mg, 2 mg
Humatrope®: 5 mg [~15 int. units], 6 mg [18 int. units], 12 mg [36 int. units], 24 mg [72 int. units]
Nutropin®: 5 mg [~15 int. units]; 10 mg [~30 int. units]
Omnitrope™: 1.5 mg [~4.5 int. units]; 5.8 mg [~17.4 int. units]
Tev-Tropin®: 5 mg [15 int. units/mL]
Saizen®: 5 mg [~15 int. units]; 8.8 mg [~26.4 int. units]
Serostim®: 4 mg [12 int. units]; 5 mg [15 int. units]; 6 mg [18 int. units]
Zorbtive®: 8.8 mg [~26.4 int. units]
Injection, solution [rDNA origin]:
Norditropin®: 5 mg/1.5 mL (1.5 mL); 15 mg/1.5 mL (1.5 mL)
Norditropin® NordiFlex®: 5 mg/1.5 mL (1.5 mL); 10 mg/1.5 mL (1.5 mL); 15 mg/1.5 mL (1.5 mL)
Nutropin AQ®: 5 mg/mL [~15 int. units/mL] (2 mL)

Somatuline® Autogel® [Can] *see* lanreotide *on page 492*

Somatuline® Depot [US] *see* lanreotide *on page 492*

Somavert® [US] *see* pegvisomant *on page 659*

Sominex® [US-OTC] *see* diphenhydramine *on page 265*

Sominex® Maximum Strength [US-OTC] *see* diphenhydramine *on page 265*

Somnote™ [US] *see* chloral hydrate *on page 172*

Som Pam [Can] *see* flurazepam *on page 366*

Sonata® [US/Can] *see* zaleplon *on page 902*

Soothe® [US-OTC] *see* artificial tears *on page 75*

Soothing Care™ Itch Relief [US-OTC] *see* pramoxine *on page 706*

sorafenib (sor AF e nib)

Synonyms BAY 43-9006; NSC-724772; sorafenib tosylate

U.S./Canadian Brand Names Nexavar® [US]

Therapeutic Category Antineoplastic Agent, Tyrosine Kinase Inhibitor; Vascular Endothelial Growth Factor (VEGF) Inhibitor

Use Treatment of advanced renal cell cancer

Usual Dosage Oral: Adults: Advanced renal cell carcinoma: 400 mg twice daily

Dosage Forms

Tablet:

Nexavar®: 200 mg

sorafenib tosylate *see* sorafenib *on this page*

sorbitol (SOR bi tole)

Therapeutic Category Genitourinary Irrigant; Laxative

Use Genitourinary irrigant in transurethral prostatic resection or other transurethral resection or other transurethral surgical procedures; diuretic; humectant; sweetening agent; hyperosmotic laxative; facilitate the passage of sodium polystyrene sulfonate through the intestinal tract

Usual Dosage Hyperosmotic laxative (as single dose, at infrequent intervals):

Children 2-11 years:

Oral: 2 mL/kg (as 70% solution)

Rectal enema: 30-60 mL as 25% to 30% solution

Children >12 years and Adults:

Oral: 30-150 mL (as 70% solution)

Rectal enema: 120 mL as 25% to 30% solution

Adjunct to sodium polystyrene sulfonate: 15 mL as 70% solution orally until diarrhea occurs (10-20 mL/2 hours) or 20-100 mL as an oral vehicle for the sodium polystyrene sulfonate resin

When administered with charcoal:

Oral:

Children: 4.3 mL/kg of 35% sorbitol with 1 g/kg of activated charcoal

Adults: 4.3 mL/kg of 70% sorbitol with 1 g/kg of activated charcoal every 4 hours until first stool containing charcoal is passed

Topical: 3% to 3.3% as transurethral surgical procedure irrigation

Dosage Forms

Solution, genitourinary irrigation: 3% (3000 mL, 5000 mL); 3.3% (2000 mL, 4000 mL)

Solution, oral: 70%

Sorbitrate® *(Discontinued)* *see* isosorbide dinitrate *on page 476*

Soriatane® [US/Can] *see* acitretin *on page 16*

Sorine® [US] *see* sotalol *on this page*

Sotacor® [Can] *see* sotalol *on this page*

sotalol (SOE ta lole)

Sound-Alike/Look-Alike Issues

sotalol may be confused with Stadol®

Betapace® may be confused with Betapace AF®

Betapace AF® may be confused with Betapace®

Synonyms sotalol hydrochloride

U.S./Canadian Brand Names Alti-Sotalol [Can]; Apo-Sotalol® [Can]; Betapace AF® [US/Can]; Betapace® [US]; CO Sotalol [Can]; Gen-Sotalol [Can]; Lin-Sotalol [Can]; Novo-Sotalol [Can]; Nu-Sotalol [Can]; PMS-Sotalol [Can]; Rho®-Sotalol [Can]; Riva-Sotalol [Can]; Rylosol [Can]; Sorine® [US]; Sotacor® [Can]

Therapeutic Category Antiarrhythmic Agent, Class II; Antiarrhythmic Agent, Class III; Beta-Adrenergic Blocker, Nonselective

Use Treatment of documented ventricular arrhythmias (ie, sustained ventricular tachycardia), that in the judgment of the physician are life-threatening; maintenance of normal sinus rhythm in patients with symptomatic atrial fibrillation and atrial flutter who are currently in sinus rhythm. Manufacturer states substitutions should not be made for Betapace AF® since Betapace AF® is distributed with a patient package insert specific for atrial fibrillation/flutter.

Usual Dosage Sotalol should be initiated and doses increased in a hospital with facilities for cardiac rhythm monitoring and assessment. Proarrhythmic events can occur after initiation of therapy and with each upward dosage adjustment.

Children: Oral: The safety and efficacy of sotalol in children have not been established

Note: Dosing per manufacturer, based on pediatric pharmacokinetic data; wait at least 36 hours between dosage adjustments to allow monitoring of QT intervals

≤2 years: Dosage should be adjusted (decreased) by plotting of the child's age on a logarithmic scale; refer to manufacturer's package labeling.

>2 years: Initial: 90 mg/m²/day in 3 divided doses; may be incrementally increased to a maximum of 180 mg/m²/day

Adults: Oral:

Ventricular arrhythmias (Betapace®, Sorine®):

Initial: 80 mg twice daily

Dose may be increased gradually to 240-320 mg/day; allow 3 days between dosing increments in order to attain steady-state plasma concentrations and to allow monitoring of QT intervals

Most patients respond to a total daily dose of 160-320 mg/day in 2-3 divided doses.

Some patients, with life-threatening refractory ventricular arrhythmias, may require doses as high as 480-640 mg/day; however, these doses should only be prescribed when the potential benefit outweighs the increased of adverse events.

Atrial fibrillation or atrial flutter (Betapace AF®): Initial: 80 mg twice daily

If the initial dose does not reduce the frequency of relapses of atrial fibrillation/flutter and is tolerated without excessive QT prolongation (not >520 msec) after 3 days, the dose may be increased to 120 mg twice daily. This may be further increased to 160 mg twice daily if response is inadequate and QT prolongation is not excessive.

Dosage Forms

Tablet: 80 mg, 80 mg [AF], 120 mg, 120 mg [AF], 160 mg, 160 mg [AF], 240 mg

Betapace® [light blue]: 80 mg, 120 mg, 160 mg, 240 mg

Betapace AF® [white]: 80 mg, 120 mg, 160 mg

Sorine® [white]: 80 mg, 120 mg, 160 mg, 240 mg

sotalol hydrochloride *see* sotalol *on previous page*

Sotradecol® [US] *see* sodium tetradecyl *on page 798*

Sotret® [US] *see* isotretinoin *on page 477*

SourceCF® [US-OTC] *see* vitamins (multiple/pediatric) *on page 896*

SourceCF® Softgels [US] *see* vitamins (multiple/oral) *on page 895*

Soyacal® *(Discontinued)* *see* fat emulsion *on page 343*

Soyalac® [US-OTC] *see* nutritional formula, enteral/oral *on page 622*

SPA *see* albumin *on page 22*

Spacol *(Discontinued)* *see* hyoscyamine *on page 441*

Spacol T/S *(Discontinued)* *see* hyoscyamine *on page 441*

Span-FF® *(Discontinued)* *see* ferrous fumarate *on page 349*

Spasmolin® *(Discontinued)* *see* hyoscyamine, atropine, scopolamine, and phenobarbital *on page 442*

Spastrin® [US] *see* belladonna, phenobarbital, and ergotamine *on page 98*

SPD417 *see* carbamazepine *on page 147*

Spectazole® [US/Can] *see* econazole *on page 289*

Spec-T® *(Discontinued)* *see* benzocaine *on page 101*

spectinomycin (spek ti noe MYE sin)

Sound-Alike/Look-Alike Issues

Trobicin® may be confused with tobramycin

Synonyms spectinomycin hydrochloride

Therapeutic Category Antibiotic, Miscellaneous

Use Treatment of uncomplicated gonorrhea

Usual Dosage I.M.:

Children:

<45 kg: 40 mg/kg/dose 1 time (ceftriaxone preferred)

≥45 kg: Refer to adult dosing

Children >8 years who are allergic to PCNS/cephalosporins may be treated with oral tetracycline

Adults:

Uncomplicated urethral, cervical, pharyngeal, or rectal gonorrhea: 2 g deep I.M. or 4 g where antibiotic resistance is prevalent 1 time; 4 g (10 mL) dose should be given as two 5 mL injections, followed by adequate chlamydial treatment (doxycycline 100 mg twice daily for 7 days)

Disseminated gonococcal infection: 2 g every 12 hours

spectinomycin hydrochloride *see* spectinomycin *on previous page*

Spectracef™ **[US]** *see* cefditoren *on page 159*

Spectrocin Plus™ *(Discontinued)* *see* bacitracin, neomycin, polymyxin B, and pramoxine *on page 92*

SPI 0211 *see* lubiprostone *on page 522*

Spiriva® **[US/Can]** *see* tiotropium *on page 845*

Spironazide® *(Discontinued)* *see* hydrochlorothiazide and spironolactone *on page 426*

spironolactone (speer on oh LAK tone)

Sound-Alike/Look-Alike Issues
Aldactone® may be confused with Aldactazide®

U.S./Canadian Brand Names Aldactone® [US/Can]; Novo-Spiroton [Can]

Therapeutic Category Diuretic, Potassium Sparing

Use Management of edema associated with excessive aldosterone excretion; hypertension; congestive heart failure; primary hyperaldosteronism; hypokalemia; cirrhosis of liver accompanied by edema or ascites

Usual Dosage To reduce delay in onset of effect, a loading dose of 2 or 3 times the daily dose may be administered on the first day of therapy. Adults: Oral:

Edema, hypokalemia: 25-200 mg/day in 1-2 divided doses
Hypertension (JNC 7): 25-50 mg/day in 1-2 divided doses
Diagnosis of primary aldosteronism: 100-400 mg/day in 1-2 divided doses
CHF, severe (with ACE inhibitor and a loop diuretic ± digoxin): 12.5-25 mg/day; maximum daily dose: 50 mg (higher doses may occasionallly be used). In the RALES trial, 25 mg every other day was the lowest maintenance dose possible.
Note: If potassium >5.4 mEq/L, consider dosage reduction.

Dosage Forms
Tablet: 25 mg, 50 mg, 100 mg
Aldactone®: 25 mg, 50 mg, 100 mg

spironolactone and hydrochlorothiazide *see* hydrochlorothiazide and spironolactone *on page 426*

Spirozide® *(Discontinued)* *see* hydrochlorothiazide and spironolactone *on page 426*

Sporanox® **[US/Can]** *see* itraconazole *on page 478*

Sportscreme® **[US-OTC]** *see* trolamine *on page 870*

SPP100 *see* aliskiren *on page 29*

Sprayzoin™ **[US-OTC]** *see* benzoin *on page 103*

Sprintec™ **[US]** *see* ethinyl estradiol and norgestimate *on page 331*

Sprycel™ **[US/Can]** *see* dasatinib *on page 233*

SPS® **[US]** *see* sodium polystyrene sulfonate *on page 797*

SRC® **Expectorant** *(Discontinued)* *see* hydrocodone, pseudoephedrine, and guaifenesin *on page 432*

Sronyx™ **[US]** *see* ethinyl estradiol and levonorgestrel *on page 325*

SSD® **[US]** *see* silver sulfadiazine *on page 786*

SSD® **AF [US]** *see* silver sulfadiazine *on page 786*

SSKI® **[US]** *see* potassium iodide *on page 702*

S.T. 37® **[US-OTC]** *see* hexylresorcinol *on page 420*

Stadol® **[US]** *see* butorphanol *on page 132*

Stadol® **NS** *(Discontinued)* *see* butorphanol *on page 132*

Staflex [US] *see* acetaminophen and phenyltoloxamine *on page 8*

Stagesic® **[US]** *see* hydrocodone and acetaminophen *on page 427*

Stalevo™ **[US]** *see* levodopa, carbidopa, and entacapone *on page 500*

StanGard® **[US]** *see* fluoride *on page 361*

StanGard® **Perio [US]** *see* fluoride *on page 361*

stannous fluoride *see* fluoride *on page 361*

stanozolol (stan OH zoe lole)
U.S./Canadian Brand Names Winstrol® [US]
Therapeutic Category Anabolic Steroid
Controlled Substance C-III
Use Prophylactic use against hereditary angioedema
Usual Dosage
Children: Acute attacks:
<6 years: 1 mg/day
6-12 years: 2 mg/day
Adults: Oral: Initial: 2 mg 3 times/day, may then reduce to a maintenance dose of 2 mg/day or 2 mg every other day after 1-3 months
Dosage Forms
Tablet:
Winstrol®: 2 mg

Starlix® [US/Can] *see* nateglinide *on page 594*

Starnoc® [Can] *see* zaleplon *on page 902*

Statex® [Can] *see* morphine sulfate *on page 578*

Staticin® (Discontinued) *see* erythromycin *on page 309*

Statobex® [Can] *see* phendimetrazine *on page 671*

Statuss™ DM [US] *see* chlorpheniramine, phenylephrine, and dextromethorphan *on page 180*

stavudine (STAV yoo deen)
Sound-Alike/Look-Alike Issues
Zerit® may be confused with Ziac®
Synonyms d4T
U.S./Canadian Brand Names Zerit® [US/Can]
Therapeutic Category Antiviral Agent
Use Treatment of HIV infection in combination with other antiretroviral agents
Usual Dosage Oral:
Newborns (Birth to 13 days): 0.5 mg/kg every 12 hours
Children:
>14 days and <30 kg: 1 mg/kg every 12 hours
≥30 kg: Refer to Adults dosing
Adults:
≥60 kg: 40 mg every 12 hours
<60 kg: 30 mg every 12 hours
Dosage Forms
Capsule:
Zerit®: 15 mg, 20 mg, 30 mg, 40 mg
Powder, for oral solution:
Zerit®: 1 mg/mL

Stelazine® (Discontinued) *see* trifluoperazine *on page 865*

Stemetil® [Can] *see* prochlorperazine *on page 716*

Sterapred® [US] *see* prednisone *on page 710*

Sterapred® DS [US] *see* prednisone *on page 710*

STI571 *see* imatinib *on page 448*

Stieprox® [Can] *see* ciclopirox *on page 188*

Stilamin® [Can] *see* somatostatin *(Canada only) on page 799*

Stimate™ [US] *see* desmopressin acetate *on page 239*

Sting-Kill [US-OTC] *see* benzocaine *on page 101*

St. Joseph® Adult Aspirin [US-OTC] *see* aspirin *on page 78*

St. Joseph® Cough Suppressant (Discontinued) *see* dextromethorphan *on page 247*

St. Joseph® Measured Dose Nasal Solution (Discontinued) *see* phenylephrine *on page 675*

Stop® [US] *see* fluoride *on page 361*

Strattera® [US/Can] *see* atomoxetine *on page 81*

Streptase® [US/Can] *see* streptokinase *on next page*

streptokinase (strep toe KYE nase)

Synonyms SK

U.S./Canadian Brand Names Streptase® [US/Can]

Therapeutic Category Fibrinolytic Agent

Use Thrombolytic agent used in treatment of recent severe or massive deep vein thrombosis, pulmonary emboli, myocardial infarction, and occluded arteriovenous cannulas

Usual Dosage I.V.:

Children: Safety and efficacy have not been not established. Limited studies have used 3500-4000 units/kg over 30 minutes followed by 1000-1500 units/kg/hour.

Clotted catheter: **Note:** Not recommended due to possibility of allergic reactions with repeated doses: 10,000-25,000 units diluted in NS to a final volume equivalent to catheter volume; instill into catheter and leave in place for 1 hour, then aspirate contents out of catheter and flush catheter with normal saline.

Adults: Antibodies to streptokinase remain for at least 3-6 months after initial dose: Administration requires the use of an infusion pump.

An intradermal skin test of 100 units has been suggested to predict allergic response to streptokinase. If a positive reaction is not seen after 15-20 minutes, a therapeutic dose may be administered.

Guidelines for acute myocardial infarction (AMI): 1.5 million units over 60 minutes

Administration:

Dilute two 750,000 unit vials of streptokinase with 5 mL dextrose 5% in water (D$_5$W) each, gently swirl to dissolve.

Add this dose of the 1.5 million units to 150 mL D$_5$W.

This should be infused over 60 minutes; an in-line filter ≥0.45 micron should be used.

Monitor for the first few hours for signs of anaphylaxis or allergic reaction. **Infusion should be slowed if blood pressure falls by 25 mm Hg or terminated if asthmatic symptoms appear.**

Following completion of streptokinase, initiate heparin, if directed, when aPTT returns to less than 2 times the upper limit of control; do not use a bolus, but initiate infusion adjusted to a target aPTT of 1.5-2 times the upper limit of control. If prolonged (>48 hours) heparin is required, infusion may be switched to subcutaneous therapy.

Guidelines for acute pulmonary embolism (APE): 3 million unit dose over 24 hours

Administration:

Dilute four 750,000 unit vials of streptokinase with 5 mL dextrose 5% in water (D$_5$W) each, gently swirl to dissolve.

Add this dose of 3 million units to 250 mL D$_5$W, an in-line filter ≥0.45 micron should be used.

Administer 250,000 units (23 mL) over 30 minutes followed by 100,000 units/hour (9 mL/hour) for 24 hours.

Monitor for the first few hours for signs of anaphylaxis or allergic reaction. **Infusion should be slowed if blood pressure is lowered by 25 mm Hg or if asthmatic symptoms appear.**

Begin heparin 1000 units/hour about 3-4 hours after completion of streptokinase infusion or when PTT is <100 seconds.

Monitor PT, PTT, and fibrinogen levels during therapy.

Thromboses: 250,000 units to start, then 100,000 units/hour for 24-72 hours depending on location.

Cannula occlusion: 250,000 units into cannula, clamp for 2 hours, then aspirate contents and flush with normal saline; **Not recommended**

streptomycin (strep toe MYE sin)

Sound-Alike/Look-Alike Issues

streptomycin may be confused with streptozocin

Synonyms streptomycin sulfate

Therapeutic Category Antibiotic, Aminoglycoside; Antitubercular Agent

Use Part of combination therapy of active tuberculosis; used in combination with other agents for treatment of streptococcal or enterococcal endocarditis, mycobacterial infections, plague, tularemia, and brucellosis

Usual Dosage Note: For I.M. administration; I.V. use is not recommended

Usual dosage range:

Children: 20-40 mg/kg/day (maximum: 1 g)

Adults: 15-30 mg/kg/day or 1-2 g/day

Indication-specific dosing:

Children: **Tuberculosis:** I.M.:

Daily therapy: 20-40 mg/kg/day (maximum: 1 g/day)

Directly observed therapy (DOT): Twice weekly: 25-30 mg/kg (maximum: 1.5 g)

Directly observed therapy (DOT): 3 times/week: 25-30 mg/kg (maximum: 1.5 g)

Adults: I.M.:

Brucellosis: 1 g/day for 14-21 days (with doxycycline, 100 mg twice daily for 6 weeks)

Endocarditis:

Enterococcal: 1 g every 12 hours for 2 weeks, 500 mg every 12 hours for 4 weeks in combination with penicillin

Streptococcal: 1 g every 12 hours for 1 week, 500 mg every 12 hours for 1 week

Mycobacterium avium **complex:** Adjunct therapy (with macrolide, rifamycin, and ethambutol): 15 mg/kg 3 times/week for first 2-3 months for severe disease

Plague: 15 mg/kg (or 1 g) every 12 hours until the patient is afebrile for at least 3 days

Tuberculosis:
Daily therapy: 15 mg/kg/day (maximum: 1 g)
Directly observed therapy (DOT): Twice weekly: 25-30 mg/kg (maximum: 1.5 g)
Directly observed therapy (DOT): 3 times/week: 25-30 mg/kg (maximum: 1.5 g)
Tularemia: 10-15 mg/kg every 12 hours (maximum: 2 g/day) for 7-10 days or until patient is afebrile for 5-7 days

Dosage Forms
Injection, powder for reconstitution: 1 g

streptomycin sulfate *see* streptomycin *on previous page*

streptozocin (strep toe ZOE sin)

Sound-Alike/Look-Alike Issues
streptozocin may be confused with streptomycin
Synonyms NSC-85998
U.S./Canadian Brand Names Zanosar® [US/Can]
Therapeutic Category Antineoplastic Agent
Use Treatment of metastatic islet cell carcinoma of the pancreas, carcinoid tumor and syndrome, Hodgkin disease, palliative treatment of colorectal cancer
Usual Dosage I.V. (refer to individual protocols): Children and Adults:
Single agent therapy: 1-1.5 g/m² weekly for 6 weeks followed by a 4-week rest period
Combination therapy: 0.5-1 g/m² for 5 consecutive days followed by a 4- to 6-week rest period
Dosage Forms
Injection, powder for reconstitution:
Zanosar®: 1 g

Stresstabs® High Potency Advanced [US-OTC] *see* vitamin B complex combinations *on page 894*

Stresstabs® High Potency Energy [US-OTC] *see* vitamin B complex combinations *on page 894*

Stresstabs® High Potency Weight [US-OTC] *see* vitamin B complex combinations *on page 894*

Striant® [US] *see* testosterone *on page 828*

Stri-dex® [US-OTC] *see* salicylic acid *on page 772*

Stri-dex® Body Focus [US-OTC] *see* salicylic acid *on page 772*

Stri-dex® Facewipes To Go™ [US-OTC] *see* salicylic acid *on page 772*

Stri-dex® Maximum Strength [US-OTC] *see* salicylic acid *on page 772*

Strifon Forte® [Can] *see* chlorzoxazone *on page 186*

Stromectol® [US] *see* ivermectin *on page 479*

StrongStart™ [US] *see* vitamins (multiple/prenatal) *on page 896*

strontium-89 chloride *see* strontium-89 *on this page*

strontium-89 (STRON shee um atey nine)

Synonyms strontium-89 chloride
U.S./Canadian Brand Names Metastron® [US/Can]
Therapeutic Category Radiopharmaceutical
Use Relief of bone pain in patients with skeletal metastases
Usual Dosage I.V.: Adults: 148 megabecquerel (4 millicurie) administered by slow I.V. injection over 1-2 minutes or 1.5-2.2 megabecquerel (40-60 microcurie)/kg; repeated doses are generally not recommended at intervals <90 days; measure the patient dose by a suitable radioactivity calibration system immediately prior to administration
Dosage Forms
Injection, solution [preservative free]:
Metastron®: 10.9-22.6 mg/mL [148 megabecquerel, 4 millicurie] (10 mL)

Strovite [US] *see* vitamin B complex combinations *on page 894*

Strovite® Advance [US] *see* vitamins (multiple/oral) *on page 895*

Strovite® Forte [US] *see* vitamins (multiple/oral) *on page 895*

Stuartnatal® Plus 3™ [OTC] *(Discontinued)* *see* vitamins (multiple/prenatal) *on page 896*

Stuart Prenatal® **[US-OTC]** *see* vitamins (multiple/prenatal) *on page 896*

SU11248 *see* sunitinib *on page 816*

suberoylanilide hydroxamic acid *see* vorinostat *on page 898*

Sublimaze® **[US]** *see* fentanyl *on page 346*

Suboxone® **[US]** *see* buprenorphine and naloxone *on page 127*

Subutex® **[US/Can]** *see* buprenorphine *on page 127*

succimer (SUKS si mer)

Synonyms DMSA
U.S./Canadian Brand Names Chemet® [US/Can]
Therapeutic Category Chelating Agent
Use Treatment of lead poisoning in children with serum lead levels >45 mcg/dL
Usual Dosage Oral: Children: 10 mg/kg/dose (or 350 mg/m^2/dose) every 8 hours for 5 days followed by 10 mg/kg/dose (or 350 mg/m^2/dose) every 12 hours for 14 days
Note: Treatment courses may be repeated, but 2-week intervals between courses is generally recommended.
Dosage Forms
Capsule:
Chemet®: 100 mg

succinylcholine (suks in il KOE leen)

Synonyms succinylcholine chloride; suxamethonium chloride
U.S./Canadian Brand Names Anectine® [US]; Quelicin® [US/Can]
Therapeutic Category Skeletal Muscle Relaxant
Use Adjunct to general anesthesia to facilitate both rapid sequence and routine endotracheal intubation and to relax skeletal muscles during surgery; to reduce the intensity of muscle contractions of pharmacologically- or electrically-induced convulsions; does not relieve pain or produce sedation
Usual Dosage I.M., I.V.: Dose to effect; doses will vary due to interpatient variability; use ideal body weight for obese patients
I.M.: Children and Adults: Up to 3-4 mg/kg, total dose should not exceed 150 mg
I.V.:
Children: **Note:** Because of the risk of malignant hyperthermia, use of continuous infusions is not recommended in infants and children
Smaller Children: Intermittent: Initial: 2 mg/kg/dose one time; maintenance: 0.3-0.6 mg/kg/dose every 5-10 minutes as needed
Older Children and Adolescents: Intermittent: Initial: 1 mg/kg/dose one time; maintenance: 0.3-0.6 mg/kg every 5-10 minutes as needed
Adults: Initial:
Short surgical procedures: 0.6 mg/kg (range 0.3-1.1 mg/kg)
Long surgical procedures:
Continuous infusion: 2.5-4.3 mg/minute; adjust dose based on response
Intermittent: Initial: 0.3-1.1 mg/kg; maintenance: 0.04-0.07 mg/kg/dose as required
Note: Initial dose of succinylcholine must be increased when nondepolarizing agent pretreatment used because of the antagonism between succinylcholine and nondepolarizing neuromuscular-blocking agents.
Dosage Forms
Injection, solution:
Anectine®: 20 mg/mL (10 mL)
Quelicin®: 20 mg/mL (5 mL, 10 mL); 100 mg/mL (10 mL)

succinylcholine chloride *see* succinylcholine *on this page*

Sucraid® **[US/Can]** *see* sacrosidase *on page 771*

sucralfate (soo KRAL fate)

Sound-Alike/Look-Alike Issues
sucralfate may be confused with salsalate
Carafate® may be confused with Cafergot®
Synonyms aluminum sucrose sulfate, basic
U.S./Canadian Brand Names Carafate® [US]; Novo-Sucralate [Can]; Nu-Sucralate [Can]; PMS-Sucralate [Can]; Sulcrate® Suspension Plus [Can]; Sulcrate® [Can]
Therapeutic Category Gastrointestinal Agent, Gastric or Duodenal Ulcer Treatment
Use Short-term (≤8 weeks) management of duodenal ulcers; maintenance therapy for duodenal ulcers
Usual Dosage Oral:
Children: Dose not established, doses of 40-80 mg/kg/day divided every 6 hours have been used

Adults:
  Stress ulcer prophylaxis: 1 g 4 times/day
  Stress ulcer treatment: 1 g every 4 hours
  Duodenal ulcer:
    Treatment: 1 g 4 times/day on an empty stomach and at bedtime for 4-8 weeks, or alternatively 2 g twice daily; treatment is recommended for 4-8 weeks in adults
    Maintenance: Prophylaxis: 1 g twice daily
Dosage Forms
  Suspension, oral: 1 g/10 mL (10 mL)
    Carafate®: 1 g/10 mL
  Tablet: 1 g
    Carafate®: 1 g

Sucrets® [US-OTC] *see* dyclonine *on page 287*

Sucrets® Cough Calmers (Discontinued) *see* dextromethorphan *on page 247*

Sucrets® Original [US-OTC] *see* hexylresorcinol *on page 420*

Sudafed® 12 Hour [US-OTC] *see* pseudoephedrine *on page 727*

Sudafed® 24 Hour [US-OTC] *see* pseudoephedrine *on page 727*

Sudafed® Children's [US-OTC] *see* pseudoephedrine *on page 727*

Sudafed® Children's Cold & Cough [US-OTC] *see* pseudoephedrine and dextromethorphan *on page 728*

Sudafed® Cold & Cough Extra Strength [Can] *see* acetaminophen, dextromethorphan, and pseudoephedrine *on page 12*

Sudafed® Decongestant [Can] *see* pseudoephedrine *on page 727*

Sudafed® Head Cold and Sinus Extra Strength [Can] *see* acetaminophen and pseudoephedrine *on page 8*

Sudafed® Maximum Strength Nasal Decongestant [US-OTC] *see* pseudoephedrine *on page 727*

Sudafed® Maximum Strength Sinus Nighttime (Discontinued) *see* triprolidine and pseudoephedrine *on page 869*

Sudafed® Multi-Symptom Sinus and Cold [US-OTC] *see* acetaminophen and pseudoephedrine *on page 8*

Sudafed® Non-Drying Sinus (Discontinued) *see* guaifenesin and pseudoephedrine *on page 406*

Sudafed PE™ [US-OTC] *see* phenylephrine *on page 675*

Sudafed® Severe Cold [US-OTC] *see* acetaminophen, dextromethorphan, and pseudoephedrine *on page 12*

Sudafed® Sinus Advance [Can] *see* pseudoephedrine and ibuprofen *on page 729*

Sudafed® Sinus & Allergy [US-OTC] *see* chlorpheniramine and pseudoephedrine *on page 178*

Sudal® 12 [US] *see* chlorpheniramine and pseudoephedrine *on page 178*

Sudex® (Discontinued) *see* guaifenesin and pseudoephedrine *on page 406*

Sudodrin [US-OTC] *see* pseudoephedrine *on page 727*

SudoGest [US-OTC] *see* pseudoephedrine *on page 727*

SudoGest Children's [US-OTC] *see* pseudoephedrine and dextromethorphan *on page 728*

Sudo-Tab® [US-OTC] *see* pseudoephedrine *on page 727*

Sufedrin® (Discontinued) *see* pseudoephedrine *on page 727*

Sufenta® [US/Can] *see* sufentanil *on this page*

sufentanil (soo FEN ta nil)
Sound-Alike/Look-Alike Issues
  sufentanil may be confused with alfentanil, fentanyl
  Sufenta® may be confused with Alfenta®, Sudafed®, Survanta®
Synonyms sufentanil citrate
U.S./Canadian Brand Names Sufentanil Citrate Injection, USP [Can]; Sufenta® [US/Can]
Therapeutic Category Analgesic, Narcotic; General Anesthetic
Controlled Substance C-II
Use Analgesic supplement in maintenance of balanced general anesthesia; primary anesthetic for induction and maintenance of anesthesia in patients undergoing major surgical procedures; epidural anesthetic in conjunction with bupivacaine in labor and delivery
(Continued)

sufentanil *(Continued)*

Usual Dosage

I.V.:

Children 2-12 years: Induction: 10-25 mcg/kg (10-15 mcg/kg most common dose) with 100% O_2; Maintenance: Up to 1-2 mcg/kg total dose

Adults: Dose should be based on body weight. **Note:** In obese patients (eg, >20% above ideal body weight), use lean body weight to determine dosage.

Surgical analgesia (surgery 1-2 hours long): Total dose: 1-2 mcg/kg; ≥75% of dose administered prior to intubation; administered with N_2O/O_2; Maintenance: 5-20 mcg as needed. Total dose should not exceed 1 mcg/kg/hour of expected surgical time.

Epidural: Adults: Analgesia: Labor and delivery: 10-15 mcg with 10 mL bupivacaine 0.125% with/without epinephrine. May repeat at ≥1-hour interval for 2 additional doses.

Dosage Forms

Injection, solution [preservative free]: 50 mcg/mL (1 mL, 2 mL, 5 mL)

Sufenta®: 50 mcg/mL (1 mL, 2 mL, 5 mL)

sufentanil citrate *see* sufentanil *on previous page*

Sufentanil Citrate Injection, USP [Can] *see* sufentanil *on previous page*

Sular® [US] *see* nisoldipine *on page 606*

sulbactam and ampicillin *see* ampicillin and sulbactam *on page 54*

sulconazole *(sul KON a zole)*

Synonyms sulconazole nitrate

U.S./Canadian Brand Names Exelderm® [US/Can]

Therapeutic Category Antifungal Agent

Use Treatment of superficial fungal infections of the skin, including tinea cruris (jock itch), tinea corporis (ringworm), tinea versicolor, and possibly tinea pedis (athlete's foot, cream only)

Usual Dosage Topical: Adults: Apply a small amount to the affected area and gently massage once or twice daily for 3 weeks (tinea cruris, tinea corporis, tinea versicolor) to 4 weeks (tinea pedis).

Dosage Forms

Cream:

Exelderm®: 1% (15 g, 30 g, 60 g)

Solution, topical:

Exelderm®: 1% (30 mL)

sulconazole nitrate *see* sulconazole *on this page*

Sulcrate® [Can] *see* sucralfate *on page 808*

Sulcrate® Suspension Plus [Can] *see* sucralfate *on page 808*

sulfabenzamide, sulfacetamide, and sulfathiazole

(sul fa BENZ a mide, sul fa SEE ta mide, & sul fa THYE a zole)

Synonyms triple sulfa

U.S./Canadian Brand Names V.V.S.® [US]

Therapeutic Category Antibiotic, Vaginal

Use Treatment of *Haemophilus vaginalis* vaginitis

Usual Dosage Intravaginal: Adults: Female: Cream: Insert one applicatorful into vagina twice daily for 4-6 days; dosage may then be decreased to $1/2$ to $1/4$ of an applicatorful twice daily

Dosage Forms

Cream, vaginal: Sulfabenzamide 3.7%, sulfacetamide 2.86%, and sulfathiazole 3.42% (78 g with applicator)

V.V.S.®: Sulfabenzamide 3.7%, sulfacetamide 2.86%, and sulfathiazole 3.42% (78 g with applicator)

sulfacetamide *(sul fa SEE ta mide)*

Sound-Alike/Look-Alike Issues

Bleph®-10 may be confused with Blephamide®

Klaron® may be confused with Klor-Con®

Synonyms sodium sulfacetamide; sulfacetamide sodium

U.S./Canadian Brand Names Bleph®-10 [US]; Carmol® Scalp [US]; Cetamide™ [Can]; Diosulf™ [Can]; Klaron® [US]; Mexar™ Wash [US]; Ovace® Wash [US]; Ovace® [US]; Rosula® NS [US]

Therapeutic Category Antibiotic, Ophthalmic

Use

Ophthalmic: Treatment and prophylaxis of conjunctivitis due to susceptible organisms; corneal ulcers; adjunctive treatment with systemic sulfonamides for therapy of trachoma

Dermatologic: Scaling dermatosis (seborrheic); bacterial infections of the skin; acne vulgaris

Usual Dosage

Children >2 months and Adults: Ophthalmic:

Ointment: Apply to lower conjunctival sac 1-4 times/day and at bedtime

Solution: Instill 1-2 drops several times daily up to every 2-3 hours in lower conjunctival sac during waking hours and less frequently at night; increase dosing interval as condition responds. Usual duration of treatment: 7-10 days

Trachoma: Instill 2 drops into the conjunctival sac every 2 hours; must be used in conjunction with systemic therapy

Children >12 years and Adults: Topical:

Acne: Apply thin film to affected area twice daily

Seborrheic dermatitis: Apply at bedtime and allow to remain overnight; in severe cases, may apply twice daily. Duration of therapy is usually 8-10 applications; dosing interval may be increased as eruption subsides. Applications once or twice weekly, or every other week may be used to prevent eruptions.

Secondary cutaneous bacterial infections: Apply 2-4 times/day until infection clears

Dosage Forms

Cream, topical:
Ovace®: 10% (30 g, 60 g)

Foam, topical:
Ovace®: 10% (50 g, 100 g)

Gel, topical:
Ovace®: 10% (30 g, 60 g)

Lotion:
Carmol® Scalp: 10% (85 g)
Klaron®: 10% (120 mL)
Ovace® Wash: 10% (180 mL, 360 mL)

Ointment, ophthalmic: 10% (3.5 g)

Pad: topical:
Rosula® NS: 10% (30s)

Soap, topical:
Mexar™ Wash: 10% (170 mL)

Solution, ophthalmic: 10% (15 mL)
Bleph®-10: 10% (5 mL)

Suspension, topical: 10% (118 mL)

sulfacetamide and prednisolone (sul fa SEE ta mide & pred NIS oh lone)

Sound-Alike/Look-Alike Issues
Blephamide® may be confused with Bleph®-10
Vasocidin® may be confused with Vasodilan®

Synonyms prednisolone and sulfacetamide

U.S./Canadian Brand Names Blephamide® [US/Can]; Dioptimyd® [Can]

Therapeutic Category Antibiotic/Corticosteroid, Ophthalmic

Use Steroid-responsive inflammatory ocular conditions where infection is present or there is a risk of infection; ophthalmic suspension may be used as an otic preparation

Usual Dosage Ophthalmic: Children >2 months and Adults:
Ointment: Apply to lower conjunctival sac 1-4 times/day
Solution, suspension: Instill 1-3 drops every 2-3 hours while awake

Dosage Forms

Ointment, ophthalmic:
Blephamide®: Sulfacetamide 10% and prednisolone 0.2% (3.5 g)

Solution, ophthalmic: Sulfacetamide 10% and prednisolone 0.25% (5 mL, 10 mL)

Suspension, ophthalmic:
Blephamide®: Sulfacetamide 10% and prednisolone 0.2% (5 mL, 10 mL)

sulfacetamide and sulfur *see* sulfur and sulfacetamide *on page 815*

sulfacetamide sodium *see* sulfacetamide *on previous page*

sulfacetamide sodium and fluorometholone
(sul fa SEE ta mide SOW dee um & flure oh METH oh lone)

Synonyms fluorometholone and sulfacetamide

U.S./Canadian Brand Names FML-S® [US]

Therapeutic Category Antibiotic/Corticosteroid, Ophthalmic

Use Steroid-responsive inflammatory ocular conditions where infection is present or there is a risk of infection

Usual Dosage Ophthalmic: Children >2 years and Adults: Instill 1 drop into affected eye(s) 4 times/day

(Continued)

sulfacetamide sodium and fluorometholone *(Continued)*

Note: Dose may be decreased but should not be discontinued prematurely; reevaluation should occur if improvement is not seen within 2 days; in chronic conditions, dosing frequency should be gradually decreased prior to discontinuing treatment

Dosage Forms

Suspension, ophthalmic:

FML-S®: Sulfacetamide sodium 10% and fluorometholone 0.1% (5 mL, 10 mL)

Sulfacet-R® [US/Can] *see* sulfur and sulfacetamide *on page 815*

sulfadiazine (sul fa DYE a zeen)

Sound-Alike/Look-Alike Issues

sulfaDIAZINE may be confused with sulfasalazine, sulfiSOXAZOLE

Tall-Man sulfa**DIAZINE**

Therapeutic Category Sulfonamide

Use Treatment of urinary tract infections and nocardiosis; adjunctive treatment in toxoplasmosis; uncomplicated attack of malaria

Usual Dosage Oral:

Asymptomatic meningococcal carriers:

Infants 1-12 months: 500 mg once daily for 2 days

Children 1-12 years: 500 mg twice daily for 2 days

Adults: 1 g twice daily for 2 days

Congenital toxoplasmosis:

Newborns and Children <2 months: 100 mg/kg/day divided every 6 hours in conjunction with pyrimethamine 1 mg/kg/day once daily and supplemental folinic acid 5 mg every 3 days for 6 months

Children >2 months: 25-50 mg/kg/dose 4 times/day

Nocardiosis: 4-8 g/day for a minimum of 6 weeks

Toxoplasmosis:

Children >2 months: Loading dose: 75 mg/kg; maintenance dose: 120-150 mg/kg/day, maximum dose: 6 g/day; divided every 4-6 hours in conjunction with pyrimethamine 2 mg/kg/day divided every 12 hours for 3 days followed by 1 mg/kg/day once daily with supplemental folinic acid

Adults: 2-6 g/day in divided doses every 6 hours in conjunction with pyrimethamine 50-75 mg/day and with supplemental folinic acid

Dosage Forms

Tablet: 500 mg

sulfadoxine and pyrimethamine (sul fa DOKS een & peer i METH a meen)

Synonyms pyrimethamine and sulfadoxine

U.S./Canadian Brand Names Fansidar® [US]

Therapeutic Category Antimalarial Agent

Use Treatment of *Plasmodium falciparum* malaria in patients in whom chloroquine resistance is suspected; malaria prophylaxis for travelers to areas where chloroquine-resistant malaria is endemic

Usual Dosage Oral: Children and Adults:

Treatment of acute attack of malaria: A single dose of the following number of Fansidar® tablets is used in sequence with quinine or alone:

2-11 months: ¼ tablet

1-3 years: ½ tablet

4-8 years: 1 tablet

9-14 years: 2 tablets

>14 years: 3 tablets

Malaria prophylaxis: A single dose should be carried for self-treatment in the event of febrile illness when medical attention is not immediately available:

2-11 months: ¼ tablet

1-3 years: ½ tablet

4-8 years: 1 tablet

9-14 years: 2 tablets

>14 years and Adults: 3 tablets

Dosage Forms

Tablet:

Fansidar®: Sulfadoxine 500 mg and pyrimethamine 25 mg

Sulfa-Gyn® *(Discontinued)* *see* sulfabenzamide, sulfacetamide, and sulfathiazole *on page 810*

Sulfamethoprim® *(Discontinued)*

sulfamethoxazole and trimethoprim (sul fa meth OKS a zole & trye METH oh prim)

Sound-Alike/Look-Alike Issues

Bactrim™ may be confused with bacitracin, Bactine®

co-trimoxazole may be confused with clotrimazole

Septra® may be confused with Ceptaz®, Sectral®, Septa®

Synonyms co-trimoxazole; SMZ-TMP; sulfatrim; TMP-SMZ; trimethoprim and sulfamethoxazole

U.S./Canadian Brand Names Apo-Sulfatrim® DS [Can]; Apo-Sulfatrim® Pediatric [Can]; Apo-Sulfatrim® [Can]; Bactrim™ DS [US]; Bactrim™ [US]; Novo-Trimel D.S. [Can]; Novo-Trimel [Can]; Nu-Cotrimox [Can]; Septra® DS [US]; Septra® Injection [Can]; Septra® [US]

Therapeutic Category Sulfonamide

Use

Oral treatment of urinary tract infections due to *E. coli*, *Klebsiella* and *Enterobacter* sp, *M. morganii*, *P. mirabilis* and *P. vulgaris*; acute otitis media in children; acute exacerbations of chronic bronchitis in adults due to susceptible strains of *H. influenzae* or *S. pneumoniae*; treatment and prophylaxis of *Pneumocystis jiroveci* pneumonitis (PCP); traveler's diarrhea due to enterotoxigenic *E. coli*; treatment of enteritis caused by *Shigella flexneri* or *Shigella sonnei*

I.V. treatment or severe or complicated infections when oral therapy is not feasible, for documented PCP, empiric treatment of PCP in immune compromised patients; treatment of documented or suspected shigellosis, typhoid fever, *Nocardia asteroides* infection, or other infections caused by susceptible bacteria

Usual Dosage Dosage recommendations are based on the trimethoprim component. Double-strength tablets are equivalent to sulfamethoxazole 800 mg and trimethoprim 160 mg.

Children >2 months:

General dosing guidelines:

Mild-to-moderate infections: Oral: 8-12 mg TMP/kg/day in divided doses every 12 hours

Serious infection:

Oral: 20 mg TMP/kg/day in divided doses every 6 hours

I.V.: 8-12 mg TMP/kg/day in divided doses every 6 hours

Acute otitis media: Oral: 8 mg TMP/kg/day in divided doses every 12 hours for 10 days

Urinary tract infection:

Treatment:

Oral: 6-12 mg TMP/kg/day in divided doses every 12 hours

I.V.: 8-10 mg TMP/kg/day in divided doses every 6, 8, or 12 hours for up to 4 days with serious infections

Prophylaxis: Oral: 2 mg TMP/kg/dose daily or 5 mg TMP/kg/dose twice weekly

Pneumocystis:

Treatment: Oral, I.V.: 15-20 mg TMP/kg/day in divided doses every 6-8 hours

Prophylaxis: Oral, 150 mg TMP/m^2/day in divided doses every 12 hours for 3 days/week; dose should not exceed trimethoprim 320 mg and sulfamethoxazole 1600 mg daily

Alternative prophylaxis dosing schedules include:

150 mg TMP/m^2/day as a single daily dose 3 times/week on consecutive days

or

150 mg TMP/m^2/day in divided doses every 12 hours administered 7 days/week

or

150 mg TMP/m^2/day in divided doses every 12 hours administered 3 times/week on alternate days

Shigellosis:

Oral: 8 mg TMP/kg/day in divided doses every 12 hours for 5 days

I.V.: 8-10 mg TMP/kg/day in divided doses every 6, 8, or 12 hours for up to 5 days

Adults:

Urinary tract infection:

Oral: One double-strength tablet every 12 hours

Duration of therapy: Uncomplicated: 3-5 days; Complicated: 7-10 days

Pyelonephritis: 14 days

Prostatitis: Acute: 2 weeks; Chronic: 2-3 months

I.V.: 8-10 mg TMP/kg/day in divided doses every 6, 8, or 12 hours for up to 14 days with severe infections

Chronic bronchitis: Oral: One double-strength tablet every 12 hours for 10-14 days

Meningitis (bacterial): I.V.: 10-20 mg TMP/kg/day in divided doses every 6-12 hours

Shigellosis:

Oral: One double strength tablet every 12 hours for 5 days

I.V.: 8-10 mg TMP/kg/day in divided doses every 6, 8, or 12 hours for up to 5 days

Travelers' diarrhea: Oral: One double strength tablet every 12 hours for 5 days

Sepsis: I.V.: 20 TMP/kg/day divided every 6 hours

Pneumocystis jiroveci:

Prophylaxis: Oral: 1 double strength tablet daily or 3 times/week

Treatment: Oral, I.V.: 15-20 mg TMP/kg/day in 3-4 divided doses

Dosage Forms The 5:1 ratio (SMX:TMP) remains constant in all dosage forms.

Injection, solution: Sulfamethoxazole 80 mg and trimethoprim 16 mg per mL (5 mL, 10 mL, 30 mL)

(Continued)

sulfamethoxazole and trimethoprim *(Continued)*

Suspension, oral: Sulfamethoxazole 200 mg and trimethoprim 40 mg per 5 mL
Tablet: Sulfamethoxazole 400 mg and trimethoprim 80 mg
Bactrim™, Septra®: Sulfamethoxazole 400 mg and trimethoprim 80 mg
Tablet, double strength: Sulfamethoxazole 800 mg and trimethoprim 160 mg
Bactrim™ DS, Septra® DS: Sulfamethoxazole 800 mg and trimethoprim 160 mg

Sulfamylon® [US] *see* mafenide *on page 524*

sulfasalazine (sul fa SAL a zeen)

Sound-Alike/Look-Alike Issues
sulfasalazine may be confused with salsalate, sulfaDIAZINE, sulfiSOXAZOLE
Azulfidine® may be confused with Augmentin®, azathioprine
Synonyms salicylazosulfapyridine
U.S./Canadian Brand Names Alti-Sulfasalazine [Can]; Azulfidine® EN-tabs® [US]; Azulfidine® [US]; Salazo-pyrin En-Tabs® [Can]; Salazopyrin® [Can]; Sulfazine EC [US]; Sulfazine [US]
Therapeutic Category 5-Aminosalicylic Acid Derivative
Use Management of ulcerative colitis; enteric coated tablets are also used for rheumatoid arthritis (including juvenile rheumatoid arthritis) in patients who inadequately respond to analgesics and NSAIDs
Usual Dosage Oral:
Children ≥2 years: Ulcerative colitis: Initial: 40-60 mg/kg/day in 3-6 divided doses; maintenance dose: 20-30 mg/kg/day in 4 divided doses
Children ≥6 years: Juvenile rheumatoid arthritis: Enteric coated tablet: 30-50 mg/kg/day in 2 divided doses; Initial: Begin with $1/4$ to $1/3$ of expected maintenance dose; increase weekly; maximum: 2 g/day typically
Adults:
Ulcerative colitis: Initial: 1 g 3-4 times/day, 2 g/day maintenance in divided doses; may initiate therapy with 0.5-1 g/day
Rheumatoid arthritis: Enteric coated tablet: Initial: 0.5-1 g/day; increase weekly to maintenance dose of 2 g/day in 2 divided doses; maximum: 3 g/day (if response to 2 g/day is inadequate after 12 weeks of treatment)
Dosage Forms
Tablet: 500 mg
Azulfidine®, Sulfazine: 500 mg
Tablet, delayed release, enteric coated: 500 mg
Azulfidine® EN-tabs®, Sulfazine EC: 500 mg

sulfatrim *see* sulfamethoxazole and trimethoprim *on previous page*

Sulfa-Trip® *(Discontinued)* *see* sulfabenzamide, sulfacetamide, and sulfathiazole *on page 810*

Sulfazine [US] *see* sulfasalazine *on this page*

Sulfazine EC [US] *see* sulfasalazine *on this page*

sulfinpyrazone (sul fin PEER a zone)

U.S./Canadian Brand Names Apo-Sulfinpyrazone® [Can]; Nu-Sulfinpyrazone [Can]
Therapeutic Category Uricosuric Agent
Use Treatment of chronic gouty arthritis and intermittent gouty arthritis
Usual Dosage Oral: Adults: 100-200 mg twice daily; maximum daily dose: 800 mg
Dosage Forms [CAN] = Canadian brand name
Tablet: 100 mg [not available in the U.S.]
Apo-Sulfinpyrazone® [CAN], Nu-Sulfinpyrazone [CAN]: 100 mg [not available in the U.S.]

sulfisoxazole (sul fi SOKS a zole)

Sound-Alike/Look-Alike Issues
sulfiSOXAZOLE may be confused with sulfaDIAZINE, sulfamethoxazole, sulfasalazine
Gantrisin® may be confused with Gastrosed™
Synonyms sulfisoxazole acetyl; sulphafurazole
Tall-Man sulfiSOXAZOLE
U.S./Canadian Brand Names Gantrisin® [US]; Novo-Soxazole [Can]; Sulfizole® [Can]
Therapeutic Category Sulfonamide
Use Treatment of urinary tract infections, otitis media, *Chlamydia*; nocardiosis
Usual Dosage Oral: Not for use in patients <2 months of age:
Children >2 months: Initial: 75 mg/kg, followed by 120-150 mg/kg/day in divided doses every 4-6 hours; not to exceed 6 g/day
Adults: Initial: 2-4 g, then 4-8 g/day in divided doses every 4-6 hours

Dosage Forms
 Suspension, oral, pediatric:
  Gantrisin®: 500 mg/5 mL
  Tablet: 500 mg

sulfisoxazole acetyl *see* sulfisoxazole *on previous page*

sulfisoxazole and erythromycin *see* erythromycin and sulfisoxazole *on page 310*

Sulfizole® [Can] *see* sulfisoxazole *on previous page*

sulfur and sulfacetamide (SUL fur & sul fa SEE ta mide)

 Synonyms sodium sulfacetamide and sulfur; sulfacetamide and sulfur; sulfur and sulfacetamide sodium
 U.S./Canadian Brand Names AVAR™ Green [US]; AVAR™ [US]; AVAR™-e Green [US]; AVAR™-e [US]; Clenia™ [US]; Plexion SCT® [US]; Plexion TS® [US]; Plexion® [US]; Rosac® [US]; Rosanil® [US]; Rosula® [US]; Sulfacet-R® [US/Can]; Suphera™ [US]; Zetacet® [US]
 Therapeutic Category Antiseborrheic Agent, Topical
 Use Aid in the treatment of acne vulgaris, acne rosacea, and seborrheic dermatitis
 Usual Dosage Topical: Children ≥12 years and Adults: Apply in a thin film 1-3 times/day. Cleansing products should be used 1-2 times/day.
 Dosage Forms
  Cleanser, topical:
   AVAR™: Sulfur 5% and sulfacetamide 10% (228 g)
   Plexion®: Sulfur 5% and sulfacetamide 10% (170 g, 340 g)
   Rosanil®: Sulfur 5% and sulfacetamide 10% (170 g, 390 g)
   Rosula®: Sulfur 5% and sulfacetamide 10% (355 mL)
  Cream, topical:
   AVAR™-e, AVAR™-e Green, Rosac®: Sulfur 5% and sulfacetamide 10% (45 g)
   Clenia™: Sulfur 5% and sulfacetamide sodium 10% (28 g)
   Plexion SCT®: Sulfur 5% and sulfacetamide sodium 10% (120 g)
   Suphera™: Sulfur 5% and sulfacetamide sodium 10% (113 g)
  Gel, topical:
   AVAR™, AVAR™ Green, Rosula®: Sulfur 5% and sulfacetamide 10% (45 g)
  Lotion, topical: Sulfur 5% and sulfacetamide 10% (25 g, 30 g, 45 g, 60 g)
   Sulfacaet-R®, Zetacet®: Sulfur 5% and sulfacetamide 10% (25 g)
  Pad [cleansing cloth]:
   Plexion®: Sulfur 5% and sulfacetamide 10% (30s, 60s)
  Suspension, topical: Sulfur 5% and sulfacetamide 10% (30 g)
   Plexion® TS, Zetacet®: Sulfur 5% and sulfacetamide 10% (30 g)
  Wash, topical: Sulfur 5% and sulfacetamide 10% (170 g, 340 g)
   Rosac®: Sulfur 1% and sulfacetamide sodium 10% (170 g)
   Clenia™, Zetacet®: Sulfur 5% and sulfacetamide 10% (170 g, 340 g)

sulfur and sulfacetamide sodium *see* sulfur and sulfacetamide *on this page*

sulindac (SUL in dak)

 Sound-Alike/Look-Alike Issues
  Clinoril® may be confused with Cleocin®, Clozaril®, Oruvail®
 U.S./Canadian Brand Names Apo-Sulin® [Can]; Clinoril® [US]; Novo-Sundac [Can]; Nu-Sundac [Can]
 Therapeutic Category Analgesic, Nonnarcotic; Nonsteroidal Antiinflammatory Drug (NSAID)
 Use Management of inflammatory disease, osteoarthritis, rheumatoid disorders, acute gouty arthritis, ankylosing spondylitis, bursitis/tendonitis of shoulder
 Usual Dosage Oral: Adults: **Note:** Maximum daily dose: 400 mg
  Osteoarthritis, rheumatoid arthritis, ankylosing spondylitis: 150 mg twice/daily
  Bursitis/tendonitis: 200 mg twice daily; usual treatment: 7-14 days
  Acute gouty arthritis: 200 mg twice daily; usual treatment: 7 days
 Dosage Forms
  Tablet: 150 mg, 200 mg
   Clinoril®: 200 mg

sulphafurazole *see* sulfisoxazole *on previous page*

Sultrin™ *(Discontinued)* *see* sulfabenzamide, sulfacetamide, and sulfathiazole *on page 810*

sumatriptan (soo ma TRIP tan)

 Sound-Alike/Look-Alike Issues
  sumatriptan may be confused with somatropin, zolmitriptan
 (Continued)

sumatriptan *(Continued)*

Synonyms sumatriptan succinate

U.S./Canadian Brand Names Apo-Sumatriptan® [Can]; CO Sumatriptan [Can]; Dom-Sumatriptan [Can]; Gen-Sumatriptan [Can]; Imitrex® DF [Can]; Imitrex® Nasal Spray [Can]; Imitrex® [US/Can]; Novo-Sumatriptan [Can]; PHL-Sumatriptan [Can]; PMS-Sumatriptan [Can]; ratio-Sumatriptan [Can]; Rhoxal-sumatriptan [Can]; Riva-Sumatriptan [Can]; Sandoz-Sumatriptan [Can]; Sumatryx [Can]

Therapeutic Category Antimigraine Agent

Use

Oral, SubQ: Acute treatment of migraine with or without aura

SubQ: Acute treatment of cluster headache episodes

Usual Dosage Adults:

Oral: A single dose of 25 mg, 50 mg, or 100 mg (taken with fluids). If a satisfactory response has not been obtained at 2 hours, a second dose may be administered. Results from clinical trials show that initial doses of 50 mg and 100 mg are more effective than doses of 25 mg, and that 100 mg doses do not provide a greater effect than 50 mg and may have increased incidence of side effects. Although doses of up to 300 mg/day have been studied, the total daily dose should not exceed 200 mg. The safety of treating an average of >4 headaches in a 30-day period have not been established.

Intranasal: A single dose of 5 mg, 10 mg, or 20 mg administered in one nostril. A 10 mg dose may be achieved by administering a single 5 mg dose in each nostril. If headache returns, the dose may be repeated once after 2 hours, not to exceed a total daily dose of 40 mg. The safety of treating an average of >4 headaches in a 30-day period has not been established.

SubQ: Up to 6 mg; if side effects are dose-limiting, lower doses may be used. A second injection may be administered at least 1 hour after the initial dose, but not more than 2 injections in a 24-hour period.

Dosage Forms

Injection, solution:

Imitrex®: 8 mg/mL (0.5 mL); 12 mg/mL (0.5 mL)

Solution, intranasal spray:

Imitrex®: 5 mg (100 µL unit dose spray device); 20 mg (100 µL unit dose spray device)

Tablet:

Imitrex®: 25 mg, 50 mg, 100 mg

sumatriptan succinate *see* sumatriptan *on previous page*

Sumatryx [Can] *see* sumatriptan *on previous page*

Summer's Eve® Anti-Itch Maximum Strength [US-OTC] *see* pramoxine *on page 706*

Summer's Eve® Medicated Douche [US-OTC] *see* povidone-iodine *on page 704*

Summer's Eve® SpecialCare™ Medicated Anti-Itch Cream *(Discontinued)* *see* hydrocortisone (topical) *on page 434*

Sumycin® *(Discontinued)* *see* tetracycline *on page 831*

Sun-Benz® [Can] *see* benzydamine *(Canada only) on page 105*

sunitinib *(su NIT e nib)*

Synonyms NSC736511; SU11248; sunitinib maleate

U.S./Canadian Brand Names Sutent® [US]

Therapeutic Category Antineoplastic Agent, Tyrosine Kinase Inhibitor; Vascular Endothelial Growth Factor (VEGF) Inhibitor

Use Treatment of gastrointestinal stromal tumor (GIST) following failure of or intolerance to imatinib; treatment of advanced renal cell cancer (RCC)

Usual Dosage Oral: Adults: Gastrointestinal stromal tumor, renal cell cancer: 50 mg once daily for 4 weeks of a 6-week treatment cycle (4 weeks on, 2 weeks off). **Note:** Dose increase or reduction should be done in increments of 12.5 mg; individualize based on safety and tolerability.

Dosage Forms

Capsule:

Sutent®: 12.5 mg, 25 mg, 50 mg

sunitinib maleate *see* sunitinib *on this page*

Supartz™ [US] *see* hyaluronate and derivatives *on page 423*

Super Dec B 100 [US-OTC] *see* vitamin B complex combinations *on page 894*

Superdophilus® [US-OTC] *see* Lactobacillus *on page 488*

Superplex-T™ [US-OTC] *see* vitamin B complex combinations *on page 894*

Super Quints 50 [US-OTC] *see* vitamin B complex combinations *on page 894*

Supeudol® [Can] *see* oxycodone *on page 640*

Suphera™ **[US]** *see* sulfur and sulfacetamide *on page 815*

Suplasyn® **[Can]** *see* hyaluronate and derivatives *on page 423*

Suppress® *(Discontinued) see* dextromethorphan *on page 247*

Suprane® **[US/Can]** *see* desflurane *on page 238*

Suprefact® **[Can]** *see* buserelin acetate *(Canada only) on page 128*

Suprefact® **Depot [Can]** *see* buserelin acetate *(Canada only) on page 128*

Surbex-T® **[US-OTC]** *see* vitamin B complex combinations *on page 894*

Surfak® **[US-OTC]** *see* docusate *on page 273*

Surgam® **[Can]** *see* tiaprofenic acid *(Canada only) on page 840*

Surgicel® **[US]** *see* cellulose, oxidized regenerated *on page 167*

Surgicel® **Fibrillar [US]** *see* cellulose, oxidized regenerated *on page 167*

Surgicel® **NuKnit [US]** *see* cellulose, oxidized regenerated *on page 167*

Surmontil® **[US]** *see* trimipramine *on page 868*

Survanta® **[US/Can]** *see* beractant *on page 106*

Sus-Phrine® *(Discontinued) see* epinephrine *on page 300*

Sustaire® *(Discontinued) see* theophylline *on page 834*

Sustiva® **[US/Can]** *see* efavirenz *on page 292*

Sutent® **[US]** *see* sunitinib *on previous page*

Su-Tuss DM [US] *see* guaifenesin and dextromethorphan *on page 402*

Su-Tuss®**-HD [US]** *see* hydrocodone, pseudoephedrine, and guaifenesin *on page 432*

suxamethonium chloride *see* succinylcholine *on page 808*

Sween Cream® **[US-OTC]** *see* vitamin A and vitamin D *on page 893*

Symadine® *(Discontinued)*

Symax SL [US] *see* hyoscyamine *on page 441*

Symax SR [US] *see* hyoscyamine *on page 441*

Symbicort® **[US/Can]** *see* budesonide and formoterol *on page 124*

Symbyax® **[US]** *see* olanzapine and fluoxetine *on page 627*

Symlin® **[US]** *see* pramlintide *on page 706*

Symmetrel® **[US/Can]** *see* amantadine *on page 38*

synacthen *see* cosyntropin *on page 217*

Synagis® **[US/Can]** *see* palivizumab *on page 646*

Synalar® **[US/Can]** *see* fluocinolone *on page 359*

Synalar-HP® **Topical** *(Discontinued) see* fluocinolone *on page 359*

Synalgos®**-DC [US]** *see* dihydrocodeine, aspirin, and caffeine *on page 259*

Synarel® **[US/Can]** *see* nafarelin *on page 587*

Syn-Diltiazem® **[Can]** *see* diltiazem *on page 261*

Synemol® **Topical** *(Discontinued) see* fluocinolone *on page 359*

Synera™ **[US]** *see* lidocaine and tetracaine *on page 508*

Synercid® **[US/Can]** *see* quinupristin and dalfopristin *on page 741*

Synphasic® **[Can]** *see* ethinyl estradiol and norethindrone *on page 328*

Syntest D.S. [US] *see* estrogens (esterified) and methyltestosterone *on page 320*

Syntest H.S. [US] *see* estrogens (esterified) and methyltestosterone *on page 320*

Synthroid® **[US/Can]** *see* levothyroxine *on page 503*

Syntocinon® **[Can]** *see* oxytocin *on page 644*

Synvisc® **[US]** *see* hyaluronate and derivatives *on page 423*

Syprine® **[US/Can]** *see* trientine *on page 865*

Syrex [US] *see* sodium chloride *on page 792*

SyringeAvitene™ **[US]** *see* collagen hemostat *on page 213*

syrup of ipecac *see* ipecac syrup *on page 470*

Systane® **[US-OTC]** *see* artificial tears *on page 75*

Systane® **Free [US-OTC]** *see* artificial tears *on page 75*

Sytobex® *(Discontinued) see* cyanocobalamin *on page 220*

T₃/T₄ liotrix *see* liotrix *on page 510*

T₄ *see* levothyroxine *on page 503*

T-20 *see* enfuvirtide *on page 297*

642® **Tablet [Can]** *see* propoxyphene *on page 723*

Tabloid® **[US]** *see* thioguanine *on page 837*

Tac™-40 Injection *(Discontinued)*

Taclonex® **[US]** *see* calcipotriene and betamethasone *on page 135*

tacrine (TAK reen)

Sound-Alike/Look-Alike Issues
Cognex® may be confused with Corgard®

Synonyms tacrine hydrochloride; tetrahydroaminoacrine; THA

U.S./Canadian Brand Names Cognex® [US]

Therapeutic Category Acetylcholinesterase Inhibitor; Cholinergic Agent

Use Treatment of mild to moderate dementia of the Alzheimer type

Usual Dosage Adults: Initial: 10 mg 4 times/day; may increase by 40 mg/day adjusted every 6 weeks; maximum: 160 mg/day; best administered separate from meal times.

Dose adjustment based upon transaminase elevations:

ALT ≤3 times ULN*: Continue titration

ALT >3 to ≤5 times ULN*: Decrease dose by 40 mg/day, resume when ALT returns to normal

ALT >5 times ULN*: Stop treatment, may rechallenge upon return of ALT to normal

*ULN = upper limit of normal

Patients with clinical jaundice confirmed by elevated total bilirubin (>3 mg/dL) should not be rechallenged with tacrine

Dosage Forms
Capsule:
Cognex®: 10 mg, 20 mg, 30 mg, 40 mg

tacrine hydrochloride *see* tacrine *on this page*

tacrolimus (ta KROE li mus)

Sound-Alike/Look-Alike Issues
Prograf® may be confused with Gengraf®

Synonyms FK506

U.S./Canadian Brand Names Prograf® [US/Can]; Protopic® [US/Can]

Therapeutic Category Immunosuppressant Agent

Use
Oral/injection: Potent immunosuppressive drug used in heart, kidney, or liver transplant recipients
Topical: Moderate-to-severe atopic dermatitis in patients not responsive to conventional therapy or when conventional therapy is not appropriate

Usual Dosage
Oral:
Children: **Notes:** Patients without preexisting renal or hepatic dysfunction have required (and tolerated) higher doses than adults to achieve similar blood concentrations. It is recommended that therapy be initiated at high end of the recommended adult I.V. and oral dosing ranges; dosage adjustments may be required. If switching from I.V. to oral, the oral dose should be started 8-12 hours after stopping the infusion. Adjunctive therapy with corticosteroids is recommended early post-transplant.
Liver transplant: Initial dose: 0.15-0.20 mg/kg/day in 2 divided doses, given every 12 hours; begin oral dose no sooner than 6 hours post-transplant
Adults: **Notes:** If switching from I.V. to oral, the oral dose should be started 8-12 hours after stopping the infusion. Adjunctive therapy with corticosteroids is recommended early post-transplant.
Heart transplant: Initial dose: 0.075 mg/kg/day in 2 divided doses, given every 12 hours; begin oral dose no sooner than 6 hours post-transplant
Kidney transplant: Initial dose: 0.2 mg/kg/day in 2 divided doses, given every 12 hours; initial dose may be given within 24 hours of transplant, but should be delayed until renal function has recovered; African-American patients may require larger doses to maintain trough concentration
Liver transplant: Initial dose: 0.1-0.15 mg/kg/day in 2 divided doses, given every 12 hours; begin oral dose no sooner than 6 hours post-transplant

I.V.: Children and Adults: **Note:** I.V. route should only be used in patients not able to take oral medications and continued only until oral medication can be tolerated; anaphylaxis has been reported. Begin no sooner than 6 hours post-transplant; adjunctive therapy with corticosteroids is recommended.

Heart transplant: Initial dose: 0.01 mg/kg/day as a continuous infusion

Kidney, liver transplant: Initial dose: 0.03-0.05 mg/kg/day as a continuous infusion

Prevention of graft-vs-host disease: 0.03 mg/kg/day as continuous infusion

Topical: Children ≥2 years and Adults: Atopic dermatitis (moderate to severe): Apply minimum amount of 0.03% or 0.1% ointment to affected area twice daily; rub in gently and completely. Discontinue use when symptoms have cleared. If no improvement within 6 weeks, patients should be reexamined to confirm diagnosis.

Dosage Forms
  Capsule:
  Prograf®: 0.5 mg, 1 mg, 5 mg
  Injection, solution:
  Prograf®: 5 mg/mL (1 mL)
  Ointment, topical:
  Protopic®: 0.03% (30 g, 60 g, 100 g); 0.1% (30 g, 60 g, 100 g)

tadalafil (tah DA la fil)

Synonyms GF196960
U.S./Canadian Brand Names Cialis® [US/Can]
Therapeutic Category Phosphodiesterase (Type 5) Enzyme Inhibitor
Use Treatment of erectile dysfunction
Usual Dosage Oral: Adults: Erectile dysfunction: 10 mg prior to anticipated sexual activity (dosing range: 5-20 mg); to be given as one single dose and not given more than once daily. **Note:** Erectile function may be improved for up to 36 hours following a single dose; adjust dose.
Dosage Forms
  Tablet:
  Cialis®: 5 mg, 10 mg, 20 mg

Tagamet® *(Discontinued)* see cimetidine *on page 189*

Tagamet® HB [Can] see cimetidine *on page 189*

Tagamet® HB 200 [US-OTC] see cimetidine *on page 189*

TAK-375 see ramelteon *on page 743*

Talacen® [US] see pentazocine and acetaminophen *on page 666*

Talwin® [US/Can] see pentazocine *on page 665*

Talwin® NX [US] see pentazocine *on page 665*

TAM see tamoxifen *on this page*

Tambocor™ [US/Can] see flecainide *on page 354*

Tamiflu® [US/Can] see oseltamivir *on page 635*

Tamofen® [Can] see tamoxifen *on this page*

tamoxifen (ta MOKS i fen)

Sound-Alike/Look-Alike Issues
  tamoxifen may be confused with pentoxifylline, Tambocor™
Synonyms ICI-46474; NSC-180973; TAM; tamoxifen citrate
U.S./Canadian Brand Names Apo-Tamox® [Can]; Gen-Tamoxifen [Can]; Nolvadex® [Can]; Nolvadex®-D [Can]; Novo-Tamoxifen [Can]; Soltamox™ [US]; Tamofen® [Can]
Therapeutic Category Antineoplastic Agent
Use Palliative or adjunctive treatment of advanced breast cancer; reduce the incidence of breast cancer in women at high risk; reduce risk of invasive breast cancer in women with ductal carcinoma *in situ* (DCIS); metastatic female and male breast cancer
Usual Dosage Adults: Oral (refer to individual protocols):
  Breast cancer:
  Metastatic (males and females) or adjuvant therapy (females): 20-40 mg/day; daily doses >20 mg should be given in 2 divided doses (morning and evening)
  Prevention (high-risk females): 20 mg/day for 5 years
  DCIS (females): 20 mg once daily for 5 years
  Note: Higher dosages (up to 700 mg/day) have been investigated for use in modulation of multidrug resistance (MDR), but are not routinely used in clinical practice
(Continued)

tamoxifen *(Continued)*

Dosage Forms
Solution, oral:
Soltamox™: 10 mg/5 mL
Tablet: 10 mg, 20 mg

tamoxifen citrate *see* tamoxifen *on previous page*

tamsulosin *(tam SOO loe sin)*

Sound-Alike/Look-Alike Issues
Flomax® may be confused with Fosamax®, Volmax®
Synonyms tamsulosin hydrochloride
U.S./Canadian Brand Names Flomax® CR [Can]; Flomax® [US/Can]
Therapeutic Category Alpha-Adrenergic Blocking Agent
Use Treatment of signs and symptoms of benign prostatic hyperplasia (BPH)
Usual Dosage Oral: Adults: BPH: 0.4 mg once daily ~30 minutes after the same meal each day; dose may be increased after 2-4 weeks to 0.8 mg once daily in patients who fail to respond. If therapy is interrupted for several days, restart with 0.4 mg once daily.
Dosage Forms
Capsule:
Flomax®: 0.4 mg

tamsulosin hydrochloride *see* tamsulosin *on this page*

Tanac® **[US-OTC]** *see* benzocaine *on page 101*

TanaCof-XR [US] *see* brompheniramine *on page 120*

Tanafed® *(Discontinued)* *see* chlorpheniramine and pseudoephedrine *on page 178*

Tanafed DMX™ [US] *see* chlorpheniramine, pseudoephedrine, and dextromethorphan *on page 183*

Tanafed DP™ [US] *see* dexchlorpheniramine and pseudoephedrine *on page 243*

Tandem® **OB [US]** *see* vitamins (multiple/prenatal) *on page 896*

Tannate-V-DM [US] *see* phenylephrine, pyrilamine, and dextromethorphan *on page 679*

Tannate 12 S [US] *see* carbetapentane and chlorpheniramine *on page 149*

Tannic-12 [US] *see* carbetapentane and chlorpheniramine *on page 149*

Tannic-12 S [US] *see* carbetapentane and chlorpheniramine *on page 149*

Tannihist-12 D *(Discontinued)* *see* carbetapentane, phenylephrine, and pyrilamine *on page 150*

Tannihist-12 RF [US] *see* carbetapentane and chlorpheniramine *on page 149*

Tanta-Orciprenaline® **[Can]** *see* metaproterenol *on page 548*

Tantum® **[Can]** *see* benzydamine *(Canada only)* *on page 105*

TAP-144 *see* leuprolide *on page 497*

Tapazole® **[US/Can]** *see* methimazole *on page 552*

Tarabine® **PFS** *(Discontinued)* *see* cytarabine *on page 226*

Tarceva® **[US/Can]** *see* erlotinib *on page 307*

Targel® **[Can]** *see* coal tar *on page 208*

Targretin® **[US/Can]** *see* bexarotene *on page 111*

Tarka® **[US/Can]** *see* trandolapril and verapamil *on page 857*

Taro-Amcinonide [Can] *see* amcinonide *on page 39*

Taro-Carbamazepine Chewable [Can] *see* carbamazepine *on page 147*

Taro-Ciprofloxacin [Can] *see* ciprofloxacin *on page 190*

Taro-Clindamycin [Can] *see* clindamycin *on page 198*

Taro-Clobetasol [Can] *see* clobetasol *on page 201*

Taro-Desoximetasone [Can] *see* desoximetasone *on page 240*

Taro-Mometasone [Can] *see* mometasone *on page 576*

Taro-Simvastatin [Can] *see* simvastatin *on page 787*

Taro-Sone® **[Can]** *see* betamethasone (topical) *on page 109*

Taro-Warfarin [Can] *see* warfarin *on page 899*

Tarsum® **[US-OTC]** *see* coal tar and salicylic acid *on page 209*

Tasmar® **[US]** *see* tolcapone *on page 849*

Tavist® **Allergy [US-OTC]** *see* clemastine *on page 198*

Tavist® **ND [US-OTC]** *see* loratadine *on page 517*

Taxol® **[US/Can]** *see* paclitaxel *on page 645*

Taxotere® **[US/Can]** *see* docetaxel *on page 272*

tazarotene (taz AR oh teen)

  U.S./Canadian Brand Names Avage™ [US]; Tazorac® [US/Can]

  Therapeutic Category Keratolytic Agent

  Use Topical treatment of facial acne vulgaris; topical treatment of stable plaque psoriasis of up to 20% body surface area involvement; mitigation (palliation) of facial skin wrinkling, facial mottled hyper-/hypopigmentation, and benign facial lentigines

  Usual Dosage Topical: **Note:** In patients experiencing excessive pruritus, burning, skin redness, or peeling, discontinue until integrity of the skin is restored, or reduce dosing to an interval the patient is able to tolerate.

  Children ≥12 years and Adults:

    Acne: Tazorac® cream/gel 0.1%: Cleanse the face gently. After the skin is dry, apply a thin film of tazarotene (2 mg/cm²) once daily, in the evening, to the skin where the acne lesions appear; use enough to cover the entire affected area

    Psoriasis: Tazorac® gel 0.05% or 0.1%: Apply once daily, in the evening, to psoriatic lesions using enough (2 mg/cm²) to cover only the lesion with a thin film to no more than 20% of body surface area. If a bath or shower is taken prior to application, dry the skin before applying. Unaffected skin may be more susceptible to irritation, avoid application to these areas.

  Children ≥17 years and Adults: Palliation of fine facial wrinkles, facial mottled hyper/hypopigmentation, benign facial lentigines: Avage™: Apply a pea-sized amount once daily to clean dry face at bedtime; lightly cover entire face including eyelids if desired. Emollients or moisturizers may be applied before or after; if applied before tazarotene, ensure cream or lotion has absorbed into the skin and has dried completely.

  Adults: Psoriasis: Tazorac® cream 0.05% or 0.1%: Apply once daily, in the evening, to psoriatic lesions using enough (2 mg/cm²) to cover only the lesion with a thin film to no more than 20% of body surface area. If a bath or shower is taken prior to application, dry the skin before applying. Unaffected skin may be more susceptible to irritation, avoid application to these areas.

  Dosage Forms

    Cream:

      Avage™: 0.1% (30 g)

      Tazorac®: 0.05% (30 g, 60 g); 0.1% (30 g, 60 g)

    Gel:

      Tazorac®: 0.05% (30 g, 100 g); 0.1% (30 g, 100 g)

Tazicef® **[US]** *see* ceftazidime *on page 163*

tazobactam and piperacillin *see* piperacillin and tazobactam sodium *on page 685*

Tazocin® **[Can]** *see* piperacillin and tazobactam sodium *on page 685*

Tazorac® **[US/Can]** *see* tazarotene *on this page*

Taztia XT™ **[US]** *see* diltiazem *on page 261*

TB skin test *see* tuberculin tests *on page 872*

3TC® **[Can]** *see* lamivudine *on page 489*

3TC *see* lamivudine *on page 489*

3TC, abacavir, and zidovudine *see* abacavir, lamivudine, and zidovudine *on page 2*

T-cell growth factor *see* aldesleukin *on page 26*

TCGF *see* aldesleukin *on page 26*

TCN *see* tetracycline *on page 831*

Td *see* diphtheria and tetanus toxoid *on page 267*

Td Adsorbed [Can] *see* diphtheria and tetanus toxoid *on page 267*

Tdap *see* diphtheria, tetanus toxoids, and acellular pertussis vaccine *on page 269*

TDF *see* tenofovir *on page 825*

Teardrops® **[Can]** *see* artificial tears *on page 75*

Tear Drop® **Solution *(Discontinued)*** *see* artificial tears *on page 75*

TearGard® **Ophthalmic Solution *(Discontinued)*** *see* artificial tears *on page 75*

Teargen® **[US-OTC]** *see* artificial tears *on page 75*

Teargen® **II [US-OTC]** *see* artificial tears *on page 75*

Tearisol® **[US-OTC]** *see* artificial tears *on page 75*

Tearisol® **[US-OTC]** *see* hydroxypropyl methylcellulose *on page 439*

Tears Again® **[US-OTC]** *see* artificial tears *on page 75*

Tears Again® **MC [US-OTC]** *see* hydroxypropyl methylcellulose *on page 439*

Tears Again® **Gel Drops**™ **[US-OTC]** *see* carboxymethylcellulose *on page 153*

Tears Again® **Night and Day**™ **[US-OTC]** *see* carboxymethylcellulose *on page 153*

Tears Naturale® **[US-OTC]** *see* artificial tears *on page 75*

Tears Naturale® **II [US-OTC]** *see* artificial tears *on page 75*

Tears Naturale® **Free [US-OTC]** *see* artificial tears *on page 75*

Tears Plus® **[US-OTC]** *see* artificial tears *on page 75*

Tears Renewed® **[US-OTC]** *see* artificial tears *on page 75*

TEAS *see* trolamine *on page 870*

Tebrazid™ **[Can]** *see* pyrazinamide *on page 733*

Tecnal C 1/2 [Can] *see* butalbital, aspirin, caffeine, and codeine *on page 131*

Tecnal C 1/4 [Can] *see* butalbital, aspirin, caffeine, and codeine *on page 131*

tegaserod (teg a SER od)

Synonyms HTF919; tegaserod maleate
U.S./Canadian Brand Names Zelnorm® [US]
Therapeutic Category Serotonin 5-HT₄ Receptor Agonist
Use Treatment of irritable bowel syndrome with constipation (IBS-C) and chronic idiopathic constipation (CIC) in women (<55 years of age) in which no alternative therapy exists
Usual Dosage Oral: Adults (<55 years of age): Females:
  IBS with constipation: 6 mg twice daily, before meals, for 4-6 weeks; may consider continuing treatment for an additional 4-6 weeks in patients who respond initially
  Chronic idiopathic constipation: 6 mg twice daily, before meals; the need for continued therapy should be reassessed periodically
Dosage Forms
  Tablet:
    Zelnorm®: 2 mg, 6 mg

tegaserod maleate *see* tegaserod *on this page*

Tega-Vert® **Oral** *(Discontinued)* *see* dimenhydrinate *on page 262*

Tegretol® **[US/Can]** *see* carbamazepine *on page 147*

Tegretol®**-XR [US]** *see* carbamazepine *on page 147*

Tekturna® **[US]** *see* aliskiren *on page 29*

Telachlor® **Oral** *(Discontinued)* *see* chlorpheniramine *on page 177*

Teladar® **Topical** *(Discontinued)*

telbivudine (tel BI vyoo deen)

Synonyms L-deoxythymidine
U.S./Canadian Brand Names Sebivo™ [Can]; Tyzeka™ [US]
Therapeutic Category Antiretroviral Agent, Reverse Transcriptase Inhibitor (Nucleoside)
Use Treatment of chronic hepatitis B with evidence of viral replication and either persistent transaminase elevations or histologically-active disease
Usual Dosage Oral: Adolescents ≥16 years and Adults: Chronic hepatitis B: 600 mg once daily
Dosage Forms
  Tablet:
    Tyzeka™: 600 mg

Teldrin® **HBP [US-OTC]** *see* chlorpheniramine *on page 177*

Teldrin® **Oral** *(Discontinued)* *see* chlorpheniramine *on page 177*

telithromycin (tel ith roe MYE sin)
Synonyms HMR 3647
U.S./Canadian Brand Names Ketek® [US/Can]
Therapeutic Category Antibiotic, Ketolide
Use Treatment of community-acquired pneumonia (mild-to-moderate) caused by susceptible strains of *Streptococcus pneumoniae* (including multidrug-resistant isolates), *Haemophilus influenzae*, *Chlamydophila pneumoniae*, *Moraxella catarrhalis*, and *Mycoplasma pneumoniae*
Usual Dosage Oral: Adults: Community-acquired pneumonia: 800 mg once daily for 7-10 days
Dosage Forms
Tablet:
Ketek®: 300 mg [not available in Canada], 400 mg
Ketek Pak™ [blister pack]: 400 mg (10s)

telmisartan (tel mi SAR tan)
U.S./Canadian Brand Names Micardis® [US/Can]
Therapeutic Category Angiotensin II Receptor Antagonist
Use Treatment of hypertension; may be used alone or in combination with other antihypertensive agents
Usual Dosage Oral: Adults: Initial: 40 mg once daily; usual maintenance dose range: 20-80 mg/day. Patients with volume depletion should be initiated on the lower dosage with close supervision.
Dosage Forms
Tablet:
Micardis®: 20 mg, 40 mg, 80 mg

telmisartan and hydrochlorothiazide (tel mi SAR tan & hye droe klor oh THYE a zide)
Synonyms hydrochlorothiazide and telmisartan
U.S./Canadian Brand Names Micardis® HCT [US]; Micardis® Plus [Can]
Therapeutic Category Antihypertensive Agent, Combination
Use Treatment of hypertension; combination product should not be used for initial therapy
Usual Dosage Oral: Adults: Replacement therapy: Combination product can be substituted for individual titrated agents. Initiation of combination therapy when monotherapy has failed to achieve desired effects:
Patients currently on telmisartan: Initial dose if blood pressure is not currently controlled on monotherapy of 80 mg telmisartan: Telmisartan 80 mg/hydrochlorothiazide 12.5 mg once daily; may titrate up to telmisartan 160 mg/hydrochlorothiazide 25 mg if needed
Patients currently on HCTZ: Initial dose if blood pressure is not currently controlled on monotherapy of 25 mg once daily: Telmisartan 80 mg/hydrochlorothiazide 12.5 mg once daily or telmisartan 80 mg/hydrochlorothiazide 25 mg once daily; may titrate up to telmisartan 160 mg/hydrochlorothiazide 25 mg if blood pressure remains uncontrolled after 2-4 weeks of therapy. Patients who develop hypokalemia may be switched to telmisartan 80 mg/hydrochlorothiazide 12.5 mg.
Dosage Forms [CAN]: Canadian brand name
Tablet:
Micardis® HCT: 40/12.5: Telmisartan 40 mg and hydrochlorothiazide 12.5 mg; 80/12.5: Telmisartan 80 mg and hydrochlorothiazide 12.5 mg; 80/25: Telmisartan 80 mg and hydrochlorothiazide 25 mg
Micardis® Plus [CAN]: 80/25: Telmisartan 80 mg and hydrochlorothiazide 25 mg [not available in the U.S.]

Telzir® [Can] *see* fosamprenavir *on page 374*

temazepam (te MAZ e pam)
Sound-Alike/Look-Alike Issues
temazepam may be confused with flurazepam, lorazepam
Restoril® may be confused with Vistaril®, Zestril®
U.S./Canadian Brand Names Apo-Temazepam® [Can]; CO Temazepam [Can]; Gen-Temazepam [Can]; Novo-Temazepam [Can]; Nu-Temazepam [Can]; PMS-Temazepam [Can]; ratio-Temazepam [Can]; Restoril® [US/Can]
Therapeutic Category Benzodiazepine
Controlled Substance C-IV
Use Short-term treatment of insomnia
Usual Dosage Oral: Adults: 15-30 mg at bedtime
Dosage Forms
Capsule: 15 mg, 30 mg
Restoril®: 7.5 mg, 15 mg, 30 mg

Temodal® [Can] *see* temozolomide *on next page*
Temodar® [US/Can] *see* temozolomide *on next page*

Temovate® **[US]** *see* clobetasol *on page 201*

Temovate E® **[US]** *see* clobetasol *on page 201*

temozolomide (te moe ZOE loe mide)

Synonyms NSC-362856; TMZ

U.S./Canadian Brand Names Temodal® [Can]; Temodar® [US/Can]

Therapeutic Category Antineoplastic Agent, Alkylating Agent

Use Treatment of adult patients with refractory anaplastic astrocytoma; newly-diagnosed glioblastoma multiforme

Usual Dosage Oral (refer to individual protocols): Adults:

Anaplastic astrocytoma (refractory): Initial dose: 150 mg/m^2/day for 5 days; repeat every 28 days. Subsequent doses of 100-200 mg/m^2/day for 5 days per treatment cycle; based upon hematologic tolerance. ANC <1000/mm^3 or platelets <50,000/mm^3 on day 22 or day 29 (day 1 of next cycle): Postpone therapy until ANC >1500/mm^3 and platelets >100,000/mm^3; reduce dose by 50 mg/m^2/day for subsequent cycle

ANC 1000-1500/mm^3 or platelets 50,000-100,000/mm^3 on day 22 or day 29 (day 1 of next cycle): Postpone therapy until ANC >1500/mm^3 and platelets >100,000/mm^3; maintain initial dose

ANC >1500/mm^3 and platelets >100,000/mm^3 on day 22 or day 29 (day 1 of next cycle): Increase dose to or maintain dose at 200 mg/m^2/day for 5 days for subsequent cycle

Glioblastoma multiforme (high-grade glioma):

Concomitant phase: 75 mg/m^2/day for 42 days with radiotherapy (60Gy administered in 30 fractions). **Note:** PCP prophylaxis is required during concomitant phase and should continue in patients who develop lymphocytopenia until recovery (common toxicity criteria [CTC] ≤1). Obtain weekly CBC.

ANC ≥1500/mm^3, platelet count ≥100,000/mm^3, and nonhematologic CTC ≤grade 1 (excludes alopecia, nausea/vomiting): Temodar® 75 mg/m^2/day may be continued throughout the 42-day concomitant period up to 49 days

Dosage modification:

ANC ≥500/mm^3 but <1500/mm^3 **or** platelet count ≥10,000/mm^3 but <100,000/mm^3 **or** nonhematologic CTC grade 2 (excludes alopecia, nausea/vomiting): Interrupt therapy

ANC <500/mm^3 **or** platelet count <10,000/mm^3 **or** nonhematologic CTC grade 3/4 (excludes alopecia, nausea/vomiting): Discontinue therapy

Maintenance phase (consists of 6 treatment cycles): Begin 4 weeks after concomitant phase completion. **Note:** Each subsequent cycle is 28 days (consisting of 5 days of drug treatment followed by 23 days without treatment). Draw CBC within 48 hours of day 22; hold next cycle and do weekly CBC until ANC >1500/mm^3 and platelet count >100,000/mm^3; dosing modification should be based on lowest blood counts and worst nonhematologic toxicity during the previous cycle.

Cycle 1: 150 mg/m^2/day for 5 days; repeat every 28 days

Dosage modification for next cycle:

ANC <1000/mm^3, platelet count <50,000/mm^3, or nonhematologic CTC grade 3 (excludes for alopecia, nausea/vomiting) during previous cycle: Decrease dose by 50 mg/m^2/day for 5 days, unless dose has already been lowered to 100 mg/m^2/day, then discontinue therapy.

If dose reduction <100 mg/m^2/day is required or nonhematologic CTC grade 4 (excludes for alopecia, nausea/vomiting), or if the same grade 3 nonhematologic toxicity occurs after dose reduction: Discontinue therapy

Cycle 2: 200 mg/m^2/day for 5 days every 28 days, unless prior toxicity, then refer to Dosage Modifications under "Cycle 1" and give adjusted dose for 5 days

Cycles 3-6: Continue with previous cycle's dose for 5 days every 28 days unless toxicity has occurred then, refer to Dosage Modifications under "Cycle 1" and give adjusted dose for 5 days

Dosage Forms

Capsule:

Temodar®: 5 mg, 20 mg, 100 mg, 140 mg, 180 mg, 250 mg

Tempra® **[Can]** *see* acetaminophen *on page 5*

Tempra® *(Discontinued)* *see* acetaminophen *on page 5*

temsirolimus (tem sir OH li mus)

Sound-Alike/Look-Alike Issues

temsirolimus may be confused with sirolimus, tacrolimus

Synonyms CCI-779; NSC-683864

U.S./Canadian Brand Names Torisel™ [US]

Therapeutic Category Antineoplastic Agent, mTOR Kinase Inhibitor

Use Treatment of advanced renal cell cancer (RCC)

Usual Dosage Note: For infusion reaction prophylaxis, premedicate with diphenhydramine 25-50 mg I.V. 30 minutes prior to infusion.

I.V.: Adults: RCC: 25 mg weekly

Dosage Forms
Injection, solution [concentrate]:
Torisel™: 25 mg/mL

tenecteplase (ten EK te plase)
Sound-Alike/Look-Alike Issues
TNKase™ may be confused with t-PA
TNK (occasional abbreviation for TNKase™) is an error-prone abbreviation (mistaken as TPA)
U.S./Canadian Brand Names TNKase™ [US/Can]
Therapeutic Category Thrombolytic Agent
Use Thrombolytic agent used in the management of acute myocardial infarction for the lysis of thrombi in the coronary vasculature to restore perfusion and reduce mortality.
Usual Dosage I.V.:
Adult: Recommended total dose should not exceed 50 mg and is based on patient's weight; administer as a bolus over 5 seconds
If patient's weight:
<60 kg, dose: 30 mg
$\geq$60 to <70 kg, dose: 35 mg
$\geq$70 to <80 kg, dose: 40 mg
$\geq$80 to <90 kg, dose: 45 mg
$\geq$90 kg, dose: 50 mg
All patients received 150-325 mg of aspirin as soon as possible and then daily. Intravenous heparin was initiated as soon as possible and aPTT was maintained between 50-70 seconds.
Dosage Forms
Injection, powder for reconstitution, recombinant:
TNKase™: 50 mg

Tenex® [US/Can] see guanfacine on page 410

teniposide (ten i POE side)
Sound-Alike/Look-Alike Issues
teniposide may be confused with etoposide
Synonyms EPT; VM-26
U.S./Canadian Brand Names Vumon® [US/Can]
Therapeutic Category Antineoplastic Agent
Use Treatment of acute lymphocytic leukemia, small-cell lung cancer
Usual Dosage I.V.:
Children: 130 mg/m^2/week, increasing to 150 mg/m^2 after 3 weeks and up to 180 mg/m^2 after 6 weeks
Acute lymphoblastic leukemia (ALL): 165 mg/m^2 twice weekly for 8-9 doses **or** 250 mg/m^2 weekly for 4-8 weeks
Adults: 50-180 mg/m^2 once or twice weekly for 4-6 weeks or 20-60 mg/m^2/day for 5 days
Small cell lung cancer: 80-90 mg/m^2/day for 5 days every 4-6 weeks
Dosage Forms
Injection, solution:
Vumon®: 10 mg/mL (5 mL)

Ten-K® (Discontinued) see potassium chloride on page 700

tenofovir (te NOE fo veer)
Synonyms PMPA; TDF; tenofovir disoproxil fumarate
U.S./Canadian Brand Names Viread® [US/Can]
Therapeutic Category Antiretroviral Agent, Reverse Transcriptase Inhibitor (Nucleotide)
Use Management of HIV infections in combination with at least two other antiretroviral agents
Usual Dosage Oral: Adults: HIV infection: 300 mg once daily
Dosage Forms
Tablet:
Viread®: 300 mg

tenofovir and emtricitabine see emtricitabine and tenofovir on page 295

tenofovir disoproxil fumarate see tenofovir on this page

tenofovir disoproxil fumarate, efavirenz, and emtricitabine see efavirenz, emtricitabine, and tenofovir on page 293

Tenolin [Can] see atenolol on page 80

Tenoretic® **[US/Can]** *see* atenolol and chlorthalidone *on page 81*

Tenormin® **[US/Can]** *see* atenolol *on page 80*

Tensilon® **[Can]** *see* edrophonium *on page 291*

Tenuate® **[Can]** *see* diethylpropion *on page 256*

Tenuate® *(Discontinued) see* diethylpropion *on page 256*

Tenuate® **Dospan**® **[Can]** *see* diethylpropion *on page 256*

Tenuate® **Dospan**® *(Discontinued) see* diethylpropion *on page 256*

Tequin® **[Can]** *see* gatifloxacin *on page 385*

Tequin® *(Discontinued) see* gatifloxacin *on page 385*

Tera-Gel™ **[US-OTC]** *see* coal tar *on page 208*

Terazol® **[Can]** *see* terconazole *on next page*

Terazol® **3 [US]** *see* terconazole *on next page*

Terazol® **7 [US]** *see* terconazole *on next page*

terazosin (ter AY zoe sin)

U.S./Canadian Brand Names Alti-Terazosin [Can]; Apo-Terazosin® [Can]; Hytrin® [Can]; Novo-Terazosin [Can]; Nu-Terazosin [Can]; PMS-Terazosin [Can]

Therapeutic Category Alpha-Adrenergic Blocking Agent

Use Management of mild to moderate hypertension; alone or in combination with other agents such as diuretics or beta-blockers; benign prostate hyperplasia (BPH)

Usual Dosage Oral: Adults:

Hypertension: Initial: 1 mg at bedtime; slowly increase dose to achieve desired blood pressure, up to 20 mg/day; usual dose range (JNC 7): 1-20 mg once daily

Dosage reduction may be needed when adding a diuretic or other antihypertensive agent; if drug is discontinued for greater than several days, consider beginning with initial dose and retitrate as needed; dosage may be given on a twice daily regimen if response is diminished at 24 hours and hypotensive is observed at 2-4 hours following a dose

Benign prostatic hyperplasia: Initial: 1 mg at bedtime, increasing as needed; most patients require 10 mg day; if no response after 4-6 weeks of 10 mg/day, may increase to 20 mg/day

Dosage Forms

Capsule: 1 mg, 2 mg, 5 mg, 10 mg

terbinafine (oral) (TER bin a feen OR al)

Sound-Alike/Look-Alike Issues

terbinafine may be confused with terbutaline

Lamisil® may be confused with Lamictal®, Lomotil®

U.S./Canadian Brand Names Lamisil® Oral [US/Can]

Therapeutic Category Antifungal Agent

Use Treatment of onychomycosis infections of the toenail or fingernail

Usual Dosage Oral: Adults:

Fingernail onychomycosis: 250 mg once daily for 6 weeks

Toenail onychomycosis: 250 mg once daily for 12 weeks

Dosage Forms

Tablet: 250 mg

Lamisil®: 250 mg

terbinafine (topical) (TER bin a feen TOP i kal)

Sound-Alike/Look-Alike Issues

terbinafine may be confused with terbutaline

Lamisil® may be confused with Lamictal®, Lomotil®

U.S./Canadian Brand Names Lamisil® Topical [US/Can]

Therapeutic Category Antifungal Agent

Use Topical antifungal for the treatment of tinea pedis (athlete's foot), tinea cruris (jock itch), and tinea corporis (ring worm); tinea versicolor (lotion)

Usual Dosage Topical: Adults:

Athlete's foot: Apply to affected area twice daily for at least 1 week, not to exceed 4 weeks

Ringworm and jock itch: Apply to affected area once or twice daily for at least 1 week, not to exceed 4 weeks

Dosage Forms

Cream: 1% (12 g, 24 g)

Lamisil® AT™: 1% (12 g)

Solution [topical spray]:
Lamisil® AT™ [OTC]: 1% (30 mL)

terbutaline (ter BYOO ta leen)

Sound-Alike/Look-Alike Issues
terbutaline may be confused with terbinafine, TOLBUTamide
U.S./Canadian Brand Names Bricanyl® [Can]
Therapeutic Category Adrenergic Agonist Agent
Use Bronchodilator in reversible airway obstruction and bronchial asthma
Usual Dosage
Children <12 years: Bronchoconstriction:
Oral: Initial: 0.05 mg/kg/dose 3 times/day, increased gradually as required; maximum: 0.15 mg/kg/dose 3-4 times/day or a total of 5 mg/24 hours
SubQ: 0.005-0.01 mg/kg/dose to a maximum of 0.3 mg/dose; may repeat in 15-20 minutes
Children ≥6 years and Adults: Bronchospasm (acute): Inhalation (Bricanyl® [CAN] MDI: 500 mcg/puff, *not labeled for use in the U.S.*): One puff as needed; may repeat with 1 inhalation (after 5 minutes); more than 6 inhalations should not be necessary in any 24 hour period. **Note:** If a previously effective dosage regimen fails to provide the usual relief, or the effects of a dose last for >3 hours, medical advice should be sought immediately; this is a sign of seriously worsening asthma that requires reassessment of therapy.
Children >12 years and Adults: Bronchoconstriction:
Oral:
12-15 years: 2.5 mg every 6 hours 3 times/day; not to exceed 7.5 mg in 24 hours
>15 years: 5 mg/dose every 6 hours 3 times/day; if side effects occur, reduce dose to 2.5 mg every 6 hours; not to exceed 15 mg in 24 hours
SubQ: 0.25 mg/dose; may repeat in 15-30 minutes (maximum: 0.5 mg/4-hour period)
Dosage Forms [CAN] = Canadian brand name
Injection, solution: 1 mg/mL (1 mL)
Powder for oral inhalation:
Bricanyl® Turbuhaler [CAN]: 500 mcg/actuation [50 or 200 metered actuations] [not available in the U.S.]
Tablet: 2.5 mg, 5 mg

terconazole (ter KONE a zole)

Sound-Alike/Look-Alike Issues
terconazole may be confused with tioconazole
Synonyms triaconazole
U.S./Canadian Brand Names Terazol® 3 [US]; Terazol® 7 [US]; Terazol® [Can]; Zazole™ [US]
Therapeutic Category Antifungal Agent
Use Local treatment of vulvovaginal candidiasis
Usual Dosage Adults: Female:
Terazol® 3, Zazole™ 0.8% vaginal cream: Insert 1 applicatorful intravaginally at bedtime for 3 consecutive days
Terazol® 7, Zazole™ 0.4% vaginal cream: Insert 1 applicatorful intravaginally at bedtime for 7 consecutive days
Terazol® 3 vaginal suppository: Insert 1 suppository intravaginally at bedtime for 3 consecutive days
Dosage Forms
Cream, vaginal: 0.4% (45 g); 0.8% (20 g)
Terazol® 7, Zazole™: 0.4% (45 g)
Terazol® 3, Zazole™: 0.8% (20 g)
Suppository, vaginal:
Terazol® 3: 80 mg (3s)

Terfluzine [Can] *see* trifluoperazine *on page 865*

teriparatide (ter i PAR a tide)

Synonyms parathyroid hormone (1-34); recombinant human parathyroid hormone (1-34); rhPTH(1-34)
U.S./Canadian Brand Names Forteo™ [US/Can]
Therapeutic Category Diagnostic Agent
Use Treatment of osteoporosis in postmenopausal women at high risk of fracture; treatment of primary or hypogonadal osteoporosis in men at high risk of fracture
Usual Dosage SubQ: Adults: 20 mcg once daily; **Note:** Initial administration should occur under circumstances in which the patient may sit or lie down, in the event of orthostasis.
Dosage Forms
Injection, solution:
Forteo®: 250 mcg/mL (3 mL)

terpin hydrate *(Discontinued)*

Terra-Cortril® **Ophthalmic Suspension** *(Discontinued)*

Terramycin® **[Can]** *see* oxytetracycline *on page 644*

Terramycin® **I.M.** *(Discontinued) see* oxytetracycline *on page 644*

Terramycin® **Oral** *(Discontinued) see* oxytetracycline *on page 644*

Terrell™ **[US]** *see* isoflurane *on page 474*

Tesamone® **Injection** *(Discontinued) see* testosterone *on this page*

Teslac® **[US/Can]** *see* testolactone *on this page*

TESPA *see* thiotepa *on page 838*

Tessalon® **[US/Can]** *see* benzonatate *on page 103*

Testim® **[US]** *see* testosterone *on this page*

Testoderm® *(Discontinued) see* testosterone *on this page*

Testoderm® **TTS** *(Discontinued) see* testosterone *on this page*

Testoderm® **With Adhesive** *(Discontinued) see* testosterone *on this page*

testolactone (tes toe LAK tone)
Sound-Alike/Look-Alike Issues
  testolactone may be confused with testosterone
U.S./Canadian Brand Names Teslac® [US/Can]
Therapeutic Category Androgen
Controlled Substance C-III
Use Palliative treatment of advanced or disseminated breast carcinoma
Usual Dosage Oral: Adults: Female: 250 mg 4 times/day for at least 3 months; desired response may take as long as 3 months
Dosage Forms
  Tablet:
    Teslac®: 50 mg

Testomar® *(Discontinued) see* yohimbine *on page 901*

Testopel® **[US]** *see* testosterone *on this page*

Testopel® **Pellet** *(Discontinued) see* testosterone *on this page*

testosterone (tes TOS ter one)
Sound-Alike/Look-Alike Issues
  testosterone may be confused with testolactone
  Testoderm® may be confused with Estraderm®
Synonyms testosterone cypionate; testosterone enanthate
U.S./Canadian Brand Names Andriol® [Can]; Androderm® [US/Can]; AndroGel® [US/Can]; Andropository [Can]; Delatestryl® [US/Can]; Depotest® 100 [Can]; Depo®-Testosterone [US]; Everone® 200 [Can]; First® Testosterone MC [US]; First® Testosterone [US]; Striant® [US]; Testim® [US]; Testopel® [US]; Virilon® IM [Can]
Therapeutic Category Androgen
Controlled Substance C-III
Use
  Injection: Androgen replacement therapy in the treatment of delayed male puberty; male hypogonadism (primary or hypogonadotropic); inoperable metastatic female breast cancer (enanthate only)
  Pellet: Androgen replacement therapy in the treatment of delayed male puberty; male hypogonadism (primary or hypogonadotropic)
  Topical (buccal system, gel, transdermal system): Male hypogonadism (primary or hypogonadotropic)
  Capsule (not available in U.S.): Androgen replacement therapy in the treatment of delayed male puberty; male hypogonadism (primary or hypogonadotropic); replacement therapy in impotence or for male climacteric symptoms due to androgen deficiency
Usual Dosage
  Adolescents and Adults: Male:
    I.M.:
      Hypogonadism: Testosterone enanthate or testosterone cypionate: 50-400 mg every 2-4 weeks (FDA-approved dosing range); 75-100 mg/week or 150-200 mg every 2 weeks (per practice guidelines)
      Delayed puberty: Testosterone enanthate: 50-200 mg every 2-4 weeks for a limited duration
      Pellet (for subcutaneous implantation): Delayed male puberty, male hypogonadism: 150-450 mg every 3-6 months

Oral: Delayed puberty, hypogonadism, or hypogonadotropic hypogonadism: Capsule (Andriol®; not available in U.S.): Initial: 120-160 mg/day in 2 divided doses for 2-3 weeks; adjust according to individual response; usual maintenance dose: 40-120 mg/day (in divided doses)

Adults:

I.M.: Female: Inoperable metastatic breast cancer: Testosterone enanthate: 200-400 mg every 2-4 weeks

Topical: Primary male hypogonadism **or** hypogonadotropic hypogonadism:

Buccal: 30 mg twice daily (every 12 hours) applied to the gum region above the incisor tooth

Transdermal system: Androderm®: Initial: Apply 5 mg/day once nightly to clean, dry area on the back, abdomen, upper arms, or thighs (do **not** apply to scrotum); dosing range: 2.5-7.5 mg/day; in nonvirilized patients, dose may be initiated at 2.5 mg/day

Gel: AndroGel®, Testim®: 5 g (to deliver 50 mg of testosterone with 5 mg systemically absorbed) applied once daily (preferably in the morning) to clean, dry, intact skin of the shoulder and upper arms. AndroGel® may also be applied to the abdomen. Dosage may be increased to a maximum of 10 g (100 mg). **Do not apply testosterone gel to the genitals.**

Dosage Forms [CAN] = Canadian brand name

Capsule, gelatin:

Andriol™ [CAN]: 40 mg (10s) [not available in the U.S.]

Gel, topical:

AndroGel®: 1.25 g/actuation (75 g); 2.5 g (30s); 5 g (30s)

Testim®: 5 g (30s)

Implant, subcutaneous:

Testopel®: 75 mg

Injection, in oil: 100 mg/mL (10 mL); 200 mg/mL (1 mL, 5 mL, 10 mL)

Depo®-Testosterone: 100 mg/mL (10 mL); 200 mg/mL (1 mL, 10 mL)

Delatestryl®: 200 mg/mL (1 mL, 5 mL)

Kit [for prescription compounding testosterone 2%]:

First® Testosterone:

Injection, in oil: Testosterone 100 mg/mL (12 mL)

Ointment: White petroleum (48 g)

First® Testosterone MC:

Injection, in oil: Testosterone 100 mg/mL (12 mL)

Cream: Moisturizing cream (48 g)

Mucoadhesive, for buccal application [buccal system]:

Striant®: 30 mg (10s)

Transdermal system:

Androderm®: 2.5 mg/day (60s); 5 mg/day (30s)

testosterone cypionate *see* testosterone *on previous page*

testosterone enanthate *see* testosterone *on previous page*

Testred® [US] *see* methyltestosterone *on page 560*

tetanus and diphtheria toxoid *see* diphtheria and tetanus toxoid *on page 267*

tetanus immune globulin (human) (TET a nus i MYUN GLOB yoo lin HYU man)

Synonyms TIG

U.S./Canadian Brand Names HyperTET™ S/D [US/Can]

Therapeutic Category Immune Globulin

Use Passive immunization against tetanus; tetanus immune globulin is preferred over tetanus antitoxin for treatment of active tetanus; part of the management of an unclean, wound in a person whose history of previous receipt of tetanus toxoid is unknown or who has received less than three doses of tetanus toxoid

Usual Dosage I.M.:

Prophylaxis of tetanus:

Children: 4 units/kg; some recommend administering 250 units to small children

Adults: 250 units

Treatment of tetanus:

Children: 500-3000 units; some should infiltrate locally around the wound

Adults: 3000-6000 units

Dosage Forms

Injection, solution [preservative free]:

HyperTET™ S/D: 250 units/mL (1 mL)

tetanus toxoid (adsorbed) (TET a nus TOKS oyd, ad SORBED)

Sound-Alike/Look-Alike Issues

Tetanus toxoid products may be confused with influenza virus vaccine and tuberculin products. Medication errors have occurred when tetanus toxoid products have been inadvertently administered instead of tuberculin skin tests (PPD) and influenza virus vaccine. These products are refrigerated and often stored in close proximity to each other.

Therapeutic Category Toxoid

Use Active immunization against tetanus when combination antigen preparations are not indicated. **Note:** Tetanus and diphtheria toxoids for adult use (Td) is the preferred immunizing agent for most adults and for children after their seventh birthday. Young children should receive trivalent DTaP (diphtheria/tetanus/acellular pertussis), as part of their childhood immunization program, unless pertussis is contraindicated, then TD is warranted.

Usual Dosage I.M.: Children ≥7 years and Adults:

Primary immunization: 0.5 mL; repeat 0.5 mL at 4-8 weeks after first dose and at 6-12 months after second dose

Routine booster dose: Recommended every 10 years

Note: In most patients, Td is the recommended product for primary immunization, booster doses, and tetanus immunization in wound management (refer to diphtheria and tetanus toxoid monograph)

Dosage Forms

Injection, suspension:

Tetanus 5 Lf units per 0.5 mL (0.5 mL)

tetanus toxoid (fluid) (TET a nus TOKS oyd FLOO id)

Sound-Alike/Look-Alike Issues

Tetanus toxoid products may be confused with influenza virus vaccine and tuberculin products. Medication errors have occurred when tetanus toxoid products have been inadvertently administered instead of tuberculin skin tests (PPD) and influenza virus vaccine. These products are refrigerated and often stored in close proximity to each other.

Synonyms tetanus toxoid plain

Therapeutic Category Toxoid

Use Indicated as booster dose in the active immunization against tetanus in the rare adult or child who is allergic to the aluminum adjuvant (a product containing adsorbed tetanus toxoid is preferred); not indicated for primary immunization

Usual Dosage

Primary immunization: Not indicated for this use.

Booster doses: I.M., SubQ: 0.5 mL every 10 years

Dosage Forms

Injection, solution:

Tetanus 4 Lf units per 0.5 mL (7.5 mL)

tetanus toxoid plain *see* tetanus toxoid (fluid) *on this page*

tetanus toxoid, reduced diphtheria toxoid, and acellular pertussis, adsorbed *see* diphtheria, tetanus toxoids, and acellular pertussis vaccine *on page 269*

tetrabenazine *(Canada only)* (tet ra BEN a zeen)

U.S./Canadian Brand Names Nitoman™ [Can]

Therapeutic Category Monoamine Depleting Agent

Use Treatment of hyperkinetic movement disorders, including Huntington chorea, hemiballismus, senile chorea, Tourette syndrome, and tardive dyskinesia

Usual Dosage Oral:

Children (limited data): Consider initiation at $1/2$ recommended adult dosage; must be titrated slowly to individualize dosage

Adults: Initial: 12.5 mg twice daily (may be given 3 times/day); may be increased by 12.5 mg/day every 3-5 days; should be titrated slowly to maximal tolerated and effective dose (dose is individualized)

Usual maximum tolerated dosage: 25 mg 3 times/day; maximum recommended dose: 200 mg/day

Note: If there is no improvement at the maximum tolerated dose after 7 days, improvement is unlikely; discontinuation should be considered.

Dosage Forms [CAN] = Canadian brand name

Tablet:

Nitoman™ [CAN]: 25 mg [not available in the U.S.]

tetracaine (TET ra kane)

Synonyms amethocaine hydrochloride; tetracaine hydrochloride

U.S./Canadian Brand Names Ametop™ [Can]; Pontocaine® Niphanoid® [US]; Pontocaine® [US/Can]

Therapeutic Category Local Anesthetic

Use Spinal anesthesia; local anesthesia in the eye for various diagnostic and examination purposes; topically applied to nose and throat for various diagnostic procedures

Usual Dosage Adults:

Ophthalmic: Short-term anesthesia of the eye: 0.5% solution: Instill 1-2 drops; prolonged use (especially for at-home self-medication) is not recommended

Injection: Spinal anesthesia: **Note:** Dosage varies with the anesthetic procedure, the degree of anesthesia required, and the individual patient response; it is administered by subarachnoid injection for spinal anesthesia.

Perineal anesthesia: 5 mg

Perineal and lower extremities: 10 mg

Anesthesia extending up to costal margin: 15 mg; doses up to 20 mg may be given, but are reserved for exceptional cases

Low spinal anesthesia (saddle block): 2-5 mg

Topical mucous membranes (rhinolaryngology): Used as a 0.25% or 0.5% solution by direct application or nebulization; total dose should not exceed 20 mg

Dosage Forms

Injection, solution: 1% [10 mg/mL] (2 mL)

Pontocaine®: 1% [10 mg/mL] (2 mL)

Injection, powder for reconstitution [preservative free]:

Pontocaine® Niphanoid®: 20 mg

Solution, ophthalmic: 0.5% [5 mg/mL] (15 mL)

Solution, topical:

Pontocaine®: 2% [20 mg/mL] (30 mL, 118 mL)

tetracaine and lidocaine *see* lidocaine and tetracaine *on page 508*

tetracaine, benzocaine, and butamben *see* benzocaine, butamben, and tetracaine *on page 103*

tetracaine hydrochloride *see* tetracaine *on this page*

Tetracap® *(Discontinued)* *see* tetracycline *on this page*

tetracosactide *see* cosyntropin *on page 217*

tetracycline (tet ra SYE kleen)

Sound-Alike/Look-Alike Issues

tetracycline may be confused with tetradecyl sulfate

achromycin may be confused with actinomycin, Adriamycin PFS®

Synonyms achromycin; TCN; tetracycline hydrochloride

U.S./Canadian Brand Names Apo-Tetra® [Can]; Nu-Tetra [Can]

Therapeutic Category Antibiotic, Ophthalmic; Antibiotic, Topical; Tetracycline Derivative

Use Treatment of susceptible bacterial infections of both gram-positive and gram-negative organisms; also infections due to *Mycoplasma*, *Chlamydia*, and *Rickettsia*; indicated for acne, exacerbations of chronic bronchitis, and treatment of gonorrhea and syphilis in patients who are allergic to penicillin; as part of a multidrug regimen for *H. pylori* eradication to reduce the risk of duodenal ulcer recurrence

Usual Dosage

Usual dosage range:

Children >8 years: Oral: 25-50 mg/kg/day in divided doses every 6 hours

Adults: Oral: 250-500 mg/dose every 6 hours

Indication-specific dosing:

Adults: Oral:

Acne: 250-500 twice daily

Chronic bronchitis, acute exacerbation: 500 mg 4 times/day

Erlichiosis: 500 mg 4 times/day for 7-14 days

Peptic ulcer disease: Eradication of *Helicobacter pylori*: 500 mg 2-4 times/day depending on regimen; requires combination therapy with at least one other antibiotic and an acid-suppressing agent (proton pump inhibitor or H₂ blocker)

Periodontitis: 250 mg every 6 hours until improvement (usually 10 days)

Vibrio cholerae: 500 mg 4 times/day for 3 days

Dosage Forms

Capsule: 250 mg, 500 mg

tetracycline hydrochloride *see* tetracycline *on this page*

tetracycline, metronidazole, and bismuth subcitrate potassium *see* bismuth, metronidazole, and tetracycline *on page 113*

tetracycline, metronidazole, and bismuth subsalicylate *see* bismuth, metronidazole, and tetracycline *on page 113*

tetrahydroaminoacrine *see* tacrine *on page 818*

tetrahydrocannabinol *see* dronabinol *on page 284*

tetrahydrocannabinol and cannabidiol *(Canada only)*
(TET ra hye droe can NAB e nol & can nab e DYE ol)

Synonyms cannabidiol and tetrahydrocannabinol; delta-9-tetrahydrocannabinol and cannabinol; GW-1000-02; THC and CBD

U.S./Canadian Brand Names Sativex® [Can]

Therapeutic Category Analgesic, Miscellaneous

Controlled Substance CDSA-II

Use Adjunctive treatment of neuropathic pain in multiple sclerosis; adjunctive treatment of moderate-to-severe pain in advanced cancer

Usual Dosage
Note: For buccal use only; spray should be directed below the tongue or on the inside of the cheeks (the site should be varied); avoid direction to the pharynx.
Buccal spray:
Initial: One spray every 4 hours to a maximum of 4 sprays.
Titration and individualization: Dosage is self-titrated by the patient. The mean daily dosage after titration in clinical trials was 5 actuations per day. Dosage should be adjusted as necessary, based on effect and tolerance. Sprays should be evenly distributed over the course of the day during initial titration. If adverse reactions, including intoxication-type symptoms, are noted the dosage should be suspended until resolution of the symptoms; a dosage reduction or extension of the interval between doses may be used to avoid a recurrence of symptoms. Retitration may be required in the event of adverse reactions and/or worsening of symptoms.

Dosage Forms [CAN] = Canadian brand name
Solution, buccal [spray]:
Sativex® [CAN]: Delta-9 tetrahydrocannabinol 27 mg/mL and cannabidiol 25 mg/mL (5.5 mL) [not available in the U.S.]

tetrahydrozoline (tet ra hye DROZ a leen)
Sound-Alike/Look-Alike Issues
Visine® may be confused with Visken®
Synonyms tetrahydrozoline hydrochloride; tetryzoline
U.S./Canadian Brand Names Eye-Sine™ [US-OTC]; Geneye® [US-OTC]; Murine® Tears Plus [US-OTC]; Optigene® 3 [US-OTC]; Tyzine® Pediatric [US]; Tyzine® [US]; Visine® Advanced Relief [US-OTC]; Visine® Original [US-OTC]
Therapeutic Category Adrenergic Agonist Agent
Use Symptomatic relief of nasal congestion and conjunctival congestion
Usual Dosage
Nasal congestion: Intranasal:
Children 2-6 years: Instill 2-3 drops of 0.05% solution every 4-6 hours as needed, no more frequent than every 3 hours
Children >6 years and Adults: Instill 2-4 drops or 3-4 sprays of 0.1% solution every 3-4 hours as needed, no more frequent than every 3 hours
Conjunctival congestion: Ophthalmic: Adults: Instill 1-2 drops in each eye 2-4 times/day
Dosage Forms
Solution, intranasal:
Tyzine®: 0.1% (15 mL, 30 mL)
Tyzine® Pediatric: 0.05% (15 mL)
Solution, ophthalmic: 0.05% (15 mL)
Eye-Sine™ [OTC], Geneye® [OTC], Optigene® 3 [OTC]: 0.05% (15 mL)
Murine® Tears Plus [OTC], Visine® Original [OTC]: 0.05% (15 mL, 30 mL)
Visine® Advanced Relief [OTC]: 0.05% (30 mL)

tetrahydrozoline hydrochloride *see* tetrahydrozoline *on this page*

Tetramune® *(Discontinued)*

Tetrasine® Extra Ophthalmic *(Discontinued)* *see* tetrahydrozoline *on this page*

Tetrasine® Ophthalmic *(Discontinued)* *see* tetrahydrozoline *on this page*

Tetra Tannate Pediatric [US] *see* chlorpheniramine, ephedrine, phenylephrine, and carbetapentane *on page 179*

tetryzoline *see* tetrahydrozoline *on previous page*

Teveten® **[US/Can]** *see* eprosartan *on page 304*

Teveten® **HCT [US/Can]** *see* eprosartan and hydrochlorothiazide *on page 305*

Teveten® **Plus [Can]** *see* eprosartan and hydrochlorothiazide *on page 305*

Tev-Tropin® **[US]** *see* somatropin *on page 799*

Texacort® **[US]** *see* hydrocortisone (topical) *on page 434*

TG *see* thioguanine *on page 837*

T-Gen® *(Discontinued)* *see* trimethobenzamide *on page 867*

THA *see* tacrine *on page 818*

thalidomide (tha LI doe mide)

Sound-Alike/Look-Alike Issues
thalidomide may be confused with flutamide
Synonyms NSC-66847
U.S./Canadian Brand Names Thalomid® [US/Can]
Therapeutic Category Immunosuppressant Agent
Use Treatment of multiple myeloma; treatment and maintenance of cutaneous manifestations of erythema nodosum leprosum (ENL)
Usual Dosage Oral:
Multiple myeloma: 200 mg once daily (with dexamethasone 40 mg daily on days 1-4, 9-12, and 17-20 of a 28-day treatment cycle)
Cutaneous ENL:
Initial: 100-300 mg/day taken once daily at bedtime with water (at least 1 hour after evening meal)
Patients weighing <50 kg: Initiate at lower end of the dosing range
Severe cutaneous reaction or patients previously requiring high dose may be initiated at 400 mg/day; doses may be divided, but taken 1 hour after meals
Maintenance: Dosing should continue until active reaction subsides (usually at least 2 weeks), then tapered in 50 mg decrements every 2-4 weeks
Patients who flare during tapering or with a history or requiring prolonged maintenance should be maintained on the minimum dosage necessary to control the reaction. Efforts to taper should be repeated every 3-6 months, in increments of 50 mg every 2-4 weeks.
Dosage Forms
Capsule:
Thalomid®: 50 mg, 100 mg, 200 mg

Thalitone® **[US]** *see* chlorthalidone *on page 185*

Thalomid® **[US/Can]** *see* thalidomide *on this page*

THAM® **[US]** *see* tromethamine *on page 871*

THC *see* dronabinol *on page 284*

THC and CBD *see* tetrahydrocannabinol and cannabidiol *(Canada only) on previous page*

Thelin™ **[Can]** *see* sitaxsentan *(Canada only) on page 790*

Theo-X® *(Discontinued)* *see* theophylline *on next page*

Theo-24® **[US]** *see* theophylline *on next page*

Theobid® *(Discontinued)* *see* theophylline *on next page*

TheoCap™ **[US]** *see* theophylline *on next page*

Theochron® **[US]** *see* theophylline *on next page*

Theochron® **SR [Can]** *see* theophylline *on next page*

Theoclear-80® *(Discontinued)* *see* theophylline *on next page*

Theoclear®**-L.A.** *(Discontinued)* *see* theophylline *on next page*

Theo-Dur® **(all products)** *(Discontinued)* *see* theophylline *on next page*

Theolair™ **[Can]** *see* theophylline *on next page*

Theolair-SR® *(Discontinued)* *see* theophylline *on next page*

Theolate *(Discontinued)* *see* theophylline and guaifenesin *on page 835*

theophylline (thee OFF i lin)

Sound-Alike/Look-Alike Issues

Theolair™ may be confused with Thiola®, Thyrolar®

Synonyms theophylline anhydrous

U.S./Canadian Brand Names Apo-Theo LA® [Can]; Novo-Theophyl SR [Can]; PMS-Theophylline [Can]; Pulmophylline [Can]; ratio-Theo-Bronc [Can]; Theo-24® [US]; TheoCap™ [US]; Theochron® SR [Can]; Theochron® [US]; Theolair™ [Can]; Uniphyl® SRT [Can]; Uniphyl® [US]

Therapeutic Category Theophylline Derivative

Use Treatment of symptoms and reversible airway obstruction due to chronic asthma, chronic bronchitis, or COPD

Usual Dosage Use ideal body weight for obese patients

I.V.: Initial: Maintenance infusion rates:

Children:

6 weeks to 6 months: 0.5 mg/kg/hour

6 months to 1 year: 0.6-0.7 mg/kg/hour

Children >1 year and Adults:

Acute bronchospasm: Approximate I.V. theophylline dosage for treatment of acute bronchospasm: **Note:** Equivalent hydrous aminophylline dosage is indicated in parentheses.

Infants 6 weeks to 6 months: 0.5 mg/kg/hour for next 12 hours

Children 6 months to 1 year: 0.6-0.7 mg/kg/hour for next 12 hours

Children 1-9 years: 0.95 mg/kg/hour (1.2 mg/kg/hour) for next 12 hours; 0.79 mg/kg/hour (1 mg/kg/hour) after 12 hours

Children 9-16 years and young adult smokers: 0.79 mg/kg/hour (1 mg/kg/hour) for next 12 hours; 0.63 mg/kg/hour (0.8 mg/kg/hour) after 12 hours

Healthy, nonsmoking adults: 0.55 mg/kg/hour (0.7 mg/kg/hour) for next 12 hours; 0.39 mg/kg/hour (0.5 mg/kg/hour) after 12 hours

Older patients and patients with cor pulmonale: 0.47 mg/kg/hour (0.6 mg/kg/hour) for next 12 hours; 0.24 mg/kg/hour (0.3 mg/kg/hour) after 12 hours

Patients with congestive heart failure or liver failure: 0.39 mg/kg/hour (0.5 mg/kg/hour) for next 12 hours; 0.08-0.16 mg/kg/hour (0.1-0.2 mg/kg/hour) after 12 hours

Approximate I.V. maintenance dosages are based upon continuous infusions; bolus dosing (often used in children <6 months of age) may be determined by multiplying the hourly infusion rate by 24 hours and dividing by the desired number of doses/day. See the following: Maintenance dose for acute symptoms:

Premature infant or newborn to 6 weeks (for apnea/bradycardia):

Oral theophylline: 4 mg/kg/day

I.V. aminophylline: 5 mg/kg/day

6 weeks to 6 months:

Oral theophylline: 10 mg/kg/day

I.V. aminophylline: 12 mg/kg/day or continuous I.V. infusion[1]

Infants 6 months to 1 year:

Oral theophylline: 12-18 mg/kg/day

I.V. aminophylline: 15 mg/kg/day or continuous I.V. infusion[1]

Children 1-9 years:

Oral theophylline: 20-24 mg/kg/day

I.V. aminophylline: 1 mg/kg/hour

Children 9-12 years, and adolescent daily smokers of cigarettes or marijuana, and otherwise healthy adult smokers <50 years:

Oral theophylline: 16 mg/kg/day

I.V. aminophylline: 0.9 mg/kg/hour

Adolescents 12-16 years (nonsmokers):

Oral theophylline: 13 mg/kg/day

I.V. aminophylline: 0.7 mg/kg/hour

Otherwise healthy nonsmoking adults:

Oral theophylline: 10 mg/kg/day (not to exceed 900 mg/day)

I.V. aminophylline: 0.5 mg/kg/hour

Cardiac decompensation, cor pulmonale, and/or liver dysfunction:

Oral theophylline: 5 mg/kg/day (not to exceed 400 mg/day)

I.V. aminophylline: 0.25 mg/kg/hour

[1]For continuous I.V. infusion, divide total daily dose by 24 = mg/kg/hour.

Oral theophylline: Initial dosage recommendation: Loading dose (to achieve a serum level of about 10 mcg/mL; loading doses should be given using a rapidly absorbed oral product **not** a sustained release product): If no theophylline has been administered in the previous 24 hours: 4-6 mg/kg theophylline

If theophylline has been administered in the previous 24 hours: administer 1/2 loading dose or 2-3 mg/kg theophylline can be given in emergencies when serum levels are not available

On the average, for every 1 mg/kg theophylline given, blood levels will rise 2 mcg/mL

Ideally, defer the loading dose if a serum theophylline concentration can be obtained rapidly. However, if this is not possible, exercise clinical judgment. If the patient is not experiencing theophylline toxicity, this is unlikely to result in dangerous adverse effects.

Oral theophylline dosage for bronchial asthma (by age):

<1 year:

Initial 3 days and second 3 days: 0.2 x (age in weeks) + 5 = mg/kg/24 hours of theophylline

Steady-state maintenance: 0.3 x (age in weeks) + 8 = mg/kg/24 hours of theophylline

1-9 years:

Initial 3 days: 16 mg/kg/24 hours of theophylline, up to a maximum of 400 mg/24 hours

Second 3 days: 20 mg/kg/24 hours of theophylline

Steady-state maintenance: 22 mg/kg/24 hours of theophylline

9-12 years:

Initial 3 days: 16 mg/kg/24 hours of theophylline, up to a maximum of 400 mg/24 hours

Second 3 days: 16 mg/kg/24 hours of theophylline, up to a maximum of 600 mg/24 hours

Steady-state maintenance: 20 mg/kg/24 hours of theophylline, up to a maximum of 800 mg/24 hours

12-16 years:

Initial 3 days: 16 mg/kg/24 hours of theophylline, up to a maximum of 400 mg/24 hours

Second 3 days: 16 mg/kg/24 hours of theophylline, up to a maximum of 600 mg/24 hours

Steady-state maintenance: 18 mg/kg/24 hours of theophylline, up to a maximum of 900 mg/24 hours

Adults:

Initial 3 days: 400 mg/24 hours

Second 3 days: 600 mg/24 hours

Steady-state maintenance: 900 mg/24 hours

Increasing dose: The dosage may be increased in approximately 25% increments at 2- to 3-day intervals so long as the drug is tolerated or until the maximum dose is reached

Maintenance dose: In children and healthy adults, a slow-release product can be used; the total daily dose can be divided every 8-12 hours

Dosage Forms

Capsule, extended release: 100 mg, 200 mg, 300 mg

TheoCap™: 125 mg, 200 mg [12 hour]

Theo-24®: 100 mg, 200 mg, 300 mg, 400 mg

Elixir: 80 mg/15 mL

Infusion [premixed in D₅W]: 200 mg (50 mL, 100 mL); 400 mg (250 mL, 500 mL); 800 mg (250 mL, 500 mL, 1000 mL)

Tablet, controlled release:

Uniphyl®: 400 mg, 600 mg

Tablet, extended release: 100 mg, 200 mg, 300 mg, 400 mg, 450 mg, 600 mg

Theochron®: 100 mg, 200 mg, 300 mg, 450 mg

theophylline and guaifenesin (thee OFF i lin & gwye FEN e sin)

Synonyms guaifenesin and theophylline

U.S./Canadian Brand Names Elixophyllin-GG® [US]

Therapeutic Category Theophylline Derivative

Use Symptomatic treatment of bronchospasm associated with bronchial asthma, chronic bronchitis, and pulmonary emphysema

Usual Dosage Oral: Adults: 16 mg/kg/day or 400 mg theophylline/day, in divided doses, every 6-8 hours

Dosage Forms

Liquid:

Elixophyllin-GG®: Theophylline 100 mg and guaifenesin 100 mg per 15 mL

theophylline anhydrous see theophylline on previous page

theophylline ethylenediamine see aminophylline on page 43

Theo-Sav® (Discontinued) see theophylline on previous page

Theospan®-SR (Discontinued) see theophylline on previous page

Theostat-80® (Discontinued) see theophylline on previous page

Theovent® (Discontinued) see theophylline on previous page

Therabid® (Discontinued)

TheraCys® [US] see BCG vaccine on page 96

Thera-Flur® (Discontinued) see fluoride on page 361

Thera-Flur-N® [US] *see* fluoride *on page 361*

Thera-Flu® Severe Cold Non-Drowsy *(Discontinued)* *see* acetaminophen, dextromethorphan, and pseudoephedrine *on page 12*

Theragran-M® Advanced Formula *(Discontinued)* *see* vitamins (multiple/oral) *on page 895*

Theragran® Heart Right™ *(Discontinued)* *see* vitamins (multiple/oral) *on page 895*

TheraPatch® Warm *(Discontinued)* *see* capsaicin *on page 145*

therapeutic multivitamins *see* vitamins (multiple/oral) *on page 895*

Theratears® [US] *see* carboxymethylcellulose *on page 153*

Thermazene® [US] *see* silver sulfadiazine *on page 786*

thiabendazole (thye a BEN da zole)
Synonyms tiabendazole
U.S./Canadian Brand Names Mintezol® [US]
Therapeutic Category Anthelmintic
Use Treatment of strongyloidiasis, cutaneous larva migrans, visceral larva migrans, dracunculiasis, trichinosis, and mixed helminthic infections
Usual Dosage Purgation is not required prior to use; drinking of fruit juice aids in expulsion of worms by removing the mucous to which the intestinal tapeworms attach themselves.

Children and Adults:
Oral: 50 mg/kg/day divided every 12 hours (if >68 kg: 1.5 g/dose); maximum dose: 3 g/day
Treatment duration:
Strongyloidiasis, ascariasis, uncinariasis: For 2 consecutive days
Cutaneous larva migrans: For 2 consecutive days; if active lesions are still present 2 days after completion, a second course of treatment is recommended.
Visceral larva migrans: For 7 consecutive days
Trichinosis: For 2-4 consecutive days; optimal dosage not established
Dracunculosis: 50-75 mg/kg/day divided every 12 hours for 3 days
Dosage Forms
Tablet, chewable:
Mintezol®: 500 mg

thiamazole *see* methimazole *on page 552*

thiamine (THYE a min)
Sound-Alike/Look-Alike Issues
thiamine may be confused with Tenormin®, Thorazine®
Synonyms aneurine hydrochloride; thiamine hydrochloride; thiaminium chloride hydrochloride; vitamin B_1
U.S./Canadian Brand Names Betaxin® [Can]
Therapeutic Category Vitamin, Water Soluble
Use Treatment of thiamine deficiency including beriberi, Wernicke encephalopathy, Korsakoff syndrome, neuritis associated with pregnancy, or in alcoholic patients; dietary supplement
Usual Dosage
Adequate Intake:
0-6 months: 0.2 mg/day
7-12 months: 0.3 mg/day
Recommended daily intake:
1-3 years: 0.5 mg
4-8 years: 0.6 mg
9-13 years: 0.9 mg
14-18 years: Female: 1 mg; Male: 1.2 mg
≥19 years: Female: 1.1 mg; Male: 1.2 mg
Pregnancy, lactation: 1.4 mg
Parenteral nutrition supplementation:
Infants: 1.2 mg/day
Adults: 6 mg/day; may be increased to 25-50 mg/day with history of alcohol abuse
Thiamine deficiency (beriberi):
Children: 10-25 mg/dose I.M. or I.V. daily (if critically ill), or 10-50 mg/dose orally every day for 2 weeks, then 5-10 mg/dose orally daily for 1 month
Adults: 5-30 mg/dose I.M. or I.V. 3 times/day (if critically ill); then orally 5-30 mg/day in single or divided doses 3 times/day for 1 month
Alcohol withdrawal syndrome: Adults: 100 mg/day I.M. or I.V. for several days, followed by 50-100 mg/day orally

Wernicke encephalopathy: Adults: Treatment: Initial: 100 mg I.V., then 50-100 mg/day I.M. or I.V. until consuming a regular, balanced diet. Larger doses may be needed in patients with alcohol abuse.

Dosage Forms
Injection, solution: 100 mg/mL (2 mL)
Tablet: 50 mg, 100 mg, 250 mg, 500 mg

thiamine hydrochloride *see* thiamine *on previous page*

thiaminium chloride hydrochloride *see* thiamine *on previous page*

thioguanine (thye oh GWAH neen)
Sound-Alike/Look-Alike Issues
6-thioguanine and 6-TG are error-prone abbreviations (associated with six-fold overdoses of thioguanine)
Synonyms 2-amino-6-mercaptopurine; NSC-752; TG; tioguanine
U.S./Canadian Brand Names Lanvis® [Can]; Tabloid® [US]
Therapeutic Category Antineoplastic Agent
Use Treatment of acute myelogenous (nonlymphocytic) leukemia; treatment of chronic myelogenous leukemia and granulocytic leukemia
Usual Dosage Total daily dose can be given at one time.
Oral (refer to individual protocols):
Infants and Children <3 years: Combination drug therapy for acute nonlymphocytic leukemia: 3.3 mg/kg/day in divided doses twice daily for 4 days
Children and Adults: 2-3 mg/kg/day calculated to nearest 20 mg or 75-200 mg/m^2/day in 1-2 divided doses for 5-7 days or until remission is attained
Dosage Forms
Tablet [scored]:
Tabloid®: 40 mg

Thiola® [US/Can] *see* tiopronin *on page 845*

thiopental (thye oh PEN tal)
Synonyms thiopental sodium
U.S./Canadian Brand Names Pentothal® [US/Can]
Therapeutic Category Barbiturate
Controlled Substance C-III
Use Induction of anesthesia; adjunct for intubation in head injury patients; control of convulsive states; treatment of elevated intracranial pressure
Usual Dosage I.V.:
Induction anesthesia:
Infants: 5-8 mg/kg
Children 1-12 years: 5-6 mg/kg
Adults: 3-5 mg/kg
Maintenance anesthesia:
Children: 1 mg/kg as needed
Adults: 25-100 mg as needed
Increased intracranial pressure: Children and Adults: 1.5-5 mg/kg/dose; repeat as needed to control intracranial pressure
Seizures:
Children: 2-3 mg/kg/dose; repeat as needed
Adults: 75-250 mg/dose; repeat as needed
Dosage Forms
Injection, powder for reconstitution:
Pentothal®: 250 mg, 400 mg, 500 mg, 1 g

thiopental sodium *see* thiopental *on this page*

thiophosphoramide *see* thiotepa *on next page*

Thioplex® *(Discontinued)* *see* thiotepa *on next page*

thioproperazine *(Canada only)* (thye oh pro PER a zeen)
U.S./Canadian Brand Names Majeptil® [Can]
Therapeutic Category Neuroleptic Agent
Use All types of acute and chronic schizophrenia, including those which did not respond to the usual neuroleptics; manic syndromes.
Usual Dosage Initial treatment: Adults: It is recommended to start treatment at a low dosage of about 5 mg/day in a single dose or in divided doses. This initial dosage is gradually increased by the same amount every
(Continued)

thioproperazine *(Canada only)* *(Continued)*

2-3 days until the usual effective dosage of 30-40 mg/day is reached. In some cases, higher dosages of 90 mg or more per day, are necessary to control the psychotic manifestations.

Children >10 years of age: Start treatment with a daily dosage of 1-3 mg following the method of treatment described for adults

Maintenance therapy: Adults and Children: Dosage should be reduced gradually to the lowest effective level, which may be as low as a few mg per day and maintained as long as necessary

Dosage Forms

Tablet, as mesylate: 10 mg

thioridazine (thye oh RID a zeen)

Sound-Alike/Look-Alike Issues

thioridazine may be confused with thiothixene, Thorazine®

Mellaril® may be confused with Elavil®, Mebaral®

Synonyms thioridazine hydrochloride

U.S./Canadian Brand Names Mellaril® [Can]

Therapeutic Category Phenothiazine Derivative

Use Management of schizophrenic patients who fail to respond adequately to treatment with other antipsychotic drugs, either because of insufficient effectiveness or the inability to achieve an effective dose due to intolerable adverse effects from those medications

Usual Dosage Oral: Adults: Schizophrenia/psychoses: Initial: 50-100 mg 3 times/day with gradual increments as needed and tolerated; maximum: 800 mg/day in 2-4 divided doses

Dosage Forms

Tablet: 10 mg, 15 mg, 25 mg, 50 mg, 100 mg, 150 mg, 200 mg

thioridazine hydrochloride *see* thioridazine *on this page*

thiosulfuric acid disodium salt *see* sodium thiosulfate *on page 798*

thiotepa (thye oh TEP a)

Synonyms TESPA; thiophosphoramide; triethylenethiophosphoramide; TSPA

Therapeutic Category Antineoplastic Agent

Use Treatment of superficial tumors of the bladder; palliative treatment of adenocarcinoma of breast or ovary; lymphomas and sarcomas; controlling intracavitary effusions caused by metastatic tumors; I.T. use: CNS leukemia/lymphoma, CNS metastases

Usual Dosage Refer to individual protocols.

Children: Sarcomas: I.V.: 25-65 mg/m^2 as a single dose every 21 days

Adults:

I.M., I.V., SubQ: 30-60 mg/m^2 once weekly

I.V.: 0.3-0.4 mg/kg by rapid I.V. administration every 1-4 weeks, **or** 0.2 mg/kg or 6-8 mg/m^2/day for 4-5 days every 2-4 weeks

High-dose therapy for bone marrow transplant: I.V.: 500 mg/m^2, up to 900 mg/m^2

I.M.: 15-30 mg in various schedules have been given

Intracavitary: 0.6-0.8 mg/kg or 30-60 mg weekly

Intrapericardial: 15-30 mg

Intrathecal: 10-15 mg or 5-11.5 mg/m^2

Dosage Forms

Injection, powder for reconstitution: 15 mg, 30 mg

thiothixene (thye oh THIKS een)

Sound-Alike/Look-Alike Issues

thiothixene may be confused with thioridazine

Navane® may be confused with Norvasc®, Nubain®

Synonyms tiotixene

U.S./Canadian Brand Names Navane® [US/Can]

Therapeutic Category Thioxanthene Derivative

Use Management of schizophrenia

Usual Dosage Oral: Adults:

Mild-to-moderate psychosis: 2 mg 3 times/day, up to 20-30 mg/day; more severe psychosis: Initial: 5 mg 2 times/day, may increase gradually, if necessary; maximum: 60 mg/day

Rapid tranquilization of the agitated patient (administered every 30-60 minutes): 5-10 mg; average total dose for tranquilization: 15-30 mg

Dosage Forms

Capsule: 1 mg, 2 mg, 5 mg, 10 mg

Navane®: 2 mg, 5 mg, 10 mg, 20 mg

thonzonium, neomycin, colistin, and hydrocortisone *see* neomycin, colistin, hydrocortisone, and thonzonium *on page 597*

Thorazine® *(Discontinued)* *see* chlorpromazine *on page 185*

Thorets [US-OTC] *see* benzocaine *on page 101*

Thrombate III® **[US/Can]** *see* antithrombin III *on page 62*

Thrombinar® *(Discontinued)* *see* thrombin (topical) *on this page*

Thrombin-JMI® **[US]** *see* thrombin (topical) *on this page*

thrombin (topical) (THROM bin, TOP i kal)

U.S./Canadian Brand Names Thrombin-JMI® [US]
Therapeutic Category Hemostatic Agent
Use Hemostasis whenever minor bleeding from capillaries and small venules is accessible
Usual Dosage Use 1000-2000 units/mL of solution where bleeding is profuse; apply powder directly to the site of bleeding or on oozing surfaces; use 100 units/mL for bleeding from skin or mucosal surfaces
Dosage Forms
Powder for reconstitution, topical:
Thrombin-JMI®: 5000 units, 20,000 units

Thrombostat® *(Discontinued)* *see* thrombin (topical) *on this page*

thymocyte stimulating factor *see* aldesleukin *on page 26*

Thymoglobulin® **[US]** *see* antithymocyte globulin (rabbit) *on page 63*

Thyrar® *(Discontinued)* *see* thyroid *on this page*

Thyrel® **TRH** *(Discontinued)*

Thyro-Block® *(Discontinued)* *see* potassium iodide *on page 702*

Thyrogen® **[US/Can]** *see* thyrotropin alpha *on this page*

thyroid (THYE roid)

Synonyms desiccated thyroid; thyroid extract; thyroid USP
U.S./Canadian Brand Names Armour® Thyroid [US]; Nature-Throid® NT [US]; Westhroid® [US]
Therapeutic Category Thyroid Product
Use Replacement or supplemental therapy in hypothyroidism; pituitary TSH suppressants (thyroid nodules, thyroiditis, multinodular goiter, thyroid cancer), thyrotoxicosis, diagnostic suppression tests
Usual Dosage Oral:
Children: Recommended pediatric dosage for congenital hypothyroidism:
0-6 months: 15-30 mg/day; 4.8-6 mg/kg/day
6-12 months: 30-45 mg/day; 3.6-4.8 mg/kg/day
1-5 years: 45-60 mg/day; 3-3.6 mg/kg/day
6-12 years: 60-90 mg/day; 2.4-3 mg/kg/day
>12 years: >90 mg/day; 1.2-1.8 mg/kg/day
Adults: Initial: 15-30 mg; increase with 15 mg increments every 2-4 weeks; use 15 mg in patients with cardiovascular disease or myxedema. Maintenance dose: Usually 60-120 mg/day; monitor TSH and clinical symptoms.
Thyroid cancer: Requires larger amounts than replacement therapy
Dosage Forms
Tablet: 30 mg, 32.5 mg, 60 mg, 65 mg, 90 mg, 120 mg, 130 mg, 180 mg, 240 mg, 300 mg
Armour® Thyroid: 15 mg, 30 mg, 60 mg, 90 mg, 120 mg, 180 mg, 240 mg, 300 mg
Nature-Throid® NT, Westhroid®: 32.5 mg, 65 mg, 130 mg, 195 mg

thyroid extract *see* thyroid *on this page*

Thyroid Strong® *(Discontinued)* *see* thyroid *on this page*

thyroid USP *see* thyroid *on this page*

Thyrolar® **[US/Can]** *see* liotrix *on page 510*

ThyroSafe™ **[US-OTC]** *see* potassium iodide *on page 702*

ThyroShield™ **[US-OTC]** *see* potassium iodide *on page 702*

thyrotropin alpha (thye roe TROH pin AL fa)

Sound-Alike/Look-Alike Issues
Thyrogen® may be confused with Thyrolar®
(Continued)

thyrotropin alpha *(Continued)*

Synonyms human thyroid stimulating hormone; TSH

U.S./Canadian Brand Names Thyrogen® [US/Can]

Therapeutic Category Diagnostic Agent

Use As an adjunctive diagnostic tool for serum thyroglobulin (Tg) testing with or without radioiodine imaging in the follow-up of patients with well-differentiated thyroid cancer

Potential clinical use:

1. Patients with an undetectable Tg on thyroid hormone suppressive therapy to exclude the diagnosis of residual or recurrent thyroid cancer
2. Patients requiring serum Tg testing and radioiodine imaging who are unwilling to undergo thyroid hormone withdrawal testing and whose treating physician believes that use of a less sensitive test is justified
3. Patients who are either unable to mount an adequate endogenous TSH response to thyroid hormone withdrawal or in whom withdrawal is medically contraindicated

Usual Dosage I.M.: Children >16 years and Adults: 0.9 mg every 24 hours for 2 doses or every 72 hours for 3 doses

For radioiodine imaging, radioiodine administration should be given 24 hours following the final Thyrogen® injection. Scanning should be performed 48 hours after radioiodine administration (72 hours after the final injection of Thyrogen®).

For serum testing, serum Tg should be obtained 72 hours after final injection of Thyrogen®.

Dosage Forms Injection, powder for reconstitution:

Thyrogen®: Four-vial kit: 1.1 mg

tiabendazole *see* thiabendazole *on page 836*

tiagabine *(tye AG a been)*

Sound-Alike/Look-Alike Issues

tiagabine may be confused with tizanidine

Synonyms tiagabine hydrochloride

U.S./Canadian Brand Names Gabitril® [US/Can]

Therapeutic Category Anticonvulsant

Use Adjunctive therapy in adults and children ≥12 years of age in the treatment of partial seizures

Usual Dosage Oral (administer with food):

Patients receiving enzyme-inducing AED regimens:

Children 12-18 years: 4 mg once daily for 1 week; may increase to 8 mg daily in 2 divided doses for 1 week; then may increase by 4-8 mg weekly to response or up to 32 mg daily in 2-4 divided doses

Adults: 4 mg once daily for 1 week; may increase by 4-8 mg weekly to response or up to 56 mg daily in 2-4 divided doses; usual maintenance: 32-56 mg/day

Patients **not** receiving enzyme-inducing AED regimens: The estimated plasma concentrations of tiagabine in patients not taking enzyme-inducing medications is twice that of patients receiving enzyme-inducing AEDs. Lower doses are required; slower titration may be necessary.

Dosage Forms

Tablet:

Gabitril®: 2 mg, 4 mg, 12 mg, 16 mg

tiagabine hydrochloride *see* tiagabine *on this page*

Tiamate® *(Discontinued) see* diltiazem *on page 261*

Tiamol® **[Can]** *see* fluocinonide *on page 360*

Tiaprofenic-200 [Can] *see* tiaprofenic acid *(Canada only) on this page*

Tiaprofenic-300 [Can] *see* tiaprofenic acid *(Canada only) on this page*

tiaprofenic acid *(Canada only)* *(tye ah PRO fen ik AS id)*

U.S./Canadian Brand Names Albert® Tiafen [Can]; Apo-Tiaprofenic® [Can]; Dom-Tiaprofenic® [Can]; Novo-Tiaprofenic [Can]; Nu-Tiaprofenic [Can]; PMS-Tiaprofenic [Can]; Surgam® [Can]; Tiaprofenic-200 [Can]; Tiaprofenic-300 [Can]

Therapeutic Category Nonsteroidal Antiinflammatory Drug (NSAID)

Use Relief of signs and symptoms of rheumatoid arthritis and osteoarthritis (degenerative joint disease)

Usual Dosage Oral: Adults:

Rheumatoid arthritis:

Tablet: Usual initial and maintenance dose: 600 mg/day in 3 divided doses; some patients may do well on 300 mg twice daily; maximum daily dose: 600 mg

Sustained release capsule: Initial and maintenance dose: 2 sustained release capsules of 300 mg once daily; Surgam® SR capsules should be swallowed whole

Osteoarthritis:
Tablet: Usual initial and maintenance dose: 600 mg/day in 2 or 3 divided doses; in rare instances patients may be maintained on 300 mg/day in divided doses; maximum daily dose: 600 mg
Sustained release capsule: Initial and maintenance dose: 2 sustained release capsules of 300 mg once daily; Surgam® SR capsules should be swallowed whole

Dosage Forms [CAN] = Canadian brand name
Capsule, sustained release: 300 mg [not available in the U.S.]
Tablet: 200 mg, 300 mg
Apo-Tiaprofenic® [CAN], Novo-Tiaprofenic [CAN], Nu-Tiaprofenic [CAN], PMS-Tiaprofenic: 200 mg, 300 mg [not available in the U.S.]
Albert® Tiafen [CAN], Dom-Tiaprofenic® [CAN], Surgam® [CAN]: 300 mg [not available in the U.S.]

Tiazac® [US/Can] *see* diltiazem *on page 261*

Tiazac® XC [Can] *see* diltiazem *on page 261*

Ticar® [US] *see* ticarcillin *on this page*

ticarcillin (tye kar SIL in)

Sound-Alike/Look-Alike Issues
Ticar® may be confused with Tigan®
Synonyms ticarcillin disodium
U.S./Canadian Brand Names Ticar® [US]
Therapeutic Category Penicillin
Use Treatment of susceptible infections such as septicemia, acute and chronic respiratory tract infections, skin and soft tissue infections, and urinary tract infections due to susceptible strains of *Pseudomonas*, and other gram-negative bacteria
Usual Dosage Note: Ticarcillin is generally given I.V., I.M. injection is only for the treatment of uncomplicated urinary tract infections and dose should not exceed 2 g/injection when administered I.M.
Usual dosage range:
Neonates: I.M., I.V.:
Postnatal age <7 days:
<2000 g: 75 mg/kg/dose every 12 hours
>2000 g: 75 mg/kg/dose every 8 hours
Postnatal age >7 days:
<1200 g: 75 mg/kg/dose every 12 hours
1200-2000 g: 75 mg/kg/dose every 8 hours
>2000 g: 75 mg/kg/dose every 6 hours
Infants and Children:
I.M.: 50-100 mg/kg/day in divided doses every 6-8 hours
I.V.: 50-300 mg/kg/day in divided doses every 4-8 hours (maximum dose: 24 g/day)
Adults: I.M., I.V.: 1-4 g every 4-6 hours
Indication-specific dosing:
Infants and Children:
Cystic fibrosis (acute pulmonary exacerbations): I.V.: 100 mg/kg every 6 hours
Systemic infection: I.V.: 200-300 mg/kg/day in divided doses every 4-6 hours
Urinary tract infections: I.M., I.V.: 50-100 mg/kg/day in divided doses every 6-8 hours
Adults:
Otitis externa (malignant): I.V.: 3 g every 4 hours with tobramycin
***Pseudomonas* infections:** I.V.: 3 g every 4 hours
Dosage Forms
Injection, powder for reconstitution:
Ticar®: 3 g

ticarcillin and clavulanate potassium (tye kar SIL in & klav yoo LAN ate poe TASS ee um)

Synonyms ticarcillin and clavulanic acid
U.S./Canadian Brand Names Timentin® [US/Can]
Therapeutic Category Penicillin
Use Treatment of lower respiratory tract, urinary tract, skin and skin structures, bone and joint, gynecologic (endometritis) and intra-abdominal (peritonitis) infections, and septicemia caused by susceptible organisms. Clavulanate expands activity of ticarcillin to include beta-lactamase producing strains of *S. aureus*, *H. influenzae*, *Bacteroides* species, and some other gram-negative bacilli
Usual Dosage Note: Timentin® (ticarcillin/clavulanate) is a combination product; each 3.1 g dosage form contains 3 g ticarcillin disodium and 0.1 g clavulanic acid.
(Continued)

ticarcillin and clavulanate potassium *(Continued)*

Usual dosage range:
Children and Adults <60 kg: I.V.: 200-300 mg of ticarcillin component/kg/day in divided doses every 4-6 hours
Children ≥60 kg and Adults: I.V.: 3.1 g (ticarcillin 3 g plus clavulanic acid 0.1 g) every 4-6 hours (maximum: 24 g of ticarcillin component/day)
Indication-specific dosing:
Children: I.V.:
Bite wounds (animal): 200 mg of ticarcillin component/kg/day in divided doses
Neutropenic fever: 75 mg of ticarcillin component/kg every 6 hours (maximum 3.1 g/dose)
Pneumonia (nosocomial): 300 mg of ticarcillin component/kg/day in 4 divided doses (maximum: 18-24 g of ticarcillin component/day)
Children ≥60 kg and Adults: I.V.:
Amnionitis, cholangitis, diverticulitis, endometritis, epididymo-orchitis, mastoiditis, orbital cellulitis, peritonitis, pneumonia (aspiration): 3.1 g every 6 hours
Liver abscess, parafascial space infections, septic thrombophlebitis: 3.1 g every 4 hours
***Pseudomonas* infections:** 3.1 g every 4 hours
Urinary tract infections: 3.1 g every 6-8 hours
Dosage Forms
Infusion [premixed, frozen]:
Timentin®: Ticarcillin 3 g and clavulanic acid 0.1 g (100 mL)
Injection, powder for reconstitution:
Timentin®: Ticarcillin 3 g and clavulanic acid 0.1 g (3.1 g, 31 g)

ticarcillin and clavulanic acid *see* ticarcillin and clavulanate potassium *on previous page*

ticarcillin disodium *see* ticarcillin *on previous page*

TICE® BCG [US] *see* BCG vaccine *on page 96*

Ticlid® [US/Can] *see* ticlopidine *on this page*

ticlopidine (tye KLOE pi deen)

Synonyms ticlopidine hydrochloride
U.S./Canadian Brand Names Alti-Ticlopidine [Can]; Apo-Ticlopidine® [Can]; Gen-Ticlopidine [Can]; Novo-Ticlopidine [Can]; Nu-Ticlopidine [Can]; Rhoxal-ticlopidine [Can]; Sandoz-Ticlopidine [Can]; Ticlid® [US/Can]
Therapeutic Category Antiplatelet Agent
Use Platelet aggregation inhibitor that reduces the risk of thrombotic stroke in patients who have had a stroke or stroke precursors. **Note:** Due to its association with life-threatening hematologic disorders, ticlopidine should be reserved for patients who are intolerant to aspirin, or who have failed aspirin therapy. Adjunctive therapy (with aspirin) following successful coronary stent implantation to reduce the incidence of subacute stent thrombosis.
Usual Dosage Oral: Adults:
Stroke prevention: 250 mg twice daily with food
Coronary artery stenting (initiate after successful implantation): 250 mg twice daily with food (in combination with antiplatelet doses of aspirin) for up to 30 days
Dosage Forms
Tablet: 250 mg
Ticlid®: 250 mg

ticlopidine hydrochloride *see* ticlopidine *on this page*

Ticon® (Discontinued) *see* trimethobenzamide *on page 867*

TIG *see* tetanus immune globulin (human) *on page 829*

Tigan® [US/Can] *see* trimethobenzamide *on page 867*

tigecycline (tye ge SYE kleen)

Synonyms GAR-936
U.S./Canadian Brand Names Tygacil™ [US]
Therapeutic Category Antibiotic, Glycylcycline
Use Treatment of complicated skin and skin structure infections caused by susceptible organisms, including methicillin-resistant *Staphylococcus aureus* and vancomycin-sensitive *Enterococcus faecalis*; treatment of complicated intra-abdominal infections
Usual Dosage I.V.: Adults:
Initial: 100 mg as a single dose
Maintenance dose: 50 mg every 12 hours

Recommended duration of therapy: Intraabdominal infections or complicated skin/skin structure infections: 5-14 days.

Dosage Forms

Injection, powder for reconstitution:

Tygacil™: 50 mg

Tikosyn® [US/Can] *see* dofetilide *on page 274*

Tilade® [US/Can] *see* nedocromil (inhalation) *on page 594*

tiludronate (tye LOO droe nate)

Synonyms tiludronate disodium

U.S./Canadian Brand Names Skelid® [US]

Therapeutic Category Bisphosphonate Derivative

Use Treatment of Paget disease of the bone in patients who have a level of serum alkaline phosphatase (SAP) at least twice the upper limit of normal, or who are symptomatic, or who are at risk for future complications of their disease

Usual Dosage Tiludronate should be taken with 6-8 oz of plain water and not taken within 2 hours of food

Oral: Adults: 400 mg (2 tablets of tiludronic acid) daily for a period of 3 months; allow an interval of 3 months to assess response

Dosage Forms

Tablet:

Skelid®: 200 mg

tiludronate disodium *see* tiludronate *on this page*

Tim-AK [Can] *see* timolol *on this page*

Time-C [US-OTC] *see* ascorbic acid *on page 76*

Time-C-Bio [US-OTC] *see* ascorbic acid *on page 76*

Timecelles® *(Discontinued)* *see* ascorbic acid *on page 76*

Timentin® [US/Can] *see* ticarcillin and clavulanate potassium *on page 841*

timolol (TIM oh lol)

Sound-Alike/Look-Alike Issues

timolol may be confused with atenolol, Tylenol®

Timoptic® may be confused with Talacen®, Viroptic®

Synonyms timolol hemihydrate; timolol maleate

U.S./Canadian Brand Names Alti-Timolol [Can]; Apo-Timol® [Can]; Apo-Timop® [Can]; Betimol® [US]; Blocadren® [US]; Gen-Timolol [Can]; Istalol™ [US]; Nu-Timolol [Can]; Phoxal-timolol [Can]; PMS-Timolol [Can]; Sandoz-Timolol [Can]; Tim-AK [Can]; Timolol GFS [US]; Timoptic-XE® [US/Can]; Timoptic® in OcuDose® [US]; Timoptic® [US/Can]

Therapeutic Category Beta-Adrenergic Blocker

Use

Ophthalmic: Treatment of elevated intraocular pressure such as glaucoma or ocular hypertension

Oral: Treatment of hypertension and angina; to reduce mortality following myocardial infarction; prophylaxis of migraine

Usual Dosage

Ophthalmic:

Children and Adults:

Solution: Initial: Instill 1 drop (0.25% solution) into affected eye(s) twice daily; increase to 0.5% solution if response not adequate; decrease to 1 drop/day if controlled; do not exceed 1 drop twice daily of 0.5% solution

Gel-forming solution (Timolol GFS, Timoptic-XE®): Instill 1 drop (either 0.25% or 0.5% solution) once daily

Adults: Solution (Istalol®): Instill 1 drop (0.5% solution) once daily in the morning

Oral: Adults:

Hypertension: Initial: 10 mg twice daily, increase gradually every 7 days, usual dosage: 20-40 mg/day in 2 divided doses; maximum: 60 mg/day

Prevention of myocardial infarction: 10 mg twice daily initiated within 1-4 weeks after infarction

Migraine headache: Initial: 10 mg twice daily, increase to maximum of 30 mg/day

Dosage Forms

Gel-forming solution, ophthalmic: 0.25% (5 mL); 0.5% (2.5 mL, 5 mL)

Timolol GFS: 0.25% (2.5 mL, 5 mL); 0.5% (2.5 mL, 5 mL)

Timoptic-XE®: 0.25% (5 mL); 0.5% (5 mL)

Solution, ophthalmic: 0.25% (5 mL, 10 mL, 15 mL); 0.5% (5 mL, 10 mL, 15 mL)

Betimol®: 0.25% (5 mL, 10 mL, 15 mL); 0.5% (5 mL, 10 mL, 15 mL)

(Continued)

timolol *(Continued)*

Istalol™: 0.5% (10 mL)
Timoptic®: 0.25% (5 mL); 0.5% (5 mL, 10 mL)
Solution, ophthalmic [preservative free]: 0.25% (0.2 mL); 0.5% (0.2 mL)
Timoptic® in OcuDose®: 0.25% (0.2 mL); 0.5% (0.2 mL)
Tablet: 5 mg, 10 mg, 20 mg
Blocadren®: 20 mg

timolol and brimonidine *see* brimonidine and timolol *(Canada only) on page 118*

timolol and dorzolamide *see* dorzolamide and timolol *on page 277*

Timolol GFS [US] *see* timolol *on previous page*

timolol hemihydrate *see* timolol *on previous page*

timolol maleate *see* timolol *on previous page*

Timoptic® [US/Can] *see* timolol *on previous page*

Timoptic® in OcuDose® [US] *see* timolol *on previous page*

Timoptic-XE® [US/Can] *see* timolol *on previous page*

Tinactin® Antifungal [US-OTC] *see* tolnaftate *on page 849*

Tinactin® Antifungal Jock Itch [US-OTC] *see* tolnaftate *on page 849*

Tinaderm [US-OTC] *see* tolnaftate *on page 849*

Tinamed® [US-OTC] *see* salicylic acid *on page 772*

TinBen® *(Discontinued)* *see* benzoin *on page 103*

Tindamax® [US] *see* tinidazole *on this page*

Ting® Cream [US-OTC] *see* tolnaftate *on page 849*

Ting® Spray Liquid [US-OTC] *see* tolnaftate *on page 849*

tinidazole (tye NI da zole)

U.S./Canadian Brand Names Tindamax® [US]
Therapeutic Category Amebicide; Antibiotic, Miscellaneous; Antiprotozoal, Nitroimidazole
Use Treatment of trichomoniasis caused by *T. vaginalis*; treatment of giardiasis caused by *G. duodenalis* (*G. lamblia*); treatment of intestinal amebiasis and amebic liver abscess caused by *E. histolytica*; treatment of bacterial vaginosis caused by *Bacteroides* spp, *Gardnerella vaginalis*, and *Prevotella* spp in nonpregnant females
Usual Dosage Oral:
Children >3 years:
Amebiasis, intestinal: 50 mg/kg/day for 3 days (maximum dose: 2 g/day)
Amebiasis, liver abscess: 50 mg/kg/day for 3-5 days (maximum dose: 2 g/day)
Giardiasis: 50 mg/kg as a single dose (maximum dose: 2 g)
Adults:
Amebiasis, intestinal: 2 g/day for 3 days
Amebiasis, liver abscess: 2 g/day for 3-5 days
Bacterial vaginosis: 2 g/day for 2 days or 1 g/day for 5 days
Giardiasis: 2 g as a single dose
Trichomoniasis: 2 g as a single dose; sexual partners should be treated at the same time
Dosage Forms
Tablet [scored]:
Tindamax®: 250 mg, 500 mg

Tinver® *(Discontinued)* *see* sodium thiosulfate *on page 798*

tinzaparin (tin ZA pa rin)

Synonyms tinzaparin sodium
U.S./Canadian Brand Names Innohep® [US/Can]
Therapeutic Category Anticoagulant (Other)
Use Treatment of acute symptomatic deep vein thrombosis, with or without pulmonary embolism, in conjunction with warfarin sodium
Usual Dosage SubQ:
Adults: 175 anti-Xa int. units/kg of body weight once daily. Warfarin sodium should be started when appropriate. Administer tinzaparin for at least 6 days and until patient is adequately anticoagulated with warfarin.
Note: To calculate the volume of solution to administer per dose: Volume to be administered (mL) = patient weight (kg) x 0.00875 mL/kg (may be rounded off to the nearest 0.05 mL)

Dosage Forms
  Injection, solution:,
    Innohep®: 20,000 anti-Xa int. units/mL (2 mL)

tinzaparin sodium *see* tinzaparin *on previous page*

tioconazole (tye oh KONE a zole)
  Sound-Alike/Look-Alike Issues
    tioconazole may be confused with terconazole
  U.S./Canadian Brand Names 1-Day™ [US-OTC]; Vagistat®-1 [US-OTC]
  Therapeutic Category Antifungal Agent
  Use Local treatment of vulvovaginal candidiasis
  Usual Dosage Adults: Vaginal: Insert 1 applicatorful in vagina, just prior to bedtime, as a single dose
  Dosage Forms
    Ointment, vaginal:
      1-Day™ [OTC], Vagistat®-1 [OTC]: 6.5% (4.6 g)

tioguanine *see* thioguanine *on page 837*

tiopronin (tye oh PROE nin)
  Sound-Alike/Look-Alike Issues
    Thiola® may be confused with Theolair™
  U.S./Canadian Brand Names Thiola® [US/Can]
  Therapeutic Category Urinary Tract Product
  Use Prevention of kidney stone (cystine) formation in patients with severe homozygous cystinuric who have urinary cystine >500 mg/day who are resistant to treatment with high fluid intake, alkali, and diet modification, or who have had adverse reactions to penicillamine
  Usual Dosage Adults: Initial dose is 800 mg/day, average dose is 1000 mg/day
  Dosage Forms
    Tablet:
      Thiola®: 100 mg

tiotixene *see* thiothixene *on page 838*

tiotropium (ty oh TRO pee um)
  Sound-Alike/Look-Alike Issues
    Spiriva® may be confused with Inspra™
  Synonyms tiotropium bromide monohydrate
  U.S./Canadian Brand Names Spiriva® [US/Can]
  Therapeutic Category Anticholinergic Agent
  Use Maintenance treatment of bronchospasm associated with COPD (bronchitis and emphysema)
  Usual Dosage Oral inhalation: Adults: Contents of 1 capsule (18 mcg) inhaled once daily using HandiHaler® device
  Dosage Forms
    Powder for oral inhalation [capsule]:
      Spiriva®: 18 mcg/capsule (5s, 30s)

tiotropium bromide monohydrate *see* tiotropium *on this page*

tipranavir (tip RA na veer)
  Synonyms PNU-140690E; TPV
  U.S./Canadian Brand Names Aptivus® [US/Can]
  Therapeutic Category Antiretroviral Agent, Protease Inhibitor
  Use Treatment of HIV-1 infections in combination with ritonavir and other antiretroviral agents; limited to highly treatment-experienced or multiprotease inhibitor-resistant patients.
  Usual Dosage Oral: Adults: 500 mg twice daily with a high-fat meal. **Note:** Coadministration with ritonavir (200 mg twice daily) is required.
  Dosage Forms
    Capsule, gelatin:
      Aptivus®: 250 mg

TipTapToe *(Discontinued)* *see* tolnaftate *on page 849*

tirofiban (tye roe FYE ban)

Sound-Alike/Look-Alike Issues
Aggrastat® may be confused with Aggrenox®, argatroban
Synonyms MK383; tirofiban hydrochloride
U.S./Canadian Brand Names Aggrastat® [US/Can]
Therapeutic Category Antiplatelet Agent
Use In combination with heparin, is indicated for the treatment of acute coronary syndrome, including patients who are to be managed medically and those undergoing PTCA or atherectomy. In this setting, it has been shown to decrease the rate of a combined endpoint of death, new myocardial infarction or refractory ischemia/repeat cardiac procedure.
Usual Dosage I.V.: Adults: Initial rate of 0.4 mcg/kg/minute for 30 minutes and then continued at 0.1 mcg/kg/minute; dosing should be continued through angiography and for 12-24 hours after angioplasty or atherectomy.
Dosage Forms
Infusion [premixed in sodium chloride]:
Aggrastat®: 50 mcg/mL (100 mL, 250 mL)
Injection, solution:
Aggrastat®: 250 mcg/mL (50 mL)

tirofiban hydrochloride *see* tirofiban *on this page*

Tiseb® [US-OTC] *see* salicylic acid *on page 772*

Tisit® [US-OTC] *see* pyrethrins and piperonyl butoxide *on page 734*

Tisit® Blue Gel [US-OTC] *see* pyrethrins and piperonyl butoxide *on page 734*

Tisseel® VH [US/Can] *see* fibrin sealant kit *on page 351*

Titralac™ [US-OTC] *see* calcium carbonate *on page 138*

Titralac® Plus [US-OTC] *see* calcium carbonate and simethicone *on page 139*

Ti-U-Lac® H [Can] *see* urea and hydrocortisone *on page 878*

tizanidine (tye ZAN i deen)

Sound-Alike/Look-Alike Issues
tizanidine may be confused with tiagabine
U.S./Canadian Brand Names Apo-Tizanidine® [Can]; Gen-Tizanidine [Can]; Zanaflex® [US/Can]
Therapeutic Category Alpha₂-Adrenergic Agonist Agent
Use Skeletal muscle relaxant used for treatment of muscle spasticity
Usual Dosage Adults: 2-4 mg 3 times/day
Usual initial dose: 4 mg, may increase by 2-4 mg as needed for satisfactory reduction of muscle tone every 6-8 hours to a maximum of three doses in any 24 hour period
Maximum dose: 36 mg/day
Dosage Forms
Capsule:
Zanaflex®: 2 mg, 4 mg, 6 mg
Tablet: 2 mg, 4 mg
Zanaflex®: 4 mg

TMC-114 *see* darunavir *on page 232*

TMP *see* trimethoprim *on page 867*

TMP-SMZ *see* sulfamethoxazole and trimethoprim *on page 813*

TMZ *see* temozolomide *on page 824*

T.N. Dickinson's® Hazelets [US-OTC] *see* witch hazel *on page 900*

TNKase™ [US/Can] *see* tenecteplase *on page 825*

TOBI® [US/Can] *see* tobramycin *on this page*

TobraDex® [US/Can] *see* tobramycin and dexamethasone *on page 848*

tobramycin (toe bra MYE sin)

Sound-Alike/Look-Alike Issues
tobramycin may be confused with Trobicin®
AKTob® may be confused with AK-Trol®
Nebcin® may be confused with Inapsine®, Naprosyn®, Nubain®
Tobrex® may be confused with TobraDex®

Synonyms tobramycin sulfate

U.S./Canadian Brand Names AKTob® [US]; PMS-Tobramycin [Can]; Sandoz-Tobramycin [Can]; TOBI® [US/Can]; Tobramycin Injection, USP [Can]; Tobrex® [US/Can]

Therapeutic Category Aminoglycoside (Antibiotic); Antibiotic, Ophthalmic

Use Treatment of documented or suspected infections caused by susceptible gram-negative bacilli including *Pseudomonas aeruginosa*; topically used to treat superficial ophthalmic infections caused by susceptible bacteria. Tobramycin solution for inhalation is indicated for the management of cystic fibrosis patients (>6 years of age) with *Pseudomonas aeruginosa*.

Usual Dosage Note: Dosage individualization is **critical** because of the low therapeutic index.

Use of ideal body weight (IBW) for determining the mg/kg/dose appears to be more accurate than dosing on the basis of total body weight (TBW). In morbid obesity, dosage requirement may best be estimated using a dosing weight of IBW + 0.4 (TBW - IBW).

Initial and periodic plasma drug levels (eg, peak and trough with conventional dosing) should be determined, particularly in critically-ill patients with serious infections or in disease states known to significantly alter aminoglycoside pharmacokinetics (eg, cystic fibrosis, burns, or major surgery).

Usual dosage range:

Infants and Children <5 years: I.M., I.V.: 2.5 mg/kg/dose every 8 hours

Children ≥5 years: I.M., I.V.: 2-2.5 mg/kg/dose every 8 hours

Note: Higher individual doses and/or more frequent intervals (eg, every 6 hours) may be required in selected clinical situations (cystic fibrosis) or serum levels document the need.

Children and Adults:

Inhalation:

Children: 40-80 mg 2-3 times/day

Adults: 60-80 mg 3 times/day

High-dose regimen: Children ≥6 years and Adults: 300 mg every 12 hours (do not administer doses <6 hours apart); administer in repeated cycles of 28 days on drug followed by 28 days off drug

Intrathecal: 4-8 mg/day

Ophthalmic: Children ≥2 months and Adults:

Ointment: Instill ¹/₂" (1.25 cm) 2-3 times/day every 3-4 hours

Solution: Instill 1-2 drops every 2-4 hours, up to 2 drops every hour for severe infections

Topical: Apply 3-4 times/day to affected area

Adults: I.M., I.V.:

Conventional: 1-2.5 mg/kg/dose every 8-12 hours; to ensure adequate peak concentrations early in therapy, higher initial dosage may be considered in selected patients when extracellular water is increased (edema, septic shock, postsurgical, and/or trauma)

Once-daily: 4-7 mg/kg/dose once daily; some clinicians recommend this approach for all patients with normal renal function; this dose is at least as efficacious with similar, if not less, toxicity than conventional dosing.

Indication-specific dosing:

Neonates: I.M., I.V.:

Meningitis:

0-7 days: <2000 g: 2.5 mg/kg every 18-24 hours; >2000 g: 2.5 mg/kg every 12 hours

8-28 days: <2000 g: 2.5 mg/kg every 8-12 hours; >2000 g: 2.5 mg/kg every 8 hours

Children:

Cystic fibrosis:

I.M., I.V.: 2.5-3.3 mg/kg every 6-8 hours; **Note:** Some patients may require larger or more frequent doses if serum levels document the need (eg, cystic fibrosis or febrile granulocytopenic patients).

Inhalation:

Standard aerosolized tobramycin: 40-80 mg 2-3 times/day

High-dose regimen (TOBI®): Children ≥6 years: See adult dosing.

Adults: I.M., I.V.:

Brucellosis: 240 mg (I.M.) daily or 5 mg/kg (I.V.) daily for 7 days; either regimen recommended in combination with doxycycline

Cholangitis: 4-6 mg/kg once daily with ampicillin

Diverticulitis, complicated: 1.5-2 mg/kg every 8 hours (with ampicillin and metronidazole)

Endocarditis prophylaxis (dental, oral, upper respiratory procedures, GI/GU procedures): 1.5 mg/kg with ampicillin (50 mg/kg) 30 minutes prior to procedure

Endocarditis or synergy (for gram-positive infections): 1 mg/kg every 8 hours (with ampicillin)

Meningitis *(Enterococcus or Pseudomonas aeruginosa):* I.V.: Loading dose: 2 mg/kg, then 1.7 mg/kg/dose every 8 hours (administered with another bacteriocidal drug)

Pelvic inflammatory disease: Loading dose: 2 mg/kg, then 1.5 mg/kg every 8 hours **or** 4.5 mg/kg once daily

Plague *(Yersinia pestis):* Treatment: 5 mg/kg/day, followed by postexposure prophylaxis with doxycycline

Pneumonia, hospital- or ventilator-associated: 7 mg/kg/day (with antipseudomonal beta-lactam or carbapenem)

Tularemia: 5 mg/kg/day divided every 8 hours for 1-2 weeks

(Continued)

tobramycin *(Continued)*

Urinary tract infection: 1.5 mg/kg/dose every 8 hours

Dosage Forms

Infusion [premixed in NS]: 60 mg (50 mL); 80 mg (100 mL)

Injection, powder for reconstitution: 1.2 g

Injection, solution: 10 mg/mL (2 mL, 8 mL); 40 mg/mL (2 mL, 30 mL, 50 mL)

Ointment, ophthalmic:
Tobrex®: 0.3% (3.5 g)

Solution for nebulization [preservative free]:
TOBI®: 60 mg/mL (5 mL)

Solution, ophthalmic: 0.3% (5 mL)
AKTob®, Tobrex®: 0.3% (5 mL)

tobramycin and dexamethasone (toe bra MYE sin & deks a METH a sone)

Sound-Alike/Look-Alike Issues
TobraDex® may be confused with Tobrex®

Synonyms dexamethasone and tobramycin

U.S./Canadian Brand Names TobraDex® [US/Can]

Therapeutic Category Antibiotic/Corticosteroid, Ophthalmic

Use Treatment of external ocular infection caused by susceptible gram-negative bacteria and steroid responsive inflammatory conditions of the palpebral and bulbar conjunctiva, lid, cornea, and anterior segment of the globe

Usual Dosage Ophthalmic: Children and Adults: Instill 1-2 drops of solution every 4 hours; apply ointment 2-3 times/day; for severe infections apply ointment every 3-4 hours, or solution 2 drops every 30-60 minutes initially, then reduce to less frequent intervals

Dosage Forms

Ointment, ophthalmic:
TobraDex®: Tobramycin 0.3% and dexamethasone 0.1% (3.5 g)

Suspension, ophthalmic:
TobraDex®: Tobramycin 0.3% and dexamethasone 0.1% (2.5 mL, 5 mL, 10 mL)

tobramycin and loteprednol etabonate *see* loteprednol and tobramycin *on page 520*

Tobramycin Injection, USP [Can] *see* tobramycin *on page 846*

tobramycin sulfate *see* tobramycin *on page 846*

Tobrex® [US/Can] *see* tobramycin *on page 846*

tocophersolan *(Discontinued)*

Today® Sponge [US-OTC] *see* nonoxynol 9 *on page 610*

Tofranil® [US/Can] *see* imipramine *on page 449*

Tofranil-PM® [US] *see* imipramine *on page 449*

tolazamide (tole AZ a mide)

Sound-Alike/Look-Alike Issues
TOLAZamide may be confused with tolazoline, TOLBUTamide
Tolinase® may be confused with Orinase®

Tall-Man TOLAZamide

U.S./Canadian Brand Names Tolinase® [Can]

Therapeutic Category Antidiabetic Agent, Oral

Use Adjunct to diet for the management of mild to moderately severe, stable, type 2 diabetes mellitus (noninsulin-dependent, NIDDM)

Usual Dosage Oral: Doses >500 mg/day should be given in 2 divided doses:

Adults:

Initial: 100-250 mg/day with breakfast or the first main meal of the day

Fasting blood sugar <200 mg/dL: 100 mg/day

Fasting blood sugar >200 mg/dL: 250 mg/day

Patient is malnourished, underweight, elderly, or not eating properly: 100 mg/day

Adjust dose in increments of 100-250 mg/day at weekly intervals to response; maximum daily dose: 1 g (doses >1 g/day are not likely to improve control)

Conversion from insulin to tolazamide

<20 units day = 100 mg/day

21- <40 units/day = 250 mg/day

≥40 units/day = 250 mg/day and 50% of insulin dose

Dosage Forms
Tablet: 100 mg, 250 mg, 500 mg

tolbutamide (tole BYOO ta mide)
Sound-Alike/Look-Alike Issues
TOLBUTamide may be confused with terbutaline, TOLAZamide
Orinase® may be confused with Orabase®, Ornex®, Tolinase®
Synonyms tolbutamide sodium
Tall-Man **TOLBUT**amide
U.S./Canadian Brand Names Apo-Tolbutamide® [Can]
Therapeutic Category Antidiabetic Agent, Oral
Use Adjunct to diet for the management of type 2 diabetes mellitus (noninsulin-dependent, NIDDM)
Usual Dosage Note: Divided doses may improve gastrointestinal tolerance
Adults: Oral: Initial: 1-2 g/day as a single dose in the morning or in divided doses throughout the day. Maintenance dose: 0.25-3 g/day; however, a maintenance dose >2 g/day is seldom required.
Dosage Forms
Tablet: 500 mg

tolbutamide sodium see tolbutamide on this page

tolcapone (TOLE ka pone)
U.S./Canadian Brand Names Tasmar® [US]
Therapeutic Category Anti-Parkinson Agent
Use Adjunct to levodopa and carbidopa for the treatment of signs and symptoms of idiopathic Parkinson disease in patients with motor fluctuations not responsive to other therapies
Usual Dosage Note: If clinical improvement is not observed after 3 weeks of therapy (regardless of dose), tolcapone treatment should be discontinued.
Oral: Adults: Initial: 100 mg 3 times/day; may increase as tolerated to 200 mg 3 times/day. **Note:** Levodopa dose may need to be decreased upon initiation of tolcapone (average reduction in clinical trials was 30%). As many as 70% of patients receiving levodopa doses >600 mg daily required levodopa dosage reduction in clinical trials. Patients with moderate-to-severe dyskinesia prior to initiation are also more likely to require dosage reduction.
Dosage Forms
Tablet:
Tasmar®: 100 mg, 200 mg

Tolectin® [US] see tolmetin on this page

Tolectin® DS (Discontinued) see tolmetin on this page

Tolinase® [Can] see tolazamide on previous page

Tolinase® (Discontinued) see tolazamide on previous page

tolmetin (TOLE met in)
Synonyms tolmetin sodium
U.S./Canadian Brand Names Tolectin® [US]
Therapeutic Category Analgesic, Nonnarcotic; Nonsteroidal Antiinflammatory Drug (NSAID)
Use Treatment of rheumatoid arthritis and osteoarthritis, juvenile rheumatoid arthritis
Usual Dosage Oral:
Children ≥2 years:
Antiinflammatory: Initial: 20 mg/kg/day in 3 divided doses, then 15-30 mg/kg/day in 3 divided doses
Analgesic: 5-7 mg/kg/dose every 6-8 hours
Adults: 400 mg 3 times/day; usual dose: 600 mg to 1.8 g/day; maximum: 2 g/day
Dosage Forms
Capsule: 400 mg
Tablet: 200 mg, 600 mg
Tolectin®: 600 mg

tolmetin sodium see tolmetin on this page

tolnaftate (tole NAF tate)
Sound-Alike/Look-Alike Issues
tolnaftate may be confused with Tornalate®
Tinactin® may be confused with Talacen®
(Continued)

tolnaftate *(Continued)*

U.S./Canadian Brand Names Blis-To-Sol® [US-OTC]; Fungi-Guard [US-OTC]; Mycocide® NS [US-OTC]; Pitrex [Can]; Podactin Powder [US-OTC]; Q-Naftate [US-OTC]; Tinactin® Antifungal Jock Itch [US-OTC]; Tinactin® Antifungal [US-OTC]; Tinaderm [US-OTC]; Ting® Cream [US-OTC]; Ting® Spray Liquid [US-OTC]

Therapeutic Category Antifungal Agent

Use Treatment of tinea pedis, tinea cruris, tinea corporis

Usual Dosage Topical: Children ≥2 years and Adults: Wash and dry affected area; spray aerosol or apply 1-3 drops of solution or a small amount of cream, or powder and rub into the affected areas 2 times/day

Note: May use for up to 4 weeks for tinea pedis or tinea corporis, and up to 2 weeks for tinea cruris

Dosage Forms

Aerosol, liquid, topical:
Tinactin® Antifungal [OTC]: 1% (60 mL, 150 mL)
Ting®: 1% (90 mL)

Aerosol, powder, topical:
Tinactin® Antifungal [OTC]: 1% (133 g)
Tinactin® Antifungal Jock Itch [OTC]: 1% (100 g, 133 g)

Cream, topical: 1% (15 g, 30 g)
Fungi-Guardl [OTC], Tinactin® Antifungal Jock Itch [OTC], Ting®l [OTC]: 1% (15 g)
Q-Naftatel [OTC], Tinactin® Antifungal [OTC]: 1% (15 g, 30 g)

Liquid, topical:
Blis-To-Sol® [OTC]: 1% (30 mL, 55 mL)
Fungi-Guard [OTC]: 1% (30 mL)

Powder, topical: 1% (45 g)
Podactin [OTC]: 1% (45 g)
Tinactin® Antifungal [OTC]: 1% (108 g)

Solution, topical: 1% (10 mL)
Mycocide® NS [OTC]: 1% (30 mL)
Tinaderm [OTC]: 1% (10 mL)

tolterodine (tole TER oh deen)

Sound-Alike/Look-Alike Issues
Detrol® may be confused with Ditropan®

Synonyms tolterodine tartrate

U.S./Canadian Brand Names Detrol® LA [US/Can]; Detrol® [US/Can]; Unidet® [Can]

Therapeutic Category Anticholinergic Agent

Use Treatment of patients with an overactive bladder with symptoms of urinary frequency, urgency, or urge incontinence

Usual Dosage Oral: Adults: Treatment of overactive bladder:
Immediate release tablet: 2 mg twice daily; the dose may be lowered to 1 mg twice daily based on individual response and tolerability
Dosing adjustment in patients concurrently taking CYP3A4 inhibitors: 1 mg twice daily
Extended release capsule: 4 mg once a day; dose may be lowered to 2 mg daily based on individual response and tolerability
Dosing adjustment in patients concurrently taking CYP3A4 inhibitors: 2 mg daily

Dosage Forms

Capsule, extended release:
Detrol® LA: 2 mg, 4 mg

Tablet:
Detrol®: 1 mg, 2 mg

tolterodine tartrate *see* tolterodine *on this page*

Tomocat® [US] *see* barium *on page 94*

Tomocat® 1000 [US] *see* barium *on page 94*

tomoxetine *see* atomoxetine *on page 81*

Tomudex® [Can] *see* raltitrexed *(Canada only) on page 743*

Tomycine® *(Discontinued)* *see* tobramycin *on page 846*

Tonocard® *(Discontinued)*

Tonojug [US] *see* barium *on page 94*

Tonopaque [US] *see* barium *on page 94*

Topamax® [US/Can] *see* topiramate *on next page*

Topamax® 200 mg Tablet *(Discontinued)* *see* topiramate *on next page*

Topicaine® **[US-OTC]** *see* lidocaine *on page 504*

Topicort® **[US/Can]** *see* desoximetasone *on page 240*

Topicort®**-LP [US]** *see* desoximetasone *on page 240*

Topicycline® **Topical *(Discontinued)*** *see* tetracycline *on page 831*

Topilene® **[Can]** *see* betamethasone (topical) *on page 109*

topiramate (toe PYRE a mate)

Sound-Alike/Look-Alike Issues
Topamax® may be confused with Tegretol®, Tegretol®-XR, Toprol-XL®

U.S./Canadian Brand Names Dom-Topiramate [Can]; Gen-Topiramate [Can]; Novo-Topiramate [Can]; PHL-Topiramate [Can]; PMS-Topiramate [Can]; ratio-Topiramate [Can]; Rhoxal-topiramate [Can]; Sandoz-Topiramate [Can]; Topamax® [US/Can]

Therapeutic Category Anticonvulsant

Use Monotherapy or adjunctive therapy for partial onset seizures and primary generalized tonic-clonic seizures; adjunctive treatment of seizures associated with Lennox-Gastaut syndrome; prophylaxis of migraine headache

Usual Dosage Oral: **Note:** Do not abruptly discontinue therapy; taper dosage gradually to prevent rebound effects. (In clinical trials, adult doses were withdrawn by decreasing in weekly intervals of 50-100 mg/day gradually over 2-8 weeks for seizure treatment, and by decreasing in weekly intervals by 25-50 mg/day for migraine prophylaxis.)

Epilepsy, monotherapy: Children ≥10 years and Adults: Partial onset seizure and primary generalized tonic-clonic seizure: Initial: 25 mg twice daily; may increase weekly by 50 mg/day up to 100 mg twice daily (week 4 dose); thereafter, may further increase weekly by 100 mg/day up to the recommended maximum of 200 mg twice daily.

Epilepsy, adjunctive therapy:

Children 2-16 years:

Partial onset seizure or seizure associated with Lennox-Gastaut syndrome: Initial dose titration should begin at 25 mg (or less, based on a range of 1-3 mg/kg/day) nightly for the first week; dosage may be increased in increments of 1-3 mg/kg/day (administered in 2 divided doses) at 1- or 2-week intervals to a total daily dose of 5-9 mg/kg/day

Primary generalized tonic-clonic seizure: Use initial dose listed above, but use slower initial titration rate; titrate to recommended maintenance dose by the end of 8 weeks

Adolescents ≥17 years and Adults:

Partial onset seizures: Initial: 25-50 mg/day (given in 2 divided doses) for 1 week; increase at weekly intervals by 25-50 mg/day until response; usual maintenance dose: 100-200 mg twice daily. Doses >1600 mg/day have not been studied.

Primary generalized tonic-clonic seizures: Use initial dose as listed above for partial onset seizures, but use slower initial titration rate; titrate upwards to recommended dose by the end of 8 weeks; usual maintenance dose: 200 mg twice daily. Doses >1600 mg/day have not been studied.

Adults: Migraine prophylaxis: Initial: 25 mg/day (in the evening), titrated at weekly intervals in 25 mg increments, up to the recommended total daily dose of 100 mg/day given in 2 divided doses

Dosage Forms
Capsule, sprinkle:
Topamax®: 15 mg, 25 mg
Tablet:
Topamax®: 25 mg, 50 mg, 100 mg, 200 mg

Topisone® **[Can]** *see* betamethasone (topical) *on page 109*

TOPO *see* topotecan *on this page*

Toposar® **[US]** *see* etoposide *on page 336*

topotecan (toe poe TEE kan)

Sound-Alike/Look-Alike Issues
Hycamtin® may be confused with Hycomine®

Synonyms hycamptamine; NSC-609699; SK and F 104864; SKF 104864; SKF 104864-A; TOPO; topotecan hydrochloride; TPT

U.S./Canadian Brand Names Hycamtin® [US/Can]

Therapeutic Category Antineoplastic Agent

Use Treatment of ovarian cancer and small cell lung cancer; cervical cancer (in combination with cisplatin)

Usual Dosage Adults (refer to individual protocols):
Metastatic ovarian cancer and small cell lung cancer: IVPB: 1.5 mg/m^2/day for 5 days; repeated every 21 days (baseline neutrophil count should be >1500/mm^3 and platelet count should be >100,000/mm^3)

(Continued)

851

topotecan *(Continued)*

Cervical cancer: IVPB: 0.75 mg/m^2/day for 3 days (followed by cisplatin 50 mg/m^2 on day 1 only, [with hydration]); repeated every 21 days (baseline neutrophil count should be >1500/mm^3 and platelet count should be >100,000/mm^3)

Dosage Forms
Injection, powder for reconstitution:
Hycamtin®: 4 mg

topotecan hydrochloride *see* topotecan *on previous page*

Toprol-XL® [US/Can] *see* metoprolol *on page 562*

Topsyn® [Can] *see* fluocinonide *on page 360*

Toradol® [US/Can] *see* ketorolac *on page 483*

Toradol® IM [Can] *see* ketorolac *on page 483*

toremifene *(tore EM i feen)*

Synonyms FC1157a; toremifene citrate
U.S./Canadian Brand Names Fareston® [US/Can]
Therapeutic Category Antineoplastic Agent
Use Treatment of advanced breast cancer; management of desmoid tumors and endometrial carcinoma
Usual Dosage Oral (refer to individual protocols): Adults: 60 mg once daily, generally continued until disease progression is observed

Dosage Forms
Tablet:
Fareston®: 60 mg

toremifene citrate *see* toremifene *on this page*

Torisel™ [US] *see* temsirolimus *on page 824*

torsemide *(TORE se mide)*

Sound-Alike/Look-Alike Issues
torsemide may be confused with furosemide
Demadex® may be confused with Denorex®
U.S./Canadian Brand Names Demadex® [US]
Therapeutic Category Diuretic, Loop
Use Management of edema associated with congestive heart failure and hepatic or renal disease; used alone or in combination with antihypertensives in treatment of hypertension; I.V. form is indicated when rapid onset is desired
Usual Dosage Oral, I.V.: Adults:
Congestive heart failure: 10-20 mg once daily; may increase gradually for chronic treatment by doubling dose until the diuretic response is apparent (for acute treatment, I.V. dose may be repeated every 2 hours with double the dose as needed). **Note:** ACC/AHA 2005 guidelines for chronic heart failure recommend a maximum daily oral dose of 200 mg; maximum single I.V. dose of 100-200 mg
Continuous I.V. infusion: 20 mg I.V. load then 5-20 mg/hour
Chronic renal failure: 20 mg once daily; increase as described above
Hepatic cirrhosis: 5-10 mg once daily with an aldosterone antagonist or a potassium-sparing diuretic; increase as described above
Hypertension: 2.5-5 mg once daily; increase to 10 mg after 4-6 weeks if an adequate hypotensive response is not apparent; if still not effective, an additional antihypertensive agent may be added

Dosage Forms
Injection, solution:
Demadex®: 10 mg/mL (2 mL, 5 mL)
Tablet: 5 mg, 10 mg, 20 mg, 100 mg
Demadex®: 5 mg, 10 mg, 20 mg, 100 mg

tositumomab I-131 *see* tositumomab and iodine I 131 tositumomab *on this page*

tositumomab and iodine I 131 tositumomab

(toe si TYOO mo mab & EYE oh dyne eye one THUR tee one toe si TYOO mo mab)

Synonyms anti-CD20-murine monoclonal antibody I-131; B1; B1 antibody; 131 I anti-B1 antibody; 131 I-anti-B1 monoclonal antibody; iodine I 131 tositumomab and tositumomab; tositumomab I-131

U.S./Canadian Brand Names Bexxar® [US]

Therapeutic Category Antineoplastic Agent, Monoclonal Antibody; Radiopharmaceutical

Use Treatment of relapsed or refractory CD20 positive, low-grade, follicular, or transformed non-Hodgkin lymphoma

Usual Dosage I.V.: Adults: Dosing consists of four components administered in 2 steps. Thyroid protective agents (SSKI, Lugol's solution or potassium iodide), acetaminophen and diphenhydramine should be given prior to or with treatment.

Step 1: Dosimetric step (Day 0):

Tositumomab 450 mg in NS 50 mL administered over 60 minutes

Iodine I 131 tositumomab (containing I-131 5.0 mCi and tositumomab 35 mg) in NS 30 mL administered over 20 minutes

Note: Whole body dosimetry and biodistribution should be determined on Day 0; days 2, 3, or 4; and day 6 or 7 prior to administration of Step 2. If biodistribution is not acceptable, do not administer the therapeutic step. On day 6 or 7, calculate the patient specific activity of iodine I 131 tositumomab to deliver 75 cGy TBD or 65 cGy TBD (in mCi).

Step 2: Therapeutic step (Day 7):

Tositumomab 450 mg in NS 50 mL administered over 60 minutes

Iodine I 131 tositumomab:

Platelets ≥150,000/mm³: Iodine I 131 calculated to deliver 75 cGy total body irradiation and tositumomab 35 mg over 20 minutes

Platelets ≥100,000/mm³ and <150,000/mm³: Iodine I 131 calculated to deliver 65 cGy total body irradiation and tositumomab 35 mg over 20 minutes

Dosage Forms

Kit [dosimetric package]:

Bexxar®: Tositumomab 225 mg/16.1 mL [2 vials], tositumomab 35 mg/2.5 mL [1 vial], and iodine I 131 tositumomab 0.1 mg/mL and 0.61mCi/mL (20 mL) [1 vial]

Kit [therapeutic package]:

Bexxar®: Tositumomab 225 mg/16.1 mL [2 vials], tositumomab 35 mg/2.5 mL [1 vial], and iodine I 131 tositumomab 1.1 mg/mL and 5.6 mCi/mL (20 mL) [1 or 2 vials]

Totacillin® **(Discontinued)** see ampicillin on page 53

total parenteral nutrition (TOE tal par EN ter al noo TRISH un)

Synonyms hyperal; hyperalimentation; parenteral nutrition; PN; TPN

Therapeutic Category Caloric Agent; Intravenous Nutritional Therapy

Use Infusion of nutrient solutions into the bloodstream to support nutritional needs during a time when patient is unable to absorb nutrients via the gastrointestinal tract, cannot take adequate nutrition orally or enterally, or have had (or are expected to have) inadequate oral intake for 7-14 days

Usual Dosage PN is a highly-individualized therapy. The following general guidelines may be used in the estimation of needs. Electrolytes, vitamins, and trace minerals should be added to TPN mixtures based on patients individualized needs.

Neonates: I.V.: **Note:** When indicated for premature neonates, start on day 1 of life if possible.

Total calories:

Term: 85-105 kcal/kg/day

Preterm (stable): 90-120 kcal/kg/day

Fluid:

<1.5 kg: 130-150 mL/kg/day

1.5-2 kg: 110-130 mL/kg/day

2-10 kg: 100 mL/kg/day

Carbohydrate (dextrose): 40% to 50 % of caloric intake; advance as tolerated

Term: Initial: 6-8 mg/kg/minute; goal: 10-14 mg/kg/minute

Premature: Initial: 6 mg/kg/minute; goal: 10-13 mg/kg/minute

Protein (amino acids):

Term: Initial: 2.5 g/kg/day; goal: 3 g/kg/day

Extremely (<1000 g) and very (<1500 g) low-birth-weight (stable): Initial: 1-1.5 g/kg/day; goal: 3.5-3.85 g/kg/day to promote utero growth rates.

Sepsis, hypoxia: Initial: 1 g/kg/day; goal: 3-3.85 g/kg/day

Fat:

Term: Initial: 0.5-1 g/kg/day (maximum: 3 g/kg/day); administer over 24 hours

Preterm: Initial: 0.25-0.5 g/kg/day (maximum: 3 g/kg/day or 1 g/kg/day if on phototherapy); administer over 24 hours

Note: Monitor triglycerides while receiving intralipids. If triglycerides >200 mg/dL, stop infusion and restart at 0.5-1g/kg/day

Heparin: 1 unit/mL of parenteral nutrition fluids should be added to enhance clearance of lipid emulsions

(Continued)

total parenteral nutrition *(Continued)*

Children: I.V.: **Note:** Give within 5-7 days if unable to meet needs orally or with enteral nutrition:

Total calories:
<6 months: 85-105 kcal/kg/day
6-12 months: 80-100 kcal/kg/day
1-7 years: 75-90 kcal/kg/day
7-12 years: 50-75 kcal/kg/day
12-18 years: 30-50 kcal/kg/day

Fluid:
2-10 kg: 100 mL/kg
>10-20 kg: 1000 mL for 10 kg plus 50 mL/kg for each kg >10
>20 kg: 1500 mL for 10 kg plus 20 mL/kg for each kg >20

Carbohydrate (dextrose): 40% to 50% of caloric intake
<1 year: Initial: 6-8 mg/kg/minute; goal: 10-14 mg/kg/minute
1-10 years: Initial: 10% to 12.5%; daily increase: 5% increments (maximum: 15 mg/kg/minute)
>10 years: Initial: 10% to 15%; daily increase: 5% increments (maximum: 8.5 mg/kg/minute)

Protein (amino acids):
1-12 months: Initial: 2-3 g/kg/day; daily increase: 1 g/kg/day (maximum: 3 g/kg/day)
1-10 years: Initial: 1-2 g/kg/day; daily increase: 1 g/kg/day (maximum: 2-2.5 g/kg/day)
>10 years: Initial: 0.8-1.5 g/kg/day; daily increase: 1 g/kg/day (maximum: 1.5-2 g/kg/day)

Fat: Initial: 1 g/kg/day; daily increase: 1 g/kg/day (maximum: 3 g/kg/day); **Note:** Monitor triglycerides while receiving intralipids.

Adults: I.V.:

Total calories: Calculate using Harris-Benedict equation or based on stress level as indicated below:
Harris-Benedict Equation (BEE):
Females: $655.1 + [(9.56 \times W) + (1.85 \times H) - (4.68 \times A)]$
Males: $66.47 + [(13.75 \times W) + (5 \times H) - (6.76 \times A)]$
Then multiply BEE x (activity factor) x (stress factor)
W = weight in kg; H = height in cm; A = age in years
Activity factor = 1.2 sedentary, 1.3 normal activity, 1.4 active, 1.5 very active
Stress factor = 1.5 for trauma, stressed, or surgical patients and underweight (to promote weight gain); 2.0 for severe burn patients

Stress level:
Normal/mild stress level: 20-25 kcal/kg/day
Moderate stress level: 25-30 kcal/kg/day
Severe stress level: 30-40 kcal/kg/day
Pregnant women in second or third trimester: Add an additional 300 kcal/day

Fluid: mL/day = 30-40 mL/kg

Carbohydrate (dextrose):
5 g/kg/day or 3.5 mg/kg/minute (maximum rate: 4-7 mg/kg/minute)
Minimum recommended amount: 400 calories/day or 100 g/day

Protein (amino acids):
Maintenance: 0.8-1 g/kg/day
Normal/mild stress level: 1-1.2 g/kg/day
Moderate stress level: 1.2-1.5 g/kg/day
Severe stress level: 1.5-2 g/kg/day
Burn patients (severe): Increase protein until significant wound healing achieved
Solid organ transplant: Perioperative: 1.5-2 g/kg/day

Dosage Forms TPN is usually compounded from optimal combinations of macronutrients (water, protein, dextrose, and lipids) and micronutrients (electrolytes, trace elements, and vitamins) to meet the specific nutritional requirements of a patient. Individual hospitals may have designated standard TPN formulas. There are a few commercially-available amino acids with electrolytes solutions; however, these products may not meet an individual's specific nutrition requirements.

Touro® CC [US] *see* guaifenesin, pseudoephedrine, and dextromethorphan *on page 408*

Touro® CC-LD [US] *see* guaifenesin, pseudoephedrine, and dextromethorphan *on page 408*

Touro® Allergy [US] *see* brompheniramine and pseudoephedrine *on page 120*

Touro® DM [US] *see* guaifenesin and dextromethorphan *on page 402*

Touro Ex® *(Discontinued)* *see* guaifenesin *on page 401*

Touro® HC [US] *see* hydrocodone and guaifenesin *on page 429*

Touro LA® [US] *see* guaifenesin and pseudoephedrine *on page 406*

tPA *see* alteplase *on page 34*

TPN *see* total parenteral nutrition *on previous page*

TPT *see* topotecan *on page 851*

TPV *see* tipranavir *on page 845*

tRA *see* tretinoin (oral) *on page 860*

trace metals (trase MET als)

Synonyms chromium; copper; iodine; manganese; molybdenum; neonatal trace metals; selenium; zinc

U.S./Canadian Brand Names Iodopen® [US]; M.T.E.-4® [US]; M.T.E.-5® [US]; M.T.E.-6® [US]; M.T.E.-7® [US]; Molypen® [US]; Multitrace™-4 Neonatal [US]; Multitrace™-4 Pediatric [US]; Multitrace™-4 [US]; Multitrace™-5 [US]; Neotrace-4® [US]; P.T.E.-4® [US]; P.T.E.-5® [US]; Pedtrace-4® [US]; Selepen® [US]

Therapeutic Category Trace Element

Use Prevention and correction of trace metal deficiencies

Usual Dosage Recommended daily parenteral dosage:

Chromium:[1]
 Infants: 0.2 mcg/kg
 Children: 0.2 mcg/kg (maximum: 5 mcg)
 Adults: 10-15 mcg
Copper:[2]
 Infants: 20 mcg/kg
 Children: 20 mcg/kg (maximum: 300 mcg)
 Adults: 0.5-1.5 mg
Manganese:[2,3]
 Infants: 1 mcg/kg
 Children: 1 mcg/kg (maximum: 50 mcg)
 Adults: 150-800 mcg
Molybdenum:[1,4]
 Infants: 0.25 mcg/kg
 Children: 0.25 mcg/kg (maximum: 5 mcg)
 Adults: 20-120 mcg
Selenium:[1,4]
 Infants: 2 mcg/kg
 Children: 2 mcg/kg (maximum: 30 mcg)
 Adults: 20-40 mcg
Zinc:
 Infants, preterm: 400 mcg/kg
 Infants, term <3 months: 250 mcg/kg
 Infants, term >3 months: 100 mcg/kg
 Children: 50 mcg/kg (maximum: 5 mg)
 Adults: 2.5-4 mg

[1]Omit in patients with renal dysfunction.
[2]Omit in patients with obstructive jaundice.
[3]Current available commercial products are not in appropriate ratios to maintain this recommendation; doses of up to 10 mcg/kg have been used.
[4]Indicated for use in long-term parenteral nutrition patients.

Dosage Forms

Injection, solution [combination products]:

M.T.E.-4®: Chromium 4 mcg, copper 0.4 mg, manganese 0.1 mg, and zinc 1 mg per mL (3 mL, 10 mL, 30 mL)

M.T.E.-4® Concentrate: Chromium 10 mcg, copper 1 mg, manganese 0.5 mg, and zinc 5 mg per mL (1 mL, 10 mL)

M.T.E.-5® [preservative free]: Chromium 4 mcg, copper 0.4 mg, manganese 0.1 mg, selenium 20 mcg, and zinc 1 mg per mL (10 mL)

M.T.E.-5® Concentrate: Chromium 10 mcg, copper 1 mg, manganese 0.5 mg, selenium 60 mcg, and zinc 5 mg per mL (1 mL, 10 mL)

M.T.E.-6® [preservative free]: Chromium 4 mcg, copper 0.4 mg, iodide 25 mcg, manganese 0.1 mg, selenium 20 mcg, and zinc 1 mg per mL (10 mL)

M.T.E.-6® Concentrate: Chromium 10 mcg, copper 1 mg, iodide 75 mcg, manganese 0.5 mg, selenium 60 mcg, and zinc 5 mg per mL (10 mL)

M.T.E.-7® [preservative free]: Chromium 4 mcg, copper 0.4 mg, iodide 25 mcg, manganese 0.1 mg, molybdenum 25 mcg, selenium 20 mcg, and zinc 1 mg per mL (10 mL)

Multitrace™-4: Chromium 4 mcg, copper 0.4 mg, manganese 0.1 mg, and zinc 1 mg per mL (10 mL)

Multitrace™-4 Neonatal: Chromium 0.85 mcg, copper 0.1 mg, manganese 0.025 mg, and zinc 1.5 mg per mL (2 mL)

Multitrace™-4 Pediatric: Chromium 1 mcg, copper 0.1 mg, manganese 0.025 mg, and zinc 1 mg per mL (3 mL)
(Continued)

trace metals *(Continued)*

Multitrace™-4 Concentrate: Chromium 10 mcg, copper 1 mg, manganese 0.5 mg, and zinc 5 mg per mL (1 mL, 10 mL)

Multitrace™-5: Chromium 4 mcg, copper 0.4 mg, manganese 0.1 mg, selenium 20 mcg, and zinc 1 mg per mL (10 mL)

Multitrace™-5 Concentrate: Chromium 10 mcg, copper 1 mg, manganese 0.5 mg, selenium 60 mcg, and zinc 5 mg per mL (1 mL, 10 mL)

Neotrace-4® [preservative free]: Chromium 0.85 mcg, copper 0.1 mg, manganese 0.025 mg, and zinc 1.5 mg per mL (2 mL)

Pedtrace-4® [preservative free]: Chromium 0.85 mcg, copper 0.1 mg, manganese 0.025 mg, and zinc 0.5 mg per mL (3 mL, 10 mL)

P.T.E.-4® [preservative free]: Chromium 1 mcg, copper 0.1 mg, manganese 0.025 mg, and zinc 1 mg per mL (3 mL)

P.T.E.-5® [preservative free]: Chromium 1 mcg, copper 0.1 mg, manganese 0.025 mg, selenium 15 mcg, and zinc 1 mg per mL (3 mL)

Trace elements pediatric: Chromium 1 mcg, copper 0.1 mg, manganese 0.03 mg, and zinc 0.5 mg per mL (10 mL)

Injection, solution [elemental equivalence]:

Chromium, as chromic chloride (hexahydrate) [preservative free]: 0.0205 mg/mL [0.004 mg/mL] (10 mL)

Copper, as cupric chloride: 1.07 mg/mL [0.4 mg/mL] (10 mL)

Iodine, as iodine sodium (Iodopen®): 0.118 mg/mL [0.1 mg/mL] (10 mL)

Manganese:

As chloride: 0.36 mg/mL [0.1 mg/mL] (10 mL)

As sulfate [preservative free]: 0.31 mg/mL [0.1 mg/mL] (10 mL)

Molybdenum, as ammonium molybdate (tetrahydrate) (Molypen®): 46 mcg/mL [25 mcg/mL] (10 mL)

Selenium, as selenious acid: 0.0654 mg/mL [0.04 mg/mL] (10 mL)

Selepen®: 0.0654 mg/mL [0.04 mg/mL] (10 mL, 30 mL) [30 mL contains benzyl alcohol]

Zinc:

As chloride: 2.09 mg/mL [1 mg/mL] (10 mL, 50 mL)

As sulfate, anhydrous [preservative free]: 2.46 mg/mL [1 mg/mL] (10 mL)

As sulfate, anhydrous, concentrate [preservative free]: 12.32 mg/mL [5 mg/mL] (5 mL)

Tracleer® [US/Can] *see* bosentan *on page 116*

Tramacet [Can] *see* acetaminophen and tramadol *on page 9*

tramadol *(TRA ma dole)*

Sound-Alike/Look-Alike Issues

tramadol may be confused with Toradol®, Trandate®, Voltaren®

Ultram® may be confused with Ultane®, Voltaren®

Synonyms tramadol hydrochloride

U.S./Canadian Brand Names Ultram® ER [US]; Ultram® [US/Can]; Zytram® XL [Can]

Therapeutic Category Analgesic, Nonnarcotic

Use Relief of moderate to moderately-severe pain

Usual Dosage Moderate-to-severe chronic pain: Oral: Adults:

Immediate release formulation: 50-100 mg every 4-6 hours (not to exceed 400 mg/day)

For patients not requiring rapid onset of effect, tolerability may be improved by starting dose at 25 mg/day and titrating dose by 25 mg every 3 days, until reaching 25 mg 4 times/day. Dose may then be increased by 50 mg every 3 days as tolerated, to reach dose of 50 mg 4 times/day.

Extended release formulations:

Ultram® ER: 100 mg once daily; titrate every 5 days (maximum: 300 mg/day)

Zytram® XL [per Canadian labeling: Not available in U.S.]: 150 mg once daily; if pain relief is not achieved may titrate by increasing dosage incrementally, with sufficient time to evaluate effect of increased dosage; generally not more often than every 7 days (maximum: 400 mg/day)

Dosage Forms [CAN] = Canadian brand name

Tablet: 50 mg

Ultram®: 50 mg

Tablet, extended release:

Ultram® ER: 100 mg, 200 mg, 300 mg

Zytram® XL [CAN]: 150 mg, 200 mg, 300 mg, 400 mg

tramadol hydrochloride *see* tramadol *on this page*

tramadol hydrochloride and acetaminophen *see* acetaminophen and tramadol *on page 9*

Trandate® [US/Can] *see* labetalol *on page 486*

trandolapril (tran DOE la pril)

U.S./Canadian Brand Names Mavik® [US/Can]

Therapeutic Category Angiotensin-Converting Enzyme (ACE) Inhibitor

Use Management of hypertension alone or in combination with other antihypertensive agents; treatment of left ventricular dysfunction after myocardial infarction

Usual Dosage Oral: Adults:

Hypertension: Initial dose in patients not receiving a diuretic: 1 mg/day (2 mg/day in black patients). Adjust dosage according to the blood pressure response. Make dosage adjustments at intervals of ≥1 week. Most patients have required dosages of 2-4 mg/day. There is a little experience with doses >8 mg/day. Patients inadequately treated with once daily dosing at 4 mg may be treated with twice daily dosing. If blood pressure is not adequately controlled with trandolapril monotherapy, a diuretic may be added.

Usual dose range (JNC 7): 1-4 mg once daily

Heart failure postmyocardial infarction or left ventricular dysfunction postmyocardial infarction: Initial: 1 mg/day; titrate patients (as tolerated) towards the target dose of 4 mg/day. If a 4 mg dose is not tolerated, patients can continue therapy with the greatest tolerated dose.

Dosage Forms

Tablet: 1 mg, 2 mg, 4 mg

Mavik®: 1 mg, 2 mg, 4 mg

trandolapril and verapamil (tran DOE la pril & ver AP a mil)

Synonyms verapamil and trandolapril

U.S./Canadian Brand Names Tarka® [US/Can]

Therapeutic Category Antihypertensive Agent, Combination

Use Combination drug for the treatment of hypertension, however, not indicated for initial treatment of hypertension; replacement therapy in patients receiving separate dosage forms (for patient convenience); when monotherapy with one component fails to achieve desired antihypertensive effect, or when dose-limiting adverse effects limit upward titration of monotherapy

Usual Dosage Dose is individualized.

Dosage Forms

Tablet, variable release:

Tarka®:

1/240: Trandolapril 1 mg [immediate release] and verapamil 240 mg [sustained release]

2/180: Trandolapril 2 mg [immediate release] and verapamil 180 mg [sustained release]

2/240: Trandolapril 2 mg [immediate release] and verapamil 240 mg [sustained release]

4/240: Trandolapril 4 mg [immediate release] and verapamil 240 mg [sustained release]

tranexamic acid (tran eks AM ik AS id)

Sound-Alike/Look-Alike Issues

Cyklokapron® may be confused with cycloSPORINE

U.S./Canadian Brand Names Cyklokapron® [US/Can]; Tranexamic Acid Injection BP [Can]

Therapeutic Category Antihemophilic Agent

Use Short-term use (2-8 days) in hemophilia patients during and following tooth extraction to reduce or prevent hemorrhage

Usual Dosage I.V.: Children and Adults: 10 mg/kg immediately before surgery, then 25 mg/kg/dose orally 3-4 times/day for 2-8 days

Alternatively:

Oral: 25 mg/kg 3-4 times/day beginning 1 day prior to surgery

I.V.: 10 mg/kg 3-4 times/day in patients who are unable to take oral

Dosage Forms

Injection, solution:

Cyklokapron®: 100 mg/mL (10 mL)

Tablet:

Cyklokapron®: 500 mg [not available in the U.S.; available from manufacturer for select cases]

Tranexamic Acid Injection BP [Can] *see* tranexamic acid *on this page*

transamine sulphate *see* tranylcypromine *on next page*

Transderm-V® [Can] *see* scopolamine derivatives *on page 778*

Transdermal-NTG® Patch *(Discontinued)* *see* nitroglycerin *on page 608*

Transderm-Nitro® [Can] *see* nitroglycerin *on page 608*

Transderm Scōp® [US] *see* scopolamine derivatives *on page 778*

Trans-Plantar® [Can] *see* salicylic acid *on page 772*

Trans-Plantar® Transdermal Patch *(Discontinued)* *see* salicylic acid *on page 772*

***trans*-retinoic acid** *see* tretinoin (topical) *on page 861*

Trans-Ver-Sal® **[US-OTC/Can]** *see* salicylic acid *on page 772*

Tranxene® **SD**™ **[US]** *see* clorazepate *on page 206*

Tranxene® **SD**™**-Half Strength [US]** *see* clorazepate *on page 206*

Tranxene® **T-Tab**® **[US]** *see* clorazepate *on page 206*

tranylcypromine (tran il SIP roe meen)

Synonyms transamine sulphate; tranylcypromine sulfate

U.S./Canadian Brand Names Parnate® [US/Can]

Therapeutic Category Antidepressant, Monoamine Oxidase Inhibitor

Use Treatment of major depressive episode without melancholia

Usual Dosage Oral: Adults: 10 mg twice daily, increase by 10 mg increments at 1- to 3-week intervals; maximum: 60 mg/day; usual effective dose: 30 mg/day

Dosage Forms
Tablet:
Parnate®: 10 mg

tranylcypromine sulfate *see* tranylcypromine *on this page*

Trasicor® **[Can]** *see* oxprenolol *(Canada only) on page 639*

trastuzumab (tras TU zoo mab)

Synonyms NSC-688097

U.S./Canadian Brand Names Herceptin® [US/Can]

Therapeutic Category Antineoplastic Agent

Use Treatment of HER-2/*neu* overexpressing metastatic breast cancer; adjuvant treatment of HER-2/*neu* overexpressing node-positive breast cancer

Usual Dosage I.V. infusion (refer to individual protocols): Adults:
Metastatic breast cancer:
Initial loading dose: 4 mg/kg infused over 90 minutes
Maintenance dose: 2 mg/kg infused over 90 minutes (can be administered over 30 minutes if prior infusions are well tolerated) weekly until disease progression
Node-positive breast cancer:
Initial loading dose: 4 mg/kg infused over 90 minutes
Maintenance dose: 2 mg/kg infused over 90 minutes (can be administered over 30 minutes if prior infusions are well tolerated) weekly for 51 weeks (total of 52 weeks)

Dosage Forms
Injection, powder for reconstitution:
Herceptin®: 440 mg

Trasylol® **[US/Can]** *see* aprotinin *on page 71*

Travatan® **[US/Can]** *see* travoprost *on next page*

Travatan® **Z [US]** *see* travoprost *on next page*

traveler's diarrhea and cholera vaccine *(Canada only)*

(TRAV uh lerz dahy uh REE uh & KOL er uh vak SEEN)

Synonyms cholera and traveler's diarrhea vaccine; enterotoxigenic *Escherichia coli* and *Vibrio cholera* vaccine; traveller's diarrhea vaccine and cholera; *Vibrio cholera* and enterotoxigenic *Escherichia coli* vaccine

U.S./Canadian Brand Names Dukoral™ [Can]

Therapeutic Category Vaccine

Use Protection against traveler's diarrhea and/or cholera in adults and children ≥2 years of age who will be visiting areas where there is a risk of contacting traveler's diarrhea caused by enterotoxigenic *E. coli* (ETEC) or cholera caused by *V. cholerae* O1 (classical and El Tor biotypes)

Usual Dosage Oral:
Cholera:
Primary immunization:
Children 2-6 years: 3 doses given at intervals of ≥1 week and completed at least 1 week prior to trip to endemic/epidemic areas; restart treatment if interval between doses >6 weeks
Children ≥6 years and Adults: 2 doses given at intervals of ≥1 week and completed at least 1 week prior to trip to endemic/epidemic areas; restart treatment if interval between doses >6 weeks
Booster:
Children 2-6 years: 1 dose after 6 months have elapsed since vaccination
Children ≥6 years and Adults: 1 dose after 2 years have elapsed since vaccination

ETEC:

Primary immunization: Children ≥2 years and Adults: 2 doses given at intervals of ≥1 week; restart treatment if interval between doses >6 weeks

Booster: Children ≥2 years and Adults:

Continued risk: 1 dose every 3 months

Renewed protection: 1 dose may be given if last booster or original immunization was <5 years ago (if >5 years, revaccinate)

Dosage Forms [CAN] = Canadian brand name

Suspension [vial]:

Dukoral™ [CAN]: 2.5 x 10^{10} of each of the following *Vibrio cholerae* O1 strains: Inaba classic (heat inactived), Inaba El Tor (formalin inactivated), Ogawa classic (heat inactivated), Ogawa classic (formalin inactivated), and 1 mg recombinant cholera toxin B subunit (rCTB) (3 mL) [not available in the U.S.]

traveller's diarrhea vaccine and cholera *see* traveler's diarrhea and cholera vaccine *(Canada only)* on previous page

travoprost (TRA voe prost)

Sound-Alike/Look-Alike Issues

Travatan® may be confused with Xalatan®

U.S./Canadian Brand Names Travatan® Z [US]; Travatan® [US/Can]

Therapeutic Category Prostaglandin, Ophthalmic

Use Reduction of elevated intraocular pressure in patients with open-angle glaucoma or ocular hypertension who are intolerant of the other IOP-lowering medications or insufficiently responsive (failed to achieve target IOP determined after multiple measurements over time) to another IOP-lowering medication

Usual Dosage Ophthalmic: Adults: Glaucoma (open angle) or ocular hypertension: Instill 1 drop into affected eye(s) once daily in the evening; do not exceed once-daily dosing (may decrease IOP-lowering effect). If used with other topical ophthalmic agents, separate administration by at least 5 minutes.

Dosage Forms

Solution, ophthalmic:

Travatan®: 0.004% (2.5 mL, 5 mL)

Travatan® Z: 0.004% (2.5 mL, 5 mL)

trazodone (TRAZ oh done)

Sound-Alike/Look-Alike Issues

Desyrel® may be confused with Demerol®, Delsym®, Zestril®

Synonyms trazodone hydrochloride

U.S./Canadian Brand Names Alti-Trazodone [Can]; Apo-Trazodone D® [Can]; Apo-Trazodone® [Can]; Desyrel® [Can]; Gen-Trazodone [Can]; Novo-Trazodone [Can]; Nu-Trazodone [Can]; PMS-Trazodone [Can]; ratio-Trazodone [Can]; Trazorel® [Can]

Therapeutic Category Antidepressant, Triazolopyridine

Use Treatment of depression

Usual Dosage Oral: Therapeutic effects may take up to 6 weeks to occur; therapy is normally maintained for 6-12 months after optimum response is reached to prevent recurrence of depression

Adults: Depression: Initial: 150 mg/day in 3 divided doses (may increase by 50 mg/day every 3-7 days); maximum: 600 mg/day

Dosage Forms Tablet: 50 mg, 100 mg, 150 mg, 300 mg

trazodone hydrochloride *see* trazodone *on this page*

Trazorel® [Can] *see* trazodone *on this page*

Trecator® [US/Can] *see* ethionamide *on page 333*

Trelstar™ [Can] *see* triptorelin *on page 870*

Trelstar™ Depot [US/Can] *see* triptorelin *on page 870*

Trelstar™ LA [US/Can] *see* triptorelin *on page 870*

Trendar® *(Discontinued)* *see* ibuprofen *on page 444*

Trental® [US/Can] *see* pentoxifylline *on page 667*

treprostinil (tre PROST in il)

Synonyms treprostinil sodium

U.S./Canadian Brand Names Remodulin® [US/Can]

Therapeutic Category Vasodilator

Use Treatment of pulmonary arterial hypertension (PAH) in patients with NYHA Class II-IV symptoms to decrease exercise-associated symptoms; to diminish clinical deterioration when transitioning from epoprostenol (I.V.)

Usual Dosage SubQ or I.V. infusion:

Adults: PAH:

Initial: New to prostacyclin therapy: 1.25 ng/kg/minute continuous; if dose cannot be tolerated, reduce to 0.625 ng/kg/minute. Increase at rate not >1.25 ng/kg/minute per week for first 4 weeks, and not >2.5 ng/kg/minute per week for remainder of therapy. Limited experience with doses >40 ng/kg/minute. **Note:** Dose must be carefully and individually titrated (symptom improvement with minimal adverse effects). Avoid abrupt withdrawal.

Transitioning from epoprostenol: I.V. Infusion: **Note:** Transition should occur in a hospital setting to follow response (eg, walking distance, sign/symptoms of disease progression). May take 24-48 hours to transition. Transition is accomplished by initiating the infusion of treprostinil, and increasing it while simultaneously reducing the dose of intravenous epoprostenol.

Transitioning from epoprostenol to treprostinil:

Step 1:
Epoprostenol: Maintain current dose
Treprostinil: Initiate at 10% initial epoprostenol dose
Step 2:
Epoprostenol: Decrease dose to 80% of starting dose
Treprostinil: Increase to 30% initial epoprostenol dose
Step 3:
Epoprostenol: Decrease dose to 60% of starting dose
Treprostinil: Increase to 50% initial epoprostenol dose
Step 4:
Epoprostenol: Decrease dose to 40% of starting dose
Treprostinil: Increase to 70% initial epoprostenol dose
Step 5:
Epoprostenol: Decrease dose to 20% of starting dose
Treprostinil: Increase to 90% initial epoprostenol dose
Step 6:
Epoprostenol: Decrease dose to 5% of starting dose
Treprostinil: Increase to 110% initial epoprostenol dose
Step 7:
Epoprostenol: Discontinue
Treprostinil: Maintain current dose plus additional 5% to 10% as needed

Dosage Forms

Injection, solution:

Remodulin®: 1 mg/mL (20 mL); 2.5 mg/mL (20 mL); 5 mg/mL (20 mL); 10 mg/mL (20 mL)

treprostinil sodium *see* treprostinil *on this page*

tretinoin and clindamycin *see* clindamycin and tretinoin *on page 200*

tretinoin and mequinol *see* mequinol and tretinoin *on page 544*

tretinoin, fluocinolone acetonide, and hydroquinone *see* fluocinolone, hydroquinone, and tretinoin *on page 360*

tretinoin (oral) (TRET i noyn, oral)

Sound-Alike/Look-Alike Issues

tretinoin may be confused with trientine

Synonyms all-*trans*-retinoic acid; ATRA; NSC-122758; Ro 5488; tRA

U.S./Canadian Brand Names Vesanoid® [US/Can]

Therapeutic Category Antineoplastic Agent

Use Induction of remission in patients with acute promyelocytic leukemia (APL), French American British (FAB) classification M3 (including the M3 variant)

Usual Dosage Oral: Children and Adults:

Remission induction: 45 mg/m²/day in 2-3 divided doses for up to 30 days after complete remission (maximum duration of treatment: 90 days)

Remission maintenance: 45-200 mg/m²/day in 2-3 divided doses for up to 12 months.

Dosage Forms
Capsule:
Vesanoid®: 10 mg

tretinoin (topical) (TRET i noyn TOP i kal)
Sound-Alike/Look-Alike Issues
tretinoin may be confused with trientine
Synonyms retinoic acid; *trans*-retinoic acid; vitamin A acid
U.S./Canadian Brand Names Avita® [US]; Rejuva-A® [Can]; Renova® [US]; Retin-A® Micro [US/Can]; Retin-A® [US/Can]; Retinova® [Can]
Therapeutic Category Retinoic Acid Derivative
Use Treatment of acne vulgaris; photodamaged skin; palliation of fine wrinkles, mottled hyperpigmentation, and tactile roughness of facial skin as part of a comprehensive skin care and sun avoidance program
Usual Dosage Topical:
Children >12 years and Adults: Acne vulgaris: Begin therapy with a weaker formulation of tretinoin (0.025% cream, 0.04% microsphere gel, or 0.01% gel) and increase the concentration as tolerated; apply once daily to acne lesions before retiring or on alternate days; if stinging or irritation develop, decrease frequency of application
Adults ≥18 years: Palliation of fine wrinkles, mottled hyperpigmentation, and tactile roughness of facial skin: Pea-sized amount of the 0.02% or 0.05% cream applied to entire face once daily in the evening
Dosage Forms
Cream, topical: 0.025% (20 g, 45 g); 0.05% (20 g, 45 g); 0.1% (20 g, 45 g)
Avita®: 0.025% (20 g, 45 g)
Renova®: 0.02% (40 g)
Retin-A®: 0.025% (20 g, 45 g); 0.05% (20 g, 45 g); 0.1% (20 g, 45 g)
Tretin-X™: 0.025% (35 g); 0.05% (35 g); 0.1% (35 g)
Gel, topical: 0.025% (15 g, 45 g)
Avita®: 0.025% (20 g, 45 g)
Retin-A®: 0.01% (15 g, 45 g); 0.025% (15 g, 45 g)
Retin-A® Micro [microsphere gel]: 0.04% (20 g, 45 g, 50 g); 0.1% (20 g, 45 g, 50 g)
Tretin-X™: 0.025% (35 g); 0.1% (35 g)

Trexall™ [US] *see* methotrexate *on page 553*

triacetin (trye a SEE tin)
Sound-Alike/Look-Alike Issues
triacetin may be confused with Triacin®
Synonyms glycerol triacetate
U.S./Canadian Brand Names Myco-Nail [US-OTC]
Therapeutic Category Antifungal Agent
Use Fungistat for athlete's foot and other superficial fungal infections
Usual Dosage Apply twice daily, cleanse areas with dilute alcohol or mild soap and water before application; continue treatment for 7 days after symptoms have disappeared
Dosage Forms
Liquid, topical:
Myco-Nail [OTC]: 25% (30 mL)

Triacin-C® *(Discontinued) see* triprolidine, pseudoephedrine, and codeine *(Canada only) on page 869*

triaconazole *see* terconazole *on page 827*

Triaderm [Can] *see* triamcinolone (topical) *on page 863*

Triafed® *(Discontinued) see* triprolidine and pseudoephedrine *on page 869*

triamcinolone acetonide, parenteral *see* triamcinolone (systemic) *on next page*

triamcinolone and nystatin *see* nystatin and triamcinolone *on page 623*

triamcinolone diacetate, oral *see* triamcinolone (systemic) *on next page*

triamcinolone diacetate, parenteral *see* triamcinolone (systemic) *on next page*

triamcinolone hexacetonide *see* triamcinolone (systemic) *on next page*

triamcinolone (inhalation, nasal) (trye am SIN oh lone in hil LA shun, NAY sal)
Sound-Alike/Look-Alike Issues
Nasacort® may be confused with NasalCrom®
(Continued)

triamcinolone (inhalation, nasal) *(Continued)*

U.S./Canadian Brand Names Nasacort® AQ [US/Can]; Nasacort® HFA [US]; Tri-Nasal® [US/Can]

Therapeutic Category Adrenal Corticosteroid

Use Nasal inhalation: Management of seasonal and perennial allergic rhinitis in patients ≥6 years of age

Usual Dosage Intranasal: Perennial allergic rhinitis, seasonal allergic rhinitis:

Nasal spray:

Children 6-11 years: 110 mcg/day as 1 spray in each nostril once daily.

Children ≥12 years and Adults: 220 mcg/day as 2 sprays in each nostril once daily

Nasal inhaler:

Children 6-11 years: Initial: 220 mcg/day as 2 sprays in each nostril once daily

Children ≥12 years and Adults: Initial: 220 mcg/day as 2 sprays in each nostril once daily; may increase dose to 440 mcg/day (given once daily or divided and given 2 or 4 times/day)

Dosage Forms

Solution, intranasal:

Tri-Nasal®: 50 mcg/inhalation (15 mL)

Suspension, intranasal:

Nasacort® AQ: 55 mcg/inhalation (16.5 g)

triamcinolone (inhalation, oral) (trye am SIN oh lone in hil LA shun, OR al)

Sound-Alike/Look-Alike Issues

TAC (occasional abbreviation for triamcinolone) is an error-prone abbreviation (mistaken as tetracaine-adrenaline-cocaine)

U.S./Canadian Brand Names Azmacort® [US]

Therapeutic Category Adrenal Corticosteroid

Use Oral inhalation: Control of bronchial asthma and related bronchospastic conditions

Usual Dosage Oral inhalation: Asthma:

Children 6-12 years: 100-200 mcg 3-4 times/day **or** 200-400 mcg twice daily; maximum dose: 1200 mcg/day

Children >12 years and Adults: 200 mcg 3-4 times/day **or** 400 mcg twice daily; maximum dose: 1600 mcg/day

Dosage Forms

Aerosol for oral inhalation:

Azmacort®: 100 mcg per actuation (20 g)

triamcinolone, oral *see* triamcinolone (systemic) *on this page*

triamcinolone (systemic) (trye am SIN oh lone sis TEM ik)

Sound-Alike/Look-Alike Issues

Kenalog® may be confused with Ketalar®

Synonyms triamcinolone acetonide, parenteral; triamcinolone diacetate, oral; triamcinolone diacetate, parenteral; triamcinolone hexacetonide; triamcinolone, oral

U.S./Canadian Brand Names Aristospan® [US/Can]; Kenalog-10® [US]; Kenalog-40® [US]; Oracort [Can]

Therapeutic Category Adrenal Corticosteroid

Use Systemic: Adrenocortical insufficiency, rheumatic disorders, allergic states, respiratory diseases, systemic lupus erythematosus (SLE), and other diseases requiring antiinflammatory or immunosuppressive effects

Usual Dosage The lowest possible dose should be used to control the condition; when dose reduction is possible, the dose should be reduced gradually. Parenteral dose is usually ⅓ to ½ the oral dose given every 12 hours. In life-threatening situations, parenteral doses larger than the oral dose may be needed.

Injection:

Acetonide:

Intraarticular, intrabursal, tendon sheaths: Adults: Initial: Smaller joints: 2.5-5 mg, larger joints: 5-15 mg

Intradermal: Adults: Initial: 1 mg

I.M.: Range: 2.5-60 mg/day

Children 6-12 years: Initial: 40 mg

Children >12 years and Adults: Initial: 60 mg

Hexacetonide: Adults:

Intralesional, sublesional: Up to 0.5 mg/square inch of affected skin

Intra-articular: Range: 2-20 mg

Oral: Adults:

Acute rheumatic carditis: Initial: 20-60 mg/day; reduce dose during maintenance therapy

Acute seasonal or perennial allergic rhinitis: 8-12 mg/day

Adrenocortical insufficiency: Range 4-12 mg/day

Bronchial asthma: 8-16 mg/day

Dermatological disorders, contact/atopic dermatitis: Initial: 8-16 mg/day

Ophthalmic disorders: 12-40 mg/day

Rheumatic disorders: Range: 8-16 mg/day

SLE: Initial: 20-32 mg/day, some patients may need initial doses ≥48 mg; reduce dose during maintenance therapy

Dosage Forms

Injection, suspension:
Kenalog-10®: 10 mg/mL (5 mL) [not for I.V. or I.M. use]
Kenalog-40®: 40 mg/mL (1 mL, 5 mL, 10 mL) [not for I.V. or intradermal use]

Injection, suspension:
Aristospan®: 5 mg/mL (5 mL); 20 mg/mL (1 mL, 5 mL) [not for I.V. use]

triamcinolone (topical) (trye am SIN oh lone TOP i kal)

Sound-Alike/Look-Alike Issues
Kenalog® may be confused with Ketalar®

U.S./Canadian Brand Names Aristocort® A [US]; Kenalog® in Orabase [Can]; Kenalog® [US/Can]; Triaderm [Can]; Triderm® [US]

Therapeutic Category Corticosteroid, Topical

Use
Oral topical: Adjunctive treatment and temporary relief of symptoms associated with oral inflammatory lesions and ulcerative lesions resulting from trauma
Topical: Inflammatory dermatoses responsive to steroids

Usual Dosage
Oral topical: Oral inflammatory lesions/ulcers: Press a small dab (about 1/4 inch) to the lesion until a thin film develops. A larger quantity may be required for coverage of some lesions. For optimal results use only enough to coat the lesion with a thin film; do not rub in.

Topical:
Cream, Ointment: Apply thin film to affected areas 2-4 times/day
Spray: Apply to affected area 3-4 times/day

Dosage Forms

Aerosol, topical:
Kenalog®: 0.2 mg/2-second spray (63 g)
Cream: 0.025% (15 g, 80 g, 454 g); 0.1% (15 g, 80 g, 454 g, 2270 g); 0.5% (15 g)
Triderm®: 0.1% (30 g, 85 g)
Lotion: 0.025% (60 mL); 0.1% (60 mL)
Ointment, topical: 0.025% (15 g, 80 g, 454 g); 0.1% (15 g, 80 g, 454 g); 0.5% (15 g)
Paste, oral, topical: 0.1% (5 g)

Triaminic® Allerchews™ [US-OTC] see loratadine on page 517

Triaminic® Cold and Allergy [Can] see chlorpheniramine and pseudoephedrine on page 178

Triaminic® Cold and Allergy (Discontinued) see chlorpheniramine and pseudoephedrine on page 178

Triaminic® Cold and Cough (Discontinued) see chlorpheniramine, pseudoephedrine, and dextromethorphan on page 183

Triaminic® Cough and Sore Throat Formula (Discontinued) see acetaminophen, dextromethorphan, and pseudoephedrine on page 12

Triaminic® Cough (Discontinued) see pseudoephedrine and dextromethorphan on page 728

Triaminic® Cough & Nasal Congestion (Discontinued) see pseudoephedrine and dextromethorphan on page 728

Triaminic® Expectorant (Discontinued)

Triaminic® Infant Thin Strips® Decongestant [US-OTC] see phenylephrine on page 675

Triaminic® Night Time Cough and Cold (Discontinued) see chlorpheniramine, pseudoephedrine, and dextromethorphan on page 183

Triaminic® Thin Strips® Cold [US-OTC] see phenylephrine on page 675

Triaminic® Thin Strips™ Cough and Runny Nose [US-OTC] see diphenhydramine on page 265

Triaminic® Thin Strips™ Long Acting Cough [US-OTC] see dextromethorphan on page 247

Triamonide® Injection (Discontinued)

triamterene (trye AM ter een)

Sound-Alike/Look-Alike Issues
triamterene may be confused with trimipramine
Dyrenium® may be confused with Pyridium®
(Continued)

triamterene *(Continued)*

U.S./Canadian Brand Names Dyrenium® [US]
Therapeutic Category Diuretic, Potassium Sparing
Use Alone or in combination with other diuretics in treatment of edema and hypertension; decreases potassium excretion caused by kaliuretic diuretics
Usual Dosage Oral: Adults: Hypertension, edema: 100-300 mg/day in 1-2 divided doses; maximum dose: 300 mg/day; usual dosage range (JNC 7): 50-100 mg/day
Dosage Forms
  Capsule:
    Dyrenium®: 50 mg, 100 mg

triamterene and hydrochlorothiazide *see* hydrochlorothiazide and triamterene *on page 427*

Triant-HC™ [US] *see* phenylephrine, hydrocodone, and chlorpheniramine *on page 678*

Triapin® *(Discontinued)*

Triatec-8 [Can] *see* acetaminophen and codeine *on page 6*

Triatec-8 Strong [Can] *see* acetaminophen and codeine *on page 6*

Triatec-30 [Can] *see* acetaminophen and codeine *on page 6*

Triavil® *(Discontinued)* *see* amitriptyline and perphenazine *on page 45*

Triaz® [US] *see* benzoyl peroxide *on page 103*

Triaz® Cleanser [US] *see* benzoyl peroxide *on page 103*

triazolam *(trye AY zoe lam)*

Sound-Alike/Look-Alike Issues
  triazolam may be confused with alprazolam
  Halcion® may be confused with halcinonide, Haldol®
U.S./Canadian Brand Names Apo-Triazo® [Can]; Gen-Triazolam [Can]; Halcion® [Can]
Therapeutic Category Benzodiazepine
Controlled Substance C-IV
Use Short-term treatment of insomnia
Usual Dosage Oral (onset of action is rapid, patient should be in bed when taking medication):
  Adults:
    Hypnotic: 0.125-0.25 mg at bedtime (maximum dose: 0.5 mg/day)
    Preprocedure sedation (dental): 0.25 mg taken the evening before oral surgery; or 0.25 mg 1 hour before procedure
Dosage Forms
  Tablet: 0.125 mg, 0.25 mg

tribavirin *see* ribavirin *on page 755*

Tri Biozene [US-OTC] *see* bacitracin, neomycin, polymyxin B, and pramoxine *on page 92*

tricalcium phosphate *see* calcium phosphate (tribasic) *on page 142*

Tricardio B [US] *see* folic acid, cyanocobalamin, and pyridoxine *on page 371*

Tri-Chlor® [US] *see* trichloroacetic acid *on this page*

Trichlor Fresh Pac™ [US] *see* trichloroacetic acid *on this page*

trichloroacetaldehyde monohydrate *see* chloral hydrate *on page 172*

trichloroacetic acid *(trye klor oh a SEE tik AS id)*

U.S./Canadian Brand Names Tri-Chlor® [US]; Trichlor Fresh Pac™ [US]
Therapeutic Category Keratolytic Agent
Use Chemical used in compounding agents for the treatment of warts, skin resurfacing (chemical peels)
Usual Dosage Topical: Apply to verruca, cover with bandage for 5-6 days, remove verruca, reapply as needed
Dosage Forms
  Liquid: 80%
    Tri-Chlor®: 80%
  Powder for reconstitution, topical: 10% (28 mL); 15% (28 mL); 20% (28 mL); 25% (28 mL); 30% (28 mL); 35% (28 mL); 40% (28 mL); 50% (28 mL)
    Trichlor Fresh Pac™: 10% (28 mL); 15% (28 mL); 20% (28 mL); 25% (28 mL); 30% (28 mL); 35% (28 mL); 40% (28 mL); 50% (28 mL)

trichloromonofluoromethane and dichlorodifluoromethane *see* dichlorodifluoromethane and trichloromonofluoromethane *on page 253*

Trichophyton skin test (trye koe FYE ton skin test)
Therapeutic Category Diagnostic Agent
Use Assess cell-mediated immunity
Usual Dosage 0.1 mL intradermally, examine reaction site in 24-48 hours; induration of ≥5 mm in diameter is a positive reaction
Dosage Forms
  Injection, solution: 1:200 (2 mL)

Tri-Clear® Expectorant *(Discontinued)*

TriCor® [US/Can] *see* fenofibrate *on page 345*

tricosal *see* choline magnesium trisalicylate *on page 187*

Tri-Cyclen® [Can] *see* ethinyl estradiol and norgestimate *on page 331*

Tri-Cyclen® Lo [Can] *see* ethinyl estradiol and norgestimate *on page 331*

Triderm® [US] *see* triamcinolone (topical) *on page 863*

Tridil® Injection *(Discontinued)* *see* nitroglycerin *on page 608*

Tridione® [US] *see* trimethadione *on page 867*

trientine (TRYE en teen)
Sound-Alike/Look-Alike Issues
  trientine may be confused with Trental®, tretinoin
Synonyms trientine hydrochloride
U.S./Canadian Brand Names Syprine® [US/Can]
Therapeutic Category Chelating Agent
Use Treatment of Wilson disease in patients intolerant to penicillamine
Usual Dosage Oral (administer on an empty stomach):
  Children <12 years: 500-750 mg/day in divided doses 2-4 times/day; maximum: 1.5 g/day
  Adults: 750-1250 mg/day in divided doses 2-4 times/day; maximum dose: 2 g/day
Dosage Forms
  Capsule:
  Syprine®: 250 mg

trientine hydrochloride *see* trientine *on this page*

triethanolamine salicylate *see* trolamine *on page 870*

triethylenethiophosphoramide *see* thiotepa *on page 838*

Trifed-C® *(Discontinued)* *see* triprolidine, pseudoephedrine, and codeine *(Canada only)* *on page 869*

trifluoperazine (trye floo oh PER a zeen)
Sound-Alike/Look-Alike Issues
  trifluoperazine may be confused with triflupromazine, trihexyphenidyl
  Stelazine® may be confused with selegiline
Synonyms trifluoperazine hydrochloride
U.S./Canadian Brand Names Apo-Trifluoperazine® [Can]; Novo-Trifluzine [Can]; PMS-Trifluoperazine [Can]; Terfluzine [Can]
Therapeutic Category Phenothiazine Derivative
Use Treatment of schizophrenia
Usual Dosage Oral:
  Children 6-12 years: Schizophrenia/psychoses: Hospitalized or well-supervised patients: Initial: 1 mg 1-2 times/day, gradually increase until symptoms are controlled or adverse effects become troublesome; maximum: 15 mg/day
  Adults:
  Schizophrenia/psychoses:
  Outpatients: 1-2 mg twice daily
  Hospitalized or well-supervised patients: Initial: 2-5 mg twice daily with optimum response in the 15-20 mg/day range; do not exceed 40 mg/day
  Nonpsychotic anxiety: 1-2 mg twice daily; maximum: 6 mg/day; therapy for anxiety should not exceed 12 weeks; do not exceed 6 mg/day for longer than 12 weeks when treating anxiety; agitation, jitteriness, or insomnia may be confused with original neurotic or psychotic symptoms
Dosage Forms
  Tablet: 1 mg, 2 mg, 5 mg, 10 mg

trifluoperazine hydrochloride *see* trifluoperazine *on this page*

trifluorothymidine *see* trifluridine *on this page*

trifluridine (trye FLURE i deen)
Sound-Alike/Look-Alike Issues
Viroptic® may be confused with Timoptic®
Synonyms F_3T; trifluorothymidine
U.S./Canadian Brand Names SAB-Trifluridine [Can]; Sandoz-Trifluridine [Can]; Viroptic® [US/Can]
Therapeutic Category Antiviral Agent
Use Treatment of primary keratoconjunctivitis and recurrent epithelial keratitis caused by herpes simplex virus types I and II
Usual Dosage Adults: Instill 1 drop into affected eye every 2 hours while awake, to a maximum of 9 drops/day, until reepithelialization of corneal ulcer occurs; then use 1 drop every 4 hours for another 7 days; do **not** exceed 21 days of treatment; if improvement has not taken place in 7-14 days, consider another form of therapy
Dosage Forms
Solution, ophthalmic: 1% (7.5 mL)
Viroptic®: 1% (7.5 mL)

Triglide™ [US] *see* fenofibrate *on page 345*

triglycerides, medium chain *see* medium chain triglycerides *on page 536*

trihexyphenidyl (trye heks ee FEN i dil)
Sound-Alike/Look-Alike Issues
trihexyphenidyl may be confused with trifluoperazine
Artane® may be confused with Altace®, Anturane®, Aramine®
Synonyms benzhexol hydrochloride; trihexyphenidyl hydrochloride
U.S./Canadian Brand Names Apo-Trihex® [Can]
Therapeutic Category Anti-Parkinson Agent; Anticholinergic Agent
Use Adjunctive treatment of Parkinson disease; treatment of drug-induced extrapyramidal symptoms
Usual Dosage Oral: Adults: Initial: 1-2 mg/day, increase by 2 mg increments at intervals of 3-5 days; usual dose: 5-15 mg/day in 3-4 divided doses
Dosage Forms
Elixir: 2 mg/5 mL
Tablet: 2 mg, 5 mg

trihexyphenidyl hydrochloride *see* trihexyphenidyl *on this page*

TriHIBit® [US] *see* diphtheria, tetanus toxoids, and acellular pertussis vaccine and *Haemophilus influenzae* b conjugate vaccine *on page 270*

Trikacide [Can] *see* metronidazole *on page 563*

Trikof-D® [US] *see* guaifenesin, pseudoephedrine, and dextromethorphan *on page 408*

TRIKOF-D® *(Discontinued)*

Tri-Kort® Injection *(Discontinued)*

Trilafon® *(Discontinued)* *see* perphenazine *on page 670*

Trileptal® [US/Can] *see* oxcarbazepine *on page 638*

Tri-Levlen® *(Discontinued)* *see* ethinyl estradiol and levonorgestrel *on page 325*

Trilisate® *(Discontinued)* *see* choline magnesium trisalicylate *on page 187*

Trilog® Injection *(Discontinued)*

Trilone® Injection *(Discontinued)*

Tri-Luma™ [US] *see* fluocinolone, hydroquinone, and tretinoin *on page 360*

TriLyte™ [US] *see* polyethylene glycol-electrolyte solution *on page 695*

Trimazide® *(Discontinued)* *see* trimethobenzamide *on next page*

trimebutine *(Canada only)* (trye me BYOO teen)
Synonyms trimebutine maleate
U.S./Canadian Brand Names Apo-Trimebutine® [Can]; Modulon® [Can]
Therapeutic Category Antispasmodic Agent, Gastrointestinal
Use Treatment and relief of symptoms associated with irritable bowel syndrome (IBS) (spastic colon). In postoperative paralytic ileus in order to accelerate the resumption of the intestinal transit following abdominal surgery.

Usual Dosage Oral: Children ≥12 years and Adults: 200 mg 3 times/day before meals
Dosage Forms [CAN] = Canadian brand name
  Tablet:
    Apo-Trimebutine® [CAN], Modulon® [CAN]: 100 mg, 200 mg [not available in the U.S.]

trimebutine maleate *see* trimebutine *(Canada only)* on previous page

trimeprazine *(Canada only)* (trye MEP re zeen)
U.S./Canadian Brand Names Panectyl® [Can]
Therapeutic Category Antihistamine
Use Perennial and seasonal allergic rhinitis and other allergic symptoms including urticaria
Usual Dosage Oral:
  Children:
    6 months to 3 years: 1.25 mg at bedtime or 3 times/day if needed
    >3 years: 2.5 mg at bedtime or 3 times/day if needed
    >6 years: Sustained release: 5 mg/day
    Adults: 2.5 mg 4 times/day (5 mg every 12-hour sustained release)
Dosage Forms
  Tablet, as tartrate: 2.5 mg, 5 mg

trimethadione (trye meth a DYE one)
Synonyms troxidone
U.S./Canadian Brand Names Tridione® [US]
Therapeutic Category Anticonvulsant, Oxazolidinedione
Use Control absence (petit mal) seizures refractory to other drugs
Usual Dosage Oral: Seizure disorders:
  Children: Initial: 25-50 mg/kg/24 hours in 3-4 equally divided doses every 6-8 hours
  Adults: Initial: 900 mg/day in 3-4 equally divided doses, increase by 300 mg/day at weekly intervals until therapeutic results or toxic symptoms appear
Dosage Forms
  Tablet, chewable:
    Tridione®: 150 mg

trimethobenzamide (trye meth oh BEN za mide)
Sound-Alike/Look-Alike Issues
  Tigan® may be confused with Tiazac®, Ticar®
Synonyms trimethobenzamide hydrochloride
U.S./Canadian Brand Names Tigan® [US/Can]
Therapeutic Category Anticholinergic Agent; Antiemetic
Use Treatment of nausea and vomiting
Usual Dosage
  Children >40 kg: Oral: 300 mg 3-4 times/day
  Adults:
    Oral: 300 mg 3-4 times/day
    I.M.: 200 mg 3-4 times/day
    Postoperative nausea and vomiting (PONV): I.M.: 200 mg, followed 1 hour later by a second 200 mg dose
Dosage Forms
  Capsule: 300 mg
    Tigan®: 300 mg
  Injection, solution: 100 mg/mL (2 mL)
    Tigan®: 100 mg/mL (2 mL [preservative free], 20 mL)

trimethobenzamide hydrochloride *see* trimethobenzamide on this page

trimethoprim (trye METH oh prim)
Sound-Alike/Look-Alike Issues
  trimethoprim may be confused with trimethaphan
  Proloprim® may be confused with Prolixin®, Protropin®
Synonyms TMP
U.S./Canadian Brand Names Apo-Trimethoprim® [Can]; Primsol® [US]; Proloprim® [US]
Therapeutic Category Antibiotic, Miscellaneous
Use Treatment of urinary tract infections due to susceptible strains of *E. coli*, *P. mirabilis*, *K. pneumoniae*, *Enterobacter* sp and coagulase-negative *Staphylococcus* including *S. saprophyticus*; acute otitis media in children; acute exacerbations of chronic bronchitis in adults; in combination with other agents for treatment of
(Continued)

trimethoprim *(Continued)*

toxoplasmosis, *Pneumocystis carinii*; treatment of superficial ocular infections involving the conjunctiva and cornea

Usual Dosage Oral:

Children: 4 mg/kg/day in divided doses every 12 hours

Adults: 100 mg every 12 hours or 200 mg every 24 hours for 10 days; longer treatment periods may be necessary for prostatitis (ie, 4-16 weeks); in the treatment of *Pneumocystis carinii* pneumonia; dose may be as high as 15-20 mg/kg/day in 3-4 divided doses

Dosage Forms

Solution, oral:

Primsol®: 50 mg/5 mL

Tablet: 100 mg

trimethoprim and polymyxin B (trye METH oh prim & pol i MIKS in bee)

Synonyms polymyxin B and trimethoprim

U.S./Canadian Brand Names PMS-Polytrimethoprim [Can]; Polytrim® [US/Can]

Therapeutic Category Antibiotic, Ophthalmic

Use Treatment of surface ocular bacterial conjunctivitis and blepharoconjunctivitis

Usual Dosage Instill 1-2 drops in eye(s) every 4-6 hours

Dosage Forms

Solution, ophthalmic: Trimethoprim 1 mg and polymyxin B 10,000 units per mL (10 mL)

Polytrim®: Trimethoprim 1 mg and polymyxin B 10,000 units per mL (10 mL)

trimethoprim and sulfamethoxazole *see* sulfamethoxazole and trimethoprim *on page 813*

trimipramine (trye MI pra meen)

Sound-Alike/Look-Alike Issues

trimipramine may be confused with triamterene, trimeprazine

Synonyms trimipramine maleate

U.S./Canadian Brand Names Apo-Trimip® [Can]; Nu-Trimipramine [Can]; Rhotrimine® [Can]; Surmontil® [US]

Therapeutic Category Antidepressant, Tricyclic (Tertiary Amine)

Use Treatment of depression

Usual Dosage Oral: Adults: 50-150 mg/day as a single bedtime dose up to a maximum of 200 mg/day outpatient and 300 mg/day inpatient

Dosage Forms

Capsule:

Surmontil®: 25 mg, 50 mg, 100 mg

trimipramine maleate *see* trimipramine *on this page*

Trimox® *(Discontinued)* *see* amoxicillin *on page 48*

Trimpex® *(Discontinued)* *see* trimethoprim *on previous page*

Tri-Nasal® [US/Can] *see* triamcinolone (inhalation, nasal) *on page 861*

Trinate [US] *see* vitamins (multiple/prenatal) *on page 896*

TriNessa™ [US] *see* ethinyl estradiol and norgestimate *on page 331*

Trinipatch® 0.2 [Can] *see* nitroglycerin *on page 608*

Trinipatch® 0.4 [Can] *see* nitroglycerin *on page 608*

Trinipatch® 0.6 [Can] *see* nitroglycerin *on page 608*

Tri-Norinyl® [US] *see* ethinyl estradiol and norethindrone *on page 328*

Trinsicon® *(Discontinued)* *see* vitamin B complex combinations *on page 894*

Triofed® Syrup *(Discontinued)* *see* triprolidine and pseudoephedrine *on next page*

Triostat® [US] *see* liothyronine *on page 510*

Tripedia® [US] *see* diphtheria, tetanus toxoids, and acellular pertussis vaccine *on page 269*

Triphasil® [US/Can] *see* ethinyl estradiol and levonorgestrel *on page 325*

Triphenyl® Expectorant *(Discontinued)*

triple antibiotic *see* bacitracin, neomycin, and polymyxin B *on page 91*

triple sulfa *see* sulfabenzamide, sulfacetamide, and sulfathiazole *on page 810*

Triposed® Syrup *(Discontinued)* *see* triprolidine and pseudoephedrine *on next page*

Tri-Previfem™ **[US]** *see* ethinyl estradiol and norgestimate *on page 331*

triprolidine and pseudoephedrine (trye PROE li deen & soo doe e FED rin)

Sound-Alike/Look-Alike Issues
Aprodine® may be confused with Aphrodyne®

Synonyms pseudoephedrine and triprolidine

U.S./Canadian Brand Names Actifed® [Can]; Allerfrim® [US-OTC]; Aprodine® [US-OTC]; Genac® [US-OTC]; Silafed® [US-OTC]; Zymine®-D [US]

Therapeutic Category Antihistamine/Decongestant Combination

Use Temporary relief of nasal congestion, decongest sinus openings, running nose, sneezing, itching of nose or throat and itchy, watery eyes due to common cold, hay fever, or other upper respiratory allergies

Usual Dosage Oral:
Liquid (Zymine®-D):
Children:
2-4 years: 1.25 mL every 4-6 hours (maximum pseudoephedrine: 60 mg/24 hours)
4-6 years: 2.5 mL every 4-6 hours (maximum pseudoephedrine: 60 mg/24 hours)
6-12 years: 2.5-5 mL every 4-6 hours (maximum pseudoephedrine: 120 mg/24 hours)
Children ≥12 years and Adults: 5-10 mL every 4-6 hours (maximum pseudoephedrine: 240 mg/24 hours)
Syrup (Allerfrim, Aprodine):
Children 6-12 years: 5 mL every 4-6 hours; do not exceed 4 doses in 24 hours
Children >12 years and Adults: 10 mL every 4-6 hours; do not exceed 4 doses in 24 hours
Tablet (Aprodine):
Children 6-12 years: 1/2 tablet every 4-6 hours; do not exceed 4 doses in 24 hours
Children >12 years and Adults: One tablet every 4-6 hours; do not exceed 4 doses in 24 hours

Dosage Forms
Liquid:
Zymine®-D: Triprolidine 1.25 mg and pseudoephedrine 45 mg per 5 mL
Syrup: Triprolidine 1.25 mg and pseudoephedrine 30 mg per 5 mL
Allerfrim® [OTC], Aprodine® [OTC], Silafed® [OTC]: Triprolidine 1.25 mg and pseudoephedrine 30 mg per 5 mL
Tablet:
Aprodine® [OTC], Genac® [OTC], Sudafed® Maximum Strength Sinus Nighttime[OTC]: Triprolidine 2.5 mg and pseudoephedrine 60 mg

triprolidine, codeine, and pseudoephedrine *see* triprolidine, pseudoephedrine, and codeine *(Canada only) on this page*

triprolidine, pseudoephedrine, and codeine *(Canada only)*
(trye PROE li deen, soo doe e FED rin, & KOE deen)

Sound-Alike/Look-Alike Issues
Triacin-C® may be confused with triacetin

Synonyms codeine, pseudoephedrine, and triprolidine; codeine, triprolidine, and pseudoephedrine; pseudoephedrine, codeine, and triprolidine; pseudoephedrine, triprolidine, and codeine; triprolidine, codeine, and pseudoephedrine

U.S./Canadian Brand Names CoActifed® [Can]; Covan® [Can]; ratio-Cotridin [Can]

Therapeutic Category Antihistamine/Decongestant/Antitussive

Controlled Substance C-V (CDSA-I)

Use Symptomatic relief of upper respiratory symptoms and cough

Usual Dosage Oral:
Children:
2-6 years: 2.5 mL 4 times/day
7-12 years: 5 mL 4 times/day **or** 1/2 tablet 4 times/day
Children >12 years and Adults: 10 mL 4 times/day **or** 1 tablet 4 times/day

Dosage Forms [CAN] = Canadian brand name
Syrup:
CoActifed® [CAN], CoVan® [CAN], ratio-Cotridin [CAN]: Triprolidine 2 mg, pseudoephedrine 30 mg, and codeine 10 mg per 5 mL [not available in the U.S.]
Tablet:
CoActifed® [CAN]: Triprolidine 4 mg, pseudoephedrine 60 mg, and codeine 20 mg (50s) [not available in the U.S.]

Tri-Pseudo® *(Discontinued) see* triprolidine and pseudoephedrine *on this page*

TripTone® *(Discontinued) see* dimenhydrinate *on page 262*

triptoraline *see* triptorelin *on next page*

triptorelin (trip toe REL in)

Synonyms AY-25650; CL-118,532; D-Trp(6)-LHRH; triptoraline; triptorelin pamoate; tryptoreline

U.S./Canadian Brand Names Trelstar™ Depot [US/Can]; Trelstar™ LA [US/Can]; Trelstar™ [Can]

Therapeutic Category Luteinizing Hormone-Releasing Hormone Analog

Use Palliative treatment of advanced prostate cancer as an alternative to orchiectomy or estrogen administration

Usual Dosage I.M.: Adults: Prostate cancer:
Trelstar™ Depot: 3.75 mg once every 28 days
Trelstar™ LA: 11.25 mg once every 84 days

Dosage Forms
Injection, powder for reconstitution:
Trelstar™ Depot: 3.75 mg
Trelstar™ LA: 11.25 mg

triptorelin pamoate see triptorelin on this page

Triquilar® [Can] see ethinyl estradiol and levonorgestrel on page 325

tris buffer see tromethamine on next page

Trisenox® [US] see arsenic trioxide on page 74

tris(hydroxymethyl)aminomethane see tromethamine on next page

trisodium calcium diethylenetriaminepentaacetate (Ca-DTPA) see diethylene triamine pentaacetic acid on page 256

Tri-Sprintec™ [US] see ethinyl estradiol and norgestimate on page 331

Tri-Statin® II Topical (Discontinued) see nystatin and triamcinolone on page 623

Tristoject® Injection (Discontinued)

Trisudex® (Discontinued) see triprolidine and pseudoephedrine on previous page

Tri-Sudo® (Discontinued) see triprolidine and pseudoephedrine on previous page

Tri-Tannate Plus® (Discontinued) see chlorpheniramine, ephedrine, phenylephrine, and carbetapentane on page 179

TriTuss® [US] see guaifenesin, dextromethorphan, and phenylephrine on page 407

TriTuss® ER [US] see guaifenesin, dextromethorphan, and phenylephrine on page 407

Trivagizole-3® [Can] see clotrimazole on page 206

Trivagizole-3® (Discontinued) see clotrimazole on page 206

trivalent inactivated influenza vaccine (TIV) see influenza virus vaccine on page 455

Tri-Vent™ DM [US] see guaifenesin, pseudoephedrine, and dextromethorphan on page 408

Tri-Vent™ DPC [US] see chlorpheniramine, phenylephrine, and dextromethorphan on page 180

Tri-Vent™ HC [US] see hydrocodone, carbinoxamine, and pseudoephedrine on page 430

Tri-Vi-Sol® [US-OTC] see vitamins (multiple/pediatric) on page 896

Tri-Vi-Sol® with Iron [US-OTC] see vitamins (multiple/pediatric) on page 896

Trivora® [US] see ethinyl estradiol and levonorgestrel on page 325

Trizivir® [US] see abacavir, lamivudine, and zidovudine on page 2

Trobicin® (Discontinued) see spectinomycin on page 803

Trocaine® [US-OTC] see benzocaine on page 101

Trocal® (Discontinued) see dextromethorphan on page 247

trolamine (TROLE a meen)

Sound-Alike/Look-Alike Issues
Myoflex® may be confused with Mycelex®

Synonyms TEAS; triethanolamine salicylate; trolamine salicylate

U.S./Canadian Brand Names Antiphlogistine Rub A-535 No Odour [Can]; Aspercreme® [US-OTC]; Flex-Power [US-OTC]; Mobisyl® [US-OTC]; Myoflex® [US-OTC/Can]; Sportscreme® [US-OTC]

Therapeutic Category Analgesic, Topical

Use Relief of pain of muscular aches, rheumatism, neuralgia, sprains, arthritis on intact skin

Usual Dosage Topical: Apply to area as needed

Dosage Forms
Cream, topical: 10% (90 g)
Aspercreme® [OTC]: 10% (5 g, 35 g, 142 g)

Flex-Power [OTC]: 10% (113 g)
Mobisyl® [OTC]: 10% (100 g, 227 g)
Myoflex® [OTC]: 10% (60 g, 120 g)
Sportscreme® [OTC]: 10% (40 g, 90 g)
Lotion, topical: 10% (180 mL)
Aspercreme® [OTC]: 10% (180 mL)
Patch, topical:
Aspercreme®: 10% (5s)

trolamine salicylate *see* trolamine *on previous page*

Trombovar® [Can] *see* sodium tetradecyl *on page 798*

tromethamine (troe METH a meen)
Sound-Alike/Look-Alike Issues
tromethamine may be confused with TrophAmine®
Synonyms tris buffer; tris(hydroxymethyl)aminomethane
U.S./Canadian Brand Names THAM® [US]
Therapeutic Category Alkalinizing Agent
Use Correction of metabolic acidosis associated with cardiac bypass surgery or cardiac arrest; to correct excess acidity of stored blood that is preserved with acid citrate dextrose (ACD); indicated in infants needing alkalinization after receiving maximum sodium bicarbonate (8-10 mEq/kg/24 hours)
Usual Dosage
Neonates and Infants: Metabolic acidosis associated with RDS: Initial: Approximately 1 mL/kg for each pH unit below 7.4; additional doses determined by changes in PaO_2, pH, and pCO_2; **Note:** Although THAM® solution does not raise pCO_2 when treating metabolic acidosis with concurrent respiratory acidosis, bicarbonate may be preferred because the osmotic effects of THAM® are greater.

Adults: Dose depends on buffer base deficit; when deficit is known: tromethamine (mL of 0.3 M solution) = body weight (kg) x base deficit (mEq/L) x 1.1
Metabolic acidosis with cardiac arrest:
I.V.: 3.6-10.8 g (111-333 mL); additional amounts may be required to control acidosis after arrest reversed
Open chest: Intraventricular: 2-6 g (62-185 mL). **Note:** Do not inject into cardiac muscle
Acidosis associated with cardiac bypass surgery: Average dose: 9 mL/kg (2.7 mEq/kg); 500 mL is adequate for most adults; maximum dose: 500 mg/kg in ≤1 hour
Excess acidity of acid citrate dextrose (ACD) blood in coronary artery surgery: 15-77 mL of 0.3 molar solution added to each 500 mL of blood
Dosage Forms
Injection, solution:
THAM®: 18 g [0.3 molar] (500 mL)

Tronolane® [US-OTC] *see* pramoxine *on page 706*

Tronolane® Suppository [US-OTC] *see* phenylephrine *on page 675*

Tropicacyl® [US] *see* tropicamide *on this page*

tropicamide (troe PIK a mide)
Synonyms bistropamide
U.S./Canadian Brand Names Diotrope® [Can]; Mydral™ [US]; Mydriacyl® [US/Can]; Tropicacyl® [US]
Therapeutic Category Anticholinergic Agent
Use Short-acting mydriatic used in diagnostic procedures; as well as preoperatively and postoperatively; treatment of some cases of acute iritis, iridocyclitis, and keratitis
Usual Dosage Ophthalmic: Children and Adults (individuals with heavily pigmented eyes may require larger doses):
Cycloplegia: Instill 1-2 drops (1%); may repeat in 5 minutes
Exam must be performed within 30 minutes after the repeat dose; if the patient is not examined within 20-30 minutes, instill an additional drop
Mydriasis: Instill 1-2 drops (0.5%) 15-20 minutes before exam; may repeat every 30 minutes as needed
Dosage Forms
Solution, ophthalmic: 0.5% (15 mL); 1% (2 mL, 15 mL)
Mydriacyl®: 1% (3 mL, 15 mL)
Mydral™, Tropicacyl®: 0.5% (15 mL); 1% (15 mL)

tropicamide and hydroxyamphetamine *see* hydroxyamphetamine and tropicamide *on page 438*

Trosec [Can] *see* trospium *on next page*

trospium (TROSE pee um)
Synonyms trospium chloride
U.S./Canadian Brand Names Sanctura® [US]; Trosec [Can]
Therapeutic Category Anticholinergic Agent
Use Treatment of overactive bladder with symptoms of urgency, incontinence, and urinary frequency
Usual Dosage Oral: Adults: 20 mg twice daily
Dosage Forms
Tablet:
Sanctura™: 20 mg

trospium chloride *see* trospium *on this page*

Trovan® *(Discontinued)*

troxidone *see* trimethadione *on page 867*

Truphylline® *(Discontinued)* *see* aminophylline *on page 43*

Trusopt® [US/Can] *see* dorzolamide *on page 277*

Truvada® [US/Can] *see* emtricitabine and tenofovir *on page 295*

trypsin, balsam peru, and castor oil (TRIP sin, BAL sam pe RUE, & KAS tor oyl)
Sound-Alike/Look-Alike Issues
Granulex® may be confused with Regranex®
Synonyms balsam peru, trypsin, and castor oil; castor oil, trypsin, and balsam peru
U.S./Canadian Brand Names Granulex® [US]; Optase™ [US]; Xenaderm™ [US]
Therapeutic Category Protectant, Topical
Use Treatment of decubitus ulcers, varicose ulcers, debridement of eschar, dehiscent wounds and sunburn; promote wound healing; reduce odor from necrotic wounds
Usual Dosage Topical: Apply a minimum of twice daily or as often as necessary
Dosage Forms
Aerosol, topical: Trypsin 0.12 mg, balsam Peru 87 mg, and castor oil 788 mg per gram (120 g)
Granulex®: Trypsin 0.12 mg, balsam Peru 87 mg, and castor oil 788 mg per gram (60 g, 120 g)
Gel, topical:
Optase™: Trypsin 0.12 mg, balsam Peru 87 mg, and castor oil 788 mg per gram (95 g)
Ointment, topical:
Allanderm-T™, Xenaderm™: Trypsin 90 USP units, balsam Peru 87 mg, and castor oil 788 mg per gram (30 g, 60 g)

tryptoreline *see* triptorelin *on page 870*

Trysul® *(Discontinued)* *see* sulfabenzamide, sulfacetamide, and sulfathiazole *on page 810*

TSH *see* thyrotropin alpha *on page 839*

TSPA *see* thiotepa *on page 838*

TST *see* tuberculin tests *on this page*

T-Stat® *(Discontinued)* *see* erythromycin *on page 309*

tuberculin purified protein derivative *see* tuberculin tests *on this page*

tuberculin skin test *see* tuberculin tests *on this page*

tuberculin tests (too BER kyoo lin tests)
Sound-Alike/Look-Alike Issues
Aplisol® may be confused with Anusol®, A.P.L.®, Aplitest®, Atropisol®
Tuberculin products may be confused with tetanus toxoid products and influenza virus vaccine. Medication errors have occurred when tuberculin skin tests (PPD) have been inadvertently administered instead of tetanus toxoid products and influenza virus vaccine. These products are refrigerated and often stored in close proximity to each other.
Synonyms mantoux; PPD; TB skin test; TST; tuberculin purified protein derivative; tuberculin skin test
U.S./Canadian Brand Names Aplisol® [US]; Tubersol® [US]
Therapeutic Category Diagnostic Agent
Use Skin test in diagnosis of tuberculosis
Usual Dosage Children and Adults: Intradermal: 0.1 mL

TST interpretation: Criteria for positive TST read at 48-72 hours (see Note below for healthcare workers):

Induration ≥5 mm: Persons with HIV infection (or risk factors for HIV infection, but unknown status), recent close contact to person with known active TB, persons with chest x-ray consistent with healed TB, persons who are immunosuppressed

Induration ≥10 mm: Persons with clinical conditions which increase risk of TB infection, recent immigrants, I.V. drug users, residents and employees of high-risk settings, children <4 years of age

Induration ≥15 mm: Persons who do not meet any of the above criteria (no risk factors for TB)

Note: A two-step test is recommended when testing will be performed at regular intervals (eg, for healthcare workers). If the first test is negative, a second TST should be administered 1-3 weeks after the first test was read.

TST interpretation (CDC guidelines) in a healthcare setting:

Baseline test: ≥10 mm is positive (either first or second step)

Serial testing without known exposure: Increase of ≥10 mm is positive

Known exposure:

≥5 mm is positive in patients with baseline of 0 mm

≥10 mm is positive in patients with negative baseline or previous screening result of ≥0 mm

Read test at 48-72 hours following placement. Test results with 0 mm induration or measured induration less than the defined cutoff point are considered to signify absence of infection with *M. tuberculosis*. Test results should be documented in millimeters even if classified as negative. Erythema and redness of skin are not indicative of a positive test result.

Dosage Forms

Injection, solution:

Aplisol®, Tubersol®: 5 TU/0.1 mL (1 mL, 5 mL)

Tubersol® [US] *see* tuberculin tests *on previous page*

Tucks® [US-OTC] *see* witch hazel *on page 900*

Tucks® Anti-Itch [US-OTC] *see* hydrocortisone (rectal) *on page 433*

Tucks® Hemorrhoidal [US-OTC] *see* pramoxine *on page 706*

Tuinal® *(Discontinued)*

Tums® [US-OTC] *see* calcium carbonate *on page 138*

Tums® E-X [US-OTC] *see* calcium carbonate *on page 138*

Tums® Extra Strength Sugar Free [US-OTC] *see* calcium carbonate *on page 138*

Tums® Smoothies™ [US-OTC] *see* calcium carbonate *on page 138*

Tums® Ultra [US-OTC] *see* calcium carbonate *on page 138*

Tur-bi-kal® [US-OTC] *see* phenylephrine *on page 675*

Tusal® *(Discontinued)*

Tusana-D [US] *see* phenylephrine, hydrocodone, and chlorpheniramine *on page 678*

Tusibron® *(Discontinued)* *see* guaifenesin *on page 401*

Tusibron-DM® *(Discontinued)* *see* guaifenesin and dextromethorphan *on page 402*

Tusnel Pediatric® [US] *see* guaifenesin, pseudoephedrine, and dextromethorphan *on page 408*

Tussafed® *(Discontinued)* *see* carbinoxamine, pseudoephedrine, and dextromethorphan *on page 152*

Tussafed® HC [US] *see* hydrocodone, phenylephrine, and guaifenesin *on page 431*

Tussafed® HCG [US] *see* hydrocodone, phenylephrine, and guaifenesin *on page 431*

Tussafin® Expectorant *(Discontinued)* *see* hydrocodone, pseudoephedrine, and guaifenesin *on page 432*

Tussend® Expectorant *(Discontinued)* *see* hydrocodone, pseudoephedrine, and guaifenesin *on page 432*

Tussend® Syrup *(Discontinued)* *see* pseudoephedrine, hydrocodone, and chlorpheniramine *on page 731*

Tussend® Tablet *(Discontinued)* *see* pseudoephedrine, hydrocodone, and chlorpheniramine *on page 731*

Tussi-12® [US] *see* carbetapentane and chlorpheniramine *on page 149*

Tussi-12® D [US] *see* carbetapentane, phenylephrine, and pyrilamine *on page 150*

Tussi-12® DS [US] *see* carbetapentane, phenylephrine, and pyrilamine *on page 150*

Tussi-12 S™ [US] *see* carbetapentane and chlorpheniramine *on page 149*

Tussigon® **[US]** *see* hydrocodone and homatropine *on page 429*

TussiNate™ **[US]** *see* hydrocodone, phenylephrine, and diphenhydramine *on page 431*

Tussionex® **[US]** *see* hydrocodone and chlorpheniramine *on page 428*

Tussi-Organidin® **DM NR [US]** *see* guaifenesin and dextromethorphan *on page 402*

Tussi-Organidin® **DM NR** *(Discontinued) see* guaifenesin and dextromethorphan *on page 402*

Tussi-Organidin® **DM-S NR [US]** *see* guaifenesin and dextromethorphan *on page 402*

Tussi-Organidin® **NR [US]** *see* guaifenesin and codeine *on page 402*

Tussi-Organidin® **S-NR [US]** *see* guaifenesin and codeine *on page 402*

Tussizone-12 RF™ **[US]** *see* carbetapentane and chlorpheniramine *on page 149*

Tuss-LA® *(Discontinued) see* guaifenesin and pseudoephedrine *on page 406*

Tusso-DF® **[US]** *see* hydrocodone and guaifenesin *on page 429*

T-Vites [US-OTC] *see* vitamins (multiple/oral) *on page 895*

TVP-1012 *see* rasagiline *on page 745*

Twelve Resin-K [US] *see* cyanocobalamin *on page 220*

Twilite® **[US-OTC]** *see* diphenhydramine *on page 265*

Twinject™ **[US/Can]** *see* epinephrine *on page 300*

Twin-K® *(Discontinued)*

Twinrix® **[US/Can]** *see* hepatitis A inactivated and hepatitis B (recombinant) vaccine *on page 416*

Two-Dyne® *(Discontinued)*

Ty21a vaccine *see* typhoid vaccine *on next page*

Tycolene [US-OTC] *see* acetaminophen *on page 5*

Tycolene Maximum Strength [US-OTC] *see* acetaminophen *on page 5*

Tygacil™ **[US]** *see* tigecycline *on page 842*

Tykerb® **[US]** *see* lapatinib *on page 494*

Tylenol® **[US-OTC/Can]** *see* acetaminophen *on page 5*

Tylenol® **8 Hour [US-OTC]** *see* acetaminophen *on page 5*

Tylenol® **Allergy Sinus [Can]** *see* acetaminophen, chlorpheniramine, and pseudoephedrine *on page 10*

Tylenol® **Allergy Sinus** *(Discontinued) see* acetaminophen, chlorpheniramine, and pseudoephedrine *on page 10*

Tylenol® **Arthritis Pain [US-OTC]** *see* acetaminophen *on page 5*

Tylenol® **Children's [US-OTC]** *see* acetaminophen *on page 5*

Tylenol® **Children's Plus Cold Nighttime** *(Discontinued) see* acetaminophen, chlorpheniramine, and pseudoephedrine *on page 10*

Tylenol® **Children's with Flavor Creator [US-OTC]** *see* acetaminophen *on page 5*

Tylenol® **Cold Day Non-Drowsy [US-OTC]** *see* acetaminophen, dextromethorphan, and pseudoephedrine *on page 12*

Tylenol® **Cold Daytime [Can]** *see* acetaminophen, dextromethorphan, and pseudoephedrine *on page 12*

Tylenol® **Cold Daytime, Children's [US-OTC]** *see* acetaminophen and pseudoephedrine *on page 8*

Tylenol® **Cold Head Congestion Daytime [US-OTC]** *see* acetaminophen, dextromethorphan, and phenylephrine *on page 11*

Tylenol® **Cold, Infants [US-OTC]** *see* acetaminophen and pseudoephedrine *on page 8*

Tylenol® **Cold Multi-Symptom Daytime [US-OTC]** *see* acetaminophen, dextromethorphan, and phenylephrine *on page 11*

Tylenol® **Decongestant [Can]** *see* acetaminophen and pseudoephedrine *on page 8*

Tylenol® **Elixir with Codeine [Can]** *see* acetaminophen and codeine *on page 6*

Tylenol® **Extra Strength [US-OTC]** *see* acetaminophen *on page 5*

Tylenol® **Flu Non-Drowsy Maximum Strength [US-OTC]** *see* acetaminophen, dextromethorphan, and pseudoephedrine *on page 12*

Tylenol® **Infants [US-OTC]** *see* acetaminophen *on page 5*

Tylenol® **Junior [US-OTC]** *see* acetaminophen *on page 5*

Tylenol® **No. 1 [Can]** *see* acetaminophen and codeine *on page 6*

Tylenol® **No. 1 Forte [Can]** *see* acetaminophen and codeine *on page 6*

Tylenol® **No. 2 with Codeine [Can]** *see* acetaminophen and codeine *on page 6*

Tylenol® **No. 3 with Codeine [Can]** *see* acetaminophen and codeine *on page 6*

Tylenol® **No. 4 with Codeine [Can]** *see* acetaminophen and codeine *on page 6*

Tylenol® **PM [US-OTC]** *see* acetaminophen and diphenhydramine *on page 7*

Tylenol® **Severe Allergy [US-OTC]** *see* acetaminophen and diphenhydramine *on page 7*

Tylenol® **Sinus [Can]** *see* acetaminophen and pseudoephedrine *on page 8*

Tylenol® **Sinus Daytime [US-OTC]** *see* acetaminophen and pseudoephedrine *on page 8*

Tylenol® **With Codeine [US]** *see* acetaminophen and codeine *on page 6*

Tylenol® **with Codeine (Elixir) *(Discontinued)*** *see* acetaminophen and codeine *on page 6*

Tylox® **[US]** *see* oxycodone and acetaminophen *on page 641*

Typherix™ [Can] *see* Salmonella typhi Vi capsular polysaccharide vaccine *(Canada only) on page 774*

Typhim Vi® **[US]** *see* typhoid vaccine *on this page*

typhoid vaccine (TYE foid vak SEEN)

Synonyms Ty21a vaccine; typhoid vaccine live oral Ty21a; Vi vaccine

U.S./Canadian Brand Names Typhim Vi® [US]; Vivotif® [US]

Therapeutic Category Vaccine, Inactivated Bacteria

Use Active immunization against typhoid fever caused by *Salmonella typhi*

Not for routine vaccination. In the United States and Canada, use should be limited to:
— Travelers to areas with a prolonged risk of exposure to *S. typhi*
— Persons with intimate exposure to a *S. typhi* carrier
— Laboratory technicians with exposure to *S. typhi*
— Travelers with achlorhydria or hypochlorhydria (Canadian recommendation)

Usual Dosage Immunization:

Oral: Children ≥6 years and Adults:

Primary immunization: One capsule on alternate days (day 1, 3, 5, and 7) for a total of 4 doses; all doses should be complete at least 1 week prior to potential exposure

Booster immunization: Repeat full course of primary immunization every 5 years

I.M.: Children ≥2 years and Adults: 0.5 mL given at least 2 weeks prior to expected exposure

Reimmunization: 0.5 mL; optimal schedule has not been established; a single dose every 2 years is currently recommended for repeated or continued exposure

Dosage Forms [CAN] = Canadian brand name

Capsule, enteric coated:

Vivotif®: Viable *S. typhi* Ty21a 2-6 x 10^9 colony-forming units and nonviable *S. typhi* Ty21a 5-50 x 10^9 bacterial cells [contains lactose and sucrose]

Injection, solution:

Typherix® [CAN]: Vi capsular polysaccharide 25 mcg/0.5 mL (0.5 mL) [derived from *S. typhi* Ty2 strain] [not available in U.S.]

Typhim Vi®: Purified Vi capsular polysaccharide 25 mcg/0.5 mL (0.5 mL, 10 mL) [derived from *S. typhi* Ty2 strain]

typhoid vaccine live oral Ty21a *see* typhoid vaccine *on this page*

Tyrodone® **Liquid *(Discontinued)*** *see* hydrocodone and pseudoephedrine *on page 430*

Tysabri® **[US]** *see* natalizumab *on page 593*

Tyzeka™ [US] *see* telbivudine *on page 822*

Tyzine® **[US]** *see* tetrahydrozoline *on page 832*

Tyzine® **Pediatric [US]** *see* tetrahydrozoline *on page 832*

506U78 *see* nelarabine *on page 595*

U-90152S *see* delavirdine *on page 235*

UAD Otic® ***(Discontinued)*** *see* neomycin, polymyxin B, and hydrocortisone *on page 597*

UCB-P071 *see* cetirizine *on page 169*

UK *see* urokinase *on page 879*

UK-88,525 *see* darifenacin *on page 232*

UK-427,857 *see* maraviroc *on page 531*

UK92480 *see* sildenafil *on page 785*

UK109496 *see* voriconazole *on page 897*

Ulcerease® [US-OTC] *see* phenol *on page 673*

Ulcidine [Can] *see* famotidine *on page 341*

ULR-LA® *(Discontinued)*

Ultane® [US] *see* sevoflurane *on page 784*

Ultiva® [US/Can] *see* remifentanil *on page 748*

Ultracaine® D-S [Can] *see* articaine and epinephrine *on page 75*

Ultracaine® D-S Forte [Can] *see* articaine and epinephrine *on page 75*

Ultracaps MT [US] *see* pancrelipase *on page 648*

Ultracet™ [US] *see* acetaminophen and tramadol *on page 9*

Ultra Freeda Iron Free [US-OTC] *see* vitamins (multiple/oral) *on page 895*

Ultra Freeda with Iron [US-OTC] *see* vitamins (multiple/oral) *on page 895*

Ultram® [US/Can] *see* tramadol *on page 856*

Ultram® ER [US] *see* tramadol *on page 856*

Ultra Mide® [US-OTC] *see* urea *on next page*

UltraMide 25™ [Can] *see* urea *on next page*

Ultramop™ [Can] *see* methoxsalen *on page 555*

Ultra NatalCare® [US] *see* vitamins (multiple/prenatal) *on page 896*

Ultraprin [US-OTC] *see* ibuprofen *on page 444*

Ultraquin™ [Can] *see* hydroquinone *on page 437*

Ultrase® [US/Can] *see* pancrelipase *on page 648*

Ultrase® MT [US/Can] *see* pancrelipase *on page 648*

Ultra Tears® [US-OTC] *see* artificial tears *on page 75*

Ultravate® [US/Can] *see* halobetasol *on page 412*

Ultravist® [US] *see* iopromide *on page 468*

Umecta® [US] *see* urea *on next page*

Unasyn® [US/Can] *see* ampicillin and sulbactam *on page 54*

undecylenic acid and derivatives (un de sil EN ik AS id & dah RIV ah tivs)

Synonyms zinc undecylenate
U.S./Canadian Brand Names Fungi-Nail® [US-OTC]
Therapeutic Category Antifungal Agent
Use Treatment of athlete's foot (tinea pedis); ringworm (except nails and scalp)
Usual Dosage Topical: Children ≥2 years and Adults: Apply twice daily to affected area for 4 weeks; apply to clean, dry area
Dosage Forms
  Solution, topical:
    Fungi-Nail® [OTC]: Undecylenic acid 25% (29.57 mL)

Unguentine® *(Discontinued)* *see* benzocaine *on page 101*

Uni-Bent® Cough Syrup *(Discontinued)* *see* diphenhydramine *on page 265*

Unicap M® [US-OTC] *see* vitamins (multiple/oral) *on page 895*

Unicap Sr® [US-OTC] *see* vitamins (multiple/oral) *on page 895*

Unicap T™ [US-OTC] *see* vitamins (multiple/oral) *on page 895*

Uni-Cof *(Discontinued)* *see* pseudoephedrine, dihydrocodeine, and chlorpheniramine *on page 730*

Unidet® [Can] *see* tolterodine *on page 850*

Uni-Dur® *(Discontinued)* *see* theophylline *on page 834*

Unipen® [Can] *see* nafcillin *on page 587*

Uniphyl® [US] *see* theophylline *on page 834*

Uniphyl® SRT [Can] *see* theophylline *on page 834*

Uni-Pro® *(Discontinued)* *see* ibuprofen *on page 444*

Uniretic® **[US/Can]** *see* moexipril and hydrochlorothiazide *on page 576*

Uni-Senna [US-OTC] *see* senna *on page 781*

Unisom®**-2 [Can]** *see* doxylamine *on page 283*

Unisom® **Maximum Strength SleepGels**® **[US-OTC]** *see* diphenhydramine *on page 265*

Unisom® **SleepTabs**® **[US-OTC]** *see* doxylamine *on page 283*

Unithroid® **[US]** *see* levothyroxine *on page 503*

Unitrol® *(Discontinued)*

Uni-tussin® *(Discontinued)* *see* guaifenesin *on page 401*

Uni-tussin® **DM** *(Discontinued)* *see* guaifenesin and dextromethorphan *on page 402*

Univasc® **[US]** *see* moexipril *on page 575*

unna's boot *see* zinc gelatin *on page 905*

unna's paste *see* zinc gelatin *on page 905*

Urabeth® *(Discontinued)* *see* bethanechol *on page 110*

Urasal® **[Can]** *see* methenamine *on page 551*

urea (yoor EE a)

Synonyms carbamide

U.S./Canadian Brand Names Amino-Cerv™ [US]; Aquacare® [US-OTC]; Aquaphilic® With Carbamide [US-OTC]; Carmol® 10 [US-OTC]; Carmol® 20 [US-OTC]; Carmol® 40 [US]; Carmol® Deep Cleaning [US]; Cerovel™ [US]; DPM™ [US-OTC]; Gormel® [US-OTC]; Keralac™ Nailstik [US]; Keralac™ [US]; Lanaphilic® [US-OTC]; Nutraplus® [US-OTC]; Rea-Lo® [US-OTC]; Ultra Mide® [US-OTC]; UltraMide 25™ [Can]; Umecta® [US]; Ureacin® [US-OTC]; Uremol® [Can]; Urisec® [Can]; Vanamide™ [US]

Therapeutic Category Diuretic, Osmotic; Topical Skin Product

Use Keratolytic agent to soften nails or skin; OTC: Moisturizer for dry, rough skin

Usual Dosage Adults:

Hyperkeratotic conditions, dry skin: Topical: Apply 1-3 times/day

Cervicitis: Vaginal: Insert 1 applicatorful in vagina at bedtime for 2-4 weeks

Dosage Forms

Cloth, topical:

Kerol™ Redi-Cloths: 42% (30s)

Cream, topical: 40% (30 g, 85 g, 199 g)

Aquacare® [OTC]: 10% (75 g)

Carmol® 20 [OTC]: 20% (90 g)

Carmol® 40: 40% (30 g, 90 g, 210 g)

Cerovel™: 40% (133 g)

DPM™ [OTC]: 20% (118 g)

Gormel® [OTC]: 20% (75 g, 120 g, 454 g, 2270 g)

Keralac™: 50% (142 g, 255 g)

Nutraplus® [OTC]: 10% (90 g, 454 g)

Rea-Lo® [OTC]: 30% (60 g, 240 g)

Ureacin®-20 [OTC]: 20% (120 g)

Vanamide™: 40% (85 g, 199 g)

Emulsion, topical:

Umecta®: 40% (120 mL, 480 mL)

Gel: 40% (15 mL)

Carmol® 40: 40% (15 mL)

Cerovel™: 40% (25 mL)

Keralac™: 50% (18 mL)

Lotion, topical: 40% (240 mL)

Aquacare® [OTC]: 10% (240 mL)

Carmol® 10 [OTC]: 10% (180 mL)

Carmol® 40: 40% (240 mL)

Cerovel™: 40% (325 mL)

Keralac™: 35% (207 mL, 325 mL)

Nutraplus® [OTC]: 10% (240 mL, 480 mL)

Ultra Mide® [OTC]: 25% (120 mL, 240 mL)

Ureacin®-10 [OTC]: 10% (240 mL)

Ointment, topical:

Aquaphilic® with Carbamide [OTC]: 10% (180 g, 480 g); 20% (480 g)

Keralac™: 50% (90 g)

(Continued)

urea *(Continued)*

Lanaphilic® [OTC]: 10% (454 g); 20% (454 g)

Shampoo, topical:

Carmol® Deep Cleaning: 10% (240 mL)

Solution, topical:

Keralac™ Nailstick: 50% (2.4 mL)

Suspension, topical:

Kerol™: 50% (284 g)

Umecta®: 40% (18 mL, 300 mL)

urea and hydrocortisone (yoor EE a & hye droe KOR ti sone)

Synonyms hydrocortisone and urea

U.S./Canadian Brand Names Carmol-HC® [US]; Ti-U-Lac® H [Can]; Uremol® HC [Can]

Therapeutic Category Corticosteroid, Topical

Use Inflammation of corticosteroid-responsive dermatoses

Usual Dosage Apply thin film and rub in well 1-4 times/day. Therapy should be discontinued when control is achieved; if no improvement is seen, reassessment of diagnosis may be necessary.

Dosage Forms

Cream:

Carmol-HC®: Urea 10% and hydrocortisone 1% (30 g)

urea, chlorophyllin, and papain *see* chlorophyllin, papain, and urea *on page 175*

Ureacin® [US-OTC] *see* urea *on previous page*

urea peroxide *see* carbamide peroxide *on page 148*

Urecholine® [US] *see* bethanechol *on page 110*

Uremol® [Can] *see* urea *on previous page*

Uremol® HC [Can] *see* urea and hydrocortisone *on this page*

Urex® [US/Can] *see* methenamine *on page 551*

Urisec® [Can] *see* urea *on previous page*

Urispas® [US/Can] *see* flavoxate *on page 354*

Uristat® [US-OTC] *see* phenazopyridine *on page 671*

Urocit®-K [US] *see* potassium citrate *on page 701*

Urodine® *(Discontinued)* *see* phenazopyridine *on page 671*

urofollitropin (yoor oh fol li TROE pin)

Synonyms follicle-stimulating hormone, human; hFSH

U.S./Canadian Brand Names Bravelle® [US/Can]; Fertinorm® H.P. [Can]

Therapeutic Category Gonadotropin; Ovulation Stimulator

Use Ovulation induction in patients who previously received pituitary suppression; development of multiple follicles with Assisted Reproductive Technologies (ART)

Usual Dosage Note: Dose should be individualized. Use the lowest dose consistent with the expectation of good results. Over the course of treatment, doses may vary depending on individual patient response.

Adults: Female:

Ovulation induction: I.M., SubQ: Initial: 150 int. units daily for the first 5 days of treatment. Dose adjustments ≤75-150 int. units can be made every ≥2 days; maximum daily dose: 450 int. units; treatment >12 days is not recommended. If response to follitropin is appropriate, hCG is given 1 day following the last dose. Withhold hCG if serum estradiol is >2000 pg/mL, if the ovaries are abnormally enlarged, or if abdominal pain occurs.

ART: SubQ: 225 int. units daily for the first 5 days; dose may be adjusted based on patient response, but adjustments should not be made more frequently than once every 2 days; maximum adjustment: 75-150 int. units; maximum daily dose: 450 int. units; maximum duration of treatment: 12 days. When a sufficient number of follicles of adequate size are present, the final maturation of the follicles is induced by administering hCG. Withhold hCG in cases where the ovaries are abnormally enlarged on the last day of therapy.

Dosage Forms

Injection, powder for reconstitution [human origin]:

Bravelle®: 75 int. units

urokinase (ur oh KYE nase)

Synonyms UK

U.S./Canadian Brand Names Abbokinase® [US]

Therapeutic Category Thrombolytic Agent

Use Thrombolytic agent for the lysis of acute massive pulmonary emboli or pulmonary emboli with unstable hemodynamics

Usual Dosage I.V.: Adults: Acute pulmonary embolism: Loading: 4400 int. units/kg over 10 minutes; mainte-nance: 4400 int. units/kg/hour for 12 hours. Following infusion, anticoagulation treatment is recommended to prevent recurrent thrombosis. Do not start anticoagulation until aPTT has decreased to less than twice the normal control value. If heparin is used, do not administer loading dose. Treatment should be followed with oral anticoagulants.

Dosage Forms

Injection, powder for reconstitution:

Abbokinase®: 250,000 int. units

Uro-KP-Neutral® **[US]** *see* potassium phosphate and sodium phosphate *on page 703*

Urolene Blue® **[US]** *see* methylene blue *on page 558*

Uro-Mag® **[US-OTC]** *see* magnesium oxide *on page 528*

Uromax® **[Can]** *see* oxybutynin *on page 639*

Uromitexan [Can] *see* mesna *on page 546*

Uroplus® **DS** *(Discontinued)*

Uroplus® **SS** *(Discontinued)*

Uroxatral® **[US]** *see* alfuzosin *on page 28*

Urso® **[Can]** *see* ursodiol *on this page*

Urso 250™ **[US]** *see* ursodiol *on this page*

ursodeoxycholic acid *see* ursodiol *on this page*

ursodiol (ur soe DYE ol)

Synonyms ursodeoxycholic acid

U.S./Canadian Brand Names Actigall® [US]; Urso 250™ [US]; Urso Forte™ [US]; Urso® DS [Can]; Urso® [Can]

Therapeutic Category Gallstone Dissolution Agent

Use Actigall®: Gallbladder stone dissolution; prevention of gallstones in obese patients experiencing rapid weight loss; Urso®: Primary biliary cirrhosis

Usual Dosage Oral: Adults:

Gallstone dissolution: 8-10 mg/kg/day in 2-3 divided doses; use beyond 24 months is not established; obtain ultrasound images at 6-month intervals for the first year of therapy; 30% of patients have stone recurrence after dissolution

Gallstone prevention: 300 mg twice daily

Primary biliary cirrhosis: 13-15 mg/kg/day in 2-4 divided doses (with food)

Dosage Forms

Capsule: 300 mg

Actigall®: 300 mg

Tablet:

Urso 250™: 250 mg

Urso Forte™: 500 mg

Urso® **DS [Can]** *see* ursodiol *on this page*

Urso Forte™ **[US]** *see* ursodiol *on this page*

UTI Relief® **[US-OTC]** *see* phenazopyridine *on page 671*

Utradol™ **[Can]** *see* etodolac *on page 335*

Uvadex® **[US/Can]** *see* methoxsalen *on page 555*

vaccinia immune globulin (intravenous) (vax IN ee a i MYUN GLOB yoo lin IN tra VEE nus)

Synonyms VIGIV

U.S./Canadian Brand Names CNJ-016™ [US]

Therapeutic Category Immune Globulin

Use Treatment of infectious complications of smallpox (vaccinia virus) vaccination, such as eczema vacci-natum, progressive vaccinia, and severe generalized vaccinia; treatment of vaccinia infections in individuals
(Continued)

vaccinia immune globulin (intravenous) *(Continued)*

with concurrent skin conditions or accidental virus exposure to eyes (except vaccinia keratitis), mouth, or other areas where viral infection would pose significant risk

Usual Dosage I.V.: Adults:

CNJ-016™ (Cangene product): 6000 units/kg; 9000 units/kg may be considered if patient does not respond to initial dose.

DynPort product: Total dose: 2 mL/kg (100 mg/kg); higher doses (200-500 mg/kg) may be considered if patient does not respond to initial recommended dose (sucrose-related renal impairment is worsened at doses ≥400 mg/kg)

Dosage Forms Injection, solution [preservative free; solvent-detergent treated]:

CNJ-016™: Cangene product: ≥50,000 units/15 mL (15 mL)

DynPort product: 50 mg/mL (50 mL)

vaccinia vaccine *see* smallpox vaccine *on page 790*

Vagifem® [US/Can] *see* estradiol *on page 313*

Vagi-Gard® [US-OTC] *see* povidone-iodine *on page 704*

Vagistat®-1 [US-OTC] *see* tioconazole *on page 845*

Vagitrol® *(Discontinued)*

valacyclovir *(val ay SYE kloe veer)*

Sound-Alike/Look-Alike Issues

valacyclovir may be confused with valganciclovir

Valtrex® may be confused with Valcyte™

Synonyms valacyclovir hydrochloride

U.S./Canadian Brand Names Valtrex® [US/Can]

Therapeutic Category Antiviral Agent

Use Treatment of herpes zoster (shingles) in immunocompetent patients; treatment of first-episode genital herpes; episodic treatment of recurrent genital herpes; suppression of recurrent genital herpes and reduction of heterosexual transmission of genital herpes in immunocompetent patients; suppression of genital herpes in HIV-infected individuals; treatment of herpes labialis (cold sores)

Usual Dosage Oral:

Adolescents and Adults: Herpes labialis (cold sores): 2 g twice daily for 1 day (separate doses by ~12 hours)

Adults:

Herpes zoster (shingles): 1 g 3 times/day for 7 days

Genital herpes:

Initial episode: 1 g twice daily for 10 days

Recurrent episode: 500 mg twice daily for 3 days

Reduction of transmission: 500 mg once daily (source partner)

Suppressive therapy:

Immunocompetent patients: 1000 mg once daily (500 mg once daily in patients with <9 recurrences per year)

HIV-infected patients (CD4 ≥100 cells/mm^3): 500 mg twice daily

Dosage Forms

Caplet:

Valtrex®: 500 mg, 1000 mg

valacyclovir hydrochloride *see* valacyclovir *on this page*

Valcyte™ [US/Can] *see* valganciclovir *on this page*

23-valent pneumococcal polysaccharide vaccine *see* pneumococcal polysaccharide vaccine (poly-valent) *on page 692*

valganciclovir *(val gan SYE kloh veer)*

Sound-Alike/Look-Alike Issues

valganciclovir may be confused with valacyclovir

Valcyte™ may be confused with Valium®, Valtrex®

Synonyms valganciclovir hydrochloride

U.S./Canadian Brand Names Valcyte™ [US/Can]

Therapeutic Category Antiviral Agent

Use Treatment of cytomegalovirus (CMV) retinitis in patients with acquired immunodeficiency syndrome (AIDS); prevention of CMV disease in high-risk patients (donor CMV positive/recipient CMV negative) undergoing kidney, heart, or kidney/pancreas transplantation

Usual Dosage Oral: Adults:
CMV retinitis:
Induction: 900 mg twice daily for 21 days (with food)
Maintenance: Following induction treatment, or for patients with inactive CMV retinitis who require maintenance therapy: Recommended dose: 900 mg once daily (with food)
Prevention of CMV disease following transplantation: 900 mg once daily (with food) beginning within 10 days of transplantation; continue therapy until 100 days posttransplantation

Dosage Forms
Tablet:
Valcyte™: 450 mg

valganciclovir hydrochloride *see* valganciclovir *on previous page*

Valisone® Scalp Lotion [Can] *see* betamethasone (topical) *on page 109*

Valisone® Topical *(Discontinued)*

Valium® [US/Can] *see* diazepam *on page 251*

Valorin [US-OTC] *see* acetaminophen *on page 5*

Valorin Extra [US-OTC] *see* acetaminophen *on page 5*

valproate semisodium *see* valproic acid and derivatives *on this page*

valproate sodium *see* valproic acid and derivatives *on this page*

valproic acid *see* valproic acid and derivatives *on this page*

valproic acid and derivatives (val PROE ik AS id & dah RIV ah tives)

Sound-Alike/Look-Alike Issues
Depakene® may be confused with Depakote®
Depakote® may be confused with Depakene®, Depakote® ER, Senokot®

Synonyms dipropylacetic acid; divalproex sodium; DPA; 2-propylpentanoic acid; 2-propylvaleric acid; valproate semisodium; valproate sodium; valproic acid

U.S./Canadian Brand Names Alti-Divalproex [Can]; Apo-Divalproex® [Can]; Apo-Valproic® [Can]; Depacon® [US]; Depakene® [US/Can]; Depakote® ER [US]; Depakote® Sprinkle [US]; Depakote® [US]; Epival® I.V. [Can]; Gen-Divalproex [Can]; Novo-Divalproex [Can]; Nu-Divalproex [Can]; PMS-Valproic Acid E.C. [Can]; PMS-Valproic Acid [Can]; Rhoxal-valproic [Can]; Sandoz-Valporic [Can]

Therapeutic Category Anticonvulsant

Use
Depacon®, Depakene®, Depakote®, Depakote® ER, Depakote® Sprinkle: Monotherapy and adjunctive therapy in the treatment of patients with complex partial seizures; monotherapy and adjunctive therapy of simple and complex absence seizures; adjunctive therapy in patients with multiple seizure types that include absence seizures
Depakote®, Depakote® ER: Mania associated with bipolar disorder; migraine prophylaxis

Usual Dosage
Seizure disorders: **Note:** Administer doses >250 mg/day in divided doses.
Oral:
Simple and complex absence seizures: Children and Adults: Initial: 15 mg/kg/day; increase by 5-10 mg/kg/day at weekly intervals until therapeutic levels are achieved; maximum: 60 mg/kg/day. Larger maintenance doses may be required in younger children.
Complex partial seizures: Children ≥10 years and Adults: Initial: 10-15 mg/kg/day; increase by 5-10 mg/kg/day at weekly intervals until therapeutic levels are achieved; maximum: 60 mg/kg/day. Larger maintenance doses may be required in younger children.
Note: Regular release and delayed release formulations are usually given in 2-4 divided doses/day; extended release formulation (Depakote® ER) is usually given once daily. Conversion to Depakote® ER from a stable dose of Depakote® may require an increase in the total daily dose between 8% and 20% to maintain similar serum concentrations. Depakote® ER is not recommended for use in children <10 years of age.
I.V.: Administer as a 60-minute infusion (≤20 mg/minute) with the same frequency as oral products; switch patient to oral products as soon as possible. Rapid infusions ≤15 mg/kg over 5-10 minutes (1.5-3 mg/kg/minute) were generally well tolerated in a clinical trial.

Mania: Adults: Oral: Initial: 750 mg/day in divided doses; dose should be adjusted as rapidly as possible to desired clinical effect; maximum recommended dosage: 60 mg/kg/day
Depakote® ER: Initial: 25 mg/kg/day given once daily; dose should be adjusted as rapidly as possible to desired clinical effect; maximum recommended dose: 60 mg/kg/day.

Migraine prophylaxis: Children ≥16 years and Adults: Oral:
Depakote® ER: 500 mg once daily for 7 days, then increase to 1000 mg once daily; adjust dose based on patient response; usual dosage range 500-1000 mg/day
Depakote® tablet: 250 mg twice daily; adjust dose based on patient response, up to 1000 mg/day
(Continued)

valproic acid and derivatives *(Continued)*

Dosage Forms Strength expressed as valproic acid.
Capsule: 250 mg
Depakene®: 250 mg
Capsule, sprinkles:
Depakote® Sprinkle: 125 mg
Injection, solution: 100 mg/mL (5 mL)
Depacon®: 100 mg/mL (5 mL)
Syrup: 250 mg/5 mL
Depakene®: 250 mg/5 mL
Tablet, delayed release:
Depakote®: 125 mg, 250 mg, 500 mg
Tablet, extended release:
Depakote® ER: 250 mg, 500 mg

valsartan (val SAR tan)

Sound-Alike/Look-Alike Issues
valsartan may be confused with losartan, Valstar™
Diovan® may be confused with Darvon®, Dioval®, Zyban®
U.S./Canadian Brand Names Diovan® [US/Can]
Therapeutic Category Angiotensin II Receptor Antagonist
Use Alone or in combination with other antihypertensive agents in the treatment of essential hypertension; treatment of heart failure (NYHA Class II-IV); reduction of cardiovascular mortality in patients with left ventricular dysfunction postmyocardial infarction
Usual Dosage Oral: Adults:
Hypertension: Initial: 80 mg or 160 mg once daily (in patients who are not volume depleted); dose may be increased to achieve desired effect; maximum recommended dose: 320 mg/day
Heart failure: Initial: 40 mg twice daily; titrate dose to 80-160 mg twice daily, as tolerated; maximum daily dose: 320 mg
Left ventricular dysfunction after MI: Initial: 20 mg twice daily; titrate dose to target of 160 mg twice daily as tolerated; may initiate ≥12 hours following MI
Dosage Forms
Tablet:
Diovan®: 40 mg, 80 mg, 160 mg, 320 mg

valsartan and amlodipine *see* amlodipine and valsartan *on page 47*

valsartan and hydrochlorothiazide (val SAR tan & hye droe klor oh THYE a zide)

Sound-Alike/Look-Alike Issues
Diovan® may be confused with Darvon®, Dioval®, Zyban®
Synonyms hydrochlorothiazide and valsartan
U.S./Canadian Brand Names Diovan HCT® [US/Can]
Therapeutic Category Antihypertensive Agent, Combination
Use Treatment of hypertension (not indicated for initial therapy)
Usual Dosage Oral: Adults: Dose is individualized (combination substituted for individual components); dose may be titrated after 3-4 weeks of therapy.
Usual recommended starting dose of valsartan: 80 mg or 160 mg once daily (maximum: 320 mg/day) when used as monotherapy in patients who are not volume depleted
Usual recommended starting dose of hydrochlorothiazide: 12.5-25 mg once daily (maximum: 25 mg/day)
Dosage Forms
Tablet:
Diovan HCT®: 80 mg/12.5 mg: Valsartan 80 mg and hydrochlorothiazide 12.5 mg; 160 mg/12.5 mg: Valsartan 160 mg and hydrochlorothiazide 12.5 mg; 160 mg/25 mg: Valsartan 160 mg and hydrochlorothiazide 25 mg; 320 mg/12.5 mg: Valsartan 320 mg and hydrochlorothiazide 12.5 mg; 320 mg/25 mg: Valsartan 320 mg and hydrochlorothiazide 25 mg

Valstar® *(Discontinued)*

Valtrex® **[US/Can]** *see* valacyclovir *on page 880*

Vamate® **Oral** *(Discontinued)* *see* hydroxyzine *on page 440*

Vanamide™ **[US]** *see* urea *on page 877*

Vanatrip® *(Discontinued)* *see* amitriptyline *on page 44*

Vancenase® **AQ 84 mcg** *(Discontinued)* *see* beclomethasone *on page 97*

Vancenase® **Pockethaler®** *(Discontinued)* *see* beclomethasone *on page 97*

Vanceril® **AEM [Can]** *see* beclomethasone *on page 97*

Vanceril® *(Discontinued)* *see* beclomethasone *on page 97*

Vancocin® **[US/Can]** *see* vancomycin *on this page*

vancomycin (van koe MYE sin)

Sound-Alike/Look-Alike Issues

vancomycin may be confused with vecuronium

I.V. vancomycin may be confused with Invanz®

Synonyms vancomycin hydrochloride

U.S./Canadian Brand Names Vancocin® [US/Can]

Therapeutic Category Antibiotic, Miscellaneous

Use Treatment of patients with infections caused by staphylococcal species and streptococcal species; used orally for staphylococcal enterocolitis or for antibiotic-associated pseudomembranous colitis produced by *C. difficile*

Usual Dosage

Usual dosage range:

Infants >1 month and Children: I.V.: 10-15 mg/kg every 6 hours

Adults:

I.V.: 2-3 g/day (20-45 mg/kg/day) in divided doses every 6-12 hours; maximum 3 g/day; **Note:** Dose requires adjustment in renal impairment

Oral: 500-100 mg/day in divided doses every 6 hours

Indication-specific dosing:

Infants >1 month and Children:

Colitis (*C. difficile*): Oral: 40 mg/kg/day in divided doses added to fluids

Infective endocarditis prophylaxis: I.V.:

Dental, oral, or upper respiratory tract surgery: 20 mg/kg 1 hour prior to the procedure. **Note:** American Heart Association (AHA) guidelines now recommend prophylaxis only in patients undergoing invasive procedures and in whom underlying cardiac conditions may predispose to a higher risk of adverse outcomes should infection occur.

GI/GU procedure: 20 mg/kg plus gentamicin 2 mg/kg 1 hour prior to surgery. **Note:** As of April 2007, routine prophylaxis no longer recommended by the AHA.

Meningitis/CNS infection:

I.V.: 15 mg/kg every 6 hours

Intrathecal: 5-20 mg/day

Susceptible gram-positive infections: I.V.: 10 mg/kg every 6 hours

Adults:

Catheter-related infections: Antibiotic lock technique: 2 mg/mL in SWFI/NS or D_5W; instill 3-5 mL into catheter port as a flush solution instead of heparin lock (**Note:** Do not mix with any other solutions.)

Hospital-acquired pneumonia (HAP): I.V.: 15 mg/kg/dose every 12 hours (American Thoracic Society [ATS] 2005 guidelines)

Infective endocarditis prophylaxis: I.V.:

Dental, oral, or upper respiratory tract surgery: 1 g 1 hour before surgery. **Note:** AHA guidelines now recommend prophylaxis only in patients undergoing invasive procedures and in whom underlying cardiac conditions may predispose to a higher risk of adverse outcomes should infection occur

GI/GU procedure: 1 g plus 1.5 mg/kg gentamicin 1 hour prior to surgery. **Note:** As of April 2007, routine prophylaxis no longer recommended by the AHA.

Meningitis (*Pneumococcus* or *Staphylococcus*):

I.V.: 30-45 mg/kg/day in divided doses every 8-12 hours **or** 500-750 mg every 6 hours (with third-generation cephalosporin for PCN-resistant *Streptococcus pneumoniae*); maximum dose: 2-3 g/day

Intrathecal: Up to 20 mg/day

Susceptible gram-positive infections: I.V.: 15-20 mg/kg/dose (usual: 750-1500 mg) every 12 hours

Dosage Forms

Capsule:

Vancocin®: 125 mg, 250 mg

Infusion [premixed in iso-osmotic dextrose]:

Vancocin®: 500 mg (100 mL); 1 g (200 mL)

Injection, powder for reconstitution: 500 mg, 1 g, 5 g, 10 g

vancomycin hydrochloride *see* vancomycin *on this page*

Vandazole™ **[US]** *see* metronidazole *on page 563*

Vanex Forte™**-D** *(Discontinued)* *see* chlorpheniramine, phenylephrine, and methscopolamine *on page 181*

Vanex-HD® *(Discontinued)* *see* phenylephrine, hydrocodone, and chlorpheniramine *on page 678*

Vaniqa™ **[US/Can]** *see* eflornithine *on page 293*

Vanos™ **[US]** *see* fluocinonide *on page 360*

Vanoxide® *(Discontinued) see* benzoyl peroxide *on page 103*

Vanoxide-HC® **[US/Can]** *see* benzoyl peroxide and hydrocortisone *on page 105*

Vanquish® **Extra Strength Pain Reliever [US-OTC]** *see* acetaminophen, aspirin, and caffeine *on page 9*

Vansil™ *(Discontinued)*

Vantin® **[US/Can]** *see* cefpodoxime *on page 162*

Vaponefrin® *(Discontinued) see* epinephrine *on page 300*

Vaprisol® **[US]** *see* conivaptan *on page 214*

VAQTA® **[US/Can]** *see* hepatitis A vaccine *on page 417*

vardenafil (var DEN a fil)

Sound-Alike/Look-Alike Issues
Levitra® may be confused with Lexiva™

Synonyms vardenafil hydrochloride

U.S./Canadian Brand Names Levitra® [US/Can]

Therapeutic Category Phosphodiesterase (Type 5) Enzyme Inhibitor

Use Treatment of erectile dysfunction

Usual Dosage Oral: Adults: Erectile dysfunction: 10 mg 60 minutes prior to sexual activity; dosing range: 5-20 mg; to be given as one single dose and not given more than once daily
Dosing adjustment with concomitant medications:
Alpha-blocker (dose should be stable at time of vardenafil initiation): Initial vardenafil dose: 5 mg/24 hours; if an alpha-blocker is added to vardenafil therapy, it should be initiated at the smallest possible dose, and titrated carefully.
Atazanavir: Maximum vardenafil dose: 2.5 mg/24 hours
Clarithromycin: Maximum vardenafil dose: 2.5 mg/24 hours
Erythromycin: Maximum vardenafil dose: 5 mg/24 hours
Indinavir: Maximum vardenafil dose: 2.5 mg/24 hours
Itraconazole:
200 mg/day: Maximum vardenafil dose: 5 mg/24 hours
400 mg/day: Maximum vardenafil dose: 2.5 mg/24 hours
Ketoconazole:
200 mg/day: Maximum vardenafil dose: 5 mg/24 hours
400 mg/day: Maximum vardenafil dose: 2.5 mg/24 hours
Ritonavir: Maximum vardenafil dose: 2.5 mg/72 hours
Saquinavir: Maximum vardenafil dose: 2.5 mg/24 hours

Dosage Forms
Tablet:
Levitra®: 2.5 mg, 5 mg, 10 mg, 20 mg

vardenafil hydrochloride *see* vardenafil *on this page*

varenicline (var e NI kleen)

Synonyms varenicline tartrate

U.S./Canadian Brand Names Champix® [Can]; Chantix™ [US]

Therapeutic Category Partial Nicotine Agonist

Use Treatment to aid in smoking cessation

Usual Dosage Oral: Adults:
Initial:
Days 1-3: 0.5 mg once daily
Days 4-7: 0.5 mg twice daily
Maintenance (week 2-12): 1 mg twice daily
Note: Start 1 week before target quit date. Patients who cannot tolerate adverse events may require temporary reduction in dose. If patient successfully quits smoking during the 12 weeks, may continue for another 12 weeks to help maintain success. If not successful in first 12 weeks, then stop medication and reassess factors contributing to failure.

Dosage Forms
Tablet, as tartrate:
Chantix™: 0.5 mg, 1 mg

varenicline tartrate *see* varenicline *on this page*

Varibar® Honey [US] *see* barium *on page 94*

Varibar® Nectar [US] *see* barium *on page 94*

Varibar® Pudding [US] *see* barium *on page 94*

Varibar® Thin Honey [US] *see* barium *on page 94*

Varibar® Thin Liquid [US] *see* barium *on page 94*

varicella, measles, mumps, and rubella vaccine *see* measles, mumps, rubella, and varicella virus vaccine *on page 533*

varicella virus vaccine (var i SEL a VYE rus vak SEEN)

Sound-Alike/Look-Alike Issues

varicella virus vaccine has been given in error (instead of the indicated varicella immune globulin) to pregnant women exposed to varicella

Synonyms chicken pox vaccine; varicella-zoster virus (VZV) vaccine (varicella); VZV vaccine (varicella)

U.S./Canadian Brand Names Varilrix® [Can]; Varivax® III [Can]; Varivax® [US]

Therapeutic Category Vaccine, Live Virus

Use Immunization against varicella in children ≥12 months of age and adults

The ACIP recommends vaccination for all children, adolescents, and adults who do not have evidence of immunity. Vaccination is especially important for:

- Persons with close contact to those at high risk for severe disease
- Persons living or working in environments where transmission is likely (teachers, child-care workers, residents and staff of institutional settings)
- Persons in environments where transmission has been reported
- Nonpregnant women of childbearing age
- Adolescents and adults in households with children
- International travelers

Postexposure prophylaxis: Vaccination within 3 days (possibly 5 days) after exposure to rash is effective in preventing illness or modifying severity of disease

Usual Dosage SubQ:

Children 12 months to 12 years: 0.5 mL; a second dose may be administered ≥3 months later

Note: The ACIP recommends that the routine childhood vaccination be 2 doses, with the first dose administered at 12-15 months of age. School age children should receive the second dose at 4-6 years of age, but it may be administered earlier provided ≥3 months have elapsed after the first dose. All children and adolescents who received only 1 dose of vaccine should receive a second dose.

Children ≥13 years to Adults: 2 doses of 0.5 mL separated by 4-8 weeks

Dosage Forms [CAN] = Canadian brand name

Injection, powder for reconstitution [preservative free]:

Varivax®: 1350 plaque-forming units (PFU)

Varivax® III [CAN]: 1350 plaque-forming units (PFU) [not available in the U.S.]

Injection, powder for reconstitution:

Valrilix® [CAN]: $10^{3.3}$ plaque-forming units (PFU) [not available in the U.S.]

varicella-zoster immune globulin (human)

(var i SEL a- ZOS ter i MYUN GLOB yoo lin HYU man)

Sound-Alike/Look-Alike Issues

varicella virus vaccine has been given in error (instead of the indicated varicella immune globulin) to pregnant women exposed to varicella.

Synonyms VZIG

U.S./Canadian Brand Names VariZIG™ [Can]

Therapeutic Category Immune Globulin

Use In pregnant women, for the prevention or reduction in severity of maternal infection within 4 days of exposure to the varicella zoster virus.

Usual Dosage I.M., I.V.: Adults: Prevention or reduction of maternal infection: 125 int. units/10 kg (minimum dose: 125 int. units; maximum dose: 625 int. units). Administer within 96 hours of exposure.

Dosage Forms [CAN = Canadian brand name]

Injection, powder for reconstitution [preservative free]:

VariZIG™ [CAN]: 125 int. units [package with diluent] [available in the U.S under expanded access protocol]

varicella-zoster virus (VZV) vaccine (varicella) *see* varicella virus vaccine *on this page*

varicella-zoster (VZV) vaccine (zoster) *see* zoster vaccine *on page 909*

Varilrix® [Can] *see* varicella virus vaccine *on this page*

Varivax® [US] *see* varicella virus vaccine *on this page*

Varivax® III [Can] *see* varicella virus vaccine *on previous page*

VariZIG™ [Can] *see* varicella-zoster immune globulin (human) *on previous page*

Vaseretic® [US/Can] *see* enalapril and hydrochlorothiazide *on page 296*

VasoClear® *(Discontinued)* *see* naphazoline *on page 590*

Vasocon® [Can] *see* naphazoline *on page 590*

Vasocon®-A *(Discontinued)*

Vasocon Regular® Ophthalmic *(Discontinued)* *see* naphazoline *on page 590*

Vasodilan® *(Discontinued)* *see* isoxsuprine *on page 477*

Vasophrinic DH [Can] *see* pseudoephedrine, hydrocodone, and chlorpheniramine *on page 731*

vasopressin (vay soe PRES in)
Sound-Alike/Look-Alike Issues
Pitressin® may be confused with Pitocin®
Synonyms ADH; antidiuretic hormone; 8-arginine vasopressin
U.S./Canadian Brand Names Pitressin® [US]; Pressyn® AR [Can]; Pressyn® [Can]
Therapeutic Category Hormone, Posterior Pituitary
Use Treatment of diabetes insipidus; prevention and treatment of postoperative abdominal distention; differential diagnosis of diabetes insipidus
Usual Dosage
Diabetes insipidus (highly variable dosage; titrated based on serum and urine sodium and osmolality in addition to fluid balance and urine output):
I.M., SubQ:
Children: 2.5-10 units 2-4 times/day as needed
Adults: 5-10 units 2-4 times/day as needed (dosage range 5-60 units/day)
Continuous I.V. infusion: Children and Adults: 0.5 milliunit/kg/hour (0.0005 unit/kg/hour); double dosage as needed every 30 minutes to a maximum of 0.01 unit/kg/hour
Intranasal: Administer on cotton pledget, as nasal spray, or by dropper
Abdominal distention: Adults: I.M.: 5 units stat, 10 units every 3-4 hours
Dosage Forms
Injection, solution: 20 units/mL (0.5 mL, 1 mL, 10 mL)
Pitressin®: 20 units/mL (1 mL)

Vasotec® [US/Can] *see* enalapril *on page 295*

Vasovist® [Can] *see* gadofosveset *(Canada only)* *on page 381*

Vaxigrip® [Can] *see* influenza virus vaccine *on page 455*

VCF™ [US-OTC] *see* nonoxynol 9 *on page 610*

VCR *see* vincristine *on page 891*

Vectibix™ [US] *see* panitumumab *on page 650*

Vectrin® *(Discontinued)* *see* minocycline *on page 571*

vecuronium (vek ue ROE nee um)
Sound-Alike/Look-Alike Issues
vecuronium may be confused with vancomycin
Norcuron® may be confused with Narcan®
Synonyms ORG NC 45
U.S./Canadian Brand Names Norcuron® [Can]
Therapeutic Category Skeletal Muscle Relaxant
Use Adjunct to general anesthesia to facilitate endotracheal intubation and to relax skeletal muscles during surgery; to facilitate mechanical ventilation in ICU patients; does not relieve pain or produce sedation
Usual Dosage Administer I.V.; dose to effect; doses will vary due to interpatient variability; use ideal body weight for obese patients
Surgery:
Neonates: 0.1 mg/kg/dose; maintenance: 0.03-0.15 mg/kg every 1-2 hours as needed
Infants >7 weeks to 1 year: Initial: 0.08-0.1 mg/kg/dose; maintenance: 0.05-0.1 mg/kg every 60 minutes as needed
Children >1 year and Adults: Initial: 0.08-0.1 mg/kg or 0.04-0.06 mg/kg after initial dose of succinylcholine for intubation; maintenance: 0.01-0.015 mg/kg 25-40 minutes after initial dose, then 0.01-0.015 mg/kg every 12-15 minutes (higher doses will allow less frequent maintenance doses); may be administered as a continuous infusion at 0.8-2 mcg/kg/minute
Pretreatment/priming: Adults: 10% of intubating dose given 3-5 minutes before initial dose

ICU: Adults: 0.05-0.1 mg/kg bolus followed by 0.8-1.7 mcg/kg/minute once initial recovery from bolus observed or 0.1-0.2 mg/kg/dose every 1 hour

Note: Children (1-10 years) may require slightly higher initial doses and slightly more frequent supplementation; infants >7 weeks to 1 year may be more sensitive to vecuronium and have a longer recovery time

Dosage Forms
Injection, powder for reconstitution: 10 mg, 20 mg

Veg-Pancreatin 4X [US-OTC] *see* pancreatin *on page 648*

Velban® *(Discontinued)* *see* vinblastine *on page 890*

Velcade® [US/Can] *see* bortezomib *on page 116*

Velivet™ [US] *see* ethinyl estradiol and desogestrel *on page 322*

Velosulin® BR (Buffered) *(Discontinued)*

venlafaxine (ven la FAX een)

U.S./Canadian Brand Names Effexor® XR [US/Can]; Effexor® [US]; Novo-Venlafaxine XR [Can]
Therapeutic Category Antidepressant, Phenethylamine
Use Treatment of major depressive disorder, generalized anxiety disorder (GAD), social anxiety disorder (social phobia), panic disorder
Usual Dosage Oral: Adults:
Depression:
Immediate-release tablets: 75 mg/day, administered in 2 or 3 divided doses, taken with food; dose may be increased in 75 mg/day increments at intervals of at least 4 days, up to 225-375 mg/day
Extended-release capsules: 75 mg once daily taken with food; for some new patients, it may be desirable to start at 37.5 mg/day for 4-7 days before increasing to 75 mg once daily; dose may be increased by up to 75 mg/day increments every 4 days as tolerated, up to a maximum of 225 mg/day
GAD, social anxiety disorder: Extended-release capsules: 75 mg once daily taken with food; for some new patients, it may be desirable to start at 37.5 mg/day for 4-7 days before increasing to 75 mg once daily; dose may be increased by up to 75 mg/day increments every 4 days as tolerated, up to a maximum of 225 mg/day
Panic disorder: Extended-release capsules: 37.5 mg once daily for 1 week; may increase to 75 mg daily, with subsequent weekly increases of 75 mg/day up to a maximum of 225 mg/day.
Note: When discontinuing this medication after more than 1 week of treatment, it is generally recommended that the dose be tapered. If venlafaxine is used for 6 weeks or longer, the dose should be tapered over 2 weeks when discontinuing its use.
Dosage Forms
Capsule, extended release:
Effexor® XR: 37.5 mg, 75 mg, 150 mg
Tablet: 25 mg, 37.5 mg, 50 mg, 75 mg, 100 mg
Effexor®: 25 mg, 37.5 mg, 50 mg, 75 mg, 100 mg

Venofer® [US/Can] *see* iron sucrose *on page 473*

Venoglobulin®-I *(Discontinued)* *see* immune globulin (intravenous) *on page 451*

Venoglobulin®-S *(Discontinued)* *see* immune globulin (intravenous) *on page 451*

Ventavis™ [US] *see* iloprost *on page 447*

Ventolin® [Can] *see* albuterol *on page 23*

Ventolin® *(Discontinued)* *see* albuterol *on page 23*

Ventolin® Diskus [Can] *see* albuterol *on page 23*

Ventolin® HFA [US/Can] *see* albuterol *on page 23*

Ventolin® Inhaler Aerosol *(Discontinued)* *see* albuterol *on page 23*

Ventrodisk [Can] *see* albuterol *on page 23*

VePesid® [US/Can] *see* etoposide *on page 336*

Veracolate [US-OTC] *see* bisacodyl *on page 112*

verapamil (ver AP a mil)

Sound-Alike/Look-Alike Issues
verapamil may be confused with Verelan®
Calan® may be confused with Colace®
Covera-HS® may be confused with Provera®
Isoptin® may be confused with Isopto® Tears
Verelan® may be confused with verapamil, Virilon®, Voltaren®
(Continued)

verapamil *(Continued)*

Synonyms iproveratril hydrochloride; verapamil hydrochloride

U.S./Canadian Brand Names Alti-Verapamil [Can]; Apo-Verap® SR [Can]; Apo-Verap® [Can]; Calan® SR [US]; Calan® [US/Can]; Chronovera® [Can]; Covera-HS® [US/Can]; Covera® [Can]; Gen-Verapamil SR [Can]; Gen-Verapamil [Can]; Isoptin® SR [US/Can]; Novo-Veramil SR [Can]; Nu-Verap [Can]; Riva-Verapamil SR [Can]; Verapamil Hydrochloride Injection, USP [Can]; Verelan® PM [US]; Verelan® [US]

Therapeutic Category Antiarrhythmic Agent, Class IV; Calcium Channel Blocker

Use Orally for treatment of angina pectoris (vasospastic, chronic stable, unstable) and hypertension; I.V. for supraventricular tachyarrhythmias (PSVT, atrial fibrillation, atrial flutter)

Usual Dosage

Children: SVT:

I.V.:

<1 year: 0.1-0.2 mg/kg over 2 minutes; repeat every 30 minutes as needed

1-15 years: 0.1-0.3 mg/kg over 2 minutes; maximum: 5 mg/dose, may repeat dose in 15 minutes if adequate response not achieved; maximum for second dose: 10 mg/dose

Oral (dose not well established):

1-5 years: 4-8 mg/kg/day in 3 divided doses **or** 40-80 mg every 8 hours

>5 years: 80 mg every 6-8 hours

Adults:

SVT: I.V.: 2.5-5 mg (over 2 minutes); second dose of 5-10 mg (~0.15 mg/kg) may be given 15-30 minutes after the initial dose if patient tolerates, but does not respond to initial dose; maximum total dose: 20 mg

Angina: Oral: Initial dose: 80-120 mg 3 times/day (elderly or small stature: 40 mg 3 times/day); range: 240-480 mg/day in 3-4 divided doses

Hypertension: Oral:

Immediate release: 80 mg 3 times/day; usual dose range (JNC 7): 80-320 mg/day in 2 divided doses

Sustained release: 240 mg/day; usual dose range (JNC 7): 120-360 mg/day in 1-2 divided doses; 120 mg/day in the elderly or small patients (no evidence of additional benefit in doses >360 mg/day).

Extended release:

Covera-HS®: Usual dose range (JNC 7): 120-360 mg once daily (once-daily dosing is recommended at bedtime)

Verelan® PM: Usual dose range: 200-400 mg once daily at bedtime

Dosage Forms

Caplet, sustained release: 120 mg, 180 mg, 240 mg

Calan® SR: 120 mg, 180 mg, 240 mg

Capsule, extended release, controlled onset: 100 mg, 200 mg, 300 mg

Verelan® PM: 100 mg, 200 mg, 300 mg

Capsule, sustained release: 120 mg, 180 mg, 240 mg, 360 mg

Verelan®: 120 mg, 180 mg, 240 mg, 360 mg

Injection, solution: 2.5 mg/mL (2 mL, 4 mL)

Tablet: 80 mg, 120 mg

Calan®: 40 mg, 80 mg, 120 mg

Tablet, extended release: 120 mg, 180 mg, 240 mg

Tablet, extended release, controlled onset:

Covera-HS®: 180 mg, 240 mg

Tablet, sustained release: 120 mg, 180 mg, 240 mg

Isoptin® SR: 120 mg, 180 mg, 240 mg

verapamil and trandolapril *see* trandolapril and verapamil *on page 857*

verapamil hydrochloride *see* verapamil *on previous page*

Verapamil Hydrochloride Injection, USP [Can] *see* verapamil *on previous page*

Verazinc® Oral *(Discontinued)* *see* zinc sulfate *on page 906*

Verdeso™ [US] *see* desonide *on page 240*

Veregen™ [US] *see* sinecatechins *on page 788*

Verelan® [US] *see* verapamil *on previous page*

Verelan® PM [US] *see* verapamil *on previous page*

Vergogel® Gel *(Discontinued)* *see* salicylic acid *on page 772*

Vergon® *(Discontinued)* *see* meclizine *on page 535*

Vermox® [Can] *see* mebendazole *on page 534*

Vermox® *(Discontinued)* *see* mebendazole *on page 534*

Versed® *(Discontinued)* *see* midazolam *on page 568*

Versel® [Can] *see* selenium sulfide *on page 780*

Versiclear™ **[US]** *see* sodium thiosulfate *on page 798*

verteporfin (ver te POR fin)
U.S./Canadian Brand Names Visudyne® [US/Can]
Therapeutic Category Ophthalmic Agent
Use Treatment of predominantly classic subfoveal choroidal neovascularization due to macular degeneration, presumed ocular histoplasmosis, or pathologic myopia
Usual Dosage Therapy is a two-step process; first the infusion of verteporfin, then the activation of verteporfin with a nonthermal diode laser.
Adults: I.V.: 6 mg/m² body surface area
Note: Treatment in more than one eye: Patients who have lesions in both eyes should be evaluated and treatment should first be done to the more aggressive lesion. Following safe and acceptable treatment, the second eye can be treated one week later. Patients who have had previous verteporfin therapy, with an acceptable safety profile, may then have both eyes treated concurrently. Treat the more aggressive lesion followed immediately with the second eye. The light treatment to the second eye should begin no later than 20 minutes from the start of the infusion.
Dosage Forms
Injection, powder for reconstitution:
Visudyne®: 15 mg

Verukan® **Solution** *(Discontinued)* *see* salicylic acid *on page 772*

Vesanoid® **[US/Can]** *see* tretinoin (oral) *on page 860*

VESIcare® **[US]** *see* solifenacin *on page 799*

Vexol® **[US/Can]** *see* rimexolone *on page 759*

VFEND® **[US/Can]** *see* voriconazole *on page 897*

Viactiv® **flavor glides [US-OTC]** *see* vitamins (multiple/oral) *on page 895*

Viactiv® **Multivitamin [US-OTC]** *see* vitamins (multiple/oral) *on page 895*

Viadur® **[US/Can]** *see* leuprolide *on page 497*

Viagra® **[US/Can]** *see* sildenafil *on page 785*

Vibramycin® **[US]** *see* doxycycline *on page 281*

Vibramycin® **I.V.** *(Discontinued)* *see* doxycycline *on page 281*

Vibra-Tabs® **[US/Can]** *see* doxycycline *on page 281*

Vibrio cholera **and enterotoxigenic** *Escherichia coli vaccine* *see* traveler's diarrhea and cholera vaccine *(Canada only) on page 858*

Vicks® **44**® **Cough Relief [US-OTC]** *see* dextromethorphan *on page 247*

Vicks® **44D Cough & Head Congestion** *(Discontinued)* *see* pseudoephedrine and dextromethorphan *on page 728*

Vicks® **44E [US-OTC]** *see* guaifenesin and dextromethorphan *on page 402*

Vicks® **44**® **Non-Drowsy Cold & Cough Liqui-Caps** *(Discontinued)* *see* pseudoephedrine and dextromethorphan *on page 728*

Vicks® **Casero**™ **Chest Congestion Relief [US-OTC]** *see* guaifenesin *on page 401*

Vicks® **Children's Chloraseptic**® *(Discontinued)* *see* benzocaine *on page 101*

Vicks® **Children's NyQuil**® *(Discontinued)* *see* chlorpheniramine, pseudoephedrine, and dextromethorphan *on page 183*

Vicks® **Chloraseptic**® **Sore Throat** *(Discontinued)* *see* benzocaine *on page 101*

Vicks® **DayQuil**® **Cold/Flu Multi-Symptom Relief [US-OTC]** *see* acetaminophen, dextromethorphan, and phenylephrine *on page 11*

Vicks® **DayQuil**® **Multi-Symptom Cold and Flu** *(Discontinued)* *see* acetaminophen, dextromethorphan, and pseudoephedrine *on page 12*

Vicks® **DayQuil**® **Sinus Pressure & Congestion Relief** *(Discontinued)*

Vicks® **Formula 44**® *(Discontinued)* *see* dextromethorphan *on page 247*

Vicks® **Formula 44**® **Pediatric Formula** *(Discontinued)* *see* dextromethorphan *on page 247*

Vicks® **Formula 44**® **Sore Throat [US-OTC]** *see* phenol *on page 673*

Vicks® **Pediatric 44**®**m** *(Discontinued)* *see* chlorpheniramine, pseudoephedrine, and dextromethorphan *on page 183*

Vicks® Pediatric Formula 44E [US-OTC] *see* guaifenesin and dextromethorphan *on page 402*

Vicks® Sinex® 12 Hour [US-OTC] *see* oxymetazoline *on page 643*

Vicks® Sinex® 12 Hour Ultrafine Mist [US-OTC] *see* oxymetazoline *on page 643*

Vicks® Sinex® Nasal Spray [US-OTC] *see* phenylephrine *on page 675*

Vicks® Sinex® UltraFine Mist [US-OTC] *see* phenylephrine *on page 675*

Vicks® Vitamin C [US-OTC] *see* ascorbic acid *on page 76*

Vicodin® [US] *see* hydrocodone and acetaminophen *on page 427*

Vicodin® ES [US] *see* hydrocodone and acetaminophen *on page 427*

Vicodin® HP [US] *see* hydrocodone and acetaminophen *on page 427*

Vicoprofen® [US/Can] *see* hydrocodone and ibuprofen *on page 430*

Vi-Daylin® ADC *(Discontinued)* *see* vitamins (multiple/pediatric) *on page 896*

Vi-Daylin® ADC + Iron *(Discontinued)* *see* vitamins (multiple/pediatric) *on page 896*

Vi-Daylin® Drops *(Discontinued)* *see* vitamins (multiple/pediatric) *on page 896*

Vi-Daylin®/F ADC *(Discontinued)* *see* vitamins (multiple/pediatric) *on page 896*

Vi-Daylin®/F ADC + Iron *(Discontinued)* *see* vitamins (multiple/pediatric) *on page 896*

Vi-Daylin®/F *(Discontinued)* *see* vitamins (multiple/pediatric) *on page 896*

Vi-Daylin®/F + Iron *(Discontinued)* *see* vitamins (multiple/pediatric) *on page 896*

Vi-Daylin® + Iron Drops *(Discontinued)* *see* vitamins (multiple/pediatric) *on page 896*

Vi-Daylin® + Iron Liquid *(Discontinued)* *see* vitamins (multiple/oral) *on page 895*

Vi-Daylin® Liquid *(Discontinued)* *see* vitamins (multiple/oral) *on page 895*

Vidaza® [US] *see* azacitidine *on page 87*

Videx® [US/Can] *see* didanosine *on page 255*

Videx® EC [US/Can] *see* didanosine *on page 255*

vigabatrin *(Canada only)* (vye GA ba trin)

U.S./Canadian Brand Names Sabril® [Can]

Therapeutic Category Anticonvulsant

Use Active management of partial or secondary generalized seizures not controlled by usual treatments; treatment of infantile spasms

Usual Dosage Oral:

Children: **Note:** Administer daily dose in 2 divided doses, especially in the higher dosage ranges:

Adjunctive treatment of seizures: Initial: 40 mg/kg/day; maintenance dosages based on patient weight:

10-15 kg: 0.5-1 g/day

16-30 kg: 1-1.5 g/day

31-50 kg: 1.5-3 g/day

>50 kg: 2-3 g/day

Infantile spasms: 50-100 mg/kg/day, depending on severity of symptoms; higher doses (up to 150 mg/kg/day) have been used in some cases.

Adults: Adjunctive treatment of seizures: Initial: 1 g/day (severe manifestations may require 2 g/day); dose may be given as a single daily dose or divided into 2 equal doses. Increase daily dose by 0.5 g based on response and tolerability. Optimal dose range: 2-3 g/day (maximum dose: 3 g/day)

Dosage Forms [CAN] = Canadian brand name

Powder for oral suspension [sachets]:

Sabril® [CAN]: 0.5 g [not available in the U.S.]

Tablet:

Sabril® [CAN]: 500 mg [not available in the U.S.]

Vigamox™ [US/Can] *see* moxifloxacin *on page 581*

VIGIV *see* vaccinia immune globulin (intravenous) *on page 879*

vinblastine (vin BLAS teen)

Sound-Alike/Look-Alike Issues

vinBLAStine may be confused with vinCRIStine, vinorelbine

Synonyms NSC-49842; vinblastine sulfate; VLB

Tall-Man vinBLAStine

Therapeutic Category Antineoplastic Agent

Use Treatment of Hodgkin and non-Hodgkin lymphoma, testicular, lung, head and neck, breast, and renal carcinomas, Mycosis fungoides, Kaposi sarcoma, histiocytosis, choriocarcinoma, and idiopathic thrombocytopenic purpura

Usual Dosage I.V. (refer to individual protocols): Children and Adults: 4-20 mg/m^2 (0.1-0.5 mg/kg) every 7-10 days **or** 5-day continuous infusion of 1.5-2 mg/m^2/day **or** 0.1-0.5 mg/kg/week

Dosage Forms
  Injection, powder for reconstitution: 10 mg
  Injection, solution: 1 mg/mL (10 mL)

vinblastine sulfate *see* vinblastine *on previous page*

Vincasar PFS® [US/Can] *see* vincristine *on this page*

vincristine (vin KRIS teen)

Sound-Alike/Look-Alike Issues
  vinCRIStine may be confused with vinBLAStine
  Oncovin® may be confused with Ancobon®

Synonyms LCR; leurocristine sulfate; NSC-67574; VCR; vincristine sulfate

Tall-Man vinCRIStine

U.S./Canadian Brand Names Vincasar PFS® [US/Can]

Therapeutic Category Antineoplastic Agent

Use Treatment of leukemias, Hodgkin disease, non-Hodgkin lymphomas, Wilms tumor, neuroblastoma, rhabdomyosarcoma

Usual Dosage Note: Doses are often capped at 2 mg; however, this may reduce the efficacy of the therapy and may not be advisable. Refer to individual protocols; orders for single doses >2.5 mg or >5 mg/treatment cycle should be verified with the specific treatment regimen and/or an experienced oncologist prior to dispensing. I.V.:

  Children ≤10 kg or BSA <1 m^2: Initial therapy: 0.05 mg/kg once weekly then titrate dose
  Children >10 kg or BSA ≥1 m^2: 1-2 mg/m^2, may repeat once weekly for 3-6 weeks; maximum single dose: 2 mg
  Neuroblastoma: I.V. continuous infusion with doxorubicin: 1 mg/m^2/day for 72 hours
  Adults: 0.4-1.4 mg/m^2, may repeat every week **or**
  0.4-0.5 mg/day continuous infusion for 4 days every 4 weeks **or**
  0.25-0.5 mg/m^2/day for 5 days every 4 weeks

Dosage Forms
  Injection, solution: 1 mg/mL (1 mL, 2 mL)
  Vincasar PFS®: 1 mg/mL (1 mL, 2 mL)

vincristine sulfate *see* vincristine *on this page*

vinorelbine (vi NOR el been)

Sound-Alike/Look-Alike Issues
  vinorelbine may be confused with vinBLAStine

Synonyms dihydroxydeoxynorvinkaleukoblastine; NVB; vinorelbine tartrate

U.S./Canadian Brand Names Navelbine® [US/Can]; Vinorelbine Injection, USP [Can]; Vinorelbine Tartrate for Injection [Can]

Therapeutic Category Antineoplastic Agent

Use Treatment of nonsmall-cell lung cancer

Usual Dosage I.V. (refer to individual protocols): Adults:
  Single-agent therapy: 30 mg/m^2 every 7 days
  Combination therapy with cisplatin: 25 mg/m^2 every 7 days (with cisplatin 100 mg/m^2 every 4 weeks); **Alternatively:** 30 mg/m^2 in combination with cisplatin 120 mg/m^2 on days 1 and 29, then every 6 weeks

Dosage Forms
  Injection, solution [preservative free]: 10 mg/mL (1 mL, 5 mL)
  Navelbine®: 10 mg/mL (1 mL, 5 mL)

Vinorelbine Injection, USP [Can] *see* vinorelbine *on this page*

vinorelbine tartrate *see* vinorelbine *on this page*

Vinorelbine Tartrate for Injection [Can] *see* vinorelbine *on this page*

Viokase® [US/Can] *see* pancrelipase *on page 648*

viosterol *see* ergocalciferol *on page 305*

Vioxx® (Discontinued)

Viracept® **[US/Can]** *see* nelfinavir *on page 595*

Viramune® **[US/Can]** *see* nevirapine *on page 601*

Viravan® **[US]** *see* phenylephrine and pyrilamine *on page 677*

Viravan®**-DM [US]** *see* phenylephrine, pyrilamine, and dextromethorphan *on page 679*

Virazole® **[US/Can]** *see* ribavirin *on page 755*

Viread® **[US/Can]** *see* tenofovir *on page 825*

Virilon® **[US]** *see* methyltestosterone *on page 560*

Virilon® **IM [Can]** *see* testosterone *on page 828*

Viroptic® **[US/Can]** *see* trifluridine *on page 866*

Viscoat® **[US]** *see* sodium chondroitin sulfate and sodium hyaluronate *on page 794*

Visicol® **[US]** *see* sodium phosphates *on page 796*

Visine-A® **[US-OTC]** *see* naphazoline and pheniramine *on page 591*

Visine® **Advanced Allergy [Can]** *see* naphazoline and pheniramine *on page 591*

Visine® **Advanced Relief [US-OTC]** *see* tetrahydrozoline *on page 832*

Visine® **L.R. [US-OTC]** *see* oxymetazoline *on page 643*

Visine® **Original [US-OTC]** *see* tetrahydrozoline *on page 832*

Visipaque™ **[US]** *see* iodixanol *on page 466*

Visken® **[Can]** *see* pindolol *on page 683*

Visken® *(Discontinued)* *see* pindolol *on page 683*

Vistacon-50® **Injection** *(Discontinued)* *see* hydroxyzine *on page 440*

Vistaquel® **Injection** *(Discontinued)* *see* hydroxyzine *on page 440*

Vistaril® **[US/Can]** *see* hydroxyzine *on page 440*

Vistazine® **Injection** *(Discontinued)* *see* hydroxyzine *on page 440*

Vistide® **[US]** *see* cidofovir *on page 189*

Visudyne® **[US/Can]** *see* verteporfin *on page 889*

Vita-C® **[US-OTC]** *see* ascorbic acid *on page 76*

Vitaball® **[US-OTC]** *see* vitamins (multiple/pediatric) *on page 896*

Vitaball® **Minis [US-OTC]** *see* vitamins (multiple/pediatric) *on page 896*

Vitaball® **Wild 'N Fruity [US-OTC]** *see* vitamins (multiple/pediatric) *on page 896*

VitaCarn® **Oral** *(Discontinued)* *see* levocarnitine *on page 499*

Vitacon Forte [US] *see* vitamins (multiple/oral) *on page 895*

Vitafol [US] *see* vitamin B complex combinations *on page 894*

Vital HN® **[US-OTC]** *see* nutritional formula, enteral/oral *on page 622*

vitamin C *see* ascorbic acid *on page 76*

vitamin D$_2$ *see* ergocalciferol *on page 305*

vitamin D$_3$ and alendronate *see* alendronate and cholecalciferol *on page 27*

vitamin D and calcium carbonate *see* calcium and vitamin D *on page 137*

vitamin A (VYE ta min aye)

Sound-Alike/Look-Alike Issues
Aquasol® may be confused with Anusol®

Synonyms oleovitamin A

U.S./Canadian Brand Names Aquasol A® [US]; Palmitate-A® [US-OTC]

Therapeutic Category Vitamin, Fat Soluble

Use Treatment and prevention of vitamin A deficiency; parenteral (I.M.) route is indicated when oral administration is not feasible or when absorption is insufficient (malabsorption syndrome)

Usual Dosage
RDA:
<1 year: 375 mcg
1-3 years: 400 mcg
4-6 years: 500 mcg*
7-10 years: 700 mcg*
>10 years: 800-1000 mcg*

Male: 1000 mcg

Female: 800 mcg

* mcg retinol equivalent (0.3 mcg retinol = 1 unit vitamin A)

Vitamin A supplementation in measles (recommendation of the World Health Organization): Children: Oral: Administer as a single dose; repeat the next day and at 4 weeks for children with ophthalmologic evidence of vitamin A deficiency:

6 months to 1 year: 100,000 units

>1 year: 200,000 units

Note: Use of vitamin A in measles is recommended only for patients 6 months to 2 years of age hospitalized with measles and its complications **or** patients >6 months of age who have any of the following risk factors and who are not already receiving vitamin A: immunodeficiency, ophthalmologic evidence of vitamin A deficiency including night blindness, Bitot spots or evidence of xerophthalmia, impaired intestinal absorption, moderate to severe malnutrition including that associated with eating disorders, or recent immigration from areas where high mortality rates from measles have been observed

Note: Monitor patients closely; dosages >25,000 units/kg have been associated with toxicity

Severe deficiency with xerophthalmia: Oral:

Children 1-8 years: 5000-10,000 units/kg/day for 5 days or until recovery occurs

Children >8 years and Adults: 500,000 units/day for 3 days, then 50,000 units/day for 14 days, then 10,000-20,000 units/day for 2 months

Deficiency (without corneal changes): Oral:

Infants <1 year: 100,000 units every 4-6 months

Children 1-8 years: 200,000 units every 4-6 months

Children >8 years and Adults: 100,000 units/day for 3 days then 50,000 units/day for 14 days

Deficiency: I.M.: **Note:** I.M. route is indicated when oral administration is not feasible or when absorption is insufficient (malabsorption syndrome):

Infants: 7500-15,000 units/day for 10 days

Children 1-8 years: 17,500-35,000 units/day for 10 days

Children >8 years and Adults: 100,000 units/day for 3 days, followed by 50,000 units/day for 2 weeks

Note: Follow-up therapy with an oral therapeutic multivitamin (containing additional vitamin A) is recommended:

Low Birth Weight Infants: Additional vitamin A is recommended, however, no dosage amount has been established

Children ≤8 years: 5000-10,000 units/day

Children >8 years and Adults: 10,000-20,000 units/day

Malabsorption syndrome (prophylaxis): Children >8 years and Adults: Oral: 10,000-50,000 units/day of water miscible product

Dietary supplement: Oral:

Infants up to 6 months: 1500 units/day

Children:

6 months to 3 years: 1500-2000 units/day

4-6 years: 2500 units/day

7-10 years: 3300-3500 units/day

Children >10 years and Adults: 4000-5000 units/day

Dosage Forms

Capsule [softgel]: 10,000 units; 25,000 units

Injection, solution:

Aquasol A®: 50,000 units/mL (2 mL)

Tablet:

Palmitate-A® [OTC]: 5000 units, 15,000 units

vitamin A acid *see* tretinoin (topical) *on page 861*

vitamin A and vitamin D (VYE ta min aye & VYE ta min dee)

Synonyms cod liver oil

U.S./Canadian Brand Names A and D® Original [US-OTC]; Baza® Clear [US-OTC]; Sween Cream® [US-OTC]

Therapeutic Category Protectant, Topical

Use Temporary relief of discomfort due to chapped skin, diaper rash, minor burns, abrasions, as well as irritations associated with ostomy skin care

Usual Dosage Topical: Apply locally with gentle massage as needed

Dosage Forms

Capsule, softgel: Vitamin A 1250 int. units and vitamin D 135 int. units; vitamin A 1250 int. units and vitamin D 130 int. units; vitamin A 5,000 int. units and vitamin D 400 int. units; vitamin A 10,000 int. units and vitamin D 400 int. units; vitamin A 10,000 int. units and vitamin D 5000 int. units; vitamin A 25,000 int. units and vitamin D 1000 int. units

(Continued)

893

vitamin A and vitamin D *(Continued)*

Cream:
Sween Cream® [OTC]: 2 g, 57 g, 85 g, 142 g, 184 g, 339 g
Ointment: 0.9 g, 5 g, 60 g, 120 g, 454 g
A and D® Original [OTC]: 45 g, 120 g, 454 g
Baza® Clear [OTC]: 50 g, 150 g, 240 g
Tablet: Vitamin A 10,000 int. units and vitamin D 400 int. units

vitamin B₁ *see* thiamine *on page 836*

vitamin B₂ *see* riboflavin *on page 756*

vitamin B₃ *see* niacin *on page 601*

vitamin B₃ *see* niacinamide *on page 602*

vitamin B₅ *see* pantothenic acid *on page 651*

vitamin B₆ *see* pyridoxine *on page 735*

vitamin B₁₂ *see* cyanocobalamin *on page 220*

vitamin B complex combinations (VYE ta min bee KOM pleks kom bi NAY shuns)

Sound-Alike/Look-Alike Issues
Nephrocaps® may be confused with Nephro-Calci®
Surbex® may be confused with Sebex®, Suprax®, Surfak®
Synonyms B complex combinations; B vitamin combinations
U.S./Canadian Brand Names Allbee® C-800 + Iron [US-OTC]; Allbee® C-800 [US-OTC]; Allbee® with C [US-OTC]; Apatate® [US-OTC]; DexFol™ [US]; Gevrabon® [US-OTC]; Kobee [US-OTC]; Metanx™ [US]; Neph-Plex® Rx [US]; Nephro-Vite® Rx [US]; Nephro-Vite® [US-OTC]; Nephrocaps® [US]; Nephron FA® [US]; Nephronex® [US]; Quin B Strong with C and Zinc [US-OTC]; Quin B Strong [US-OTC]; Rena-Vite RX [US]; Rena-Vite [US-OTC]; Renal Caps [US]; Senilezol [US]; Stresstabs® High Potency Advanced [US-OTC]; Stresstabs® High Potency Energy [US-OTC]; Stresstabs® High Potency Weight [US-OTC]; Strovite [US]; Super Dec B 100 [US-OTC]; Super Quints 50 [US-OTC]; Superplex-T™ [US-OTC]; Surbex-T® [US-OTC]; Vitafol [US]; Z-Bec® [US-OTC]
Therapeutic Category Vitamin, Water Soluble
Use Supplement for use in the wasting syndrome in chronic renal failure, uremia, impaired metabolic functions of the kidney, dialysis; labeled for OTC use as a dietary supplement
Usual Dosage Oral: Adults:
Dietary supplement: One tablet daily
Apatate® liquid: One teaspoonful daily, 1 hour prior to mid-day meal
Gevrabon® liquid: Two tablespoonsful (30 mL) once daily; shake well before use
Renal patients: One tablet or capsule daily between meals; take after treatment if on dialysis
Nephron FA®: Two tablets once daily, between meals
Dosage Forms Content varies depending on product used. For more detailed information on ingredients in these and other multivitamins, please refer to package labeling.

vitamin E (VYE ta min ee)

Sound-Alike/Look-Alike Issues
Aquasol E® may be confused with Anusol®
Synonyms d-alpha tocopherol; dl-alpha tocopherol
U.S./Canadian Brand Names Alph-E [US-OTC]; Alph-E-Mixed [US-OTC]; Aquasol E® [US-OTC]; Aquavit-E® [US-OTC]; d-Alpha-Gems™ [US-OTC]; E-Gems Elite® [US-OTC]; E-Gems Plus® [US-OTC]; E-Gems® [US-OTC]; Ester-E™ [US-OTC]; Gamma E-Gems® [US-OTC]; Gamma-E Plus [US-OTC]; High Gamma Vitamin E Complete™ [US-OTC]; Key-E® Kaps [US-OTC]; Key-E® [US-OTC]
Therapeutic Category Vitamin, Fat Soluble; Vitamin, Topical
Use Dietary supplement
Usual Dosage Vitamin E may be expressed as alpha-tocopherol equivalents (ATE), which refer to the biologically active (R) stereoisomer content. Oral:
Recommended daily allowance (RDA):
Infants (adequate intake; RDA not establshed):
≤6 months: 4 mg
7-12 months: 6 mg
Children:
1-3 years: 6 mg; upper limit of intake should not exceed 200 mg/day
4-8 years: 7 mg; upper limit of intake should not exceed 300 mg/day
9-13 years: 11 mg; upper limit of intake should not exceed 600 mg/day
14-18 years: 15 mg; upper limit of intake should not exceed 800 mg/day

Adults: 15 mg; upper limit of intake should not exceed 1000 mg/day
Pregnant female:
≤18 years: 15 mg; upper level of intake should not exceed 800 mg/day
19-50 years: 15 mg; upper level of intake should not exceed 1000 mg/day
Lactating female:
≤18 years: 19 mg; upper level of intake should not exceed 800 mg/day
19-50 years: 19 mg; upper level of intake should not exceed 1000 mg/day

Vitamin E deficiency:
Children (with malabsorption syndrome): 1 unit/kg/day of water miscible vitamin E (to raise plasma tocopherol concentrations to the normal range within 2 months and to maintain normal plasma concentrations)
Adults: 60-75 units/day
Prevention of vitamin E deficiency: Adults: 30 units/day
Cystic fibrosis, beta-thalassemia, sickle cell anemia may require higher daily maintenance doses:
Children:
Cystic fibrosis: 100-400 units/day
Beta-thalassemia: 750 units/day
Adults: Sickle cell: 450 units/day
Dosage Forms
Capsule: 400 int. units, 1000 int. units
Key-E® Kaps [OTC]: 200 int. units, 400 int. units
Capsule, softgel: 200 int. units, 400 int. units, 600 int. units, 1000 int. units
Alph-E [OTC], Aqua Gem E® [OTC]: 200 int. units, 400 int. units
Alph-E-Mixed [OTC]: 200 int. units, 400 int. units, 1000 int. units
d-Alpha-Gems™ [OTC], E-Gems Elite® [OTC], Ester-E™ [OTC]: 400 int. units
E-Gems® [OTC]: 30 int. units, 100 int. units, 200 int. units, 400 int. units, 600 int. units, 800 int. units, 1000 int. units, 1200 int. units
E-Gems Plus® [OTC]: 200 int. units, 400 int. units, 800 int. units
Gamma E-Gems® [OTC]: 90 int. units
Gamma-E Plus [OTC], High Gamma Vitamin E Complete™ [OTC]: 200 int. units
Cream: 50 int. units/g (60 g), 100 int. units/g (60 g), 1000 int. units/120 g (120 g), 30,000 int. units/57 g (57g)
Key-E® [OTC]: 30 int. units/g (60 g, 120 g, 600 g)
Lip balm:
E-Gem® Lip Care: 1000 int. units/tube
Oil, oral/topical: 100 int. units/0.25 mL, 1150 units/0.25 mL, 28,000 int. units/30 mL
Alph-E [OTC]: 28,000 int. units/30 mL
E-Gems® [OTC]: 100 units/10 drops
Ointment, topical:
Key-E® [OTC]: 30 units/g (60 g, 120 g, 480 g)
Powder:
Key-E® [OTC]: 700 int. units per 1/4 teaspoon
Solution, oral drops: 15 int. units/0.3 mL
Aquasol E® [OTC], Aquavit-E [OTC]: 15 int. units/0.3 mL
Suppository, rectal/vaginal:
Key-E® [OTC]: 30 int. units (12s, 24s)
Tablet: 100 int. units, 200 int. units, 400 int. units, 500 int. units
Key-E® [OTC]: 200 int. units, 400 int. units

vitamin G *see* riboflavin *on page 756*

vitamin K₁ *see* phytonadione *on page 681*

vitamins (multiple/injectable) (VYE ta mins, MUL ti pul/in JEK ti bal)
U.S./Canadian Brand Names Infuvite® Adult [US]; Infuvite® Pediatric [US]; M.V.I. Adult™ [US]; M.V.I® Pediatric [US]
Therapeutic Category Vitamin
Use Nutritional supplement in patients receiving parenteral nutrition or requiring intravenous administration
Usual Dosage I.V.: Not for direct infusion
Children: ≥3 kg to 11 years: Pediatric formulation: 5 mL/day added to TPN or ≥100 mL of appropriate solution
Children >11 years and Adults: Adult formulation: 10 mL/day added to TPN or ≥500 mL of appropriate solution
Dosage Forms Content varies depending on product used. For more detailed information on ingredients in these and other multivitamins, please refer to package labeling.

vitamins (multiple/oral) (VYE ta mins, MUL ti pul/OR al)
Sound-Alike/Look-Alike Issues
Theragran® may be confused with Phenergan®
(Continued)

vitamins (multiple/oral) *(Continued)*

Synonyms multiple vitamins; therapeutic multivitamins; vitamins, multiple (oral); vitamins, multiple (therapeutic); vitamins, multiple with iron

U.S./Canadian Brand Names Androvite® [US-OTC]; Centamin [US-OTC]; Centrum® Performance™ [US-OTC]; Centrum® Silver® [US-OTC]; Centrum® [US-OTC]; Diatx®Zn [US]; Drinkables® MultiVitamins [US-OTC]; Freedavite [US-OTC]; Geri-Freeda [US-OTC]; Geriation [US-OTC]; Geritol Complete® [US-OTC]; Geritol Extend® [US-OTC]; Geritol® Tonic [US-OTC]; Glutofac®-MX [US]; Glutofac®-ZX [US]; Gynovite® Plus [US-OTC]; Hemocyte Plus® [US]; Hi-Kovite [US-OTC]; Iberet® [US-OTC]; Iberet®-500 [US-OTC]; Monocaps [US-OTC]; Myadec® [US-OTC]; Ocuvite® Adult 50+ [US-OTC]; Ocuvite® Adult [US-OTC]; Ocuvite® Extra® [US-OTC]; Ocuvite® Lutein [US-OTC]; Ocuvite® [US-OTC]; Olay® Vitamins Complete Women's 50+ [US-OTC]; Olay® Vitamins Complete Women's [US-OTC]; One-A-Day® 50 Plus Formula [US-OTC]; One-A-Day® Active Formula [US-OTC]; One-A-Day® All Day Energy [US-OTC]; One-A-Day® Cholesterol Plus™ [US-OTC]; One-A-Day® Essential Formula [US-OTC]; One-A-Day® Maximum Formula [US-OTC]; One-A-Day® Men's Health Formula [US-OTC]; One-A-Day® Weight Smart [US-OTC] ; One-A-Day® Women's Formula [US-OTC]; Optivite® P.M.T. [US-OTC]; PreserVision® AREDS [US-OTC]; PreserVision® Lutein [US-OTC]; Quintabs [US-OTC]; Quintabs-M [US-OTC]; Replace with Iron [US-OTC]; Replace [US-OTC]; Repliva 21/7™ [US]; SourceCF® Softgels [US]; Strovite® Advance [US]; Strovite® Forte [US]; T-Vites [US-OTC]; Ultra Freeda Iron Free [US-OTC]; Ultra Freeda with Iron [US-OTC]; Unicap M® [US-OTC]; Unicap Sr® [US-OTC]; Unicap T™ [US-OTC]; Viactiv® flavor glides [US-OTC]; Viactiv® Multivitamin [US-OTC]; Vitacon Forte [US]; Xtramins [US-OTC]

Therapeutic Category Vitamin

Use Prevention/treatment of vitamin and mineral deficiencies; labeled for OTC use as a dietary supplement

Usual Dosage Oral: Adults: Daily dose of adult preparations varies by product. Generally, 1 tablet or capsule or 5-15 mL of liquid per day. Consult package labeling. Prescription doses may be higher for burn or cystic fibrosis patients.

Dosage Forms Content varies depending on product used. For more detailed information on ingredients in these and other multivitamins, please refer to package labeling.

vitamins, multiple (oral) *see* vitamins (multiple/oral) *on previous page*

vitamins (multiple/pediatric) (VYE ta mins, MUL ti pul/pe de AT rik)

Synonyms children's vitamins; multivitamins/fluoride

U.S./Canadian Brand Names ADEKs [US-OTC]; AquADEKs™ [US-OTC]; Centrum Kids® Complete [US-OTC]; Centrum Kids® Dora the Explorer™ Complete [US-OTC]; Centrum Kids® Rugrats® Complete [US-OTC]; Centrum Kids® SpongeBob™ SquarePants Complete [US-OTC]; Flintstones® Complete [US-OTC]; Flintstones® Plus Iron [US-OTC]; Flintstones™ Gummies [US-OTC]; Flintstones™ Plus Immunity Support [US-OTC]; Flintstones™ Sour Gummies [US-OTC]; My First Flintstones® [US-OTC]; MyKidz Iron FL™ [US-OTC]; One-A-Day® Kids Bugs Bunny and Friends Complete [US-OTC]; One-A-Day® Kids Scooby-Doo! Complete [US-OTC]; One-A-Day® Kids Scooby-Doo! Plus Calcium [US-OTC]; One-A-Day® Scooby-Doo! Gummies [US-OTC]; Poly-Vi-Flor® With Iron [US]; Poly-Vi-Sol® with Iron [US-OTC]; Poly-Vi-Sol® [US-OTC]; SourceCF® [US-OTC]; Tri-Vi-Sol® with Iron [US-OTC]; Tri-Vi-Sol® [US-OTC]; Vitaball® Minis [US-OTC]; Vitaball® Wild 'N Fruity [US-OTC]; Vitaball® [US-OTC]

Therapeutic Category Vitamin

Use Prevention/treatment of vitamin deficiency; products containing fluoride are used to prevent dental caries; labeled for OTC use as a dietary supplement

Usual Dosage Daily dose varies by product; refer to package insert for specific product labeling

Dosage Forms Content varies depending on product used. For more detailed information on ingredients in these and other multivitamins, please refer to package labeling.

vitamins (multiple/prenatal) (VYE ta mins, MUL ti pul/pree NAY tal)

Sound-Alike/Look-Alike Issues

PreCare® may be confused with Precose®

Synonyms prenatal vitamins

U.S./Canadian Brand Names A-Free Prenatal [US]; Advanced NatalCare® [US]; Advanced-RF NatalCare® [US]; Aminate Fe-90 [US]; Cal-Nate™ [US]; CareNatal™ DHA [US]; Citracal® Prenatal +DHA [US]; Citracal® Prenatal 90+DHA [US]; Daily Prenatal [US]; Duet® [US]; Duet™ DHA [US]; Icar™ Prenatal [US]; KPN Prenatal [US]; Mini-Prenatal [US]; NataCaps™ [US]; NataChew™ [US]; NataFort® [US]; NatalCare® GlossTabs™ [US]; NatalCare® PIC Forte [US]; NatalCare® PIC [US]; NatalCare® Plus [US]; NatalCare® Rx [US]; NatalCare® Three [US]; NataTab™ CFe [US]; NataTab™ FA [US]; NataTab™ Rx [US]; NutriNate® [US]; NutriSpire™ [US]; PreCare Premier™ [US]; PreCare® Conceive™ [US]; PreCare® Prenatal [US]; PreCare® [US]; Prenatal AD [US]; Prenatal H [US]; Prenatal MR 90 Fe™ [US]; Prenatal MTR with Selenium [US]; Prenatal Plus [US]; Prenatal Rx 1 [US]; Prenatal U [US]; Prenatal Z [US]; Prenate DHA™ [US]; Prenate Elite™ [US]; PrimaCare® One [US]; PrimaCare® [US]; StrongStart™ [US]; Stuart Prenatal® [US-OTC]; Tandem® OB [US]; Trinate [US]; Ultra NatalCare® [US]

Therapeutic Category Vitamin

Use Nutritional supplement for use prior to conception, during pregnancy, and postnatal (in lactating and nonlactating women)

Usual Dosage Oral: Adults:

Capsule, tablet: One daily

Powder: 4 teaspoonfuls/day; given once daily or in divided doses; mix 1 teaspoonful in 1 ounce of water

Dosage Forms Content varies depending on product used. For more detailed information on ingredients in these and other multivitamins, please refer to package labeling.

vitamins, multiple (therapeutic) *see* vitamins (multiple/oral) *on page 895*

vitamins, multiple with iron *see* vitamins (multiple/oral) *on page 895*

Vitaneed™ **[US-OTC]** *see* nutritional formula, enteral/oral *on page 622*

Vitelle™ **Irospan**® *(Discontinued)* *see* ferrous sulfate and ascorbic acid *on page 350*

Vitrase® **[US]** *see* hyaluronidase *on page 424*

Vitrasert® **[US/Can]** *see* ganciclovir *on page 383*

Vitrax® **[US]** *see* hyaluronate and derivatives *on page 423*

Vitussin [US] *see* hydrocodone and guaifenesin *on page 429*

Vi vaccine *see* typhoid vaccine *on page 875*

Vivactil® **[US]** *see* protriptyline *on page 727*

Viva-Drops® **[US-OTC]** *see* artificial tears *on page 75*

Vivaglobin® **[US]** *see* immune globulin (subcutaneous) *on page 452*

Vivarin® **[US-OTC]** *see* caffeine *on page 133*

Vivelle® **[US]** *see* estradiol *on page 313*

Vivelle-Dot® **[US]** *see* estradiol *on page 313*

Vivitrol™ **[US]** *see* naltrexone *on page 590*

Vivonex® **[US-OTC]** *see* nutritional formula, enteral/oral *on page 622*

Vivonex® **T.E.N. [US-OTC]** *see* nutritional formula, enteral/oral *on page 622*

Vivotif® **[US]** *see* typhoid vaccine *on page 875*

VLB *see* vinblastine *on page 890*

VM-26 *see* teniposide *on page 825*

Volmax® *(Discontinued)* *see* albuterol *on page 23*

Voltaren® **[US/Can]** *see* diclofenac *on page 253*

Voltaren Ophtha® **[Can]** *see* diclofenac *on page 253*

Voltaren Ophthalmic® **[US]** *see* diclofenac *on page 253*

Voltaren Rapide® **[Can]** *see* diclofenac *on page 253*

Voltaren®-**XR [US]** *see* diclofenac *on page 253*

VoLumen™ **[US]** *see* barium *on page 94*

Voluven® **[Can]** *see* hetastarch *on page 420*

voriconazole (vor i KOE na zole)

Synonyms UK109496

U.S./Canadian Brand Names VFEND® [US/Can]

Therapeutic Category Antifungal Agent

Use Treatment of invasive aspergillosis; treatment of esophageal candidiasis; treatment of candidemia (in nonneutropenic patients); treatment of disseminated *Candida* infections of the skin and viscera; treatment of serious fungal infections caused by *Scedosporium apiospermum* and *Fusarium* spp (including *Fusarium solani*) in patients intolerant of, or refractory to, other therapy

Usual Dosage

Usual dosage ranges:

Children ≥12 years and Adults:

Oral: 100-300 mg every 12 hours

I.V.: 6 mg/kg every 12 hours for 2 doses; followed by maintenance dose of 4 mg/kg every 12 hours

Indication-specific dosing: Children ≥12 years and Adults:

Aspergillosis (invasive), scedosporiosis, fusariosis: I.V.: Initial: Loading dose: 6 mg/kg every 12 hours for 2 doses; followed by maintenance dose of 4 mg/kg every 12 hours

(Continued)

voriconazole (Continued)

Candidemia and other deep tissue *Candida* infections: I.V.: Initial: Loading dose 6 mg/kg every 12 hours for 2 doses; followed by maintenance dose of 3-4 mg/kg every 12 hours

Endophthalmitis, fungal: I.V.: 6 mg/kg every 12 hours for 2 doses, then 200 mg orally twice daily

Esophageal candidiasis: Oral:

Patients <40 kg: 100 mg every 12 hours; maximum: 300 mg/day

Patients ≥40 kg: 200 mg every 12 hours; maximum: 600 mg/day

Note: Treatment should continue for a minimum of 14 days, and for at least 7 days following resolution of symptoms.

Conversion to oral dosing:

Patients <40 kg: 100 mg every 12 hours; increase to 150 mg every 12 hours in patients who fail to respond adequately

Patients ≥40 kg: 200 mg every 12 hours; increase to 300 mg every 12 hours in patients who fail to respond adequately

Dosage adjustment in patients unable to tolerate treatment:

I.V.: Dose may be reduced to 3 mg/kg every 12 hours

Oral: Dose may be reduced in 50 mg increments to a minimum dosage of 200 mg every 12 hours in patients weighing ≥40 kg (100 mg every 12 hours in patients <40 kg)

Dosage adjustment in patients receiving concomitant CYP450 enzyme inducers or substrates:

Cyclosporine: Reduce cyclosporine dose by $\frac{1}{2}$ and monitor closely.

Efavirenz: Oral: Increase maintenance dose of voriconazole to 400 mg every 12 hours and reduce efavirenz dose to 300 mg once daily

Phenytoin:

I.V.: Increase maintenance dosage to 5 mg/kg every 12 hours

Oral: Increase dose to 400 mg every 12 hours in patients ≥40 kg (200 mg every 12 hours in patients <40 kg)

Dosage Forms

Injection, powder for reconstitution:

VFEND®: 200 mg

Powder for oral suspension:

VFEND®: 200 mg/5 mL

Tablet:

VFEND®: 50 mg, 200 mg

vorinostat (vor IN oh stat)

Synonyms NSC-701852; SAHA; suberoylanilide hydroxamic acid

U.S./Canadian Brand Names Zolinza™ [US]

Therapeutic Category Antineoplastic Agent, Histone Deacetylase Inhibitor

Use Treatment of relapsed or refractory cutaneous T-cell lymphoma (CTCL)

Usual Dosage Oral: Adults: Cutaneous T-cell lymphoma: 400 mg once daily

Dosage adjustment for intolerance: Reduce dose to 300 mg once daily; may further reduce to 300 mg daily for 5 consecutive days per week

In clinical trials, **dose reductions** were instituted for the following adverse events: Increased serum creatinine, decreased appetite, hypokalemia, leukopenia, nausea, neutropenia, thrombocytopenia, and vomiting. Vorinostat was **discontinued** for the following adverse events: Anemia, angioneurotic edema, weakness, chest pain, exfoliative dermatitis, DVT, ischemic stroke, lethargy, pulmonary embolism, and spinal cord injury.

Dosage Forms

Capsule:

Zolinza™: 100 mg

VoSol® *(Discontinued)* see acetic acid on page 14

VoSol® HC [US] see acetic acid, propylene glycol diacetate, and hydrocortisone on page 14

VoSpire ER® [US] see albuterol on page 23

VP-16 see etoposide on page 336

VP-16-213 see etoposide on page 336

V-Tann [US] see phenylephrine and pyrilamine on page 677

Vumon® [US/Can] see teniposide on page 825

Vusion™ [US] see miconazole and zinc oxide on page 567

V.V.S.® [US] see sulfabenzamide, sulfacetamide, and sulfathiazole on page 810

vWF:RCof see antihemophilic factor/von Willebrand factor complex (human) on page 60

Vytone® [US] see iodoquinol and hydrocortisone on page 467

Vytorin® **[US]** *see* ezetimibe and simvastatin *on page 339*

Vyvanse™ **[US]** *see* lisdexamfetamine *on page 511*

VZIG *see* varicella-zoster immune globulin (human) *on page 885*

VZV vaccine (varicella) *see* varicella virus vaccine *on page 885*

VZV vaccine (zoster) *see* zoster vaccine *on page 909*

warfarin (WAR far in)

Sound-Alike/Look-Alike Issues
Coumadin® may be confused with Avandia®, Cardura®, Compazine®, Kemadrin®
Synonyms warfarin sodium
U.S./Canadian Brand Names Apo-Warfarin® [Can]; Coumadin® [US/Can]; Gen-Warfarin [Can]; Jantoven™ [US]; Novo-Warfarin [Can]; Taro-Warfarin [Can]
Therapeutic Category Anticoagulant (Other)
Use Prophylaxis and treatment of thromboembolic disorders (eg, venous, pulmonary) and embolic complications arising from atrial fibrillation or cardiac valve replacement; adjunct to reduce risk of systemic embolism (eg, recurrent MI, stroke) after myocardial infarction
Usual Dosage Note: New labeling identifies genetic factors which may increase patient sensitivity to warfarin. Specifically, genetic variations in the proteins CYP2C9 and VKORC1, responsible for warfarin's primary metabolism and pharmacodynamic activity, respectively, have been identified as predisposing factors associated with decerased dose requirement and increased bleeding risk. A genotyping test is available, and may provide important guidance on initiation of anticoagulant therapy.
Oral:
  Adults: Initial dosing must be individualized. Consider the patient (hepatic function, cardiac function, age, nutritional status, concurrent therapy, risk of bleeding) in addition to prior dose response (if available) and the clinical situation. Start 2-5 mg daily for 2 days. Adjust dose according to INR results; usual maintenance dose ranges from 2-10 mg daily (individual patients may require loading and maintenance doses outside these general guidelines).
  Note: Lower starting doses may be required for patients with hepatic impairment, poor nutrition, CHF, elderly, high risk of bleeding, or patients who are debilitated, or those with reduced function genomic variants of the catabolic enzymes CYP2C9 (*2 or *3 alleles) or VKORC1 (-1639 polymorphism). Higher initial doses may be reasonable in selected patients (ie, receiving enzyme-inducing agents and with low risk of bleeding).
  I.V.: Adults: 2-5 mg/day administered as a slow bolus injection
Dosage Forms
Injection, powder for reconstitution:
  Coumadin®: 5 mg
Tablet: 1 mg, 2 mg, 2.5 mg, 3 mg, 4 mg, 5 mg, 6 mg, 7.5 mg, 10 mg
  Coumadin®, Jantoven™: 1 mg, 2 mg, 2.5 mg, 3 mg, 4 mg, 5 mg, 6 mg, 7.5 mg, 10 mg

warfarin sodium *see* warfarin *on this page*

Wartec® **[Can]** *see* podofilox *on page 693*

Wart-Off® **Maximum Strength [US-OTC]** *see* salicylic acid *on page 772*

4-Way® **12 Hour [US-OTC]** *see* oxymetazoline *on page 643*

4 Way® **Fast Acting [US-OTC]** *see* phenylephrine *on page 675*

4 Way® **Menthol [US-OTC]** *see* phenylephrine *on page 675*

4 Way® **No Drip [US-OTC]** *see* phenylephrine *on page 675*

4-Way® **Saline Moisturizing Mist [US-OTC]** *see* sodium chloride *on page 792*

WelChol® **[US/Can]** *see* colesevelam *on page 212*

Wellbutrin® **[US/Can]** *see* bupropion *on page 127*

Wellbutrin XL™ **[US/Can]** *see* bupropion *on page 127*

Wellbutrin SR® **[US]** *see* bupropion *on page 127*

Wellcovorin® *(Discontinued)* *see* leucovorin *on page 496*

Westcort® **[US/Can]** *see* hydrocortisone (topical) *on page 434*

Westhroid® **[US]** *see* thyroid *on page 839*

40 Winks® *(Discontinued)* *see* diphenhydramine *on page 265*

Winpred™ **[Can]** *see* prednisone *on page 710*

WinRho SD® *(Discontinued)*

WinRho® **SDF [US/Can]** *see* Rh₀(D) immune globulin *on page 753*

Winstrol® **[US]** *see* stanozolol *on page 805*

witch hazel (witch HAY zel)
Synonyms hamamelis water
U.S./Canadian Brand Names Dickinson's® Witch Hazel [US-OTC]; Preparation H® Cleansing Pads [Can]; Preparation H® Medicated Wipes [US-OTC]; T.N. Dickinson's® Hazelets [US-OTC]; Tucks® [US-OTC]
Therapeutic Category Astringent
Use After-stool wipe to remove most causes of local irritation; temporary management of vulvitis, pruritus ani and vulva; help relieve the discomfort of simple hemorrhoids, anorectal surgical wounds, and episiotomies
Usual Dosage Apply to anorectal area as needed
Dosage Forms
Liquid, topical: 100% (120 mL, 480 mL)
Dickinson's® Witch Hazel [OTC]: 100% (60 mL, 240 mL, 480 mL)
Pads: 50% (100s)
Dickinson's® Witch Hazel [OTC]: 50% (20s, 50s, 100s)
Preparation H® Medicated Wipes [OTC]: 50% (8s, 48s)
T.N. Dickinson's® Hazelets [OTC]: 50% (50s, 60s)
Tucks® [OTC]: 50% (12s, 40s, 100s)

Wolfina® *(Discontinued)*

Wound Wash Saline™ **[US-OTC]** *see* sodium chloride *on page 792*

WR-2721 *see* amifostine *on page 40*

WR-139007 *see* dacarbazine *on page 227*

WR-139013 *see* chlorambucil *on page 172*

WR-139021 *see* carmustine *on page 155*

Wycillin® **[Can]** *see* penicillin G procaine *on page 663*

Wycillin *(Discontinued)* *see* penicillin G procaine *on page 663*

Wydase® *(Discontinued)* *see* hyaluronidase *on page 424*

Wygesic® *(Discontinued)* *see* propoxyphene and acetaminophen *on page 723*

Wymox® *(Discontinued)* *see* amoxicillin *on page 48*

Wytensin® **[Can]** *see* guanabenz *on page 410*

Wytensin® *(Discontinued)* *see* guanabenz *on page 410*

Xalatan® **[US/Can]** *see* latanoprost *on page 494*

Xanax® **[US/Can]** *see* alprazolam *on page 32*

Xanax TS™ **[Can]** *see* alprazolam *on page 32*

Xanax XR® **[US]** *see* alprazolam *on page 32*

Xatral **[Can]** *see* alfuzosin *on page 28*

Xeloda® **[US/Can]** *see* capecitabine *on page 144*

Xenaderm™ **[US]** *see* trypsin, balsam peru, and castor oil *on page 872*

Xenical® **[US/Can]** *see* orlistat *on page 633*

Xerac AC™ **[US]** *see* aluminum chloride hexahydrate *on page 36*

Xibrom™ **[US]** *see* bromfenac *on page 119*

Xifaxan™ **[US]** *see* rifaximin *on page 758*

Xigris® **[US/Can]** *see* drotrecogin alfa *on page 285*

XiraTuss™ *(Discontinued)* *see* carbetapentane, phenylephrine, and chlorpheniramine *on page 150*

Xodol® 5/300 **[US]** *see* hydrocodone and acetaminophen *on page 427*

Xodol® 7.5/300 **[US]** *see* hydrocodone and acetaminophen *on page 427*

Xodol® 10/300 **[US]** *see* hydrocodone and acetaminophen *on page 427*

Xolair® **[US/Can]** *see* omalizumab *on page 628*

Xolegel™ **[US/Can]** *see* ketoconazole *on page 482*

Xopenex® **[US/Can]** *see* levalbuterol *on page 498*

Xopenex HFA™ **[US]** *see* levalbuterol *on page 498*

XPECT™ **[US-OTC]** *see* guaifenesin *on page 401*

Xpect-HC™ **[US]** *see* hydrocodone and guaifenesin *on page 429*

XPECT-PE™ **[US]** *see* guaifenesin and phenylephrine *on page 404*

X-Prep® *(Discontinued)* *see* senna *on page 781*

X-Seb T® Pearl [US-OTC] *see* coal tar and salicylic acid *on page 209*

X-Seb T® Plus [US-OTC] *see* coal tar and salicylic acid *on page 209*

Xtramins [US-OTC] *see* vitamins (multiple/oral) *on page 895*

Xylocaine® **[US/Can]** *see* lidocaine *on page 504*

Xylocaine® MPF [US] *see* lidocaine *on page 504*

Xylocaine® MPF With Epinephrine [US] *see* lidocaine and epinephrine *on page 506*

Xylocaine® Viscous [US] *see* lidocaine *on page 504*

Xylocaine® With Epinephrine [US/Can] *see* lidocaine and epinephrine *on page 506*

Xylocard® [Can] *see* lidocaine *on page 504*

Xyrem® [US/Can] *see* sodium oxybate *on page 795*

Xyzal® [US] *see* levocetirizine *on page 500*

Y-90 ibritumomab *see* ibritumomab *on page 443*

Y-90 zevalin *see* ibritumomab *on page 443*

Yasmin® [US/Can] *see* ethinyl estradiol and drospirenone *on page 323*

Yaz [US] *see* ethinyl estradiol and drospirenone *on page 323*

yellow fever vaccine (YEL oh FEE ver vak SEEN)
U.S./Canadian Brand Names YF-VAX® [US/Can]
Therapeutic Category Vaccine, Live Virus
Use Induction of active immunity against yellow fever virus, primarily among persons traveling or living in areas where yellow fever infection exists
Usual Dosage SubQ: Children ≥9 months and Adults: One dose (0.5 mL) ≥10 days before travel; Booster: Every 10 years
Dosage Forms
Injection, powder for reconstitution [17D-204 strain]:
YF-VAX®: ≥4.74 Log_{10} plaque-forming units (PFU) per 0.5 mL dose

YF-VAX® [US/Can] *see* yellow fever vaccine *on this page*

YM087 *see* conivaptan *on page 214*

YM-08310 *see* amifostine *on page 40*

Yocon® [US/Can] *see* yohimbine *on this page*

Yodoxin® [US] *see* iodoquinol *on page 467*

yohimbine (yo HIM bine)
Sound-Alike/Look-Alike Issues
Aprodyne® may be confused with Aprodine®
Yocon® may be confused with Zocor®
Synonyms yohimbine hydrochloride
U.S./Canadian Brand Names Aphrodyne® [US]; PMS-Yohimbine [Can]; Yocon® [US/Can]
Therapeutic Category Miscellaneous Product
Usual Dosage Oral: Adults:
Male erectile impotence: 5.4 mg tablet 3 times/day have been used. If side effects occur, reduce to $^1/_2$ tablet (2.7 mg) 3 times/day followed by gradual increases to 1 tablet 3 times/day. Results of therapy >10 weeks are not known.
Orthostatic hypotension: Doses of 12.5 mg/day have been utilized; however, more research is necessary
Dosage Forms
Tablet: 5.4 mg
Aphrodyne®, Yocon®: 5.4 mg

yohimbine hydrochloride *see* yohimbine *on this page*

Yohimex™ *(Discontinued)* *see* yohimbine *on this page*

Yutopar® Injection *(Discontinued)*

Z4942 *see* ifosfamide *on page 447*

Zaditen® [Can] *see* ketotifen *on page 484*

Zaditor® **[US-OTC/Can]** *see* ketotifen *on page 484*

zafirlukast (za FIR loo kast)

Sound-Alike/Look-Alike Issues
Accolate® may be confused with Accupril®, Accutane®, Aclovate®

Synonyms ICI-204,219

U.S./Canadian Brand Names Accolate® [US/Can]

Therapeutic Category Leukotriene Receptor Antagonist

Use Prophylaxis and chronic treatment of asthma in adults and children ≥5 years of age

Usual Dosage Oral:
Children <5 years: Safety and effectiveness have not been established
Children 5-11 years: 10 mg twice daily
Children ≥12 years and Adults: 20 mg twice daily

Dosage Forms
Tablet:
Accolate®: 10 mg, 20 mg

Zagam® *(Discontinued)*

zaleplon (ZAL e plon)

U.S./Canadian Brand Names Sonata® [US/Can]; Starnoc® [Can]

Therapeutic Category Hypnotic, Nonbenzodiazepine (Pyrazolopyrimidine)

Controlled Substance C-IV

Use Short-term (7-10 days) treatment of insomnia (has been demonstrated to be effective for up to 5 weeks in controlled trial)

Usual Dosage Oral: Adults: 10 mg at bedtime (range: 5-20 mg); has been used for up to 5 weeks of treatment in controlled trial setting

Dosage Forms
Capsule:
Sonata®: 5 mg, 10 mg

Zanaflex® **[US/Can]** *see* tizanidine *on page 846*

zanamivir (za NA mi veer)

U.S./Canadian Brand Names Relenza® [US/Can]

Therapeutic Category Antiviral Agent, Inhalation Therapy

Use Treatment of uncomplicated acute illness due to influenza virus A and B in patients who have been symptomatic for no more than 2 days; prophylaxis against influenza virus A and B

Usual Dosage Oral inhalation:
Children ≥5 years and Adults: Prophylaxis (household setting): Two inhalations (10 mg) once daily for 10 days. Begin within 1 ¹/₂ days following onset of signs or symptoms of index case.
Children ≥7 years and Adults: Treatment: Two inhalations (10 mg total) twice daily for 5 days. Doses on first day should be separated by at least 2 hours; on subsequent days, doses should be spaced by ~12 hours. Begin within 2 days of signs or symptoms.
Adolescents and Adults: Prophylaxis (community outbreak): Two inhalations (10 mg) once daily for 28 days. Begin within 5 days of outbreak.

Dosage Forms
Powder for oral inhalation:
Relenza®: 5 mg/blister (20s)

Zanosar® **[US/Can]** *see* streptozocin *on page 807*

Zantac® **[US/Can]** *see* ranitidine *on page 744*

Zantac 75® **[US-OTC/Can]** *see* ranitidine *on page 744*

Zantac 150™ **[US-OTC]** *see* ranitidine *on page 744*

Zantac® **EFFERdose**® **[US]** *see* ranitidine *on page 744*

Zantryl® *(Discontinued) see* phentermine *on page 674*

Zapzyt® **[US-OTC]** *see* benzoyl peroxide *on page 103*

Zapzyt® **Acne Wash [US-OTC]** *see* salicylic acid *on page 772*

Zapzyt® **Pore Treatment [US-OTC]** *see* salicylic acid *on page 772*

Zarontin® **[US/Can]** *see* ethosuximide *on page 333*

Zaroxolyn® **[US/Can]** *see* metolazone *on page 562*

Zartan® *(Discontinued)* see cephalexin *on page 167*

Zavesca® [US/Can] see miglustat *on page 570*

Zazole™ [US] see terconazole *on page 827*

Z-Bec® [US-OTC] see vitamin B complex combinations *on page 894*

Z-chlopenthixol see zuclopenthixol *(Canada only) on page 909*

Z-Cof™ DM [US] see guaifenesin, pseudoephedrine, and dextromethorphan *on page 408*

Z-Cof HC [US] see phenylephrine, hydrocodone, and chlorpheniramine *on page 678*

Z-Cof LA™ [US] see guaifenesin and dextromethorphan *on page 402*

ZD1033 see anastrozole *on page 56*

ZD1694 see raltitrexed *(Canada only) on page 743*

ZD1839 see gefitinib *on page 385*

ZDV see zidovudine *on next page*

ZDV, abacavir, and lamivudine see abacavir, lamivudine, and zidovudine *on page 2*

Zeasorb®-AF [US-OTC] see miconazole *on page 566*

Zebeta® [US/Can] see bisoprolol *on page 114*

Zebutal™ [US] see butalbital, acetaminophen, and caffeine *on page 130*

Zefazone® *(Discontinued)*

Zegerid® [US] see omeprazole and sodium bicarbonate *on page 629*

Zelapar™ [US] see selegiline *on page 780*

zeldox see ziprasidone *on page 907*

Zelnorm® [US] see tegaserod *on page 822*

Zemaira® [US] see alpha$_1$-proteinase inhibitor *on page 32*

Zemplar® [US/Can] see paricalcitol *on page 653*

Zemuron® [US/Can] see rocuronium *on page 764*

Zenapax® [US/Can] see daclizumab *on page 228*

Zenchent™ [US] see ethinyl estradiol and norethindrone *on page 328*

zeneca 182,780 see fulvestrant *on page 378*

Zephiran® [US-OTC] see benzalkonium chloride *on page 100*

Zephrex LA® *(Discontinued)* see guaifenesin and pseudoephedrine *on page 406*

Zerit® [US/Can] see stavudine *on page 805*

ZerLor™ [US] see acetaminophen, caffeine, and dihydrocodeine *on page 10*

Zestoretic® [US/Can] see lisinopril and hydrochlorothiazide *on page 512*

Zestril® [US/Can] see lisinopril *on page 512*

Zetacet® [US] see sulfur and sulfacetamide *on page 815*

Zetar® [US-OTC] see coal tar *on page 208*

Zetia™ [US] see ezetimibe *on page 339*

Zevalin® [US/Can] see ibritumomab *on page 443*

Ziac® [US/Can] see bisoprolol and hydrochlorothiazide *on page 114*

Ziagen® [US/Can] see abacavir *on page 2*

Ziana™ [US] see clindamycin and tretinoin *on page 200*

ziconotide (zi KOE no tide)

U.S./Canadian Brand Names Prialt® [US]

Therapeutic Category Analgesic, Nonnarcotic; Calcium Channel Blocker, N-Type

Use Management of severe chronic pain in patients requiring intrathecal (I.T.) therapy and who are intolerant or refractory to other therapies

Usual Dosage I.T.: Adults: Chronic pain: Initial dose: ≤2.4 mcg/day (0.1 mcg/hour)

Dose may be titrated by ≤2.4 mcg/day (0.1 mcg/hour) at intervals ≤2-3 times/week to a maximum dose of 19.2 mcg/day (0.8 mcg/hour) by day 21; average dose at day 21: 6.9 mcg/day (0.29 mcg/hour). A faster titration should be used only if the urgent need for analgesia outweighs the possible risk to patient safety.

(Continued)

ziconotide *(Continued)*

Dosage Forms
Injection, solution [preservative free]:
Prialt®: 25 mcg/mL (20 mL); 100 mcg/mL (1 mL, 2 mL, 5 mL)

zidovudine *(zye DOE vyoo deen)*

Sound-Alike/Look-Alike Issues
azidothymidine may be confused with azathioprine, aztreonam
Retrovir® may be confused with ritonavir
AZT is an error-prone abbreviation (mistaken as azathioprine, aztreonam)

Synonyms azidothymidine; compound S; ZDV

U.S./Canadian Brand Names Apo-Zidovudine® [Can]; AZT™ [Can]; Retrovir® [US/Can]

Therapeutic Category Antiviral Agent

Use Treatment of HIV infection in combination with at least two other antiretroviral agents; prevention of maternal/fetal HIV transmission as monotherapy

Usual Dosage
Prevention of maternal-fetal HIV transmission:
Neonatal: **Note:** Dosing should begin 8-12 hours after birth and continue for the first 6 weeks of life.
Oral:
Full-term infants: 2 mg/kg/dose every 6 hours
Infants ≥30 weeks and <35 weeks gestation at birth: 2 mg/kg/dose every 12 hours; at 2 weeks of age, advance to 2 mg/kg/dose every 8 hours
Infants <30 weeks gestation at birth: 2 mg/kg/dose every 12 hours; at 4 weeks of age, advance to 2 mg/kg/dose every 8 hours
I.V.: Infants unable to receive oral dosing:
Full term: 1.5 mg/kg/dose every 6 hours
Infants ≥30 weeks and <35 weeks gestation at birth: 1.5 mg/kg/dose every 12 hours; at 2 weeks of age, advance to 1.5 mg/kg/dose every 8 hours
Infants <30 weeks gestation at birth: 1.5 mg/kg/dose every 12 hours; at 4 weeks of age, advance to 1.5 mg/kg/dose every 8 hours
Maternal: Oral (per AIDS info guidelines): 100 mg 5 times/day **or** 200 mg 3 times/day **or** 300 mg twice daily. Begin at 14-34 weeks gestation and continue until start of labor.
During labor and delivery, administer zidovudine I.V. at 2 mg/kg as loading dose followed by a continuous I.V. infusion of 1 mg/kg/hour until the umbilical cord is clamped
Treatment of HIV infection:
Children 6 weeks to 12 years:
Oral: 160 mg/m^2/dose every 8 hours (maximum: 200 mg every 8 hours); some Working Group members use a dose of 180 mg/m^2 to 240 mg/m^2 every 12 hours when using in drug combinations with other antiretroviral compounds, but data on this dosing in children is limited
I.V. continuous infusion: 20 mg/m^2/hour
I.V. intermittent infusion: 120 mg/m^2/dose every 6 hours
Adults:
Oral: 300 mg twice daily or 200 mg 3 times/day
I.V.: 1 mg/kg/dose administered every 4 hours around-the-clock (5-6 doses/day)

Dosage Forms
Capsule:
Retrovir®: 100 mg
Injection, solution [preservative free]:
Retrovir®: 10 mg/mL (20 mL)
Syrup:
Retrovir®: 50 mg/5 mL
Tablet: 300 mg
Retrovir®: 300 mg

zidovudine, abacavir, and lamivudine *see* abacavir, lamivudine, and zidovudine *on page 2*

zidovudine and lamivudine *(zye DOE vyoo deen & la MI vyoo deen)*

Sound-Alike/Look-Alike Issues
Combivir® may be confused with Combivent®, Epivir®
AZT is an error-prone abbreviation (mistaken as azathioprine, aztreonam)

Synonyms lamivudine and zidovudine

U.S./Canadian Brand Names Combivir® [US/Can]

Therapeutic Category Antiviral Agent

Use Treatment of HIV infection when therapy is warranted based on clinical and/or immunological evidence of disease progression

Usual Dosage Oral: Children ≥12 years and Adults: One tablet twice daily
   Note: Because this is a fixed-dose combination product, avoid use in patients requiring dosage reduction including children <12 years of age, renally-impaired patients with a creatinine clearance ≤50 mL/minute, hepatic impairment, or those patients experiencing dose-limiting adverse effects.
   Dosage Forms
      Tablet:
         Combivir®: Zidovudine 300 mg and lamivudine 150 mg

Zilactin® [Can] *see* lidocaine *on page 504*

Zilactin-L® [US-OTC] *see* lidocaine *on page 504*

Zilactin®-B [US-OTC/Can] *see* benzocaine *on page 101*

Zilactin Baby® [Can] *see* benzocaine *on page 101*

Zilactin Toothache and Gum Pain® [US-OTC] *see* benzocaine *on page 101*

zileuton (zye LOO ton)
   U.S./Canadian Brand Names Zyflo CR™ [US]; Zyflo® [US]
   Therapeutic Category 5-Lipoxygenase Inhibitor
   Use Prophylaxis and chronic treatment of asthma in children ≥12 years of age and adults
   Usual Dosage Oral:
      Children <12 years: Safety and effectiveness have not been established
      Children ≥12 years and Adults:
      Zyflo®: 600 mg 4 times/day
      Zyflo CR™: 1200 mg twice daily.
   Dosage Forms
      Tablet:
         Zyflo®: 600 mg
      Tablet, extended release:
         Zyflo CR™: 600 mg

Zinacef® [US/Can] *see* cefuroxime *on page 165*

zinc *see* trace metals *on page 855*

Zincate® [US] *see* zinc sulfate *on next page*

zinc chloride (zink KLOR ide)
   Therapeutic Category Trace Element
   Use Cofactor for replacement therapy to different enzymes; helps maintain normal growth rates, normal skin hydration, and senses of taste and smell
   Usual Dosage Clinical response may not occur for up to 6-8 weeks
      Supplemental to I.V. solutions:
      Premature Infants <1500 g, up to 3 kg: 300 mcg/kg/day
      Infants (full term) and Children ≤5 years: 100 mcg/kg/day
      Adults:
         Stable with fluid loss from small bowel: 12.2 mg zinc/L TPN or 17.1 mg zinc/kg (added to 1000 mL I.V. fluids) of stool or ileostomy output
         Metabolically stable: 2.5-4 mg/day; add 2 mg/day for acute catabolic states
   Dosage Forms
      Injection, solution: 1 mg/mL (10 mL, 50 mL)

zinc diethylenetriaminepentaacetate (Zn-DTPA) *see* diethylene triamine penta-acetic acid *on page 256*

Zincfrin® [Can] *see* phenylephrine and zinc sulfate *(Canada only) on page 677*

zinc gelatin (zink JEL ah tin)
   Synonyms dome paste bandage; unna's boot; unna's paste; zinc gelatin boot
   U.S./Canadian Brand Names Gelucast® [US]
   Therapeutic Category Protectant, Topical
   Use As a protectant and to support varicosities and similar lesions of the lower limbs
   Usual Dosage Topical: Apply externally as an occlusive boot
   Dosage Forms
      Bandage: 3" x 10 yards; 4" x 10 yards
      Gelucast®: 3" x 10 yards; 4" x 10 yards

zinc gelatin boot *see* zinc gelatin *on this page*

Zincofax® [Can] *see* zinc oxide *on this page*

Zincon® [US-OTC] *see* pyrithione zinc *on page 737*

zinc oxide (zink OKS ide)

Synonyms base ointment; lassar's zinc paste

U.S./Canadian Brand Names Ammens® Medicated Deodorant [US-OTC]; Balmex® [US-OTC]; Boudreaux's® Butt Paste [US-OTC]; Critic-Aid Skin Care® [US-OTC]; Desitin® Creamy [US-OTC]; Desitin® [US-OTC]; Zincofax® [Can]

Therapeutic Category Topical Skin Product

Use Protective coating for mild skin irritations and abrasions; soothing and protective ointment to promote healing of chapped skin, diaper rash

Usual Dosage Topical: Infants, Children, and Adults: Apply as required for affected areas several times daily

Dosage Forms

Cream:
Balmex® [OTC]: 11.3% (60 g, 120 g, 480 g)
Ointment, topical: 20% (30 g, 60 g, 454 g); 40% (120 g)
Desitin® [OTC]: 40% (30 g, 60 g, 90 g, 120 g, 270 g, 480 g)
Desitin® Creamy [OTC]: 10% (60 g, 120 g)

Paste, topical:
Boudreaux's® Butt Paste [OTC]: 16% (30 g, 60 g, 120 g, 480 g)
Critic-Aid Skin Care® [OTC]: 20% (71 g, 170 g)

Powder, topical:
Ammens® Medicated Deodorant [OTC]: 9.1% (187.5 g, 330 g)

zinc oxide and miconazole nitrate *see* miconazole and zinc oxide *on page 567*

zinc sulfate (zink SUL fate)

Sound-Alike/Look-Alike Issues
ZnSO$_4$ is an error-prone abbreviation (mistaken as morphine sulfate)

U.S./Canadian Brand Names Anuzinc [Can]; Orazinc® [US-OTC]; Rivasol [Can]; Zincate® [US]

Therapeutic Category Electrolyte Supplement, Oral

Use Zinc supplement (oral and parenteral); may improve wound healing in those who are deficient

Usual Dosage

RDA: Oral:
Birth to 6 months: 3 mg elemental zinc/day
6-12 months: 5 mg elemental zinc/day
1-10 years: 10 mg elemental zinc/day
≥11 years: 15 mg elemental zinc/day

Zinc deficiency: Oral:
Infants and Children: 0.5-1 mg elemental zinc/kg/day divided 1-3 times/day; somewhat larger quantities may be needed if there is impaired intestinal absorption or an excessive loss of zinc
Adults: 110-220 mg zinc sulfate (25-50 mg elemental zinc)/dose 3 times/day
Parenteral TPN: I.V.:
Infants (premature, birth weight <1500 g up to 3 kg): 300 mcg/kg/day
Infants (full-term) and Children ≤5 years: 100 mcg/kg/day
Adults:
Acute metabolic states: 4.5-6 mg/day
Metabolically stable: 2.5-4 mg/day
Stable with fluid loss from the small bowel: 12.2 mg zinc/L of TPN solution, or an additional 17.1 mg zinc (added to 1000 mL I.V. fluids) per kg of stool or ileostomy output

Dosage Forms

Capsule: 220 mg
Orazinc® [OTC], Zincate®: 220 mg
Injection, solution [preservative free]: 1 mg elemental zinc/mL (10 mL); 5 mg elemental zinc/mL (5 mL)
Tablet: 110 mg
Orazinc® [OTC]: 110 mg

zinc sulfate and phenylephrine *see* phenylephrine and zinc sulfate *(Canada only)* *on page 677*

zinc undecylenate *see* undecylenic acid and derivatives *on page 876*

Zinecard® [US/Can] *see* dexrazoxane *on page 245*

Ziox™ [US] *see* chlorophyllin, papain, and urea *on page 175*

Ziox 405™ [US] *see* chlorophyllin, papain, and urea *on page 175*

ziprasidone (zi PRAS i done)

Synonyms zeldox; ziprasidone hydrochloride; ziprasidone mesylate
U.S./Canadian Brand Names Geodon® [US]
Therapeutic Category Antipsychotic Agent
Use Treatment of schizophrenia; treatment of acute manic or mixed episodes associated with bipolar disorder with or without psychosis; acute agitation in patients with schizophrenia
Usual Dosage Adults:
  Bipolar mania: Oral: Initial: 40 mg twice daily (with food)
    Adjustment: May increase to 60 or 80 mg twice daily on second day of treatment; average dose 40-80 mg twice daily
  Schizophrenia: Oral: Initial: 20 mg twice daily (with food)
    Adjustment: Increases (if indicated) should be made no more frequently than every 2 days; ordinarily patients should be observed for improvement over several weeks before adjusting the dose
    Maintenance: Range 20-100 mg twice daily; however, dosages >80 mg twice daily are generally not recommended
  Acute agitation (schizophrenia): I.M.: 10 mg every 2 hours **or** 20 mg every 4 hours; maximum: 40 mg/day; oral therapy should replace I.M. administration as soon as possible
Dosage Forms
  Capsule:
    Geodon®: 20 mg, 40 mg, 60 mg, 80 mg
  Injection, powder for reconstitution:
    Geodon®: 20 mg

ziprasidone hydrochloride *see* ziprasidone *on this page*
ziprasidone mesylate *see* ziprasidone *on this page*
Zithromax® [US/Can] *see* azithromycin *on page 88*
Zithromax® TRI-PAK™ *see* azithromycin *on page 88*
Zithromax® Z-PAK® *see* azithromycin *on page 88*
ZM-182,780 *see* fulvestrant *on page 378*
Zmax™ [US] *see* azithromycin *on page 88*
Zn-DTPA *see* diethylene triamine penta-acetic acid *on page 256*
ZNP® Bar [US-OTC] *see* pyrithione zinc *on page 737*
Zocor® [US/Can] *see* simvastatin *on page 787*
Zoderm® [US] *see* benzoyl peroxide *on page 103*
Zofran® [US/Can] *see* ondansetron *on page 630*
Zofran® ODT [US/Can] *see* ondansetron *on page 630*
Zoladex® [US/Can] *see* goserelin *on page 399*
Zoladex® LA [Can] *see* goserelin *on page 399*
zoledronate *see* zoledronic acid *on this page*

zoledronic acid (zoe le DRON ik AS id)

Synonyms CGP-42446; NSC-721517; zoledronate
U.S./Canadian Brand Names Aclasta® [Can]; Reclast® [US]; Zometa® [US/Can]
Therapeutic Category Bisphosphonate Derivative
Use Treatment of hypercalcemia of malignancy, multiple myeloma, bone metastases of solid tumors, Paget disease of bone, postmenopausal osteoporosis
Usual Dosage I.V.: Adults:
  Hypercalcemia of malignancy (albumin-corrected serum calcium ≥12 mg/dL) (Zometa®): 4 mg (maximum) given as a single dose. Wait at least 7 days before considering retreatment. Dosage adjustment may be needed in patients with decreased renal function following treatment.
  Multiple myeloma or metastatic bone lesions from solid tumors (Zometa®): 4 mg every 3-4 weeks
    Note: Patients should receive a daily calcium supplement and multivitamin containing vitamin D
  Paget disease (Reclast®, Aclasta® [not available in U.S.]): 5 mg infused over at least 15 minutes. **Note:** Data concerning retreatment is not available, but may be considered. Patients should receive a daily calcium supplement and multivitamin containing vitamin D.
Dosage Forms [CAN] = Canadian brand name
  Infusion, solution [premixed]:
    Aclasta® [CAN]): 5 mg (100 mL) [not available in the U.S.]
    Relcast®: 5 mg (100 mL)
  (Continued)

zoledronic acid (Continued)
Injection, solution:
Zometa®: 4 mg/5 mL (5 mL)

Zolicef® **(Discontinued)** see cefazolin on page 158

Zolinza™ [US] see vorinostat on page 898

zolmitriptan (zohl mi TRIP tan)
Sound-Alike/Look-Alike Issues
zolmitriptan may be confused with sumatriptan
Synonyms 311C90
U.S./Canadian Brand Names Zomig-ZMT™ [US]; Zomig® Nasal Spray [Can]; Zomig® Rapimelt [Can]; Zomig® [US/Can]
Therapeutic Category Antimigraine Agent; Serotonin Agonist
Use Acute treatment of migraine with or without aura
Usual Dosage Oral:
Children: Safety and efficacy have not been established
Adults: Migraine:
Tablet: Initial: ≤2.5 mg at the onset of migraine headache; may break 2.5 mg tablet in half
Orally-disintegrating tablet: Initial: 2.5 mg at the onset of migraine headache
Nasal spray: Initial: 1 spray (5 mg) at the onset of migraine headache
Note: Use the lowest possible dose to minimize adverse events. If the headache returns, the dose may be repeated after 2 hours; do not exceed 10 mg within a 24-hour period. Controlled trials have not established the effectiveness of a second dose if the initial one was ineffective
Dosage Forms
Solution, nasal spray [single dose]:
Zomig®: 5 mg/0.1 mL (0.1 mL)
Tablet:
Zomig®: 2.5 mg, 5 mg
Tablet, orally disintegrating
Zomig-ZMT™: 2.5 mg, 5 mg

Zoloft® [US/Can] see sertraline on page 783

zolpidem (zole PI dem)
Sound-Alike/Look-Alike Issues
Ambien® may be confused with Ambi 10®
Synonyms zolpidem tartrate
U.S./Canadian Brand Names Ambien CR™ [US]; Ambien® [US]
Therapeutic Category Hypnotic, Nonbarbiturate
Controlled Substance C-IV
Use
Ambien®: Short-term treatment of insomnia (with difficulty of sleep onset)
Ambien CR™: Short-term treatment of insomnia (with difficulty of sleep onset and/or sleep maintenance)
Usual Dosage Oral: Adults:
Ambien®: 10 mg immediately before bedtime; maximum dose: 10 mg
Ambien CR™: 12.5 mg immediately before bedtime
Dosage Forms
Tablet: 5 mg, 10 mg
Ambien®: 5 mg, 10 mg
Tablet, extended release:
Ambien CR™: 6.25 mg, 12.5 mg

zolpidem tartrate see zolpidem on this page

Zometa® [US/Can] see zoledronic acid on previous page

Zomig® [US/Can] see zolmitriptan on this page

Zomig® Nasal Spray [Can] see zolmitriptan on this page

Zomig® Rapimelt [Can] see zolmitriptan on this page

Zomig-ZMT™ [US] see zolmitriptan on this page

Zomorph® [Can] see morphine sulfate on page 578

Zonalon® [US/Can] see doxepin on page 279

Zonegran® [US/Can] see zonisamide on next page

zonisamide (zoe NIS a mide)
U.S./Canadian Brand Names Zonegran® [US/Can]
Therapeutic Category Anticonvulsant, Sulfonamide
Use Adjunct treatment of partial seizures in children >16 years of age and adults with epilepsy
Usual Dosage Oral: Children >16 years and Adults: Adjunctive treatment of partial seizures: Initial: 100 mg/day; dose may be increased to 200 mg/day after 2 weeks. Further dosage increases to 300 mg/day and 400 mg/day can then be made with a minimum of 2 weeks between adjustments, in order to reach steady state at each dosage level. Doses of up to 600 mg/day have been studied, however, there is no evidence of increased response with doses above 400 mg/day.
Dosage Forms
Capsule: 25 mg, 50 mg, 100 mg
Zonegran®: 25 mg, 100 mg

zopiclone *(Canada only)* (ZOE pi clone)
U.S./Canadian Brand Names Alti-Zopiclone [Can]; Apo-Zopiclone® [Can]; CO Zopiclone [Can]; Dom-Zopiclone [Can]; Gen-Zopiclone [Can]; Imovane® [Can]; Novo-Zopiclone [Can]; Nu-Zopiclone [Can]; PMS-Zopiclone [Can]; RAN™-Zopiclone [Can]; Ratio-Zopiclone [Can]; Rhovane® [Can]; Rhoxal-zopiclone [Can]; Riva-Zopiclone [Can]; Sandoz-Zopiclone [Can]
Therapeutic Category Hypnotic
Use Symptomatic relief of transient and short-term insomnia
Usual Dosage Administer just before bedtime: Oral: Adults: 5-7.5 mg
Patients with chronic respiratory insufficiency: 3.75 mg; may increase up to 7.5 mg with caution in appropriate cases
Dosage Forms [CAN] = Canadian brand name
Tablet: 5 mg, 7.5 mg [not available in the U.S.]
Apo-Zopiclone® [CAN], Gen-Zopiclone [CAN], Imovane® [CAN], Novo-Zopiclone [CAN], Nu-Zopiclone [CAN], PMS-Zopiclone [CAN], Rhovane® [CAN], Rhoxal-zopiclone [CAN]: 5 mg, 7.5 mg

Zorbtive® [US] *see* somatropin *on page 799*

Zorcaine™ [US/Can] *see* articaine and epinephrine *on page 75*

ZORprin® [US] *see* aspirin *on page 78*

Zostavax® [US] *see* zoster vaccine *on this page*

zoster vaccine (ZOS ter vak SEEN)
Synonyms shingles vaccine; varicella-zoster (VZV) vaccine (zoster); VZV vaccine (zoster)
U.S./Canadian Brand Names Zostavax® [US]
Therapeutic Category Vaccine
Use Prevention of herpes zoster (shingles) in patients ≥60 years of age
Usual Dosage SubQ: Adults ≥60 years: 0.65 mL administered as a single dose; there is no data to support readministration of the vaccine
Dosage Forms
Injection, powder for reconstitution [preservative free]
Zostavax®: 19,400 plaque-forming units (PFU)

Zostrix® [US-OTC/Can] *see* capsaicin *on page 145*

Zostrix®-HP [US-OTC/Can] *see* capsaicin *on page 145*

Zosyn® [US] *see* piperacillin and tazobactam sodium *on page 685*

Zovia™ [US] *see* ethinyl estradiol and ethynodiol diacetate *on page 324*

Zovirax® [US/Can] *see* acyclovir *on page 17*

Ztuss™ Tablet [US] *see* hydrocodone, pseudoephedrine, and guaifenesin *on page 432*

Ztuss™ ZT [US] *see* hydrocodone and guaifenesin *on page 429*

zuclopenthixol acetate *see* zuclopenthixol *(Canada only)* *on this page*

zuclopenthixol *(Canada only)* (zoo kloe pen THIX ol)
Synonyms Z-chlopenthixol; zuclopenthixol acetate; zuclopenthixol decanoate; zuclopenthixol dihydrochloride
U.S./Canadian Brand Names Clopixol-Acuphase® [Can]; Clopixol® Depot [Can]; Clopixol® [Can]
Therapeutic Category Antipsychotic Agent
Use Management of schizophrenia; acetate injection is intended for short-term acute treatment; decanoate injection is for long-term management; dihydrochloride tablets may be used in either phase
(Continued)

zuclopenthixol *(Canada only)* *(Continued)*

Usual Dosage Adults:

Oral: Zuclopenthixol dihydrochloride: Initial: 20-30 mg/day in 2-3 divided doses; usual maintenance dose: 20-40 mg/day; maximum daily dose: 100 mg

I.M.:

Zuclopenthixol acetate: 50-150 mg; may be repeated in 2-3 days; no more than 4 injections should be given in the course of treatment; maximum dose during course of treatment: 400 mg (maximum treatment period: 2 weeks)

Transfer of patients from I.M. acetate (Acuphase®) to oral (tablets):
50 mg = 20 mg daily
100 mg = 40 mg daily
150 mg = 60 mg daily

Zuclopenthixol decanoate: 100 mg by deep I.M. injection; additional I.M. doses of 100-200 mg may be given over the following 1-4 weeks; maximum weekly dose: 600 mg; usual maintenance dose: 150-300 mg every 2 weeks

Transfer of patients from oral (tablets) to I.M. decanoate (depot):
≤20 mg daily = 100 mg every 2 weeks
25-40 mg daily = 200 mg every 2 weeks
50-75 mg daily = 300 mg every 2 weeks
>75 mg/day = 400 mg every 2 weeks

Transfer of patients from I.M. acetate (Acuphase®) to I.M. decanoate (depot):
50 mg every 2-3 days = 100 mg every 2 weeks
100 mg every 2-3 days = 200 mg every 2 weeks
150 mg every 2-3 days = 300 mg every 2 weeks

Dosage Forms [CAN] = Canadian brand name

Injection:

Clopixol Acuphase® [CAN]: 50 mg/mL [zuclopenthixol 42.5 mg/mL] (1 mL, 2 mL) [not available in the U.S.]
Clopixol® Depot [CAN]: 200 mg/mL [zuclopenthixol 144.4 mg/mL] (10 mL) [not available in the U.S.]

Tablet:

Clopixol® [CAN]: 10 mg, 25 mg, 40 mg [not available in the U.S.]

zuclopenthixol decanoate *see* zuclopenthixol *(Canada only)* on previous page

zuclopenthixol dihydrochloride *see* zuclopenthixol *(Canada only)* on previous page

Zyban® **[US/Can]** *see* bupropion on page 127

Zydone® **[US]** *see* hydrocodone and acetaminophen on page 427

Zyflo® **[US]** *see* zileuton on page 905

Zyflo CR™ **[US]** *see* zileuton on page 905

Zylet™ **[US]** *see* loteprednol and tobramycin on page 520

Zyloprim® **[US/Can]** *see* allopurinol on page 30

Zymar™ **[US/Can]** *see* gatifloxacin on page 385

Zymase® *(Discontinued)* *see* pancrelipase on page 648

Zymine®**-D [US]** *see* triprolidine and pseudoephedrine on page 869

Zyprexa® **[US/Can]** *see* olanzapine on page 626

Zyprexa® **Zydis**® **[US/Can]** *see* olanzapine on page 626

Zyrtec® **[US]** *see* cetirizine on page 169

Zyrtec-D 12 Hour® **[US]** *see* cetirizine and pseudoephedrine on page 169

Zytram® **XL [Can]** *see* tramadol on page 856

Zyvox® **[US]** *see* linezolid on page 509

Zyvoxam® **[Can]** *see* linezolid on page 509

APPENDIX

Visit the**Point** http://thepoint.lww.com/QL2008 for exclusive access to:

Apothecary/Metric Conversions

Pounds/Kilograms Conversion

Temperature Conversion

Pharmaceutical Manufacturers and Distributors

Vitamin Products

Refer to the inside front cover of this book for your online access code.

ABBREVIATIONS & SYMBOLS COMMONLY USED IN MEDICAL ORDERS

Abbreviation	From	Meaning
<		less than
>		greater than
≤		less than or equal to
≥		greater than or equal to
a̅a̅, aa	ana	of each
AA		Alcoholics Anonymous
ABG		arterial blood gases
ac	ante cibum	before meals or food
ACA		Adult Children of Alcoholics
ACLS		advanced cardiac life support
ad	ad	to, up to
a.d.	aurio dextra	right ear
ADHD		attention-deficit/hyperactivity disorder
ADLs		activities of daily living
ad lib	ad libitum	at pleasure
AIDS		acquired immune deficiency syndrome
AIMS		Abnormal Involuntary Movement Scale
a.l.	aurio laeva	left ear
ALS		amyotrophic lateral sclerosis
AM	ante meridiem	morning
AMA		against medical advice
amp		ampul
amt		amount
aq	aqua	water
aq. dest.	aqua destillata	distilled water
ARC		AIDS-related complex
ARDS		adult respiratory distress syndrome
ARF		acute renal failure
a.s.	aurio sinister	left ear
ASAP		as soon as possible
ASA-PS		American Society of Anesthesiologists - Physical Status
		P1: Normal, healthy patient
		P2: Patient having mild systemic disease
		P3: Patient having severe systemic disease
		P4: Patient having severe systemic disease which is a constant threat to life
		P5: Moribund patient; not expected to survive without the procedure
		P6: Patient declared brain-dead; organs being removed for donor purposes
a.u.	aures utrae	each ear
AUC		area under the curve
BDI		Beck Depression Inventory
bid	bis in die	twice daily
BLS		basic life support
bm		bowel movement
BMI		body mass index
bp		blood pressure
BPH		benign prostatic hyperplasia
BPRS		Brief Psychiatric Rating Scale
BSA		body surface area
c̲	cong	a gallon
c̅	cum	with
CA		cancer
CABG		coronary artery bypass graft
CAD		coronary artery disease
cal		calorie
cap	capsula	capsule
CBT		cognitive behavioral therapy
cc		cubic centimeter
CCL		creatinine clearance
CF		cystic fibrosis

(continued)

Abbreviation	From	Meaning
CGI		Clinical Global Impression
CIE		chemotherapy-induced emesis
CIV		continuous I.V. infusion
cm		centimeter
CNS		central nervous system
comp	compositus	compound
cont		continue
COPD		chronic obstructive pulmonary disease
CRF		chronic renal failure
CT		computed tomography
d	dies	day
DBP		diastolic blood pressure
d/c		discontinue
dil	dilue	dilute
disp	dispensa	dispense
div	divide	divide
DOE		dyspnea on exertion
DSC		discontinued
DSM-IV		Diagnostic and Statistical Manual
DTs		delirium tremens
dtd	dentur tales doses	give of such a dose
DVT		deep vein thrombosis
Dx		diagnosis
ECG		electrocardiogram
ECT		electroconvulsive therapy
EEG		electroencephalogram
elix, el	elixir	elixir
emp		as directed
EPS		extrapyramidal side effects
ESRD		end stage renal disease
et	et	and
EtOH		alcohol
ex aq		in water
f, ft	fac, fiat, fiant	make, let be made
FDA		Food and Drug Administration
FMS		fibromyalgia syndrome
g	gramma	gram
GA		Gamblers Anonymous
GABA		gamma-aminobutyric acid
GAD		generalized anxiety disorder
GAF		Global Assessment of Functioning Scale
GERD		gastroesophageal reflux disease
GFR		glomerular filtration rate
GITS		gastrointestinal therapeutic system
gr	granum	grain
gtt	gutta	a drop
GVHD		graft versus host disease
h	hora	hour
HAM-A		Hamilton Anxiety Scale
HAM-D		Hamilton Depression Scale
hs	hora somni	at bedtime
HSV		herpes simplex virus
HTN		hypertension
IBD		inflammatory bowel disease
IBS		irritable bowel syndrome
ICH		intracranial hemorrhage
IHSS		idiopathic hypertrophic subaortic stenosis
I.M.		intramuscular
IOP		intraocular pressure
IU		international unit
I.V.		intravenous
kcal		kilocalorie
kg		kilogram
KIU		kallikrein inhibitor unit
L		liter

APPENDIX

Abbreviation	From	Meaning
LAMM		L-α-acetyl methadol
liq	liquor	a liquor, solution
LVH		left ventricular hypertrophy
M	misce	mix; Molar
MADRS		Montgomery Asbery Depression Rating Scale
MAOIs		monoamine oxidase inhibitors
mcg		microgram
MDEA		3,4-methylene-dioxy amphetamine
m. dict	more dictor	as directed
MDMA		3,4-methylene-dioxy methamphetamine
mEq		milliequivalent
mg		milligram
mixt	mixtura	a mixture
mL		milliliter
mm		millimeter
mM		millimolar
MMSE		mini mental status examination
MPPP		l-methyl-4-proprionoxy-4-phenyl pyridine
MR		mental retardation
MRI		magnetic resonance image
MS		multiple sclerosis
NF		National Formulary
NKA		no known allergies
NMS		neuroleptic malignant syndrome
no.	numerus	number
noc	nocturnal	in the night
non rep	non repetatur	do not repeat, no refills
NPO		nothing by mouth
NSAID		nonsteroidal antiinflammatory drug
NV		nausea and vomiting
O, Oct	octarius	a pint
OA		osteoarthritis
OCD		obsessive-compulsive disorder
o.d.	oculus dexter	right eye
o.l.	oculus laevus	left eye
o.s.	oculus sinister	left eye
o.u.	oculo uterque	each eye
PANSS		Positive and Negative Symptom Scale
PAT		paroxysmal artrial tachycardia
pc, post cib	post cibos	after meals
PCP		phencyclidine
PD		Parkinson disease
PE		pulmonary embolus
per		through or by
PID		pelvic inflammatory disease
PM	post meridiem	afternoon or evening
P.O.	per os	by mouth
PONV		postoperative nausea and vomiting
P.R.	per rectum	rectally
prn	pro re nata	as needed
PSVT		paroxysmal supraventricular tachycardia
PTA		prior to admission
PTSD		post-traumatic stress disorder
PUD		peptic ulcer disease
pulv	pulvis	a powder
PVD		peripheral vascular disease
q		every
qad	quoque alternis die	every other day
qd		every day, daily
qh	quiaque hora	every hour
qid	quater in die	four times a day
qod		every other day
qs	quantum sufficiat	a sufficient quantity
qs ad		a sufficient quantity to make
qty		quantity

(continued)

Abbreviation	From	Meaning
qv	quam volueris	as much as you wish
RA		rheumatoid arthritis
REM		rapid eye movement
Rx	recipe	take, a recipe
rep	repetatur	let it be repeated
s̄	sine	without
sa	secundum artem	according to art
SAH		subarachnoid hemorrhage
sat	sataratus	saturated
SBE		subacute bacterial endocarditis
SBP		systolic blood pressure
SIADH		syndrome of inappropriate antidiuretic hormone secretion
sig	signa	label, or let it be printed
SL		sublingual
SLE		systemic lupus erythematosus
SOB		shortness of breath
sol	solutio	solution
solv		dissolve
s̄s̄, ss	semis	one-half
sos	si opus sit	if there is need
SSKI		saturated solution of potassium iodide
SSRIs		selective serotonin reuptake inhibitors
stat	statim	at once, immediately
STD		sexually transmitted disease
SubQ		subcutaneous
supp	suppositorium	suppository
SVT		supraventricular tachycardia
Sx		symptom
syr	syrupus	syrup
tab	tabella	tablet
tal		such
TCA		tricyclic antidepressant
TD		tardive dyskinesia
tid	ter in die	three times a day
TKO		to keep open
TPN		total parenteral nutrition
tr, tinct	tincture	tincture
trit		triturate
tsp		teaspoonful
Tx		treatment
u.d., ut dict		as directed
ULN		upper limits of normal
ung	unguentum	ointment
URI		upper respiratory infection
USAN		United States Adopted Names
USP		United States Pharmacopeia
UTI		urinary tract infection
v.o.		verbal order
VTE		venous thromboembolism
VZV		varicella zoster virus
w.a.		while awake
x3		3 times
x4		4 times
YBOC		Yale Brown Obsessive-Compulsive Scale
YMRS		Young Mania Rating Scale

NORMAL LABORATORY VALUES FOR ADULTS

Automated Chemistry (CHEMISTRY A)

Test	Values	Remarks
SERUM / PLASMA		
Acetone	Negative	
Albumin	3.2-5 g/dL	
Alcohol, ethyl	Negative	
Aldolase	1.2-7.6 IU/L	
Ammonia	20-70 mcg/dL	Specimen to be placed on ice as soon as collected
Amylase	30-110 units/L	
Bilirubin, direct	0-0.3 mg/dL	
Bilirubin, total	0.1-1.2 mg/dL	
Calcium	8.6-10.3 mg/dL	
Calcium, ionized	2.24-2.46 mEq/L	
Chloride	95-108 mEq/L	
Cholesterol, total	≤200 mg/dL	Fasted blood required --- normal value affected by dietary habits. This reference range is for a general adult population
HDL cholesterol	40-60 mg/dL	Fasted blood required --- normal value affected by dietary habits
LDL cholesterol	<160 mg/dL	If triglyceride is >400 mg/dL, LDL cannot be calculated accurately (Friedewald equation). Target LDL-C depends on patient's risk factors.
CO_2	23-30 mEq/L	
Creatine kinase (CK) isoenzymes		
CK-BB	0%	
CK-MB (cardiac)	0%-3.9%	
CK-MM (muscle)	96%-100%	

CK-MB levels must be both ≥4% and 10 IU/L to meet diagnostic criteria for CK-MB positive result consistent with myocardial injury.

Test	Values	Remarks
Creatine phosphokinase (CPK)	8-150 IU/L	
Creatinine	0.5-1.4 mg/dL	
Ferritin	13-300 ng/mL	
Folate	3.6-20 ng/dL	
GGT (gamma-glutamyltranspeptidase)		
male	11-63 IU/L	
female	8-35 IU/L	
GLDH	To be determined	
Glucose (preprandial)	<115 mg/dL	Goals different for diabetics
Glucose, fasting	60-110 mg/dL	Goals different for diabetics
Glucose, nonfasting (2-h postprandial)	<120 mg/dL	Goals different for diabetics
Hemoglobin A_{1c}	<8	
Hemoglobin, plasma free	<2.5 mg/100 mL	
Hemoglobin, total glycosylated (Hb A_1)	4%-8%	
Iron	65-150 mcg/dL	
Iron binding capacity, total (TIBC)	250-420 mcg/dL	
Lactic acid	0.7-2.1 mEq/L	Specimen to be kept on ice and sent to lab as soon as possible
Lactate dehydrogenase (LDH)	56-194 IU/L	
Lactate dehydrogenase (LDH) isoenzymes		
LD_1	20%-34%	
LD_2	29%-41%	
LD_3	15%-25%	
LD_4	1%-12%	
LD_5	1%-15%	

Test	Values	Remarks
Flipped LD_1/LD_2 ratios (>1 may be consistent with myocardial injury) particularly when considered in combination with a recent CK-MB positive result		
Lipase	23-208 units/L	
Magnesium	1.6-2.5 mg/dL	Increased by slight hemolysis
Osmolality	289-308 mOsm/kg	
Phosphatase, alkaline		
adults 25-60 y	33-131 IU/L	
adults ≥61 y	51-153 IU/L	
infancy-adolescence	Values range up to 3-5 times higher than adults	
Phosphate, inorganic	2.8-4.2 mg/dL	
Potassium	3.5-5.2 mEq/L	Increased by slight hemolysis
Prealbumin	>15 mg/dL	
Protein, total	6.5-7.9 g/dL	
SGOT (AST)	<35 IU/L (20-48)	
SGPT (ALT) (10-35)	<35 IU/L	
Sodium	134-149 mEq/L	
Thyroid stimulating hormone (TSH)		
adult ≤20 y	0.7-6.4 mIU/L	
21-54 y	0.4-4.2 mIU/L	
55-87 y	0.5-8.9 mIU/L	
Transferrin	>200 mg/dL	
Triglycerides	45-155 mg/dL	Fasted blood required
Troponin I	<1.5 ng/mL	
Urea nitrogen (BUN)	7-20 mg/dL	
Uric acid		
male	2-8 mg/dL	
female	2-7.5 mg/dL	

APPENDIX

Test	Values	Remarks
CEREBROSPINAL FLUID		
Glucose	50-70 mg/dL	
Protein	15-45 mg/dL	CSF obtained by lumbar puncture

Note: Bloody specimen gives erroneously high value due to contamination with blood proteins

URINE		
(24-hour specimen is required for all these tests unless specified)		
Amylase	32-641 units/L	The value is in units/L and **not** calculated for total volume
Amylase, fluid (random samples)		Interpretation of value left for physician, depends on the nature of fluid
Calcium	Depends upon dietary intake	
Creatine		
male	150 mg/24 h	Higher value on children and during pregnancy
female	250 mg/24 h	
Creatinine	1000-2000 mg/24 h	
Creatinine clearance (endogenous)		
male	85-125 mL/min	A blood sample must accompany urine specimen
female	75-115 mL/min	
Glucose	1 g/24 h	
5-hydroxyindoleacetic acid	2-8 mg/24 h	
Iron	0.15 mg/24 h	Acid washed container required
Magnesium	146-209 mg/24 h	
Osmolality	500-800 mOsm/kg	With normal fluid intake
Oxalate	10-40 mg/24 h	
Phosphate	400-1300 mg/24 h	
Potassium	25-120 mEq/24 h	Varies with diet; the interpretation of urine electrolytes and osmolality should be left for the physician
Sodium	40-220 mEq/24 h	
Porphobilinogen, qualitative	Negative	
Porphyrins, qualitative	Negative	
Proteins	0.05-0.1 g/24 h	
Salicylate	Negative	
Urea clearance	60-95 mL/min	A blood sample must accompany specimen
Urea N	10-40 g/24 h	Dependent on protein intake
Uric acid	250-750 mg/24 h	Dependent on diet and therapy
Urobilinogen	0.5-3.5 mg/24 h	For qualitative determination on random urine, send sample to urinalysis section in Hematology Lab
Xylose absorption test		
children	16%-33% of ingested xylose	
FECES		
Fat, 3-day collection	<5 g/d	Value depends on fat intake of 100 g/d for 3 days preceding and during collection
GASTRIC ACIDITY		
Acidity, total, 12 h	10-60 mEq/L	Titrated at pH 7

BLOOD GASES

	Arterial	Capillary	Venous
pH	7.35-7.45	7.35-7.45	7.32-7.42
pCO$_2$ (mm Hg)	35-45	35-45	38-52
pO$_2$ (mm Hg)	70-100	60-80	24-48
HCO$_3$ (mEq/L)	19-25	19-25	19-25
TCO$_2$ (mEq/L)	19-29	19-29	23-33
O$_2$ saturation (%)	90-95	90-95	40-70
Base excess (mEq/L)	-5 to +5	-5 to +5	-5 to +5

HEMATOLOGY

Complete Blood Count

Age	Hgb (g/dL)	Hct (%)	MCV (fL)	MCH (pg)	MCHC (%)	RBC (mill/mm^3)	RDW	PLTS (x 10^3/mm^3)
0-3 d	15.0-20.0	45-61	95-115	31-37	29-37	4.0-5.9	<18.0	250-450
1-2 wk	12.5-18.5	39-57	86-110	28-36	28-38	3.6-5.5	<17.0	250-450
1-6 mo	10.0-13.0	29-42	74-96	25-35	30-36	3.1-4.3	<16.5	300-700
7 mo - 2 y	10.5-13.0	33-38	70-84	23-30	31-37	3.7-4.9	<16.0	250-600
2-5 y	11.5-13.0	34-39	75-87	24-30	31-37	3.9-5.0	<15.0	250-550
5-8 y	11.5-14.5	35-42	77-95	25-33	31-37	4.0-4.9	<15.0	250-550
13-18 y	12.0-15.2	36-47	78-96	25-35	31-37	4.5-5.1	<14.5	150-450
Adult male	13.5-16.5	41-50	80-100	26-34	31-37	4.5-5.5	<14.5	150-450
Adult female	12.0-15.0	36-44	80-100	26-34	31-37	4.0-4.9	<14.5	150-450

WBC and Diff

Age	WBC (x 10³/mm³)	Segs	Bands	Eos	Basos	Lymphs	Atypical Lymphs	Monos	# of NRBCs
0-3 d	9.0-35.0	32-62	10-18	0-2	0-1	19-29	0-8	5-7	0-2
1-2 wk	5.0-20.0	14-34	6-14	0-2	0-1	36-45	0-8	6-10	0
1-6 mo	6.0-17.5	13-33	4-12	0-3	0-1	41-71	0-8	4-7	0
7 mo - 2 y	6.0-17.0	15-35	5-11	0-3	0-1	45-76	0-8	3-6	0
2-5 y	5.5-15.5	23-45	5-11	0-3	0-1	35-65	0-8	3-6	0
5-8 y	5.0-14.5	32-54	5-11	0-3	0-1	28-48	0-8	3-6	0
13-18 y	4.5-13.0	34-64	5-11	0-3	0-1	25-45	0-8	3-6	0
Adults	4.5-11.0	35-66	5-11	0-3	0-1	24-44	0-8	3-6	0

Erythrocyte Sedimentation Rates and Reticulocyte Counts

Sedimentation rate, Westergren

Children	0-20 mm/hour
Adult male	0-15 mm/hour
Adult female	0-20 mm/hour

Sedimentation rate, Wintrobe

Children	0-13 mm/hour
Adult male	0-10 mm/hour
Adult female	0-15 mm/hour

Reticulocyte count

Newborns	2%-6%
1-6 mo	0%-2.8%
Adults	0.5%-1.5%

NORMAL LABORATORY VALUES FOR CHILDREN

CHEMISTRY		Normal Values
Albumin	0-1 y	2.0-4.0 g/dL
	1 y - adult	3.5-5.5 g/dL
Ammonia	Newborns	90-150 mcg/dL
	Children	40-120 mcg/dL
	Adults	18-54 mcg/dL
Amylase	Newborns	0-60 units/L
	Adults	30-110 units/L
Bilirubin, conjugated, direct	Newborns	<1.5 mg/dL
	1 mo - adult	0-0.5 mg/dL
Bilirubin, total	0-3 d	2.0-10.0 mg/dL
	1 mo - adult	0-1.5 mg/dL
Bilirubin, unconjugated, indirect		0.6-10.5 mg/dL
Calcium	Newborns	7.0-12.0 mg/dL
	0-2 y	8.8-11.2 mg/dL
	2 y - adult	9.0-11.0 mg/dL
Calcium, ionized, whole blood		4.4-5.4 mg/dL
Carbon dioxide, total		23-33 mEq/L
Chloride		95-105 mEq/L
Cholesterol	Newborns	45-170 mg/dL
	0-1 y	65-175 mg/dL
	1-20 y	120-230 mg/dL
Creatinine	0-1 y	≤0.6 mg/dL
	1 y - adult	0.5-1.5 mg/dL
Glucose	Newborns	30-90 mg/dL
	0-2 y	60-105 mg/dL
	Children to Adults	70-110 mg/dL
Iron	Newborns	110-270 mcg/dL
	Infants	30-70 mcg/dL
	Children	55-120 mcg/dL
	Adults	70-180 mcg/dL
Iron binding	Newborns	59-175 mcg/dL
	Infants	100-400 mcg/dL
	Adults	250-400 mcg/dL
Lactic acid, lactate		2-20 mg/dL
Lead, whole blood		<10 mcg/dL
Lipase	Children	20-140 units/L
	Adults	0-190 units/L
Magnesium		1.5-2.5 mEq/L
Osmolality, serum		275-296 mOsm/kg
Osmolality, urine		50-1400 mOsm/kg

CHEMISTRY		Normal Values
Phosphorus	Newborns	4.2-9.0 mg/dL
	6 wk to 19 mo	3.8-6.7 mg/dL
	19 mo to 3 y	2.9-5.9 mg/dL
	3-15 y	3.6-5.6 mg/dL
	>15 y	2.5-5.0 mg/dL
Potassium, plasma	Newborns	4.5-7.2 mEq/L
	2 d - 3 mo	4.0-6.2 mEq/L
	3 mo - 1 y	3.7-5.6 mEq/L
	1-16 y	3.5-5.0 mEq/L
Protein, total	0-2 y	4.2-7.4 g/dL
	>2 y	6.0-8.0 g/dL
Sodium		136-145 mEq/L
Triglycerides	Infants	0-171 mg/dL
	Children	20-130 mg/dL
	Adults	30-200 mg/dL
Urea nitrogen, blood	0-2 y	4-15 mg/dL
	2 y - adult	5-20 mg/dL
Uric acid	Male	3.0-7.0 mg/dL
	Female	2.0-6.0 mg/dL

ENZYMES

Alanine aminotransferase (ALT) (SGPT)	0-2 mo	8-78 units/L
	>2 mo	8-36 units/L
Alkaline phosphatase (ALKP)	Newborns	60-130 units/L
	0-16 y	85-400 units/L
	>16 y	30-115 units/L
Aspartate aminotransferase (AST)	Infants	18-74 units/L
(SGOT)	Children	15-46 units/L
	Adults	5-35 units/L
Creatine kinase (CK)	Infants	20-200 units/L
	Children	10-90 units/L
	Adult Male	0-206 units/L
	Adult Female	0-175 units/L
Lactate dehydrogenase (LDH)	Newborns	290-501 units/L
	1 mo - 2 y	110-144 units/L
	>16 y	60-170 units/L

BLOOD GASES

	Arterial	Capillary	Venous
pH	7.35-7.45	7.35-7.45	7.32-7.42
pCO_2 (mm Hg)	35-45	35-45	38-52
pO_2 (mm Hg)	70-100	60-80	24-48
HCO_3 (mEq/L)	19-25	19-25	19-25
TCO_2 (mEq/L)	19-29	19-29	23-33
O_2 saturation (%)	90-95	90-95	40-70
Base excess (mEq/L)	-5 to +5	-5 to +5	-5 to +5

THYROID FUNCTION TESTS

T_4 (thyroxine)	1-7 d	10.1-20.9 mcg/dL
	8-14 d	9.8-16.6 mcg/dL
	1 mo - 1 y	5.5-16.0 mcg/dL
	>1 y	4.0-12.0 mcg/dL
FTI	1-3 d	9.3-26.6
	1-4 wk	7.6-20.8
	1-4 mo	7.4-17.9
	4-12 mo	5.1-14.5
	1-6 y	5.7-13.3
	>6 y	4.8-14.0
T_3 by RIA	Newborns	100-470 ng/dL
	1-5 y	100-260 ng/dL
	5-10 y	90-240 ng/dL
	10 y - adult	70-210 ng/dL
T_3 uptake		35%-45%
TSH	Cord	3-22 μIU/mL
	1-3 d	<40 μIU/mL
	3-7 d	<25 μIU/mL
	>7 d	0-10 μIU/mL

ACQUIRED IMMUNODEFICIENCY SYNDROME (AIDS) — LAB TESTS AND APPROVED DRUGS FOR HIV INFECTION AND AIDS-RELATED CONDITIONS

This list of tests is not intended in any way to suggest patterns of physician's orders, nor is it complete. These tests may support possible clinical diagnoses or rule out other diagnostic possibilities. Each laboratory test relevant to AIDS is listed and weighted. Two symbols (**) indicate that the test is diagnostic, that is, documents the diagnosis if the expected is found. A single symbol (*) indicates a test frequently used in the diagnosis or management of the disease. The other listed tests are useful on a selective basis with consideration of clinical factors and specific aspects of the case.

Acid-Fast Stain
Acid-Fast Stain, Modified, *Nocardia* Species
Antimicrobial Susceptibility Testing, Fungi
Antimicrobial Susceptibility Testing, Mycobacteria
Arthropod Identification
Babesiosis Serological Test
Bacteremia Detection, Buffy Coat Micromethod
Bacterial Culture, Blood
Bacterial Culture, Bronchoscopy Specimen
Bacterial Culture, Sputum
Bacterial Culture, Stool
Bacterial Culture, Throat
Bacterial Culture, Urine, Clean Catch
Beta$_2$-Microglobulin
Blood and Fluid Precautions, Specimen Collection
Bronchial Washings Cytology
Bronchoalveolar Lavage Cytology
Brushings Cytology
Candida Antigen
Candidiasis Serologic Test
Cat Scratch Disease Serology
CD4/CD8 Enumeration
Cerebrospinal Fluid Cytology
Cryptococcal Antigen Titer
Cryptosporidium Diagnostic Procedures
Cytomegalic Inclusion Disease Cytology
Cytomegalovirus Antibody
Cytomegalovirus Antigen Detection
Cytomegalovirus Culture
Cytomegalovirus DNA Detection
Darkfield Examination, Syphilis
Electron Microscopy
Folic Acid, Serum
Fungal Culture, Biopsy or Body Fluid
Fungal Culture, Blood
Fungal Culture, Cerebrospinal Fluid
Fungal Culture, Sputum
Fungal Culture, Stool
Fungal Culture, Urine
Hemoglobin A$_2$
Hepatitis B Surface Antigen
Herpes Cytology
Herpes Simplex Virus Antigen Detection
Herpes Simplex Virus Culture
Histopathology
Histoplasmosis Antibody
Histoplasmosis Antigen
**HIV-1/HIV-2 Serology
HTLV-I/II Antibody
*Human Immunodeficiency Virus Culture
*Human Immunodeficiency Virus DNA Amplification

India Ink Preparation
Inhibitor, Lupus, Phospholipid Type
KOH Preparation
Leishmaniasis Serological Test
Leukocyte Immunophenotyping
Lymphocyte Transformation Test
Microsporidia Diagnostic Procedures
Mycobacteria by DNA Probe
Mycobacterial Culture, Biopsy or Body Fluid
Mycobacterial Culture, Cerebrospinal Fluid
Mycobacterial Culture, Cutaneous and Subcutaneous Tissue
Mycobacterial Culture, Sputum
Mycobacterial Culture, Stool
Neisseria gonorrhoeae Culture and Smear
Nocardia Culture
Ova and Parasites, Stool
*p24 Antigen
Platelet Count
Pneumocystis carinii Preparation
Pneumocystis Immunofluorescence
Polymerase Chain Reaction
Red Blood Cell Indices
Risks of Transfusion
Skin Biopsy
Sputum Cytology
Toxoplasmosis Serology
VDRL, Serum
Viral Culture
Viral Culture, Blood
Viral Culture, Body Fluid
Viral Culture, Central Nervous System Symptoms
Viral Culture, Dermatological Symptoms
Viral Culture, Tissue
Virus, Direct Detection by Fluorescent Antibody
White Blood Count

CURRENTLY APPROVED ANTIRETROVIRAL DRUGS

Antiretroviral Drugs

Generic Name	Synonyms	Brand Name
FUSION INHIBITOR		
enfuvirtide	T-20	Fuzeon®
NONNUCLEOSIDE REVERSE TRANSCRIPTASE INHIBITORS (NNRTIs)		
delavirdine	DLV	Rescriptor®
efavirenz	EFV	Sustiva®
nevirapine	NVP	Viramune®
NUCLEOTIDE ANALOG REVERSE TRANSCRIPTASE INHIBITORS (NtARTIs)		
adefovir	bis-POM PMPA	Preveon®
tenofovir		Viread®
PROTEASE INHIBITORS (PIs)		
amprenavir	APV	Agenerase®
atazanavir sulfate	ATV	Reyataz®
darunavir		Prezista®
fosamprenavir calcium	FOS-APV	Lexiva®
indinavir	IND	Crixivan®
lopinavir and ritonavir	LPV/RTV	Kaletra®
nelfinavir mesylate	NFV	Viracept®
ritonavir	RTV	Norvir®
saquinavir mesylate	SQV	Invirase®
tipranavir	TPV	Aptivus®
NUCLEOSIDE REVERSE TRANSCRIPTASE INHIBITORS (NRTIs)		
abacavir sulfate	ABC	Ziagen®
abacavir and lamivudine	ABC + 3TC	Epzicom®
abacavir, zidovudine, and lamivudine	ABC + AZT + 3TC	Trizivir®
didanosine	dideoxyinosine, ddI	Videx®
emtricitabine	FTC	Emtriva®
enteric coated didanosine	ddI EC	Videx® EC
lamivudine	3TC	Epivir®
lamivudine and zidovudine		Combivir®
stavudine	d4T	Zerit®
tenofovir disoproxil fumarate	TDF	Viread®
tenofovir disoproxil fumarate and emtricitabine		Truvada®
zalcitabine	dideoxycytidine, ddC	Hivid®
zidovudine	azidothymidine, AZT, ZDV	Retrovir®
COMBINATION PRODUCTS		
efavirenz, emtricitabine and tenofovir disoproxil fumarate		Atripla™
Entry Inhibitors - CCR5 co-receptor antagonist		
maraviroc		Selzentry®

DRUGS USED TO TREAT COMPLICATIONS OF HIV / AIDS

Brand Name	Generic Name (Synonym)	Use
Abelcet®, Ambisome®	amphotericin B, ABLC	Antifungal for aspergillosis
Bactrim®, Septra®	sulfamethoxazole and trimethoprim, SMZ/TMP	Antiprotozoal antibiotic for *Pneumocystis carinii* pneumonia treatment and prevention
Biaxin®	clarithromycin	Antibiotic for *Mycobacterium avium* prevention and treatment
Cytovene®	ganciclovir, DHPG	Antiviral for CMV retinitis
DaunoXome®	daunorubicin citrate (liposomal)	Chemotherapy for Kaposi sarcoma
Diflucan®	fluconazole	Antifungal for candidiasis, crytococcal meningitis
Doxil®	doxorubicin (liposomal)	Chemotherapy for Kaposi sarcoma
Eraxis™	anidulafungin	Antifungal (intravenous), used to treat *Candida* infections in the esophagus (candidiasis), blood stream (candidemia), and other forms of *Candida* infections, including abdominal abscesses and peritonitis (inflammation of the lining of the abdominal cavity)
Famvir®	famciclovir	Antiviral for herpes
Foscavir®	foscarnet	Antiviral for herpes, CMV retinitis
Gamimune® N	immune globulin, gamma globulin, IGIV	Immune booster to prevent bacterial infections in children
Intron® A	interferon alfa-2b	Karposi sarcoma, hepatitis C
Marinol®	dronabinol	Treat appetite loss
Megace®	megestrol acetate	Treat appetite and weight loss
Mepron®	atovaquone	Antiprotozoal antibiotic for *Pneumocystis carinii* pneumonia treatment and prevention
Mycobutin®	rifabutin	Antimycobacterial antibiotic for *Mycobacterium avium* prevention
NebuPent®	pentamidine	Antiprotozoal antibiotic for *Pneumocystis carinii* pneumonia prevention
Neutrexin®	trimetrexate glucuronate and leucovorin	Antiprotozoal antibiotic for *Pneumocystis carinii* pneumonia treatment
Panretin® Gel	alitretinoin gel 0.1%	AIDS-related Karposi sarcoma
Procrit®, Epogen®	erythropoetin, EPO	Treat anemia related to AZT therapy
Roferon-A®	interferon alfa-2a	Karposi sarcoma and hepatitis C
Serostim®	somatropin rDNA	Treat weight loss
Sporanox®	itraconazole	Antifungal for blastomycosis, histoplasmosis, aspergillosis, and candidiasis
Taxol®	paclitaxel	Karposi sarcoma
Valcyte™	valganciclovir	Antiviral for CMV retinitis
VFEND®	voriconazole	Antifungal for invasive aspergillosis and serious fungal infections due to *Fusarium sporotrichoides and Scedosporium apiospermum*, and Esophageal Candidiasis
Vistide®	cidofovir, HPMPC	Antiviral for CMV retinitis
Vitrasert® Implant	ganciclovir insert	Antiviral for CMV retinitis
Vitravene® Intravitreal Injectable	fomivirsen sodium injection	Antiviral for CMV retinitis
Zithromax®	azithromycin	Antibiotic for *Mycobacterium avium*

CHEMOTHERAPY REGIMENS

5 + 2

Use: Leukemia, acute myeloid (induction)
Regimen:
Cytarabine: I.V.: 100-200 mg/m^2/day continuous infusion days 1-5
  [total dose/cycle = 500-1000 mg/m^2]
with
Daunorubicin: I.V.: 45 mg/m^2/day days 1 and 2 [total dose/cycle = 90 mg/m^2]

7 + 3 (Daunorubicin)

Use: Leukemia, acute myeloid (induction)
Regimen:
Cytarabine: I.V.: 100 mg/m^2/day continuous infusion days 1-7 [total dose/cycle = 700 mg/m^2]
Daunorubicin: I.V.: 45 mg/m^2/day days 1-3 [total dose/cycle = 135 mg/m^2]
Administer one cycle only

7 + 3 (Idarubicin)

Use: Leukemia, acute myeloid (induction)
Regimen:
Cytarabine: I.V.: 100-200 mg/m^2/day continuous infusion days 1-7
  [total dose/cycle = 700-1400 mg/m^2]
Idarubicin: I.V.: 12 mg/m^2/day days 1-3 [total dose/cycle = 36 mg/m^2]
Administer one cycle only

7 + 3 (Mitoxantrone)

Use: Leukemia, acute myeloid (induction)
Regimen:
Cytarabine: I.V.: 100-200 mg/m^2/day continuous infusion days 1-7
  [total dose/cycle = 700-1400 mg/m^2]
Mitoxantrone: I.V.: 12 mg/m^2/day days 1-3 [total dose/cycle = 36 mg/m^2]
Administer one cycle only

7 + 3 + 7

Use: Leukemia, acute myeloid
Regimen:
Cytarabine: I.V.: 100 mg/m^2/day continuous infusion days 1-7 [total dose/cycle = 700 mg/m^2]
Daunorubicin: I.V.: 50 mg/m^2/day days 1-3 [total dose/cycle = 150 mg/m^2]
Etoposide: I.V.: 75 mg/m^2/day days 1-7 [total dose/cycle = 525 mg/m^2]
Repeat cycle every 21 days; up to 3 cycles may be given based on individual response

8 in 1 (Brain Tumors)

Use: Brain tumors

Regimen: Note: Multiple variations are listed below.

Variation 1:

Methylprednisolone: I.V.: 300 mg/m^2 every 6 hours day 1 (3 doses)
[total dose/cycle = 900 mg/m^2]

Vincristine: I.V.: 1.5 mg/m^2 (maximum 2 mg) day 1 [total dose/cycle = 1.5 mg/m^2]

Lomustine: Oral: 75 mg/m^2 day 1 [total dose/cycle = 75 mg/m^2]

Procarbazine: Oral: 75 mg/m^2 day 1; 1 hour after methylprednisolone and vincristine
[total dose/cycle = 75 mg/m^2]

Hydroxyurea: Oral: 3000 mg/m^2 day 1; 2 hours after methylprednisolone and vincristine
[total dose/cycle = 3000 mg/m^2]

Cisplatin: I.V.: 90 mg/m^2 day 1; 3 hours after methylprednisolone and vincristine
[total dose/cycle = 90 mg/m^2]

Cytarabine: I.V.: 300 mg/m^2 day 1; 9 hours after methylprednisolone and vincristine
[total dose/cycle = 300 mg/m^2]

Dacarbazine: I.V.: 150 mg/m^2 day 1; 12 hours after methylprednisolone and vincristine
[total dose/cycle = 150 mg/m^2]

Repeat cycle every 14 days

Variation 2:

Methylprednisolone: I.V.: 300 mg/m^2 every 6 hours day 1 (3 doses)
[total dose/cycle = 900 mg/m^2]

Vincristine: I.V.: 1.5 mg/m^2 (maximum 2 mg) day 1 [total dose/cycle = 1.5 mg/m^2]

Lomustine: Oral: 75 mg/m^2 day 1 [total dose/cycle = 75 mg/m^2]

Procarbazine: Oral: 75 mg/m^2 day 1; 1 hour after methylprednisolone and vincristine
[total dose/cycle = 75 mg/m^2]

Hydroxyurea: Oral: 3000 mg/m^2 day 1; 2 hours after methylprednisolone and vincristine
[total dose/cycle = 3000 mg/m^2]

Cisplatin: I.V.: 60 mg/m^2 day 1; 3 hours after methylprednisolone and vincristine
[total dose/cycle = 60 mg/m^2]

Cytarabine: I.V.: 300 mg/m^2 day 1; 9 hours after methylprednisolone and vincristine
[total dose/cycle = 300 mg/m^2]

Cyclophosphamide: I.V.: 300 mg/m^2 day 1; 12 hours after methylprednisolone and vincristine
[total dose/cycle = 300 mg/m^2]

Repeat cycle every 14 days

8 in 1 (Retinoblastoma)

Use: Retinoblastoma

Regimen:

Vincristine: I.V.: 1.5 mg/m^2 day 1 [total dose/cycle = 1.5 mg/m^2]

Methylprednisolone: I.V.: 300 mg/m^2 day 1 [total dose/cycle = 300 mg/m^2]

Lomustine: Oral: 75 mg/m^2 day 1 [total dose/cycle = 75 mg/m^2]

Procarbazine: Oral: 75 mg/m^2 day 1 [total dose/cycle = 75 mg/m^2]

Hydroxyurea: Oral: 1500 mg/m^2 day 1 [total dose/cycle = 1500 mg/m^2]

Cisplatin: I.V.: 60 mg/m^2 day 1 [total dose/cycle = 60 mg/m^2]

Cytarabine: I.V.: 300 mg/m^2 day 1 [total dose/cycle = 300 mg/m^2]

Repeat cycle every 28 days

AAV (DD)

Use: Wilms Tumor

Regimen:

Dactinomycin: I.V.: 15 mcg/kg/day days 1-5 of weeks 0, 13, 26, 39, 52, 65
[total dose/cycle = 450 mcg/kg]

Doxorubicin: I.V.: 20 mg/m^2/day days 1-3 of weeks 6, 19, 32, 45, 58
[total dose/cycle = 300 mg/m^2]

Vincristine: I.V.: 1.5 mg/m^2 day 1 of weeks 0-10, 13, 14, 26, 27, 39, 40, 52, 53, 65, 66
[total dose/cycle = 31.5 mg/m^2]

ABVD
Use: Lymphoma, Hodgkin disease
Regimen:
Doxorubicin: I.V.: 25 mg/m^2/day days 1 and 15 [total dose/cycle = 50 mg/m^2]
Bleomycin: I.V.: 10 units/m^2/day days 1 and 15 [total dose/cycle = 20 units/m^2]
Vinblastine: I.V.: 6 mg/m^2/day days 1 and 15 [total dose/cycle = 12 mg/m^2]
Dacarbazine: I.V.: 375 mg/m^2/day days 1 and 15 [total dose/cycle = 750 mg/m^2]
Repeat cycle every 28 days

AC
Use: Breast cancer
Regimen: Note: Multiple variations are listed below.

Variation 1: AC (conventional):
Doxorubicin: I.V.: 60 mg/m^2 day 1 [total dose/cycle = 60 mg/m^2]
Cyclophosphamide: I.V.: 600 mg/m^2 day 1 [total dose/cycle = 600 mg/m^2]
Repeat cycle every 21 days

Variation 2:
Cyclophosphamide: Oral: 200 mg/m^2/day days 3-6 [total dose/cycle = 800 mg/m^2]
Doxorubicin: I.V.: 40 mg/m^2 day 1 [total dose/cycle = 40 mg/m^2]
Repeat cycle every 3 weeks for 3 cycles, then every 4 weeks

AC/Paclitaxel (Sequential)
Use: Breast cancer
Regimen: Note: Multiple variations are listed below.

Variation 1: AC + Paclitaxel (conventional):
Doxorubicin: I.V.: 60 mg/m^2 day 1 [total dose/cycle = 60 mg/m^2]
Cyclophosphamide: I.V.: 600 mg/m^2 day 1 [total dose/cycle = 600 mg/m^2]
Repeat cycle every 21 days for 4 cycles

followed by
Paclitaxel: I.V.: 175 mg/m^2 day 1 [total dose/cycle = 175 mg/m^2]
Repeat cycle every 21 days for 4 cycles

Variation 2: AC + Paclitaxel (dose dense):
Doxorubicin: I.V.: 60 mg/m^2 day 1 [total dose/cycle = 60 mg/m^2]
Cyclophosphamide: I.V.: 600 mg/m^2 day 1 [total dose/cycle = 600 mg/m^2]
Filgrastim: SubQ: 5 mcg/kg/day days 3-10 [total dose/cycle = 40 mcg/kg]
Repeat cycle every 14 days for 4 cycles

followed by
Paclitaxel: I.V.: 175 mg/m^2 day 1 [total dose/cycle = 175 mg/m^2]
Filgrastim: SubQ: 5 mcg/kg/day days 3-10 [total dose/cycle = 40 mcg/kg]
Repeat cycle every 14 days for 4 cycles

AC-Paclitaxel-Trastuzumab
Use: Breast cancer
Regimen: Note: Multiple variations are listed below.
   Variation 1:
   Doxorubicin: I.V.: 60 mg/m^2 day 1 [total dose/cycle = 60 mg/m^2]
   Cyclophosphamide: I.V.: 600 mg/m^2 day 1 [total dose/cycle = 600 mg/m^2]
   Repeat cycle every 21 days for 4 cycles
   followed by
   Paclitaxel: I.V.: 175 mg/m^2 day 1 [total dose/cycle = 175 mg/m^2]
   Trastuzumab: I.V.: 4 mg/kg (loading dose) day 1 (cycle 1 only) [total dose/cycle = 4 mg/kg]
   followed by I.V.: 2 mg/kg/day days 8 and 15 (cycle 1) [total dose/cycle = 4 mg/kg]
   then I.V.: 2 mg/kg/day days 1, 8, 15 (cycles 2, 3, 4) [total dose/cycle = 6 mg/kg]
   Repeat cycle every 21 days for 4 cycles
   followed by
   Trastuzumab: I.V.: 2 mg/kg weekly for 40 weeks
   Variation 2:
   Doxorubicin: I.V.: 60 mg/m^2 day 1 [total dose/cycle = 60 mg/m^2]
   Cyclophosphamide: Oral: 600 mg/m^2 day 1 [total dose/cycle = 600 mg/m^2]
   Repeat cycle every 21 days for 4 cycles
   followed by
   Paclitaxel: I.V.: 80 mg/m^2 day 1 week 13 [total dose/cycle = 80 mg/m^2]
   Trastuzumab: I.V.: 4 mg/kg (loading dose) day 1 week 13 only [total dose/cycle = 4 mg/kg]
   followed by
   Paclitaxel: I.V.: 80 mg/m^2 weekly [total dose/cycle = 80 mg/m^2]
   Trastuzumab: I.V.: 2 mg/kg/weekly [total dose/cycle = 2 mg/kg]
   Repeat cycle every week for 11 cycles
   followed by
   Trastuzumab: I.V.: 2 mg/kg/weekly for 40 weeks

ACAV (J)
Use: Wilms tumor
Regimen:
   Dactinomycin: I.V.: 15 mcg/kg/day days 1-5 of weeks 0, 13, 26, 39, 52, 65
      [total dose/cycle = 450 mcg/kg]
   Cyclophosphamide: I.V.: 10 mg/kg/day days 1-3 of weeks 0, 6, 13, 19, 26, 32, 39, 45, 52, 58, 65
      [total dose/cycle = 330 mg/kg]
   Doxorubicin: I.V.: 20 mg/m^2/day days 1-3 of weeks 6, 19, 32, 45, 58
      [total dose/cycle = 300 mg/m^2]
   Vincristine: I.V.: 1.5 mg/m^2 day 1 of weeks 0-10, 13, 14, 19, 20, 26, 27, 32, 33, 39, 40, 45, 52, 53, 56, 57, 65, 66
      [total dose/cycle = 42 mg/m^2]

AD
Use: Soft tissue sarcoma
Regimen:
   Doxorubicin: I.V.: 60 mg/m^2/day day 1 [total dose/cycle = 60 mg/m^2]
   Dacarbazine: I.V.: 250 mg/m^2 days 1-5 [total dose/cycle = 1250 mg/m^2]
   Repeat cycle every 21 days

AI
Use: Soft tissue sarcoma
Regimen: Note: Multiple variations are listed below.
   Variation 1:
   Doxorubicin: I.V.: 25 mg/m^2/day continuous infusion days 1, 2, 3 [total dose/cycle = 75 mg/m^2]
   Ifosfamide: I.V.: 2 g/m^2/day days 1-5 [total dose/cycle = 10 g/m^2]
   Mesna: I.V.: 400 mg/m^2 day 1
   followed by I.V.: 1200 mg/m^2/day continuous infusion days 1-5 [total dose/cycle = 6400 mg/m^2]
   Repeat cycle every 3 weeks
   Variation 2:
   Doxorubicin: I.V.: 30 mg/m^2/day continuous infusion days 1, 2, 3 [total dose/cycle = 90 mg/m^2]
   Ifosfamide: I.V.: 2.5 g/m^2/day days 1-4 [total dose/cycle = 10 g/m^2]
   Mesna: I.V.: 500 mg/m^2 day 1
   followed by I.V.: 1500 mg/m^2/day continuous infusion days 1-4 [total dose/cycle = 6500 mg/m^2]
   Filgrastim: SubQ: 5 mcg/kg/day days 5 through ANC recovery
   Repeat cycle every 3 weeks

AP

Use: Endometrial Cancer
Regimen:
    Doxorubicin: I.V.: 60 mg/m^2 day 1 [total dose/cycle = 60 mg/m^2]
    Cisplatin: I.V.: 60 mg/m^2 day 1 [total dose/cycle = 60 mg/m^2]
    Repeat cycle every 21-28 days

AV (EE)

Use: Wilms Tumor
Regimen:
    Dactinomycin: I.V.: 15 mcg/kg/day days 1-5 of weeks 0, 5, 13, 26 [total dose/cycle = 300 mcg/kg]
    Vincristine: I.V.: 1.5 mg/m^2/dose day 1 of weeks 1-10, and days 1 and 5 of weeks 13 and 26
        [total dose/cycle = 21 mg/m^2]

AV (K)

Use: Wilms tumor
Regimen:
    Dactinomycin: I.V.: 15 mcg/kg/day days 1-5 of weeks 0, 5, 13, 22, 31, 40, 49, 58
        [total dose/cycle = 600 mcg/kg]
    Vincristine: I.V.: 1.5 mg/m^2/dose day 1 of weeks 0-10, 15-20, 24-29, 33-38, 42-47, 51-56, 60-65
        [total dose/cycle = 70.5 mg/m^2]

AV (L)

Use: Wilms tumor
Regimen:
    Dactinomycin: I.V.: 15 mcg/kg/day days 1-5 of weeks 0 and 5 [total dose/cycle = 150 mcg/kg]
    Vincristine: I.V.: 1.5 mg/m^2 day 1 of weeks 0-10 [total dose/cycle = 16.5 mg/m^2]

AV (Wilms tumor)

Use: Wilms tumor
Regimen:
    Dactinomycin: I.V.: 15 mcg/kg/day days 1-5 of weeks 0, 13, 26, 39, 52, 65
        [total dose/cycle = 450 mcg/kg]
    Vincristine: I.V.: 1.5 mg/m^2/dose day 1 of weeks 1-8, 13, 14, 26, 27, 39, 40, 52, 53, 65, 66
        [total dose/cycle = 27 mg/m^2]

AVD

Use: Wilms tumor
Regimen:
    Dactinomycin: I.V.: 15 mcg/kg/day days 1-5 of weeks 0, 13, 26, 39, 52, 65
        [total dose/cycle = 450 mcg/kg]
    Doxorubicin: I.V.: 60 mg/m^2/day day 1 of weeks 6, 19, 32, 45, 58
        [total dose/cycle = 300 mg/m^2]
    Vincristine: I.V.: 1.5 mg/m^2 day 1 of weeks 1-8, 13, 14, 26, 27, 39, 40, 52, 53, 65, 66
        [total dose/cycle = 27 mg/m^2]

BEACOPP

Use: Lymphoma, Hodgkin disease
Regimen:
    Bleomycin: I.V.: 10 units/m^2 day 8 [total dose/cycle = 10 units/m^2]
    Etoposide: I.V.: 100 mg/m^2/day days 1-3 [total dose/cycle = 300 mg/m^2]
    Doxorubicin: I.V.: 25 mg/m^2 day 1 [total dose/cycle = 25 mg/m^2]
    Cyclophosphamide: I.V.: 650 mg/m^2 day 1 [total dose/cycle = 650 mg/m^2]
    Vincristine: I.V.: 1.4 mg/m^2 (maximum 2 mg) day 8 [total dose/cycle = 1.4 mg/m^2; maximum 2 mg]
    Procarbazine: Oral: 100 mg/m^2/day days 1-7 [total dose/cycle = 700 mg/m^2]
    Prednisone: Oral: 40 mg/m^2/day days 1-14 [total dose/cycle = 560 mg/m^2]
    Repeat cycle every 21 days

BEP (Ovarian Cancer)
Use: Ovarian cancer
Regimen:
Bleomycin: I.V.: 20 units/m^2 (maximum 30 units) day 1 [total dose/cycle = 20 units/m^2]
Etoposide: I.V.: 75 mg/m^2/day days 1-5 [total dose/cycle = 375 mg/m^2]
or 75 mg/m^2/day days 1-4 (if received prior radiation therapy) [total dose/cycle = 300 mg/m^2]
Cisplatin: I.V.: 20 mg/m^2/day days 1-5 [total dose/cycle = 100 mg/m^2]
Repeat cycle every 3 weeks for 4 cycles

BEP (Ovarian Cancer, Testicular Cancer)
Use: Ovarian cancer; Testicular cancer
Regimen:
Bleomycin: I.V.: 30 units/day days 2, 9, 16 [total dose/cycle = 90 units]
Etoposide: I.V.: 100 mg/m^2/day days 1-5 [total dose/cycle = 500 mg/m^2]
or 120 mg/m^2/day days 1-3 [total dose/cycle = 360 mg/m^2]
Cisplatin: I.V.: 20 mg/m^2/day days 1-5 [total dose/cycle = 100 mg/m^2]
Repeat cycle every 21 days

BEP (Testicular Cancer)
Use: Testicular cancer
Regimen: Note: Multiple variations are listed below.
Variation 1:
Bleomycin: I.V.: 30 units/day days 2, 9, 16 [total dose/cycle = 90 units]
Etoposide: I.V.: 100 mg/m^2/day days 1-5 [total dose/cycle = 500 mg/m^2]
Cisplatin: I.V.: 20 mg/m^2/day days 1-5 [total dose/cycle = 100 mg/m^2]
Repeat cycle every 21 days
Variation 2:
Bleomycin: I.V.: 30 units once weekly [total dose/cycle = 90 units]
Etoposide: I.V.: 120 mg/m^2/day days 1, 3, 5 [total dose/cycle = 360 mg/m^2]
Cisplatin: I.V.: 20 mg/m^2/day days 1-5 [total dose/cycle = 100 mg/m^2]
Repeat cycle every 21 days
Variation 3:
Bleomycin: I.V.: 30 units/day days 1, 8, 15 [total dose/cycle = 90 units]
Etoposide: I.V.: 165 mg/m^2/day days 1-3 [total dose/cycle = 495 mg/m^2]
Cisplatin: I.V.: 50 mg/m^2/day days 1, 2 [total dose/cycle = 100 mg/m^2]
Repeat cycle every 21 days

Bevacizumab-Fluorouracil-Leucovorin
Use: Colorectal cancer
Regimen:
Bevacizumab: I.V.: 5 mg/kg/day days 1, 15, 29, 43 [total dose/cycle = 20 mg/kg]
Leucovorin: I.V.: 500 mg/m^2/day days 1, 8, 15, 22, 29, 36 [total dose/cycle = 3000 mg/m^2]
Fluorouracil: I.V.: 500 mg/m^2/day days 1, 8, 15, 22, 29, 36 [total dose/cycle = 3000 mg/m^2]
Repeat cycle every 56 days

Bevacizumab-Irinotecan-Fluorouracil-Leucovorin
Use: Colorectal cancer
Regimen:
Bevacizumab: I.V.: 5 mg/kg/day days 1, 15, 29 [total dose/cycle = 15 mg/kg]
Irinotecan: I.V.: 125 mg/m^2/day days 1, 8, 15, 22 [total dose/cycle = 500 mg/m^2]
Fluorouracil: I.V.: 500 mg/m^2/day days 1, 8, 15, 22 [total dose/cycle = 2000 mg/m^2]
Leucovorin: I.V.: 20 mg/m^2/day days 1, 8, 15, 22 [total dose/cycle = 80 mg/m^2]
Repeat cycle every 42 days

Bicalutamide + LHRH-A
Use: Prostate cancer
Regimen:
Bicalutamide: Oral: 50 mg/day [total dose/cycle = 50 mg] **with**
Goserelin acetate: SubQ: 3.6 mg day 1 [total dose/cycle = 3.6 mg] **or**
Leuprolide depot: I.M.: 7.5 mg day 1 [total dose/cycle = 7.5 mg]
Repeat cycle every 28 days

BIP

Use: Cervical cancer
Regimen:

Bleomycin: I.V.: 30 units continuous infusion day 1 [total dose/cycle = 30 units]
Cisplatin: I.V.: 50 mg/m^2 day 2 [total dose/cycle = 50 mg/m^2]
Ifosfamide: I.V.: 5 g/m^2 continuous infusion day 2 [total dose/cycle = 5 g/m^2]
Mesna: I.V.: 6 g/m^2 continuous infusion over 36 hours day 2 (start with ifosfamide) [total dose/cycle = 6 g/m^2]
Repeat cycle every 21 days

BOLD

Use: Melanoma
Regimen:

Dacarbazine: I.V.: 200 mg/m^2/day days 1-5 [total dose/cycle = 1000 mg/m^2]
Vincristine: I.V.: 1 mg/m^2/day days 1 and 4 [total dose/cycle = 2 mg/m^2]
Bleomycin: I.V.: 15 units/day days 2 and 5 [total dose/cycle = 30 units]
Lomustine: Oral: 80 mg day 1 [total dose/cycle = 80 mg]
Repeat cycle every 4 weeks

BOLD (Melanoma)

Use: Melanoma
Regimen: Note: Multiple variations are listed below.

Variation 1:

Bleomycin: SubQ: 7.5 units/day days 1 and 4 (cycle 1 only) **followed by** SubQ: 15 units/day days 1 and 4
   (subsequent cycles) [total dose/cycle = 45 units; maximum total dose (all cycles) = 400 units]
Vincristine: I.V.: 1 mg/m^2/day days 1 and 5 [total dose/cycle = 2 mg/m^2]
Lomustine: Oral: 80 mg/m^2 (maximum 150 mg/dose) day 1 [total dose/cycle = 80 mg/m^2]
Dacarbazine: I.V.: 200 mg/m^2/day (maximum 400 mg/dose) days 1-5
   [total dose/cycle = 1000 mg/m^2; maximum 2000 mg]
Repeat cycle every 4-6 weeks

Variation 2:

Bleomycin: I.V.: 15 units/day days 1 and 4 [total dose/cycle = 30 units]
Vincristine: I.V.: 1 mg/m^2/day days 1 and 5 [total dose/cycle = 2 mg/m^2]
Lomustine: Oral: 80 mg/m^2 (maximum 150 mg/dose) day 1 [total dose/cycle = 80 mg/m^2]
Dacarbazine: I.V.: 200 mg/m^2/day days 1-5 [total dose/cycle = 1000 mg/m^2]
Repeat cycle every 4 weeks

Variation 3:

Bleomycin: I.V.: 15 units/day days 1 and 4 [total dose/cycle = 30 units]
Vincristine: I.V.: 1 mg/m^2 day 1 [total dose/cycle = 1 mg/m^2]
Lomustine: Oral: 80 mg/m^2 day 3 (odd numbered cycles) [total dose/cycle = 80 mg/m^2; every other cycle]
Dacarbazine: I.V.: 200 mg/m^2/day days 1-5 [total dose/cycle = 1000 mg/m^2]
Repeat cycle every 4 weeks

BOLD + Interferon

Use: Melanoma
Regimen: Note: Multiple variations are listed below.

Variation 1:

Bleomycin: I.V.: 15 units/day days 2 and 5 [total dose/cycle = 30 units]
Vincristine: I.V.: 1 mg/m^2/day days 1 and 4 [total dose/cycle = 2 mg/m^2]
Lomustine: Oral: 80 mg day 1 [total dose/cycle = 80 mg]
Dacarbazine: I.V.: 200 mg/m^2/day days 1-5 [total dose/cycle = 1000 mg/m^2]
Interferon Alfa-2b: SubQ: 3 million units/day days 8-49 (cycles 1 and 2)
   [total dose through day 49 = 126 million units]
followed by SubQ: 6 million units 3 times/week (beginning day 50 and subsequent cycles)
   [total dose/cycle = 72 million units]
Repeat cycle every 4 weeks

Variation 2:

Bleomycin: I.V.: 30 units days 1 [total dose/cycle = 30 units]

Vincristine: I.V.: 2 mg day 1 [total dose/cycle = 2 mg]

Lomustine: Oral: 80 mg day 1 [total dose/cycle = 80 mg]

Dacarbazine: I.V.: 700 mg/m^2 day 1 [total dose/cycle = 700 mg/m^2]

Interferon Alfa-2b: SubQ: 3 million units 3 times/week [total dose/cycle = 36 million units]

Repeat cycle every 4 weeks

Variation 3:

Bleomycin: I.V.: 15 units/day days 2 and 5 [total dose/cycle = 30 units]

Vincristine: I.V.: 1-2 mg/day days 1 and 4 [total dose/cycle = 2-4 mg]

Lomustine: Oral: 80 mg day 1 [total dose/cycle = 80 mg]

Dacarbazine: I.V.: 200 mg/m^2/day days 1-5 [total dose/cycle = 1000 mg/m^2]

Interferon Alfa-2b: SubQ: 6 million units 3 times/week, for 6 doses, starting day 8
[total dose/cycle = 36 million units]

Repeat cycle every 4 weeks

Variation 4:

Bleomycin: I.V.: 15 units/day days 2 and 5 [total dose/cycle = 30 units]

Vincristine: I.V.: 1 mg/m^2/day (maximum 2 mg/dose) days 1 and 4 [total dose/cycle = 2 mg/m^2]

Lomustine: Oral: 80 mg day 1 [total dose/cycle = 80 mg]

Dacarbazine: I.V.: 200 mg/m^2/day days 1-5 [total dose/cycle = 1000 mg/m^2]

Interferon Alfa-2b: SubQ: 3 million units/day days 8, 10, 12, 15, 17, 19 [total dose/cycle = 18 million units]

Repeat cycle every 4 weeks

Bortezomib-Doxorubicin (Liposomal)

Use: Multiple myeloma

Regimen:

Bortezomib: I.V.: 1.3 mg/m^2/day days 1, 4, 8, 11
[total dose/cycle = 5.2 mg/m^2]

Doxorubicin (liposomal): I.V.: 30 mg/m^2 day 4 [total dose/cycle = 30 mg/m^2]

Repeat cycle every 21 days for up to 8 cycles

CA

Use: Leukemia, acute myeloid

Regimen:

Cytarabine: I.V.: 3000 mg/m^2 every 12 hours days 1 and 2 (4 doses)
[total dose/cycle = 12,000 mg/m^2]

Asparaginase: I.M.: 6000 units/m^2 at hour 42 [total dose/cycle = 6000 units/m^2]

Repeat cycle every 7 days for 2 or 3 cycles

CABO

Use: Head and neck cancer

Regimen:

Cisplatin: I.V.: 50 mg/m^2 day 4 [total dose/cycle = 50 mg/m^2]

Methotrexate: I.V.: 40 mg/m^2/day days 1 and 15 [total dose/cycle = 80 mg/m^2]

Bleomycin: I.V.: 10 units/day days 1, 8, and 15 [total dose/cycle = 30 units]

Vincristine: I.V.: 2 mg/day days 1, 8, and 15 [total dose/cycle = 6 mg]

Repeat cycle every 21 days

CAD/MOPP/ABV
Use: Lymphoma, Hodgkin disease
Regimen:
CAD:
Lomustine: Oral: 100 mg/m² day 1 [total dose/cycle = 100 mg/m²]
Melphalan: Oral: 6 mg/m²/day days 1-4 [total dose/cycle = 24 mg/m²]
Vindesine: I.V.: 3 mg/m²/day days 1 and 8 [total dose/cycle = 6 mg/m²]
MOPP:
Mechlorethamine: I.V.: 6 mg/m²/day days 1 and 8 [total dose/cycle = 12 mg/m²]
Vincristine: I.V.: 1.4 mg/m²/day days 1 and 8 [total dose/cycle = 2.8 mg/m²]
Procarbazine: Oral: 100 mg/m²/day days 1-14 [total dose/cycle = 1400 mg/m²]
Prednisone: Oral: 40 mg/m²/day days 1-14 [total dose/cycle = 560 mg/m²]
ABV:
Doxorubicin: I.V.: 25 mg/m²/day days 1 and 14 [total dose/cycle = 50 mg/m²]
Bleomycin: SubQ: 6 units/m²/day days 1 and 14 [total dose/cycle = 12 units/m²]
Vinblastine: I.V.: 2 mg/m² continuous infusion days 4-12 and 18-26 [total dose/cycle = 36 mg/m²]
CAD is administered first, then MOPP begins on day 29 or day 37 following CAD. ABV is administered on day 29 following MOPP; CAD recycles on day 29 following ABV.

CAF
Use: Breast cancer
Regimen: Note: Multiple variations are listed below.
Variation 1:
Cyclophosphamide: Oral: 100 mg/m²/day days 1-14 [total dose/cycle = 1400 mg/m²]
Doxorubicin: I.V.: 30 mg/m²/day days 1 and 8 [total dose/cycle = 60 mg/m²]
Fluorouracil: I.V.: 500 mg/m²/day days 1 and 8 [total dose/cycle = 1000 mg/m²]
Repeat cycle every 28 days
Variation 2:
Cyclophosphamide: Oral: 100 mg/m²/day days 1-14 [total dose/cycle = 1400 mg/m²]
Doxorubicin: I.V.: 25 mg/m²/day days 1 and 8 [total dose/cycle = 50 mg/m²]
Fluorouracil: I.V.: 500 mg/m²/day days 1 and 8 [total dose/cycle = 1000 mg/m²]
Repeat cycle every 28 days

CAP
Use: Bladder Cancer
Regimen:
Cyclophosphamide: I.V.: 400 mg/m² day 1 [total dose = 400 mg/m²]
Doxorubicin: I.V.: 40 mg/m² day 1 [total dose = 40 mg/m²]
Cisplatin: I.V.: 60 mg/m² day 1 [total dose = 60 mg/m²]
Repeat cycle every 21 days

Capecitabine + Docetaxel (Breast Cancer)
Use: Breast cancer
Regimen: Note: Multiple variations are listed below.
Variation 1:
Capecitabine: Oral: 1250 mg/m² twice daily days 1-14 [total dose/cycle = 35,000 mg/m²]
Docetaxel: I.V.: 75 mg/m² day 1 [total dose/cycle = 75 mg/m²]
Repeat cycle every 3 weeks
Variation 2:
Capecitabine: Oral: 1000 mg/m² twice daily days 2-15 [total dose/cycle = 28,000 mg/m²]
Docetaxel: I.V.: 75 mg/m² day 1 [total dose/cycle = 75 mg/m²]
Repeat cycle every 3 weeks
Variation 3:
Capecitabine: Oral: 937.5 mg/m² twice daily days 2-15 [total dose/cycle = 26,250 mg/m²]
Docetaxel: I.V.: 60 mg/m² day 1 [total dose/cycle = 60 mg/m²]
Repeat cycle every 3 weeks

Capecitabine + Docetaxel (Gastric Cancer)

Use: Gastric cancer

Regimen: Note: Multiple variations are listed below.

Variation 1:

Capecitabine: Oral: 1000 mg/m^2 twice daily days 1-14 [total dose/cycle = 28,000 mg/m^2]

Docetaxel: I.V.: 75 mg/m^2 day 1 [total dose/cycle = 75 mg/m^2]

Repeat cycle every 3 weeks

Variation 2:

Capecitabine: Oral: 1000 mg/m^2 twice daily days 1-14 [total dose/cycle = 28,000 mg/m^2]

Docetaxel: I.V.: 36 mg/m^2 days 1 and 8 [total dose/cycle = 72 mg/m^2]

Repeat cycle every 3 weeks

Capecitabine + Docetaxel (Nonsmall Cell Lung Cancer)

Use: Lung cancer, nonsmall cell

Regimen: Note: Multiple variations are listed below.

Variation 1:

Capecitabine: Oral: 1000 mg/m^2 twice daily days 1-14 [total dose/cycle = 28,000 mg/m^2]

Docetaxel: I.V.: 36 mg/m^2 days 1 and 8 [total dose/cycle = 72 mg/m^2]

Repeat cycle every 3 weeks

Variation 2:

Capecitabine: Oral: 625 mg/m^2 twice daily days 5-18 [total dose/cycle = 17,500 mg/m^2]

Docetaxel: I.V.: 36 mg/m^2 days 1, 8, 15 [total dose/cycle = 108 mg/m^2]

Repeat cycle every 4 weeks

Capecitabine + Lapatinib

Use: Breast cancer

Regimen:

Capecitabine: Oral: 1000 mg/m^2 twice daily days 1-14 [total dose/cycle = 28,000 mg/m^2]

Lapatinib: Oral: 1250 mg/day days 1-21 [total dose/cycle = 26,250 mg]

Repeat cycle every 3 weeks

Carbo-Tax (Adenocarcinoma)

Use: Adenocarcinoma, unknown primary

Regimen:

Paclitaxel: I.V.: 135 mg/m^2 infused over 24 hours day 1 [total dose = 135 mg/m^2]

followed by:

Carboplatin: I.V.: Target AUC 7.5 [total dose = AUC = 7.5]

Repeat cycle every 21 days

Carbo-Tax (Nonsmall Cell Lung Cancer)

Use: Lung cancer, nonsmall cell

Regimen:

Paclitaxel: I.V.: 135-215 mg/m^2 infused over 24 hours day 1 [total dose/cycle = 135-215 mg/m^2] **or**

175 mg/m^2 infused over 3 hours day 1 [total dose/cycle = 175 mg/m^2] **followed by:**

Carboplatin: I.V.: Target AUC 7.5 [total dose/cycle = AUC = 7.5]

Repeat cycle every 21 days

Carbo-Tax (Ovarian Cancer)

Use: Ovarian cancer
Regimen: Note: Multiple variations are listed below.
Variation 1:
Paclitaxel: I.V.: 135 mg/m^2 infused over 24 hours day 1 [total dose/cycle = 135 mg/m^2] **or**
175 mg/m^2 over 3 hours day 1 [total dose/cycle = 175 mg/m^2]
followed by:
Carboplatin: I.V.: Target AUC 5 [total dose/cycle = AUC = 5]
Repeat cycle every 21 days
Variation 2:
Paclitaxel: I.V.: 175 mg/m^2 day 1 [total dose/cycle = 175 mg/m^2]
Carboplatin: I.V.: AUC 7.5 day 1 [total dose/cycle = AUC = 7.5]
Repeat cycle every 21 days
Variation 3:
Paclitaxel: I.V.: 185 mg/m^2 day 1 [total dose/cycle = 185 mg/m^2]
Carboplatin: I.V.: AUC 6 day 1 [total dose/cycle = AUC = 6]
Repeat cycle every 21 days

CaT (Nonsmall Cell Lung Cancer)

Use: Lung cancer, nonsmall cell
Regimen: Note: Multiple variations are listed below.
Variation 1:
Paclitaxel: I.V.: 175 mg/m^2 day 1 [total dose/cycle = 175 mg/m^2] **or**
135 mg/m^2 continuous infusion day 1 [total dose/cycle = 135 mg/m^2]
Carboplatin: I.V.: AUC 7.5 day 1 or 2 [total dose/cycle = AUC = 7.5]
Repeat cycle every 21 days
Variation 2:
Paclitaxel: I.V.: 225 mg/m^2 day 1 [total dose/cycle = 225 mg/m^2]
Carboplatin: I.V.: AUC 6 day 1 [total dose/cycle = AUC = 6]
Repeat cycle every 21 days

CaT (Ovarian Cancer)

Use: Ovarian cancer
Regimen:
Paclitaxel: I.V.: 175 mg/m^2 day 1 [total dose/cycle = 175 mg/m^2] **or**
135 mg/m^2 continuous infusion day 1 [total dose/cycle = 135 mg/m^2]
Carboplatin: I.V.: AUC 7.5 day 1 or 2 [total dose/cycle = AUC = 7.5]
Repeat cycle every 21 days

CAVE

Use: Lung cancer, small cell
Regimen:
Cyclophosphamide: I.V.: 750 mg/m^2 day 1 [total dose/cycle = 750 mg/m^2]
Doxorubicin: I.V.: 50 mg/m^2 day 1 [total dose/cycle = 50 mg/m^2]
Vincristine: I.V.: 1.4 mg/m^2 (maximum 2 mg) day 1 [total dose/cycle = 1.4 mg/m^2]
Etoposide: I.V.: 60-100 mg/m^2/day days 1-3 [total dose/cycle = 180-300 mg/m^2]
Repeat cycle every 21 days

CAV-P/VP

Use: Neuroblastoma
Regimen:
Course 1, 2, 4, 6:
Cyclophosphamide: I.V.: 70 mg/kg/day days 1 and 2 [total dose/cycle = 140 mg/kg]
Doxorubicin: I.V.: 25 mg/m^2/day continuous infusion days 1-3 [total dose/cycle = 75 mg/m^2]
Vincristine: I.V.: 0.033 mg/kg/day continuous infusion days 1-3 [total dose/cycle = .099 mg/kg]
Vincristine: I.V.: 1.5 mg/m^2 day 9
Course 3, 5, 7:
Etoposide: I.V.: 200 mg/m^2/day days 1-3 [total dose/cycle = 600 mg/m^2]
Cisplatin: I.V.: 50 mg/m^2/day days 1-4 [total dose/cycle = 200 mg/m^2]

CC
Use: Ovarian cancer
Regimen:
   Carboplatin: I.V.: Target AUC 5-7.5 day 1 [total dose/cycle = AUC = 5-7.5]
   Cyclophosphamide: I.V.: 600 mg/m^2 day 1 [total dose/cycle = 600 mg/m^2]
   Repeat cycle every 28 days

CCCDE (Retinoblastoma)
Use: Retinoblastoma
Regimen:
   Cyclophosphamide: I.V.: 150 mg/m^2/day days 1-7 [total dose/cycle = 1050 mg/m^2]
   Cyclophosphamide: Oral: 150 mg/m^2/day days 22-28, 43-49 [total dose/cycle = 2100 mg/m^2]
   Doxorubicin: I.V.: 35 mg/m^2/day days 10 and 52 [total dose/cycle = 70 mg/m^2]
   Cisplatin: I.V.: 90 mg/m^2/day days 8, 50, 71 [total dose/cycle = 270 mg/m^2]
   Etoposide: I.V.: 150 mg/m^2/day continuous infusion days 29-31, 73-75
      [total dose/cycle = 900 mg/m^2]

CCDDT (Neuroblastoma)
Use: Neuroblastoma
Regimen:
   Cyclophosphamide: I.V.: 40 mg/kg/day days 1 and 2 [total dose/cycle = 80 mg/kg]
   Cisplatin: I.V.: 20 mg/m^2/day days 1-5 [total dose/cycle = 100 mg/m^2]
   Teniposide: I.V.: 100 mg/m^2 day 7 [total dose/cycle = 100 mg/m^2]
   Doxorubicin: I.V.: 60 mg/m^2 day 1 [total dose/cycle = 60 mg/m^2]
   Dacarbazine: I.V.: 250 mg/m^2/day days 1-5 [total dose/cycle = 1250 mg/m^2]
   Repeat cycle every 21-28 days

CCDT (Melanoma)
Use: Melanoma
Regimen:
   Dacarbazine: I.V.: 220 mg/m^2/day days 1-3, every 21-28 days [total dose/cycle = 660 mg/m^2]
   Carmustine: I.V.: 150 mg/m^2 day 1, every 42-56 days [total dose/cycle = 150 mg/m^2]
   Cisplatin: I.V.: 25 mg/m^2/day days 1-3, every 21-28 days [total dose/cycle = 75 mg/m^2]
   Tamoxifen: Oral: 20 mg/day (use of tamoxifen is optional)

CCT (Neuroblastoma)
Use: Neuroblastoma
Regimen:
   Cyclophosphamide: I.V.: 40 mg/kg/day days 1 and 2 [total dose/cycle = 80 mg/kg]
   Cisplatin: I.V.: 20 mg/m^2/day days 22-26 [total dose/cycle = 100 mg/m^2]
   Teniposide: I.V.: 100 mg/m^2 day 28 [total dose/cycle = 100 mg/m^2]
   Repeat every 42 days for 3 cycles

CDDP/VP-16
Use: Brain tumors
Regimen:
   Cisplatin: I.V.: 90 mg/m^2 day 1 [total dose/cycle = 90 mg/m^2]
   Etoposide: I.V.: 150 mg/m^2/day days 3 and 4 [total dose/cycle = 300 mg/m^2]
   Repeat cycle every 21 days

CE (Neuroblastoma)
Use: Neuroblastoma
Regimen:
   Carboplatin: I.V.: 500 mg/m^2/day days 1 and 2 [total dose/cycle = 1000 mg/m^2]
   Etoposide: I.V.: 100 mg/m^2/day days 1-3 [total dose/cycle = 300 mg/m^2]
   Repeat cycle every 21-28 days

CE (Retinoblastoma)

Use: Retinoblastoma
Regimen:
Etoposide: I.V.: 100 mg/m^2/day days 1-5 [total dose/cycle = 500 mg/m^2]
Carboplatin: I.V.: 160 mg/m^2/day days 1-5 [total dose/cycle = 800 mg/m^2]
Repeat cycle every 21 days

CE-CAdO

Use: Neuroblastoma
Regimen:
Carboplatin: I.V.: 160 mg/m^2/day days 1-5 [total dose/cycle = 800 mg/m^2]
Etoposide: I.V.: 100 mg/m^2/day days 1-5 [total dose/cycle = 500 mg/m^2] **or**
Carboplatin: I.V.: 200 mg/m^2/day days 1-3 [total dose/cycle = 600 mg/m^2]
Etoposide: I.V.: 150 mg/m^2/day days 1-3 [total dose/cycle = 450 mg/m^2] **and**
Cyclophosphamide: I.V.: 300 mg/m^2/day days 1-5 [total dose/cycle = 1500 mg/m^2]
Doxorubicin: I.V.: 60 mg/m^2 day 5 [total dose/cycle = 60 mg/m^2]
Vincristine: I.V.: 1.5 mg/m^2/day days 1 and 5 [total dose/cycle = 3 mg/m^2]
Repeat cycle every 21 days

CEF

Use: Breast cancer
Regimen:
Cyclophosphamide: Oral: 75 mg/m^2/day days 1-14 [total dose/cycle = 1050 mg/m^2]
Epirubicin: I.V.: 60 mg/m^2/day days 1 and 8 [total dose/cycle = 120 mg/m^2]
Fluorouracil: I.V.: 500 mg/m^2/day days 1 and 8 [total dose/cycle = 1000 mg/m^2]
Repeat cycle every 28 days

CEPP(B)

Use: Lymphoma, non-Hodgkin
Regimen:
Cyclophosphamide: I.V.: 600-650 mg/m^2/day days 1 and 8 [total dose/cycle = 1200-1300 mg/m^2]
Etoposide: I.V.: 70-85 mg/m^2/day days 1-3   [total dose/cycle = 210-255 mg/m^2]
Procarbazine: Oral: 60 mg/m^2/day days 1-10 [total dose/cycle = 600 mg/m^2]
Prednisone: Oral: 60 mg/m^2/day days 1-10 [total dose/cycle = 600 mg/m^2]
Bleomycin: I.V.: 15 units/m^2/day days 1 and 15 (bleomycin is sometimes omitted)
   [total dose/cycle = 30 units/m^2]
Repeat cycle every 28 days

Cetuximab-Irinotecan

Use: Colorectal cancer
Regimen: Note: Multiple variations are listed below.
   Variation 1:
   Cycle 1:
   Cetuximab: I.V.: 400 mg/m^2 (loading dose) day 1 (week 1, cycle 1 only) [total loading dose = 400 mg/m^2]**followed**
      by I.V.: 250 mg/m^2/day days 8, 15, 22, 29, 36 [total dose/cycle 1 = 1650 mg/m^2]
   Irinotecan: I.V.: 125 mg/m^2/day days 1, 8, 15, 22 [total dose/cycle = 500 mg/m^2]
   Subsequent cycles:
   Cetuximab: I.V.: 250 mg/m^2/day days 1, 8, 15, 22, 29, 36 [total dose/cycle = 1500 mg/m^2]
   Irinotecan: I.V.: 125 mg/m^2/day days 1, 8, 15, 22 [total dose/cycle = 500 mg/m^2]
   Repeat cycle every 42 days
   Variation 2:
   Cycle 1:
   Cetuximab: I.V.: 400 mg/m^2 (loading dose) day 1 (week 1, cycle 1 only)
      [total loading dose = 400 mg/m^2]
      followed by I.V.: 250 mg/m^2/day days 8 and 15 (cycle 1) [total dose/cycle 1 = 900 mg/m^2]
   Irinotecan: I.V.: 350 mg/m^2 day 1 [total dose/cycle = 350 mg/m^2]
   Subsequent cycles:
   Cetuximab: I.V.: 250 mg/m^2/day days 1, 8, 15, [total dose/cycle = 750 mg/m^2]
   Irinotecan: I.V.: 350 mg/m^2 day 1 [total dose/cycle = 350 mg/m^2]
   Repeat cycle every 21 days

CEV

Use: Rhabdomyosarcoma
Regimen:
Carboplatin: I.V.: 500 mg/m² day 1 [total dose/cycle = 500 mg/m²]
Epirubicin: I.V.: 150 mg/m² day 1 [total dose/cycle = 150 mg/m²]
Vincristine: I.V.: 1.5 mg/m²/day days 1 and 7 [total dose/cycle = 3 mg/m²]
Repeat cycle every 21 days

CF

Use: Head and neck cancer
Regimen: Note: Multiple variations are listed below.
Variation 1:
Cisplatin: I.V.: 100 mg/m² day 1 [total dose/cycle = 100 mg/m²]
Fluorouracil: I.V.: 1000 mg/m²/day continuous infusion days 1-4 [total dose/cycle = 4000 mg/m²]
Repeat cycle every 3-4 weeks
Variation 2:
Cisplatin: I.V.: 100 mg/m² day 1 [total dose/cycle = 100 mg/m²]
Fluorouracil: I.V.: 1000 mg/m²/day continuous infusion days 1-5 [total dose/cycle = 5000 mg/m²]
Repeat cycle every 3 or 4 weeks
Variation 3:
Cisplatin: I.V.: 60 mg/m² day 1 [total dose/cycle = 60 mg/m²]
Fluorouracil: I.V.: 800 mg/m²/day continuous infusion days 1-5 [total dose/cycle = 4000 mg/m²]
Repeat cycle every 14 days
Variation 4:
Cisplatin: I.V.: 20 mg/m²/day days 1-5 [total dose/cycle = 100 mg/m²]
Fluorouracil: I.V.: 200 mg/m²/day days 1-5 [total dose/cycle = 1000 mg/m²]
Repeat cycle every 3 weeks
Variation 5:
Cisplatin: I.V.: 80 mg/m²/day continuous infusion day 1 [total dose/cycle = 80 mg/m²]
Fluorouracil: I.V.: 800 mg/m²/day continuous infusion days 2-6 [total dose/cycle = 4000 mg/m²]
Repeat cycle every 3 weeks
Variation 6:
Cisplatin: I.V.: 75 mg/m² day 1 [total dose/cycle = 75 mg/m²]
Fluorouracil: I.V.: 1000 mg/m²/day continuous infusion days 1-4 [total dose/cycle = 4000 mg/m²]
Repeat cycle every 4 weeks
Variation 7:
Cisplatin: I.V.: 120 mg/m² day 1 [total dose/cycle = 120 mg/m²]
Fluorouracil: I.V.: 1000 mg/m²/day continuous infusion days 1-5 [total dose/cycle = 5000 mg/m²]
Repeat cycle every 3 weeks
Variation 8:
Cisplatin: I.V.: 25 mg/m²/day continuous infusion days 1-4 [total dose/cycle = 100 mg/m²]
Fluorouracil: I.V.: 1000 mg/m²/day days 1-4 [total dose/cycle = 4000 mg/m²]
Repeat cycle every 3 weeks
Variation 9:
Fluorouracil: I.V.: 350 mg/m²/day continuous infusion days 1-5 [total dose/cycle = 1750 mg/m²]
Cisplatin: I.V.: 50 mg/m² day 6 [total dose/cycle = 50 mg/m²]
Repeat cycle every 3 weeks
Variation 10:
Cisplatin: I.V.: 5 mg/m²/day continuous infusion days 1-14 [total dose/cycle = 70 mg/m²]
Fluorouracil: I.V.: 200 mg/m²/day continuous infusion days 1-14 [total dose/cycle = 2800 mg/m²]
With concurrent radiation therapy, cycle does not repeat

CFP

Use: Breast cancer
Regimen:
Cyclophosphamide: I.V.: 150 mg/m²/day days 1-5 [total dose/cycle = 750 mg/m²]
Fluorouracil: I.V.: 300 mg/m²/day days 1-5 [total dose/cycle = 1500 mg/m²]
Prednisone: Oral: 30 mg/day days 1-14 (cycle 1 only)
    followed by Oral: 20 mg/day days 15-21 (cycle 1 only)
    followed by Oral: 10 mg daily thereafter as maintenance
    [total dose/cycle = 700 mg in cycle 1; 350 mg in subsequent cycles]
Repeat cycle every 35 days

CHAMOCA (Modified Bagshawe Regimen)

Use: Gestational trophoblastic tumor

Regimen: Note: Multiple variations are listed below.

Variation 1:

Hydroxyurea: Oral: 500 mg every 6 hours, for 4 doses, day 1 (start at 6 AM)
[total dose/cycle = 2000 mg]

Dactinomycin: I.V.: 0.2 mg/day days 1-3 (give at 7 PM) **followed by** 0.5 mg/day days 4 and 5 (give at 7 PM) [total dose/cycle = 1.6 mg]

Cyclophosphamide: I.V.: 500 mg/m^2/day days 3 and 8 (give at 7 PM)
[total dose/cycle = 1000 mg/m^2]

Vincristine: I.V.: 1 mg/m^2 (maximum 2 mg) day 2 (give at 7 AM) [total dose/cycle = 1 mg/m^2; maximum 2 mg]

Methotrexate: I.V. bolus: 100 mg/m^2 day 2 (give at 7 PM) **followed by** 200 mg/m^2 continuous infusion over 12 hours day 2 [total dose/cycle = 300 mg/m^2]

Leucovorin: I.M.: 14 mg every 6 hours for 6 doses days 3-5 (begin at 7 PM on day 3; start 24 hours after the start of methotrexate)
[total dose/cycle = 84 mg]

Doxorubicin: I.V.: 30 mg/m^2 day 8 (give at 7 PM) [total dose/cycle = 30 mg/m^2]

Repeat cycle every 18 days or as toxicity permits (cycle may be repeated 10 days after last treatment)

Variation 2:

Hydroxyurea: Oral: 500 mg every 12 hours, for 4 doses, days 1 and 2 (usually started in early morning)
[total dose/cycle = 2000 mg]

Dactinomycin: I.V.: 10 mcg/kg/day days 5, 6, 7 [total dose/cycle = 30 mcg/kg]

Vincristine: I.V.: 1 mg/m^2 day 3 [total dose/cycle = 1 mg/m^2]

Methotrexate: I.V. bolus: 100 mg/m^2 day 3 **followed by** I.V.: 200 mg/m^2 continuous infusion over 12 hours day 3
[total dose/cycle = 300 mg/m^2]

Leucovorin: I.M.: 10 mg/m^2 every 12 hours, for 4 doses, days 4 and 5 (start 24 hours after the start of methotrexate)
[total dose/cycle = 40 mg/m^2]

Cyclophosphamide: I.V.: 600 mg/m^2 day 5
[total dose/cycle = 600 mg/m^2]

Doxorubicin: I.V.: 30 mg/m^2 day 10 [total dose/cycle = 30 mg/m^2]

Repeat cycle every 3 weeks

Variation 3:

Hydroxyurea: Oral: 500 mg every 12 hours, for 4 doses, days 1 and 2 (usually started in early morning)
[total dose/cycle = 2000 mg/m^2]

Vincristine: I.V.: 1 mg/m^2 day 3 [total dose/cycle = 1 mg/m^2]

Methotrexate: I.V. bolus: 100 mg/m^2 day 3 **followed by** 200 mg/m^2 continuous infusion over 12 hours day 3 [total dose/cycle = 300 mg/m^2]

Leucovorin: I.M.: 14 mg every 6 hours, for 6 doses, days 4, 5, 6 (start 24 hours after start of methotrexate)
[total dose/cycle = 84 mg]

Dactinomycin: I.V.: 0.2 mg/day days 2, 3, 4 **followed by** I.V.: 0.5 mg/day days 5 and 6 [total dose/cycle = 1.6 mg]

Cyclophosphamide: I.V.: 500 mg/m^2 day 4
[total dose/cycle = 500 mg/m^2]

Doxorubicin: I.V.: 30 mg/m^2 day 9 [total dose/cycle = 30 mg/m^2]

Melphalan: I.V.: 6 mg/m^2 day 9 [total dose/cycle = 6 mg/m^2]

Repeat cycle approximately every 3 weeks

Variation 4:

Hydroxyurea: Oral: 500 mg 4 times/day, for 4 doses, day 1
[total dose/cycle = 2000 mg/m^2]

Vincristine: I.V.: 1 mg/m^2 day 2 [total dose/cycle = 1 mg/m^2]

Methotrexate: I.V. bolus: 100 mg/m^2 day 2 **followed by** 200 mg/m^2 continuous infusion over 12 hours day 2 [total dose/cycle = 300 mg/m^2]

Leucovorin: I.M.: 14 mg every 6 hours, for 6 doses, days 3, 4, 5 (start 24 hours after the start of methotrexate)
[total dose/cycle = 84 mg]

Dactinomycin: I.V.: 0.2 mg days 1, 2, 3, then 0.5 mg days 4 and 5 [total dose/cycle = 1.6 mg]

Cyclophosphamide: I.V.: 500 mg/m^2 day 3
[total dose/cycle = 500 mg/m^2]

Cyclophosphamide: I.V.: 300 mg/m^2 on day 8
[total dose/cycle = 300 mg/m^2]

Doxorubicin: I.V.: 30 mg/m^2 day 8 [total dose/cycle = 30 mg/m^2]

Repeat cycle approximately every 3 weeks

CHAMOMA (Bagshawe Regimen)
Use: Gestational trophoblastic tumor
Regimen:
Hydroxyurea: Oral: 500 mg every 12 hours, for 4 doses, days 1 and 2
   [total dose/cycle = 2000 mg]
Vincristine: I.V.: 1 mg/m^2 day 3 [total dose/cycle = 1 mg/m^2]
Methotrexate: I.V. bolus: 100 mg/m^2 day 3 **followed by** I.V.: 200 mg/m^2 continuous infusion over 12 hours day 3
   [total dose/cycle = 300 mg/m^2]
Leucovorin: I.M.: 12 mg/m^2 every 12 hours, for 4 doses, days 4 and 5 (start 12 hours after the end of methotrexate
   infusion)
   [total dose/cycle = 48 mg/m^2]
Dactinomycin: I.V.: 10 mcg/kg/day days 5, 6, 7 [total dose/cycle = 30 mcg/kg]
Cyclophosphamide: I.V.: 600 mg/m^2 day 5
   [total dose/cycle = 600 mg/m^2]
Doxorubicin: I.V.: 30 mg/m^2 day 10 [total dose/cycle = 30 mg/m^2]
Melphalan: I.V.: 6 mg/m^2 day 10 [total dose/cycle = 6 mg/m^2]
Repeat cycle approximately every 3 weeks

ChIVPP
Use: Lymphoma, Hodgkin disease
Regimen:
Chlorambucil: Oral: 6 mg/m^2/day (maximum 10 mg) days 1-14 [total dose/cycle = 84 mg/m^2]
Vinblastine: I.V.: 6 mg/m^2/day (maximum 10 mg) days 1 and 8 [total dose/cycle = 12 mg/m^2]
Procarbazine: Oral: 100 mg/m^2/day (maximum 150 mg) days 1-14
   [total dose/cycle = 1400 mg/m^2]
Prednisone: Oral: 40-50 mg/m^2/day days 1-14 [total dose/cycle = 560-700 mg]
Repeat cycle every 28 days

CHL + PRED
Use: Leukemia, chronic lymphocytic
Regimen:
Chlorambucil: Oral: 0.4 mg/kg/day for 1 day every other week; increase initial dose of 0.4 mg/kg by 0.1 mg/kg every
   2 weeks until toxicity or disease control is achieved
Prednisone: Oral: 100 mg/day for 2 days every other week

CHOP
Use: Lymphoma, non-Hodgkin
Regimen: Note: Multiple variations are listed below.
Variation 1:
Cyclophosphamide: I.V.: 750 mg/m^2 day 1 [total dose/cycle = 750 mg/m^2]
Doxorubicin: I.V.: 50 mg/m^2 day 1 [total dose/cycle = 50 mg/m^2]
Vincristine: I.V.: 1.4 mg/m^2 (maximum 2 mg) day 1 [total dose/cycle = 1.4 mg/m^2]
Prednisone: Oral: 100 mg/day days 1-5 [total dose/cycle = 500 mg]
or 50 mg/m^2/day days 1-5 [total dose/cycle = 250 mg/m^2]
or 100 mg/m^2/day days 1-5 [total dose/cycle = 500 mg/m^2]
Repeat cycle every 21 days
Variation 2:
Cyclophosphamide: I.V.: 750 mg/m^2 day 1 [total dose/cycle = 750 mg/m^2]
Doxorubicin: I.V.: 50 mg/m^2 day 1 [total dose/cycle = 50 mg/m^2]
Vincristine: I.V.: 2 mg day 1 [total dose/cycle = 2 mg]
Prednisone: Oral: 75 mg/day days 1-5 [total dose/cycle = 375 mg]
Repeat cycle every 21 days
Variation 3:
Cyclophosphamide: I.V.: 750 mg/m^2/day days 1 and 8 [total dose/cycle = 1500 mg/m^2]
Doxorubicin: I.V.: 25 mg/m^2/day days 1 and 8 [total dose/cycle = 50 mg/m^2]
Vincristine: I.V.: 1.4 mg/m^2/day (maximum 2 mg) days 1 and 8 [total dose/cycle = 2.8 mg/m^2]
Prednisone: Oral: 50 mg/m^2/day days 1-8 [total dose/cycle = 400 mg/m^2]
Repeat cycle every 28 days
Variation 4 (mini-CHOP):
Cyclophosphamide: I.V.: 250 mg/m^2/day days 1, 8, 15 [total dose/cycle = 750 mg/m^2]
Doxorubicin: I.V.: 16.7 mg/m^2/day days 1, 8, 15 [total dose/cycle = 50.1 mg/m^2]
Vincristine: I.V.: 0.67 mg/day days 1, 8, 15 [total dose/cycle = 2.01 mg]
Prednisone: Oral: 75 mg/day days 1-5 [total dose/cycle = 375 mg]
Repeat cycle every 21 days

CI (Neuroblastoma)

Use: Neuroblastoma
Regimen:
Ifosfamide: I.V.: 1500 mg/m^2/day days 1-3 [total dose/cycle = 4500 mg/m^2]
Mesna: I.V.: 500 mg/m^2 every 3 hours, for 3 doses each day, days 1-3 [total dose/cycle = 4500 mg/m^2]
Carboplatin: I.V.: 400 mg/m^2 day 4 [total dose/cycle = 400 mg/m^2]
Repeat cycle every 21-28 days

CISCA

Use: Bladder cancer
Regimen:
Cyclophosphamide: I.V.: 650 mg/m^2 day 1 [total dose = 650 mg/m^2]
Doxorubicin: I.V.: 50 mg/m^2 day 1 [total dose = 50 mg/m^2]
Cisplatin: I.V.: 100 mg/m^2 day 2 [total dose = 100 mg/m^2]
Repeat cycle every 21-28 days

Cisplatin-Docetaxel

Use: Bladder cancer
Regimen:
Cisplatin: I.V.: 30 mg/m^2 day 1 [total dose/cycle = 30 mg/m^2]
Docetaxel: I.V.: 40 mg/m^2 day 4 [total dose/cycle = 40 mg/m^2]
Repeat cycle weekly for 8 weeks

Cisplatin-Fluorouracil

Use: Cervical cancer
Regimen: Note: Multiple variations are listed below.
Variation 1:
Cisplatin: I.V.: 75 mg/m^2 day 1 [total dose/cycle = 75 mg/m^2]
Fluorouracil: I.V.: 1000 mg/m^2/day continuous infusion days 1-4 (96 hours)
    [total dose/cycle = 4000 mg/m^2]
Repeat cycle every 21 days
Variation 2:
Cisplatin: I.V.: 50 mg/m^2 day 1 starting 4 hours before radiotherapy [total dose/cycle = 50 mg/m^2]
Fluorouracil: I.V.: 1000 mg/m^2/day continuous infusion days 2-5 (96 hours)
    [total dose/cycle = 4000 mg/m^2]
Repeat cycle every 28 days

Cisplatin + Pemetrexed

Use: Malignant pleural mesothelioma
Regimen:
Pemetrexed: I.V.: 500 mg/m^2 infused over 10 minutes day 1 [total dose/cycle = 500 mg/m^2]
Cisplatin: I.V.: 75 mg/m^2 infused over 2 hours (start 30 minutes after pemetrexed)
    [total dose/cycle = 75 mg/m^2]
Repeat cycle every 21 days

Cisplatin-Vinorelbine

Use: Cervical cancer
Regimen:
Cisplatin: I.V.: 80 mg/m^2 day 1 [total dose/cycle = 80 mg/m^2]
Vinorelbine: I.V.: 25 mg/m^2/day days 1 and 8 [total dose/cycle = 50 mg/m^2]
Repeat cycle every 21 days

CMF

Use: Breast cancer

Regimen: Note: Multiple variations are listed below.

Variation 1:

Methotrexate: I.V.: 40 mg/m^2/day days 1 and 8 [total dose/cycle = 80 mg/m^2]

Fluorouracil: I.V.: 600 mg/m^2/day days 1 and 8 [total dose/cycle = 1200 mg/m^2]

Cyclophosphamide: Oral: 100 mg/m^2/day days 1-14 [total dose/cycle = 1400 mg/m^2]

Repeat cycle every 28 days

Variation 2 (>60 years of age):

Methotrexate: I.V.: 30 mg/m^2 days 1 and 8 [total dose/cycle = 60 mg/m^2]

Fluorouracil: I.V.: 400 mg/m^2 days 1 and 8 [total dose/cycle = 800 mg/m^2]

Cyclophosphamide: Oral: 100 mg/m^2 days 1-14 [total dose/cycle = 1400 mg/m^2]

Repeat cycle every 28 days

CMF-IV

Use: Breast cancer

Regimen:

Cyclophosphamide: I.V.: 600 mg/m^2 day 1 [total dose/cycle = 600 mg/m^2]

Methotrexate: I.V.: 40 mg/m^2 day 1 [total dose/cycle = 40 mg/m^2]

Fluorouracil: I.V.: 600 mg/m^2 day 1 [total dose/cycle = 600 mg/m^2]

Repeat cycle every 21 or 28 days

CMFP

Use: Breast cancer

Regimen:

Cyclophosphamide: Oral: 100 mg/m^2/day days 1-14 [total dose/cycle = 1400 mg/m^2]

Methotrexate: I.V.: 30 or 40 mg/m^2/day days 1 and 8 [total dose/cycle = 60 or 80 mg/m^2]

Fluorouracil: I.V.: 400 or 600 mg/m^2/day days 1 and 8 [total dose/cycle = 800 or 1200 mg/m^2]

Prednisone: Oral: 40 mg/m^2/day days 1-14 [total dose/cycle = 560 mg/m^2]

Repeat cycle every 28 days

CMFVP (Cooper Regimen, VPCMF)

Use: Breast cancer

Regimen:

Cyclophosphamide: Oral: 2 mg/kg/day days 1-252 [total dose/cycle = 504 mg/kg]

Methotrexate: I.V.: 0.7 mg/kg day 1, weeks 1-8, 10, 12, 14, 16, 18, 20, 22, 24, 26, 28, 30, 32, 34, 36
[total dose/cycle = 15.4 mg/kg]

Fluorouracil: I.V.: 12 mg/kg day 1, weeks 1-8, 10, 12, 14, 16, 18, 20, 22, 24, 26, 28, 30, 32, 34, 36
[total dose/cycle = 264 mg/kg]

Vincristine: I.V.: 0.035 mg/kg (maximum 2 mg) day 1, weeks 1-5, 8, 12, 16, 20, 24, 28, 32, 36
[total dose/cycle = 0.455 mg/kg]

Prednisone: Oral: 0.75 mg/kg/day days 1-10, taper off over next 40 days

Administer one cycle only

CMV

Use: Bladder cancer

Regimen:

Cisplatin: I.V.: 100 mg/m^2 infused over 4 hours (start 12 hours after methotrexate) day 2
[total dose = 100 mg/m^2]

Methotrexate: I.V.: 30 mg/m^2/day days 1 and 8 [total dose = 60 mg/m^2]

Vinblastine: I.V.: 4 mg/m^2/day days 1 and 8 [total dose = 8 mg/m^2]

Repeat cycle every 21 days

CNF

Use: Breast cancer

Regimen: Note: Multiple variations are listed below.

Variation 1:

Cyclophosphamide: I.V: 500 mg/m^2 day 1 [total dose/cycle = 500 mg/m^2]

Mitoxantrone: I.V.: 10 mg/m^2 day 1 [total dose/cycle = 10 mg/m^2]

Fluorouracil: I.V.: 500 mg/m^2 day 1 [total dose/cycle = 500 mg/m^2]

Repeat cycle every 21 days

Variation 2:

Cyclophosphamide: I.V.: 500-600 mg/m^2 day 1 [total dose/cycle = 500-600 mg/m^2]

Fluorouracil: I.V.: 500-600 mg/m^2 day 1 [total dose/cycle = 500-600 mg/m^2]

Mitoxantrone: I.V.: 10-12 mg/m^2 day 1 [total dose/cycle = 10-12 mg/m^2]

Repeat cycle every 21 days

CNOP

Use: Lymphoma, non-Hodgkin

Regimen:

Cyclophosphamide: I.V.: 750 mg/m^2 day 1 [total dose/cycle = 750 mg/m^2]

Mitoxantrone: I.V.: 10 mg/m^2 day 1 [total dose/cycle = 10 mg/m^2]

Vincristine: I.V.: 1.4 mg/m^2 day 1 [total dose/cycle = 1.4 mg/m^2]

Prednisone: Oral: 50 mg/m^2/day days 1-5 [total dose/cycle = 250 mg/m^2]

Repeat cycle every 21 days

CO

Use: Retinoblastoma

Regimen:

Cyclophosphamide: I.V.: 10 mg/kg/day days 1-3 [total dose/cycle = 30 mg/kg]

Vincristine: I.V.: 1.5 mg/m^2 day 1 [total dose/cycle = 1.5 mg/m^2]

Repeat cycle every 21 days

CODOX-M

Use: Lymphoma, non-Hodgkin

Regimen:

Cytarabine: I.T.: 70 mg/day days 1 and 3 [total dose/cycle = 140 mg]

Cyclophosphamide: I.V.: 800 mg/m^2 day 1, then 200 mg/m^2/day days 2-5
[total dose/cycle = 1600 mg/m^2]

Vincristine: I.V.: 1.5 mg/m^2/day days 1 and 8 (cycle 1); days 1, 8, 15 (cycle 3) [total dose/cycle = 3-4.5 mg/m^2]

Doxorubicin: I.V.: 40 mg/m^2 day 1 [total dose/cycle = 40 mg/m^2]

Methotrexate:

I.T.: 12 mg day 15 [total dose/cycle = 12 mg]

I.V.: 1200 mg/m^2 loading dose then 240 mg/m^2/hour for 23 hours day 10
[total dose/cycle = 6720 mg/m^2]

Leucovorin: I.V.: 192 mg/m^2 day 11 then 12 mg/m^2 every 6 hours until methotrexate level <5 X 10^{-8}M (begin 36
hours after the start of methotrexate infusion)

Sargramostim: SubQ: 7.5 mcg/kg/day day 13 until ANC >1000 cells/mm^3

Repeat cycle when ANC >1000 cells/mm^3

CODOX-M/IVAC

Use: Lymphoma, non-Hodgkin (Burkitt)

Regimen:

CODOX-M

Cyclophosphamide: I.V.: 800 mg/m^2/day days 1 and 2 [total dose/cycle = 1600 mg/m^2]

Vincristine: I.V.: 1.4 mg/m^2/day (maximum 2 mg) days 1 and 10
  [total dose/cycle = 2.8 mg/m^2; maximum 4 mg/cycle]

Doxorubicin: I.V.: 50 mg/m^2 day 1 [total dose/cycle = 50 mg/m^2]

Methotrexate: I.V.: 3 g/m^2 day 10 [total dose/cycle = 3 g/m^2]

Leucovorin: I.V.: 200 mg/m^2 day 11

followed by: Oral, I.V.: 15 mg/m^2 every 6 hours until methotrexate level <0.1 Mmol/L

Cytarabine: I.T.: 50 mg/day days 1 and 3 [total dose/cycle = 100 mg]

Methotrexate: I.T.: 12 mg day 1 [total dose/cycle = 12 mg]

Filgrastim: SubQ: Dose not specified, days 3-8 and day 12 until ANC >1000 cells/mm^3

Cycle alternates with IVAC (cycles begin when ANC >1000 cells/mm^3)

Note: Hydrocortisone 50 mg may be added to intrathecal therapy to reduce the incidence of side effects/chemical arachnoiditis.

IVAC:

Ifosfamide: I.V.: 1500 mg/m^2/day days 1-5 [total dose/cycle = 7500 mg/m^2]

Mesna: I.V.: 1500 mg/m^2/day (in divided doses) days 1-5 [total dose/cycle = 7500 mg/m^2]

Etoposide: I.V.: 60 mg/m^2/day days 1-5 [total dose/cycle = 300 mg/m^2]

Cytarabine: I.V.: 2 g/m^2 every 12 hours, for 4 doses, days 1 and 2 [total dose/cycle = 8 g/m^2]

Methotrexate: I.T.: 12 mg day 5 [total dose/cycle = 12 mg]

Filgrastim: SubQ: Dose not specified, day 6 until ANC >1000 cells/mm^3

Cycle alternates with CODOX-M (cycles begin when ANC >1000 cells/mm^3)

Note: Hydrocortisone 50 mg may be added to intrathecal therapy to reduce the incidence of side effects/chemical arachnoiditis.

COMLA

Use: Lymphoma, non-Hodgkin

Regimen:

Cyclophosphamide: I.V.: 1500 mg/m^2 day 1 [total dose/cycle = 1500 mg/m^2]

Vincristine: I.V.: 1.4 mg/m^2/day (maximum 2 mg) days 1, 8, 15 [total dose/cycle = 4.2 mg/m^2]

Methotrexate: I.V.: 120 mg/m^2/day days 22, 29, 36, 43, 50, 57, 64, 71
  [total dose/cycle = 960 mg/m^2]

Leucovorin: Oral: 25 mg/m^2 every 6 hours for 4 doses (beginning 24 hours after each methotrexate dose)
  [total dose/cycle = 800 mg/m^2]

Cytarabine: I.V.: 300 mg/m^2/day days 22, 29, 36, 43, 50, 57, 64, 71
  [total dose/cycle = 2400 mg/m^2]

Repeat cycle every 85 days

COMP

Use: Lymphoma, Hodgkin disease; Lymphoma, non-Hodgkin disease

Regimen:

Cyclophosphamide: I.V.: 1200 mg/m^2 day 1, cycle 1 [total dose/cycle = 1200 mg/m^2]
  followed by 1000 mg/m^2 day 1 on subsequent cycles [total dose/cycle = 1000 mg/m^2]

Vincristine: I.V.: 2 mg/m^2/day (maximum 2 mg) days 3, 10, 17, 24, cycle 1
  [total dose/cycle = 8 mg/m^2]
  followed by 1.5 mg/m^2/day days 1 and 4, on subsequent cycles
  [total dose/cycle = 3 mg/m^2]

Methotrexate: I.V.: 300 mg/m^2 day 12 [total dose/cycle = 300 mg/m^2]

Prednisone: Oral: 60 mg/m^2/day (maximum 60 mg) days 3-30 then taper over next 7 days, cycle 1
  [total dose/cycle = 1680 mg/m^2 + taper dose over 7 days]
  followed by 60 mg/m^2 (maximum 60 mg) days 1-5, on subsequent cycles [total dose/cycle = 300 mg/m^2]

Maintenance cycles repeat every 28 days

COP-BLAM

Use: Lymphoma, non-Hodgkin

Regimen:

Cyclophosphamide: I.V.: 400 mg/m^2 day 1 [total dose/cycle = 400 mg/m^2]

Vincristine: I.V.: 1 mg/m^2 day 1 [total dose/cycle = 1 mg/m^2]

Prednisone: Oral: 40 mg/m^2/day days 1-10 [total dose/cycle = 400 mg/m^2]

Bleomycin: I.V.: 15 mg day 14 [total dose/cycle = 15 mg]

Doxorubicin: I.V.: 40 mg/m^2 day 1 [total dose/cycle = 40 mg/m^2]

Procarbazine: Oral: 100 mg/m^2/day days 1-10 [total dose/cycle = 1000 mg/m^2]

COPE or Baby Brain I

Use: Brain tumors

Regimen:

Cycle A:

Vincristine: I.V.: 0.065 mg/kg/day (maximum 1.5 mg) days 1 and 8 [total dose/cycle = 0.13 mg/kg]

Cyclophosphamide: I.V.: 65 mg/kg day 1 [total dose/cycle = 65 mg/kg]

Cycle B:

Cisplatin: I.V.: 4 mg/kg day 1 [total dose/cycle = 4 mg/kg]

Etoposide: I.V.: 6.5 mg/kg/day days 3 and 4 [total dose/cycle = 13 mg/kg]

Repeat cycle every 28 days in the following sequence: AABAAB

COPP (C MOPP)

Use: Lymphoma, non-Hodgkin

Regimen:

Cyclophosphamide: I.V.: 450-650 mg/m^2/day days 1 and 8 [total dose/cycle = 900-1300 mg/m^2]

Vincristine: I.V.: 1.4-2 mg/m^2/day (maximum 2 mg) days 1 and 8 [total dose/cycle = 2.8-4 mg/m^2]

Procarbazine: Oral: 100 mg/m^2/day days 1-14 [total dose/cycle = 1400 mg/m^2]

Prednisone: Oral: 40 mg/m^2/day days 1-14 [total dose/cycle = 560 mg/m^2]

Repeat cycle every 3-4 weeks

CP (Leukemia)

Use: Leukemia, chronic lymphocytic

Regimen:

Chlorambucil: Oral: 30 mg/m^2 day 1 [total dose/cycle = 30 mg/m^2]

Prednisone: Oral: 80 mg/day days 1-5 [total dose/cycle = 400 mg]

Repeat cycle every 14 days

CP (Ovarian Cancer)

Use: Ovarian cancer

Regimen:

Cyclophosphamide: I.V.: 750 mg/m^2 day 1 [total dose/cycle = 750 mg/m^2]

Cisplatin: I.V.: 75 mg/m^2 day 1 [total dose/cycle = 75 mg/m^2]

Repeat cycle every 21 days

CT

Use: Ovarian cancer

Regimen:

Cisplatin: I.V.: 75 mg/m^2 day 2 [total dose/cycle = 75 mg/m^2]

Paclitaxel: I.V.: 135 mg/m^2 continuous infusion day 1 [total dose/cycle = 135 mg/m^2]

Repeat cycle every 21 days

CV
Use: Retinoblastoma
Regimen:
    Cyclophosphamide: I.V.: 300 mg/m^2 [total dose/cycle = 300 mg/m^2]
    Vincristine: I.V.: 1.5 mg/m^2 [total dose/cycle = 1.5 mg/m^2]
    Repeat weekly for 6 weeks
    followed by:
    Cyclophosphamide: I.V.: 200 mg/m^2 [total dose/cycle = 200 mg/m^2]
    Vincristine: I.V.: 1.5 mg/m^2 [total dose/cycle = 1.5 mg/m^2]
    Repeat weekly for 42 weeks

CVD
Use: Melanoma
Regimen:
    Cisplatin: I.V.: 20 mg/m^2/day days 2-5 [total dose/cycle = 80 mg/m^2]
    Vinblastine: I.V.: 1.6 mg/m^2/day days 1-5 [total dose/cycle = 8 mg/m^2]
    Dacarbazine: I.V.: 800 mg/m^2 day 1 [total dose/cycle = 800 mg/m^2]
    Repeat cycle every 21 days

CVP (Leukemia)
Use: Leukemia, chronic lymphocytic
Regimen: Note: Multiple variations are listed below.
    Variation 1:
    Cyclophosphamide: Oral: 400 or 300 mg/m^2/day days 1-5
        [total dose/cycle = 2000 or 1500 mg/m^2]
    Vincristine: I.V.: 1.4 mg/m^2 (maximum 2 mg) day 1 [total dose/cycle = 1.4 mg/m^2]
    Prednisone: Oral: 100 mg/m^2/day days 1-5 [total dose/cycle = 500 mg/m^2]
    Repeat cycle every 21 days
    Variation 2:
    Cyclophosphamide: I.V.: 800 mg/m^2 day 1 [total dose/cycle = 800 mg/m^2]
    Vincristine: I.V.: 1.4 mg/m^2 (maximum 2 mg) day 1 [total dose/cycle = 1.4 mg/m^2]
    Prednisone: Oral: 100 mg/m^2/day days 1-5 [total dose/cycle = 500 mg/m^2]
    Repeat cycle every 21 days

CVP (Lymphoma, non-Hodgkin)
Use: Lymphoma, non-Hodgkin
Regimen:
    Cyclophosphamide: Oral: 400 mg/m^2/day days 1-5 [total dose/cycle = 2000 mg/m^2]
    Vincristine: I.V.: 1.4 mg/m^2 day 1 [total dose/cycle = 1.4 mg/m^2]
    Prednisone: Oral: 100 mg/m^2/day days 1-5 [total dose/cycle = 500 mg/m^2]
    Repeat cycle every 21 days

Cyclophosphamide + Doxorubicin
Use: Prostate cancer
Regimen:
    Doxorubicin: I.V.: 40 mg/m^2 day 1 [total dose/cycle = 40 mg/m^2]
    Cyclophosphamide: I.V.: 800-2000 mg/m^2 day 1 [total dose/cycle = 800-2000 mg/m^2]
    Filgrastim: SubQ: 5 mcg/kg/day days 2-10 (or until ANC >10,000 cells/μL)
        [total dose/cycle = 45 mcg/kg or ANC >10,000 cells/μL]
    Repeat cycle every 21 days

Cyclophosphamide + Estramustine
Use: Prostate cancer
Regimen:
    Cyclophosphamide: Oral: 2 mg/kg/day days 1-14 [total dose/cycle = 28 mg/kg]
    Estramustine: Oral: 10 mg/kg/day days 1-14 [total dose/cycle = 140 mg/kg]
    Repeat cycle every 28 days

Cyclophosphamide + Etoposide
Use: Prostate cancer
Regimen:
Cyclophosphamide: Oral: 100 mg/day days 1-14 [total dose/cycle = 1400 mg]
Etoposide: Oral: 50 mg/day days 1-14 [total dose/cycle = 700 mg]
Repeat cycle every 28 days

Cyclophosphamide + Vincristine + Dexamethasone
Use: Prostate cancer
Regimen:
Cyclophosphamide: Oral: 250 mg/day days 1-14 [total dose/cycle = 3500 mg]
Vincristine: I.V.: 1 mg/day days 1, 8, 15 [total dose/cycle = 3 mg]
Dexamethasone: Oral: 0.75 mg twice daily days 1-14 [total dose/cycle = 21 mg]
Repeat cycle every 28 days

CYVADIC
Use: Sarcoma
Regimen:
Cyclophosphamide: I.V.: 500 mg/m^2 day 1 [total dose/cycle = 500 mg/m^2]
Vincristine: I.V.: 1.4 mg/m^2/day days 1 and 5 [total dose/cycle = 2.8 mg/m^2]
Doxorubicin: I.V.: 50 mg/m^2 day 1 [total dose/cycle = 50 mg/m^2]
Dacarbazine: I.V.: 250 mg/m^2/day days 1-5 [total dose/cycle = 1250 mg/m^2]
Repeat cycle every 21 days

DA
Use: Leukemia, acute myeloid (induction)
Regimen: Induction:
Daunorubicin: I.V.: 45 mg/m^2/day days 1-3 [total dose/cycle = 135 mg/m^2]
Cytarabine: I.V.: 100 mg/m^2/day continuous infusion days 1-7 [total dose/cycle = 700 mg/m^2]

Dacarbazine-Carboplatin-Aldesleukin-Interferon
Use: Melanoma
Regimen:
Dacarbazine: I.V.: 750 mg/m^2/day days 1 and 22 [total dose/cycle = 1500 mg/m^2]
Carboplatin: I.V.: 400 mg/m^2/day days 1 and 22 [total dose/cycle = 800 mg/m^2]
Aldesleukin: SubQ: 4,800,000 units every 8 hours days 36 and 57
[total dose/cycle = 28,800,000 units]
then 4,800,000 units every 12 hours days 37 and 58 [total dose/cycle = 19,200,000 units]
then 4,800,000 units/day days 38 to 40, 43 to 47, 50 to 54, 59 to 61, 65 to 68, 71 to 75
[total dose/cycle = 120,000,000 units]
Interferon alpha-2a: SubQ: 6,000,000 units days 38, 40, 43, 45, 47, 50, 52, 54, 59, 61, 64, 66, 68, 71, 73, 75
[total dose/cycle = 96,000,000 units]
Repeat cycle every 78 days for 3 cycles

Dartmouth Regimen
Use: Melanoma
Regimen: Note: Multiple variations are listed below.
Variation 1:
Cisplatin: I.V.: 25 mg/m^2/day days 1-3 [total dose/cycle = 75 mg/m^2]
Dacarbazine: I.V.: 220 mg/m^2/day days 1-3 [total dose/cycle = 660 mg/m^2]
Carmustine: I.V.: 150 mg/m^2 day 1 (every other cycle) [total dose/cycle = 150 mg/m^2; every other cycle]
Tamoxifen: Oral: 10 mg twice daily (begin 1 week before chemotherapy) [total dose/cycle = 420 mg]
Repeat cycle every 21 days

Variation 2:
Carmustine: I.V.: 150 mg/m² day 1 [total dose/cycle = 150 mg/m²]
Cisplatin: I.V.: 25 mg/m²/day days 1, 2, 3, 22, 23, 24 [total dose/cycle = 150 mg/m²]
Dacarbazine: I.V.: 220 mg/m²/day days 1, 2, 3, 22, 23, 24 [total dose/cycle = 1320 mg/m²]
Tamoxifen: Oral: 10 mg twice daily days 1-42 [total dose/cycle = 840 mg]
Repeat cycle every 42 days

Variation 3:
Carmustine: I.V.: 150 mg/m² day 1 [total dose/cycle = 150 mg/m²]
Cisplatin: I.V.: 25 mg/m²/day days 1, 2, 3, 22, 23, 24 [total dose/cycle = 150 mg/m²]
Dacarbazine: I.V.: 220 mg/m²/day days 1, 2, 3, 22, 23, 24 [total dose/cycle = 1320 mg/m²]
Tamoxifen: Oral: 160 mg/day days -6-0 (cycle 1 only) [total dose/cycle = 840 mg]
followed by: Oral: 40 mg/day days 1-42 [total dose/cycle = 1680 mg]
Repeat cycle every 42 days

Variation 4:
Carmustine: I.V.: 150 mg/m² day 1 [total dose/cycle = 150 mg/m²]
Cisplatin: I.V.: 25 mg/m²/day days 1, 2, 3, 29, 30, 31 [total dose/cycle = 150 mg/m²]
Dacarbazine: I.V.: 220 mg/m²/day days 1, 2, 3, 29, 30, 31 [total dose/cycle = 1320 mg/m²]
Tamoxifen: Oral: 10-20 mg twice daily days 1-56 [total dose/cycle = 1120-2240 mg]
Repeat cycle every 56 days

DAT
Use: Leukemia, acute myeloid (induction)
Regimen: Induction:
Daunorubicin: I.V. bolus: 45 mg/m²/day days 1-3 [total dose/cycle = 135 mg/m²]
Cytarabine: I.V. bolus: 200 mg/m² [total dose/cycle = 200 mg/m²]
Thioguanine: Oral: 100 mg/m²/day days 1-7 [total dose/cycle = 700 mg/m²]

DAV
Use: Leukemia, acute myeloid
Regimen:
Daunorubicin: I.V.: 60 mg/m²/day days 3-5 [total dose/cycle = 180 mg/m²]
Cytarabine: I.V.: 100 mg/m²/day continuous infusion days 1 and 2
[total dose/cycle = 200 mg/m²] **followed by** 100 mg/m² every 12 hours days 3-8 (12 doses)
[total dose/cycle = 1200 mg/m²]
Etoposide: I.V.: 150 mg/m²/day days 6-8 [total dose/cycle = 450 mg/m²]
Administer one cycle only

DHAP
Use: Lymphoma, non-Hodgkin
Regimen: Note: Multiple variations are listed below.
Variation 1:
Dexamethasone: I.V. or Oral: 40 mg/day days 1-4 [total dose/cycle = 160 mg]
Cisplatin: I.V.: 100 mg/m² day 1 [total dose/cycle = 100 mg/m²]
Cytarabine: I.V.: 2000 mg/m² every 12 hours for 2 doses day 2 (begins at the end of the cisplatin infusion)
[total dose/cycle = 4000 mg/m²]
Repeat cycle every 3-4 weeks for 6-10 cycles (salvage therapy) or 1-2 cycles (mobilization prior to high-dose
therapy with peripheral hematopoietic progenitor cell support)
Variation 2:
Dexamethasone: I.V. or Oral: 40 mg/day days 1-4 [total dose/cycle = 160 mg]
Oxaliplatin: I.V.: 130 mg/m² day 1 [total dose/cycle = 130 mg/m²]
Cytarabine: I.V.: 2000 mg/m² every 12 hours for 2 doses day 2 [total dose/cycle = 4000 mg/m²]
Repeat cycle every 3 weeks

Docetaxel (Weekly)
Use: Prostate cancer
Regimen:
> Docetaxel: I.V.: 40 mg/m^2 days 1, 8, 15 [total dose/cycle = 120 mg/m^2]
> Repeat cycle every 4 weeks

Docetaxel-Cisplatin
Use: Lung cancer, nonsmall cell
Regimen:
> Docetaxel: I.V.: 75 mg/m^2 day 1 [total dose/cycle = 75 mg/m^2]
> Cisplatin: I.V.: 75 mg/m^2 day 1 [total dose/cycle = 75 mg/m^2]
> Repeat cycle every 21 days

Docetaxel-Cisplatin-Fluorouracil
Use: Head and neck cancer, gastric adenocarcinoma
Regimen:
> Docetaxel: I.V.: 75 mg/m^2 day 1 [total dose/cycle = 75 mg/m^2]
> Cisplatin: I.V.: 75 mg/m^2 day 1 [total dose/cycle = 75 mg/m^2]
> Fluorouracil: I.V.: 750 mg/m^2/day continuous infusion days 1-5 [total dose/cycle = 3750 mg/m^2]
> Repeat cycle every 21 days (for 4 cycles for head and neck cancer)

Docetaxel-Prednisone
Use: Prostate cancer
Regimen:
> Docetaxel: I.V.: 75 mg/m^2 day 1 [total dose/cycle = 75 mg/m^2]
> Prednisone: Oral: 5 mg twice daily [total dose/cycle = 210 mg]
> Repeat cycle every 21 days for up to 10 cycles

Docetaxel-Thalidomide
Use: Prostate cancer
Regimen:
> Docetaxel: I.V.: 30 mg/m^2/day days 1, 8, 15 [total dose/cycle = 90 mg/m^2]
> Thalidomide: Oral: 200 mg daily (at bedtime) [total dose/cycle = 5600 mg]
> Repeat cycle every 28 days

Dox-CMF (Sequential)
Use: Breast cancer
Regimen:
> Doxorubicin: I.V.: 75 mg/m^2 day 1 [total dose/cycle = 75 mg/m^2]
> Repeat cycle every 21 days for 4 cycles
> **followed by** (after completing Cycle 4)
> Cyclophosphamide: I.V.: 600 mg/m^2 day 1 [total dose/cycle = 600 mg/m^2]
> Methotrexate: I.V.: 40 mg/m^2 day 1 [total dose/cycle = 40 mg/m^2]
> Fluorouracil: I.V.: 600 mg/m^2 day 1 [total dose/cycle = 600 mg/m^2]
> Repeat cycle every 21 days for 8 cycles

Doxorubicin + Ketoconazole
Use: Prostate cancer
Regimen:
> Doxorubicin: I.V.: 20 mg/m^2 continuous infusion day 1 [total dose/cycle = 20 mg/m^2]
> Ketoconazole: Oral: 400 mg 3 times/day days 1-7 [total dose/cycle = 8400 mg]
> Repeat cycle every 7 days

Doxorubicin + Ketoconazole/Estramustine + Vinblastine
Use: Prostate cancer
Regimen:
    Doxorubicin: I.V.: 20 mg/m^2/day days 1, 15, 29 [total dose/cycle = 60 mg/m^2]
    Ketoconazole: Oral: 400 mg 3 times/day days 1-7, 15-21, 29-35
        [total dose/cycle = 25,200 mg]
    Estramustine: Oral: 140 mg 3 times/day days 8-14, 22-28, 36-42
        [total dose/cycle = 8820 mg]
    Vinblastine: I.V.: 5 mg/m^2/day days 8, 22, 36 [total dose/cycle = 15 mg/m^2]
    Repeat cycle every 8 weeks

Doxorubicin (Liposomal)-Vincristine-Dexamethasone
Use: Multiple myeloma
Regimen: Note: Multiple variations are listed below.
    Variation 1:
    Doxorubicin, liposomal: I.V.: 40 mg/m^2 day 1 [total dose/cycle = 40 mg/m^2]
    Vincristine: I.V.: 2 mg day 1 [total dose/cycle = 2 mg]
    Dexamethasone: Oral or I.V.: 40 mg/day days 1-4 [total dose/cycle = 160 mg]
    Repeat cycle every 4 weeks
    Variation 2:
    Doxorubicin, liposomal: I.V.: 40 mg/m^2 day 1 [total dose/cycle = 40 mg/m^2]
    Vincristine: I.V.: 1.4 mg/m^2 (maximum 2 mg) day 1 [total dose/cycle = 1.4 mg/m^2; maximum 2 mg]
    Dexamethasone: Oral: 40 mg/day days 1-4 [total dose/cycle = 160 mg]
    Repeat cycle every 4 weeks

DTPACE
Use: Multiple myeloma
Regimen:
    Dexamethasone: Oral: 40 mg/day days 1-4 [total dose/cycle = 160 mg]
    Thalidomide: Oral: 400 mg/day [total dose/cycle = 11,200-16,800 mg]
    Cisplatin: I.V.: 10 mg/m^2/day continuous infusion days 1-4 [total dose/cycle = 40 mg/m^2]
    Doxorubicin: I.V.: 10 mg/m^2/day continuous infusion days 1-4 [total dose/cycle = 40 mg/m^2]
    Cyclophosphamide: I.V.: 400 mg/m^2 continuous infusion days 1-4
        [total dose/cycle = 1600 mg/m^2]
    Etoposide: I.V.: 40 mg/m^2 continuous infusion days 1-4 [total dose/cycle = 160 mg/m^2]
    Repeat cycle every 4-6 weeks

DVP
Use: Leukemia, acute lymphocytic
Regimen: Induction:
    Daunorubicin: I.V.: 25 mg/m^2/day days 1, 8, and 15 [total dose/cycle = 75 mg/m^2]
    Vincristine: I.V.: 1.5 mg/m^2/day (maximum 2 mg) days 1, 8, 15, and 22
        [total dose/cycle = 6 mg/m^2]
    Prednisone: Oral: 60 mg/m^2/day days 1-28 then taper over next 14 days
        [total dose/cycle = 1680 mg/m^2 + taper over next 14 days]
    Administer single cycle; used in conjunction with intrathecal chemotherapy

EAP
Use: Gastric cancer
Regimen:
    Etoposide: I.V.: 120 mg/m^2/day days 4-6 [total dose/cycle = 360 mg/m^2]
    Doxorubicin: I.V.: 20 mg/m^2/day days 1 and 7 [total dose/cycle = 40 mg/m^2]
    Cisplatin: I.V.: 40 mg/m^2/day days 2 and 8 [total dose/cycle = 80 mg/m^2]
    Repeat cycle every 22-28 days

ECF

Use: Gastric cancer
Regimen:
Epirubicin: I.V.: 50 mg/m^2 day 1 [total dose/cycle = 50 mg/m^2]
Cisplatin: I.V.: 60 mg/m^2 day 1 [total dose/cycle = 60 mg/m^2]
Repeat cycle every 3 weeks
Fluorouracil: I.V.: 200 mg/m^2/day continuous infusion for up to 6 months
   [total dose/cycle = 36,000 mg/m^2]

EC (Nonsmall Cell Lung Cancer)

Use: Lung cancer, nonsmall cell
Regimen:
Etoposide: I.V.: 120 mg/m^2/day days 1-3 [total dose/cycle = 360 mg/m^2]
Carboplatin: I.V.: AUC 6 day 1 [total dose/cycle = AUC = 6]
Repeat cycle every 21-28 days

EC (Small Cell Lung Cancer)

Use: Lung cancer, small cell
Regimen: Note: Multiple variations are listed below.
Variation 1:
Etoposide: I.V.: 100-120 mg/m^2/day days 1-3 [total dose/cycle = 300-360 mg/m^2]
Carboplatin: I.V.: 325-400 mg/m^2 day 1 [total dose/cycle = 325-400 mg/m^2]
Repeat cycle every 28 days
Variation 2:
Etoposide: I.V.: 120 mg/m^2/day days 1-3 [total dose/cycle = 360 mg/m^2]
Carboplatin: I.V.: AUC 6 day 1 [total dose/cycle = AUC = 6]
Repeat cycle every 21-28 days

EE

Use: Wilms tumor
Regimen:
Dactinomycin: I.V.: 15 mcg/kg/day days 1-5 of weeks 0, 5, 13, 24 [total dose/cycle = 300 mcg/kg]
Vincristine: I.V.: 1.5 mg/m^2 day 1 of weeks 1-10, 13, 14, 24, 25 [total dose/cycle = 21 mg/m^2]

EE-4A

Use: Wilms tumor
Regimen:
Dactinomycin: I.V.: 45 mcg/kg day 1 of weeks 0, 3, 6, 9, 12, 15, 18
   [total dose/cycle = 315 mcg/kg]
Vincristine: I.V.: 2 mg/m^2 day 1 of weeks 1-10, 12, 15, 18 [total dose/cycle = 26 mg/m^2]

EFP

Use: Gastric cancer
Regimen: Note: Multiple variations are listed below.
Variation 1:
Etoposide: I.V.: 90 mg/m^2/day days 1, 3, 5 [total dose/cycle = 270 mg/m^2]
Fluorouracil: I.V.: 900 mg/m^2/day (20-hour infusion) days 1-5 [total dose/cycle = 4500 mg/m^2]
Cisplatin: I.V.: 20 mg/m^2/day days 1-5 [total dose/cycle = 100 mg/m^2]
Repeat cycle every 24-28 days

Variation 2:
Etoposide: I.V.: 100 mg/m^2/day days 1, 3, 5 [total dose/cycle = 300 mg/m^2]
Fluorouracil: I.V.: 800 mg/m^2/day (12-hour infusion) days 1-5 [total dose/cycle = 4000 mg/m^2]
Cisplatin: I.V.: 20 mg/m^2/day days 1-5 [total dose/cycle = 100 mg/m^2]
Repeat cycle every 3 weeks

ELF
Use: Gastric cancer
Regimen:
Leucovorin calcium: I.V.: 300 mg/m^2/day days 1-3, [total dose/cycle = 900 mg/m^2] **followed by:**
Etoposide: I.V.: 120 mg/m^2/day days 1-3, [total dose/cycle = 360 mg/m^2] **followed by:**
Fluorouracil: I.V.: 500 mg/m^2/day days 1-3 [total dose/cycle = 1500 mg/m^2]
Repeat cycle every 21-28 days

EMA 86
Use: Leukemia, acute myeloid
Regimen:
Mitoxantrone: I.V.: 12 mg/m^2/day days 1-3 [total dose/cycle = 36 mg/m^2]
Etoposide: I.V.: 200 mg/m^2/day continuous infusion days 8-10 [total dose/cycle = 600 mg/m^2]
Cytarabine: I.V.: 500 mg/m^2/day continuous infusion days 1-3 and 8-10
    [total dose/cycle = 3000 mg/m^2]
Administer one cycle only

EMA/CO
Use: Gestational trophoblastic tumor
Regimen: Note: Multiple variations are listed below.
Variation 1:
Etoposide: I.V.: 100 mg/m^2/day days 1 and 2 [total dose/cycle = 200 mg/m^2]
Methotrexate: I.V.: 300 mg/m^2 continuous infusion over 12 hours day 1 [total dose/cycle = 300 mg/m^2]
Dactinomycin: I.V. push: 0.5 mg/day days 1 and 2 [total dose/cycle = 1 mg]
Leucovorin: Oral, I.M.: 15 mg twice daily for 2 days (start 24 hours after the start of methotrexate) days 2 and 3
    [total dose/cycle = 60 mg]
Alternate weekly with:
Cyclophosphamide: I.V.: 600 mg/m^2 day 1
    [total dose/cycle = 600 mg/m^2]
Vincristine: I.V. push: 0.8 mg/m^2 (maximum 2 mg) day 1 [total dose/cycle = 0.8 mg/m^2]
Repeat cycle every 2 weeks

Variation 2:
Dactinomycin: I.V.: 0.5 mg/day days 1 and 2 [total dose/cycle = 1 mg]
Etoposide: I.V.: 100 mg/m^2/day days 1 and 2 [total dose/cycle = 200 mg/m^2]
Methotrexate: I.V. bolus: 100 mg/m^2 then 200 mg/m^2 continuous infusion over 12 hours day 1
    [total dose/cycle = 300 mg/m^2]
Leucovorin: Oral, I.M.: 15 mg every 12 hours for 4 doses (start 24 hours after methotrexate) days 2 and 3
    [total dose/cycle = 60 mg]
Vincristine: I.V.: 1 mg/m^2 day 8 [total dose/cycle = 1 mg/m^2]
Cyclophosphamide: I.V.: 600 mg/m^2 day 8
    [total dose/cycle = 600 mg/m^2]
Repeat cycle every 2 weeks

Variation 3:
Dactinomycin: I.V.: 0.5 mg/day days 1 and 2 [total dose/cycle = 1 mg]
Etoposide: I.V.: 100 mg/m^2/day days 1 and 2 [total dose/cycle = 200 mg/m^2]
Methotrexate: I.V.: 300 mg/m^2 continuous infusion over 12 hours day 1 [total dose/cycle = 300 mg/m^2]
Leucovorin: Oral, I.M.: 15 mg every 12 hours for 4 doses (start 24 hours after start of methotrexate) days 2 and 3
    [total dose/cycle = 60 mg]
Vincristine: I.V.: 1 mg/m^2 day 8 [total dose/cycle = 1 mg/m^2]
Cyclophosphamide: I.V.: 600 mg/m^2 day 8
    [total dose/cycle = 600 mg/m^2]
Repeat cycle every 2 weeks

APPENDIX

EMA/CO *(continued)*

Variation 4:

Dactinomycin: I.V.: 0.35 mg/m^2/day days 1 and 2 [total dose/cycle = 0.7 mg/m^2]

Etoposide: I.V.: 100 mg/m^2/day days 1 and 2 [total dose/cycle = 200 mg/m^2]

Methotrexate: I.V. bolus: 100 mg/m^2 then 200 mg/m^2 continuous infusion over 12 hours day 1
[total dose/cycle = 300 mg/m^2]

Leucovorin: Oral, I.M.: 15 mg every 12 hours for 4 doses (start 24 hours after start of methotrexate) days 2 and 3
[total dose/cycle = 60 mg]

Vincristine: I.V.: 1 mg/m^2 day 8 [total dose/cycle = 1 mg/m^2]

Cyclophosphamide: I.V.: 600 mg/m^2 day 8
[total dose/cycle = 600 mg/m^2]

Repeat cycle every 2 weeks

Variation 5 (patients with brain metastases):

Dactinomycin: I.V.: 0.5 mg/day days 1 and 2 [total dose/cycle = 1 mg]

Etoposide: I.V.: 100 mg/m^2/day days 1 and 2 [total dose/cycle = 200 mg/m^2]

Methotrexate: I.V.: 1 g/m^2 continuous infusion over 12 hours day 1 [total dose/cycle = 1 g/m^2]

Leucovorin: I.M.: 20 mg/m^2 every 6 hours for 12 doses (start 24 hours after start of methotrexate) days 2, 3, 4
[total dose/cycle = 240 mg/m^2]

Vincristine: I.V.: 1 mg/m^2 day 8 [total dose/cycle = 1 mg/m^2]

Cyclophosphamide: I.V.: 600 mg/m^2 day 8
[total dose/cycle = 600 mg/m^2]

Repeat cycle every 2 weeks

Variation 6 (patients with brain metastases):

Dactinomycin: I.V.: 0.5 mg/day days 1 and 2 [total dose/cycle = 1 mg]

Etoposide: I.V.: 100 mg/m^2/day days 1 and 2 [total dose/cycle = 200 mg/m^2]

Methotrexate: I.V.: 1 g/m^2 continuous infusion over 12 hours day 1 [total dose/cycle = 1 g/m^2]

Leucovorin: Oral, I.M.: 30 mg every 12 hours for 6 doses (start 32 hours after start of methotrexate) days 2, 3, 4
[total dose/cycle = 180 mg/m^2]

Vincristine: I.V.: 1 mg/m^2 day 8 [total dose/cycle = 1 mg/m^2]

Cyclophosphamide: I.V.: 600 mg/m^2 day 8

[total dose/cycle = 600 mg/m^2]

Repeat cycle every 2 weeks

Variation 7:

Dactinomycin: I.V.: 0.5 mg/day days 1 and 2 [total dose/cycle = 1 mg]

Etoposide: I.V.: 100 mg/m^2/day days 1 and 2 [total dose/cycle = 200 mg/m^2]

Methotrexate: I.V.: 1 g/m^2 continuous infusion over 24 hours day 1 [total dose/cycle = 1 g/m^2]

Leucovorin: Oral, I.M.: 15 mg every 8 hours for 9 doses (start 32 hours after start of methotrexate) days 2, 3, 4
[total dose/cycle = 135 mg/m^2]

Vincristine: I.V.: 1 mg/m^2 day 8 [total dose/cycle = 1 mg/m^2]

Cyclophosphamide: I.V.: 600 mg/m^2 day 8
[total dose/cycle = 600 mg/m^2]

Repeat cycle every 2 weeks

Variation 8 (patients with lung metastases):

Dactinomycin: I.V.: 0.5 mg/day days 1 and 2 [total dose/cycle = 1 mg]

Etoposide: I.V.: 100 mg/m^2/day days 1 and 2 [total dose/cycle = 200 mg/m^2]

Methotrexate: I.V. bolus: 100 mg/m^2 then 200 mg/m^2 continuous infusion over 12 hours day 1
[total dose/cycle = 300 mg/m^2]

Leucovorin: Oral, I.M.: 15 mg every 12 hours for 4 doses (start 24 hours after methotrexate) days 2 and 3
   [total dose/cycle = 60 mg]

Vincristine: I.V.: 1 mg/m^2 day 8 [total dose/cycle = 1 mg/m^2]

Cyclophosphamide: I.V.: 600 mg/m^2 day 8
   [total dose/cycle = 600 mg/m^2]

Methotrexate: I.T.: 10 mg day 1 (every other cycle) [total dose/cycle = 10 mg, every other cycle]

Repeat cycle every 2 weeks

Variation 9 (patients with lung metastases):

Dactinomycin: I.V.: 0.5 mg/day days 1 and 2 [total dose/cycle = 1 mg]

Etoposide: I.V.: 100 mg/m^2/day days 1 and 2 [total dose/cycle = 200 mg/m^2]

Methotrexate: I.V. bolus: 100 mg/m^2 then 200 mg/m^2 continuous infusion over 12 hours day 1
   [total dose/cycle = 300 mg/m^2]

Leucovorin: Oral, I.M.: 15 mg every 12 hours for 4 doses (start 24 hours after start of methotrexate) days 2 and 3
   [total dose/cycle = 60 mg]

Vincristine: I.V.: 1 mg/m^2 day 8 [total dose/cycle = 1 mg/m^2]

Cyclophosphamide: I.V.: 600 mg/m^2 day 8
   [total dose/cycle = 600 mg/m^2]

Methotrexate: I.T.: 12.5 mg day 8 [total dose/cycle = 12.5 mg]

Repeat cycle every 2 weeks

EP (Adenocarcinoma)

Use: Adenocarcinoma, unknown primary

Regimen:

   Cisplatin: I.V.: 60-100 mg/m^2 day 1 [total dose = 60-100 mg/m^2]

   Etoposide: I.V.: 80-100 mg/m^2/day days 1-3 [total dose = 240-300 mg/m^2]

   Repeat cycle every 21 days

EP (Nonsmall Cell Lung Cancer)

Use: Lung cancer, nonsmall cell

Regimen:

   Etoposide: I.V.: 80-120 mg/m^2/day days 1-3 [total dose/cycle = 240-360 mg/m^2]

   Cisplatin: I.V.: 80-100 mg/m^2 day 1 [total dose/cycle = 80-100 mg/m^2]

   Repeat cycle every 21-28 days

EP (Small Cell Lung Cancer)

Use: Lung cancer, small cell

Regimen: Note: Multiple variations are listed below.

   Variation 1:

   Etoposide: I.V.: 100 mg/m^2/day days 1-3 [total dose/cycle = 300 mg/m^2]

   Cisplatin: I.V.: 100 mg/m^2 day 1 [total dose/cycle = 100 mg/m^2]

   Repeat cycle every 21 days

   Variation 2:

   Etoposide: I.V.: 80 mg/m^2/day days 1-3 [total dose/cycle = 240 mg/m^2]

   Cisplatin: I.V.: 80 mg/m^2 day 1 [total dose/cycle = 80 mg/m^2]

   Repeat cycle every 21-28 days

EP (Testicular Cancer)

Use: Testicular cancer
Regimen: Note: Multiple variations are listed below.
Variation 1:
Etoposide: I.V.: 100 mg/m²/day days 1-5 [total dose/cycle = 500 mg/m²]
Cisplatin: I.V.: 20 mg/m²/day days 1-5 [total dose/cycle = 100 mg/m²]
Repeat cycle every 21 days
Variation 2:
Etoposide: I.V.: 120 mg/m²/day days 1-3 [total dose/cycle = 360 mg/m²]
Cisplatin: I.V.: 20 mg/m²/day days 1-5 [total dose/cycle = 100 mg/m²]
Repeat cycle every 3 or 4 weeks
Variation 3:
Etoposide: I.V.: 120 mg/m²/day days 1, 3, 5 [total dose/cycle = 360 mg/m²]
Cisplatin: I.V.: 20 mg/m²/day days 1-5 [total dose/cycle = 100 mg/m²]
Repeat cycle every 3 weeks

EP/EMA

Use: Gestational trophoblastic tumor
Regimen: Note: Multiple variations are listed below.
Variation 1:
Etoposide: I.V.: 150 mg/m² day 1 [total dose/cycle = 150 mg/m²]
Cisplatin: I.V.: 25 mg/m² infused over 4 hours for 3 consecutive doses, day 1
  [total dose/cycle = 75 mg/m²]
Alternate weekly with:
Etoposide: I.V.: 100 mg/m² day 1 [total dose/cycle = 100 mg/m²]
Methotrexate: I.V.: 300 mg/m² infused over 12 hours day 1 [total dose/cycle = 300 mg/m²]
Dactinomycin: I.V. push: 0.5 mg day 1 [total dose/cycle = 0.5 mg]
Leucovorin: Oral, I.M.: 15 mg twice daily for 2 days (start 24 hours after the start of methotrexate) days 2, 3
  [total dose/cycle = 60 mg]
Variation 2:
Dactinomycin: I.V.: 0.5 mg/day days 1 and 2 [total dose/cycle = 1 mg]
Etoposide: I.V.: 100 mg/m²/day days 1 and 2 [total dose/cycle = 200 mg/m²]
Methotrexate: I.V.: 300 mg/m² continuous infusion over 12 hours day 1 [total dose/cycle = 300 mg/m²]
Leucovorin: Oral, I.M.: 15 mg every 12 hours for 4 doses (start 24 hours after the start of methotrexate) days 2 and
  3 [total dose/cycle = 60 mg]
Etoposide: I.V.: 150 mg/m² day 8 [total dose/cycle = 150 mg/m²]
Cisplatin: I.V.: 75 mg/m² day 8 [total dose/cycle = 75 mg/m²]
Repeat cycle every 2 weeks

EP/PE

Use: Lung cancer, nonsmall cell
Regimen:
Etoposide: I.V.: 120 mg/m²/day days 1-3 [total dose/cycle = 360 mg/m²]
Cisplatin: I.V.: 60-120 mg/m² day 1 [total dose/cycle = 60-120 mg/m²]
Repeat cycle every 21-28 days

EPOCH

Use: Lymphoma, non-Hodgkin
Regimen:
Etoposide: I.V.: 50 mg/m²/day continuous infusion days 1-4 [total dose/cycle = 200 mg/m²]
Vincristine: I.V.: 0.4 mg/m²/day continuous infusion days 1-4 [total dose/cycle = 1.6 mg/m²]
Doxorubicin: I.V.: 10 mg/m²/day continuous infusion days 1-4 [total dose/cycle = 40 mg/m²]
Cyclophosphamide: I.V.: 750 mg/m² day 6 [total dose/cycle = 750 mg/m²]
Prednisone: Oral: 60 mg/m²/day days 1-6 [total dose/cycle = 360 mg/m²]
Repeat cycle every 21 days

ESHAP

Use: Lymphoma, non-Hodgkin
Regimen: Note: Multiple variations are listed below.

Variation 1:
Etoposide: I.V.: 40 mg/m^2/day days 1-4 [total dose/cycle = 160 mg/m^2]
Methylprednisolone: I.V.: 250-500 mg/day days 1-5 [total dose/cycle = 1250-2500 mg]
Cytarabine: I.V.: 2000 mg/m^2 day 5 [total dose/cycle = 2000 mg/m^2]
Cisplatin: I.V.: 25 mg/m^2/day continuous infusion days 1-4 [total dose/cycle = 100 mg/m^2]
Repeat cycle every 21-28 days

Variation 2:
Etoposide: I.V.: 40 mg/m^2/day days 1-4 [total dose/cycle = 160 mg/m^2]
Methylprednisolone: I.V.: 500 mg/day days 1-5 [total dose/cycle = 2500 mg]
Cytarabine: I.V.: 2000 mg/m^2 day 5 [total dose/cycle = 2000 mg/m^2]
Cisplatin: I.V.: 25 mg/m^2/day continuous infusion days 1-4 [total dose/cycle = 100 mg/m^2]
Repeat cycle every 21-28 days

Variation 3:
Etoposide: I.V.: 60 mg/m^2/day days 1-4 [total dose/cycle = 240 mg/m^2]
Methylprednisolone: I.V.: 500 mg/day days 1-4 [total dose/cycle = 2000 mg]
Cytarabine: I.V.: 2000 mg/m^2 day 5 [total dose/cycle = 2000 mg/m^2]
Cisplatin: I.V.: 25 mg/m^2/day continuous infusion days 1-4 [total dose/cycle = 100 mg/m^2]
Repeat cycle every 21 days

Estramustine + Docetaxel

Use: Prostate cancer
Regimen: Note: Multiple variations are listed below.

Variation 1:
Docetaxel: I.V.: 20-80 mg/m^2 day 2 [total dose/cycle = 20-80 mg/m^2]
Estramustine: Oral: 280 mg 3 times/day days 1-5 [total dose/cycle = 4200 mg]
Repeat cycle every 21 days

Variation 2:
Docetaxel: I.V.: 20-80 mg/m^2 day 2 [total dose/cycle = 20-80 mg/m^2]
Estramustine: Oral: 14 mg/kg/day days 1-21 [total dose/cycle = 294 mg/kg]
Repeat cycle every 21 days

Variation 3:
Docetaxel: I.V.: 35 mg/m^2/day days 2 and 9 [total dose/cycle = 70 mg/m^2]
Estramustine: Oral: 420 mg 3 times/day for 4 doses, then 280 mg 3 times/day for 5 doses days 1, 2, 3, 8, 9, and 10 [total dose/cycle = 6160 mg]
Repeat cycle every 21 days

Variation 4:
Docetaxel: I.V.: 60 mg/m^2 day 2 cycle 1 [total dose/cycle = 60 mg/m^2]
followed by: I.V.: 60-70 mg/m^2 day 2 (subsequent cycles) [total dose/cycle = 60-70 mg/m^2]
Estramustine: Oral: 280 mg 3 times/day days 1-5 [total dose/cycle = 4200 mg]
Repeat cycle every 21 days for up to 12 cycles

Estramustine + Docetaxel + Calcitriol

Use: Prostate cancer
Regimen:

Cycle 1:
Calcitriol: Oral: 60 mcg (in divided doses) day 1 [total dose/cycle = 60 mcg]
Estramustine: Oral: 280 mg 3 times/day days 1-5 [total dose/cycle = 4200 mg]
Docetaxel: I.V.: 60 mg/m^2 day 2 [total dose/cycle = 60 mg/m^2]
Treatment cycle is 21 days

Subsequent cycles:
Calcitriol: Oral: 60 mcg (in divided doses) day 1 [total dose/cycle = 60 mcg]
Estramustine: Oral: 280 mg 3 times/day days 1-5 [total dose/cycle = 4200 mg]
Docetaxel: I.V.: 70 mg/m^2 day 2 [total dose/cycle = 70 mg/m^2]
Repeat cycle every 21 days for up to 12 cycles

Estramustine + Docetaxel + Carboplatin

Use: Prostate cancer
Regimen:
Docetaxel: I.V.: 70 mg/m^2 day 2 [total dose/cycle = 70 mg/m^2]
Estramustine: Oral: 280 mg 3 times/day days 1-5 [total dose/cycle = 4200 mg]
Carboplatin: I.V.: Target AUC 5 day 2 [total dose/cycle = AUC = 5]
Repeat cycle every 3 weeks

Estramustine + Docetaxel + Hydrocortisone

Use: Prostate cancer
Regimen:
Docetaxel: I.V.: 70 mg/m^2 day 2 [total dose/cycle = 70 mg/m^2]
Estramustine: Oral: 10 mg/kg/day days 1-5 [total dose/cycle = 50 mg/kg]
Hydrocortisone: Oral: 40 mg daily [total dose/cycle = 840 mg]
Repeat cycle every 3 weeks

Estramustine + Docetaxel + Prednisone

Use: Prostate cancer
Regimen:
Estramustine: Oral: 280 mg 3 times/day days 1-5 and days 7-11 [total dose/cycle = 8400 mg]
Docetaxel: I.V.: 70 mg/m^2 day 2 [total dose/cycle = 70 mg/m^2]
Prednisone: Oral: 10 mg daily [total dose/cycle = 210 mg]
Repeat cycle every 21 days for up to 6 cycles

Estramustine + Etoposide

Use: Prostate cancer
Regimen: Note: Multiple variations are listed below.
Variation 1:
Estramustine: Oral: 15 mg/kg/day days 1-21 [total dose/cycle = 315 mg/kg]
Etoposide: Oral: 50 mg/m^2/day days 1-21 [total dose/cycle = 1050 mg/m^2]
Repeat cycle every 4 weeks
Variation 2:
Estramustine: Oral: 10 mg/kg/day days 1-21 [total dose/cycle = 210 mg/kg]
Etoposide: Oral: 50 mg/m^2/day days 1-21 [total dose/cycle = 1050 mg/m^2]
Repeat cycle every 4 weeks
Variation 3:
Estramustine: Oral: 140 mg 3 times/day days 1-21 [total dose/cycle = 8820 mg]
Etoposide: Oral: 50 mg/m^2/day days 1-21 [total dose/cycle = 1050 mg/m^2]
Repeat cycle every 4 weeks

Estramustine + Vinorelbine

Use: Prostate cancer
Regimen: Note: Multiple variations are listed below.
Variation 1:
Estramustine: Oral: 140 mg 3 times/day days 1-14 [total dose/cycle = 5880 mg]
Vinorelbine: I.V.: 25 mg/m^2/day days 1 and 8 [total dose/cycle = 50 mg/m^2]
Repeat cycle every 21 days
Variation 2:
Estramustine: Oral: 280 mg 3 times/day days 1-3
    [total dose/cycle = 2520 mg/m^2]
Vinorelbine: I.V.: 15 or 20 mg/m^2 day 2 [total dose/cycle = 15 or 20 mg/m^2]
Repeat cycle weekly for 8 weeks, then every other week

EV

Use: Prostate cancer
Regimen: Note: Multiple variations are listed below.
   Variation 1:
   Estramustine: Oral: 10 mg/kg/day days 1-42
      [total dose/cycle = 420 mg/kg]
   Vinblastine: I.V.: 4 mg/m^2/day days 1, 8, 15, 22, 29, 36
      [total dose/cycle = 24 mg/m^2]
   Repeat cycle every 8 weeks
   Variation 2:
   Estramustine: Oral: 600 mg/m^2/day days 1-42
      [total dose/cycle = 25,200 mg/m^2]
   Vinblastine: I.V.: 4 mg/m^2/day days 1, 8, 15, 22, 29, 36 [total dose/cycle = 24 mg/m^2]
   Repeat cycle every 8 weeks

EVA

Use: Lymphoma, Hodgkin disease
Regimen:
   Etoposide: I.V.: 100 mg/m^2/day days 1-3 [total dose/cycle = 300 mg/m^2]
   Vinblastine: I.V.: 6 mg/m^2 day 1 [total dose/cycle = 6 mg/m^2]
   Doxorubicin: I.V.: 50 mg/m^2 day 1 [total dose/cycle = 50 mg/m^2]
   Repeat cycle every 28 days

FAC

Use: Breast cancer
Regimen: Note: Multiple variations are listed below.
   Variation 1:
   Fluorouracil: I.V.: 500 mg/m^2/day days 1 and 8 [total dose/cycle = 1000 mg/m^2]
      or 500 mg/m^2 day 1 [total dose/cycle = 500 mg/m^2]
   Doxorubicin: I.V.: 50 mg/m^2 day 1 [total dose/cycle = 50 mg/m^2]
   Cyclophosphamide: I.V.: 500 mg/m^2 day 1 [total dose/cycle = 500 mg/m^2]
   Repeat cycle every 21-28 days
   Variation 2:
   Fluorouracil: I.V.: 200 mg/m^2/day days 1-3 [total dose/cycle = 600 mg/m^2]
   Doxorubicin: I.V.: 40 mg/m^2 day 1 [total dose/cycle = 40 mg/m^2]
   Cyclophosphamide: I.V.: 400 mg/m^2 day 1 [total dose/cycle = 400 mg/m^2]
   Repeat cycle every 28 days
   Variation 3:
   Fluorouracil: I.V.: 400 mg/m^2/day days 1 and 8 [total dose/cycle = 800 mg/m^2]
   Doxorubicin: I.V.: 40 mg/m^2 day 1 [total dose/cycle = 40 mg/m^2]
   Cyclophosphamide: I.V.: 400 mg/m^2 day 1 [total dose/cycle = 400 mg/m^2]
   Repeat cycle every 28 days
   Variation 4:
   Fluorouracil: I.V.: 600 mg/m^2/day days 1 and 8 [total dose/cycle = 1200 mg/m^2]
   Doxorubicin: I.V.: 60 mg/m^2 day 1 [total dose/cycle = 60 mg/m^2]
   Cyclophosphamide: I.V.: 600 mg/m^2 day 1 [total dose/cycle = 600 mg/m^2]
   Repeat cycle every 28 days
   Variation 5:
   Fluorouracil: I.V.: 300 mg/m^2/day days 1 and 8 [total dose/cycle = 600 mg/m^2]
   Doxorubicin: I.V.: 30 mg/m^2 day 1 [total dose/cycle = 30 mg/m^2]
   Cyclophosphamide: I.V.: 300 mg/m^2 day 1 [total dose/cycle = 300 mg/m^2]
   Repeat cycle every 28 days

FAM

Use: Gastric cancer; Pancreatic cancer
Regimen: Note: Multiple variations are listed below.

Variation 1:
Fluorouracil: I.V.: 600 mg/m^2/day days 1, 8, 29, 36 [total dose/cycle = 2400 mg/m^2]
Doxorubicin: I.V.: 30 mg/m^2/day days 1 and 29 [total dose/cycle = 60 mg/m^2]
Mitomycin C: I.V.: 10 mg/m^2 day 1 [total dose/cycle = 10 mg/m^2]
Repeat cycle every 8 weeks

Variation 2:
Fluorouracil: I.V.: 600 mg/m^2/day days 29-32 [total dose/cycle = 2400 mg/m^2]
Doxorubicin: I.V.: 50 mg/m^2 day 1 [total dose/cycle = 50 mg/m^2]
Mitomycin: I.V.: 10 mg/m^2 day 3 [total dose/cycle = 10 mg/m^2]
Repeat cycle every 8 weeks

Variation 3:
Fluorouracil: I.V.: 500 mg/m^2/day days 1, 8, 21, 28 [total dose/cycle = 2000 mg/m^2]
Doxorubicin: I.V.: 30 mg/m^2/day days 1 and 21 [total dose/cycle = 60 mg/m^2]
Mitomycin: I.V.: 10 mg/m^2 day 1 [total dose/cycle = 10 mg/m^2]
Repeat cycle every 6 weeks

Variation 4:
Fluorouracil: I.V.: 275 mg/m^2/day days 1-5, and 36-40 [total dose/cycle = 2750 mg/m^2]
Doxorubicin: I.V.: 30 mg/m^2/day days 1 and 36 [total dose/cycle = 60 mg/m^2]
Mitomycin: I.V.: 10 mg/m^2 day 1 [total dose/cycle = 10 mg/m^2]
Repeat cycle every 10 weeks

Variation 5:
Fluorouracil: I.V.: 600 mg/m^2/day days 1, 8, 22, 29 [total dose/cycle = 2400 mg/m^2]
Doxorubicin: I.V.: 30 mg/m^2/day days 1 and 22 [total dose/cycle = 60 mg/m^2]
Mitomycin I.V.: 10 mg/m^2 day 1 [total dose/cycle = 10 mg/m^2]
Repeat cycle every 6 weeks

FAMe

Use: Gastric cancer
Regimen:
Fluorouracil: I.V.: 325 mg/m^2/day days 1-5 and 36-40 [total dose/cycle = 3250 mg/m^2]
Doxorubicin: I.V.: 40 mg/m^2 days 1 and 36 [total dose/cycle = 80 mg/m^2]
Lomustine: Oral: 110 mg/m^2 day 1 [total dose/cycle = 110 mg/m^2]
Repeat cycle every 10 weeks

FAMTX

Use: Gastric cancer
Regimen: Note: Multiple variations are listed below.

Variation 1:
Methotrexate: I.V.: 1500 mg/m^2 day 1 [total dose/cycle = 1500 mg/m^2]
Fluorouracil: I.V.: 1500 mg/m^2 (1 hour after methotrexate) day 1 [total dose/cycle = 1500 mg/m^2]
Leucovorin: Oral: 15 mg/m^2 every 6 hours for 48 hours (start 24 hours after methotrexate) day 2
  [total dose/cycle = 120 mg/m^2]
Doxorubicin: I.V.: 30 mg/m^2 day 15 [total dose/cycle = 30 mg/m^2]
Repeat cycle every 28 days

Variation 2:
Methotrexate: I.V.: 1500 mg/m^2 day 1 [total dose/cycle = 1500 mg/m^2]
Fluorouracil: I.V.: 1500 mg/m^2 (1 hour after methotrexate) day 1 [total dose/cycle = 1500 mg/m^2]
Leucovorin: Oral: 30 mg/m^2 every 6 hours for 8 doses (start 24 hours after methotrexate)
  [total dose/cycle = 240 mg/m^2] **followed by** 30 mg/m^2 every 6 hours for 8 more doses if 24-hour methotrexate
  level ≥2.5 mol/L [total dose/cycle = 480 mg/m^2]
Doxorubicin: I.V.: 30 mg/m^2 day 15 [total dose/cycle = 30 mg/m^2]
Repeat cycle every 28 days

Variation 3:
Methotrexate: I.V.: 1000 mg/m^2 day 1 [total dose/cycle = 1000 mg/m^2]
Fluorouracil: I.V.: 1500 mg/m^2 (1 hour after methotrexate) day 1 [total dose/cycle = 1500 mg/m^2]
Leucovorin: Oral: 15 mg every 6 hours for 8 doses (start 24 hours after methotrexate)
  [total dose/cycle = 120 mg/m^2]
Doxorubicin: I.V.: 30 mg/m^2 day 15 [total dose/cycle = 30 mg/m^2]
Repeat cycle every 28 days

F-CL

Use: Colorectal cancer
Regimen: Note: Multiple variations are listed below.
    Variation 1 (Mayo Regimen):
    Fluorouracil: I.V.: 425 mg/m^2/day days 1-5 [total dose/cycle = 2125 mg/m^2]
    Leucovorin: I.V.: 20 mg/m^2/day days 1-5 [total dose/cycle = 100 mg/m^2]
    Repeat cycle every 28 days
    Variation 2:
    Fluorouracil: I.V.: 400 mg/m^2/day days 1-5 [total dose/cycle = 2000 mg/m^2]
    Leucovorin: I.V.: 20 mg/m^2/day days 1-5 [total dose/cycle = 100 mg/m^2]
    Repeat cycle every 28 days
    Variation 3:
    Fluorouracil: I.V.: 500 mg/m^2 day 1 [total dose/cycle = 500 mg/m^2]
    Leucovorin: I.V.: 20 mg/m^2 (2-hour infusion) day 1
        [total dose/cycle = 20 mg/m^2] **or** 500 mg/m^2 (2-hour infusion) day 1 [total dose/cycle = 500 mg/m^2]
    Repeat cycle weekly
    Variation 4:
    Fluorouracil: I.V.: 600 mg/m^2 weekly for 6 weeks [total dose/cycle = 3600 mg/m^2]
    Leucovorin: I.V.: 500 mg/m^2 (3-hour infusion) weekly for 6 weeks [total dose/cycle = 3000 mg/m^2]
    Repeat cycle every 8 weeks
    Variation 5:
    Fluorouracil: I.V.: 600 mg/m^2 weekly for 6 weeks [total dose/cycle = 3600 mg/m^2]
    Leucovorin: I.V.: 500 mg/m^2 weekly for 6 weeks [total dose/cycle = 3000 mg/m^2]
    Repeat cycle every 8 weeks
    Variation 6:
    Fluorouracil: I.V.: 600 mg/m^2 weekly [total dose/cycle = 600 mg/m^2]
    Leucovorin: I.V.: 500 mg/m^2 (2-hour infusion) weekly [total dose/cycle = 500 mg/m^2]
    Repeat cycle weekly
    Variation 7:
    Fluorouracil: I.V.: 2600 mg/m^2 continuous infusion day 1 [total dose/cycle = 2600 mg/m^2]
    Leucovorin: I.V.: 500 mg/m^2 continuous infusion day 1 [total dose/cycle = 500 mg/m^2]
    Repeat cycle weekly
    Variation 8:
    Fluorouracil: I.V.: 2600 mg/m^2 continuous infusion day 1 [total dose/cycle = 2600 mg/m^2]
    Leucovorin: I.V.: 300 mg/m^2 (maximum 500 mg) continuous infusion day 1
        [total dose/cycle = 300 mg/m^2; maximum 500 mg]
    Repeat cycle weekly
    Variation 9:
    Fluorouracil: I.V.: 2600 mg/m^2 continuous infusion once weekly for 6 weeks
        [total dose/cycle = 15,600 mg/m^2]
    Leucovorin: I.V.: 500 mg/m^2 weekly for 6 weeks [total dose/cycle = 3000 mg/m^2]
    Repeat cycle every 8 weeks
    Variation 10:
    Fluorouracil: I.V.: 2300 mg/m^2 continuous infusion day 1 [total dose/cycle = 2300 mg/m^2]
    Leucovorin: I.V.: 50 mg/m^2 continuous infusion day 1 [total dose/cycle = 50 mg/m^2]
    Repeat cycle weekly
    Variation 11:
    Fluorouracil: I.V.: 200 mg/m^2/day continuous infusion days 1-14 [total dose/cycle = 2800 mg/m^2]
    Leucovorin: I.V.: 5 mg/m^2/day days 1-14 [total dose/cycle = 70 mg/m^2]
    Repeat cycle every 28 days
    Variation 12:
    Cycle 1:
    Fluorouracil: I.V.: 200 mg/m^2/day continuous infusion for 4 weeks
        [total dose/cycle = 5600 mg/m^2]
    Leucovorin: I.V.: 20 mg/m^2/day days 1, 8, 15, 22 [total dose/cycle = 80 mg/m^2]
    Treatment cycle is 6 weeks
    Subsequent cycles:
    Fluorouracil: 200 mg/m^2 continuous infusion days 1 and 21 [total dose/cycle = 4200 mg/m^2]
    Leucovorin: I.V.: 20 mg/m^2/day days 1, 8, 15 [total dose/cycle = 60 mg/m^2]
    Repeat cycle every 4 weeks

FAP

Use: Gastric cancer
Regimen:
    Fluorouracil: I.V.: 300 mg/m^2/day days 1-5 [total dose/cycle = 1500 mg/m^2]
    Doxorubicin: I.V.: 40 mg/m^2 day 1 [total dose/cycle = 40 mg/m^2]
    Cisplatin: I.V.: 60 mg/m^2 day 1 [total dose/cycle = 60 mg/m^2]
    Repeat cycle every 5 weeks

FEC
Use: Breast cancer
Regimen:
Fluorouracil: I.V.: 500 mg/m^2 day 1 [total dose/cycle = 500 mg/m^2]
Cyclophosphamide: I.V.: 500 mg/m^2 day 1 [total dose/cycle = 500 mg/m^2]
Epirubicin: I.V.: 100 mg/m^2 day 1 [total dose/cycle = 100 mg/m^2]
Repeat cycle every 21 days

FIS-HAM
Use: Leukemia, acute lymphocytic; Leukemia, acute myeloid
Regimen:
Fludarabine: I.V.: 15 mg/m^2/day every 12 hours days 1, 2, 8, 9 [total dose/cycle = 120 mg/m^2]
Cytarabine: I.V.: 750 mg/m^2/day every 3 hours days 1, 2, 8, 9 [total dose/cycle = 24,000 mg/m^2]
Mitoxantrone: I.V.: 10 mg/m^2/day days 3, 4, 10, 11 [total dose/cycle = 40 mg/m^2]

FL
Use: Prostate cancer
Regimen: Note: Multiple variations are listed below.
Variation 1:
Flutamide: Oral: 250 mg every 8 hours [total dose/cycle = 21,000 mg]
Leuprolide acetate: SubQ: 1 mg/day [total dose/cycle = 28 mg]
Repeat cycle every 28 days
Variation 2:
Flutamide: Oral: 250 mg every 8 hours [total dose/cycle = 67,500 mg]
Leuprolide acetate depot: I.M.: 22.5 mg day 1 [total dose/cycle = 22.5 mg]
Repeat cycle every 3 months

FLAG
Use: Leukemia, acute myeloid
Regimen:
Fludarabine: I.V.: 30 mg/m^2/day days 1-5 [total dose/cycle = 150 mg/m^2]
Cytarabine: I.V.: 2 g/m^2/day days 1-5 (3.5 hours after end of fludarabine infusion)
      [total dose/cycle = 10 g/m^2]
Filgrastim: SubQ: 5 mcg/kg day 1
      [total dose/cycle = 5 mcg/kg] **followed by** 300 mcg daily until ANC >500-1000 cells/mcL postnadir
      [total dose/cycle = 40-7800 mcg/kg]
Repeat cycle every 3-4 weeks

FLAG-IDA
Use: Leukemia, acute myeloid
Regimen:
Fludarabine: I.V.: 30 mg/m^2/day days 1-5 [total dose/cycle = 150 mg/m^2]
Cytarabine: I.V.: 2 g/m^2/day days 1-5 [total dose/cycle = 10 g/m^2]
Idarubicin: I.V.: 10 mg/m^2/day days 1, 2, 3
      [total dose/cycle = 30 mg/m^2]
Filgrastim: 5 mcg/kg from day 6 until neutrophil recovery
Administer one cycle only

FLOX (Nordic FLOX)
Use: Colorectal cancer
Regimen:
Oxaliplatin: I.V.: 85 mg/m^2 day 1 [total dose/cycle = 85 mg/m^2]
Fluorouracil: I.V.: 500 mg/m^2/day days 1 and 2 [total dose/cycle = 1000 mg/m^2]
Leucovorin: I.V.: 60 mg/m^2/day days 1 and 2
      [total dose/cycle = 120 mg/m^2]
Repeat cycle every 2 weeks

Fludarabine-Cyclophosphamide-Rituximab
Use: Leukemia, chronic lymphocytic
Regimen:
Cycle 1:
Rituximab: I.V.: 375 mg/m² day 1 [total dose/cycle = 375 mg/m²]
Fludarabine: I.V.: 25 mg/m²/day days 2, 3, 4 [total dose/cycle = 75 mg/m²]
Cyclophosphamide: I.V.: 250 mg/m²/day days 2, 3, 4 [total dose/cycle = 750 mg/m²]
Treatment cycle is every 4 weeks
Cycles 2-6:
Rituximab: I.V.: 500 mg/m² day 1 [total dose/cycle = 500 mg/m²]
Fludarabine: I.V.: 25 mg/m²/day days 1, 2, 3 [total dose/cycle = 75 mg/m²]
Cyclophosphamide: I.V.: 250 mg/m²/day days 1, 2, 3 [total dose/cycle = 750 mg/m²]
Repeat cycle every 4 weeks

Fludarabine-Rituximab
Use: Leukemia, chronic lymphocytic
Regimen:
Rituximab: I.V.: 375 mg/m²/day days 1 and 4 (cycle 1); [total dose/cycle 1 = 750 mg/m²] day 1 (cycles 2-6)
  [total dose/cycle = 375 mg/m²]
Fludarabine: I.V.: 25 mg/m²/day days 1-5 [total dose/cycle = 125 mg/m²]
Repeat cycle every 4 weeks

Fluorouracil + Carboplatin
Use: Head and neck cancer
Regimen: Note: Multiple variations are listed below.
Variation: 1:
Fluorouracil: I.V.: 600 mg/m²/day continuous infusion days 1-4 [total dose/cycle = 2400 mg/m²]
Carboplatin: I.V.: 70 mg/m²/day days 1-4 [total dose/cycle = 280 mg/m²]
Repeat cycle every 3 weeks for 3 cycles
Variation: 2:
Carboplatin: I.V.: 400 mg/m² day 1 [total dose/cycle = 400 mg/m²]
Fluorouracil: I.V.: 1000 mg/m²/day continuous infusion days 1-4 [total dose/cycle = 4000 mg/m²]
Repeat cycle every 28 days

FOIL
Use: Colorectal cancer
Regimen:
Irinotecan: I.V.: 175 mg/m² day 1 [total dose/cycle = 175 mg/m²]
Oxaliplatin: I.V.: 100 mg/m² day 1 [total dose/cycle = 100 mg/m²]
Leucovorin: I.V.: 200 mg/m² day 1 [total dose/cycle = 200 mg/m²]
Fluorouracil: I.V.: 3800 mg/m²/day continuous infusion days 1 and 2 [total dose/cycle = 7600 mg/m²]
Repeat cycle every 14 days

FOLFOX 1
Use: Colorectal cancer
Regimen:
Oxaliplatin: I.V.: 130 mg/m² day 1 (every other cycle) [total dose/cycle = 130 mg/m²]
Leucovorin: I.V.: 500 mg/m²/day days 1 and 2 [total dose/cycle = 1000 mg/m²]
Fluorouracil: I.V.: 1.5-2 g/m²/day continuous infusion days 1 and 2 [total dose/cycle = 3-4 g/m²]
Repeat cycle every 14 days

FOLFOX 2
Use: Colorectal cancer
Regimen:
Oxaliplatin: I.V.: 100 mg/m² day 1 [total dose/cycle = 100 mg/m²]
Leucovorin: I.V.: 500 mg/m²/day days 1 and 2 [total dose/cycle = 1000 mg/m²]
Fluorouracil: I.V.: 1.5-2 g/m²/day continuous infusion days 1 and 2 [total dose/cycle = 3-4 g/m²]
Repeat cycle every 14 days

FOLFOX 3

Use: Colorectal cancer
Regimen:

Oxaliplatin: I.V.: 85 mg/m^2 day 1 [total dose/cycle = 85 mg/m^2]
Leucovorin: I.V.: 500 mg/m^2/day days 1 and 2 [total dose/cycle = 1000 mg/m^2]
Fluorouracil: I.V.: 1.5-2 g/m^2/day continuous infusion days 1 and 2 [total dose/cycle = 3-4 g/m^2]
Repeat cycle every 14 days

FOLFOX 4

Use: Colorectal cancer
Regimen:

Oxaliplatin: I.V.: 85 mg/m^2 day 1 [total dose/cycle = 85 mg/m^2]
Leucovorin: I.V.: 200 mg/m^2/day days 1 and 2 [total dose/cycle = 400 mg/m^2]
Fluorouracil: I.V. bolus: 400 mg/m^2/day days 1 and 2
  [total dose/cycle = 800 mg/m^2] **followed by** 600 mg/m^2 CIVI (over 22-hour) days 1 and 2
  [total dose/cycle = 1200 mg/m^2]
Note: Bolus fluorouracil and CIVI are both given on each day.
Repeat cycle every 14 days

FOLFOX 6

Use: Colorectal cancer
Regimen:

Oxaliplatin: I.V.: 100 mg/m^2 day 1 [total dose/cycle = 100 mg/m^2]
Leucovorin: I.V.: 400 mg/m^2 day 1 [total dose/cycle = 400 mg/m^2]
Fluorouracil: I.V. bolus: 400 mg/m^2 day 1 [total dose/cycle = 400 mg/m^2] **followed by** 2.4-3 g/m^2 continuous
  infusion (46 hours) extending over days 1 and 2 [total dose/cycle = 2.4-3 g/m^2]
Repeat cycle every 14 days

FOLFOX 7

Use: Colorectal cancer
Regimen:

Oxaliplatin: I.V.: 130 mg/m^2 day 1 [total dose/cycle = 130 mg/m^2]
Leucovorin: I.V.: 400 mg/m^2 day 1 [total dose/cycle = 400 mg/m^2]
Fluorouracil: I.V. bolus: 400 mg/m^2 day 1
  [total dose/cycle = 400 mg/m^2] **followed by** 2.4 g/m^2 continuous infusion (46 hours) extending over days 1 and
  2 [total dose/cycle = 2.4 g/m^2]
Repeat cycle every 14 days

FU HURT

Use: Head and neck cancer
Regimen:

Hydroxyurea: Oral: 1000 mg every 12 hours for 11 doses days 0-5 [total dose/cycle = 11,000 mg]
Fluorouracil: I.V.: 800 mg/m^2/day continuous infusion (start AM after admission) days 1-5
  [total dose/cycle = 4000 mg/m^2]
Paclitaxel: I.V.: 5-25 mg/m^2/day continuous infusion days 1-5 [total dose/cycle = 25-125 mg/m^2]
Filgrastim: SubQ: 5 mcg/kg/day days 6-12 (start ≥12 hours after completion of fluorouracil infusion)
5-7 cycles may be administered

FU/LV

Use: Colorectal cancer
Regimen:

Fluorouracil: I.V.: 400 mg/m^2/day days 1-5
  [total dose/cycle = 2000 mg/m^2]
Leucovorin: I.V.: 20 mg/m^2/day days 1-5 [total dose/cycle = 100 mg/m^2]
Repeat cycle every 28 days

FU/LV/CPT-11

Use: Colorectal cancer
Regimen: Note: Multiple variations are listed below.

Variation: 1:
Irinotecan: I.V.: 350 mg/m^2 day 1 [total dose/cycle = 350 mg/m^2]
Leucovorin: I.V.: 20 mg/m^2/day days 22-26 [total dose/cycle = 100 mg/m^2]
Fluorouracil: I.V.: 425 mg/m^2/day days 22-26 [total dose/cycle = 2125 mg/m^2]
Repeat cycle every 6 weeks

Variation: 2:
Irinotecan: I.V.: 80 mg/m^2 day 1 [total dose/cycle = 80 mg/m^2]
Fluorouracil: I.V.: 2300 mg/m^2 continuous infusion day 1 [total dose/cycle = 2300 mg/m^2]
Leucovorin: I.V.: 500 mg/m^2 day 1 [total dose/cycle = 500 mg/m^2]
Repeat cycle weekly **or**
Irinotecan: I.V.: 180 mg/m^2 day 1 [total dose/cycle = 180 mg/m^2]
Leucovorin: I.V.: 200 mg/m^2/day days 1 and 2 [total dose/cycle = 400 mg/m^2]
Fluorouracil: I.V.: 400 mg/m^2/day days 1 and 2 [total dose/cycle = 800 mg/m^2]
followed by 600 mg/m^2/day continuous infusion days 1 and 2 [total dose/cycle = 1200 mg/m^2]
Repeat cycle every 2 weeks

Variation 3:
Irinotecan: I.V.: 175 mg/m^2 day 1 [total dose/cycle = 175 mg/m^2]
Leucovorin: I.V.: 250 mg/m^2 day 2 [total dose/cycle = 250 mg/m^2]
Fluorouracil: I.V.: 950 mg/m^2 day 2 [total dose/cycle = 950 mg/m^2] **or**
Irinotecan: I.V.: 200 mg/m^2 day 1 [total dose/cycle = 200 mg/m^2]
Leucovorin: I.V.: 250 mg/m^2 day 2 [total dose/cycle = 250 mg/m^2]
Fluorouracil: I.V.: 850 mg/m^2 day 2 [total dose/cycle = 850 mg/m^2]
Repeat cycle every other week

FU/LV/CPT-11 (Saltz Regimen)

Use: Colorectal cancer
Regimen:
Fluorouracil: I.V.: 500 mg/m^2/day days 1, 8, 15, 22 [total dose/cycle = 2000 mg/m^2]
Leucovorin: I.V.: 20 mg/m^2/day days 1, 8, 15, 22 [total dose/cycle = 80 mg/m^2]
Irinotecan: I.V.: 125 mg/m^2/day days 1, 8, 15, 22 [total dose/cycle = 500 mg/m^2]
Repeat cycle every 42 days

FUP

Use: Gastric cancer
Regimen:
Fluorouracil: I.V.: 1000 mg/m^2/day continuous infusion days 1-5 [total dose/cycle = 5000 mg/m^2]
Cisplatin: I.V.: 100 mg/m^2 day 2 [total dose/cycle = 100 mg/m^2]
Repeat cycle every 28 days

FZ

Use: Prostate cancer
Regimen: Note: Multiple variations are listed below.

Variation 1:
Flutamide: Oral: 250 mg every 8 hours [total dose/cycle = 21,000 mg]
Goserelin acetate: SubQ: 3.6 mg day 1 [total dose/cycle = 3.6 mg]
Repeat cycle every 28 days

Variation 2:
Flutamide: Oral: 250 mg every 8 hours [total dose/cycle = 67,500 mg]
Goserelin acetate: SubQ: 10.8 mg day 1 [total dose/cycle = 10.8 mg]
Repeat cycle every 3 months

GC

Use: Lung cancer, nonsmall cell
Regimen:
Gemcitabine: I.V.: 1000 mg/m^2/day days 1, 8, 15 [total dose/cycle = 3000 mg/m^2]
Cisplatin: I.V.: 100 mg/m^2 day 1 **or** 2 **or** 15 [total dose/cycle = 100 mg/m^2]
Repeat cycle every 28 days for 2-6 cycles

Gemcitabine/Capecitabine

Use: Biliary adenocarcinoma; Pancreatic cancer

Regimen:
Gemcitabine: I.V.: 1000 mg/m^2/day days 1 and 8 [total dose/cycle = 2000 mg/m^2]
Capecitabine: Oral: 650 mg/m^2 twice daily days 1-14 [total dose/cycle = 18,200 mg/m^2]
Repeat cycle every 21 days

Gemcitabine-Carboplatin (Bladder Cancer)

Use: Bladder cancer

Regimen:
Gemcitabine: I.V.: 1000 mg/m^2/day days 1 and 8
   [total dose/cycle = 2000 mg/m^2]
Carboplatin: I.V.: AUC 5 day 1 [total dose/cycle = AUC = 5]
Repeat cycle every 21 days for up to 6 cycles

Gemcitabine-Carboplatin (Nonsmall Cell Lung Cancer)

Use: Lung cancer, nonsmall cell

Regimen:
Gemcitabine: I.V.: 1000 or 1100 mg/m^2/day days 1 and 8
   [total dose/cycle = 2000 or 2200 mg/m^2]
Carboplatin: I.V.: AUC 5 day 8 [total dose/cycle = AUC = 5]
Repeat cycle every 28 days

Gemcitabine-Cis

Use: Lung cancer, nonsmall cell

Regimen: Note: Multiple variations are listed below.
   Variation 1:
Gemcitabine: I.V.: 1000-1200 mg/m^2/day days 1, 8, 15 [total dose/cycle = 3000-3600 mg/m^2]
Cisplatin: I.V.: 100 mg/m^2 day 2 **or** 15 [total dose/cycle = 100 mg/m^2]
Repeat cycle every 28 days
   Variation 2:
Gemcitabine: I.V.: 1000-1200 mg/m^2/day 1, 8, 15 [total dose/cycle = 3000-3600 mg/m^2]
Cisplatin: I.V.: 100 mg/m^2 day 1 **or** 2 **or** 15 [total dose/cycle = 100 mg/m^2]
Repeat cycle every 28 days

Gemcitabine-Cisplatin

Use: Bladder cancer

Regimen:
Gemcitabine: I.V.: 1000 mg/m^2/day days 1, 8, 15 [total dose/cycle = 3000 mg/m^2]
Cisplatin: I.V.: 70 mg/m^2 day 2 [total dose/cycle = 70 mg/m^2]
Repeat cycle every 28 days for 6 cycles

Gemcitabine-Docetaxel (Bladder Cancer)

Use: Bladder cancer

Regimen:
Docetaxel: I.V.: 40 mg/m^2/day days 1 and 8 [total dose/cycle = 80 mg/m^2]
Gemcitabine: 800 mg/m^2/day days 1 and 8 [total dose/cycle = 1600 mg/m^2]
Repeat cycle every 21 days for up to 6 cycles

Gemcitabine-Docetaxel (Sarcoma)

Use: Osteosarcoma; Soft tissue sarcoma

Regimen:
Gemcitabine: I.V.: 675 mg/m^2/day days 1 and 8 [total dose/cycle = 1350 mg/m^2]
Docetaxel: I.V.: 100 mg/m^2 day 8 [total dose/cycle = 100 mg/m^2]
Repeat cycle every 21 days

Gemcitabine-Erlotinib

Use: Pancreatic cancer

Regimen:

Cycle 1:

Gemcitabine: I.V.: 1000 mg/m^2/day days 1, 8, 15, 22, 29, 36, 43 (cycle 1 only) [total dose/cycle 1 = 7000 mg/m^2]
Erlotinib: Oral: 100 mg once daily days 1-56 [total dose/cycle 1 = 5600 mg]
Treatment cycle is 56 days

Subsequent cycles:

Gemcitabine: I.V.: 1000 mg/m^2/day days 1, 8, 15 [total dose/cycle = 3000 mg/m^2]
Erlotinib: Oral: 100 mg once daily days 1-28 [total dose/cycle = 2800 mg]
Repeat cycle every 28 days

Gemcitabine/Irinotecan

Use: Pancreatic cancer

Regimen:

Gemcitabine: I.V.: 1000 mg/m^2/day days 1 and 8 [total dose/cycle = 2000 mg/m^2]
Irinotecan: I.V.: 100 mg/m^2/day days 1 and 8 [total dose/cycle = 200 mg/m^2]
Repeat cycle every 21 days

Gemcitabine-Paclitaxel

Use: Ovarian cancer

Regimen:

Paclitaxel: I.V.: 80 mg/m^2 infused over 60 minutes days 1, 8, 15
    [total dose/cycle = 240 mg/m^2]
Gemcitabine: I.V.: 1000 mg/m^2/day (start at end of paclitaxel infusion) days 1, 8, 15
    [total dose/cycle = 3000 mg/m^2]
Repeat cycle every 4 weeks

Gemcitabine-Vinorelbine

Use: Lung cancer, nonsmall cell

Regimen: Note: Multiple variations are listed below.

Variation 1:

Gemcitabine: I.V.: 1200 mg/m^2/day days 1 and 8 [total dose/cycle = 2400 mg/m^2]
Vinorelbine: I.V.: 30 mg/m^2/day days 1 and 8 [total dose/cycle = 60 mg/m^2]
Repeat cycle every 21 days for 6 cycles

Variation 2:

Gemcitabine: I.V.: 1000 mg/m^2/day days 1, 8, 15 [total dose/cycle = 3000 mg/m^2]
Vinorelbine: I.V.: 20 mg/m^2/day days 1, 8, 15 [total dose/cycle = 60 mg/m^2]
Repeat cycle every 28 days for 6 cycles

GEMOX

Use: Biliary adenocarcinoma

Regimen:

Gemcitabine: I.V.: 1000 mg/m^2 day 1 [total dose/cycle = 1000 mg/m^2]
Oxaliplatin: I.V.: 100 mg/m^2 day 2 [total dose/cycle = 100 mg/m^2]
Repeat cycle every 2 weeks

HDMTX (Osteosarcoma)

Use: Osteosarcoma

Regimen:

Methotrexate: I.V.: 12 g/m^2/week for 2-12 weeks [total dose/cycle = 24-144 g/m^2]
Leucovorin calcium rescue: Oral, I.V.: 15 mg/m^2 every 6 hours (beginning 30 hours after the beginning of the 4-hour methotrexate infusion) for 10 doses; **serum methotrexate levels must be monitored**
    [total dose/cycle = 150 mg/m^2]

HIPE-IVAD

Use: Neuroblastoma
Regimen:
Cisplatin: I.V.: 40 mg/m^2/day days 1-5 [total dose/cycle = 200 mg/m^2]
Etoposide: I.V.: 100 mg/m^2/day days 1-5 [total dose/cycle = 500 mg/m^2]
Ifosfamide: I.V.: 3 g/m^2/day days 21-23 [total dose/cycle = 9 g/m^2]
Mesna: I.V.: 3 g/m^2/day continuous infusion days 21-23 [total dose/cycle = 9 g/m^2]
Vincristine: I.V.: 1.5 mg/m^2 day 21 [total dose/cycle = 1.5 mg/m^2]
Doxorubicin: I.V.: 60 mg/m^2 day 23 [total dose/cycle = 60 mg/m^2]
Repeat cycle every 28 days

Hyper-CVAD (Leukemia, Acute Lymphocytic)

Use: Leukemia, acute lymphocytic
Regimen: Note: Multiple variations are listed below.

Variation 1:

Cycle A: (Cycles 1, 3, 5, and 7):
Cyclophosphamide: I.V.: 300 mg/m^2 every 12 hours, for 6 doses, days 1-3 [total dose/cycle = 1800 mg/m^2]
Mesna: I.V.: 1200 mg/m^2/day continuous infusion days 1-3 [total dose/cycle = 3600 mg/m^2]
Vincristine: I.V.: 2 mg/day days 4 and 11 [total dose/cycle = 4 mg]
Doxorubicin: I.V.: 50 mg/m^2 day 4 [total dose/cycle = 50 mg/m^2]
Dexamethasone: (route not specified): 40 mg/day days 1-4 and 11-14 [total dose/cycle = 320 mg]

Cycle B: (Cycles 2, 4, 6, and 8)
Methotrexate: I.V.: 1 g/m^2 continuous infusion day 1 [total dose/cycle = 1 g/m^2]
Leucovorin: (route not specified): 15 mg every 6 hours, for 8 doses (start 12 hours after end of methotrexate
   infusion) [total dose/cycle = 120 mg]
Cytarabine: I.V.: 3 g/m^2 every 12 hours, for 4 doses, days 2 and 3 [total dose/cycle = 12 g/m^2]
Methylprednisolone: I.V.: 50 mg twice daily, for 6 doses, days 1-3 [total dose/cycle = 300 mg/m^2]
Repeat every 6 weeks in the following sequence: ABABABAB

CNS Prophylaxis
Methotrexate: I.T.: 12 mg/day day 2 [total dose/cycle = 12 mg]
   or 6 mg/day into Ommaya day 2 [total dose/cycle = 6 mg]
Cytarabine: I.T.: 100 mg day 8 [total dose/cycle = 100 mg]
Repeat cycle every 3 weeks

Maintenance (POMP)
Mercaptopurine: Oral: 50 mg 3 times/day [total dose/cycle = 4200-4650 mg]
Vincristine: I.V.: 2 mg day 1 [total dose/cycle = 2 mg]
Methotrexate: Oral: 20 mg/m^2/day days 1, 8, 15, 22 [total dose/cycle = 80 mg/m^2]
Prednisone: Oral: 200 mg/day days 1-5 [total dose/cycle = 1000 mg/m^2] **or**
Mercaptopurine: I.V.: 1 g/m^2/day days 1-5 [total dose/cycle = 5 g/m^2]
Vincristine: I.V.: 2 mg day 1 [total dose/cycle = 2 mg]
Methotrexate: I.V.: 10 mg/m^2/day days 1-5 [total dose/cycle = 50 mg/m^2]
Prednisone: Oral: 200 mg/day days 1-5 [total dose/cycle = 1000 mg/m^2]
Repeat cycles every month for 2 years

Variation 2:

Cycle A: (Cycles 1, 3, 5, and 7)
Cyclophosphamide: I.V.: 300 mg/m^2 every 12 hours, for 6 doses, days 1-3 [total dose/cycle = 1800 mg/m^2]
Mesna: I.V.: 600 mg/m^2/day continuous infusion days 1-3 [total dose/cycle = 1800 mg/m^2]
Vincristine: I.V.: 2 mg/day days 4 and 11 [total dose/cycle = 4 mg]
Doxorubicin: I.V.: 50 mg/m^2 day 4 [total dose/cycle = 50 mg/m^2]
Dexamethasone: Oral, I.V.: 40 mg/day days 1-4 and 11-14 [total dose/cycle = 320 mg]

Cycle B: (Cycles 2, 4, 6, and 8)

Methotrexate: I.V.: 1 g/m^2 continuous infusion day 1 [total dose/cycle = 1 g/m^2]

Leucovorin: I.V.: 50 mg (start 12 hours after end of methotrexate infusion)

followed by: I.V.: 15 mg every 6 hours, for 8 doses [total dose/cycle = 170 mg]

Cytarabine: I.V.: 3 g/m^2 every 12 hours, for 4 doses, days 2 and 3 [total dose/cycle = 12 g/m^2]

Repeat every 6 weeks in the following sequence: ABABABAB

CNS Prophylaxis

Methotrexate: I.T.: 12 mg day 2 [total dose/cycle = 12 mg]

   or 6 mg into Ommaya day 2 [total dose/cycle = 6 mg]

Cytarabine: I.T.: 100 mg day 7 [total dose/cycle = 100 mg]

Repeat cycle every 3 weeks

Variation 3:

Cycle A: (Cycles 1, 3, 5, and 7)

Cyclophosphamide: I.V.: 300 mg/m^2 every 12 hours, for 6 doses, days 1-3 [total dose/cycle = 1800 mg/m^2]

Mesna: I.V.: 600 mg/m^2/day continuous infusion days 1-3 [total dose/cycle = 1800 mg/m^2]

Vincristine: I.V.: 2 mg/day days 4 and 11 [total dose/cycle = 4 mg]

Doxorubicin: I.V.: 50 mg/m^2 continuous infusion day 4 [total dose/cycle = 50 mg/m^2]

Dexamethasone: Oral, I.V.: 40 mg/day days 1-4 and 11-14 [total dose/cycle = 320 mg]

Cycle B: (Cycles 2, 4, 6, and 8)

Methotrexate: I.V.: 200 mg/m^2 day 1

followed by I.V.: 800 mg/m^2 continuous infusion day 1 [total dose/cycle = 1 g/m^2]

Leucovorin: I.V.: 50 mg (start 12 hours after end of methotrexate infusion)

followed by: I.V.: 15 mg every 6 hours, for 8 doses [total dose/cycle = 170 mg/m^2]

Cytarabine: I.V.: 3 g/m^2 every 12 hours, for 4 doses, days 2 and 3 [total dose/cycle = 12 g/m^2]

Repeat every 6 weeks in the following sequence: ABABABAB

CNS Prophylaxis

Methotrexate: I.T.: 12 mg day 2 [total dose/cycle = 12 mg]

   or 6 mg into Ommaya day 2 [total dose/cycle = 6 mg]

Cytarabine: I.T.: 100 mg day 7 **or** 8 [total dose/cycle = 100 mg]

Repeat cycle every 3 weeks for 6 or 8 cycles

Maintenance (POMP)

Mercaptopurine: Oral: 50 mg 3 times/day [total dose/cycle = 4200-4650 mg]

Vincristine: I.V.: 2 mg day 1 [total dose/cycle = 2 mg]

Methotrexate: Oral, I.V.: 20 mg/m^2/day days 1, 8, 15, 22 [total dose/cycle = 80 mg/m^2]

Prednisone: Oral: 200 mg/day days 1-5 [total dose/cycle = 1000 mg/m^2] **or**

Mercaptopurine: I.V.: 1 g/m^2/day days 1-5 [total dose/cycle = 5 g/m^2]

Vincristine: I.V.: 2 mg day 1 [total dose/cycle = 2 mg]

Methotrexate: I.V.: 10 mg/m^2/day days 1-5 [total dose/cycle = 50 mg/m^2]

Prednisone: Oral: 200 mg/day days 1-5 [total dose/cycle = 1000 mg]

Repeat cycles every month (except months 7 and 11 or 9 and 12) for 2 years

Intensification

Etoposide: I.V.: 100 mg/m^2/day days 1-5 [total dose/cycle = 500 mg/m^2]

Pegaspargase: I.V.: 2500 units/m^2 day 1 [total dose/cycle = 2500 units/m^2]

Given during months 9 and 12 of maintenance

   or

Methotrexate: I.V.: 100 mg/m^2/day days 1, 8, 15, 22 [total dose/cycle = 400 mg/m^2]

Asparaginase: I.V.: 20,000 units/day days 2, 9, 16, 23 [total dose/cycle = 80,000 units]

Given during months 7 and 11 of maintenance

Variation 4:

Cycle A: (Cycles 1, 3, 5, and 7)

Cyclophosphamide: I.V.: 300 mg/m^2 every 12 hours, for 6 doses, days 1-3 [total dose/cycle = 1800 mg/m^2]

Mesna: I.V.: 600 mg/m^2/day continuous infusion days 1-3 [total dose/cycle = 1800 mg/m^2]

Hyper-CVAD (Leukemia, Acute Lymphocytic) *(continued)*

Vincristine: I.V.: 2 mg/day days 4 and 11 [total dose/cycle = 4 mg]

Doxorubicin: I.V.: 50 mg/m^2 day 4 [total dose/cycle = 50 mg/m^2]

Dexamethasone: (route not specified): 40 mg/day days 1-4 and 11-14 [total dose/cycle = 320 mg]

Cycle B: (Cycles 2, 4, 6, and 8)

Methotrexate: I.V.: 200 mg/m^2 day 1

followed by I.V.: 800 mg/m^2 continuous infusion day 1 [total dose/cycle = 1 g/m^2]

Leucovorin: (route not specified): 15 mg every 6 hours, for 8 doses (start 24 hours after end of methotrexate infusion) [total dose/cycle = 120 mg]

Cytarabine: I.V.: 3 g/m^2 every 12 hours, for 4 doses, days 2 and 3 [total dose/cycle = 12 g/m^2]

Repeat every 6 weeks in the following sequence: ABABABAB

CNS Prophylaxis

Methotrexate: I.T.: 12 mg day 2 [total dose/cycle = 12 mg]

Cytarabine: I.T.: 100 mg day 8 [total dose/cycle = 100 mg]

Repeat cycle every 3 weeks for 4-8 cycles

Maintenance (POMP)

Mercaptopurine: Oral: 50 mg 3 times/day [total dose/cycle = 4200-4650 mg]

Vincristine: I.V.: 2 mg day 1 [total dose/cycle = 2 mg]

Methotrexate: Oral: 20 mg/m^2/day days 1, 8, 15, 22 [total dose/cycle = 80 mg/m^2]

Prednisone: Oral: 200 mg/day days 1-5 [total dose/cycle = 1000 mg/m^2]
    or

Mercaptopurine: I.V.: 1 g/m^2/day days 1-5 [total dose/cycle = 5 g/m^2]

Vincristine: I.V.: 2 mg day 1 [total dose/cycle = 2 mg]

Methotrexate: I.V.: 10 mg/m^2/day days 1-5 [total dose/cycle = 50 mg/m^2]

Prednisone: Oral: 200 mg/day days 1-5 [total dose/cycle = 1000 mg]
    or

Interferon alfa: SubQ: 5 million units/m^2 daily [total dose/cycle = 140-155 million units/m^2]

Cytarabine: SubQ: 10 mg daily [total dose/cycle = 280-310 mg]

Repeat cycles every month for 2 years

Variation 5:

Cycle A: (Cycles 1, 4, 6, and 8)

Cyclophosphamide: I.V.: 300 mg/m^2 every 12 hours, for 6 doses, days 1-3 [total dose/cycle = 1800 mg/m^2]

Mesna: I.V.: 600 mg/m^2/day continuous infusion days 1-3 [total dose/cycle = 1800 mg/m^2]

Vincristine: I.V.: 2 mg/day days 4 and 11 [total dose/cycle = 4 mg]

Doxorubicin: I.V.: 50 mg/m^2 continuous infusion day 4 [total dose/cycle = 50 mg/m^2]

Dexamethasone: Oral, I.V.: 40 mg/day days 1-4 and 11-14 [total dose/cycle = 320 mg]

Cycle B: (Cycles 3, 5, 7, and 9)

Methotrexate: I.V.: 200 mg/m^2 day 1

followed by I.V.: 800 mg/m^2/day continuous infusion day 1 [total dose/cycle = 1 g/m^2]

Leucovorin: I.V.: 50 mg (start 12 hours after end of methotrexate infusion)

followed by: I.V.: 15 mg every 6 hours, for 8 doses [total dose/cycle = 170 mg]

Cytarabine: I.V.: 3 g/m^2 every 12 hours, for 4 doses, days 2 and 3 [total dose/cycle = 12 g/m^2]

Cycle C: Liposomal daunorubicin/cytarabine (Cycles 2):

Daunorubicin, liposomal: I.V.: 150 mg/m^2/day days 1 and 2 [total dose/cycle = 300 mg/m^2]

Cytarabine: I.V.: 1.5 g/m^2/day continuous infusion days 1 and 2 [total dose/cycle = 3 g/m^2]

Prednisone: Oral: 200 mg/day days 1-5 [total dose/cycle = 1000 mg]

Administer in the following sequence: ACBABABA (Cycle C does not repeat)

CNS Prophylaxis
Methotrexate: I.T.: 12 mg day 2 [total dose/cycle = 12 mg]
  or 6 mg into Ommaya day 2 [total dose/cycle = 6 mg]
Cytarabine: I.T.: 100 mg day 7 **or** 8 [total dose/cycle = 100 mg]
Repeat cycle every 3 weeks for 6 or 8 cycles
Maintenance (POMP)
Mercaptopurine: I.V.: 1 g/m^2/day days 1-5 [total dose/cycle = 5 g/m^2]
Vincristine: I.V.: 2 mg day 1 [total dose/cycle = 2 mg]
Methotrexate: I.V.: 10 mg/m^2/day days 1-5 [total dose/cycle = 50 mg/m^2]
Prednisone: Oral: 200 mg/day days 1-5 [total dose/cycle = 1000 mg]
Repeat cycles monthly, except months 6, 7, 18, 19 for 3 years
Intensification
Methotrexate: I.V.: 100 mg/m^2/day days 1, 8, 15, 22 [total dose/cycle = 400 mg/m^2]
Asparaginase: I.V.: 20,000 units/day days 2, 9, 16, 23 [total dose/cycle = 80,000 units]
Given during months 6 and 18 of maintenance
Cyclophosphamide: I.V.: 300 mg/m^2 every 12 hours, for 6 doses, days 1-3 [total dose/cycle = 1800 mg/m^2]
Mesna: I.V.: 600 mg/m^2/day continuous infusion days 1-3 [total dose/cycle = 1800 mg/m^2]
Vincristine: I.V.: 2 mg/day days 4 and 11 [total dose/cycle = 4 mg]
Doxorubicin: I.V.: 50 mg/m^2/day continuous infusion day 4 [total dose/cycle = 50 mg/m^2]
Dexamethasone: Oral, I.V.: 40 mg/day days 1-4 and 11-14 [total dose/cycle = 320 mg]
Given during months 7 and 19 of maintenance

Hyper-CVAD (Lymphoma, non-Hodgkin)
Use: Lymphoma, non-Hodgkin
Regimen:
  Cycle A: (Cycles 1, 3, 5, and 7)
  Cyclophosphamide: I.V.: 300 mg/m^2 every 12 hours, for 6 doses, days 1-3 [total dose/cycle = 1800 mg/m^2]
  Vincristine: I.V.: 2 mg/day days 4 and 11 [total dose/cycle = 4 mg]
  Doxorubicin: I.V.: 25 mg/m^2/day continuous infusion days 4 and 5 [total dose/cycle = 50 mg/m^2]
  Dexamethasone: Oral, I.V.: 40 mg/m^2/day days 1-4 and 11-14 [total dose/cycle = 320 mg]
  Cycle B: (Cycles 2, 4, 6, and 8)
  Methotrexate: I.V.: 200 mg/m^2 day 1
    followed by 800 mg/m^2 continuous infusion day 1 [total dose/cycle = 1 g/m^2]
  Leucovorin: Oral: 50 mg
    followed by Oral: 15 mg every 6 hours, for 8 doses (start 24 hours after end of methotrexate infusion)
    [total dose/cycle = 170 mg]
  Cytarabine: I.V.: 3 g/m^2 every 12 hours, for 4 doses, days 2 and 3 [total dose/cycle = 12 g/m^2]
  Repeat every 6 weeks in the following sequence: ABABABAB

Hyper-CVAD (Multiple Myeloma)
Use: Multiple myeloma
Regimen:
  Cyclophosphamide: I.V.: 300 mg/m^2 every 12 hours, for 6 doses, days 1-3 [total dose/cycle = 1800 mg/m^2]
  Mesna: I.V.: 600 mg/m^2/day continuous infusion days 1-3 [total dose/cycle = 1800 mg/m^2]
  Doxorubicin: I.V.: 25 mg/m^2/day continuous infusion days 4 and 5 [total dose/cycle = 50 mg/m^2]
  Vincristine: I.V.: 1 mg/day continuous infusion days 4 and 5
    followed by I.V.: 2 mg day 11 [total dose/cycle = 4 mg]
  Dexamethasone: Oral, I.V.: 20 mg/day days 1-5 and 11-14 [total dose/cycle = 180 mg/m^2]
  Repeat cycle once if ≥50% reduction in myeloma protein
  Maintenance
  Cyclophosphamide: Oral: 125 mg/m^2 every 12 hours, for 10 doses, days 1-5 [total dose/cycle = 1250 mg/m^2]
  Dexamethasone: Oral: 20 mg/m^2/day days 1-5 [total dose/cycle = 100 mg/m^2]
  Repeat maintenance cycle every 5 weeks

Hyper-CVAD + Imatinib
Use: Leukemia, acute lymphocytic
Regimen:
Cycle A: (Cycles 1, 3, 5, and 7)
Imatinib: Oral: 400 mg/day days 1-14 [total dose/cycle = 5600 mg]
Cyclophosphamide: I.V.: 300 mg/m^2 every 12 hours, for 6 doses, days 1-3
   [total dose/cycle = 1800 mg/m^2]
Mesna: I.V.: 600 mg/m^2/day continuous infusion days 1-3 [total dose/cycle = 1800 mg/m^2]
Vincristine: I.V.: 2 mg/day days 4 and 11 [total dose/cycle = 4 mg]
Doxorubicin: I.V.: 50 mg/m^2/day continuous infusion day 4 [total dose/cycle = 50 mg/m^2]
Dexamethasone: Oral, I.V.: 40 mg/day days 1-4 and 11-14 [total dose/cycle = 320 mg]
Cycle B: (Cycles 2, 4, 6, and 8)
Imatinib: Oral: 400 mg/day days 1-14 [total dose/cycle = 5600 mg]
Methotrexate: I.V.: 1 g/m^2/day continuous infusion day 1 [total dose/cycle = 1 g/m^2]
Leucovorin: I.V.: 50 mg then 15 mg every 6 hours, for 8 doses (start 12 hours after end of methotrexate infusion)
   [total dose/cycle = 170 mg]
Cytarabine: I.V.: 3 g/m^2 every 12 hours, for 4 doses, days 2 and 3 [total dose/cycle = 12 g/m^2]
Repeat every 6 weeks in the following sequence: ABABABAB
CNS Prophylaxis
Methotrexate: I.T.: 12 mg/day day 2 [total dose/cycle = 12 mg]
   or 6 mg into Ommaya day 2 [total dose/cycle = 6 mg/day]
Cytarabine: I.T.: 100 mg/day day 7 or 8 [total dose/cycle = 100 mg/day]
Repeat cycle every 3 weeks for 3 or 4 cycles
Maintenance (POMP)
Imatinib: Oral: 600 mg/day [total dose/cycle = 18,000 mg]
Vincristine: I.V.: 2 mg day 1 [total dose/cycle = 2 mg]
Prednisone: Oral: 200 mg/day days 1-5 [total dose/cycle = 1000 mg/m^2]
Repeat cycles every month (except months 6 and 13) for 13 months
Intensification
Imatinib: Oral: 400 mg/day days 1-14 [total dose/cycle = 5600 mg]
Cyclophosphamide: I.V.: 300 mg/m^2 every 12 hours, for 6 doses, days 1-3 [total dose/cycle = 1800 mg/m^2]
Mesna: I.V.: 600 mg/m^2/day continuous infusion days 1-3 [total dose/cycle = 1800 mg/m^2]
Vincristine: I.V.: 2 mg/day days 4 and 11 [total dose/cycle = 4 mg]
Doxorubicin: I.V.: 50 mg/m^2/day continuous infusion day 4 [total dose/cycle = 50 mg/m^2]
Dexamethasone: I.V. or Oral: 40 mg/day days 1-4 and 11-14 [total dose/cycle = 320 mg]
Cycle is given in months 6 and 13 during maintenance

Hyper-CVAD + Rituximab
Use: Lymphona, non-Hodgkin (Mantle cell)
Regimen:
Cycle A: (Cycles 1, 3, 5, [and 7, if needed])
Rituximab: I.V.: 375 mg/m^2 day 1 [total dose/cycle = 375 mg/m^2]
Cyclophosphamide: I.V.: 300 mg/m^2 every 12 hours, for 6 doses, days 2-4
   [total dose/cycle = 1800 mg/m^2]
Mesna: I.V.: 600 mg/m^2 continuous infusion days 2-4 [total dose/cycle = 1800 mg/m^2]
Vincristine: I.V.: 1.4 mg/m^2 (maximum 2 mg) days 5 and 12 [total dose/cycle = 2.8 mg/m^2; maximum 4 mg]
Doxorubicin: I.V.: 16.7 mg/m^2 continuous infusion days 5-7 [total dose/cycle = 50.1 mg/m^2]
Dexamethasone: Oral, I.V.: 40 mg/day days 2-5 and 12-15 [total dose/cycle = 320 mg]
Cycle B: (Cycles 2, 4, 6, [and 8, if needed])
Rituximab: I.V.: 375 mg/m^2 day 1 [total dose/cycle = 375 mg/m^2]
Methotrexate: I.V.: 200 mg/m^2 day 2
followed by I.V.: 800 mg/m^2 continuous infusion day 2 [total dose/cycle = 1000 mg/m^2]
Leucovorin: Oral: 50 mg (start 12 hours after end of methotrexate infusion)
followed by Oral: 15 mg every 6 hours, for 8 doses [total dose/cycle = 170 mg]
Cytarabine: I.V.: 3 g/m^2 every 12 hours, for 4 doses, days 3 and 4 [total dose/cycle = 12 g/m^2]
Repeat every 6 weeks in the following sequence: ABABABAB

ICE (Lymphoma, non-Hodgkin)

Use: Lymphoma, non-Hodgkin
Regimen:
Etoposide: I.V.: 100 mg/m^2/day days 1-3 [total dose/cycle = 300 mg/m^2]
Carboplatin: I.V.: AUC 5 (maximum 800 mg) day 2 [total dose/cycle = AUC = 5]
Ifosfamide: I.V.: 5000 mg/m^2 continuous infusion day 2 [total dose/cycle = 5000 mg/m^2]
Mesna: I.V.: 5000 mg/m^2 continuous infusion day 2 [total dose/cycle = 5000 mg/m^2]
Filgrastim: SubQ: 5 mcg/kg/day days 5-12 (cycles 1 and 2 only) [total dose/cycle = 40 mcg/kg]
followed by SubQ: 10 mcg/kg/day day 5 through completion of leukaphoresis (cycle 3 only)
Repeat cycle every 2 weeks for 3 cycles

ICE (Sarcoma)

Use: Osteosarcoma; Soft tissue sarcoma
Regimen:
Ifosfamide: I.V.: 1500 mg/m^2/day days 1-3 [total dose/cycle = 4500 mg/m^2]
Carboplatin: I.V.: 300-635 mg/m^2 day 3 [total dose/cycle = 300-635 mg/m^2]
Etopside: I.V.: 100 mg/m^2/day days 1-3 [total dose/cycle = 300 mg/m^2]
Mesna: I.V.: 500 mg/m^2 prior to each ifosfamide, and every 3 hours for 2 more doses/day days 1-3
    [total dose/cycle = 4500 mg/m^2]
Repeat cycle every 21-28 days

ICE-T

Use: Soft tissue sarcoma; Breast cancer
Regimen:
Ifosfamide: I.V.: 1250 mg/m^2/day days 1, 2, 3 [total dose/cycle = 3750 mg/m^2]
Carboplatin: I.V.: 300 mg/m^2 day 1 [total dose/cycle = 300 mg/m^2]
Etopside: I.V.: 80 mg/m^2/day days 1, 2, 3 [total dose/cycle = 240 mg/m^2]
Paclitaxel: I.V.: 175 mg/m^2 day 4 [total dose/cycle = 175 mg/m^2]
Mesna: I.V.: 250 mg prior to ifosfamide day 1-3
followed by: Oral: 500 mg at 4 and 8 hours after ifosfamide days 1-3
    [total dose/cycle = I.V. 750 mg; Oral 3000 mg]
    or
Mesna: I.V.: 1250 mg/m^2/day over 6 hours, days 1-3 [total dose/cycle = 3750 mg/m^2]
Repeat cycle every 28 days

Idarubicin, Cytarabine, Etoposide (ICE Protocol)

Use: Leukemia, acute myeloid
Regimen:
Idarubicin: I.V.: 6 mg/m^2/day days 1-5 [total dose/cycle = 30 mg/m^2]
Cytarabine: I.V.: 600 mg/m^2/day days 1-5 [total dose/cycle = 3000 mg/m^2]
Etoposide: I.V.: 150 mg/m^2/day days 1-3 [total dose/cycle = 450 mg/m^2]
Administer one cycle only

Idarubicin, Cytarabine, Etoposide (IDA-Based BF12)

Use: Leukemia, acute myeloid
Regimen: Induction:
Idarubicin: I.V.: 5 mg/m^2/day days 1-5 [total dose/cycle = 25 mg/m^2]
Cytarabine: I.V.: 2000 mg/m^2 every 12 hours days 1-5 (10 doses)
    [total dose/cycle = 20,000 mg/m^2]
Etoposide: I.V.: 100 mg/m^2/day days 1-5 [total dose/cycle = 500 mg/m^2]
Second cycle may be given based on individual response; time between cycles not specified

IE

Use: Soft tissue sarcoma
Regimen:
Etoposide: I.V.: 100 mg/m^2/day days 1-3 [total dose/cycle = 300 mg/m^2]
Ifosfamide: I.V.: 2500 mg/m^2/day days 1-3 [total dose/cycle = 7500 mg/m^2]
Mesna: I.V.: 500 mg/m^2 prior to ifosfamide, after ifosfamide, and every 4 hours for 3 more doses (total of 5
    doses/day) days 1-3
    [total dose/cycle = 7500 mg/m^2]
Repeat cycle every 28 days

IL-2 + IFN

Use: Melanoma

Regimen:

Cisplatin: I.V.: 20 mg/m²/day days 1-4 [total dose/cycle = 80 mg/m²]

Vinblastine: I.V.: 1.6 mg/m²/day days 1-4 [total dose/cycle = 6.4 mg/m²]

Dacarbazine: I.V.: 800 mg/m² day 1 [total dose/cycle = 800 mg/m²]

Aldesleukin: I.V.: 9 million units/m²/day continuous infusion days 1-4
[total dose/cycle = 36 million units/m²]

Interferon alfa-2b: SubQ: 5 million units/m²/day days 1-5, 7, 9, 11, 13
[total dose/cycle = 45 million units/m²]

Repeat cycle every 21 days

IMVP-16

Use: Lymphoma, non-Hodgkin

Regimen:

Ifosfamide: I.V.: 4 g/m² continuous infusion over 24 hours day 1 [total dose/cycle = 4 g/m²]

Mesna: I.V.: 800 mg/m² bolus prior to ifosfamide, then 4 g/m² continuous infusion over 12 hours concurrent with
ifosfamide; then 2.4 g/m² continuous infusion over 12 hours after ifosfamide infusion day 1
[total dose/cycle = 7.2 g/m²]

Methotrexate: I.V.: 30 mg/m²/day days 3 and 10 [total dose/cycle = 60 mg/m²]

Etoposide: I.V.: 100 mg/m²/day days 1-3 [total dose/cycle = 300 mg/m²]

Repeat cycle every 21-28 days

Interleukin 2-Interferon Alfa 2

Use: Renal cell cancer

Regimen:

Weeks 1 and 4:

Aldesleukin: SubQ: 20 million units/m² 3 times weekly [total dose/cycle = 120 million units/m²]

Interferon alfa: SubQ: 6 million units/m² once weekly [total dose/cycle = 12 million units/m²]

Weeks 2, 3, 5, and 6:

Aldesleukin: SubQ: 5 million units/m² 3 times weekly [total dose/cycle = 60 million units/m²]

Interferon alfa: SubQ: 6 million units/m² 3 times weekly [total dose/cycle = 72 million units/m²]

Repeat cycle every 56 days

Interleukin 2-Interferon Alfa 2-Fluorouracil

Use: Renal cell cancer

Regimen:

Weeks 1 and 4:

Aldesleukin: SubQ: 20 million units/m² 3 times weekly [total dose/cycle = 120 million units/m²]

Interferon alfa: SubQ: 6 million units/m² once weekly [total dose/cycle = 12 million units/m²]

Weeks 2 and 3:

Aldesleukin: SubQ: 5 million units/m² 3 times weekly [total dose/cycle = 30 million units/m²]

Weeks 5-8:

Interferon alfa: SubQ: 9 million units/m² 3 times weekly [total dose/cycle = 108 million units/m²]

Fluorouracil: I.V.: 750 mg/m² once weekly [total dose/cycle = 3000 mg/m²]

Repeat cycle every 56 days

IPA

Use: Hepatoblastoma

Regimen:

Ifosfamide: I.V.: 500 mg/m^2 day 1 [total dose/cycle = 500 mg/m^2] **followed by**
1000 mg/m^2/day continuous infusion days 1-3 [total dose/cycle = 3000 mg/m^2]
Cisplatin: I.V.: 20 mg/m^2/day days 4-8 [total dose/cycle = 100 mg/m^2]
Doxorubicin: I.V.: 30 mg/m^2/day continuous infusion days 9 and 10 [total dose/cycle = 60 mg/m^2]
Repeat cycle every 21 days

Irinotecan/Cisplatin

Use: Esophageal cancer

Regimen:

Cisplatin: I.V.: 30 mg/m^2/day days 1, 8, 15, 22 [total dose/cycle = 120 mg/m^2]
Irinotecan: I.V.: 65 mg/m^2/day days 1, 8, 15, 22 [total dose/cycle = 260 mg/m^2]
Repeat cycle every 6 weeks

IVAC

Use: Lymphoma, non-Hodgkin

Regimen:

Ifosfamide: I.V.: 1500 mg/m^2/day days 1-5 [total dose/cycle = 7500 mg/m^2]
Etoposide: I.V.: 60 mg/m^2/day days 1-5 [total dose/cycle = 300 mg/m^2]
Cytarabine: I.V.: 2 g/m^2 every 12 hours days 1 and 2 [total dose/cycle = 8 g/m^2]
Mesna: I.V.: 360 mg/m^2 every 3 hours days 1-5 [total dose/cycle = 14,400 mg/m^2]
Methotrexate: I.T.: 12 mg day 5 [total dose/cycle = 12 mg]
Sargramostim: SubQ: 7.5 mcg/kg day 7 until ANC >1000 cells/mm^3
Repeat when ANC >1000 cells/mm^3

Larson Regimen

Use: Leukemia, acute lymphocytic

Regimen: Induction:

Cyclophosphamide: I.V.: 1200 mg/m^2 day 1 [total dose/cycle = 1200 mg/m^2]
Daunorubicin: I.V.: 45 mg/m^2/day days 1-3 [total dose/cycle = 135 mg/m^2]
Vincristine: I.V.: 2 mg/day days 1, 8, 15, 22 [total dose/cycle = 8 mg]
Prednisone: Oral or I.V.: 60 mg/m^2/day days 1-21 [total dose/cycle = 1260 mg/m^2]
Asparaginase: SubQ: 6000 units/m^2/day days 5, 8, 11, 15, 18, 22
    [total dose/cycle = 36,000 units/m^2]
Administer one cycle only

Lenalidomide-Dexamethasone

Use: Multiple myeloma

Regimen:

Lenalidomide: Oral: 25 mg/day days 1-21 [total dose/cycle = 525 mg]
Dexamethasone: Oral: 40 mg/day days 1-4, 9-12, 17-20 (cycles 1, 2, 3, 4) [total dose/cycle = 480 mg]
Dexamethasone: Oral: 40 mg/day days 1-4 (cycles 5 and beyond) [total dose/cycle = 160 mg]
Repeat cycle every 28 days

Linker Protocol

Use: Leukemia, acute lymphocytic

Regimen:

Remission induction:

Daunorubicin: I.V.: 50 mg/m^2/day days 1-3 [total dose/cycle = 150 mg/m^2]

Vincristine: I.V.: 2 mg/day days 1, 8, 15, 22 [total dose/cycle = 8 mg]

Prednisone: Oral: 60 mg/m^2/day days 1-28 [total dose/cycle = 1680 mg/m^2]

Asparaginase: I.M.: 6000 units/m^2/day days 17-28 [total dose/cycle = 72,000 units/m^2]

If residual leukemia in bone marrow on day 14:

Daunorubicin: I.V.: 50 mg/m^2 day 15 [total dose/cycle = 50 mg/m^2]

If residual leukemia in bone marrow on day 28:

Daunorubicin: I.V.: 50 mg/m^2 days 29 and 30 [total dose/cycle = 100 mg/m^2]

Vincristine: I.V.: 2 mg/day days 29 and 36 [total dose/cycle = 4 mg]

Prednisone: Oral: 60 mg/m^2/day days 29-42 [total dose/cycle = 840 mg/m^2]

Asparaginase: I.M.: 6000 units/m^2/day days 29-35 [total dose/cycle = 42,000 units/m^2]

Consolidation therapy:

Treatment A (cycles 1, 3, 5, and 7)

Daunorubicin: I.V.: 50 mg/m^2/day days 1 and 2 [total dose/cycle = 100 mg/m^2]

Vincristine: I.V.: 2 mg/day days 1 and 8 [total dose/cycle = 4 mg]
Prednisone: Oral: 60 mg/m^2/day days 1-14 [total dose/cycle = 840 mg/m^2]

Asparaginase: I.M.: 12,000 units/m^2/day days 2, 4, 7, 9, 11, 14
  [total dose/cycle = 72,000 units/m^2]

Treatment B (cycles 2, 4, 6, and 8)

Teniposide: I.V.: 165 mg/m^2/day days 1, 4, 8, 11 [total dose/cycle = 660 mg/m^2]

Cytarabine: I.V.: 300 mg/m^2/day days 1, 4, 8, 11 [total dose/cycle = 1200 mg/m^2]
Treatment C (cycle 9)

Methotrexate: I.V.: 690 mg/m^2 continuous infusion day 1 (over 42 hours)
  [total dose/cycle = 690 mg/m^2]
Leucovorin: I.V.: 15 mg/m^2 every 6 hours for 12 doses (start at end of methotrexate infusion)
  [total dose/cycle = 180 mg/m^2]

Administer remission induction regimen for one cycle only. Repeat consolidation cycle every 28 days

LOPP

Use: Lymphoma, Hodgkin disease

Regimen:

Chlorambucil: Oral: 10 mg/day days 1-10 [total dose/cycle = 100 mg]

Vincristine: I.V.: 1.4 mg/m^2/day (maximum 2 mg) days 1 and 8 [total dose/cycle = 2.8 mg/m^2]

Procarbazine: Oral: 100 mg/m^2/day days 1-10 [total dose/cycle = 1000 mg/m^2]
Prednisone: Oral: 25 mg/m^2/day (maximum 60 mg) days 1-14
  [total dose/cycle = 350 mg/m^2] **or**

Prednisolone: Oral: 25 mg/m^2/day (maximum 60 mg) days 1-14 [total dose/cycle = 350 mg/m^2]

Repeat cycle every 28 days

M-2

Use: Multiple myeloma
Regimen:

Vincristine: I.V.: 0.03 mg/kg (maximum 2 mg) day 1 [total dose/cycle = 0.03 mg/kg]
Carmustine: I.V.: 0.5-1 mg/kg day 1 [total dose/cycle = 0.5-1 mg/kg]
Cyclophosphamide: I.V.: 10 mg/kg day 1 [total dose/cycle = 10 mg/kg]
Melphalan: Oral: 0.25 mg/kg/day days 1-4 [total dose/cycle = 1 mg/kg] **or** 0.1 mg/kg/day days 1-7
   or 1-10 [total dose/cycle = 0.7 or 1 mg/kg]
Prednisone: Oral: 1 mg/kg/day days 1-7
   [total dose/cycle = 7 mg/kg]
Repeat cycle every 35-42 days

MACOP-B

Use: Lymphoma, non-Hodgkin
Regimen:

Methotrexate: I.V. bolus: 100 mg/m^2 weeks 2, 6, 10
   followed by 300 mg/m^2 over 4 hours weeks 2, 6, 10 [total dose/cycle = 1200 mg/m^2]
Doxorubicin: I.V.: 50 mg/m^2 weeks 1, 3, 5, 7, 9, 11 [total dose/cycle = 300 mg/m^2]
Cyclophosphamide: I.V.: 350 mg/m^2 weeks 1, 3, 5, 7, 9, 11 [total dose/cycle = 2100 mg/m^2]
Vincristine: I.V.: 1.4 mg/m^2 (maximum 2 mg) weeks 2, 4, 6, 8, 10, 12
   [total dose/cycle = 8.4 mg/m^2; maximum 12 mg]
Bleomycin: I.V.: 10 units/m^2 weeks 4, 8, 12 [total dose/cycle = 30 units/m^2]
Prednisone: Oral: 75 mg/day for 12 weeks, then taper over 2 weeks
Leucovorin calcium: Oral: 15 mg/m^2 every 6 hours, for 6 doses (beginning 24 hours after methotrexate) weeks 2, 6,
   10 [total dose/cycle = 270 mg/m^2]
Administer one cycle

MAID

Use: Soft tissue sarcoma
Regimen:

Mesna: I.V.: 2500 mg/m^2/day continuous infusion days 1-4 [total dose/cycle = 10,000 mg/m^2]
Doxorubicin: I.V.: 20 mg/m^2/day continuous infusion days 1-3 [total dose/cycle = 60 mg/m^2]
Ifosfamide: I.V.: 2500 mg/m^2/day continuous infusion days 1-3 [total dose/cycle = 7500 mg/m^2]
Dacarbazine: I.V.: 300 mg/m^2/day continuous infusion days 1-3 [total dose/cycle = 900 mg/m^2]
Repeat cycle every 21-28 days

m-BACOD

Use: Lymphoma, non-Hodgkin
Regimen:

Methotrexate: I.V.: 200 mg/m^2/day days 8 and 15 [total dose/cycle = 400 mg/m^2]
Leucovorin calcium: Oral: 10 mg/m^2 every 6 hours for 8 doses (beginning 24 hours after each methotrexate dose)
   days 9 and 16 [total dose/cycle = 160 mg/m^2]
Bleomycin: I.V.: 4 units/m^2 day 1 [total dose/cycle = 4 units/m^2]
Doxorubicin: I.V.: 45 mg/m^2 day 1 [total dose/cycle = 45 mg/m^2]
Cyclophosphamide: I.V.: 600 mg/m^2 day 1 [total dose/cycle = 600 mg/m^2]
Vincristine: I.V.: 1 mg/m^2 day 1 [total dose/cycle = 1 mg/m^2]
Dexamethasone: Oral: 6 mg/m^2/day days 1-5 [total dose/cycle = 30 mg/m^2]
Repeat cycle every 21 days

Melphalan-Prednisone-Thalidomide

Use: Multiple myeloma
Regimen:

Melphalan: Oral: 4 mg/m^2/day days 1-7 [total dose/cycle = 28 mg/m^2]
Prednisone: Oral: 40 mg/m^2/day days 1-7 [total dose/cycle = 280 mg/m^2]
Thalidomide: Oral: 100 mg/day days 1-28 [total dose/cycle = 2800 mg]
Repeat cycle every 28 days for 6 cycles
followed by
Thalidomide: Oral: 100 mg daily (as maintenance)

MF
Use: Breast cancer
Regimen:
Methotrexate: I.V.: 100 mg/m^2/day days 1 and 8 [total dose/cycle = 200 mg/m^2]
Fluorouracil: I.V.: 600 mg/m^2/day (start 1 hour after methotrexate) days 1 and 8 [total dose/cycle = 1200 mg/m^2]
Leucovorin: Oral, I.V.: 10 mg/m^2 every 6 hours for 6 doses (start 24 hours after methotrexate)
[total dose/cycle = 60 mg/m^2]
Repeat cycle every 28 days for 12 cycles

MINE
Use: Lymphoma, non-Hodgkin
Regimen:
Mesna: I.V.: 1.33 g/m^2/day concurrent with ifosfamide dose, then 500 mg orally (4 hours after each ifosfamide
infusion) days 1-3 [total dose/cycle = 3.99 g/m^2/1500 mg]
Ifosfamide: I.V.: 1.33 g/m^2/day days 1-3 [total dose/cycle = 3.99 mg/m^2]
Mitoxantrone: I.V.: 8 mg/m^2 day 1 [total dose/cycle = 8 mg/m^2]
Etoposide: I.V.: 65 mg/m^2/day days 1-3 [total dose/cycle = 195 mg/m^2]
Repeat cycle every 28 days

MINE-ESHAP
Use: Lymphoma, non-Hodgkin
Regimen:
Mesna: I.V.: 1.33 g/m^2 concurrent with ifosfamide dose, then 500 mg orally (4 hours after ifosfamide) days 1-3
[total dose/cycle = 4 g/m^2/1500 mg]
Ifosfamide: I.V.: 1.33 g/m^2/day days 1-3 [total dose/cycle = 4 g/m^2]
Mitoxantrone: I.V.: 8 mg/m^2 day 1 [total dose/cycle = 8 mg/m^2]
Etoposide: I.V.: 65 mg/m^2/day days 1-3 [total dose/cycle = 195 mg/m^2]
Repeat cycle every 21 days for 6 cycles, followed by
3-6 cycles of ESHAP

mini-BEAM
Use: Lymphoma, Hodgkin disease
Regimen:
Carmustine: I.V.: 60 mg/m^2 day 1 [total dose/cycle = 60 mg/m^2]
Etoposide: I.V.: 75 mg/m^2/day days 2-5 [total dose/cycle = 300 mg/m^2]
Cytarabine: I.V.: 100 mg/m^2 every 12 hours days 2-5 (8 doses) [total dose/cycle = 800 mg/m^2]
Melphalan: I.V.: 30 mg/m^2 day 6 [total dose/cycle = 30 mg/m^2]
Repeat cycle every 4-6 weeks

Mitomycin-Vinblastine
Use: Breast cancer
Regimen:
Mitomycin: I.V.: 20 mg/m^2 day 1 [total dose/cycle = 20 mg/m^2]
Vinblastine: I.V.: 0.15 mg/kg/day days 1 and 21 [total dose/cycle = 0.3 mg/kg]
Repeat cycle every 6-8 weeks

Mitoxantrone + Hydrocortisone
Use: Prostate cancer
Regimen:
Mitoxantrone: I.V.: 14 mg/m^2 day 1 [total dose/cycle = 14 mg/m^2]
Hydrocortisone: Oral: 40 mg daily [total dose/cycle = 840 mg]
Repeat cycle every 3 weeks

MM
Use: Leukemia, acute lymphocytic (maintenance)
Regimen:
Mercaptopurine: Oral: 50-75 mg/m^2/day days 1-7 [total dose/cycle = 350-525 mg/m^2]
Methotrexate: Oral, I.V.: 20 mg/m^2 day 1 [total dose/cycle = 20 mg/m^2]
Repeat cycle every 7 days

MOP

Use: Brain tumors
Regimen:
Mechlorethamine: I.V.: 6 mg/m^2/day days 1 and 8 [total dose/cycle = 12 mg/m^2]
Vincristine: I.V.: 1.5 mg/m^2/day (maximum 2 mg) days 1 and 8 [total dose/cycle = 3 mg/m^2]
Procarbazine: Oral: 100 mg/m^2/day days 1-14 [total dose/cycle = 1400 mg/m^2]
Repeat cycle every 28 days

MOPP (Lymphoma, Hodgkin Disease)

Use: Lymphoma, Hodgkin disease
Regimen: Note: Multiple variations are listed below.

Variation 1:
Mechlorethamine: I.V.: 6 mg/m^2/day days 1 and 8 [total dose/cycle = 12 mg/m^2]
Vincristine: I.V.: 1.4 mg/m^2/day days 1 and 8 [total dose/cycle = 2.8 mg/m^2]
Procarbazine: Oral: 100 mg/m^2/day days 1-14 [total dose/cycle = 1400 mg/m^2]
Prednisone: Oral: 40 mg/m^2/day days 1-14 (cycles 1 and 4) [total dose/cycle = 560 mg/m^2]
Repeat cycle every 28 days for 6-8 cycles

Variation 2:
Mechlorethamine: I.V.: 6 mg/m^2/day (maximum 15 mg) days 1 and 8
   [total dose/cycle = 12 mg/m^2]
Vincristine: I.V.: 1.4 mg/m^2/day (maximum 2 mg) days 1 and 8 [total dose/cycle = 2.8 mg/m^2]
Procarbazine: Oral: 100 mg/m^2/day days 1-10 [total dose/cycle = 1000 mg/m^2]
Prednisone: Oral: 25 mg/m^2/day (maximum 60 mg) days 1-14
   [total dose/cycle = 350 mg/m^2] **or**
Prednisolone: Oral: 25 mg/m^2/day (maximum 60 mg) days 1-14 [total dose/cycle = 350 mg/m^2]
Repeat cycle every 28 days

Variation 3:
Mechlorethamine: I.V.: 6 mg/m^2/day days 1 and 8 [total dose/cycle = 12 mg/m^2]
Vincristine: I.V.: 1.4 mg/m^2/day days 1 and 8 [total dose/cycle = 2.8 mg/m^2]
Procarbazine: Oral: 50 mg day 1, 100 mg day 2, 100 mg/m^2/day days 3-14
   [total dose/cycle = 150 mg / 1200 mg/m^2]
Prednisone: Oral: 40 mg/m^2/day days 1-14 [total dose/cycle = 560 mg/m^2]
Repeat cycle every 28 days

Variation 4:
Mechlorethamine: I.V.: 6 mg/m^2/day days 1 and 8 [total dose/cycle = 12 mg/m^2]
Vincristine: I.V.: 1.4 mg/m^2/day days 1 and 8 [total dose/cycle = 2.8 mg/m^2]
Procarbazine: Oral: 50 mg day 1, 100 mg day 2, 100 mg/m^2/day days 3-10
   [total dose/cycle = 150 mg / 800 mg/m^2]
Prednisone: Oral: 40 mg/m^2/day days 1-14 [total dose/cycle = 560 mg/m^2]
Repeat cycle every 28 days

Variation 5:
Mechlorethamine: I.V.: 6 mg/m^2/day days 1 and 8 [total dose/cycle = 12 mg/m^2]
Vincristine: I.V.: 1.4 mg/m^2/day days 1 and 8 [total dose/cycle = 2.8 mg/m^2]
Procarbazine: Oral: 50 mg/m^2 day 1, then 100 mg/m^2/day days 2-14
   [total dose/cycle = 1350 mg/m^2]
Prednisone: Oral: 40 mg/m^2/day days 1-14 [total dose/cycle = 560 mg/m^2]
Repeat cycle every 28 days

MOPP (Medulloblastoma)

Use: Brain tumors
Regimen:
Mechlorethamine: I.V.: 3 mg/m^2/day days 1 and 8 [total dose/cycle = 6 mg/m^2]
Vincristine: I.V.: 1.4 mg/m^2/day (maximum 2 mg) days 1 and 8 [total dose/cycle = 2.8 mg/m^2]
Prednisone: Oral: 40 mg/m^2/day days 1-10 [total dose/cycle = 400 mg/m^2]
Procarbazine: Oral: 50 mg day 1 [total dose = 50 mg] **followed by**
100 mg day 2 [total dose = 100 mg] **followed by**
100 mg/m^2/day days 3-10 [total dose = 800 mg/m^2]
Repeat cycle every 28 days

MOPP/ABV Hybrid

Use: Lymphoma, Hodgkin disease
Regimen:
Mechlorethamine: I.V.: 6 mg/m² day 1 [total dose/cycle = 6 mg/m²]
Vincristine: I.V.: 1.4 mg/m² (maximum 2 mg) day 1 [total dose/cycle = 1.4 mg/m²]
Procarbazine: Oral: 100 mg/m²/day days 1-7 [total dose/cycle = 700 mg/m²]
Prednisone: Oral: 40 mg/m²/day days 1-14 [total dose/cycle = 560 mg/m²]
Doxorubicin: I.V.: 35 mg/m² day 8 [total dose/cycle = 35 mg/m²]
Bleomycin: I.V.: 10 units/m² day 8 [total dose/cycle = 10 units/m²]
Vinblastine: I.V.: 6 mg/m² day 8 [total dose/cycle = 6 mg/m²]
Repeat cycle every 28 days

MOPP/ABVD

Use: Lymphoma, Hodgkin disease
Regimen: Note: Multiple variations are listed below.

Variation 1:
Mechlorethamine: I.V.: 6 mg/m²/day days 1 and 8 [total dose/cycle = 12 mg/m²]
Vincristine: I.V.: 1.4 mg/m²/day (maximum 2 mg) days 1 and 8 [total dose/cycle = 2.8 mg/m²]
Procarbazine: I.V.: 100 mg/m²/day days 1-14 [total dose/cycle = 1400 mg/m²]
Prednisone: Oral: 40 mg/m²/day days 1-14 (during cycles 1, 4, 7, and 10 only)
    [total dose/cycle = 560 mg/m²]
Doxorubicin: I.V.: 25 mg/m²/day days 29 and 43 [total dose/cycle = 50 mg/m²]
Bleomycin: I.V.: 10 units/m²/day day 29 and 43 [total dose/cycle = 20 units/m²]
Vinblastine: I.V.: 6 mg/m²/day days 29 and 43 [total dose/cycle = 12 mg/m²]
Dacarbazine: I.V.: 375 mg/m²/day days 29 and 43 [total dose/cycle = 750 mg/m²]
Repeat cycle every 56 days

Variation 2:
Mechlorethamine: I.V.: 6 mg/m²/day days 1 and 8 [total dose/cycle = 12 mg/m²]
Vincristine: I.V.: 1.4 mg/m²/day (maximum 2 mg) days 1 and 8 [total dose/cycle = 2.8 mg/m²]
Procarbazine: I.V.: 100 mg/m²/day days 1-14 [total dose/cycle = 1400 mg/m²]
Prednisone: Oral: 40 mg/m²/day days 1-14 (during cycles 1 and 7 only)
    [total dose/cycle = 560 mg/m²]
Doxorubicin: I.V.: 25 mg/m²/day days 29 and 43 [total dose/cycle = 50 mg/m²]
Bleomycin: I.V.: 10 units/m²/day days 29 and 43 [total dose/cycle = 20 units/m²]
Vinblastine: I.V.: 6 mg/m²/day days 29 and 43 [total dose/cycle = 12 mg/m²]
Dacarbazine: I.V.: 375 mg/m²/day days 29 and 43 [total dose/cycle = 750 mg/m²]
Repeat cycle every 56 days

Variation 3:
Mechlorethamine: I.V.: 6 mg/m²/day days 1 and 8 [total dose/cycle = 12 mg/m²]
Vincristine: I.V.: 1.4 mg/m²/day (maximum 2 mg) days 1 and 8 [total dose/cycle = 2.8 mg/m²]
Procarbazine: I.V.: 100 mg/m²/day days 1-14 [total dose/cycle = 1400 mg/m²]
Prednisone: Oral: 40 mg/m²/day days 1-14 (every cycle) [total dose/cycle = 560 mg/m²]
Doxorubicin: I.V.: 25 mg/m²/day days 29 and 43 [total dose/cycle = 50 mg/m²]
Bleomycin: I.V.: 10 units/m²/day days 29 and 43 [total dose/cycle = 20 units/m²]
Vinblastine: I.V.: 6 mg/m²/day days 29 and 43 [total dose/cycle = 12 mg/m²]
Dacarbazine: I.V.: 375 mg/m²/day days 29 and 43 [total dose/cycle = 750 mg/m²]
Repeat cycle every 56 days

Variation 4:
MOPP Regimen:
Mechlorethamine: I.V.: 6 mg/m²/day days 1 and 8 [total dose/cycle = 12 mg/m²]
Vincristine: I.V.: 1.4 mg/m²/day (maximum 2 mg) days 1 and 8 [total dose/cycle = 2.8 mg/m²]
Procarbazine: I.V.: 100 mg/m²/day days 1-14 [total dose/cycle = 1400 mg/m²]
Prednisone: Oral: 25 mg/m²/day days 1-14 [total dose/cycle = 350 mg/m²]

ABVD Regimen:
Doxorubicin: I.V.: 25 mg/m²/day days 1 and 15 [total dose/cycle = 50 mg/m²]
Bleomycin: I.V.: 6 units/m²/day days 1 and 15 [total dose/cycle = 12 units/m²]
Vinblastine: I.V.: 6 mg/m²/day days 1 and 15 [total dose/cycle = 12 mg/m²]
Dacarbazine: I.V.: 250 mg/m²/day days 1 and 15 [total dose/cycle = 500 mg/m²]
Each regimen cycle is 28 days. Administer regimens in alternating fashion as follows: 2 cycles of MOPP alternating
    with 2 cycles of ABVD for a total of 8 cycles

Variation 5 (pediatrics):
Mechlorethamine: I.V.: 6 mg/m^2/day days 1 and 8 [total dose/cycle = 12 mg/m^2]
Vincristine: I.V.: 1.4 mg/m^2/day days 1 and 8 [total dose/cycle = 2.8 mg/m^2]
Procarbazine: Oral: 100 mg/m^2/day days 1-14 [total dose/cycle = 1400 mg/m^2]
Prednisone: Oral: 40 mg/m^2/day days 1-14 [total dose/cycle = 560 mg/m^2]
Doxorubicin: I.V.: 25 mg/m^2/day days 29 and 42 [total dose/cycle = 50 mg/m^2]
Bleomycin: I.V.: 10 units/m^2/day days 29 and 42 [total dose/cycle = 20 units/m^2]
Vinblastine: I.V.: 6 mg/m^2/day days 29 and 42 [total dose/cycle = 12 mg/m^2]
Dacarbazine: I.V.: 150 mg/m^2/day days 29-33 [total dose/cycle = 750 mg/m^2]
Repeat cycle evey 56 days for 4 cycles
Variation 6 (pediatrics):
Mechlorethamine: I.V.: 6 mg/m^2/day days 1 and 8 [total dose/cycle = 12 mg/m^2]
Vincristine: I.V.: 1.4 mg/m^2/day days 1 and 8 [total dose/cycle = 2.8 mg/m^2]
Procarbazine: Oral: 100 mg/m^2/day days 1-14 [total dose/cycle = 1400 mg/m^2]
Prednisone: Oral: 40 mg/m^2/day days 1-14 [total dose/cycle = 560 mg/m^2]
Doxorubicin: I.V.: 25 mg/m^2/day days 29 and 42 [total dose/cycle = 50 mg/m^2]
Bleomycin: I.V.: 10 units/m^2/day days 29 and 42 [total dose/cycle = 20 units/m^2]
Vinblastine: I.V.: 6 mg/m^2/day days 29 and 42 [total dose/cycle = 12 mg/m^2]
Dacarbazine: I.V.: 375 mg/m^2/day days 29 and 43 [total dose/cycle = 750 mg/m^2]
Repeat cycle evey 56 days for 4 cycles

MP (Multiple Myeloma)
Use: Multiple myeloma
Regimen:
Melphalan: Oral: 8-10 mg/m^2/day days 1-4 [total dose/cycle = 32-40 mg/m^2]
Prednisone: Oral: 40-60 mg/m^2/day days 1-4 [total dose/cycle = 160-240 mg/m^2]
Repeat cycle every 28-42 days

MP (Prostate Cancer)
Use: Prostate cancer
Regimen:
Mitoxantrone: I.V.: 12 mg/m^2 day 1 [total dose/cycle = 12 mg/m^2]
Prednisone: Oral: 5 mg twice daily [total dose/cycle = 210 mg]
Repeat cycle every 21 days

MTX/6-MP/VP (Maintenance)
Use: Leukemia, acute lymphocytic
Regimen:
Methotrexate: Oral: 20 mg/m^2 weekly [total dose/cycle = 80 mg/m^2]
Mercaptopurine: Oral: 75 mg/m^2/day [total dose/cycle = 2250 mg/m^2]
Vincristine: I.V.: 1.5 mg/m^2 day 1 [total dose/cycle = 1.5 mg/m^2]
Prednisone: Oral: 40 mg/m^2/day days 1-5 [total dose/cycle = 200 mg/m^2]
Repeat monthly for 2-3 years

MTX-CDDPAdr
Use: Osteosarcoma
Regimen:
Cisplatin: I.V.: 75 mg/m^2 day 1 of cycles 1-7 [total dose/cycle = 75 mg/m^2]
    then 120 mg/m^2 day 1 cycles 8-10 [total dose/cycle = 120 mg/m^2]
Doxorubicin: I.V.: 25 mg/m^2/day days 1-3 of cycles 1-7 [total dose/cycle = 75 mg/m^2]
Methotrexate: I.V.: 12 g/m^2/day days 21 and 28 [total dose/cycle = 24 g/m^2]
Leucovorin calcium rescue: I.V.: 20 mg/m^2 every 3 hours (beginning 16 hours after completion of methotrexate) for
    8 doses, then orally every 6 hours for 8 doses [total dose/cycle = 640 mg/m^2]

MV
Use: Leukemia, acute myeloid
Regimen: Induction:
Mitoxantrone: I.V.: 10 mg/m^2/day days 1-5 [total dose/cycle = 50 mg/m^2]
Etoposide: I.V.: 100 mg/m^2/day days 1-5 [total dose/cycle = 500 mg/m^2]
Second cycle may be given based on individual response; time between cycles not specified

M-VAC (Bladder Cancer)

Use: Bladder cancer

Regimen: Note: Multiple variations are listed below.

Variation 1:
Methotrexate: I.V.: 30 mg/m²/day days 1, 15, 22 [total dose/cycle = 90 mg/m²]
Vinblastine: I.V.: 3 mg/m²/day days 2, 15, 22 [total dose/cycle = 9 mg/m²]
Doxorubicin: I.V.: 30 mg/m² day 2 [total dose/cycle = 30 mg/m²]
Cisplatin: I.V.: 70 mg/m² day 2 [total dose/cycle = 70 mg/m²]
Repeat cycle every 4 weeks

Variation 2:
Methotrexate: I.V.: 40 or 50 mg/m²/day days 1, 15, 22 [total dose/cycle = 120 or 150 mg/m²]
Vinblastine: I.V.: 4 or 5 mg/m²/day days 2, 15, 22 [total dose/cycle = 12 or 15 mg/m²]
Doxorubicin: I.V.: 40 or 50 mg/m² day 2 [total dose/cycle = 40 or 50 mg/m²]
Cisplatin: I.V.: 100 mg/m² day 2 [total dose/cycle = 100 mg/m²]
Repeat cycle every 4 weeks

Variation 3:
Methotrexate: I.V.: 30 mg/m²/day days 1, 15, 22 [total dose/cycle = 90 mg/m²]
Vinblastine: I.V.: 3 mg/m² day 2 [total dose/cycle = 3 mg/m²]
Doxorubicin: I.V.: 30 mg/m² day 2 [total dose/cycle = 30 mg/m²]
Cisplatin: I.V.: 70 mg/m² day 2 [total dose/cycle = 70 mg/m²]
Repeat cycle every 4 weeks

Variation 4:
Methotrexate: I.V.: 60 mg/m² day 1 [total dose/cycle = 60 mg/m²]
followed by 30 mg/m² day 16 [total dose/cycle = 30 mg/m²]
Vinblastine: I.V.: 4 mg/m²/day days 2 and 16 [total dose/cycle = 8 mg/m²]
Doxorubicin: I.V.: 60 mg/m² day 2 [total dose/cycle = 60 mg/m²]
Cisplatin: I.V.: 100 mg/m² day 2 [total dose/cycle = 100 mg/m²]
Repeat cycle every 23 days

Variation 5:
Methotrexate: I.V.: 30 mg/m²/day days 1, 16, 23 [total dose/cycle = 90 mg/m²]
Vinblastine: I.V.: 4 mg/m²/day days 1, 16, 23 [total dose/cycle = 12 mg/m²]
Doxorubicin: I.V.: 60 mg/m² day 2 [total dose/cycle = 60 mg/m²]
Cisplatin: I.V.: 100 mg/m² day 2 [total dose/cycle = 100 mg/m²]
Repeat cycle every 23 days

Variation 6:
Methotrexate: I.V.: 30 or 35 mg/m² day 1 [total dose/cycle = 30 or 35 mg/m²]
Vinblastine: I.V.: 3 or 3.5 mg/m² day 2 [total dose/cycle = 3 or 3.5 mg/m²]
Doxorubicin: I.V.: 30 or 35 mg/m² day 2 [total dose/cycle = 30 or 35 mg/m²]
Cisplatin: I.V.: 70 or 80 mg/m² day 2 [total dose/cycle = 70 or 80 mg/m²]
Repeat cycle every 2 weeks

Variation 7:
Methotrexate: I.V.: 30 mg/m² day 1 [total dose/cycle = 30 mg/m²]
Vinblastine: I.V.: 3 mg/m² day 2 [total dose/cycle = 3 mg/m²]
Doxorubicin: I.V.: 30 mg/m² day 2 [total dose/cycle = 30 mg/m²]
Cisplatin: I.V.: 70 mg/m² day 2 [total dose/cycle = 70 mg/m²]
Repeat cycle every 14 days

Variation 8:
Methotrexate: I.V.: 30 mg/m²/day days 1, 15, 22 [total dose/cycle = 90 mg/m²]
Vinblastine: I.V.: 3 mg/m²/day days 1, 15, 22 [total dose/cycle = 9 mg/m²]
Doxorubicin: I.V.: 45 mg/m² day 2 [total dose/cycle = 45 mg/m²]
Cisplatin: I.V.: 70 mg/m² day 2 [total dose/cycle = 70 mg/m²]
Repeat cycle every 4 weeks

Variation 9:
Methotrexate: I.V.: 40 mg/m²/day days 1 and 15 [total dose/cycle = 80 mg/m²]
Vinblastine: I.V.: 4 mg/m²/day days 1, 16, 23 [total dose/cycle = 12 mg/m²]
Doxorubicin: I.V.: 60 mg/m² day 2 [total dose/cycle = 60 mg/m²]
Cisplatin: I.V.: 100 mg/m² day 2 [total dose/cycle = 100 mg/m²]
Repeat cycle every 23 days

Variation 10:
Methotrexate: I.V.: 30 mg/m²/day days 1, 15, 22 [total dose/cycle = 90 mg/m²]
Vinblastine: I.V.: 3 mg/m²/day days 1, 16, 22 [total dose/cycle = 9 mg/m²]
Doxorubicin: I.V.: 30 mg/m² day 1 [total dose/cycle = 30 mg/m²]
Cisplatin: I.V.: 70 mg/m² day 1 [total dose/cycle = 70 mg/m²]
Repeat cycle every 4 weeks

Variation 11:
Methotrexate: I.V.: 30 mg/m²/day days 1, 15, 22 [total dose/cycle = 90 mg/m²]
Vinblastine: I.V.: 3 mg/m²/day days 2, 15, 22 [total dose/cycle = 9 mg/m²]
Doxorubicin: I.V.: 30 mg/m² day 2 [total dose/cycle = 30 mg/m²]
Cisplatin: I.V.: 70 mg/m² day 2 [total dose/cycle = 70 mg/m²]
Leucovorin: Oral: 15 mg every 6 hours for 4 doses, days 2, 16, 23
    [total dose/cycle = 180 mg]
Repeat cycle every 4 weeks

Variation 12:
Methotrexate: I.V.: 30 mg/m^2/day days 1 and 15 [total dose/cycle = 60 mg/m^2]
Vinblastine: I.V.: 3 mg/m^2/day days 2 and 15 [total dose/cycle = 6 mg/m^2]
Doxorubicin: I.V.: 30 or 40 mg/m^2 day 3 [total dose/cycle = 30 or 40 mg/m^2]
Cisplatin: I.V.: 70 mg/m^2 day 2 [total dose/cycle = 70 mg/m^2]
Repeat cycle every 4 weeks
Variation 13:
Methotrexate: I.V.: 30 mg/m^2/day days 1 and 15 [total dose/cycle = 60 mg/m^2]
Vinblastine: I.V.: 3 mg/m^2/day days 2 and 15 [total dose/cycle = 6 mg/m^2]
Doxorubicin: I.V.: 30 or 40 mg/m^2 day 2 [total dose/cycle = 30 or 40 mg/m^2]
Cisplatin: I.V.: 70 mg/m^2 day 2 [total dose/cycle = 70 mg/m^2]
Repeat cycle every 4 weeks

M-VAC (Breast Cancer)
Use: Breast cancer
Regimen:
Methotrexate: I.V.: 30 mg/m^2/day days 1, 15, 22 [total dose/cycle = 90 mg/m^2]
Vinblastine: I.V.: 3 mg/m^2/day days 2, 15, 22 [total dose/cycle = 9 mg/m^2]
Doxorubicin: I.V.: 30 mg/m^2 day 2 [total dose/cycle = 30 mg/m^2]
Cisplatin: I.V.: 70 mg/m^2 day 2 [total dose/cycle = 70 mg/m^2]
Leucovorin: Oral: 10 mg every 6 hours for 6 doses days 2, 16, 23
    [total dose/cycle = 180 mg]
Repeat cycle every 4 weeks

M-VAC (Cervical Cancer)
Use: Cervical cancer
Regimen:
Methotrexate: I.V.: 30 mg/m^2/day days 1, 15, 22 [total dose/cycle = 90 mg/m^2]
Vinblastine: I.V.: 3 mg/m^2/day days 2, 15, 22 [total dose/cycle = 9 mg/m^2]
Doxorubicin: I.V.: 30 mg/m^2 day 2 [total dose/cycle = 30 mg/m^2]
Cisplatin: I.V.: 70 mg/m^2 day 2 [total dose/cycle = 70 mg/m^2]
Repeat cycle every 4 weeks

M-VAC (Endometrial Cancer)
Use: Endometrial cancer
Regimen:
Methotrexate: I.V.: 30 mg/m^2/day days 1, 15, 22 [total dose/cycle = 90 mg/m^2]
Vinblastine: I.V.: 3 mg/m^2/day days 2, 15, 22 [total dose/cycle = 9 mg/m^2]
Doxorubicin: I.V.: 30 mg/m^2/day day 2 [total dose/cycle = 30 mg/m^2]
Cisplatin: I.V.: 70 mg/m^2/day day 2 [total dose/cycle = 70 mg/m^2]
Repeat cycle every 4 weeks

M-VAC (Head and Neck Cancer)
Use: Head and neck cancer
Regimen:
Methotrexate: I.V.: 30 mg/m^2/day days 1, 15, 22 [total dose/cycle = 90 mg/m^2]
Vinblastine: I.V.: 3 mg/m^2/day days 2, 15, 22 [total dose/cycle = 9 mg/m^2]
Doxorubicin: I.V.: 30 mg/m^2 day 2 [total dose/cycle = 30 mg/m^2]
Cisplatin: I.V.: 70 mg/m^2 day 2 [total dose/cycle = 70 mg/m^2]
Repeat cycle every 4 weeks

MVPP
Use: Lymphoma, Hodgkin disease
Regimen:
Mechlorethamine: I.V.: 6 mg/m^2/day days 1 and 8 [total dose/cycle = 12 mg/m^2]
Vinblastine: I.V.: 4 mg/m^2/day days 1 and 8 [total dose/cycle = 8 mg/m^2]
Procarbazine: Oral: 100 mg/m^2/day days 1-14 [total dose/cycle = 1400 mg/m^2]
Prednisone: Oral: 40 mg/m^2/day days 1-14 [total dose/cycle = 560 mg/m^2]
Repeat cycle every 4-6 weeks

N4SE Protocol

Use: Neuroblastoma
Regimen:
Vincristine: I.V.: 0.05 mg/kg/day days 1 and 2 [total dose/cycle = 0.1 mg/kg]
Doxorubicin: I.V.: 15 mg/m²/day days 1 and 2 [total dose/cycle = 30 mg/m²]
Cyclophosphamide: I.V.: 30 mg/kg/day days 1 and 2 [total dose/cycle = 60 mg/kg]
Fluorouracil: I.V.: 1 mg/kg/day days 3, 8, 9 [total dose/cycle = 3 mg/kg]
Cytarabine: I.V.: 3 mg/kg/day days 3, 8, 9 [total dose/cycle = 9 mg/kg]
Hydroxyurea: Oral: 40 mg/kg/day days 3, 8, 9 [total dose/cycle = 120 mg/kg]
Repeat cycle every 21-28 days

N6 Protocol

Use: Neuroblastoma
Regimen:
Course 1, 2, 4, 6
Cyclophosphamide: I.V.: 70 mg/kg/day days 1 and 2 [total dose/cycle = 140 mg/kg]
Doxorubicin: I.V.: 25 mg/m²/day continuous infusion days 1-3 [total dose/cycle = 75 mg/m²]
Vincristine: I.V.: 0.033 mg/kg/day continuous infusion days 1-3 [total dose/cycle = 0.099 mg/kg]
Vincristine: I.V.: 1.5 mg/m² day 9 [total dose/cycle = 1.5 mg/m²]
Course 3, 5, 7
Etoposide: I.V.: 200 mg/m²/day days 1-3 [total dose/cycle = 600 mg/m²]
Cisplatin: I.V.: 50 mg/m²/day days 1-4 [total dose/cycle = 200 mg/m²]

NFL

Use: Breast cancer
Regimen: Note: Multiple variations are listed below.
Variation 1:
Mitoxantrone: I.V.: 12 mg/m² day 1 [total dose/cycle = 12 mg/m²]
Fluorouracil: I.V.: 350 mg/m²/day days 1-3 [total dose/cycle = 1050 mg/m²]
Leucovorin: I.V.: 300 mg/m²/day days 1-3 [total dose/cycle = 900 mg/m²]
Repeat cycle every 21 days
Variation 2:
Mitoxantrone: I.V.: 10 mg/m² day 1 [total dose/cycle = 10 mg/m²]
Fluorouracil: I.V.: 1000 mg/m²/day continuous infusion days 1-3 [total dose/cycle = 3000 mg/m²]
Leucovorin: I.V.: 100 mg/m²/day days 1-3 [total dose/cycle = 300 mg/m²]
Repeat cycle every 21 days

OPA

Use: Lymphoma, Hodgkin disease
Regimen:
Vincristine: I.V.: 1.5 mg/m²/day (maximum 2 mg) days 1, 8, 15 [total dose/cycle = 4.5 mg/m²]
Prednisone: Oral: 60 mg/m²/day days 1-15 in 3 divided doses [total dose/cycle = 900 mg/m²]
Doxorubicin: I.V.: 40 mg/m²/day days 1 and 15 [total dose/cycle = 80 mg/m²]
Second cycle may be given based on individual response; time between cycles not specified

OPEC

Use: Neuroblastoma
Regimen:
Vincristine: I.V.: 1.5 mg/m² day 1 [total dose/cycle = 1.5 mg/m²]
Cyclophosphamide: I.V.: 600 mg/m² day 1 [total dose/cycle = 600 mg/m²]
Cisplatin: I.V.: 100 mg/m² day 2 [total dose/cycle = 100 mg/m²]
Teniposide: I.V.: 150 mg/m² day 4 [total dose/cycle = 150 mg/m²]
Repeat cycle every 21 days

OPEC-D
Use: Neuroblastoma
Regimen:
  Vincristine: I.V.: 1.5 mg/m^2 day 1 [total dose/cycle = 1.5 mg/m^2]
  Cyclophosphamide: I.V.: 600 mg/m^2 day 1 [total dose/cycle = 600 mg/m^2]
  Doxorubicin: I.V.: 40 mg/m^2 day 1 [total dose/cycle = 40 mg/m^2]
  Cisplatin: I.V.: 100 mg/m^2 day 2 [total dose/cycle = 100 mg/m^2]
  Teniposide: I.V.: 150 mg/m^2 day 4 [total dose/cycle = 150 mg/m^2]
  Repeat cycle every 21 days

OPPA
Use: Lymphoma, Hodgkin disease
Regimen:
  Vincristine: I.V.: 1.5 mg/m^2/day (maximum 2 mg) days 1, 8, 15 [total dose/cycle = 4.5 mg/m^2]
  Prednisone: Oral: 60 mg/m^2/day days 1-15 in 3 divided doses [total dose/cycle = 900 mg/m^2]
  Doxorubicin: I.V.: 40 mg/m^2/day days 1 and 15 [total dose/cycle = 80 mg/m^2]
  Procarbazine: Oral: 100 mg/m^2/day days 1-15 in 2 or 3 divided doses
      [total dose/cycle = 1500 mg/m^2]
  Second cycle may be given based on individual response; time between cycles not specified

PAC (CAP)
Use: Ovarian cancer
Regimen:
  Cisplatin: I.V.: 50 mg/m^2 day 1 [total dose/cycle = 50 mg/m^2]
  Doxorubicin: I.V.: 50 mg/m^2 day 1 [total dose/cycle = 50 mg/m^2]
  Cyclophosphamide: I.V.: 1000 mg/m^2 day 1 [total dose/cycle = 1000 mg/m^2]
  Repeat cycle every 21 days for 8 cycles

PA-CI
Use: Hepatoblastoma
Regimen: Note: Multiple variations are listed below.
  Variation 1:
  Cisplatin: I.V.: 90 mg/m^2 day 1 [total dose/cycle = 90 mg/m^2]
  Doxorubicin: I.V.: 20 mg/m^2/day continuous infusion days 2-5 [total dose/cycle = 80 mg/m^2]
  Repeat cycle every 21 days
  Variation 2:
  Cisplatin: I.V.: 20 mg/m^2/day days 1-4 [total dose/cycle = 80 mg/m^2]
  Doxorubicin: I.V.: 100 mg/m^2 continuous infusion day 1 [total dose/cycle = 100 mg/m^2]
  Repeat cycle every 21-28 days

Paclitaxel, Carboplatin, Bevacizumab
Use: Lung cancer, nonsquamous, nonsmall cell
Regimen:
  Paclitaxel: I.V.: 200 mg/m^2 infused over 3 hours day 1 [total dose/cycle = 200 mg/m^2]
  followed by
  Carboplatin: I.V.: Target AUC 6 day 1 [total dose/cycle = AUC = 6]
  followed by
  Bevacizumab: I.V.: 15 mg/kg day 1 [total dose/cycle = 15 mg/kg]
  Repeat cycle every 21 days for 6 cycles

Paclitaxel, Carboplatin, Etoposide
Use: Adenocarcinoma, unknown primary
Regimen:
  Paclitaxel: I.V.: 200 mg/m^2 infused over 1 hour day 1 [total dose/cycle = 200 mg/m^2] **followed by:**
  Carboplatin: I.V.: Target AUC 6 [total dose/cycle = AUC = 6]
  Etoposide: Oral: 50 mg/day, days 1, 3, 5, 7, 9 **and** 100 mg/day days 2, 4, 6, 8, 10 [total dose/cycle = 750 mg/day]
  Repeat cycle every 21 days

Paclitaxel-Carboplatin-Gemcitabine
Use: Bladder cancer
Regimen:
Paclitaxel: I.V.: 200 mg/m^2 day 1 [total dose/cycle = 200 mg/m^2]
Gemcitabine: I.V.: 1000 mg/m^2/day days 1 and 8 [total dose/cycle = 2000 mg/m^2]
Carboplatin: I.V.: AUC 5 day 1 [total dose/cycle = AUC = 5]
Repeat cycle every 21 days

Paclitaxel + Estramustine + Carboplatin
Use: Prostate cancer
Regimen:
Paclitaxel: I.V.: 100 mg/m^2 day 3 each week [total dose/cycle = 400 mg/m^2]
Estramustine: Oral: 10 mg/kg/day days 1-5 each week [total dose/cycle = 200 mg/kg]
Carboplatin: I.V.: Target AUC 6 day 3 [total dose/cycle = AUC = 6]
Repeat cycle every 28 days

Paclitaxel + Estramustine + Etoposide
Use: Prostate cancer
Regimen:
Paclitaxel: I.V.: 135 mg/m^2 day 2 [total dose/cycle = 135 mg/m^2]
Estramustine: Oral: 280 mg 3 times/day days 1-14 [total dose/cycle = 11,760 mg]
Etoposide: Oral: 100 mg/day days 1-14   [total dose/cycle = 1400 mg]
Repeat cycle every 21 days

Paclitaxel-Ifosfamide-Cisplatin
Use: Testicular cancer
Regimen:
Paclitaxel: I.V.: 250 mg/m^2 continuous infusion day 1 [total dose/cycle = 250 mg/m^2]
Ifosfamide: I.V.: 1500 mg/m^2/day days 2-5 [total dose/cycle = 6000 mg/m^2]
Cisplatin: I.V.: 25 mg/m^2/day days 2-5   [total dose/cycle = 100 mg/m^2]
Mesna: I.V.: 500 mg/m^2 prior to ifosfamide and every 4 hours for 2 doses, days 2-5 [total dose/cycle = 6000 mg/m^2]
Repeat cycle every 21 days for 4 cycles

Paclitaxel-Vinorelbine
Use: Breast cancer
Regimen: Note: Multiple variations are listed below.
Variation 1:
Paclitaxel: I.V.: 135 mg/m^2 day 1 [total dose/cycle = 135 mg/m^2]
Vinorelbine: I.V.: 30 mg/m^2 day 1 [total dose/cycle = 30 mg/m^2]
Repeat cycle every 21 days
Variation 2:
Paclitaxel: I.V.: 150 mg/m^2 day 1 [total dose/cycle = 150 mg/m^2]
Vinorelbine: I.V.: 25 mg/m^2 day 1 [total dose/cycle = 25 mg/m^2]
Repeat cycle every 21 days
Variation 3:
Paclitaxel: I.V.: 135 mg/m^2 day 1 [total dose/cycle = 135 mg/m^2]
Vinorelbine: I.V.: 30 mg/m^2/day days 1 and 8 [total dose/cycle = 60 mg/m^2]
Repeat cycle every 28 days

PC (Bladder Cancer)
Use: Bladder cancer
Regimen:
Paclitaxel: I.V.: 200 mg/m^2 or 225 mg/m^2 day 1 [total dose/cycle = 200 or 225 mg/m^2]
Carboplatin: I.V.: AUC 5-6 day 1 [total dose/cycle = AUC = 5-6]
Repeat cycle every 21 days

PC (Nonsmall Cell Lung Cancer)
Use: Lung cancer, nonsmall cell
Regimen: Note: Multiple variations are listed below.
Variation 1:
Paclitaxel: I.V.: 175-225 mg/m² day 1 [total dose/cycle = 175-225 mg/m²]
Carboplatin: I.V.: Target AUC 5-7 day 1 [total dose/cycle = AUC = 5-7]
Repeat cycle every 21 days for 2-8 cycles
Variation 2:
Paclitaxel: I.V.: 175 mg/m² day 1 [total dose/cycle = 175 mg/m²]
Cisplatin: I.V.: 80 mg/m² day 1 [total dose/cycle = 80 mg/m²]
Repeat cycle every 21 days
Variation 3:
Paclitaxel: I.V.: 135 mg/m² continuous infusion day 1 [total dose/cycle = 135 mg/m²]
Carboplatin: I.V.: AUC 7.5 day 2 [total dose/cycle = AUC = 7.5]
Repeat cycle every 21 days
Variation 4:
Paclitaxel: I.V.: 135 mg/m² continuous infusion day 1 [total dose/cycle = 135 mg/m²]
Cisplatin: I.V.: 75 mg/m² day 2 [total dose/cycle = 75 mg/m²]
Repeat cycle every 21 days

PCE
Use: Adenocarcinoma, unknown primary
Regimen:
Paclitaxel: I.V.: 200 mg/m² day 1 [total dose/cycle = 200 mg/m²]
Carboplatin: I.V.: AUC = 6 day 1 [total dose/cycle = AUC = 6]
Etoposide: Oral: 50 mg/day days 1, 3, 5, 7, 9 **and** Oral: 100 mg/day days 2, 4, 6, 8, 10 [total dose/cycle = 750 mg]
Repeat cycle every 3 weeks

PCV
Use: Brain tumors
Regimen:
Lomustine: Oral: 110 mg/m² day 1 [total dose/cycle = 110 mg/m²]
Procarbazine: Oral: 60 mg/m²/day days 8-21 [total dose/cycle = 840 mg/m²]
Vincristine: I.V.: 1.4 mg/m²/day (maximum 2 mg) days 8 and 29 [total dose/cycle = 2.8 mg/m²; maximum 4 mg]
Repeat cycle every 6-8 weeks

PE
Use: Prostate cancer
Regimen: Note: Multiple variations are listed below.
Variation 1:
Paclitaxel: I.V.: 30-35 mg/m²/day continuous infusion (given in 2-3 divided doses daily) either days 1-4 or days 2-5 [total dose/cycle = 120-140 mg/m²]
Estramustine: Oral: 600 mg/m²/day days 1-21 [total dose/cycle = 12,600 mg/m²]
Repeat cycle every 21 days
Variation 2:
Paclitaxel: I.V. 60-107 mg/m² infused over 3 hours weekly for 6 weeks [total dose/cycle = 360-642 mg/m²]
Estramustine: Oral: 280 mg twice daily 3 days/week for 6 weeks [total dose/cycle = 3360 mg]
Repeat cycle every 8 weeks
Variation 3:
Paclitaxel: I.V. 150 mg/m²/day days 2, 9, 16 [total dose/cycle = 450 mg/m²]
Estramustine: Oral: 280 mg 3 times/day days 1, 2, 3, 8, 9, 10, 15, 16, 17 [total dose/week = 7560 mg/m²]
Repeat cycle every 4 weeks
Variation 4:
Paclitaxel: I.V.: 100 mg/m²/day days 2, 9, and 16 [total dose/cycle = 300 mg/m²]
Estramustine: Oral: 280 mg 3 times/day days 1, 2, 3, 8, 9, 10, 15, 16, 17 [total dose/cycle = 7560 mg]
Repeat cycle every 4 weeks

PE-CAdO
Use: Neuroblastoma
Regimen:
Cisplatin: I.V.: 100 mg/m^2 day 1 [total dose/cycle = 100 mg/m^2]
Teniposide: I.V.: 160 mg/m^2 day 3 [total dose/cycle = 160 mg/m^2]
alternating with
Cyclophosphamide: I.V.: 300 mg/m^2/day days 1-5 [total dose/cycle = 1500 mg/m^2]
Doxorubicin: I.V.: 60 mg/m^2 day 5 [total dose/cycle = 60 mg/m^2]
Vincristine: I.V.: 1.5 mg/m^2/day days 1 and 5 [total dose/cycle = 3 mg/m^2]
Repeat cycle every 21 days

PFL (Colorectal Cancer)
Use: Colorectal cancer
Regimen:
Cisplatin: I.V.: 25 mg/m^2/day continuous infusion days 1-5 [total dose/cycle = 125 mg/m^2]
Fluorouracil: I.V.: 800 mg/m^2/day continuous infusion days 2-5 [total dose/cycle = 3200 mg/m^2]
Leucovorin calcium: I.V.: 500 mg/m^2/day continuous infusion days 1-5
[total dose/cycle = 2500 mg/m^2]
Repeat cycle every 28 days

PFL (Head and Neck Cancer)
Use: Head and neck cancer
Regimen: Note: Multiple variations are listed below.
Variation 1:
Cisplatin: I.V.: 25 mg/m^2/day continuous infusion days 1-5 [total dose/cycle = 125 mg/m^2]
Fluorouracil: I.V.: 800 mg/m^2/day continuous infusion days 2-6 [total dose/cycle = 4000 mg/m^2]
Leucovorin: I.V.: 500 mg/m^2/day continuous infusion days 1-6 [total dose/cycle = 3000 mg/m^2]
Repeat cycle every 28 days
Variation 2:
Cisplatin: I.V.: 100 mg/m^2 day 1 [total dose/cycle = 100 mg/m^2]
Fluorouracil: I.V.: 600-1000 mg/m^2/day continuous infusion days 1-5
[total dose/cycle = 3000-5000 mg/m^2]
Leucovorin: Oral: 50 mg/m^2 every 4-6 hours days 1-6 [total dose/cycle = 1200-1800 mg/m^2]
Repeat cycle every 21 days

PFL + IFN
Use: Head and neck cancer
Regimen:
Cisplatin: I.V.: 100 mg/m^2 day 1 [total dose/cycle = 100 mg/m^2]
Fluorouracil: I.V.: 640 mg/m^2/day continuous infusion days 1-5 [total dose/cycle = 3200 mg/m^2]
Leucovorin calcium: Oral: 100 mg every 4 hours days 1-5 [total dose/cycle = 3000 mg/m^2]
Interferon alfa-2b: SubQ: 2 x 10^6 units/m^2 days 1-6 [total dose/cycle = 12 x 10^6 units/m^2]

POC
Use: Brain tumors
Regimen:
Prednisone: Oral: 40 mg/m^2/day days 1-14 [total dose/cycle = 560 mg/m^2]
Vincristine: I.V.: 1.5 mg/m^2/day (maximum 2 mg) days 1, 8, 15 [total dose/cycle = 4.5 mg/m^2]
Lomustine: Oral: 100 mg/m^2 day 1 [total dose/cycle = 100 mg/m^2]
Repeat cycle every 6 weeks

POG-8651

Use: Osteosarcoma

Regimen:

(Surgery at week 10)

Methotrexate: I.V.: 12 g/m² weeks 0, 1, 5, 6, 13, 14, 18, 19, 23, 24, 37, 38
[total dose/cycle = 144 g/m²]

Leucovorin: (route not specified): 15 mg every 6 hours for 10 doses, weeks 0, 1, 5, 6, 13, 14, 18, 19, 23, 24, 37, 38
[total dose/cycle = 1800 mg]

Doxorubicin: I.V.: 37.5 mg/m²/day day 1 and weeks 2, 7, 25, 28 and 30 mg/m² days 1, 2, 3, week 20
[total dose/cycle = 390 mg/m²]

Cisplatin: I.V.: 60 mg/m²/day days 1, 2, weeks 2, 7, 25, 28
[total dose/cycle = 480 mg/m²]

Cyclophosphamide: I.V.: 600 mg/m²/day days 1, 2, 3, weeks 15, 31, 34, 39, 42
[total dose/cycle = 9000 mg/m²]

Bleomycin: I.V.: 15 units/m²/day days 1, 2, 3, weeks 15, 31, 34, 39, 42
[total dose/cycle = 225 units/m²]

Dactinomycin: I.V.: 0.6 mg/m²/day days 1, 2, 3, weeks 15, 31, 34, 39, 42
[total dose/cycle = 9 mg/m²]

OR

(Surgery at week 0)

Methotrexate: I.V.: 12 g/m² weeks 3, 4, 8, 9, 13, 14, 18, 19, 23, 24, 37, 38
[total dose/cycle = 144 g/m²]

Leucovorin: (route not specified): 15 mg every 6 hours for 10 doses, weeks 3, 4, 8, 9, 13, 14, 18, 19, 23, 24, 37, 38
[total dose/cycle = 1800 mg]

Doxorubicin: I.V.: 37.5 mg/m²/day days 1, 2, weeks 5, 10, 25, 28, and 30 mg/m² days 1, 2, 3, week 20
[total dose/cycle = 390 mg/m²]

Cisplatin: I.V.: 60 mg/m²/day days 1, 2, weeks, 5, 10, 25, 28
[total dose/cycle = 480 mg/m²]

Cyclophosphamide: I.V.: 600 mg/m²/day days 1, 2, 3, weeks 15, 31, 34, 39, 42
[total dose/cycle = 9000 mg/m²]

Bleomycin: I.V.: 15 units/m²/day days 1, 2, 3, weeks 15, 31, 34, 39, 42
[total dose/cycle = 225 mg/m²]

Dactinomycin: I.V.: 0.6 mg/m²/day days 1, 2, 3, weeks 15, 31, 34, 39, 42
[total dose/cycle = 9 mg/m²]

POMP

Use: Leukemia, acute lymphocytic

Regimen: Maintenance:

Mercaptopurine: Oral: 50 mg 3 times/day [total dose/cycle = 4200-4650 mg]

Methotrexate: Oral: 20 mg/m² once weekly [total dose/cycle = 80 mg/m²]

Vincristine: I.V.: 2 mg day 1 [total dose/cycle = 2 mg]

Prednisone: Oral: 200 mg/day days 1-5 [total dose/cycle = 1000 mg]

Repeat cycle monthly for 2 years

Pro-MACE-CytaBOM

Use: Lymphoma, non-Hodgkin

Regimen:

Prednisone: Oral: 60 mg/m²/day days 1-14 [total dose/cycle = 840 mg/m²]
Doxorubicin: I.V.: 25 mg/m² day 1 [total dose/cycle = 25 mg/m²]
Cyclophosphamide: I.V.: 650 mg/m² day 1 [total dose/cycle = 650 mg/m²]
Etoposide: I.V.: 120 mg/m² day 1 [total dose/cycle = 120 mg/m²]
Cytarabine: I.V.: 300 mg/m² day 8 [total dose/cycle = 300 mg/m²]
Bleomycin: I.V.: 5 units/m² day 8 [total dose/cycle = 5 units/m²]
Vincristine: I.V.: 1.4 mg/m² (maximum 2 mg) day 8 [total dose/cycle = 1.4 mg/m²]
Methotrexate: I.V.: 120 mg/m² day 8 [total dose/cycle = 120 mg/m²]
Leucovorin: Oral: 25 mg/m² every 6 hours for 4 doses (start 24 hours after methotrexate) day 9
[total dose/cycle = 100 mg/m²]
Repeat cycle every 21 days

PVA (POG 8602)

Use: Leukemia, acute lymphocytic

Regimen:

Induction:

Prednisone: Oral: 40 mg/m^2/day (maximum 60 mg) days 0-28 (given in 3 divided doses)
[total dose/cycle = 1160 mg/m^2]

Vincristine: I.V.: 1.5 mg/m^2/day (maximum 2 mg) days 0, 7, 14, and 21
[total dose/cycle = 6 mg/m^2; maximum 8]

Asparaginase: I.M.: 6000 units/m^2 3 times per week for 2 weeks
[total dose/cycle = 36,000/units/m^2]

Intrathecal therapy (triple): Days 0 and 22

Leucovorin: route and dose not specified: single dose 24 hours after every intrathecal treatment days 1 and 23

Administer one cycle only

CNS consolidation:

Mercaptopurine: Oral: 75 mg/m^2/day days 29-43 [total dose/cycle = 1125 mg/m^2]

Intrathecal therapy (triple): Days 29 and 36

Leucovorin: route and dose not specified: single dose 24 hours after every intrathecal treatment days 30 and 37

Administer one cycle only

Intensification:

Regimen A:

Methotrexate: I.V.: 1000 mg/m^2 continuous infusion over 24 hours day 1 [total dose/cycle = 1000 mg/m^2]

Cytarabine: I.V.: 1000 mg/m^2 continuous infusion over 24 hours day 1 (start 12 hours after methotrexate)
[total dose/cycle = 1000 mg/m^2]

Leucovorin: I.M., I.V., or Oral: 30 mg/m^2 at 24 and 36 hours after the start of methotrexate
[total dose/cycle = 60 mg/m^2]

followed by 3 mg/m^2 at 48, 60, and 72 hours after the start of methotrexate
[total dose/cycle = 9 mg/m^2]

Repeat cycle every 3 weeks for 6 cycles (administered weeks 7, 10, 13, 16, 19, 22)

Intrathecal therapy (triple): Weeks 9, 12, 15, and 18

Leucovorin: route and dose not specified: single dose 24 hours after every intrathecal treatment weeks 9, 12, 15, 18
or

Regimen B:

Methotrexate: I.V.: 1000 mg/m^2 continuous infusion over 24 hours day 1 [total dose/cycle = 1000 mg/m^2]

Cytarabine: I.V.: 1000 mg/m^2 continuous infusion over 24 hours day 1 (start 12 hours after methotrexate)
[total dose/cycle = 1000 mg/m^2]

Leucovorin: I.M., I.V., or Oral: 30 mg/m^2 at 24 and 36 hours after the start of methotrexate
[total dose/cycle = 60 mg/m^2]

followed by 3 mg/m^2 at 48, 60, and 72 hours after the start of methotrexate
[total dose/cycle = 9 mg/m^2]

Repeat cycle every 12 weeks for 6 cycles (administer weeks 7, 19, 31, 43, 55, 67)

Intrathecal therapy (triple): Weeks 9, 12, 15, and 18

Leucovorin: route and dose not specified: single dose 24 hours after every intrathecal treatment weeks 9, 12, 15, 18

Maintenance:

Regimen A:

Methotrexate: I.M.: 20 mg/m^2 weekly, weeks 25-156 [total dose/cycle = 2640 mg/m^2]

Mercaptopurine: Oral: 75 mg/m^2 daily, weeks 25-156 [total dose/cycle = 69,300 mg/m^2]

Intrathecal therapy (triple): Every 8 weeks, weeks 26-105

Leucovorin: route and dose not specified: single dose 24 hours after every intrathecal treatment weeks 26-105

Prednisone: Oral: 40 mg/m^2/day (maximum 60 mg) days 1-7 (given in 3 divided doses), weeks 8, 17, 25, 41, 57, 73, 89, 105
[total dose/cycle = 2240 mg/m^2; maximum 3360 mg]

Vincristine: I.V.: 1.5 mg/m^2/day (maximum 2 mg) day 1, weeks 8, 9, 17, 18, 25, 26, 41, 42, 57, 58, 73, 74, 89, 90, 105, 106
[total dose/cycle = 24 mg/m^2; maximum 32 mg]
or

Regimen B:

Methotrexate: I.M.: 20 mg/m^2 weekly, weeks 22-28, 34-40, 46-52, 58-64 [total dose/cycle = 560 mg/m^2]

Mercaptopurine: Oral: 75 mg/m^2 daily for 7 weeks, weeks 22-28, 34-40, 46-52, 58-64
[total dose/cycle = 14,700 mg/m^2]

followed by
Methotrexate: I.M.: 20 mg/m^2 weekly, weeks 70-156 [total dose/cycle = 1720 mg/m^2]
Mercaptopurine: Oral: 75 mg/m^2 daily, weeks 70-156 [total dose/cycle = 45,150 mg/m^2]
Intrathecal therapy (triple): Every 8 weeks, weeks 26-105
Leucovorin: route and dose not specified: single dose 24 hours after every intrathecal treatment weeks 26-105
Prednisone: Oral: 40 mg/m^2/day (maximum 60 mg) days 1-7 (given in 3 divided doses), weeks 8, 17, 25, 41, 57, 73, 89, 105 [total dose/cycle = 2240 mg/m^2]
Vincristine: I.V.: 1.5 mg/m^2/day (maximum 2 mg) day 1, weeks 8, 9, 17, 18, 25, 26, 41, 42, 57, 58, 73, 74, 89, 90, 105, 106 [total dose/cycle = 24 mg/m^2; maximum 32 mg]

PVB
Use: Testicular cancer
Regimen: Note: Multiple variations are listed below.
Variation 1:
Cisplatin: I.V.: 20 mg/m^2/day days 1-5 [total dose/cycle = 100 mg/m^2]
Vinblastine: I.V.: 0.2 mg/kg/day days 1 and 2 [total dose/cycle = 0.4 mg/kg]
Bleomycin: I.V.: 30 units/day days 2, 9, 16 [total dose/cycle = 90 units]
Repeat cycle every 3 weeks
Variation 2:
Cisplatin: I.V.: 20 mg/m^2/day days 1-5 [total dose/cycle = 100 mg/m^2]
Vinblastine: I.V.: 0.15 mg/kg/day days 1 and 2 [total dose/cycle = 0.3 mg/kg]
Bleomycin: I.V.: 30 units days 2, 9, 16 [total dose/cycle = 90 units]
Repeat cycle every 3 weeks
Variation 3:
Cisplatin: I.V.: 20 mg/m^2/day days 1-5 [total dose/cycle = 100 mg/m^2]
Vinblastine: I.V.: 6 mg/m^2/day days 1 and 2 [total dose/cycle = 12 mg/m^2]
Bleomycin: I.M.: 30 units/day days 2, 9, 16 [total dose/cycle = 90 units]
Repeat cycle every 3 weeks

PVDA
Use: Leukemia, acute lymphocytic
Regimen: Induction:
Prednisone: Oral: 60 mg/m^2/day days 1-28 [total dose/cycle = 1680 mg/m^2]
Vincristine: I.V.: 1.5 mg/m^2/day days 1, 8, 15, 22 [total dose/cycle = 6 mg/m^2]
Daunorubicin: I.V.: 25 mg/m^2/day days 1, 8, 15, 22 [total dose/cycle = 100 mg/m^2]
Asparaginase: I.M., SubQ, or I.V.: 5000 units/m^2/day days 1-14
    [total dose/cycle = 70,000 units/m^2]
Administer one cycle only; used in conjunction with intrathecal chemotherapy

R-CHOP
Use: Lymphoma, non-Hodgkin
Regimen:
Rituximab: I.V.: 375 mg/m^2 day 1 [total dose/cycle = 375 mg/m^2]
Cyclophosphamide: I.V.: 750 mg/m^2 day 1 [total dose/cycle = 750 mg/m^2]
Doxorubicin: I.V.: 50 mg/m^2 day 1 [total dose/cycle = 50 mg/m^2]
Vincristine: I.V.: 1.4 mg/m^2 (maximum 2 mg) day 1 [total dose/cycle = 1.4 mg/m^2; maximum 2 mg]
Prednisone: Oral: 40 mg/m^2/day days 1-5 [total dose/cycle = 200 mg/m^2]
Repeat cycle every 21 days

R-CVP
Use: Lymphoma, non-Hodgkin
Regimen:
Rituximab: I.V.: 375 mg/m^2 day 1 [total dose/cycle = 375 mg/m^2]
Cyclophosphamide: I.V.: 750 mg/m^2 day 1 [total dose/cycle = 750 mg/m^2]
Vincristine: I.V.: 1.4 mg/m^2 day 1 [total dose/cycle = 1.4 mg/m^2]
Prednisolone: Oral: 40 mg/m^2/day days 1-5 [total dose/cycle = 200 mg/m^2]
Repeat cycle every 21 days

Regimen A1
Use: Neuroblastoma
Regimen:
Cyclophosphamide: I.V.: 1.2 g/m^2 day 1 [total dose/cycle = 1.2 g/m^2]
Vincristine: I.V.: 1.5 mg/m^2 day 1 [total dose/cycle = 1.5 mg/m^2]
Doxorubicin: I.V.: 40 mg/m^2 day 3 [total dose/cycle = 40 mg/m^2]
Cisplatin: I.V.: 90 mg/m^2 day 5 [total dose/cycle = 90 mg/m^2]
Repeat cycle every 28 days

Regimen A2
Use: Neuroblastoma
Regimen:
Cyclophosphamide: I.V.: 1.2 g/m^2 day 1 [total dose/cycle = 1.2 g/m^2]
Etoposide: I.V.: 100 mg/m^2/day days 1-5 [total dose/cycle = 500 mg/m^2]
Doxorubicin: I.V.: 40 mg/m^2 day 3 [total dose/cycle = 40 mg/m^2]
Cisplatin: I.V.: 90 mg/m^2 day 5 [total dose/cycle = 90 mg/m^2]
Repeat cycle every 28 days

RICE
Use: Lymphoma, non-Hodgkin
Regimen:
Rituximab: I.V.: 375 mg/m^2/day days -2 and 1 (cycle 1) [total dose/cycle = 750 mg/m^2]
Rituximab: I.V.: 375 mg/m^2 day 1 (cycles 2 and 3) [total dose/cycle = 375 mg/m^2]
Etoposide: I.V.: 100 mg/m^2/day days 3-5 [total dose/cycle = 300 mg/m^2]
Carboplatin: I.V.: AUC = 5 (maximum 800 mg) day 4 [total dose/cycle = AUC = 5]
Ifosfamide: I.V.: 5000 mg/m^2 continuous infusion day 4 [total dose/cycle = 5000 mg/m^2]
Mesna: I.V.: 5000 mg/m^2 continuous infusion day 4 [total dose/cycle = 5000 mg/m^2]
Filgrastim: SubQ: 5 mcg/kg/day days 7-14 (cycles 1 and 2) [total dose/cycle = 40 mcg/kg]
Filgrastim: SubQ: 10 mcg/kg/day days 7-14 (cycle 3) [total dose/cycle = 80 mcg/kg]
Repeat cycle every 2 weeks

Stanford V
Use: Lymphoma, Hodgkin disease
Regimen:
Mechlorethamine: I.V.: 6 mg/m^2 day 1 [total dose/cycle = 6 mg/m^2]
Doxorubicin: I.V.: 25 mg/m^2/day days 1 and 15 [total dose/cycle = 50 mg/m^2]
Vinblastine: I.V.: 6 mg/m^2/day days 1 and 15 [total dose/cycle = 12 mg/m^2]
Vincristine: I.V.: 1.4 mg/m^2/day (maximum 2 mg) days 8 and 22 [total dose/cycle = 2.8 mg/m^2; maximum 4 mg]
Bleomycin: I.V.: 5 units/m^2/day days 8 and 22 [total dose/cycle = 10 units/m^2]
Etoposide: I.V.: 60 mg/m^2/day days 15 and 16 [total dose/cycle = 120 mg/m^2]
Prednisone: Oral: 40 mg/m^2 every other day for 9 weeks
    followed by tapering of dose by 10 mg every other day, beginning at week 10
Repeat cycle every 28 days, for 3 cycles

TAC

Use: Breast cancer
Regimen: Note: Multiple variations are listed below.
Variation 1:
Docetaxel: I.V.: 75 mg/m^2 day 1 [total dose/cycle = 75 mg/m^2]
Doxorubicin: I.V.: 50 mg/m^2 day 1 [total dose/cycle = 50 mg/m^2]
Cyclophosphamide: I.V.: 500 mg/m^2 day 1 [total dose/cycle = 500 mg/m^2]
Repeat cycle every 3 weeks
Variation 2:
Docetaxel: I.V.: 60 mg/m^2 day 1 [total dose/cycle = 60 mg/m^2]
Doxorubicin: I.V.: 60 mg/m^2 day 1 [total dose/cycle = 60 mg/m^2]
Cyclophosphamide: I.V.: 600 mg/m^2 day 1 [total dose/cycle = 600 mg/m^2]
Repeat cycle every 3 weeks

TAD

Use: Leukemia, acute myeloid
Regimen:
Daunorubicin: I.V.: 60 mg/m^2/day days 3-5 [total dose/cycle = 180 mg/m^2]
Cytarabine: I.V.: 100 mg/m^2/day continuous infusion days 1 and 2
[total dose/cycle = 200 mg/m^2] **followed by** 100 mg/m^2/day every 12 hours days 3-8
[total dose/cycle = 1200 mg/m^2]
Thioguanine: Oral: 100 mg/m^2/day every 12 hours days 3-9 [total dose/cycle = 1400 mg/m^2]
Administer one cycle only

Tamoxifen-Epirubicin

Use: Breast cancer
Regimen:
Tamoxifen: Oral: 20 mg daily [total dose/cycle = 560 mg]
Epirubicin: I.V.: 50 mg/m^2/day days 1 and 8 [total dose/cycle = 100 mg/m^2]
Repeat epirubicin cycle every 28 days for 6 cycles; continue tamoxifen for 4 years

TCF

Use: Esophageal cancer
Regimen:
Paclitaxel: I.V.: 175 mg/m^2 day 1 [total dose/cycle = 175 mg/m^2]
Cisplatin: I.V.: 20 mg/m^2/day days 1-5 for Cycles 1, 2, 3 [total dose/cycle = 100 mg/m^2]
then 15 mg/m^2/day days 1-5 [total dose/cycle = 75 mg/m^2]
Fluorouracil: I.V.: 750 mg/m^2/day continuous infusion days 1-5 [total dose/cycle = 3750 mg/m^2]
Repeat cycle every 28 days

TEX (Capecitabine + Docetaxel + Epirubicin)

Use: Breast cancer
Regimen:
Capecitabine: Oral: 1000 mg/m^2 twice daily days 1-14 [total dose/cycle = 28,000 mg/m^2]
Docetaxel: I.V.: 75 mg/m^2 day 1 [total dose/cycle = 75 mg/m^2]
Epirubicin: I.V.: 75 mg/m^2 day 1 [total dose/cycle = 75 mg/m^2]
Repeat cycle every 3 weeks

Thalidomide + Dexamethasone

Use: Multiple myeloma

Regimen: Note: Multiple variations are listed below.

Variation 1:

Thalidomide: Oral: 100 mg/day days 1-28 [total dose/cycle = 2800 mg]

Dexamethasone: Oral: 40 mg/day days 1-4 [total dose/cycle = 160 mg]

Repeat cycle every 28 days

Variation 2:

Thalidomide: Oral: 200 mg/day days 1-14 cycle 1

followed by 400 mg/day days 15-28 cycle 1 [total dose/cycle = 8400 mg]

Thalidomide: Oral: 400 mg/day days 1-28 (subsequent cycles) [total dose/cycle = 11,200 mg]

Dexamethasone: Oral: 20 mg/m^2/day days 1-4, 9-12, and 17-20 cycle 1 (subsequent cycles) [total dose/cycle = 240 mg/m^2]

Dexamethasone: Oral: 20 mg/m^2/day days 1-4 (subsequent cycles) [total dose/cycle = 80 mg/m^2]

Repeat cycle every 28 days

Variation 3:

Thalidomide: Oral: 100 mg/day days 1-7, 150 mg/day days 8-14, 200 mg/day days 15-21, 250 mg/day days 22-28, and 300 mg/day days 29-35 (cycle 1) [total dose/cycle = 7000 mg]

Thalidomide: Oral: 300 mg/day days 1-35 (subsequent cycles) [total dose/cycle = 10,500 mg]

Dexamethasone: Oral: 20 mg/m^2/day days 1-4, 9-12, and 17-20 [total dose/cycle = 240 mg/m^2]

Repeat cycle every 35 days

Variation 4:

Thalidomide: Oral: 200 mg/day days 1-28 [total dose/cycle = 5600 mg]

Dexamethasone: Oral: 40 mg/day days 1-4, 9-12, and 17-20 (odd cycles) [total dose/cycle = 480 mg]

Dexamethasone: Oral: 40 mg/day days 1-4 (even cycles) [total dose/cycle = 160 mg]

Repeat cycle every 28 days

TIP

Use: Esophageal cancer; Head and neck cancer

Regimen:

Paclitaxel: I.V.: 175 mg/m^2 day 1 [total dose/cycle = 175 mg/m^2]

Ifosfamide: I.V.: 1000 mg/m^2/day days 1-3 [total dose/cycle = 3000 mg/m^2]

Mesna: I.V.: 400 mg/m^2/day before ifosfamide days 1-3

plus 200 mg/m^2 4 hours after ifosfamide days 1-3 [total dose/cycle = 1800 mg/m^2]

Cisplatin: I.V.: 60 mg/m^2 day 1 [total dose/cycle = 60 mg/m^2]

Repeat cycle every 21-28 days

Trastuzumab-Paclitaxel

Use: Breast cancer

Regimen:

Paclitaxel: I.V.: 175 mg/m^2 day 1 [total dose/cycle = 175 mg/m^2]

Trastuzumab: I.V.: 4 mg/kg (loading dose) day 1 cycle 1 [total dose/cycle = 4 mg/kg]

Trastuzumab: I.V.: 2 mg/kg/day days 8 and 15 (cycle 1) [total dose/cycle = 4 mg/kg]

followed by 2 mg/kg/day days 1, 8, 15 (subsequent cycles) [total dose/cycle = 6 mg/kg]

Repeat cycle every 21 days for at least 6 cycles

Tretinoin/Idarubicin

Use: Leukemia, acute promyelocytic

Regimen: Note: Multiple variations are listed below.

Variation 1: Induction:

Tretinoin: Oral: 45 mg/m^2/day day 1 up to 90 days [total dose/cycle = up to 4050 mg/m^2]

≤20 years: 25 mg/m^2/day day 1 up to 90 days [total dose/cycle = up to 2250 mg/m^2]

Idarubicin: I.V.: 12 mg/m^2/day days 2, 4, 6, 8 [total dose/cycle = 48 mg/m^2]

Consolidation: Course 1:

Idarubicin: I.V.: 5 mg/m^2/day days 1-4 [total dose/cycle = 20 mg/m^2] **or**

Idarubicin: I.V.: 7 mg/m^2/day days 1-4 [total dose/cycle = 28 mg/m^2]

Tretinoin: Oral: 45 mg/m^2/day days 1-15 [total dose/cycle = 675 mg/m^2]

Course 2:

Mitoxantrone: I.V.: 10 mg/m^2/day days 1-5 [total dose/cycle = 50 mg/m^2]

or

Mitoxantrone: I.V.: 10 mg/m^2/day days 1-5 [total dose/cycle = 50 mg/m^2]

Tretinoin: Oral: 45 mg/m^2/day days 1-15 [total dose/cycle = 675 mg/m^2]

Course 3:

Idarubicin: I.V.: 12 mg/m^2 day 1 [total dose/cycle = 12 mg/m^2] **or**

Idarubicin: I.V.: 12 mg/m^2/day days 1-2 [total dose/cycle = 24 mg/m^2]

Tretinoin: Oral: 45 mg/m^2/day days 1-15 [total dose/cycle = 675 mg/m^2]

Administer courses sequentially at 1-month intervals for 3 months

Maintenance:

Mercaptopurine: Oral: 50 mg/m^2 daily [total dose/cycle = 4500 mg/m^2 (90 days)]

Methotrexate: I.M.: 15 mg/m^2 weekly [total dose/cycle = 180 mg/m^2]

Tretinoin: Oral: 45 mg/m^2/day days 1-15 [total dose/cycle = 675 mg/m^2]

Repeat every 3 months for 2 years

Variation 2: Induction:

Tretinoin: Oral: 45 mg/m^2/day day 1 up to 90 days [total dose/cycle = up to 4050 mg/m^2]

<15 years: 25 mg/m^2/day day 1 up to 90 days [total dose/cycle = up to 2250 mg/m^2]

Idarubicin: I.V.: 12 mg/m^2/day days 2, 4, 6, and 8 [total dose/cycle = 48 mg/m^2]

Consolidation: Course 1:

Idarubicin: I.V.: 5 mg/m^2/day days 1-4 [total dose/cycle = 20 mg/m^2]

Course 2:

Mitoxantrone: I.V.: 10 mg/m^2/day days 1-5 [total dose/cycle = 50 mg/m^2]

Course 3:

Idarubicin: I.V.: 12 mg/m^2 day 1 [total dose/cycle = 12 mg/m^2]

Administer courses sequentially at 1-month intervals for 3 months

Maintenance:

Mercaptopurine: Oral: 90 mg/m^2 daily [total dose/cycle = 8100 mg/m^2]

Methotrexate: I.M.: 15 mg/m^2 weekly [total dose/cycle = 180 mg/m^2]

Tretinoin: Oral: 45 mg/m^2/day days 1-15 [total dose/cycle = 675 mg/m^2]

Repeat every 3 months for 2 years

TVTG

Use: Leukemia, acute lymphocytic; Leukemia, acute myeloid

Regimen:

Topotecan: I.V.: 1 mg/m^2/day continuous infusion days 1-5 [total dose/cycle = 5 mg/m^2]

Vinorelbine: I.V.: 20 mg/m^2/day days 0, 7, 14, 21 [total dose/cycle = 80 mg/m^2]

Thiotepa: I.V.: 15 mg/m^2 day 2 [total dose/cycle = 15 mg/m^2]

Gemcitabine: I.V.: 3600 mg/m^2 day 7 [total dose/cycle = 3600 mg/m^2]

Dexamethasone: Oral or I.V.: 45 mg/m^2/day days 7-14 (given in 3 divided doses)

[total dose/cycle = 315 mg/m^2]

Repeat cycle when ANC >500 cells/mcL and platelet count >75,000 cells/mcL

VAC (Retinoblastoma)

Use: Retinoblastoma

Regimen:

Vincristine: I.V.: 1.5 mg/m^2 day 1 [total dose/cycle = 1.5 mg/m^2]

Dactinomycin: I.V.: 0.015 mg/kg/day days 1-5 [total dose/cycle = 0.075 mg/kg]

Cyclophosphamide: I.V.: 200 mg/m^2/day days 1-5 [total dose/cycle = 1000 mg/m^2]

VAC (Rhabdomyosarcoma)
Use: Rhabdomyosarcoma
Regimen:
Induction (weeks 1-17):
Vincristine: I.V. push: 1.5 mg/m^2 (maximum 2 mg) day 1 of weeks 1-13, then one dose at week 17
Dactinomycin: I.V. push: 0.015 mg/kg/day (maximum 0.5 mg) days 1-5, of weeks 1, 4, 7, 17
Cyclophosphamide: I.V.: 2.2 g/m^2 day 1 of weeks 1, 4, 7, 10, 13, 17
Continuation (weeks 21-44):
Vincristine: I.V. push: 1.5 mg/m^2 (maximum 2 mg) day 1 of weeks 21-26, 30-35, 39-44
Dactinomycin: I.V. push: 0.015 mg/kg/day (maximum 0.5 mg) days 1-5 of weeks 21, 24, 30, 33, 39, 42
Cyclophosphamide: I.V.: 2.2 mg/m^2 day 1 of weeks 21, 24, 30, 33, 39, 42

VAC Alternating With IE (Ewing Sarcoma)
Use: Ewing sarcoma
Regimen:
Cycle A: (Odd numbered cycles)
Cyclophosphamide: I.V.: 1200 mg/m^2 day 1 (followed by mesna; dose not specified)
[total dose/cycle = 1200 mg/m^2]
Vincristine: I.V.: 2 mg/m^2 (maximum 2 mg) day 1
[total dose/cycle = 2 mg/m^2; maximum 2 mg]
Doxorubicin: I.V.: 75 mg/m^2 day 1, for 5 cycles (maximum cumulative dose: 375 mg/m^2)
[total dose/cycle = 75 mg/m^2; maximum cumulative dose: 375 mg/m^2]
Dactinomycin: I.V.: 1.25 mg/m^2 day 1, begin cycle 11 (after reaching maximum cumulative doxorubicin dose)
[total dose/cycle = 1.25 mg/m^2]
Cycle B: (Even numbered cycles)
Ifosfamide: I.V.: 1800 mg/m^2/day days 1-5 (given with mesna) [total dose/cycle = 9000 mg/m^2]
Etoposide: I.V.: 100 mg/m^2/day days 1-5 [total dose/cycle = 500 mg/m^2]
Alternate Cycles A and B, administering a cycle every 3 weeks (alternating in the following sequence: ABABAB for 17 cycles

VAC Pulse
Use: Rhabdomyosarcoma
Regimen:
Vincristine: I.V.: 2 mg/m^2/dose (maximum 2 mg/dose) every 7 days for 12 weeks
[total dose/cycle = 24 mg/m^2]
Dactinomycin: I.V.: 0.015 mg/kg/day (maximum 0.5 mg/day) days 1-5, every 3 months for 5 courses
Cyclophosphamide: Oral, I.V.: 10 mg/kg/day for 7 days, repeat every 6 weeks

VAD
Use: Multiple myeloma
Regimen:
Vincristine: I.V.: 0.4 mg/day continuous infusion days 1-4 [total dose/cycle = 1.6 mg]
Doxorubicin: I.V.: 9 mg/m^2/day continuous infusion days 1-4 [total dose/cycle = 36 mg/m^2]
Dexamethasone: Oral: 40 mg/day days 1-4, 9-12, 17-20 [total dose/cycle = 480 mg]
Repeat cycle every 28-35 days

VAD/CVAD
Use: Leukemia, acute lymphocytic
Regimen:
Induction:
Vincristine: I.V.: 0.4 mg continuous infusion/day days 1-4, 24-27 [total dose/cycle = 3.2 mg]
Doxorubicin: I.V.: 12 mg/m^2/day continuous infusion days 1-4, 24-27
[total dose/cycle = 96 mg/m^2]
Dexamethasone: Oral: 40 mg/day days 1-4, 9-12, 17-20, 24-27, 32-35, 40-43 [total dose/cycle = 960 mg]
Cyclophosphamide: I.V.: 1 g/m^2 day 24 [total dose/cycle = 1 g/m^2]
Administer one cycle only

VATH

Use: Breast cancer
Regimen:
Vinblastine: I.V.: 4.5 mg/m^2 day 1 [total dose/cycle = 4.5 mg/m^2]
Doxorubicin: I.V.: 45 mg/m^2 day 1 [total dose/cycle = 45 mg/m^2]
Thiotepa: I.V.: 12 mg/m^2 day 1 [total dose/cycle = 12 mg/m^2]
Fluoxymesterone: Oral: 10 mg 3 times/day days 1-21 [total dose/cycle = 630 mg]
Repeat cycle every 21 days

VBAP

Use: Multiple myeloma
Regimen:
Vincristine: I.V.: 1 mg day 1 [total dose/cycle = 1 mg]
Carmustine: I.V.: 30 mg/m^2 day 1 [total dose/cycle = 30 mg/m^2]
Doxorubicin: I.V.: 30 mg/m^2 day 1 [total dose/cycle = 30 mg/m^2]
Prednisone: Oral: 100 mg/day days 1-4 [total dose/cycle = 400 mg]
Repeat cycle every 21 days

VBMCP

Use: Multiple myeloma
Regimen:
Vincristine: I.V.: 1.2 mg/m^2 (maximum 2 mg) day 1 [total dose/cycle = 1.2 mg/m^2; maximum 2 mg]
Carmustine: I.V.: 20 mg/m^2 day 1 [total dose/cycle = 20 mg/m^2]
Melphalan: Oral: 8 mg/m^2/day days 1-4 [total dose/cycle = 32 mg/m^2]
Cyclophosphamide: I.V.: 400 mg/m^2 day 1 [total dose/cycle = 400 mg/m^2]
Prednisone: Oral: 40 mg/m^2/day days 1-7 (all cycles) [total dose/cycle = 280 mg/m^2]
followed by 20 mg/m^2/day days 8-14 (first 3 cycles only) [total dose/cycle = 140 mg/m^2]
Repeat cycle every 35 days

VBP (PVB)

Use: Testicular cancer
Regimen:
Vinblastine: I.V.: 0.15 mg/kg/day days 1 and 2 [total dose/cycle = 0.3 mg/kg]
Bleomycin: I.V.: 30 units/day days 2, 9, 16 [total dose/cycle = 90 units]
Cisplatin: I.V.: 20 mg/m^2/day days 1-5 [total dose/cycle = 100 mg/m^2]
Repeat cycle every 21 days for 4 cycles

VC

Use: Lung cancer, nonsmall cell
Regimen: Note: Multiple variations are listed below.
Variation 1:
Vinorelbine: I.V.: 25 mg/m^2/day days 1, 8, 15, 22 [total dose/cycle = 100 mg/m^2]
Cisplatin: I.V.: 100 mg/m^2 day 1 [total dose/cycle = 100 mg/m^2]
Repeat cycle every 28 days
Variation 2:
Vinorelbine: I.V.: 30 mg/m^2 weekly [total dose/cycle = 180 mg/m^2]
Cisplatin: I.V.: 120 mg/m^2/day days 1 and 29, then once ever 6 weeks

VCAP

Use: Multiple myeloma
Regimen:
Vincristine: I.V.: 1 mg/m^2 (maximum 1.5 mg) day 1 [total dose/cycle = 1 mg/m^2]
Cyclophosphamide: Oral: 125 mg/m^2/day days 1-4 [total dose/cycle = 500 mg/m^2]
Doxorubicin: I.V.: 30 mg/m^2 day 1 [total dose/cycle = 30 mg/m^2]
Prednisone: Oral: 60 mg/m^2/day days 1-4 [total dose/cycle = 240 mg/m^2]
Repeat cycle every 21 days for 6-12 months

VD
Use: Breast cancer
Regimen:
Vinorelbine: I.V.: 25 mg/m^2/day days 1 and 8 [total dose/cycle = 50 mg/m^2]
Doxorubicin: I.V.: 50 mg/m^2 day 1 [total dose/cycle = 50 mg/m^2]
Repeat cycle every 3 weeks

Vinorelbine-Gemcitabine
Use: Lung cancer, nonsmall cell
Regimen:
Vinorelbine: I.V.: 20 mg/m^2/day days 1, 8, 15 [total dose/cycle = 60 mg/m^2]
Gemcitabine: I.V.: 800 mg/m^2/day days 1, 8, 15 [total dose/cycle = 2400 mg/m^2]
Repeat cycle every 28 days

VIP (Etoposide) (Testicular Cancer)
Use: Testicular cancer
Regimen: Note: Multiple variations are listed below.
Variation 1:
Etoposide: I.V.: 75 mg/m^2/day days 1-5 [total dose/cycle = 375 mg/m^2]
Ifosfamide: I.V.: 1200 mg/m^2/day days 1-5 [total dose/cycle = 6000 mg/m^2]
Cisplatin: I.V.: 20 mg/m^2/day days 1-5 [total dose/cycle = 100 mg/m^2]
Mesna: I.V.: 400 mg day 1 only
followed by 1200 mg/day continuous infusion days 1-5 [total dose/cycle = 6400 mg]
Repeat cycle every 21 days for 4 cycles
Variation 2:
Etoposide: I.V.: 100 mg/m^2/day days 1-5 [total dose/cycle = 500 mg/m^2]
Ifosfamide: I.V.: 1200 mg/m^2/day days 1-5 [total dose/cycle = 6000 mg/m^2]
Cisplatin: I.V.: 20 mg/m^2/day days 1-5 [total dose/cycle = 100 mg/m^2]
Mesna: I.V.: 200 mg/m^2 every 4 hours, for 3 doses each day, days 1, 2, 3 [total dose/cycle = 1800 mg/m^2]
Repeat cycle every 21 days
Variation 3:
Ifosfamide: I.V.: 2500 mg/m^2/day days 1 and 2 [total dose/cycle = 5000 mg/m^2]
Mesna: I.V.: 2400 mg/m^2/day days 1 and 2 [total dose/cycle = 4800 mg/m^2]
Etoposide: I.V.: 100 mg/m^2/day days 3, 4, and 5 [total dose/cycle = 300 mg/m^2]
Cisplatin: I.V.: 40 mg/m^2/day days 3, 4, and 5 [total dose/cycle = 120 mg/m^2]
Repeat cycle every 21 days
Variation 4:
Etoposide: I.V.: 75 mg/m^2/day days 1-5 [total dose/cycle = 375 mg/m^2]
Ifosfamide: I.V.: 1200 mg/m^2/day days 1-5 [total dose/cycle = 6000 mg/m^2]
Cisplatin: I.V.: 20 mg/m^2/day days 1-5 [total dose/cycle = 100 mg/m^2]
Mesna: I.V.: 120 mg/m^2 day 1 only
followed by 1200 mg/m^2/day continuous infusion days 1-5 [total dose/cycle = 6120 mg/m^2]
Repeat cycle every 21 days for 4 cycles

VIP (Small Cell Lung Cancer)
Use: Lung cancer, small cell
Regimen:
Etoposide: I.V.: 75 mg/m^2/day days 1-4 [total dose/cycle = 300 mg/m^2]
Ifosfamide: I.V.: 1200 mg/m^2/day days 1-4 [total dose/cycle = 4800 mg/m^2]
Cisplatin: I.V.: 20 mg/m^2/day days 1-4 [total dose/cycle = 80 mg/m^2]
Mesna: I.V.: 300 mg/m^2 day 1 only
followed by 1200 mg/m^2/day continuous infusion days 1-4 [total dose/cycle = 5100 mg/m^2]
Repeat cycle every 21 days

VIP (Vinblastine) (Testicular Cancer)

Use: Testicular cancer

Regimen: Note: Multiple variations are listed below.

Variation 1:

Vinblastine: I.V.: 0.11 mg/kg/day days 1 and 2 [total dose/cycle = 0.22 mg/kg]

Ifosfamide: I.V.: 1200 mg/m^2/day days 1-5 [total dose/cycle = 6000 mg/m^2]

Cisplatin: I.V.: 20 mg/m^2/day days 1-5 [total dose/cycle = 100 mg/m^2]

Mesna: I.V.: 400 mg day 1

followed by 1200 mg/day continuous infusion days 1-5 [total dose/cycle = 6400 mg]

Repeat cycle every 21 days for 4 cycles

Variation 2:

Vinblastine: I.V.: 6 mg/m^2/day days 1 and 2 [total dose/cycle = 12 mg/m^2]

Ifosfamide: I.V.: 1500 mg/m^2/day days 1-5 [total dose/cycle = 7500 mg/m^2]

Cisplatin: I.V.: 20 mg/m^2/day days 1-5 [total dose/cycle = 100 mg/m^2]

Mesna: I.V.: 300 mg/m^2 3 times/day days 1-5 [total dose/cycle = 4500 mg/m^2]

Repeat cycle every 21 days for 4 cycles

VM

Use: Breast cancer

Regimen: Note: Multiple variations are listed below.

Variation 1:

Mitomycin: I.V.: 10 mg/m^2 days 1 and 28, for 2 cycles [total dose/cycle = 20 mg/m^2]

followed by I.V.: 10 mg/m^2 day 1 only for subsequent cycles [total dose/cycle = 10 mg/m^2]

Vinblastine: I.V.: 5 mg/m^2/day days 1, 14, 28, 42, for 2 cycles [total dose/cycle = 20 mg/m^2]

followed by 5 mg/m^2/day days 1 and 21 [total dose/cycle = 10 mg/m^2]

Repeat cycle every 6-8 weeks

Variation 2:

Mitomycin: I.V.: 10 mg/m^2/day days 1 and 28, for 2 cycles [total dose/cycle = 20 mg/m^2]

followed by 10 mg/m^2 day 1 only for subsequent cycles [total dose/cycle = 10 mg/m^2]

Vindesine: I.V.: 2 mg/m^2/day days 1, 14, 28, 42, for 2 cycles [total dose/cycle = 8 mg/m^2]

followed by I.V.: 2 mg/m^2/day days 1 and 21 for subsequent cycles [total dose/cycle = 4 mg/m^2]

Repeat cycle every 6-8 weeks

VP (Small Cell Lung Cancer)

Use: Lung cancer, small cell

Regimen:

Etoposide: I.V.: 100 mg/m^2/day days 1-4 [total dose/cycle = 400 mg/m^2]

Cisplatin: I.V.: 20 mg/m^2/day days 1-4 [total dose/cycle = 80 mg/m^2]

Repeat cycle every 21 days

V-TAD

Use: Leukemia, acute myeloid

Regimen:

Induction:

Etoposide: I.V.: 50 mg/m^2/day days 1-3 [total dose/cycle = 150 mg/m^2]

Thioguanine: Oral: 75 mg/m^2/day every 12 hours days 1-5 [total dose/cycle = 750 mg/m^2]

Daunorubicin: I.V.: 20 mg/m^2/day days 1 and 2 [total dose/cycle = 40 mg/m^2]

Cytarabine: I.V.: 75 mg/m^2/day continuous infusion days 1-5 [total dose/cycle = 375 mg/m^2]

Up to 3 cycles may be given based on individual response; time between cycles not specified

XelOx

Use: Colorectal cancer

Regimen: Note: Multiple variations are listed below.

Variation 1:
Oxaliplatin: I.V.: 130 mg/m^2 day 1 [total dose/cycle = 130 mg/m^2]
Capecitabine: Oral: 2500 mg/m^2/day days 1-14 [total dose/cycle = 35,000 mg/m^2]
Repeat cycle every 21 days

Variation 2:
Oxaliplatin: I.V.: 85 mg/m^2/day day 1 [total dose/cycle = 85 mg/m^2]
Capecitabine: Oral: 3500 mg/m^2/day days 1-7 [total dose/cycle = 24,500 mg/m^2]
Repeat cycle every 14 days

Variation 3:
Oxaliplatin: I.V.: 50-80 mg/m^2/day days 1, 8, 22, and 29 [total dose/cycle = 200-320 mg/m^2]
Capecitabine: Oral: 1650 mg/m^2/day days 1-14 and 22-35 [total dose/cycle = 46,200 mg/m^2]

Variation 4:
Oxaliplatin: I.V.: 70 mg/m^2/day days 1 and 8 [total dose/cycle = 140 mg/m^2]
Capecitabine: Oral: 2000 mg/m^2/day days 1-14 [total dose/cycle = 28,000 mg/m^2]
Repeat cycle every 21 days

Variation 5:
Oxaliplatin: I.V.: 120 mg/m^2 day 1 [total dose/cycle = 120 mg/m^2]
Capecitabine: Oral: 2500 mg/m^2/day days 1-14 [total dose/cycle = 35,000 mg/m^2]
Repeat cycle every 21 days

Variation 6:
Oxaliplatin: I.V.: 85 mg/m^2 day 1 [total dose/cycle = 85 mg/m^2]
Capecitabine: Oral: 2500 mg/m^2/day days 1-7 [total dose/cycle = 17,500 mg/m^2] **or**
Capecitabine: Oral: 3000 mg/m^2/day days 1-7 [total dose/cycle = 21,000 mg/m^2] **or**
Capecitabine: Oral: 3500 mg/m^2/day days 1-7 [total dose/cycle = 24,500 mg/m^2] **or**
Capecitabine: Oral: 4000 mg/m^2/day days 1-7 [total dose/cycle = 28,000 mg/m^2]
Repeat cycle every 14 days

CHEMOTHERAPY REGIMEN INDEX

Eye

Gastrointestinal

Genitourinary

Prostate Cancer
Bicalutamide + LHRH-A *on page 933*
Cyclophosphamide + Doxorubicin *on page 949*
Cyclophosphamide + Estramustine *on page 949*
Cyclophosphamide + Etoposide *on page 950*
Cyclophosphamide + Vincristine + Dexamethasone *on page 950*
Docetaxel (Weekly) *on page 952*
Docetaxel-Prednisone *on page 952*
Docetaxel-Thalidomide *on page 952*
Doxorubicin + Ketoconazole *on page 952*
Doxorubicin + Ketoconazole/Estramustine + Vinblastine *on page 953*
Estramustine + Docetaxel *on page 959*
Estramustine + Docetaxel + Calcitriol *on page 959*
Estramustine + Docetaxel + Carboplatin *on page 960*
Estramustine + Docetaxel + Hydrocortisone *on page 960*
Estramustine + Docetaxel + Prednisone *on page 960*
Estramustine + Etoposide *on page 960*
Estramustine + Vinorelbine *on page 960*
EV *on page 961*
FL *on page 964*
FZ *on page 967*
Mitoxantrone + Hydrocortisone *on page 980*
MP (Prostate Cancer) *on page 983*
Paclitaxel + Estramustine + Carboplatin *on page 988*
Paclitaxel + Estramustine + Etoposide *on page 988*
PE *on page 989*

Renal Cell Cancer
Interleukin 2-Interferon Alfa 2 *on page 976*
Interleukin 2-Interferon Alfa 2-Fluorouracil *on page 976*

Testicular Cancer
BEP (Ovarian Cancer, Testicular Cancer) *on page 933*
BEP (Testicular Cancer) *on page 933*
EP (Testicular Cancer) *on page 958*
Paclitaxel-Ifosfamide-Cisplatin *on page 988*
PVB *on page 993*
VBP (PVB) *on page 999*
VIP (Etoposide) (Testicular Cancer) *on page 1000*
VIP (Vinblastine) (Testicular Cancer) *on page 1001*

Wilms Tumor
AAV (DD) *on page 929*
ACAV (J) *on page 931*
AV (EE) *on page 932*
AV (K) *on page 932*
AV (L) *on page 932*
AV (Wilms Tumor) *on page 932*
AVD *on page 932*
EE *on page 954*
EE-4A *on page 954*

Gynecologic
Cervical Cancer
BIP *on page 934*
Cisplatin-Fluorouracil *on page 944*
Cisplatin-Vinorelbine *on page 944*
M-VAC (Cervical Cancer) *on page 985*

Endometrial Cancer
AP *on page 932*
M-VAC (Endometrial Cancer) *on page 985*

Gestational Trophoblastic Neoplasm
CHAMOCA (Modified Bagshawe Regimen) *on page 942*
CHAMOMA (Bagshawe Regimen) *on page 943*
EMA/CO *on page 955*
EP/EMA *on page 958*

Head and Neck Cancer

Hematologic/Leukemia

Lung

Nonsmall Cell

Small Cell

Lymphoid Tissue (Lymphoma)

Lymphoma, Hodgkin Disease

Lymphoma, Non-Hodgkin

Lymphoma, Non-Hodgkin (Burkitt)
CODOX-M/IVAC *on page 947*

Lymphoma, Non-Hodgkin (Mantle cell)
Hyper-CVAD + Rituximab *on page 974*

Malignant Pleural Mesothelioma
Cisplatin + Pemetrexed *on page 944*

Myeloma

Multiple Myeloma
Bortezomib-Doxorubicin (Liposomal) *on page 935*
Doxorubicin (Liposomal)-Vincristine-Dexamethasone *on page 953*
DTPACE *on page 953*
Hyper-CVAD (Multiple Myeloma) *on page 973*
Lenalidomide-Dexamethasone *on page 977*
M-2 *on page 979*
Melphalan-Prednisone-Thalidomide *on page 979*
MP (Multiple Myeloma) *on page 983*
Thalidomide + Dexamethasone *on page 996*
VAD *on page 998*
VBAP *on page 999*
VBMCP *on page 999*
VCAP *on page 999*

Sarcoma
CYVADIC *on page 950*
VAC Alternating With IE (Ewing Sarcoma) *on page 998*

Osteosarcoma
Gemcitabine-Docetaxel (Sarcoma) *on page 968*
HDMTX (Osteosarcoma) *on page 969*
ICE (Sarcoma) *on page 975*
MTX-CDDPAdr *on page 983*
POG-8651 *on page 991*

Rhabdomyosarcoma
CEV *on page 941*
VAC (Rhabdomyosarcoma) *on page 998*
VAC Pulse *on page 998*

Soft Tissue Sarcoma
AD *on page 931*
AI *on page 931*
Gemcitabine-Docetaxel (Sarcoma) *on page 968*
ICE (Sarcoma) *on page 975*
ICE-T *on page 975*
IE *on page 975*
MAID *on page 979*

Skin

Melanoma
BOLD *on page 934*
BOLD (Melanoma) *on page 934*
BOLD + Interferon *on page 934*
CCDT (Melanoma) *on page 939*
CVD *on page 949*
Dacarbazine-Carboplatin-Aldesleukin-Interferon *on page 950*
Dartmouth Regimen *on page 950*
IL-2 + IFN *on page 976*

HERBS AND COMMON NATURAL AGENTS

The authors have chosen to include this list of natural products and their reported uses. Due to limited scientific evidence to support these uses, the information provided here is not intended as a cure for any disease, and should not be construed as curative or healing. In addition, the reader is strongly encouraged to seek other references that discuss this information in more detail, and that discuss important issues such as contraindications, warnings, precautions, adverse reactions, and interactions.

PROPOSED CLAIMS

Herb	Reported Uses
Acetyl-L-carnitine (ALC)	Alzheimer disease; cerebral ischemia; depression; diabetic peripheral neuropathy; fragile X syndrome; infertility; Parkinson disease; Peyronie disease; tuberculosis
Adrenal extract	Depression; fatigue; stress; fibromyalgia
Aloe (*Aloe supp*)	Aphthous stomatitis; cancer (prevention); constipation; diabetes; genital herpes; gingivitis; healing agent for wounds, minor burns, and other minor skin irritations; psoriasis vulgaris; ulcerative colitis
Alpha-Lipoic acid	Alcohol-induced liver damage; chemotherapy and radiation (adjunct); circulation; diabetes, diabetic peripheral neuropathy; insulin resistance; drug-induced cardiotoxicity; glaucoma; hypertension; multiple sclerosis; neuralgias; prevention of cataracts; prevention of neurologic disorders, including stroke
Androstenedione	Athletic performance (enhancement)
Aortic extract	Circulation structure, function, and integrity (arteries and veins); prevention of vascular disease including atherosclerosis, cerebral and peripheral arterial insufficiency, varicose veins, hemorrhoids, and vascular retinopathies such as macular degeneration
Arabinoxylane	Chemotherapy-induced leukopenia; immune system enhancement (antiviral and anticancer activity); HIV infection
Arginine	Adrenoleukodystrophy (ALD); angina; burns; cardiovascular disease; chronic heart failure; circulation; critical illness; dental pain; erectile dysfunction; gastrointestinal cancer surgery; growth hormone reserve test/pituitary disorder diagnosis; heart protection during CABG; hypercholesterolemia; hypertension; immune support; inborn errors of urea synthesis; inflammatory bowel disease; increases lean body mass; male infertility; MELAS syndrome; migraine headache; myocardial infarction; peripheral vascular disease/claudication; pre-eclampsia; pressure ulcers; recovery after surgery; sexual vitality and enhancement; transplants; wound healing
Artichoke (*Cynara scolymus*)	Bile flow; dyspepsia (non-ulcer); eczema and other dermatologic problems; hepatic protection/stimulation; hypercholesterolemia; indigestion; irritable bowel syndrome (IBS)
Ashwagandha (*Withania somnifera*)	Adaptogen/tonic (promote wellness); chemotherapy and radiation (adjunct); diabetes (type 2); diuresis; hypercholesterolemia; longevity/anti-aging; osteoarthritis; Parkinson disease; stress, fatigue, nervous exhaustion
Astragalus (*Astragalus membranaceus*) [Milk Vetch]	Adaptogen/tonic (promote wellness); antiviral activity; athletic performance (enhancement); burns; chemotherapy and radiation (adjunct); coronary artery disease; diabetes; heart failure; immune support; liver protection; mental performance; multiple sclerosis; otitis media; renal failure; smoking cessation; tissue oxygenation; tuberculosis
Bacopa (*Bacopa monniera*)	Anxiety; Alzheimer disease/senility; epilepsy; irritable bowel syndrome (IBS); memory enhancement and improvement of cognitive function
Beta-Carotene	Asthma; breast cancer; carotenoid deficiency; cataract prevention; cervical dysplasia; chromosome damage (reduction); chronic obstructive pulmonary disease (COPD); coronary heart disease (risk reduction; in combination); cystic fibrosis; diabetes; diabetes, type 2; esophageal cancer; gastric cancer; immune support; LDL oxidation (decrease in males); macular degeneration; night blindness; oral leukoplakia; osteoarthritis; photoprotection (erythropoietic protoporphyria); prevention of lung cancer; pregnancy related complications
Betaine hydrochloride	Cardiovascular disease (in homocystinuric patients); cholesterol levels; digestive aid (hypochlorhydria and achlorhydria); hyperhomocysteinemia; hyperhomocysteinemia (in chronic renal failure patients); rosacea; steatohepatitis (nonalcoholic); weight loss
Bifidobacterium bifidum (*bifidus*)	Atopic dermatitis; constipation; Crohn disease; diarrhea; gastrointestinal microflora recolonization (anaerobic); immune function; irritable bowel syndrome (IBS); pouchitis; ulcerative colitis

(continued)

Herb	Reported Uses
Bilberry (*Vaccinium myrtillus*)	Circulation, peripheral; diabetes; diarrhea; dysmenorrhea; fibrocystic breast disease (FBD); hemorrhoids; ophthalmologic disorders (antioxidant) including myopia, diminished acuity, glaucoma, dark adaptation, macular degeneration, night blindness, diabetic retinopathy, cataracts; peptic ulcer disease; scleroderma; vascular disorders including varicose veins, capillary permeability/stability, phlebitis
Biotin (Vitamin H)	Brittle nails; diabetes; diabetic peripheral neuropathy; pregnancy supplementation; seborrheic dermatitis; total parenteral nutrition (TPN); uncombable hair syndrome
Bismuth	Diarrhea; ulcers
Bitter melon (*Momordica charantia*)	Antiviral; cancer; diabetes, including impaired glucose tolerance (IGT)
Black cohosh (*Cimicifuga racemosa*)	Arthritis; menopause symptoms (including vasomotor); premenstrual syndrome (PMS); mild depression
Bladderwrack (*Fucus vesiculosus*)	Anticoagulant; antioxidant; bacterial and fungal infections; cancer; diabetes; fibrocystic breast disease (FBD); hypothyroidism; nutrient (rich source of iodine, potassium, magnesium, calcium, and iron)
Boron	Cognitive function improvement; osteoarthritis; osteoporosis; rheumatoid arthritis; vaginitis
Boswellia (*Boswellia serrata*)	Antiinflammatory; arthritis; asthma; Crohn disease; ulcerative colitis
Branched-chain amino acids (BCAAs)	Amyotrophic latreal sclerosis; anorexia; cirrhosis; hepatic encephalopathy; muscle development and lean body mass (increase); tardive dyskinesia
Bromelain (*Anas comosus*)	Arthritis (antiinflammatory; proteolytic); burn debridement; cancer; cervical dysplasia; chronic obstructive pulmonary disease (COPD); digestive enzyme; osteoarthritis of the knee; sinusitis; steatorrhea; urinary tract infection (UTI)
Bupleurum (*Bupleurum falcatum*)	Brain damage (minimal, children); chronic inflammatory disease; fatigue; hepatic protection; hepatitis; systemic lupus erythematosus (SLE); thrombocytopenic purpura
Calcium	Antacid; black widow spider bite; blood pressure regulation; bone loss; bone stress injury prevention; cancer prevention; colon cancer (distal); colorectal adenomas (recurrence); growth; hypercholesterolemia; hyperkalemia; hypermagnesemia; hyperparathyroidism; hyperphosphatemia; hypertension; kidney stones; lead toxicity; osteomalacia/rickets; poison ivy (topical; lactate form); premenstrual syndrome (PMS); pregnancy; pregnancy-induced hypertension; prevention of osteoporosis; weight loss
Calendula (*Calendula officinalis*)	Antibacterial, antifungal, antiviral, antiprotozoal; radiation dermatitis; skin inflammation; wound-healing
Caprylic acid	Antifungal/antiyeast; candidiasis; Crohn disease; dysbiosis; epilepsy (children)
Carnitine	Angina; athletic performance (enhancement); attention deficit hyperactivity disorder (ADHD); congestive heart failure (CHF); diabetes; HIV/AIDS; hypercholesterolemia; hyperlipoproteinemia; hyperthyroidism; male infertility; myocardial infarction; obesity; renal failure/dialysis; weight loss
Cascara (*Rhamnus purshiana*)	Laxative
Cat's claw (*Uncaria tomentosa*)	Allergies; antiinflammatory; antimicrobial (antibacterial, antifungal, antiviral); antioxidant; arthritis; cancer; cervical dysplasia; Crohn disease; diverticulitis; endometriosis; fibromyalgia; immune support; multiple sclerosis; rosacea; systemic lupus erythematosus (SLE)
Cayenne (*Capsicum annuum, Capsicum frutescens*)	Antiinflammatory and analgesic (topical); cardiovascular circulatory support; cluster headache; digestive stimulant; fibromyalgia; postherpetic neuralgia; pruritus; rhinitis
Chamomile, German (*Matricaria chamomilla, Matricaria recutita*)	Carminative, antispasmodic; insomnia (mild sedative); anxiolytic; colic; common cold; diaper rash; diarrhea (children); indigestion; minor injury (topical antiinflammatory); nausea/vomiting; oral health (as mouth rinse/gargle); stress/anxiety; teething; uterine tonic; vaginitis
Chasteberry (*Vitex agnus-castus*)	Acne vulgaris; cervical dysplasia; corpus luteum insufficiency; hyperprolactinemia and insufficient lactation; cyclic mastalgia; menopause; menorrhagia; menstrual disorders including amenorrhea, endometriosis, premenstrual syndrome (PMS); rosacea
Chitosan	Dental plaque; hyperlipidemia; renal failure; weight loss; wound healing

(continued)

Herb	Reported Uses
Chlorophyll	Antiinflammatory, antioxidant, and wound-healing properties; bacteriostatic; cancer; chemoprevention; herpes simplex, herpes zoster; odor absorbent/suppressant (breath freshener, toothpaste, mouthwash, and deodorant); pancreatitis; protectant; rheumatoid arthritis
Chondroitin sulfate	Coronary artery disease; interstitial cystitis; iron absorption enhancement; ophthalmologic uses; osteoarthritis; psoriasis
Chromium	Atherosclerosis; diabetes, type 1; diabetes, type 2; glaucoma; hypercholesterolemia; hypertriglyceridemia; hypothyroidism; immunosuppression; premenstrual syndrome (PMS); weight loss
Clove (*Syzygium aromaticum*)	Antiseptic; analgesic (toothache and teething); mosquito repellent
Coenzyme Q_{10}	Acute myocardial infarction; AIDS; Alzheimer disease; angina; cancer (preventive); cardiomyopathy; cardioprotection during surgery; chemotherapy (adjunct); chronic fatigue syndrome; congestive heart failure (CHF); exercise performance; fibromyalgia; gingivitis; hypercholesterolemia; hypertension; HMG-CoA reductase inhibitors (may cause depletion of this nutraceutical); migraine; mitochondrial disease and Kearns-Sayre syndrome; multiple sclerosis; muscular dystrophy; Parkinson disease; periodontal disease; renal failure; weight loss
Coleus (*Coleus forskohlii*)	Antiinflammatory action after cardiopulmonary bypass; asthma and allergies; eczema; glaucoma; hypertension and congestive heart failure (CHF); psoriasis
Collagen (Type II)	Arthritis (rheumatoid and osteo); burns (first- and second-degree); ulcers (pressure, venous stasis, diabetic); surgical and traumatic wounds; wound healing (topical)
Colostrum	Antiviral (mild); athletic performance (enhancement); body composition; cryptosporidiosis; diarrhea; immune support; prevention of NSAID-induced GI injury; shigellosis; sore throat; upper respiratory tract infection
Conjugated linoleic acid (CLA)	Cancer; muscle development and lean body mass (increase); obesity; oxidative stress and inflammatory disease in obese men
Copper	Age related macular degeneration; anemia; atherosclerosis; copper deficiency; growth promotion; marasmus; osteoporosis; plaque prevention; rheumatoid arthritis
Cordyceps (*Cordyceps sinensis*)	Adaptogen/tonic (promote wellness); antioxidant; chemotherapy and radiation (adjunct); endurance and stamina; fibromyalgia; hepatoprotection; hyperlipidemia; lung, liver, and kidney function (general support); sexual vitality (males and females); tissue oxygenation; fatigue; immunomodulator
Cranberry (*Vaccinium macrocarpon*)	Achlorhydria and B_{12} absorption; antioxidant; bacterial and fungal infections; cancer (prevention); *H. pylori* infection; nephrolithiasis (preventive); plaque; urinary tract infection, including prevention
Creatine	Enhancement of athletic performance (energy production and protein synthesis for muscle building); congestive heart failure (CHF); GAMT deficiency; Huntington disease; McArdle disease; muscular dystrophy; Parkinson disease
Cyclo-hispro	Diabetes, type 2; hypoglycemia
Dandelion (*Taraxacum officinale*)	Leaf used as a diuretic; root used for disorders of bile secretion (choleretic), appetite stimulation, dyspepsia
Dehydroepiandrosterone (DHEA)	Adrenal insufficiency; AIDS; antiaging; cardiovascular disease; cervical cancer; chronic fatigue syndrome; cocaine withdrawal; dementia; depression; diabetes, type 2; erectile dysfunction; fatigue; fibromyalgia; induction of labor; infertility; libido; lupus; obesity; psoriasis; rheumatoid arthritis; schizophrenia; Sjogren syndrome
Devil's claw (*Harpagophytum procumbens*)	Antiinflammatory; back pain; osteoarthritis, gout, and other inflammatory conditions
Docosahexaenoic acid (DHA)	Alzheimer disease; angina pectoris; arrhythmias; asthma; attention deficit disorder and attention deficit hyperactivity disorder (ADD/ADHD); bipolar disorder; cancer (prevention); cardiovascular disease; coronary heart disease (risk reduction); Crohn disease; cystic fibrosis; depression; diabetes; diabetes, type 2; dysmenorrhea; eczema; hypercholesterolemia; hypertension; hypertriglyceridemia; IgA nephropathy; immune support; infant eye/brain development; lupus; nephrotic syndrome; pre-eclampsia; prevention of graft failure after heart bypass surgery; protection from cyclosporine toxicity in organ transplant patients; psoriasis; rheumatoid arthritis; schizophrenia; stroke (risk reduction); ulcerative colitis
Dong quai (*Angelica sinensis*)	Anemia; energy enhancement (particularly in females); hypertension; menopause, dysmenorrhea, premenstrual syndrome (PMS), and amenorrhea; menorrhagia; phytoestrogen; pulmonary hypertension

Herb	Reported Uses
Echinacea (*Echinacea purpurea, Echinacea angustifolia*)	Antibacterial (topical; boils, abscesses, tonsillitis, poison ivy); antiviral; arthritis (*E. augustifolia*); genital herpes; immune support (cold and other upper respiratory infections); otitis media; radiation associated leucopenia; upper respiratory infection
Elder (*Sambucus nigra, Sambucus canadensis*)	Berry used as an antiviral, antioxidant, and for influenza; flower used as an antiinflammatory, colds and influenza, diaphoretic, diuretic, fever, sinusitis, and sore throat
Evening primrose (*Oenothera biennis*)	Amenorrhea; atopic dermatitis; attention deficit disorder (ADD); depression; diabetes; diabetic peripheral neuropathy; eczema, dermatitis, and psoriasis; endometriosis; fatigue; fibrocystic breast disease (FBD); hypercholesterolemia; irritable bowel syndrome; mastalgia; menorrhagia; multiple sclerosis; obesity; omega-6 fatty acid supplementation; premenstrual syndrome (PMS) and menopause; pre-eclampsia; rheumatoid arthritis; Raynaud phenomenon; rosacea; scleroderma
Eyebright (*Euphrasia officinalis*)	Conjunctivitis; eye fatigue; catarrh of the eyes; hepatoprotection
Fenugreek (*Trigonella foenum-graecum*)	Diabetes; hypercholesterolemia
Feverfew (*Tanacetum parthenium*)	Antiinflammatory, rheumatoid arthritis; migraine headache (preventive); muscle soreness
Fish oils	Acne vulgaris; angina pectoris; arrhythmias; asthma; bipolar disorder; cancer (prevention); cardiac death (sudden; preventive); cardiac support (general; proposed benefits); cardiovascular disease; circulation; cognitive performance; colon cancer; coronary heart disease (preventive); Crohn disease; cystic fibrosis; depression; diabetes; diabetes, type 2; dysmenorrhea; eczema, psoriasis; fatigue; headache; heart disease and heart attack (risk reduction), including women; herpes simplex 2; hypercholesterolemia; hypertension; hypertriglyceridemia; IgA nephropathy; immune support; infant eye/brain development; lupus; memory enhancement; multiple sclerosis; nephrotic syndrome; pre-eclampsia; premenstrual syndrome (PMS); prevention of graft failure after heart bypass surgery; protection from cyclosporine toxicity in organ transplant patients; rheumatoid arthritis; rosacea; schizophrenia; scleroderma; stroke (risk reduction); ulcerative colitis
Flaxseed oil	Acne vulgaris; arthritis (rheumatoid); asthma; breast cancer; constipation; coronary heart disease (risk reduction); cyclic mastalgia; diabetes; hemorrhoids; HIV/AIDS; hyperlipidemia; lupus nephritis; hypertension; menopausal symptoms; multiple sclerosis; omega-3 essential fatty acid source (cell wall and cellular membrane structure; cholesterol transport and oxidation); premenstrual syndrome (PMS); prostaglandins production; psoriasis; stroke (risk reduction); systemic lupus erythematosus (SLE)
Folic acid	Alcoholism; anemia; atherosclerosis; cancer prevention (colon and breast); cervical dysplasia; coronary heart disease (risk reduction); coronary restenosis (rate reduction by decreasing plasma homocysteine levels); Crohn disease; dementia and Alzheimer disease (risk reduction); depression; homocysteine; gingivitis; methotrexate toxicity; nitrate tolerance; osteoporosis; pregnancy (prevention of birth defects) and lactation; schizophrenia (risk reduction, by decreasing homocysteine levels); ulcer, aphthous; vitiligo
Garcinia (*Garcinia cambogia*)	Exercise performance; pancreatic function (supportive) and glucose regulation; weight loss
Garlic (*Allium sativum*)	Antimicrobial (bacterial and fungal); antioxidant (practitioners should be aware that aged garlic extracts have been reported to improve this benefit); atherosclerosis; cancer (prevention); coagulation (mild inhibitor of platelet-activating factor); cryptococcal meningitis; hyperlipidemia; hypertension; immune support; peripheral vascular disease; tick repellant; upper respiratory tract infection
Ginger (*Zingiber officinale*)	Antiemetic, for nausea and vomiting in pregnancy; motion sickness; antiinflammatory (musculoskeletal); diverticulitis; indigestion/heartburn; osteoarthritis
Ginkgo (*Ginkgo biloba*)	Acute ischemic stroke; Alzheimer disease, dementia; asthma; chemotherapy (adjunct); chronic cochleovestibular disorders; depression; epilepsy; gastric cancer; glaucoma; headaches; intermittent claudication; macular degeneration; memory enhancement; mountain sickness; multiple sclerosis; Parkinson disease; peripheral blood flow (cerebral vascular disease, peripheral vascular insufficiency, impotence, tinnitus, and depression); premenstrual syndrome (PMS); quality of life; Raynaud phenomenon; retinopathy; seasonal affective disorder (SAD); tinnitus; vertigo; vitiligo; seizures; sexual dysfunction (antidepressant-induced)
Ginseng, Panax (*Panax ginseng*)	Adrenal tonic; diabetes; physical and mental performance, [energy enhancement], chemotherapy and radiation (adjunct); immune support

(continued)

Herb	Reported Uses
Ginseng, Siberian (*Eleutherococcus senticosus*)	Adaptogen/tonic (promote wellness); athletic performance (enhancement); stress (decreased fatigue); immune support
Glucosamine	Chronic venous insufficiency; inflammatory bowel disease; osteoarthritis and joint structure support; rheumatoid arthritis and other inflammatory conditions; temporomandibular joint (TMJ)
Glutamine	Alcoholism; athletic performance (enhancement); cancer (adjunct); catabolic wasting; chemotherapy (prevention of adverse effects); critical illness; fibromyalgia; HIV infection (adjunct); HIV wasting; immune support; peptic ulcer disease; postsurgical healing; ulcerative colitis and other inflammatory bowel diseases
Glutathione	Antioxidant, chemoprotection; hepatoprotection (alcohol-induced liver damage); immune support; male infertility; peptic ulcer disease; peripheral artery disease
Golden seal (*Hydrastis canadensis*)	Fever; gallbladder; heart failure; immune stimulation; malaria (chloroquine resistant); mucous membrane tonifying (used in inflammation of mucosal membranes); gastritis; antimicrobial (antibacterial/antifungal); bronchitis, cystitis, and infectious diarrhea; narcotic concealment (urine analysis); sinusitis; sore throat; trachoma; urinary tract infection (UTI)
Gotu kola (*Centella asiatica*)	Anxiety; connective tissue (support); diabetic microangiopathy; hemorrhoids (topical); macular degeneration; memory enhancement; psoriasis; venous insufficiency; wound healing (topical)
Grapefruit seed (*Citrus paradisi*)	Antifungal, antibacterial, antiparasitic; diarrhea; diverticulitis; eczema; endometriosis; heart disease; irritable bowel syndrome (IBS); rosacea; sinusitis; sore throat; ulcerative colitis; urinary tract infection (UTI)
Grape seed (*Vitis vinifera*)	Agitation (aromatherapy); allergies, antiinflammatory, asthma; antioxidant; cardiovascular health; chloasma; circulation, platelet aggregation inhibitor, capillary fragility, arterial/venous insufficiency (intermittent claudification, varicose veins); gingivitis; glaucoma; macular degeneration; multiple sclerosis; Parkinson disease; scleroderma; sun protection
Green tea (*Camellia sinensis*)	Antioxidant; cancer and cardiovascular disease (preventive); chemotherapy and radiation (adjunct); diabetes; diarrhea; gingivitis; human T-cell lymphocytic virus; hypercholesterolemia; hypertension; hypertriglyceridemia; macular degeneration; photoprotection; platelet-aggregation inhibitor; weight loss
Ground ivy (*Hedera helix*)	Croup; mucolytic; upper respiratory congestion and cough
Guggul (*Commiphora mukul*)	Acne vulgaris; hypercholesterolemia; hypothyroidism; osteoarthritis; rheumatoid arthritis; weight loss
Gymnema (*Gymnema sylvestre*)	Diabetes, blood sugar regulation; hyperlipidemia
Hawthorn (*Crataegus oxyacantha*)	Angina, hypotension, hypertension, peripheral vascular disease, tachycardia; cardiotonic; congestive heart failure
Hops (*Humulus lupulus*)	Sedative/hypnotic (mild)
Horse chestnut (*Aesculus hippocastanum*)	Scleroderma; venous insufficiency (varicose veins, hemorrhoids, deep venous thrombosis, lower extremity edema [oral and topical])
Horsetail (*Equisetum arvense*)	Diuretic; high mineral content (including silicic acid); bone and connective tissue strengthening, including osteoporosis
Huperzine A (*Huperzia serrata*)	Myasthenia gravis; senile dementia and Alzheimer disease
Hydroxymethyl butyrate (HMB)	AIDS wasting; athletic performance (enhancement); muscle damage
5-Hydroxytryptophan (5-HTP)	Anxiety; cerebellar ataxia; depression; fibromyalgia; headache; migraine; schizophrenia; sleep disorders, insomnia (stimulates the production of melatonin); weight loss/obesity
Inositol hexaphosphate (IP-6)	Cancer (preventive); intermittent claudication
Iodine	Bacterial conjunctivitis; bladder irrigation; bowel irrigation; cancer; cognitive function; corpus vitreous degeneration; fibrocystic breast disease (FBD); filarial lymphoedema; goiter (preventive); Graves disease; hypothyroidism; molluscum; mucolytic; ophthalmia neonatorum (preventive); oral intubation; periodontitis/gingivitis; pneumonia; postcesarean endometriosis; renal pelvic instillation sclerotherapy; skin disinfectant (wound cleansing); thyrotoxicosis; water purification

APPENDIX

(continued)

Herb	Reported Uses
Ipriflavone	Prevention of osteoporosis (men and women); menopausal symptoms
Iron	ACE inhibitor associated cough; anemia; attention deficit hyperactivity disorder (ADHD); cognitive performance; menorrhagia; pregnancy; restless legs syndrome
Isoflavones (soy)	Benign prostatic hyperplasia (BPH); bone mineral density (increase); cancer (preventive); cardiovascular effects; cervical dysplasia; chemotherapy (adjunct); cognitive function; diarrhea; endometriosis; hypercholesterolemia; menopausal symptoms; menstrual migraine; osteoarthritis; osteoporosis; premenstrual syndrome (PMS); weight loss
Kava kava (*Piper methysticum*)	Fibromyalgia; insomnia; anxiety/stress, skeletal muscle relaxation, postischemic episodes; muscle soreness
Lactobacillus acidophilus	Allergies; bacterial vaginosis; constipation; diarrhea (infantile); eczema (preventive); gastrointestinal microflora recolonization; hepatic encephalopathy; hypercholesterolemia; immune support; irritable bowel syndrome (IBS); lactose intolerance; vaginal candidiasis
Lavender (*Lavendula officinalis*)	Anxiety; cancer; depression; dementia; hypnotic/sleep; perineal discomfort following childbirth; spasmolytic (oral); wound healing including minor burns (topical)
Lemon balm/Melissa (*Melissa officinalis*)	Agitation in dementia; antiviral (oral herpes virus); anxiety; attention deficit hyperactivity disorder (ADHD); cognitive performance; colitis; dyspepsia; sedation (pediatrics); sleep quality; teething (topical)
Licorice (*Glycyrrhiza glabra*)	Adrenal insufficiency (licorice); aphthous ulcers/canker sores; atopic dermatitis; body fat mass reduction; Crohn disease; croup; expectorant and antitussive (licorice); familial Mediterranean fever (FMF); gastrointestinal ulceration (DGL chewable products); herpes simplex; hyperkalemia; viral hepatitis
Liver extract	Chronic fatigue syndrome; liver tonic
Lutein	Cataracts; colon cancer; macular degeneration; pre-eclampsia
Lycopene	Asthma (exercise induced); atherosclerosis; cancer (preventive; especially lung and prostate); macular degeneration
Lysine	Angina pectoris; growth and development (children); herpes simplex; osteoporosis; ulcer, aphthous
Magnesium	Arrhythmias/torsades de pointes; asthma; attention deficit hyperactivity disorder (ADHD); cardiovascular disease; circulation; colic (magnesium salt); congestive heart failure (CHF); constipation; coronary artery disease; diabetes; dysmenorrhea; epilepsy; fatigue; fibromyalgia (magnesium salt); gallbladder (magnesium salt); hearing loss; heart disease; hypertension; hypoglycemia; insomnia; kidney stones; migraine headache; mitral valve prolapse (MVP); multiple sclerosis; muscle cramps; nervousness; neuropathic pain; osteoporosis; pre-eclampsia/eclampsia; premenstrual syndrome (PMS); stress/anxiety
Malic acid	Aluminum toxicity; fibromyalgia
Manganese	Diabetes; epilepsy; menstrual symptoms; osteoporosis
Marshmallow (*Althaea officinalis*)	Cough; croup; mucilaginous, demulcent; peptic ulcer disease; skin inflammatory conditions; sore throat
Mastic (*Pistacia lentiscus*)	Dental plaque; *H. pylori* inhibitor; peptic ulcer disease
Melatonin	Alzheimer disease (sleep disorders); benzodiazepine tapering; bipolar disorder; cancer; chemotherapy adverse effects; depression (sleep disturbances); glaucoma; headache prevention; HIV/AIDS; hypertension; insomnia; jet lag; oxidative stress in dialysis patients (preventive); Parkinson disease; periodic limb movement disorder; preoperative sedation/anxiolysis; Rett syndrome; schizophrenia (sleep disorders); seasonal affective disorder (SAD); seizure disorders; skin damage; sleep disturbances; stroke; tardive dyskinesia; thrombocytopenia
Methionine	Acetaminophen toxicity; liver detoxification
Methyl sulfonyl methane (MSM)	Allergies; analgesia; arthritis (osteo and rheumatoid); interstitial cystitis; lupus; seasonal allergic rhinitis
Milk thistle (*Silybum marianum*)	*Amanita phalloides* mushroom toxicity; antidote for poisoning by Death Cup mushroom; antioxidant (specifically hepatic cells), liver diseases including acute/chronic hepatitis, jaundice, and stimulation of bile secretion/cholagogue; chemotherapy and radiation (adjunct); cirrhosis; constipation; diabetes; eczema; gallbladder; halitosis; hepatoprotection, including drug toxicities (ie, phenothiazines, butyrophenones, ethanol, and acetaminophen); hyperlipidemia; hyperthyroidism; psoriasis; rosacea
Modified citrus pectin (MCP)	Anticarcinogenic; diarrhea; hypercholesterolemia; prostate cancer
Muira puama (*Ptychopetalum olacoides*)	Athletic performance (enhancement); erectile dysfunction; sexual vitality (males)

(continued)

Herb	Reported Uses
N-Acetyl cysteine (NAC)	Acetaminophen toxicity; acute respiratory distress syndrome (ARDS); acute respiratory infection; angina; asthma (mucolytic, antioxidant); bronchitis; cancer; cardioprotection (during chemotherapy); chemotherapy adverse effects; chronic obstructive pulmonary disease (COPD); fatigue; glutathione production; heavy metal detoxification; HIV/AIDS; hyperthyroidism; hypothyroidism; influenza prevention; macular degeneration; multiple sclerosis; myocardial infarction; nephropathy (preventive); Parkinson disease; polycystic ovarian syndrome; renal impairment; scleroderma; sepsis; Sjogren syndrome; systemic lupus erythematosus (SLE)
Nicotinamide adenine dinucleotide (NADH)	Chronic fatigue syndrome; dementia; diabetes, type 1; hepatitis; Parkinson disease; stamina and energy
Olive leaf (*Olea europaea*)	Acne vulgaris; antibacterial; antifungal, antiviral; Crohn disease; diabetes; diarrhea; diverticulitis; eczema; endometriosis; hypertension; multiple sclerosis; scleroderma; ulcerative colitis; urinary tract infection (UTI)
Pancreatic extract	Antiinflammatory; cancer (adjunct); celiac disease; digestive disturbances; food allergies; immune complex diseases; malabsorption
Para-Aminobenzoic acid (PABA)	Peyronie disease; scleroderma; vitiligo
Parsley (*Petroselinum crispum*)	Halitosis; antibacterial, antifungal
Passion flower (*Passiflora spp*)	Congestive heart failure (CHF); hyperthyroidism; insomnia (sedative)
Peppermint (*Mentha piperita*)	Brain injury (aromatherapy); carminative, spasmolytic; colic; cough; dyspepsia; indigestion; irritable bowel syndrome; motion sickness; nasal congestion; postherpetic neuralgia; postoperative nausea (inhalation); tension headache (topical)
Phenylalanine	Reward deficiency syndrome in addiction; analgesic; depression; pain; Parkinson disease; vitiligo
Phosphatidyl choline (PC)	Alcohol-induced liver damage; Alzheimer disease; gallstones; hepatitis; hypercholesterolemia; tardive dyskinesia
Phosphatidyl serine (PS)	Alzheimer disease; depression; memory enhancement
Potassium	Bone loss; cardiac arrhythmias; congestive heart failure (CHF); hypercalciuria; hypertension; kidney stones; QT prolongation
Pregnenolone	Arthritis; hormone precursor (DHEA, cortisol, progesterone, estrogens, and testosterone); mental performance
Progesterone	Breast cancer (preventive); dysmenorrhea; endometriosis; infertility; menopause symptoms; osteoporosis; premenstrual syndromes (PMS)
Psyllium (*Plantago ovata, Plantago isphagula*)	Anal fissures; bulk-forming laxative (containing 10% to 30% mucilage); colon cancer; colonoscopy preparation; diarrhea; flatulence; halitosis; hemorrhoids; hypercholesterolemia; hyperglycemia; induction of labor; inflammatory bowel disease; irritable bowel syndrome (IBS); obesity
Pygeum (*Pygeum africanum, Prunus africana*)	Benign prostatic hyperplasia (BPH)
Pyruvate	Athletic performance (enhancement); hyperlipidemia; photoaging; weight loss
Quercetin	Allergies; asthma; atherosclerosis; cardiovascular disease; cataracts; peptic ulcer disease; prostatitis; sinusitis
Red clover (*Trifolium pratense*)	Benign prostatic hyperplasia (BPH); endometriosis; hypercholesterolemia; liver and kidney detoxification (liquid extract); menopause symptoms (proprietary extract contains 4 phytoestrogens); menorrhagia; osteoporosis; prostate cancer
Red yeast rice (*Monascus purpureus*)	Hypercholesterolemia
Rehmannia (*Rehmannia glutinosa*)	Aplastic anemia (adjuvant); rheumatoid arthritis; Sheehan syndrome; systemic lupus erythematosus (SLE)
Reishi (*Ganoderma lucidum*)	Chemotherapy and radiation (adjunct); hypertension; seizure disorder; immune support; fatigue; chronic hepatitis B; coronary heart disease; diabetes type 2; poisoning; postherpetic neuralgia; proteinuria
SAMe (S-adenosyl methionine)	Attention deficit hyperactivity disorder (ADHD); cardiovascular disease; cholestasis; depression; fibromyalgia; headache; insomnia; liver disease; osteoarthritis; rheumatoid arthritis

(continued)

Herb	Reported Uses
Saw palmetto (*Serenoa repens*)	Androgenetic alopecia (topical); benign prostatic hyperplasia (BPH)
Schisandra (*Schizandra chinensis*)	Adaptogen/tonic (to promote wellness); hepatic protection and detoxification; chemotherapy and radiation (adjunct); endurance, stamina, and work performance (enhancement); decreases fatigue
Selenium	Acne vulgaris (with vitamin E); AIDS; atherosclerosis; bronchial asthma; burns; cancer (preventive); cardiomyopathy; cataracts; chemotherapy and radiation (adjunct); chromosome damage (reduction); circulation; cystic fibrosis; dandruff; dialysis; eczema; epilepsy; esophageal cancer; gastric cancer; hemorrhoids; herpes simplex 1 and 2; hypothyroidism; infection; infertility; intracranial pressure symptoms; low birth weight; lymphedema; macular degeneration; myotonic dystrophy; pancreatitis; pre-eclampsia; prostate cancer (preventive); psoriasis; sepsis; thyroid conditions; tinea capitis; tinea versicolor; ulcerative colitis
Senna (*Cassia senna*)	Laxative
Shark cartilage	Analgesia; cancer therapy; macular degeneration; osteoarthritis, rheumatoid arthritis; psoriasis
Spleen extract	Chemotherapy and radiation (adjunct); cold/flu; fatigue; spleen function (supportive)
Stinging nettle (*Urtica dioica*)	Leaf used for allergic rhinitis, allergy and hay fever symptoms, arthritis, joint pain, sinusitis, and uric acid excretion; root used for benign prostatic hyperplasia (BPH)
St John's wort (*Hypericum perforatum*)	Antibacterial, antiinflammatory (topical: minor wounds, infections, bruises, muscle soreness, and sprains); antiviral; atopic dermatitis; mild to moderate depression, depression (children); seasonal affective disorder (SAD); melancholia; stress and anxiety; obsessive compulsive disorder (OCD); perimenopausal symptoms; premenstrual syndrome (PMS); social phobia; somatoform disorders
Taurine	Congestive heart failure (CHF); cystic fibrosis; diabetes; energy; gallbladder; hypercholesterolemia; hypertension; iron deficiency anemia; liver disease; myotonic dystrophy; nutritional supplement (infant formula); nutritional support (TPN); obesity; seizure disorders; surgery; vaccine adjunct; vision problems
Tea tree (*Melaleuca alternifolia*)	**Not for ingestion**; acne vulgaris; antifungal, antibacterial; mouthwash for dental and oral health; burns, cuts, scrapes, insect bites
Thyme (*Thymus vulgaris*)	Alopecia areata; antifungal; cough (upper respiratory origin); croup; dental plaque; inflammatory skin disorders
Thymus extract	Fatigue; food allergies; immune support; otitis media; respiratory tract infection; sinusitis; systemic lupus erythematosus (SLE)
Thyroid extract	Fatigue; immune support; fibromyalgia; hypothyroidism
Tocotrienols	Atherosclerosis; cancer (preventive); heart disease; hypercholesterolemia; skin (supportive, protective)
Tribulus (*Tribulus terrestris*)	Athletic performance (enhancement), sexual vitality; coronary artery disease; infertility
Turmeric (*Curcuma longa*)	Antioxidant; antiinflammatory; antirheumatic, hypercholesterolemia; cancer; cholelithiasis prevention; dysmenorrhea; dyspepsia; HIV; muscle soreness; peptic ulcer disease; scabies; uveitis
Tylophora (*Tylophora asthmatica*)	Allergies; asthma
Tyrosine	Alzheimer disease; attention deficit disorder and attention deficit hyperactivity disorder (ADD/ADHD); cocaine cravings; depression; hypertension; hypothyroidism; narcolepsy; phenylketonuria (PKU); Rett syndrome; schizophrenia; stress; substance abuse
Uva-Ursi (*Arctostaphylos uva-ursi*)	Hyperpigmentation; urinary tract infections and kidney stone prevention
Valerian (*Valeriana officinalis*)	Anxiety; hyperthyroidism; insomnia (sedative/hypnotic); premenstrual syndrome (PMS), menopause; restless motor syndromes and muscle spasms
Vanadium	Diabetes, type 1; diabetes, type 2; hypercholesterolemia; hypoglycemia
Vinpocetine	Acute ischemic stroke; cognitive function; Alzheimer disease and senility; hearing impairment; joint disorders; urinary incontinence

(continued)

Herb	Reported Uses
Vitamin A (Retinol)	Acne vulgaris; acute promyelocytic leukemia; AIDS; cancer (preventive); cataract preventive; cervical dysplasia; circulation; cold/influenza; Crohn disease; diarrhea; diverticulitis; eczema; esophageal cancer; fibrocystic breast disease (FBD); gastric cancer; glaucoma; hemorrhoids; immune function; infant mortality; iron deficiency anemia; malaria; measles; menorrhagia; night blindness; otitis media; photorefractive keratectomy; pneumonia; polp prevention; pregnancy related complications; premenstrual syndrome (PMS); psoriasis; rosacea; skin cancer preventive; sore throat; ulcerative colitis; urinary tract infection (UTI); weight loss; wound healing; xerophthalmia
Vitamin B_1 (Thiamine)	Alcoholism; Alzheimer disease; anemia (megaloblastic); cancer; cataract prevention; congestive heart failure (CHF); Crohn disease; diabetes; Didmoad (Wolfram) syndrome; fibromyalgia; heart failure (cardiomyopathy); insomnia; metabolic disorders; neurological conditions (Bell palsy, trigeminal neuralgia, sciatica, sensory neuropathies); psychiatric illness; pyruvate dehydrogenase deficiency (PDH); total parenteral nutrition (TPN)
Vitamin B_2	Anemia; anorexia/bulimia; cataracts; depression; esophageal cancer; ethylmalonic encephalopathy; malaria; migraine; neonatal jaundice; pre-eclampsia
Vitamin B_3	Acne vulgaris (4% niacinamide topical gel); atherosclerosis; cataracts; coronary disease (preventive); diabetes, type 1; diabetes, type 2; hyperlipidemia (hypercholesterolemia, hypertriglyceridemia); impaired glucose tolerance; intermittent claudication; myocardial infarction (risk reduction); osteoarthritis; pellagra; Raynaud phenomenon; rheumatoid arthritis; schizophrenia;
Vitamin B_5 (Pantothenic acid)	Adrenal support; allergies; arthritis; athletic performance (enhancement); attention deficit hyperactivity disorder (ADHD); constipation; hyperlipidemia (pantethine, but not pantothenic acid, lowers cholesterol and triglycerides); osteoarthritis; rheumatoid arthritis; wound healing
Vitamin B_6 (Pyridoxine)	Akathisia; Alzheimer disease; angioplasty; arthritis; asthma; attention deficit hyperactivity disorder (ADHD); autism; birth outcomes; cardiovascular disease; carpal tunnel syndrome; coronary heart disease (risk reduction); coronary restenosis (rate reduction by lowering plasma homocysteine levels); dementia (risk reduction); depression (associated with oral contraceptives); diabetic peripheral neuropathy; epilepsy, B_6-dependant; headache; hereditary sideroblastic anemia; homocysteine (reduction); hyperkinetic syndrome; insomnia; kidney stones; lactation suppression; monosodium glutamate (MSG) sensitivity; nausea and vomiting (in pregnancy); peptic ulcer disease; premenstrual syndrome (PMS); pyridoxine dependent seizures in newborns; tardive dyskinesia
Vitamin B_{12} (Cobalamin)	AIDS; angioplasty; asthma; atherosclerosis (due to homocysteine elevation); breast cancer; coronary heart disease; coronary restenosis (rate reduction by lowering plasma homocysteine levels); Crohn disease; dementia and Alzheimer disease (risk reduction); depression; diabetic peripheral neuropathy; fatigue; homocysteine (reduction); Imerslund-Grasbeck disease; male infertility; megaloblastic anemia; memory loss; multiple sclerosis; pernicious anemia; sickle cell disease; sulfite sensitivity
Vitamin B complex-25	See individual B vitamins
Vitamin C	AIDS; alkaptonuria; allergies; Alzheimer disease; asthma; atherosclerosis; cancer; cardiovascular disease (negative report); cataracts; cervical dysplasia; chromosome damage (reduction); circulation; cold; constipation; coronary heart disease (preventive, in patients laking lipid-lowering agents); Crohn disease; diabetes; diabetes, type 2; diverticulitis; eczema; endometriosis; fatigue; fever; fibrocystic breast disease (FBD); fibromyalgia; gallbladder disease (risk reduction); gingivitis; glaucoma; herpes simplex virus 1 and 2; immune support; iron absorption enhancement; irritable bowel syndrome (IBS); LDL oxidation (decrease in males); macular degeneration; multiple sclerosis; myocardial infarction (risk reduction); nitrate tolerance (preventive); osteoporosis; otitis media; Parkinson disease; peptic ulcer disease; plaque; pregnancy; psoriasis; reflex sympathetic dystrophy (preventive); sinusitis; sore throat; stress/anxiety; stroke (preventive); sunburn; ulcerative colitis; urinary tract infection (UTI); vaginitis; wound healing
Vitamin D	Cancer; Crohn disease; diabetes; epilepsy (during anticonvulsant therapy); fall prevention; familial hypophosphatemia; fanconi syndrome; hearing loss; hepatic osteodystrophy; hypertension; hypocalcemia; multiple sclerosis; muscle weakness; Myelodysplastic syndrome; osteogenesis imperfecta; osteomalacia; osteoporosis; prostate cancer; proximal myopathy; psoriasis; renal osteodystrophy; rheumatoid arthritis; rickets; scleroderma; seasonal affective disorder (SAD); senile warts; tooth retention

APPENDIX

(continued)

Herb	Reported Uses
Vitamin E	Acne vulgaris (with selenium); Alzheimer disease; anemia; angina; arterial elasticity; atherosclerosis; Benign prostatic hyperplasia (BPH); bladder cancer; breast cancer; cancer (preventive); cardiovascular disease; cataracts; cervical dysplasia; chromosome damage (reduction); circulation; colon cancer (preventive); congestive heart failure; diabetes; diabetes, type 2; dyslipidemias; dysmenorrhea; eczema; endometriosis; epilepsy; esophageal caner; fibrocystic breast disease (FBD); G6PD deficiency; gallbladder; gastric cancer; glomerulosclerosis (kidney disease); hemorrhoids; hyperlipidemia; immune support; intermittent claudication; LDL oxidation (decrease in males); macular degeneration; multiple sclerosis; myocardial infarction (risk reduction); neurotoxicity; osteoarthritis; Parkinson disease; peptic ulcer disease; peripheral circulation; photorefractive keratectomy; platelet aggregation; premenstrual syndrome (PMS); prostate cancer; psoriasis; respiratory infection (preventive); rheumatoid arthritis; scleroderma; steatohepatitis; sunburn; systemic lupus erythematosus; tardive dyskinesia; ulcerative colitis
Vitamin K	Osteoporosis; synthesis of blood clotting factors; warfarin toxicity
White oak (*Quercus alba*)	Antiinflammatory (mild: throat and mouth as a soothing agent)
White willow (*Salix alba*)	Antipyretic; antiinflammatory; headache; low back pain; osteoarthritis
Wild yam (*Dioscorea villosa*)	Female vitality (conversion to progesterone in the body is poor); hyperlipidemia; menopause
Yohimbe (*Pausinystalia yohimbe*)	Autonomic failure; platelet aggregation inhibition; sexual side effects of SSRIs; sexual vitality (men and women); male erectile dysfunction; xerostomia (psychotropic drug induced)
Zinc	Acne vulgaris; alopecia areata; aphthous ulcers; attention deficit hyperactivity disorder (ADHD); benign prostatic hyperplasia (BPH); beta-thalassemia; cirrhosis; closed head injuries; cognitive deficits (children); common cold; Crohn disease; dandruff; diabetes; diabetic neuropathy; diaper rash; diarrhea; diverticulitis; Down syndrome; exercise performance; fungal infections; gastric ulcer healing; Gilbert syndrome; halitosis; hepatic encephalopathy; hepatitis C; herpes simplex; HIV/AIDS; hyperlipidemia; immune support; infertility; kwashiorkor; leg ulcers; leprosy; lower respiratory tract infection (children); macular degeneration; malaria; mucositis; muscle cramps; osteoporosis; otitis media; parasite infection; plaque/gingivitis; poisoning (arsenic); pregnancy; prostatitis (chronic); rheumatoid arthritis; sexual vitality (men); sickle cell anemia; skin conditions, eczema, psoriasis; sore throat; stomatitis; taste perception; tinnitus; trichomoniasis; ulcerative colitis; viral warts; Wilson disease; wound healing

NEW DRUGS ADDED SINCE LAST EDITION

Brand Name	Generic Name	Use
Altabax™	retapamulin	Treatment of impetigo
Atripla™	efavirenz, emtricitabine, and tenofovir	Treatment of HIV infection
Azasite™	azithromycin	Bacterial conjunctivitis
Brovana™	arformoterol	Chronic obstructive pulmonary disease (COPD)
Divigel®	estradiol	Topical gel for hormone replacement
Duetact™	pioglitazone and glimepiride	Type 2 diabetes
Duodote™	atropine and pralidoxime	Organophosphorous nerve agent poisoning
Elaprase™	idursulfase	Treatment of Hunter syndrome (MPS II)
Endometrin®	progesterone	Embryo implantation support
Evamist™	estradiol	Menopausal symptoms
Exforge®	amlodipine and valsartan	Hypertension
Implanon™	etonogestrel	Prevention of pregnancy
Invega™	paliperidone	Treatment of schizophrenia
Janumet™	sitagliptin and metformin	Type 2 diabetes
Januvia™	sitagliptin	Type 2 diabetes
Letairis™	ambrisentan	Pulmonary arterial hypertension
NeoProfen®	ibuprofen	Patent ductus arteriosus (PDA)
Neupro®	rotigotine	Parkinson disease
Noxafil®	posaconazole	Oral antifungal
Omnaris™	ciclesonide	Treatment of allergic rhinitis
Oracea™	doxycycline	Inflammatory rosacea
Selzentry™	maraviroc	Treatment of HIV-1 infection
Soliris™	eculizumab	Paroxysmal nocturnal hemoglobinuria
Tekturna®	aliskiren	Treatment of hypertension
Torisel™	temsirolimus	Advanced renal cell carcinoma
Tykerb®	lapatinib	Advanced breast cancer
Tyzeka™	telbivudine	Treatment of chronic hepatitis b
Vectibix™	panitumumab	Treatment of metastasized colorectal cancer
Veregen™	sinecatechins	Topical green tea extract for treatment of external genital and perianal warts
Vivaglobin®	immune globulin	Subcutaneous formulation for patients with primary immune deficiency
Vyvanse™	lisdexamfetamine	A prodrug of dextroamphetamine for ADHD
Xyzal®	levocetirizine	Allergic rhinitis and chronic urticaria
Zolinza™	vorinostat	Skin cancer
----	influenza vaccine, H5N1	Vaccine against the H5N1 influenza virus (avian or bird flu)

PENDING DRUGS OR DRUGS IN CLINICAL TRIALS

Proposed Brand Name or Synonym	Generic Name	Use
AP23573	deforolimus	Cancer
Arcoxia®	etoricoxib	Osteoarthritis
Entereg®	alvimopan	Opioid-induced bowel dysfunction
Isentres™	raltegravir	HIV
Isovorin™	levofolinic acid	Osteogenic sarcoma, colorectal cancer
Kiacta™ (formerly Fibrillex™)	eprodisate	Amyloid A amyloidosis
Kuvan™	sapropterin	Phenylketonuria
MCC	mycobacterial cell wall-DNA complex	Bladder cancer
NBI-34060	indiplon	Insomnia
Orplanta®	satraplatin	Prostate cancer
Pristiq™	desvenlafaxine	Depression, perimenopausal symptoms
Provenge™	sipuleucel-T	Prostate cancer
RSD1235	vernakalant	Atrial fibrillation
Spera™	satraplatin	Prostate cancer
Surfaxin™	lucinactant	Respiratory distress syndrome
Treanda™	bendamustine	Chronic lymphocytic leukemia
Trexima™	sumatriptan succinate and naproxen sodium	Migraine
Xiaflex®	clostridial collagenase	Dupuytren contracture
Zimulti® (formerly Acomplia™)	rimonabant	Weight loss agent

INDICATION/THERAPEUTIC CATEGORY INDEX

Antibiotic, Topical

Estrogen and Androgen Combination

Keratolytic Agent

Aminoquinoline (Antimalarial)

AMENORRHEA

Diagnostic Agent

Ergot Alkaloid and Derivative

Gonadotropin

Progestin

AMMONIACAL URINE

Urinary Acidifying Agent

AMMONIA INTOXICATION

Ammonium Detoxicant

AMYLOIDOSIS

Mucolytic Agent

AMYOTROPHIC LATERAL SCLEROSIS (ALS)

Anticholinergic Agent

Cholinergic Agent

Miscellaneous Product

Skeletal Muscle Relaxant

ANAPHYLACTIC SHOCK

Adrenergic Agonist Agent

ANAPHYLACTIC SHOCK (PROPHYLAXIS)

Plasma Volume Expander

ANEMIA

Anabolic Steroid

Androgen

Antineoplastic Agent

Colony-Stimulating Factor

Electrolyte Supplement, Oral

ANESTHESIA (GENERAL)

ANESTHESIA (LOCAL)

ANESTHESIA (OPHTHALMIC)

Local Anesthetic

ANGINA PECTORIS

Beta-Adrenergic Blocker

Antiarrhythmic Agent, Miscellaneous

ARSENIC POISONING

Chelating Agent

ARTHRITIS

Analgesic, Topical

Antiinflammatory Agent

Gold Compound

Immunosuppressant Agent

Monoclonal Antibody

Nonsteroidal Antiinflammatory Drug (NSAID)

Nonsteroidal Antiinflammatory Drug (NSAID), COX-2 Selective

ARTHRITIS (RHEUMATOID)

Antirheumatic, Disease Modifying

ASCARIASIS

Anthelmintic

ASCITES

Diuretic, Loop

Diuretic, Miscellaneous

Diuretic, Potassium Sparing

Diuretic, Thiazide

ASPERGILLOSIS

Antifungal Agent

Local Anesthetic

BITES (SNAKE)

Antivenin

BITES (SPIDER)

Antivenin

Electrolyte Supplement, Oral

Skeletal Muscle Relaxant

BLADDER IRRIGATION

Antibacterial, Otic

Antibacterial, Topical

BLASTOMYCOSIS

Antifungal Agent

BLEPHARITIS

Antifungal Agent

BLEPHAROSPASM

Ophthalmic Agent, Toxin

BOTULISM

Immune Globulin

Anticholinergic Agent

Beta₂-Adrenergic Agonist Agent

Bronchodilator

Expectorant

Mast Cell Stabilizer

Theophylline Derivative

BRUCELLOSIS

Antibiotic, Aminoglycoside

Antitubercular Agent

Tetracycline Derivative

BULLOUS SKIN DISEASE

Antibacterial, Topical

Gold Compound

Immunosuppressant Agent

BURNS

Antibacterial, Topical

Antifungal Agent, Parental

Antifungal Agent, Parenteral

Antifungal Agent, Systemic

Antifungal/Corticosteroid

Drug-induced Neuritis, Treatment Agent

Echinocandin

CANKER SORE

Antiinfective Agent, Oral

Antiinflammatory Agent, Locally Applied

Local Anesthetic

Protectant, Topical

CARCINOMA

Androgen

Antiandrogen

Antineoplastic Agent

Antineoplastic Agent, Alkylating Agent

Antineoplastic Agent, Anthracycline

Antineoplastic Agent, Antibiotic

Antineoplastic Agent, Antimetabolite

Antineoplastic Agent, Antimicrotubular

Antineoplastic Agent, Estrogen Receptor Antagonist

Antineoplastic Agent, Hormone (Antiestrogen)

Antineoplastic Agent, Miscellaneous

Antineoplastic Agent, Monoclonal Antibody

Antineoplastic Agent, mTOR Kinase Inhibitor

Antineoplastic Agent, Natural Source (Plant) Derivative

Antineoplastic Agent, Tyrosine Kinase Inhibitor

Antineoplastic, Tyrosine Kinase Inhibitor

Antiviral Agent

Biological Response Modulator

Contraceptive, Progestin Only

Epidermal Growth Factor Receptor (EGFR) Inhibitor

Estrogen and Androgen Combination

Estrogen Derivative

Vitamin

Vitamin, Fat Soluble

CEREBRAL PALSY

Skeletal Muscle Relaxant

CEREBROVASCULAR ACCIDENT (CVA)

Antiplatelet Agent

Fibrinolytic Agent

CHICKENPOX

Antiviral Agent

Vaccine, Live Virus

CHOLELITHIASIS

Gallstone Dissolution Agent

CHOLERA

Vaccine

CHOLESTASIS

Vitamin, Fat Soluble

CHOLINESTERASE INHIBITOR POISONING

Antidote

CHORIORETINITIS

Adrenal Corticosteroid

Immunosuppressant Agent

Vitamin D Analog

Vitamin, Fat Soluble

CISPLATIN TOXICITY

Antidote

Antifungal Agent

CLAUDICATION

Blood Viscosity Reducer Agent

CMV RETINITIS

Antiviral Agent

COCCIDIOIDOMYCOSIS

Antifungal Agent

COLD

Cough and Cold Combination

COLD SORE

Antiviral Agent

COLITIS (ULCERATIVE)

5-Aminosalicylic Acid Derivative

Antiinflammatory Agent

COLLAGEN DISORDERS

Adrenal Corticosteroid

COLONIC EVACUATION

Laxative

COMMON COLD

Antitussive

Antitussive/Decongestant

Decongestant/Anticholingeric Combination

Expectorant

Expectorant/Decongestant/Antitussive

Sympathomimetic

CONDYLOMA ACUMINATUM

Antiviral Agent

Biological Response Modulator

Immune Response Modifier

Keratolytic Agent

CONGENITAL SUCRASE-ISOMALTASE
DEFICIENCY

Enzyme

CONGESTION

Antihistamine

Antihistamine/Decongestant/Antitussive

Antitussive

Antitussive/Decongestant/Expectorant

Cough and Cold Combination

Decongestant

CONGESTION (NASAL)

Adrenergic Agonist Agent

Expectorant/Decongestant

Sympathomimetic

CONGESTIVE HEART FAILURE

Adrenergic Agonist Agent

Alpha-Adrenergic Blocking Agent

Angiotensin-Converting Enzyme (ACE) Inhibitor

Beta-Adrenergic Blocker

Cardiac Glycoside

Cardiovascular Agent, Other

Diuretic, Loop

CONSTIPATION (CHRONIC IDIOPATHIC)

Gastrointestinal Agent, Miscellaneous

COPROPORPHYRIA

Beta-Adrenergic Blocker

CORNEAL EDEMA

Lubricant, Ocular

COUGH

Antihistamine/Antitussive

Antihistamine/Decongestant/Antitussive

Antihistamine/Decongestant/Antitussive/Expectorant

Antitussive

Antitussive/Decongestant

Antitussive/Decongestant/Expectorant

Antitussive/Expectorant

Cough Preparation

Expectorant/Decongestant/Antitussive

CROHN DISEASE

5-Aminosalicylic Acid Derivative

Monoclonal Antibody

CROUP

Adrenergic Agonist Agent

CRYPTOCOCCOSIS

Antifungal Agent

Antifungal Agent, Systemic

CRYPTORCHIDISM

Gonadotropin

DEBRIDEMENT OF CALLOUS TISSUE

Keratolytic Agent

DEBRIDEMENT OF ESCHAR

Protectant, Topical

DECUBITUS ULCERS

Enzyme

Enzyme, Topical Debridement

Protectant, Topical

DEEP VEIN THROMBOSIS (DVT)

Anticoagulant (Other)

Factor Xa Inhibitor

Low Molecular Weight Heparin

DEMENTIA

Acetylcholinesterase Inhibitor

Antidepressant, Tricyclic (Tertiary Amine)

Benzodiazepine

Cholinergic Agent

Ergot Alkaloid and Derivative

Phenothiazine Derivative

DIABETES INSIPIDUS

Hormone, Posterior Pituitary

Vasopressin Analog, Synthetic

DIABETES MELLITUS, INSULIN-DEPENDENT (IDDM)

Antidiabetic Agent

Antidiabetic Agent, Insulin

Insulin, Intermediate-Acting

DIABETES MELLITUS, NONINSULIN-DEPENDENT (NIDDM)

Antidiabetic Agent

Antidiabetic Agent (Biguanide)

Antidiabetic Agent, Dipeptidyl Peptidase IV (DPP-IV) Inhibitor

Antidiabetic Agent, Incretin Mimetic

Antidiabetic Agent, Oral

DIVERTICULITIS

Amebicide

Aminoglycoside (Antibiotic)

Antibiotic, Miscellaneous

Antiprotozoal

DRACUNCULIASIS

DRUG DEPENDENCE (OPIOID)

DRY EYES

DRY MOUTH

DRY SKIN

ENCEPHALITIS (HERPESVIRUS)

Antiviral Agent

ENDOCARDITIS TREATMENT

Aminoglycoside (Antibiotic)

Antibiotic, Miscellaneous

Antifungal Agent

Cephalosporin (First Generation)

Penicillin

Quinolone

ENDOMETRIOSIS

Androgen

Contraceptive, Oral

Contraceptive, Progestin Only

Hormone, Posterior Pituitary

Progestin

END-STAGE RENAL DISEASE (ESRD)

Phosphate Binder

ENURESIS

Antidepressant, Tricyclic (Tertiary Amine)

Antispasmodic Agent, Urinary

Vasopressin Analog, Synthetic

ENZYME DEFICIENCY

Enzyme

EPICONDYLITIS

Nonsteroidal Antiinflammatory Drug (NSAID)

EPIDERMAL GROWTH FACTOR RECEPTOR (EGFR)

Antineoplastic Agent, Monoclonal Antibody

Epidermal Growth Factor Receptor (EGFR) Inhibitor

EPILEPSY

Anticonvulsant

Anticonvulsant, Miscellaneous

Anticonvulsant, Oxazolidinedione

Anticonvulsant, Sulfonamide

Barbiturate

FEVER

Antipyretic

FIBROCYSTIC BREAST DISEASE

Androgen

FIBROCYSTIC DISEASE

Vitamin, Fat Soluble

HYPERAMMONEMIA

Ammonium Detoxicant

HYPERCALCEMIA

Bisphosphonate Derivative

Chelating Agent

Polypeptide Hormone

HYPERCHOLESTEROLEMIA

Antihyperlipidemic Agent, Miscellaneous

Antilipemic Agent, 2-Azetidinone

HYPERPARATHYROIDISM

Calcimimetic

Vitamin D Analog

HYPERPHOSPHATEMIA

Electrolyte Supplement, Oral

Phosphate Binder

HYPERPIGMENTATION

Topical Skin Product

HYPERPLASIA, VULVAR SQUAMOUS

Estrogen Derivative

HYPERPROLACTINEMIA

Anti-Parkinson Agent (Dopamine Agonist)

Ergot Alkaloid and Derivative

Ergot-like Derivative

HYPERTENSION

Adrenergic Agonist Agent

Alpha-Adrenergic Agonist

Alpha-Adrenergic Blocking Agent

Alpha-/Beta- Adrenergic Blocker

Angiotensin II Antagonist Combination

Angiotensin II Receptor Antagonist

Angiotensin II Receptor Blocker Combination

Angiotensin-Converting Enzyme (ACE) Inhibitor

Beta-Adrenergic Blocker, Nonselective

Beta Blocker, Beta1 Selective

Calcium Channel Blocker

Ganglionic Blocking Agent

Miscellaneous Product

Rauwolfia Alkaloid

Renin Inhibitor

Selective Aldosterone Blocker

Vasodilator

HYPERTENSION (ARTERIAL)

Beta-Adrenergic Blocker

HYPERTENSION (CEREBRAL)

Barbiturate

Diuretic, Osmotic

HYPERTENSION (CORONARY)

Vasodilator

HYPERTENSION (EMERGENCY)

Antihypertensive Agent

HYPERTENSION (OCULAR)

Alpha2-Adrenergic Agonist Agent, Ophthalmic

Beta-Adrenergic Blocker

HYPERTHERMIA (MALIGNANT)

Skeletal Muscle Relaxant

Barbiturate

Benzodiazepine

Hypnotic

Hypnotic, Nonbarbiturate

Hypnotic, Nonbenzodiazepine

Hypnotic, Nonbenzodiazepine (Pyrazolopyrimidine)

INSULIN-LIKE GROWTH FACTOR-1 DEFICIENCY (IGF-1 DEFICIENCY)

Growth Hormone

INTERMITTENT CLAUDICATION

Platelet Aggregation Inhibitor

INTERSTITIAL CYSTITIS

Analgesic, Urinary

Urinary Tract Product

INTRACRANIAL PRESSURE

Barbiturate

Diuretic, Osmotic

IRIDOCYCLITIS

Adrenal Corticosteroid

LICHEN SIMPLEX CHRONICUS

Antidepressant, Tricyclic (Tertiary Amine)

Topical Skin Product

LUNG SURFACTANT

Lung Surfactant

LYME DISEASE

Cephalosporin (Third Generation)

Macrolide (Antibiotic)

Penicillin

Tetracycline Derivative

LYMPHOMA

Antineoplastic Agent

Antineoplastic Agent, Histone Deacetylase Inhibitor

MALODORS

Gastrointestinal Agent, Miscellaneous

MANIA

Anticonvulsant

Antimanic Agent

Phenothiazine Derivative

MAPLE SYRUP URINE DISEASE

Vitamin, Water Soluble

MARFAN SYNDROME

Rauwolfia Alkaloid

MAROTEAUX-LAMY SYNDROME

Enzyme

MASTOCYTOSIS

Histamine H2 Antagonist

Mast Cell Stabilizer

MEASLES
Vaccine, Live Virus

MEASLES (RUBEOLA)
Immune Globulin

MECONIUM ILEUS
Mucolytic Agent

MELANOMA
Antineoplastic Agent

Antiviral Agent

Biological Response Modulator

MELASMA (FACIAL)
Corticosteroid, Topical

Depigmenting Agent

Retinoic Acid Derivative

MENINGITIS (TUBERCULOUS)
Antibiotic, Aminoglycoside

Antitubercular Agent

MENINGOCOCCAL DISEASE
Vaccine

MENOPAUSE
Ergot Derivative

Estrogen and Androgen Combination

Estrogen and Progestin Combination

Estrogen Derivative

MENORRHAGIA

Androgen

MERCURY POISONING

Chelating Agent

METHANOL POISONING

Intravenous Nutritional Therapy

METHEMOGLOBIN

Antidote

Vitamin, Water Soluble

METHOTREXATE POISONING

Folic Acid Derivative

MIGRAINE

Analgesic, Nonnarcotic

Antimigraine Agent

MYCOSIS (FUNGOIDES)

Psoralen

MYDRIASIS

Adrenergic Agonist Agent

Adrenergic Agonist Agent, Ophthalmic

Anticholinergic/Adrenergic Agonist

Anticholinergic Agent

MYELODYSPLASTIC SYNDROME (MDS)

Angiogenesis Inhibitor

Antineoplastic Agent, Antimetabolite (Pyrimidine)

Immunosuppressant Agent

Tumor Necrosis Factor (TNF) Blocking Agent

MYELOMA

Antineoplastic Agent

Proteasome Inhibitor

MYOCARDIAL INFARCTION

Anticoagulant (Other)

Antiplatelet Agent

Beta-Adrenergic Blocker

Fibrinolytic Agent

Thrombolytic Agent

Vasodilator

MYOCARDIAL REINFARCTION

Antiplatelet Agent

Beta-Adrenergic Blocker

Vasodilator

MÉNIÈRE DISEASE

Antihistamine

Antidepressant, Tricyclic (Tertiary Amine)

OCULAR INFLAMMATORY

Antibiotic/Corticosteroid, Ophthalmic

OCULAR INJURY

Nonsteroidal Antiinflammatory Drug (NSAID)

OCULAR REDNESS

Adrenergic Agonist Agent

Antihistamine/Decongestant Combination

ONYCHOMYCOSIS

Antifungal Agent

OPHTHALMIC DISORDERS

Adrenal Corticosteroid

OPHTHALMIC SURGICAL AID

Ophthalmic Agent, Miscellaneous

OPIATE WITHDRAWAL (NEONATAL)

Analgesic, Narcotic

OPIOID DEPENDENCE

Analgesic, Narcotic

OPIOID POISONING

Antidote

ORGANOPHOSPHATE PESTICIDE POISONING

Anticholinergic Agent

Antidote

ORGANOPHOSPHOROUS POISONING

Anticholinergic Agent

Nonsteroidal Antiinflammatory Drug (NSAID), COX-2 Selective

OSTEODYSTROPHY

Vitamin D Analog

OSTEOMALACIA

Vitamin D Analog

OSTEOMYELITIS

Antibiotic, Miscellaneous

Antifungal Agent, Systemic

Carbapenem (Antibiotic)

Cephalosporin (First Generation)

Cephalosporin (Second Generation)

Cephalosporin (Third Generation)

Penicillin

OSTEOSARCOMA

Antineoplastic Agent

OSTOMY CARE

Protectant, Topical

OTITIS EXTERNA

Adrenal Corticosteroid

Aminoglycoside (Antibiotic)

Antibacterial, Otic

Antibacterial, Topical

Antibiotic/Corticosteroid, Otic

Antibiotic, Miscellaneous

Antibiotic, Otic

Cephalosporin (Third Generation)

Otic Agent, Analgesic

Otic Agent, Antiinfective

Otic Agent, Ceruminolytic

Quinolone

OTITIS MEDIA

Antibiotic, Carbacephem

Antibiotic/Corticosteroid, Otic

Antibiotic, Miscellaneous

Antibiotic, Otic

Cephalosporin (First Generation)

Analgesic, Nonnarcotic

Analgesic, Opioid

PAIN (ANOGENITAL)

Anesthetic/Corticosteroid

Local Anesthetic

PAIN (BONE)

Radiopharmaceutical

PAIN (DIABETIC NEUROPATHY NEURALGIA)

Analgesic, Topical

PAIN (LUMBAR PUNCTURE)

Analgesic, Topical

PAIN (MUSCLE)

Analgesic, Topical

PAIN (NEUROPATHIC)

Analgesic, Miscellaneous

PAROXYSMAL NOCTURNAL HEMOGLOBINURIA (PNH)

Monoclonal Antibody

Monoclonal Antibody, Complement Inhibitor

PAROXYSMAL SUPRAVENTRICULAR TACHYCARDIA (PSVT)

Antiarrhythmic Agent, Class IV

Diagnostic Agent

PELLAGRA

Vitamin, Water Soluble

PELVIC INFLAMMATORY DISEASE (PID)

Aminoglycoside (Antibiotic)

Cephalosporin (Second Generation)

Cephalosporin (Third Generation)

Macrolide (Antibiotic)

Penicillin

Quinolone

PHEOCHROMOCYTOMA (DIAGNOSIS)

Alpha-Adrenergic Agonist

PHEOCHROMOCYTOMA (TREATMENT)

Alpha-Adrenergic Blocking Agent

Beta-Adrenergic Blocker

Diagnostic Agent

Tyrosine Hydroxylase Inhibitor

PILONIDAL CYST WOUNDS

Enzyme, Topical Debridement

PINWORMS

Anthelmintic

PITUITARY FUNCTION TEST (GROWTH HORMONE)

Diagnostic Agent

PITYRIASIS (ROSEA)

Corticosteroid, Topical

PREMATURE LUTEINIZING HORMONE (LH) SURGES

Antigonadotropic Agent

PREMENSTRUAL DYSPHORIC DISORDER (PMDD)

Antidepressant, Selective Serotonin Reuptake Inhibitor

PREOPERATIVE SEDATION

Antihistamine

Barbiturate

Benzodiazepine

General Anesthetic

PRIMARY IMMUNE DEFICIENCY (PID)

Immune Globulin

PRIMARY PULMONARY HYPERTENSION (PPH)

Platelet Inhibitor

PROCTITIS

5-Aminosalicylic Acid Derivative

PUBERTY (DELAYED)

PUBERTY (PRECOCIOUS)

PULMONARY ARTERIAL HYPERTENSION (PAH)

PULMONARY ARTERY HYPERTENSION (PAH)

PULMONARY EMBOLI

PULMONARY EMBOLISM

PULMONARY TUBERCULOSIS

PURPURA

Cephalosporin (First Generation)

Cephalosporin (Second Generation)

Cephalosporin (Third Generation)

Cold Preparation

Decongestant

Decongestant/Analgesic

Decongestant/Anticholingeric Combination

Expectorant/Decongestant

Macrolide (Antibiotic)

Penicillin

Quinolone

Sulfonamide

Sympathomimetic

Tetracycline Derivative

SJÖGREN SYNDROME

Cholinergic Agent

STATUS EPILEPTICUS

Anticonvulsant

Barbiturate

Benzodiazepine

Hydantoin

STOMATITIS

Local Anesthetic

Skin and Mucous Membrane Agent

STRABISMUS

Cholinesterase Inhibitor

Ophthalmic Agent, Toxin

STROKE

Antiplatelet Agent

Fibrinolytic Agent

SUDECK ATROPHY

Calcium Channel Blocker

SUNBURN

Nonsteroidal Antiinflammatory Drug (NSAID)

SURFACE ANTISEPTIC

Antibacterial, Topical

SURGICAL AID (OPHTHALMIC)

Ophthalmic Agent, Viscoelastic

SWEATING

Alpha-Adrenergic Blocking Agent

SWIMMER'S EAR

Antibiotic/Corticosteroid, Otic

Otic Agent, Analgesic

TOOTHACHE

TOPICAL ANESTHESIA

TOURETTE DISEASE

Antipsychotic Agent, Butyrophenone

Neuroleptic Agent

Phenothiazine Derivative

TOXICITY, NONSPECIFIC (TREATMENT)

Antacid

Antidote

Diuretic, Osmotic

TOXOPLASMOSIS

Antibiotic, Miscellaneous

Folic Acid Antagonist (Antimalarial)

QUICK LOOK DRUG BOOK

Top 200 Prescribed Tablets and Capsules with Images

The Quick Look Drug Book 2008 Top 200 Prescribed Drugs insert displays actual color photographs of the most commonly prescribed tablets and capsules.

Drugs are listed alphabetically by generic name, and, where applicable, the trade name is listed. Dosages appear under each individual image.

Use the white scale at the bottom of each image to determine the actual size. The distance between each division on the scale is equivalent to 1/8 inch or 3.175 mm.

Acetaminophen and Codeine

(generic)

300/15 mg 300/30 mg

300/60 mg 325/15 mg

325/30 mg 325/60 mg

Albuterol

(generic)

2 mg 4 mg

Alendronate

Fosamax®

5 mg 10 mg

35 mg 40 mg

70 mg

Allopurinol

(generic)

100 mg 300 mg

Alprazolam

(generic)

0.25 mg 0.5 mg

1 mg 2 mg

Amitriptyline

(generic)

10 mg	25 mg
50 mg	75 mg
100 mg	150 mg

Amlodipine and Benazepril

Lotrel®

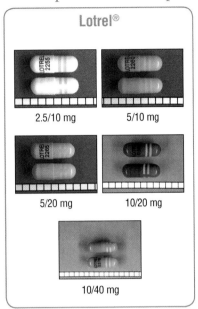

2.5/10 mg	5/10 mg
5/20 mg	10/20 mg
10/40 mg	

Amlodipine

Norvasc®

2.5 mg	5 mg
10 mg	

Amoxicillin

(generic)

250 mg	250 mg
400 mg	500 mg
500 mg	875 mg

Amoxicillin and Clavulanate Potassium

(generic)

200/28.5 mg 400/57 mg

500/125 mg 875/125 mg

Aripiprazole

Abilify®

5 mg 10 mg

15 mg 20 mg

30 mg

Atenolol

(generic)

25 mg 50 mg

100 mg

Atorvastatin

Lipitor®

10 mg 20 mg

40 mg 80 mg

Azithromycin

Zithromax® Z-PAK®

250 mg

(generic)

| 250 mg | 600 mg |

Bupropion

Wellbutrin XL®

| 150 mg | 300 mg |

Carvedilol

Coreg®

| 3.125 mg | 6.25 mg |
| 12.5 mg | 25 mg |

Cefdinir

Omnicef®

300 mg

Celecoxib

Celebrex™

| 100 mg | 200 mg |

400 mg

Cephalexin

(generic)

| 250 mg | 500 mg |

Cetirizine

Zyrtec®

5 mg   10 mg

Ciprofloxacin

(generic)

250 mg   500 mg

750 mg

Citalopram

(generic)

10 mg   20 mg

40 mg

Clonazepam

(generic)

0.5 mg   1 mg

2 mg

Clonidine

(generic)

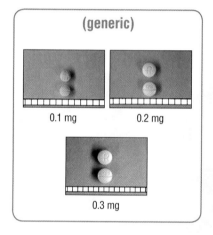

0.1 mg   0.2 mg

0.3 mg

Cyclobenzaprine

(generic)

10 mg

Desloratadine

Clarinex®

5 mg

Dextroamphetamine and Amphetamine

Adderall XR®

5 mg   10 mg

15 mg   20 mg

25 mg   30 mg

Diazepam

(generic)

2 mg   5 mg

10 mg

Digoxin

Digitek®

125 mcg   250 mcg

Diltiazem

Cartia XT™

120 mg   180 mg

240 mg   300 mg

Donepezil

Aricept®

5 mg   10 mg

Doxycycline

(generic)

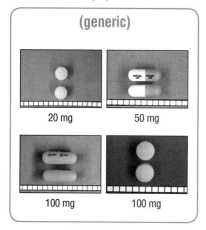

20 mg   50 mg

100 mg   100 mg

Duloxetine

Cymbalta®

20 mg   30 mg

60 mg

Enalapril

(generic)

2.5 mg   5 mg

10 mg   20 mg

Escitalopram

Lexapro™

5 mg   10 mg

20 mg

Esomeprazole

Nexium®

20 mg   40 mg

Estrogens
(Conjugated/Equine)

Premarin®

0.3 mg   0.45 mg

0.625 mg   0.9 mg

1.25 mg

Eszopiclone

Lunesta™

1 mg   2 mg

3 mg

Ethinyl Estradiol
and Drospirenone

Yasmin®

0.03/3 mg

Ethinyl Estradiol
and Norgestimate

Ortho Tri-Cyclen® Lo

multiple dosages

Tri-Sprintec® 28

multiple dosages

Ezetimibe

Zetia™

10 mg

Ezetimibe and Simvastatin

Vytorin™

10/10 mg   10/20 mg

10/40 mg   10/80 mg

Fenofibrate

TriCor®

48 mg   54 mg

145 mg   160 mg

Fluconazole

(generic)

50 mg   100 mg

150 mg   200 mg

Fluoxetine

(generic)

10 mg   20 mg

40 mg

Folic Acid

(generic)

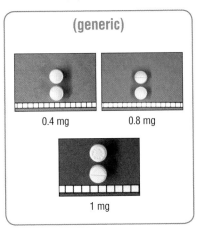

0.4 mg   0.8 mg

1 mg

Furosemide

(generic)

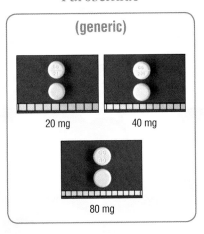

20 mg   40 mg

80 mg

Gabapentin

(generic)

100 mg   100 mg

300 mg   300 mg

400 mg   400 mg

600 mg   800 mg

Glipizide

(generic)

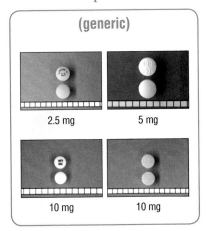

2.5 mg   5 mg

10 mg   10 mg

Glyburide

(generic)

1.25 mg

1.5 mg

2.5 mg

3 mg

5 mg

6 mg

Hydrochlorothiazide

(generic)

12.5 mg

25 mg

50 mg

Hydrochlorothiazide and Triamterene

(generic)

25/37.5 mg

25/37.5 mg

25/50 mg

50/75 mg

Hydrocodone and Acetaminophen

(generic)

2.5/500 mg

5/500 mg

5/500 mg

7.5/500 mg

7.5/650 mg

7.5/750 mg

10/325 mg

10/500 mg

| 10/650 mg | 10/660 mg |

Ibuprofen

(generic)

| 200 mg | 400 mg |
| 600 mg | 800 mg |

Irbesartan

Avapro®

| 75 mg | 150 mg |
| 300 mg | |

Irbesartan and Hydrochlorothiazide

Avalide®

| 150/12.5 mg | 300/12.5 mg |

Isosorbide Mononitrate

Imdur®

| 30 mg | 60 mg |
| 120 mg | |

(generic)

| 10 mg | 20 mg |
| 30 mg | 60 mg |

120 mg

Lamotrigine

Lamictal®

5 mg

25 mg

25 mg

100 mg

150 mg

200 mg

Lansoprazole

Prevacid®

15 mg

30 mg

Levofloxacin

Levaquin®

250 mg

500 mg

750 mg

Levothyroxine

(generic)

25 mcg

50 mcg

75 mcg

88 mcg

100 mcg

112 mcg

125 mcg

137 mcg

150 mcg

175 mcg

200 mcg

300 mcg

Levoxyl®

25 mcg

50 mcg

75 mcg

88 mcg

100 mcg

112 mcg

125 mcg

137 mcg

150 mcg

175 mcg

200 mcg

Synthroid®

25 mcg

50 mcg

75 mcg

88 mcg

100 mcg

112 mcg

125 mcg

137 mcg

150 mcg

175 mcg

200 mcg

300 mcg

Lisinopril

(generic)

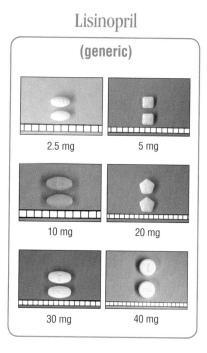

2.5 mg

5 mg

10 mg

20 mg

30 mg

40 mg

Lisinopril and Hydrochlorothiazide

(generic)

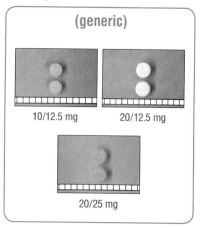

10/12.5 mg

20/12.5 mg

20/25 mg

Lorazepam

(generic)

0.5 mg   1 mg

2 mg

Losartan

Cozaar®

25 mg   50 mg

100 mg

Losartan and Hydrochlorothiazide

Hyzaar®

50/12.5 mg   100/25 mg

Lovastatin

(generic)

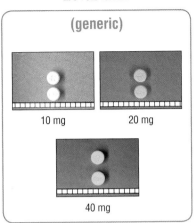

10 mg   20 mg

40 mg

Meclizine

(generic)

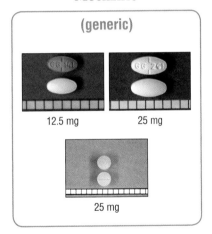

12.5 mg   25 mg

25 mg

Meloxicam

Mobic®

7.5 mg   15 mg

Memantine

Namenda™

| 5 mg | 10 mg |

Metformin

(generic)

| 500 mg | 500 mg |
| 750 mg | 850 mg |
| 1000 mg |

Methylphenidate

Concerta®

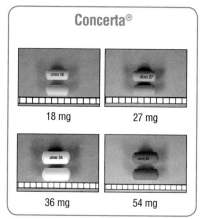

| 18 mg | 27 mg |
| 36 mg | 54 mg |

Metoprolol

(generic)

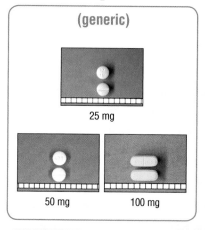

| 25 mg |
| 50 mg | 100 mg |

Toprol-XL®

| 25 mg | 50 mg |
| 100 mg | 200 mg |

Montelukast

Singulair®

4 mg   5 mg

10 mg

Naproxen

(generic)

220 mg   250 mg

275 mg   375 mg

375 mg   500 mg

500 mg   550 mg

Niacin

Niaspan®

500 mg   750 mg

1000 mg

Olanzapine

Zyprexa®

2.5 mg   5 mg

7.5 mg   10 mg

15 mg   20 mg

Olmesartan

Benicar™

5 mg

20 mg

40 mg

Olmesartan and Hydrochlorothiazide

Benicar HCT™

20/12.5 mg

40/12.5 mg

40/25 mg

Omeprazole

(generic)

10 mg

20 mg

Oxycodone and Acetaminophen

(generic)

5/325 mg

5/500 mg

7.5/500 mg

10/325 mg

10/650 mg

Pantoprazole

Protonix®

20 mg

40 mg

Paroxetine

(generic)

10 mg	20 mg
30 mg	40 mg

Penicillin V Potassium

(generic)

250 mg	500 mg

Phenytoin

(generic)

100 mg

Pioglitazone

Actos™

15 mg	30 mg
45 mg	

Potassium Chloride

(generic)

8 mEq	10 mEq
10 mEq	20 mEq

Klor-Con® M20

20 mEq

Pravastatin

Pravachol®

10 mg 20 mg

40 mg 80 mg

Prednisone

(generic)

1 mg 2.5 mg

5 mg 10 mg

20 mg 50 mg

Pregabalin

Lyrica®

25 mg 50 mg

75 mg

Promethazine

(generic)

25 mg 50 mg

Propoxyphene and Acetaminophen

(generic)

50/325 mg 65/650 mg

100/650 mg

Quetiapine

Seroquel®

25 mg   50 mg

100 mg   200 mg

300 mg   400 mg

Quinapril

(generic)

5 mg   10 mg

20 mg   40 mg

Rabeprazole

Aciphex®

20 mg

Raloxifene

Evista®

60 mg

Ramipril

Altace™

1.25 mg   2.5 mg

5 mg   10 mg

Ranitidine

(generic)

75 mg   150 mg

300 mg

Risedronate

Actonel®

5 mg   30 mg

35 mg

Risperidone

Risperdal®

0.25 mg   0.5 mg

1 mg   2 mg

3 mg   4 mg

Rosiglitazone

Avandia®

2 mg   4 mg

8 mg

Rosuvastatin

Crestor®

5 mg   10 mg

20 mg   40 mg

Sertraline

(generic)

50 mg   100 mg

Zoloft®

25 mg   50 mg

100 mg

Sildenafil

Viagra™

25 mg   50 mg

100 mg

Simvastatin

Zocor®

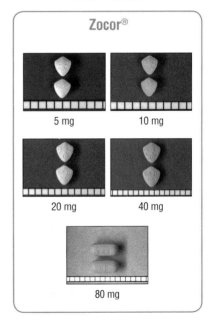

5 mg   10 mg

20 mg   40 mg

80 mg

Sulfamethoxazole and Trimethoprim

(generic)

400/80 mg   800/160 mg

Sumatriptan

Imitrex®

25 mg   50 mg

100 mg

Tadalafil

Cialis®

10 mg   20 mg

Tamsulosin

Flomax®

0.4 mg

Temazepam

(generic)

15 mg   30 mg

Tiotropium

Spiriva® HandiHaler®

18 mcg

Tolterodine

Detrol® LA

2 mg   4 mg

Topiramate

Topamax®

15 mg	25 mg
25 mg	50 mg
100 mg	200 mg

Tramadol

(generic)

50 mg

Trazodone

(generic)

| 50 mg | 100 mg |

150 mg

Valacyclovir

Valtrex®

| 500 mg | 1 g |

Valproic Acid and Derivatives

Depakote®

| 125 mg | 250 mg |

500 mg

Depakote® ER

250 mg   500 mg

Valsartan

Diovan®

40 mg   80 mg

160 mg   320 mg

Valsartan and Hydrochlorothiazide

Diovan HCT®

80/12.5 mg   160/12.5 mg

160/25 mg

Venlafaxine

Effexor XR®

37.5 mg   75 mg

Verapamil

(generic)

40 mg   80 mg

120 mg   120 mg

180 mg   180 mg

240 mg   240 mg

240 mg   360 mg

Warfarin

(generic)

1 mg

2 mg

2.5 mg

3 mg

4 mg

5 mg

6 mg

7.5 mg

10 mg

Coumadin®

2 mg

2.5 mg

3 mg

4 mg

5 mg

7.5 mg

10 mg

Zolpidem

Ambien®

5 mg

10 mg